FOUNDATIONS OF OSTEOPATHIC MEDICINE

THIRD EDITION

FOUNDATIONS OF

OSTEOPATHIC MEDICINE

Published under the auspices of the American Osteopathic Association

THIRD EDITION

EXECUTIVE EDITOR

ANTHONY G. CHILA, D.O., F.A.A.O. *dist*, **F.C.A.**
Professor
Department of Family Medicine
College of Osteopathic Medicine
Ohio University
Athens, Ohio

SECTION EDITORS

JANE E. CARREIRO, D.O.
Associate Professor and Chair
Department of Osteopathic Manipulative Medicine
University of New England
College of Osteopathic Medicine
Biddeford, Maine

DENNIS J. DOWLING, D.O., F.A.A.O.
Attending Physician and Director of Manipulative Medicine
Physical Medicine and Rehabilitation Department
Nassau University Medical Center
East Meadow, New York

Director of Osteopathic Manipulative Medicine Assessment
The National Board of Osteopathic Medical Examiners
Clinical Skills Testing Center
Conshohocken, Pennsylvania

RUSSELL G. GAMBER, D.O., M.P.H.
Professor, Department of Osteopathic Manipulative Medicine
University of North Texas Health Science Center at
Fort Worth
Texas College of Osteopathic Medicine
Fort Worth, Texas

JOHN C. GLOVER, D.O., F.A.A.O.
Professor and Chair
Department of Osteopathic Manipulative Medicine
Touro University-California
College of Osteopathic Medicine
Vallejo, California

ANN L. HABENICHT, D.O., F.A.A.O., F.A.C.O.F.P.
Professor, Department of Osteopathic Manipulative Medicine
Chicago College of Osteopathic Medicine
Midwestern University
Downers Grove, Illinois

JOHN A. JEROME, PH.D., B.C.F.E.
Associate Professor of Clinical Medicine
Department of Osteopathic Medicine
Michigan State University
East Lansing, Michigan

Pain Psychologist
Lansing Neurosurgery and The Spine Center
East Lansing, Michigan

MICHAEL M. PATTERSON, PH.D. (RETIRED)
Nova Southeastern University College of Osteopathic
Medicine
Fort Lauderdale, Florida

FELIX J. ROGERS, D.O., F.A.C.O.I.
Downriver Cardiology Consultants
Trenton, Michigan

MICHAEL A. SEFFINGER, D.O., F.A.A.F.P.
Associate Professor
Family Medicine/Osteopathic Manipulative Medicine
Chair, Department of Neuromusculoskeletal Medicine/
Osteopathic Manipulative Medicine
College of Osteopathic Medicine of the Pacific
Western University of Health Sciences
Pomona, California

FRANK H. WILLARD, PH.D.
Professor of Anatomy
Department of Anatomy
University of New England
College of Osteopathic Medicine
Biddeford, Maine

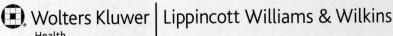

Wolters Kluwer | Lippincott Williams & Wilkins
Health

Philadelphia • Baltimore • New York • London
Buenos Aires • Hong Kong • Sydney • Tokyo

Acquisitions Editor: Charles W. Mitchell
Product Manager: Jennifer Verbiar
Designer: Steven Druding
Compositor: SPi Technologies

Third Edition

Library of Congress Cataloging-in-Publication Data
Foundations of osteopathic medicine. — 3rd ed. / published under the auspices of the American Osteopathic Association; executive editor, Anthony G. Chila; section editors, Jane E. Carreiro . . . [et al.].
   p. ; cm.
Rev. ed. of: Foundations for osteopathic medicine / executive editor, Robert C. Ward. 2nd ed. c2003.
Includes bibliographical references and index.
ISBN 978-0-7817-6671-5 (alk. paper)
1. Osteopathic medicine.   2. Osteopathic medicine—Philosophy.   I. Chila, Anthony G.   II. American Osteopathic Association.   III. Foundations of osteopathic medicine.
[DNLM: 1. Osteopathic Medicine—methods. WB 940]
RZ342.F68 2011
615.5'33—dc22

                                                    2010028827

DISCLAIMER

DEDICATION

This third edition of Foundations of Osteopathic Medicine *is dedicated to two individuals who made very significant contributions to the development of osteopathic medical research. Common threads bound their careers together: dedication to better understanding of the scientific basis of osteopathic medicine; complementary relationship in Basic Science and Clinical Science research; and sustained support of the research effort of the American Academy of Osteopathy, an affiliate body of the American Osteopathic Association. Their respective years of passage span the time between the release of the second and third editions of this text.*

WILLIAM L. JOHNSTON, DO, FAAO

February 17, 1921–June 10, 2003

It is with sadness that I announce the passing of William L. Johnston, DO, and commemorate his numerous achievements. As Editor-in-Chief of the American Osteopathic Association (AOA) and having served on the AOA Bureau of Research, I have had the opportunity to work with truly outstanding people. Dr Johnston, with whom I collaborated for more than 20 years, was certainly one of those individuals.

I consider Dr Johnston a mentor in the truest sense of the word. He introduced me to research involving osteopathic principles and practice in a meaningful way. I met Dr Johnston at the Michigan State University College of Osteopathic Medicine (MSU–COM), East Lansing, when I was a young physician assuming a new role as vice chairman of the Bureau of Research. I was thoroughly impressed with the breadth and depth of his understanding of osteopathic medicine, particularly the focus he believed was needed in future research.

An outstanding teacher and, more important, an original and profound thinker, Dr Johnston was a professional who got things done. Truly, he was an original and special man who deserves every accolade that can be applied to such a professional. I am sure I am but one individual who will write a memoriam about Dr Johnston.

When I became the AOA's Editor-in-Chief, I decided to name new members to *JAOA*'s Editorial Advisory Board. I needed a mentor to guide my choices. I wanted someone who had the respect of the profession and who understood what is meant by osteopathic principles and practice at the deepest level.

I found that the individual I needed was already on the Editorial Advisory Board. He was a go-to individual for many of my questions concerning osteopathic medicine. When he spoke at our Editorial Advisory Board meetings, the room became quiet and all attention was directed toward him. Everything Dr Johnston said was meaningful and important and sometimes enormously funny in the way he had of bringing reality to the table.

All in the osteopathic medical profession will miss Dr Johnston. I know that the faculty and students at MSU–COM will deeply miss him. And I will personally feel the void left by one so large in knowledge and personal responsibility.

Dr Johnston's family was blessed to have had his loving presence. I am sure that he will remain firmly in their minds and deep in their hearts for the remainder of their lives and will most likely live on for generations to come. A finer, more dedicated osteopathic physician committed to this profession, its research, and education would be difficult to find.

ALBERT F. KELSO, PHD, DSCI (HON)

November 19, 1917–January 29, 2009

It was with a great sense of loss that we inform you of the death of Albert F. Kelso, PhD. Dr. Kelso was more than just a colleague and fellow Academy member. Dr. Kelso received a Doctor of Philosophy degree from Loyola University Graduate School in 1959 and later received a Doctor of Science (Hon) from Kirksville College of Osteopathic Medicine in 1970. Dr. Kelso was also a student at the Institute of Medicine in Chicago as well as the University of Chicago.

Beginning in the mid-40s, Dr. Kelso worked as a biology and physiology instructor, professor, and department chair at George Williams College and the Chicago College of Osteopathic Medicine. By 1975, he was involved in research serving as the director of research affairs as well as a research professor in osteopathic medicine. It was in 1974 when he first became a research consultant on the AAO's Louisa Burns Clinical Observation Committee where he still gave counsel until his passing. He was awarded the American Osteopathic Association's 1981 Louisa Burns Memorial Lecture, "Planning, Developing and Conducting Osteopathic Clinical Research." Dr. Kelso was honored as the 2005 recipient of the ACADEMY AWARD in recognition of his outstanding commitment to the osteopathic medical profession, supporting its philosophy, principles, and practices.

As a representative of the Association of Colleges of Osteopathic Medicine, Dr. Kelso served on the National Society of Medical Research in addition to serving as a representative to the Medical Legal Council of the Illinois State Medical Society, Medical Records and Right to Privacy through 1982. Dr. Kelso was an educational consultant for the AOA's Committee on Colleges and served on their Council of Osteopathic Educational Development. Since 1981, he served as an editorial referee for the Journal of the AOA, and he was an associate editor of the definitive textbook, Foundations of Osteopathic Medicine, which was published in 1997.

Dr. Kelso was author or contributing author on several publications and has many abstracts and papers printed in a variety of medical journals. He was a member of many notable professional societies such as the American Academy of Osteopathy, American Osteopathic Association, American Physiologic Society, and the Illinois Society for Medical Research.

We know that his passing will leave a void not only in our lives but also in the hearts of all those who knew him.

GILBERT E. D'ALONZO, JR, DO

CONTENTS

PART I: FOUNDATIONS

Section 1

Overview of the Osteopathic Medical Profession 3
Section Editor: Michael A. Seffinger, DO, FAAFP

Section 2

Basic Sciences 53
Section Editors: Frank H. Willard, PhD, and
John A. Jerome, PhD, BCFE

PART II: THE PATIENT ENCOUNTER

Section Editor: Felix J. Rogers, DO, FACOI

PART III: APPROACH TO THE SOMATIC COMPONENT

Section Editors: Ann L. Habenicht, DO, FAAO,
Dennis J. Dowling, DO, FAAO, Russell G. Gamber, DO, MPH,
and John C. Glover, DO, FAAO

Section 1

Basic Evaluation 401

    Ehrenfeuchter

35. Segmental Motion Testing 431
    Ehrenfeuchter

36. Postural Considerations in Osteopathic Diagnosis and
    Treatment 437
    Kuchera

Section 2

Osteopathic Considerations of Regions   484

37. Head and Suboccipital Region 484
    Heinking, Kappler, Ramey

38. Cervical Region 513
    Heinking, Kappler

39. Thoracic Region and Rib Cage 528
    Hruby

40. Lumbar Region 542
    Heinking

41. Pelvis and Sacrum 575
    Heinking, Kappler

42. Lower Extremities 602
    Kuchera

43. Upper Extremities 640
    Heinking

44. Abdominal Region 660
    Hruby

Section 3

Osteopathic Manipulative Treatment   669

TRADITIONAL APPROACHES

45. Thrust (High Velocity/Low Amplitude) Approach;
    "The Pop" 669
    Hohner, Cymet

46. Muscle Energy Approach 682
    Ehrenfeuchter

47. Myofascial Release Approach 698
    O'Connell

48. Osteopathy in the Cranial Field 728
    King

49. Strain and Counterstrain Approach 749
    Glover, Rennie

50. Soft Tissue/Articulatory Approach 763
    Ehrenfeuchter

51. Lymphatics Approach 786
    Kuchera

CONTEMPORARY APPROACHES

52. Representative Models 809
    Dowling

    A. Balanced Ligamentous Tension and
       Ligamentous Articular Strain 809
       Crow

    B. Facilitated Positional Release 813
       Dowling

    C. Progressive Inhibition of Neuromuscular
       Structures 820
       Dowling

    D. Functional Technique 831
       Johnston

    E. Visceral Manipulation 845
       Lossing

    F. Still Technique 849
       Van Buskirk

    G. Chapman's Approach 853
       Fossum, Kuchera, Devine, Wilson

    H. Fulford Percussion 866
       Yadava

PART IV: APPROACH TO OSTEOPATHIC PATIENT MANAGEMENT

Section Editors: Jane E. Carreiro, DO, Anthony G. Chila, DO, FAAO dist, FCA., and John C. Glover, DO, FAAO

CONTRIBUTORS

Peter Adler-Michaelson, D.O., Ph.D.
Clinical Professor, Osteopathic Medicine
Michigan State University
College of Osteopathic Medicine
East Lansing, Michigan

Margaret Aguwa, D.O., M.P.H., F.A.C.O.F.P.
Professor of Family and Community Medicine
Associate Dean, Community Outreach and
    Clinical Research
College of Osteopathic Medicine
Michigan State University
East Lansing, Michigan

David A. Baron, M.S.Ed., D.O.
Professor and Chair
Department of Psychiatry
Temple University School of Medicine
Philadelphia, Pennsylvania

Bruce P. Bates, D.O., F.A.C.O.F.P.
Chair of Family Medicine
College of Osteopathic Medicine
University of New England
Biddeford, Maine

Per Gunnar Brolinson, D.O.
Professor of Sports Medicine
Virginia College of Osteopathic Medicine
Blacksburg, Virginia

Richard Butler, D.O.
Associate Professor of Internal Medicine
Virginia Tech Carilion School of Medicine
Director of Osteopathic Medical Education
Program Director, Osteopathic Internal Medicine
Carilion Clinic
Roanoke, Virginia

Robert A. Cain, D.O.
Clinical Professor of Pulmonary Medicine
College of Osteopathic Medicine
Ohio University
Athens, Ohio
Director of Medical Education
Grandview Hospital
Dayton, Ohio

Roberto Cardarelli, D.O., M.P.H., F.A.A.F.P.
Associate Professor of Family Medicine
Director, Primary Care Research Institute
University of North Texas Health Science Center
Plaza Medical Center
Forth Worth, Texas

William Thomas Crow, D.O., F.A.A.D.
Director, FPI NMM Integrated Residency
Department of Graduate Medical Education
Florida Hospital East Orlando
Orlando, Florida

Tyler C. Cymet, D.O.
Associate Vice President for Medical Education
The American Association of Colleges of
    Osteopathic Medicine
Chevy Chase, Maryland

Gilbert E. D'Alonzo, Jr., D.O.
Professor of Medicine
Department of Pulmonary and Critical Care
Temple University School of Medicine
Attending Physician
Department of Pulmonary and Critical Care
Temple University Hospital
Philadelphia, Pennsylvania

Brian Degenhardt, D.O.
Assistant Vice President for Osteopathic Research
Director, Center of Advancement of Osteopathic Research
    Methodologies (CORM)
A.T. Still Research Institute
Kirksville, Missouri

William H. Devine, D.O
Clinical Professor and Chair of Osteopathic Manipulation
Arizona College of Osteopathic Medicine
Midwestern University
Glendale, Arizona

Walter C. Ehrenfeuchter, D.O., F.A.A.O.
Professor and Chairman of Osteopathic Manipulative Medicine
Philadelphia College of Osteopathic Medicine,
    Georgia Campus
Suwanee, Georgia

Mitchell L. Elkiss, D.O.
Associate Professor of Neurology
College of Osteopathic Medicine
Michigan State University
East Lansing, Michigan
Attending Neurologist
Department of Internal Medicine
Providence-St. John Hospital
Smithfield, Michigan
Department of Neurology
Botsford General Hospital
Farmington Hills, Michigan

Hugh Ettlinger, D.O., F.A.A.O.
Associate Professor of Osteopathic Manipulative Medicine
New York College of Osteopathic Medicine
Old Westbury, New York
Director, Neuromusculoskeletal Medicine and Osteopathic
    Manipulative Medicine
St. Barnabas Hospital
Bronx, New York

William A. Falls, Ph.D.
Professor and Associate Dean of Radiology
College of Osteopathic Medicine
Michigan State University
East Lansing, Michigan

William M. Foley, D.O.
Assistant Professor of Osteopathic Manipulative Medicine
College of Osteopathic Medicine
University of New England
Biddeford, Maine
Instructor of Family Medicine and Community Health
University of Massachusetts
Worcester, Massachusetts

Brian H. Foresman, D.O.
Director, Sleep Medicine and Circadian Biology Program
Indiana University School of Medicine
Indianapolis, Indiana

Christian Fossum, D.O.
Assistant Professor
Department of Osteopathic Manipulative Medicine
Associate Director
A.T. Still Research Institute
Kirksville, Missouri

Marcel P. Fraix, D.O.
Assistant Professor of Physical Medicine and Rehabilitation and
    Osteopathic Manipulative Medicine
College of Osteopathic Medicine of the Pacific
Western University of Health Sciences
Pomona, California

Wolfgang G. Gilliar, D.O., F.A.A.P.M.R.
Professor and Chair of Osteopathic Manipulative Medicine
New York College of Osteopathic Medicine
New York Institute of Technology
Old Westbury, New York

Rebecca E. Giusti, D.O.
Assistant Professor of Family Medicine
Department of Osteopathic Manipulative Medicine
Western University of Health Sciences
Pomona, California

Thomas Glonek, Ph.D.
Professor of Osteopathic Manipulative Medicine
Midwestern University
Assistant Chair of the Research and Education of the Michael Reese
    Medical Staff
Michael Reese Hospital
Chicago, Illinois

Thomas A. Goodwin, D.O.
Clinical Assistant Professor
Family and Community Medicine
College of Osteopathic Medicine
Michigan State University
East Lansing, Michigan

Marilyn R. Gugliucci, Ph.D., A.G.H.E.F, G.S.A.F, A.G.S.F.
Director of Geriatric Education and Research
Department of Geriatric Medicine
University of New England College of Osteopathic Medicine
Biddeford, Maine

Mary Anne Morelli Haskell, D.O.
Associate Professor of Osteopathic Manipulative Medicine
Western University
Pomona, California

Kurt P. Heinking, D.O., F.A.A.O.
Chair of Osteopathic Manipulative Medicine
Chicago College of Osteopathic Medicine
Midwestern University
Downers Grove, Illinois
Department of Family Medicine
Hinsdale Hospital
Hinsdale, Illinois
LaGrange Hospital
LaGrange, Illinois

John G. Hohner, D.O., F.A.A.O.
Associate Professor of Osteopathic Manipulative Medicine
Chicago College of Osteopathic Medicine
Midwestern University
Downers Grove, Illinois

Kari Hortos, D.O.,
Associate Dean and Professor of Internal Medicine
College of Osteopathic Medicine
Michigan State University
Clinton Township, Michigan

Raymond J. Hruby, D.O., M.S., F.A.A.O.
Professor of Osteopathic Manipulative Medicine
College of Osteopathic Medicine of the Pacific
Western University of Health Sciences
Pomona, California

John M. Jones III, D.O.
Professor of Family Medicine, Chair
Osteopathic Principles and Practice Department
William Carey University College of Osteopathic Medicine
Hattiesburg, Mississippi

Rose J. Julius, D.O.
Philadelphia, Pennsylvania

Robert E. Kappler, D.O., F.A.A.O.
Professor of Osteopathic Manipulative Medicine
Midwestern University Chicago College of Osteopathic Medicine
Downers Grove, Illinois

Brian E. Kaufman, D.O.
Adjunct Clinical Professor of Osteopathic Manipulative Medicine
College of Osteopathic Medicine
University of New England
Biddeford, Maine
Goodall Hospital
Sanford, Maine

Hollis H. King, D.O., Ph.D.
Associate Professor of Osteopathic Manipulative Medicine
Texas College of Osteopathic Medicine
University of North Texas Health Science Center
Fortworth, Texas
Associate Executive Director
Osteopathic Research Center
University of North Texas Health Science Center
Fortworth, Texas

Michael L. Kuchera, D.O., F.A.A.O.
Professor of Osteopathic Manipulative Medicine
Clinical Director, Center for Chronic Disorders of Aging
Philadelphia College of Osteopathic Medicine
Philadelphia, Pennsylvania

Alyse Ley, D.O.
Assistant Professor
Associate Director
Psychiatry Residency Education
Department of Psychiatry
College of Human Medicine
College of Osteopathic Medicine
Michigan State University
East Lansing, Michigan

James A. Lipton, D.O., F.A.A.O., F.A.A.P.M.R.
Physical Medicine and Rehabilitation
Sentara Virginia Beach General Hospital
Hampton, Virginia

Kenneth Lossing, D.O.
San Rafael, California

John M. McPartland, D.O.
Assistant Clinical Professor of Osteopathic Manipulative Medicine
Michigan State University
East Lansing, Michigan

Jed Magen, D.O.
Chair, Department of Psychiatry
College of Human Medicine
College of Osteopathic Medicine
Michigan State University
East Lansing, Michigan

Miriam V. Mills, M.D., F.A.A.P.
Clinical Professor of Osteopathic Manipulative
    Medicine
Oklahoma State University Center for Health Sciences
Tulsa, Oklahoma

Kenneth E. Nelson, D.O., F.A.A.O, F.AC.O.F.P.
Professor of Osteopathic Manipulative Medicine, Family Medicine and
    Biochemistry
Chicago College of Osteopathic Medicine
Midwestern University
Downers Grove, Illinois

Natalie A. Nevins, D.O., M.S.H.P.E.
Clinical Associate Professor of Family Medicine
Western University of Health Sciences
Pomona, California
Director of Medical Education
Family Practice Residency Program
Downey Regional Medical Center
Downey, California

Karen J. Nichols, D.O., F.A.C.O.I.
Dean
Chicago College of Osteopathic Medicine
Midwestern University
Downers Grove, Illinois

Judith A. O'Connell, D.O., F.A.A.O.
Clinical Professor of Osteopathic Manipulative Medicine
School of Osteopathic Medicine
Pikesville College
Pikesville, Kentucky
Chairperson
Department of Osteopathic Manipulative Medicine
Grandview Medical Center
Dayton, Ohio

Gerald Guy Osborn, D.O., M.Phil., D.F.A.C.N., D.F.A.P.A.
Professor and Chair of Psychiatry and
    Behavioral Medicine
Associate Dean for International Medicine
DeBusk College of Osteopathic Medicine
Lincoln Memorial University
Harrogate, Tennessee

Barbara E. Peterson, D. Litt. (Hon)
American Academy of Osteopathy
Evanston, Illinois

Kenneth A. Ramey, D.O.
Assistant Professor, OPP
Department of Osteopathic Principles and Practices
Rocky Vista University
Parker, Colorado

Paul R. Rennie, D.O., F.A.A.O.
Associate Professor and Department Chair
Department of Osteopathic Manipulative Medicine
Touro University Nevada College of
    Osteopathic Medicine
Henderson, Nevada

Jesus Sanchez, Jr., D.O., M.S.H.P.E.
Assistant Professor of Neuromusculoskeletal Medicine and Osteopathic
    Manipulative Medicine
College of Osteopathic Medicine of the Pacific
Western Univesity of Health Sciences
Pomona, California
Assistant Director of Medical Education
Department of Medical Training
Downey Regional Medical Center
Downey, California

Brent W. Sanderlin, D.O.
Seton Family of Doctors at Hays
Kyle, Texas

Stephen M. Scheinthal, D.O., F.A.C.N.
Associate Professor, and Chief
Geriatric Behavioral Health
Department of Psychiatry
University of Medicine and Dentistry
School of Osteopathic Medicine
Cherry Hill, New Jersy

Howard Schubiner, M.D.
Clinical Professor of Internal Medicine
Wayne State University School of Medicine
Detroit, Michigan
Director, Mind Body Medicine Program
Department of Internal Medicine
Providence Hospital
St. John's Health System
Southfield, Michigan

Nicette Sergueef, D.O.
Associate Professor
Department of Osteopathic Manipulative Medicine
Chicago College of Osteopathic Medicine
Midwestern University
Downers Grove, IL

Harriet H. Shaw, D.O.
Clinical Professor of Osteopathic Manipulative
    Medicine
Oklahoma State University Center for Health Sciences
Staff Physician
Department of Osteopathic Manipulative Medicine
Oklahoma State University Medical Center
Tulsa, Oklahoma

Michael B. Shaw, D.O.
Assistant Clinical Professor of Surgery
Oklahoma State University
Tulsa, Oklahoma
Attending Physician
Department of Ear, Nose, and Throat
Southcrest Hospital
Tulsa, Oklahoma

Paul R. Standley, Ph.D.
Professor of Basic Medical Sciences
College of Medicine
University of Arizona
Phoenix, Arizona

Karen M. Steele, D.O., F.A.A.O.
Professor and Associate Dean of Osteopathic
    Medical Education
Department of Osteopathic Principles and Practices
West Virginia School of Osteopathic Medicine
Lewisburg, West Virginia

Scott T. Stoll, D.O., Ph.D.
University of North Texas Health Science Center
Texas College of Osteopathic Medicine
Department of Osteopathic Manipulative Medicine
Fort Worth, Texas

Melicien Tettambel, D.O., F.A.A.O., F.A.C.O.O.G.
Professor and Chair of Osteopathic Principles and Practice
College of Osteopathic Medicine
Pacific Northwest University
Yakima, Washington

Lex C. Towns, Ph.D.
Professor and Head of Anatomy
Pacific Northwest University of Health Sciences
Yakima, Washington

Beth A. Valashinas, D.O.
Assistant Professor of Rheumatology
University of North Texas Health Science Center
Fort Worth, Texas

Richard L. Van Buskirk, D.O., Ph.D., F.A.A.O.
Sarasota, Florida

Deborah A. Wagenaar, D.O, M.S.
Associate Professor
Director, Medical Education
Department of Psychiatry
Michigan State University
East Lansing, Michigan

Robert C. Ward, D.O., F.A.A.O.
Professor Emeritus
Osteopathic Manipulative Medicine and Family Medicine
Michigan State University College of Osteopathic Medicine
East Lansing, Michigan

Michael R. Wells, Ph.D.
Associate Professor and Chairman
Department of Biomechanics and Bioengineering
New York College of Osteopathic Medicine
New York Institute of Technology
Old Westbury, New York

J. Michael Wieting, D.O.
Professor of Osteopathic Principles and Practices
DeBusk College of Osteopathic Medicine
Lincoln Memorial University
Harrogate, Tennessee

Kendall Wilson, D.O.
Vice Chair, Member at Large
Doctor of Osteopathy, West Virginia School of
    Osteopathic Medicine
Physician, Family Medicine
Lewisburg, West Virginia

Suzanne G. Wilson, RN
Mount Clemens General Hospital
Mount Clemens, Michigan

Robert D. Wurster, D.O.
Professor
Department of Physiology
Loyola University Medical Center
Maywood, Illinois

Rajiv L. Yadava, D.O.
Des Peres Hospital
St. Louis, Missouri

PREFACE

This third edition of *Foundations of Osteopathic Medicine* (FOM3) is built on a years-long commitment by members of the osteopathic medical profession and the American Osteopathic Association (AOA). An informal proposal for a textbook began 30 or more years ago by the Educational Council on Osteopathic Principles (ECOP). The effort at that time was directed toward development of a longitudinal curriculum in Osteopathic Principles and Practice (OPP). Historically, other such forums had also discussed additional alternatives. The concept and plan for the text as it emerged were developed within the Bureau of Research of the AOA. It was the Bureau's decision to term this activity the "Osteopathic Principles Textbook Project". The Board of Trustees and House of Delegates of the AOA provided financial support for its development, and the project was launched in July 1990. Under the pioneering leadership of Executive Editor Robert C. Ward, DO, FAAO, the first and second editions of this text appeared in 1997 and 2003, respectively. Doctor Ward's decision not to continue led to search and selection of a new executive editor. It was with some trepidation that I accepted this great responsibility in late 2006. Personal friendship with Dr. Ward over many years helped to assuage concern, and transitioning in responsibility occurred between Dr. Ward and I began in November 2006. Formal meetings with Lippincott Williams & Wilkins (LWW) personnel and section editors for FOM3 occurred at Philadelphia, PA (LWW corporate offices) in January 2007 and Chicago, IL (AOA Headquarters) in October 2008. The remainder of work to conclusion of the FOM3 project was carried out via a series of teleconferences and ongoing electronic communication.

The process of review and revision was carried out in a careful and thoughtful manner. Particular attention was given to change in the construct and delivery of health care in recent years. From this viewpoint, the traditional and present positions of the osteopathic medical profession were analyzed. Also factored into discussions was the rapid growth in numbers and student bodies of colleges of osteopathic medicine. This entailed consideration of contemporary curricular tendencies in the numerous institutions. The overall decision reached was that FOM3 should be prepared and viewed as a resource applicable to all phases of osteopathic medical education. As in previous editions, recognition is given to addressing the needs of students and practitioners. The format chosen emphasizes the approach to the patient. The organization of the text is given in the following overview.

PART I: FOUNDATIONS

Section 1: Overview of the Osteopathic Medical Profession

The number of chapters in this section is doubled from previous editions. The role of the ECOP in developing the Osteopathic Five Models is elaborated in *Osteopathic Philosophy*. This effort considers the manifestation of the models (Biomechanical; Respiratory-Circulatory; Metabolic; Neurological; Behavioral) in three components of a philosophy of medicine (Health, Disease, Patient Care). New chapters are *Osteopathic Education and Regulation* and *International Osteopathic Medicine and Osteopathy*.

Section 2: Basic Sciences

Two major changes characterize this section: The five models of patient diagnosis, treatment, and management frequently used by osteopathic physicians provide the background for this section. As a result, all but three of the chapters in *Basic Science and Behavioral Science* (FOM2) have been completely rewritten or replaced by new material. In addition, consolidation into one section reflects a strong belief that integration of body and mind lies at the heart of osteopathic medicine.

A complete explanation of the significance of these changes is provided in Chapter 5.

PART II: THE PATIENT ENCOUNTER

A completely new emphasis is found in this contribution to FOM3. Authors point out that in the initial patient encounter, patient rapport is as important as the gathering of historical information. It is acknowledged that several clinical issues represent public health problems of such magnitude that all physicians must participate in detection and treatment (e.g., cancer, hypertension, hypercholesterolemia). Effective patient management occurs best within the largest possible context, including cultural, socioeconomic, and religious/spiritual issues.

PART III: APPROACH TO THE SOMATIC COMPONENT

A reorganization of concept characterizes the change represented in PART III. Fundamental methods remain, as do osteopathic considerations for the various regions of the body. Methods, however, receive a very different perspective. Designation as *Traditional Approaches* or *Contemporary Approaches* portrays the present-day teaching emphases in the various colleges of osteopathic medicine. Patient Vignettes are found throughout. These are presented as commonly encountered clinical complaints and serve as a means of reinforcing the value of skillful palpation, establishment of an appropriate palpatory diagnosis, and a rationale for the selection of osteopathic manipulative intervention.

Section 1: Basic Evaluation

Palpation, Screening Examination, Segmental Motion Testing, and Posture continue to define fundamental approaches to patient assessment.

Section 2: Osteopathic Considerations of Regions

Following precedents from FOM1 and FOM2, the various body regions are discussed with a view to facilitating the use of contemporary medical information in the establishment of an osteopathic medical approach to diagnosis, treatment, and management of clinical presentations.

Section 3: Osteopathic Manipulative Treatment

Traditional Approaches

Represented here are the methods of osteopathic manipulative intervention uniformly taught at all colleges of osteopathic medicine: *Thrust (HV/LA); "The Pop"; Muscle Energy; Myofascial Release; Osteopathy in the Cranial Field; Strain/Counterstrain; Soft Tissue/Articulatory; Lymphatics.*

This group of methods was determined during various consultations and discussions held with the ECOP during its meetings, 2007–2009.

Contemporary Approaches

In the broader perspective of osteopathic theory and practice, various other methods are being developed, refined, and taught. Not all are regularly taught at colleges of osteopathic medicine. Representatives of this group of methods are *Balanced Ligamentous Tension/ Ligamentous Articular Strain; Facilitated Positional Release; Progressive Inhibition of Neuromuscular Structures; Functional Technique; Visceral Manipulation; Still Technique; Chapman's Approach; Fulford Percussion.*

Whether *Traditional* or *Contemporary*, all approaches described in FOM3 reflect the components of the osteopathic medical profession's definition of *Somatic Dysfunction:* Impaired or altered function of related components of the somatic (body framework) system: skeletal, arthrodial, and myofascial structures, and related vascular, lymphatic, and neural elements. The systematic use of palpation in the process of palpatory diagnosis remains the hallmark expression of osteopathic medical practice.

PART IV: APPROACH TO OSTEOPATHIC PATIENT MANAGEMENT

Another completely new emphasis is found in this contribution to FOM3. It is well recognized that the curricula of many colleges of osteopathic medicine utilize case-based learning modules, which may employ various formats. Represented here is a selection of commonly encountered clinical presentations found in individuals from the young to the elderly. The entities chosen for presentation do not constitute a comprehensive listing, but serve as guides to the development of the thought processes of the osteopathic medical student and practitioner. Patient Vignettes are used to demonstrate an osteopathic medical approach to diagnosis, treatment, and management of each situation. Further, the applicability of the five models of patient diagnosis, treatment, and management is given specific attention within the context of the clinical presentation.

PART V: APPROACHES TO OSTEOPATHIC MEDICAL RESEARCH

Continued refinement of the focus for osteopathic medical research has defined five components: *Foundations; Priorities; Development/ Support; Biobehavioral; Future.* The osteopathic medical profession has made many original contributions to the study of its premises. There is, in society at large, generous recognition of such. More effort is needed in validation of Osteopathic Manipulative Treatment (OMT). With pending changes in the health care delivery system in coming years, documentation of efficacy of OMT in promoting and maintaining health would be a most welcome contribution. Although not the exclusive expression of osteopathic medical practice, elucidation of knowledge about efficacy would significantly enhance the appreciation of this approach in attaining and maintaining health. This, after all, was the vision of Andrew Taylor Still.

The goal of the editorial team of FOM3 has been to continue to build on the work of our predecessors in FOM1 and FOM2. Change as introduced in this text seeks to acknowledge present trends in the educational formats and styles used in colleges of osteopathic medicine and their various programs. In doing so, it is hoped that the result offers the contemporary expression of osteopathic medical practice. It can only be certain that, with pending changes in health care delivery, future editions of this text will also seek to improve upon this effort.

It has been a privilege to serve.

ANTHONY G. CHILA, DO, FAAO *dist*, FCA
Executive Editor

FOREWORD

As Editor-in-Chief of the American Osteopathic Association, I again have the pleasure to present another edition of *Foundations of Osteopathic Medicine*. This third edition has uniqueness. It is a robust revision of an already strong textbook that has embraced the guiding principle and goal of teaching osteopathic medical students to think like osteopathic physicians. So instead of trying to create an "encyclopedic cookbook" that educates students on how to treat patients for every conceivable illness, this textbook concentrates on providing a solid foundation and clear examples that illustrate how osteopathic physicians think through patients' problems.

To that end, we replaced the section on individual specialties with 17 new chapters in Part IV on problem-based learning. It is not intended for these chapters to be all-encompassing. Instead, each chapter involves a case example of how osteopathic principles and practice can be applied to patient care using existing osteopathic evidence and experience. We hope that faculty at osteopathic colleges and universities use and build on these chapters to provide their students with solid examples on how to apply the fundamentals of osteopathic medicine to daily patient care.

Additionally, the third edition has been strengthened with revisions made to the chapters on osteopathic manipulative treatment techniques (Part III) to concentrate on the techniques that are universally taught at osteopathic medical schools. However, there has been a preservation of the second edition's effort to expose osteopathic medical students to as many OMT techniques as possible by placing eight lesser used treatments in Chapter 52, which is titled "Contemporary Approaches."

Also central to this textbook are osteopathic medicine's five models of treatment, which are introduced in Chapter 5 and applied throughout Part IV. Equally critical to understanding and appreciating the Foundation's major themes are Chapter 1 on osteopathic philosophy and Part II on the patient encounter. Together, these chapters will lead students to understand how to think and practice osteopathically and use the rest of the textbook more effectively.

One can not help but to believe that all physicians may benefit from various sections in this textbook. I have expressed before how I have uncovered both scientific and clinical information that has helped me understand and practice pulmonary and critical care medicine using osteopathic principles and practices.

Importantly, the American Association of Colleges of Osteopathic Medicine's Educational Council on Osteopathic Principles (ECOP) was consulted throughout the process of revising this textbook. As with the first two editions of Foundations, ECOP's glossary of terminology is included as an appendix to the third edition.

The Foundations textbook was the vision of Howard M. Levine, D.O., and the first two editions that were edited by Robert C. Ward, D.O. Through their persistent commitment to the osteopathic medical profession, this textbook came to life and flourished. This third edition would not have been possible without its executive editor, Anthony G. Chila, D.O., who dedicated four years of his life to planning and executing this revision. He has been a model of diligence and diplomacy, working with 10 dedicated section editors, all highly accomplished within the osteopathic medical profession, nearly 80 authors and numerous peer reviewers. To ensure that he could devote the necessary time and concentrated effort to this edition, Dr. Chila made such sacrifices as passing on the reins of the editorship of the American Academy of Osteopathy Journal. Combining his skills as a leader with his expertise in osteopathic medicine, Dr. Chila commanded and received the respect of the numerous contributors to Foundations and pulled them together to work as a team.

More than anyone else, Dr. Chila identified the new and guiding vision for the third edition. He inspired the other leaders and contributors, and he kept the entire complex process on track and on time. Dr. Chila paid careful attention to the needs of the faculty at our colleges and universities, making sure that he received feedback from ECOP on the plans and outcome of this edition.

On a personal note, I have known Tony for nearly thirty years, and I have admired him for the countless contributions he has made to osteopathic medicine. When I asked him to take this challenge on, he accepted without hesitation. As his colleague and as Editor-in-Chief of AOA Publications, I view the third edition of *Foundations of Osteopathic Medicine* as among Tony's greatest legacies to the osteopathic profession and to medicine in general. I am proud of what he has done to make this edition even more relevant than previous editions for educating both current and future DOs to think like osteopathic physicians.

GILBERT E. D'ALONZO, D.O.
Editor-in-Chief, AOA Publications
American Osteopathic Association

ACKNOWLEDGMENTS

The work involved in preparation of this third edition of *Foundations of Osteopathic Medicine* (FOM3) was a dedicated effort by many individuals. In accomplishing their various tasks, all contributed to a cohesive product representing another level of development for this text. Grateful appreciation is extended to the following:

SECTION EDITORS

Jane E. Carreiro, DO
Anthony G. Chila, DO, FAAO *dist*, FCA
Dennis J. Dowling, DO, FAAO
Russell G. Gamber, DO, MPH
John C. Glover, DO, FAAO
Ann L. Habenicht, DO, FAAO
John A. Jerome, PhD, BCFE
Michael M. Patterson, PhD
Felix J. Rogers, DO, FACOI
Michael A. Seffinger, DO, FAAFP
Frank H. Willard, PhD

In establishing a new direction for FOM3, the *Section Editors* readily acknowledged the accomplishments and effort of contributors to the second edition of this text (FOM2). Specific recommendation was made to allow for online access to Section VI of FOM2 (*Clinical Specialties*). This offers demonstrable continuity between the second and third editions of this text.

In the matter of reformulating the content approach of this third edition of FOM3, the *Section Editors* also sought to express appreciation to former authors whose contributions helped shape the conceptual expression of the text:

David A. Baron, MSEd, DO
Ronald H. Bradley, DO, PhD
Boyd R. Buser, DO
Thomas A. Cavalieri, DO
Shawn Centers, DO
Eileen L. DiGiovanna, DO, FAAO
Norman Gevitz, PhD
Philip E. Greenman, DO, FAAO
Deborah M. Heath, DO, MD(H)
James B. Jensen, DO
Lauritz A. Jensen, DO
H. James Jones, DO
Edna M. Lay, DO, FAAO
John C. Licciardone, DO, MS, MBA
Alexander S. Nicholas, DO, FAAO
Donald R. Noll, DO
David A. Patriquin, DO, FAAO
Ronald P. Portanova, PhD
Bernard R. Rubin, DO
Mark Sandhouse, DO
Stanley Schiowitz, DO, FAAO
Richard J. Snow, DO, MPH
Harvey Sparks Jr., MD, PhD
Sarah A. Sprafka, PhD
Robert J. Theobald Jr., PhD
Terri Turner, DO
Colleen Vallad-Hix, DO
Elaine M. Wallace, DO
Mary C. Williams, DO
John M. Willis, DO
Robert D. Wurster, PhD

The artwork of William A. Kuchera, DO, FAAO

EDUCATIONAL COUNCIL ON OSTEOPATHIC PRINCIPLES (ECOP)

This Council is comprised of the Departmental Chairpersons of the various Colleges of Osteopathic Medicine. During the years 2007–2010, support of the FOM3 Project was generously given by members of ECOP and its subgroups. Presentations on behalf of FOM3 were facilitated by Chairpersons John C. Glover, DO, FAAO (2007–2009) and David C. Mason, DO, FACOFP (2009–2010).

During the life of the project, at different times, members of ECOP were presented material in preparation and asked for their comment and critique. Special thanks for her initiative and leadership in this activity is given to Kendi Hensel, DO, PhD.

LIPPINCOTT WILLIAMS & WILKINS

Charles W. Mitchell, Acquisitions Editor
Jennifer Verbiar, Product Manager
Nancy Peterson, Development Editor

THE AMERICAN OSTEOPATHIC ASSOCIATION

John Crosby, JD, Executive Director, American Osteopathic Association
Gilbert E. D'Alonzo, Jr., MS, DO, FACOI, Editor-in-Chief, Publications, American Osteopathic Association
Michael Fitzgerald, Director of Publications and Publisher

STUDENT REVIEWERS

The following Student Physicians gave generously of their time in providing comments and reviews of various sections of FOM3. Appreciation is extended to these future leaders in practice and publication.

UNIVERSITY OF NORTH TEXAS HEALTH SCIENCE CENTER AT FORT WORTH
TEXAS COLLEGE OF OSTEOPATHIC MEDICINE

Delukie, Ali; Luu, Huy; Sprys, Michael (2009)

Ashraf, Hossain; Dunn, Angela; Lehmann, Amber; Martinez, Vanessa; Shanafelt (Peer), Christie (2010)

Curtis, Sarah; Knitig, Christopher; Stovall, Bradley (2011)

MIDWESTERN UNIVERSITY
CHICAGO COLLEGE OF OSTEOPATHIC MEDICINE

Hohner, Elita L. (2012)

WESTERN UNIVERSITY OF HEALTH SCIENCES
COLLEGE OF OSTEOPATHIC MEDICINE OF THE PACIFIC

Bae, Esther (2011)
Harms, Sarah (2012)

PHILADELPHIA COLLEGE OF OSTEOPATHIC MEDICINE

Malka, Eli (2013)

SPECIAL THANKS

Special thanks to Samantha D. Dutrow and Cathy J. Bledsoe for their contributions to Chapter 30, "Health Promotion and Maintenance"

The Arizona College of Osteopathic Medicine—Midwestern University supported the *Chapman's Think Tank Retreat* which was held at Glendale, AZ in September, 2006. Contributors to this effort were Loren H. Rex, DO and Linos Cidros, ATC. Proofreading and critical suggestions were provided by Gary A. Fryer, PhD, BSc (Osteo) and Eliah Malka. These contributors helped pave the way for publication of FOM3 PART III, Chapter 52G; *Chapman's Approach*.

Foundations

1

Osteopathic Philosophy

MICHAEL A. SEFFINGER, HOLLIS H. KING, ROBERT C. WARD, JOHN M. JONES, III, FELIX J.
ROGERS, AND MICHAEL M. PATTERSON

KEY CONCEPTS

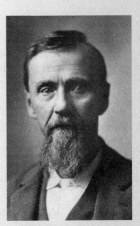

- Osteopathic philosophy forms the foundation for the practice of osteopathic medicine, which is a comprehensive and scientifically based school of medicine.
- Classic osteopathic philosophy was articulated by the founder of the profession, Dr. Andrew Taylor Still, and his direct students.
- Classic osteopathic philosophy expresses Dr. Still's understanding of health and disease and his approach to patient care.
- Various aspects of osteopathic philosophy and principles have ancient historical roots, but, as a unified set of concepts, the philosophy represents a unique approach to health and patient care.
- The expression and emphasis of osteopathic philosophy and its tenets continue to evolve over time.
- Irvin M. Korr, Ph.D., eloquently expressed the tenets of osteopathic philosophy to generations of osteopathic students, physicians, and scientists as a professor at several osteopathic colleges throughout the latter half of the 20th century.
- The Educational Council of Osteopathic Principles of the American Association of Colleges of Osteopathic Medicine developed a Glossary of Osteopathic Terminology and identified the fundamental osteopathic approaches to patient care.
- Osteopathic principles guide osteopathic physicians toward a health-oriented, patient-centered approach to health care.

INTRODUCTION

Osteopathic philosophy, deceptively simple in its presentation, forms the basis for osteopathic medicine's distinctive approach to health care. The philosophy acts as a unifying set of ideas for the organization and application of scientific knowledge to patient care. Through the philosophy, this knowledge is organized in relation to all aspects of health (physical, mental, emotional, and spiritual). A patient-centered focus, using health-oriented principles of patient care and unique skills, including hands-on manual diagnosis and treatment, guide the application of that knowledge. These concepts form the foundation for practicing osteopathic medicine.

Viewpoints and attitudes arising from osteopathic principles give osteopathic physicians an important template for clinical problem solving, health restoration and maintenance, and patient education. In the 21st century, this viewpoint is particularly useful as practitioners from a wide variety of disciplines confront increasingly complex physical, psychological, social, ethical, and spiritual problems affecting individuals, families, and populations from a wide variety of cultures and backgrounds.

THE EDUCATIONAL COUNCIL ON OSTEOPATHIC PRINCIPLES

In the contemporary era, the evolution, growth, and teaching of osteopathic philosophy have been coordinated through the Educational Council on Osteopathic Principles (ECOP) of the American

Association of Colleges of Osteopathic Medicine. This organization consists of the chairs of the departments of osteopathic principles and practice from each osteopathic medical school. It is the "expert panel" in the osteopathic medical profession in regard to osteopathic manipulative medicine and osteopathic philosophy and principles. These osteopathic physicians are considered leading-edge thinkers in terms of osteopathic philosophy and principles.

One of ECOP's charges is to obtain consensus on the usage of terms within the profession. *The Glossary of Osteopathic Terminology* was first published in 1981 (1) and is updated annually. The latest edition is available through the American Association of Colleges of Osteopathic Medicine and the American Osteopathic Association (AOA) websites; the 2009 edition is reprinted in the appendix to this textbook. The 2009 Glossary includes the following definition of osteopathic philosophy:

A concept of health care supported by expanding scientific knowledge that embraces the concept of the unity of the living organism's structure (anatomy) and function (physiology). Osteopathic philosophy emphasizes the following principles:

1. The human being is a dynamic unit of function
2. The body possesses self-regulatory mechanisms that are self-healing in nature
3. Structure and function are interrelated at all levels
4. Rational treatment is based on these principles

One of the products of ECOP's work was the development of a uniquely osteopathic curriculum for medical education that was founded upon a health-oriented, patient-centered perspective and focused on restoration, enhancement, and maintenance of normal physiologic processes (2). When utilizing a health-oriented perspective, it is crucial to restrain from focusing solely on that which is dysfunctional or impeding function, but to also acknowledge the physiologic adaptive response pattern that can be facilitated to enhance the patient's capacity to maintain or restore optimal function and health. Physiology texts (e.g., Vander) describe ten basic coordinated body functions, namely:

1. Control of posture and body movement
2. Respiration
3. Circulation
4. Regulation of water and electrolyte balance
5. Digestion and absorption of nutrients and elimination of wastes
6. Metabolism and energy balance
7. Protective mechanisms
8. The sensory system
9. Reproduction
10. Consciousness and behavior

The ECOP group combined these into five basic integrative and coordinated body functions and coping strategies that were considered in a context of healthful adaptation to life and its circumstances:

1. Posture and motion, including fundamental structural and biomechanical reliability
2. Gross and cellular respiratory and circulatory factors
3. Metabolic processes of all types, including endocrine-mediated, immune-regulatory, and nutritionally related biochemical processes
4. Neurologic integration, including central, peripheral, autonomic, neuroendocrine, neurocirculatory, and their reflex relationships
5. Psychosocial, cultural, behavioral, and spiritual elements

USING THE FIVE MODELS IN PATIENT ASSESSMENT AND TREATMENT

These five coordinated body functions have been referred to as "five models," referring to the fact that they represent particular approaches to the patient. The conceptual models are perspectives by which one might view the patient. This is analogous to viewing a patient through a lens; by altering the focal length of the lens one could view different aspects of the patient and gain various perspectives on the patient's struggle to maintain health. This would open many avenues for diagnosis, treatment, and management, including the use of palpatory diagnosis and osteopathic manipulative treatment (OMT). It is important to keep in mind that the five models are merely expressions of our physiological functions that maintain health and play key roles in adaptation to stressors as well as in recovery and repair from illness and disease.

The musculoskeletal system can be viewed as the core that links these five coordinated body functions.

Figure 1.1 depicts the musculoskeletal system as the core or hub of a five-spoked wheel. Careful observation and educated palpation help make the musculoskeletal system a natural entry point for both diagnosis and treatment. Importantly, the musculoskeletal system often reflects numerous signs relating to internal diseases. The models provide a framework for interpreting the significance of somatic dysfunction within the context of objective and subjective clinical information. These models therefore guide the osteopathic

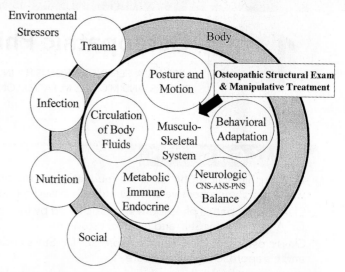

Figure 1-1 Osteopathic philosophy of health displayed as the coordinated activity of five basic body functions, integrated by the musculoskeletal system, adapting to environmental stressors. Evaluation and treatment of the musculoskeletal system is performed in light of its ability to affect not only the five functions but also ultimately the person's own ability to adapt to internal and external stressors.

practitioner's approach to diagnosis and treatment. Typically, a combination of models will be appropriate for an individual patient. The combination chosen is modified by the patient's differential diagnosis, comorbidities, and other therapeutic regimens.

The five-model concept has been used in osteopathic postgraduate manual medicine courses for over 35 years (3), in osteopathic manual medicine texts (4), and in osteopathic postgraduate education journals (5,6). In 2006, the World Health Organization recognized the osteopathic five-model concept as a unique osteopathic contribution to world health care (Personal Communication, Jane Carreiro, DO, AOA representative to the World Health Organization, 2006). The five models are:

- Biomechanical model
- Respiratory-Circulatory model
- Neurological model
- Metabolic-Energy model
- Behavioral model

Regional anatomical approaches to the patient were presented initially in the writings of Dr. Andrew Taylor Still, MD, DO. In considering an osteopathic visual and palpatory structural evaluation and treatment approach to the various body regions, ECOP considered that as the muscles and joints of the trunk and extremities are primarily involved in posture and motion, addressing them would be within the perspective of the Biomechanical model; addressing the costal cage and diaphragms, being that they are responsible for the movements associated with thoracic respiration and return of venous and lymph to the heart for recirculation, are considered as part of the Respiratory-Circulatory model; assessment and treatment of the abdominopelvic regions represent the Metabolic-Energy model as this is where our internal organs that process food, convert it to usable energy, and discard metabolic by-products (waste) reside; assessing and treating the head and spinal regions represent the Neurological model; addressing the patient's lifestyle, environmental stressors, values, and choices represents the Behavioral model. Table 1.1 outlines the five models as applied to assessment and treatment.

TABLE 1.1

Osteopathic Approaches to Patient Care

Model	Anatomical Correlates	Physiological Functions
Biomechanical	Postural muscles, spine, and extremities	Posture and motion
Respiratory-Circulatory	Thoracic inlet, thoracic and pelvic diaphragms, tentorium cerebelli, costal cage	Respiration, circulation, venous, and lymphatic drainage
Metabolic-Energy	Internal organs, endocrine glands	Metabolic processes, homeostasis, energy balance, regulatory processes; immunological activities and inflammation and repair; digestion, absorption of nutrients, removal of waste; reproduction
Neurological	Head (organs of special senses), brain, spinal cord, autonomic nervous system, peripheral nerves	Control, coordination, and integration of body functions; protective mechanisms; sensation
Behavioral	Brain	Psychological and social activities, e.g., anxiety, stress, work, family; habits, e.g., sleep, drug abuse, sexual activities, exercise; values, attitudes, beliefs

Biomechanical Model

The Biomechanical model views the patient from a structural or mechanical perspective. Alterations of postural mechanisms, motion, and connective tissue compliance, regardless of etiology, often impede vascular, lymphatic, and neurologic functions. As the structural integrity and function of the musculoskeletal system is interactive and interdependent with the neurologic, respiratory-circulatory, metabolic, and behavioral structural components and functions of the patient, this model considers that a structural impediment causing, or being caused by, a dysfunction of muscles, joints, and/or connective tissue, can compromise vascular or neurologic structures and therefore affect associated metabolic processes and/or overt behaviors. Depending on the person's adaptive capabilities, this can lead to disturbances in various body functions, including mental functions, as well as decrease the patient's homeostatic capacity. The person's ability to adapt to, or recover from, insults and stressors, or prevent further breakdown, becomes further compromised. Social activity is often adversely affected and economic consequences follow. The biomechanical perspective leads the osteopathic physician to assess the patient for a structural impediment, and upon removal of the impediment, that is, by correction of somatic dysfunction through application of OMT, enable the patient to regain associated structural, vascular, neurologic, metabolic, and behavioral functions. The objective is to optimize the patient's adaptive potential through restoration of structural integrity and function.

For example, a patient who is in an automobile accident often sustains a whiplash-type injury and subsequently has difficulty moving her neck, shoulders, and low back. If there is trauma to the costal cage, rib motion is impeded and breathing becomes difficult as well. Due to the lack of motion and muscle spasms, the patient begins to feel shooting pains into her arms, or pins and needles in her thumb and index fingers. She gets lightheaded and dizzy upon standing, loses her appetite, cannot maintain her exercise routine, has difficulty sleeping, and therefore cannot concentrate on studying or doing her work very well. Her structural problems have caused motion restrictions that have affected her four other main physiological functions, that is, the other four domains of health. Alleviation of her somatic dysfunction enables restoration of her normal posture and motion and improvement in her breathing and blood circulation; she begins to eat well again, restarts her exercise program, and sleeps through the night to awaken refreshed, energetic, and able to concentrate. She can study and do her work once again.

Respiratory-Circulatory Model

Approaching the patient from the perspective of the Respiratory-Circulatory model entails focusing on respiratory and circulatory components of the homeostatic response in pathophysiological processes. This includes central as well as peripheral processes that are involved in the dynamic interaction between these two paramount functions, that is, central neural control, cerebral spinal fluid flow, arterial supply, venous and lymphatic drainage, as well as pulmonary and cardiovascular function. Additionally, this model views the interaction between respiratory-circulatory functions and musculoskeletal, neurologic, metabolic, and behavioral functions as they affect the patient's adaptive response and total homeostatic or health potential. Evaluation and treatment is geared toward maximizing the capacity and efficiency of respiratory-circulatory functions in order to maximize the patient's health potential. The respiratory-circulatory model concerns itself with the maintenance of extra- and intracellular environments through the unimpeded delivery of oxygen and nutrients and the removal of cellular waste products. Tissue stress interfering with the flow or circulation of any body fluid can affect tissue health. OMT within this model addresses dysfunction in respiratory mechanics, circulation, and the flow of body fluids.

A case in point is the patient with pneumonia. In this condition, an infection occurs in the lung, there is congestion of fluids in the lungs, and respiration is compromised. Often, each breath causes pain. The nervous system communicates this information to the musculoskeletal system that accommodates and responds by decreasing respiratory motion in the costal cage and upper back in the area of the infected lung tissue and irritated pleura. These changes in the musculoskeletal system can be palpated and treated with osteopathic manipulation to relax the tense muscles and provide some comfort, as well as helping to mobilize the congested fluids in the lungs. The pneumonia also affects the patient's metabolism and energy level. Fighting an infection such as this is exhausting and the patient complains of fatigue, loss of appetite, and has increased need for sleep. Social interactions are adversely affected. So, all five domains of health are affected and need to be addressed as part of the management plan for this patient. Getting the patient's respiration and circulation of fluids back into normal order is the primary goal, which will improve function of all of the other body functions in a coordinated fashion. Thus, the osteopathic physician would focus on treating the pneumonia with antibiotics, rehydrating the patient with intravenous fluids and restoring normal motion and function of the costal cage, diaphragm, and thoracic and cervical spine with OMT as appropriate.

Neurological Model

The Neurologic model views the patient's problems in terms of aberrancies or impairments of neural function that are caused by or cause pathophysiologic responses in structural, respiratory-circulatory structures and functions, metabolic processes, and behavioral activities. More specifically, the Neurological model considers the influence of spinal facilitation, proprioceptive function, the autonomic nervous system, and activity of nociceptors (pain fibers) on the function of the neuroendocrine immune network. Of particular importance is the relationship between the somatic and the visceral (autonomic) systems. Therapeutic application of OMT within this model focuses on the reduction of mechanical stresses, balance of neural inputs, and the elimination of nociceptive drive. The goal of treatment in this model is to re-establish normal (optimal) neural function. Restoration or optimization of neural integrative and regulatory functions will improve efficiency in associated structural, vascular, metabolic, and behavioral functions. This will help to maximize the patient's adaptive potential and regain optimal health.

An example patient for whom using a neurological focus for evaluation and management would be advantageous is one with peristalsis, or lack of intestinal motion, after general anesthesia and abdominal surgery. Through neurological reflexes, the paraspinal back and neck muscles tighten. The intestines fill with gas, which, due to lack of intestinal motility, expand within the abdominal cavity causing distension, pain, and sometimes nausea and vomiting. The patient is not able to eat or pass the gas through the rectum, cannot sleep, ambulate, or take full breaths. The lungs partially collapse and breathing becomes difficult. All five domains of health are compromised. Treatment entails OMT to release the paraspinal tensions and spasms that decreases sympathetic hyperactivity and increases parasympathetic activity, ultimately restoring normal intestinal motility. Sometimes, nasogastric suction is helpful as well. Intravenous fluids may be needed to hydrate the patient. Once the nervous system functions normally once again, metabolic, respiratory, and motion functions return to normal as well. The patient returns to normal activity, and normal diet and sleep cycles also are restored.

Metabolic-Energy Model

In viewing the patient from the perspective of the Metabolic-Energy model, focus is placed upon the metabolic and energy-conserving aspects of the homeostatic adaptive response. This includes evaluation and treatment of cellular, tissue, and organ systems as they relate to each other's energy demand and consumption as well as production of work or products. The role of the musculoskeletal system and the connective tissues of the body in pathophysiological processes are important as they are accessible to palpation and manipulation. Efficient posture and motion, arterial supply, venous and lymphatic drainage, CSF fluid mechanics, neurologic, endocrine and immune functions, and prudent behaviors, balanced emotions, and proper nutrition are the keystones of energy conservation and efficiency of metabolic functions. Improving the functions of any of these components will aid the total body energy economy. This will maximize the patient's adaptive resources and ability to successfully respond and adapt to stressors.

The Metabolic-Energy model recognizes that the body seeks to maintain a balance between energy production, distribution, and expenditure. This aids the body in its ability to adapt to various stressors, including immunological, nutritional, and psychological types. The body's ability to restore and maintain health requires energy-efficient response to infectious agents and repair of injuries. Proper nutrition enables normal biochemical processes, cellular functions, and neuromusculoskeletal activity. Additionally, injuries to the musculoskeletal system tax the body's energy economy. Physical activity promotes optimum cardiovascular function, but an inefficient musculoskeletal system increases the body's allostatic load or burden. Therapeutic application of OMT within this model addresses somatic dysfunction that has the potential to dysregulate the production, distribution or expenditure of energy, increase allostatic load, or interfere with immunological and endocrinological regulatory functions. Another therapeutic application using this model includes prescribing medications to improve and stabilize metabolic and systemic functions.

A patient with congestive heart failure has to conserve energy so as not to further strain the heart. Any compromise of efficient posture and motion will place too high of an energy demand on the failing heart, increasing the congestion in the lungs and edema in the feet. So, if the patient stumbles and sprains his ankle, the difficulty in ambulating with only one good leg can cause significant worsening of the congestive heart failure. Breathing becomes more difficult and appetite becomes decreased. The nervous system relays information from the struggling heart to the surrounding musculoskeletal system, which creates muscle tensions and stiffness in the costal cage and cervical and thoracic spinal joints. The patient is unable to lie down or sleep well. Again, all five domains of health are affected. The primary goal of treatment is to relieve the burden on the failing heart, that is, fix the sprained ankle and support the patient's motion needs in the meantime. Fluid and salt intake need to be closely controlled. Medications that help to excrete the excess fluids from the body and strengthen the heart contractility are typically needed as well as bed rest until the heart regains its strength. Once the metabolic-energy expenditure needs are addressed, respiration-circulation, posture and motion, neurological function, and behavioral activities are subsequently restored.

Behavioral Model

The Behavioral model recognizes that the assessment of a patient's health includes assessing his or her mental, emotional, and spiritual state of being as well as personal lifestyle choices. Health is often affected by environmental, socioeconomic, cultural, and hereditary factors and the various emotional reactions and psychological stresses with which patients contend. Environmentally induced trauma and toxicities, inactivity and lack of exercise, use of addictive substances, and poor dietary choices all serve to diminish a patient's adaptive capacity, rendering the patient vulnerable to opportunistic organisms and/or organ and system failure.

The osteopathic physician uses the behavioral perspective to consider that the musculoskeletal system expresses feelings and emotions, and stress manifests in increased neuromuscular tension. Somatic dysfunction affects the musculoskeletal system's reaction to biopsychosocial stressors. OMT is employed within this model with the goal of improving the body's ability to effectively manage, compensate, or adapt to these stressors. The osteopathic physician utilizes compassionate, caring, and education skills to help patients maximize their coping capabilities and improve healthy lifestyle and behavioral choices. The whole person—body, mind, and spirit—is considered in the individualized management plan. Psychological, social, cultural, behavioral, and spiritual elements are addressed within the management plan as needed. In addition to providing care for the cause of diseases, the patient's perspective of needing palliative and remedial care is also addressed. In addition, the Behavioral model entails providing patient education on health, disease and lifestyle choices, mental outlook, and preventive care.

A patient with chronic obstructive pulmonary disease (emphysema) from tobacco abuse is a patient for whom the behavioral perspective plays a primary role in osteopathic management. After decades of smoking at least one pack of cigarettes per day, the lungs undergo anatomical change and can no longer exchange carbon dioxide for oxygen appropriately. This alters many metabolic processes throughout the body that rely on this gas exchange. Vascular functions are compromised since oxygen is not delivered appropriately to the tissues and carbon dioxide builds up creating an acidic environment that is toxic to normal cells. Neurologic functions, that is, brain activity, suffer from this altered metabolic milieu. Musculoskeletal structures and functions throughout the body undergo adaptation, that is, the barrel-shaped costal cage formed by patients with emphysema due to retained air in the lungs. There are further changes in the behavioral realm. The patient who cannot breathe efficiently becomes short of breath, anxious, and agitated easily, insecure, and loses self-confidence. He or she cannot tolerate exercise or exertion. Sleep is disturbed and difficult as the patient can only get rest in the seated position, or propped up on two or more pillows in bed, which is not comfortable for the low back after several hours. Work and social relations are compromised, often leading to disability and isolation. Smoking is an addictive behavior that requires the patient to exert considerable willpower, courage, and perseverance in order to overcome the habit. Medications may be needed to help the patient gain control over the addiction. The osteopathic physician and the entire professional health care team, including family and friends, need to encourage the patient to work toward the goal of restoration of health by removal of the offending agent (tobacco and its related chemicals), offering medications to improve lung function, and providing much-needed psychological support. The primary treatment for the disease is for the patient to stop smoking and allow the body to heal itself. OMT to improve compliance of the costal cage can reduce the physical burden of breathing that is typically labored and exhausting to the muscles of respiration. The cervical paraspinal muscles become hypertonic and painful, which can be relieved with OMT. In this instance, OMT is an adjunct to the primary treatment, which is behavioral in nature. Often, OMT enables the physician to obtain trust and build rapport with the patient, enabling a partnership that facilitates the achievement of the mutual goal of ridding the patient of the smoking habit.

OSTEOPATHIC PRINCIPLES AS PRACTICE GUIDELINES

The contributions of A.T. Still and the osteopathic medical profession affect many aspects of general patient care. First, irrespective of diagnoses or practitioner, the patient is of central importance. Second, a competent differential diagnosis is essential. This includes all aspects of the person (body, mind, and spirit), as shown in Box 1.1. Third, clinical activities integrate realistic expectations with measurable outcomes. Finally, and ideally, patient-oriented educational efforts pragmatically address both personal and family-related concerns. The patient is ultimately responsible for long-term self-health care. Emphasis is on health restoration and disease prevention.

Irvin M. Korr, Ph.D., a prominent and well-respected scientist, philosopher, and educator reasoned (7):

> [There are] three major components of our indwelling health care system, each comprising numerous component systems. In the order in which humans became aware of them, they are (a) the healing (remedial, curative, palliative, recuperative, rehabilitative) component; (b) the component that defends against threats from the external environment; and (c) the homeostatic, health-maintaining component. These major component systems, of course, share subcomponents and mechanisms.

Health Restoration and Disease Prevention

Although osteopathically oriented medical care emphasizes competent comprehensive patient management, it also places importance on restoration of well being appropriate for the patient's age and health potential. This includes addressing:

- Physical, mental, and spiritual components
- Personal safety, such as wearing seat belts
- Sufficient rest and relaxation
- Proper nutrition
- Regular aerobic, stretching and strengthening exercises
- Maintaining rewarding social relationships
- Avoidance of tobacco and other abused substances
- Eliminating or modifying abusive personal, interpersonal, family, and work-related behavior patterns
- Avoidance of environmental radiation and toxins

When the internal health care system is permitted to operate optimally, without impediment, its product is what we call health. Its natural tendency is always toward health and the recovery of health. Indeed, the personal health care system is the very source of health, upon which all externally applied measures depend for their beneficial effects. The internal health care system, in effect, makes its own diagnoses, issues its own prescriptions, draws upon its own vast pharmacy, and in most situations, administers each dose without side effects. Health and healing, therefore, come from within. It is the patient who gets well, and not the practitioner or the treatment that makes [him or her] well.

In caring for the whole person, the well-grounded osteopathic physician goes beyond the presenting complaint, beyond relief of symptoms, beyond identification of the disease and treatment of the impaired organ, malfunction, or pathology, important as they are to total care. The osteopathic physician also explores those factors in the person and the person's life that may have contributed to the illness and that, appropriately modified, compensated, or eliminated, would favor recovery, prevent recurrence, and improve health in general.

The physician then selects that factor or combination of factors that are readily subject to change and that would be of sufficient impact to shift the balance toward recovery and enhancement of health. The possible factors include such categories as the biological (e.g., genetic, nutritional), psychological, behavioral (use, neglect, or abuse of body and mind; interpersonal relationships; habits; etc.), sociocultural, occupational, and environmental. Some of these factors, especially some of the biological [ones], are responsive to appropriate clinical intervention, some are responsive only to social or governmental action, and still others require changes by patients themselves. Osteopathic whole-person care, therefore, is a collaborative relationship between patient and physician.

It is obvious that some of the most deleterious factors are difficult or impossible for patient and physician to change or eliminate. These include (at least at present) genetic factors (although some inherited predispositions can be mitigated by lifestyle change). They include also such items as social convention, lifelong habits (e.g., dietary and behavioral), widely shared beliefs, prejudices, misconceptions and cultural doctrines, attitudes, and values. Others, such as the quality of the physical or socioeconomic environments, may require concerted community, national, and even international action.

Focus falls, therefore, upon those deleterious factors that are favorably modifiable by personal and professional action, and that, when appropriately modified or eliminated, mitigate the health-impairing effects of the less changeable factors. Improvement of body mechanics by osteopathic manipulative treatment is a major consideration when dealing with these complex interactions.

Korr explored the implications of what he called "our personal health care systems" and how that concept guides the doctor-patient relationship:

> This principle has important implications for the respective responsibilities of patient and physician and for their relationship. Since each person is the owner and hence the guardian of his or her own personal health care system, the ultimate source of health and healing, the primary responsibility for one's

health is each individual's. That responsibility is met by the way the person lives, thinks, behaves, nourishes himself or herself, uses body and mind, relates to others, and the other factor usually called lifestyle. Each person must be taught and enabled to assume that responsibility.

> It is the physician's responsibility, while giving palliative and remedial attention to the patient's immediate problem, to support each patient's internal health care system, to remove impediments to its competence, and above all, to do it no harm. It is also the responsibility of physicians to instruct patients on how to do the same for themselves and to strive to motivate them to do so, especially by their own example.

> The relationship between patient and osteopathic physician is therefore a collaborative one, a partnership, in maintaining and enhancing the competence of the patient's personal health care system. The maintenance and enhancement of health is the most effective and comprehensive form of preventive medicine, for health is the best defense against disease (7).

In 2002, an ad hoc interdisciplinary task force of osteopathic educators, philosophers, and researchers proposed osteopathic principles for patient care (8):

1. **The Patient Is the Focus for Health Care**—All osteopathic physicians, irrespective of the specialty of the practitioner, are trained to focus on the individual patient. The relationship between clinician and patient is a partnership in which both parties are actively engaged. The osteopathic physician is an advocate for the patient, supporting his or her efforts to optimize the circumstances to maintain, improve, or restore health.

2. **The Patient Has the Primary Responsibility for His or Her Health**—While the physician is the professional charged with the responsibility to assist a patient in being well, the physician can no more impart health to another person than he or she can impart charm, wisdom, wit, or any other desirable trait. Although the patient–physician relationship is a partnership, and the physician has significant obligations to the patient, ultimately the patient has primary responsibility for his or her health. The patient has inherent healing powers and must nurture these through diet and exercise as well as adherence to appropriate advice in regard to stress, sleep, body weight, and avoidance of abuse.

3. **An Effective Treatment Program for Patient Care**—An effective treatment program for patient care is founded on the above tenets and incorporates evidence-based guidelines, optimizes the patient's natural healing capacity, addresses the primary cause of disease, and emphasizes health maintenance and disease prevention. The emphasis on the musculoskeletal system as an integral part of patient care is one of the defining characteristics of osteopathic medicine.

When applied as part of a coherent philosophy of the practice of medicine, these tenets represent a distinct and necessary approach to health care. Evidence-based guidelines should be used to encourage those treatments with proven efficacy and to discourage those that are not beneficial, or even harmful. Osteopathic medicine embraces the concept of evidence-based medicine as part of a valuable reformation of clinical practice.

Andrew Taylor Still told his students "the object of the doctor is to seek health; anyone can find disease." This precept provides a useful orientation in patient care. An emphasis on health rather than disease helps to promote optimism. It may facilitate efforts to engage the patient as an active participant in recovery from illness. It may also encourage the realization that no single treatment approach is successful for every patient. Rather, optimal approaches will use diet, exercise, medications, manipulative treatment, surgery, or other modalities according to the needs and wishes of the patient and the skill and aptitude of the practitioner (8).

In end-stage conditions, it is recognized that treatment may be only palliative, remedial, and supportive. The AOA position paper on end-of-life care promotes compassionate and humanistic care tailored to the needs of each individual patient and his or her family.

Osteopathically oriented problem solving and treatment plans help guide the application of osteopathic principles in medical, behavioral, and surgical care. In 1987, ECOP developed guidelines for use by osteopathic physicians in developing an osteopathic management plan (2). The extent to which palpatory diagnosis and manipulative treatment are specifically useful interventions for a wide variety of neuromusculoskeletal problems remains to be seen through research. However, since many clinical presentations commonly interfere with a patient's ability to meet the requirements of normal daily activities (including appropriate exercise), it stands to reason that improving the efficiency of the neuromusculoskeletal system would benefit each patient. "There is a somatic component in all clinical situations. The somatic component is addressed to the extent that it influences patient well-being. Conceptually, osteopathic manipulative treatment is designed to address both structural abnormalities and self-regulatory capabilities" (2).

HOW IT ALL BEGAN

Andrew Taylor Still, M.D., D.O. (Fig. 1.1) (1828–1917), was an American frontier doctor who was convinced that 19th century patient care was severely inadequate. This resulted in an intense desire on his part to improve surgery, obstetrics, and the general treatment of diseases, placing them on a more rational and scientific basis.

As his perspectives and clinical understanding evolved, Still created an innovative system of diagnosis and treatment with two major emphases. The first highlights treatment of physical and mental ailments (i.e., diseases) while emphasizing the normalization of body structures and functions. Its hallmark was a detailed knowledge of anatomy that became the basis for much of his diagnostic and clinical work, most notably palpatory diagnosis and manipulative treatment. The second emphasizes the importance of health and well being in its broadest sense, including mental, emotional, and spiritual health, and the avoidance of alcohol and drugs and other negative health habits.

ORIGINS OF OSTEOPATHIC PHILOSOPHY

Historically, Still was not the first to call attention to inadequacies of the health care of his time; Hippocrates (c. 460–c. 377 B.C.E.), Galen (c. 130–c. 200), and Sydenham (1624–1689) were others. Each, in his own way, criticized the inadequacies of existing medical practices while focusing contemporary thinking on the patient's natural ability to heal.

In addition, Still was deeply influenced by a number of philosophers, scientists, and medical practitioners of his time. There is also evidence he was well versed in the religious philosophies

and concepts of the Methodist, Spiritualist, and Universalist movements of the period (9).

Following the loss of three children to spinal meningitis in 1864, Still immersed himself in the study of the nature of health, illness, and disease (10). His goal was to discover definitive methods for curing and preventing all that ailed his patients. He implicitly believed there was "a God of truth," and that "All His works, spiritual and material, are harmonious. His law of animal life is absolute. So wise a God had certainly placed the remedy within the material house in which the spirit of life dwells." Furthermore, he believed he could access these natural inherent remedies "… by adjusting the body in such a manner that the remedies may naturally associate themselves together, hear the cries, and relieve the afflicted" (10). In this quest, he combined contemporary philosophical concepts and principles with existing scientific theories. Always a pragmatist, Still accepted aspects of different philosophies, concepts, and practices that worked for him and his patients. He then integrated them with personal discoveries of his own from in-depth studies of anatomy, physics, chemistry, and biology (9). The result was the formulation of his new philosophy and its applications. He called it "Osteopathy."

Still's moment of clarity came on June 22, 1874. He writes, "I was shot, not in the heart, but in the dome of reason" (10). "Like a burst of sunshine the whole truth dawned on my mind, that I was gradually approaching a science by study, research, and observation that would be a great benefit to the world" (10). He realized that all living things, especially humans, were created by a perfect God. If humans were the embodiment of perfection, then they were fundamentally made to be healthy. There should be no defect in their structures and functions.

Since he believed that "the greatest study of man is man," he dissected numerous cadavers to test his hypothesis (10). He believed that if he could understand the construction (anatomy) of the human body, he would comprehend Nature's laws and unlock the keys to health. Still found no flaws in the concepts of the body's well-designed structure, proving to himself that his own hypothesis was correct.

A corollary to Still's revelation was that the physician does not cure diseases. In his view, it was the job of the physician to correct structural disturbances so the body works normally, just as a mechanic adjusts his machine. In *Research and Practice* he wrote,

The God of Nature is the fountain of skill and wisdom and the mechanical work done in all natural bodies is the result of absolute knowledge. Man cannot add anything to this perfect work nor improve the functioning of the normal body…. Man's power to cure is good as far as he has a knowledge of the right or normal position, and so far as he has the skill to adjust the bones, muscles and ligaments and give freedom to nerves, blood, secretions and excretions, and no farther. We credit God with wisdom and skill to perform perfect work on the house of life in which man lives. It is only justice that God should receive this credit and we are ready to adjust the parts and trust the results (11).

While Still practiced the orthodox medicine of his day from 1853 to 1879, including the use of oral medications such as purgatives, diuretics, stimulants, sedatives, and analgesics, and externally applied salves and plasters, once he began using his new philosophical system he virtually ceased using drugs. This occurred after several years where he experimented with combinations of drugs and manipulative treatment. In addition, he compared his results with those of patients who received no treatment at all (10). After several years' experience, he became convinced that his mechanical corrections consistently achieved the same or better results without using medications.

It was at that point that Still philosophically divorced himself from the orthodox practices of 19th century medicine (10). He writes, "Having been familiar myself for years with all their methods and having experimented with them I became disheartened and dropped them" (11). His unerring faith in the natural healing capabilities of the mechanically adjusted body formed the foundation for his new philosophy.

Unsure of what to call his new hands-on approach in the early years, Still at times referred to himself as a "magnetic healer" and "lightning bone-setter" (9,12). In the 1880s, Still began publicly using the term "osteopathy" as the chosen name for his new profession (5,9,13). He writes, "Osteopathy is compounded of two words, osteon, meaning bone, (and) pathos, (or) pathine, to suffer. I reasoned that the bone, 'Osteon,' was the starting point from which I was to ascertain the cause of pathological conditions, and so I combined the 'Osteo' with the 'pathy' and had as a result, Osteopathy" (10).

As the name osteopathy implies, Still used the bony skeleton as his reference point for understanding clinical problems and their pathological processes. On the surface, he was most interested in anatomy. On the other hand, he taught that there is more to the skeleton than 206 bones attached together by ligaments and connective tissue. In his discourses, Still would describe the anatomy of the arterial supply to the femur, for example, trace it back to the heart and lungs, and relate it to all of the surrounding and interrelated nerves, soft tissues, and organs along the way (Fig. 1.2). He would then demonstrate how the obstruction of arterial flow anywhere along the pathway toward the femur would result in pathophysiologic changes in the bone, producing pain or dysfunction.

He writes of his treatment concepts: "Bones can be used as levers to relieve pressure on nerves, veins and arteries" (10). This can be understood in the context that vascular and neural structures pass between bones or through orifices (foramina) within a bone. These are places where they are most vulnerable to bony compression and disruption of their functions. In addition, fascia is a type of connective tissue that attaches to bones. Fascia also envelops all muscles, nerves, and vascular structures. When strained or twisted by overuse or trauma myofascial structures not only restrict bony mobility, but also compress neurovascular structures and disturb their functions. By using the bones as manual levers, bony or myofascial entrapments of nerves or vascular structures can be removed, thus restoring normal nervous and vascular functions.

As Korr explained, "Even at the time of the founding of the osteopathic profession in 1892, the available knowledge in the sciences of physiology, biochemistry, microbiology, immunology, and pathology was meager. Indeed, immunology, biochemistry, and various other neurosciences and biomedical sciences had yet to appear as distinct disciplines. Therefore, these principles could only be expressed as aphorisms, embellished perhaps with conjectures about their biological basis" (7).

Beyond Neuromusculoskeletal Diagnosis and Treatment

The osteopathic medical profession is not only a neuromusculoskeletal-oriented diagnostic and treatment system, it is also a comprehensive and scientifically based school of medicine that embraces a philosophy. In answer to the question, "What is osteopathy?" Still stated, "It is a scientific knowledge of anatomy and physiology in the hands of a person of intelligence and skill, who can apply that knowledge to the use of man when sick or wounded by strains, shocks, falls, or mechanical derangement or injury of any kind to the body" (14) (Fig. 1.3).

Furthermore, osteopathy had a greater calling. In what could be considered a mission statement, Still wrote, "The object of Osteopathy is to improve upon the present systems of surgery, midwifery, and treatment of general diseases" (10).

The primary ideological components that distinguish one philosophy of healing from another are that system's concepts of what constitutes health, disease, and patient care. The following sections delineate how osteopathic philosophy has evolved and expressed itself in regards to these three concepts.

Classical osteopathic philosophy is described in Box 1.2.

CLASSIC OSTEOPATHIC PHILOSOPHY OF HEALTH

Health Is a Natural State of Harmony

Still believed health to be the natural state of the human being. In his own words:

> Osteopathy is based on the perfection of Nature's work. When all parts of the human body are in line we have health. When they are not the effect is disease. When the parts are readjusted disease gives place to health. The work of the osteopath is to adjust the body from the abnormal to the normal, then the abnormal conditions give place to the normal and health is the result of the normal condition (11).

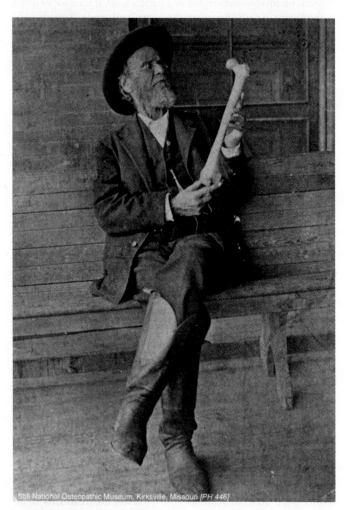

Figure 1-2 A.T. Still analyzing a human femur as he ponders the principles of osteopathy. (Still National Osteopathic Museum, Kirksville, MO.)

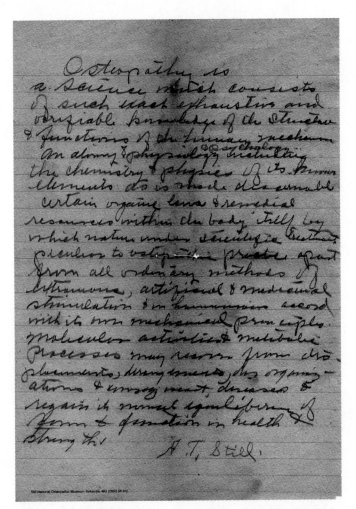

Figure 1-3 Handwritten definition of osteopathy by A.T. Still, M.D., D.O. (Still National Osteopathic Museum, Kirksville, MO.)

Classical Osteopathic Philosophy

A.T. Still's fundamental concepts of osteopathy can be organized in terms of health, disease, and patient care.

Health

1. Health is a natural state of harmony.
2. The human body is a perfect machine created for health and activity.
3. A healthy state exists as long as there is normal flow of body fluids and nerve activity.

Disease

4. Disease is an effect of underlying, often multifactorial causes.
5. Illness is often caused by mechanical impediments to normal flow of body fluids and nerve activity.
6. Environmental, social, mental, and behavioral factors contribute to the etiology of disease and illness.

Patient Care

7. The human body provides all the chemicals necessary for the needs of its tissues and organs.
8. Removal of mechanical impediments allows optimal body fluid flow, nerve function, and restoration of health.
9. Environmental, cultural, social, mental, and behavioral factors need to be addressed as part of any management plan.
10. Any management plan should realistically meet the needs of the individual patient.

Mechanics and Health

Still's concept of a healthy person is insightful. It places his belief of the importance of structural and mechanical integrity within the perspective of a comprehensive view of a human being within society:

> When complete, he is a self-acting, individualized, separate personage, endowed with the power to move, and mind to direct in locomotion, with a care for comfort and a thought for his continued existence in the preparation and consumption of food to keep him in size and form to suit the duties he may have to perform (14).

Still believed that life exists as a unification of vital forces and matter. Since the body is controlled by the mind to exhibit purposeful motion in attaining the needs and goals of the organism, he stated that "Osteopathy … is the law of mind, matter and motion" (10). Once Still accepted that motion is an inherent quality of life itself, it was a small step to inquiring into what is moving and how it moves. Through his in-depth study of anatomy, he could see the interdependent relationships among different tissues and their component parts. He observed that each part developed as the body was moving, growing, and developing from embryo to fetus to newborn and throughout life. Thus, each tissue, organ, and structure is designed for motion. "As motion is the first and only evidence of life, by this thought we are conducted to the machinery through which life works to accomplish these results" (15).

If "life is matter in motion" (14), then what is the effect on a body part that is not moving? Still reasoned that a lack of motion is not conducive to life or health. "[The osteopath's] duties as a philosopher admonish him that life and matter can be united, and that that union cannot continue with any hindrance to free and absolute motion" (14). Further, he boldly states that the practice of osteopathy "covers all phases of disease and it is the law that keeps life in motion" (10).

Normal Nerve Activity and Flow of Body Fluids

A machine cannot run without proper lubrication, fuel, and mechanisms to remove the by-products of combustion. In teaching his students, Still identified each component of the body's intricate mechanisms as he knew them. In the process, he discussed various forces that he reasoned create motion and maintain life. He explained how lubricating and nourishing fluids flow through the arteries, veins, lymphatics, and nerves. He also noted that they turn over by-products of metabolism through the venous and lymphatic systems. "The human body is a machine run by the unseen force called life, and that it may be run harmoniously it is necessary that there be liberty of blood, nerves and arteries from their generating point to their destination" (10).

Another component of Still's machine concept was the power source. He identified the brain as the dynamo, the electric battery that keeps the body moving and working:

> The brain furnishes nerve-action and forces to suit each class of work to be done by that set of nerves which is to construct forms and to keep blood constantly in motion in the arteries and from all parts back to the heart through the veins that it may be purified, renewed, and re-enter circulation (14).

CLASSIC OSTEOPATHIC PHILOSOPHY OF DISEASE

Disease Is an Effect of an Underlying Cause or Causes

From the time of Hippocrates through the first half of the 20th century, diseases were identified primarily through simple and complex descriptions of symptoms and signs. Many afflictions were without clear etiology. In spite of our current greater levels of knowledge and understanding, this is still true in many cases.

Still taught that disease is the effect of an abnormal anatomic state with subsequent physiologic breakdown and decreased host adaptability. Germs were first discovered in the 17th century with the invention of the microscope, but the germ theory of disease was not accepted until Pasteur provided convincing scientific evidence in the mid-19th century. However, experienced clinicians like Still, as well as an emerging group of laboratory scientists, saw germs as opportunists to decreased host function, not as primary causes of disease in themselves. They speculated that infections resulted from an interaction between the degree of virulence and quantity of the infecting agent and the level of host immunity.

Still also realized that there were multifactorial components to disease processes (16,17). He believed that disease was a combination of influences arising from decreased host adaptability and adverse environmental conditions. He recognized that symptoms often were a manifestation of nerves irritated by pathophysiologic processes commonly created by an accumulation of fluids (congestion and inflammation). This diminished the patient's ability to adapt to the environment (10). Additionally, Still was keenly aware of the deleterious effects of environmentally induced trauma, or abrupt changes in the atmosphere, causing physical or emotional "shock" or inertia, and therefore obstructing normal metabolic processes, body fluids, and nerve activity (11).

Mechanical Impediments to Flow of Body Fluids and Nerve Activity

Still's study of pathology found that in all forms of disease there is mechanical interruption of normal circulation of body fluids and nerve force to and from cells, tissues, and organs (11). "Sickness is an effect caused by the stoppage of some supply of fluid or quality of life" (10). He understood that it is the combination of free circulation of wholesome blood and motor, nutrient, and sensory nerve activity that creates tissues and organs, and facilitates their growth, maintenance, and repair. Through cadaver dissection studies he reasoned that strains, twists, or distortions in fascia, ligaments, or muscle fibers surrounding the small capillaries and nerve bundles could very well be the cause of ischemia and congestion by mechanical obstruction, interruption, or impediment to normal flow of vital fluids.

Still understood that the flow of body fluids was under the control of the nerves that innervated the blood vessel walls, adjusting the diameter of the vessels and thus controlling the amount and rate of blood flow to the tissues and organs. "While the vascular and nervous systems are dependent upon each other, it must be remembered that the bloodstream is under the control of the nervous system, not only indirectly through the heart, but directly through the vasoconstrictor and vasodilator nerve fibers, which regulate the caliber and rhythm of the blood vessels" (17). Still writes, "All diseases are mere effects, the cause being a partial or complete failure of the nerves to properly conduct the fluids of life" (10). Although he emphasized that "the rule of the artery is absolute, universal, and it must be unobstructed, or disease will result" (10), he also pointed out the importance of unimpeded flow of lymphatics: "[W]e must keep the lymphatics normal all the time or see confused Nature in the form of disease. We strike at the source of life and death when we go to the lymphatics" (14). However, even if the blood and the lymph are flowing normally, Still pointed out that "the cerebro spinal fluid is the highest known element that is contained in the human body, and unless the brain furnishes this fluid in abundance a disabled condition of the body will remain. He who is able to reason will see that this great river of life must be tapped and the withering field irrigated at once, or the harvest of health be forever lost" (15).

Holistic Aspects—Environmental and Biopsychosocial Etiologies

For the most part, Still described the origins of disease and illness as a result of "anatomic disturbances followed by physiologic discord." However, at the same time, he acknowledged the potential detrimental influences of heredity, lifestyle, environmental conditions, contagious diseases, inactivity and other personal behavior choices, and psychological and social stress on health (14,16,17).

Still also recognized that substance abuse (e.g., alcohol and opium) as well as poor sanitation, personal hygiene, and dietary indiscretion, lack of exercise or fitness all contributed to illness and disease. He lectured passionately against the social forces that promulgated these deleterious behaviors and social situations, including slavery and economic inequities. Indeed, he spoke from personal experience as he and his family members suffered from these challenging social circumstances during the pioneer days of the 19th century Midwest.

CLASSIC OSTEOPATHIC PHILOSOPHY AND PATIENT CARE

The Body Provides Its Own Drug Store

Like many others, Still observed that some people are more susceptible to epidemic diseases than others. It was also recognized that host resistance to disease is more apparent in certain individuals (18) who have so-called natural immunity that is either inherited or acquired (19,20). Still believed that promoting free flow of arterial blood to an infected area would enable "Nature's own germicide" to eradicate the infectious agent (11). Still's philosophy places complete trust in the innate self-healing ability of the body. Removing all hindrances to health was not enough, however, as it was incumbent upon the physician to ensure that the body's natural chemicals were able to work effectively in alleviating any pathophysiologic processes (10).

Medications

I was born and raised to respect and confide in the remedial power of drugs, but after many years of practice in close conformity to the dictations of the very best medical authors and in consultation with representatives of the various schools, I failed to get from drugs the results hoped for and I was face to face with the evidence that medication was not only untrustworthy but was dangerous (11).

Initially, Still conceived of the osteopathic medical profession as "a system of healing that reaches both internal and external diseases by manual operation and without drugs" (10). Although he stated, "Osteopathy is a drugless science," he clarified this statement by explaining that he believed that drugs "should not be used as remedial agents," since the medications of his era only addressed symptoms or abnormal bodily responses to an unknown cause. In osteopathy, there is no place for injurious medications, whose risks outweigh their benefits, especially if safer and equally effective alternatives exist.

Specifically, Still was against the irrational use of drugs that (a) showed no benefit, (b) had proven to be harmful, and (c) had no proven relationship to the cause of disease processes. He accepted anesthetics, poison antidotes, and a few others that had proven beneficial. "Osteopathy has no use for drugs as remedies, but a great use for chemistry when dealing with poisons and antidotes" (21). Still supports his reasons by listing the life-threatening risks of using drugs commonly employed in the late 19th century, namely: calomel, digitalis, aloe, morphine, chloral hydrate, veratrine, pulsatilla, and sedatives (10). Still persuasively argued that a detailed physical examination, with focus on the neuromusculoskeletal system, followed by a well-designed manipulative treatment, often removes impediments to motion and function. Where he differed from others was his view that manipulative treatment should always be used before deciding that the body had failed in its own efforts.

Vaccinations

Jenner introduced the smallpox vaccine in the 17th century with considerable success. Still acknowledged this by stating, "I believe the philosophy of fighting one infection with another infectious substance that could hold the body immune by long and continuous possession is good and was good" (14). Without disrespect to Jenner, he described shortcomings of Jenner's methods, pointing out that there were many patients on whom the vaccine did not work or who became disabled or fatally ill. He stated his belief that there is a less harmful method of vaccination and requested that Jenner's methods be improved.

Still's rejection of drugs and vaccinations showed up in the initial mission statement for the American School of Osteopathy (ASO) (11). However, in 1910, even while he was president, the school changed its stance and accepted vaccinations and serums as part of osteopathic practices.

First and foremost, Still clearly believed that the osteopathic physician should strive to help the patient's body release its own medicine for a particular problem. He writes:

> The brain of man was God's drug store, and had in it all liquids, drugs, lubricating oils, opiates, acids, and antacids, and every quality of drugs that the wisdom of God thought necessary for human happiness and health (21).

The Mechanical Approach to Treating the Cause of Disease

Still reasoned that the cause of most diseases was mechanical; therefore, treatment must follow the laws of mechanics. As a consequence, he used manipulative approaches designed to release bony and soft tissue barriers to nervous and circulatory functions in order to improve chances for healing. He claimed that mobilization of these structures improved the outcomes of his patients (11). However, manipulation procedures were not only applied to relieve musculoskeletal strains and injuries, but to treat internal organ diseases as well. For example, he found characteristic paraspinal muscle rigidity and other abnormal myofascial tensions in patients with infectious diseases. He noted improvement in the health of these patients as well when the musculoskeletal and myofascial impediments to normal physiologic processes were alleviated. In a majority of cases, the patient's condition was seemingly cured, leading him to believe that the mechanical aspects of dysfunction or disease were vitally important (11). Still thus proposed that in all diseases, mobilization of all the spinal joints not in their proper positional and functional relationships was necessary to ensure proper nerve activity and blood and lymph flow throughout the body. This included everything from the occiput to the coccyx, and indicated adjustment of the pelvis, clavicles, scapulae, costal cage, and diaphragm.

Comprehensive Treatment

While heavily committed to the use of palpatory diagnosis and manipulative treatment, Dr. Still continued many other aspects of patient care. He practiced surgery and midwifery (obstetrics), although little is documented about specific activities.

His patient education strategies highlighted moderation. He included advice for removing noxious or toxic substances from the diet and environment and behavioral adjustments such as adding exercises and stopping smoking. He also admonished his patients for abusing alcohol, opium, and heroin.

Mental illness and stress-related problems were also important to Still (10,11). He wrote about the role the physician can take in providing emotional support and encouragement to patients with end-stage medical problems. He described the importance of giving hope to patients and, at the same time, providing them with a realistic approach to managing their clinical condition (11).

Individualized Treatment

Each person is treated as a unique individual, not as a disease entity. Still taught that the history and physical evaluation of each person would turn up unhealthy self-care behaviors or circumstances and parts of the body not moving normally; the combination interferes with the body's natural ability to heal itself. The treatment would need to be tailored specifically for each patient's particular needs.

The classical philosophy of osteopathic medicine formed the foundation upon which contemporary osteopathic patient care is based. The contemporary "five models of osteopathic care" can be understood in the context of the classical osteopathic philosophy of health, disease, and patient care, as depicted in Table 1.2.

HISTORICAL DEVELOPMENT OF OSTEOPATHIC CONCEPTS

Exactly how much influence previous or contemporary philosophies and practices had on Still is purely speculative, since he never discussed specific attachments for any particular philosopher or scientist. The writings of contemporary philosophers of science and biology, like Herbert Spencer (1820–1903) and Alfred Russel Wallace (1823–1913), resonated with those of Still (9). They promoted the theories of evolution and the interdependence of the environment and the organism in all biologic processes, including the origins of disease. They also promoted the concepts of

> ### TABLE 1.2
>
> #### Osteopathic Five Models in the Context of the Three Domains of a Philosophy of Medicine
>
> | Models | Health | Disease | Patient Care[a] |
> |---|---|---|---|
> | Biomechanical | Efficient and effective posture and motion throughout the musculoskeletal system | Somatic dysfunction; inefficient posture; joint motion restrictions or hyper mobility; instability | Alleviate somatic dysfunction utilizing osteopathic palpatory diagnosis and OMT to restore normal motion and function throughout the body |
> | Respiratory-Circulatory | Efficient and effective arterial supply, venous and lymphatic drainage to and from all cells; effective respiration | Vascular compromise, edema, tissue congestion; poor gas exchange | Remove mechanical impediments to respiration and circulation and relieve congestion and edema by improving venous and lymphatic drainage |
> | Neurological | Efficient and effective sensory processing, neural integration and control, autonomic balance, central and peripheral nervous functions | Abnormal sensation, imbalance of autonomic functions, central and peripheral sensitization/malfunction; pain syndromes | Restore normal sensation, neurological processes and control; alleviate pain |
> | Metabolic-Energy | Efficient and effective cellular metabolic processes, energy expenditure and exchange, endocrine and immune regulation and control | Energy loss, fatigue, ineffective metabolic processes, toxic waste buildup, inflammation, infection, poor wound healing, poor nutrition; adverse response to medication; loss of endocrine control of vital functions | Restore efficient metabolic processes and bioenergetics, alleviate inflammation, infection, restore healing and repair functions and endocrine control |
> | Behavioral | Efficient and effective mental, emotional and spiritual functions, healthy lifestyle choices and activities, good social support system | Ineffective function due to drug abuse, environmental chemical exposure or trauma, poor lifestyle choices (i.e., inactivity, dietary indiscretions); inability to adapt to stress or environmental challenges | Assess and treat the whole person—physical, psychological, social, cultural, behavioral and spiritual aspects; collaborative partnership; individualized patient care and self-responsibility for healthy lifestyle choices |
>
> [a]Utilizing combinations of osteopathic manipulative medicine, medications, surgery, and education as appropriate.

the interdependence of structure and function, the importance of differentiating cause and effect, and emphasized the unity of the organism and interrelatedness of its parts. Throughout his life, however, Still maintained that his discoveries and thoughts were based on personal observation, experimentation, applications of factual knowledge, and the power of reasoning. After nearly 50 years of developing his concepts, he stated:

> I have explored by reading and inquiry much that has been written on kindred subjects, hoping to get something on this great law written by the ancient philosophers, but I come back as empty as I started (10).

A number of scholars and educators have attempted to trace both the historical development and the evolution of thoughts and practices that may have influenced Still's thinking (18–20,22–26). In general, the authors compare Still's ideas with well-known discourses passed on principally through Western cultural ideas. In 1901, Littlejohn, one of Still's students who became a faculty member at the ASO and founder of two osteopathic colleges, wrote, "Osteopathy did not invent a new anatomy or physiology or construct a new pathology. It has built upon the foundation of sciences already deeply seated in the philosophy of truth, chemistry, anatomy and physiology, a new etiology of diseases, gathering together, adding to and reinforcing natural methods of treating disease that have been accumulating since the art of healing began" (18). However, other students of A.T. Still disagreed with this perspective. C.M.T. Hulett, emphatically stated that "Osteopathy is a new system of thought, a new philosophy of life" (27). Whereas Littlejohn (22) finds the foundation of osteopathy in Greek and

Roman medicine, G.D. Hulett (20) and Downing (23) trace the origins of various osteopathic concepts to the philosophy and practice of medicine found in other ancient writings, such as those of the Ptolemies, Brahmins, Chinese, and Hebrews. All agree on the further development of medicine throughout Europe as a precursor to American osteopathic medical practice. Northup compares osteopathy to the concepts of Hippocrates and the Cnidian schools (26). Korr contrasts the contributions of Asclepian and Hygeian roots (25). Whereas G.D. Hulett (20) and Korr (25) describe osteopathy as part of an *evolution* of the philosophy of medicine, Lane (19) and Northup (26) consider it a *reformation* of medical theory and practice.

Still's use of spinal manipulation had many precedents. Schiötz and Cyriax (28) and Lomax (29), among many, document the use of manual treatments for millennia. Hippocrates discussed "subluxations" or minor displacements of vertebra in his treatise "On the Articulations" and the manual adjustments used to correct them (30). In the 18th and 19th centuries, many American and European practitioners acknowledged that there are relationships among displaced or "subluxed" vertebrae and "irritated" spinal nerves in relation to both musculoskeletal and visceral disorders (31).

EVOLUTION OF OSTEOPATHIC PHILOSOPHY

In his unique way, Still integrated many of these concepts into his new system and molded it into a distinctive medical school curriculum that continues to evolve to this day. Still was adamant that he did not expect his students and colleagues to take what he advocated as dogma. He taught, "You must reason. I say reason, or you will finally fail in all enterprises. Form your own opinions, select all facts you can obtain. Compare, decide, then act. Use no man's opinion; accept his works only" (14). He urged his students to study, test, and improve upon his ideas.

An example of this evolution is a shift from Still's early, and virtually exclusive, emphasis on anatomy to a more inclusive stress on primary physiologic functions that strengthen his concepts. Initially, Littlejohn (22), and later, Burns (32), Cole (33,33a), Denslow (34), and Korr (35,36), promoted integrative neurophysiologic and neuroendocrine concepts.

Whereas Littlejohn interpreted Still's concepts in light of 19th century physiologic theories, Burns, Cole, Denslow, and Korr pioneered distinctive osteopathic approaches to physiologic investigations, making significant scientific contributions. Korr was particularly influential in interpreting osteopathic concepts in light of the rapidly developing science of physiology in the 20th century (Box 1.3). He has been referred to as "the second great osteopathic philosopher" (37) (Figs. 1.4 and 1.5).

Korr's Explication of Osteopathic Principles

For the first edition of this text, Korr wrote an "Explication of Osteopathic Principles," which was his last published work. It is included here to demonstrate how he was able to use the osteopathic philosophy and tenets to organize and apply 20th century scientific knowledge to patient care:

> At this stage of your medical training, you have become familiar with osteopathic principles and can recite them in their usual brief, maxim form. The purpose of this section is to explore more fully the meaning, biological foundations, and clinical implications of the founding principles of osteopathic medicine.

Irvin Korr, Ph.D.

Irvin Korr, Ph.D., received his physiology degree from Princeton University. Most of his teaching and research career was spent at the Kirksville College of Osteopathic Medicine in Missouri, with later appointments at both Michigan State University College of Osteopathic Medicine and The Texas College of Osteopathic Medicine (University of North Texas). A multitalented individual, Korr was an accomplished violinist, sometimes playing chamber music with Albert Einstein, who was in residence at the time of his postgraduate training. He published extensively with several colleagues, including J.S. Denslow, A.D. Krems, Martin J. Goldstein, Price E. Thomas, Harry M. Wright, and Gustavo S.L. Appeltauer. In 1947, Korr's initial publication, with Denslow and Krems, focused on facilitation of neural impulses in motoneuron pools. Original research papers followed this on dermal autonomic activity, electrical skin resistance, and trophic function of nerves (36). As Korr gained insight into Still's concepts, he lectured widely and published a number of important treatises tying osteopathic concepts together with proven physiologic models that emphasized the important roles played by the neuromusculoskeletal system. Whereas Still emphasized a focus on bones as the starting place from which he was to discern the cause of pathology, Korr expanded this concept to include the integrative activity of the spinal cord and its relationships with the musculoskeletal and the sympathetic nervous systems (36). Similar to Still, however, Korr often referred to the neuromusculoskeletal system as the "Primary Machinery of Life."

For 50 years, Irwin M. Korr, scientist, philosopher, and humanist, has led and inspired several generations of osteopathic physicians and educators. His final treatise on osteopathic philosophy was written for the first edition of this text published in 1997. Upon reflection on the osteopathic principles, Korr stated "It is to the credit and honor of the osteopathic profession that it contributed cogent elaboration of the principles, developed effective methods for their implementation, built a system of practice upon those principles, and disclosed much about their basis in biological mechanisms through research (7)."

Remember that these principles began to evolve centuries ago, even before the time of Hippocrates. However, their basis in animal and, more specifically, human biology did not begin to become evident through research until late in the 19th century. The origin of these principles, therefore, was largely empirical; that is, they were the product of thoughtful and widely shared observations of ill and injured people. For example, it could hardly escape notice, even in primitive societies, that people (and animals) recovered from illness and wounds healed without intervention and, therefore, some natural indwelling healing power must be at work.

Even at the time of the founding of the osteopathic profession in 1892, the available knowledge in the sciences of physiology, biochemistry, microbiology, immunology, and pathology was meager. Indeed, immunology, biochemistry, and various other neurosciences and biomedical sciences had yet to appear as distinct disciplines. Therefore, these principles could only be expressed as aphorisms, embellished perhaps with conjectures about their biological basis. It is to the credit and honor of the osteopathic profession that it contributed cogent elaboration of the principles, developed effective methods for their implementation, built a system of practice upon those principles, and

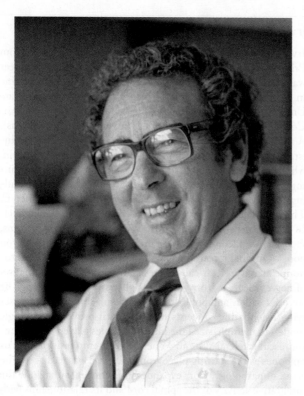

Figure 1-4 Irwin M. Korr, Ph.D. (1909–2004), "The second great osteopathic philosopher."

disclosed much about their basis in biological mechanisms through research.

In view of the enormous amount of biomedical knowledge recorded throughout the 20th century, it is timely to examine the principles that guide osteopathic practice in the light of that knowledge and to explore their relevance to clinical practice and to current and future health problems. What follows is an effort in that direction, without detailed reference to individual research.

THE PERSON AS A WHOLE

The Body

The principle of the unity of the body, so central to osteopathic practice, states that every part of the body depends on other parts for maintenance of its optimal function and even of its integrity. This interdependence of body components is mediated by the communication systems of the body: exchange of substances via circulating blood and other body fluids and exchange of nerve impulses and neurotransmitters through the nervous system.

The circulatory and nervous systems also mediate the regulation and coordination of cellular, tissue, and organ functions and thus the maintenance of the integrity of the body as a whole. The organized and integrated collaboration of the body components is reflected in the concept of homeostasis, the maintenance of the relative constancy of the internal environment in which all the cells live and function.

In view of this interdependence and exchange of influences, it is inevitable that dysfunction or failure of a major body component will adversely affect the competence of other organs and tissues and, therefore, one's health.

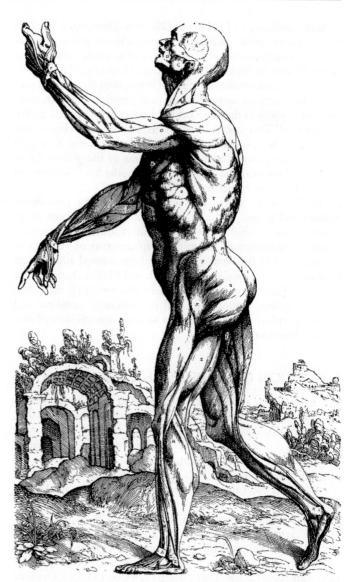

Figure 1-5 I.M. Korr, Ph.D., like A.T. Still, M.D., D.O., emphasized the role of the musculoskeletal system as The Primary Machinery of Life. This is a drawing by the renowned anatomist, Vesalius (1514–1564), depicting the muscles of the body in a dramatic pose. (Vesalius, Andreas De humani corporis fabrica plate 25 (Liber I) Basileae, [Ex officina Joannis Oporini, 1543]. Courtesy of the National Library of Medicine.)

The Person

Important and valid as is the concept of body unity, it is incomplete in that it is, by implication, limited to the physical realm. Physicians minister not to bodies but to individuals, each of whom is unique by virtue of his or her genetic endowment, personal history, and the variety of environments in which that history has been lived.

The person, obviously, is more than a body, for the person has a mind, also the product of heredity and biography. Separation of body and mind, whether conceptually or in practice, is an anachronistic remnant of such dualistic thinking as that of the 17th century philosopher-scientist, René Descartes. It was his belief that body and mind are separate domains, one publicly visible and palpable, the other invisible, impalpable, and private. This dualistic concept is anachronistic because, while it is almost universally rejected as a concept, it is still acted out in much of clinical practice and in biomedical research.

Clinical and biomedical research (as well as everyday experience) has irrefutably shown that body and mind are so inseparable, so pervasive to each other, that they can be regarded—and treated—as a single entity. It is now widely recognized (whether or not it is demonstrated in practice) that what goes on (or goes wrong) in either body or mind has repercussions in the other. It is for reasons such as these that I prefer unity of the person to unity of the body, conveying totally integrated humanity and individuality.

The Person as Context

Phenomena assigned to mind (consciousness, thought, feelings, beliefs, attitudes, etc.) have their physiological and behavioral counterparts; conversely, bodily and behavioral changes have psychological concomitants, such as altered feelings and perceptions. It must be noted, however, that it is the person who is feeling, perceiving, and responding not the body or the mind. It is you who feels well, ill, happy, or sad, and not your body or mind. What goes on in body and mind is conditioned by who the person is and their entire history.

In short, the person is far more than the union of body and mind, in the same sense that water is more than the union of hydrogen and oxygen. Nothing that we know about either oxygen or hydrogen accounts for the three states of water (liquid, solid, and gas), their respective properties, the boiling and freezing points, viscosity, and so forth. Water incorporates yet transcends oxygen and hydrogen. To understand water, we must study water and not only its components. In the same way, at an enormously more complex level, the person comprises yet transcends body and mind.

Moreover, once hydrogen and oxygen are joined to form water, they become subject to the laws that govern water. In the same but infinitely more complex sense, it is you who makes up your mind, changes your mind, trains and enriches your mind, and puts it to work. It is you who determines from moment to moment whether and in what way you will express, through your body, what is in or on your mind.

Thus the person is the context, the environment, in which all the body parts live and function and in which the mind finds expression. Everything about the person—genetics, history from conception to the present moment, nutrition, use and abuse of body and mind, parental and school conditioning, physical and sociocultural environments, and so on—enters into determining the quality of physical and mental function. The better the quality of the environment provided by the person for the mental and bodily components, the better they will function. For example, someone who has a peptic ulcer is not ill because of the ulcer. The ulcer exists because of an unfavorable internal environment.

In conclusion, just as the proper study of mankind is man (Alexander Pope), so is the study of human health and illness also man. As will become evident, the principle of the unity of the person leads naturally to the next principle.

THE PLACE OF THE MUSCULOSKELETAL SYSTEM IN HUMAN LIFE

The Means of Expression of Our Humanity and Individuality

Structure determines function, structure and function are reciprocally interrelated, and similar aphorisms have traditionally represented another osteopathic principle. That principle recognizes the special place of the musculoskeletal system among the body systems and its relation to the health of the person. We examine now the basis for the osteopathic emphasis on the musculoskeletal system in total health care.

Human life is expressed in human behavior, in humans doing the things that humans do. And whatever humans do, they do with the musculoskeletal system. That system is the ultimate instrument for carrying out human action and behavior. It is the means through which we manifest our human qualities and our personal uniqueness—personality, intellect, imagination, creativity, perceptions, love, compassion, values, and philosophies. The most noble ethical, moral, or religious principle has value only insofar as it can be overtly expressed through behavior.

That expression is made possible by the coordinated contractions and relaxations of striated muscles, most of them acting upon bones and joints. The musculoskeletal system is the means through which we communicate with each other, whether it be by written, spoken, or signed language, or by gesture or facial expression. Agriculture, industry, technology, literature, the arts and sciences—our very civilization—are the products of human action, interaction, communication, and behavior, that is, by the orchestrated contractions and relaxations of the body's musculature.

Relation to the Body Economy

The musculoskeletal system is the most massive system in the community of body systems. Its muscular components are collectively the largest consumer in the body economy. This is true not only because of their mass, but because of their high energy requirements. Furthermore, those requirements may vary widely from moment to moment according to what the person is doing, with what feelings, and in what environments.

The high and varying metabolic requirements of the musculoskeletal system are met by the cardiovascular, respiratory, digestive, renal, and other visceral systems. Together, they supply the required fuels and nutrients, remove the products of metabolism, and control the composition and physical properties of the internal environment. In servicing the musculoskeletal system in this manner, these organ systems are at the same time servicing each other (and, of course, the nervous system).

The nervous system is also, to a great degree, occupied with the musculoskeletal system, that is, with behavior and motor control. Indeed, most of the fibers in the spinal nerves are those converging impulses to and from the muscles and other components of the musculoskeletal system. In addition, the nervous system, its autonomic components, and the circulatory system mediate communication and exchange of signals and substances between the soma and the viscera. In this way, visceral, metabolic, and endocrine activity is continually tuned to moment-to-moment requirements of the musculoskeletal system, that is, to what the person is doing from moment to moment.

Consequences of Visceral Dysfunction

Impairment or failure of some visceral function or of communication between the musculoskeletal system and the viscera is reflected in the musculoskeletal system. When the resulting dysfunction is severe and diffuse, motor activity and even maintenance of posture are difficult or impossible and automatically imposed.

The Musculoskeletal System as Source of Adverse Influences on Other Systems

In view of the rich afferent input of the musculoskeletal system into the central nervous system and its rich interchange of substances with other systems through the body fluids, it is inevitable that structural and functional disturbances in the musculoskeletal system will have repercussions elsewhere in the body.

Such structural and functional disturbances may be of postural, traumatic, or behavioral origin (neglect, misuse, or abuse by the person). Further, it must be appreciated that the human framework is, compared with other (quadruped) mammals, uniquely unstable and vulnerable to compressive, torsional, and shearing forces, because of the vertical configuration, higher center of gravity, and the comparatively small, bipedal base.

The human musculoskeletal system, therefore, is the frequent source of aberrant afferent input to the central nervous system and its autonomic distribution, with at least potential consequences to visceral function. Which organs, blood vessels, etc. are at risk is determined by the site of the musculoskeletal dysfunction and the part(s) of the central nervous system, (e.g., spinal segments) into which it discharges its sensory impulses.

When a dysfunction or pathology has developed in a visceral organ, that disturbance is reflected in segmentally related somatic tissues. Viscus and soma become linked in a vicious circle of afferent and efferent impulses, which sustain and exacerbate the disturbance. Appropriate treatment of the somatic component reduces its input to the vicious circle and may even interrupt that circle with therapeutic effect.

Importance of the Personal Context

Whether or not visceral or vasomotor consequences of somatic dysfunction occur, and with what consequences to the person, depends on other factors in the person's life, such as the genetic, nutritional, psychological, behavioral, sociocultural, and environmental. As research has shown, however, the presence of somatic dysfunction and the accompanying reflex and neurotrophic effects exaggerate the impact of other detrimental factors on the person's health. Effective treatment of the musculoskeletal dysfunction shields the patient by reducing the deleterious effects of the other factors. Such treatment, therefore, has preventive as well as therapeutic benefits.

Such treatment directed to the musculoskeletal system assumes even greater and often crucial significance when it is recognized that the other kinds of harmful factors, such as those enumerated above, are not readily subject to change and may even require social or governmental intervention. The musculoskeletal system, however, is readily accessible and responsive to OMT. I view these considerations as the rationale for OMT and its strategic role in total health care.

Finally, the osteopathic philosophy and the unity of the person concept enjoin the physician to treat the patient as a whole and not merely the affected parts. Hence, appropriate corrective attention should also be given to other significant risk factors that are subject to change by both patient and physician.

OUR PERSONAL HEALTH CARE SYSTEMS

The Natural Healing Power

Appreciation, even in ancient times, of our inherent recuperative, restorative, and rehabilitative powers is reflected in the Latin phrase, *vis medicatrix naturae* (nature's healing force). We recover from illnesses, fevers drop, blood clots and wounds heal, broken bones reunite, infections are overcome, skin eruptions clear up, and even cancers are known to occasionally undergo spontaneous remission. But miraculous as is the healing power (and appreciated

as it was until we became more impressed by human-made miracles and breakthroughs), the other, more recently revealed components of the health care system with which each of us is endowed are no less marvelous.

The Component System That Defends against Threats from Without

This component includes, among others, immune mechanisms that defend us against the enormous variety and potency of foreign organisms that invade our bodies, wreaking damage and even bringing death. These same immune mechanisms guard us against those of our own cells that become foreign and malignant as the result of mutation. Included also are the mechanisms that defend against foreign and poisonous substances that we may take in with our food and drink or that enter through the skin and lungs, by disarming them, converting them to innocuous substances, and eliminating them from the body. They defend us (until overwhelmed) even against the toxic substances that we ourselves introduce into the atmosphere, soil, water, or more directly into our own bodies.

Mechanisms That Defend against Changes in the Internal Environment

We humans are exposed to, and adapt to, wide variations in physical and chemical properties of our environment (e.g., temperature, barometric pressure, oxygen, and carbon dioxide concentrations) and sustain ourselves with chemically diverse food and drink. But the cells of our body can function and survive only in the internal environment of interstitial fluids that maintain body functions within relatively narrow limits as regards variations in chemical composition, temperature, tissue, osmotic pressure, pH, etc.

This phenomenon, called homeostasis, is based on thousands of simultaneously dynamic equilibria occurring throughout the body. Examples include rates of energy consumption and replenishment by the cells. Homeostasis constancy and quick restoration of constancy must be accomplished regardless of the variations in the external environment, composition of food and drink, and the moment-to-moment activities of the person. It is accomplished by an enormously complex array of regulatory mechanisms that continually monitor and control respiratory, circulatory, digestive, renal, metabolic, and countless other functions and processes. Maintenance of optimal environments for cellular function is essential to health. The homeostatic mechanisms may, therefore, be viewed as the health maintenance system of the body.

Commentary

These, then, are the three major components of our indwelling health care system, each comprising numerous component systems. In the order in which humans became aware of them, they are (a) the healing (remedial, curative, palliative, recuperative, rehabilitative) component; (b) the component that defends against threats from the external environment; and (c) the homeostatic, health-maintaining component. These major component systems, of course, share subcomponents and mechanisms.

When the internal health care system is permitted to operate optimally, without impediment, its product is what we call health. Its natural tendency is always toward health and the recovery of health. Indeed, the personal health care system is the very source of health, upon which all externally applied measures depend for their beneficial effects. The internal health care system, in effect, makes its own diagnoses, issues its own prescriptions, draws upon its own vast pharmacy, and in most situations, administers each dose without side effects.

Health and healing, therefore, come from within. It is the patient who gets well, and not the practitioner or the treatment that makes them well.

THE THREE PRINCIPLES AS GUIDES TO MEDICAL PRACTICE

The Unity of the Person

In caring for the whole person, the well-grounded osteopathic physician goes beyond the presenting complaint, beyond relief of symptoms, beyond identification of the disease and treatment of the impaired organ, malfunction, or pathology, important as they are to total care. The osteopathic physician also explores those factors in the person and the person's life that may have contributed to the illness and that, appropriately modified, compensated, or eliminated, would favor recovery, prevent recurrence, and improve health in general.

The physician then selects that factor or combination of factors that are readily subject to change and that would be of sufficient impact to shift the balance toward recovery and enhancement of health. The possible factors include such categories as the biological (e.g., genetic, nutritional), psychological, behavioral (use, neglect, or abuse of body and mind; interpersonal relationships; habits; etc.), sociocultural, occupational, and environmental. Some of these factors, especially some of the biological, are responsive to appropriate clinical intervention, some are responsive only to social or governmental action, and still others require changes by patients themselves. Osteopathic whole-person care, therefore, is a collaborative relationship between patient and physician.

The Place of the Musculoskeletal System in Human Biology and Behavior: The Strategic Role of Osteopathic Manipulative Treatment

It is obvious that some of the most deleterious factors are difficult or impossible for patient and physician to change or eliminate. These include (at least at present) genetic factors (although some inherited predispositions can be mitigated by lifestyle change). They include also such items as social convention, lifelong habits (e.g., dietary and behavioral), widely shared beliefs, prejudices, misconceptions and cultural doctrines, attitudes, and values. Others, such as the quality of the physical or socioeconomic environments, may require concerted community, national, and even international action.

Focus falls, therefore, upon those deleterious factors that are favorably modifiable by personal and professional action, and that, when appropriately modified or eliminated, mitigate the health-impairing effects of the less changeable factors. Improvement of body mechanics by OMT is a major consideration when dealing with these complex interactions.

OUR PERSONAL HEALTH CARE SYSTEMS

This principle has important implications for the respective responsibilities of patient and physician and for their relationship. Since each person is the owner and hence the guardian of his or her own personal health care system, the ultimate source of health and healing, the primary responsibility for one's health is each individual's. That responsibility is met by the way the person lives, thinks, behaves, nourishes himself or herself, uses body and mind, relates to others, and the other factor usually called lifestyle. Each person must be taught and enabled to assume that responsibility.

It is the physician's responsibility, while giving palliative and remedial attention to the patient's immediate problem, to support each patient's internal health care system, to remove impediments to its competence, and above all, to do it no harm. It is also the responsibility of physicians to instruct patients on how to do the same for themselves and to strive to motivate them to do so, especially by their own example.

The relationship between patient and osteopathic physician is therefore a collaborative one, a partnership, in maintaining and enhancing the competence of the patient's personal health care system. The maintenance and enhancement of health is the most effective and comprehensive form of preventive medicine, for health is the best defense against disease. As stated by Still, "To find health should be the object of the doctor. Anyone can find disease."

Relevance to the Current and Future Health of the Nation

The preventive strategy of health maintenance and health enhancement, intrinsic to the osteopathic philosophy, is urgently needed by our society today. One of the greatest burdens on the nation's health care system and on the national economy is in the care of victims of the chronic degenerative diseases, such as heart disease, cancer, stroke, and arthritis, which require long-term care.

The incidence of these diseases has increased and will continue to increase well into the next century as the average age of our population continues to increase. The widely accepted (but usually unspoken) assumption that guides current practice (and national policy) is that the chronic degenerative diseases are an inevitable aspect of the aging process; that is, that aging is itself pathological. It is now increasingly apparent, however, that the increase of their incidence with age is because the longer one lives, the greater the toll taken by minor, seemingly inconsequential, inconspicuous, treatable impairments, and modifiable contributing factors in and around the person. They are, therefore, largely the natural culmination of less-than-favorable lifestyles, and, hence, they are largely preventable.

The great national tragedy is that, while the nation's health care system is so extensively and expensively absorbed in the care of millions of older adult victims of chronic disease (at per capita cost 3.5 times that of persons under the age of 65 years), tens of millions of younger people and children are living on and embarking on life paths that will culminate in the same diseases. The health care system simply must move upstream to move people from pathogenic to salutary paths. And the osteopathic profession can show the way.

The osteopathic profession has a historic opportunity to make an enormous contribution to the enhancement of the health of our nation. It can do this by giving leadership in addressing this great tragedy by bringing its basic strategy of whole-person, health-oriented care to bear on the problem and demonstrating its effectiveness in practice.

Having reviewed and enlarged on the principles of osteopathic medicine, their meaning, biological foundations, and clinical implications, it seems appropriate to propose a definition of osteopathic medicine. The author offers the following: Osteopathic medicine is a system of medicine that is based on the continually deepening and expanding understanding of (a) human nature; (b) those components of human biology that are centrally relevant to health, namely the inherent regulatory, protective, regenerative, and recuperative biological mechanisms, whose combined effect is consistently in the direction of the maintenance, enhancement, and recovery of health; and (c) the factors in and around the person that both favorably and unfavorably affect those mechanisms.

The practice of osteopathic medicine is, essentially, the potentiation of the intrinsic health-maintaining and health-restoring resources of the individual. The methods and agents employed are those that are effective in enhancing the favorable factors and diminishing or eliminating the unfavorable factors affecting each individual. Osteopathic medical practice necessarily includes the application of palliative and remedial measures, but always on the condition that they do no harm to the patient's own health-maintaining and health-restoring resources. This stipulation governing the choice of methods and agents is based on the recognition that all therapeutic methods depend on the patient's own recuperative power for their effectiveness and are valueless without it and that health and the recovery of health come from within.

The art and science of osteopathic medicine are expressed in the identification and selection of those factors in each individual that are accessible and amenable to change and that, when changed, would most decisively potentate the person on health-supporting resources.

> Osteopathic physicians give special emphasis to factors originating in the musculoskeletal system, for the following reasons:
>
> 1. The vertical human framework (a) is highly vulnerable to compressive (gravitational), torsional, and shearing forces, and (b) encases the entire central nervous system.
> 2. Since the massive, energy-demanding system has rich two-way communication with all other body systems, it is, because of its vulnerability, a common and frequent source of impediments to the functions of other systems.
> 3. These impediments exaggerate the physiological impact of other detrimental factors in the person's life, and, through the central nervous system, focus it on specific organs and tissues.
> 4. The musculoskeletal impediments (somatic dysfunctions) are readily accessible to the hands and responsive to the manipulative and other methods developed and refined by the osteopathic medical profession.

The Definition of Osteopathy

Osteopathic philosophy has been defined various ways over the years. To get a better sense of the evolution of the osteopathic philosophy since its inception, it is instructive to follow how it has been defined over time. In his autobiography, Still gave a "technical" definition as follows:

> Osteopathy is that science which consists of ... knowledge of the structure and functions of the human mechanism ... by which nature under the scientific treatment peculiar to osteopathic practice ... in harmonious accord with its own mechanical principles, ... may recover from displacements, disorganizations, derangements, and consequent disease and regain its normal equilibrium of form and function in health and strength. (10)

Besides Still, several other American osteopathic scholars wrote treatises on osteopathic philosophy and principles (19,20,23, 24,33,33a,38–44). Each author had his or her own definition and explanation of osteopathic philosophy. There have been several attempts over the past century to obtain consensus, or agreement,

on a unifying definition and clearly stated tenets or principles that govern the practice of osteopathic medicine.

According to Littlejohn, the first consensus definition of osteopathy, among multiple faculty members representing several osteopathic medical schools, was published in 1900 (18). After Still passed away in 1917, the AOA House of Delegates passed a resolution that the A.T. Still Research Institute, under the direction of Louisa Burns, D.O. at the time, would publish an updated version of the most popular textbook on osteopathic principles in print, adding current scientific knowledge in support of the philosophy. The book was passed around to all the osteopathic colleges for input and consensus. In 1922, this consensus based textbook was published by the A.T. Still Research Institute as a revised edition of the classic textbook by G.D. Hulett initially written at the turn of the 20th century (20). By this time in medical thought, it was widely accepted that cellular level activity was a strong determinant of health or disease states. In an attempt to update osteopathic philosophy in light of emerging concepts in cellular biology, the authors applied Still's mechanistic viewpoint to cellular physiology. The following passage not only illustrates this approach but also demonstrates the desire of the profession to state osteopathic philosophy and principles in terms of concise tenets based on contemporary scientific knowledge:

> The osteopathic view of the cell ... is largely covered by the following statements:
>
> - Normal structure is essential to normal function.
> - Normal function is essential if normal structure is to be maintained.
> - Normal environment is essential to normal function and structure, though some degree of adaptation is possible for a time, even under abnormal conditions.
>
> In the human body, with its diversified functions, we may add also:
>
> - The blood preserves and defends the cells of the body.
> - The nervous system unifies the body in its activities.
> - Disease symptoms are due either to failure of the organism to meet adverse circumstances efficiently, or to structural abnormalities.
> - Rational methods of treatment are based upon an attempt to provide normal nutrition, innervation, and drainage to all tissues of the body, and these depend chiefly upon the maintenance of normal structural relations (20).

The addition of medications in the practices of osteopathic physicians and surgeons over the years affected how the philosophy was stated. For example, in 1948 the faculty at the College of Osteopathic Physicians and Surgeons in Los Angeles added the following phrase to their basic osteopathic principles statement: "Like a machine, the body can function efficiently only when in proper adjustment and when its chemical needs are satisfied either by food or medical substances" (45). Further evolution occurred in 1953 when the faculty of the Kirksville College of Osteopathy and Surgery agreed on the following:

> Osteopathy, or Osteopathic Medicine, is a philosophy, a science, and an art. Its philosophy embraces the concept of the unity of body structure and function in health and disease. Its science includes the chemical, physical, and biological sciences related to the maintenance of health and the prevention, cure, and alleviation of disease. Its art is the application of the philosophy and the science in the practice of osteopathic medicine and surgery in all its branches and specialties.

Health is based on the natural capacity of the human organism to resist and combat noxious influences in the environment and to compensate for their effects—to meet, with adequate reserve, the usual stresses of daily life, and the occasional severe stresses imposed by extremes of environment and activity. Disease begins when this natural capacity is reduced, or when it is exceeded or overcome by noxious influences.

Osteopathic medicine recognizes that many factors impair this capacity and the natural tendency toward recovery, and that among the most important of these factors are the local disturbances or lesions of the musculoskeletal system. Osteopathic medicine is therefore concerned with liberating and developing all the resources that constitute the capacity for resistance and recovery, thus recognizing the validity of the ancient observation that the physician deals with a patient as well as a disease (46).

They then combined several concepts and restated them as four principles:

The osteopathic concept emphasizes four general principles from which are derived an etiological concept, a philosophy and a therapeutic technic that are distinctive, but not the only features of osteopathic diagnosis and treatment.

1. The body is a unit.
2. The body possesses self-regulatory mechanisms.
3. Structure and function are reciprocally inter-related.
4. Rational therapy is based upon an understanding of body unity, self-regulatory mechanisms, and the inter-relationship of structure and function (46).

Over the ensuing 40 years, advances in the biologic sciences elucidated many mechanisms in support of the concept that optimal health calls for integration of countless functions ranging from the molecular to the behavioral level. When this integration breaks down, dysfunction and disease commonly follow. Infectious and metabolic diseases, as well as diseases of aging and genetics, are frequent examples. Interdisciplinary fields of study have been developed to investigate and delineate the complex interactions of numerous coordinated body functions in health and disease. Psychoneuroimmunology, for example, provides substantial evidence linking mind, body, and spiritual activities with a wide variety of biologic observations (47–50).

Clinical applications of the advances in molecular, cellular, neurologic, and behavioral sciences, combined with the decreased emphasis on mechanical factors within osteopathic medical practice, demanded a new consensus statement. Using the 1953 Kirksville faculty statement as a beginning, the associate editors of the first edition of this text (1997) stated

Health is the adaptive and optimal attainment of physical, mental, emotional, and spiritual well-being. It is based on our natural capacity to meet, with adequate reserves, the usual stresses of daily life and the occasional severe stresses imposed by extremes of environment and activity. It includes our ability to resist and combat noxious influences in our environment and to compensate for their effects. One's health at any given time depends on many factors including his or her polygenetic inheritance, environmental influences, and adaptive response to stressors (51).

The editors modified the four key principles of osteopathic philosophy as follows:

1. The body is a unit; the person is a unit of body, mind, and spirit.

2. The body is capable of self-regulation, self-healing, and health maintenance.
3. Structure and function are reciprocally interrelated.
4. Rational treatment is based upon an understanding of the basic principles of body unity, self-regulation, and the interrelationship of structure and function (51).

In July 2008, the AOA House of Delegates adopted a policy statement accepting these four tenets as stated.

In order to represent an increasingly diverse group of osteopathic physicians, the AOA adopted a general statement regarding osteopathic medicine. Since 1991, the official AOA definition of *osteopathic medicine* has been reviewed periodically. The latest rendition defines Osteopathic Medicine.

A complete system of medical care with a philosophy that combines the needs of the patient with current practice of medicine, surgery and obstetrics; that emphasizes the interrelationship between structure and function; and that has an appreciation of the body's ability to heal itself.

SUMMARY

Based on a health-oriented medical philosophy, osteopathic medicine uses a number of concepts to implement its principles. The neuromusculoskeletal system is used as a common point of reference because it directly relates the individual to the physical environment on a day-to-day basis. The practitioner's primary roles are to:

- Address primary cause(s) of disease using available evidence-based practices
- Enhance the patient's healing capacity
- Individualize patient management plans with an emphasis on health restoration and disease prevention
- Use palpatory diagnosis and manipulative treatment to focus on and affect somatic signs of altered structural, mechanical, and physiologic states

Osteopathic philosophy is meant to guide osteopathic physicians in the best use of scientific knowledge to optimize health and diminish disease processes. Upon founding his profession and school, Still expressed the hope that "the osteopath will take up the subject and travel a few miles farther toward the fountain of this great source of knowledge and apply the results to the relief and comfort of the afflicted who come for counsel and advice" (14). It is the intention of the authors to organize current medical knowledge and place it on a foundation of osteopathic philosophy. We do this in order to provide the osteopathic medical student with a road map that will lead to the further study of the science of osteopathy and the practice of the highest quality patient-centered health care possible.

REFERENCES

1. Ward R, Sprafka S. Glossary of osteopathic terminology. *J Am Osteopathic Assoc* 1981;80(8):552–567.
2. Educational Council on Osteopathic Principles. Core Curriculum Outline. Washington, DC: American Association of Colleges of Osteopathic Medicine; Approved by the Council of Deans, 1987.
3. Sirica CM, ed. *Current Challenges to M.D.s and D.O.s.* New York, NY: Josiah Macy, Jr Foundation, 1996:114–120.
4. Greenman PE. *Principles of Manual Medicine.* 3rd Ed. Philadelphia, PA: Lippincott, Williams and Wilkins, 2003.

5. Hruby RJ. Pathophysiologic models: aids to the selection of manipulative techniques. *AAO J* 1991;1(3):8–10.

6. Hruby RJ. Pathophysiologic models and the selection of osteopathic manipulative techniques. *J Osteopath Med* 1992;6(4):25–30.

7. Korr IM. An explication of osteopathic principles. In: Ward RC, exec ed. *Foundations for Osteopathic Medicine*. Baltimore, MD: Williams & Wilkins, 1997:7–12.

8. Rogers FJ, D'Alonzo GE, Glover J, et al. Proposed tenets of osteopathic medicine and principles for patient care. *J Am Osteopath Assoc* 2002;102(2):63–65.

9. Trowbridge C. *Andrew Taylor Still*. Kirksville, MO: Thomas Jefferson University Press, Northeast Missouri State University, 1991:95–140.

10. Still AT. *Autobiography of Andrew T. Still*. Rev ed. Kirksville, MO: Published by the author, 1908. Distributed, Indianapolis: American Academy of Osteopathy.

11. Still AT. *Osteopathy Research and Practice*. Seattle, WA: Eastland Press, 1992. Originally published by the author; 1910.

12. Still CE Jr. *Frontier Doctor Medical Pioneer*. Kirksville, MO: Thomas Jefferson University Press, Northeast Missouri State University, 1991.

13. Hildreth AG. *The Lengthening Shadow of Dr. Andrew Taylor Still*. Macon, MO: Privately published, 1942. Reprinted and distributed, Kirksville, MO: Osteopathic Enterprises, Inc.

14. Still AT. *The Philosophy and Mechanical Principles of Osteopathy*. Kirksville, MO: Original copyright by the author, 1892. Then, Kansas City, MO: 1902. Reprinted, Kirksville, MO: Osteopathic Enterprises, 1986.

15. Still AT. *Philosophy of Osteopathy*. Kirksville, MO: 1899. Reprinted, Academy of Applied Osteopathy, Carmel, CA, 1946.

16. Booth ER. Summation of causes in disease and death. *J Am Osteopath Assoc* 1902;2(2):33–41.

17. Lyne ST. Osteopathic philosophy of the cause of disease. *J Am Osteopath Assoc* 1904;3(12):395–403. Reprinted in *J Am Osteopath Assoc* 2000;100(3):181–189.

18. Littlejohn JM. Osteopathy: an independent system co-extensive with the science and art of healing. *J Am Osteopath Assoc* 1901;1. Reprinted in *J Am Osteopath Assoc* 2000;100(1):14–26.

19. Lane MA. *Dr. A.T. Still. Founder of Osteopathy*. Chicago, IL: The Osteopathic Publishing Co., 1918.

20. Hulett GD. *A Text Book of the Principles of Osteopathy*. 5th Ed. Pasadena, CA: A.T. Still Research Institute, 1922.

21. Schnucker RV, ed. *Early Osteopathy: In the Words of A.T. Still*. Kirksville, MO: Thomas Jefferson University Press, Northeast Missouri State University, 1991.

22. Littlejohn JM. The physiological basis of the therapeutic law. *J Sci Osteopath* 1902;3(4).

23. Downing CH. *Osteopathic Principles in Disease*. Originally published, San Francisco, CA: Ricardo J. Orozco, 1935. Reprinted and published, Newark, OH: American Academy of Osteopathy, 1988.

24. Page LE. *Principles of Osteopathy*. Kansas City, MO: Academy of Applied Osteopathy, 1952.

25. Korr IM. The osteopathic role in medical evolution. *The DO*. Nov, 1973.

26. Northup GW. *Osteopathic Medicine: An American Reformation*. Chicago, IL: American Osteopathic Association, 1979.

27. Hulett CMT. Relation of osteopathy to other systems. *J Am Osteopath Assoc* 1901;1:227–233.

28. Schiötz, EH, Cyriax J. *Manipulation. Past and Present*. London, England: William Heinemann Medical Books, Ltd, 1975.

29. Lomax E. Manipulative therapy: a historical perspective from ancient times to the modern era. In: Goldstein M, ed. *The Research Status of Spinal Manipulative Therapy*. Bethesda, MD: U.S. Dept. of Health, Education and Welfare, 1975:11–17. NIH publication 76-998.

30. Adams F. *The Genuine Works of Hippocrates*. First published his translation in 1849, then again in 1886, and again in 1929. However, the published editions that are usually available today were published in Philadelphia, PA: Williams & Wilkins, 1939.

31. Harris JD, McPartland JM. Historical perspectives of manual medicine. In: Stanton DF, Mein EA, eds. *Physical Med Rehabil Clin N Am* 1996;7(4): 679–692.

32. Burns L. *Pathogenesis of Visceral Disease Following Vertebral Lesions*. Chicago, IL: American Osteopathic Association, 1948.

33. Beal MC, ed. *The Cole Book of Papers Selected From the Writings and Lectures of Wilbur V. Cole, D.O., F.A.A.O.* Newark, OH: American Academy of Osteopathy, 1969.

33a. Hoag JM, Cole WV, Bradford SG, eds. *Osteopathic Medicine*. New York, NY: McGraw-Hill, 1969.

34. Beal MC, ed. *Selected Papers of John Stedman Denslow, DO*. Indianapolis, IN: American Academy of Osteopathy, 1993.

35. Korr IM. *The Neurobiologic Mechanisms of Manipulative Therapy*. New York, NY: Plenum Press, 1977.

36. Peterson B, ed. *The Collected Papers of Irvin M. Korr*. Colorado Springs, CO: The American Academy of Osteopathy (currently in Indianapolis, IN), 1979.

37. Jones JM. Osteopathic philosophy. In: Gallagher RM, Humphrey FJ. eds. *Osteopathic Medicine: A Reformation in Progress*. New York, NY: Churchill Livingstone, 2001.

38. McConnell CP, Teall CC. *The Practice of Osteopathy*. 3rd Ed. Kirksville, MO: The Journal Printing Co., 1906.

39. Tasker D. *Principles of Osteopathy*. Los Angeles, CA: Baumgardt Publishing Co., 1903.

40. Burns L. *Studies in the Osteopathic Sciences: Basic Principles*, Vol I. Los Angeles, CA: Occident Printery, 1907.

41. Downing CH. *Principles and Practice of Osteopathy*. Kansas City, MO: Williams Publishing Co., 1923.

42. Barber E. *Osteopathy Complete*. Kansas City, MO: Hudson-Kimberly Publishing, 1898.

43. Booth ER. *History of Osteopathy and Twentieth Century Medical Practice*. Cincinnati, OH: Jennings and Graham, 1905.

44. Hildreth AG. *The Lengthening Shadow of Andrew Taylor Still*. Macon, MO and Paw Paw, MI: Privately published by Mrs. AG Hildreth and Mrs. AE Van Vleck, 1942.

45. College of Osteopathic Physician and Surgeons documents, 1948. University of California at Irvine, Library Archives, Special Collections.

46. Special Committee on Osteopathic Principles and Osteopathic Technic, Kirksville College of Osteopathy and Surgery. An interpretation of the osteopathic concept. Tentative formulation of a teaching guide for faculty, hospital staff and student body. *J Osteopath* 1953;60(10):7–10.

47. Felton DL. Neural influence on immune responses: underlying suppositions and basic principles of neural-immune signaling. *Prog Brain Res* 2000;122.

48. Pert CB. *Molecules of Emotion: The Science Behind Mind-Body Medicine*. New York, NY: Touchstone, Simon and Schuster, 1997.

49. Damasio A. *The Feeling of What Happens: Body and Emotion in the Making of Consciousness*. New York, NY: Harcourt, 1999.

50. Dossey L. *Prayer Is Good Medicine: How to Reap the Healing Benefits of Prayer*. San Francisco, CA: HarperCollins, 1996.

51. Seffinger MA. Development of osteopathic philosophy. In: Ward RC, exec ed. *Foundations for Osteopathic Medicine*. Baltimore, MD: Williams & Wilkins, 1997:3–7.

Major Events in Osteopathic History

BARBARA E. PETERSON

KEY CONCEPTS

- The origin of osteopathic medicine is the story of a search for improvement in the system of health care.
- Growth of the osteopathic profession followed a philosophy enunciated by Andrew Taylor Still.
- The establishment of an osteopathic educational process was influenced by individuals not only in the United States but also from other countries.
- Andrew Taylor Still did not intend to establish a separate profession for the practice of medicine but sought acceptance of his ideas within teaching programs of traditional medicine.
- The growth of osteopathic professional organizations was made necessary by concerted resistance from the organizations of traditional medicine.
- The continued demonstration of strength and growth by the osteopathic profession led to recognition by state and federal governments.
- The need to provide expanded teaching of osteopathic theory, methods, and practice led to the development of hospitals, primary care emphasis, and the implementation of specialty training programs.

INTRODUCTION

Osteopathic medicine has from its beginning been a profession based on ideas and tenets that have lasted through all sorts of adversity and have been credited with bringing the profession to its present level of success. The previous chapter outlines in some detail the growth of these ideas. It is perhaps significant that the profession's founder never wrote clinical manuals, only books of philosophy (1–4).

It is striking that these ideas, still quoted extensively today (5), came not from universities or medical centers but from the creative problem solving of an informally educated American frontier doctor named Andrew Taylor Still. Looking back more than a century, it seems surprising that his ideas were so controversial when first put forward. But perhaps history has caught up with this eccentric, inventive man.

ANDREW TAYLOR STILL

The story of Andrew Taylor Still is worth knowing in detail but must be told superficially. He was born in a log cabin in Virginia in 1828, the year Andrew Jackson was elected president (Fig. 2.1). Still's family were farmers, as most people were then; his father was also a Methodist circuit rider who preached and treated people's ills. He later would teach his five sons to be doctors in the usual frontier apprentice system of the time.

Still's mother came from a family that was nearly all wiped out by a Shawnee Indian massacre (6), and it must have seemed a supreme irony when in 1851 she and her husband moved to Kansas as missionaries to the descendants of these same Indians. However, the family course first took them to Tennessee and then to Missouri, where they also were frontier missionaries.

Still had the sketchy education of a frontier child (3) but he was an inventive person and liked to read. Eventually, he would become familiar with many of the major practical and ideological trends

of his time. But learning to survive had to come first; Missouri and Kansas were true frontiers. The Stills first eked out a living by hunting for food and making some of their clothes from animal skins. The family also plowed their land claim and established a farm while the father rode a circuit among scattered settlers, ministering to minds and bodies. It was a lifestyle that gave substance to the word "survivor" (7).

Still would later say how important animal dissection had been as a preparation for study of human anatomy. He also recorded another prophetic childhood experience in his *Autobiography*:

> One day, when about ten years old, I suffered from a headache. I made a swing of my father's plow-line between two trees; but my head hurt too much to make swinging comfortable, so I let the rope down to about eight or ten inches of the ground, threw the end of a blanket on it, and I lay down on the ground and used the rope for a swinging pillow. Thus I lay stretched on my back, with my neck across the rope. Soon I became easy and went to sleep, got up in a little while with the headache gone. As I knew nothing of anatomy at this time, I took no thought of how a rope could stop headache and the sick stomach which accompanied it. After that discovery I roped my neck whenever I felt one of those spells coming on (3).

To the end of his life, Still continued to "rope his neck" (Fig. 2.2). In his old age, he would lie down daily with his neck on a version of a Chinese pillow, known among country folk as a "saint's rest"—a wooden frame with a leather strap suspended across it—giving the same effect as a plow rope suspended between two trees. In his middle years, he discovered other crude but effective methods for self-treatment, notably a croquet ball upon which he would lie down at the correct point when the problem was in his back rather than his neck (Mrs. J.S. Denslow [Dr. Still's granddaughter], personal communication, 1972).

In the 1840s, the issue of slavery divided the Methodist church and the Stills stayed with the northern (abolitionist) branch.

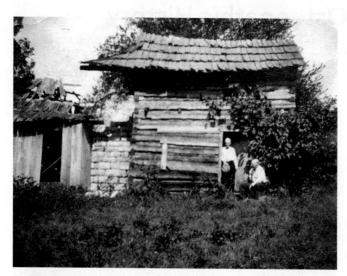

Figure 2-1   A.T. Still's birthplace: a one-room log cabin near Jonesville, Virginia. Preserved and displayed at the A.T. Still Museum on the campus of A.T. Still University in Kirksville, MO. (Still National Osteopathic Museum, Kirksville, MO.)

By the early 1850s, most of the family had moved to Kansas, including Still and his young wife. At that time Still began seriously to read and practice medicine with his father. They gave the Indians "such drugs as white men used [and] cured most of the cases [they] met" (3).

In 1855, the government forced the Shawnees farther west, and Kansas became a virtual war zone as both abolitionist and proslavery settlers rushed in. The fate of Kansas as a free state depended on a popular vote. The Stills chose to be active abolitionists. Still recalled:

> I could not do otherwise, for no man can have delegated to him by statute a just right to any man's liberty, either on account of race or color. With these truths before me I entered all combats for the abolition of slavery at home and abroad, and soon had a host of bitter political enemies, which resulted in many thrilling and curious adventures (3).

The Stills met John Brown and fought, under the command of Jim Lane, two of the abolitionist leaders active on the western frontier. There are numerous stories of "abolitionist encounters" during the pre-Civil War days (8–10). The struggle lasted, said Still, until Abraham Lincoln "wrote the golden words: 'Forever free, without regard to race or color.' I will add–or sex" (3).

The territorial political situation was volatile and confusing, with even the elections seemingly decided by gun battles. There are many accounts of "bloody Kansas" in the pre-Civil War period, including those in early osteopathic writings. But somehow a free state legislature was elected in 1857, and Still was a proud member of that group (11).

Still's first wife, née Mary Margaret Vaughn, died in 1859, leaving three children. In late 1860, Still married a young schoolteacher who had learned to mix prescriptions for her physician father and who was prepared by her background to accept Still's medical and spiritual speculations (8). It was a most important partnership; Mary Elvira Turner Still was to support her husband and family through the long period of doubt and disgrace that preceded successful establishment of the osteopathic profession and again through the heady days of unexpected success. But all this was in the future.

When the Civil War officially began, Still enlisted first in a cavalry division of a force assigned to Jim Lane. Later, he organized a company of Kansas militia, which was in turn consolidated with other militia battalions. He was commissioned a major and saw active combat; some experiences are recounted in his *Autobiography* (3). He also served as a military surgeon, though he had been listed as a hospital steward on the official record (12). His unit was disbanded in October 1864, and Still went home to resume normal civilian life.

It was not exactly a joyful homecoming. In February 1864, his three children had died of cerebrospinal meningitis, despite the best efforts of the physicians called to help. All around him, Still saw people who had become addicted to alcohol or morphine, and he considered that these were "habits, customs, and traditions no better than slavery in its worst days" (3).

Mainstream Civil War medicine still depended heavily on purging, bloodletting, and an armamentarium of medicines that could only be characterized as violent. On both sides, there were

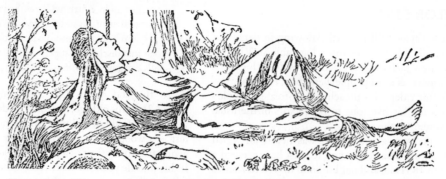

Figure 2-2   Like many physicians before and after him, Dr. A.T. Still applied his new philosophy first to himself and then to his patients. In a famous early anecdote, he stopped a headache by suspending his neck across a low-lying rope swing. He later applied self-adjustments of spinal joint dysfunction to abate an attack of "flux" (bloody dysentery). After he was successful at curing 17 children of the same affliction by adjusting their spinal joint dysfunctions, he realized he was onto something worthwhile. (From Still AT. *Autobiography of Andrew T. Still*. Rev Ed. Kirksville, MO: Published by the author, 1908. Distributed, Indianapolis: American Academy of Osteopathy.)

many more casualties from sickness than from battle injuries (13). A history of American medicine recounts:

> Even the most erudite and experienced physician had few effective medicines at his command. Some of those which were effective were unknown to the poorly educated practitioner; others he knew not how to use. The short list of effective agents in the 1870s included the anesthetics (ether, chloroform, and nitrous oxide); opium and its alkaloids (morphine was first used extensively during the Civil War to ease the pain of the wounded); digitalis, which was used chiefly for cardiac edema [congestive heart failure]; ergot, to stimulate uterine contractions and to control postpartum hemorrhage; mercury in the form of an inunction for syphilis and in the form of calomel to purge and salivate; various cathartics of botanical origin; iron, usually in the form of Blaud's pills for anemia; quinine for malaria; amyl nitrite, which was first recommended for the relief of angina pectoris by Sir Thomas Lauder Brunton in 1867 but was still not well known in 1876; sulfur ointment for the itch (scabies); green vegetables or citrus fruit for the prevention or treatment of scurvy. These various medicines were administered either by mouth, by rectum, by inhalation, or by application to the skin. The hypodermic syringe had been introduced by the French surgeon Pravaz in 1851. He employed it to inject "chloride of iron" into vascular tumors to coagulate their contents. Although it was subsequently used for other restricted purposes, the danger of infection limited its use until the physician had learned how to prevent infections by the preparation of sterile solutions (14).

This description of the *best* of the armamentarium available was recorded about a decade after the Civil War. The urban populations certainly benefited most from these breakthroughs; frontier doctors and their patients were very much worse off. Still agonized over the situation:

> My sleep was well nigh ruined; by day and night I saw legions of men and women staggering to and fro, all over the land, crying for freedom from habits of drugs and drink.... I dreamed of the dead and dying who were and had been slaves of habit. I sought to know the cause of so much death, bondage, and distress among my race.... I who had had some experience in alleviating pain found medicine a failure. Since my early life I had been a student of nature's book. In my early days in windswept Kansas I had devoted my attention to the study of anatomy. I became a robber in the name of science. Indian graves were desecrated and the bodies of the sleeping dead exhumed in the name of science. Yes, I grew to be one of those vultures with the scalpel, and studied the dead that the living might be benefited. I had printed books, but went back to the great book of nature as my chief study (3).

He also wrote that he attended a course of lectures at a Kansas City medical school that was long defunct at the time of writing (15).

The next decade of Still's life was devoted to a search for a better way. He farmed, and he invented a butter churn and a version of a grain reaper. More children were born, the sons and daughter who would eventually become prominent in the profession their father was soon to found.

The search for a better way had many potential bypaths. The post-Civil War period was a time of great diversity in the healing professions, both in terms of how one became identified as a physician and how one approached the practice (16). In the mid-19th century, there were no licensing boards and only scattered state laws governing medical practice. There were a few medical schools but there were no standard curricula. Most physicians, especially on the frontiers, were trained as apprentices, doing some reading and serving as a physician's assistant for an unstated length of time.

A majority of physicians followed a standard pattern, heavily influenced by the "heroic medicine" of Benjamin Rush, who said that "there is but one disease in the world" and that it was treatable by "depletion," which translated as bloodletting, blistering, and purging. One influential textbook writer, John Esten Cooke, wrote that:

> All diseases, particularly fevers, arose from cold or malaria, which weakened the heart and thus produced an accumulation of blood in the vena cavae and in the adjoining large veins of the liver. Consequently, calomel and other cathartics which acted on that organ were the cure. "If calomel did not salivate and opium did not constipate, there is no telling what we could do in the practice of physic" (17).

Calomel and other mercury compounds were still listed as late as 1899 in the first Merck's manual, along with opium and morphine and many alcohol-based compounds (18). The practice of "heroic" dosing was well established and well defended. By the time of the Civil War, the system was also called "allopathy," now defined as "that system of therapeutics in which diseases are treated by producing a condition incompatible with or antagonistic to the condition to be cured or alleviated" (19).

The damage caused by the "heroic" techniques was obvious to thinkers before Still, and there were alternative systems of medicine available for consideration. Home remedies and Indian herbal preparations were a basic choice, and this lore was substantial and widely used (17). Numerous resources for botanic preparations were available as well; many of these manuals were widely circulated.

Homeopathy was a major influence in the 19th century. Articulated by Samuel Hahnemann (1755–1843), it was a system of therapy in which "diseases are treated by drugs which are capable of producing in healthy persons symptoms like those of the disease to be treated, the drug being administered in minute doses" (19,20). Eclecticism was another choice, described as "a once popular system of medicine which treats diseases by the application of single remedies to known pathologic conditions, without reference to nosology, special attention being given to developing indigenous plant remedies" (16). Magnetic healing, which "combined spiritualism and healing by seeking to restore the balance of an invisible magnetic fluid circulating throughout the body" (16), and its variants that attempted to use electrical current to restore health were employed. The water cure, movements emphasizing hygiene, antialcoholism or temperance, fresh air and sunlight, nutritional programs, and physical education and popular versions of mental healing, including hypnotism, spiritualism (table rapping), and phrenology, were additional alternatives. And, there were the bonesetters.

At least two of these methods attracted Still and he linked his name to each for a time. A professional card in the Still Museum in Kirksville, Missouri, identifies Still as a "lightning bone-setter." In 1874, he advertised himself in Kirksville as a "magnetic healer," possibly because he was persuaded by "the metaphor of the harmonious balance of the interaction of body parts and the unobstructed flow of body fluids" (16).

After a decade of study, in 1874, Still "flung to the breeze the banner of osteopathy" (3). He did not say precisely what that meant—perhaps a decision, perhaps a sudden coming together of creative thought—but it was followed by attempts to present his findings at Baker University, an institution his family had helped to found (21). He could not get a hearing. Furthermore, he was ejected from the Methodist church on the basis that only Christ

Figure 2-3   The American School of Osteopathy in the 1890s with Dr. A.T. Still sitting on a rail on the porch. (Still National Osteopathic Museum, Kirksville, MO.)

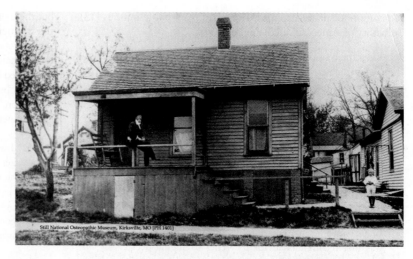

was allowed to heal by the laying on of hands. Still's description of that experience makes it clear that his "laying on of hands" was therapeutic manipulation.

During the next year, Still spent some time with his brother, who had become addicted to morphine through medical treatment. This experience, added to the uselessness of medications in saving his family and others, roused in Still a hatred for the drugs of the day. This enmity sometimes appeared to be nearly absolute, even when the armamentarium of drugs began to move from harmful toward helpful (1–4,22). However, there is evidence in his own writings that he sometimes used topical medications. For example, for snakebites, he washed the wounds with spirits of ammonia, and washed areas bitten by a dog with hydrophobia/rabies with a diluted sulfuric acid solution, and used alcohol to wash a spasmodic tetanic joint (4).

Late in 1875, Still moved from Kansas to Kirksville, Missouri, where he spent the rest of his life. For several years, Still used Kirksville as a base to conduct a marginal itinerant practice (23). His practice evolved as he gained experience, so that the main treatment modality became manipulation. Although this treatment included some of the traditions of magnetic healing and bone setting, it emphasized detailed knowledge of anatomy and body mechanics so that treatment could be said to restore normal function. He held that the body is an efficient chemical laboratory that, in health, makes all the "drugs" it naturally needs. The object of treatment was to discover what caused the sickness and remove the interference so that the body could heal itself (2).

By 1887, enough patients came to Kirksville so that Still could stop his itinerant practice. Word of dramatic successful outcomes

began to spread via the newspapers and word of mouth, and once that happened, the burden of practice quickly became heavy. Still began to think about teaching others his methods; unlike many alternative practitioners of his day, he never intended to keep therapeutic secrets to himself or to grow rich from his methods. There were abortive attempts first to train apprentices and then to teach a class of operators to assist in the practice of osteopathy. The attempts were unsuccessful largely because the students lacked Still's detailed knowledge of anatomy and bodily function.

The term "osteopathy" was coined by Still in about 1889. The story is told (24) that, when challenged because this word was not in the dictionary, Still replied, "We are going to put it there." The word became for Still and his followers a symbol for medical reform, for a science that would refocus medicine on the restoration of normal function. Osteopathy aimed to work with and facilitate the natural machinery of the body for normal and reparative function, rather than working against it, as seemed to be the case with purgatives, emetics, bloodletting, and addictive drugs.

PROFESSIONAL EDUCATION AND GROWTH

First School

The first successful school where osteopathy was taught, the American School of Osteopathy, was chartered in May 1892 and opened that fall with a class of about 21 men and women, including members of Still's family and other local people (Figs. 2.3 and 2.4). The faculty consisted of Still and Dr. William Smith, a physician

Figure 2-4   The first class of the American School of Osteopathy had five women (1892). (Still National Osteopathic Museum, Kirksville, MO.)

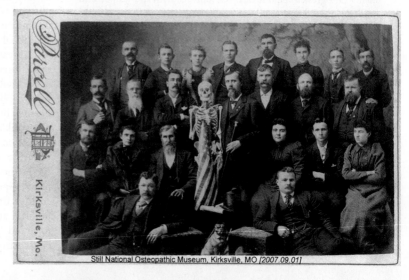

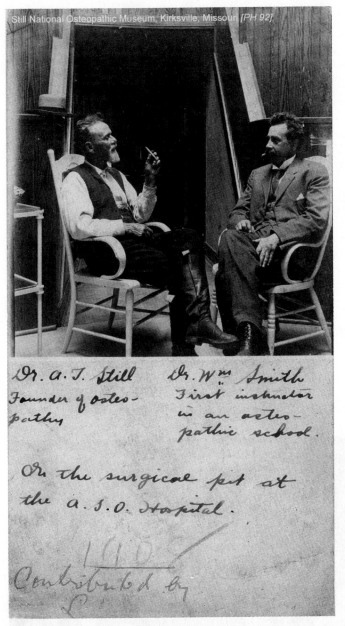

Figure 2-5 A.T. Still, M.D., (left) and William Smith, M.D., were the inaugural faculty of the newly founded American School of Osteopathy in 1892. (Still National Osteopathic Museum, Kirksville, MO.)

trained in Edinburgh, Scotland, who taught anatomy in exchange for learning osteopathy (Fig. 2.5)

The goal, as stated in the revised (1894) charter for the school, was "to improve our present system of surgery, obstetrics, and treatment of diseases generally, and [to] place the same on a more rational and scientific basis, and to impart information to the medical profession." The charter would have permitted granting the doctor of medicine (MD) degree, but Still insisted on a distinctive recognition for graduates, DO, for diplomate in osteopathy (later doctor of osteopathy) (25).

The first course was just a few months long; most of the students voluntarily returned for a second year of additional training. By 1894, the course was 2 years long, two terms of 5 months each. In addition to their study of anatomy, students worked in the clinic under experienced operators, at first only under Still but later under graduates as well.

During the last 5 years of the 19th century, the growth of both the clinic and the school was spectacular. Patients came from near and distant places, having heard by word of mouth or by printed accounts of near-miraculous cures. There were enough such "miracles" that the osteopathic profession was widely promoted by grateful patients. A significant number of early DOs were either former patients or family members of patients who came to their studies with a kind of evangelical fervor. The town of Kirksville prospered and came to regard Still, who once was ridiculed, as a citizen of immense importance. He was lavishly praised, and he lived to see his statue, with the inscription "The God I Worship Demonstrates All His Work," erected in the town square (26,27) (Fig. 2.6).

Data on numbers of enrolled students illustrate the school's dramatic growth. In October 1895, there were 28 students. By the following summer, there were 102. By 1900, there were over 700 students, with a faculty of 18 (25) (Fig. 2.7). By the turn of the century, there were also more than a dozen "daughter" schools founded by graduates of the original school (28). Some of the schools were well organized under the model established by Still; others were established as diploma mills with the anticipation of generating large incomes for the persons establishing them. Still considered many of these to be for training "engine wipers" who were incapable or inexperienced in the practice of osteopathy. Many of these closed as standards were established by the American Osteopathic

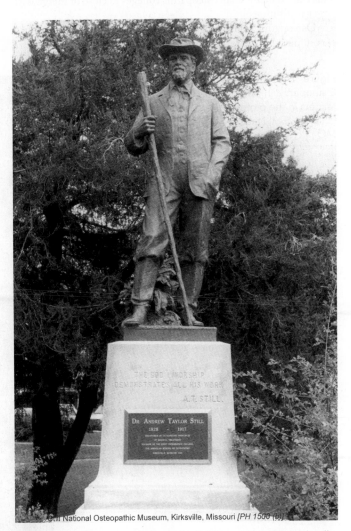

Figure 2-6 The statue dedicated in 1917 to A.T. Still in Kirksville, MO, still stands today in the town square. (Still National Osteopathic Museum, Kirksville, MO.)

Association (AOA) and by state licensure; by 1910, only eight remained.

Conflict with the American Medical Association

Medical education in the late 19th century was not well regulated. Many schools—allopathic, eclectic, homeopathic, and osteopathic—had virtually no entrance requirements except tuition payments, and many schools were for-profit institutions. Licensing laws had not yet reached a stage where they were effective in setting educational standards. The American Medical Association (AMA), founded in 1847 and later a powerful influence on raising educational standards, was weak and in need of reorganization in the 1890s.

A new, reorganized AMA, observing that there were too many doctors, made its first order of business, under a revised constitution, the regulation of medical education. Its Council on Medical Education was formed in 1904, with a charge (among others) to improve the academic requirements for medical schools. This was fulfilled by rating all medical schools as class A (approved), B (probation), or C (unapproved) and making the findings available to state licensing boards (29).

Even before the AMA formed its Council on Medical Education, the young AOA had adopted standards of its own for approval of osteopathic colleges (1902) and began inspections (1903) (30). This caused many small osteopathic colleges to close or merge with larger institutions.

Osteopathic schools were not included in the first AMA survey but they were included in the influential Flexner Report,

published in 1910 (31). After this report, which harshly condemned osteopathic schools along with many medical schools, more marginal schools closed, and the surviving ones converted to a not-for-profit status. Few of the schools established for teaching black physicians survived this period (32) and all but two or three of the schools for women closed (33,34). State licensing boards began to enforce stricter requirements; this probably was a more decisive influence than the Flexner Report (16, 35).

Curriculum

Many medical schools formed affiliations with universities; by doing so, they gained both experienced science faculty and stable funding. This was not an option for osteopathic institutions at that time, and they faced a difficult dilemma: raise entry standards and lose major portions of tuition payments, which represented their only income, or adopt a "go slow" attitude. They chose the latter, which meant that they were perhaps 2 decades behind in the educational reforms that many agreed were desirable (36). AOA standards did increase the required length of osteopathic curricula to 3 years in 1905 and to 4 years in 1915 (30).

The profession responded officially to external criticism by pointing out the differences between osteopathic and orthodox medical education. However, when there was an opportunity to raise general standards, as came about in the 1930s, the profession did so. By the mid-1930s, osteopathic colleges were requiring at least 2 years of college before matriculation; in 1954, 3 years were required; by 1960, over 70% of students had either baccalaureate

Figure 2-7 The faculty of the American School of Osteopathy in 1899. Several soon thereafter became leaders in the profession and founded new osteopathic colleges. (Still National Osteopathic Museum, Kirksville, MO.)

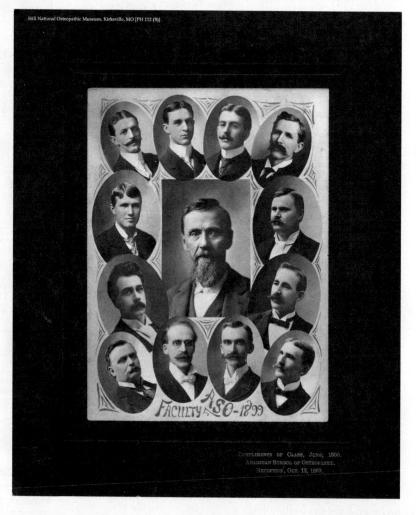

or advanced degrees prior to entry (36). At present, virtually all students enter colleges of osteopathy with at least baccalaureate degrees; many have advanced degrees as well.

Curriculum content similarly grew and changed with the times. An 1899–1900 Kirksville catalogue describes the school's course of study as follows (37):

> The course of study extends over two years and is divided into four terms of five months each, as shown in Table 2.1.

The major difference between this 1899–1900 curriculum and that of an allopathic medical school of the same period, in addition to the distinctive osteopathic content, was the exclusion of *materia medica* (pharmacology).

Early in osteopathic history, a difference appeared between so-called lesion osteopaths and broad osteopaths: those who limited their therapeutic practice essentially to manipulation and those who used all the tools available to medicine, including *materia medica*.

Still practiced midwifery (obstetrics) and surgery; both were taught under his guidance. Indeed, when the issue of surgery became controversial among later DOs, Still's son provided an affidavit

---

TABLE 2.1

Description of Course of Study by Term

Term	Topics
1	• Descriptive anatomy, including osteology, syndesmology, and myology • Lectures on histology, illustrated by microstereopticon • Principles of general inorganic chemistry, physics, and toxicology
2	• Descriptive and regional anatomy with demonstrations • Didactic and laboratory work in histology • Physiology and physiological demonstrations • Physiological chemistry and urinalysis • Principles of osteopathy • Clinical demonstrations in osteopathy
3	• Demonstrations in regional anatomy • Physiology and physiological demonstrations • Lectures on pathology illustrated by microstereopticon • Symptomatology • Bacteriology • Physiological psychology • Clinical demonstrations in osteopathy and osteopathic diagnosis and therapeutics
4	• Symptomatology • Surgery • Didactic and laboratory work in pathology • Psychopathology and psychotherapeutics • Gynecology • Obstetrics • Hygiene and public health • Venereal diseases • Medical jurisprudence • Dietetics • Clinical demonstrations • Osteopathic and operative clinics

---

concerning his father's practice (38). As already noted, Still remained skeptical about using or teaching any form of pharmaceutical therapy.

Still's general opposition to drugs did not prevent some early DOs from using them for treatment. Quite a few had been trained as MDs before they came to osteopathic schools; others went on to earn MD degrees after they became DOs; still others simply decided to use all the adjunctive treatments available. Most "broad" osteopaths felt that after new safer medications were developed it was consistent with being a completely trained physician to incorporate them into osteopathic practice. The most direct early confrontation came in 1897 when a DO-MD opened the short-lived Columbian School of Osteopathy in Kirksville, with the announced intention of offering DO and MD degrees upon graduation from a course in manipulation, surgery, and *materia medica*. The competitive and personal issues in this case extended beyond the academic questions and the school closed after graduating only three classes (25). The issue was professionally divisive for many years thereafter.

Adjunctive treatments became a major subject of debate within the AOA and the Associated Colleges of Osteopathy (now the American Association of Colleges of Osteopathic Medicine) for many years. The question finally was resolved in favor of the "broad" osteopaths, not by consensus over the idea but by recognizing that state licensing laws required fuller training. In 1916, against the direct protest of Still (39), the trustees revoked a previous year's action condemning individuals and colleges that taught drug therapy, effectively opening the way for the colleges to form their own curricula. The profession's great success in using manipulative treatment during the 1918 influenza epidemic (40) probably slowed the integration of *materia medica* into the osteopathic curriculum. However, by the late 1920s, it became officially permissible to institute courses in "comparative therapeutics," of which pharmacology was one subheading (36). By the mid-1930s, the integration was complete. The change was validated as drugs were greatly improved, making it possible to offer pharmaceutical treatment where benefits outweighed risks.

Curricular improvement continued as clinical teaching facilities grew and as budgets permitted the hiring of full-time faculty, particularly in the basic sciences. While instruction by physicians in active practice was an advantage for students who were developing clinical skills, the basic sciences and laboratory-based research required faculty who could give these interests their full attention. All the colleges had full-time basic science faculty by the time the first osteopathic medical school became affiliated with a major American university; such affiliations had been the route by which allopathic schools had strengthened their basic science teaching earlier in the 20th century.

One other curricular improvement deserves mention. For many years, teachers of osteopathic principles and practice developed courses in their area of expertise as traditions within their individual schools, sometimes jealously guarded and always zealously defended. In 1968, a small intercollegiate group of osteopathic principles professors met for the first time. The initial agenda was a response to the new initiative of uniform medical coding, in light of a movement to change the term "osteopathic lesion" to "somatic dysfunction." This change had to be discussed and agreed upon as part of preparation for diagnostic coding. The group continued to meet and it became known as the Educational Council on Osteopathic Principles; later, it became affiliated with the American Association of Colleges of Osteopathic Medicine. Its agenda grew to include a uniform glossary of osteopathic terminology (a current edition is included at the back of this text); systematic development of agreement about the content of a multidisciplinary, problem-based, and patient-oriented osteopathic principles curriculum; and finally, this textbook, *Foundations of Osteopathic Medicine*. Its continuing role also includes development of osteopathic-oriented questions for national board/licensure and specialty board examinations.

Research

On one level, since its earliest days, osteopathic medicine has been a profession based on a research question: "Can we find a better way?" Osteopathic manipulation developed as an experimental approach to clinical conditions that did not respond to the conventional treatments of the time, and its practical success became the empirical research results that led to another level: the questions of "why" and "what if" appropriate to laboratory study. Medical research, in parallel with medical education, underwent a process of developing new traditions and controls, as well as better equipment, all of which would shape future clinical studies.

Laboratory studies began among osteopathic physicians almost as soon as there was an organized osteopathic school (41). Study of the scientific questions raised by osteopathic manipulative practice has never been easy; the difficulty can be illustrated by one obvious clinical question: "What is a manipulative placebo?" In spite of these and other difficulties, a number of significant accomplishments have been recorded (42). Part V of this book offers an extensive survey of osteopathic research efforts from past to present.

Growth of the Profession's Schools

Enthusiastic graduates of the first osteopathic college—for reasons evangelistic or pecuniary—quickly began to establish new schools throughout the country. Some of these were short-lived because they were unable to meet the rising standards of the AOA. Others merged with stronger institutions and survived in a new organization. Still others strengthened their positions and survived. This was the general trend for medical education in the 19th century, and the smaller schools, whether allopathic, osteopathic, or homeopathic, had similar closures, consolidations, or rebuilding.

As noted previously, by 1910 only eight of the early osteopathic schools were still in operation. Six of these have survived into the new millennium; all have had complicated histories of name changes, relocations, charter changes, mergers, and affiliations with other educational institutions. The five original schools still accredited (28) are

- Kirksville College of Osteopathic Medicine, successor to the first school (1892)
- Philadelphia College of Osteopathic Medicine (1898)
- Chicago College of Osteopathic Medicine at Midwestern University (1900)
- University of Health Sciences, College of Osteopathic Medicine, Kansas City (1916)—there had been an osteopathic college in Kansas City as early as 1895
- Des Moines University, College of Osteopathic Medicine and Surgery (1905)—there had been a school in Des Moines as early as 1898

One school, the College of Osteopathic Physicians and Surgeons, Los Angeles, has survived as a medical school (University of California at Irvine School of Medicine). The California conflict and merger in the 1960s, described briefly under "State Licensure," resulted not only in the change of an osteopathic college to an allopathic college but also in a revival of interest in osteopathic education in the profession. The first new educational focus was in Michigan, and it began not only a new tradition in osteopathic education but also became an impetus for nationwide growth that continues to this day (43).

In 1964, the Michigan Association of Osteopathic Physicians and Surgeons committed itself to develop a new, independently funded college of osteopathic medicine. This initiative occurred because more than 1,000 osteopathic physicians practiced in the state, representing about 5% of the state's physician total and providing care for about 20% of the state's patients. None of these DOs had received their education in the state. In 1969, 18 students enrolled in the first class at a new campus in Pontiac, Michigan. Within 2 years, it was clear that a program of such complexity could not survive financially as a freestanding institution. A number of strong supporters in the Michigan legislature, and Michigan's governor, were willing to support a bill for state funding with one major stipulation: the college had to be integrated with an existing, accredited university program. After complex negotiations, the program transferred to the campus of Michigan State University in 1971, where it became the first university-based osteopathic college.

After this affiliation proved successful, 20 more osteopathic schools (some public, some private) were developed over the next 38 years. In 2009, 26 colleges were accredited by the AOA for predoctoral osteopathic education (28). See Table 4.2 for a list of these colleges and Chapter 4 in this section for the current scope and status of osteopathic education and regulation.

STATE LICENSURE

Closely related to the issue of educational standards was licensure under increasingly strict state laws.

The first legislative recognition of osteopathic practice came from Vermont in 1896 (44), where graduates of the American School of Osteopathy, Kirksville, were accorded the right to practice in that state. Missouri had a successful bill as early as 1895, but it was vetoed by the governor; what was hailed as a better bill was passed and signed into law in March 1897 (22,45).

Such laws as these, greeted with much rejoicing, made tremendous growth possible in the osteopathic profession in states where legislation provided a friendly welcome. Osteopathic history includes numerous stories about legal action against DOs for practicing without a valid license, David-and-Goliath encounters of DOs with MD-dominated legislatures, and testimony or influence offered by prominent people who were osteopathic patients. These colorful tales were the war stories of an energetic first generation of DOs, who managed to secure legislative rights to at least limited practice in a majority of states.

Registration and licensure were related (but often different) matters. Some states provided for the formation of separate osteopathic licensing boards, some permitted the addition of an osteopathic representative to an existing or composite board, and a few permitted DOs to apply through a medical board without osteopathic representation.

The roles of these boards were not immediately clear at the time of their formation. There was opposition on ideological grounds even to the idea of licensure. Some populists, not partisan to either osteopathic or allopathic physicians, said that medical licensure was in itself discriminatory. Others said that licensing would interfere with freedom of medical research. Some social Darwinists went so far as to say that if the poor died of their own foolishness in choosing bad medical practitioners, the species would improve (32).

By 1901, however, every state had some form of legislation requiring at least registration, with a diploma from an accepted school, or a state examination of some type. When the Missouri board began to function in 1903, the first certificate it issued was to Still (46).

Licensure to practice a full scope of medicine was another matter, and in most places, it was related first to the content of the osteopathic curriculum and later to the results of examinations. Again using Missouri as an example, by 1897, the subjects taught had expanded to include anatomy, physiology, surgery, midwifery, histology, chemistry, urinalysis, toxicology, pathology, and symptomatology. Everything was included except *materia medica* and academic consciences were temporarily satisfied. By 1937, however, only 26 states had any provision to provide unlimited licenses to DOs.

In some states, DOs were ineligible to apply because their education did not meet specific criteria. As late as 1937, osteopathic standards did not meet preprofessional college requirements in 16 states; in 8 states, a year's internship was needed. Originally, DOs who took examinations under medical or composite boards showed a much lower pass rate. Whether this was a difference in osteopathic curricula or an educational deficiency, as it was argued, in due course, the curricula were altered and the pass rates increased. The major changes were addition of more basic science courses, more faculty, and larger clinical facilities (36).

After World War II, a major effort was made to change the old limited practice laws. These efforts, along with major changes in osteopathic education, enabled the enactment of new practice laws for all 50 states (47).

A final dramatic chapter in the American licensing story of the osteopathic professional came when the California Osteopathic Association agreed in 1961 to merge with the California Medical Association, and the College of Osteopathic Physicians and Surgeons, Los Angeles, became the California College of Medicine. Qualified and consenting DOs were conferred MD degrees as a preparation for a referendum approved by voters in 1962, which discontinued new licensure of DOs in that state (36,43).

A new state osteopathic group, Osteopathic Physicians and Surgeons of California, was chartered by the AOA. This group fought against the referendum but lost; they then began a long legal battle that culminated in a 1974 decision by the California Supreme Court that licensure of DOs must be resumed (36,43,48). A new college was chartered in that state, and professional continuity was restored (43).

By the end of the 20th century, state licensure could be attained in various ways: through the standard national osteopathic licensing examination and/or through the standard national medical licensing examination, depending on state requirements. Some states maintained separate osteopathic and allopathic licensing boards; many were composite boards. Graduate education required for new licenses still varied from state to state. In every state, however, as well as in a number of foreign countries, it was possible for DOs to be licensed for unlimited practice.

OSTEOPATHIC ORGANIZATION

The AOA began as a student organization in Kirksville, under the name American Association for the Advancement of Osteopathy, in 1897. Its present name was adopted in 1901 (49). The second national association was the Associated Colleges of Osteopathy (now the American Association of Colleges of Osteopathic Medicine), formed in 1898. Both groups sought to protect and raise standards for education and practice of DOs. The AOA became the regulatory group, no longer under student control; the Associated Colleges became a discussion and consensus group for faculty and officers of the schools.

In 1907, the first organization devoted to osteopathic research began, though the first recorded osteopathic research was done almost a decade earlier (41). The AOA played a vital role in encouraging and supporting osteopathic research. Money for research has never been plentiful; a major portion of the support for osteopathic research, especially in earlier days, had come from financial contributions by DOs themselves. More recently, qualified researchers have been recipients of public grant funds, but the role of AOA-affiliated research organizations has been essential for start-up projects.

State (divisional) and local (district) osteopathic organizations were established to serve DOs in their own localities. When the AOA grew too large for general membership meetings, state societies began (in 1920) to name representatives to serve in an AOA House of Delegates. That body, thereafter, became the chief policy-making group for the osteopathic profession. A board of trustees, elected by the house, oversaw the implementation of those policies, a role it still fills. Students participate as voting members of delegations from the states in which their schools are located; are appointed to AOA boards, bureaus, and committees; and also have a number of organizations of their own.

A major early effort of the AOA was to produce a code of ethics; this was accomplished in 1904. A participant in those deliberations observed that the problem was not because anyone really wished to practice unethically, but rather that on some points it was difficult to agree upon what was ethical (50). To put this in perspective, the issue of advertising was a hard-fought question among all professionals at that time. The question was resolved by declaring advertising unethical except for brief professional card listings. By the 1990s, advertising by professionals was ultimately considered ethical, though not of course to condone unfounded claims.

Over time, many osteopathic organizations grew from starting points as various as special tasks, geographic or school affinity, and practice interest. A current guide to all AOA-recognized osteopathic organizations is available online, which is updated annually (51). These include state and regional osteopathic medical associations, specialty groups, osteopathic colleges, nonpractice affiliates, accredited hospital and health care facilities, and AOA-supported programs.

The AOA has always been the umbrella group that recognizes and coordinates its efforts on behalf of the profession. The AOA itself has many important functions. Through its bureaus, councils, and committees, it is the osteopathic accrediting organization for undergraduate, graduate, and continuing medical education and for health care facilities. It certifies specialists in all fields, through a network of specialty boards and its own central bureau. Research grants and related projects, as well as educational meetings, are arranged through AOA bureaus and councils.

Staff, directed by elected officers and trustees, provide professional services including maintenance of central records on all DOs, public and legislative education, member services, educational activities including publications and conventions, and coordinated special efforts on a variety of concerns. Position papers on various topics are approved by the House of Delegates and presented as the profession's position on questions of public health and professional interest.

In addition to activities of the AOA itself, a network of divisional and affiliate societies is recognized by the AOA. Certain major "subumbrella" organizations have networks of their own: the associations of osteopathic colleges, health care organizations, licensing groups, and foundations.

Specialty colleges, distinct from the certifying boards, conduct educational affairs and recognize their own members' achievements through fellowships and other awards. State (divisional) and local (district) societies typically deal with state legislative and regulatory affairs, conduct educational programs, and provide a variety of member services.

Colleges typically have student and alumni groups, student chapters of certain specialty organizations, fraternities and sororities, and a variety of special interest groups. Many of the physicians' and students' organizations have auxiliary organizations for spouses.

All organizations recognized by the AOA accept such ongoing controls as approval of any changes in basic documents and designation of how many representatives (if any) are sent to the AOA House of Delegates for voice and vote in professional policy affairs.

FEDERAL GOVERNMENT RECOGNITION

The first major attempt by the AOA to obtain federal government recognition was during World War I when it tried to gain commissions for DOs as military physicians (40). This effort was unsuccessful in spite of active support by such prominent advocates as the former president of the United States, Theodore Roosevelt (52).

At that time, an examination was set, and it was understood that if DOs (along with MDs) took this and passed it, they could be commissioned as medical officers. About 25 DOs took the examination and were recommended for commissions. The surgeon general unilaterally ruled that only MDs were eligible. Bills were then introduced (1917) in both the House of Representatives and the Senate to correct this inequity. The bills were referred to the Military Affairs Committees, and hearings were held. The committee then referred the issue to the surgeon general, who in his statement of opposition claimed that regular physicians would withhold their services if DOs were allowed to serve. The bills remained in committee without resolution until the end of the war. Meanwhile, DOs served as regular soldiers, unable to use their medical training.

The situation remained uncorrected when World War II began. Again there were efforts to obtain commissions for DOs, this time emphasizing regulatory rather than legislative barriers (40,53). DOs were deferred rather than drafted, waiting for the possibility to serve in a medical capacity that never came. Ironically, the DOs left behind became family physicians to the thousands of the patients left by the MDs in military service, which enhanced the public's view of DOs as full-service physicians.

The pressure for federal recognition continued after World War II ended and in 1956 a new law specifically provided for the appointment of DOs as commissioned officers in the nation's military medical corps. However, implementation of that law was blocked for another 10 years until the Vietnam conflict created another special need for military physicians. The first DO was finally commissioned in May 1966. The next year the AMA withdrew its long-standing opposition and DOs were included in the doctor draft. It was another 16 years, in 1983, before the first DO was promoted to be a flag officer in the U.S. military medical corps (30).

Acceptance of DOs as medical officers in the U.S. Civil Service was accomplished in 1963. Careers in this field became possible after that date. Nearly every federal recognition for DOs came after a long and difficult fight. Among the important federal recognitions were the following (30,36):

1951: The U.S. Public Health Service first awarded renewable teaching grants to each of the six osteopathic colleges.
1957: The AOA was recognized by the U.S. Office of Education, Department of Health, Education and Welfare (DHEW), as the accrediting body for osteopathic education.
1963: The Health Professions Educational Assistance Act included a provision for matching construction grants for osteopathic colleges and loans to osteopathic students.

1966: The AOA was designated by the DHEW (now the Department of Health and Human Services [DHHS]) as the official accrediting body for hospitals under Medicare.
1967: The AOA was recognized by the National Commission on Accrediting as the accrediting agency for all facets of osteopathic education.
1983: The first osteopathic flag officer in the U.S. military was appointed.
1997: The first osteopathic surgeon general of the army was appointed.

The U.S. Postal Service commemorated a stamp in 1972 in honor of the 75th anniversary of the founding of the AOA; it was also the 80th anniversary of the first osteopathic medical school and nearly a century since Still "flung to the breeze the banner of osteopathy" in 1874 (Fig. 2.8).

The AOA continues to maintain a presence in Washington, DC, where it attempts to ensure inclusion of DOs and osteopathic institutions as active partners in all legislative and regulatory initiatives.

SPECIALTIES AND HOSPITALS

Perhaps the first osteopathic activity in what now is called a medical specialty began only 3 years after Wilhelm Roentgen announced the discovery of radiographs. The second x-ray machine west of the Mississippi was installed in Kirksville in 1898. With it, Dr. William Smith formulated a method to inject a radiopaque substance in cadaveric veins and arteries to demonstrate the normal pattern of circulation. Two articles were published late that year, one in the *Journal of Osteopathy*, a Kirksville journal associated with the American School of Osteopathy, and the other in the fledgling *American X-Ray Journal*. These were reprinted for modern reference in AOA publications in 1974 (54). When formal certifying boards for osteopathic specialties were organized, radiology was the first (1939) (30).

Along with these events came the long story of the development of osteopathic hospitals, internships, residencies, specialty organizations, specialty standards, examinations, and recognition for those standards. By the 1990s, a full complement of specialties, training programs, and certifying boards were well established in the osteopathic profession, including a board recognizing osteopathic manipulative medicine, now referred to as neuromusculoskeletal medicine. At the same time, the profession was unknowingly developing what would come to be the most needed type of practice for the 1990s: primary care.

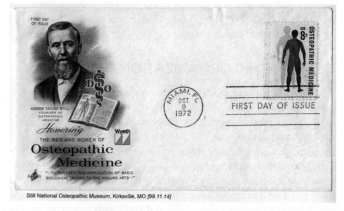

Figure 2-8 In 1972, an osteopathic medicine commemorative stamp was issued by the U.S. Postal Service. (Still National Osteopathic Museum, Kirksville, MO.)

Throughout its history, osteopathic clinical education has taken place in primary care settings: community hospitals and clinics. The profession has supported very few academic medical centers. By the 1990s, this disadvantage became an advantage because of the profession's success in producing primary care physicians, including many willing to work in underserved communities.

Many factors have been cited as influential in the choice of practice type and venue, but the chief ones seem to be undergraduate experiences and role models (55). Students trained in academic medical centers tend to have only subspecialists as role models and their clinical contacts tend to be cases typically referred to tertiary medical centers. Meanwhile, osteopathic students have continued to have regular contact with community clinics and hospitals and have many faculty role models who are primary care physicians.

For instance, rural clinics, long a mainstay of clinical education for the Kirksville college and later for other osteopathic schools, have become a model for primary care education (56). In the last decade of the 20th century, the osteopathic profession found itself in the enviable role of adviser on how to replicate its educational processes in other places.

As with medicine in general, hospitals had their share of developmental problems in the 19th century. Inadequate facilities and staff, infection, disagreement over who should get patient fees, social stigma, and hospital ownership all entered the picture. By about 1900, however, with the growth of an educated nursing profession and a new sense of sanitation, hospitals began to be—at the very least—safe. Many small institutions were privately owned by surgeons who furnished hotel services and nursing for their own patients. New general hospitals began to appeal to patients other than the poor, and patient fees began to help with hospital development (35).

There were osteopathic hospitals early in the 20th century; at the time of Flexner's inspection, Kirksville had the largest, with 54 beds. Chicago had 20 beds; the Pacific College, 15; Boston, 10; and Philadelphia, 3. No others were listed in that report (36). Eventually, the numbers and size of osteopathic hospitals grew, but few reached the size and diversity of specialties that characterized the academic medical centers associated with university medical schools. However, the osteopathic profession did set hospital standards, first for the training of interns and residents and then for accreditation of the institutions themselves.

The growth of osteopathic hospitals was especially marked in the period during and after World War II when MD-run hospitals did not permit DOs to join their medical staffs. When U.S. government programs were approved to help with construction of hospitals, osteopathic institutions participated along with MD-run institutions. Many community teaching hospitals were constructed during those years.

In 1954, a landmark court decision in Audrain County, Missouri, made it illegal for public hospitals to deny staff membership and admitting privileges to qualified DOs. This initiated a series of changes in areas outside California, where DOs had been in charge of a segregated building at the Los Angeles County Hospital since 1928 (43). By the 1960s, most public hospitals were open to DOs; by the 1980s, most private hospitals were open as well.

By the 1990s, with medical residencies open to both MDs and DOs, the need for a network of osteopathic hospitals for training purposes was much reduced. Mechanisms were adopted to recognize training that took place in allopathic institutions as acceptable for osteopathic board certification. This is now possible either by affiliation of the MD institution with an accredited osteopathic college or by direct AOA accreditation of the training institution (51).

By 1999, osteopathic graduate training institutes were the standard, linking resources through hospital–college consortiums.

Reorganization of the health care system itself made these changes necessary. Payment mechanisms led to the formation of large networks of health care providers, including hospitals, outpatient facilities, home care, extended and long-term care, and multiple independent contractors and physician organizations. Community hospitals, including many osteopathic institutions, were merged with larger groups or simply closed. The lines between osteopathic and allopathic hospitals blurred as both came under the umbrella of managed care organizations.

In a case of history repeating itself, economic factors control health care delivery, and the profit motive is once again a respectable part of medical practice. This is placed against a call for serious reform of medical education and better distribution of primary care physicians. The goal is to provide excellence in patient care and in physician education while seeking through corporate management tools the funds to survive in a competitive environment.

SUMMARY

At the start of the 21st century, the "parallel and distinctive" osteopathic profession is respected in many quarters for a variety of reasons. First and foremost is the osteopathic emphasis on primary care. This arose not only from the earlier circumstances of training opportunities and role models but also from the profession's traditional whole-person philosophy.

Additionally, there has been a rebirth of interest in manual medicine and other osteopathic methods. In most osteopathic colleges and graduate education programs, there is increased emphasis on historic tenets and clinical skills. The profession's horizons have been expanded by a global emphasis of its own and an interest in international groups devoted to manual medicine (57–60).

Osteopathic physicians have gained a positive voice in public affairs. In the public arena, DOs are regarded as "parallel and distinctive" in regulatory and legislative affairs, and the profession is consulted on most matters of public health policy. The profession has also launched clinical initiatives in such categories as women's health, minority health care, and pediatric end-of-life care. Continued emphasis on preventive care and health maintenance is in line with traditional osteopathic values. An ambitious strategic plan launched in 2001 by the AOA formalized some of these emphases and added others, including international recognition of United States–trained DOs, an AOA Center for International Affairs, and a new World Osteopathic Medical Association (61).

One of the dedicatees of this volume, George W. Northup, wrote in 1988:

> Today, the practice of medicine needs as never before the guiding light of a fundamental philosophy. It needs to recognize the action and interaction of all body systems. It should apply known truths and explore new frontiers founded on the osteopathic profession's basic philosophy.... Dr Still did not say he was giving the world a philosophy that should act as a guide to the future. Rather, in his book, *The Philosophy of Osteopathy*, he stated his desire was "... to give the world a start in a philosophy that may be a guide to the future" (62).

The purpose of medical history has long been a subject for discussion. At its best and fullest, it can be said to "provide a wonderful schooling in prudence" (63). The caution follows that the historical record must be "considered in terms of its own circumstances and standards. This demands insight into the viewpoints, thoughts, emotions, reactions, and likes and dislikes of people of the past." Such insight requires a more thorough study than an introductory chapter can offer.

Some care has been taken to offer to the interested student a list of references that can facilitate deepened insights. But beyond these readings, there is much more to explore and understand.

REFERENCES

Note: Concerning references 40 and 52: A number of interesting anecdotal accounts were published in JAOA by various authors: 18:247–248, Jan 1919; 18:277–278 and 18:299–302, Feb 1919; 18:335–338 and 18:357–368, Mar 1919; 18:396–398 and 18:415–418, Apr 1919. Also: An attempt was made by the editors of the publication Osteopathic Physician to quantify treatment results. See OP 34:1–2, Dec 1918 and 36:1, Jul 1919. Some suggestive details on type of treatment also were published and reprinted in Time Capsule, The DO 1980;(Jan):31–36. See also Booth ER: History of Osteopathy and Twentieth Century Medical Practice, 1924 edition.

1. Still AT. *The Philosophy and Mechanical Principles of Osteopathy.* Kansas City, MO: Hudson-Kimberly Publishing Co., 1892 and 1902.
2. Still AT. *Philosophy of Osteopathy.* Kirksville, MO: Author, 1899.
3. Still AT. *Autobiography of Andrew T. Still with a History of the Discovery and Development of the Science of Osteopathy.* Rev Ed., Kirksville, MO: Published by the author, 1908.
4. Still AT. *Osteopathy, Research and Practice.* Kirksville, MO: Published by the author, 1910.
5. Gallagher RM, Humphrey FJ II, Micozzi MS, eds. *Osteopathic Medicine: A Reformation in Progress.* London, England: Churchill Livingstone, 2001.
6. Brown JM, Woodworth RB. *The Captives of Abb's Valley; a Legend of Frontier Life.* New ed. Staunton, VA: Printed for the author by the McClure Co., 1942.
7. Dick E. *The Sod-House Frontier.* Lincoln, NE: Johnsen Publishing Co., 1954.
8. Trowbridge C. *Andrew Taylor Still, 1828–1917.* Kirksville, MO: Thomas Jefferson University Press, Northeast Missouri State University, 1991.
9. Thomas JL, ed. *Slavery Attacked: The Abolitionist Crusade.* Englewood Cliffs, NJ: Prentice-Hall, 1965.
10. Monaghan J. *Civil War on the Western Border, 1854–1865.* New York, NY: Bonanza Books, 1965.
11. Eldridge SW. First free-state legislature. In: *Recollections of Early Days in Kansas; Publications of the Kansas State Historical Society.* Vol II. Topeka, KS: Kansas State Printing Plant, 1920:149–158.
12. A.T. Still Pension File. Still National Osteopathic Museum, Kirksville, MO.
13. Duffy J. *From Humors to Medical Science; A History of American Medicine.* 2nd Ed. Urbana, IL: University of Illinois Press, 1993.
14. Bordley J, Harvey AM. *Two Centuries of American Medicine, 1776–1976.* Philadelphia, PA: WB Saunders Co., 1976:97.
15. Laughlin GM. Asks if A.T. Still was ever a doctor. *Osteopath Physician* 1909;15(Jan):8.
16. Osborn GG. The beginning: nineteenth century medical sectarianism. In: Humphrey RM, Gallagher FJ, eds. *Osteopathic Medicine: A Reformation in Progress.* London, England: Churchill Livingstone, 2001: 3–26.
17. Pickard ME, Buley RC. *The Midwest Pioneer; His Ills, Cures & Doctors.* Crawfordsville, IN: R.E. Banta, 1945.
18. *Merck's 1899 Manual of the Materia Medica, Together with a Summary of Therapeutic Indications and a Classification of Medicaments; a Ready-Reference Pocket Book for the Practicing Physician.* New York, NY: Merck & Co., 1899. Reprinted in facsimile by Merck & Co., 1999.
19. *Dorland's Illustrated Medical Dictionary.* 26th ed. Philadelphia, PA: WB Saunders Co., 1981.
20. Danciger E. *The Emergence of Homeopathy; Alchemy into Medicine.* London, England: Century Hutchinson Ltd, 1987.
21. Ebright HK. *The History of Baker University.* Baldwin, KS: Published by the University, 1951.

22. Schnucker RV, ed. *Early Osteopathy in the Words of A.T. Still.* Kirksville, MO: Thomas Jefferson University Press, Northeast Missouri State University, 1991.
23. Still CE. A.T. Still: the itinerant years. In: From the Archives. *The DO* 1975;(Mar):27–30.
24. Riley GW. Following osteopathic principles. In: Hildreth AG, ed. *The Lengthening Shadow of Dr. Andrew Taylor Still.* Macon, MO: Published by the author, 1938:411–435.
25. Walter GW. *The First School of Osteopathic Medicine; A Chronicle, 1892–1992.* Kirksville, MO: Thomas Jefferson University Press, Northeast Missouri State University, 1992.
26. Violette EM. *History of Adair County.* Kirksville, MO: Denslow History Co., 1911:253.
27. Still CE Jr. *Frontier Doctor, Medical Pioneer; The Life and Times of A.T. Still and His Family.* Kirksville, MO: Thomas Jefferson University Press, Northeast Missouri State University, 1991.
28. Historic reference of osteopathic colleges. American Osteopathic Association. Available at: http://history.osteopathic.org/collegehist.shtml. Accessed December 20, 2009.
29. Johnson V, Weiskotten HG. *A History of the Council on Medical Education and Hospitals of the American Medical Association.* Chicago, IL: American Medical Association, 1960.
30. Important dates in osteopathic history. American Osteopathic Association. Available at: http://history.osteopathic.org/timeline.shtml. Accessed December 20, 2009.
31. Flexner A. *Medical Education in the United States and Canada; a Report to the Carnegie Foundation for the Advancement of Teaching.* Boston, MA: Merrymount Press, 1910.
32. Morais HM. The history of the Negro in medicine. In: *International Library of Negro Life and History.* Vol 4. The Association for the Study of Negro Life and History. New York, NY: Publishers Co., 1968.
33. Lopate C. *Women in Medicine.* Published for the Josiah Macy, Jr. Foundation. Baltimore, MD: Johns Hopkins Press, 1968.
34. Walsh MR. *Doctors Wanted: No Women Need Apply; Sexual Barriers in the Medical Profession.* New Haven, CT: Yale University Press, 1977.
35. Starr P. *The Social Transformation of American Medicine.* New York, NY: Basic Books, 1982.
36. Gevitz N. *The D.O.s: Osteopathic Medicine in America.* Baltimore, MD: Johns Hopkins University Press, 1982:75–87. 2nd Ed, 2004.
37. *Catalogue of the American School of Osteopathy, Session of 1899–1900.* Kirksville, MO; seventh annual announcement.
38. The memoirs of Dr. Charles Still; IV. A postscript. In: From the Archives. *The DO.* 1975;(Jun):25–26.
39. Booth ER. *History of Osteopathy and Twentieth-Century Medical Practice.* Cincinnati, OH: Printed for the author by the Caxton Press, 1924.
40. Gevitz N. The sword and the scalpel: the osteopathic 'war' to enter the Military Medical Corps, 1916–1966. *J Am Osteopath Assoc* 1998(May); 279–286.
41. Peterson B. How old is osteopathic research? In: Time Capsule. *The DO.* 1978;(Dec):24–26.
42. Cole WV. Historical basis for osteopathic theory and practice. In: Northup GW, ed. *Osteopathic Research: Growth and Development.* Chicago, IL: American Osteopathic Association, 1987:57.
43. Reinsch S, Seffinger MA, Tobis JS. *The Merger: MDs and DOs in California.* Xlibris press, www.xlibris.com, 2009.
44. A Vermont story and Contacts with the law. In: From the Archives. *The DO.* 1972;(Nov):46–50.
45. Hildreth AG. *The Lengthening Shadow of Dr Andrew Taylor Still.* Macon, MO: Published by the author, 1938.
46. The Old Doctor gets first certificate. *J Osteopathy.* 1904;11(Jan):28.
47. Ross-Lee B, Wood DL. Osteopathic medical education. In: Sirica CM, ed. *Osteopathic Medicine: Past, Present and Future.* New York, NY: Josiah Macy, Jr. Foundation, 1996.
48. Frymann VM. Alexander Tobin, 1921–1992. In: *The Collected Papers of Viola M. Frymann, DO.* Indianapolis, IN: American Academy of Osteopathy, 1996.
49. Students form association. American Osteopathic Association. Available at: http://history.osteopathic.org/aoa.shtml. Accessed December 20, 2009.

50. Evans AL. The beginnings of the AOA (1928 manuscript). In: From the Archives. *The DO.* 1972;(Sep):34–38.

51. American Osteopathic Association. Available at: http://www.osteopathic.org. Accessed December 20, 2009.

52. They passed the exam, but they could not serve: the DO doughboys. In: From the Archives. *The DO.* 1975;(Aug):39–46.

53. How DOs gained commissions. In: Time Capsule. *The DO.* 1980;(Apr): 25–32.

54. 1898: Radiology in Kirksville. In: Time Capsule. *J Am Osteopath Assoc* 1974;74(Oct):167–172.

55. Rodos JJ, Peterson B. *Proposed Strategies for Fulfilling Primary Care Manpower Needs; a White Paper Prepared for the National Advisory Council, National Health Service Corps, U.S. Public Health Service.* Rockville, MD: National Health Service Corps, 1990.

56. Blondell RD, Smith IJ, Byrne ME, Higgins CW. Rural health, family practice, and area health education centers: a national study. *Fam Med.* 1989;3(May–Jun):183–186.

57. Svoboda J. C'mon, take your medicine—global. *The DO* 2000(Dec):56–58.

58. Vitucci N. Healing hands around the world. *The DO* 2002(Mar):36–40.

59. Vitucci N. Finding common ground. *The DO* 2002(Mar):42–45.

60. Kuchera ML. Global alliances: advancing research and the evidence base. *J Am Osteopath Assoc* 2002;102:5–7.

61. AOA's annual report: 2000–01 and beyond. *The DO* 2001;(Sep):65– 70.

62. Northup GW. Mission accomplished? *J Am Osteopath Assoc* 1988;9(Sep). Reprinted in Beal MC, ed. *1995–96 Yearbook: Osteopathic Vision.* Indianapolis, IN: American Academy of Osteopathy, 1996:124.

63. Rosen G. Purposes and values of medical history. In: Galdston I, ed. *On the Utility of Medical History.* New York, NY: International Universities Press, 1957:11–19.

3

Osteopathic Education and Regulation

BRUCE P. BATES

KEY CONCEPTS

- Characteristics of preparation for osteopathic medical school include personality development, experience in health care and service, knowledge of osteopathic philosophy and history, presence of a good support system, and a college degree.
- The osteopathic medical school application and selection process views the applicant as a whole person and considers personal and professional attributes in addition to grades and test scores.
- The Colleges of Osteopathic Medicine are accredited by the Commission on Osteopathic College Accreditation of the American Osteopathic Association.
- Osteopathic medical school curriculum entails preclinical basic science education and clinical skill development, including training in osteopathic palpatory diagnosis and manual treatment.
- Osteopathic clinical training includes experiential learning in accredited hospitals and clinics associated with the colleges.
- Osteopathic education engenders lifelong learning and professional commitment.

Preparation to appreciate and utilize the knowledge, attitude, and skills to be an osteopathic physician begins well before entry into an osteopathic medical school. An appreciation for the philosophical basis and key tenets of the profession noted in Chapter 1 is an obvious base. An understanding of the major historical events recounted previously allows one to appreciate the challenges that the profession has overcome to achieve its current professional standing. These underpinnings set the stage for the growth and development of individuals desirous of becoming osteopathic physicians.

ASPIRATIONS AND PREPARATION

Traditionally, men have sought careers in medicine, including osteopathic medicine, at rates greater than women. Since the 1990s, there has been a significant narrowing of that gap from less than 30% in the 1980s to 50/50 by 2004 (1) (Fig. 3.1). The aspirations for entering a career in medicine include sociodemographic factors (family income, parental careers, and parental education) and personality-career fit characteristics (2). Family role models and expectations have long been known to influence career choice in numerous professions. This is true of medicine as well. For example, having a parent of the same gender who was a doctor is as predictive of having medical career aspirations as is years of preparation in the biological sciences, math, and foreign languages (2). This is especially true for women. Men, unlike women, also need a social or altruistic personality in order to aspire to a medical career (2). Based on the Holland Personality—Occupation Typology, those aspiring to be physicians are best described by three personality types—investigative, artistic, and social. The investigative personality tends to be analytical, curious, methodological, and precise. The artistic individual tends to be expressive, nonconforming, original, and introspective; and the social individual enjoys working with and helping others.

Thus, it is not surprising that the characteristics expected of students seeking to enter the osteopathic profession mirror

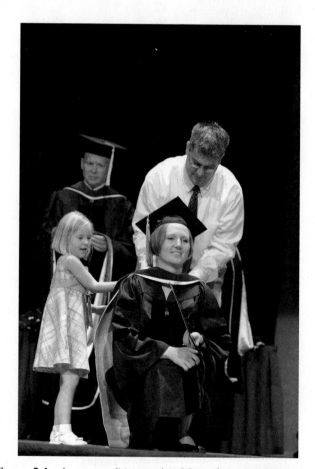

Figure 3-1 As per tradition at the COM of the Pacific at Western University of Health Sciences graduation ceremonies, graduate Lynsey Drew, D.O. receives her doctor's hood from her family supporters, her husband and daughter, as Board of Trustees Vice-Chairman Richard A. Bond, D.O., DrPH, FAAFP, looks on from afar. Photo courtesy of Western University of Health Sciences.

these same elements. While particular details may vary between individual schools, all expect a strong grounding in the sciences such as Biology/Zoology, Chemistry, Physics, and English. Firm academic preparation is necessary to aspire to being an osteopathic physician. The 2006 application cycle saw MCAT scores for applicants averaging 8.02 verbal, 7.72 physical, and 8.30 biology with an average GPA of 3.38. Those actually selected for matriculation in 2007 scored slightly higher: MCAT averaging 8.52 verbal, 8.18 physical, 8.82 biology, with mean GPA of 3.45 (3).

While grades provide a convenient comparison score, and applicants must meet the minimums of preparatory education noted above, osteopathic schools also look for additional factors. Applicants should demonstrate additional challenging academic preparation, experience with the health care system, direct knowledge of the profession, awareness of the sociopolitical aspects of medical practice in general and the osteopathic medical profession specifically, and evidence of leadership in service. Osteopathic medical schools have a long tradition of accepting nontraditional students. These students bring a richness of experience and perspective to their class, classmates, and career choices. These students comprise approximately 25% of the osteopathic student body across the country (3).

Osteopathic physicians differ from allopathic physicians in their philosophical approach to patients. Beyond the use of manipulative treatments, patient-centered care has been the hallmark of osteopathic medicine since its inception. Such an approach is gaining popularity across the health professions. A recent study by the Maine Medical Assessment Foundation and the University of North Carolina noted that osteopathic physicians were easily distinguished from allopathic physicians by their verbal interactions with patients. Osteopathic physicians were more personal, likely to use the patient's first name, explain etiologic factors, and discuss social, family, and emotional impact of illnesses (4). Similar personality and behavioral characteristics are sought in applicants to osteopathic schools and expected throughout the professional development of the osteopathic physician.

APPLICATION PROCESS

The application process begins well before the submission of application documents to the osteopathic school of choice. The applicant begins with a well-designed course of study, contributions of leadership in service to community and others, experiences in health care settings, and participation in scholarly activities such as research and writing. If the applicant is a second career applicant, similar attributes are expected to complement the life experience as evidence of the pursuit of continued intellectual and academic rigor. All candidates should develop ongoing mentoring relationships with professors and osteopathic physicians to facilitate the candidate's understanding of the career they have chosen to seek and to allow the character and individualism of the candidate to be defined.

Twenty-five out of twenty-six osteopathic medical schools utilize the American Association of Colleges of Osteopathic Medicine Application Service (AACOMAS). This centralized service allows the applicant to file a single electronic application. AACOMAS then verifies, standardizes, compiles, and distributes the electronic application to each of the osteopathic schools designated by the applicant. Osteopathic medical schools utilize a holistic approach to the applicant and look beyond the GPA and MCAT scores submitted. Each school has a secondary application process to identify those applicants best suited to the mission and goals of the individual school. Letters of recommendation,

experiences in the health professions, and knowledge of and experience with osteopathic medicine are important features considered in the secondary application process. Personal statements and interviews may be vital considerations. The personal and professional fit for the applicant and the school are crucial to the attainment of mutual success.

Successful candidates demonstrate achievement in the required prerequisite course work including growth in meeting challenges of increasing academic rigor. The profession of osteopathic medicine focuses on the whole person and the prospective student must demonstrate the ability to relate to individuals and to society as well as being intellectually sound. Evidence of character traits such as honesty, reliability, and commitment is sought. Leadership in service-beyond-self is desired. Likewise, experience and knowledge with the health care system and osteopathic medicine in particular, within the context of the sociopolitical aspect of medical practice, complements a candidate's successful application (Table 3.1).

CURRICULUM

The American Osteopathic Association (AOA) Commission on Osteopathic College Accreditation (COCA) is the accrediting agency of predoctoral osteopathic education. It is recognized by the United States Department of Education. Accreditation means that a college or a school of osteopathic medicine has appropriately identified its mission, has secured the necessary resources to accomplish that mission, currently shows evidence of accomplishing that mission, and may be expected to continue to do so. Accreditation requires each school or college to undergo continuing self-study and periodic peer evaluation to ensure its continued performance within the standards established by the COCA. The president of the AOA appoints the members of the commission, but the COCA is otherwise self-determining as to the standards it defines and the assessment of achievement necessary to award accreditation status to an individual school. Once a school is accredited, ongoing reassessments are required to maintain accreditation status. Accreditation is a necessary step for a school's graduates to be eligible for residency training and licensure. COCA currently accredits 26 colleges of osteopathic medicine offering instruction at 32 locations in 23 states (Table 3.2).

AOA-accredited schools have met or exceeded standards determined by COCA in seven areas:

1. Organization Administration and Finance
2. Faculty and instruction
3. Curriculum
4. Student Services
5. Performance and evaluation
6. Research and Scholarly Activity; and
7. Facilities

Each of these areas has specific guidelines determined by COCA that are available online through the AOA predoctoral accreditation website (http://www.osteopathic.org/index.cfm?PageID=acc_predoc). The evaluation of compliance with these guidelines is determined through self-study reports and on-site reviews by members of the COCA registry of evaluators.

The standards for accreditation require each College of Osteopathic Medicine (COM) to have a clearly defined mission statement including goals and objectives appropriate to osteopathic medical education that address teaching, research, service, including osteopathic clinical service, and student achievement (5). The COM may implement its curriculum utilizing different curriculum models. The particular curriculum is the prerogative of the individual schools within the COCA guidelines. Two frequently used

TABLE 3.1

Characteristics of Applicants to Osteopathic Medical School

Requirements	Personal Qualities	Achievements
• At least 3 y of college education in biology, chemistry, physics, English	• Honest, reliable, responsible	• Demonstrated success in challenging academic college courses
• Medical College Admissions Test	• Family support and encouragement	• Most have at least a bachelor's degree
• Personal statement	• Investigative, social and artistic personality	• Experience with health care system
• Letters of recommendation, including at least one from an osteopathic physician	• Second career (25%)	• Direct knowledge of the osteopathic profession (e.g., shadowing a D.O.)
• Secondary college application		• Awareness of the sociopolitical aspects of osteopathic medical practice
• Interviews		• Evidence of leadership and community service
		• Research experience

models are the discipline-based and system-based models. The former is organized around specific academic and practice specialties such as internal medicine, obstetrics, and family medicine and the basic science disciplines, such as physiology and anatomy. The latter is organized around body systems such as the cardiovascular or reproductive systems and attempts to integrate the disciplines through the study of those body systems. Newer models include case-based, evidence-based, problem-based and independent study models. Each school may choose a variety of methods to achieve its specific mission and goals. Thus, schools may vary in the amount of emphasis placed on such teaching methods as small group exercises, problem-based learning, didactic lecturing or on particular elements of the curriculum such as research, rural medicine, or primary care, depending on the mission of the particular school (6).

Since each school may employ different methods in its curriculum, it is imperative that the student have a good understanding of his or her learning style and seek an environment that is conducive to that learning style. Independent and experiential learners may thrive in a problem-based environment, whereas traditional learners may do better in a discipline-based curriculum. In any event, the medical student will evolve a learning style that is increasingly driven by adult learning theory. One of the most difficult transitions that most medical students encounter is away from the teacher-driven academic learning and evaluation environment. In that environment, the instructor likely determines the student's more concrete assignments, readings, and testing parameters. As students progress through medical education, there is transition to adult learning methods in which the learner must assume increasing responsibilities for learning. This is often based on a case-oriented need-to-know basis but requires a discipline on the part of the learner to secure the best evidence for the query.

AACOM

The growth and acceptance of the profession has been impressive. As colleges developed, it became clear that a single avenue of advocacy for osteopathic education, development and integration educational paradigms, and a forum for collegial collaboration would benefit the profession. In 1898, the American Association of Colleges of Osteopathic Medicine was founded to lend support and assistance to the nation's osteopathic medical schools. This association serves as the unifying voice of the colleges through proactive advocacy. It fosters collaboration and innovation among its member colleges particularly with its membership councils that bring interest groups together on issues of professional education. It provides a centralized service for data collection and analysis including the online application service. The AACOM develops national initiatives to promote and raise awareness of osteopathic medical education.

Led by the Board of Deans that includes the dean of each Osteopathic school, the AACOM includes 11 councils to encourage interest groups ranging from information technology and library services to financial officers, student affairs personnel, development officers, researchers, and more. These include the following:

■ Council of Development and Alumni Relations Professionals
■ Council of Fiscal Officers
■ Council for Information and Technology
■ Council of Medical Admissions Officers
■ Council of Osteopathic Librarians
■ Council of Osteopathic Medical Student Services Officers
■ Council of Osteopathic Student Government Presidents
■ Council of Researchers
■ Council of Student Financial Aid Administrators

TABLE 3.2

Osteopathic Medical Schools Accredited by the AOA COCA as of December 2009

Year Established	Name and Location	City, State	Type
1892	A.T. Still University of Health Sciences/Kirksville College of Osteopathic Medicine (**ATSU/KCOM**);	Kirksville, MO	Private
	A.T. Still University, School of Osteopathic Medicine in Arizona (**ATSU-SOMA**)[a], founded in 2008	Mesa, AZ	
1898	Des Moines University-College of Osteopathic Medicine (**DMU-COM**)	Des Moines, IA	Private
1899	Philadelphia College of Osteopathic Medicine (**PCOM**)	Philadelphia, PA;	Private
	Philadelphia College of Osteopathic Medicine (**Georgia-PCOM**), founded in 2004	Suwanee, GA	
1900	Midwestern University/Chicago College of Osteopathic Medicine of (**MWU/CCOM**)	Downers Grove, IL	Private
	Midwestern University/Arizona College of Osteopathic Medicine of (**MWU/AzCOM**), founded in 1995	Glendale, AZ	
1916	Kansas City University of Medicine and Biosciences—College of Osteopathic Medicine (**KCUMB-COM**)	Kansas City, MO	Private
1966	University of North Texas Health Science Center at Fort Worth, Texas College of Osteopathic Medicine (**UNTHSC**)	Ft. Worth, TX	Public
1969	Michigan State University College of Osteopathic Medicine (**MSUCOM**)	East Lansing, MI	Public
1970	Oklahoma State University Center for Health Sciences College of Osteopathic Medicine (**OSU-COM**)	Tulsa, OK	Public
1974	West Virginia School of Osteopathic Medicine (**WVSOM**)	Lewisburg, WV	Public
1975	Ohio University College of Osteopathic Medicine (**OU-COM**)	Athens, OH	Public
1976	University of New England, College of Osteopathic Medicine (**UNE/COM**)	Biddeford, ME	Private
1976	University of Medicine and Dentistry of New Jersey, School of Osteopathic Medicine (**UMDNJ-SOM**)	Stratford, NJ	Public
1977	Western University of Health Sciences, College of Osteopathic Medicine of the Pacific (**COMP**)	Pomona, CA	Private
1977	New York College of Osteopathic Medicine (**NYCOM**), of the New York Institute of Technology	Old Westbury, Long Island, NY	Private
1979	Nova Southeastern University College of Osteopathic Medicine (**NSU-COM**)	Fort Lauderdale, FL	Private
1992	Lake Erie College of Osteopathic Medicine (**LECOM**)	Erie, PA	Private
	Lake Erie College of Osteopathic Medicine–Bradenton (**LECOM–Bradenton**), founded in 2003	Bradenton, FL	
1996	Touro University College of Osteopathic Medicine (**TUCOM**)	Mare Island, Vallejo, CA;	Private
	Touro University College of Osteopathic Medicine–Nevada (**TUCOM–NV**), founded in 2003	Las Vegas, NV	
1997	Pikeville College School of Osteopathic Medicine (**PCSOM**)	Pikeville, KY	Private
2000	Edward Via Virginia College of Osteopathic Medicine (**VCOM**)	Blacksburg, VA	Private
2006	Lincoln Memorial University DeBusk College of Osteopathic Medicine (**LMU-DCOM**)[a]	Harrogate, TN	Private
2007	Rocky Vista University College of Osteopathic Medicine (**RVUCOM**)[a]	Parker, CO	Private
2007	Pacific Northwest University of Health Sciences College of Osteopathic Medicine (**PNWU-COM**)[a]	Yakima, WA	Private
2008	Touro College of Osteopathic Medicine (**TouroCOM**)[a]	New York, NY	Private
2009	William Carey University College of Osteopathic Medicine (**WCU-COM**)[a]	Hattiesburg, MS	Private

[a]Provisional Accreditation until the college graduates its first class.

- Educational Council on Osteopathic Principles (ECOP); and
- Marketing and Communication Advisory Council

Aided by the Board of Deans of AACOM, the Society of Osteopathic Medical Educators and its member councils, the AACOM promotes educational development, research initiatives, and membership services for students, educators and colleges, and professional advocacy for all the colleges of osteopathic medicine. (see AACOM web page at www.aacom.org)

ECOP, which was established in 1969 under the leadership of Ira Rumney, D.O., and Norm Larson, D.O., serves as the cooperative voice for the teaching of osteopathic principles and practices for the member colleges of AACOM. ECOP consists of the chairs, or designees, from the departments at the osteopathic colleges that oversee the teaching of the structural diagnosis and osteopathic manipulative treatment (OMT) portion of the curriculum. It develops and promotes the improvement of curricula in these areas as well as best practices across the continuum of education. As an initial publication of its work, the ECOP developed a *Glossary of Osteopathic Terminology* in 1981 which it updates and regularly publishes, and which is used worldwide. In 1987, the Council of Deans approved the ECOP consensus document: Core Curriculum in Osteopathic Principles Education for the AACOM colleges. ECOP was a critical impetus for the establishment of the *Foundations for Osteopathic Medicine* textbook, and its members perform vital roles as authors, editors, and peer reviewers for each edition.

SCHOLARSHIP AND RESEARCH

Osteopathic medical schools have always fostered research among the faculty of the schools and to a lesser extent the students and residents engaged in the programs of the colleges. However, the emphasis has always focused on patient care; research has not been as much of the focus as it is with allopathic schools. Scholarship and research are necessary for the advancement of the credibility and visibility of the profession. The profession also has an obligation to contribute to the fund of knowledge and application of research to the milieu of medical care. Therefore, the standards for colleges of osteopathic medicine, and osteopathic postgraduate training have increasingly emphasized research and scholarship skills as desired traits in applicants, students, faculty, and residents. Many schools seek students with research backgrounds, and a few offer value-added PhD and Masters level programs to complement the offerings available to students and practitioners of osteopathic medicine. Nowhere is this more important than in the fundamental research accorded to OMT. A firm evidence-based research track in this important modality and translational research into its effective implementation remains as a core challenge to the profession. Furthermore, it appears that competitive specialty and subspecialty training programs increasingly value residents with a firm understanding of research and a record of scholarly achievement. Even students without aspirations in a research career are well served by a basic understanding of research design and interpretation. The rapid advancements in the practice of medicine require the practitioner of the future to be able to critically appraise the voluminous literature to determine its validity and application to the patients who come under the care of an osteopathic physician. Evidence-based medicine—the practice of medicine according to the best available information—is a standard of practice expected by hospitals, insurance carriers, and patients. In the meantime, practicing physicians are confronted with a large amount of information

from various sources. Some of this is tainted by commercialism or self-promotion. Some is critical information that makes a significant contribution to the outcomes of care. Much of what appears in print or in online resources is irrelevant, inaccurate, or mediocre. The ability to successfully differentiate these to improve the delivery of patient-oriented care demands that the practitioners of osteopathic medicine attain a level of competency in this critical area.

PRECLINICAL CURRICULUM

Classically, osteopathic medical schools have viewed the curriculum in two parts—each dependent on the other. The first portion of the curriculum encompasses the acquisition of basic knowledge and skills in the sciences and the fundamental development of attitudes and skills in clinical practice. This is typically 2 years in length. While the emphasis is on securing a base of knowledge, most schools also work to expose students to fundamental patient care skills in physical examination and medical documentation during this phase of education. The AOA COCA requires the various colleges to stipulate the course of instruction designed to address the educational objectives, the resources and the faculty available for offering this instruction and for assessing the students' achievement of these objectives. This includes the integration of osteopathic philosophy, principles, and practices throughout the entire curriculum. Many osteopathic schools also include introductory exposure to patients in this first 2 years through observerships and limited practicums. This allows the emphasis to remain on acquiring the skills necessary for a focus on the person/the patient in addition to the acquisition of basic skills and knowledge.

CLINICAL CURRICULUM

Traditionally, the clinical curriculum of medical schools has included experiential learning in hospitals and clinics associated with the medical school. This has occurred largely during the last 2 years of the osteopathic medical school curriculum. Because of its emphasis in primary care and community-based care, the osteopathic profession has always utilized a number of community-based and affiliated sites to secure the best educational opportunities for its graduates. This diversity of training sites has served the profession to ensure exposure to a number of venues of care, from tertiary-care hospitals to rural clinics and private practices. While many allopathic schools have found the maintenance of a central academic medical center difficult, the osteopathic profession has reached out to community-based training as consistent with the mission and goals of most osteopathic medical schools. Many studies, including the GPEP (General Professional Education of the Physician) report and the Pew Foundation have noted that training in tertiary-care centers alone leads to a large percentage of students choosing to be tertiary-care doctors as they are exposed to those role models. Mentoring and role models in primary care can best be served in nontertiary care models including community hospitals and private practices. The AOA COCA standards recognize this and note that such training must be a cooperative venture between the training locales and the college. The college must define the educational objectives and appoint the faculty of the affiliated distant sites. Most important, the college must establish clinical core competencies to be acquired and a methodology to ensure they are being met in preparation for the graduates' entry into postdoctoral (residency) programs. This can be assessed through a variety of tools including standardized patients, skills' testing clerkship exams, and clerkship training evaluation. The clinical experience curriculum is referred to as the clerkships curriculum. It is often divided into the core clerkship and the elective clerkship curriculum at the discretion of the college. The core clerkship includes the basic requirements designed and administered by the COM in such disciplines as family medicine, obstetrics, pediatrics, internal medicine, and surgery. This phase is usually offered during the third year. Students are frequently given latitude to select specialties and training locales on an elective basis with the permission of the COM in their fourth year. This allows the student an opportunity to pursue additional training in an area of interest, to supplement previous experiences, and to explore postgraduate opportunities for residency training.

COMLEX—USA

All osteopathic students must pass three of the four parts of the National Board of Osteopathic Medical Examiners, Inc. (NBOME) Comprehensive Osteopathic Medical Licensing Examination (COMLEX-USA) to graduate from an accredited osteopathic school. COMLEX-USA Level 1 concentrates on the assessment of basic science and clinical science knowledge through a variety of computer-accessed case-based questions. This is typically administered online at the end of the preclinical portion of the curriculum at the end of year two of the traditional curriculum. COMLEX-USA Level 2 CE (cognitive evaluation) similarly assesses case-based knowledge in clinical presentations and is typically administered online at the conclusion of the core clinical curriculum, usually at the end of the core clerkships of year three of the traditional curriculum. In addition, students must pass the COMLEX-USA PE (Performance Evaluation) wherein standardized patients are used to assess the student skills and competencies in two domains. The first domain is the humanistic domain concentrating on the physician-patient interaction emphasizing interpersonal and communication skills. The second is the biophysical domain concentrating on the skill of the patient interview, the physical examination, the selection and performance of OMT, and the writing of medical notes documenting the patient care encounter. In the COMLEX-USA level 2 PE process, communication and performance is emphasized, while in COMLEX-USA level 1 and

COMLEX-USA level 2 CE, knowledge acquisition and decision making is emphasized.

The USA COMLEX-USA offers a third exam at the end of the first year of postgraduate training (COMLEX-USA level 3 CE) that is the final step in meeting state examination requirements for licensure. This examination places an emphasis on case analysis, diagnostic choices, and patient management (Table 3.3).

The allopathic profession offers similar examinations entitled the United States Medical Licensing Exam (USMLE). This exam is divided into three sections like the COMLEX-USA. These may not be substituted for the COMLEX-USA requirements. Some students choose to also take the USMLE equivalent examinations believing that this may be advantageous to them in the pursuit of residency. Comparisons between allopathic and osteopathic education requirements are listed in Table 3.4.

POSTDOCTORAL

For many years, the osteopathic and allopathic professions had no requirement for additional training beyond the years of medical school. Only a few graduates apprenticed with experienced doctors. In the early 1950s, a formal program of additional training became commonplace as a 1-year internship through the general wards of care in a hospital. The young graduate was in place (interned) in the hospital for a year of intensive tutelage at the hands of a group of experienced physicians. Gradually becoming more formalized postgraduate training expanded to longer periods of time in areas of specialization. This often required the aspiring specialist to live at the hospital (thus the term resident) and to be available for service and learning at all times. Living quarters and perhaps a small stipend was provided if the resident was fortunate. As medicine grew even more complex, both the AMA and the AOA developed criteria and standards to govern the content and duration of these residencies. For the AMA, the oversight body for these residencies became the Accreditation Council for Graduate Medical Education (ACGME) and its Residency Review Committees. For the AOA, it became the Council on Postdoctoral Training (COPT) and its Program and Trainee Review Committee (PTRC) and the Committee on Osteopathic Postdoctoral Training Institutions Committee.

TABLE 3.3

Content Emphasis for each COMLEX Licensing Examination[a] and Year Taken During Osteopathic Medical Education

Content Emphasis	Level 1 Second Year	Level 2-CE Third Year	Level 2-PE Fourth Year	Level 3 PGY-1
Basic and Clinical Science Knowledge	x			
Case-Based Knowledge and Decision Making		x		
Communication and Osteopathic Skill Performance			x	
Case Analysis, Diagnostic Choices, and Patient Management				x

[a] Aspects of each component exist as a part of each exam. For further information, see the NBOME web site at http://www.nbome.org/docs/comlexBOI.pdf, accessed Dec.18, 2009.

CE, cognitive evaluation; PE, performance evaluation; PGY, postgraduate year

TABLE 3.4

Osteopathic versus Allopathic Education

Category	Osteopathic	Allopathic
Premedical Education	University Degree or equivalent education	University Degree or equivalent education
Medical School Duration	4 y	4 y
Degree	D.O.	M.D.
Residency	AOA or ACGME Approved (3–5 y)	ACGME Approved (3–5 y)
Licensing Exam	COMLEX	USMLE
Board Certification	AOA and/or ACGME	ACGME

COPT AND OPTI

Postdoctoral education is the prerogative of the individual specialties. Each osteopathic specialty has a board that defines the requirements of training for that specialty. These must be within the guidelines and oversight of the basic standards of the COPT. These basic standards are enforced through program inspections, self-study, and reviews by the PTRC. Every osteopathic residency must be a member of an osteopathic postgraduate training consortium known as an OPTI (Osteopathic Postgraduate Training Institution). These OPTIs provide a source of expertise and cooperative education by incorporating member hospitals, COMs, and residencies into a collective entity to design, implement, and assess the delivery of quality osteopathic postdoctoral education and experiences to member programs and its residents. Cooperative activities require the incorporation of osteopathic principles, OMT, faculty development, didactic education, program assessment, peer review, and resident support services between programs and with COMs. The AOA promotes attainment of six basic core competencies in all its residencies, including application of osteopathic philosophy and principles in practice and appropriate utilization of OMT (Table 3.5).

Graduates of osteopathic schools may choose to seek postgraduate training in a number of venues and disciplines. Graduates are selected for ACGME programs, military programs and COPT-approved programs. The COPT will give osteopathic recognition to those ACGME programs that meet COPT standards on an individual basis. Although there is no official designation recognizing approval by both the COPT and the ACGME, these are often referred to as "dual approved." Approximately 38% of the 3,462 members of the 2008 osteopathic medical student graduating class chose COPT-approved osteopathic programs with 82% achieving their first-choice placement (8). Another 13% of osteopathic graduates were accepted into AOA positions after failing to match in a program (post match "scramble"); thus, a total of 51% of the 2008 graduating class matched in AOA internship or first-year residency positions (8). The remainder matched in ACGME or military programs. Those who do select nonosteopathic programs may request approval from the COPT but must meet stringent programmatic guidelines to gain approval.

RESIDENCY SEARCH AND SELECTION

The search for a residency necessitates the careful consideration of a career track. Osteopathic students are encouraged not to track too early to a specialty area. Many students find their initial expectation for specialty to change often during the medical school time. It is not uncommon to become enamored of each specialty as one proceeds through the clerkship years. Thus, the best option for most students is to seek preparation as a generalist. The best specialists are first and foremost well-prepared generalists. Both core clerkships and elective clerkships allow students to explore various fields of practice and potential sites for later residencies.

Students typically obsess over grades as they prepare to seek residency training. While course grades and standardized

TABLE 3.5

AOA CORE Competencies

1. Osteopathic Philosophy and Principles (OPP) and Osteopathic Manipulative Medicine (OMM)[a]
2. Medical knowledge and OPP/OMM
3. Patient Care and OPP/OMM
4. Interpersonal and Communication Skills and OPP/OMM
5. Professionalism and OPP/OMM
6. Practice-based Learning and Improvement and OPP/OMM
7. Systems Based Practice and OPP/OMM

[a]The NBOME has integrated the Osteopathic philosophy and principles competency into all of the other six core competencies in its national board examinations.

Source: AOA Accreditation Document for Osteopathic Postdoctoral Institutions and the Basic Document for Postdoctoral Training Programs.

test scores like the NBOME are important, studies show other characteristics are equally, if not more important (9). These divide into three categories: performance on service (clerkship), personal characteristics, and the COM academic record. Academic performance is important and students should strive for excellence, but residency directors are more likely to select candidates they have encountered on service in their hospital during clerkship time. If the student has not been on service in that hospital, then the same service at a similar hospital known to the residency director becomes important. This allows residency directors to assess the character, work ethic, professional responsibility, and reliability of the applicant. These characteristics are important to residencies due to the necessity of interdependency and teamwork. Secondly, directors tend to seek evidence of intellectual curiosity and leadership. This can be demonstrated by the service record of the student during medical school and by a record of scholarship in research or publication. The "student performance letter" a.k.a. "the dean's letter" and the other letters of recommendation are viewed as less informative to most residency directors.

Students interview at a number of residency programs during clerkship time and select programs to apply to based upon a number of personal and professional factors and their feeling as to the likelihood of acceptance. Once a student selects the programs, it is necessary to complete the ERAS (Electronic Residency Application Service) forms online via the internet. This also involves submitting various supporting documents, letters of recommendation, and transcripts. There are specific deadlines for these and students are well advised to work with their individual schools to begin this process well in advance. Similar to selecting a COM, students should consider the quality of the program as well as personal quality of life issues in selecting a residency. Physicians are likely to practice near their site of final training, where they grew up or where their significant other grew up.

Residents are chosen by a computer match process. The military programs, osteopathic programs, and allopathic programs all use a similar process. Programs list their preferred candidates in order. The applicants list their programs in order of preference. The computer then selects candidates by matching these preferences through an algorithm established by the oversight committees for the respective programs. The military programs are the first to match and those candidates are removed from the pool. The osteopathic and allopathic matches occur separately. Once a student matches with a program, the match is considered ethically made and both sides are expected to adhere to the results. Prematch deals are considered unethical and are frowned upon. Once the match is confirmed, contracts are signed and registered with the AOA for osteopathic programs. Should a student not "match" there is a period following that seeks to connect the unmatched student and program. Many excellent programs have unmatched positions. This is especially true in primary care. Allopathic programs may try to fill those unmatched spots with foreign graduates.

When a residency is completed, a physician may choose to enter a subspecialty. This may be a fellowship or "plus one" program depending on the nature of the program and the oversight organization or board. It may not be necessary to complete the entire residency to qualify for a fellowship, but a substantial part must be completed. Thus, an osteopathic physician may complete a portion of general surgery residency and apply for a fellowship in urologic surgery or complete an internal medicine residency and apply for a cardiology fellowship. Likewise, a resident might complete a family medicine residency and choose to do a plus 1 year in osteopathic manipulative medicine. The specifics of these options vary from specialty to specialty and are the prerogative of the specialty. Details are available from the various specialty organizations.

BOARDS

Generically, the term "boards" refers to the examinations that are taken to demonstrate the acquisition of a basic competency. "National boards" refer to the NBOME- or the USMLE-generated examinations given during osteopathic medical school and the first part of postgraduate training. As a physician progresses through training and into practice, additional boards may be required. At the conclusion of residency or fellowship, a physician is termed board eligible. This means that the physician has met the requirements of preparatory training and experience to take the examination that may include written exams, practical exams, and record reviews at the discretion of the specialty. Once the examination is successfully completed, the physician is now considered "boarded" or certified in the discipline. The specialty may impose other criteria in addition to the examination. Specialty board certification is usually time limited and the applicant must meet certain continuing study and reexamination standards as the specialty may specify.

LICENSURE

In the United States, licensure is the prerogative of the licensing boards of the state or jurisdiction in which one chooses to practice. Licensing requirements are stipulated by the state and, at a minimum, include requirements for graduation from an accredited school, a specified length of postgraduate training and the passage of a recognized board exam. States vary on the amount of postgraduate training required from 1 to 3 years. All states recognize the NBOME COMLEX-USA examination. States may impose additional requirements such as attestations as to character, criminal background checks, review of the physicians data bank, and letters of reference. These requirements may change over time and contact with the various state licensing boards is recommended. States may have a single licensing board or have separate osteopathic and allopathic boards. Licensure allows the practitioner to practice generally within the state but does not specify the scope of practice, nor guarantee acceptance by a hospital or inclusion in an insurance carrier's panel of providers. These privileges are discussed later.

Once granted, licensure is for a specific period of time and must be periodically renewed with evidence of continued education and capacity to practice as specified by individual states. States have the option to reciprocate licensure with other states if the requirements are deemed equivalent. This varies from state to state and should not be assumed. Typically, the military requires licensure in at least one state in order to practice in a military facility. An individual may hold licensure in more than one state.

Osteopathic physicians may be eligible for licensure in other countries. There are an expanding number of countries accepting the osteopathic physicians trained under the AOA guidelines. In some cases, there are not any laws or regulations pertaining to osteopathic physicians because no individual has ever applied. The AOA or particular jurisdiction should be contacted for specific requirements.

CREDENTIALS AND PRIVILEGING

The sum total of a physician's educational history, degrees, awards, residency completion, licensure, and boards constitutes the credentials of a physician. These credentials provide documentation of the achievements of the physician. In many ways, they serve as surrogate evidence of competency or the ability to practice. Various organizations use these credentials along with other information to determine acceptance of the individual physician into the organization and to determine the extent or scope of activities the physician will be allowed within the organization. This right to practice a certain scope of activities is termed privileging—the physician is given the privilege of practicing the activity.

Privileging is the prerogative of a specific organization. Different hospitals and insurance carriers may grant different privileges to the same physician based on their own needs and assessment of the credentials. For example, a physician may have the privilege of doing endoscopies at one hospital in town but not another. Physicians, and particularly residents, should maintain a log of their activities to demonstrate familiarity and currency with diagnostic entities and medical procedures. This will serve to bolster their credentials for privileges when requesting the right to do procedures or attend to patients with certain types of illnesses.

CONTINUING MEDICAL EDUCATION

Continuing medical education (CME) allows a physician to update and refresh an information base that is increasingly challenged with advancing knowledge, techniques, and skills. The ability to interpret and utilize new information is a critical skill for physicians. Licensing boards, specialty societies, and privileging organizations expect physicians to keep current. As such they specify the amount and type of continuing education expected. This may vary from state to state and organization to organization. The nature, content, and amount required are the prerogative of the individual state or member organization. Members of the AOA are afforded a tracking service to maintain a record of CME attendance.

The AOA Council on Continuing Medical Education recognizes continuing education in four categories:

1. Category 1A includes formal osteopathically sponsored and delivered educational programs and osteopathic medical school teaching
2. Category 1B includes osteopathic scholarly production and osteopathic student precepting
3. Category 2A includes formal nonosteopathic continuing education programs
4. Category 2B includes self-study readings and presentation at society meetings

The members of the AOA are expected to accomplish 120 hours of CME in each 3-year cycle of which at least 30 hours are expected in category 1A. Physicians who are certified are expected to maintain 150 total hours including 50 hours of Category 1A credit per 3-year cycle in their primary specialty. Individual states may require specific content hours such as medical liability hours or HIV hours to maintain licensure. Each specialty may impose additional expectations for CME as well (10).

PROFESSIONAL ORGANIZATIONS

Osteopathic physicians enjoy a special place in their communities. Being a physician is both a privilege and an obligation. It is a privilege due to the esteem and trust placed in physicians. It is an obligation due to the responsibility to meet standards of care in an ethical manner and in the best interest of the patient.

Osteopathic physicians are expected to contribute to the advancement, visibility, and credibility of the profession. They can do this as community leaders and as participants in various professional organizations. This includes, but is not limited to, the AOA, the state osteopathic society, and the applicable specialty organization. Just being a member is not enough. True membership includes contributing knowledge, time, energy, and financial resources to promote osteopathic education, political

---

TABLE 3.6

The Osteopathic Oath

I do hereby affirm my loyalty to the profession I am about to enter. I will be mindful always of my great responsibility to preserve the health and the life of my patients, to retain their confidence and respect both as a physician and a friend who will guard their secrets with scrupulous honor and fidelity, to perform faithfully my professional duties, to employ only those recognized methods of treatment consistent with good judgment and with my skill and ability, keeping in mind always nature's laws and the body's inherent capacity for recovery.

I will be ever vigilant in aiding in the general welfare of the community, sustaining its laws and institutions, not engaging in those practices which will in any way bring shame or discredit upon myself or my profession. I will give no drugs for deadly purpose to any person though it be asked of me.

I will endeavor to work in accord with my colleagues in a spirit or progressive co-operation, and never by word or by act cast imputations upon them or the rightful practices.

I will look with respect and esteem upon all who have taught me my art. To my college I will be loyal and strive always for its best interests and for the interests of the students who will come after me. I will be ever alert to further the application of basic biologic truths to the healing arts and to develop the principles of osteopathy which were first enunciated by Andrew Taylor Still.

advocacy, and membership services. This is clear in the osteopathic oath (Table 3.6) all graduates recite at graduation and in the Osteopathic Pledge (Table 3.7) that practicing physicians recite to renew their commitment to the profession in mind, body, and spirit.

TABLE 3.7

Osteopathic Pledge of Commitment

I pledge to:

Provide compassionate, quality care to my patients;

Partner with them to promote health;

Display integrity and professionalism throughout my career;

Advance the philosophy, practice, and science of osteopathic medicine;

Continue lifelong learning;

Support my profession with loyalty in action, word, and deed; and

Live each day as an example of what an osteopathic physician should be.

REFERENCES

1. American Association of Medical Colleges. U.S. Medical School Applicants and Students 1982 to 2007-08. Available at: http://www.aamc.org/data/facts/charts1982to2007.pdf. Accessed July 5, 2010.
2. Anthony JS. Exploring the factors that influence men and women to form medical career aspirations. *J Coll Stud Develop* 1998;39(5):417.
3. American Association of Colleges of Osteopathic Medicine (AACOM). *Osteopathic Medical Education Information Book*. Chevy Chase, MD: AACOM; 2010.
4. Carey TS, Motyka TM, Garrett JM, et al. Do osteopathic physicians differ in patient interaction from allopathic physicians? An empirically derived approach. *J Am Osteopath Assoc* 2003;103(7):313–318.
5. Accreditation of Colleges of Osteopathic Medicine; Colleges of Osteopathic Medicine Standards and Procedures. Chicago, IL: American Osteopathic Association; 2007.
6. Teitelbaum HS. Osteopathic medical education in the united states: improving the future of medicine. A report jointly sponsored by the American Association of Colleges of Osteopathic Medicine and the American Osteopathic Association. Washington, DC; June 2005. Available at: http://www.aacom.org/resources/bookstore/Pages/OMEinUS-report.aspx. Accessed December 18, 2009.
7. Cruser A, Dubin B, Brown SK, et al. Biomedical research competencies for osteopathic medical students. *Osteopath Med Prim Care* 2009;13;3:10.
8. Freeman E and Lischka TA. Osteopathic graduate medical education. *J Am Osteopath Assoc*. 2009;109(3):135–145.
9. Bates BP. Selection criteria for applicants in primary care osteopathic graduate medical education. *J Am Osteopath Assoc*. 2002;102:621–626.
10. American Osteopathic Association, CME Accreditation. Available at http://www.do-online.org/index.cfm?pageID=acc_cmemain. Accessed July 25, 2010.

4 International Osteopathic Medicine and Osteopathy

JANE E. CARREIRO AND CHRISTIAN FOSSUM (NORWAY)

KEY CONCEPTS

- Internationally, the practice and training of osteopathic medicine evolved differently influenced by the particular political and socioeconomic conditions within different countries.
- The principles of osteopathy and the practice of osteopathic manipulative techniques are employed by limited-license practitioners and fully licensed medical physicians throughout the world.
- American-trained osteopathic physicians practice *osteopathic medicine* and use osteopathic manipulative *treatment* as a component of *comprehensive patient care*.
- The international osteopathic community has adopted the term "osteopath" to describe osteopathic clinicians with limited medical training and practice, and "osteopathic physician" to describe osteopathic clinicians with full medical training and practice.

INTRODUCTION

Osteopathic medicine was established in America in the last decade of the 19th century. Before the beginning of the 20th century, American osteopathic physicians traveled abroad and began disseminating and practicing osteopathy worldwide. American-trained osteopathic physicians have unlimited practice rights throughout the United States and in several countries around the world. However, not all countries offer full unlimited practice rights to osteopathic physicians. In addition, many countries have osteopathic colleges for students who do not want to become, or cannot become, physicians or surgeons, but are content with having a limited osteopathic manual therapy scope of practice. Thus, there are many foreign-trained osteopaths who practice abroad as well as in the United States; most have licenses to practice some form of manual therapy, but many do not have a formal license to practice osteopathy or osteopathic medicine.

Although Dr. A. T. Still intended his principles of osteopathy to be an extension of traditional medical training and practice, he was met with significant resistance from the medical establishment in the United States Nevertheless, in a relatively short period of time, the principles and practice he discovered had spread throughout the world, taking on different faces in different countries.

Currently, the principles of osteopathy and the practice of osteopathic manipulative techniques are employed by limited-license osteopaths as well as by fully licensed osteopathic physicians throughout the world (World Osteopathic Health Organization, 2004). In some countries, including the United States of America, licensed MDs have studied and use osteopathic philosophy, principles, and osteopathic manipulative treatment as well. The evolution of the training and scope of practice of osteopathic practitioners has been influenced by the specific cultural, economic, and political factors in individual countries. These varied influences have resulted in the emergence of two recognized models of osteopathic training and practice: osteopathic physicians and osteopaths.

An osteopathic physician is defined as a person with full, unlimited medical practice rights who has achieved the nationally recognized academic and professional standards within his or her country to diagnose and provide treatment based upon the principles of osteopathic philosophy. An osteopath is defined as a person with limited practice rights who has achieved the nationally recognized academic and professional standards within her or his country to independently practice diagnosis and treatment based upon the principles of osteopathic philosophy.

Individual countries establish the national academic and professional standards for osteopathic practitioners within their countries (Educational Council on Osteopathic Principles, Personal Communication, 2002, 2003; World Osteopathic Health Organization, 2004). Within the last 5 years, two organizations have been formed to help establish standardization within the international osteopathic community. These organizations, the International Osteopathic Alliance (OIA) and the World Osteopathic Health Organization (WOHO), are working together to promote the training and practice rights of osteopathic physicians and osteopaths.

The common denominator existing between the osteopathic professions in different countries is the practice of osteopathic philosophy and principles through the utilization of osteopathic manipulation. Although osteopathic physicians and osteopaths share a core curriculum and core competencies defined by the World Health Organization's *Guidelines for the Training and Practice of Osteopathy*, there are still significant differences in education, clinical competency, and scope of practice between the two recognized groups.

In the United States, osteopathic medicine is established and legally recognized as the purview of osteopathic physicians. The United Kingdom legally recognizes both osteopathic physicians and osteopaths but refers to them both as "osteopaths." Australia and New Zealand have legislation governing the practice of osteopathy by limited-license osteopaths; however, licensed physicians may practice osteopathic techniques without additional qualification.

In addition, there are many other countries in which osteopathy and osteopathic medicine are not recognized as legal, independent professions, or they fall under the scope of practice of another profession. Depending upon the country, American-trained DOs may need to meet licensing requirements of both medical and osteopathic bodies. This chapter presents an overview of the development of the international osteopathic profession from a chronological standpoint.

EARLY OSTEOPATHIC EDUCATION AND ITS IMPACT ON GLOBALIZATION

The student body at the ASO in its first decade of existence also had international representation from countries such as the Canada, the British Isles (United Kingdom, Scotland, and Ireland), Australia, New Zealand, and the Indian Territories. Several of these international students would later become instrumental in bringing osteopathy to countries outside of the United States. They were educated in a curriculum entrenched with Still's founding philosophy and a manipulative-focused practice, and this is what they brought with them when establishing the profession in countries outside of the United States. They identified with the term "Osteopath" and their designated degree was the DO which stood for "Diplomate in Osteopathy." This tradition continues in numerous countries with many osteopaths (see previous definition) believing themselves to be closer to Still's original idea of a diplomate.

OSTEOPATHIC MEDICINE AND MANUAL MEDICINE IN THE INTERNATIONAL MEDICAL ARENA

The philosophy of osteopathy was a relatively innovative perspective on health care when Dr. Still introduced it in the 19th century. While the whole-body/mind-body paradigms cast a different light on healthcare in the new millennium, the philosophy of osteopathy and the structure-function models which it employs, remain uniquely health centered rather than disease centered. So while osteopathic philosophy continues to retain its unique position, the manipulative techniques used in osteopathic practice fall under the larger discipline of manual medicine.

The application of hands-on techniques to the body for the treatment of disease and promotion of health is ancient. After World War II (WWII), manual medicine in its modern form was in common practice in many countries. The Fédération Internationale de Médecine Manuelle was founded in 1958 as a federation of national societies of physicians who practice Manual/Musculoskeletal Medicine (FIMM, Personal Communication, 2008). Membership in FIMM was, and is, based on national affiliation, with each country having a single national professional organization holding membership. North America had a single organization NAAMM, the North American Academy of Manual Medicine holding membership. Only MDs were allowed membership in NAAMM and attendance at their meetings. In 1977, NAAMM changed its by-laws to allow DOs into the organization. They also wanted access to osteopathic educators.

That year, the annual meeting of the NAAMM was held in Williamsburg, VA. Paul Kimberly, D.O., and Philip Greenman, D.O., were invited to the meeting as attendees. At the instigation of John Mennell, M.D., one of the power leaders of NAAMM, Drs. Kimberly and Greenman were invited to a luncheon meeting with the Board of Directors of NAAMM to discuss osteopathic physicians providing manual medicine courses to the NAAMM membership. Mennell felt that the best place to hold such educational opportunities for the NAAMM members would be at Michigan State University, as it was the only university with both an MD and a DO medical school and could handle the political fallout of such an arrangement (P.E. Greenman, *personal communication*, 2008). Because NAAMM was the organization that was part of FIMM, DO membership in NAAMM automatically carried membership in FIMM. Paul Kimberly was the first DO to gain membership in NAAMM, and Greenman was the second. Subsequently, three DOs served as presidents of NAAMM:

Robert C. Ward, D.O.; Allen W. Jacobs, D.O.; Ph.D., and Philip E. Greenman, D.O. Arguably, these leaders helped change the relationship between MDs and DOs practicing any of the disciplines related to musculoskeletal medicine. In the early 1990s, NAAMM merged with the American Academy of Orthopedic Medicine, the organization that was to continue as the North American representative member of FIMM.

In 1998, The FIMM Congress was held in Australia. Michael Kuchera, D.O., then Professor at the Kirksville College of Osteopathic Medicine, was instrumental in accomplishing two major things for the American Osteopathic community (P.E. Greenman, *personal communication*, 2008). Following the merger of NAAMM and AAOM in the early 1990s, AAOM represented both the United States and Canada. At this Congress, Kuchera was able to negotiate a new arrangement whereby the AAOM represented the United States of America, and the American Academy of Osteopathy (AAO) would represent Canada. Therefore, any member of the AAO automatically became a member of FIMM. Subsequently, this arrangement was used by an American-trained DO to argue parity with MDs and gain practice rights in New Zealand. In the mid-1990s, the AAOM folded leaving the AAO as FIMM's sole North American member.

Individual physician members can join the International Academy for Manual/Musculoskeletal Medicine (IAMMM), which was established in 2008. IAMMM's mission is to enhance and develop scientific approaches that focus on musculoskeletal-related problems and to encourage collaboration between scientists and teachers, based on individual membership, thereby creating a scientific platform independent of National Society interest and representation.

CANADA

Shortly after the opening of the American School of Osteopathy, Osteopathic Medicine quickly spread to Canada with the appearance of the first Canadian DO in 1899. The Ontario Osteopathic Association was chartered in 1901, the Western Canada Osteopathic Association in 1923, and the Canadian Osteopathic Association in 1926. In 1925, 200 American-trained DOs were in practice in Ontario. At the present time, 21 American-trained DOs are registered with the Canadian Osteopathic Association, although not all of those are in full time practice.

In Canada, as in the United States, medical licensure is governed by the State or Province. Each province is free to establish its own standards for the registration of physicians, and for recognizing the equivalency of foreign-issued diplomas. As a result, Canadian-trained MDs do not enjoy full reciprocity of practice rights between provinces. The same is true for American-trained MDs or DOs.

There are three national medical organizations of importance to Osteopathic physicians in Canada: the Medical Council of Canada (MCC), the College of Family Physicians of Canada (CFPC), and the Royal College of Physicians and Surgeons of Canada (RCPSC).

The MCC is primarily responsible for establishing and maintaining a certification process that in theory, should allow interprovincial reciprocity of accredited physicians. All Canadian medical school graduates complete the two-part MCC qualifying examination. In this regard, it has a role similar to the USMLE or COMLEX process. American-trained DOs have had access to the MCC examinations since 1991. MCC certification is a requirement for licensure in many, but not all, provinces. Some provinces require that all foreign-trained physicians, including American-trained MDs, take these examinations.

The CFPC is responsible for accrediting family medicine residencies in Canada and for certifying graduates of Canadian family medicine residency programs through an examination process. Two American-trained DOs have completed family medicine residencies in Canada and achieved CFPC certification (CCFP), most recently in 1989. Unfortunately, in 1990, the College rescinded the ability of American-trained DOs to take their examinations, which effectively made them ineligible to apply for residency programs. Recent contact with this organization suggests that beginning in 2009, American-trained DOs will again have access to these examinations.

The RCPSC has the same role for all other specialists that the CFPC has for family physicians. The RCPSC has been intransigent in opening their examination process to foreign-trained physicians, including American MDs. Several provinces have made Royal College certification a requirement for provincial registration for specialists. This has led to a significant barrier in the ability of the provinces to recruit foreign specialists, and many provinces are now enacting regulations to "bypass" the RCPSC certification requirements.

In Canada, the equivalent of the U.S. State Medical Board is the provincial College of Physicians and Surgeons (CPS), which is responsible for physician registration and discipline. The standards for physician registration are established by the provincial ministry of health with significant influence from the respective provincial CPS. Box 4-1 provides an overview of Canadian provincial status.

Not surprisingly, given the needs of a growing and aging population, the demands of new technologies, and the changing practice profiles of new graduates, there is now a serious shortage of physicians across the country. This has led to new opportunities for progress for the Canadian Osteopathic Association, in partnership with the Council on International Osteopathic Medical Education and Affairs of the American Osteopathic Association.

Another condition existing in Canada which differs from the United States of America is the presence of osteopaths who are not trained as physicians. With respect to this, educational and legislative issues remain regarding practice rights and licensure.

UNITED KINGDOM

A key figure in the globalization was John Martin Littlejohn (1865–1947). He was educated at Glasgow University, Scotland, in divinity, law, oriental languages, and political history (Collins, 2005). In 1892, Littlejohn decided to immigrate to the United States for health-related reasons. He enrolled at Columbia University in New York where he studied political theory, political economy, and finance, resulting in the publication of his Ph.D. thesis (Collins, 2005; Littlejohn, 1895). In 1894, he accepted the position as President of the Amity College in Iowa Springs, IA, an educational establishment granting degrees in Arts, Science, Philosophy, and Letters. In 1897 while at College Springs, Littlejohn began traveling to Kirksville, MO, to receive treatment from Still for his throat condition. Impressed with the results, he decided to take up the study of osteopathy (Hall, 1952a). While still a student he was appointed Professor of Physiology, Psychology, and Dietetics, and eventually in 1898 he was appointed as Dean of Faculty of the ASO (Booth, 1924; Collins, 2005; Hall, 1952a). Within a year of his appointments, he had written and published three textbooks on the subject of physiology and inaugurated two osteopathic journals. After graduating from the ASO in 1900, Littlejohn left for Chicago where he and his brother established the American College of Osteopathic Medicine and Surgery, a name chosen because its founders believed that osteopathy was a system of medicine and should be so recognized (Littlejohn, 1924). This may have been the first time the term "osteopathic medicine" was officially used.

Overview of Canadian Provincial Status

British Columbia
There are two pathways for DO registration in British Columbia. The first recognizes the COMLEX examinations and two years of AOA-certified postgraduate training. The DO has a limited license and is restricted from performing surgery and obstetrics. This pathway is primarily intended for the DO that wishes to establish an OMT focused practice. The second pathway requires completion of the MCC examinations and at least one year of postgraduate training in that province. The DO will then receive an unrestricted license.

Alberta
The DO candidate is required to complete the MCC examinations. AOA-certified residencies are recognized. There has been informal interest expressed in considering the COMLEX as an alternative to the MCC examinations.

Saskatchewan
A board exists separate from the provincial College for the registration of DOs, although it has not been active for many years. DOs are registered by the board to practice "osteopathy," although that is not clearly defined. Interest has been expressed by the Ministry of Health in updating regulations.

Manitoba
As of 2002, American-trained DOs are eligible for registration in Manitoba.

Ontario
In 1926, the "Drugless Practitioners Act" was proclaimed as a "temporary" measure for the registration of American-trained DOs. As the title suggests, the scope of practice was severely limited. Under these conditions, osteopathic practice in Ontario has dwindled severely, in spite of many years of political lobbying on behalf of Ontario DOs and their patients. Action in Ontario has been the focus of activity by the Canadian and American Osteopathic Associations for the past several years and the results are beginning to be seen. In theory, American-trained DOs have been recognized as eligible for registration in Ontario by the Ontario government since the passage of the Medicine Act (Bill 55) in 1991. However, those sections that relate to osteopathic physicians were not "proclaimed" into law, on the objection of the CPS at that time. Nevertheless in the mid-1990s, two American-trained DOs were granted unlimited licensure by exception. In November 2002, the Ministry of Health announced that a new "Fast Track Assessment Program" would be initiated for the registration of qualifying foreign-trained physicians, including American-trained MDs and DOs. As of this writing, the regulations under which this will operate are still unclear.

Quebec
American-trained DOs have been eligible for registration in Quebec for approximately 30 years. The candidate also must pass a French language proficiency examination and complete one year of postgraduate training in the province, although this can be at the fellowship level. MCC certification and Royal College certification are not necessary. Unfortunately, the title protection that exists for MDs does not exist for DOs with the result that the title use is not restricted in that province.

(continued)

New Brunswick:

DOs are eligible for full registration in New Brunswick. There is a pathway that extends reciprocity to a DO with Maine licensure.

Nova Scotia

As of 2002, full registration for American-trained DOs is similar to that extended to American-trained MDs.

Prince Edward Island

At the moment, PEI is the only Canadian province without a current or anticipated registration pathway for American-trained Osteopathic physicians.

Newfoundland

As of 2002, the College has committed itself to seeing that the government establishes a registration pathway for American-trained DOs, although it is anticipated that this may take a couple of years.

Territories (Yukon, Northwest, Nunavut)

In most instances, the Territories will grant registration to any physician that qualifies for licensure in any other province.

Canadian Armed Services

American-trained DOs are eligible for service with the Canadian Armed Services, including scholarship opportunities, although to date this has never happened.

There are several conditions in Canada that have influenced the ability of American-trained DOs to gain licensure. The first has to do with manpower. In the early 1990s, Canada's health ministers were faced with a situation of spiraling health care costs, and a seemingly inexhaustible source of physicians. It was felt that one of the primary drivers of medical costs was an excess of physician manpower. Measures were taken to impede the ability of foreign-trained physicians to acquire licensure in most provinces and Canadian medical school enrollment was reduced by 15% on average. In this environment, it was very difficult for the Canadian Osteopathic Association to make headway in promoting full-practice rights for American-trained DOs in those provinces in which it did not already exist.

Osteopathy as a subject was introduced in the United Kingdom through a series of talks given by Littlejohn in 1898, 1899, and 1900 to the Society of Science, Letters, and Arts in London (Hall, 1952a). William Smith, M.D., D.O., a member of the first graduating class of the ASO and its first anatomy teacher, returned to the British Isles in 1901 to practice osteopathy, and in 1902 he was followed by several other early ASO graduates: L. Lillard Walker, Franz Joseph Horn, and Jay Dunham. By 1910, there were so many U.S.-trained osteopaths in Great Britain that the British Osteopathic Society was formed, which in 1911 became the British Osteopathic Association (Beal, 1950; Collins, 2005).

As early as 1903, Littlejohn held talks with Walker and Horn about establishing a school of osteopathy in Great Britain. These plans did not materialize until Littlejohn returned to the United Kingdom for good in 1913. The British School of Osteopathy (BSO) was incorporated in London in 1917 as a nonprofit organization to train osteopaths, although neither the degree nor the profession was recognized by legislation. Its 4-year curriculum, excluding pharmacology and surgery, was completed in 1921 (McKone, 2001). Access to hospitals, dissection laboratories,

and other aspects of physician training were denied. In the early 1920s, the BSO's faculty consisted purely of graduates from U.S. osteopathic schools under the Deanship of John Martin Littlejohn (Hall, 1952b). As graduates were produced from the BSO, this situation gradually changed, and by the early 1930s a large proportion of the faculty was U.K. trained (Littlejohn, 1931). In 1946, the London College of Osteopathy was opened to provide a postgraduate osteopathic training program to medical doctors. This 18-month program provided medical doctors with core training in osteopathic principles, practices, and techniques. Graduates of the London College became members of the British Institute of Manual Medicine and with the formation of FIMM in 1958, MDs trained at the London College of Osteopathy were granted membership. For 20 years, they remained the only osteopathic physicians in FIMM (P.E. Greenman, *personal communication*, 2008).

In 1936, a voluntary registry was established for the osteopathic profession and the designation MRO (Member of the Registry of Osteopaths) could be secured by individuals meeting the required qualifications. The osteopathic profession made several unsuccessful attempts to secure regulation and legislation between the arrival of Littlejohn and the arrival of the 1990s. Finally, the Osteopaths Act was finally passed by the House of Lords in 1993 granting Statutory Self-regulation to the profession and control of the titles "Osteopath" and "Osteopathic Physician." The entire profession underwent revalidation to ensure that minimal criteria for practice were met. The General Council and Register of Osteopaths were abolished and the General Osteopathic Council (GOsC) was established to oversee educational standards, professional development, and patient safety issues. The GosC is the regulating body for all individuals practicing osteopathy or osteopathic medicine in the United Kingdom. Registration with the GosC is now required for the legal practice of osteopathy in the United Kingdom; this includes medical doctors practicing osteopathic medicine. Additionally, osteopathic schools in the United Kingdom need to have a recognized qualification status from the GosC in order to provide their graduates entry to its register. In early 2008, there were almost 4,000 registered osteopaths in the United Kingdom. American-trained DOs wishing to practice as full-scope osteopathic physicians would need to meet licensing criteria for both the GosC and the General Medical Council. Those wishing to practice as limited-license osteopaths would need to be accepted by the GOsC only.

AUSTRALIA

Osteopathy spread to Australia and New Zealand via two mechanisms. In the later 1890s and early 1900s, osteopaths who had trained in the United States carried their training "down under," creating an osteopathic profession. After the first and second world wars, manual medicine was introduced to the established medical profession and became a medical discipline under the international umbrella of FIMM. This created parallel pathways for the development of osteopathy in Australia and New Zealand.

Between 1909 and 1913, several early graduates from the American School of Osteopathy returned to Australia to practice osteopathy (Hawkins and O'Neill, 1990). The growth of the osteopathic profession was slow, and as in the United Kingdom, unwelcomed by the medical community. These émigrés founded a professional association in the state of Victoria modeled after the American Osteopathic Association. Although U.K.-trained osteopaths soon arrived in the country, only American-trained DOs were allowed membership in the Australian Osteopathic Association

(AusOA) until the late 1920s. In the early 1930s, a medical doctor who had graduated from the BSO emigrated to Australia and was allowed entry into the AusOA group. Other BSO graduates used this acknowledgement of the BSO training as a successful argument for inclusion in the association. By the 1940s, several private colleges provided osteopathic training, but because of the unregulated nature of the profession, the quality of these courses was variable (Cameron, 1998; Hawkins and O'Neill, 1990). In 1974, the Australian Federal Government Health Minister commissioned an inquiry into chiropractic, osteopathy, homeopathy, and naturopathy, which resulted in a report published in 1977. This report influenced the development of osteopathy in Australia, officially limiting osteopathy's scope of practice to manipulative therapy and primarily the management of musculoskeletal conditions (Cameron, 1998).

During the 1980s, programs in osteopathy as a limited manual therapy practice and osteopathic medicine for physicians developed on parallel pathways. Philip Greenman, D.O., a Professor at Michigan State University, was invited to Australia in 1986 to present a paper to the annual meeting of the Australian Association of Physical and Rehabilitative Medicine. At the suggestion of Vladimir Janda, M.D., the Department of Physiotherapy at the University of Brisbane invited Dr. Greenman to present a 5-day course on Muscle Energy technique to their senior practitioners and faculty. In 1992, Greenman was invited by the Australian Society of Rehabilitation, MDs that did musculoskeletal medicine with heavy emphasis on manipulation, to provide two courses, one on muscle energy and the other on HVLA. He was also invited by the AusOA to provide the same two courses to the osteopathic community. Interestingly, these courses were held separately, although the table trainers for all four courses were from the faculty of one of the osteopathic colleges.

In 1986, the first federally funded course in osteopathy commenced at the Phillip Institute of Technology in Melbourne, Victoria (which later merged with the Royal Melbourne Institute of Technology). This course provided training for manual medicine practitioners, not physicians. As of 1995, the course awarded double degrees to its graduates; graduates from any of the Australian colleges are awarded a Bachelor of Science (Clinical Science) and a Master of Health Science (Osteopathy) (Cameron, 1998). Until the first part of the 21st century, a joint board of chiropractors and osteopaths in each territory awarded licenses. Today, each territory has an osteopathic board to oversee licensing issues for osteopaths. The Australian Osteopathic Association (AOA or AusOA) was founded as a professional society to promote osteopathy, and in 1991 it became the federal body representing osteopaths in Australia. American-trained DOs wishing to have limited practice rights would need to meet the criteria of the osteopathic licensing board in that territory. Those wishing to practice full-scope osteopathic medicine need to meet the criteria of both the Medical and the Osteopathic boards.

NEW ZEALAND

Until the mid-1990s, most osteopaths practicing in New Zealand (N.Z.) received their training in Australia or the United Kingdom. A voluntary registry existed and there was no legislation regarding training or practice. In the late 1990s, the first full-time accredited training program was created at UNITEC in Auckland. David Patriquin, D.O., who was on faculty at Ohio University College of Osteopathic Medicine, became the program's inaugural principal. In 2003, the Health Practitioners Competence Assurance Act was passed establishing the Osteopathic Council of New Zealand to regulate the training and practice of osteopathy in N.Z. (The legal status of osteopathy and its educational structure in New Zealand is similar to that in Australia.)

As in Australia, there was some attempt to advance the American model of osteopathic medicine in N.Z. in the 1980s. Philip Greenman, D.O., was invited by Barrie Tait, M.D., Department of Rheumatology at the University of Dunedin, New Zealand, to be a Visiting Professor for 6 months. The purpose was to assist Dr. Tait in the preparation of an 18-month diploma course in Musculoskeletal Medicine for the Family Medicine Practitioners in the New Zealand system (P.E. Greenman, *personal communication*, 2008). This required that Dr. Greenman obtain a medical qualification from N.Z. in order to participate in patient care both in the ambulatory and the hospital environment. He was the first American DO in the Medical Registry of New Zealand. His qualification was based upon his Professorship at Michigan State University and having a license to practice medicine and surgery from the state of New York. Since that time, other American DOs have gained registry in N.Z. With the inception of the Osteopathic Council, it is unclear whether American-trained DOs wishing to practice full-scope osteopathic medicine need to meet the criteria of both the Medical Registry and the Osteopathic Council. Dr. Greenman helped develop a 6-month diploma course for physicians, which continues to this day. It was also the model adopted by two universities in Australia (P.E. Greenman, Personal Communication, 2008).

CONTINENTAL EUROPE

Initially, osteopathy came to continental Europe after WWII when practitioners trained in America and England immigrated to the continent. Random conferences and courses featuring visiting osteopathic practitioners were held separately for physicians and therapists. Beginning in 1957, faculty from various COMs and the Sutherland Cranial Teaching Foundation were invited to present at conferences and hold courses throughout Europe. The courses were often segregated between physiotherapists and physicians. Over time, this became the norm, rather than the exception, and by the late 1980s, there were many schools of osteopathy scattered throughout Western Europe catering to either physiotherapists or physicians. A rare few of these schools established quality assurance for the examination process by relying upon teachers from other schools to evaluate their students; however, most schools implemented their own curriculums and evaluation processes without objective checks or standardization. As the international osteopathic profession began to come together in the early 1990s, there was a strong movement within both communities to establish a core curriculum and objective, standardized assessment tools.

In most of post-World War II Europe, the practice of manual medicine was incorporated into standard medical training and many countries had national manual medicine societies. Over the following decades, these societies were given the role of standardizing curriculum and practice, becoming the credentialing bodies in their countries. By the 1990s, manual medicine training tended to be a secondary specialty of medical training in Western Europe, rather than primary, with family practitioners and orthopedic surgeons making up the bulk of the providers. Beginning in the early 1970s, physicians practicing in the Netherlands, Sweden, Czechoslovakia, and much of Eastern Europe were exposed to the Gaymann-Lewit technique. Fritz Gaymann and Karel Lewit developed this manual medicine approach that was based upon Fred Mitchell's muscle energy system that Gaymann learned during a prolonged visit to the United States (P.E. Greenman, *personal communication*, 2008). Later physicians were exposed to the osteopathic approach through their involvement with FIMM. In 1979, faculty members from Michigan State University, Kirksville, Chicago, and Texas were invited to the Canary Islands to present a basic course on osteopathic manipulative techniques to the leadership of the German Manual Medicine Society (DGMM). Under the German medical training structure, the DGMM is the equivalent of a specialty college that grants board certification. In August of that year, MSUCOM offered the first basic course in osteopathic technique to MDs. During the 1980s and 1990s, faculty from the various COMs were recruited to develop and deliver basic courses in osteopathic techniques in Germany, Switzerland, France, Belgium, and the Netherlands. By the mid-1990s, many of the manual medicine societies in these countries had affiliate organizations of M.D.-trained osteopathic physicians with shared prerequisites, curriculum, and standards for examination. Nevertheless, osteopathic medicine was not recognized as a profession but as a manual medicine subspecialty available to trained physicians.

In 1998, the European Union Health Administration included osteopathy in a resolution accepting alternative and complementary medicines, although specifics of education and practice were not incorporated. Initiatives have been taken by the European Union, the Forum for Osteopathic Regulation in Europe, the European Registry of Osteopathic Physicians, the World Health Organization, the WOHO, and the Osteopathic International Alliance to promote the regulation of practice and training based on minimum competencies. Although over the years individual American-trained DOs have obtained licensure to practice medicine in European countries, full reciprocity with the United States does not exist for American DOs or MDs. Application for licensure is made on an individual basis.

The following is an overview of osteopathy in Europe by country.

FRANCE

In 1951, the French School of Osteopathy (Ecole Francaise d'Osteopathie) was opened in Paris as a postgraduate training course for physical therapists and medical doctors. The faculty mainly consisted of individuals from the United Kingdom, and because osteopathy was illegal in France, the school was forced to move to the United Kingdom in 1965 (T. Dummer, *personal communication*, 1999). It was initially hosted by the British College of Naturopathy and Osteopathy, but remained a French-speaking part-time course for health professionals. In 1968, the school relocated to Maidstone, England, and in 1971 became the Ecole Europeenne d'Osteopathie. Until 1974, the school functioned solely as a French-speaking part-time course. That same year, it opened its full-time English-speaking 4-year program and became the European School of Osteopathy (Collins, 2005; T. Dummer, *personal communication*, 1999). The school continued its French-speaking part-time course until 1987. The postgraduate part-time course of the Ecole Francaise d'Osteopathie became a model of osteopathic training for nonmedical health care professionals in France in the 1980s and 1990s. During this time, many schools opened throughout France and with them several voluntary registries. The registries tended to be associated with a school or area, and each had its own criteria and standards for training and practice. In 2002, the practice of osteopathy by nonphysicians was recognized in France, and as of 2008 standards for competency rules governing curriculum and scope of practice had been developed (Ducaux, 2008).

Robert Maigne was a French MD who studied at the London School of Osteopathy while Myron Beal, D.O., FAAO was on faculty. Maigne was active in FIMM and brought an osteopathic perspective to that group. In 1975 Myron Magen, D.O., the dean of MSUCOM met with Maigne and other FIMM representatives to negotiate attendance of America DOs at their meetings. In 1977, Robert Ward and Philip Greenman were the first American-trained DOs to attend a FIMM meeting. This was done by special invitation. At that meeting, Greenman and Ward established relationships with Karel Lewit (Czech), Vladimir Janda (Czech), and Heinz-Deiter Neumann (German), leaders in the manual medicine world, which provided the foundation for future collaborations. French physicians were able to obtain osteopathic training through periodic lecture, workshops, and presentations. Several groups were established to provide osteopathic training opportunities for their members after completion of a FIMM-recognized certificate in manual medicine. In France in 1998, the Diploma of Manual Medicine and Osteopathy was developed for medical doctors. Reportedly 13 of the medical universities in France may grant this diploma (Baecher, 1999).

BELGIUM

In 1998, the Belgian Parliament brought forth a bill, which was passed in 1999, to recognize the practice of osteopathy. Standards for training nonphysician osteopaths were also developed. The practice of osteopathic medicine was not specifically covered in the bill, although MD physicians trained in manual medicine may use osteopathic techniques as part of their scope of practice. There is no specific provision for American-trained DOs to obtain full practice rights in Belgium however (AAO International Affairs Committee, 2000).

GERMANY

German law allows medical doctors to practice osteopathic medicine as part of their scope of practice. Medical doctors are trained as osteopathic physicians through programs that share core competencies with the U.S. osteopathic schools and are recognized by the German Manual Medicine Association, the OIA, and the World Osteopathic Health Organization. Graduates of these programs are affiliated with one of the osteopathic medical associations such as the Deutsch German Society for Osteopathic Medicine and the Deutsch American Association of Osteopathy. The European Register for Osteopathic Physicians was created in 2003, and currently osteopathic physician groups in France, Germany, and Switzerland share a common standard for training and examination. At the time of this writing, American-trained DOs have been able to obtain license to practice medicine in Germany.

In Germany, both part-time and full-time training programs are available for physiotherapists and other nonmedical professionals. Some of these are affiliated with universities and offer the equivalent of bachelor or master degrees. There are also several voluntary registries and societies for practicing osteopaths. Nonphysician osteopaths may practice osteopathy under the rules governing heilpractika (traditional healers), although osteopathy as a profession is not legislated.

SWITZERLAND

As in Germany, the practice of osteopathic medicine falls within the scope of practice of Swiss manual medicine physicians.

The Swiss Society of Osteopathic Physicians was formed in 2003. It adapted the same curriculum for osteopathic medicine as is used by the German medical groups. Physiotherapists in Switzerland can enter full-time and part-time programs to train as osteopaths. Several cantons have recognized the practice of osteopathy by non-physicians, but specifics of training and scope of practice have not yet been finalized. In 2007, the various registries for the osteopathic medical profession came together to try to create a single cohesive group that could legislate more effectively (Rudolf, 2008).

RUSSIA

Manual medicine is a component of medical training in Russia. Osteopathic philosophy and practice was brought to Russia via U.S.- and U.K.-trained osteopaths and osteopathic physicians such as Viola Frymann. Currently, the practice of osteopathic medicine falls under the purview medical doctors in Russia, although there is no specific legislation. There are schools in St. Petersburg, Moscow, and Vladivostok. The programs are designed for fully trained physicians and generally last 2 to 3 years. U.S.-trained DOs can apply for licensure with a sponsor such as a hospital, business, or school.

JAPAN

Osteopathic philosophy, principles, and techniques were introduced to Japan in the early 1900s. There is at least one Japanese book preserved from 1910, written by Yamada, which describes natural methods of healing, with a focus on manual therapy that includes mention of osteopathy. The study of osteopathy in Japan was promoted by post-World War II lay healers and bonesetters, as well as by oriental medical doctors and acupuncturists. In the 1970s and 1980s, small groups of Japanese traveled to England and America to attend introductory seminars in osteopathy, and osteopaths from England and osteopathic physicians from America were invited to Japan to give short seminars introducing osteopathy to a variety of professionals as well as the lay public.

In 1986, Viola Frymann, D.O., F.A.A.O., and President Philip Pumerantz, Ph.D., representing the College of Osteopathic Medicine of the Pacific in Pomona, CA, presented a 3-day seminar in Tokyo, which was the beginning of the development of formal training programs. Shortly thereafter, representing the Kirksville College of Osteopathic Medicine in Missouri, President Fred Tinning, Ph.D., and Michael Kuchera, D.O., F.A.A.O., visited Tokyo and presented seminars and appealed to the Japanese government to allow osteopathic medicine to become a regulated and accepted practice. John Jones, D.O., also visited the Japanese government with the same plea a few years later, but, also, to no avail.

In the mid-1990s, the first college of osteopathy, the Japan College of Osteopathy, was established. It consists of a three-year curriculum and graduates are granted the Diplomate in Osteopathy degree. Since there is no Japanese osteopathic licensing board or regulating body, its graduates practice osteopathic manual therapy under the auspices of another professional license, such as bonesetter or oriental medical doctor.

There are many supportive osteopathic associations in Japan. From 1996 to 1998, through the AAO, Michael Seffinger, D.O., facilitated the collaboration among three of the larger societies. Along with consultation from Dr. Frymann and members of the AAO International Affairs Committee, he encouraged the formation of the Japan Osteopathic Federation (JOF). The JOF was incorporated in 1998. It immediately implemented a formal training program and certification mechanism in order to establish a self-regulating body for the practice of osteopathy in Japan. Applicants that meet the criteria for certification are given the status of Member of the Registry of Osteopathy—Japan (MRO-J) designation, which entitles them to participate in JOF-sponsored seminars and courses. Members are licensed professionals who have taken a prescribed number of hours of a variety of osteopathic manipulation courses, and passed standardized written, oral, and practical examinations. There are over 400 members of the JOF and over 150 certified (MRO-J) Japanese osteopaths.

The osteopathic profession in Japan is growing slowly but steadily. Although most of the proponents and leaders have been licensed professionals from other disciplines, this past decade has witnessed an increase in foreign-trained DOs emerging as leaders, developers, and organizers of the profession. In 2008, for instance, a Japanese native and graduate of Still University, Kirksville College of Osteopathic Medicine in America, opened a second college of the osteopathic medical profession, Atlas College of Osteopathy, near Tokyo. Several Japanese have graduated from the British osteopathic schools and are back in Japan helping to teach and develop the profession. Additionally, several Japanese MD, led by long-time proponents of the osteopathic medical profession, and an orthopedic surgeon in Tokyo who learned the osteopathic medical profession through decades of seminars both in Japan and abroad, practice osteopathic manual therapy in various parts of the country.

REFERENCES

The Journal of Osteopathy. Vol IV. London: British School of Osteopathy, 1932.

The origin and development of osteopathy in Great Britain. The General Council & Register of Osteopaths, Ltd. London, The General Council & Register of Osteopaths, Ltd., 1956.

Baecher R. *Update on Osteopathic Medicine in France*. American Academy of Osteopathy, 1999.

Beal MC. *The London College of Osteopathy*. Indianapolis, IN: Academy of Applied Osteopathy, 1950.

Booth, E. *History of Osteopathy and 20th Century Medical Practice*. 2nd Ed. Cincinnati, OH: Press of Jennings and Graham, 1924.

Cameron M. A comparison of osteopathic history, education and practice in Australia and the United States of America. *Aust Osteopath Med Rev* 1998;2:6–12.

Collins, M. *Osteopathy in Britain: The First Hundred Years*. London: BookSurge publishing, 2005.

Ducaux B. *French Standards for Practice of Osteopathy by Non-physicians*. World Osteopathic Health Organization, 2008.

Hall T. *The contribution of John Martin Littlejohn to osteopathy*. London: The Osteopathic Publishing Co. Ltd., 1952a.

Hall T. The littlejohn memorial. *Osteopath Q* 1952b;5:101–107.

Hawkins P, O'Neill A. *Osteopathy in Australia*. Bundoora: PIT Press, 1990.

International Affairs Committee. *Update International Osteopathic Profession*. Indianapolis: American Academy of Osteopathy, 2000.

Littlejohn JM. Osteopathy in Great Britain. *The Reflex* 1924.

Littlejohn JM. *The Political theory of the Schoolmen and Grotius*. Current Press, 1895.

Littlejohn J. *The Journal of Osteopathy*. Vol II[3]. London: British School of Osteopathy, 1931.

McKone, L. *Osteopathic Medicine—Philosophy, Principles, and Practice*. Oxford: Blackwell Science, 2001.

Rudolf, T. *World Osteopathic Health Organization, Update osteopathy and osteopathic medicine in Switzerland*, 2008.

World Osteopathic Health Organization. *Osteopathic Glossary*, 2004.

5 Introduction: The Body in Osteopathic Medicine—the Five Models of Osteopathic Treatment

FRANK H. WILLARD AND JOHN A. JEROME

The Basic Science section of the third edition of the Foundations for Osteopathic Medicine has two major changes from the first two editions. First, to form the background for this edition of the Foundations, we have adopted the five models of patient diagnosis, treatment, and management frequently used by osteopathic clinicians.

The five models are:

1. Biomechanical model
2. Respiratory-Circulatory model
3. Neurological model
4. Metabolic-Energy model
5. Behavioral model

These five models are commonly used in physical evaluation, diagnosis, treatment, and patient management. A detailed explanation of the five models and their application in osteopathic medicine can be found in Chapter 1 of this edition of the Foundations. To best provide an understanding of the five models, all but three of the chapters in the Basic Science and Behavioral Science sections from the second edition have been completely rewritten or replaced by new material. In addition, the Basic Science chapters and the Behavioral Science chapters have been consolidated into one section, a move that reflects the editor's strong belief that the integration of body and mind lies at the heart of osteopathic medicine.

ORGANIZATION OF MATERIAL IN THE BASIC SCIENCE SECTION

Chapter 06: The Concepts of Anatomy

The Basic Science section begins with a chapter on anatomy since this discipline, of all sciences, is most fundamental to osteopathic medicine. This chapter represents a consolidation of the two anatomy chapters from the previous editions of the Foundations text. The authors (L. Towns and W. Falls) have articulated four concepts that underpin the study of anatomy. A sound knowledge of anatomy is paramount to understanding the application of the five models in osteopathic medicine.

Chapter 07: The Fascial System of the Body

This chapter specifically focuses on the fascias of the body, which play an important role in palpatory diagnosis and osteopathic manipulative treatment. The fascias are also particularly significant within the concepts of the biomechanical and respiratory/circulatory models. Yet while fascia is typically referred to in textbooks of anatomy and manual medicine, it is very rarely defined. To add insult to injury, anatomy texts often decompose fascia sheets into small isolated regions with various eponyms. In attempt to answer these needs, the authors (F.H. Willard, C. Fossum, and P.R. Standley) offer a pragmatic definition of fascia that can easily be applied to any tissue in the body in an effort to determine whether it should be termed fascia or not. Chapter 7 also attempts to consolidate all fascias into four primary fascial layers in the human body; the composition of each layer based on its distribution and function. This approach emphasizes the unity of fascia in the body. Finally, the chapter surveys some of the major cell types present in fascia and reviews their functions, including the very interesting myofibocyte.

Chapter 08: Biomechanics of the Musuloskeletal System

The chapter on biomechanics by M. Wells has been included in its entirety from the second edition of the Foundations text. The chapter succinctly applies the rules of biomechanics to the muscles, bones, and joints of the musculoskeletal system in a way that is most helpful in understanding the biomechanical model in osteopathic medicine.

Chapter 09: Somatic Dysfunction, Spinal Facilitation, and Viscerosomatic Integration

Central to the concept of osteopathic medicine is somatic dysfunction and its influence on the spinal cord, termed spinal facilitation. Somatic dysfunction plays a key role in the biomechanical and neurologic models and strongly influences the respiratory/circulatory, metabolic-energy, and behavioral models. Working from their previous chapters that appeared in the first and second editions of Foundations, the authors (M. Patterson and Robert D. Wurster) have updated and expanded the concept of somatic dysfunction and its influences on both the somatic and the visceral systems of the body.

Chapter 10: Autonomic Nervous System

The link between the somatic and the visceral systems of the body is very strong and has a major impact on the all of the five treatment models. This link lies at the heart of many referred pain patterns as well as the referral of dysfunction patterns between the musculoskeletal and the visceral systems; between visceral organs in the various body cavities; and between various musculoskeletal tissues. Understanding this link requires practical knowledge of the anatomy of the autonomic nervous system; the bridge between the somatic and visceral tissues. The chapter on the Autonomic Nervous System present in the previous two editions of this text provides a map for translating clinical findings into diagnostics using the integration of the somatic and visceral nervous system. For that reason, the chapter has been retained in the third edition of Foundations; however, the author (F.H. Willard) has significantly revised the figures to allow correlations with *Grant's Atlas of Human Anatomy* (A.M. Agur and A.F. Dalley. *Grant's Atlas of Anatomy.* Philadelphia, PA: Lippincott Williams & Wilkins, 2009).

Chapter 11: Physiological Rhythms/Oscillations

The human body has many intrinsic oscillating rhythms, some of which well-trained osteopathic physicians can detect through palpation. In Chapter 11, the authors (T. Glonek, N. Sergueef, and K. Nelson) examine the myriad of oscillating rhythms known to exist in a human. These rhythms are central to the respiratory/circulatory model in osteopathic medicine. The authors also describe their work using the noninvasive instrumentation of human subjects to record multiple oscillating rhythms as well as study the possible modification of specific rhythms using osteopathic techniques of manipulative medicine.

Chapter 12: Anatomy and Physiology of the Lymphatic System

A major component of the respiratory/circulatory model is the movement of low-pressure fluids through the tissues of the body. A key component of low-pressure fluid dynamics is the lymphatic system. A new chapter summarizing current knowledge of lymphatic system anatomy and physiology has been added to this edition of the Foundations. The authors (H. Ettlinger and F. Willard) begin by describing the movement of lymphatic fluid into the terminal lymphatic vessels. This is followed by a discussion of the anatomy of the lymphatic vascular system and the physiology of movement of lymph. The significance of osteopathic manipulative treatment and its potential effects on the lymphatic system forms the final portions of this chapter.

Chapter 13: Mechanics of Respiration

The respiratory/circulatory model relies on the mechanical movement of the body walls to perfuse the lungs with air and to assist in moving fluid in and out of tissue. Over the past 10 to 15 years, research has greatly altered the understanding of the biomechanics of the respiratory muscles. To address these issues, Chapter 13, "The Mechanics of Respiration" was added to this section in this third edition of Foundations. In this chapter, the author (F. Willard) presents a review of the major groups of primary respiratory muscles and their influence on the fibroelastic cylinder that represents the thoracoabdominal wall. The chapter ends with a discussion of the thoracoabdominal diaphragm and its role in both respiration and movement of lymphatic fluid from the abdominal cavity.

Chapter 14: Touch

Nothing is as important to the skilled osteopathic physician as the concept of touch. The joining of two individuals through physical contact facilitates diagnosis, treatment, and trust; it is central to each of the five models. With this in mind, a chapter devoted to the physical and emotional aspects of touch has been added to this third edition of Foundations. In this chapter, the authors (F. Willard, J. Jerome, and M. Elkiss) examine the significance of touch for the osteopathic physician and the patient. The physical process of touch from the peripheral receptor to the representation of touch information on the cerebral cortex is reviewed. A distributed network of information processing is described that can function to integrate somesthetic stimuli with primary senses such as visual or auditory to develop an emerging image representing the touch, the touched object or the significance of the touch. Further interactions of this network with areas of prefrontal cortex allow the formation of a palpatory or tactile memory. All of palpatory diagnosis is predicated on previously formed tactile memories; acquiring these memories is a process critical to the development of skills in the osteopathic physician-in-training. The chapter concludes by demonstrating how this distributed cortical network integrates emotional components of our brain to place a meaningful balance on the experience of touch and how this can be very impactful on

the physician-patient relationship thereby significantly influencing the outcome of treatment protocols.

Chapter 15: Nociception and Pain: The Essence of Pain Lies Mainly in the Brain

Pain can impact all aspects of the five models in osteopathic medicine. Pain can influence muscle tone and alter mechanical function. It can sensitize areas of the nervous system creating enhanced painful states. Pain can influence breathing and alter heart rate, changing circulatory mechanics. Pain can induce the secretion of stress response hormones vastly impacting systemic metabolism. Finally, pain influences psychological states and behavior; the concept of "self and other" changes in extreme states of pain. Our knowledge of acute and chronic pain and their etiologies is changing rapidly; thus, this edition of the Foundations has a completely rewritten chapter on pain mechanisms. The authors (F. Willard and J. Jerome) begin with the origin of nociception in peripheral tissue and follow the process through the spinal cord and brainstem to the forebrain and the emergence of the feelings of pain. This chapter should provide an important back ground for the osteopathic physician to understand the origin of pain in their patient as well as their patient's response to the presence of this pain.

Chapter 16: Chronic Pain Management

A pain pattern, once it has become chronic, can be very difficult to manage. As the knowledge of chronic pain etiologies grows, treatment possibilities expand. For this reason, the Chronic Pain Management chapter has been completely rewritten from the previous editions. The authors (M. Elkiss and J. Jerome) build the chapter on the basic science of pain perception and neuronal sensitization described in Chapter 15. An emphasis is placed on the integrated response of the neuromusculoskeletal, endocrine, and immune systems to states of chronic pain. The close relationship between the development chronic pain and that of depression is considered. Finally, the role of osteopathic assessment of chronic pain is described as a dynamic process using multifaceted approaches centered on the behavioral model and having a strong focus on the place of the patient in their life cycle.

Chapter 17: Psychoneuroimmunology— Basic Mechanisms

In the past 20 years, the understanding of the relationship between physical and psychosocial stressors and specific disease states has expanded rapidly. It is now apparent that a patient's general health—somatic, visceral, and psychosocial—can suffer significantly in response to chronic or uncontrolled activation of a complex stress response system—a situation termed allostasis to separate it from the normal homeostatic functions of the body. The first edition of Foundations reviewed the hypothalamic-pituitary-adrenal axis and the neuroendocrine immune basis of stress-related disease, while the second edition extended this concept of allostasis into the clinical realm. In the third edition, the author, J. Jerome expands on earlier versions with new information to emphasize the strong relationship between inescapable stressors and the progressive deterioration of homeostasis, which manifests as worsening of various musculoskeletal, visceral, and psychiatric diseases. In essence, dysregulation in the behavioral model can have significant impact on all four of the other models especially the metabolic model; therefore, a particular emphasis is placed in this chapter on the behavioral and psychiatric manifestations of stress and their impact on the general health of the patient.

Chapter 18: Psychoneuroimmunology— Stress Management

Stress management involved a multifaceted approach to the patient physical and psychological status. In this chapter, the authors (J. Jerome and G. Osborn) build on the basic material outlined in Chapter 18 to develop a distinctly osteopathic approach to stress management, taking into consideration somatic dysfunctions as well as psychological stressors. The chapter uses the behavioral model to develop insights into the treatment and management of depression, anxiety, alcohol abuse, and insomnia from an osteopathic prospective.

Chapter 19: Life Stages—Basic Mechanisms

Understanding the impact of disease across the life cycle of a human involves knowledge of the composition of human life stages and their changing profiles from preterm to geriatric stages. In essence, this process represents the penultimate application of the five models of osteopathic medicine. Each stage in life is impacted by genetic and environmental factors; as the life stages change, the susceptibility to disease changes. For this reason, the final chapter in the basic science section is a survey of the life stages in human development, dealing with growth from birth to death. The authors (J. Megan, A. Ley, D. Wagenaar, and S. Scheinthald) meticulously examine the prenatal, infant, school-aged, adolescent, adult, and geriatric stages of life. At each stage in the life cycle, the unique vulnerabilities inherent in the associated physiological changes in each of the first four models are tied to the changes occurring in behavioral model. Viewed through this continuum of life, a better appreciation of human health and disease can be developed.

SUMMARY

The material in the basic science section of the third edition of the Foundations for Osteopathic Medicine has been chosen to provide a background understanding of the five models used in diagnosis, treatment, and management by osteopathic physicians. The journey begins with anatomy, fascia, biomechanics, respiration, lymphatics, and oscillating rhythms from which it progresses through such neurological items as somatic dysfunction, viscerosomatic integration, touch, nociception, and acute and chronic pain to end with a strong emphasis on the behavioral model. Knowledge of this material will best provide the future students of osteopathic medicine with the foundations of their profession.

6

The Concepts of Anatomy

LEX TOWNS, ALLEN W. JACOBS AND WILLIAM M. FALLS (SECOND EDITION)

KEY CONCEPTS

- Early developmental events are reflected in the organization of the adult body.
- Common cellular anatomy imposes anatomical constraints on body structure and function.
- Movement is a defining feature of the living state.
- Body unity is imposed by those structures that interconnect distant parts of the body.

INTRODUCTION

Understanding anatomy is fundamental to the rational practice of medicine. To assess health and disease, physicians must have a detailed knowledge of the structures of the body. A physician's comprehensive anatomical knowledge may be restricted to the particular body area or functional system that he or she uses in a specialized practice. However, effective physicians, even those in specialized practices, need and use a working knowledge of the reciprocal, interactive nature of the body's structure and function. Osteopathic physicians need sufficient knowledge of body structure and function to understand how focal destructive causes may not only lead to localized effects but may also contribute to more subtle, widespread, or distant degenerative, morbid events. The reward for mastering anatomy is to develop the ability to practice medicine—especially osteopathic medicine—in a more intelligent, predictable, and effective manner.

This chapter does not attempt to thoroughly review anatomy. Numerous excellent books and programs are available on human anatomy, and the effective methods of teaching anatomy vary from school to school. The purpose of this chapter is to provide the beginning student with some conceptual bases to guide the study of anatomy and thereby to help maximize the positive impact of anatomical knowledge on the eventual osteopathic medical practice.

Learning the seemingly enormous amount of anatomical detail can be daunting—the oft-repeated "drinking from a fire house" metaphor comes to mind—but there are some simplifying ideas that, if clearly understood, will make the task of comprehending anatomy both easier and more durable. Here, we introduce *four concepts* that we intend to assist in the mental organization of the anatomy of the body: *first*, early developmental events are reflected in the organization of the adult body; *second*, common cellular anatomy imposes anatomical constraints on body structure and function; *third*, movement is a defining feature of the living state; and *fourth*, body unity is imposed by those structures which interconnect distant parts of the body.

We will generally focus on the musculoskeletal system in this overview. However, the principles to be described apply throughout the study of anatomy, and we will point out some instances of more universal application.

NEUROMUSCULOSKELETAL DEVELOPMENT

Understanding the developmental history of the body is the first topic that truly assists the learning of gross anatomy. Principles of gross anatomy—general rules of where structures are and how they relate to other structures—are predicated on the way the body develops. Thus, understanding general developmental events will greatly enhance the comprehension and retention of the anatomy of the mature form.

At about four weeks of gestation, the embryo is a flat disc composed of three cell layers. The outer layer, ectoderm, will form principally skin and most of the nervous system. The middle layer, mesoderm, will form mainly muscles and bones, and the inner layer, endoderm, will form most of the internal organs. All organs and tissues of the body will develop by differentiation and growth of these three cell layers.

As development continues, the cells of the middle layer—called mesenchyme at this early stage—begin to form into a series of bilaterally symmetric clusters of cells; each cluster is called a somite. The formation of pairs of somites begins in the cervical region and proceeds caudally until about 38 separate pairs of somites are formed. The mature organization of the musculoskeletal system is a direct reflection of the embryologic development of segmental somites.

Each somite differentiates into two parts: a sclerotome and a dermomyotome (Fig. 6.1). The sclerotome will form the bones and cartilages of the axial skeleton (vertebrae and ribs), and two things form from the dermomyotome: the "dermo" part becomes the dermis of the skin and the myotome will form the axial muscles (muscles of the trunk).

As somites form in the middle layer of embryonic cells, related developmental events are taking place in the overlying ectoderm. The ectoderm becomes grooved in the midline, and the edges of the groove then move together until a tube is formed. The tube—now called the neural tube—is the embryonic precursor of the spinal cord. Ectodermal tissue adjacent to the neural tube is called the neural crests and is the precursor of elements of the peripheral nervous system.

As each somite of the trunk forms, there is a simultaneous segmentation of the adjacent part of the neural tube. Sensory and motor nerves of a specific part of the developing spinal cord will be segmentally related to an adjacent developing somite. Thus, a close correspondence is maintained between the developing segments of the body wall and the central nervous system (CNS) (Figs. 6.2 and 6.3). While the close coherence between the spinal cord and the truncal musculoskeletal system is maintained by these developmental events, anticipating topics of visceral-somatic relationships to be discussed below, it is useful to point out that there is also a relationship between the developing thoracic and abdominopelvic organs and the spinal cord. As a result, the nervous

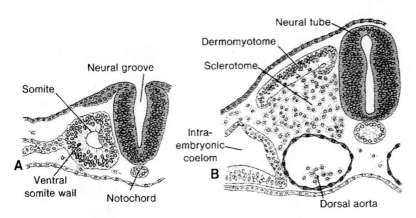

Figure 6-1 A and **B.** Transverse sections showing differentiation of a somite in relation to development of neural tube.

system provides the link between the somatic tissue of the trunk (i.e., bones and muscles) and the viscera (i.e., heart or gastrointestinal system). This segmental relationship between the body wall and internal organs is hypothesized to be the underlying mechanism for referred pain—perceiving pain on the body wall (i.e., chest pain) when the tissue damage is in an internal organ (i.e., cardiac ischemia).

Development of the Trunk

Segmentation—the result of embryonic somitic and neural development—is most obvious in the adult through levels of the thorax and abdomen. Each thoracic myotome will further divide into an epimere and hypomere. The mesenchymal cells in the epimere become the deep back muscles in the adult, while the mesenchymal cells in the hypomere become the muscles of the anterolateral wall of the thorax and abdomen (Fig. 6.3).

A typical transverse section through the thoracic region demonstrates the basic segmental organization (Figs. 6.3 and 6.4). Throughout the thoracic region, each segmental level is organized symmetrically about a central axis composed of the vertebra and spinal cord. Emanating from the spinal cord at each segmental level will be a pair of spinal nerves that distribute principally to the skin, bones, and muscles derived from that segment's dermomyotome.

The typical spinal nerve is formed by the union of the ventral (motor) and dorsal (sensory) roots just lateral to the spinal cord. Within a short distance, each spinal nerve divides to form a posterior primary ramus and an anterior primary ramus (Fig. 6.4). Each ramus contains both sensory and motor nerve fibers. The posterior primary rami of thoracic and lumbar spinal nerves are distributed to the deep ("true") back muscles, the joints which the muscles functionally move and the skin over these muscles. The anterior primary ramus in the thoracic and lumbar regions innervates the muscles of the body wall (i.e., intercostal and abdominal muscles) and the skin of the thorax and abdomen. The pattern of thoracic and abdominal nerve distribution is clinically demonstrated as the dermatomes—restricted areas of the skin served by individual spinal nerves (Fig. 6.5).

As will be typical throughout the body, there is also a segmentation of blood supply to the thoracic and abdominal wall that is similar to segmentation of muscles and nerves. For example, in the thoracic region, the aorta gives rise to right and left posterior intercostal arteries, which supply the thoracic and abdominal walls segmentally (Fig. 6.4). This area of supply includes the skin, superficial and deep fascia, intercostal and abdominal musculature, ribs, vertebrae, and paravertebral musculature. This parallel segmentation of nerves and vessels is readily seen on the inferior surface of each rib where a neurovascular bundle, which includes the intercostal nerve, artery, and vein (as well as segmental intercostal lymphatics) is located (Fig. 6.4). These structures supply and drain the muscle, connective tissue, and skin within and over the thorax and abdomen.

The segmental pattern of neurovascular distribution in the thorax and abdomen is an example of developmental segmentation that

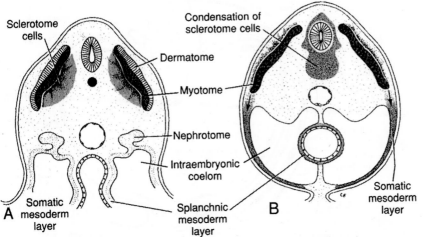

Figure 6-2 A and **B.** Transverse actions showing migration of cells from sclerotome and myotome during development.

Figure 6-3 **A** and **B.** Transverse sections showing segmental nerve from developing spinal cord and innervating developing musculature of thorax and abdomen.

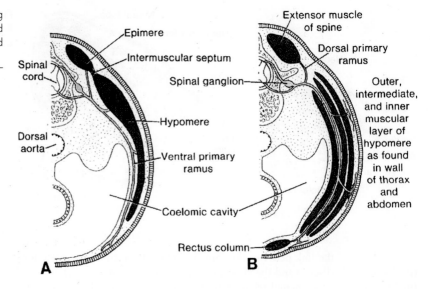

Development of the Upper and Lower Limbs

Segmentation and the results of early embryonic segmentation are not as readily apparent in the adult limbs. Nevertheless, keeping the original segmentation in mind will help you understand the overall anatomy of the limbs. The anatomy of the upper and lower limbs is comparable. The limbs are divided into four major parts. The upper limb is divided into the shoulder (shoulder girdle), arm, forearm, and hand; while the lower limb consists of the pelvic girdle, thigh, leg, and foot.

The upper and lower limbs develop from localized enlargements of mesenchyme—limb buds; the limb buds of the upper limb develop from lower cervical and upper thoracic segments (C5-C8 and T1), while the lower limb buds develop from lower lumbar and upper sacral segments (L2-L5 and S1 and S2). The hypomere of the mesenchyme at each of these levels will form bone, connective tissue, and muscle of the limb. As the limb bud expands, anterior primary rami of spinal nerves grow into the developing limb, thus maintaining a segmental correspondence between the developing limb and the spinal cord (Fig. 6.6). However, through differential limb growth and development (e.g., mesenchymal cells from different segments combining to form a single muscle in the adult), the initial segmental representation of the embryo is modified in the adult.

The bones of the upper and lower limbs arise *in situ* in the developing limb buds. They begin as mesenchyme that condenses and differentiates into hyaline cartilage models of the future bones. These cartilaginous models eventually ossify through a complex process of endochondral ossification. Limb musculature is also derived from mesenchyme but, unlike that which form the bones, muscle mesenchyme is derived from somites adjacent to the developing neural tube and migrates into the limb bud from the hypomere where it condenses adjacent to the developing bones (Fig. 6.6). As the limb elongates, the muscular tissue splits into flexor (anterior) and extensor (posterior) components. Initially, the muscles of the limbs are segmental in character, but in time, they fuse, migrate, and are composed of muscle tissue from several segments. Upper limb buds are opposite neural tube (spinal cord) segments C5-C8 and T1 while lower limb buds lie opposite segments L2-L5 and S1 and S2.

As the limbs grow, posterior and anterior branches derived from anterior primary rami of spinal nerves penetrate into the

Figure 6-4 Transverse section illustrating contents of a segmental level through the thorax.

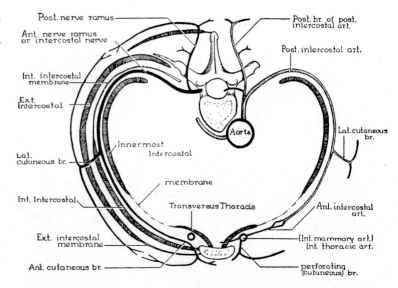

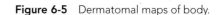

Figure 6-5 Dermatomal maps of body.

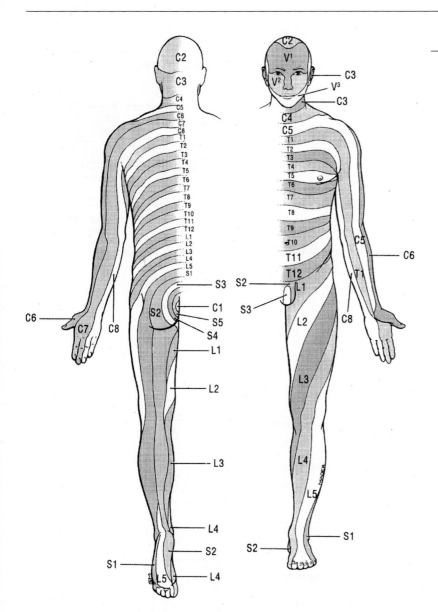

developing muscles (Fig. 6.6). Posterior branches enter extensor musculature while anterior branches enter flexor musculature. With continued development, the posterior and anterior branches from each anterior primary ramus unite to form large posterior and anterior nerves. This union of the original segmental posterior and anterior branches from each anterior primary ramus is the basis for the formation of the brachial and lumbosacral plexuses (Fig. 6.7A, C, D & E) and comes about with the fusion of segmental muscles. The large posterior and anterior nerves are represented in the adult upper limb as the radial nerve supplying extensor musculature, while the median and ulnar nerves innervate flexor musculature (Fig. 6.7A & C). In the adult lower limb, the large posterior and anterior nerves are represented as the femoral and common fibular nerves supplying extensor musculature and the tibial nerve supplying flexor musculature (Fig. 6.7D & E). Contact between nerves and differentiating muscle cells is a prerequisite for complete functional muscle differentiation. The segmental spinal nerves also provide sensory innervation of the limb dermatomes. The original segmental dermatomal pattern is modified with growth of the limbs, but an orderly sequence is present in the adult (Fig. 6.8).

While the development of the upper and lower limbs is similar, there one major difference: the limbs rotate in opposite directions. The upper limb rotates 90 degrees laterally so that the elbow points posteriorly, the extensor musculature lies on lateral and posterior surfaces while the flexor musculature lies on anterior and medial surfaces, and the thumb lies laterally on the anterior facing palm. The lower limb rotates 90 degrees medially so that the knee points anteriorly, the extensor muscles are on the anterior surface while the flexor muscles are on the posterior surface, and the big toe is medial.

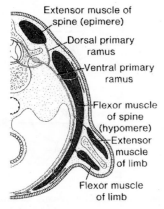

Figure 6-6 Transverse section showing that muscles (as well as bone and connective tissues) of developing limbs maintain segmental innervation from developing spinal cord.

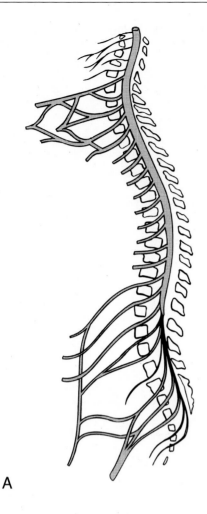

A

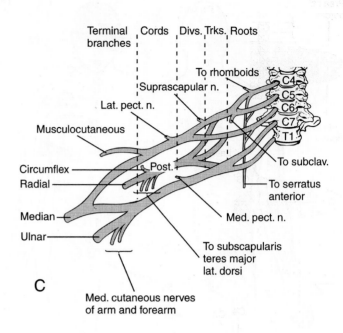

Terminal branches | Cords | Divs. | Trks. | Roots

To rhomboids
Suprascapular n.
Lat. pect. n.
Musculocutaneous
Circumflex
Radial
Post.
Median
Ulnar
To subclav.
To serratus anterior
Med. pect. n.
To subscapularis teres major lat. dorsi
Med. cutaneous nerves of arm and forearm

C4
C5
C6
C7
T1

C

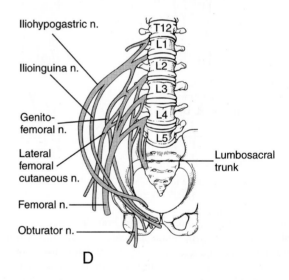

Iliohypogastric n.
Ilioinguina n.
Genito-femoral n.
Lateral femoral cutaneous n.
Femoral n.
Obturator n.

T12
L1
L2
L3
L4
L5

Lumbosacral trunk

D

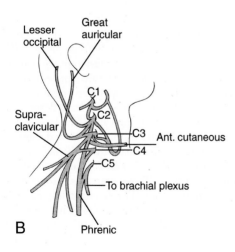

Lesser occipital
Great auricular
Supra-clavicular
C1
C2
C3
C4
C5
Ant. cutaneous
To brachial plexus
Phrenic

B

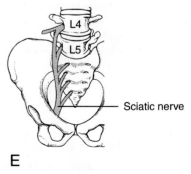

L4
L5

Sciatic nerve

E

Figure 6-7   Spinal cord and plexuses. **A.** Sagittal view of spinal cord and plexuses. **B.** Cervical plexus. **C.** Brachial plexus. **D.** Lumbar plexus. **E.** Sacral plexus.

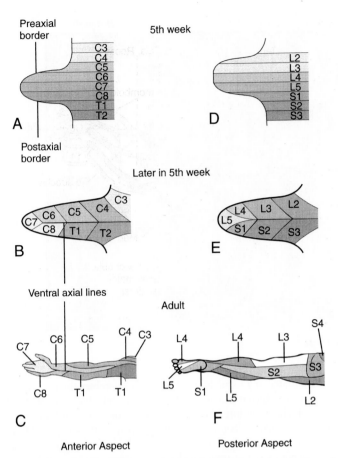

Figure 6-8 Developing dermatomal patterns in upper **(A–C)** and lower **(D–F)** limbs. **A–C.** Anterior view, upper limb. **D** and **F.** Posterior view, lower limb. **A, B, D,** and **E.** Limb buds in embryo. **C** and **F.** Adult limbs.

These rotations, thus, determine the functions that the limbs will perform in the adult. In the limbs, deep fascia and intermuscular septa connecting with bone separate or compartmentalize groups of muscles (more on this below). The muscles in each compartment share similar functions, developmental histories, nerve and arterial supply as well as venous and lymphatic drainage.

MUSCULOSKELETAL MICROSCOPIC ANATOMY

As discussed above, understanding segmental developmental events provides an organizational framework by which to comprehend and utilize knowledge of the mature musculoskeletal system. Similarly, a basic understanding of the tissues of the musculoskeletal system provides a conceptual framework through which to understand the mechanisms of health and disease as manifest in body movements. The cellular and extracellular components of the musculoskeletal system are generally classified into two groups: connective tissue and muscle.

Connective Tissue

The connective tissues of the body are derived from mesenchyme. These developing tissues (connective tissue, bone, and cartilage) contain cells (fibroblasts, osteoblasts, and chondroblasts), which produce a matrix of ground substance and fibers that surround the cells. Each type of connective tissue has a unique arrangement of cell types within a specific matrix of ground substance and fibers. By changing these three elements (cells, ground substance, and fibers), the variable composition and consistency of each type of connective tissue in the musculoskeletal system is produced. Thus, all connective tissue can be classified on the basis of the arrangement of these three elements.

Loose connective tissue forms an open meshwork of cells (fibrocytes; fibroblasts) and fibers (collagen, elastic, reticular), with a large amount of fat cells and ground substance in between. Loose connective tissue also surrounds neurovascular bundles and fills the spaces between individual muscles and fascial planes (Fig. 6.9).

Dense fibrous connective tissue is composed predominantly of collagen fiber bundles and is classified as regular or irregular on the basis of the arrangement of the closely packed collagen. Collagen fibers in dense regular connective tissue show a regular arrangement and run in the same direction. Dense regular connective tissue forms the substance of periosteum, tendons, and ligaments. Irregular connective tissue (e.g., periosteum and deep fascia) is composed of collagen fibers that lack such a consistent pattern (Fig. 6.10).

Cartilage and Bone

Cartilage and bone are highly specialized connective tissues in which the ground substance of the matrix is predominant over the cellular and fibrous elements, and thus, cartilage and bone can have a texture that is considerably different from that of dense connective tissue.

The chondroblast is responsible for producing the ground substance and fibers of the three types of cartilage: hyaline (articular; found in synovial joints), elastic (found in the external ear, auditory tube, larynx, and epiglottis), and fibrous (found in intervertebral disks). These three cartilage types vary in histological makeup on the basis of their ground substance and predominant fiber type (collagen or elastin) and are avascular (Figs. 6.11–6.13).

The osteocytes of bone are maintained in a rigid matrix, which is calcified and reinforced by connective tissue fibers, which are produced by the osteoblasts. The structural unit of bone, the osteon (Haversian system), is formed by concentric lamellae of bone surrounding a microscopic neurovascular bundle in the Haversian canal. The osteocytes are located within microscopic spaces (lacunae) between the concentric bone matrix lamellae and extend processes into the matrix (Fig. 6.14).

Skeletal Muscle

As described above, skeletal muscle tissue is derived from mesenchyme and is highly modified for the specific function of contraction. The individual skeletal muscle cells (fibers) are arranged in a regular systematic manner to facilitate contraction when stimulated by a nerve impulse. The microscopic appearance of skeletal muscle presents a classic banding pattern, which represents the internal organization of the protein contractile elements in each muscle fiber (Fig. 6.15). The highly differentiated cytoarchitecture of muscle tissue relates closely to the inability of the muscle tissue to heal following injury.

Response to Injury

The inherent capacity of the musculoskeletal system to heal and repair following injury is a direct reflection of the histological organization of connective tissue. At the macroscopic level, the connective tissue invests the neurovascular bundles, which supply specific parts of the body. At the microscopic level, the capillary beds are

Figure 6-9 Cellular elements of loose connective tissue.

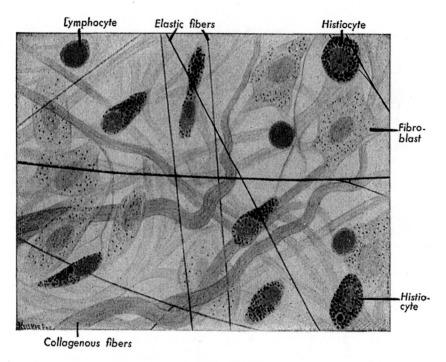

located within the open meshwork of loose connective tissue and nourish the cellular elements of the tissue. These cells in turn produce the ground substance and fibers of the connective tissue. Following injury, a complex biochemical reaction results in stimulating the inherent capacity of healing and repair. In general, the more

differentiated any tissue is (i.e., the less it resembles the embryonic tissue from which it was derived), the less capable that tissue is of cell division and, therefore, the less able the tissue is to heal via mitotic addition of new cells following injury. Because of its highly differentiated nature, skeletal muscle and cartilage often repair as a scar mainly composed of irregular dense connective tissue. Bone represents a major exception to this rule. Since bone is actively remodeling in the living state, it will rapidly form a scar following injury and then gradually remodel the scar into the normal architecture of the adult bone. A corollary of this principle on differentiation can be seen in cancerous tissue. Generally, differentiated cells have to dedifferentiate in order to become a malignancy. The more undifferentiated a cell becomes, the more potential it has to divide; thus, some of the most dangerous malignancies are anaplastic lesions in which cells appear to return to a primitive, embryonic-looking state.

FUNCTION OF THE MUSCULOSKELETAL SYSTEM

Understanding the function of the musculoskeletal system remains at the heart of osteopathic medical practice and, so, constitutes a significant portion of most anatomy courses. The musculoskeletal system is approximately 75% of the body mass; this vast system gives stability in health, provides clues to dysfunction and disease, and offers a mode of treatment to support the patient who is diseased or stressed. Osteopathic physicians must understand well the function of the individual components of the musculoskeletal system. This function is seen from two fundamental, complementary perspectives: What action or function does a muscle (joint, bone, ligament, etc.) produce? And, which muscle (joint, bone, ligament, etc.) produces a specific action or function?

Understanding the rule of function in the musculoskeletal system leads inevitably to a series of questions predicated on more complex structural and functional interrelationships: How might dysfunction of the muscle (or other musculoskeletal component) affect total body efficiency and health? How might dysfunction of some visceral element degrade the structural or functional integrity of the musculoskeletal system? And, how are these dysfunctions

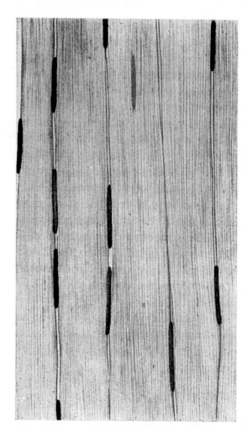

Figure 6-10 Cellular elements of dense, regular fibrous connective tissue. Dark fibroblast nuclei lie between bundles of regularly arranged collagen fibers.

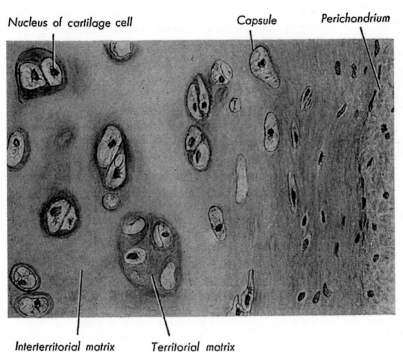

Nucleus of cartilage cell   Capsule   Perichondrium

Interterritorial matrix   Territorial matrix

Figure 6-11 Cellular elements of hyaline (articular) cartilage.

segmentally related to other tissues and organ system? These questions form the core of rational osteopathic medical practice.

Muscle Function

A muscle normally contracts because it is stimulated by a motor nerve. A single motor nerve fiber innervates more than one skeletal muscle fiber. The nerve fiber and all the muscle fibers it innervates are called the motor unit (Fig. 6.16). In general, small muscles that react quickly (e.g., extraocular muscles) have ten or fewer muscle fibers innervated by a single nerve fiber. In contrast, large muscles that do not require fine CNS control (e.g., deep back muscles) may have up to one thousand muscle fibers in a motor unit. When a muscle is resting, some motor units are always discharging. It may

Figure 6-12 Cellular elements of elastic cartilage.

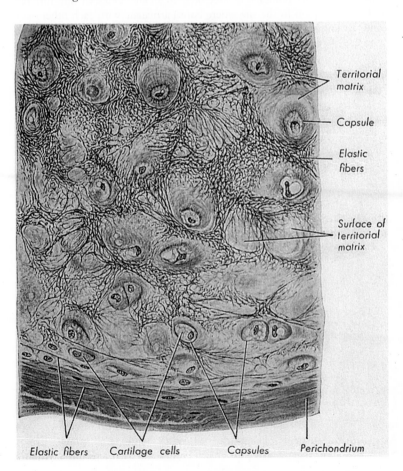

Territorial matrix

Capsule

Elastic fibers

Surface of territorial matrix

Elastic fibers   Cartilage cells   Capsules   Perichondrium

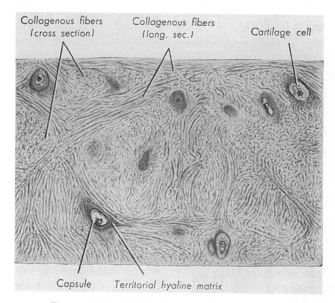

Figure 6-13 Cellular elements of fibrocartilage.

not be the same motor units at each instance in time. This type of motor activity (muscle tone) is the background for muscular contraction in the performance of a purposeful movement.

When most muscles contract, their fibers act through tendons on moveable bones to get the desired action (Fig. 6.17). Movements result in the activation of motor units in some muscles and the simultaneous relaxation of motor units in other muscles. Movement that comes about from muscle contraction causes the muscles to change in length. When this occurs, tension created within the muscle remains constant and the contraction is called isotonic. If movement does not occur as a result of muscle contraction and muscle length stays constant with elevated tension generated within the muscles, the contraction is called isometric (e.g., posterior compartment muscles of the leg in standing). Isotonic contractions may be concentric (shortening of the muscle) or eccentric (lengthening of the muscle).

Most movements require the combined action of several muscles. The term prime mover is used for those muscles that act directly to bring about the desired movement. Every muscle, which acts on a joint, is paired with another muscle that has the opposite action on the same joint. These muscles are antagonists of each other (e.g., muscles that flex the elbow and muscles that extend the elbow are antagonists of each other). During any movement around a joint, both agonist and antagonists are contracting—the agonist contracts more forcefully to produce movement, but the antagonist maintains some tonus that does not significantly block the action of the agonist, but helps to stabilize the movement. There are times when prime movers and antagonists contract together and are called fixators. This occurs to stabilize a joint or hold a part of the body in an appropriate position. Muscles, which contract at the same time to produce a movement are called synergists. These can be either muscles that aid the agonist in the performance of the desired action or antagonist muscles that contract at the same time as an agonist and thereby prevent unwanted movement that would be counterproductive to the desired action. Individual muscles should not always be considered as units with a single function, and different parts of the same muscle may have different, even antagonistic, actions (e.g., the trapezius).

The function of most skeletal muscles is to produce movement of bones relative to each other. For example, contraction of the arm muscles will cause flexion of extension of the elbow. While emphasis to this point has focused on muscles and bones, we now turn our attention to the site where bones articulate with each other—the joints.

Figure 6-14 Transverse section showing cellular elements of compact bone.

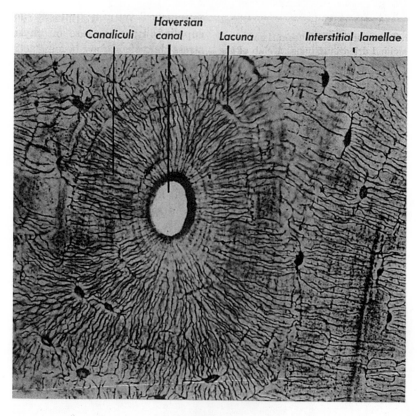

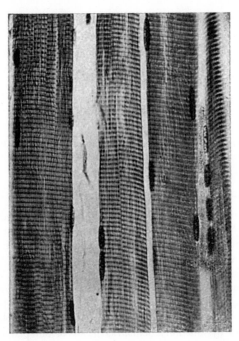

Figure 6-15 Longitudinal section of skeletal muscle showing classic banding pattern found in individual fibers.

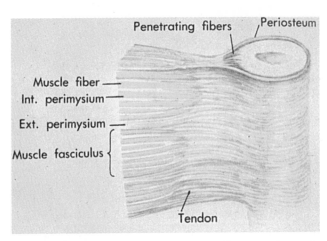

Figure 6-17 Diagrammatic representation of how muscle attaches to bone.

Synovial and Nonsynovial Joints

All synovial joints of the body are freely movable and similar in structure. The "typical" synovial joint is exemplified in Figure 6.18. The articular surfaces of the two bones, which form the joint, are covered by hyaline (articular) cartilage, which is specifically modified for the function of articular motion. The two articular surfaces are separated by a monolayer of synovial fluid in the joint cavity. The joint capsule is composed of two layers. The unique inner layer of the joint capsule is the synovial membrane, which lines the fibrous outer layer. This membrane secretes the synovial fluid, which lubricates the internal joint surfaces and the articular hyaline cartilage. The uniqueness of this membrane is that it is derived from mesenchyme. However, microscopically and functionally, this tissue is similar to epithelial tissue, which is an ectodermal derivative.

Each synovial joint is stabilized by specific ligaments. Ligaments may be classified as capsular or accessory. A capsular ligament is a part of the fibrous outer layer of the joint capsule while accessory ligaments are either located within the joint cavity (intracapsular) or outside the joint capsule, separated from the fibrous outer layer (extracapsular). All ligaments are histologically composed of dense regular fibrous connective tissue and have microscopic, structural, and functional continuity with the periosteum of adjacent bone. Some joints (temporomandibular joint or knee joint, for example) are even more specialized as they have the unique feature of either a disk or a meniscus (incomplete disk) within the joint cavity (Fig. 6.19). The fibrocartilaginous disk provides for additional support and stability as it separates the two hyaline cartilage articular surfaces.

Synovial joints are commonly classified according to the shape of the articular surfaces and/or the movements, which are permitted. None of the articular surfaces are truly flat. Biomechanically, these joint surfaces permit motion, which is described as spin, roll, or slide (Fig. 6.20). Spin represents rotation about the longitudinal axis of a bone. Roll is the result of decreasing and increasing the angle between the two bones at an articulation. Slide is the result of a translatory motion of one bone gliding/sliding on the other at the joint. Specific details regarding the classification system and individual synovial joints can be found in any anatomy textbook.

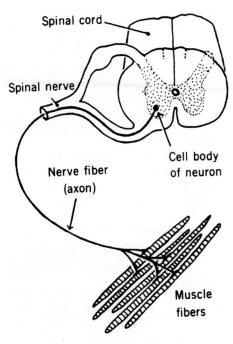

Figure 6-16 A motor unit.

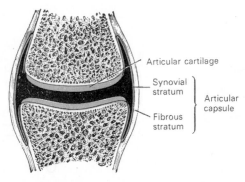

Figure 6-18 Typical synovial joint.

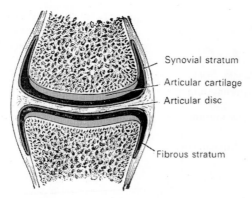

Figure 6-19 Synovial joint with an articular disc.

Synovial stratum
Articular cartilage
Articular disc

Fibrous stratum

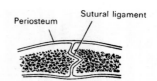

Periosteum   Sutural ligament

Figure 6-21 A suture is an example of a fibrous joint.

Nonsynovial joints are subdivided into fibrous and cartilaginous types. These joints where the articulating bones are directly connected by either fibrous tissue or cartilage have no free surface for movement, but provide for strength and stability between adjacent bones. The fibrous joints include the sutures of the skull (Fig. 6.21), teeth in the mandible and maxilla, and the distal tibiofibular joint. The fibrocartilaginous intervertebral disks between adjacent vertebral bodies and the pubic symphysis (Fig. 6.22) are examples of cartilaginous joints.

The sutures of the skull provide a classic example of the interrelationship between structure and function. Each suture (joint) between adjacent cranial bones uniquely provides support and mobility. Unlike the freely moveable synovial joints, the sutures are highly restricted to slight gliding motion. However, motion loss/restriction is the clinically significant factor in describing somatic dysfunction of the joint.

Cranial bone motion is also influenced by the tension of the cranial dura mater, which covers the brain and forms the internal lining of the skull. Cranial dura mater consists of two layers: periosteal and meningeal. The periosteal layer is the periosteal lining of the cranium and there is histological continuity of this layer with the fibrous tissue (sutural ligament) at each cranial suture. The meningeal layer of cranial dura mater has continuity with the spinal dura mater (thecal sac) at the foramen magnum of the occipital bone (Fig. 6.23). The direct effect of these connective tissues on cranial bone motion has been described by Sutherland as the reciprocal tension membrane.

In summary, synovial and nonsynovial joints exemplify the osteopathic concept of the inter-relationship between structure and function. Synovial joints, which are freely moveable, allow for the body to have mobility and greater range of motion. The

nonsynovial joints (fibrous and cartilaginous) provide strength and stability within a limited range of motion.

Joint Play

The voluntary movement of synovial joints is accommodated by joint play as described by Mennell. Joint play is defined as a small but precise amount of movement (<1/8″), which is independent of the action of voluntary muscle function. The normal, easy, voluntary range of active motion at a synovial joint is dependent upon the integrity of joint play. Joint play is only present in the living synovial joint. The movement of joint play can only be demonstrated by passive examination. Each synovial joint has one or more joint play movements. Joint dysfunction is defined as the loss of joint play and therefore a limitation of the voluntary range of motion at a synovial joint. Joint dysfunction is a component of somatic dysfunction (acute or chronic), which is diagnosed in the evaluation of the neuromusculoskeletal system. The restoration of joint play appears to be the basis for the success of synovial joint mobilization using direct or indirect action treatment techniques in osteopathic manipulation.

BODY UNITY

Although to this point we have emphasized the segmental and cellular nature of the human body, in reality, the body is one unified structure. The various regional anatomical and cellular components of the neuromusculoskeletal system—derived embryological from somites and associated neural precursors—are bound together and unified into a functional whole by arteries, veins, lymphatics, nerves, circulating factors, and fascia.

It has not been customary in modern medicine to point out that the human is a complex, unified organism made up of many overlapping, interconnected systems. Recently, conventional medicine has attempted to reassemble its various specialties and subspecialties, each focused on a body region or functional system, into a holistic understanding of health and disease. Nevertheless, the structure of medicine retains much of its compartmentalization; it is difficult for even the most thoughtful physician, particularly those in a demanding specialty practice, to step back routinely and holistically assess a patient.

A physician's understanding of body unity and the propensity to view the patient holistically is heightened by remembering a basic unifying principle: although the body is made up of many structurally and functionally discrete elements, the elements

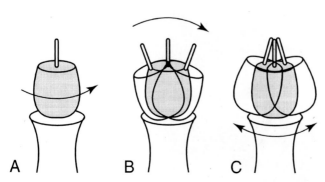

Figure 6-20 Motion at a synovial joint. **A.** Spin. **B.** Roll. **C.** Slide.

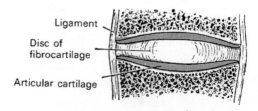

Ligament
Disc of fibrocartilage
Articular cartilage

Figure 6-22 A symphysis is an example of a cartilaginous joint.

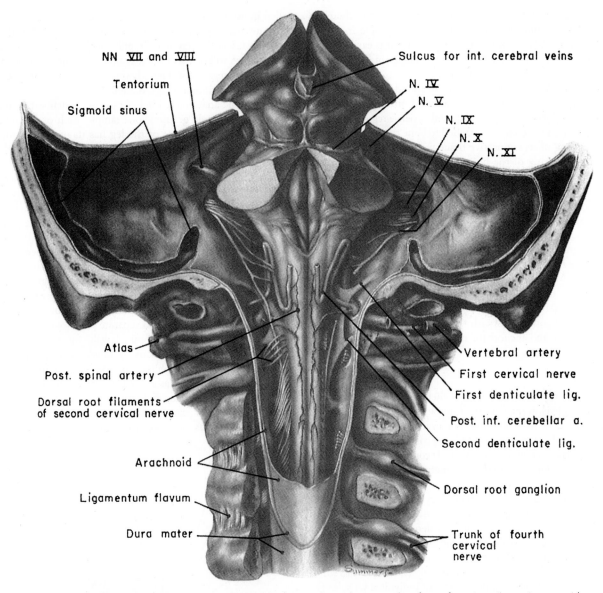

Figure 6-23   Area of foramen magnum. Cranial dura mater lines the internal surface of cranium, is continuous with fibrous tissue of sutures, and is continuous with spinal dura mater of foramen magnum.

are linked together by a number of connectors. As such, these connectors make up a significant portion of the study of medicine in general and the study of anatomy in particular.

The "connectors" are easily listed; they are connective tissue, the nervous system, the endocrine system, and the vascular and lymphatic systems. The circulatory system serves distant body parts and, among other things, provides a means of communication. The nervous system, although it is traditionally divided into component parts—central, peripheral, autonomic, and enteric—is one continuous, functional entity. The nervous system constantly receives external and internal stimuli filters, sorts and integrates those stimuli, and then produces the coordinated contraction of muscles and/or secretion of glands in response to those stimuli. The nervous system can even impel muscular contraction and/or glandular secretion independent of external stimulation. The endocrine and immune systems, interconnected to each other and to the nervous systems, also bring tissues distant from each other under unified, coordinated control. Indeed, contemporary analyses

suggest that, as the endocrine, immune and nervous systems all use a common set of messengers (e.g., norepinephrine, neuropeptide Y, cholecystokinin, and many others), that they be considered one overlapping system by which body unity is established and maintained.

Connective Tissue

As described above, connective tissue is one important component of the musculoskeletal system. Connective tissue serves both to isolate individual elements of the body and to unify adjacent and distant structures. Connective tissue begins at the molecular level and extends to the gross, macroscopic level.

Connective tissue binds organ to organ, muscle to bone, and bone to bone and literally is the fundamental connector that allows structural and functional systems to be physically grouped into a unified package. Without connective tissue, the body is a dissociated mass of dying cells. It is the connective tissue, most of it a proteinaceous extracellular matrix, that enforces form and thereby permits function. Connective tissue plays a critical role in body health and disease, but ironically it is so pervasive it is easily overlooked in the study of anatomy, in the maintenance of health, and in the diagnosis and treatment of disease.

Individual skeletal muscle fibers are surrounded by a delicate network of fine connective tissue. At each end of the muscle, this connective tissue forms a tendon composed of dense regular fibrous connective tissue. The tendon is attached to bone through a microscopic interlacing of its connective tissue with the periosteal connective tissue covering of the bone (Fig. 6.17). Each muscle has two parts: a predominant connective tissue at its ends, which attach to bones and a predominance of muscle tissue in its functional contractile belly. The change to connective tissue at its ends provides the muscle a firm attachment to bone.

The musculotendinous junction represents the point at which there is a significant change in the histological composition of skeletal muscle from predominantly muscle fibers to predominantly collagen fibers. Muscle contraction exerts force on the musculotendinous junction and then the tendon, which moves a bone at a joint. The connective tissue of the joint and joint capsule is then connected to and continuous with the connective tissue that surrounds the muscle and anchors the muscle to bone.

Fascia

Fascia is as rather generalized term for sheets or layers of connective tissue that envelop specific structures and segregate one structure, organ, or area from another. For example, throughout the body, there is a subcutaneous layer of loose connective tissue called the superficial fascia (Figs. 6.9 and 6.24). It contains collagen fibers that connect the skin to underlying structures as well as variable amounts of fat. Superficial fascia serves to increase skin mobility, acts as a thermal insulator, and stores energy for metabolic use.

As will be seen in Chapter 7 on the Fascial System, enveloping deep fascia will be defined as irregular dense connective tissue. Deep fascia is the dense connective tissue envelope (also composed primarily of collagen fibers) that both connects and separates individual muscles of the limbs and trunk. Individual muscles are surrounded by a deep fascia. This deep fascia of individual muscles is continuous with the deep fascia that connects muscle to bone and with the deep fascia that ensheaths and separates groups of muscles of similar location and function (e.g., anterior thigh muscles). The deep fasciae passing between muscle groups in the limbs are

called intermuscular septa. The deep fasciae of muscle groups and intermuscular septa are, in turn, continuous with a tightly adhering deep fascia that completely encircles all of the muscles of the limb, and, as will be mentioned again below, the deep fascia encasing different regions of the body represents a mass of tissue that is everywhere continuous (Figs. 6.25–6.27).

At a basic anatomical level, these fasciae define the individual muscles and muscle groups. For example, each of the muscles in the anterior compartment of the leg has its own investing fascia. The entire group is bounded laterally by a wall of fascia, the anterior crural septum, medially by fascia that is continuous with the periosteum of the tibia, and anteriorly by the encasing deep fascia of the leg. As is typical, the blood and nervous supply to these muscles, as well as venous and lymphatic return, is principally contained within this fascial compartment. These fasciae collectively define the anterior compartment. More importantly, they enhance the extensor functions of the muscles, while simultaneously providing protection, support, and separation from other muscle groups. The fasciae define the normal, healthy limit of the group; they tend to constrain destructive states and prevent the spread of bleeding, infection, tumor growth, etc. into adjacent compartments.

Fascial compartments also separate muscles of the trunk. The muscles of the anterior abdominal wall, for example, are easily divided into planes and groups by tough enveloping fascia. The external oblique, internal oblique, transversus abdominis, and rectus abdominis are delineable as a group and from one another not only by their attachments and orientations but also by the tight-fitting sheets of fascia that enclose them. Planes of fascia are also found in the subcutaneous space, external to the deep fascia that bounds

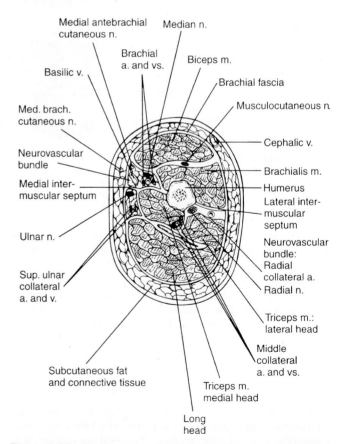

Figure 6-25 Transverse section through the arm. Neurovascular bundles are found between skeletal muscles in anterior and posterior compartments.

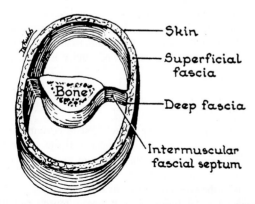

Figure 6-24 Diagrammatic representation of a transverse section through the arm, illustrating the organization of superficial and deep fascia. Deep fascia divides the arm into compartments by way of intermuscular septa.

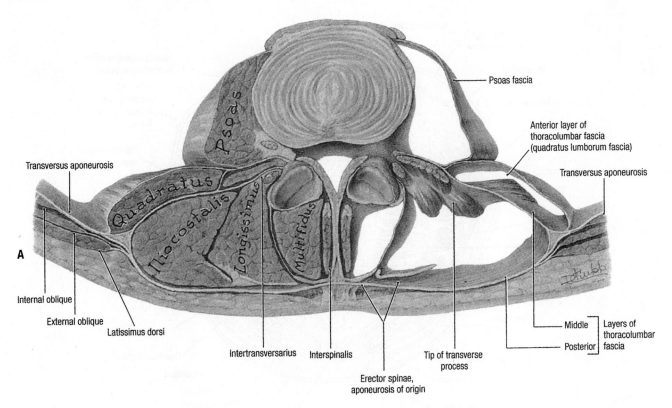

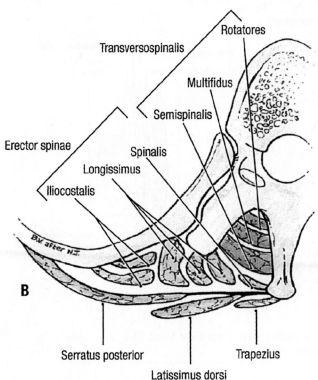

Figure 6-26 Transverse section through the back, illustrating the organization of deep fascia. The deep fascia serves to divide the back into compartments for muscles of similar function.

the surfaces of the muscles. Understanding the placement of these fasciae is important in a variety of medical and surgical settings.

Peripheral nerves, blood, and lymph vessels lie in loose connective tissue fascia between muscles. This fascia serves to bind together these nerves and vessels and collectively the components form the neurovascular bundle (Fig. 6.25).

While fascia tends to separate and isolate groups of muscle of similar location and function, many of the layers of fascia, whether subcutaneous or investing, merge together and/or have common points of attachment. The fascia that separate and ensheathe the external and internal abdominal obliques merge posteriorly with the thick, connective tissue thoracolumbar fascia; they are

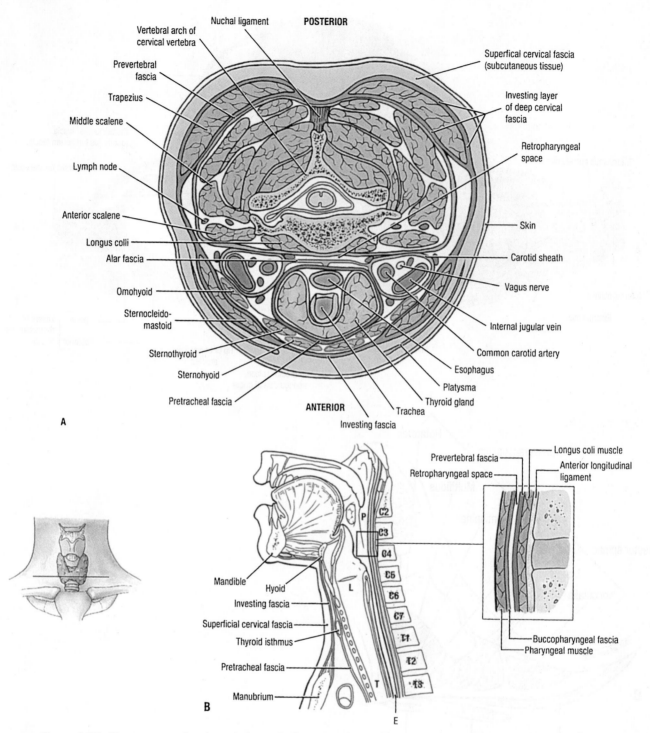

Figure 6-27 Transverse section through the neck, illustrating the organization of the deep fascia. The deep fascia divides the neck into muscular, visceral, and neurovascular compartments.

continuous upward, encasing and separating the erector spinae, the deep muscles of the back. Anteriorly, the fasciae of the abdominal muscles merge, split, and are reflected to contribute to the inguinal anatomy and abdominal aponeurosis. These fasciae are continuous with connective tissue sheets that flow over the crest of the pelvis and become the fascia lata of the thigh. The fascia of the thigh is continuous, in turn, with the crural fascia of the leg. As a consequence of the widespread continuity of fascia, distortion or damage to fascia in one area can have effects in a distant, seemingly unrelated area.

The subcutaneous fasciae are also continuous from one body region to another. The deep layer of superficial fascia of the abdomen (Scarpa fascia) defines a space that is more or less continuous from the flank onto the abdominal wall. It continues inferiorly into the perineum, where it is the superficial perineal space (bounded by Colles and dartos fascia, continuations of Scarpa fascia). Fluid or infection in the abdominal subcutaneous space can, thus, spread to the lumbar area or into the perineum.

The importance of the two-faceted aspect of fascia, that it at once not only separates and segregates but is also continuous structure to structure and area to area, should not be overlooked. This pervasive connector (along with muscle and bone) helps to regionalize the body and also connects region to region. Such a dualism is apparent in many physical manifestations of both health and disease.

Arteries

Two structural entities, arteries and nerves, are important for the health and maintenance of any organ or area. Arteries supply nutrients, oxygen, and a variety of immune and endocrine regulatory substances to the area of their distribution. Nerves provide ongoing neural control of skeletal and smooth muscle and glandular tissue as well as deliver trophic or regulatory factors to the muscles or organs that they innervate. The rule of supply illustrates a major source for maintenance of health or, conversely, origin of pathology when disrupted.

Few statements are more cogent than A.T. Still's insightful dictum, "The rule of the artery is supreme." An adequate blood supply during varying physiological conditions is a prerequisite for health of an organ or region. Conversely, compromise to the blood supply often leads to diminished functional capacity, cascading, in turn, toward disease. The osteopathic physician must work to ensure continued blood supply in the healthy state and, when treating injury or disease, should attempt to enhance arterial supply to affected regions. One important condition of compromise is bleeding due to trauma or disease. The physician must have sufficient understanding of anatomy to be able to halt hemorrhage quickly and subsequently restore adequate blood flow to ischemic areas. But the physician must also be able to recognize the clinical signs of ischemia due to blockage of arterial supply and work to relieve the blockage.

To optimize strategies that continue arterial supply (and vigor) in the healthy state, and to use appropriate therapeutic interventions in disease or injury to restore adequate blood supply, a physician must have an accurate knowledge of the arterial supply to an area. Consistent with rule 1 above, it is not sufficient simply to know the name of the artery that provides supply; rather, the passage of the arterial supply must be placed in the context of surrounding muscles, bones, organs, lymphatics, fascia, etc.

One of the goals of an osteopathic approach to medical treatment is, first, to recognize which piece of surrounding tissue might be compressing an artery and, having visualized the mechanical impediment to blood flow, adopt appropriate therapies to relieve the compression and thereby restore normal flow. Similarly, the osteopathic physician works to recognize in the healthy individual those areas or organs that might be at risk for reduced blood flow caused by lifestyle, activities, posture, obesity, etc. and adopt a treatment plan to maintain health in zones at risk.

Nerves

As do arteries, nerves also supply vital components to every portion of the body. First, nerves supply control; they are a major component of the body's homeostatic mechanisms. Nerve cell bodies in the CNS send nerve fibers to control contraction of smooth (involuntary) muscles and skeletal (voluntary) muscles and to control secretion of glands. Nerves also provide sensory input; they convey either exteroceptive input concerning physical forces that impinge on the body or interoceptive feedback about the status of the internal milieu. Nerve fibers also supply chemical materials from the CNS to the periphery and vice versa. Through the mechanism of axoplasmic transport, trophic (growth promoting) chemicals are manufactured in the neuron cell body and carried to target muscles

or organs where, after release into the synaptic space, they are taken into the target tissue and there promote healthy function. These substances can be small molecules (e.g., amino acids), well-known neurotransmitters (acetylcholine or serotonin), and more complex molecules also associated with other physiologic functions (substance-P, calcitonin gene-related polypeptide, somatostatin, glucagon, and vasoactive intestinal peptide are examples). Passing in the opposite direction, chemicals from the muscle or organ can cross the synapse, be taken up into the axon terminal, and be transported retrogradely to the neuron cell bodies where the chemicals can then alter basic neuronal function. Thus, a bidirectional communication is established fostering the exchange of information between the nervous system and the somatic and visceral tissues of the body.

As described above, individual peripheral nerves have specific segmental relationship to the CNS and, thence, to the entire body. The segmental origin of nerves is pertinent to three general targets of innervation: skin, muscles, and internal organs. The dermatomal (skin) innervation pattern is relatively straightforward. Pain or sensory loss over some specific dermatomal zone leads the physician to inferences about the integrity of restricted areas of the CNS or nerves near their origin. Innervation of the skin of the limbs becomes a bit more complicated because the sensory nerves from specific spinal cord segments are drawn together into specific cutaneous nerves that contain sensory fibers from more than one segment. A specific peripheral nerve (e.g., the medial cutaneous nerve of the forearm) will contain fibers from two or more segments (in this case C8 and T1), although those fibers will distribute at their termination in the skin in a dermatomal pattern. Here, the notion is that the examining physician must have sufficient understanding of anatomy to be able to differentiate sensory disturbances that arise in a particular peripheral nerve (peripheral neuropathy) as opposed to an entire segmental level as occurs in a radicolopathy.

The innervation pattern of muscles is particularly pertinent to osteopathic medicine because changes in the tone, texture, or function of a muscle may be related to the segmental source of nerve supply to that muscle. The innervation of muscles of the trunk is relatively simple and follows a pattern similar to that of the dermatomes. Nerve fibers to the muscles of the limbs, on the other hand, arise from the spinal cord and are woven through complex networks (the brachial plexus and lumbosacral plexus) that combine fibers from several spinal cord segments into motor nerves that typically serve functional groups of muscles. A physician must understand innervation of limb muscles well enough to reconstruct those nerve fibers from their termination, through the plexus to their spinal cord origin. As with the sensory nerves, the goal for the physician is to be able to differentiate motor losses due to compromise of a distal, peripheral nerve versus losses associated with lesion of one or more spinal cord segments or associated spinal nerves.

The internal viscera receive abundant autonomic nerve supply, and the sensory innervation to the internal viscera that signals functional status, distention, and pain typically accompanies the autonomic innervation to the target organ. The pattern by which this autonomic and sensory nerve supply arises from the spinal cord or brainstem and passes to target tissue is presented in Chapter 10, The Autonomic Nervous System. The key point to be made, however, is that because of developmental and maturational events, an organ in the adult may come to be relatively distant from its embryonic, segmental origin having pulled its nerve supply with it, however. Thus, changes in that organ will be sensed by nerve fibers that report to the part of the developed neural tube (i.e., the spinal cord or brainstem) that was adjacent to its embryonic, segmental origin. As a result, changes in a particular visceral organ may appear as pain to the body surface some distance from the organ. And, the painful or altered input from an organ can alter the somatic and autonomic outflow from that part of the spinal cord, too. For example, aberrant sensory feedback from a diseased organ can produce changes in muscle tonus or sympathetic function at a seemingly unrelated site. Conversely, painful sensory input from localized musculoskeletal misalignment may produce alteration in autonomic outflow from the related segmental zone of the spinal cord and may disturb function in an internal organ some distance away from that segment. In a very general way, internal organs map to the body surface and vice versa. The osteopathic physician must understand both the general segmental origin and the anatomical pathway by which autonomic nerve fibers and the accompanying sensory nerve fibers pass to the various internal organs and must be alert to the implications of pain and musculoskeletal changes as diagnostic clues and treatment options.

Nerves supply important functional and trophic control to all parts of the body. An important aspect of osteopathic medical practice is to recognize and treat conditions that alter nerve supply to a region or organ. The success of palpation and treatments in recognizing and relieving compression or irritation to nerves and the effectiveness of maintenance of nerve traffic by healthy lifestyles depend directly on how well the physician understands the route that nerves take from their origin to their destination.

Veins and Lymphatics

While the arterial supply is the only means by which fluid and blood cellular components are taken to an area, two pathways remove fluids and blood cells from a region. The venous network collects the deoxygenated blood from the capillary bed; the lymphatic channels drain the relatively cell-free extracellular fluid that accumulates outside the vascular system. Compromise to either of these return channels leads to edema in the affected area: more fluid goes in than comes out.

To alleviate edema, the osteopathic physician may choose to use protocols to enhance venous and/or lymphatic return. The strategy selected depends, of course, on the medical condition of the patient as well as on a thorough knowledge of the anatomy of the venous and lymphatic systems. As with the arterial system, the knowledge of anatomy places venous and lymphatic channels into the context of surrounding organs, muscles, bones, fascia, etc., usually by appreciating those structures on the basis of subtle palpable or surface landmarks.

Peripheral venous channels tend to be somewhat variable, with considerable anastomoses. For general medical application, it is acceptable to understand the overall pattern of peripheral venous drainage and concentrate one's effort on the larger, more predictable central veins. Understanding the anastomoses of peripheral venous channels is useful in the treatment of the venous system. For example, venous anastomoses offer therapeutic strategies for the physician as alternate routes of venous drainage are established. Understanding the routes of venous anastomoses is vital also to correctly diagnosing pathology as significant venous blood flow through some anastomoses is unusual and may indicate a pathological condition. Most venous blood from the gastrointestinal system, for example, is drained through the portal venous system to the liver. But most of the blood from the lower half of the body wall and lower limbs drains into the inferior vena cava. There are some small, usually insignificant anastomoses between these two major venous channels. However, in disease states when large amounts of blood are shunted from the portal system to the caval system, these anastomotic vessels become enlarged. Internal anal hemorrhoids or esophageal varices are engorgements of these anastomotic vessels

and indicate shunting of blood from the portal venous system to the vena caval system and may, thus, indicate blockage of venous drainage to the liver—so-called portal hypertension—that results when the liver is diseased.

The rule of venous drainage is to know by which veins an area is typically drained of blood, by what routes blood drains if the typical route is blocked, and where the veins lie relative to the surrounding structures. This knowledge can assist in designing a plan for restoration of normal function in a patient suffering with edematous conditions.

Arteries bring blood into tissue, in capillary beds a filtrate of plasma, ions, and proteins are extruded into the extracellular spaces. Although veins will absorb some of this fluid, much protein is retained in the tissues. Removal of the protein is the job of the lymphatic system as will be discussed in Chapter 12 on the Lymphatic System.

Lymphatic channels are typically even more variable than veins in their gross morphology; knowing general patterns and spatial relations of lymph drainage is usually sufficient. Although they are less well defined anatomically, they are important to understand. As with venous return, selecting osteopathic approaches to treatment of edema assumes a working knowledge of the location of lymph channels and how to augment lymphatic flow. Lymph collects into blind-ended endothelial tubes in the periphery. These channels throughout the body merge into ever-larger channels, are filtered at predictable intervals by lymph nodes, and finally converge on (usually) two large lymphatic ducts in the root of the neck. These two lymphatic ducts then empty into the venous system near the heart.

As the lymphatic system has no centrally located, intrinsic pump as that seen in the circulatory system, fluid is moved from peripheral to central regions by osmotic pressure, skeletal muscular contractions, external pressure, pressure differences between the thorax and the abdomen, as well as by contraction of smooth muscle surrounding the lymphatic collecting vessels. There are various techniques to increase lymphatic return. When using techniques of muscle contraction or applying local pressure or lymphatic pump mechanisms, one needs prerequisite knowledge of the anatomy of lymphatic flow.

In addition to returning extracellular fluid to the general circulation, the lymphatic system and the lymph nodes are often indicators of disease. The lymphoid system houses important cells of the immune system. As a result of infection, lymphocytes proliferate and are sequestered in lymph nodes, where they attack pathogens (bacteria, viruses, etc.) in the lymph. Because of this important immune function, lymph nodes draining an infected area are often swollen and palpable.

Cancer in an organ will often metastasize to adjacent lymph nodes and will also cause node enlargement. It is crucial, therefore, that the examining physician understand the potential significance of enlarged lymph nodes. For example, breast cancer may metastasize to the lymph nodes on the lateral thoracic wall or in the axilla that drain lymph from the breast. Or, illustrating a less obvious anatomical relationship, an enlarged node above the clavicle in the root of the neck may indicate disease of the stomach. When enlarged lymph nodes are detected, the examining physician can use knowledge of the anatomical pattern by which lymph drains to infer the source of a disease process.

SUMMARY

The body, so often represented as a group of discrete regions or functional systems, is in reality an integrated whole. The integration of the body region to region and system to system is accomplished by a series of connectors. Some of these connectors, the endocrine and immune systems, are more commonly included in the context of physiology, biochemistry, or immunology. The nervous system, the vascular system, and the lymphatics are also important connectors, the structural components of which are part of anatomical disciplines. Finally, the visible connective tissues of the body, and particularly the fascia, are great physical connectors that bind organs or muscles into larger groups.

Coherent medical practice requires attention to the connected nature of the unified human organism. Typically, one disturbing force (a localized injury, lesion, or infection) causes a cascade of altered structural and functional changes in other areas or systems. Similarly, the treatment of localized disease or injury must be not only localized but must also attempt to bring the whole organism into healthy equilibrium. Planned treatments must account for not only the effect of the treatment protocol on the target site or organ system, but also the so-called side effect alterations brought about in distant, relatively healthy systems by the treatment.

Observe the obvious examples of body unity. Take time to appreciate the connected nature of the body. For didactic reasons, the body is traditionally disassembled into component parts or regions such as bones, muscles, vessels, nerves, thorax, gastrointestinal system, or upper limb. Yet it is important to be able mentally to reconstruct the intact specimen. The fundamental idea of holistic medicine is predicated on this.

SUGGESTED READINGS

Magoun HI. *Osteopathy in the Cranial Field*. 3rd Ed. Kirksville, MO: The Journal Printing Company, 1976.

Mennell J. *Joint Pain*. Boston, MA: Little, Brown & Company, 1964.

Still AT. *Autobiography of A.T. Still*. Kirksville, MO: Published by the author, 1897:219.

7

The Fascial System of the Body

FRANK H. WILLARD, CHRISTIAN FOSSUM, AND PAUL R. STANDLEY

KEY CONCEPTS

- Fascial is a unitary body system with a function that can be described as supportive, protective and healing in nature.
- Fascia is composed of irregular connective tissue that can have varying densities.
- Four fundamental layers of fascia can be described: a layer of pannicular fascia covering the body, a denser layer of investing fascia surrounding the musculoskeletal system of the axial and appendicular body, a complex series of meningeal fascial layers surrounding the central nervous system and a fatty layer of visceral fascial surrounding the body cavities and organ systems.
- Fascia has a dynamic aspect imparted by its cellular components especially the fibroblast and the myofibroblast

INTRODUCTION

Definition

Fascia is the connective tissue that unites all aspects of the body. While by definition it functions as packing tissue and organ system cushioning (Clemente, 1985; Standring, 2008), its cellular composition suggests that it is also critical for metabolic activity and immune surveillance (Cormack, 1987; see Chapter 6). Unfortunately, there is much confusion in the literature concerning the components of fascial, its architecture, and the distribution of fascia within the body (see discussion in Fasel et al., 2007). At the time of this writing, there did not appear to be any publication in which fascia is treated as a definable organ system in the body. This poses a problem when trying to decide which tissues actually belong to fascia and which are really part of another organ system such as a tendon, ligament, or joint capsule. Early writings described fascia in a broad sense as being everywhere interconnected and serving a packing function (Anderson and Makins, 1890); however, more recent studies, performed to solve surgical issues, have taken a more fractionated approach (e.g., Garcia-Armengol et al., 2008). *Gray's Anatomy* describes fascia as the "dissectable, fibrous connective tissue of the body, other than the specifically organized structures tendons, aponeuroses, and ligaments, are called fasciae" (Gray, 1948). This definition of fascia was introduced under C.M. Goss as editor of the American version of *Gray's Anatomy* in 1948, and it was maintained by Clemente in the most recent edition (Clemente, 1985). This definition is relatively clear in its exclusion of tendons, ligaments, and aponeurosis from the term *fascia*; it also goes on to describe the investing nature of most fascia providing a packing substance around muscles, tendon, ligaments, and aponeuroses as well as visceral organs. A similar definition of fascia is offered in the English version of *Gray's Anatomy* (Standring, 2008), where fascia is also described as having collagenous fibers that are generally interwoven as opposed to the parallel array of fibers seen in tendons, ligaments, and aponeuroses. In this chapter, we will offer a slightly expanded definition of fascia as a system (a) complete with blood supply, fluid drainage, and innervations and thus the largest organ system in the body, (b) composed of irregularly arranged fibrous elements of varying density, and (c) involved in tissue protection and healing of surrounding systems. As consistent with the definition in *Gray's Anatomy*, tendons, ligaments, and aponeuroses are excluded from the term *fascia* based on

their histological composition. We will then examine the cells and extracellular substance that constitute fascia. We will conclude with a discussion of the dynamics of fascia and its role in tissue repair.

Previous Studies of Fascia

In recent times, there has been a strong resurgence of interest in both basic and applied science research in fascia. Traditionally, the view has been that the fascias are inconsequential residues that are less important than the tissues with which they are associated (Benjamin, 2009). The term *fascia*, derived from Latin for *band* or *bandage*, emerged in its anatomical and medical usage in the 16th and 18th centuries. The sometimes vague and inconsistent descriptions of fascia in anatomy and across languages resulted in the publication of two anatomy texts in the 1930s solely devoted to the anatomy of the fascial planes (Gallaudet, 1931; Singer, 1935). Subsequently, based on developmental approaches involving studies of the sequential development of visceral changes as observed in closely graded series of human embryos, fetuses, newborn infants, and adults, a detailed investigation of the adult fascia was done (Hayes, 1950). It highlighted the process of development and organ migration producing different types of fascia in a predictable and confirmable pattern, referring to it as *migration fascia*. It also described the fascia resulting from fusion of the primitive mesenteries as *fusion fascia* and the *parietal fascia* as intrinsic to the structures in the wall of the developing abdominopelvic cavity (Hayes, 1950). This was probably one of the first attempts at linking embryological development and growth to the anatomy of the adult fascia. Innervation of the deep fascia in both human and animals in the form of nerve terminations consisting of free endings and simple small encapsulated endings was described around the same time (Stilwell, 1956), and it was proposed that they may have a kinesthetic function as well as contributing to pain transmission. Based on such observations and experimentations, it became more obvious that the fascia, rather than being an inert structure, with a passive function, is a very active tissue playing an important role in the economy of the body, and in health and disease (Snyder, 1956). Despite the advancement in the anatomical knowledge of the fascia, some confusion still remains on the proper terminology. Efforts has been made in recent years to standardize anatomical terminology with the introduction and constant revision of the *Nomina*

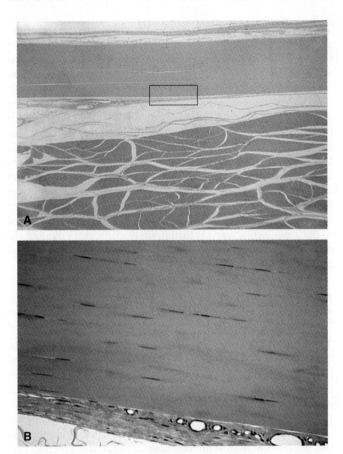

Figure 7-1 Photomicrographs of dense, regular connective tissue as seen in (A) a tendon (B) a ligament.

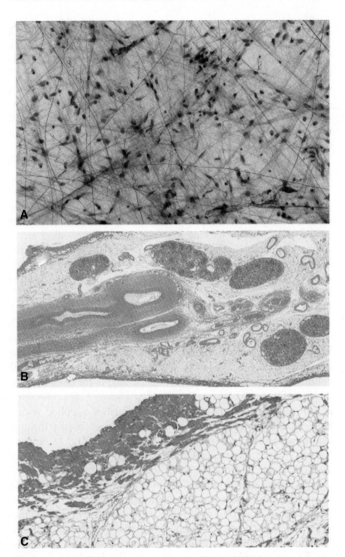

Figure 7-2 Forms of connective tissue typically found in fascia. **A.** This is a loose connective (areolar) tissue spread demonstrating a fairly random arrangement of collagenous and elastic fibers. (Taken from the University of New England, Histology Site.) **B.** This is a cross-section taken through mesentery demonstrating a thin layer of dense, irregular collagenous fibers underlying the mesothelium with a central core of adipose tissue surrounding several vessels and lymph nodes. Note the thickened tunica adventitia of the vessels. (Taken from the University of Michigan Histology Site.) **C.** This is a magnified view of the mesentery border showing the thin layer of dense irregular collagenous fibers underlying the single cell layer of mesothelium.

Anatomica, but despite this, adequate descriptions of fascial structures from an anatomical point of view are still lacking (Ercoli et al., 2005; Skandalakis et al., 2006).

Overview of Fascia

Tendons, ligaments, and joint capsules are generally composed of dense connective tissue with regularly arranged fibrous elements designed to meet specific functional requirements such as to resist pull, shear, or compressive stress in a given direction (Fig. 7.1). These elements typically have definable anatomical borders where tendons, ligaments, or joint capsules attach to surrounding structures. Conversely, by its very nature, fascia lacks this specificity in design; it packs the spaces around organ systems and interconnects between systems seemingly without providing specific functions (Fig. 7.2). This lack of specificity is best suited by an irregular arrangement of fibrous elements capable of resisting pull or stretch in multiple different directions. The irregular construction of fascial tissue also facilitates its continuity from one region of the body to another without forming the precise borders seen with such structures as tendons and ligaments of joint capsules. Thus, perimysium (fascia) is anatomically continuous with peritendium, which is anatomically continuous with perosteum on bone. All of these structures lack the well-defined border such as exists at a myotendonous border or an endthesis where muscle joins tendon and tendon joins bone, respectively.

The lack of precise borders seen in the fascial tissue allows it to form long planes spanning multiple organ systems or compartments surrounding one or more muscles. When entering fascial compartments, neurovascular bundles—which themselves are surrounded by irregular dense connective tissue fascial wrappings—course along or through fascial planes that would otherwise represent obstacles if composed of highly organized regularly arranged fibrous elements such as seen in a aponeurosis, tendon, ligament, or joint capsule. Lymphatic flow, which would be quickly interrupted if forced through tissue with precise boundaries, can flow easily through lymphatic vessels distributed in the irregular tissue of the fascial plane.

As with any other organ system, fascia has an innervation (see the section "Innervation of the Fascia"). As vessels course through fascial planes, they are typically accompanied by small-caliber nerve fibers. Some of these fibers contain catecholamines and belong to the autonomic nervous system (Bevan et al., 1980; Burnstock, 1980), whereas others are somatic nerve fibers (Stilwell, 1956), many of which contain neuropeptides (Walsh and McWilliams, 2006) and belong to sensory systems (also see Chapter 15 on Nociception). Endings from these fibers have a basal release of catecholamine and neuropeptide into the vessel wall and surrounding tissue. These compounds exert control over the vasculature and determine, in part, the texture of the tissue and the trafficking of white blood cells through the tissue.

Finally, like any other organ system of the body, fascia has definitive functions and capabilities. Most organ systems, including both musculoskeletal organs and visceral organs, are surrounded by a fascial capsule from which septae arise and penetrate into the organ often subdividing it into functionally distinct regions; this imparts fascia with a packing function as well as providing access routes for metabolic channels. In essence, fascia is acting as the skeleton for the specific organ system. As the body moves, so do its organs; to avoid friction and injury healthy fascia layers distort easily, tolerating stretch in multiple planes, and thereby providing a distensible cushion that allows organs to glide by each other while protecting more delicate fluid channels. Supplying each organ will be one or more neurovascular bundles and numerous lymphatic drainage routes; each of these communicates with the organ through its fascial layers. Thus, fascia is providing a movable conduit through which the neurovascular lifeline for the metabolic activity of the organ system passes.

Generally, all layers of fascia are themselves supplied with a well-organized blood supply and fluid drainage routes through venous and lymphatic channels (see Chapter 12 on Lymphatic System). Given the irregular arrangement of the fibrous nature of fascia, it is quick to initiate repair following injury and often will rapidly form a scar or callous. Thus, it plays an important role in wound healing and tissue repair. Although long thought to be relatively motionless—one prominent textbook of histology defines fascia as "non-contractile connective tissue"—recent evidence is beginning to demonstrate a slow contractile nature to fascial tissue. This contractile nature appears to be closely related the tissue repair process and will be discussed at the end of this chapter.

Architecture of Fascia

General Approach

Several attempts at describing the fascias of the body have been published (Benjamin, 2009; Gallaudet, 1931; Singer, 1935). Numerous discrepancies exist concerning which layers are considered fascia and how many subdivisions exist for each layer. Unfortunately, the lack of a clear definition of fascia has prevented any resolution of such arguments (Fasel et al., 2007; Skandalakis et al., 2006; Wendell-Smith, 1997). In this chapter, using irregular connective tissue as a histological definition, we will describe a system of four primary layers that cover the axial portion of the body. Modification of this fundamental plan will allow accommodation of the limbs.

The four primary layers in the torso are arranged as a series of concentric tubes. Starting with the outermost layer of fascia, it is best termed the *panniculus* or *panniculus adiposus*: a term used by Singer (Singer, 1935) in his treatise on fascia and strongly urged for general usage by Last (Last, 1978) in his textbook. This is an overall layer of fascia that covers the entire body and is exposed by removing the epidermis and dermis. Although the pannicular layer can be subdivided into several additional layers regionally in the body, for the sake of this chapter it will be considered as a primary layer. Deep to the pannicular layer is the *axial fascia* of the torso.

This layer gives rise to the investing fascia or epimysium of the axial muscles of the body and is continuous with the appendicular (investing) fascia in the extremity. As with the pannicular layer, the axial layer is subdivided; however, again in this chapter it will be treated as a primary layer. Internal to the axial fascia are two additional layers: the first surrounds the neural structures and is termed *meningeal fascia* and the second surrounds all body cavities and is best termed *visceral fascia*. In considering the limbs, the pannicular layer extends outward covering the entire surface of the limb. Under the pannicular layer, a fascial layer of similar composition to the axial fascia is present surrounding the muscles of the extremity and can be termed *appendicular fascia*, it lies deep to the pannicular fascia and invests the appendicular muscles. Regional names often relate the fascia to a specific muscle such as deltoid fascia. Internal to the appendicular fascia is the intramuscular septum housing the neurovascular bundles; this septal layer is thought to be derived from developmentally the axial fascia at the base of the limb.

FOUR PRIMARY LAYERS OF FASCIA

Pannicular Fascia

The outermost layer is the pannicular fascia (reviewed in Clemente, 1985). This superficial layer is derived from the somatic mesenchyme and surrounds the entire body with the exception of its orifices such as the orbits, nasal passages, and the oral and aboral openings. It is composed of both loose and dense irregular connective tissue with a highly variable fat content (Fig. 7.3). While the outermost portion of this layer is typically invaded by adipose tissue, the inner portion is membranous in nature and generally very adherent to the outer portion except over the abdomen where the two can be easily separated by blunt dissection. The thickness of the pannicular layer is highly variable in the human population. In the region of the head and neck, humans have several thin muscles embedded in the pannicular fascia; these are the platysma (Fig. 7.4) and associated facial muscles innervated by the facial nerve. Pannicular fascia covers both the axial and appendicular body.

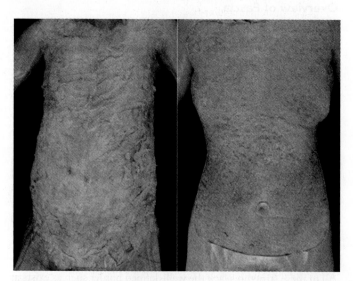

Figure 7-3   The pannicular layer of fascia. This is an anterior view of the thorax and abdomen of a male and a female cadaver. The body on the left is that of a 54-year-old male and on the right a 54-year-old female. Both specimens have had the dermis removed to reveal the pannicular layer of fascia. (Used with permission from the Willard/Carreiro Collection.)

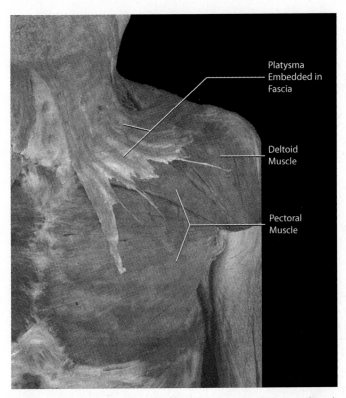

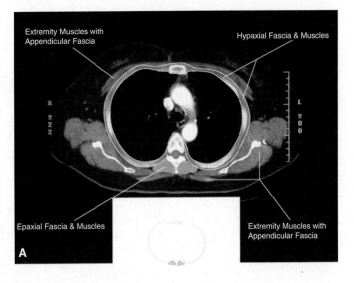

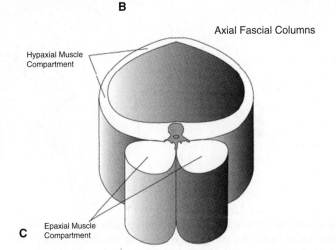

Figure 7-4 This is an anterior view of the upper thorax and neck illustrating the platysma, a pannicular muscle, embedded in the pannicular fascia and separated from the underlying muscles. The deltoid and pectoral muscles are extremity muscles and are normally embedded in fascia derived from the extremity. The investing fascia of the extremity has been cleaned off of the deltoid and pectoral muscles. (Used with permission from the Willard/Carreiro Collection.)

A complex relationship exists where the extremities meet the axial portion of the body. The muscles of the upper extremity form a hood that extends medially from the humerus and scapula, coursing deep to the pannicular fascia to reach their attachments on or near the midline. Each muscle is surrounded by appendicular fascia (also termed *deep investing fascia of the muscle*). The appendicular muscles and their associated fascia pass between the pannicular layer and the axial fascia layers until they can make an attachment. Therefore, these large wing-shaped muscles, such as the trapezius, latissimus dorsi, rhomboideus, and pertoralis muscles, have to reach to the spinous process on the posterior midline or the sternum or ribs anteriorly for their attachment to the torso.

Axial and Appendicular Fascia

Internal to the pannicular layer is the axial or investing fascia (*deep fascia* as described in Clemente, 1985); it is also derived from somatic mesenchyme and is fused to the panniculus peripherally and extends deep into the body surrounding the hypaxial and epaxial muscles (see the chapter on Anatomy). This layer forms the epimysium of skeletal muscle, the periosteum of bone, and the peritendon of the tendons. The axial layer can be depicted as two tubes of fascia separated centrally by the vertebral column (notochord in the embryo; Fig. 7.5): the anterior tube surrounds the hypaxial muscles and attaches to the vertebral column at the transverse process. The hypaxial muscles include the longus and scalene muscles in the cervical region, the intercostals muscles in the thoracic region and the oblique and rectus muscles in the abdominal

Figure 7-5 This is an axial plane spiral CT taken through a male thorax. The white outline surrounding the axial muscles—hypaxial and epaxial—marks the course of the axial fascia. (Used with permission from the Willard/Carreiro Collection.)

region. The posterior tube of axial fascia surrounds the epaxial muscles and is attached to the transverse processes. At each level, the vertebral spinous process divides the epaxial fascial tube into two "half-tubes" (Fig. 7.5). The paraspinal muscles of the back are contained in the smaller "half-tube" of the epaxial fascia.

Axial fascia extends into the extremities as the intermuscular septum and the appedicular fascia investing individual muscles (Fig. 7.6). The fascial sheath that surrounds the neurovascular bundles such as the brachial plexus and lumbosacral plexus extends outward to form the intermuscular septum in which branches of the neurovascular bundle will course as they progress distally in the extremity.

The arrangement of fascias within the body wall is made very complex by the attachment of the limbs. The muscles of the upper extremity, such as the pectoralis, trapezius, serratus anterior, and latissimus dorsi muscles, form long wing-like expansions that wrap over the torso to attach to the midline of the body or to structures that ultimately attach to the midline such as the thoracolumbar fascia (Fig. 7.7). These extremity muscles pass internal to the panniculus of fascia and external to the axial fascia as they embrace the axial body wall. Each muscle is surrounded by a layer of investing or appendicular fascia. The arrangement of these fascia sheets is visualized in the two dissections illustrated in Figures 7.8–7.12. In Figure 7.8, the

Figure 7-6 The fascia surrounding the neurovascular bundle in the axial portion of the body extends outward into the extremity. (Taken from L. H. Mathers, R. A. Chase, J. Dolph, E. F. Glasgow, and J. A. Gosling. *Clinical Anatomy Principles*, St Louis: Mosby, 1996.)

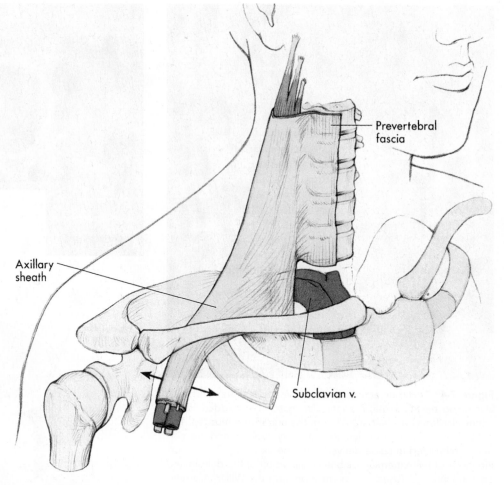

Prevertebral fascia

Axillary sheath

Subclavian v.

epidermis and dermis have been removed to expose the underlying pannicular fascia. An elongated rectangular window (outline) was opened into the pannicular fascia to expose the investing fascia (appendicular fascia) of the pectoral muscles. In Figure 7.9 the window was enlarged and divided into two portions, the medial portion still has appendicular fascia covering the muscle, but in the lateral portion the investing appendicular fascia has been removed to expose the pectoralis muscle. With the inferolateral border of the pectoral muscle elevated (Fig. 7.10), the investing (appendicular) fascia separates it from the serratus anterior can be visualized. To expose the

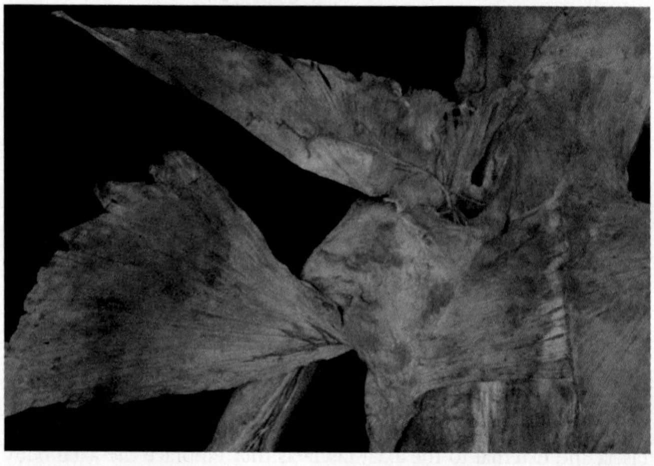

Figure 7-7 Wing-like arrangement of the trapezius and latissimus dorsi. (Used with permission from the Willard/Carreiro Collection.)

axial investing fascia of the intercostals muscles, the pectoral major and serratus anterior muscles and their investing appendicular fascia must be removed (Fig. 7.11). In this figure, the pectoralis major and serratus anterior muscles have been removed to expose the intercostals muscles and their thin layer of investing axial fascia (note that the pectoralis minor muscle is still attached). Finally, Figure 7.12 shows the exposed intercostals muscles by carefully dissecting away all axial fascia.

Meningeal Fascia

The third fascial layer is meningeal fascia, which surrounds the nervous system (Fig. 7.13). This layer, including the dura and the underlying leptomeninges, derives from the primitive meninx that surrounds the embryonic nervous system. Specifically the spinal meninges is most likely derived from the somatic mesoderm, while the brainstem meninges arises from cephalic mesoderm and the telecephalic meninges from the neural crest (Catala, 1998). Meningeal fascia terminates with the development of the epineurium that surrounds the peripheral nerve.

Visceral Fascia

The fourth fascial layer is visceral fascia and is by far the most complex of the four main layers of fascia. Embryologically, this layer of fascia is derived from the splanchnic tissue and thus surrounds the body cavities—pleural, pericardial, and peritoneal. The visceral layer follows the visceral pleura and peritoneum and provides the conduit for neurovascular bundles entering the visceral organs as well as a drainage route out of the organ. On the midline of the body, the visceral fascia forms a thickened mediastium that extends from the cranial base into the pelvic cavity (Fig. 7.12).

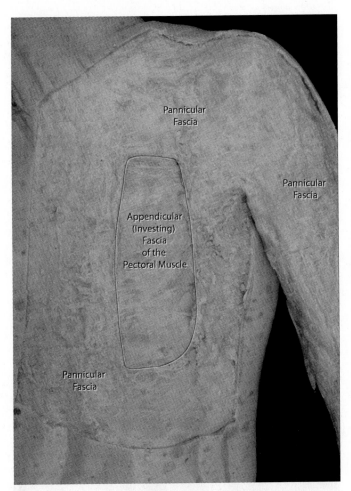

Figure 7-8 This is a photograph of a male with the epidermis and dermis removed to expose the pannicular fascia on the chest wall. A vertical window has been cut in the pannicular fascia to expose the underlying appendicular fascia. (Used with permission from the Willard/Carreiro Collection.)

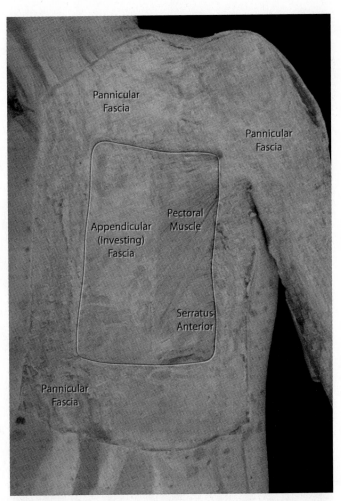

Figure 7-9 The fascia of the anterior chest wall. A window has been cut in the pannicular fascia on the left side of the window the appendicular fascia investing the pectoralis major is seen. On the right side of the window this fascia has been removed to demonstrate the muscle. (Used with permission from the Willard/Carreiro Collection.)

In the cranial region, visceral fascia surrounds the pharynx and its attachment to the cranial base. Superiorly, visceral fascia includes the pharyngobasalar and pharyngobuccal fascia and, as such, fuses to the cranial base surrounding the attachments of the superior constrictor muscles (Last, 1978). Cervical visceral fascia extends inferiorly into the neck surrounding the nasopharynx, orophaynx, and remaining cervical viscera. Thus, at the cranial base, cervical fascia has a flared opening surrounding the nasal passageways and the mouth (Fig. 7.14, Sections 22 and 46)

In the neck, visceral fascia incorporates such regional fascias as pretracheal, retropharyngeal, and alar (carotid sheath) fascias as well as the fascia surrounding the thyroid cartilage and thyroid gland (Fig. 7.14, Section 66 and 86). Thus, visceral fascia can be conceived of as a continuous vertical sleeve lying internal to the hyoid muscles, anterior to the longus muscles and extending into the thorax (Fig. 7.15).

Upon entering the thorax, the visceral fascia is forced to accommodate the two pleural cavities; this it does by flattening on to the thoracic wall where it is termed *endothoracic fascia*. Centrally, visceral fascia expands in bulk and forms the packing substance of the mediastinum (Fig. 7.-15). In the mediastinum, visceral fascia surrounds the great vessels of the heart and thickens to become the fibrous pericardium anteriorly. Posteriorly, the visceral fascia forms a loose matrix surrounding the aorta, esophagus, trachea, primary bronchi, and the thoracic duct. This matrix is very loose to allow distension of the esophagus upon swallowing. No significant condensations of fascia are present in this region. Finally, visceral fascia surrounds the bronchi as they pass through the root of the lung; this fascia becomes continuous with the stroma of the airways.

Visceral fascia also accompanies the esophagus into the abdominal cavity. Here, the visceral layer spreads outward to surround the peritoneum where it is termed *endoabdominal fascia* posteriorly and *transversalis fascia* anteriorly. The endoabdominal fascia thickens significantly along the posterior midline and forms a column analogous to the mediastinum of the thoracic (Fig. 7.16). As in the thorax, the abdominal mediastinum contains the major vascular and neural channels. Extensions of the abdominal mediastinal fascia pass into the mesogastrium, mesentery and mesocolon to reach the visceral organs of the abdomen. It is along this pathway that the blood supply, innervation, and lymphatic channels reach the peritoneal organs. This situation is remarkably similar to that seen with the mediastinum of the thorax, the root of the lung, and the lung tissue. The endoabdominal (visceral) fascia is especially thick surrounding the kidneys where it forms a perirenal fat pad termed *Gerota's fascia* (Fig. 7.17).

In the pelvic basin, the endoabdominal fascia becomes continuous with the endopelvic fascia, which then surrounds the inferior region of the peritoneum. The inferior border of the endopelvic

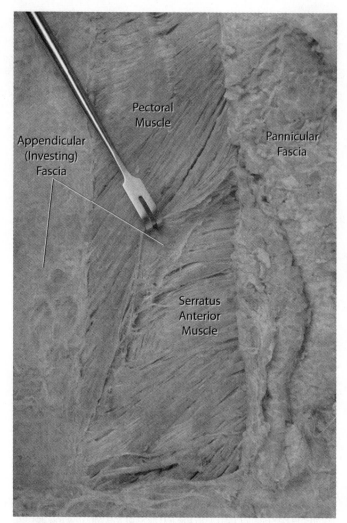

Figure 7-10 The fascia of the anterior chest wall. A window has been cut in the pannicular fascia as described in figure 7-9. The inferolateral border of the pectoralis major muscle has been elevated to reveal the investing appendicular fascia separating this muscle from the underlying anterior serratus. (Used with permission from the Willard/Carreiro Collection.)

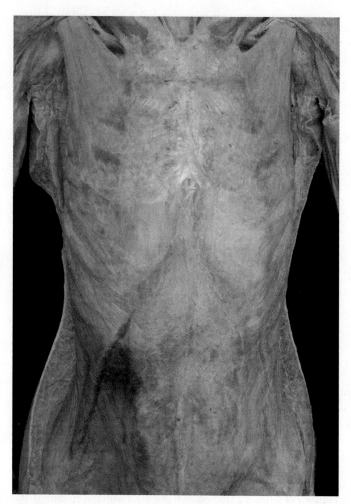

Figure 7-11 The pectoralis major muscle has been removed exposing the underlying axial fascia that surrounds the sternum, ribs, and intercostal muscles. The pectoralis minor is still in place on this female specimen. (Used with permission from the Willard/Carreiro Collection.)

fascia is the pelvic diaphragm composed of the levator ani and coccygeus muscles. Inferior to the pelvic diaphragm is the ischorectal (ischoanal) fossa; it is packed with pannicular fascia (Fig. 7.18). The anterior and inferior border of the endopevic fascia fills the retropubic space surrounding the base of the urinary bladder. As in the thorax and abdomen, the endopelvic fascia thickens on the midline where it again forms a mediastinum surrounding the rectum, reproductive organs, and urinary bladder. Similar to the mediastinum in the thorax and abdomen, the endopelvic fascia serves as a conduit through which the major organ systems in the pelvic basin receive their blood supply and innervations as well as their lymphatic drainage. In the female, extensions of the pelvic mediastinal component of the visceral fascia form the core of the broad ligament and condensations of this visceral fascia form the transverse cervical ligament of the uterus.

In summary, visceral fascia can be traced from the cranial base into the pelvic cavity. It forms the packing surrounding the body cavities where it is compressed against the somatic body wall. It also forms the packing around visceral organs, many of which it reaches by passing along the suspensory ligaments such as the mesenteries. This fascia also functions as a conduit for the neurovascular

and lymphatic bundles as they radiate outward from the thoracic, abdominal, and pelvic mediastinum to reach the specific organs.

Visceral Ligaments

A note here is necessary concerning the used of the word *ligament* when referring to structures found in the body cavity. Visceral ligaments are in no sense of the word similar to the ligaments seen in somatic body parts. Ligaments in the somatic portion of the body are structures that join bone to bone and are composed of dense, regular connective tissue, which itself is surrounded by a thin periligamentum of investing fascia, typically part of the axial or appendicular fascia. The word *ligament* used for structures found in body cavities such as pulmonary ligaments, Trietz ligament, transverse cervical ligament or broad ligament refers to a loose condensation of visceral fascia (irregular connective tissue of varying density) in some cases surrounded by a thin serous membrane. Visceral ligaments generally cannot bear as much strain as somatic ligaments nor are they as clearly defined on dissection. Unlike ligaments in somatic tissue, visceral ligaments typically function to carry blood supply and innervations to an organ system or to loosely anchor an organ in the body cavity. Visceral

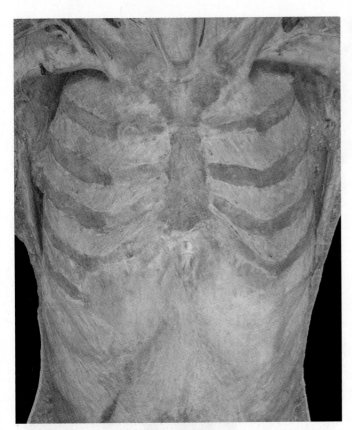

Figure 7-12   The axial fascia has been removed to expose the sternum, ribs, and intercostal muscles. (Used with permission from the Willard/Carreiro Collection.)

ligaments also need to be distinguished from fibrotic adhesions that typically develop secondary to irritation and inflammation.

Adhesions

Fibrotic adhesions derive from areas of chronic inflammation (Wynn, 2008). Activated immune cells release cytokines that stimulate fibrocytes to generate additional collagen during the repair process (some of the mechanisms involved in this process will be described in a later section of this chapter). The collagen laid down is irregular in arrangement and is thus similar to fascia in its construction. When excessive, these bands of increased collagen can form adhesions that can reach pathological proportions. Adhesions can occur in any region of the body either visceral or somatic. In the abdomen and pelvis, adhesions can envelope the tubular bowel and be strong enough to obstruct movement within its lumen or interfere with reproductive organ functions. Similarly, adhesions forming in and around synovial sheaths in the carpal tunnel can interfere with movement of the digital flexor tendons.

Innervation of the Fascia

It has been proposed that the fascia plays an important role in musculoskeletal biomechanics, peripheral motor coordination, proprioception, regulation of posture and as a potential pain generator (Langevin, 2008; Langevin and Sherman, 2007; Stecco et al., 2007). Central to these roles is the innervation and the cellular-mediated contractility of the fascia. Reports suggest that the fascia is richly innervated, and abundant free and encapsulated nerve endings have been described at a number of anatomical sites (Benjamin, 2009). These include the thoracolumbar fascia, the

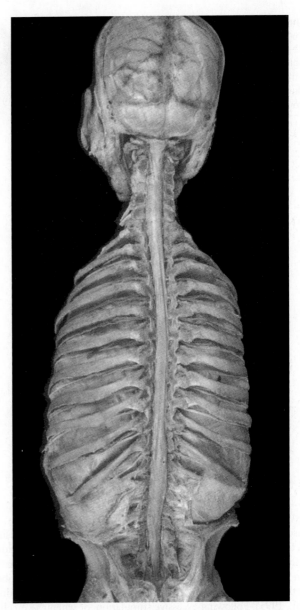

Figure 7-13   The paraspinal muscles have been removed and a total laminectomy preformed to expose the spinal dural sac. In addition, the occipital bone was removed to demonstrate the cranial dura. (Used with permission from the Willard/Carreiro Collection.)

bicipital aponeuroses, and the crural fascia (Palmieri et al., 1986; Sanchis-Alfonso and Rosello-Sastre, 2000; Staubesand and Li, 1996; Stecco et al., 2006, 2007; Stilwell, 1957; Tanaka and Ito, 1977; Yahia et al., 1992). These nerve endings are particularly numerous around vessels, but are also distributed homogeneously throughout the fibrous components of the fascia (Stecco et al., 2008). Besides the identified Ruffini, Pacini, and Golgi-Mazzoni corpuscles and their possible proprioceptive role (Schleip, 2003a; Stecco et al., 2007; Yahia et al., 1992), some of the nerve fibers associated with the fascia are adrenergic and likely to be involved in controlling local blood flow (Benjamin, 2009). This is supported by reports that when intrafascial nerve fibers were subjected to morphological evaluation, they exhibited characteristics typical of autonomic nerve fibers (Stecco et al., 2008).

As for the proposed proprioceptive role, the fascia should be considered in close association with its related muscles. When

Figure 7-14 Cervical Visceral Fascia. These images are a series of four cervical CT sections from one individual with the visceral fascia indicated by shading. This fascia begins as a flared opening (section 22 and 46) attached to the cranial base and consolidates into a continuous column of irregular connective tissue as it descends through the neck (sections 66 and 86).

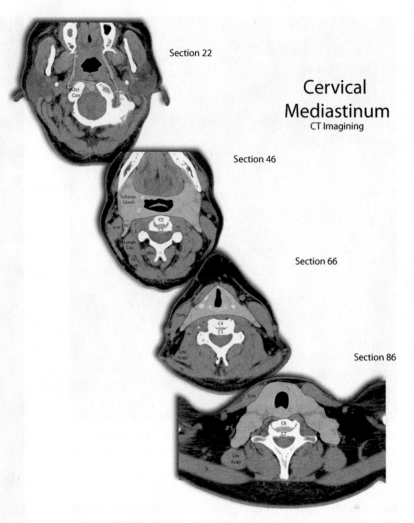

muscles contract, their tension is transmitted to the fascia causing traction of it, possibly activating nerve terminals embedded in the fascia (Stecco et al., 2007, 2008). The degree of innervation may also change in patients with chronic pain, as described in thoracolumbar fascia in patients with back pain (Bednar et al., 1995). Following excessive stimulation, or when the mechanoreceptors are stretched beyond their physiological limit, they

have the ability of becoming nociceptors (Stecco et al., 2007). It has also been suggested that manual loading of fascia as in various manual medicine modalities may cause changes through activation of these receptors (Lundon, 2007; Schleip, 2003a,b). Despite the recent advances in knowledge concerning the innervation of the fascia, our understanding of it is still very incomplete (Benjamin, 2009).

COMPONENTS OF FASCIA

Fascia is composed connective tissue with varying densities of irregularly arranged collagenous fiber. As such, the components of fascia are the items typically found in irregular connective tissue.

Cellular Elements

Fibroblasts

Fascia supports connective, biochemical, and biophysical associations between itself and underlying muscles, bones, and organs. Fibroblasts are the principal cell type of fascia; they synthesize and secrete cytokines (e.g., interleukins [ILs], interferons, growth factors, etc.) as well as connective tissue extracellular matrix proteins (ECMPs) such as collagen, fibronectin, and others (Fig. 7.19). Fibroblasts also secrete and maintain connective tissue ground substance containing glycosaminoglycans, proteoglycans, hyaluronic acid, and glycoproteins. This ground substance provides the medium through which exchange of molecules between

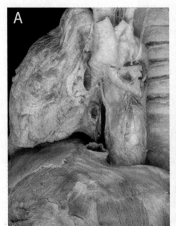

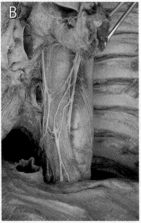

Figure 7-15 The mediastinum: visceral fascia. In A, the esophagus, vagus nerve and aorta are still embedded in the visceral fascia while in B, the visceral fascia has been removed to expose these organs. (Used with permission from the Willard/Carreiro Collection.)

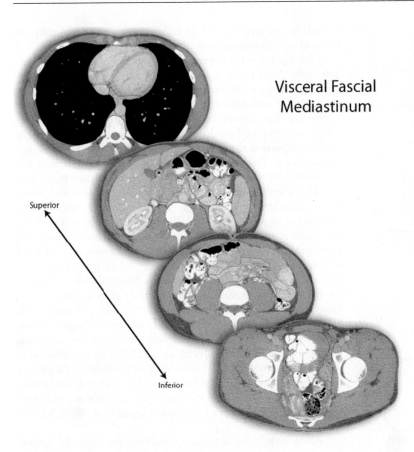

Visceral Fascial
Mediastinum

Figure 7-16 This is a series of four axial plane CT scans taken through the thorax, abdomen and pelvis of a patient. The visceral fascia has been outlined and faintly shade in each image.

blood, lymph, and tissue cells takes place thereby making fibroblast secretions deliverable both locally and systemically.

The shape of the fibroblast is dependent on the environment with which it is located; elongate or fusiform cell shapes are seen when the cell is at rest such as occurs in mature connective tissue where the cell is typically entangled in thick bundle of collagen fibers. The stellate cell shape is seen when fibroblasts are grown in tissue culture or are present in either immature or healing tissue or in a fibrotic tissue (Rhee and Grinnell, 2007). Fibroblast shape is also sensitive to the tension in the tissue; in the quiescent state, cells have spindle shapes with long dendritic process; however, when mechanically stressed, these cells round up becoming stellate in shape (Grinnell et al., 2003; Langevin et al., 2005).

Some fibroblasts are of mesenchymal origin, similar to osteocytes and chondrocytes; however, other fibroblasts, particularly those found in the connective tissue layers of visceral organs such as lung, liver, and kidney, arise from a process of transformation

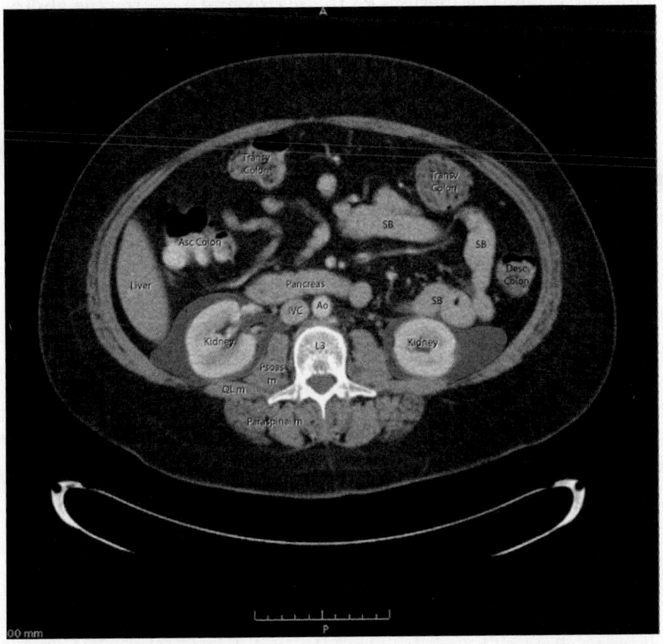

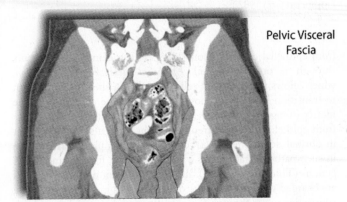

Pelvic Visceral
Fascia

Figure 7-18 The fascias of the pelvis. The levator ani separates the endopelvic fascia (lighter shading) that surrounds the pelvic viscera from the pannicular fascia of the ischiorectal fossa (darker shading). (Used with permission from the Willard/Carreiro Collection.)

Figure 7-17 The perirenal fascia. The perirenal pad of fat and fascia has been outlined and faintly shaded.

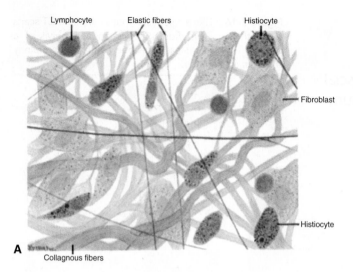

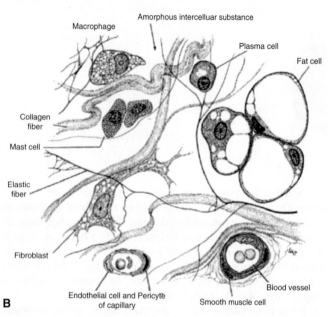

Figure 7-19 Histological sections of loose connective tissue demonstrating the fibrous and cellular components. (Figure **A** taken from Kelley DE, Wood RL, Enders AC. *Bailey's Textbook of Microscopic Anatomy.* Baltimore, MD: Williams & Wilkins, 1984; Figure **B** taken from Cormack DH. *Ham's Histology.* Philadelphia, PA: J.B. Lippincott Co., 1987.)

from epithelial cells (Neilson, 2006). This metamorphosis occurs through a process termed *Epithelial–Mesenchymal Transition*, which allows the polarized cells located in a sheet of epithelium to transition into highly motile cells inside the connective tissue matrix (Yang and Weinberg, 2008). The formation of fibroblasts from epithelial cells is currently thought to be a significant event in normal developmental processes as well as play a critical role in such pathological processes as tissue repair, fibrosis, and oncogenesis (Thiery et al., 2009). Regardless of their origin, fibroblasts are charged with maintenance of homeostasis in the matrix of the connective tissue through the production and remodeling of both fibers and the extracellular matrix (Laurent et al., 2007). Part of this task also involves monitoring and maintaining the appropriate degree of tension in the connective tissues (Grinnell et al., 2003; Tomasek et al., 2002) and the chemical quality of the tissue. Thus

fibroblasts are capable of both mechanoreception (responsive to tension) and chemoreception (responsive to growth factors).

Fibroblasts exist in the extracellular matrix of the fascia. A primary role of the fascia and its ECMPs is to endow cells and tissues with their specific mechanical and physiochemical properties. As such, the extracellular matrix represents a three-dimensional scaffolding that supports cellular adhesion and tissue-specific functions. Since imposed mechanical loads physically affect the fascia, it plays important simultaneous roles of force sensor as well as a transmitter of force input generated by muscle contractions and by external forces including osteopathic manipulative techniques (OMTs). Fibroblasts can detect the change in tension and generate an adaptive response, which can involve contraction and the secretion of large quantities of collagen. Thus, fascia itself may also be capable of smooth muscle-like contractions, thereby influencing underlying musculoskeletal dynamics and displaying the existence of true (i.e., skeletal muscle-independent) fascial tone (Hinz et al., 2004; Schleip et al., 2005). Osteopathic Manipulative Techniques are hypothesized to mediate corrections of such fascial hypertonicity and/or abnormal tissue collagen crosslinking (Gupta et al., 1998) which may occur postinjury or during prolonged immobilization. Therefore, due to their location within the trafficking ground substance, their ability to secrete ECMPs and mediators of pain and inflammation, and the ability to generate and transduce force input, fibroblasts have been thought to be uniquely poised to be targets of soft tissue injuries, myofascial release, and other Osteopathic Manipulative Techniques (Eagan et al., 2007; Meltzer and Standley, 2007).

Along with changing tension, fibroblasts also respond to growth factors and inflammatory substances secreted into the matrix from epithelial cells, mast cells, macrophages, and lymphocytes. Numerous cell types found in connective tissue, such as macrophages, mast cell, epithelial cells, and fibroblasts, produce transforming growth factor-beta (TGF-β) (Laurent et al., 2007). Similar to physical stress, activation of fibroblasts by TGF-β or inflammatory compounds leads to the expression of as many as 150 genes (Laurent et al., 2007). An end result of this process is the production of collagen and differentiation of the fibroblast into a myofibroblast with focal cellular adhesions to the matrix and a contractile ability (see the section "Myofibroblasts").

Fibroblasts form a distinct network in connective tissue. The long thin processes of the cell make contact with those of other fibroblasts creating a three-dimensional network within the tissue. Control of the formation of dendritic processes and their coupling with other fibroblast processes appears to lie with the balance of growth factors in the tissue. These factors, such as platelet-derived growth factor and lysophosphotidic acid, act on the fibroblast through a family of small g-proteins involving Rho and Rac (Grinnell et al., 2003). The gap junction protein, connexin 43, has been detected at points where fibroblast process make contact, yet, to date, gap junctions, as seen with electron microscopy, have not been visualized at these points of contact between fibroblast processes. However, the presence of the connexin protein on these processes raises the interesting possibility that the fibroblasts have an interconnected communications network throughout connective tissue that functions through the membrane-bound connexin proteins. The concept of an interconnected cellular network among fibroblasts would not be out of context since similar networks are seen between mature osteocytes (mesenchymal-derived cells) located in bone as well as between fibroblasts located around bundles of collagen fibers in tendons. In both bone and tendon, these cellular networks function to detect mechanical stress and orchestrate an adaptive response by the tissue (Banes et al., 1995).

Myofibroblasts

Myofibroblasts are differentiated fibroblasts that share many cellular and biochemical similarities with smooth muscle cells. These cells can arise from fibroblasts in connective tissue (Fig. 7.21); however, they also can be derived from epithelial cells or endothelial cells through a transformation process. In addition, a circulating fibroblast like-bone marrow stem cell capable of forming myofibroblasts has been described (Wynn, 2008) and in liver, stellate cells along the margins of the sinusoids transform into myofibroblasts.

Histochemically, myofibroblasts express a number of specific markers used to differentiate them from undifferentiated fibroblasts. These include alpha smooth muscle actin (αSMA), cadherin II (Ehrlich et al., 2006), and paladin 4lg (Ronty et al., 2006). In some tissues, myofibroblasts play longstanding resident roles of support and immunology. For example, myofibroblasts normally function to maintain and regulate shape of crypts and villi in the alimentary tract but can also act as stem cells and as atypical antigen-presenting cells. They lend structural support to tissues and perform paracrine/endocrine functions. In most other tissues, myofibroblasts exist in the short term to facilitate wound healing. After injury, myofibroblasts resemble many aspects of a smooth muscle cell and, when activated, migrate to sites of damaged tissues and synthesize cytokines and ECMPs to facilitate healing (Hinz, 2007). Signals for fibroblast to myofibroblast differentiation include biomechanical strain and a variety of cytokines, most notably TGF-β (Fig. 7.20). In response to mechanical strain, fibroblasts acquire contractile stress fibers (Werner and Grose, 2003) composed of cytoplasmic actins. At this stage, a unique phenotype, the protomyofibroblast, appears to exist. These cells begin the process connecting to ECMPs via stress fibers and to other cells via N-cadherin-type adherens junctions (Hinz et al., 2004). Normally, at the conclusion of tissue repair, the reconstructed ECMPs (produced by matured myofibroblasts) take over the mechanical load, leading to the lack of further need for resident myofibroblasts (Tomasek et al., 2002). Increased interstitial fluid flow increases fibroblast to myofibroblast differentiation, collagen production, and alignment and fibroblast proliferation. These observations lead to the speculation that enhanced lymphatic drainage may play a role in fibrogenesis and fascial repair by promoting interstitial fluid flow (Hinz et al., 2004). Expression of αSMA allows for significant contractile ability (Hinz et al., 2001). This process appears to be irreversible and be regulated at the level of Rho/Rho kinase-mediated inhibition

of myosin light chain phosphatase (Tomasek et al., 2006). If this occurs throughout the fascia, then the hypothesis that fascia is capable of contraction may have its origin in the recruitment and/or differentiation of fibroblasts to myofibroblasts (Schleip et al., 2005). Since myofibroblasts express gap junctions, cell: cell communication is facilitated and potential syncitial behavior, such as coordinated contraction of large sheets of myofibroblasts (Gabbiani et al., 1971) lends further support that fascia has the capacity for myofascial-mediated contraction that is propagated and reinforced cell to cell.

Macrophages

Several types of cells typically found in connective tissue appear to have the ability to activate fibroblasts, enhance fibrosis, and most likely increase the transformation of these cells into myofibroblasts. The first of these cell types is the fixed macrophage or histiocyte (Fig. 7.14); these cells represent the major link between the fascia system and the immune system. Macrophages are derived from circulating monocytes that have migrated into the tissue. Once in the tissue, monocytes differentiate into one of three main lineages: tissue macrophages (histiocytes such as is seen in fascia, Kuppfer cells in the liver, and microglia in the central nervous system), myeloid dendritic cells such as is found in the skin and gut lining, or osteoclasts in bone. Cellular debris or proinflammatory cytokines in the surrounding extracellular matrix activate tissue macrophages. Activation increases macrophage phagocytic capabilities and their secretory activity, producing additional cytokines. Taken together, macrophages and monocytes are the largest producer of tumor necrosis factor-α (TNF-α) (Papadakis and Targan, 2000). In addition, activated macrophages express more class II MHC molecules and are more potent antigen-presenting cells than resting macrophages. Migration of additional macrophages into injured tissue is further enhanced by proinflammatory substances. Importantly, activated tissue macrophages release TGF-β1, which promotes the proliferation and differentiation of collagen-producing cells such as fibroblasts and myofibroblasts (Kisseleva and Brenner, 2008). These processes predispose to increased fibrosis and scar or adhesion formation.

Mast Cells

Scattered throughout connective tissue and typically associated with neurovascular bundles are histamine-containing mast cells. The precursors of these histamine-containing cells are generated by hematopoietic stem cells in bone marrow. Contrary to histamine-containing basophils, the precursors of the mast cells enter the circulation in an immature form and do not complete their maturation until they enter the peripheral tissue. Mast cells are heterogeneous with at least two populations identifiable by staining, one group contains trypase and favors visceral organs in their distribution and the other group contains multiple protease enzymes and is more often found in connective tissue such as dermis. Commonly associated with the response to parasite invasion, mast cells are known to have other functions in connective tissue as well. These granule-laden cells are capable of phagocytosis and the production of proinflamatory cytokines. Mast cells express FcεRI, a receptor that binds the Fc portion of the IgE antibody. When IgE binds to the cell, a degranulation process is initiated resulting in the release of a host of biologically active agents such as histamine, heparin, chondroitin sulfates, neutral proteases (trypase), acid hydrolases, capthepsin G, and carboxypeptidase (Galli, 1993). The location of the mast cell in connective tissue facilitates the delivery of its active agents to fibroblasts. Connective tissue mast cells have been identified as carrying prefabricated stores of TNF-α, a potent proinflammatory

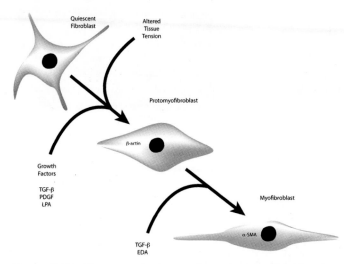

Figure 7-20 The stages in the transformation of a fibroblast into a myofibroblast.

compound that stimulates fibroblasts and results in fibrosis (Galli, 1993). Mast cell have been reported in increased numbers in tissue undergoing fibrosis (Metcalfe et al., 1997), but their role in tissue healing is not yet clarified. Thus, along with macrophages, mast cells appear to be capable of activating fibroblasts and enhancing the fibrosis occurring in and about an inflammatory event.

Extracellular Matrix Components

Connective tissue is composed of two major extracellular components: the first is a fibrous component responsible for the toughness of connective tissue and the second is the gel-like ground substance into which the cells and fibers are embedded. The most prevalent of the fibers present in connective tissue are those constructed of collagen molecules.

Collagen Fibers

Collagen is an insoluble fibrous protein, each fibrous molecule of which is made up of three pro-α-chains of amino acids woven together in a triple helix. The collagen molecules are woven together in a periodic manner as illustrated in Figure 7.21. Variations in the types of amino acids utilized in the α-chains create at least 27 described variants of collagen (Kavitha and Thampan, 2008). Differing collagens types are found in diverse tissue reflecting their various functions (Table 7.1). Major forms in the human body are types I, II, and III.

Although individual collagen molecules are synthesized intracellularly, the fibrils are assembled in the extracellular medium surrounding the cell. Collagen is produced by fibroblasts and myofibroblasts as well as by some forms of epithelial cells (Tabata et al., 2008). Activated monocyte also act as a potential source of collagen. Common factors that can enhance the production of collagen include acetaldehyde, a breakdown product of alcohol, radiation, ascorbic acid and, glucose (type III collagen only). Growth factors such as TGF-β and PDGF increase collagen synthesis, while TNF-α (originally named *cachexin*) suppresses collagen

synthesis. Minerals such as calcium and hormones such as estrogen enhance collagen synthesis, while parathyroid hormone decreases collagen synthesis (Kavitha and Thampan, 2008).

Elastic Fibers

Similar to collagen, elastin is a water-insoluble protein molecule, derived from tropoelastin. This precursor protein is synthesized in the cell and assembled into fibrils in the extracellular matrix. However, unlike collagen, tropoelastin is an amorphous substance and an additional molecule, a microfibril, has to be produced and secreted in order for elastic fibers to form. The microfibril acts as scaffolding into which the tropoelastin molecules are placed.

Elastic fibers are distensible and will rebound when released from a stressor; thus, as the percentage of elastin increases, the connective tissue becomes more resilient. Examples include the ligamentum flavum in the spine and the elastic layers present in the larger arteries.

Laminin and Fibronectin

To maintain healthy and responsive connective tissue, there must be a mechanism for linking its cellular components to the surrounding environment. This involves several glycoprotein molecules of which laminin and fibronectin are key representative examples. These molecules function, in part, to link the cytoskeleton of the cell to the fibrous skeleton—collagenous and elastic—of the surrounding connective tissue. Laminin and fibronectin are secreted from fibrocytes and bind with integrins (adhesion molecules) located on the membranes of cells as well as to matrix components such as collagen, fibrin, and heparin sulfate proteoglycons. In this manner, the cell attaches to the surrounding extracellular matrix and the resulting complex determines cell shape and facilitates cell migration through the matrix as well as enhancing the cells' responsiveness to stressors within the matrix.

Integrins initiate cell signaling processes leading to changes in cell function (Schwartz and DeSimone, 2008). Thus, integrins, by transmitting force across the cell membrane, represent a major

Figure 7-21   A diagram summarizing the formation and periodic nature of collagen fibrils. (Taken from Cormack DH. *Ham's Histology*. Philadelphia, PA: J.B. Lippincott Co., 1897.)

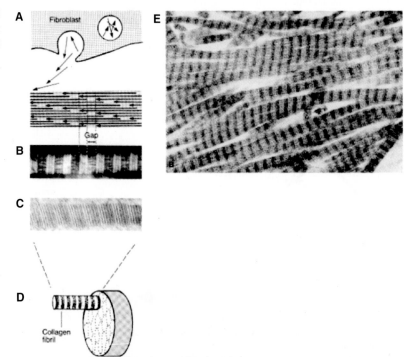

TABLE 7.1

Summary of collagen types along with their structure and function

Classes of Collagen	Collagen Type	Tissue Distribution	Ultrastructure	Site of Synthesis	Function
Fibril-forming collagens	I	Dermis, bone, tendon, teeth, fascia, sciera, organ capsules, fibrous cartilage	Densely packed thick fibrils with marked variation in diameter	Fibroblast, osteoblast, odontoblast	Resistance to tension
	II	Hyaline and elastic cartilage, intervertebral disc, vitreous	No fibers, very thin fibrils embedded in ground substance	Chondroblast	Resistance to tension
	III	Bone, skin, smooth muscle, arteries, uterus, kidney, lung, tendon, periosteum, endoneurium	Loosely packed thin fibrils with more uniform diameter	Fibroblast, smooth muscle cells, Schwann cells, hepatocytes, mesenchymal cells	Structural maintenance in expansile organs, wound healing, mediate attachments of tendon, ligament, and periosteum to bone cortex
	V	Skin, bone, tendon, synovial, membrane, liver, vascular tissue, placenta, teeth	Form quarter staggered fibrils	Fibroblats, osteoblasts	Control of fiber diameter
	XI	Cartilaginous tissue	Form quarter staggered fibrils	Chondrocytes	Control of fiber diameter
Fibril-associated collagens	IX	Uniform throughout cartilage matrix, vitreous humor	Covalently crosslinked to type II collagen fibrils	Chondrocytes	Contributor of mechanical stability and resistance to swelling of type II collagen framework
	XII	Ligament, tendon, perichondrium, periosteum, periodontal ligament, reticular dermis	Covalently crosslinked to type I collagen fibrils	Fibroblast, myoblast	Control of fiber diameter and interaction of proteoglycans
	XIV	Codistribued with type I	Covalently crosslinked to collagen fibrils	Fibroblast, myoblast, oteoblasts, endoneural and perineural cells	Control of fiber diameter and interaction or proteoglycans
	XVI	Skin and cartilage		Fibroblasts, keratinocytes	Maintenance, organization, and interaction of fibrillar structures in the ECM
Network forming collagens	IV	Basement membranes		Fibroblasts	Separates tissue compartments, surrounds many cell types (e.g., Smooth muscle cells and nerve cells), plays a role in regulation of cell growth, migration, and differentiation.

(continued)

TABLE 7.1		*(Continued)*		
Filamentous collagens	VI	Ubiquitous in connective tissue, concentrated in particular and adjacent to basement membranes of myofibers, blood vessels and intramuscular nerves	Fibroblasts, macrophages	Cell attachment, differentiation, suppression of apoptosis and as an anchoring meshwork for ECM structures
Short-chain collagens	VIII	Cornea and vascular tissue	Smooth muscle cells	Stimulates smooth muscle cell migration, invasion and binding in vascular tissue
	X	Hyaline cartilage	Chondrocytes	Possibly endochondral ossification and indirectly hematopoiesis
	XIII	Blood vessel wall, glomeruli of kidney, myotendinous junction	Fibroblasts, osteoblasts	
Long-chain collagens	VII	Skin basement membrane	Keratinocytes, fibroblasts	Secures basement membrane to adjacent connective tissue matrix

Sources: Liu et al., 1995; Culav et al., 1999; Hou et al., 2000; Kassner et al., 2004; Eble et al., 2006; Zou et al., 2008; Schnorr et al., 2008.

link between external mechanical force applied to the extracellular matrix and the cell and the initiation of movement and metabolic changes within the cell (Katsumi et al., 2004). This process has been termed *mechanotransduction* and is a feature of fibroblasts, chondrocytes, and osteoblasts. Importantly, stress and strain placed on the connective tissue can be transferred, through its fibrous component, to the cell membrane and cell cytoplasm. The time frame on this response is relatively rapid; changes in integrin composition can be noted in stressed cells within tens of seconds to tens of minutes after the onset of the stressor.

Mechanotransduction, leading to intracellular signal transduction, plays numerous roles in normal development, the maintenance of health and the ontogeny of disease, particularly in the aging process (Silver et al., 2003; Wu et al., 2009). Aging can impair the ability of skeletal muscle to respond to altered load and tension; the pathophysiological causes of these changes appear to involve intracellular signaling transduction pathways sensitive to mechanotransduction at the cell surface. Similarly, synovial joints respond best to cyclic stimulation; this quality is mediated by mechanotransduction and diminished in the aging joint. Additional age-related changes in mechanotransduction in the cardiovascular and respiratory systems underlie the onset of the loss of compliance in the heart as well as endothelial cell and smooth muscle dysfunction in the vasculature. Age-related loss in control of smooth muscle cell contraction, leading to airway hypersensitivity and hyperreactivity, is possibly related to a decreased sensitivity to tension in the airway walls, a result of the slow loss of mechanotransduction in the airway smooth muscle. Finally, age-related loss of contact between fibroblasts process and collagen fibers in the dermis results

in diminishing mechanotransduction and is thought to be related to decreasing resilience of skin with age (Wu et al., 2009).

Growth Factors Associated with Fibrosis

Transforming Growth Factor-β

Extensive cell-to-cell communication is necessary in all tissues in order to maintain normal homeostatic activities and to respond appropriately to any allostatic challenge. Cytokines represent a group of soluble mediators intimately involved in regulating cell function in health and disease. The TGF family is a major group of cytokines regulating the growth and differentiation of cells as well as cellular response to stress and injury including programmed cell death. TGF-β, one of several members of the TGF family, is a protein secreted in an inactive form, which is subsequently activated through proteolysis. Numerous cell types produce TGF-β; however, a very significant reserve of TGF-β in tissue comes from blood platelets. The receptors for TGF-β are members of a kinase family and initiate signal transduction pathways in the receiving cell (Massagué, 1996). TGF-β plays a significant role in the normal development and maturation of tissues and in tissue healing subsequent to injury as well as in tissue remodeling leading to fibrosis and oncogenesis (August and Suthanthiran, 2006; Border and Noble, 1994; Kitisin et al., 2007; Sporn et al., 1986).

The function of TGF-β is dependent on the specific tissue in which it is located and the surrounding extracellular milieu. Thus, activated TGF-β can either inhibit or stimulate cell proliferation based on environmental factors; however, in most situations, it appears to repress cell division and enhance differentiation

(Massague, 1990). It is also chemoattractive to immune cells and enhances the deposition of extracellular matrix by activating fibroblasts (reviewed in Border and Noble, 1994). Interestingly, TGF-β is also capable of autoinduction of its own production from connective tissue cells such as macrophages. In inflamed tissue, TGF-β can inhibit the production of TNF-α and IL-1 and suppress free radical production by macrophages, giving it an anti-inflammatory role.

TGF-β is extensively involved in wound repair and overproduction of TGF-β is a key feature in tissue fibrosis (Barrientos et al., 2008). Acute injury presents with a transient increase in TGF-β; however, chronic reinjury results in overproduction of TGF-β and subsequent tissue fibrosis. Elevated levels of TGF-β are seen in disease states and during chemotherapy and are thought to be responsible for the resulting tissue fibrosis in the liver and lung (Kisseleva and Brenner, 2008).

TISSUE DYNAMICS: FIBROSIS AND TISSUE REPAIR

Fibrosis involves the proliferation extracellular matrix material replacing or overgrowing the parachymal tissue resulting the scarring and hardening of the organ. Typically, it develops from a chronic inflammatory state and can occur in such organs as kidney, liver, and lung as well as in muscle and tendon (Wynn, 2008). In acute tissue injury, transient expression of TGF-β leads to the development of myofibroblasts and the synthesis of collagen, both processes beneficial to normal wound repair. However, persistent irritation of the tissue sustains the production of growth factors as TGF-β leading to the persistence of myofibroblasts and the excessive secretion of collagen, processes fostering the buildup of fibrotic scars.

That myofibroblasts normally disappear from newly repaired sites support its role in wound repair, and this process is one of spontaneous and widespread myofibroblasts apoptosis—also termed *programmed cell death* (Carlson et al., 2003). Therefore, proapoptotic molecules such as nitric oxide (NO) signal the end of the reparative stage, and their premature presence could lead to incomplete repair by premature loss of load-bearing myofibroblasts and the ECMP they secrete. In cases where normal apoptosis does not occur, fibroblasts as well as myofibroblasts proliferate leading to fibrosis. The increased secretion of ECMPs by these cells, while affording tissue repair, also potentiates tensile strength and may ultimately restrict the very structures it aims to repair and protect. In fact, fascial restrictions, palpable by clinicians, are the very sites targeted by several osteopathic manipulative techniques (Osteopathic Manipulative Techniques) including direct and indirect myofascial release techniques. Proliferative fasciitis is associated with activated pericytes (fibroblast-like cells found lying along blood vessels), which appear to act as additional sources of fibroblasts and/or myofibroblasts. Presence of additional myofibroblasts, in turn, would perpetuate enhanced fascial tension and exacerbate inflammatory cytokine production. In addition to ECMPs, myofibroblasts also express and secrete numerous cytokines including the interleukins and others. Given that fascia has been shown to support blood cell flow through channels (fascial extensions of inferiorly based fasciocutaneous flaps exhibit erythrocyte flow in vascular channels of the deep fascia; Bhattacharya et al., 2005), it is theorized that fascia-derived cytokines have the ability to be delivered systemically by hematogenous movement. PGE$_2$ and PGEFr-α have been identified in association with nodular myofibroblasts in the fascia of patients with Dupuytren disease. Therefore, molecules such as these with vasoactive capacity may also play key roles in the recruitment and/or differentiation of myofibroblasts as well as

distribution of myofibroblast-derived cytokines to distant tissues such as brain, lung, heart, or kidney. If true, this could be a mechanism by which Osteopathic Manipulative Techniques targeting fascia in specific anatomical locations could effect change at distant sites (Eagan et al., 2007; Meltzer and Standley, 2007).

Clinically, anti-inflammatory cytokines may play cardinal roles in Osteopathic Manipulative Techniques efficacy as they reduce edema, increase range of motion (ROM), and decrease analgesic requirements (Andoh et al., 2005; Glover and Rennei, 2003; Meltzer and Standley, 2007; Nemet et al., 2002). Relevant to this notion, equibiaxial strain of tendon fibroblasts (3.5% beyond L∘) for 2 hours resulted in increased ATP release and inhibition IL-1β expression (Tsuzaki et al., 2003). Since IL-1β is proinflammatory, such fibroblast strain may set in motion a cascade of events to attenuate proinflammatory as well as stimulate anti-inflammatory signaling pathways. Other reports have shown that biophysical perturbation (in the form of shear stress) decreased expression of a number of inflammatory biomarkers (e.g., IL-1α, IL-14, IL-15, IL-16, and the IL-13 receptor) in endothelial cells (Chen et al., 2001), a process that may be attributed to upregulation of the transcription factors NF-κB and AP-1 (Resnick and Gimbrone, 1995).

Fascial Response to Stress

The mechanisms by which the fascia generates and responds to biomechanical strain are not clearly elucidated and are likely multifaceted. Mechanosignaling could result from normal movements, injury, Osteopathic Manipulative Techniques, or other stimuli and appears to rely on ion channel gating, integrins, focal adhesions, or by αSMA itself (Goffin et al., 2006). Mechanical deformation of cell shape stretches cells in one or more axes. Types of stretch range from pressure that can be positive (e.g., increased blood vessel flow) or negative (e.g., hypertonic extracellular fluid [ECF]-induced cell shrinking), flow over a cell surface (e.g., shear forces such as seen in vascular endothelial cells), cell elongation (e.g., as seen in muscle cells and various fibroblasts), and bending (e.g., as seen in normal bone cells (Brown, 2000). Fibroblasts and myofibroblasts respond in multiple ways to a wide variety of biophysical perturbations. While integrins and their receptors appear to be critical for some aspects of "outside-in signaling" as reported for ligamentous fibroblasts (Hannafin et al., 2006; Khalsa et al., 2004), strain is sensed at the cellular level by integrin-independent alterations in membrane ion conductances (Yang et al., 2004). Mechanogated ion channels have been reported, and a subset that conducts calcium and that is blocked by the lanthanide gadolinium (Gd) has been termed *stretch-activated calcium channels* (SACCs; see Gupta et al., 1998). Potential roles for calcium in strain-regulated fibroblast function have been reported. For example, palmar fascia responded to mechanical stress by significantly increasing tissue intracellular free calcium concentration (Gupta et al., 1998). In other studies, gingival fibroblasts were stretched in vitro to 1% or 2.8% beyond resting length. While the 1% group showed no intracellular free calcium changes, the 2.8% group displayed a significant increase in free calcium followed by calcium oscillations with a frequency of 2,000/s. These oscillations appear to involve extracellular calcium flux through SACCs in a process that required intact actin scaffolding (Arora et al., 1994).

A Role for Actin in Mechanotransduction

Disruption of polymerized actin, whose expression is greatly elevated upon fibroblast differentiation into myofibroblasts, inhibited strain-induced intracellular Ca^{2+} release as reported in several studies (Arora et al., 1994; Mohanty and Li, 2002; Wang et al., 2005). These data highlight the potential importance of the actin cytoskeleton in cosensing biophysical strain and perhaps themselves being responsible for changes in SACC conductance observed with strain. The precise role of actin in mediating these responses is unclear, but likely involves the ability of mechanically activated Src (a nonreceptor tyrosine kinase; Wang et al., 2005). Specifically, when actin (by cytochalasin D) or microtubules (by the antineoplastic agent nocodazole) were disrupted, force-induced changes in endothelial cell Src activation were blocked. The directional Src activation observed (i.e., pointing in the opposite direction to the applied stretching of the cell) may aid in the release of cell tension, thus serving as a feedback mechanism for cells to adapt to mechanical perturbations. That others have shown SACC activation to be dependent upon an intact actin cytoskeleton (Arora et al., 1994; Ko et al., 2001; Mohanty and Li, 2002) suggests that injuries and Osteopathic Manipulative Techniques strain could be mechanotransduced cellularly by actin/SACC association.

Direction of the Strain

In addition to strain frequency, magnitude and duration of recent in vitro data suggest that strain direction differentially regulates fibroblast growth, ion conductances, and gene expression. For example, human dermal fibroblasts strained multiaxially caused cellular alignment in a manner perpendicular to the strain vector. However, uniaxial shear stress did not affect cells in this regard (Neidlinger-Wilke et al., 2001). Cultured fibroblasts also responded to uniaxial strain with increased thymidine incorporation (signifying DNA replication) and collagen incorporation of labeled proline. Importantly, both these measures *decreased* significantly in fibroblasts strained biaxially (Berry et al., 2003). Fibroblasts depolarized (by increasing nonspecific inward cation current) when compressed, but hyperpolarized when stretched uniaxially between two patch pipettes (Kamkin et al., 2003). Others reported that smooth muscle responded to hyposmotic ECF-induced cell stretch (yielding multiaxial strain) with increased inward calcium current within one minute. This response was not however repeatable if cells were stretched uniaxially between two electrodes (Xu et al., 2000). When C2C12 myotubes were strained multiaxially, ribosomal S6 kinase phosphorylation increased significantly, a response found to be actin dependent since cytochalasin D blocked it. Interestingly, this study also reported that myotubes stretched multiaxially responded with increased p70 signaling, and this was Gd (and therefore SACC) insensitive. Conversely, uniaxial strain of these cells increased protein kinase B expression, a response that was Gd sensitive (Hornberger et al., 2005). Taken together, these data strongly suggest that fascial fibroblasts and myofibroblasts are capable of discerning among various strain directions and responding accordingly with differential stretch-activated calcium channel signaling. Data from these studies suggest mechanisms by which uni- and multiaxial fascia-directed Osteopathic Manipulative Techniques might yield distinct clinical outcomes.

Cyclic stretch of aortic tissue cultures increased mitogen-activated protein kinase (MAPK) phosphorylation. This process led to extracellular signal-regulated kinase-1 and kinase-2 transfer to the nucleus where they phosphorylated transcription factors including NF-κB and AP-1 (Lehoux et al., 2000). Since these factors are responsible for IL-6 and IL-8 expression (Andoh et al., 2005), they may be involved in strain regulation of fibroblast IL and other cytokine secretion. These data further suggest a mechanism (i.e., MAPK) by which strain stimulates fibroblast proliferation (Berry et al., 2003; Standley et al., 1999, 2001). Fibroblast

proliferation, while often thought of as contributing to tissue congestion, edema, and other proinflammatory processes, could also serve as a mechanism by which myofascial release (MFR) and other manual medicine techniques (MMT) result in long-term positive treatment outcomes. This would be accomplished by further (and potentially sustained) enhancement of cytokine pools from actively proliferating fascial fibroblasts and correction of dysfunctional ECMP crosslinking as has been postulated by others (Gupta et al., 1998). Alternatively, long-term efficacy could result from MFR-induced release of apoptotic cytokines (e.g., NO; see Dodd et al., 2006) causing selective fibroblast death from injury sites and removal of fibrotic materials responsible for pain and attenuated ROM. It has been reported that fibroblasts themselves respond to various strain types by increasing secretion of several ILs, while decreasing secretion of others (Eagan et al., 2007; Meltzer and Standley, 2007). In fact, in vitro modeling of repetitive motion strains increases while addition of modeled counterstrain decreases inflammatory IL secretion. Whether this process involves fibroblast to myofibroblast differentiation has not been reported. Clinically, activation of anti-inflammatory cytokines (and/or attenuation of proinflammatory ones) could account for increased ROM of injured tissues and joints, decreased edema, and decreased need for analgesics in manners dependent upon fibroblast growth responses.

SUMMARY

Fascia is defined as irregular connective tissue that plays a role in surrounding and protecting the organ systems of the body.

Four distinct layers of fascia were presented: pannicular, axial (appendicular), meningeal, and visceral.

The components of fascia were presented with particular emphasis place on the myofibroblasts.

The dynamic aspect of fascia was discussed.

REFERENCES

Anderson W, Makins GH. The planes of subperitoneal and subpleural connective tissue, with their connections. *J Anat Physiol* 1890;25(pt 1): 78–86.

Andoh A, Zhang Z, Inatomi O, et al. Interleukin-22, a member of the IL-10 subfamily, induces inflammatory responses in colonic subepithelial myofibroblasts. *Gastroenterology* 2005;129(3):969–984.

Arora PD, Bibby KJ, McCulloch CA. Slow oscillations of free intracellular calcium ion concentration in human fibroblasts responding to mechanical stretch. *J Cell Physiol* 1994;161(2):187–200.

August P, Suthanthiran M. Transforming growth factor beta signaling, vascular remodeling, and hypertension. *N Engl J Med* 2006;354(25):2721–2723.

Banes AJ, Tsuzaki M, Yamamoto J, et al. Mechanoreception at the cellular level: the detection, interpretation, and diversity of responses to mechanical signals. *Biochem Cell Biol* 1995;73(7–8):349–365.

Barrientos S, Stojadinovic O, Golinko MS, et al. Growth factors and cytokines in wound healing. *Wound Repair Regen* 2008;16(5):585–601.

Bednar DA, Orr FW, Simon GT. Observations on the pathomorphology of the thoracolumbar fascia in chronic mechanical back pain: a microscopic study. *Spine* 1995;20(10):1161–1164.

Benjamin M. The fascia of the limbs and back—a review. *J Anat* 2009;214(1): 1–18.

Berry CC, Cacou C, Lee DA, et al. Dermal fibroblasts respond to mechanical conditioning in a strain profile dependent manner. *Biorheology* 2003;40 (1–3):337–345.

Bevan JA, Bevan RD, Duckles SP. Adrenergic regulation of vascular smooth muscle. In: Bohr DF, Somlyo AP, Sparks HV, Geiger SR, eds. *Handbook of Physiology: Section 2, The Cardiovascular System: Volume II, Vascular Smooth Muscle.* Bethesda, MD: American Physiology Society, 1980:515–566.

Bhattacharya V, Watts RK, Reddy GR. Live demonstration of microcirculation in the deep fascia and its implication. *Plast Reconstr Surg* 2005;115(2):458–463.

Border WA, Noble NA. Transforming growth factor beta in tissue fibrosis. *N Engl J Med* 1994;331(19):1286–1292.

Brown TD. Techniques for mechanical stimulation of cells in vitro: a review. *J Biomech* 2000;33(1):3–14.

Burnstock G. Cholinergic and purinergic regulation of blood vessels. *Handbook of Physiology* Sec. 2; Vol II. 1980:567–612.

Carlson MA, Longaker MT, Thompson J. Wound splinting regulates granulation tissue survival. *J Surg Res* 2003;110(1):304–309.

Catala M. Embryonic and fetal development of structures associated with the cerebro-spinal fluid in man and other species. Part I: The ventricular system, meninges and choroid plexuses. *Arch Anat Cytol Pathol* 1998;46(3):153–169.

Chen BP, Li YS, Zhao Y, et al. DNA microarray analysis of gene expression in endothelial cells in response to 24-h shear stress. *Physiol Genomics* 2001;7(1):55–63.

Clemente CD. *Gray's Anatomy of the Human Body*. Philadelphia, PA: Lea & Febiger, 1985.

Cormack DH. *Ham's Histology*. 9th Ed. Philadelphia. PA: J.B. Lippincott Co., 1987.

Dodd JG, Good MM, Nguyen TL, et al. In vitro biophysical strain model for understanding mechanisms of osteopathic manipulative treatment. *J Am Osteopath Assoc* 2006;106(3):157–166.

Eagan TS, Meltzer KR, Standley PR. Importance of strain direction in regulating human fibroblast proliferation and cytokine secretion: a useful in vitro model for soft tissue injury and manual medicine treatments. *J Manipulative Physiol Ther* 2007;30(8):584–592.

Ehrlich HP, Allison GM, Leggett M. The myofibroblast, cadherin, alpha smooth muscle actin and the collagen effect. *Cell Biochem Funct* 2006;24(1):63–70.

Ercoli A, Delmas V, Fanfani F, et al. Terminologia Anatomica versus unofficial descriptions and nomenclature of the fasciae and ligaments of the female pelvis: a dissection-based comparative study. *Am J Obstet Gynecol* 2005;193(4):1565–1573.

Fasel JH, Dembe JC, Majno PE. Fascia: a pragmatic overview for surgeons. *Am Surg* 2007;73(5):451–453.

Gabbiani G, Ryan GB, Majne G. Presence of modified fibroblasts in granulation tissue and their possible role in wound contraction. *Experientia* 1971;27(5):549–550.

Gallaudet BB. *A Description of the Planes of Fascia of the Human Body with Special Reference to the Fascias of the Abdomen, Pelvis and Perineum*. New York, NY: Columbia University Press, 1931; 76.

Galli SJ. New concepts about the mast cell. *N Engl J Med* 1993;328:257–265.

Garcia-Armengol J, Garcia-Botello S, Martinez-Soriano F, et al. Review of the anatomic concepts in relation to the retrorectal space and endopelvic fascia: Waldeyer's fascia and the rectosacral fascia. *Colorectal Dis* 2008;10(3):298–302.

Glover JC, Rennei PR. Strain and counterstrain techniques. In: Ward R, ed. *Foundations for Osteopathic Medicine*. 2nd Ed. Philadelphia, PA: Lippincott, Williams & Wilkins, 2003:1002–1016.

Goffin JM, Pittet P, Csucs G, et al. Focal adhesion size controls tension-dependent recruitment of alpha-smooth muscle actin to stress fibers. *J Cell Biol* 2006;172(2):259–268.

Gray H. *Anatomy of the Human Body*. 25th Ed. Philadelphia, PA: Lea & Febiger, 1948.

Grinnell F, Ho CH, Tamariz E, et al. Dendritic fibroblasts in three-dimensional collagen matrices. *Mol Biol Cell* 2003;14(2):384–395.

Gupta R, Allen F, Tan V, et al. The effect of shear stress on fibroblasts derived from Dupuytren's tissue and normal palmar fascia. *J Hand Surg Am* 1998;23(5):945–950.

Hannafin JA, Attia EA, Henshaw R, et al. Effect of cyclic strain and plating matrix on cell proliferation and integrin expression by ligament fibroblasts. *J Orthop Res* 2006;24(2):149–158.

Hayes MA. Abdominopelvic fascia. *Am J Anat* 1950;87(1):119–161.

Hinz B. Formation and function of the myofibroblast during tissue repair. *J Invest Dermatol* 2007;127(3):526–537.

Hinz B, Celetta G, Tomasek JJ, et al. Alpha-smooth muscle actin expression upregulates fibroblast contractile activity. *Mol Biol Cell* 2001;12(9):2730–2741.

Hinz B, Pittet P, Smith-Clerc J, et al. Myofibroblast development is characterized by specific cell-cell adherens junctions. *Mol Biol Cell* 2004;15(9):4310–4320.

Hornberger TA, Armstrong DD, Koh TJ, et al. Intracellular signaling specificity in response to uniaxial vs. multiaxial stretch: implications for mechanotransduction. *Am J Physiol Cell Physiol* 2005;288(1):C185–C194.

Kamkin A, Kiseleva I, Isenberg G. Activation and inactivation of a non-selective cation conductance by local mechanical deformation of acutely isolated cardiac fibroblasts. *Cardiovasc Res* 2003;57(3):793–803.

Katsumi A, Orr AW, Tzima E, et al. Integrins in mechanotransduction. *J Biol Chem* 2004;279(13):12001–12004.

Kavitha O, Thampan RV. Factors influencing collagen biosynthesis. *J Cell Biochem* 2008;104(4):1150–1160.

Khalsa PS, Ge W, Uddin MZ, et al. Integrin alpha2beta1 affects mechanotransduction in slowly and rapidly adapting cutaneous mechanoreceptors in rat hairy skin. *Neuroscience* 2004;129(2):447–459.

Kisseleva T, Brenner DA. Mechanisms of fibrogenesis. *Exp Biol Med (Maywood)* 2008;233(2):109–122.

Kitisin K, Saha T, Blake T, et al. TGF-beta signaling in development. *Sci STKE* 2007;2007(399):cm1.

Ko KS, Arora PD, Bhide V, et al. Cell-cell adhesion in human fibroblasts requires calcium signaling. *J Cell Sci* 2001;114(pt 6):1155–1167.

Langevin HM. Potential role of fascia in chronic musculoskeletal pain. In: Audette JF, Bailey A, eds. *Integrative Pain Medicine*. Totowa, NJ: Humana Press, 2008:123–132.

Langevin HM, Bouffard NA, Badger GJ, et al. Dynamic fibroblast cytoskeletal response to subcutaneous tissue stretch ex vivo and in vivo. *Am J Physiol Cell Physiol* 2005;288(3):C747–C756.

Langevin HM, Sherman KJ. Pathophysiological model for chronic low back pain integrating connective tissue and nervous system mechanisms. *Med Hypotheses* 2007;68(1):74–80.

Last RJ. *Anatomy: Regional and Applied*. 6th Ed. Edinburgh: Churchill Livingstone, 1978.

Laurent GJ, Chambers RC, Hill MR, et al. Regulation of matrix turnover: fibroblasts, forces, factors and fibrosis. *Biochem Soc Trans* 2007;35(pt 4):647–651.

Lehoux S, Esposito B, Merval R, et al. Pulsatile stretch-induced extracellular signal-regulated kinase 1/2 activation in organ culture of rabbit aorta involves reactive oxygen species. *Arterioscler Thromb Vasc Biol* 2000;20(11):2366–2372.

Lundon K. The effect of mechanical load on soft connective tissues. In: *Functional Soft-Tissue Examination and Treatment by Manual Methods*. Boston, MA: Bartlett and Jones Publishers, 2007:15–30.

Massague J. The transforming growth factor-beta family. *Annu Rev Cell Biol* 1990;6:597–641.

Massagué J. TGFβ signaling: Receptors, transducers, and mad proteins. *Cell* 1996;85(7):947–950.

Meltzer KR, Standley PR. Modeled repetitive motion strain and indirect osteopathic manipulative techniques in regulation of human fibroblast proliferation and interleukin secretion. *J Am Osteopath Assoc* 2007;107(12):527–536.

Metcalfe DD, Baram D, Mekori YA. Mast cells. *Physiol Rev* 1997;77(4):1033–1079.

Mohanty MJ, Li X. Stretch-induced Ca(2+) release via an IP(3)-insensitive Ca(2+) channel. *Am J Physiol Cell Physiol* 2002;283(2):C456–C462.

Neidlinger-Wilke C, Grood ES, Wang JHC, et al. Cell alignment is induced by cyclic changes in cell length: studies of cells grown in cyclically stretched substrates. *J Orthop Res* 2001;19(2):286–293.

Neilson EG. Mechanisms of disease: fibroblasts—a new look at an old problem. *Nat Clin Pract Nephrol* 2006;2(2):101–108.

Nemet D, Hong S, Mills PJ, et al. Systemic vs. local cytokine and leukocyte responses to unilateral wrist flexion exercise. *J Appl Physiol* 2002;93(2):546–554.

Palmieri G, Panu R, Asole A, et al. Macroscopic organization and sensitive innervation of the tendinous intersection and the lacertus fibrosus of the biceps brachii muscle in the ass and horse. *Arch Anat Histol Embryol* 1986;69:73–82.

Papadakis KA, Targan SR. Tumor necrosis factor: biology and therapeutic inhibitors. *Gastroenterology* 2000;119(4):1148–1157.

Resnick N, Gimbrone MA Jr. Hemodynamic forces are complex regulators of endothelial gene expression. *FASEB J* 1995;9(10):874–882.

Rhee S, Grinnell F. Fibroblast mechanics in 3D collagen matrices. *Adv Drug Deliv Rev* 2007;59(13):1299–1305.

Ronty MJ, Leivonen SK, Hinz B, et al. Isoform-specific regulation of the actin-organizing protein palladin during TGF-beta1-induced myofibroblast differentiation. *J Invest Dermatol* 2006;126(11):2387–2396.

Sanchis-Alfonso V, Rosello-Sastre E. Immunohistochemical analysis for neural markers of the lateral retinaculum in patients with isolated symptomatic patellofemoral malalignment. A neuroanatomic basis for anterior knee pain in the active young patient. *Am J Sports Med* 2000;28(5):725–731.

Schleip R. Fascial plasticity: a new neurobiological explanation: part 1. *J Bodyw Mov Ther* 2003a;7(1):11–19.

Schleip R. Fascial plasticity—a new neurobiological explanation: part 2. *J Bodyw Mov Ther* 2003b;7(2):104–116.

Schleip R, Klingler W, Lehmann-Horn F. Active fascial contractility: Fascia may be able to contract in a smooth muscle-like manner and thereby influence musculoskeletal dynamics. *Med Hypotheses* 2005;65(2):273–277.

Schwartz MA, DeSimone DW. Cell adhesion receptors in mechanotransduction. *Curr Opin Cell Biol* 2008;20(5):551–556.

Silver FH, DeVore D, Siperko LM. Invited review: role of mechanophysiology in aging of ECM: effects of changes in mechanochemical transduction. *J Appl Physiol* 2003;95(5):2134–2141.

Singer E. Fascia of the human body and their relations to the organs they envelop. Philadelphia, PA: Williams and Wilkins, 1935.

Skandalakis PN, Zoras O, Skandalakis JE, et al. Transversalis, endoabdominal, endothoracic fascia: who's who? *Am Surg* 2006;72(1):16–18.

Snyder G. Fascia—applied anatomy and physiology. In: *Academy of Applied Osteopathy Yearbook.* 1956.

Sporn MB, Roberts AB, Wakefield LM, et al. Transforming growth factor-β: biological function and chemical structure. *Science* 1986;233(4763):532–534.

Standley PR, Obards TJ, Martina CL. Cyclic stretch regulates autocrine IGF-I in vascular smooth muscle cells: implications in vascular hyperplasia. *Am J Physiol* 1999;276(4 pt 1):E697–E705.

Standley PR, Stanley MA, Senechal P. Activation of mitogenic and antimitogenic pathways in cyclically stretched arterial smooth muscle. *Am J Physiol Endocrinol Metab* 2001;281(6):E1165–E1171.

Standring S. *Gray's Anatomy: The Anatomical Basis of Clinical Practice.* 40th Ed. Edinburgh: Elsevier Churchill Livingston, 2008.

Staubesand J, Li Y. Zum feinbau der fascia cruris mit Besonderer Berucksichtigung epi- und intrafasziale Nerven. *Manuelle Medizin* 1996;34:196–200.

Stecco C, Gagey O, Macchi V, et al. Tendinous muscular insertions onto the deep fascia of the upper limb. First part: anatomical study. *Morphologie* 2007;91(292):29–37.

Stecco C, Porzionato A, Lancerotto L, et al. Histological study of the deep fasciae of the limbs. *J Bodyw Mov Ther* 2008;12(3):225–230.

Stecco C, Porzionato A, Macchi V, et al. Histological characteristics of the deep fascia of the upper limb. *Ital J Anat Embryol* 2006;111(2):105–110.

Stilwell DL. The nerve supply of the vertebral column and its associated structures in the monkey. *Anat Rec* 1956;125:139–169.

Stilwell DL. Regional variations in the innervation of deep fasciae and aponeuroses. *Anat Rec* 1957;127(4):635–648.

Tabata T, Kawakatsu H, Maidji E, et al. Induction of an epithelial integrin alphavbeta6 in human cytomegalovirus-infected endothelial cells leads to activation of transforming growth factor-beta1 and increased collagen production. *Am J Pathol* 2008;172(4):1127–1140.

Tanaka S, Ito T. Histochemical demonstration of adrenergic fibers in the fascia periosteum and retinaculum. *Clin Orthop Relat Res* 1977;126: 276–281.

Thiery JP, Acloque H, Huang RY, et al. Epithelial-mesenchymal transitions in development and disease. *Cell* 2009;139(5):871–890.

Tomasek JJ, Gabbiani G, Hinz B, et al. Myofibroblasts and mechano-regulation of connective tissue remodelling. *Nat Rev Mol Cell Biol* 2002;3(5): 349–363.

Tomasek JJ, Vaughan MB, Kropp BP, et al. Contraction of myofibroblasts in granulation tissue is dependent on Rho/Rho kinase/myosin light chain phosphatase activity. *Wound Repair Regen* 2006;14(3):313–320.

Tsuzaki M, Bynum D, Almekinders L, et al. ATP modulates load-inducible IL-1beta, COX 2, and MMP-3 gene expression in human tendon cells. *J Cell Biochem* 2003;89(3):556–562.

Walsh DA, McWiliams F. Tachykinins and the cardiovascular system. *Curr Drug Targets* 2006;7(8):1031–1042.

Wang Y, Botvinick EL, Zhao Y, et al. Visualizing the mechanical activation of Src. *Nature* 2005;434(7036):1040–1045.

Wendell-Smith CP. Fascia: an illustrative problem in international terminology. *Surg Radiol Anat* 1997;19(5):273–277.

Werner S, Grose R. Regulation of wound healing by growth factors and cytokines. *Physiol Rev* 2003;83(3):835–870.

Wu M, Fannin J, Rice KM, et al. Effect of aging on cellular mechanotransduction. *Ageing Res Rev* 2009.

Wynn TA. Cellular and molecular mechanisms of fibrosis. *J Pathol* 2008;214(2):199–210.

Xu WX, Li Y, Wu LR, et al. Effects of different kinds of stretch on voltage-dependent calcium current in antrial circular smooth muscle cells of the guinea-pig. *Sheng Li Xue Bao* 2000;52(1):69–74.

Yahia LH, Rhalmi S, Newman N, et al. Sensory innervation of the human thoracolumbar fascia. *Acta Orthop Scand* 1992;63:195–197.

Yang G, Crawford RC, Wang JH. Proliferation and collagen production of human patellar tendon fibroblasts in response to cyclic uniaxial stretching in serum-free conditions. *J Biomech* 2004;37(10):1543–1550.

Yang J, Weinberg RA. Epithelial-mesenchymal transition: at the crossroads of development and tumor metastasis. *Dev Cell* 2008;14(6):818–829.

8 Biomechanics

MICHAEL R. WELLS

KEY CONCEPTS

- Biomechanics describes the relationship between structure and function.
- Motion and forces in three-dimensional space can be divided into components with a magnitude of action in each dimension.
- Stress, strain, and force moments are terms used to describe how forces act on objects and how objects respond to those forces.
- The biomaterial properties of tissues such as bone, cartilage, muscles, tendons, and ligaments, are based on a hierarchy of biomechanical properties from the molecular, cellular, tissue, and gross anatomic levels.
- Tissues are constantly remodeling in response to the stresses placed upon them.
- Excessive stresses or inadequate responses to them (loss of homeostasis) result in injury or disease in tissues.
- The basic biomaterial properties and remodeling capacity (adaptability) of tissues change with age, generally to render them more vulnerable to stresses and injury.
- The gross biomechanical properties of the skeleton are defined by bony structure and the attachment of muscles and tendons that produce forces across joints.
- The primary motions at the surfaces of articulations are gliding (translation), rotation, rolling, compression, and distraction.
- Basic properties of joint kinetics can be described by measuring the forces produced by muscles and the length of moment arms acting across joints.
- The elastic properties of muscles, tendons, and ligaments allow them to store energy in some phases of movements for release during others.
- Normal movement in the spinal column is a composite of smaller motions of individual vertebrae. Restrictions of movement in one area can result in a compensatory increased mobility in others.
- The orientation of intervertebral joint facets in the spine, in association with the direction of spinal muscle contraction, produces a motion coupling of vertebral movement. These coupling relationships differ over areas of the spine.
- It is necessary to consider the biomechanical relationships of the body as a whole when attempting to define the consequences of injury or altered function of a body segment.

BIOMECHANICS DESCRIBES THE RELATIONSHIP BETWEEN STRUCTURE AND FUNCTION

The inter-relationship of structure and function in the body is one of the basic principles of the osteopathic medical profession. The science of biomechanics is dedicated to describing this relationship more generally in biologic systems. This can apply to the organism as a whole (as with kinesiology) or even on a subcellular level (as with microtubular transport mechanisms). The approach to the mechanics of biologic systems is similar to the mechanics of inanimate objects and consists largely of how they respond to forces applied to them. When struck with a hammer, an object may shatter or absorb the force and be accelerated into movement. The response will depend upon a variety of factors including the material comprising the object, the object's shape, internal structure, where and how the force is applied, and so forth. The response of the human body to either externally or internally applied forces can be described similarly, as it must obey the same basic laws of physics. However, the human body and other biologic systems have extremely intricate structural arrangements of highly variable materials down to the molecular level. This can make the accurate

biomechanical modeling of even simple movements very challenging. Additionally, the body also has the essential biologic ability to adapt and structurally remodel itself according to the stresses placed upon it. Some of these adaptations, as in the mechanical properties of tissues, can occur relatively rapidly. This "moving target" property can add an additional layer of difficulty for accurate description.

The capacity of the body to adapt appropriately to environmental stress will make the difference between health and disease. The goal of the osteopathic physician is to assist the body in regaining a balance with the stressors of the patient's environment, usually at multiple levels of consideration. From a biomechanical standpoint, this may involve the correction of somatic dysfunctions or to break cycles of inappropriate responses that have produced them. In doing so, the primary biomechanical considerations for the osteopathic physician must include broad characteristics encompassing both biomaterial characteristics of tissues and the primary mechanical operation of the body as a unit. As opposed to other medical disciplines, this must include a literal "feel" for the characteristics of tissues in addition to figurative "feel" for the understanding of body mechanics derived from a knowledge of anatomy. The primary goal of this chapter is to assist the reader in obtaining this latter knowledge. For this reason, an emphasis will be placed on basic biomaterial and biomechanical concepts rather than mathematical modeling of properties. As with other chapters in this volume, this chapter is intended to be a summary of biomechanical concepts that are of particular relevance to those who study osteopathic medicine. More comprehensive discussions may be readily obtained from texts on particular topics. It will be assumed that the reader has a basic working knowledge of gross anatomy and the concepts relating anatomy to function.

Motion and Forces Can Be Described as Components With a Magnitude in Each Dimension of Three-Dimensional Space

The strategy for describing the mechanics of biologic materials begins with the same terms and methods employed to describe inanimate objects. The process of interest is broken down into components that can be measured and characterized. These components and their properties are then incorporated into models (often mathematical) that can be used to describe the system and predict its reaction to defined stresses. The terminology used is common to areas of mechanical sciences and can be categorized into terms related to:

1. Dimensions and movement in three-dimensional space
2. The nature of applied forces
3. Properties of biomaterials

Objects and Movements in Three-Dimensional Space Can Be Described as Components in Each of the Three Dimensions

An object can be described by the magnitude of its size in each of its dimensions (length, width, height; Fig. 8.1). Similarly, simple movement (translation) of an object in three-dimensional space can be described as three different components (*vectors*) of movement

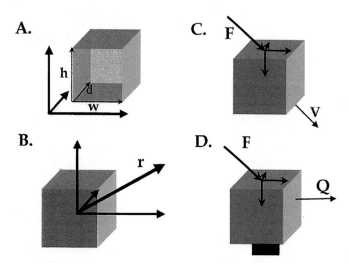

Figure 8-1 **A.** An object in three-dimensional space (axes) can be described by the length vectors (height [*h*], width [*w*], depth [*d*]). **B.** The motion of an object can be described as three separate primary vectors of velocity. The actual movement of the object is represented by the resultant vector (*r*). **C.** A force (*F*) that is applied to an object may also be represented by separate force vectors in each dimension directed into the object. The object may be moved in a direction (*v*) by the force. **D.** If one component of the accelerating force is resisted, the object will move in a new direction (*Q*), determined by the magnitude of the remaining vector components.

(up/down, back and forth, in and out relative to the page) that can occur simultaneously. Vectors will have a magnitude and direction similar to describing the dimensions of an object, except that the magnitude of movement is expressed as velocity (meters per second). Vector components are shown on an axis system (Fig. 8.1) that is used to model three-dimensional space. By describing the vectors of movement in each of these three dimensions, the motion of the object can be characterized. The actual path of the object is referred to as the *resultant velocity vector*. Biomechanical analysis uses similar vector systems to describe most parameters in space, such as velocity, acceleration, and pressure.

Beyond simple models, the properties of each component of a resultant vector can become increasingly complex. For example, an object of irregular shape will require more than a simple length measurement in each dimension to describe it. Similarly, an object moving in space may also rotate about an axis. Because of this, even relatively simple movements of body segments may require sophisticated mathematical modeling to describe the movement.

Applied Forces Can Also Be Expressed as Three-Dimensional Vectors

Applied *forces*, such as a manipulative thrust, are essentially *pressure* (force per unit area) applied to an object. By definition, forces act to accelerate an object of a given mass. Accordingly, an object at rest must have a force applied to it in order to achieve movement through acceleration. An object moving at a constant velocity will require no forces to sustain movement, unless other forces (e.g., friction) are acting to resist the movement. The object's resistance to change of velocity (*inertia*) is also described as the force required to accelerate it from rest (zero velocity) or to decelerate it from movement.

The magnitude of forces and associated force vectors is used to describe external pressures applied to the body and internal forces like those generated in muscles to achieve limb movement. Force magnitudes are expressed as the mass of the object times the acceleration ($F = ma$). The metric unit of force is a newton (N) or 1 kg accelerated to a velocity of 1 m/s each second (kg × m/s²). Like velocity, forces are characterized as a combination of vector components of a certain magnitude in each of the three axes defining space (Fig. 8.1). The *resultant force* is the sum of the individual force vectors. The manner in which the object might be moved or mobilized by the force will depend upon which of the vector components are resisted and which are not (Fig. 8.1). Similarly, a resultant force vector arising from a manipulative thrust would be characterized by describing force components not only directly into the body, but also in lateral directions (rostral, caudal, medial, or lateral) as well as rotational components. Mobilization of body segments by the force will depend upon which components of the thrust meet with direct resistance and obviously how the body is positioned. In biomechanics, it is important to characterize the different components that a force may have in order to understand the ensuing reaction of the material or body structures.

Moments Are Forces that Act at a Distance and/or Produce Rotation of an Object

Forces that act to produce rotation of an object about an axis, or in two-dimensional models, a center point (Fig. 8.2), are called *force moments* (also *moment* or *torque*). The magnitude of a force moment is the product of the force applied and the distance of application from the center of rotation (force × distance). The latter distance is referred to as the *moment arm*. This is essentially a process of using a lever to produce rotation about an axis. Because of this relationship, it is important to note that moments of the same magnitude may

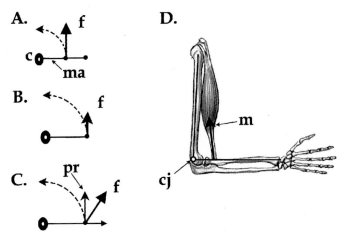

Figure 8-2   Force moments on an object such as a door. **A.** A force (f) applied at a distance (moment arm, *ma*) in the middle of the door can produce rotation (*dotted arrow*) around a center or axis (*c*) located at the hinge. The moment is the force applied times the distance (*d*) from the center (*f* × *d*). A smaller force acting on a longer moment arm at the doorknob (**B**) will produce the same moment (*f* × *d*). **C.** If the force is applied in a direction other than directly against the moment arm, only part (*pr*) of the force will be used to produce the rotation. **D.** In the body, force moments are generated by muscle contraction forces (*m*) that produce rotation of a mobile body segment about a center in the joint (*cj*).

be produced by increasing the force applied while proportionately reducing the moment arm or vice versa (Fig. 8.2). A common example of the properties of force moments can be obtained from pushing open a door (Fig. 8.2). Pushing the door open at the handle usually is relatively easy (low force), because of the long distance (moment arm) between the handle and the center of rotation at the hinge. Note, however, that opening the door at the handle requires a relatively large distance of movement (large displacement). Attempting to push the door open at a point near the hinge (short moment arm) is much more difficult (greater force), but requires less displacement to open the door. Note also that the direction or angle at which the push is applied to the door will determine how much of the force applied is actually used to push the door open (2). This rotation component of the applied force is at a right angle to the surface of the door (directly into the door) at any instant. The remaining force component will be in a direction along the surface of the door. For the same opening force to be maintained, the direction of the applied force must change constantly to move in a circle with the door.

The strategy of changing the force or the length of the moment arm and the direction at which forces are applied is often employed in body mechanics and in manipulation techniques, depending upon the need for more or less force at the cost of greater or lesser displacement.

Moments are used in the biomechanical modeling of body motion because most movements are composites of rotational movements of individual body segments around joints. Force moments are generated from the contraction of muscles attached between two body segments causing the movement of the more mobile segment around a center of rotation (Fig. 8.2). The center of rotation is usually near the articulation surface in the less mobile segment. The moment arm of the contracting force is related to the distance of the muscle insertion on the mobile segment from the center of rotation. In simple biomechanical models of body movement, this

center of rotation in the joint is usually shown as immobile. In actual movements, both segments may be mobile and motions within the joint may also occur to change the center of rotation.

Stresses Are Forces Applied to Objects in Various Orientations

The characteristics of forces applied to an object are described as *stresses* (Fig. 8.3). The magnitude of basic stresses is described as force applied over a defined unit of object surface area or pressure. This may be described as pounds per square inch (psi) or in the metric form, pascals (N per square m). Particular types of stresses are identified to describe their relationship to the object acted upon (Fig. 8.3). For convenience, stresses are usually described for an object that is immobilized or constrained, such that the object must resist the stress and not undergo acceleration or movement other than deformation (see "Strain Is Deformation Produced by Stress," later in the chapter). *Tension* is a force applied perpendicularly outward from the surface of an object (pull), such that the object would be elongated or stretched. *Compression* stress is a force applied perpendicularly inward (push) to the surface of an object, such that the object would be shortened or compressed. *Shear stresses* are forces applied parallel to the surface of an object. *Torsion stresses* are rotation-like forces, which, on a constrained object, act to twist it about a neutral axis (i.e., an axis that would not be translated or moved by the force). *Bending* is also technically a rotation-like force (or coupled coactive forces) that acts to fold or bend an appropriately constrained object along a neutral axis. The sum of all stresses on an object is termed *load*.

BEHAVIOR OF MATERIALS SUBJECTED TO FORCES

The Behavior of an Object or Material May Be Isotropic or Anisotropic

While stresses may originate from external forces applied to an object's surfaces, they are also transmitted from the area of contact through the entire substance comprising the object. The primary

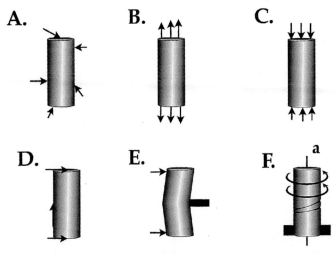

Figure 8-3   **A.** Stresses are forces acting from various orientations relative to the object. Stresses are named according to their action upon the object. **B.** Tensile stresses act to stretch an object. **C.** Compressive stresses compact the object. **D.** Shear stresses act parallel to the surface of an object. **E.** Bending stress acts to fold an object about an axis. **F.** Torsion stresses twist an object about an axis.

factors affecting the transmission of forces through an object are its shape and material composition including infrastructure. The characteristics of the material composition of the object will determine if the object can be accelerated or rotated by a stress of sufficient magnitude or physically broken by it. The shape of an object may dramatically affect the manner in which it responds to similar stresses exerted in different places on the object. An object, such as a sphere of homogenous composition, will respond in the same way to a particular type and magnitude of stress applied to any point on its surface. This type of object is referred to as *isotropic* in relation to stresses. Objects having a nonuniform surface shape (such as an irregular cube) or heterogeneous composition will respond to the same stress differently depending upon the point of application. These objects or materials are referred to as *anisotropic*. Most biologic structures fall into this category.

As with surface characteristics, the internal structure or composition of an object will also determine its response characteristics to stresses. The object's composition and molecular infrastructure determine how a force applied to a particular location is transmitted to the remainder of the object's mass. In objects that have an anisotropic internal composition, such as biologic materials, localized internal stresses are often the primary determinant of the toleration of the material for stresses of a particular magnitude and orientation of a stress. As discussed subsequently, bone, muscle, tendons, and ligaments have a linear cellular/molecular structure that causes the response to loads to differ dramatically depending upon the orientation of the applied stress.

Strain Is Deformation Produced by Stress

As muscles contract, they apply primary localized tensile stresses to bone to accelerate the mobile segment(s) and to stabilize the immobile segment(s). Under this condition, the applied stresses produce a change in the shape of the bone or object (*deformation*). The magnitude of deformation produced by stress is referred to as *strain*. The actual deformation of an object will depend upon the same factors defining stress distribution (internal composition and infrastructure) and is characterized as a sum of different strain vectors. These vectors are usually named for the type of stress producing them (e.g., tensile strain, compressive strain, etc.). Many different strain vectors may be produced within an object by a particular type of stress. A simple example is a bending stress that produces tensile strain on the side of the object opposite the neutral axis and compressive strain in the direction of bending (Fig. 8.4). A similar condition exists with strain on a spinal disc with bending between segments.

The Elastic Modulus Shows the Relationship Between Stress and Strain

While it can generally be assumed that increases in stress on an object will produce an increase in strain, the relationship is not direct, particularly for biologic materials. The relationship between the amount of a particular stress applied to an object and the resulting deformation or strain is shown by a stress/strain curve (Fig. 8.5). In this instance, a material is subjected to a defined stress such as tension. In this model, the strain may be quantified as the change in length of the object (as with a tendon or ligament). A similar result could be obtained by the displacement of the center of a bending load (as with a bone). Stress/strain relationships for most materials have a linear region (elastic behavior) in which increasing stress produces a corresponding amount of deformation (Fig. 8.5). Reducing the stress or unloading of the object will allow it to return

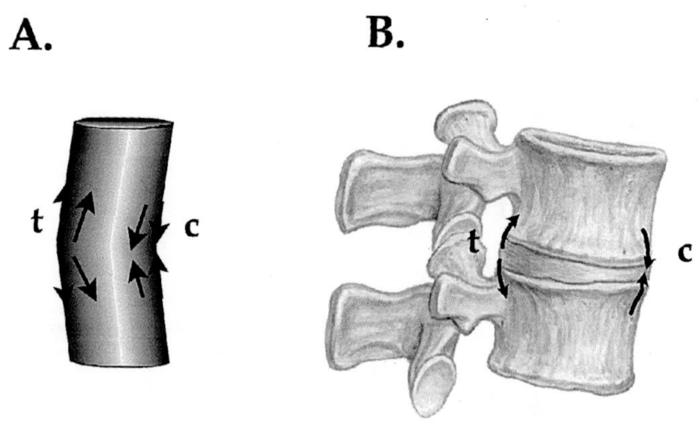

Figure 8-4 **A.** Bending strain produces tensile stress (*t*) on one side of an object and compressive stress (*c*) on the other. **B.** This same principle applies directly to biologic materials, such as spinal discs.

to its former shape without a permanent change in shape. In this elastic area of the stress/strain curve, the slope of the line (stress/strain) is termed the *elastic modulus*. The elastic modulus is also a quantitative description of *stiffness*, a term commonly associated with the amount of force necessary to bend an object.

When an applied stress is greater than that defined by the elastic area (Fig. 8.5), a permanent deformation of the material or plasticity will result. The plastic behavior area of the curve ends with the material *failure* or breaking of the object. Materials may also be described as *brittle* or *ductile* depending upon the amount of deformation they can undergo before failure. *Brittle* objects such as glass will undergo little deformation before they break (fail), and the pieces after breaking retain their shape such that pieces will fit together to produce a puzzlelike reproduction of the object with little deformation. *Ductile* materials such as a copper wire will have a permanently altered shape beyond their elastic region and after failure. Many factors other than basic structure of a material may significantly affect the stress/strain relationship. The most common of these are temperature and the rate at which a stress is applied.

Viscoelasticity Is the Combination of Elastic and Viscous Properties of Materials in Response to Stress

The rate at which a stress is applied can be a particularly important determinant in the response of materials that exhibit a combination of both elastic and viscous behavior in response to an applied stress. Viscous behavior can be described as resistance to flow, such as that observed with cold syrup. Viscosity in biologic materials arises largely, but not completely, from the resistance of their water content to flow into and out of the material with applied stress. For example, spaces between molecules of collagen in ligaments contain a large amount of water with salts and other small relatively mobile molecules. Tensile stress (stretching) of the ligament will decrease the available space between collagen molecules, forcing the fluid between them out of the ligament. This process is similar to stretching a wet sponge (Fig. 8.6). If the structure is stretched rapidly, there is an increasing resistance to fluid movement out of (and into) these spaces, since this requires time. The time required for fluids to move out of intermolecular spaces acts to slow the rate of deformation of an elastic material. This alters the elastic and plastic regions of the stress/strain curve. In combination with

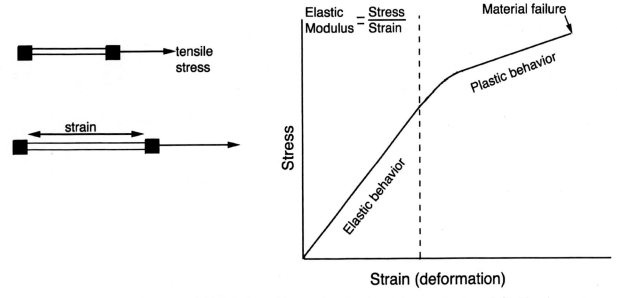

Figure 8-5 A stress/strain curve **(right)** of an object undergoing increasing tensile stress **(left)**. The change in length can be used as a measure of strain. The curve has an area of elastic behavior, in which a release of stress will allow the object to return to its original shape. In this area, the stress/strain relationship can be expressed as elastic modulus. With increasing stress, the material has permanent deformation or plastic behavior, followed by material failure.

the elastic properties of the material, this behavior is described as *viscoelasticity*. This property is usually modeled as a spring acting in parallel to a resistance provided by a fluid compartment (Fig. 8.6).

Besides the flow of small molecules from intermolecular spaces, frictional resistance due to molecular movement and ionic interactions between molecules also contributes to the viscosity

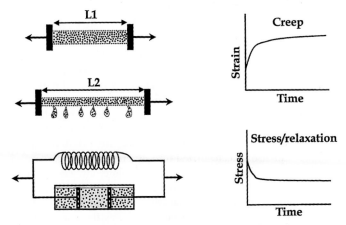

Figure 8-6 **Left.** Viscoelastic behavior occurs when a material containing a mobile fluid phase is stretched (or compressed) from a resting length (*L1*) to force fluid out of an elastic matrix similar to a sponge to a greater length (*L2*). This can be modeled schematically **(bottom)** as a spring in parallel with a fluid containing resistance compartment with porous baffles. **Right.** Time-dependent viscoelastic behavior of a material under tensile stress. Creep **(top)** is a measure of deformation (strain) over time with stress (stretch force) held constant. Stress/relaxation **(bottom)** is a measure of stress over time with strain held constant. (Portions of this figure have been adapted from Carlstedt CA, Nordin M. Biomechanics of tendons and ligaments. In: Nordin M, Frankel VH, eds. *Basic Biomechanics of the Musculoskeletal System.* 2nd Ed. Philadelphia, PA: Lea & Febiger, 1989:59–74, with permission.)

in a material. These molecular interactions, along with the elastic properties of the material, are important in the return of water and other small molecules back into the matrix, again much as a sponge reabsorbs fluid after being squeezed. This recovery process is important if the biomaterial properties of the tissue are to be maintained under repeated loading. Additionally, since viscoelastic behavior involves the movement of small molecules and the interaction between molecules, temperature can significantly affect this property.

Viscoelastic properties can produce significant alteration of material behavior when the rate of loading is too fast for the fluid exchange to occur. Under these conditions, a material may exhibit a higher elastic modulus (i.e., appear stiffer or more brittle) under high loading rates, as compared to the same load applied over a longer period of time. If a viscoelastic material is stretched rapidly and the load is sustained after the initial loading period, there will be a rapid initial deformation of the material followed by a slower deformation as the remaining fluid in the matrix reaches a new equilibrium at a slower rate (Fig. 8.6). Two types of measurements are used to describe this property. First, if the material is subjected to an initial load, such as tensile stress (Fig. 8.6), which is then maintained, the material will stretch to an initial length and then more slowly increase in length as the more resistant fluid in the matrix effuses. The slower phase after the initial stretch is called *creep*.

Another measurement looks at the load necessary to maintain a constant deformation or, in the case of Figure 8.6, the length of the material. As the matrix reaches equilibrium, the load necessary to maintain the length will decrease. This property is referred to as *stress/relaxation*.

Because of their high water and solute content, bone, muscle, ligament, tendon, and other biologic materials have viscoelastic properties that are important for their function. Due to the differences in the cellular structure and the matrix between cells in these materials, the actual viscoelastic properties of these tissues differ markedly.

Fatigue is the Failure of a Material as a Result of Repeated Stress

Fatigue is a multifaceted term that is used to describe material failure after repeated application of stresses that, if applied individually, would not produce failure. In nonbiologic materials such as metals, a significant part of fatigue failure can result from the accumulated breakdown of crystalline structure as the result of repeated stress, such as breaking a steel or copper wire by repeated bending. In biologic systems, the process of fatigue failure becomes more complicated, because of the ability to repair and adapt materials to repeated stress. For example, bone under repeated stress may undergo microfractures in its structure (see the following section). Depending upon the frequency of the stress and the ability of the bone to repair these microfractures, the bone may suffer a fatigue fracture or adapt to the stress by increasing its mass.

PROPERTIES OF BIOLOGIC MATERIALS: BONE

Bone Is an Anisotropic Material Comprising Osteons

Mechanical models describing nonbiologic materials are difficult to apply to biologic systems directly, due in part to their complicated structure. The response of biologic materials to stresses is determined by structural properties layered down to the subcellular level. Still, the material properties of bone structure as a whole are clearly traceable from tissue structure (1). Bone consists of connective tissue cells organized and embedded in a highly mineralized extracellular matrix. Although lower than other tissues, this matrix also contains significant amounts of water and other small molecules, giving bone viscoelastic material properties. The basic unit of organization is the osteon or haversian system. These systems consist of concentric rings of bone cells or osteocytes around a central cavity (the haversian canal) through which the blood vessels and nerves supplying the bone travel (Fig. 8.7). The osteons are arranged in a dense, regular pattern around the shaft of long bones to form cortical or compact bone. The border between osteons is the *cement line*. The cement line is structurally weaker than the substance of the circularly oriented osteons and can often be identified microscopically as the site of failure of bone tissue under high stresses (2). Osteocyte lacunae may also be a site of structural weakness (3). Beneath the cortical layer of compact bone is a central core of more porous bone (termed cancellous, trabecular, or spongy bone), with lacunae comprising the marrow space. While the structure of cancellous bone may initially appear as a random mesh of thin bone, it can be readily shown that areas of organization do exist and contribute to the structural stability of the bone as a whole by distributing stresses internally in the bone structure (4) (Fig. 8.7).

Bones Are Structured to Resist the Primary Functional Stresses Placed Upon Them

As might be expected, the highly organized cellular and gross structure of bone causes it to behave in an anisotropic manner to applied stresses. The outward structure and infrastructure of bones are organized to resist the major stresses to which they are subjected under normal physiologic conditions. For the structure of a long bone such as the tibia, the compressive loading lengthwise will require much higher stress before failure compared to a stress of similar magnitude applied perpendicularly to the long axis. In this manner, from the subcellular to gross structure, bone represents one of the most obvious examples of the structure-to-function relationship. This anisotropic behavior also defines the manner in

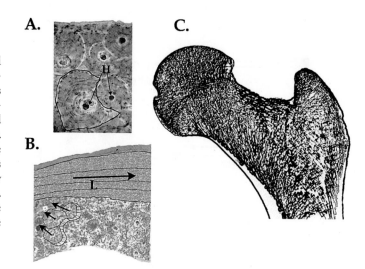

Figure 8-7 Histologic and structural properties of bone. **A.** Compact bone structure is organized into cylinder-shaped osteons with haversian canals (*H*) that are separated by a cement line (*outline*). **B.** In long bones, osteons are oriented longitudinally along the axis of the bone and surrounded by circumferentially oriented lamellar bone (*L*). Both surround a marrow space that contains marrow and cancellous bone. **C.** The organization cancellous bone is not random in structures such as the femur, where the trabeculae (*black*) help to distribute stresses through the internal structure of the bone.

which bones will undergo material failure when excessive stresses are placed upon them.

Different Stress Vectors Produce Varying Types of Bone Failure (Fracture)

The material failure (fracture) of bone can be observed clinically for all major categories of stresses, with the mechanism of material failure varying with type of loading (1). Also, the viscoelastic behavior of bone gives it sensitivity to loading rate. At rapid loading rates, bone appears stiffer as the movement of fluid and molecular friction increasingly resists deformation. This causes bone to store more energy before failure. When bone does fail at high loading rates, its more brittle behavior makes it more likely to fragment, much like shattering glass (comminuted fracture) (5). Accordingly, fractures can also be categorized into different types according to the energy absorbed with the resulting failure, low energy, high energy, and very high energy. Higher-energy fractures (automobile accidents, gunshot wounds) are typically accompanied by bone fragmentation and soft soft-tissue damage, as the energy stored under rapid loading is dissipated with biomaterial failure.

Under physiologic conditions, bones will experience a combination of stress vectors at the same time and failures may result from the combination rather than a particular stress type. However, fractures do begin in the stress component direction most prone to failure according to the material properties of the bone. This allows the description of some types of fracture resulting from particular stress categories. Muscles pulling on bone typically generate tensile stress fractures. The tensile fracture of the calcaneus adjacent to the Achilles tendon insertion is a frequent example (Fig. 8.8). Compression fractures are most commonly found in the vertebral column, which is subject to high compressive load and a weakening of the bones with age. Shear forces act parallel to bone surfaces, typically at articulations, where bones are in contact. Shear fractures can

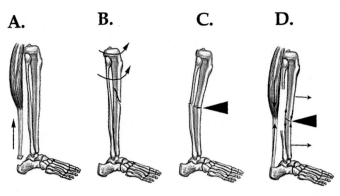

Figure 8-8 Examples of fracture types resulting from a material failure due to a primary stress component. **A.** Tensile fracture of the calcaneus. **B.** Spiral fracture from torsional stress of the tibia. **C.** Bending stress fracture. **D.** Example of how muscle contraction forces can act to counter bending stress. Bending stress produces tensile forces on one side of the tibia and compressive stress on the other (see fig 8.4). Muscle contraction can act to counter the tensile component by producing a compressive moment. (Portions of this figure have been adapted from Gollnick PD, Matoba H. The muscle fiber composition of skeletal muscle as a predictor of athletic success. An overview. *Am J Sports Med.* 1984;12:212–217, with permission.)

occur under conditions of compression loading of a joint, coupled with a shear or a lateral force across the articulation with a failure of the joint bony plateau. Bending and torsional loading produce multiple types of material stresses on bone depending upon the direction of the loading. As described earlier, bending of an object produces tensile stress on one side of an object and compression on the other (Fig. 8.4). Bone is weaker in tension than compression, so bone material failure begins upon the tensile stress side (Fig. 8.8). Immature bone, which is less calcified and more ductile, may be more sensitive to compression and fractures may occur on the compressive side first. Torsional loading (Fig. 8.8), or usually twisting around the long axis of bones, produces shear stresses around the neutral axis while compression and tension loading are diagonal to the axis. The resulting failure (spiral fracture) is initially due to shear stress followed by tensile stress failure along a diagonal axis. As should be expected, if there are weaknesses in the bone structure, such as during rehabilitation after injury, failure will occur at the weakest point or at the site of bony defect with bending loads.

The biomaterial failure of bone under stresses is greatly influenced by the attachment and contraction of muscles. Muscle activity can decrease or counter stresses produced on bone by altering the direction of the resultant stress vectors to those to which bone may be more tolerant. Figure 8.8 shows how muscle activity may alter a bending or tensile stress to produce compression stress. As bone is very resistant to compressive stress (such as weight on the long axis of the tibia), this redistribution of stress can be important to avoiding stress fracture. Consequently, the physiologic tiring of muscle during strenuous exercise can contribute significantly to fractures because the protective mechanism is lost.

While sudden, large stresses are usually associated with bone fracture, failure of the material itself can result from repetitive loading over a period of time. This fatigue-type fracture of bone involves an accumulation of smaller failures within the bone microstructure and is dependent upon the magnitude, frequency, and rate of loading. Even low-level repetitive loads may produce fatigue microfractures in bone (6). In living bone, these microfractures will be repaired by cellular reactions to the injury. If the fatigue process

outpaces the repair, failure will eventually occur as a repetitive stress fracture. A common example of this is the fatigue fracture of metatarsal bones in long-distance runners (7).

Bone Remodels Its Structure in Response to Stress and Depends upon Stresses to Maintain Its Material Properties

In the presence of stresses, bone can alter size, shape, and structure to withstand stresses placed upon it. The unusual corollary to this property is that bone must be subjected to stress in order to maintain its biomaterial properties. The underlying principle of this process in bone has been expressed as Wolff law, which states that bone is increased where needed and resorbed where not needed (8). The resorption of bone under conditions of reduced usage or immobilization (9) is of particular concern clinically, since mechanical stress on bone is reduced during casting or in more limited conditions, such as weightlessness in space travel (10). Immobilization results in the resorption of periosteal and subperiosteal bone (11) and a decrease in bone strength and stiffness (12). Conversely, the hypertrophy (13,14) and increase in density of bone (15) may be observed in normal bones in response to strenuous exercise. Both hypertrophy and resorption of bone may be observed around implant screws and plates used to surgically stabilize bone defects or to attach prosthetic joints (16).

Bone properties also are altered with aging, with a progressive loss of bone density and size (17,18). This is independent of the condition of osteoporosis. The result is a decrease in bone strength and stiffness and altered stress/strain properties, including an increase in brittleness and a reduction in energy storage capacity. These properties make bones more susceptible to material failure under high stress conditions with increasing age.

ARTICULAR CARTILAGE

The Surfaces of Contact Between Bones in Synovial Joints Is Hyaline Cartilage

There are three identified primary types of cartilage in the human body: hyaline cartilage, fibrocartilage, and elastic cartilage. Hyaline cartilage covers the surface of the articulations of almost all diarthrodial joints and will be the focus of our description of basic biomaterial properties of cartilage. Cartilage has some similarity to bone in that it consists of cells (chondrocytes) surrounded by an extensive extracellular matrix that they secrete. However, cartilage is avascular; lacking blood vessels, lymph channels, or nerves within its matrix; and the matrix secreted is not calcified as in bone. The extracellular matrix of cartilage consists primarily of collagen (type II), proteoglycans, and 60% to 87% water with inorganic salts and other minor matrix proteins and lipids (19,20). The collagen and proteoglycans form the major structural elements of cartilage, and these interact extensively on a molecular level with the smaller molecules, including water. The interaction of these elements with each other within cartilage and their interaction with the water in the matrix determine the primary biomaterial properties of cartilage.

The major collagen and proteoglycan structural element on the cartilage of articular surfaces is not randomly organized and can be divided into histologic zones that differ in cellular organization from the surface to the underlying subchondral bone (20) (Fig. 8.9). The orientation of collagen fibril bundles within the matrix differs between the layers (Fig. 8.9) with a tangential orientation at the surface, random organization in the middle zone, and radial

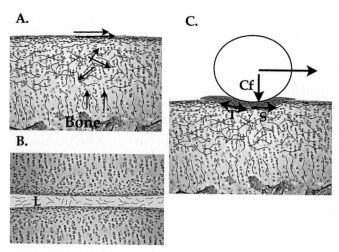

Figure 8-9 **A.** Schematic of the orientation (*arrows*) of collagen fibrils (*drawn lines*) in articular cartilage. The orientation varies from the articular surface to the bone interface. **B.** Representation of cartilage surface separated by a thin layer of lubricating fluid (*L*) that prevents direct surface contact. **C.** With a compressive force on the surface (*cf*), additional fluid is exuded and the matrix is compressed. Lateral movement produces tensile (*t*) and shear (*s*) stress on the cartilage surface and matrix components.

orientation near the subchondral bone surface. This orientation provides the basic structural framework for the cartilage and resistance to the loads placed upon it. Depending upon the particular joint function, the primary stresses may be compression, which, as the joint moves, contributes to shear and tensile stresses on the cartilage surfaces (Fig. 8.9).

Cartilage Has Significant Viscoelastic Properties That Are Essential to Its Function

The collagen and proteoglycan structural elements of cartilage have spaces between them filled with water, salts, and other small molecules, forming a matrix with viscoelastic properties as previously described. Further, the structural elements contain molecules such as hyaluronic acid and have ionically charged groups throughout their structure. This property allows them to strongly bind water and inorganic salt within the cartilaginous matrix. The cartilage matrix has properties of flexibility from a pliable, porous collagen superstructure containing small molecules that can be forced out, but with some molecular and ionic interaction based resistance to the efflux. The properties of this matrix allow a viscoelastic behavior in which the cartilage allows rapid, but declining deformation (cushioning) in response to compressive loads followed by creep or stress/relaxation (21) (Fig. 8.7). The slower deformation will continue until equilibrium is reached between the load and the forces resisting it within the matrix. The differing mechanical properties of the layers of articular cartilage interact dynamically to reach equilibrium in response to a sustained compressive force (22).

On a tissue level more closely related to normal function, the viscoelastic response of cartilage can be explained by a compressive stress that produces a rapid efflux of fluid forced out of the extracellular matrix directly beneath it and in areas immediately adjacent to it (Fig. 8.9). The resistance to this efflux of fluid is dependent upon the effective porosity or space available in the cartilage matrix for fluid to move. Other resistance to matrix deformation includes the internal friction generated by movement

between long polymer molecules such as collagen and attached proteoglycans and the ionic binding of these chains to the water and other small molecules. The time required for the fluid phase to reach a full equilibrium between cartilage layers under the applied load may require hours (21). However, because of the elasticity of the collagenous structural elements and ionic interactions with the small molecules of the matrix, this fluid exchange is reversible and supplies a pumping action of nutrients into and waste products out of cartilage in addition to normal diffusion. This action is particularly important because of the avascular nature of cartilage.

Articular Cartilage Has Several Properties That Act to Prevent Wear Damage

Under physiologic conditions, cartilage surfaces of joints contact each other under a variety of loading conditions while showing little wear. This occurs in spite of the fact that joint surfaces are not perfectly smooth. The prevention of wear is due in part to a system of lubrication of synovial articular surfaces provided by synovial fluid and the properties of the cartilage itself. Fluids lubricate surfaces by preventing their direct contact (Fig. 8.9). The first level of lubrication of joint surfaces is the absorption of lubricin, a glycoprotein in synovial fluid that is absorbed onto articular surfaces. This provides a thin boundary of lubricant on the joint surface. The synovial fluid itself also provides a thin film of fluid between the joint surfaces that can be redistributed under loading conditions. Further, during loading, the fluid extruded as a result of the compressive deformation of the cartilage will provide a fluid layer to separate the opposed surfaces (23).

Under normal conditions, the fluid-lubricating properties of the joint will prevent the direct contact of uneven sections or asperities of joint surfaces to contact each other. If contact does occur, wear of the joint surfaces or interfacial wear (mechanical removal of material from a solid surface) may occur. This may consist of abrasion of the joint surface because of contact of uneven elements of the surface or small fragments of joint surfaces may adhere to each other and be dislodged. The efficient lubricating properties of normal joint usually preclude interfacial wear, but it may occur in damaged or degenerated joints (22).

Cartilage Wear May Result from Several Different Mechanisms, Including Intrinsic Changes with Aging

While cartilage can be damaged as a result of traumatic injury as in shearing stress applied to the meniscal cartilage of the knee, the mechanisms of abnormal wear are not as clear. Hypotheses of the mechanism of cartilage wear include the disruption of the structural molecules of the cartilage matrix through repeated stress (24,25) and the alteration of the matrix content under the same conditions. As with bone, rapid loading of a viscoelastic matrix increases the stiffness of cartilage, and the loss of the fluid component of the matrix will also increase stiffness. This loss of fluid may include soluble proteoglycans from the cartilage surface that are important in the maintenance of its properties. Under conditions of rapidly repeated high-impact loading, the fluid forced from the matrix that would normally provide a cushioning effect cannot be reabsorbed in time to cushion subsequent impacts. This may also produce plastic deformation of cartilage surfaces that does not sufficiently recover for smooth surface contact upon subsequent loading. The increased stiffness and deformation of the matrix increases the likelihood of mechanical wear in addition to rendering the subchondral bone surface more vulnerable to damage.

Cartilage wear may also be complicated by the limited capacity of cartilage to repair or regenerate. This property gives it a limited capacity to adapt to stress. In conjunction with repeated stresses and minor injuries, a cycle of damage, wear, and insufficient recovery may occur, leading to joint degeneration and/or osteoarthritis. The inability of cartilage to recover during repeated high stress loads may be one source of macroscopic structural defects observed in cartilage (26) and responsible for the high incidence of specific joint degeneration and the development of osteoarthritis in persons with certain occupations (football players and dancers).

The intrinsic composition and properties of cartilage also change with age (27). The matrix composition changes and permeability increases, decreasing cartilage stiffness and rendering it less resistant to rapid loading. Along with the accumulation of injuries from which the tissue cannot recover, these age-related changes may contribute to the increased incidence of joint degeneration with age.

LIGAMENTS AND TENDONS

Ligaments and Tendons Are Dense, Regular Connective Tissue with a High Resistance to Tensile Loading

Ligaments and tendons, along with joint capsules, surround the articulations of the skeletal system. Their functions are, in the case of ligaments and joint capsules, to structurally connect, stabilize, and guide the bones forming the articulation (28). They may also act as a sensor for joint position and strain for the joint. Tendons connect muscle to bone and transmit forces from muscle to bone to produce motion. Both tendons and ligaments are classified as dense, regular connective tissues. They have sparse cellular elements and abundant extracellular matrix in a highly organized array. The extracellular matrix is rich in collagen and water with a small amount of elastin, again producing a viscoelastic behavior under stress. The collagen molecules are linked together in lengthwise overlapping arrays to microfibrils, which are in turn combined in similar overlapping arrays to form fibrils, then fibers, and bundles of fibers to form the macroscopic tendon (Fig. 8.10). This successive parallel linkage down to the molecular level makes ligaments and tendons capable of handling high tensile loads. The arrangement of fibrils

in ligament tissue is less parallel than tendon and accounts for its higher resistance to tensile loading in orientations other than along the tissue axis. The collagen molecules are also linked to each other by crosslinks. While there are some important biomechanical differences between ligaments and tendons, most of their properties are basically similar and will be described together here.

The Primary Biomaterial Characteristics of Ligaments and Tendons Are Described by Elastic Modulus and Viscoelastic Properties

The primary stress response characteristics of ligaments and tendons are described by their modulus of elasticity properties. Under tensile loading (stretch), ligaments and tendons exhibit a modulus of elasticity that is variable with load (Fig. 8.10). Under low loading, there is a relatively large increase in length in response to the load applied (low elastic modulus). This is attributed to lengthening as the result of macromolecular "slack" within the collagen fiber structure that offers less resistance to an imposed load. As the slack is taken up, fibers slide relative to each other and fluid is extruded from the matrix. The elastic modulus then increases (stiffness increases) gradually with increasing load and shows a linear response up to the point where failure begins. The behavior of tendons and ligaments is similar except for ligament tissue such as the ligamentum flavum of the spinal column, where a high elastic content produces a different pattern of the elastic modulus.

The extracellular matrix of tendons and ligaments between the collagen fibrils has proteoglycans, a high water content, and other small ionically charged molecules that can interact with structural elements. This matrix is comparatively more porous than cartilage or bone, and is structured to resist tensile rather than compressive stresses. The viscoelastic properties become evident at high loading rates, where the tissue will demonstrate increased stiffness and offer increased resistance to tensile stress (stretch). As with cartilage, repeated tensile loading in cycles can result in a slow increase in elastic stiffness due to plastic deformation (29,30). This plastic deformation is presumably due to molecular deformation in the fibrous structural elements of the tendon or ligament, and also to the inability of fluid and small charged molecules to reequilibrate within the molecular structure.

Ligaments and tendons also demonstrate the viscoelastic properties of stress or load relaxation and creep. To characterize these properties, the tissue is placed under a tensile load (stretch) within the linear region of the elastic modulus and maintained at a constant length (stress relaxation) or a constant load (creep). Ligament and tendon tissue adjusts its molecular structure and fluid distribution to the load primarily within the first 6 to 8 hours, but will continue over a period of months. The creep phenomenon is used clinically as plaster casts or braces are employed to place a constant load to correct a soft-tissue deformity, such as some spinal curvatures (31).

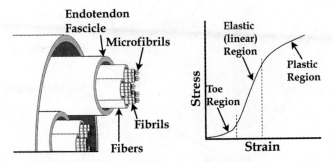

Figure 8-10 Left. Schematic view of the structural organization of tendon. Microfibrils are the smallest component consisting of collagen molecules. Microfibrils are organized into fibrils that are grouped into fibers. Fibers are grouped into fascicles that comprise the tendon. **Right.** Idealized version of a stress/strain curve for tendon under tensile stress. The toe region is a nonlinear behavior attributed to the "slack" between collagen molecules. The elastic region has a linear relationship between stress and strain. In the plastic region, permanent deformation occurs, eventually resulting in failure.

Material Failure of Ligaments and Tendons Is Preceded by Microfailure of the Molecular Structural Elements

Overall failure of the ligament or tendon is usually sudden and preceded by the microfailure of the attachments between collagen fibers within the tissue and loss of the ability of the tendon or ligament to recover its length. With tendon and ligament, it is also important to distinguish eventual failure due to a sustained load (creep failure) from sustained cyclic loading and unloading (fatigue failure). Both are important biomaterial properties for tendon and ligament. As with bone, a smaller degree of microfailure may occur within the range of physiologic loading, suggesting that repeated stress may lead to declining strength or fatigue over time (32). There may be a range of damage depending upon the total deformation and extent of partial failure. Inflammation resulting from such damage is associated with tendonitis (32).

Failure of both tendons and ligaments may also occur at the bone interface. The site of failure may depend upon the loading rate (33). Tendons, with their attached muscles, typically have a higher tensile strength than muscle, and rupture of muscle is more common than tendon. The instability of the joint that may result from tendon, or especially ligament, damage can contribute to and be complicated by damage to the joint capsule. This damage and associated abnormal loading patterns may contribute to osteoarthritis (31).

Ligaments and Tendons Can Adapt to Stresses

Like other tissue, ligament and tendon structurally remodel in response to the stresses placed upon them within the limits of damage (32). They become stronger and stiffer with increased stress and weaker and less stiff with a reduction in stress (34). Physical training can increase the strength of tendons and ligaments along with the ligament-bone interface (35,36). Immobilization (such as from casting) can decrease the strength and stiffness of ligaments. While reconditioning can occur, it can require a considerable length of time (34,37).

The Properties and Structure of Ligaments and Tendons Change with Age

During maturation, the number and quality of crosslinks increases in the collagen of ligaments and tendons and fibril diameter increases as well (38), producing increased tensile strength. The mechanical properties of collagen reach a maximum with maturation and begin to decrease with age (39). The collagen content of ligaments and tendons decreases as well. This loss of collagen results in a decrease in strength, stiffness, and the amount of deformation required to produce to failure (40). However, the overall biomechanical properties of tendon remain reasonably constant with age (41). The amount of time required for tissue repair and reconditioning (discussed previously) will also increase. Other physiologic factors, such as pregnancy, can also affect the biomechanical properties of ligaments and tendons (31,40).

SKELETAL MUSCLE

Skeletal Muscle Provides the Forces for Body Movement

Since a more complete description of muscle is given elsewhere in this volume, only those elements essential to understanding the biomechanical aspects of muscle tissue will be given here. Of the three types of muscle tissue, skeletal muscle is the most abundant tissue in the body, accounting for 40% of body weight (42). The forces necessary to provide movement to the body are provided by the contraction of skeletal muscles acting across joints. These contractions may produce dynamic work or participate in static maintenance of posture. While subcellular units known as *sarcomeres* are the source of muscle contraction, the basic contractile unit of skeletal muscle as a tissue is the *muscle fiber*. The fiber may range in size from 10 to 100 μm in diameter and between 1 and 30 cm in length (43).

The metabolic and contractile properties of muscle fibers may differ according to the physiologic demands placed upon them as described subsequently.

Both Contractile Elements and Connective Tissue Contribute to the Biomechanical Properties of Muscle

Muscle may be histologically and mechanically described as bundles of contractile elements in a series of connective tissue sheaths (Fig. 8.11). The basic unit of the contractile/connective tissue relationship is an individual muscle fiber surrounded by a connective tissue sheath, the *endomysium*. This basic unit of skeletal muscle is then organized into fascicles or groups of fibers by a thicker connective tissue sheath, the *perimysium*. Finally, groups of muscle fascicles are organized into the entire muscle itself and covered by the epimysium, which surrounds the entire structure. The epimysium and loose connective tissue form the fascial planes between muscles. The connective tissue sheaths are continuous with each other and the muscle tendon and/or attachments to bone. Both connective tissue and the contractile elements contribute to the biomechanical properties of muscle. The contractile elements provide active energy expending forces with some elastic and viscoelastic properties, while the connective tissue contributes passive elastic and viscoelastic influences on the pattern of force transduction to the skeleton.

The Basic Relationship Between Nerve and Muscle Is Defined by the Motor Unit

Muscle fibers contract in response to acetylcholine released by motor nerves. An individual motor neuron, with the muscle fibers contacted by it, forms a motor unit. The size of motor units may vary dramatically between muscles and within the muscle itself. The motor neuron generates an action potential lasting 1 to 2 ms that produces a contraction of all of the muscle fibers in a motor unit in an "on-off" fashion. The response of the motor unit

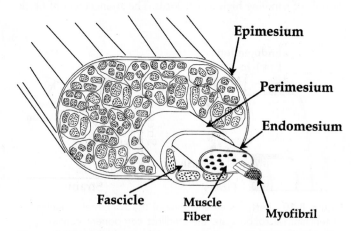

Figure 8-11 Schematic of the structural organization of a muscle. The basic subcellular unit of the muscle is the myofibril. Collections of myofibrils are present in muscle cells (muscle fibers). Muscle fibers are organized into fascicles and groups of fascicles make up the muscle. The connective tissue coverings of the muscle include the endomysium that surrounds muscle fibers, the perimysium surrounding muscle fascicles, and the epimysium surrounding the entire muscle.

to a single action potential is termed a *twitch,* the basic unit of recordable muscle activity. The time required for a motor unit to fully contract and then return to resting length is variable (from 10 to 100 ms) according to fiber type, but in all cases much longer than a nerve action potential. If additional nerve stimulation occurs before the contraction phase of the twitch has ended, contraction can be maintained and increased in a process called *summation.* The limit of summation, such that contraction is maintained and does not increase with a greater frequency of stimulation, is called *tetanic contraction* or *tetany.* The force of contraction of the muscle as a whole may be further regulated by increasing or decreasing the number of motor units used to produce the contraction, a process termed *recruitment.* In this way, the nervous system may control the force of muscle contraction by the size and number of motor units employed to produce the contraction and the frequency of activation of motor units.

Types of Muscle Contraction Are Defined by the Movements Occurring During Contraction

Dynamic muscle contractions in the processes of producing movement can be classified as *concentric* and *eccentric.* Concentric contractions produce movement in the direction of muscle contraction (Fig. 8.12), while eccentric contractions act to decelerate or resist movement, as in slowly placing an object down rather than letting it fall. Muscles also produce contractions without substantial movement, as in static posture against gravity. This type of contraction is termed *isometric,* as no change in muscle length occurs during contraction. Another term, *isotonic* contraction, refers to muscle contraction with a change in length under constant tension.

The Mechanical Properties of Contractile Elements and Their Connective Tissue in Muscle Is Described as a Musculotendinous Unit

The force production characteristics of a muscle as a whole are a combination of the material properties of its contractile

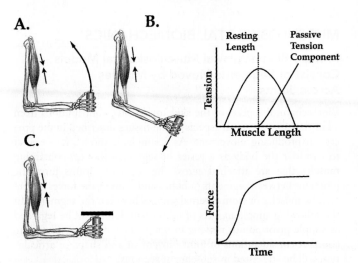

Figure 8-12 Left. Types of muscle contraction. **A.** Concentric. **B.** Eccentric. **C.** Isometric. **Right. Top**—Muscle tension relationship to muscle length. The greatest active tension is near the muscle-resting length. The passive tension component from stretch of connective tissue increases beyond the resting length. **Bottom**—Force-time relationship of muscle contraction. The time lag in reaching maximum force is related to the elasticity of tissue components.

components, the connective tissue that surrounds them (and the whole muscle), and the tendon of its insertion. From a mechanical viewpoint, this combination is a *musculotendinous unit* (44). The contractile elements add a rapid tensile load on the connective tissue elements, which in turn respond according to their elastic and viscoelastic properties as described earlier. As with ligaments and tendons alone, this will mean that there is rapid component to stretch, produced in this case by contraction, followed by a slower change in length as the connective tissue elements reach equilibrium with the contracting force (Fig. 8.12).

The connective tissues surrounding the muscle and its tendon have elastic properties that can store energy with stretch like a rubber band. In the process of muscle contraction, the tendon and connective tissue are stretched. The energy is released by moving a body segment or by stretching the contractile elements as the muscle relaxes. The elasticity also helps to keep the muscle prepared for contraction by reducing slackening of contractile elements, preventing passive overstretch of muscle fibers, thereby reducing the danger of injury. This energy storage also occurs as muscles are stretched under load. The muscle contractile elements may also have some elasticlike properties of energy storage (45,46).

The sum of the interaction of the contractile elements and elastic elements of muscle contraction can be demonstrated in the force-time curve of muscle contraction (Fig. 8.12). While the tension or force of contraction of the muscle fibers may reach maximum within a relatively short time, a much longer time is required for this tension to be transferred through the elastic components. Because of this time lag, the active contraction process must be long enough in time for the full transfer of tension to occur.

Many Factors, Such as Length, Load, and Temperature, May Affect the Force Produced by Muscle Contraction

The force of muscle contraction can be affected by various mechanical factors, including length-tension relationships, load-velocity, and force-time properties (43). Other significant factors may include temperature, muscle fatigue, and prestretching. The length-tension property of a muscle as a whole (Fig. 8.12) involves both the active contractile elements and the passive connective tissue elements (47). The maximum force or tension produced by contractile elements, such as the muscle fiber, is obtained at near its resting length. Contraction at lengths beyond or smaller than the resting length results in reduced tension production by the muscle fiber. This is a result of intrinsic properties of muscle fiber sarcomeres. For the muscle as a whole, reducing or increasing the muscle length from its resting position will reduce the tension produced by contractile elements. However, increasing muscle length will also produce a passive tension as a result of stretching the connective tissue elements, although the contractile force is reduced. The passive component of stretch, which is readily detectable by passively stretching a relaxed limb, will eventually become the dominant source of resistance or tension as muscle length increases, effectively protecting the muscle from overstretch. (Fig. 8.12).

Applied Loads Affect the Velocity of Muscle Contraction

The relationship of the load applied to a muscle and the velocity with which it contracts defines the load-velocity property of muscle contraction. The shortening of muscles contracting concentrically is most rapid with no external load and progressively slows with increasing external loads (48). The shortening velocity will reach zero as the load reaches the maximum contraction force of the muscle (isometric contraction) and then reverse to a lengthening velocity with eccentric contraction. As might be expected, eccentric contraction lengthening velocity increases with increasing external load.

A Rise in Temperature Can Increase the Efficiency of Muscle Contraction

In the process of contraction, muscle efficiency is usually no more than 20% to 25% in the translation of chemical energy into useful work, with the majority of the energy being dissipated as heat (42). Even so, the heat dissipation can have positive effects on muscle contraction properties by increasing temperature. As would be attained through a warm-up procedure, temperature increases usually arise from increased blood flow and the production of heat by the muscle itself from metabolic reactions and friction generated by the sliding of molecules past each other in the contractile and elastic elements. Within physiologic ranges, increases in temperature will increase the conduction velocity across the muscle fiber membrane (sarcolemma) (48), increasing the rate of contraction and increasing the rate at which the muscle can be stimulated. This can mean an increase in the production of muscle force. A rise in temperature can also increase enzymatic activity related to muscle metabolism and increase the efficiency of muscle contraction. The viscoelastic properties of the musculotendinous unit are also affected by rises in temperature, generally increasing the elasticity of the collagen, decreasing stiffness, and enhancing the extensibility of the unit. While these basic biomechanical properties of muscle tissue change with temperature to enhance the contractile properties of the musculotendinous unit, the effects from stretching or "warming up" prior to activity are much more complex and not completely understood (49,50). The physiologic aspects of stretch (or release) involve highly significant neural components and reflexes beyond the biomechanical properties of the tissues alone.

Muscle Fatigue Properties Are Affected by the Muscle Fiber Type(s) Comprising the Muscle

Fatigue of muscle with prolonged contraction activity results from the depletion of the nutrients and oxygen required to produce adenosine triphosphate (ATP) as an energy supply from either aerobic or anaerobic glycolysis. The result is a decrease in force production by the muscle eventually to total cessation (42). The rate at which a muscle will reach fatigue can vary according to the types of muscle fibers it contains. Muscle fiber types are distinguished by the rate at which ATP can be made available to the sarcomeres for contraction and the metabolic pathways through which ATP is generated. The rate of availability of ATP directly affects the rate of contraction or twitch time of a muscle fiber. Accordingly, muscle fiber types can be classified as slow or fast twitch. Two primary metabolic pathways involved to generate ATP (oxidative or glycolytic) further divide these two basic types of contractile behavior. Using these properties, three primary muscle fiber types are distinguished including type I or slow-twitch oxidative fibers, type IIA, fast-twitch oxidative-glycolytic fibers, and type IIB, fast-twitch glycolytic fibers. These different fiber types have varying degrees of contraction time, resistance to fatigue, and a dependence on aerobic or anaerobic metabolism. As their names suggest, type I fibers have slower contraction rates, and, with a metabolism directed toward aerobic pathways, are resistant to fatigue. They are relatively small in diameter and produce a relatively low amount of tension per fiber.

These properties make this fiber type well suited for prolonged low-intensity work (51). Type IIA fibers are fast contracting and rich in aerobic and anaerobic (glycolytic) enzymes with a moderate resistance to fatigue. They appear to be intermediate between type I and type IIB in their capacity for contractile force and resistance to fatigue. Type IIB fibers are fast contracting, rely primarily on glycolytic pathways, and may fatigue rapidly. However, they have a large fiber diameter and can produce relatively large amounts of tension.

Muscles May Have Some Ability to Change Their Fiber Type According to Demand

Most muscles are of mixed fiber types with the proportion of fiber types determined by the nerve innervating the muscle (52,53). The overall distribution of muscle fiber types in the muscles of the body appears to have a strong genetic component (42,51,54). The fiber type can be changed with nerve stimulation (55), suggesting that patterns of activity may alter fiber metabolism. Some changes in fiber types may also occur with physical training, but much of this change is a result of increases in the cross-sectional area of the fiber type corresponding to the activity rather than an actual change in fiber type (54,56). The extent to which actual alterations in the type of muscle fiber occur as a result of activity demand therefore remains unclear.

Muscle Adapts to Physiologic Demands

Although the extent of fiber type change under physiologic conditions is unclear, muscle will clearly remodel according to the stresses placed upon it. Muscle atrophies with disuse and hypertrophies with increased use. Studies of muscle atrophy in both animal and clinical studies suggest that early dynamic motion after debilitating injury may be important in the minimization of atrophy, particularly of type I muscle fibers (57,58). Electric stimulation may also prevent some of this fiber loss (56). Hypertrophy of muscle with physical training is generally the result of increases in the cross-sectional area of all muscle fibers (58,59).

MUSCULOSKELETAL BIOMECHANICS

Primary Biomechanical Musculoskeletal Models Consist of Segments Moved by Muscles Across Joints

Biomechanical aspects of the skeleton involve contributions from all of the biomechanical aspects of the tissues described in the process of producing movement. As a simplistic model, it is easiest to consider the body as a series of segments (bones) containing muscles that are attached across the segments. Joints form the junctions between segments or bones and transfer the forces generated by muscles or from external sources between the segments. In the following simple models of movement, joints will be regarded as simple pivot points, moving in one plane (coplanar). The more complex considerations of joint movement and shape of articulation will be addressed in subsequent sections.

Force Moments Are Used to Describe Models of Musculoskeletal Movement

Using the simple model used for the descriptions of moments earlier in the chapter, a joint, such as the elbow (Fig. 8.13), becomes a rotation system with the flexor system and the extensors using the

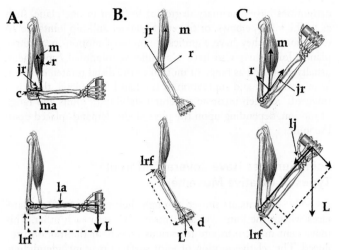

Figure 8-13 Schematic of basic joint moments and their variation with movement. Sections on top represent muscle contraction moments. Figures on the bottom show moments generated by the load. **A.** Right angle resistance to a load (*l*). **Top.** Moments about the joint center (*c*) include the moment arm of the muscle (*ma*) that is moved by a resisting component (*r*) of the muscle contraction force (*m*), this is resisted by the load **(bottom)** acting on a load moment arm (*la*). Joint reaction forces include the portion of the muscle force directed into the joint (*jr*) and a moment generated from the load into the joint with a center of rotation about the muscle insertion (*lrf, dotted lines displaced*). **B.** At extension, the angle of muscle pull directs more of the muscle force into the joint **(top)** and a portion of the load force (*l*) moment pulls out on the joint as a distracting force (*d*). **C.** In a flexed position, the muscle moment **(top)** is divided into the resisting component (*r*) and a joint reaction distracting force away from the joint (*jr*). A portion of the load force **(bottom)** now is directed into the joint (*lj*).

joint as a center of rotation to move the distal limb and any load on the limb. In mathematical modeling of joint function, the description of such movements is a system of balanced moments produced by the load on the limb and muscle contraction forces. Characterizing movement in this way becomes particularly important as other aspects of joint function (noncoplanar movement, movement within the joint) and more mechanically complicated joint types are modeled.

As a distal segment moves relative to a more proximal segment, the distal segment will rotate about the instant center of the joint or center of rotation (*c*, Fig. 8.13). The effective distance from the center of the joint's rotation to where the force is acting (muscle insertion) is the *moment arm* (*ma*) for the muscle. The product of the force applied from the muscle and the moment arm (force × distance) is the *moment* (or torque) used to resist a load on the distal limb. For concentric contraction to occur, this moment of resistance must exceed the moment produced by the load (distance to the load from *c* × weight). In a more complete model, the weight of the limb must also be considered. Note also that if the load moment is resisted by the pull of the muscle, there is also a center of rotation created at the point of muscle insertion about which the load exerts a moment into the joint (*lrf*, Fig. 8.13). Together with the portion of the muscle contraction force directed into the joint (discussed subsequently), this becomes part of the *joint reaction force* that applies a stress to the joint during movement.

Muscle Moments Necessary to Resist a Load Vary with Joint Position

As can be seen from Figure 8.13, although the length moment arm does not change, the proportion of muscle contraction force (vector) that is applied to resist the load will vary as the limb is flexed. With the joint fully extended, most of the muscle contraction force vector is directed into the joint. This muscle component force also contributes to the joint reaction force and may be particularly important in the stabilization of load-bearing joints, such as the knee. The relative size of the joint reaction and load-resistive forces can be expressed by simple trigonometric functions in mathematical models, but it is sufficient here to be aware of how these forces change with joint position. In this model, the portion of the muscle contraction vector used to resist the load increases as the angle of tendon is closer to a right angle (Fig. 8.13A, orthogonal) to the forearm. Beyond this point, a portion of the load vector becomes directed into the joint (Fig. 8.13C) reducing the effective load on the muscle, but placing stress on the joint and more proximal segments. In the flexed position, the angle of pull by the muscle directs a portion of the muscle contraction force against this load into the joint.

Muscle Moments Are Also Transferred Across Joints by Tendons

Muscle forces are also conveyed to distal segments across joints by tendons. In joints associated with the knee, hands, and feet, tendons cross the joint(s) to produce a "pulley" effect (Fig. 8.14). In this arrangement, as in the knee, the distance between the center of rotation of the joint and the tendon defines the moment arm for the contracting muscle.

The wheel and axle mechanism (60) is an instructive related model used to achieve rotary movements (Fig. 8.14). In this case, muscle contraction forces are applied to the opposite sides of a segment to produce rotation about an axis. The length moment arm in this case is the distance to the center of rotation. This mechanism is used widely throughout the body to achieve rotation of limbs and the body, as in rotation of the head, torso, or shoulder. As with simple flexors and extensors, muscles producing rotational

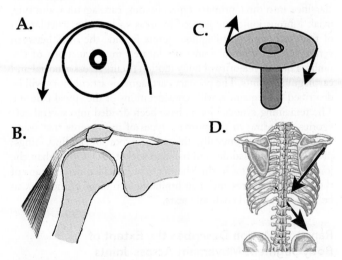

Figure 8-14 Strategies of muscles and tendons pulling across joints. **A.** A pulleylike mechanism in which the direction of pull is changed. **B.** A similar mechanism is used in knee extension. **C.** A wheel and axle mechanism in which coactive forces act to rotate an axle, such as the shoulders **(D)** relative to the spine.

components work in pairs and significant clinical problems may arise from imbalances in function of the pair.

Muscle Moments Generally Have a Low Mechanical Advantage

As suggested in the examples that have been given, the lever arrangement of muscle insertions and joints in limbs is such that a comparatively small distance of muscle contraction can produce a large displacement of the load at the expense of needing large muscle contraction forces. This is described as having a low mechanical advantage. The relative mechanical advantage is a function of the position of the muscle origin and insertion on the two bony segments relative to the joint. Because both the moment arm (distance, d) and the contraction force (f) equally contribute to the moment ($f \times d$) producing the movement or resistance, small differences in the moment arm can produce significant changes in the amount of muscle contraction required. As origins and insertions of muscles and segment lengths vary markedly between individuals, the ability to produce different types of movement using the same muscle contraction force will also differ.

While muscles must create large forces to produce movements at a low mechanical advantage, distally applied loads, such as to the hand acting through the elbow, have a comparatively large moment arm (Fig. 8.13) and require less force to produce large moments about the joint. This will be true of manipulative forces placed distally for purposes of applying passive stretch to muscles and joints. It is a useful principle, but must be approached with caution, since large, potentially damaging force moments can be generated.

Joint Structure Defines How Movements Can Occur Between Body Segments

Beyond movement models that regard joints as simple pivot points for the transfer muscle forces between body segments, the next level of modeling must consider the structure of these intersegmental contacts. In fact, the directions of movement that can occur between body segments are largely defined by the structure of the joints between them. Joints are classified according to the type of tissue they contain and their structure. On a tissue level, joints are classified into three primary types: fibrous, cartilaginous, and synovial. Fibrous joints are located in areas such as the articulations of the skull, while cartilaginous joints include the discs between vertebrae, and synovial joints are located in articulations of the limbs. The vast majority of body motion occurs across synovial and cartilaginous joints. The primary cartilaginous articulations will be described subsequently, with considerations of the spinal column. The remaining synovial joints have been divided into several categories according to the primary types of movements that occur across them. Anatomically, the major types are gliding, hinge, pivot, condyloid, saddle, and ball and socket (61). Other than the joints described later in this chapter, more detailed descriptions of these joint structures and their limitations on range of motion can be found in general anatomic texts.

Range of Motion Describes the Extent of Body Segment Movement Across Joints

Movements are usually described as occurring in one of the primary body planes (frontal, sagittal, or transverse). The extent of joint motion in a plane defines its *range of motion* in that plane, usually in degrees. Although all synovial joints may have some minor range of motion in all three planes, most joints in the

extremities have a primary degree of freedom in one plane, such as in the knees, elbows, or fingers. Shoulder and hip joints are an exception, as they have significant ranges of motion in all three planes. Joints may also have a significant rotational component, usually expressed as range of motion of the distal rotated element, as in pronation and supination of the hand. In general, there is a trade-off between intrinsic structural stability of joints and range of motion, depending upon the physiologic demands placed upon the joint.

Joint Surfaces Have Several Different Types of Relative Movement

As body segments are moved through their range of motion, surfaces within the joint will also move relative to each other. This movement may contribute to various aspects of the motion produced. The relative motion of joint surfaces may include gliding, rolling, rotation, compression, or distraction (Fig. 8.15), or a combination of these movements. Gliding (also referred to as translation or sliding) represents a movement of one surface relative to another without a rotational component. In rolling, one surface of the articulation rolls over the other, like a ball rolling over a surface. Rotation (spinning) consists of one joint surface spinning on the surface of the other without a translational component. Compression represents force pushing the joint surfaces together, while distraction tends to pull the surfaces apart.

Movements between articular surfaces in a joint can occur in consistent combinations (coupled) such that one type of motion is always accompanied by another. This motion coupling can occur for movements within the same articulation (see the upcoming example given under "The Knee") or in another joint that is part of an articulation complex (see the example given with "The Elbow" later in the chapter) (62). A disruption of one part of a coupled motion will affect the other and can produce dysfunction of the joint or joint complex. An example of this is a coupling of the elbow complex where there is a coupling of the intra-articular

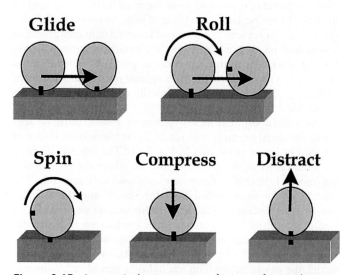

Figure 8-15 Intra-articular movement of joint surfaces relative to each other. In gliding (also referred to as "sliding" or "translation"), surfaces move without rotation. In rolling, one surface rotates and translates over the other at a distance equal to the arc of the rotating surface. In spinning, one surface rotates on the other without translation. Compression and distraction are opposing vertical forces on the joint.

motions of humeroulnar and humeroradial joints during flexion/ extension movements (see "The Elbow"). Coupling of articular surface motions within the joint also depends upon which segment of the joint is mobile (62). An example of this difference is the articular surface movement of the knee during weight bearing versus swing phase (see "The Knee"). Significant alterations in the relative movements of joint surfaces can produce problems in joints, including abnormal wear and dislocation.

The Instant Center Defines the Center of Rotation of a Body Segment at Any Given Time

In order to study movement within a joint during functional movement, both the motion of the surfaces relative to each other and the shape of the articulating surfaces must be considered. As one segment moves in a joint such as the knee, the center of rotation located within the joint at any instant will have zero velocity. Because the femoral condyles and tibial plane are not spheric surfaces and translational movement can occur within the joint, the center of rotation of the leg will change as the leg is extended. To determine properties such as the length of the moment arm under these circumstances, the center of rotation must be redefined as *instant center* of rotation joint at any given time (63). The instant center can be defined clinically from sequential roentgenograms or other pictures of movement using the intersection of lines from defined points from the joint segments. This technique can be important for identifying abnormal joint movement. It should be noted, however, that displacement of the instant center can occur in all three dimensions simultaneously. Roentgenograms or other planar depictions of joint motion can be misleading. From a functional point of view, changes in the location of the instant center will change the relative magnitude of the contraction-force vectors of the muscle tendon acting across a joint. This can result in weakness or abnormal stresses within the joint.

SOME PROPERTIES OF SPECIFIC JOINT ARTICULATIONS

The previous discussions in this chapter have focused on the biomechanical properties of tissues and models of forces acting to create movements or stresses on body segments. We will now consider how these properties apply to some of the primary articulation systems in the body. The biomechanical aspects to be considered are not intended to be comprehensive.

THE KNEE

The knee joins two of the body's longest moment arms (the thigh and leg) in a joint consisting of two primary articulations, the tibiofemoral joint and the patellofemoral joint (Fig. 8.16). Because of its location and weight-bearing properties, the knee sustains relatively high load forces and is particularly susceptible to injury. Stability of the knee is obtained from the internal and external ligaments, joint capsule, and muscles acting across the joint. The cartilage menisci act to distribute the compressive stresses between the condyles of the femur and the tibial plateau.

The Knee Has One Primary Range of Motion in the Sagittal Plane

Although the knee joint itself has some range of motion in all three planes of motion, its primary range of motion is in the

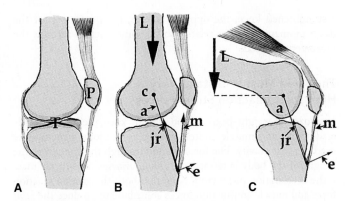

Figure 8-16 A. The knee joint consists of the tibiofibular (*t*) and patellofibular joints (*p*). **B.** Moments produced by the load (*L*) of body weight require little muscle activity with the knee extended, but are maintained by a muscle contraction force through the patellar tendon (*m*), which produces moments through a moment arm (*a*) to the instant center of rotation of the joint (*c*). The moment is divided by the angle of muscle pull into a joint reaction force (*jr*) and an extending component (*e*). **C.** With the knee flexed, the body weight produces a moment through the joint (*c*) that must be resisted by the extending component (*e*). In this instance, the patella increases the distance of the tendon from the femur to provide a more advantageous angle for the muscle contraction force on the tibia. This increases the proportion of the extension moment. Note that the position of the center of rotation (*c*) has changed slightly.

sagittal plane where a range from full extension to full flexion is approximately 140 degrees (63). Motion in the transverse plane (internal and external rotation) and frontal planes (abduction and adduction) is dependent upon the positioning of the tibia relative to the femur. In the transverse and frontal planes, full extension of the knee precludes almost all motion due to an interlocking of the femoral and tibial condyles, while range of motion increases as the knee is flexed. Maximal internal and external rotation is possible with the knee flexed at approximately 90 degrees ranging from a neutral position to 45 degrees of external rotation and 30 degrees of internal rotation. In the frontal plane, passive adduction and abduction is obtained at approximately 30 degrees of flexion, but it is only a few degrees in either direction (63).

Primary Muscle Forces Through the Knee Are Conducted Through the Hamstrings and the Patellar Tendon

The primary muscle forces through the joint occur through the quadriceps tendon and hamstrings. The hamstrings use the knee joint as a primary lever in flexing, while the quadriceps use the patellar tendon system as a pulley with the center of rotation within the femoral condyles (Fig. 8.16). As with other hinge-type joints, in a basic biomechanical model, muscle contraction forces are divided primarily into a joint reaction force directed into the joint and a force moment that acts to move the mobile segment. In extension of the knee, the moment that acts to straighten the knee pulls on the leg through the patella and tendon. This will act to rotate the tibial plateau relative to the condyles of the femur. Presuming a constant muscle force, this component of moment decreases or mechanical advantage decreases in proportion to the joint reaction force as extension proceeds (Fig. 8.16). This decrease is to some extent compensated by the movement of the patella and the shape of the femoral condyles as described subsequently. With flexing a straightened knee, the opposite is true; the proportion of the flexor moment increases relative to the joint reaction force as the movement proceeds.

The Knee Must Withstand Very High Joint Reaction Stress Forces

In a load- or weight-bearing model of the knee, the leg is considered stable, and muscle contraction forces and joint structure are used to resist gravity. The force exerted through the knee from the weight of the body is termed the *ground reaction force* (body mass × the acceleration of gravity). Note that both the ground reaction force and muscle contraction forces contribute to produce the *joint reaction force* or total force directed into the joint as described previously. These combined forces, along with the impact of landing from activities such as jumping, can produce very high compressive and other stress forces on the knee joint surfaces.

If the knee is fully extended, most of the ground reaction force is directed through the bone structure of the femur and tibia (a moment arm through the joint of almost zero), and minimal or no muscle contraction force is required to resist the ground reaction force. This changes as the knee is bent, and at 90 degrees of flexion, extensor muscle reaction forces must resist the ground reaction force consisting of the body weight acting at a distance of almost the entire length of the femur. At this angle, the extensor muscles have a relatively small moment arm. Accordingly, a very high muscle contraction force in excess of body weight must be exerted to resist a moment of this magnitude. The knee joint has several mechanisms to help compensate for the rather low mechanical advantage of muscle contraction forces in this situation.

The Application of Muscle Contraction Forces to Movement Across the Knee Is Affected by the Structural Properties of the Joints

Beyond the basic segment model, there are basic structural properties of the knee that change the mechanical advantage muscles across the joint. These primary structural properties include the patellofemoral joint and the shape and movement of the femoral condyles. The patella and tendon act to increase the moment arm for the quadriceps by increasing the effective distance of the tendon from the center of rotation of the joint, thereby increasing the component of the muscle contraction force vector acting to straighten the joint (Fig. 8.16). This adds mechanical advantage to the extensor muscle contraction forces in a partially flexed knee. The gliding (sliding) motion of the patella between the medial and the lateral femoral facets also alters the moment arm over the range of motion of the knee. Additionally, the patella acts to distribute this force over the surface of the femoral condyles.

The primary properties of the femoral condyles that affect the mechanics of movement include the noncircular shape of the condyles and their movement on the tibial plateau (Fig. 8.16). The shape of the femoral condyles is such that the center of rotation of the joint changes through the knee's range of motion, giving a greater moment arm to extensor forces as the knee is flexed. This can be important in resisting the high forces such as body weight with a partially flexed knee. In addition to a noncircular shape, the femoral condyles also have differences in their effective diameters with the medial being larger. This produces a coupling of flexion and extension with a rotational component to the knee (called the screw-home mechanism), such that flexion is accompanied by an internal rotation component and extension is accompanied

by external rotation of the femoral condyles relative to the tibial plateau (64). This provides additional stability to the joint in certain circumstances.

The Intra-articular Movements of the Knee Depend Upon Which Surface Is Moving and Load Bearing

The femoral condyles also glide (slide, translate) on the tibial plateau as the knee is moved (described previously). These structural properties of the femoral condyles can act to change the center of rotation as the joint progresses through its range of motion and alters the effective moment arm length through which the muscle contraction forces are acting. The relative movements of the joint surfaces in the knee give an example of how motion coupling can depend upon the load status of the joint and which joint surface is mobile (62). In walking, as the leg swings forward (swing phase), the femoral condyles and tibial plateau are not under the compressive load of the body. The movement is a gliding motion of the tibial plateau coupled with a rolling of the tibia on the femoral condyles in the same direction. When the leg is placed on the ground with the knee partially flexed and then extended as the body is moved forward (see "Normal Locomotion (Gait) Employs the Entire Body for Efficiency of Movement" later in the chapter), the tibial plateau is stable relative to the femoral condyles. The motion of the joint surfaces now consists of a gliding and rolling of the femoral condyles on the tibia in opposite directions. This is an example of how compressive forces and segment stabilization change articular surface motion. This can have important implications in surface damage and dysfunction.

Knee Joint Structure and the Movement of Joint Surfaces Promote Efficiency of Movement

Through their structure and interaction during movement, the patellofemoral joint and femoral condyles contribute to the efficient use of muscle contraction forces for movement and joint stability by changing the moment arm (mechanical advantage) of the contracting muscles in the process of extending or flexing the knee. This has important consequences for movement through the knee and load bearing. The effective use of these structural properties is dependent upon internal joint movement and the joint stability provided by soft tissues. For this reason, soft-tissue injury or changes producing either a lack of or excess of internal "play" in the knee joint can contribute to serious problems with joint function.

THE HIP

The Hip Is a Load-Bearing Ball-and-Socket Joint with Ranges of Motion in All Three Planes

The relatively rigid ball-and-socket arrangement of the hip joint between the head of the femur and the acetabulum provides greater intrinsic stability compared to joints such as the knee. In addition to stability, the ball-and-socket structure of the hip allows greater range of motion in all three planes of body movement. Motion in the sagittal plane is greatest with approximately 140 degrees of flexion and 15 degrees of extension from a neutral position. The range of abduction is approximately 30 degrees and adduction 25 degrees. External rotation from a flexed position is approximately 90 degrees and internal rotation approximately 70 degrees. Rotation decreases with extension due to soft-tissue restrictions (65).

The Angular Alignment of the Articular Components Is Important for Normal Hip Function

The angular structure of the joint relative to the pelvis, femoral shaft, and knee joint can vary significantly between individuals and have a great influence on the biomechanics of the lower limb. In the relationship of the joint surface to the pelvis, the location of the acetabulum places the plane of its opening angled 40 degrees posterior to a sagittal plane and 60 degrees lateral to a transverse plane (Fig. 8.17). Both the femoral head and the acetabulum have roughly spheric surfaces of contact. The relationship of the femoral head through its neck with the femoral shaft is important in the biomechanics of hip function and load-bearing stress on the neck. It is an important determinant of the effective moment arms of the muscles producing movement across the joint. The angle of inclination of the neck to the shaft (Fig. 8.17) is approximately 125 degrees, but may vary between 90 and 135 degrees. This angle offsets the femoral shaft from the pelvis laterally. The angle in a transverse plane between lines drawn through the femoral head and greater trochanter and between the medial and the lateral condyles (angle of anteversion) determines the normal relationship of the primary plane of movement of the knee to the hip. It is normally about 12 degrees but can vary widely (65). An angle of greater than 12 degrees tends to produce internal compensatory rotation of the leg during gait, while an angle of less than 12 degrees produces an external rotation. These compensations are made to maintain the stability of the hip. They are common in children and usually outgrown (65).

Models of Hip Function Balance Ground Reaction, Joint, and Muscle Contraction Forces

Biomechanical models of the hip can be used to illustrate some of the important aspects of the structure-function relationship of the joint. Stability of the hip joint is maintained through the alignment of the body over the joint (Fig. 8.18), the joint capsule, and capsular ligaments and muscle contraction to counteract remaining ground force moments. The relative magnitude of forces applied into and across the hip joint can be considered through a model of a single leg stance with the body center of mass (or gravity) balanced (i.e., located on an axis of alignment) over one hip joint (Fig. 8.18). In this balanced condition, little or no muscle contraction forces are necessary to maintain equilibrium, as in the knee. The joint reaction force or force directed into the joint will equal the ground reaction force produced by the weight of the body above the hip. In an unbalanced state, the body center of

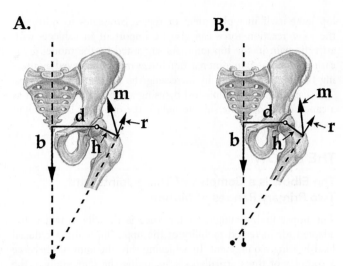

Figure 8-18 A simple coplanar model of a single leg stance moment in balance. **A.** In the balanced state, the body weight (*b*) is balanced over the foot (not shown), which would be at the intersection of the *dotted lines*. In this balance, the body weight (*b*) acts as a force applied on a moment arm (*d*) through the center of rotation in the femoral head to produce a body moment (*b* × *d*). This is balanced by the rotational component (*r*) of the muscle contraction force (*m*) acting over a moment arm through the femur (*h*) to produce a muscle contraction moment (*r* × *h*). For balance to be maintained (*b* × *d*) = (*r* × *h*). **B.** The balanced condition can be disturbed by a shift of the body and a slight change of the angle of pull by the muscle (*m*). To restore balance, the moment (*r*) must be increased or altered so that the moments can be rebalanced.

mass is no longer directly over the bony structure and produces an unbalanced moment about the center of rotation of the hip joint. To restore equilibrium, the force of the contracting abductor muscles must generate an equal force moment across the hip in the direction opposite of the moment generated by the body weight. By measuring the length of the moment arms for muscle contraction in the body and knowing the body weight, the approximate resisting moment of muscle contraction can be calculated along with the joint reaction component produced.

Note that in this model, the angle of the femoral neck will affect the relative lengths of the moment arms (or the angle of pull) by muscles. This will directly influence the muscle contraction forces required to resist the body weight moment and the proportion of the contraction force directed into the joint. This is why an abnormal angle of the femoral neck can adversely affect hip function and the stresses on the joint.

Hip Joint Function Requires High Muscle Contraction Forces and the Ability to Withstand High Joint Reaction Forces

As with the knee, it can be seen that hip stability under load-bearing conditions can require high muscle contraction forces because of a relatively short moment arm through which the muscle forces are applied. As a combination of ground reaction force and the portion of the muscle contraction forces directed into the joint, the joint reaction forces are also high relative to the body weight. Calculations suggest that under these conditions, the muscle contraction force is approximately twice the body weight and the joint reaction force almost three times the body weight (66,67). Joint reaction forces are important in consideration of stresses on the

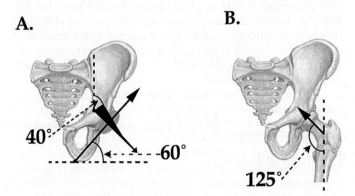

Figure 8-17 A. Angle of the opening of the acetabulum. The opening is oriented 60 degrees lateral to a transverse plane and 40 degrees posterior to a sagittal plane. **B.** The angle between the femoral neck and the shaft is approximately 125 degrees.

hip joint itself in replacement or repair. Strategies to minimize the joint reaction force can also be important in subjects with arthritic pain in the hip joint. As suggested by the model given earlier, a reduction in joint reaction forces may be achieved by altering the angle of the hip by increasing the muscle moment arms. This can also be accomplished by using a support device, such as a cane on the opposite side, to reduce the opposing body weight moment.

THE ELBOW

The Elbow Is a Complex of Three Joints with Two Primary Ranges of Motion

The upper limb analogue of the knee is the elbow, which has adapted for increased mobility of the upper limb and a reduced load-bearing requirement. In achieving this, the joint has become a complex of three articulations, including the humeroulnar, the humeroradial, and the proximal radioulnar joints (Fig. 8.19). The joint complex allows two primary ranges of motion: flexion-extension and pronation-supination. Flexion and extension occur across the humeroulnar and humeroradial joints, which act as a hinged joint. The normal range of motion in flexion-extension is approximately 140 degrees, with limits established by the angular characteristics of the bony components (68). The axis of motion passes through the middle of the trochlea and is principally a gliding motion (69) up to the last 5 to 10 degrees of flexion, where rolling occurs. Pronation and supination occur at the humeroradial and proximal radioulnar joints. The reported normal range of motion varies between studies (68) with the American Academy of Orthopaedic Surgeons (70) reporting an average of 70 degrees of pronation and 85 degrees of supination. The range of motion required for typical daily activities of both flexion-extension and pronation-supination can be performed between a much more limited range (71).

Much of the elbow joint's stability during normal use is supplied by the shape of the articulating surfaces. Of the three articulations, the humeroulnar articulation supplies the primary anterior-posterior stability, although the radiohumeral articulation can contribute to stability from posterior dislocation at flexion of 90 degrees or more. Beyond the bony stability of the joint, the ligaments and joint capsules around the elbow provide remaining stability and the interosseous membrane binds the radial and ulnar shafts together.

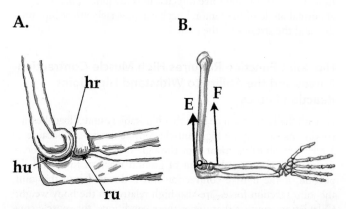

Figure 8-19   A. The elbow joint complex consists of the humeroulnar (*hu*), humeroradial (*hr*), and proximal radioulnar joints. **B.** The primary flexor (*F*) and extensor (*E*) moments across the joint.

Basic Functions of the Elbow Can Be Described by Simple Joint Moments

The basic biomechanics of the elbow can be described largely as a system of simple levers or joint moments as suggested earlier in the section on basic mechanics of joint systems (Figs. 8.13 and 8.19). Muscle forces act at a low mechanical advantage to achieve a large movement. Due to disadvantageous vector angles through some of their range, relatively high muscle contraction forces are required. These muscle contraction forces typically generate large joint reaction force components that act through the bony elements to stabilize the elbow. These joint reaction forces may exceed body weight even during normal activities.

The Elbow Complex Provides an Example of Dysfunctions from the Coupling of Intra-articular Motion

As a joint complex, the elbow provides a reasonably simple example of coupling relationships of intra-articular joint motions that, when disrupted, can produce dysfunction. During flexion-extension movements, the humeroulnar joint has a primary gliding motion that is accompanied by a movement of the head of the radius on the capitulum of the humerus. This produces a smaller proximal and distal gliding of the proximal radius in the radial notch of the ulna (62). The extent of this latter movement is greatest when the joint is half-flexed. Although this motion is not a primary component of the segmental motion, its disruption can produce pain and dysfunction in the joint during movement. It is therefore important to understand the coupled movements of the complex as well as the individual articulations. More complicated examples can occur in more extensive joint chains such as in the spine and feet.

THE SHOULDER

The Shoulder Is a Complex of Four Joints with Different Properties

The shoulder consists of a complex of four articulations: the glenohumeral, acromioclavicular, sternoclavicular, and scapulothoracic articulations (Fig. 8.20). Of these, the scapulothoracic articulation is not a true articulation, but an indirect attachment of the scapula to the thoracic wall indirectly through muscles. The shoulder complex acts in concert with contributions from each joint to produce movement through greater than a hemisphere of range. The glenohumeral joint is a basic ball-and-socket joint, but has much less intrinsic stability than its lower limb analogue at the hip. The reduced stability is reflected by the structure of the articulating surfaces of the joint. The area of the glenoid fossa that contacts the humerus is only one third to one fourth the size of the joint surface of the humeral head (72).

This allows a more circular range of motion relative to the scapula, but at the cost of intrinsic structural stability of the joint. Although some vertical structural support may be derived from the overlying acromion process and attached clavicle, the glenohumeral joint is reliant, to a great degree, on soft-tissue structures (ligaments, tendons, joint capsules, and muscles) for stability (73). During function, the glenohumeral joint primarily rotates, but rolling and translation may also take place. This translation may increase substantially with soft-tissue injury or dislocation.

The scapula attaches to the thoracic skeleton through a chain of two articulations, the acromioclavicular and sternoclavicular joints. The acromioclavicular joint between the clavicle and the proximal

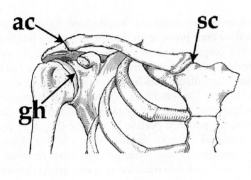

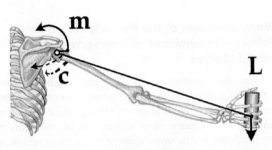

Figure 8-20   Top. Front view of the shoulder complex consisting of the glenohumeral (*gh*) acromioclavicular (*ac*), and sternoclavicular (*sc*) articulations. The scapulothoracic junction is not a true articulation, but describes the relationship of the scapula and thorax as can be seen in the lower figure. **Bottom.** An example of the differences in the moment arms of shoulder muscles (*m*) and a load (*L*) in a lift with the shoulder abducted and arm extended. Co-contracting muscles (*c, dotted arrows*) are important to stabilize the shoulder complex during such tasks.

acromion of the scapula has a meniscus of cartilage, a thick fibrous capsule, and supporting ligaments that stabilize the joint and allows the scapula motion in three planes (74). These planes include a vertical axis (protraction and retraction) and transverse axes in the frontal and sagittal planes. The proximal end of the clavicle (sternoclavicular joint) is stabilized by a fibrocartilage, meniscus-containing, articulation capsule and ligaments to the sternum and 1st rib. The joint allows protraction and retraction, elevation and depression, and rotation of the clavicle relative to the sternum.

The concept of a scapulothoracic articulation involves a description of the movement of the scapula relative to the thorax as limited by its muscular attachments and the clavicular chain. This structural arrangement allows a wide range of motion of the scapula including protraction retraction, elevation, depression, and rotation. Movement of the scapula involves the translocation of the entire glenohumeral joint, contributing substantially to the range of motion of the arm. A simple example is the contribution of scapular motion to the elevation of the arm. In this circumstance the scapula rotates to elevate the shoulder and the glenohumeral joint as the arm is raised.

Shoulder Range of Motion Is Usually Described for the Entire Joint Complex Rather than Individual Joints

With the complex interaction of the individual articulations, the range of motion of the shoulder is usually described for the complex as a whole. From a resting position at the side, the range of motion in the shoulder complex is typically described in the context of range of elevation of the shoulder or movement of the humerus away from the thorax in any of the three primary planes. Forward flexion and abduction are approximately 180 degrees, and in the plane of the scapula may exceed 180 degrees. Backward elevation or extension is approximately 60 degrees. Other motions including bringing the humerus in adduction beyond the midline limit of the body in an upward direction is approximately 75 degrees (70). Horizontal flexion in a transverse plane at 90 degrees of abduction is approximately 135 degrees, with horizontal extension of 45 degrees. Rotation about the long axis of the humerus varies with the degree of arm elevation, but in general, both internal and external rotation can be approximately 90 degrees, with a total range of 180 degrees (74).

The Glenohumeral Joint Depends upon Muscle Stabilizing Forces to Resist Distal Loads

Because of the relative lack of structural stability of the glenohumeral joint, soft-tissue connections through the joint must play a greater role in its stability. In addition to the joint capsule and ligamentous connections, muscle contraction forces that essentially hold the joint together become more important in resisting the loads placed on the distal upper limb. The use of force-coupling arrangements in the muscles of the rotator cuff is particularly important in this process. In force coupling, muscles of the rotator cuff act in concert to produce offsetting moments (a net joint reaction force) to stabilize the joint (Fig. 8.20) as elevation is produced. The actual calculations of joint reaction forces under these circumstances are difficult due to the large numbers of muscles involved in arrangements that will vary according to the plane of motion. Estimates of these forces suggest magnitudes near body weight (75). It is also important to note that the low mechanical advantage of muscles in the shoulder compared to the moment arm of a load in the hand of an extended arm requires very high contraction forces (Fig. 8.20). The low mechanical advantage of shoulder muscles under loading and the dependency of the joint on soft tissues for stability make the shoulder particularly vulnerable to injury.

THE SPINE

The spine as a whole represents an extremely complicated system of articulations and bony segments that act to protect the spinal cord while providing a basic support axis for the upper body. The structure and motion of spinal segments differs substantially over the spinal column. Due to this complexity and variation, only some basic principles of spinal biomechanics can be covered here.

Spinal Motion Segments Consist of Two Vertebrae and Associated Soft Tissues

The functional unit of the spine or motion segment consists of two vertebrae and their associated soft tissues (Fig. 8.21). The segment is functionally and physically divided into anterior and posterior segments. The anterior portion consists of the vertebral body, the disc between them, and the longitudinal ligaments (Fig. 8.21). The posterior segment consists of the vertebral arches, the articulations between the facets, the transverse and spinous processes, and the ligaments binding them together. Besides containing the spinal cord and associated structures, the architecture of the posterior segment acts to guide and limit the motion that can occur between the vertebrae of the segment. The anterior segment of the unit is the primary load-bearing section, with the vertebral bodies and the

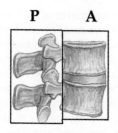
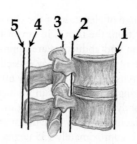

Figure 8-21 Left. A basic motion segment of the lumbar spine divided into anterior (*A*) and posterior (*P*) portions. The anterior portion contains the vertebral bodies, the spinal disc, and the anterior longitudinal (*1*) and posterior longitudinal (*2*) ligaments **(right)**. The posterior portion contains the vertebral canal, the bony segments associated with it, and associated ligaments including the ligamentum flavum (*3*), the interspinous ligament (*4*), and the supraspinous ligament (*5*). Other soft-tissue structures (e.g., capsular ligaments, etc.) are not shown.

intervening disc increasing in size in the lower segments to sustain greater loading stress. Load bearing in the posterior segment can be significant when the spine is hyperextended (76) and during forward bending coupled with rotation (77).

The Bony Structure of the Spine Is Supported by an Intricate Arrangement of Soft Tissues

The soft-tissue support for the spinal column consists of the ligaments, joint capsules, and muscles that connect to the transverse and spinous processes of the vertebrae as part of the posterior motion segments. The primary ligaments include the anterior and posterior ligaments, the ligamentum flavum, the supraspinous and interspinous ligaments (Fig. 8.21), and the intertransverse ligaments, all of which provide intrinsic support for the spinal column. The capsular ligaments for the facet articulations also contribute to stability and limitation of motion. The ligaments have a high collagen content except for the ligamentum flavum, which has a high elastin content. The ligaments add stability and store energy during movement of the spinal column. For example, flexion primarily stretches the interspinous ligaments, capsular ligaments, and the ligamentum flavum. These store energy like an elastic band and can be used for subsequent recovery to a neutral position. Other ligaments similarly participate in lateral bending and rotation.

Intervertebral Discs Are Structured to Cushion and Distribute Stresses between Vertebrae

The intervertebral discs sustain and distribute primarily compressive loading of the vertebrae and restrict excessive motion. The disc consists of a tough outer covering of fibrocartilage, the annulus fibrosus, bounded above and below by a plate of hyaline cartilage adjacent to the vertebrae. The collagen fibers of the annulus fibrosus are arranged in concentric layers and differing orientations to the vertical axis of ±30 degrees in a cross-hatched arrangement. This covering encloses a gelatinous inner core, the nucleus pulposus, that acts to distribute and redirect stresses and store energy, similar to a partially inflated ball. The nucleus pulposus contains a water-binding glycosaminoglycan gel (80% to 88% water) (78) that becomes progressively less hydrated with age (79). This change can reduce the elasticity, ability to store energy, and stress loading distribution properties of the disc and make it less capable of resisting loads.

In the unloaded condition, longitudinal ligaments and the ligamenta flava exert pressure on the disc to create a prestress condition (80). Compressive stress on the disc through the vertebral bodies creates a circumferential tensile stress that is resisted by the annular fibers of the annulus fibrosus. During motions such as flexion bending, the vertebrae rotate forward, creating compression stress and some strain (bulging) on the anterior disc and tensile stress on the posterior portion of the disc (Fig. 8.4). Rotation produces torsional stress on the disc, which is also redistributed through its structure. These strain patterns allow vertebral movement under load, and redistribution of forces across the vertebral-disc interface, to minimize localized extremes in stress.

The Bony Structure of the Posterior Segment Is a Primary Determinant of Intervertebral Ranges of Motion

Aside from their connection through the vertebral bodies and the intervening disc, the vertebrae interact structurally through the facets of intervertebral joints in the posterior portion of the motion segment. Under most circumstances, vertebral movement is restricted by the orientation of these facets relative to the vertebral column and each other (Fig. 8.22). Exceptions include particular regions of the spinal column, where articulations with structures such as the skull, ribs, or sacrum may add additional constraints on vertebral movement. The orientation of intervertebral facets changes throughout the spinal column (81) and the actual angle of the facets may vary significantly between individuals. The orientation of intervertebral facets also acts to produce additional directional components (motion coupling, as described in the next section) in vertebral motion during basic movement, such as flexion, extension, rotation, and lateral flexion.

The primary variation in facet orientation can be defined in the transverse and frontal planes. A positive angle deviation from the transverse plane indicates that the facets are oriented above

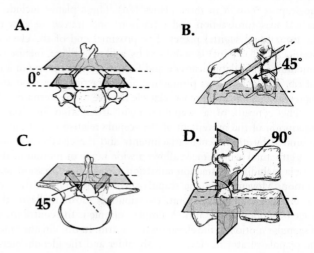

Figure 8-22 The orientation of intervertebral joint facets in the frontal and transverse planes relative to the spinal column. In the cervical vertebrae (**A, B**), the surfaces of the facets on either side are parallel to each and to a frontal plane (**A**), but inclined at 45 degrees above a transverse plane through a vertebra as viewed from the side (**B**). In the lumbar spine (**C, D**), the surfaces of the facets are oriented at 45 degrees to the frontal plane (**C**) and 90 degrees above a transverse plane as shown from the side (**D**). The facet orientations restrict the mobility of intervertebral movement and define the motion-coupling characteristics.

a horizontal (transverse) plane through the body (Fig. 8.22). Positive deviation in the frontal plane effectively describes the orientation of the facet surfaces on each side of the vertebra relative to each other, although the angle is defined relative to a frontal plane (Fig. 8.22). The atlas and axis have facets that are almost parallel to the transverse plane, with the remaining facets of the cervical vertebrae oriented at a 45-degree angle to the transverse plane and parallel to the frontal plane (Fig. 8.22). The alignment of the C3-C7 vertebrae allows flexion, extension, lateral flexion, and rotation (82). This can be compared to the facets of thoracic vertebrae that are oriented 60 degrees from the transverse plane and 20 degrees from the frontal plane. This allows lateral bending, rotation, and some flexion and extension. The lumbar vertebrae have facets oriented 90 degrees to the transverse plane and 45 degrees to the frontal plane. This allows almost no rotation, but flexion, extension, and lateral bending. The lumbosacral joints do allow more rotation (83), with facets oriented more obliquely to the transverse plane.

The Motion of the Spine Is a Composite of Small Movements in Individual Vertebrae and Coupling Between Vertebrae

The kinematic and kinetic considerations of spinal movements are particularly complicated, since overall movements are a composite of comparatively small movements of each vertebral segment. Each vertebra has some degree of rotation or translation in each of its transverse, sagittal, and longitudinal axes (or 6 degrees of freedom in movement). This movement is largely limited by the intervertebral joint facet orientations. These orientations vary markedly over the spinal column (81). Flexion-extension movements are greatest in the cervical, lower thoracic, and lumbar spine; rotation is greatest in the cervical and upper thoracic spine; and lateral bending is greatest in the cervical spine and more evenly distributed over remaining vertebrae.

It should be noted here that the convention in osteopathic medicine is to describe rotation of a vertebra as the direction in which the anterior part of the vertebral body or anterior segment rotates. In some biomechanical texts, rotation of the vertebra is described as the direction in which the posterior segment or spinous process rotates. Even though these conventions describe the same rotary motion, they are on opposite sides of the center of rotation and therefore the inverse of each other. This difference can become particularly confusing in relation to descriptions of motion coupling between vertebrae over the spine (discussed subsequently). The osteopathic convention will be used here, unless specific reference is made to the spinous process. Another caveat of the descriptions of vertebral movements given is that active, muscle contraction-based movement characteristics may or may not be similar to movements produced by external forces (e.g., manipulations). This should be taken into account in comparisons of these characteristics as described in the chapters on manipulation.

Physiologically normal movements of the spinal column in any of the primary directions (flexion-extension, lateral bending, rotation) produce additional motion vectors in the vertebrae as a consequence of the orientation of the intervertebral facets and other articulations (Fig. 8.23). This coupling may include motions of lateral bending (flexion), rotation, and translation in several axes simultaneously, although only major coupling relationships are typically noted as clinically significant. The coupling can differ markedly over the spine and only a limited description will be given here. In the thoracic region, rotation is coupled with lateral flexion. This is greatest in the upper thoracic region, with the vertebrae rotating toward the same side as the lateral flexion (81). In the lumbar

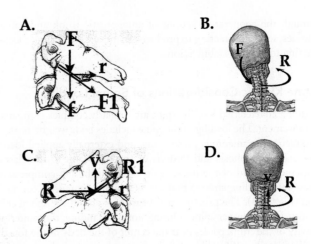

Figure 8-23 Motion coupling as influenced by the orientation of intervertebral facets in cervical vertebrae. **A.** A lateral flexing force (*F*) on the side of the vertebrae acting to move the upper vertebrae relative to the bottom will be redirected by the facets in a new direction (*F1*). The divided moment will have a remaining flexing component (*f*) and a rotational component (*r*) that will add (couple) rotation (*R*) of the vertebrae to the flexing movement **(B). C.** A rotational force (*R*) on one vertebra is redirected by the facets to glide in a new direction (*R1*). R1 has both a vertical (*v*) and a remaining rotational component (*r*) (vectors). The vertical component will cause the side of the vertebra to lift upward and produces lateral flexion on the opposite side **(D).** However, in isolated rotation movements, this flexing moment is restricted to produce vertical translation (telescoping) of the cervical spine, particularly at the C1-C2 joint.

spine, rotation is also coupled with lateral flexion, but the vertebrae rotate in a direction opposite the lateral flexion. Additional motion coupling in the cervical spine is described subsequently.

Overall Range of Motion of the Spine Varies Widely Between Individuals

The composite nature of spinal movements along with individual structural and soft-tissue differences help to explain a great variation in the range of motion in individuals. There are also significant variations in spinal range of motion with age and sex (84). This makes the listing of normal values without specification of these factors of little clinical significance. Difficulties in defining normal ranges of motion also derive from a large capacity of the spine to produce compensatory changes in movement to achieve a similar net movement. In this strategy, a limitation of movement that exists in the structural aspects of one area of the spinal column can be alleviated by a compensatory greater mobility in other areas (85). For example, the movement of the spinal column is also accompanied by motion in the pelvis. In body flexion, the initial 50 to 60 degrees of motion occurs in the lumbar spine with little contribution from the thoracic vertebra due to the orientation of the facets and the rib cage. Additional flexion is accomplished by the tilting of the pelvis.

Restriction of movement in the lumbar spine can be replaced, to some extent, by greater and earlier tilting of the pelvis. The movement of the pelvis also contributes to lateral bending and rotation of the trunk, and may be used similarly to compensate for restrictions.

As in other multiple-articulation chains, movements of the spine are accomplished through complex interactions of agonist and antagonist muscle groups. Movement aspects are accomplished through the cooperative actions of antagonistic trunk and spinal muscles, some contracting to produce the movement, others cocontracting to provide stabilization.

Some Kinetic Considerations of Spinal Loading

Loading characteristics of the spine are similarly complex compared to movement. The loading of the spine includes body weight, muscle contraction, ligamentous prestressing, and externally applied loads. The natural kyphosis and lordosis of the spine add to the elastic resistance to load of the discs, again by redistributing compressive stress into bending stresses that can be resisted by muscle contraction (Fig. 8.24). The primary load-bearing region of the spinal column is in the lumbar spine. During normal standing, the center of gravity of the trunk passes near the center of the body of the fourth lumbar vertebra (86). This distribution and the static load on the spine can be altered appreciably by the angle of the pelvis. Tilting the pelvic angle (sacral angle) forward from its normal 30 degrees to the transverse plane accentuates the lumbar lordosis. Tilting backward from the normal angle flattens the lumbar lordosis. Both movements affect the lever arm of the body weight on the spine and require compensatory muscle activity to resist. This also creates greater loads on the lumbar spine during sitting versus relaxed standing (87). Reorientation of the spine from its normal curvature also produces stresses on the discs by changing the alignment of the vertebrae.

The Orientation of the Spine During Lifting Can Influence the Distribution of Stress on the Lumbar Spine

Lifting an object places added stress on the spine by creating an added load at a distance from the center of support in the spine (Fig. 8.24). The stress on the lumbar vertebrae by the load is primarily a function of the distance of the load from the vertebrae (moment arm or lever arm) and the weight of the load. Bending the body forward adds distance from the body, whether or not

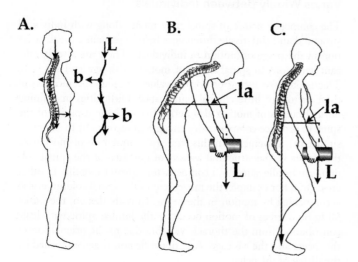

Figure 8-24 **A.** The normal curvatures of the spine *in situ* and in a model **(right)** will split vertical compression components into bending forces (*b*) that can be counteracted with muscle contraction. **B.** Force moments on the back are larger if an object is further from the vertebrae being compressed. The force moment is a product of the load (*L*) and the load arm (*la*). This compressive force alone is not dependent upon the bending of the knees **(C)**, but bending of the knees can help to shorten the load arm.

the knees are bent (82). Contraction of back muscles and to some degree, intra-abdominal pressure must counterbalance the forward-bending forces. In consideration of posture in lifting, the lumbar spine has less resistance to bending compared to direct compressive forces (88) and lateral flexion or flexion combined with axial rotation (87) increases pressure on lumbar discs. This further suggests that a vertical lifting position of the spine is preferred to reduce pressures on lumbar discs.

The Cervical Spine Has Some Unique Structural Properties and Biomechanical Properties

The cervical spine and its articulation with the skull have some special biomechanical and structural properties that require special consideration. It has five of seven vertebrae that are described as more or less typical, except for the presence of the transverse foramen for the vertebral artery in C3-C6. The grooving of the transverse process for the exit of the cervical nerves lends to further structural weakness. Both the presence of the vertebral artery and the comparative structural weakness of the transverse process suggest reason for caution with high-velocity manipulations of this region. This is particularly true for older adults in whom both soft tissue and bone biomechanical properties add weakness to this region. Other structural differences in the C3-C6 vertebrae include more prominent uncinate processes and thinner intervertebral discs. Because of this, uncinate processes may also play a role in guiding and limiting cervical motion (89).

The Atlas and Axis Have Additional Structural Properties That Define Their Range of Movement

The atypical vertebrae (C1 and C2) have unique bony structures that limit their mobility. The atlas (C1) has no true vertebral body or disc, but an anterior arch with an articulating surface for the dens of the axis (C2). The atlas articulates with the skull in two superior facets that have a semicircular shape. This limits the motion of the skull relative to the atlas to almost no rotation. The inferior facets of the atlas articulate with C2 almost parallel to the transverse plane. The axis, with its superior protrusion, the dens, provides an axis of rotation for C1. Posterior translation of the dens within the vertebral foramen is prevented by ligamentous support from the cruciform ligament. It also contains two superior, convex-shaped facets for articulation, with two slightly convex-shaped articulations (62) of the atlas that affect motion coupling in rotation.

These structural properties help to make the cervical region the most mobile region of the spine. The range of motion at the atlanto-occipital articulation is approximately 10 to 15 degrees of flexion extension and 8 degrees of lateral bending (81,89). Axial rotation is largely precluded by the structure of the articulation and is transferred to the C1-C2 articulation. The C1-C2 interface is the most mobile segment of the spine with about 47 degrees of axial rotation, or almost 50% of the axial rotation capability of the entire cervical spine (90). Flexion-extension is limited to 10 degrees, and little or no lateral bending occurs. Throughout the cervical spine, the combined range of motion is approximately 145 degrees of flexion-extension, 180 degrees of axial rotation, and 90 degrees of lateral flexion (89).

Motion Coupling of the Cervical Spine Includes Transverse and Vertical Translation and Rotation

Motion coupling of the cervical spine also has some important characteristics in addition to those mentioned earlier due to its unique anatomy. Flexion-extension is coupled with transverse translation, particularly at the C1-C2 interface (89,91). As discussed previously, lateral flexion (side bending) tends to rotate the spinous process away (vertebral body toward) from the direction of bending (Fig. 8.23) (81). Isolated rotation produces a vertical translation, or telescoping, of the cervical spine due to the orientation of the facets and restriction of flexor moments (Fig. 8.23).

Increased Mobility of the Cervical Spine Is Accompanied by Reduced Stability

The high range of motion in the cervical spine is accompanied by a lower intrinsic stability, but reduced load compared to the lumbar spine. This makes the cervical spine and associated soft- tissue support particularly vulnerable to excessive dynamic loading, with flexion-extension injuries the most common. As in other areas of the spine, restriction of movement in the cervical spine usually results in an increased compensatory mobility of other areas to achieve a functional range of motion. As a result, restriction of motion at one level, due to injury or a brace, may produce increased motion (and increased stress) at other levels (83,92). This consideration can be important in the determination of symptom-cause relationships in the diagnosis of spinal dysfunction.

BIOMECHANICAL CONSIDERATIONS OF THE BODY AS A UNIT

Normal Locomotion (Gait) Employs the Entire Body for Efficiency of Movement

Motions of the body incorporate the individual biomechanical properties of soft and hard tissues and kinematic aspects of the individual articulations into complicated movement processes. A particularly good example of this integration can be found in normal ambulation or gait (Fig. 8.25). Gait may be described as a controlled falling with propulsion. In this process, the center of mass of the body is subjected to relatively small vertical displacements. The actual energy expended is distributed over many muscle

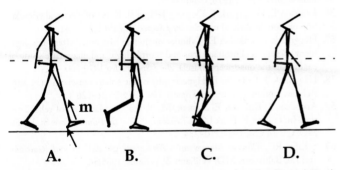

Figure 8-25 Basic gait patterns using computer-generated (Peak Performance Technologies, Inc., Englewood, CO) stick figures of an individual in normal gait. The gait cycle arbitrarily begins with the contact of one heel with the floor (**A**). The force of the body weight and motion on the heel (*arrow*) is decelerated by the anterior muscle group of the leg (*m, arrow*) through the ankle. **B.** Body weight is transferred to the supporting leg, which supports the body with slight knee flexion. **C.** The moving leg is swung forward and the supporting leg is slightly extended (*arrow*) to raise the body center of mass to its high point (*dotted line*). **D.** The body is propelled forward by plantar flexion of the supporting leg to be "caught" with the heel strike of the moving leg and the cycle begins for the opposite side.

groups beyond the legs and by subtle, but significant movements. In normal gait, one leg is moved forward while the weight of the body is supported by the opposing leg (swing phase) (Fig. 8.25). In the swing phase of the leg, the foot goes from plantar flexion to dorsal flexion. The knee is flexed and then extended, the hip moves from extension to flexion, and the pelvis rotates and changes its tilt as muscles of the lower spine and trunk are used to generate power.

Swinging the opposing arm will assist in compensating balance and rotation moments through the trunk. The body is propelled forward and its center of mass moved slightly upward and then forward and down to be "caught" by the heel strike of the extended leg. As the heel hits a surface, the foot rocks down and is decelerated by the anterior muscle groups of the leg. The knee, which initially is almost completely extended, begins to flex and becomes progressively loaded as the body weight is transferred from the opposing leg. The opposing hip and pelvis are then rotated forward to begin the process for the opposite side. Small adjustments, such as increasing the tilt of the trunk and head in the direction of progression, bring the center of mass of the body forward and assist in increasing the rate of movement.

This basic process, grossly simplified here, can reflect one of the most frequently encountered examples of the ability of the body to adapt to injury or degenerative processes. Compensatory gait patterns can vary widely according to the underlying cause, but always have an underlying biomechanical rationale, even though these adaptations may themselves produce problems. In a typical example, an injury to the knee or foot on one side may produce a compensatory shift of the body center of mass over the opposing limb. This will produce pain, stress injuries, or palpable dysfunctions in the opposite knee, back, hip, or even neck, if body posture has been significantly affected. Some aspects of these compensatory adjustments may survive the healing of the original injury, particularly if the recuperative process has been lengthy. This emphasizes the importance of the subject's history and careful observation and knowledge of mechanical body function in the diagnosis and treatment of somatic dysfunctions.

REFERENCES

1. Nordin M, Frankel VH. Biomechanics of bone. In: Nordin M, Frankel VH, eds. *Basic Biomechanics of the Musculoskeletal System.* 2nd Ed. Philadelphia, PA: Lea & Febiger, 1989:3–27.
2. Dempster WT, Coleman RF. Tensile strength of bone along and across the grain. *J Appl Physiol* 1960;16:355–360.
3. Reilly GC. Observations of microdamage around osteocyte lacunae in bone. *J Biomech* 2000;33:1131–1134.
4. Siffert RS, Levy RN. Trabecular patterns and the internal architecture of bone. *Mt Sinai J Med* 1981;48:221–229.
5. Sammarco J, Burstein A, Davis W, et al. The biomechanics of torsional fractures: the effect of loading on ultimate properties. *J Biomech* 1971;4: 113–117.
6. Carter DR, Hayes WC. Compact bone fatigue damage. A microscopic examination. *Clin Orthop* 1977;127:265–274.
7. Korpelainen R, Orava S, Karpakka J, et al. Risk factors for recurrent stress fractures in athletes. *Am J Sports Med* 2001;29:304–10.
8. Wolff, J. *The Law of Bone Remodeling.* In: Maquet P, Furlong R, trans. Berlin, Germany: Springer-Verlag, 1986, originally published in 1870.
9. Schneider VS, McDonald J. Skeletal calcium homeostasis and counter measures to prevent disuse osteoporosis. *Calc Tissue Int* 1984;36(suppl 1): 5141–5144.
10. Zerath E. Effects of microgravity on bone and calcium homeostasis. *Adv Space Res* 1998;21:1049–1058.
11. Jenkins DP, Cochran TH. Osteoporosis: the dramatic effect of disuse of an extremity. *Clin Orthop* 1969;64:128–134.

12. Kazarian LE, vonGierke HE. Bone loss as a result of immobilization and chelation. Preliminary results in Macaca mulatta. *Clin Orthop* 1969;65:67–75.

13. Huddleston AL, Rockwell D, Kulund DN, et al. Bone mass in lifetime tennis athletes. *JAMA* 1980;244:1107–1109.

14. Woo SL, Kuei SC, Amiel D, et al. The effect of prolonged physical training on the properties of long bone: a study of Wolff's law. *J Bone Joint Surg Am* 1981;63(5):780–787.

15. Morris FL, Naughton GA, Gibbs JL, et al. Prospective ten-month exercise intervention in premenarchal girls: positive effects on bone and lean mass. *J Bone Mineral Res* 1997;9:1453–1462.

16. Burstein AH, Currey J, Frankel VH, et al. Bone strength. The effect of screw holes. *J Bone Joint Surg* 1972;54A:1143–1156.

17. Smith EL, Gilligan C. Physical activity effects on bone metabolism. *Calcif Tissue Int* 1991;49(suppl):S50–S54.

18. Wilmore JH. The aging of bone and muscle. *Clin Sports Med* 1991;10:231–44.

19. Armstrong CG, Mow VC. Variations in the intrinsic mechanical properties of human articular cartilage with age, degeneration, and water content. *J Bone Joint Surg* 1982;64A:88–94.

20. Poole AR, Kojima T, Yasuda T, et al. Composition and structure of articular cartilage: a template for tissue repair. *Clin Orthop* 2001;391(suppl):S26–33.

21. Mow VC, Kuei SC, Lai WM, et al. Biphasic creep and stress relaxation of articular cartilage in compression: theory and experiments. *J Biomech Eng* 1980;102:73–84.

22. Mow VC, Proctor CS, Kelly MA. Biomechanics of articular cartilage. In: Nordin M, Frankel VH, eds. *Basic Biomechanics of the Musculoskeletal System*. 2nd Ed. Philadelphia, PA: Lea & Febiger, 1989:31–58.

23. Mansour JM, Mow VC. The permeability of articular cartilage under compressive strain and at high pressures. *J Bone Joint Surg* 1976;58A:509–516.

24. Freeman MAR. The fatigue of cartilage in the pathogenesis of osteoarthrosis. *Acta Orthop Scand* 1975;46:323–328.

25. Weightman B, Kempson G. Load carriage. In: Freeman MAR, ed. *Adult Articular Cartilage*. 2nd Ed. Tunbridge Wells, UK: Pitman Medical, 1979:291–329.

26. Meachim G, Fergie IA. Morphological patterns of articular cartilage fibrillation. *J Pathol* 1975;115:231–240.

27. Inerot S, Heinegard D, Audell L, et al. Articular-cartilage proteoglycans in aging and osteoarthritis. *Biochem J* 1978;169:143.

28. Frank CB, Shrive, NG. Ligament. In: Nigg BM, Herzog W, eds. *Biomechanics of the Musculoskeletal System*. 2nd Ed. New York, NY: John Wiley & Sons, 1999:107–126.

29. Viidik A. Elasticity and tensile strength of the anterior cruciate ligament in rabbits as influenced by training. *Acta Physiol Scand* 1968;74:372–380.

30. Schatzmann L, Brunner P, Staubli HU. Effect of cyclic preconditioning on the tensile properties of human quadricep tendons and patellar ligaments. *Knee Surg Sports Traumatol Arthrosc* 1998;6(suppl 1):556–561.

31. Carlstedt CA, Nordin M. Biomechanics of tendons and ligaments. In: Nordin M, Frankel VH, eds. *Basic Biomechanics of the Musculoskeletal System*. 2nd Ed. Philadelphia, PA: Lea & Febiger, 1989:59–74.

32. Herzog W, Gal J. Tendon. In: Nigg BM, Herzog W, eds. *Biomechanics of the Musculoskeletal System*. 2nd Ed. New York, NY: John Wiley & Sons, 1999:127–147.

33. Noyes FR, Grood ES. The strength of the anterior cruciate ligament in humans and Rhesus monkeys. Age-related and species-related changes. *J Bone Joint Surg* 1976;58A:1074–1082.

34. Noyes FR. Functional properties of knee ligaments and alterations induced by immobilization. *Clin Orthop* 1977;123:210–242.

35. Hayashi K. Biomechanical studies of the remodeling of knee joint tendons and ligaments. *J Biomech* 1996;29:707–716.

36. Kannus P, Jozsa L, Natri A, et al. Effects of training, immobilization and remobilization on tendons. *Scand J Med Sci Sports* 1997;7:67–71.

37. Yasuda K, Hayashi K. Changes in biomechanical properties of tendons and ligaments from joint disuse. *Osteoarthritis Cartilage* 1999;7:122–129.

38. Parry DAD, Barnes GRG, Craig AS. A comparison of the size distribution of collagen fibrils in connective tissues as a function of age and a possible relation between fibril size distribution and mechanical properties. *Proc R Soc Lond [Biol]* 1978;203:305–321.

39. Viidik A, Danielsen CC, Oxlund H. Fourth International Congress of Biorheology Symposium on Mechanical Properties of Living Tissues: on fundamental and phenomenological models, structure and mechanical properties of collagen, elastic and glycosaminoglycan complexes. *Biorheology* 1982;19:437–451.

40. Zernicke RF, Judex S. Adaptation of biological materials to exercise, disuse, and aging. In: Nigg BM, Herzog W, eds. *Biomechanics of the Musculoskeletal System*. 2nd Ed. New York, NY: John Wiley & Sons, 1999:189–204.

41. Johnson GA, Tramaglini DM, Levine RE, et al. Tensile and viscoelastic properties of human patellar tendon. *J Orthop Res* 1994;12:796–803.

42. Guyton AC, Hall JE. *Textbook of Medical Physiology*. 9th Ed. Philadelphia, PA: WB Saunders Co., 1996.

43. Pitman MI, Peterson L. Biomechanics of skeletal muscle. In: Nordin M, Frankel VH, eds. *Basic Biomechanics of the Musculoskeletal System*. 2nd Ed. Philadelphia, PA: Lea & Febiger, 1989:89–111.

44. Hill AV. *First and Last Experiments in Muscle Mechanics*. Cambridge, England: Cambridge University Press, 1970.

45. Cavanagh PR, Komi PV. Electromechanical delay in human muscle under concentric and eccentric contractions. *Eur J Appl Physiol* 1973;42:159–163.

46. Ciullo JV, Zarins B. Biomechanics of the musculotendinous unit: relation to athletic performance and injury. *Clin Sports Med* 1983;2:71–86.

47. Crawford GNC, James NT. The design of muscles. In: Owen R, Goodfellow J, Bullough P, eds. *Scientific Foundations of Orthopaedics and Traumatology*. London, England: William Heinemann, 1980:67–74.

48. Phillips CA, Petrofsky JS. *Mechanics of Skeletal and Cardiac Muscle*. Springfield, IL: Charles C Thomas Publisher, 1983.

49. Stanish WP. Neurophysiology of stretching. In: D'Ambrosio I, Drey O, eds. *Prevention and Treatment of Running Injuries*. Thorofare, NJ: Chas B Leach, 1982.

50. Taylor DC, Dalton JD Jr, Seaber AV, et al. Viscoelastic properties of muscle-tendon units. The biomechanical effects of stretching. *Am J Sports Med* 1990;18:300–309.

51. Gollnick PD, Matoba H. The muscle fiber composition of skeletal muscle as a predictor of athletic success. An overview. *Am J Sports Med* 1984;12:212–217.

52. Buller AJ, Eccles JC, Eccles RM. Differentiation of fast and slow muscles in the cat hind limb. *J Physiol* 1960;150:399–416.

53. Dubowitz V. Change in enzyme pattern after cross-innervation of fast and slow skeletal muscle. *Nature* 1967;214:840–841.

54. Jansson E, Sjodin B, Tesch P. Changes in muscle fibre type distribution in man after physical training. A sign of fiber type transformation. *Acta Physiol Scand* 1978;104:235–237.

55. Munsat TL, McNeal D, Waters R. Effects of nerve stimulation on human muscle. *Arch Neurol* 1976;33:608–617.

56. Eriksson E, Häggmark T, Kiessling KH, et al. Effect of electrical stimulation on human skeletal muscle. *Int J Sports Med* 1981;2:18–22.

57. Häggmark T, Eriksson E. Cylinder or mobile cast brace after knee ligament surgery: a clinical analysis and morphologic and enzymatic study of changes in the quadriceps muscle. *Am J Sports Med* 1979;7:48–56.

58. Häggmark T, Eriksson E. Hypertrophy of the soleus muscle in man after Achilles tendon rupture. *Am J Sports Med* 1979;7:121–126.

59. Arvisdson I, Eriksson E, Pitman, M. Neuromuscular basis of rehabilitation. In: Hunter E, Funk J, eds. *Rehabilitation of the Injured Knee*. St. Louis, MO: CV Mosby, 1984:210–234.

60. Schafer RC. *Clinical Biomechanics: Musculoskeletal Actions and Reactions*. 2nd Ed. Baltimore, MD: Williams & Wilkins, 1987:54–55.

61. Van De Graaff KM. *Human Anatomy*. 4th Ed. Dubuque, IA: William C Brown, 1997:197–200.

62. Warwick R, Williams PL. Arthrology. In: *Gray's Anatomy*. 35th Ed. Philadelphia, PA: WB Saunders Co., 1973:389–471.

63. Nordin M, Frankel VH. Biomechanics of the knee. In: Nordin M, Frankel VH, eds. *Basic Biomechanics of the Musculoskeletal System*. 2nd Ed. Philadelphia, PA: Lea & Febiger, 1989:115–133.

64. Helfet AJ. Anatomy and mechanics of movement of the knee joint. In: Helfet A, ed. *Disorders of the Knee*. Philadelphia, PA: JB Lippincott Co., 1974:1–17.

65. Nordin M, Frankel VH. Biomechanics of the hip. In: Nordin M, Frankel VH, eds. *Basic Biomechanics of the Musculoskeletal System*. 2nd Ed. Philadelphia, PA: Lea & Febiger, PA, 1989:135–161.

66. Rydell NW. Forces acting on the femoral head prosthesis. A study on strain gauge supplied prostheses in living persons. *Acta Orthop Scand Suppl* 1966;88:1–132.

67. English TA, Kilvington M. In vivo records of hip loads using a femoral implant with telemetric output (a preliminary report). *J Biomed Eng* 1979;1:111–115.

68. Zuckerman JD, Matsen FA. Biomechanics of the elbow. In: Nordin M, Frankel VH, eds. *Basic Biomechanics of the Musculoskeletal System.* 2nd Ed. Philadelphia, PA: Lea & Febiger, 1989:249–260.

69. London JT. Kinematics of the elbow. *J Bone Joint Surg* 1981;63A:529–535.

70. American Academy of Orthopaedic Surgeons. *Joint Motion. Method of Measuring and Recording.* Chicago, IL: American Academy of Orthopaedic Surgeons, 1965. Reprinted by the British Orthopaedic Association, 1966.

71. Morrey BF, Askew LJ, An KN, Chao EY. A biomechanical study of normal elbow motion. *J Bone Joint Surg* 1981;63A:872–877.

72. Saha AK. Dynamic stability of the glenohumeral joint. *Acta Orthop Scand* 1971;42:491–505.

73. Bigliani LU, Kelkar R, Flatow EL, et al. Glenohumeral stability. Biomechanical properties of passive and active stabilizers. *Clin Orthop* 1996;330:13–30.

74. Zuckerman JD, Matsen FA. Biomechanics of the shoulder. In: Nordin M, Frankel VH, eds. *Basic Biomechanics of the Musculoskeletal System.* 2nd Ed. Philadelphia, PA: Lea & Febiger, 1989:225–247.

75. Poppen NK, Walker PS. Forces at the glenohumeral joint in abduction. *Clin Orthop* 1978;135:165–170.

76. King AI, Prasad P, Ewing CL. Mechanism of spinal injury due to caudocephalad acceleration. *Orthop Clin North Am* 1975;6:19–31.

77. El-Bohy AA, King AI. Intervertebral disc and facet contact pressure in axial torsion. In: Lantz SA, King AI, eds. *Advances in Bioengineering.* New York, NY: American Society of Mechanical Engineers, 1986:26–27.

78. Gower WE, Pedrini, V. Age related variations in protein-polysaccharides from human nucleus pulposus, annulus fibrosus and costal cartilage. *J Bone Joint Surg* 1969;51A:1154–1162.

79. Urban JPG, McMullin JF. Swelling pressure of the intervertebral disc: influence of proteoglycan and collagen contents. *Biorheology* 1985;22:145–157.

80. Nachemson A. Lumbar intradiscal pressure. *Acta Orthop Scand Suppl* 1960;43:1–140.

81. White AA, Panjabi MM. *Clinical Biomechanics of the Spine.* Philadelphia, PA: JB Lippincott Co., 1978.

82. Lindh M. Biomechanics of the lumbar spine. In: Nordin M, Frankel VH, eds. *Basic Biomechanics of the Musculoskeletal System.* 2nd Ed. Philadelphia, PA: Lea & Febiger, 1989;183–207.

83. Lumsden R, Morris JM. An in vivo study of axial rotation and immobilization at the lumbosacral joint. *J Bone Joint Surg* 1968;50A:1591–1602.

84. Moll JMH, Wright V. Normal range of spinal mobility. An objective study. *Ann Rheum Dis* 1971;30:381–386.

85. Panjabi MM. The stabilizing system of the spine. Part I. Function, dysfunction, adaptation, and enhancement. *J Spinal Disord* 1992;5:383–389.

86. Asmussen E, Klausen K. Form and function of the erect human spine. *Clin Orthop* 1962;25:55–63.

87. Andersson GBJ, Örtengren R, Nachemson A. Intradiskal pressure, intra-abdominal pressure and myoelectric back muscle activity related to posture and loading. *Clin Orthop* 1977;129:156–164.

88. Lin HS, Liu YK, Adams KH. Mechanical response of the lumbar intervertebral joint under physiological (complex) loading. *J Bone Joint Surg* 1978;60A:41–55.

90. Shapiro I, Frankel VH. Biomechanics of the cervical spine. In: Nordin M, Frankel VH, eds. *Basic Biomechanics of the Musculoskeletal System.* 2nd Ed. Philadelphia, PA: Lea & Febiger, 1989:209–224.

91. Crisco JJ 3rd, Panjabi MM, Dvorak J. A model of the alar ligaments of the upper cervical spine in axial rotation. *J Biomech* 1991;24:607–614.

92. Oda T, Panjabi MM, Crisco JJ III. Three-dimensional translational movements of the upper cervical spine. *J Spinal Disord* 1991;4:411–419.

93. Norton PL, Brown T. The immobilizing efficiency of back braces. Their effect on the posture and motion of the lumbosacral spine. *J Bone Joint Surg* 1957;39A:111–139.

9

Somatic Dysfunction, Spinal Facilitation, and Viscerosomatic Integration

MICHAEL M. PATTERSON AND ROBERT D. WURSTER

KEY CONCEPTS

- The osteopathic lesion (somatic dysfunction) was conceived as one of the primary factors influencing body economy and the root of many diseases.
- Louisa Burns and her colleagues performed many studies on the effects of somatic dysfunction on visceral function, thus showing many somatovisceral influences well before they were generally recognized by the scientific and medical communities.
- Reflexes have an afferent arm bringing impulses to the central nervous system (CNS), a central arm within the CNS and an efferent are taking impulses to peripheral structures.
- While usually thought of as simple hardwired pathways, reflexes are actually complex interconnections influenced by many factors such as ascending messages, descending influences from higher centers, and general CNS excitability.
- Somatovisceral and viscerosomatic reflexes are one of the main integrating mechanisms of body function, closely tying somatic and visceral organs together to achieve integrated function.
- In general, sympathetic control from the brain is often localized to specific visceral organs, suggesting that the brain, through the sympathetic nervous system, can selectively influence specific organ function.
- Manipulative treatment of somatic structures can influence sympathetic function and hence visceral function through the somatovisceral reflex networks.
- Sensitization is a process that occurs in spinal gray matter neurons (interneurons) and results in an increased excitability of the involved neurons, thus increasing the gain of the input pathway.
- Long-term sensitization is a longer-lasting form of excitability increase in the reflex pathways that can last for hours and often occurs with the same stimuli as sensitization.
- Presumably permanent changes of reflex excitability can occur in reflex pathways with inhibitory cell death and new synapse formation.
- Neurons exhibit a continuous flow of intra-axonal substances both away from and toward the cell body. This flow has been shown to include transport of proteins across the synapse from nerve cell to nerve cell and from nerve cell to end organ.

> The human body is a machine run by the unseen force called life, and that it may be run harmoniously it is necessary that there be liberty of blood, nerves, and arteries from the generating point to destination (1).

INTRODUCTION

This chapter presents the neurophysiological basis for viscerosomatic and somatovisceral interactions so vital to both function and to the diagnostic and treatment modalities of manual medicine. In addition, the research work of Denslow and Korr on spinal excitability is outlined. This work laid the foundation for the osteopathic profession's modern views of the osteopathic lesion, now known as the somatic dysfunction. The basis of spinal cord excitability changes that underlie chronic and neuropathic pain syndromes is also discussed as it relates to somatic dysfunction. However, the neurophysiology of pain is considered in Chapter 16. Implications for somatic dysfunction of trophic nerve functions are presented, and possible implications of Osteopathic Manipulative Treatment (OMT) for trophic function presented.

The foundations of the osteopathic profession, laid by its founder, Andrew Taylor Still, M.D., D.O., recognize that the state of health

is a continuum from complete breakdown to perfect function. One of Still's basic beliefs about function was that the body was a totally integrated unit, its structures working together harmoniously to produce a state of health. Lacking that harmonious function, the body produced conditions promoting loss of health, or disease. Implicit in these assumptions is the idea that the various parts of the body are functionally interconnected, allowing for necessary adaptations when demands on the body change. This view necessitates that the supply and maintenance organs, mainly the visceral structures, are functionally connected with the primary energy consumer of the body, the musculoskeletal system. This interrelationship has long been neglected in medical practice. The communicating systems of the body, including the immune, endocrine, and neural systems, provide this interconnectedness. When a problem develops in the integrating systems of the body, function cannot help but be compromised, and the stage is set for a lowered state of health, and eventually disease, to occur.

The field of neurophysiology is important to the physician. A thorough knowledge of anatomy and the structural relationships within the body is vital. The physician must also know how these structures function and relate to each other. He or she needs a basis for providing the patient with a rational course of treatment, especially manipulative treatment. The physician must be aware of what palpatory diagnosis is telling him or her about the underlying state of the body, and therefore of the person. Many excellent neurophysiology texts are available that outline the basics of the field.

This chapter does not attempt to give an overview of the entire field or all the areas of special interest to the osteopathic physician. It focuses on the integration of somatic and visceral function through the reflex pathways and relates these interactions to their specific neural basis. Functional alterations in reflex pathways that can disrupt integration are reviewed, along with the nonimpulse-based or trophic function of the nervous system, and how this provides a means of two-way communication within the body not dependent on the better-understood neural impulse–based communication. These aspects of the integrative activity of the nervous system are important in the osteopathic clinical experience and the role of manipulative treatment in health care. As Still recognized before the turn of the century, proper function necessitates the free interaction and integration of all body systems. Rational treatment of functional problems likewise requires an understanding of how these interactions occur and what can alter their function.

NEUROPHYSIOLOGY IN THE OSTEOPATHIC PROFESSION

The search for mechanisms underlying the efficacy of osteopathic methods began with the founding of the osteopathic profession. Although Still did not pursue what we would call organized research, he certainly was a fine researcher. He constantly questioned his observations and searched for better ways to find health and ameliorate disease. His early students at the American School of Osteopathy soon began to actively investigate the basis for the treatments they were developing. Their observations resulted in the formulation of the concept of the osteopathic lesion (now known as the somatic dysfunction). The osteopathic lesion was a set of palpatory cues and signs that indicated a functional disturbance in the body that predisposed it to disease. The early pioneers of the profession believed that somatic dysfunctions were primary causes of clinical breakdowns that resulted in the many manifestations of disease, either by themselves or by allowing, through reduced function, microorganisms to overwhelm the body defenses. When viewed in this perspective, the statement by Still that "all diseases are mere effects, the cause being a partial or complete failure of the nerves to properly conduct the fluids of life" (1) is more meaningful.

Still believed that various types of diseases were not entities unto themselves but were the result of the body's efforts to regain optimal function in the face of adverse influences, which is a view that is becoming more strongly supported by the current idea of the "illness response" (2,3) this being the initial quick immune response to pathogenic invasion, which can, ironically be triggered by psychological stressors. Thus, the events that led to the disruption of the body's normal function became the primary events to treat in the osteopathic physician's efforts to remove the influences resulting in clinical illness. The osteopathic lesion was viewed as one of the primary factors influencing body function and was amenable to physical manipulations. In addition, Still and his students realized that the body was of necessity an integrated unit; the visceral systems were tightly connected to the somatic systems. They felt strongly that visceral disturbances would cause manifestations in the somatic structures and that somatic disturbances would cause visceral dysfunctions. This reciprocal relationship became very important in the profession's thinking, clinical practice, and research endeavors.

Early research efforts in the profession largely aimed at providing evidence for the somatic problems identified as the osteopathic lesion and the effects of these dysfunctions on various aspects

of function (4). In their efforts to find objective measures of the osteopathic lesion, researchers at the American School of Osteopathy used skiography, an early form of x-ray, to look at bony placement and circulatory function as early as 1898. Another early research thrust was the effects of somatic disturbances on visceral function. Louisa Burns began research in this area early in the 1900s with studies on dogs that showed that stimulation of the lower dorsal region increased muscle contraction in the stomach and intestines but that steady pressure for a time tended to inhibit such contractions (4). Burns eventually became head of the A.T. Still Research Institute in Chicago and produced a body of research suggesting that strains produced in the vertebral column would, over time, have definite and reproducible effects on visceral function and morphology. Aided later by Wilber Cole, effects of somatic strains on neural endplate function controlling visceral organs were found and documented by neural stains. In addition, Cole (5) was able to well delineate the pathways for the effects of somatic influences on visceral function. The early research efforts of the osteopathic profession by Burns, Cole, and others were attempts to describe the effects of somatic disturbances on visceral function and the effects of manipulative treatment on immune and general function, among other things. They established a firm interest in the profession on the interrelationships between somatic and visceral function.

Beginning in the late 1930s, a new era of research in osteopathic medicine began. In an effort to enhance the profession's reputation, J.S. Denslow began a program of research at the Kirksville College of Osteopathy and Surgery that was to span 40 years and add much to the understanding of the methods of manipulative treatment. With his colleagues, Denslow (6) used the then cutting-edge technology of electromyographic (EMG) recording to obtain objective evidence of specific alterations in somatic function that correlated almost exactly to palpatory findings. Joined by Irvin M. Korr (7) in 1945, Denslow used the EMG technology to show that one of the underlying causes of palpatory findings was, indeed, altered muscle excitability. Korr then interpreted these findings in terms of neural function and the concept of the facilitated segment was developed as an underpinning of the osteopathic lesion. The research of the Kirksville group (see discussion later in this chapter) firmly placed the interactions between somatic and visceral structures in the forefront of the underpinnings of osteopathic clinical practice and philosophy. It became obvious that the interactions between visceral and somatic structures were important in health maintenance and disease processes. These interactions also provided an explanatory framework for the impact of manipulative treatment as not only influencing somatic function but also having a real and often vital effect on visceral function. Thus, this chapter will focus on the interactions between visceral and somatic structures and how they are organized. In addition, the alterations in spinal cord function that can occur with somatic input and its influence on visceral function will be discussed. Understanding these interactions and alterations, beginning with the organization of the basic reflex arc, is important in understanding the value of osteopathic treatment techniques and the neural basis of health.

THE REFLEX

In 1905, Charles Sherrington (8) published *The Integrative Action of the Nervous System*. This classic text represented current knowledge about the fundamental aspects of how the nervous system handled and integrated information. Over the ensuing years, considerably more has been learned about the function of the nervous system and how it integrates the many functions of the body. A great deal is known about how the basic structural unit of the nervous system, the neuron, interacts with other cells through synaptic structures and the release of neurotransmitters and neuromodulators. The billions of neurons and glial cells that make up the nervous system are organized into functional groups, often with widely differing structural and functional characteristics. Many of the neurons are involved in networks that respond to stimuli impinging on or even originating in the body, which results in commands to muscles and glands that produce activity or secretions. These networks, the reflexes, have been more fully analyzed in recent years. What were previously considered to be almost autonomous units of function are actually complex and interactive aspects of an organizational whole. The reflex has been found to be anything but a static unit of input/output relationships, but rather it is an active and ever-changing mosaic. The characteristics of reflex function are modulated by messages from other areas of the nervous system and by activity of the endocrine and immune systems. In fact, reflexes must not be viewed as separate entities but as parts of various programs that control motor and secretory actions. Thus, an individual reflex may serve differing functions depending on which control program is operating (9). However, for purposes of analysis, reflexes have usually been isolated for study, a practice that has erroneously led many students to view reflexes as simple and unchanging entities.

Structure

The common concept of the reflex is basically one of a relationship between an input stimulus to the body and an output action to either a muscle or a secretory organ. Sherrington (8) viewed the reflex as an input/output relationship between information coming into the body and a response to that information. He viewed a reflex as always inherited and innately given. The concept of a reflex includes an afferent or incoming limb from a sensory receptor, which is a central component in the spinal cord or brain. It also includes an output (efferent) limb that is usually a motor component to either somatic (musculoskeletal) or visceral structures terminating in synaptic connections that may either activate or inhibit activity in these structures (Fig. 9.1).

The usual concept of the reflex suggests that the reflex limbs are fairly well defined and limited primarily to one input and one output channel, with little interaction with other reflex networks (Figs. 9.2 and 9.3). Almost all reflex networks can be influenced by a wide variety of other excitatory and inhibitory signals, including those coming from higher or lower levels of the central nervous system (CNS). The picture of a reflex as a simple message pathway from the patellar tendon that causes the quadriceps femoris muscle to contract, resulting in a knee jerk, is a vast oversimplification of the interactions that occur when a stimulus causes a response. The tendon tap reflex, exemplified by the patellar tap/knee jerk reflex activation, is, however, a prime example of the simplest reflex structure.

The tendon tap, or myotatic reflex, is a monosynaptic reflex. It is the only monosynaptic reflex present in the human. The stimulus of a tap to a tendon stretches the muscle attached to the tendon, which in turn stretches the muscle spindle organs in the muscle. Neural signals, or action potentials, are sent from the spindle organs to the spinal cord on the incoming, or afferent, limb of the reflex. In this case, the signals travel through the spinal cord on the axons from the spindles directly to the motoneurons that innervate the muscle that was stretched. They make synaptic contact with the motoneurons causing them to generate action potentials that travel over the efferent, or outgoing, limb of the reflex network back to the muscle, which causes it to contract.

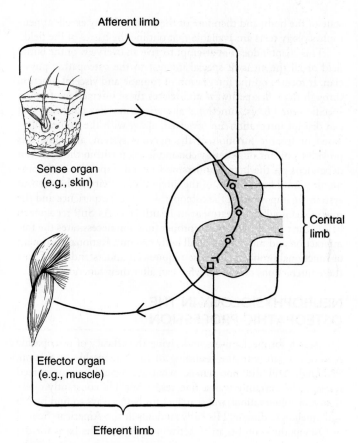

Figure 9-1 Schematic of reflex as it is usually envisioned, with afferent, central, and efferent limbs.

It would be a simple picture if this was all that happened. However, the incoming axons send off branches that go to other neurons in the spinal cord that, in turn, send axons to the motoneurons of the antagonist of the stretched muscle. These axons provide signals that inhibit the motoneurons innervating the antagonist

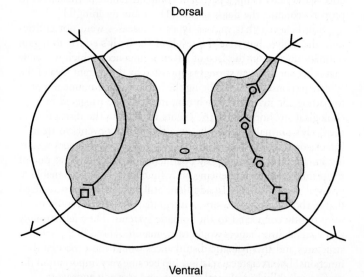

Figure 9-2 A common, mistaken concept of how a reflex is constructed. Afferent limb simply connects with central limb, which activates efferent limb. **Left**, monosynaptic reflex; **right**, polysynaptic reflex. Actual complexity is better represented in Figure 7.3.

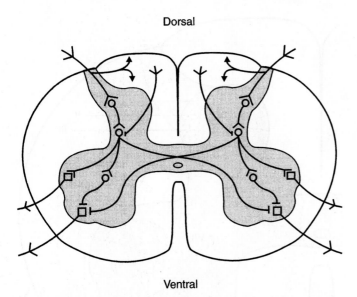

Dorsal

Ventral

Figure 9-3 Schematic of neural interactions at the spinal level, indicating the complexity of even simple reflexes. Input to the spinal cord sends collaterals up and down the cord and is acted on by ascending and descending influences, as well as input from the opposite side of the cord. Input courses through several synapses and interneurons before acting (in thoracolumbar cord) on both somatic and sympathetic motoneurons. In cervical and sacral cord areas, parasympathetic pathways are involved.

muscle. When the stretched muscle contracts, the antagonist muscle is inhibited to allow a smooth movement to occur. In addition, other branches from the incoming axons go up the spinal cord to other spinal areas (e.g., to the arms if the patellar reflex was stimulated), to the brainstem, as well as down the spinal cord to lower spinal centers. What appeared to be a simple reflex network has become a complex set of pathways within the spinal cord and brainstem. In addition, pathways from both above and below the level of the input axons can directly influence the basic excitability of the motoneurons involved and, hence, alter the reflex activity observed when the tendon is tapped. Indeed, when elicited clinically, the tendon tap reflex is used as a porthole into the nervous system to see how it is functioning, and the clinician is not usually interested in that reflex per se. In fact, the main purpose of using the tendon tap reflex clinically is to test the excitability of the motoneurons, as a function of both local and distant influences.

SOMATOSOMATIC

Although the tendon tap reflex is used a great deal clinically, the most familiar of the spinal reflexes are the defensive reflexes, such as the withdrawal movements of a limb to a noxious stimulus. These somatosomatic reflexes occur when some stimulus is applied to a somatic structure. This initiates a volley of neural activity (often nociceptive) through the afferent limb of the reflex to the spinal cord. The afferent input activity flows through synapses into the interneurons of the spinal cord central gray, and finally into the ventral horn motoneurons. These motoneurons then cause somatic muscle contraction. The reflexes have at least one interneuron between the sensory input in the dorsal horn of the cord and the motoneurons of the ventral horn (Fig. 9.3). They are named from the origin of the information and the locus of action, both somatic.

Many somatosomatic reflexes have been documented and studied. The simple somatosomatic reflexes are exemplified by defensive

withdrawal actions such as when accidentally touching a hot object and the arm jerks back. Very complex activities, such as the righting reflexes that occur, for example, when a cat is dropped upside down and lands on its feet are also found, but even these reflexes do not occur in isolation; as with the myotatic reflexes, they are accompanied by a spread of activity throughout the nervous system.

VISCEROVISCERAL

A second type of reflex is the viscerovisceral reflex, in which sensory input from a visceral structure causes activity in a visceral organ. These reflexes are involved, for example, in distention of the gut that results in increased contraction of the gut muscle. Viscerovisceral reflexes involve afferent activity flowing from the receptors into the spinal cord through interneurons to produce efferent or outflow activity within the sympathetic and/or parasympathetic motoneurons.

REFLEX INTERACTIONS

We might expect to find that afferent input from somatic structures has some influence on visceral organs and that input from visceral structures has some effect on somatic organs. Somatovisceral and viscerosomatic reflexes have been known for many years but, until recently, have received little attention from the research and medical community. However, these types of reflex interactions are very important for the practice and understanding of osteopathic palpatory diagnosis and treatment and for the integration of body function.

A familiar example of a viscerosomatic reflex is pain and muscle tightness in the left shoulder with onset of a myocardial infarction (MI). The nociceptive input from the compromised myocardium (a visceral structure) is exciting not only the pathways that are interpreted as shoulder pain (a somatic structure) but is also causing the motoneurons supplying the shoulder muscles to become active. In a classic study, Eble (10) showed several such reflexes by stimulating visceral structures and recording somatic muscle activity. He demonstrated that stimulation of various visceral structures produced somatic muscle activity.

Conversely, activity in a somatic structure can alter visceral function. In a number of studies over the last several years, Sato (11) clearly demonstrated the effect of somatic stimulation on various visceral functions, ranging from heart rate to adrenal output. These studies have also shown that some of these reflex interactions occur directly in the spinal cord. With others, the afferent activity from the somatic stimulation travels up the spinal cord to the brainstem, resulting in a cascade of activity from the brainstem back down to the spinal autonomic motoneurons.

In both viscerosomatic and somatovisceral reflex networks, activity resulting from the stimulation of a structure can have either an excitatory or an inhibitory influence on the motoneurons involved. For example, stimulation of the belly skin usually results in inhibition of gut activity (a somatovisceral reflex) but increases heart rate.

In daily life, the body's somatic system is active. The skeletal muscles are the machines that carry out activities. The visceral organs are the means by which the energy demands and maintenance of the muscles are met and by which waste is disposed of. Without a continuous and highly integrated communication between these two systems, the body could not continue to achieve a balance among:

Its energy needs and supply
The amount of blood necessary to carry nutrients and waste and fulfill the demands of the muscles and bones
Supply and demand in general

The neural connections represented by these reflex systems are one of the primary ways this integration is carried out.

For the osteopathic physician, the viscerosomatic and somatovisceral reflexes are of extreme importance. When using palpatory diagnosis to detect subtle problems in function, whether it be tissue texture changes, motion characteristics, or temperature variations of the body, the physician is sensing clues from the musculoskeletal system, skin, muscles, and fascias. These clues reflect not only aspects of these tissues but also functional characteristics of the underlying visceral organs and tissues through the viscerosomatic reflex networks. When the physician uses manipulative treatment to correct somatic dysfunctions, underlying visceral function is affected through the somatovisceral reflex networks. Thus, for both palpation and treatment, an understanding of reflex function is necessary.

NEURAL BASIS FOR REFLEX INTERACTIONS

Evidence is accumulating about the neural basis of viscerosomatic and somatovisceral interactions. When a stimulus is applied, afferent input from either visceral or somatic structures flows into the spinal cord along the dorsal roots and enters the upper areas of the spinal gray matter. The spinal gray matter is commonly divided into ten layers, first documented on cytoarchitectural evidence by Rexed (12) (Fig. 9.4). Large-diameter, cutaneous afferent input that signals nonnociceptive stimuli enters the spinal gray of the dorsal horn and terminates primarily in layers III and IV. Nociceptive afferents from both somatic and visceral structures enter the cord and send branches rostrally and caudally in Lissauer's tract that runs along the apex of the dorsal horn. Branches of this nociceptive input then terminate in layers I, II, V, VII, and X. Layers I and V display an especially tremendous overlap of the input from somatic and visceral nociceptors (13).

It now appears that in most areas of the spinal cord, practically every interneuron that receives input from a visceral nociceptor also receives input from a somatic source. It also appears that almost 80% of interneurons that receive input from somatic structures also receive visceral input. Presently, there is no evidence for any ascending pathway that transmits only visceral sensory signals from the spinal cord to the brain. This raises the question of how an individual can distinguish visceral from somatic pain or sensation at all. In many cases, visceral pain is felt as a diffuse and poorly localized sensation and is referred to somatic structures. The overlap of somatic and visceral input explains the referral of visceral pain to somatic structures, which is designated as referred pain.

Impulses arriving from visceral structures and converging onto interneurons also receiving somatic afferents activate ascending pathways to the brain that result in the perception of pain in the somatic structure. In addition, more somatic than visceral input occurs because the viscera are much more sparsely innervated with sensory receptors. This suggests that visceral input has much more diffuse functional effects than the corresponding somatic afferents do. For example, it appears that many of the somatic C fibers terminate primarily in focal areas of layer II of the cord. Visceral C fibers extend for several segments and give off collaterals at regular intervals. Only about 10% of the inflow into the thoracolumbar spinal cord comes from visceral structures (14). This sparse innervation but wide distribution of visceral afferents may be the basis for the diffuse nature of most visceral pain. The evidence indicates that the widespread effects of visceral input are due more to functional (spread of activity through networks) than anatomic (many collateral branches) divergence (15). Figure 9.5 shows the afferent

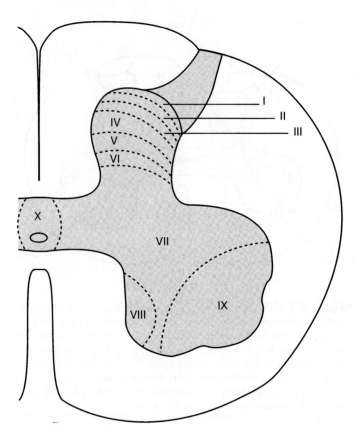

Figure 9-4 Rexed layers. Laminae at the L7 segment of a cat spinal cord. From Rexed B. The cytoarchitectonic organization of the spinal cord in the cat. *J Comp Neurol* 1952;96:415–495, with permission.

terminations of somatic and visceral afferent fibers in the various levels of the spinal cord.

The overlap of input onto common interneurons within the gray matter of the spinal cord is also the basis for the activation of somatic muscle activity seen with visceral disturbances. The excitatory drive provided onto common interneurons by visceral input activates not only sympathetic outflow back to visceral structures but also motoneurons (both alpha and gamma) that innervate skeletal musculature. The result is a tonic activation of skeletal muscles in the referral area of visceral input. This is the viscerosomatic reflex manifestation, or splinting, that is seen, for example, in appendicitis.

These relationships also underlie the reverse phenomenon, that of the somatovisceral reflex, in which somatic input alters sympathetic and parasympathetic outflow. The data on the convergence of somatic and visceral input are beginning to explain the interrelations between visceral and somatic structures, especially when nociceptive input is activated.

There are descending influences on the activity of both somatic and visceral reflex pathways. In many of the reflex loops driven by both visceral and somatic input, there is a strong effect of descending pathways on the long-lasting excitability of the reflex outflow. These descending influences can maintain the excitability of the reflex for extended periods. They may account for some of the long-term increases in sensitivity, muscle contractions, and hyperexcitable sympathetic output seen especially with visceral disturbances. Likewise, the long-lasting descending influences can be inhibitory, resulting in lowered somatic or autonomic outflow. For example, the effects of rib-raising techniques (a somatic stimulation) on

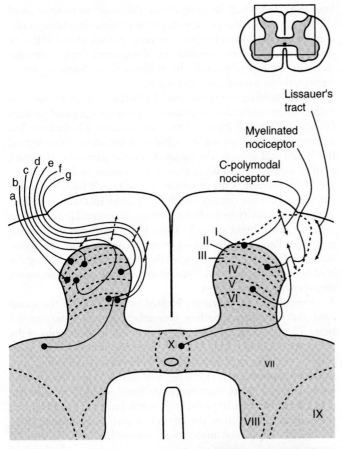

Figure 9-5 Terminal patterns of primary afferent collaterals in the transverse plane of spinal cord. **Left**, primary afferent terminations of axons not associated with nociception. *A*, C-low-threshold mechanoreceptor; *B*, innocuous cooling receptor; *C*, A hair afferent; *D*, G-1 and G-2 hair receptors; *E*, slowly adapting type I and II afferents; *F*, primary and secondary muscle spindle afferents; *G*, Golgi tendon organ. The *arrow* indicates that the parent axon bifurcates and ascends and descends the spinal cord for 17 segments giving off collaterals along this course. **Right**, nociceptor afferents from both somatic and visceral structures. Both visceral and somatic A and C fiber nociceptor afferents terminate in Rexed lamina I, II, V, and to some extent in VII and X. Lamina are indicated on the right and outlined by *dotted lines*. From Light AR. *The Initial Processing of Pain and Its Descending Control: Spinal and Trigeminal Systems.* Basel, Switzerland: Karger, 1992:88, with permission.

sympathetic outflow seem to be primarily inhibitory through the descending brain influences, resulting in decreased vasoconstriction and better fluid flow in the thoracic area (16).

Although much of our information on the activation of sympathetic afferents by skeletal input has come from nociceptive input, there is evidence that sympathetic output can also be strongly driven independent of nociception by muscle proprioceptors. For example, Kaufman (17) has shown large effects on sympathetic outflow driven by alteration of proprioceptive input from muscles. Pickar and his colleagues have also found evidence for somatosympathetic reflex interactions from the low back (18). Thus, the evidence for activation and control of sympathetic activity by somatic input strongly suggests a basis for musculoskeletal activity in the regulation of body function through somatovisceral reflexes. Likewise, recent research by Jou and Foreman (19)

has shown that cardiac efferents can have dramatic influences on muscle activity, supporting the role of viscerosomatic reflex connections as underlying the effectiveness of palpatory diagnosis in visceral disease states.

However, the direct interactions through the spinal cord of visceral and somatic inputs are not the only important means of interactions. Goehler and her colleagues have delineated a strong vagal to brain input that is primary in signaling pathogenic disturbances in the gut (20–22). The vagus is a very potent signaler for the very short latency first immune response to impending infections. The total response to vagal signals involves autonomic, somatic, and psychological responses that prepare the body to fight the infection. Called the bottom-up response, it prepares the whole system for defense. Interestingly, the same response can occur from the "top down" being triggered by psychological stress (21). The complexity of visceral, somatic, and psychological interactions is truly remarkable and only beginning to be understood.

CARDIAC CONTROL

We will now consider a model of viscerosomatic and somatovisceral interactions shown in cardiac control. Neural input from somatic structures may affect neural activity to both somatic and visceral structures. A good example of the interaction between somatic afferents and autonomic outflow is the control of the heart. As with most visceral structures, the heart receives its autonomic innervation from both sympathetic and parasympathetic nerves.

SYMPATHETIC INNERVATION OF THE HEART

Excitation of the cardiac sympathetic nerves (Fig. 9.6) causes the following effects:

Increased heart rate
Increased atrial and ventricular contractility
Decreased conduction time from the atrium to the ventricle

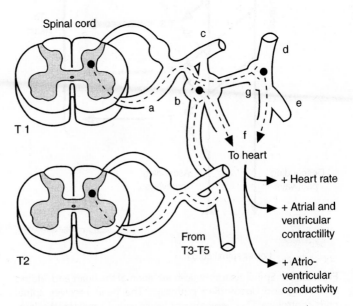

Figure 9-6 Sympathetic innervation of heart. *A*, ventral root; *B*, stellate ganglion; *C*, spinal nerve; *D*, vagosympathetic trunk; *E*, vagus nerve; *F*, cardiac nerves; *G*, middle cervical ganglion.

The heart's spinal innervation is associated with spinal cord levels from T1 to about T5, with T2 probably contributing the most (Fig. 9.7).

The preganglionic fibers leave the spinal cord via the ventral roots and course a short distance in the spinal nerves (Fig. 9.6). The preganglionic fibers then exit the spinal nerves to enter the adjoining sympathetic chain ganglia. Most preganglionic sympathetic fibers controlling the heart course though the stellate ganglion to the middle cervical ganglion. There, they excite ganglion cells that send their axons, the postganglionic fibers, via the cardiac nerves, to innervate:

Pacemaker cells
Myocardium
Conductile system
Coronary arteries

The first paravertebral ganglion associated with the heart is the stellate ganglion, where some preganglionic axons excite ganglion cells whose axons also run directly to the heart (23).

Segmental-like innervation to different portions of the heart does not seem to occur (24). In other words, a particular spinal level (e.g., T4), sends its sympathetic influences to most areas of the heart, not to one area. One should be cautious in relating problems in one portion of the heart to problems associated with one spinal level. However, different spinal segmental levels innervate different organs, for example, heart versus lungs. Some degree of segmental-like innervation does occur.

Understanding the spinal cord levels that control the heart is helpful in understanding responses of spinal cord–injured patients (Fig. 9.7) (25,26). With spinal cord lesions above T1, the brain has no control of the heart via the spinal cord and sympathetic nerves, but it can still activate the parasympathetic pathways. However, marked cardiac alterations may occur via reflexes mediated by sensory input that enters the spinal cord below the C8 level. For example, input from the urinary bladder may cause markedly increased sympathetic activity to the heart. Patients with spinal lesions below T1 have some brain control of the heart via descending spinal pathways. Patients with lesions below T5 rarely show any spinal reflexes influencing the heart from the spinal afferents entering the cord below the lesion level. Specific levels of the spinal cord innervate specific visceral organs.

Sympathetic motoneurons located in both sides of the spinal cord and their corresponding sympathetic nerves innervate the heart. There are some quantitative differences in the regions of the heart that are innervated (24). For example, stimulation of sympathetic preganglionic nerves from both sides of the spinal cord causes increases in heart rate. The right side has a greater influence on heart rate and the sinoatrial node function. Both sides innervate the atrioventricular node, both ventricles, and atria. However, sympathetic output from the left spinal cord has a greater effect on cardiac output and myocardial contractility (24,26). Visceral organs receive asymmetrical autonomic control from the left and right sides of the spinal cord.

Several different descending spinal pathways can affect autonomic outflow from the spinal cord. Many of these pathways are located in the lateral funiculus of the spinal cord. Both anatomic (27) and physiologic (28) evidence suggests that the descending spinal pathways are organized according to a viscerotropic pattern. Localized lesions of the spinal cord, or portions of the descending spinal pathways, may result in loss of brain control of one particular visceral organ, which also suggests that the brain has the potential to separately control different visceral organs (Fig. 9.8).

PARASYMPATHETIC INNERVATION OF THE HEART

Parasympathetic innervation of the heart is via the vagus nerve that causes the following (Fig. 9.9):

Decreased heart rate
Slowed atrioventricular conduction

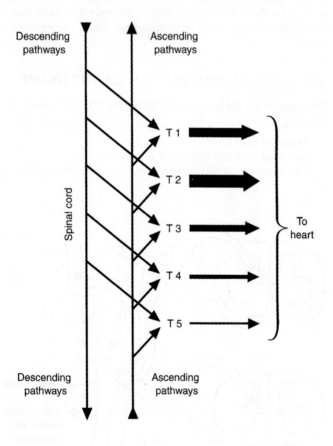

Figure 9-7 Spinal sympathetic innervation of the heart and related ascending and descending pathways. The heart receives spinal cord control via T1-T5 spinal cord levels with T2 making the largest functional contribution. Lesions above T1 and below T5 block brain control of cardiac sympathetic activity and reflex responses to ascending afferent activation, respectively.

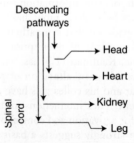

Figure 9-8 Viscerotropic organization of the descending spinal pathways controlling autonomic outflow.

Decreased atrial contraction

Limited decrease of ventricular contractility

The cardiac vagal fibers travel in the cervical vagus nerve (vago-sympathetic trunk) into the thorax where they separate from the vagus nerve to form the cardiac nerves. These cardiac vagal nerves have their cell bodies in the medulla, that is, the nucleus ambiguous and the dorsomotor nucleus (29–33).

These two medullary regions may subserve different cardiac functions. For example, the nucleus ambiguous may mediate heart rate while the dorsomotor nucleus regulates ventricular contractility (31). Not only are there regions of the brainstem controlling cardiac function that seem to be distinct from those controlling gastrointestinal function and other visceral organs, but different brainstem regions may also control separate cardiac functions.

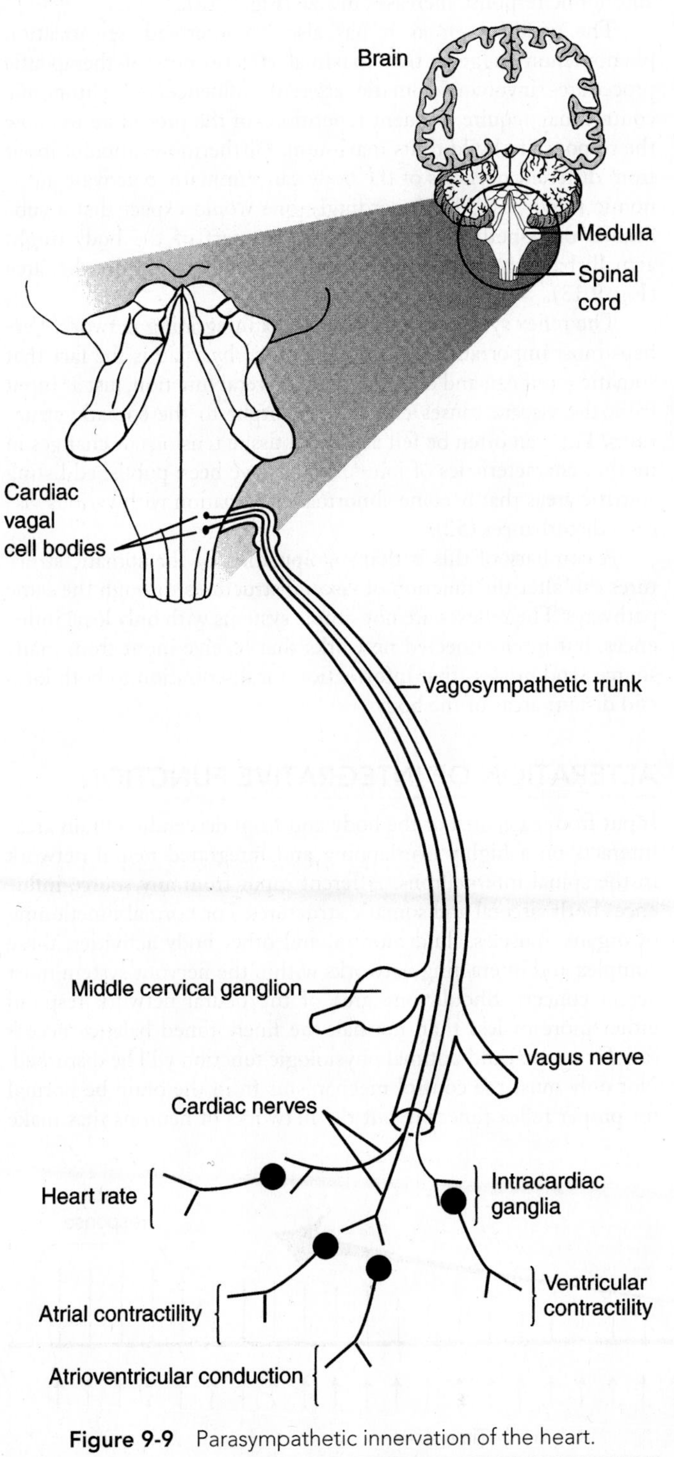

VISCERAL FUNCTION CONTROL

Cardiovascular function can be reflexively controlled by somatic afferents via the somatosympathetic reflexes. These reflexes may be mediated at the spinal cord level or via suprasegmental connections. The spinal somatosympathetic reflexes demonstrate dependency on segmental organization. These sympathetic reflex responses at one segmental level are larger if the somatic afferent activity enters at the same spinal level than if it enters at adjoining levels (34,35). These reflexes also demonstrate laterality, because they are larger for ipsilateral reflexes than for contralateral reflexes (Fig. 9.10).

Visceral afferents can also influence somatic reflexes, and muscle tone may be altered by visceral input. Many of these reflex possibilities are very important for osteopathic palpatory diagnosis and treatment because they provide mechanisms for the use of muscle tone as an indicator of visceral disturbances. The work by Eble (36) showed activation of skeletal muscles with stimulation of visceral structures, and Schoen and Finn (37) reported EMG activity in shoulder muscles of the cat following experimental MI. The cardiac viscerosomatic reflex has an influence on somatic musculature (19).

Not only can there be activity from somatic or visceral structures that influences the opposite structures, but another type of activity, independent of the brain or spinal cord, may also occur. Recently, neural activity has been recorded from *in vitro* sympathetic ganglion cells and intracardiac ganglion cells, demonstrating considerable action potential activity even when the neuronal connections to the CNS are severed (29,31–33). These observations suggest that the autonomic ganglia may function as little brains within peripheral ganglia and the heart. These ganglia may have the neural circuitry to act almost independently and have the ability to integrate intrinsic cardiocardiac reflexes as well as information from the CNS. However, the functional roles of these peripheral nervous system interactions are presently unknown (Fig. 9.11).

The possibility of little brains within the autonomic ganglia presents many more possibilities. If visceral afferents have reflexes

Figure 9-9 Parasympathetic innervation of the heart.

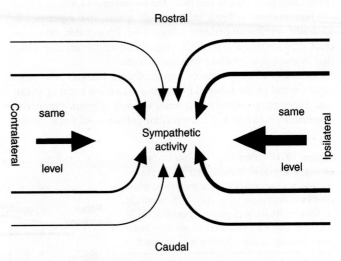

Figure 9-10 Laterality of cardiac sympathetic control and segmental organization of spinal sympathetic reflexes.

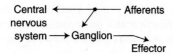

Figure 9-11 Afferent reflex control of autonomic effectors may be mediated via reflexes within peripheral autonomic ganglia as well as via CNS connections.

within the autonomic ganglia, somatic afferents could also have reflex connections within them. Some somatic afferent fibers pass through the autonomic ganglia. It is possible that somatic afferents influence sympathetic activity not only to the somatic structure but also to visceral structures such as the heart. Activation of somatic afferents might cause reflex alteration of cardiac function via direct ganglionic reflexes as well as via the CNS-mediated reflexes. Likewise, visceral afferents might activate sympathetic ganglion cells with axons supplying somatic structures (38–41). The therapeutic implications of reflexes within autonomic ganglia may be important.

INTERACTIONS OF SOMATIC AFFERENTS AND BARORECEPTOR CONTROL OF AUTONOMIC ACTIVITY

Blood pressure and cardiac function are reflexively controlled through alteration of autonomic activity mediated by arterial blood pressure afferent receptors called baroreceptors. Increased arterial blood pressure excites baroreceptor activity, which is carried to the brainstem via the glossopharyngeal and vagus nerves. In the brainstem, the baroreceptor afferent activity eventually leads to excitation of the medullary cardiac vagal cell bodies. It also leads to inhibition of the sympathetic activity to the cardiovascular system via descending brainstem/spinal pathways (42). Baroreceptor reflexes involving the cardiac vagus nerves have parallel inhibitory effects on the sinoatrial node (slowing heart rate) and atrioventricular node (slowing atrioventricular conduction) (43).

Although these baroreceptor reflexes have powerful influences on cardiovascular function, they also interact with other spinal reflexes, especially from small, high-threshold, afferent fibers. With activation of these spinal afferents, reflex changes in sympathetic activity (somatosympathetic reflexes) occur at the spinal cord level and through suprasegmental reflexes involving ascending and then descending pathways to and from the brainstem (44,45).

Baroreceptor reflexes inhibit both spinal and supraspinally mediated somatosympathetic reflexes (46). Presumably, other visceral afferents that also mediate sympathetic reflexes are also inhibited by these powerful baroreceptor reflexes.

Somatic afferent activity can modulate baroreceptor reflex vagal control of the heart. Baroreceptor activation excites the cardiac vagus nerve activity. However, somatic afferent stimulation attenuates or blocks the baroreceptor influence of vagal cardiac

nerves. Somatic afferents and baroreceptors compete for control of autonomic activity. The ascending and descending pathways for these reflexes have been localized in the dorsal portion of the lateral funiculus of the spinal cord (47–49).

Summation Characteristics of Somatovisceral Reflexes

Somatovisceral reflexes demonstrate temporal and spatial summation as indicated by the wind-up phenomenon and the effect of input from different parts of the body. These somatovisceral reflexes do not reach their maximal activity immediately (50). Rather, when stimulated at a slow repetition rate, these reflexes exhibit wind-up. With each repetition of the stimulation up to about 20 times, the autonomic response increases in size (Fig. 9.12).

The wind-up, or as it has also been termed, sensitization phenomenon suggests that maximal effectiveness of therapeutic procedures involving somatic afferent influences on autonomic control may require frequent repetitions of the procedure to allow the response to build to its maximum. Furthermore, afferent input from different portions of the body can summate to activate autonomic responses (51). Accordingly, one would expect that a subliminal or noneffective stimulus to one part of the body might actually have an effect if combined with stimulation to another area (Fig. 9.13).

The reflex system is truly a complex integrating network. Perhaps most important for the osteopathic physician is the fact that somatic input can and does influence visceral function, just as input from the viscera causes changes in output to the somatic structures. This can often be felt as altered tissue tensions or changes in motion characteristics of joints. Maps have been published listing somatic areas that become abnormal to palpation with various visceral disturbances (52).

A corollary of this is that manipulation of the somatic structures can alter the function of visceral structures through the same pathways. The reflexes are not simple systems with only local influences, but interconnected networks that receive input from many sources and process that information for distribution to both local and distant areas of the body.

ALTERATION OF INTEGRATIVE FUNCTION

Input from each area of the body and from descending brain areas interacts on a highly overlapping and integrated neural network in the spinal interneurons. Afferent input from any source influences both visceral and somatic structures. For normal functioning of organs, muscles, fluid motion, and other body activities, these complex and interacting networks within the nervous system must act in concert. Should one area of the neural network respond either more or less than normal, the finely tuned balance necessary for normal and optimal physiologic function will be disturbed. Not only must the control mechanisms from the brain be normal for proper reflex function, but the networks of neurons that make

Figure 9-12 Wind-up or sensitization. When a stimulus is repeated at a rate of once every second or two, response to stimulus may continue to grow for 20 seconds or more. Finally, a stable response level is reached that can continue at an increased level as long as the stimulus is continued.

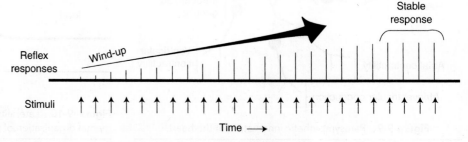

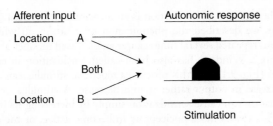

Figure 9-13 Summation of autonomic responses. Input from two different locations adds together to produce a larger autonomic response than either input produces when it occurs alone.

up the reflexes must also be acting normally. Unfortunately, these networks themselves can be altered, resulting in a loss of proper function.

Although Sherrington postulated that reflexes are innately given, evidence is accumulating that the function of reflex networks can be influenced by many factors. They are subject to both short-term and long-term changes that can have consequences for the health of the individual.

In the early and mid-1940s, Denslow et al. (53–55) were among the first to show the results of changes in the integrative function of reflex networks in humans. They performed a series of studies on normal, young adult volunteers to determine whether the reflex excitabilities at various spinal levels of the body were stable and comparable. They measured how much stimulation it took to evoke muscle activity (EMG) in the paraspinal muscles of the back at several levels of the thoracic spine.

They found that, on the average, reflex excitability to pressure on the spinous processes was highest in the upper thoracic area and lowest in the midlumbar area. Although decreased excitability from the upper thoracic to the lower lumbar areas was seen overall in the subjects studied, practically all individuals studied had areas that were very highly excitable, responding to small amounts of pressure on the spinous process at that spinal level. In normal areas, in contrast, even a fairly heavy pressure in the spinous processes did not produce any muscle activity in the associated muscles. The highly excitable areas were characterized by not only the increased muscle activity to pressure on the spinous process but also often by pain and tenderness in the area. The areas of increased sensitivity to stimulation were not uniform from individual to individual and were long lasting (some cases remaining almost the same for years). In most cases, the individual did not realize that any change was present.

These long-lasting, low-threshold areas to afferent input could be activated not only by stimulating tissues at the same level of the spinal cord but also by stimulating other areas of the back or even by providing a psychological stress to the individual. With remote input, such as pressure on a spinous process four vertebrae away from the level of the low-threshold area, the muscles at the level of the input remained silent while those at the level of the low threshold became active. The same pattern occurred with psychological stressors. The normal areas remained silent, but the low-threshold areas showed muscle activity.

In later studies, Denslow and co-workers (56,57) found that not only was muscle activity affected but so were the activities of visceral organs through altered sympathetic output. Here, again, the interrelatedness of the somatic and visceral portions of the body was shown.

Although many otherwise normal subjects had low-threshold or high-excitability areas, it became evident from subject-to-subject variability, and from further data showing that the excitability

increases often accompanied injury and disease, that the excitability changes were not a normal state. They represented areas of neural function that were operating out of synchrony with other areas of the neural system, causing the organs served by those neural supplies also to be out of synchrony with the total body function.

Korr (7) suggested that these low-threshold spinal reflexes represented pathways that were being held in a hyperexcited state, perhaps by continued bombardment of input. He termed these areas the facilitated segment (although "segment" is a misnomer), as the areas rarely follow dermatomal boundaries. He pointed out that they acted to magnify input to the area from any source and to cause a magnified outflow to the organs innervated by that level of the spinal cord. Thermographic studies were also conducted (56,57). Not only did the skeletal muscles respond in an exaggerated fashion in the low-threshold areas but the sympathetic outflow also increased. Such areas of abnormally increased excitability or decreased threshold within the otherwise normal areas of the spinal cord must act to decrease the overall integration of body function. No matter the source of input to a facilitated spinal area, the neural outflow would be exaggerated relative to the same response at other spinal levels. Such a situation lasting over time can have only undesirable consequences for total body function.

Beginning and Maintenance of Reflex Facilitation

The finding that facilitated or low-threshold areas could continue for long periods of time and the fact that these areas were not the same between individuals suggested that some process could occur that would establish these chronically hyperactive areas. Initial speculation suggested that the hyperexcitability was maintained by tonic afferent input. Most input from either somatic or visceral structures, however, decreases dramatically with activities such as sleep or other forms of relaxation. Why should the hyperexcitability continue even with the loss of afferent activity? What is the nature of the neural processing within the reflex pathways to afferent stimuli that might explain the appearance of regions of hyperexcitability? More recent studies have provided some answers that have a bearing on how changes in reflex excitability can at times be an adaptive process and at times a detrimental one.

ALTERATION OF REFLEX EXCITABILITY

The concept of the reflex as a simple, unchanging, static input/output relationship is oversimplified. Although he characterized reflex function as innately given, even Sherrington recognized that reflex excitability could be momentarily altered by influences such as signals from higher brain structures or by rapid and repeated use, which, he noted, caused reflex fatigue. The notion that reflexes are fundamentally unchanging, static input/output relationships is still widespread despite the fact that it is now clear that the excitability of spinal reflex pathways can be altered by many influences. These changes can range from short-lasting, fleeting changes to very long-lasting ones that may even become permanent. These long-lasting alterations may well be the basis for the changes shown by Denslow in his studies of human motoneuron excitability and for the facilitated state hypothesized by Korr. These threats to functional integration of the body may be related to the effects of nociceptive stimuli at the periphery.

ALTERATION OF NOCICEPTIVE INPUT

Inflammation from strong stimulation of the skin or other peripheral somatic or visceral structures produces a set of changes in the sensory receptors of the organ that dramatically alters the amount of neural activity sent to the spinal cord (58). Most tissues are innervated by various sensory receptors, such as:

Touch
Temperature
Stretch
Nociceptors

The nociceptors are composed primarily of naked (unmyelinated) nerve endings that respond to potentially tissue-damaging stimuli. In the hollow visceral organs, they respond to stretch or dilation of the organ, for example. These receptors send impulses through thin myelinated (group III or A) or unmyelinated (group IV or C) fibers into the spinal gray matter, where they synapse primarily in Rexed layers I and V. When activity occurs in these pathways, the resulting sensation is usually discomfort or pain, although the input may be blocked (by other neural activity) from reaching the areas of the brainstem where they are appreciated as pain. However, even though a nociceptive input to the spinal cord does not reach the conscious level, it may affect the dynamics of the spinal pathways (59).

Once a stimulus sufficiently strong to activate nociceptive input begins, impulses travel into the spinal cord via the dorsal roots. At the branches of the peripheral neurons, the afferent impulses invade the afferent branches and are conveyed back out to the nerve terminals where they cause release of various peptides into the surrounding tissues. The sites of peptide release may be some distance from the original stimulus. The result of this release is the start of a cascade of events that leads to involvement of the sympathetic postganglionic nerve terminals and to the release of serum from the surrounding capillaries. Prostaglandins released from the sympathetic nerve terminals continue the serum release that leads to local inflammation.

This process begins the healing process, although it may be sufficiently severe that the healing process is retarded (60). The inflammation also produces dramatic changes in the characteristics of the local nociceptors in the area. Schmidt (58) demonstrated in the cat knee joint that the number of nociceptors responding to a stretch stimulation may be between 3,000 and 4,000 after inflammation. In contrast, even severe stretch of the normal joint may cause only 400 nociceptors to fire. Also, the receptive fields of the active nociceptors enlarge dramatically in the inflamed area, and the threshold to activation significantly decreases. The result of an inflammatory process (or a strong stimulus that produces tissue damage) will be to lower nociceptor thresholds and dramatically increase input to the spinal cord. Peripheral events can lead to dramatic changes in the amount of stimuli caused by changes in the peripheral receptors.

What happens to spinal reflex networks when stimulus input changes? In the normal reflex pathway, repeated activation of the pathway by a weak afferent input results in a temporary decrease in the output of the network. Sherrington described this short-term decrease in reflex pathway excitability as reflex fatigue. This process, now termed habituation, has been studied extensively and is a characteristic of polysynaptic reflex pathways in the spinal cord and brainstem.

Habituation is characterized by a decrease in output from a neural pathway that has repeated stimulus input of a mild to moderate intensity. A stimulus may initially produce a response of a certain magnitude, but if the stimulus is repeated several times, the response decreases. If the stimulus is then terminated, the response returns to its initial level in a matter of seconds to minutes (61). The process of habituation is a ubiquitous phenomenon, occurring in almost all animals and in all mammalian reflex pathways except the monosynaptic myotatic reflex. It is a necessary part of the neural integration, because it allows nonessential stimuli to be muted in their effects on the nervous system.

The opposite of habituation is an increase in reflex excitability. Earlier, we described the phenomenon of wind-up, in which a stimulus repeated several times causes an increased number of neural firings. Wind-up has also been called sensitization in earlier studies (Fig. 9.12). In this process, a repetitive stimulus can cause an increase in output rather than a decrease. A stimulus causing habituation can cause sensitization simply by increasing its intensity. This causes more nociceptors to become active, or the same nociceptors to produce more impulses. Like habituation, sensitization can occur within a matter of seconds, and it can also dissipate in a matter of seconds when the stimulus is terminated (61).

Both habituation and sensitization have been extensively studied at the cellular level. In the mammal, both occur within the spinal central gray matter in the interneuron pathways. They are probably subserved by two different sets of interneurons, which then synapse on the motoneurons of both the sympathetic and the somatic systems. Both sensitization and habituation are apparently presynaptic processes that either inhibit (habituation) or enhance (sensitization) the release of neurotransmitter with each activation of the presynaptic terminal (62). They are independent of descending influences from higher nervous centers. Both processes can be demonstrated in humans with spinal cord transections.

Habituation and sensitization are different processes but occur at the synaptic level and can occur over a few seconds of sensory input. Although the process of sensitization may not be a unitary one (because there may be more than one form of sensitization), when the initiating stimulus is terminated, both processes do appear to dissipate in a fairly short time.

Habituation allows the organism to damp the response to nonthreatening stimuli, while sensitization allows the individual to respond more forcefully to a stimulus that is stronger and thus threatens tissue damage. These two processes are valuable in maintaining the organism in its everyday existence. Under normal conditions, the opposing processes of habituation and sensitization function to maintain a balance between overreaction and underreaction to normal stimuli. When the inflammation process occurs, whether it is a minimal or a maximal inflammation, the balances of habituation and sensitization are disrupted. The normal damping effects of habituation are shifted toward the sensitization process. This is caused by the larger and more extreme responses of the peripheral receptors to what would usually be a nonthreatening stimulus. The result is a larger-than-normal motor output to both the visceral and the somatic structures innervated by the affected reflex pathways and, thus, to an overresponse to stimuli. The process disrupts the normal integration of physiologic function.

Once the process of sensitization has begun, often over a few seconds of strong input, a secondary process begins to occur. Sensitization dissipates a few seconds or minutes after the stimulus is gone. A longer-lasting process, termed long-term sensitization, begins to develop in the reflex pathways once sensitization has been in place for several minutes. This process precludes the excitability of the neural pathways from returning to normal for some time, often hours.

The effects of this process can often be seen in laboratory experiments when bursts of stimulation are given followed by an occasional stimulus pulse to test the responsiveness of the reflex system. After initial sensitization and the rapid decrease of reflex excitability after stimulus termination, the response being tracked does not return to its prestimulation baseline but remains a small but significant amount above the base level. This hyperexcitability does not decay for varying amounts of time depending on the time and strength of the stimulus. Unlike sensitization, long-term sensitization is thought to be a postsynaptic event, possibly involving the elaboration of proteins in the postsynaptic neuron that remain active for some time after the initiating event.

Recently, Mantyh et al. (63) have shown dramatic changes in the substance P receptors and even structural reorganization of the dendrites of spinal interneurons after nociceptive input. These changes could be the basis for long-term sensitization. Long-term sensitization involves a different mechanism than the short-term process does and can have effects that far outlast the originating stimulus.

Once a stimulus has acted on a reflex network for a longer time, the results can be even more dramatic. For many years, a process known as spinal fixation has been known but not fully recognized. First shown in anesthetized animals, spinal fixation was manifest as remaining active leg flexion after 3 to 4 hours of limb flexion secondary to a cerebella lesion. The lesion produced disrupted outflow from the postural centers in the cerebellum, resulting in sustained flexion of a leg. When the spinal cord was sectioned immediately after the lesion, the limb dropped to the usual flaccid paralysis of the animal. However, if the spinal cord was allowed to remain intact for 3 to 4 hours after the lesion and then transected, the limb remained flexed to some extent. The explanation was that the strong outflow from the injured cerebellum caused a hyperexcitability to develop in the target interneurons of the cord that remained active after spinal transection and resulted in continued motor activity.

In the mid-1960s, research showed that the minimal time necessary for the fixation of this excitability was approximately 45 minutes. Animals receiving the spinal transection within 35 minutes showed no remaining flexion, but those having 45 minutes between lesion and transection showed remaining flexion (64). This effect has now been shown to occur not only as a result of a cerebella lesion but also with stimulation of the skin of the hind limb, and it has also been shown to occur in either intact or animals with spinal transection (65–67). The change in the spinal reflexes produced by the cerebella lesion was caused not by pain or nociceptive input but by changes in outflow from the postural centers.

This, along with more recent research, shows that changes in the reflex functions can occur with both nociceptive and nonnociceptive input, although nociceptive input produces the changes more quickly than nonnociceptive input does. Reflex excitability changes can be influenced by many factors, including:

Stress prior to stimulation
Length and severity of stimulation
Whether the spinal cord is intact or sectioned

The changes have been traced for 3 days to 3 weeks after only 45 minutes of fairly intense nociceptive stimulation and may last even longer. With intense stimulus input, the effect is seen after as little as 20 minutes of stimulation (68). Obviously, strong input, especially nociceptive in nature, can have rapid and long-lasting effects on the excitability of reflex circuits. Although the locus of the changes seen in fixation is not yet known, it seems likely that the alterations observed are processes akin to long-term sensitization but which last a much longer time. It appears that the fixation process is also dependent on the elaboration of proteins in the postsynaptic cells and that it would affect the responsiveness of those cells not only to the original input but also to all input to the cell.

Another line of evidence of long-lasting increases in reflex excitability comes from studies of peripheral inflammation that show that there are peripheral effects of inflammation on afferent input and receptive fields. Continued afferent input from peripheral inflammation produces dramatic changes in the responsiveness of spinal interneurons. Interneurons on which afferent fibers from affected nociceptors synapse begin to respond much more easily to input from a variety of sources, such as touch, pressure, and even the movement of distant muscles. These dramatic changes in excitability also last for long periods (days and weeks) and develop during the initial inflammatory episode (69,70).

Knowing something about the mechanisms of the changes may allow us to restore more normal function. Dubner, Ruda, and Gold (71,72) summarized a series of intracellular changes that are linked to the excitability alterations seen with the inflammation process. The cells activated by nociceptive input from inflamed peripheral structures begin to show enhanced activation of specific parts of the postsynaptic cell membrane called *N*-methyl *D*-aspartate receptors. When these receptors become more active, the excitability of the cell is increased. If cellular activation continues even longer, changes in the activity of genes within the neuron are seen. A class of genes called intermediate-early genes, c-fos, and c-jun, become more active, causing increased dynorphin release within the cell. Dynorphin is a substance that causes increased cell excitation. With more of it being produced, the cell is then held in a hyperexcitable state. Wolpaw (73) provided strong evidence that excitability increases and decreases can be produced not only by nociceptive input to the spinal circuits, but also by nonnociceptive input. In Wolpaw's studies, both increased and decreased spinal reflex excitability were produced by long-term input that was nonnociceptive. Thus, it is beginning to appear that spinal circuits can be altered rapidly by nociceptive input, and more slowly by nonnociceptive input.

Other studies have begun to show that a fourth type of spinal circuit excitability alteration can occur. With heightened excitability over several days, a process begins to occur in the interneuron cell body that finally destroys the cell. Although both inhibitory and excitatory interneurons should theoretically be affected by this process, it appears that inhibitory interneurons are affected primarily (74). Thus, after the long-term excitability increases of the fixation type are established, continued activation of the pathways may result in the loss of inhibitory interneurons. This is certainly an almost permanent event. However, it is apparently not the end of the story. In some cases where inhibitory interneurons have been lost, there may be new excitatory synapses actually formed to replace the lost inhibitory synapses (75). These two additional processes would further shift the balance of excitation in the spinal cord toward enhanced excitability, perhaps permanently.

We have outlined four steps that have been shown to occur in the spinal cord reflex circuitry to alter the excitability of those pathways:

Sensitization
Long-term sensitization
Fixation
Loss of inhibitory interneurons/new excitatory synapse formation

These four overlapping and progressive stages in spinal excitability alterations are underlain by different neural processes, ranging from simple synaptic transmission alterations to complex changes in the genetic function of the cell. With increased understanding of the underlying processes involved, it may be possible to find ways to stop or even reverse them and, hence, re-establish normal excitability in an affected region. In addition, the restoration of normal input to an affected spinal area would have an ameliorative effect on the function. However, at present, little is known about how to reverse the effects of these excitability alterations.

These four steps are a progression from short-term to long-term and even permanent alterations of spinal excitability. It seems almost certain that these steps underlie the changes recorded by Denslow et al. (53) and interpreted by Korr (7) as the facilitated segment. They saw these alterations as having widespread and often grave consequences for the patient. Although they had no way to understand the basis of the facilitated segment at that time, they rightly viewed these alterations in function as a real threat to the health and function of the patient. An area of spinal reflex pathways that are either temporarily or permanently in a state of increased excitability would respond to all input in an exaggerated way, with the result that the organs or tissues innervated by those areas of the spinal cord would receive exaggerated neural drive. Thus, the affected tissues, somatic or visceral, would be driven to respond in a fashion that was not in harmony with the rest of the body. Over time, this increased drive on the tissues would be expected to take a toll on the functional ability of the tissues and could result in premature breakdown or loss of normal function.

It is also evident that areas of increased spinal excitability would respond to central commands in an inappropriate way. This could be the reason why some people respond to stress with heart palpitations while others respond with gastric distress. The abnormally excitable area of the cord would be the one to respond with abnormal drive onto the innervated tissues, resulting in clinical manifestations not seen in other tissues. Thus, a clinical problem may be the result of a long-standing facilitated area of the spinal cord.

In addition to spinal circuit changes, it is now becoming apparent that nociceptive input may cause changes in the brainstem and even in the cortical areas that could account for many of the usual symptoms seen with chronic pain. Indeed, there is evidence that in the prefrontal cortex, cortical neurons analogous to the spinal inhibitory interneurons may be destroyed with some types of pain input (76). The probable result of these changes in the brainstem and even cortex that may be analogous to those seen in the spinal cord will be to alter the ability of the system to respond to environmental stress, and may predispose to disease, altered immune function, and depressive states.

Thus, the spinal excitability alterations first seen by Denslow and Korr seem to be underlain by a series of progressively longer-lasting spinal circuit alterations that result in altered outflow to central brain areas and to both somatic and visceral tissues innervated by that area. As noted above, the restoration of normal input to the area from somatic and visceral tissues would almost surely help normalize the function of the affected areas in all but extreme cases. The restoration of normal tissue function by manipulative procedures would be expected to help restore normal function in the spinal circuits. Thus, given an altered reflex network, that area can no longer respond in concert with other networks, producing diminished functional integration, and beginning the loss of health associated with disease.

NONIMPULSE-BASED INTEGRATION

Neurons not only convey impulses throughout the body to integrate function, but there is also a steady stream of material flowing from the neural cell body out the axon and dendrites (anterograde flow) as well as a flow of materials from the periphery of the nerve back to the cell body (retrograde flow). These flows are called axoplasmic flow. Anterograde flow transports materials from where they are manufactured in the cell body down a complex microtubular structure within the axon. Materials to supply rebuilding of the axon walls, to resupply the transmitter substances, and so forth are carried on this system. The most common clinical effects of the loss of this transport system can be seen when neural contact is withdrawn from an end organ, such as when a muscle is denervated by cutting its motor nerve (a relatively common occurrence). Not only does the muscle cease to contract, but unless the nerve regrows again to contact the muscle, the muscle fibers eventually lose their ability to contract. They change their structure to that of noncontractile connective tissue. Likewise, if an end organ is damaged, its nerve supply often retracts and the synapses are lost. The end organ supplies something to the nerve that allows the synapses to remain viable.

A great deal of study has been done on the uptake of substances supplied by the end organ to nerve terminals. A family of substances known as nerve growth factor (NGF) is essential to continued nerve contact with an end organ and for continued viability of contacts between nerves higher up the chain. If the end organ does not supply NGF, the synaptic contact is lost.

This factor is also essential in development, allowing appropriate nerves to reach and establish contact with the appropriate end organs. Loss of appropriate NGF causes deterioration of the nerve and its contacts. NGF is elaborated in the end organ and taken up by the presynaptic membranes, where it is transported up the axon to the cell body (retrograde transport). There, it regulates the function of the nerve and the nerve's ability to maintain synaptic contacts. Many other substances can be taken up and transported to the cell body, but not all of them are helpful to nerve function. The tetanus toxin, tetanospasmin, is made in peripheral structures after infection by the Clostridium tetani bacterium. The toxin is taken up by nerve terminals and transported to the CNS, where it affects neural function, causing the clinical signs of tetanus.

Many common nerve-tracing techniques rely on the ability of the neuron to take up substances and transport them from the periphery of the nerve to the cell body. For example, horseradish peroxidase is used as a nerve tracer by injecting it into the area of nerve terminals, where it is taken into the cell and transported up the axon, eventually filling the cell body and even dendrites. A fixative can then be used to turn the horseradish peroxidase a dark brown-black, providing an easily visualized portrait of the cell. Many other dyes and materials are commonly used in this way to visualize nerve cells.

Although much is known about the NGF family and some other substances and about the actual transport mechanisms within the axon, less is known about the delivery of substances to end organs through transport from cell body to axon (anterograde flow), such as what is delivered to keep a muscle functional. In 1967, Korr et al. (77) published the results of a study that showed that amino acids placed on the cell bodies of the hypoglossal nucleus on the floor of the fourth ventricle were incorporated into the cell body and transported down the axon to the tongue muscle, where they were delivered into the muscle fibers. Later work showed that not only was the material transported but it was also transported at several different rates of flow. That study and others since have shown that flow rates within an axon vary from as slow as 0.5 mm/d to as fast as 400 mm/d. The observed rates are (78):

Slow (0.52 mm/d)
Medium (25 mm/d)
Fast (up to 400 mm/d)
Very fast (up to 2,000 mm/d)

While his work on transynatic flow of proteins was at first not taken seriously, in 1971, Grafstein (79), previously one of Korr's most vocal critics, published data supporting protein transport across synapses in the optic system. There is currently much data supporting both anterograde and retrograde transport of materials across synapses throughout the nervous system (80–83).

Although much of the anterogradely transported materials are related to support of the neuron and synaptic functions (such as supply of neurotransmitter components), materials delivered by the nerve to its end organ are necessary for either its function or continued existence (84).

Thus, the nervous system is not only the network for rapid communications within the body, but it also serves as a vast network for a far slower two-way communication between the central nervous structures and every part of the body. Disruption of this slow transport of materials has consequences for continued function that may not be immediately evident but that range from subtle to disastrous. Complete withdrawal of NGF or of the materials delivered by the nerve to its end organ may result in loss of function. Disturbance of the flow of materials in either direction results in less than optimal function of the organs involved (85).

Many questions remain about the two-way communication of axoplasmic flow. What substances are being delivered? How necessary are they? What do the materials transported from the periphery to the nerve cell bodies do to the function of the cell or of the entire CNS? Are there crucial times for delivery of nerve factors to end organs for proper development? However these questions are answered, it is important to recognize the vast integrating nature of the nonimpulse-based transport systems of the nervous system and the importance of proper function of this system.

Many things have been shown to affect the material flow within the nerve cells. Even small pressure on axons can impede proper axoplasmic flow. A sustained increased number of impulses carried by the neuron (as in those originating in facilitated areas of the cord) may decrease flow rates. Improper supplies of nutrients and oxygen to the cell body or axon alter the flow. The occurrence of the tissue tensions and fluid flow disturbances often associated with somatic dysfunctions can be factors in altering axoplasmic flows. The somatic dysfunctions treated with the use of manipulation would be expected to have a positive effect on the flow of materials in axons of the area and, hence, to improve body function and integration.

CONCLUSION

In the normal, integrative function of the nervous system, a great number of influences obviously act on any neural pathway. Afferent input activates reflex outflow. Descending activities from higher nervous centers modulate excitability of interneurons. Ascending influences from lower spinal areas increase or decrease activity. Psychological effects are played out on all levels of the neuraxis. The nerves deliver the materials necessary for normal function to their end organs, while the end organs send the substances necessary for continued synaptic viability to the nerves.

These influences come together to determine the moment-to-moment excitability of any area of the CNS and to determine overall outflow to both somatic and visceral structures. If all of these influences are working in harmony, optimally integrated function can be expected from the various organs. If, however, one area is in a hyperexcitable state, the output from that area of the system will not be in harmony with the output of the other areas. In that case, the optimal function is disrupted and the individual becomes increasingly prone to loss of function and disease.

The long-term alterations in spinal reflex excitability (now well demonstrated by various studies) seem almost certain to underlie the alterations demonstrated by Denslow and his colleagues.

These breaks in the normal integration of the nervous system were shown to affect both visceral and somatic structures. The interaction between visceral and somatic input in the spinal cord provides the basis for that common effect. The changes shown in response to nociceptive input can easily account for the long-lasting nature of the facilitation identified in those studies. The facilitation was hypothesized by Korr to be the basis for the somatic dysfunctions long recognized by the osteopathic profession.

Because the neurons involved in the altered excitability are interneurons (the neurons on which a variety of different pathways synapse), the data also support the effects of excitability changes on both somatic and autonomic outflow. The inputs from both visceral and somatic structures end on common interneurons. When the excitability of those interneurons is altered, the outflow to all structures innervated by motoneurons to which those interneurons connect is affected.

The reflex networks of the nervous system are not at all static, genetically determined entities. They are a vast network of highly interconnected pathways that are continually changing to meet local needs and to maintain integration of function. These processes allow the delicate moment-to-moment integration that characterizes optimal functional capacity. The integration, however, can be turned against the very system it serves. When abnormal or very strong input occurs, the result can be a long-term disruption of the normal excitatory/inhibitory balances and a shift to excessive excitability (or in some cases, to excessive inhibition). The result, in either case, is the loss of functional integration and a decrease in functional capacity of the individual.

There are many factors that influence the total function of the individual, including their:

  Accumulated effects of life
  Habits
  Living environment
  Food
  Psychological and spiritual makeup and state

The role of the state of the nervous system is but one of the factors influencing the total health of the person. Because it affects all organs and structures with which it communicates, an area of central excitation or facilitation delivers the effects of all other stressors on the individual to the end organs. In essence, it is the final common factor in communicating with the end organ. Most of the other stressors in life are difficult to change, and the osteopathic physician has little impact on or control over them. However, the physician can directly affect the course of the facilitation and its effects by recognizing that it occurs and by using modalities, especially manipulative treatment, that alter it.

Rational therapy dictates the normalization of afferent input as quickly as possible. In chronic situations, use methods to reduce the abnormal input to allow the body to restore normal balances of excitation and inhibition as fully as possible. In this way, the goal of total osteopathic treatment, to optimize each individual's function and to restore the individual's dynamic functional balance of optimal health, can be brought closer to reality.

REFERENCES

1. Still AT. *Autobiography of A. T. Still*. Kirksville, MO: Published by the author, 1897.
2. Watkins LR, Maier SF. The pain of being sick: implications of immune-to-brain communication for understanding pain. *Annu Rev Psychol* 2000;51:29–57.
3. Watkins LR, Maier SF. Implications of immune-to-brain communication for sickness and pain. *Proc Natl Acad Sci USA* 1999;96(14):7710–7713.

4. Northup GW, ed. *Osteopathic Research: Growth and Development*. Chicago, IL: American Osteopathic Association, 1987.

5. Cole WV. The osteopathic lesion syndrome. In: *American Academy of Osteopathy Yearbook*. Indianapolis, IN: American Academy of Osteopathic Medicine, 1951:149–178.

6. Denslow JS. *The Early Years of Research at the Kirksville College of Osteopathic Medicine*. Kirksville, MO: Kirksville College of Osteopathic Medicine Press, 1982.

7. Korr IM. The neural basis of the osteopathic lesion. *J Am Osteopath Assoc* 1947;46:191–198.

8. Sherrington CS. *The Integrative Action of the Nervous System*. New Haven, CT: Yale University Press, 1905.

9. Wurster RD. Program control of circulatory behavior. *Behav Brain Sci* 1986;9:305.

10. Eble JN. Patterns of response of the paravertebral musculature to visceral stimuli. *Am J Physiol* 1960;198:429–433.

11. Sato A. Reflex modulation of visceral functions by somatic afferent activity. In: Patterson MM, Howell JN, eds. *The Central Connection: Somatovisceral/Viscerosomatic Interaction*. Indianapolis, IN: American Academy of Osteopathic Medicine, 1992;53–72.

12. Rexed B. The cytoarchitectonic organization of the spinal cord in the cat. *J Comp Neurol* 1952;96:415–495.

13. DeGroat WC. Spinal cord processing of visceral and somatic nociceptive input. In: Patterson MM, Howell JN, eds. *The Central Connection: Somatovisceral/Viscerosomatic Interaction*. Indianapolis, IN: American Academy of Osteopathic Medicine, 1992;47–71.

14. Cervero R, Foreman RD. Sensory innervation of the viscera. In: Loewy AD, Spyer KM, eds. *Central Regulation of Autonomic Functions*. New York, NY: Oxford University Press, 1990.

15. Cervero F. Visceral and spinal components of viscero-somatic interactions. In: Patterson MM, Howell JN, eds. *The Central Connection: Somatovisceral/Viscerosomatic Interaction*. Indianapolis, IN: American Academy of Osteopathic Medicine, 1992;77–85.

16. Sato A. The somatosympathetic reflexes: their physiological and clinical significance. In: Goldstein M, ed. *The Research Status of Manipulative Therapy*. Bethesda, MD: National Institutes of Health, 1975:163–172.

17. Hill JM, Adreani CM, Kaufman MP. Muscle reflex stimulates sympathetic postganglionic efferents innervating *triceps surae* muscles of cats. *Am J Physiol* 1996;271(1 pt 2):H38–H43.

18. Kang Y, Kenney M, Spratt K, et al. Somatosympathetic reflexes from the low back in the anesthetized cat. *J Neurophysiol* 2003;90(4):2548–2559.

19. Jou JC, Farber JP, Qin C, et al. Afferent pathways for cardiac-somatic motor reflexes in rats. *Am J Physiol Regul Integr Comp Physiol* 2001;281: R2096–R2102.

20. Goehler LE, Gaykema RP, Hansen MK, et al. Vagal immune-to-brain communication: a visceral chemosensory pathway. *Auton Neurosci* 2000; 85(1–3):49–59.

21. Goehler LE. Vagal complexity: substrate for body-mind connections? *Bratisl Lek Listy* 2006;107(8):275–276.

22. Maier SF, Goehler LE, Fleshner M, et al. The role of the vagus nerve in cytokine-to-brain communication. *Ann N Y Acad Sci* 1998;840:289–300.

23. Hopkins D, Armour J. Localization of sympathetic postganglionic and parasympathetic preganglionic neurons which innervate different regions of the dog heart. *J Comp Neurol* 1984;229:186–198.

24. Norris J, Foreman R, Wurster R. Responses of the canine heart to stimulation of the first five ventral thoracic roots. *Am J Physiol* 1974;227:912.

25. Wurster R, Randall W. Cardiovascular responses to bladder distension in patients with spinal transection. *Am J Physiol* 1975;228:1288–1292.

26. Wurster R. Spinal sympathetic control of the heart. In: Randall WC, ed. *Neural Regulation of the Heart*. New York, NY: Oxford University Press, 1976:157–186.

27. Chung K, Chung J, LaVelle F, et al. The anatomical localization of descending pressor pathways in the cat spinal cord. *Neurosci Lett* 1979;15:71–75.

28. Barman S, Wurster R. Visceromotor organization within descending spinal sympathetic pathways. *Circ Res* 1975;37:209–214.

29. Geis G, Kozelka J, Wurster R. Organization and reflex control of vagal cardiomotor neurons. *J Auton Nerv Syst* 1981;5:63–73.

30. Geis G, Wurster R. Horseradish peroxidase localization of cardiac vagal preganglionic somata. *Brain Res Brain Res Rev* 1980;182:1930.

31. Geis G, Wurster R. Cardiac responses during stimulation of dorsal motor nucleus and nucleus ambiguus in the cat. *Circ Res* 1980;46:606–611.

32. Kalia M, Mesulam M. Brainstem projections of sensory and motor components of the vagus complex in the cat. II: Laryngeal, tracheobronchial, pulmonary, cardiac, and gastrointestinal branches. *J Comp Neurol* 1980;193:467–508.

33. Hopkins D, Armour J. Medullary cells of origin of physiologically identified cardiac nerves in the dog. *Brain Res Bull* 1982;8:359–365.

34. Beacham W, Perl E. Background and reflex discharge of sympathetic preganglionic neurons in the spinal cat. *J Physiol* 1964;172:400–416.

35. Beacham W, Perl E. Characteristics of a spinal sympathetic reflex. *J Physiol* 1964;173:431–448.

36. Eble JN. Patterns of response of the paravertebral musculature to visceral stimuli. *Am J Physiol* 1960;198(2):429–433.

37. Schoen RE, Finn WE. A model for studying a viscerosomatic reflex induced by myocardial infarction in the cat. *J Am Osteopath Assoc* 1978;78(1): 122–123.

38. Amour J. Activity of in situ stellate ganglion neurons of dogs recorded extracellularly. *Can J Physiol Pharmacol* 1986;64:101–111.

39. Amour J. Activity of in situ middle cervical ganglion neurons in dogs, using extracellular recording techniques. *Can J Physiol Pharmacol* 1985;63: 704–716.

40. Boznjak Z, Kampine J. Intracellular recordings from the stellate ganglion of the cat. *J Physiol* 1982;324:273–283.

41. Gagliardi M, Randall W, Bieger D, et al. Activity of in vivo canine cardiac plexus neurons. *Am J Physiol* 1988;255:789–800.

42. Terui N, Koizumi K. Responses of cardiac vagus and sympathetic nerve to excitation of somatic and visceral nerves. *J Auton Nerv Syst* 1984;10: 73–91.

43. O'Toole M, Wurster R, Phillips J, et al. Parallel baroreceptor control of sinoatrial rate and atrioventricular conduction. *Am J Physiol* 1984;246:H149–H153.

44. Koizumi K, Brooks C. The integration of autonomic system reactions: discussion of autonomic reflexes, their control and their association with somatic reactions. *Ergeb Physiol Biol Chem Exp Pharmakol* 1972;67:168.

45. Sato A, Schmidt R. Somatosympathetic reflexes: Afferent fibers, central pathways, discharge characteristics. *Physiol Rev* 1973;53:916–947.

46. Barman S, Wurster R. Interaction of descending sympathetic pathways and afferent nerves. *Am J Physiol* 1978;234:H223–H229.

47. Geis G, Wurster R. Localization of ascending inotropic and chronotropic pathways in the cat. *Circ Res* 1981;49:711–717.

48. Kozelka J, Christy G, Wurster R. Somato-autonomic reflexes in anesthetized and unanesthetized dogs. *J Auton Nerv Syst* 1982;5:63–70.

49. Kozelka J, Chung J, Wurster R. Ascending spinal pathways mediating somato-cardiovascular reflexes. *J Auton Nerv Syst* 1981;3:171–175.

50. Chung J, Webber C, Wurster R. Ascending spinal pathways for the somatosympathetic A and C reflex. *Am J Physiol* 1979;237:H342–H347.

51. Chung J, Wurster R. Neurophysiological evidence for spatial summation in the CNS from unmyelinated afferent fibers. *Brain Res* 1978;153:596–601.

52. Te Poorten BA. Spinal palpatory diagnosis of visceral disease. *Osteopath Ann* 1979:52–53.

53. Denslow JS, Korr IM, Krems AD. Quantitative studies of chronic facilitation in human motoneuron pools. *Am J Physiol* 1947;105(2):229–238.

54. Denslow JS. The central excitatory state associated with postural abnormalities. *J Neurophysiol* 1942;5(5):393–402.

55. Denslow JS. An analysis of the variability of spinal reflex thresholds. *J Neurophysiol* 1944;7(July):207–215.

56. Korr IM, Thomas PE, Wright HM. Patterns of electrical skin resistance in man. *J Neural Transm* 1958;17:77–96.

57. Wright HM. Local and regional variations in cutaneous vasomotor tone of the human trunk. *J Neural Transm* 1960;22:34–52.

58. Schmidt RF. Neurophysiological mechanisms of arthritic pain. In: Patterson MM, Howell JN, eds. *The Central Connection: Somatovisceral/Viscerosomatic Interaction*. Indianapolis, IN: American Academy of Osteopathic Medicine, 1992:130–151.

59. Schmidt RF. Nociception and pain. In: Schmidt RF, Thews G, eds. *Human Physiology*. Heidelberg, Germany: Springer-Verlag, 1987.

60. Payan DG. Peripheral neuropeptides, inflammation, and nociception. In: Willard FH, Patterson MM, eds. *Nociception and the Neuroendocrine-Immune*

Connection. Indianapolis, IN: American Academy of Osteopathic Medicine, 1994:34–42.

61. Groves P, Thompson R. Habituation: a dual-process theory. *Psychol Rev* 1970;77(5):419–450.

62. Kandel ER, Brunelli M, Byrne J, et al. A common presynaptic locus for the synaptic changes underlying short-term habituation and sensitization of the gill-withdrawal reflex in aplysia. *Cold Spring Harbor Symposium on Quantitative Biology.* 1977;40:465–482.

63. Mantyh PW, DeMaster E, Malhotra A, et al. Receptor endocytosis and dendrite reshaping in spinal neurons after somatosensory stimulation. *Science* 1995;268:1629–1632.

64. Chamberlain TJ, Halick P, Gerard RW. Fixation of experience in the rat spinal cord. *J Neurophysiol* 1963;26:662–673.

65. Steinmetz JE, Cervenka J, Robinson C, et al. Fixation of spinal reflexes in rats by central and peripheral sensory input *J Comp Psychol* 1981;95:548–555.

66. Steinmetz JE, Patterson MM. Fixation of spinal reflex alterations in spinal rats by sensory nerve stimulation. *Behav Neurosci* 1985;99(1):97–108.

67. Patterson MM, Steinmetz JE. Long-lasting alterations of spinal reflexes: A potential basis for somatic dysfunction. *J Am Osteopath Assoc* 1986;2:38–42.

68. Patterson MM. Spinal fixation: long-term alterations in spinal reflex excitability. In: Patterson MM, Grau JW, eds. *Spinal Cord Plasticity: Alterations in Reflex Function.* Boston, MA: Kluwer Academic Publishers, 2001:77–100.

69. Willis WD. Mechanisms of central sensitization of nociceptive dorsal horn neurons. In: Patterson MM, Grau JW, eds. *Spinal Cord Plasticity: Alterations in Reflex Function.* Boston, MA: Kluwer Academic Publishers, 2001:127–162.

70. Coderre TJ. Noxious stimulus-induced plasticity in spinal cord dorsal horn: Evidence and insights on mechanisms obtained using the formalin test. In: Patterson MM, Grau JW, eds. *Spinal Cord Plasticity: Alterations in Reflex Function.* Boston, MA: Kluwer Academic Publishers, 2001:163–184.

71. Dubner R, Ruda MA. Activity-dependent neuronal plasticity following tissue injury and inflammation. *Trends Neurosci* 1992;15(3):96–103.

72. Dubner R, Gold M. The neurobiology of pain. *Proc Natl Acad Sci USA* 1999;96(July):7627–7630.

73. Wolpaw JR. Spinal cord plasticity in the acquisition of a simple motor. In: Patterson MM, Grau JW, eds. *Spinal Cord Plasticity: Alterations in Reflex Function.* Boston, MA: Kluwer Academic Publishers, 2001:101–126.

74. Mayer DJ, Mao J, Holt J, et al. Cellular mechanisms of neuropathic pain, morphine tolerance, and their interactions. *Proc Natl Acad Sci USA* 1999;96(July):7731–7736.

75. Woolf CJ, Saler MW. Neuronal plasticity: Increasing the gain in pain. *Science* 2000;288:1765–1768.

76. Grachev ID, Fredrickson BE, Apkarian AV. Abnormal brain chemistry in chronic back pain: An in vivo proton magnetic resonance spectroscopy study. *Pain* 2000;89(1):7–18.

77. Korr IM, Wilkinson PN, Chornock FW. Axonal delivery of neuroplasmic components to muscle cells. *Science* 1967;155(760):342–345.

78. Korr IM, ed. *The Neurobiologic Mechanisms in Manipulative Therapy.* New York, NY: Plenum Publishing, 1978.

79. Grafstein B. Transneuronal transfer of radioactivity in the central nervous system. *Science* 1971;172(979):177–179.

80. Schwab ME, Thoenen H. Retrograde axonal and transsynaptic transport of macromolecules: physiological and pathophysiological importance. *Agents Actions* 1977;7(3):361–368.

81. Regalado MP, Terry-Lorenzo RT, Waites CL, et al. Transsynaptic signaling by postsynaptic synapse-associated protein 97. *J Neurosci* 2006;26(8):2343–2357.

82. Vizzard MA, Brisson M, de Groat WC. Transneuronal labeling of neurons in the adult rat central nervous system following inoculation of pseudorabies virus into the colon. *Cell Tissue Res* 2000;299(1):9–26.

83. Banati RB. Brain plasticity and microglia: is transsynaptic glial activation in the thalamus after limb denervation linked to cortical plasticity and central sensitisation? *J Physiol Paris* 2002;96(3–4):289–299.

84. Korr IM. The spinal cord as organizer of disease process: axonal transport and neurotrophic function in relation to somatic dysfunction. *J Am Osteopath Assoc* 1981;80(7):451–459.

85. De Vos KJ, Grierson AJ, Ackerley S, et al. Role of axonal transport in neurodegenerative diseases. *Annu Rev Neurosci* 2008;31:151–173.

10

Autonomic Nervous System

FRANK H. WILLARD

KEY CONCEPTS

- The two components of the peripheral nervous system are somatic and autonomic.
- The somatic component provides innervation of the skeletal muscle; while the influence of autonomic portion, representing the predominant component, is seen on almost all other tissues in body.
- Organization of the autonomic nervous system is similar to the somatic nervous system, including the following roles: receiving afferent fibers, processing information in central circuits, and forming output to connective tissue cells, smooth muscle cells, secretory cells, and immune cells.
- The distinctive feature of the autonomic nervous system is the two-step output pathway involving centrally located preganglionic neurons and peripherally located ganglionic neurons.
- There are two anatomically, biochemically, and functionally distinct divisions of the peripheral autonomic nervous system: sympathetic and parasympathetic, with dual effects on many organ systems.
- Innervation of the visceral organs occurs through the great autonomic plexus that extends from the base of neck through the thorax, diaphragm, and abdomen and terminates in the pelvis.
- The great autonomic plexus is supplied with parasympathetic fibers from the vagus and pelvic splanchnic nerves and sympathetic fibers from the thoracic, lumbar, and sacral splanchnic nerves.
- The central origin and importance of sympathetic and parasympathetic innervation for organ systems in the head, neck, thorax, abdomen, and pelvis.
- The origin and importance of sympathetic innervation for the peripheral vasculature.
- The primary afferent innervation of organ systems is instrumental in controlling the output of the autonomic nervous system.
- Neuropeptide markers in afferent nerve fibers and small-caliber, primary afferent fibers involved with detection of nociceptive stimuli.

Our daily existence depends on the coordinated activities of our internal organ systems. A major factor in orchestrating the diverse functions of these internal structures is the autonomic nervous system. Through an extensive network of connections, the autonomic nervous system helps maintain the normal rhythm of activity in the visceral organs, adjusting their output to accommodate any external challenge. The limbic structures of the brain control the autonomic nervous system through the hypothalamus. The hypothalamus itself is closely integrated into a complex network involving the endocrine and immune systems. This conglomerate of interlocking systems, with its pervasive influence on our physiology and psychology, is called the neuroendocrine-immune network.

The terminology used to describe the part of the nervous system usually not under voluntary control varies widely. Since the 18th century, different terms have been used by researchers in different countries. None of these terms refers to the exact same group of structures or functions. Examples include:

Vegitive nervensystem
Grand symapathique
Ganglionic nervous system
Visceral nervous system

The two most commonly used terms are vegetative and autonomic nervous system. For a thorough discussion of the history of terminology concerning this system, see Clarke and Jacyna (1). The present chapter uses the term autonomic nervous system to refer to all components of the nervous system using preganglionic and ganglionic neurons as an efferent pathway. This definition excludes

only the neuromuscular junctions between the ventral horn of the spinal cord (and a few cranial nuclei) and the skeletal muscle.

The clinical importance of understanding the circuits of the autonomic nervous system cannot be overstated. Almost all communication between neurons in these circuits occurs via synaptic transmission. This process depends on the production, distribution, and recognition of specific neurochemicals. Most pharmaceutical agents, either as a desired first action or as an undesired side effect, affect these metabolic and stereologic events. Knowledge of nervous system structure, function, and chemistry is a necessity for the educated use of these substances and the intelligent approach to the maintenance of health.

The autonomic nervous system is sensitive to events occurring in somatic tissue such as cutaneous and musculoskeletal systems. The autonomic and somatic nervous systems are interlocked through numerous somatovisceral and viscerosomatic reflexes. Visceral symptoms may be the primary manifestations of somatic dysfunction and vice versa. This chapter examines the organization of the autonomic nervous system and its afferent component and emphasizes the pattern of innervation reaching the major organs of the thoracoabdominopelvic viscera and the segmental representation of these organs in the spinal cord.

ORGANIZATION OF THE AUTONOMIC NERVOUS SYSTEM

The autonomic nervous system has components in both the central and the peripheral nervous systems (PNS) (Fig. 10.1).

The major autonomic components of the central nervous system (CNS) include:

> Limbic forebrain
> Hypothalamus
> Several brainstem nuclei
> Intermediolateral cell column of the spinal cord

The autonomic components of the PNS include numerous ganglia (collections of neuron cell bodies located outside of the CNS) and a network of fibers distributed to all tissues of the body with the exception of the hyaline cartilages, the centers of the intervertebral disks, and the parenchymal tissues of the CNS. This review focuses on the peripheral distribution of the autonomic nervous system.

Peripheral Nervous Systems

The axons from neurons located in the CNS enter the periphery through spinal and cranial nerves. The peripheral portion of the nervous system can be divided into two fundamental parts based on the target structures of efferent fibers. Axons derived from the somatic component of the PNS innervate skeletal muscle. Axons derived from the autonomic component of the PNS enter the periphery and form complex interwoven plexuses containing clusters of cell bodies called ganglia. Neurons in these ganglia innervate all other targets, including:

> Smooth muscle
> Cardiac muscle
> Glands
> Connective tissue
> Cells in the immune system

This fundamental division in the PNS also reflects differential methods in cellular communication. The mechanism of transmission in the neuromuscular junction of the somatic system involves ionotrophic principles (2). This mechanism uses the ion-gated channels to quickly depolarize the cell membrane, a process referred to as fast transmission. Conversely, chemical signaling in the autonomic PNS uses metabotrophic principles and volume transmission (3), the diffusion of transmitter substance away from axonal vesicles, as well as fast synaptic transmission. The metabotrophic methods of signaling usually involve a neuromodulator that binds to a membrane receptor, activating second-messenger pathways within the target cell. These methods are also called slow transmission and often lead to altered gene expression. To further understand the distinction between somatic and visceral PNSs, compare the typical neural circuitry present in reflex arcs.

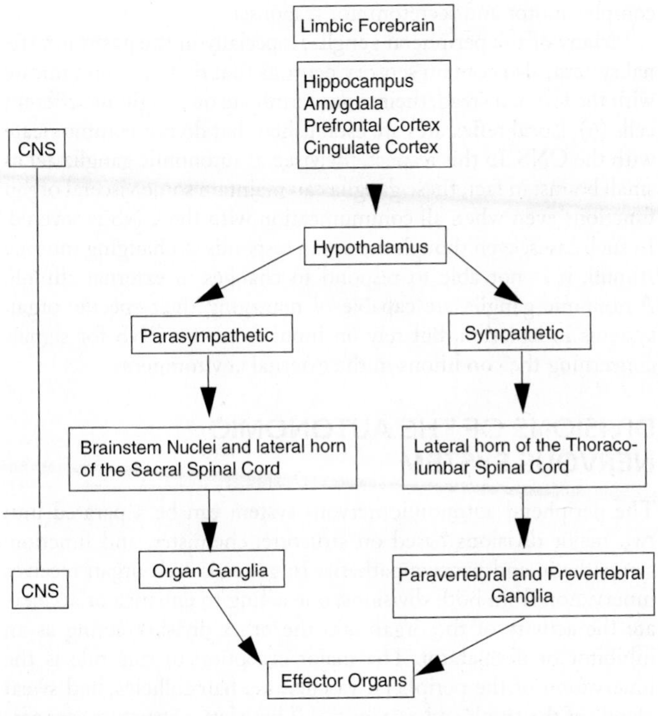

SOMATIC REFLEX ARC

Input and output for the peripheral somatic nervous system occur through spinal and cranial nerves. Figure 10.2 diagrams a typical spinal nerve, illustrating the basic circuitry of the somatic reflex arc. In its simplest form, the reflex arc contains a primary afferent neuron in a ganglion and a centrally located motor neuron connected by a synaptic junction. Because only one synapse separates the input from the output, this circuit is called a monosynaptic reflex. The cell body of the primary sensory neuron is located in the dorsal root ganglia or in the peripheral ganglia of a cranial nerve. The peripheral process of the sensory neuron is directed outward along a spinal or cranial nerve to reach its target in the peripheral tissue. This process either acts as a receptor end organ itself or is attached to one located in skin, muscle, or connective tissue. Each sensory neuron also has a central process (axon) that extends into the dorsal horn of the spinal cord or into the brainstem.

Two fundamental types of primary afferent neurons are present in sensory ganglia. One class of sensory neuron features a large cell body with a myelinated process; this kind of cell forms the A-afferent or large-caliber fiber system and is involved in proprioception or discriminative mechanoreception (4). Conversely, other sensory neurons have small cell bodies, with lightly myelinated or unmyelinated processes. These cells form the B-afferent or small-caliber fiber system and are involved in crude touch and nociception (4) (see Chapters 7 and 8 for additional discussion of this concept).

Figure 10-1 General organization of the autonomic nervous system.

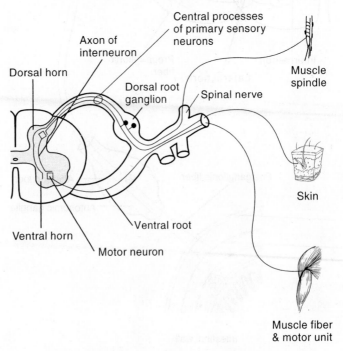

Figure 10-2 Components of somatic reflex arc.

The second component of the monosynaptic reflex arc, the motor neuron, has a cell body in the ventral horn of the spinal cord or a brainstem nucleus. Motor neuron axons leave the CNS in the ventral root of a spinal nerve or in a cranial nerve, eventually innervating its effector organ, skeletal muscle, through a neuromuscular synaptic junction. These monosynaptic reflex connections occur between the largest sensory neurons (the A-afferent system) and ventral horn motor neurons innervating skeletal muscle.

All other somatic reflexes involve the presence of interneurons situated between the central processes of the sensory neuron and the motoneurons; several synaptic connections must be traversed to complete the arc. Such circuits are called disynaptic or polysynaptic reflex arcs. The polysynaptic reflexes involve input from both A-afferent and B-afferent systems. Although the addition of interneurons into the circuit slows the conduction of information through these reflex arcs, it greatly facilitates the construction of more complex circuits and, consequently, more complicated behavior patterns in response to sensory information.

AUTONOMIC REFLEX ARC

Input and output for the peripheral autonomic nervous system occur via spinal, cranial, and splanchnic (visceral) nerves. Figure 10.3

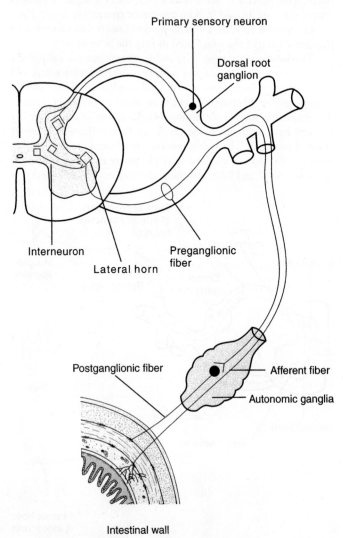

Primary sensory neuron

Dorsal root ganglion

Interneuron

Lateral horn

Preganglionic fiber

Postganglionic fiber

Afferent fiber

Autonomic ganglia

Intestinal wall

Figure 10-3 Components of visceral reflex arc.

is a diagram of a typical spinal nerve and its connections with a splanchnic nerve. The afferent neuron has a peripheral process ending in a visceral organ or a blood vessel, a cell body located in the dorsal root ganglia, and a central process that terminates in the dorsal horn of spinal cord. This central process terminates on interneurons that, in turn, innervate the effector (motor or pseudomotor) neurons in the gray matter of the spinal cord or brainstem. The effector or preganglionic neurons are found in the lateral horn of the spinal cord or in specific brainstem nuclei; their myelinated preganglionic axons terminate on ganglionic neurons located outside the CNS. These peripheral neurons are found either in encapsulated ganglia in the fascia of the body wall or in ganglia embedded in the fascia surrounding a specific organ. Unmyelinated, postganglionic axons travel from peripheral ganglia to cellular targets in visceral organs. The presence of two sequential neurons in the output pathway is a critical feature distinguishing the autonomic from somatic PNSs. The sensory neurons of these two systems are otherwise very similar in morphology and function.

Ganglionic neurons of the autonomic system are found primarily in three locations (Fig. 10.4):

1. The paravertebral ganglia or sympathetic trunk lying along the side of the spinal cord.
2. The prevertebral ganglia or collateral ganglia scattered in several clusters associated with the large vessels of the abdominal cavity.
3. In isolated ganglia or hypogastric ganglia embedded in the adventitial tissue of specific visceral organs of the pelvis.

These ganglia contain a variety of chemically differentiated neurons producing numerous neuroregulators. The ratio between pre- and postganglionic neurons has been reported to range from 1:2 to 1:196 for sympathetic ganglia and 1:1 to 1:6,000 for parasympathetic ganglia (5). This arrangement of a few central neurons influencing effector organs through a large battery of chemically distinct, postganglionic neurons is divergent in nature. As such, it allows for a limited number of input channels to initiate numerous, complex motor and secretomotor responses.

Many of the peripheral ganglia, especially in the gastrointestinal system, also contain sensory neurons that do not communicate with the CNS; instead, their axons terminate on ganglionic efferent cells (6). Local reflex arcs are established that do not communicate with the CNS. In this respect, the visceral autonomic ganglia act as small brains; in fact, these ganglia can maintain some visceral organ functions even when all communication with the CNS is severed. In such cases, even though the organ responds to changing internal stimuli, it is not able to respond to changes in external stimuli. Autonomic ganglia are capable of managing their specific organ systems in isolation, but rely on input from the CNS for signals concerning the conditions in the external environment.

DIVISIONS OF THE AUTONOMIC NERVOUS SYSTEM

The peripheral autonomic nervous system can be separated into two major divisions based on structure, chemistry, and function: sympathetic and parasympathetic. In general, each organ receives innervation from both divisions, one acting to enhance or accelerate the activity of the organ and the other division acting as an inhibitor or decelerator. The major exception to this rule is the innervation of the peripheral vasculature, hair follicles, and sweat glands of the trunk and extremities. These latter structures are serviced solely by the sympathetic system. However, in this situation, cholinergic fibers arising in the sympathetic ganglia are involved in at least hair follicle and sweat gland innervation, if not the peripheral vasculature (7). These fibers have been termed the sympathetic cholinergic system. The distribution of the sympathetic nervous system is illustrated in Figure 10.4 and that of the parasympathetic nervous system in Figure 10.5.

A morphologic distinction between sympathetic and parasympathetic systems is seen in the arrangement of their ganglia. In general, the ganglionic neurons of the sympathetic nervous system are located in the paravertebral and prevertebral ganglia with the exception of scattered ganglia found in the hypogastric plexus of the pelvis. Those of the parasympathetic nervous system are found in ganglia located on either cranial nerves or organ walls. The preganglionic axons of the sympathetic system tend to be short, reaching only to the paravertebral and prevertebral ganglia, and the postganglionic axons, which reach to the visceral organs, are longer. The situation is reversed in the parasympathetic system where the preganglionic axons tend to be long (extending all the way to the ganglia in the organ wall) and the postganglionic axons

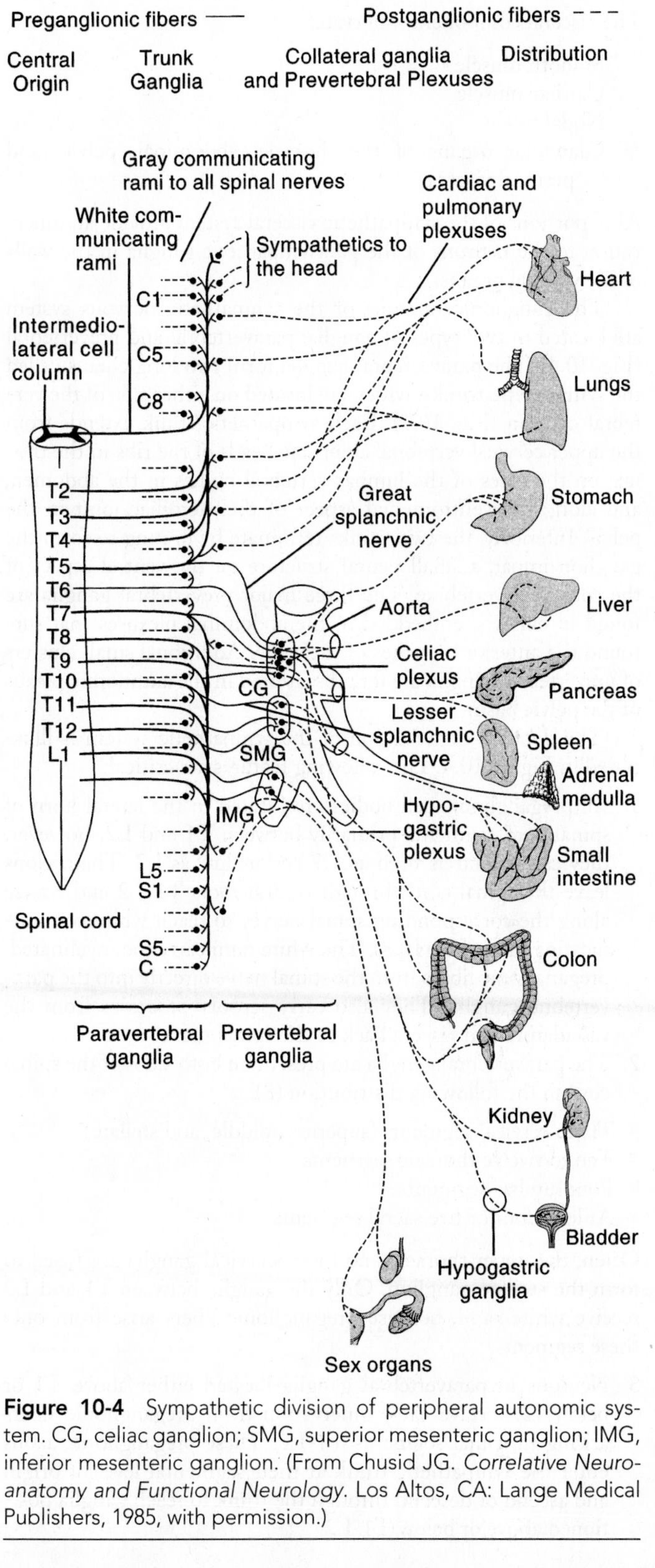

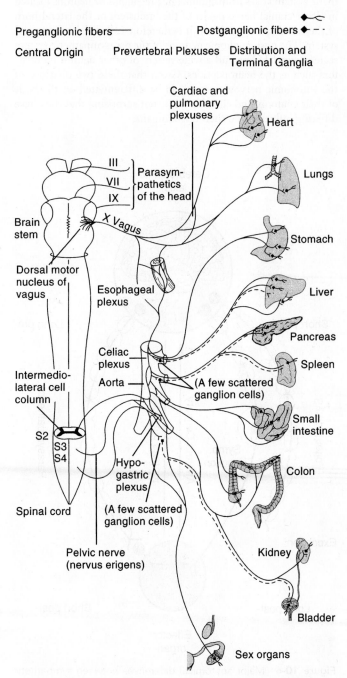

Figure 10-4 Sympathetic division of peripheral autonomic system. CG, celiac ganglion; SMG, superior mesenteric ganglion; IMG, inferior mesenteric ganglion. (From Chusid JG. *Correlative Neuroanatomy and Functional Neurology.* Los Altos, CA: Lange Medical Publishers, 1985, with permission.)

Figure 10-5 Parasympathetic division of peripheral autonomic system. (From Chusid JG. *Correlative Neuroanatomy and Functional Neurology.* Los Altos, CA: Lange Medical Publishers, 1985, with permission.)

tend to be short (confined to a distribution along the organ wall) (Fig. 10.6).

This distinction between the major divisions of the autonomic nervous system is further reflected in their chemistry. The sympathetic system arises from cholinergic preganglionic neurons located in the lateral horn of the thoracic and lumbar spinal cord; it is also called the thoracolumbar system. In general, the postganglionic neurons of the sympathetic system are adrenergic and secrete norepinephrine. However, there are important exceptions. For example, some cholinergic ganglionic neurons contribute to the innervation of the hair follicles and sweat glands as well as possibly innervating the vasculature in skeletal muscle (7). The parasympathetic system arises from cholinergic preganglionic neurons located in either cranial nerve nuclei of the brainstem or the lateral horn of the sacral spinal cord, and it is therefore called the craniosacral system. The postganglionic neurons of the parasympathetic system secrete acetylcholine and a wide variety of other neuron modulators such as the neuropeptides. Given that these two divisions of the autonomic nervous system can be differentiated on the basis of their anatomy and chemistry, it is not surprising that they have differing influences on their target organs.

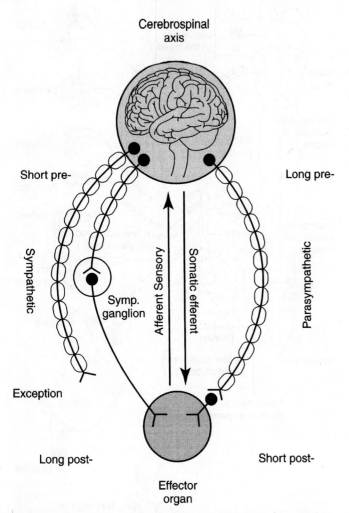

Figure 10-6 Major anatomical differences between sympathetic and parasympathetic divisions of autonomic system. (From Harati Y. Anatomy of the spinal and peripheral autonomic nervous system. In: Low PA, ed. *Clinical Autonomic Disorders*. Boston, MA: Little, Brown and Company, 1993, with permission.)

Sympathetic Autonomic Nervous System

The sympathetic autonomic nervous system has two major components: vascular and visceral. The vascular component is associated with the spinal nerves and innervates:

Fascia
Smooth muscle of vasculature
Smooth muscle of hair follicles
Secretory cells in the sweat glands of the skin

The visceral component innervates:

Smooth muscle
Cardiac muscle
Nodal tissue
Glandular organs of the thoracic, abdominal, pelvic, and perineal viscera

Also, portions of the sympathetic visceral system provide an innervation to the neurons of the parasympathetic ganglia in the walls of the visceral organs.

The ganglionic neurons of the sympathetic nervous system are located in two types of ganglia: paravertebral and prevertebral (Fig. 10.4). The paravertebral ganglia form two long chains called the sympathetic trunks, which are located on either side of the vertebral column (Fig. 10.7). Each sympathetic trunk extends from the upper cervical vertebrae along the heads of the ribs in the thorax, on the sides of the lumbar vertebral bodies in the abdomen, and along the ventromedial aspect of the sacroiliac joint in the pelvis. Inferiorly, the two trunks terminate by uniting to form the ganglion impar, a small neural structure on the ventral aspect of the coccygeal vertebrae. The three major prevertebral ganglia are found in clusters, embedded in the abdominal plexuses that surround the anterior branches of the aorta. Additional small clusters of prevertebral ganglia are found scattered in the autonomic plexus of the pelvic basin.

The detailed organization of the sympathetic system is illustrated in Figure 10.4. The following features are critical:

1. All preganglionic cell bodies are located in the lateral horn of spinal cord segments primarily between T1 and L2; however, they can extend as high as C7 and as low as L3. Their axons leave the spinal cord through ventral roots T1-L2 and course along the corresponding spinal nerves to reach white communicating rami (Fig. 10.8). The white rami carry the myelinated, preganglionic fibers from the spinal nerve directly into the paravertebral ganglia. They also carry sensory processes from the vasculature and viscera back to the spinal nerve.

2. The paravertebral ganglia are present on both sides of the spinal cord in the following distribution (8):

■ Three cervical segments (superior, middle, and stellate)
■ Ten to twelve thoracic segments
■ Four lumbar segments
■ At least four or five sacral segments

Often, the upper thoracic and lower cervical ganglia are fused to form the stellate ganglion. Only the ganglia between T1 and L2 receive white rami, because preganglionic fibers arise from only these segments.

3. Neurons in paravertebral ganglia located either above T1 or below L2 receive their innervation from preganglionic fibers arising in spinal segments T1-L2. These preganglionic axons enter the sympathetic trunk at their segmental level of origin and ascend or descend through the trunk to reach ganglia positioned above or below T1-L2.

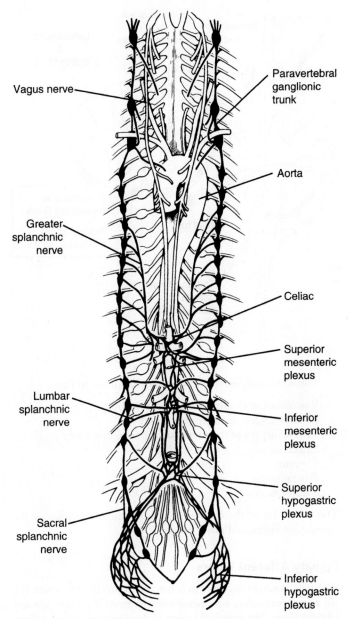

Vagus nerve

Paravertebral
ganglionic
trunk

Aorta

Greater
splanchnic
nerve

Celiac

Superior
mesenteric
plexus

Lumbar
splanchnic
nerve

Inferior
mesenteric
plexus

Superior
hypogastric
plexus

Sacral
splanchnic
nerve

Inferior
hypogastric
plexus

Figure 10-7 Paravertebral ganglia (sympathetic trunk) lying along median axis of body. (From Rohen JW, Yokochi C. *Color Atlas of Anatomy.* New York, NY: Igaku-Shoin Medical Publishers, 1983, with permission.)

4. Ganglionic neurons destined to innervate blood vessels, smooth muscles, and glands of the skin are found in all the paravertebral ganglia. Their postganglionic axons gain access to spinal nerves by passing over gray rami (Fig. 10.8). All paravertebral ganglia give rise to gray rami; each spinal nerve receives at least one gray ramus. The postganglionic axons follow the spinal nerves distally before shifting to assume a position in the fascia along the wall of a blood vessel.

5. Ganglionic neurons with axons innervating thoracic, abdominal, and pelvic viscera are found in the three cervical ganglia, the upper five thoracic paravertebral ganglia, and the prevertebral ganglia. These are the celiac and the superior and inferior mesenteric ganglia, as well as small scattered ganglia in the pelvic plexus. These prevertebral ganglia receive their preganglionic axons through thoracic, lumbar, and sacral splanchnic nerves.

The term splanchnic refers to the viscera; splanchnic nerves are simply visceral nerves. Thoracic, lumbar, and sacral splanchnic nerves carry sympathetic fibers and pelvic splanchnic nerves carry parasympathetic fibers.

The sympathetic ganglia receive information from the CNS through the axons of the preganglionic neurons. A preganglionic axon of the sympathetic system has a number of options after passing through a white ramus between T1 and L2 to enter a paravertebral ganglion:

1. It can innervate a ganglionic neuron in the paravertebral ganglion at its spinal cord level of entry.
2. It can pass either up or down in the sympathetic trunk to innervate ganglionic neurons located at levels not serviced by white rami.
3. It can proceed through the paravertebral ganglia without forming synaptic contacts, join a thoracic, lumbar, or sacral splanchnic nerve, and subsequently innervate neurons in one of the retroperitoneal prevertebral ganglia.

These options are diagrammed in Figure 10.8, which illustrates a typical thoracic spinal segment and its accompanying spinal nerve and paravertebral ganglia. The significance of these innervation patterns is further considered as the innervation of specific organs is examined.

Parasympathetic Autonomic Nervous System

The parasympathetic autonomic nervous system, unlike its sympathetic counterpart, innervates only visceral organs and blood vessels in the:

Head and neck
Thorax
Abdomen
Pelvis

The parasympathetic nervous system lacks a division innervating the peripheral vasculature of the extremities and trunk. It is divided into two portions: cranial and sacral. These are based on the location of its preganglionic neurons (Figs. 10.5 and 10.9). The cranial portion consists of several brainstem nuclei and their preganglionic nerves. Cranial nerves III, VII, and IX give rise to parasympathetic preganglionic fibers that innervate ganglia located in the:

Orbit (ciliary ganglion)
Sphenopalatine fossa (sphenopalatine ganglion)
Inferior temporal fossa (otic ganglion)
Floor of the mouth (submandibular and sublingual ganglia)

Cranial nerve X, the vagus nerve, innervates ganglia in the organs of the cervical, thoracic, and superior portions of the abdominal viscera.

The vagus nerve is a significant source of parasympathetic innervation to the thoracic and upper abdominal viscera. It enters the thoracic cavity along the upper portion of the mediastinal wall and passes posterior to the root of the lung to gain a position on the walls of the esophagus. Vagal branches are given off to the cardiac and pulmonary plexuses and to the esophageal plexus. Through the upper portion of the vagus, the nucleus ambiguus of the medulla contributes innervation to the pharynx, larynx, and skeletal muscle portion of the upper esophagus. Preganglionic vagal fibers from the dorsal motor nucleus of the medulla terminate in ganglia on the walls of each organ beginning in the upper esophagus and extending to the splenic flexure of the colon. From these ganglia,

Figure 10-8 Neuronal circuitry present in typical peripheral thoracic spinal segment. (From Harati Y. Anatomy of the spinal and peripheral autonomic nervous system. In: Low PA, ed. *Clinical Autonomic Disorders*. Boston, MA: Little, Brown and Company, 1993, with permission.)

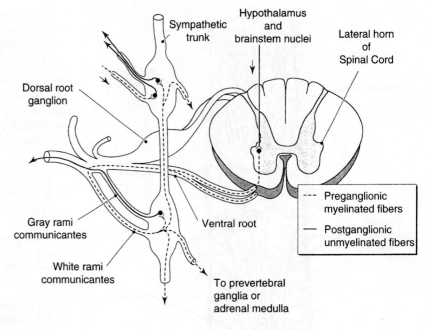

postganglionic fibers arise and course in and around the smooth muscle layers and glands of the organ. The left and right trunks of the vagus rotate around the esophagus (due to the fetal rotation of the gut), forming the anterior and posterior trunks of the vagus, respectively. At the distal end of the esophagus, these two trunks slip through the esophageal hiatus of the diaphragm riding in the fatty adventitial fascia of the esophageal walls. Although the identity of the vagus nerve is lost as its axons join the celiac plexus, its preganglionic fibers continue in the celiac and superior mesenteric plexus eventually reaching the full extent of these two corresponding neurovascular territories. The vagal preganglionic axons reach only as far inferiorly as the splenic flexure of the colon.

The lower portion of the gastrointestinal tract located distal to the splenic flexure, as well as the pelvic viscera, receives their parasympathetic innervation from the pelvic splanchnic nerves. These latter nerves form the sacral component of the parasympathetic nervous system. The preganglionic neurons are located in the lateral horn of spinal cord segments S2-S4. Their axons exit the spinal cord by traveling in the sacral nerve roots. As these roots pass through the endopelvic fascia, small pelvic splanchnic nerves branch off. These branches quickly join the inferior hypogastric plexus (pelvic plexus), which is also located in the endopelvic fascia. Through this plexus, the preganglionic axons can reach the visceral organs of the pelvic basin such as the urinary bladder, the internal reproductive organs, and the rectum. By ascending along the hypogastric plexus, these axons also enter the inferior mesenteric plexus of the abdomen. From the inferior mesenteric plexus, these preganglionic axons follow the vascular branches of the inferior mesenteric artery to service structures such as the descending and sigmoid colon. The preganglionic axons of the vagus and of the pelvic splanchnic nerves terminate in ganglia located in the walls of the abdominopelvic viscera. Short, postganglionic axons invade the organ to terminate in layers of smooth muscle and in surrounding glands. The pattern of parasympathetic innervation of the visceral organs continues in an uninterrupted manner through the abdominopelvic cavity even though the source of this innervation shifts from cranial origins to sacral origins at the splenic flexure of the large bowel.

The autonomic nervous system provides input to the:

Vasculature and fascias throughout the body
Visceral organs of the head and neck
Visceral organs of the thoracoabdominopelvic cavity
Spleen
Thymus
Bone marrow
Lymph modes

The remainder of the chapter focuses on the innervation of the vasculature, fascia, and major organs.

Primary Afferent Fibers

The autonomic nervous system is not strictly an efferent system (9). All nerves containing autonomic efferent axons also carry primary afferent fibers. The principal targets of these primary afferent fibers are the:

Dorsal horn of the spinal cord from approximately T1-L2 and S2-4
Solitary nucleus of the vagal complex in the medulla

Although the majority of primary afferent fibers in autonomic nerves are of the small-caliber variety (B-afferent system), a few larger, myelinated fibers are also present (A-afferent system). In general, the input over visceral afferent fibers to the medullary brainstem involves the non-noxious regulation of organ function. Conversely, many of the primary afferent fibers targeting the spinal cord have the characteristics of nociceptive fibers. They produce neuropeptides such as substance-P and calcitonin gene–related polypeptide and respond to nociceptive stimuli. In addition, some are capable of eliciting a neurogenic inflammatory response in the surrounding tissue (10,11). Nociceptive input from these fibers to the spinal cord can facilitate spinal segments. This initiates vasomotor changes and alters the output to somatic musculature (viscerosomatic reflexes) and refers pain to the somatic structures (12,13). (The relationship of the visceral afferent fibers to viscerosomatic reflexes is reviewed elsewhere in this text.)

REGIONAL DISTRIBUTION OF THE AUTONOMIC NERVOUS SYSTEM

Trunk and Limbs

Peripheral Vasculature

The vascular tree is divided into four different types of vessels based on their distinctive functions (14):

1. Conduit vessels comprise the arterial system prior to arterioles.
2. Resistance vessels represent arterioles.
3. Exchange vessels are capillaries.
4. Capacitance vessels consist of veins.

Most aspects of the vascular tree receive an innervation that controls the resistance of these vessels to blood flow (7,14,15). Different types of axons in these vascular nerves can be identified by their neurochemistry. Sensory fibers, coursing in the vascular nerves, typically contain neuropeptides such as substance-P and calcitonin gene–related polypeptide. Efferent axons in the peripheral autonomic nerves can be (14):

> Adrenergic
> Cholinergic
> Histaminergic
> Purinergic

In general, the adrenergic fibers function as constrictors, contracting smooth muscle in the tunica media and increasing the resistance in the peripheral vasculature. These norepinephrine-containing fibers arise from the paravertebral ganglia of the sympathetic nervous system and innervate all vasculature of the body. Cholinergic fibers are much fewer in number in most tissue and are vasodilating in nature. These nerves are of mixed origin, and most often arise from the parasympathetic ganglia innervating the vasculature in the head and neck and the visceral organs of the thorax, abdomen, and pelvis. Cholinergic vasodilator fibers, innervating blood vessels in the extremities, arise in the sympathetic trunk of some mammals; however, the importance of this system is in humans is not known (16). Purinergic and histaminergic axons also mediate relaxation of vascular wall smooth muscle, but their origin and role in vasodilation are not clear (14).

The sympathetic innervation of blood vessels in muscle and skin is accomplished by preganglionic neurons located in the lateral horn of spinal segments T2 through L2-L3. Their axons leave the spinal cord in the ventral roots and pass through white rami to innervate neurons located in the paravertebral ganglia (Fig. 10.8). Vasomotor neurons present in the paravertebral ganglia give rise to axons that leave the ganglia over the gray rami to rejoin the spinal nerves. In this way, they reach the somatic peripheral tissue where they innervate blood vessels, sweat glands, and hair follicles. A topographic map of the vasculature in the body is contained within paravertebral ganglia such that (17,18):

1. The vasomotor fibers to the head and neck come from spinal segments T1-T4. Their axons travel superiorly in the sympathetic trunk to reach the cervical ganglia. Postganglionic axons follow the carotid vascular tree to reach the head and neck. Segments T1-T2 provide innervation for the brain and meninges; T2-T4 provides innervation to the vasculature of the face and neck.
2. The vasomotor fibers to the upper extremity come from spinal segments T5-T7. Their axons course superiorly in the sympathetic trunk to reach the upper thoracic and lower cervical ganglia. Postganglionic axons join the spinal nerves of the brachial plexus to reach the vasculature of the upper extremity.
3. The vasomotor fibers to the lower extremity come from spinal segments T10 through L2-L3. Their axons descend in the sympathetic trunk to reach the lower lumbar and sacral ganglia. Postganglionic axons join the spinal nerves of the lumbosacral plexus to reach the vasculature of the lower extremity.

Sympathetic fibers course along the outer border of the tunica media of the artery and secrete their neuroregulators into the extracellular fluids surrounding the vascular smooth muscle. Most sympathetic fibers release norepinephrine from small swellings along the terminal distribution of the axon. This neuromodulator interacts with its specific receptors on the vascular smooth muscle cell membranes. Both α- and β-adrenergic receptors are present on these plasma membranes (19). Activation of α-adrenoceptors leads to contraction of the smooth muscle cells and vasoconstriction, while activation of the β-adrenoceptors mediates relaxation of the muscle cell, resulting in vasodilatation. In general, the α-adrenoceptors predominate on the smooth muscle of resistance vessels; therefore, adrenergic stimulation yields vasoconstriction in skeletal muscle.

Additional control of skeletal muscle resistance arteries is accomplished through numerous endothelium-derived substances such as the vasodilator nitric oxide or the vasoconstrictors prostacyclin, endothelin, and angiotensin (20). The tone in the vessel wall is the product of a complex interaction of these vasoactive substances (21). Neurally mediated, active vasodilation of cutaneous capillary bed is well established in the literature (16). Sympathetic cholinergic fibers do not appear to innervate the cutaneous vascular tree; instead, a nonadrenergic, noncholinergic vasodilatory mechanism exists for these vessels (22). Neurally mediated, active vasodilation of skeletal muscle vascular beds appears to be doubtful and has recently been questioned (16).

Along with the efferent innervation of the vascular tree, afferent or sensory fibers also course in the walls of the blood vessels. Little is known of the sensory feedback to the spinal cord provided by these fibers. The nomenclature of these afferent fibers is confusing because it is not clear whether they are somatic or visceral afferent fibers. Jinkins et al. (23) have termed the vascular afferent fibers found in somatic tissue somatosympathetic fibers because they course through somatic tissue but are related to the autonomic nervous system. However, because these afferent fibers are generally small caliber and contain an array of neuropeptides such as substance-P, much of the information they carry is most likely related to nociceptive stimuli. The normal, baseline release of neuropeptides such as substance-P from these fibers may play an important role in maintaining vascular tone (24). Thus, the small-caliber, primary afferent fibers appear to have additional homeostatic functions in the peripheral tissue beyond that of nociception.

When irritated, some of these small-caliber, sensory axons can secrete quantities of substance-P (a proinflammatory, vasodilatory neuropeptide) into the surrounding tissue. This release of an inflammatory agent from a peripheral nerve terminal is involved in initiating the processes of neurogenic inflammation and edema (25). Neurogenic inflammation is a critical component in inflammatory joint disease, which suggests an important role for the small-caliber, primary afferent fibers in these diseases (26).

An interaction between sensory axons and sympathetic neurons appears to occur in the peripheral tissues. Sympathetic adrenergic terminals often end in close association with the peripheral processes of sensory neurons. Secretion of norepinephrine can increase the levels of prostaglandins E_2 and I_2 in the tissue (27). Prostaglandins are irritating to many small-caliber, primary afferent fibers. Sufficient sympathetic discharge therefore can result in a nociceptive input to the spinal cord. In addition, evidence strongly suggests that small-caliber, primary afferent fibers can become sensitized to sympathetic nervous system activity (27). This interaction between sympathetic efferent axons and primary afferent neurons is a possible mechanism for sympathetically dependent hyperalgesia such as that present in reflex sympathetic dystrophy (28).

Sweat Glands and Connective Tissue

Along with innervating the vasculature, the peripheral autonomic fibers also provide an innervation to sweat glands and fascia. Sweat glands receive an exclusively cholinergic innervation from the sympathetic trunk ganglia; these fibers are termed the sympathetic cholinergic system (15). The cholinergic fibers stimulate secretory activity in the gland.

Small-caliber, neuropeptide-containing, primary afferent fibers innervate all forms of connective tissue. These fibers often course in close association with adrenergic sympathetic axons and blood vessels. A close relationship between these fibers and the connective tissue components of the fascia is seen in such tissue as the:

Cranial dura (29,30)
Gastrointestinal tract (31)
Synovium of diarthrodial joints (32)

In several locations, such as joints, these fibers have been demonstrated to play a role in modulating the cellular components (mast cells) of the connective tissue and to contribute to the maintenance of tissue integrity (32,33). Finally, the interaction of these two fiber types appears to play an important role in the maintenance of normal vascular tone in connective tissue (24).

Head and Neck

The autonomic innervation of the head and neck arises from two general sources: sympathetic and parasympathetic. The sympathetic innervation originates in the intermediolateral nucleus of the upper thoracic segments (T1-T4) of the spinal cord, and their ganglionic neurons are located in the cervical sympathetic ganglia of the neck. Postganglionic fibers from the superior cervical ganglion enter the head following the course of the carotid and vertebral arteries and the jugular vein. The parasympathetic innervation originates from several nuclei in the brainstem, and the ganglionic neurons are located in these ganglia (Fig. 10.9):

Ciliary sphenopalatine
Otic
Geniculate

Recently, additional parasympathetic ganglia located on the walls of the internal carotid artery have been described (34–36). The autonomic innervation of the cranial viscera, the function of these nerves, and the neurology of their dysfunction are amply described elsewhere (17,37–40).

The third cranial nerve contains parasympathetic axons that arise in the Edinger-Westphal nucleus of the midbrain and innervate the ciliary ganglion of the eye (Fig. 10.9). These axons are responsible for constricting the pupil through the pupillary sphincter muscles and contracting the ciliary body to thicken the lens in the accommodation reflex. The facial (VII) cranial nerve carries parasympathetic preganglionic axons from the superior salivatory and lacrimal nuclei in the pontine region of the brainstem. These secretomotor and vasomotor axons course along the superficial petrosal nerve to reach the sphenopalatine ganglion. Postganglionic axons follow branches of the trigeminal nerve to reach the lacrimal gland and mucosal glands of the nasal and oral cavities. Preganglionic axons from the superior salivatory nucleus also follow

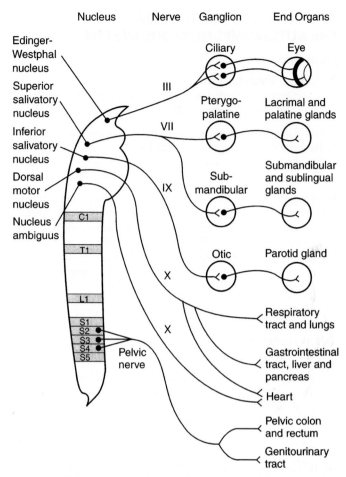

Figure 10-9 Summary of parasympathetic nervous system emphasizing distribution of cranial nerves III, VII, IX, and X. (From Barron KD, Chokroverty S. Anatomy of the autonomic nervous system: brain and brainstem. In: Low PA, ed. *Clinical Autonomic Disorders.* Boston, MA: Little, Brown and Company, 1993, with permission.)

the chorda tympani, a branch of the facial nerve, to reach the submandibular and sublingual ganglia. Postganglionic axons from these ganglia supply the salivary glands on the floor of the mouth. The glossopharyngeal nerve carries secretomotor and vasomotor axons from the inferior salivatory nucleus located at the pontomedullary border to the otic ganglion. These latter axons pass over the lesser petrosal nerve. Postganglionic axons from the otic ganglion extend to the parotid gland over branches of the third division of the trigeminal nerve.

Cranial nerve X, the vagus, is the largest of the parasympathetic nerves. It supplies preganglionic parasympathetic innervation of the viscera in the thorax and abdomen to the level of the splenic flexure in the transverse colon. Efferent vagal axons arise in the dorsal motor nucleus and nucleus ambiguous of the medulla. The vagus is largely a sensory nerve; afferent fibers outnumber efferent fibers in the mammalian vagus by more than 10:1 (41). These sensory fibers include the afferent innervation of the thoracoabdominal viscera and the general sensory innervation of the:

Pharynx
Larynx
Skin of the ear
External auditory meatus
External surface of the tympanic membrane

The cell bodies for these afferent fibers are located in the two nuclei of the vagus: the superior (jugular) ganglion and the inferior ganglion. Their central brainstem targets include the nucleus solitarius, nucleus ambiguous, and spinal trigeminal nucleus.

An area of much recent interest is the autonomic innervation of the vascular and dural systems in the head. Preganglionic sympathetic input to the cranial vasculature and dura arises in the upper thoracic spinal segments. Those controlling the vasculature of the brain and meninges are located in segments T1-2, and those involved with the vasculature of the face and neck are located in T2-T4 (17). Ganglionic neurons are located in the superior cervical sympathetic ganglion and in small ganglia embedded in the fibers of the internal carotid nerve (18). Their axons course along the carotid arteries; those going to the cerebral vessels and dura form the well-developed internal carotid nerve. Within the dura, the adrenergic fibers diverge away from the vasculature to form a dense plexus within the connective tissue substrate of the dura itself (30). The extensive autonomic innervation may play a role in regulating the metabolic activity of the dural tissue. The sympathetic innervation of the dura and associated vasculature is of interest due to its proposed role in the cause of migraine headache (42).

Parasympathetic axons innervating the cerebral vasculature arise in these ganglia: sphenopalatine, otic, and internal carotid (36,43–45). Axons from the ganglia contain acetylcholine and neuropeptides such as vasoactive intestinal polypeptide and neuropeptide-Y, among others (35,46). The axons form a delicate plexus wrapped around cerebral arteries as they travel through the subarachnoid space. Primary afferent fibers containing neuropeptides such as substance-P and calcitonin gene–related polypeptide are also present in the plexus surrounding the cerebral vessels. These fibers arise in the ophthalmic and maxillary divisions of the trigeminal ganglion (47) and constitute the "trigeminovascular system" (48). Similar primary afferent fibers containing substance-P and calcitonin gene–related polypeptide have been described in the dura mater (30). Some of these fibers form free endings and are postulated to have trophic relationships with the connective tissue cells in the dura such as the fibroblast and mast cells. Release of these proinflammatory peptides has been indicated in the pathogenesis of certain inflammatory headaches such as the migraine and cluster varieties (49,50).

Thorax

A large autonomic plexus of fibers extends from the superior mediastinum inferiorly through the posterior mediastinum and continues into the abdominopelvic cavity, using the esophageal hiatus of the diaphragm as a conduit (Fig. 10.10). In total, this complex arrangement of fibers is best termed the thoracic plexus, although it has several regionally named components. The thoracic plexus is derived from the vagus nerve and its branches and from splanchnic branches from the paravertebral ganglia. The thoracic plexus is located near the midline and divided approximately into two parts: superior and inferior. Superiorly, this complex arrangement of fibers contains the interwoven cardiac and pulmonary plexuses that are distributed around the great vessels of the heart and the large airways. Inferiorly, it contains the esophageal plexus wrapped around the esophagus as it courses through the posterior mediastinum. Figure 10.11 is a schematic diagram illustrating the thoracic plexus. Branches from this autonomic plexus in the thorax supply the following with afferent and efferent nerves:

Heart
Trachea

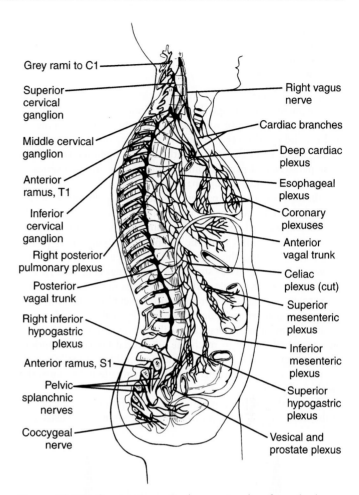

Figure 10-10 Great autonomic plexus extending from the lower cervical region through the thorax and abdomen to reach the pelvis. (From Bannister LH, Berry MM, Collins P, et al., eds. *Gray's Anatomy.* New York, NY: Churchill Livingstone, 1995, with permission.)

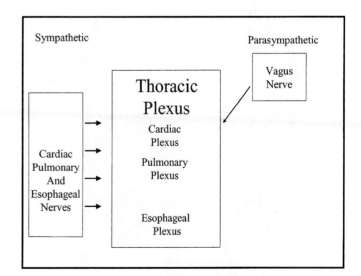

Figure 10-11 A schematic diagram illustrating the thoracic plexus and its associated systems. The thoracic, cardiac, pulmonary, and esophageal nerves are a source of sympathetic postganglionic fibers into the plexus. The vagus nerve is a source of parasympathetic preganglionic fibers to the plexus. Organ ganglia for the parasympathetic system will be found within the parts of the thoracic plexus.

Bronchi
Lungs
Esophagus
Thoracic duct

Sympathetic innervation of the thoracic viscera arises in spinal cord segments T1 through T5 or T6. Axons from these preganglionic neurons synapse with ganglionic neurons in the superior, middle, and inferior cervical ganglia as well as in the sympathetic trunk ganglia T1 to T5-T6. Sympathetic postganglionic axons from these paravertebral ganglia join the thoracic plexus via a series of small, delicate cardiac, pulmonary, and esophageal nerves. Within the thoracic plexus, sympathetic cardiac and pulmonary nerves descend through the superior mediastinum joining with similarly named parasympathetic branches from the vagus and recurrent laryngeal nerves. They form the complex cardiopulmonary plexus of fibers surrounding the great vessels of the heart (Fig. 10.12) and the vasculature and airway structures of the lungs (Fig. 10.13). The individual superior, middle, and inferior cardiac nerves of the sympathetic trunk and vagus are extremely inconsistent in actual form (51). The esophageal sympathetic nerves arise from the thoracic paravertebral ganglia and course diagonally downward across the thoracic vertebral bodies to reach the adventitial fascia surrounding the esophagus in the posterior mediastinum. Here, they join with the main trunks of the vagus nerve (parasympathetic) to form the esophageal plexus.

The mixing of parasympathetic and sympathetic axons begins in the most superior aspect of the thoracic autonomic plexus as it extends upward into the cervical region. Scattered communicating branches unite the vagus and recurrent laryngeal nerves with the sympathetic trunk. Therefore, even at the most superior aspect of the plexus, there are no pure sympathetic or parasympathetic nerves. Also, all fibers in the plexus contain a mixture of afferent and efferent axons, so the plexus cannot be considered a purely efferent structure either.

Cardiovascular Plexus

The cardiac plexus represents a region of the thoracic plexus closely related to the innervation of the heart. The cardiac plexus consists of a mixture of sympathetic and parasympathetic fibers (as well as afferent fibers) woven around the great vessels of the heart (Fig. 10.12). Sympathetic input to the cardiac plexus arises from preganglionic neurons located in the nucleus intermediolateralis of the lateral horn of the spinal cord extending from segments T1 to T5. This column of spinal cord neurons contains a topographic map of the heart. The ventricular innervation is represented in the higher thoracic segments, but the atrial representation is found in the lower segments (52). This inverted cardiac map results from the embryologic origin of the heart; the ventricular system forms superior to the atrial system (53). The preganglionic axons of the spinal cord neurons enter the sympathetic trunk by passing over white rami in the upper thoracic segments. Once in the trunk, most of these fibers ascend to reach their ganglionic neurons located primarily in the two to three cervical ganglia. Variable numbers of cervical and thoracic sympathetic cardiac nerves leave the cervical and upper thoracic ganglia, course through the fascia of the mediastinum, and join the cardiac branches of the vagus to form the cardiac plexus. This plexus is primarily located on the walls of the pulmonary arterial tree (54).

The parasympathetic input to the cardiac plexus arises from preganglionic neurons in the dorsal motor nucleus of the vagus and the nucleus ambiguus of the medulla (55,56). These preganglionic axons leave the vagus nerve over its variable (one to three) cardiac branches beginning in the neck and extending into the superior mediastinum. The axons target a parasympathetic ganglion embedded in the cardiac plexuses, termed Wristberg ganglion. Short cholinergic axons from these ganglia reach the sinoatrial (SA) and atrioventricular (AV) nodes and course in the myocardium of the ventricles. The parasympathetic innervation of the ventricular wall is much less dense than that of the sympathetic fibers (57).

From the cardiac plexus, sympathetic adrenergic and parasympathetic cholinergic, postganglionic axons form a rich network of fibers distributed along the coronary vasculature, coursing throughout the myocardium of the atria and ventricles, and reaching the SA and AV nodes (57). The innervation of the intrinsic nodal system of the heart is bilaterally asymmetric; the right side of the plexus favors the SA node but the left side of the plexus tends to target the AV node. Thus, stimulation of the sympathetic fibers on the left side accelerates cardiac output but is arrhythmogenic because it is directed to the AV node (58). A similar reaction is obtained by cooling the right sympathetic fibers, indicating that cardiac activity is influenced by the balance of activity between the two sympathetic inputs (58). Stimulation of the parasympathetic vagal fibers tends to stabilize heart rate. It appears that the balance of tonic neural activity occurring in the vagus and sympathetic systems influences, in part, heart rate and volume output.

Cardiac afferent nerves are an important consideration in understanding reflex control of the heart, patterns of referred cardiac

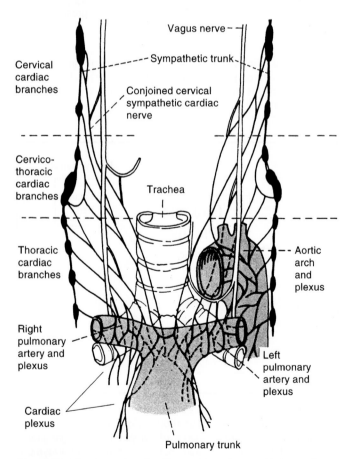

Figure 10-12 Nerve supply of heart. (From Bonica JJ. General considerations of pain in the chest. In: Bonica JJ, ed. *The Management of Pain.* Philadelphia, PA: Lea & Febiger, 1990, with permission.)

(Figure labels:) Vagus nerve; Sympathetic trunk; Cervical cardiac branches; Conjoined cervical sympathetic cardiac nerve; Cervicothoracic cardiac branches; Trachea; Thoracic cardiac branches; Aortic arch and plexus; Right pulmonary artery and plexus; Left pulmonary artery and plexus; Cardiac plexus; Pulmonary trunk

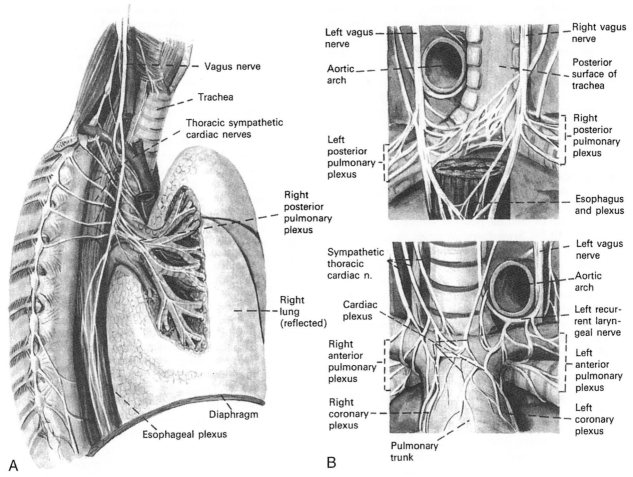

Figure 10-13 Innervation of lung. (From Bonica JJ. General considerations of pain in the chest. In: Bonica JJ, ed. *The Management of Pain*. Philadelphia, PA: Lea & Febiger, 1990:981, with permission.)

pain, and patterns of cardiac-facilitated segments. Small-caliber, primary afferent fibers are distributed throughout the (59–61):

Myocardium
Coronary vasculature
Roots of its great vessel
Parietal pericardium

There are at least two different pathways for these cardiac sensory fibers. Those coursing with the sympathetic nerves have their cell bodies located in dorsal root ganglia extending from C6 to T7, and their central processes terminate in the dorsal horn of the spinal cord (62,63). Sensory axons coursing with the parasympathetic nerves have cell bodies located in the nodose ganglion of the vagus nerve and central processes that terminate in the solitary nucleus of the medulla. In addition to the autonomic nerves supplying an afferent innervation of the pericardium, afferent fibers reach this structure over the phrenic nerve as well. These phrenic afferent fibers enter the spinal cord over segments C3-C5.

Along with the dual origin of sensory nerves, there is a differential distribution of these two sensory pathways in the cardiovascular system. The afferent fibers of the vagus nerve terminate in the (61):

Ascending aorta
Aortic arch
Pulmonary trunk

Arterial walls
Atrial walls
Atrioventricular valve
Ventricular walls

The afferent fibers from the sympathetic nerves reach the (60):

Atrial walls
Pulmonary arteries
Atrioventricular and aortic valves
Parietal peritoneum

Afferent fibers from both systems reach the coronary arteries. Those from the vagus extend to a more distal level of the vasculature closer to the apex of the heart than do afferent fibers associated with the sympathetic nervous system. Both Aδ- and C-afferent fibers are present in the heart (64). Many of these fibers contain neuropeptides such as substance-P or calcitonin gene–related polypeptide that are typical of small-caliber, primary afferent fibers. At least one population of these cardiac C-fibers has the physiologic properties of nociceptive axons.

In general, the afferent fibers coursing with the sympathetic nerves are involved with cardiac nociception, and those following the parasympathetic nerves are mainly involved in reflexogenic regulation of heart functions through their brainstem connection (62). Section of the sympathetic nerves to the heart can relieve cardiac pain in the chest, arms, and neck (65). These cardiac afferent fibers enter the spinal cord over a range of segments from C6 to T7, but the influence of these nerves can extend at least two segments below T7 (66). The signs of segmental facilitation due to cardiac disease can present in the vicinity of the cervicothoracic junction and extend downward through at least T9 (67). Importantly, the nociceptive afferent fibers reaching the dorsal horn of the spinal cord influence neurons with concomitant somatic receptive fields. This viscerosomatic convergence of nociceptive information provides an explanation for the referral of pain from cardiac structures to the body wall and extremity (68).

Respiratory Plexus

The airways of the respiratory system receive their innervation through the large pulmonary plexus that surrounds the pulmonary artery and extends onto the posterior surface of the trachea and bronchi (Fig. 10.13). Sympathetic preganglionic neurons that contribute to this plexus are located in the lateral horn of spinal segments T2-T7, and their ganglionic neurons are located in the cervical and first four thoracic ganglia. Postganglionic axons from these ganglia course through cardiac and esophageal nerves from the sympathetic trunk to reach the pulmonary plexus. These adrenergic axons primarily target the glandular tissue surrounding the bronchi and bronchioles; little direct adrenergic innervation of the bronchial musculature has been noted. β-adrenergic receptors are present on the glandular cells and on bronchial smooth muscle cells. Stimulation of the β-adrenergic, sympathetic nervous system leads to bronchial dilation and the release of a more viscous secretion (69).

The vagus nerve is the source of parasympathetic innervation for the respiratory airways. After entering the thorax, the vagus shifts posteriorly in the mediastinum to pass behind the root of the lung. Anterior and posterior pulmonary branches are given off that contribute to the pulmonary plexus. Parasympathetic ganglia located in the walls of the airways receive preganglionic fibers from these vagal branches. Postganglionic parasympathetic fibers course in the arteriobronchial tree to terminate around bronchial smooth musculature, mucosal glands, and blood vessels. Stimulation of these cholinergic fibers causes (69):

Bronchoconstriction
Hypersecretion of a serous secretion
Vasodilation

The pulmonary plexus and ganglia contain intrinsic neurons, i.e., cells whose processes remain in the peripheral tissue and do not innervate the CNS. Such cells are called interneurons. Some of these cells produce a variety of neuropeptides, among which is vasoactive intestinal polypeptide, a potent bronchodilator (70). In addition, several neuropeptides corelease with norepinephrine from sympathetic terminals and with acetylcholine from parasympathetic terminals. These ubiquitous neuropeptides have recently gained considerable interest due to their role in controlling the diameter of the bronchial lumen and the initiation of bronchial wall inflammation (71).

Small-caliber, primary afferent fibers are also present in the pulmonary plexus. These fibers provide sensory information to the brainstem via the vagus and to the spinal cord via the sympathetic trunk. This information is involved in reflex arcs related to:

Sneezing
Coughing
Bronchospasms
Pulmonary congestion

Many of these fibers, and particularly the smallest of them, contain neuropeptides such as substance-P and calcitonin gene–related polypeptide, among others. Irritation of these sensory fibers results in the release of proinflammatory substances, leading to neurogenic edema and inflammation in the lung. Substance-P, released from these sensory axons into the pulmonary parenchyma, is a potent bronchoconstrictor, vasodilator, and secretagogue (72).

Activation of these primary afferent nociceptors can also facilitate segments in the spinal cord extending from the cervical region into the low thoracic cord (67). The extended range of activation most likely relates to the wide distribution of the central processes of these primary afferent fibers. Changes in spinal cord activity are seen in response to pulmonary afferent stimulation. Electrical stimulation of inflamed tracheobronchial mucosa produces a decrease in electrical skin resistance in the T2-5 dermatomes followed by cutaneous hyperalgesia hours later (65). Unlike the heart, pain from the lungs and bronchial tree is carried in the vagal fibers as well as in the spinal afferent fibers. Lung tumors can refer pain to the skin around the ear (73), which is a region of the head innervated by small cutaneous branches of the vagus nerve. Electrical stimulation of the laryngeal and tracheal mucosa refers pain to the neck, and similar irritation of the bronchial tree refers pain to the anterior chest wall. Section of the vagus nerve below the recurrent laryngeal branch ameliorates the pain (74), suggesting that the nerve is the conduit for this referred pain.

The costal parietal pleura receive an afferent innervation derived from the intercostal nerves of the thorax. The mediastinal pleura are innervated by sensory fibers from the phrenic nerve, and diaphragmatic pleura is innervated by twigs from the intercostal nerves (65). The parietal plural membrane is sensitive to noxious stimuli. The visceral pleura in the lungs receive sympathetic and sensory fibers from the autonomic plexuses surrounding the bronchi, but is insensitive to pain (65).

Esophageal Plexus

The esophagus extends from an upper sphincter region located at the inferior border of the pharynx to a lower sphincter region located at the border of the stomach. Along its route, the body of the esophagus is lodged in the loose connective tissues of the superior and posterior mediastinum.

The upper esophageal sphincter is mainly derived from the cricopharyngeus and thyropharyngeus muscles (together they compose the inferior pharyngeal constrictor), which receive their innervation from the pharyngeal plexus composed of the superior laryngeal and pharyngeal branches of the vagus nerve (75). The body of the esophagus is surrounded by a plexus of autonomic nerves derived from the inferior laryngeal branch of the vagus and esophageal branches of the sympathetic trunk (76). The superior portion of the esophagus is a mixture of skeletal and smooth muscle, although the lower portion is composed of smooth muscle only. The preganglionic parasympathetic innervation to the superior portion of the esophagus (skeletal muscle portion) is derived from the nucleus ambiguous. The smooth muscle of the esophagus is derived primarily from the dorsal motor nucleus of the vagus nerve (77). The left and right vagal trunks approach the esophagus at the root of the lung and form an elaborate plexus, which follows this structure through the esophageal hiatus in the diaphragm. The postganglionic parasympathetic neurons are contained in two intrinsic ganglia in the walls of the esophagus: Auerbach's, or the myenteric plexus; and Meissner's, or the submucosal plexus. Sympathetic preganglionic neurons are located in the intermediolateral nucleus of spinal cord segments ranging from T2 to T8 (78):

Cervical esophageal portion T2-T4
Thoracic esophageal portion T3-T6
Abdominal portion T5-T8

The preganglionic axons synapse in the cervical and upper thoracic sympathetic ganglia. Small esophageal branches, derived from the cervical to fourth and fifth thoracic ganglia and carrying postganglionic sympathetic fibers, join the vagal plexus along the walls of the esophagus (78).

At rest, the cricopharyngeus and thyropharyngeus muscles maintain a tonic contraction driven by the vagal fibers from the nucleus ambiguous (75). During swallowing, the tonic vagal drive is inhibited and the upper esophageal sphincter relaxes. Peristalsis in the upper portion (skeletal muscle portion) of the esophagus is driven by the nucleus ambiguous of the vagus nerve (75), although that in the body and lower portion of the esophagus is driven by the dorsal motor nucleus of the vagus. The relaxation of the lower esophageal sphincter is accomplished by the nitrergic neurons in Aurbach's plexus driven by the dorsal motor nucleus of the vagus nerve (79).

Afferent fibers from the esophageal walls follow the vagus nerve back to the solitary nucleus of the medulla. They also follow the sympathetic fibers back to the dorsal horn of the upper segment of the spinal cord (80). Vagal afferent fibers ending in the solitary nucleus of the medulla contribute to a visceroviseral reflex arc by synapsing on premotor neurons of the nucleus ambiguous and preganglionic neurons of the dorsal motor nucleus of the vagus nerve (75). The premotor neurons subsequently innervate the motor neurons of the nucleus ambiguous. The premotor neurons form the central pattern generator for organized movements of the esophagus such as swallowing (79). The spinal afferent fibers from the esophagus contribute to the referral of pain. These afferent fibers innervate spinal segments that also receive afferent information from the:

Heart
Pulmonary tree
Chest
Upper back and torso

Esophageal pain can refer substernally (heartburn) or posteriorly through the back into the area of the scapula (81). Referred pain from the esophagus has numerous patterns, the more common of which are gripping, pressing, boring, or stabbing (82).

Aortic Plexus

The thoracic aorta has an intimate relationship with both divisions of the autonomic nervous system. Sympathetic input and sensory fibers reach the superior thoracic aorta through cardiac and pulmonary nerves as well as by following direct branches from the sympathetic trunk. The inferior thoracic aorta receives branches of the thoracic splanchnic nerves. The preganglionic sympathetic axons arise in the upper five thoracic spinal segments and the postganglionic fibers arise from the upper five thoracic paravertebral ganglia. Once on the wall of the aorta, these fibers form an adrenergic plexus in the adventitial tissue. Afferent fibers from this large, elastic artery follow the sympathetic nerves back to the upper five thoracic spinal segments (65). This observation accounts for the referral of pain from the thoracic aorta to the thoracic spinal segments, resulting in their subsequent facilitation. Vagal cardiac nerves traverse the walls of the aorta as they descend toward their targets. Small twigs from these branches provide afferent as well as parasympathetic efferent innervation (Fig. 10.14).

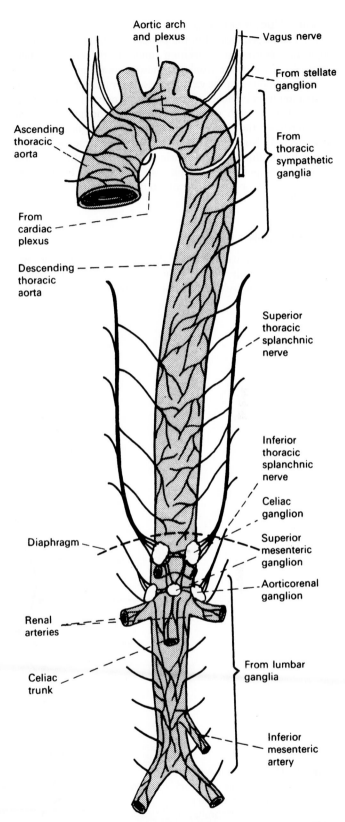

Figure 10-14 Innervation of thoracic and abdominal aorta. (From Bonica JJ. General considerations of pain in the chest. In: Bonica JJ, ed. *The Management of Pain.* Philadelphia, PA: Lea & Febiger, 1990:979, with permission.)

Thoracic Duct Innervation

The thoracic duct, located in the posterior mediastinum near the esophagus, receives an innervation similar to the vascular innervation elsewhere in the trunk. Its muscular walls receive cholinergic innervation from the vagus nerve and sympathetic adrenergic innervation from branches of the intercostal nerves in a segmental pattern. The eleventh thoracic ganglion and the left splanchnic nerve innervate the cisterna chyli, which is the origin of the thoracic duct (83). Norepinephrine and epinephrine act to increase the flow of lymph through the thoracic duct (84). The effect of these adrenergic compounds on lymph vessels appears to be mediated through α-receptors on the smooth muscle cells of the lymph vessel wall (85).

Abdominopelvic Region

The thoracic plexus passes through the diaphragm to continue inferiorly in the abdominopelvic cavity as the abdominopelvic plexus. This plexus is a massive network of fibers lying along the midline astride the aorta and extending from the abdominal diaphragm to the pelvic diaphragm.

At the level of the abdominal diaphragm, the plexus has two major components: parasympathetic and sympathetic. The two vagal trunks and their associated branches, representing the parasympathetic component, enter the abdomen riding on the walls of the esophagus. The sympathetic component (or thoracic splanchnic nerves) passes directly through the crura of the diaphragm or under the medial arcuate ligament to enter the abdomen. Once in the abdominal cavity, the vagal trunks and thoracic splanchnic nerves unite around the aortic prevertebral ganglia. The resultant abdominopelvic plexus of fibers follows the abdominal aorta to the pelvic brim and bifurcates slightly above the sacral promontory, and the resulting two divisions of the plexus descend into the pelvic basin (Fig. 10.15). Throughout the abdomen, the plexus contains both sympathetic and parasympathetic axons and also has numerous afferent fibers. Toward the inferior end of the abdominopelvic plexus, additional sympathetic contributions arise in the lumbar and sacral splanchnic nerves, although additional parasympathetic

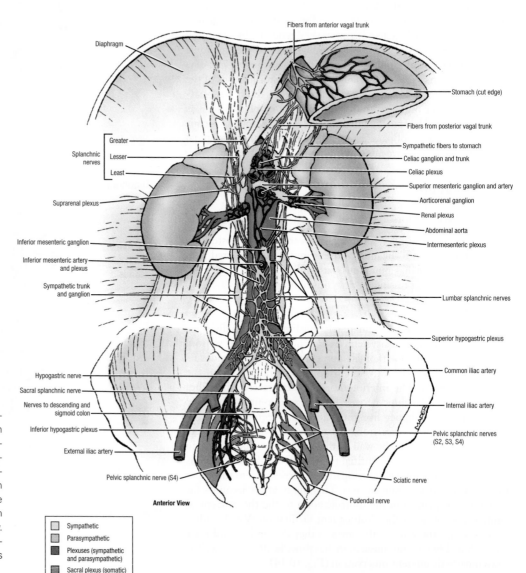

Figure 10-15 The great abdominopelvic plexus. This diagram illustrates the position of the prevertebral and paravertebral sympathetic ganglia in the abdominopelvic plexus. The plexus lies in the visceral fascia surrounding the abdominal aorta. (Figure taken from A. M. Agur and A. F. Dalley. *Grant's Atlas of Anatomy.* Philadelphia, PA: Lippincott Williams & Wilkins, 2009.)

contributions come from the pelvic splanchnic nerves in the pelvic basin.

Like the thoracic plexus, the abdominopelvic plexus can be divided into several geographical regions. Along the abdominal aorta, the major prevertebral ganglia mark out differing territories:

Celiac
Superior mesenteric
Inferior mesenteric

The superior hypogastric plexus lies between the inferior mesenteric plexus and the sacral promontory. Below the sacral promontory, the plexus splits to pass laterally around the pelvic organs. This region is called the inferior hypogastric plexus or, simply, the pelvic plexus. Frequently, the fibers of the superior hypogastric plexus unite into a few large cords in the region directly over the sacral promontory and just prior to bifurcation into the two inferior hypogastric plexuses. These cords are often referred to in the surgical literature as the presacral nerve (86). Although the abdominal autonomic nervous system has regional names, in reality the components blend together to form one great abdominopelvic plexus. The abdominal portion of this great plexus supplies efferent and afferent nerves to the organs of the abdominal cavity including the gastrointestinal organs, spleen, and kidneys. The pelvic portion of this plexus supplies the rectum, urinary organs, and reproductive organs. In addition to the organs, the abdominopelvic plexus also innervates the vasculature of the abdominopelvic cavity.

Gastrointestinal Tract

The gastrointestinal system receives a complex pattern of extrinsic innervation involving splanchnic nerves derived from the thoracolumbar and sacral portions of the spinal cord and the terminal portion of the vagus and pelvic splanchnic nerves (Figs. 10.4 and 10.5). These nerves form a complex network of fibers lying along the abdominal aorta and extending from the thoracoabdominal diaphragm to the pelvic diaphragm (Fig. 10.15). This elaborate plexus, like its visceral blood supply, can be divided into three zones based on embryologic partitions of the gastrointestinal system:

Celiac (foregut)
Superior mesenteric (midgut)
Inferior mesenteric (hindgut)

A complex network of intrinsic fibers and neurons called the enteric nervous system is found within the walls of the gut. The enteric or intrinsic neural system controls the activity of gut smooth muscle and glands. In turn, it is modulated by the extrinsic fibers from the CNS via the sympathetic and parasympathetic nerves. Numerous sensory feedback loops exist in the gastrointestinal system. Afferent fibers within the luminal surface and gut wall form short feedback loops within the enteric nervous system. Longer feedback loops connect the gut to the prevertebral ganglia, and still longer loops connect the gut with the spinal cord and brainstem (6,13,87–90). Figure 10.16 is a schematic diagram of the abdominopelvic plexus demonstrating its input from sympathetic and parasympathetic sources.

The gastrointestinal tract has a special pattern of sympathetic innervation that differs significantly from that of the thoracic viscera. Preganglionic fibers arise in the lateral horn of spinal segments T9-L2, but they do not terminate in the paravertebral ganglia. Instead, they pass through a series of thoracic, lumbar, and sacral splanchnic nerves (branches off of the sympathetic truck) to reach the prevertebral sympathetic ganglia on the anterior wall of the abdominal aorta (Fig. 10.15).

The major prevertebral ganglia are distributed around the three abdominal arteries:

Celiac
Superior mesenteric
Inferior mesenteric

Anatomical authorities subdivide the celiac ganglia into numerous parts based on its location about the celiac artery and aorta; however, from a practical perspective, it is simpler to consider it as one anatomical unit. Also, the celiac and superior mesenteric ganglia are often fused together into an inseparable mass surrounding the trunks of their two arteries. An older term for this arrangement is the solar plexus. Additional clusters of sympathetic ganglia neurons are found scattered in the hypogastric plexus as it enters the pelvic basin.

Neurons in each prevertebral ganglion give rise to postganglionic fibers that innervate abdominal and pelvic viscera. These axons travel to their target organs by hitchhiking on abdominal and pelvic arteries. Each prevertebral ganglion innervates a different region of the viscera.

Celiac Ganglia

The celiac ganglionic mass surrounds the celiac trunk. It is often fused to the superior mesenteric ganglia to form one large, complex mass. When carefully dissected, the precise shape of the ganglion complex is very irregular and defies meaningful classification (51). The celiac ganglia receive afferent fibers from the thoracic splanchnic nerves (T5-T9). In turn, it supplies postganglionic sympathetic axons to the vascular territory of the celiac artery including the (Figs. 10.17 and 10.18):

Distal esophagus
Stomach

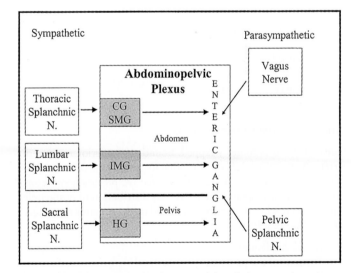

Figure 10-16 A schematic diagram of the abdominopelvic plexus illustrating its ganglia and sources of input. Thoracic, lumbar, and sacral splanchnic nerves for the sympathetic trunk carry sympathetic preganglionic fibers to the paravertebral ganglia located in the plexus. Postganglionic axons from the paravertebral ganglia target the intrinsic enteric ganglia of the organ walls. Parasympathetic fibers arise in the vagus nerve superiorly and the pelvic splanchnic nerves inferiorly. These fibers also target the intrinsic enteric ganglia located on the organ walls. CG, celiac ganglion; SMG, superior mesenteric ganglion; IMG, inferior mesenteric ganglion; HG, Hypogastric ganglion.

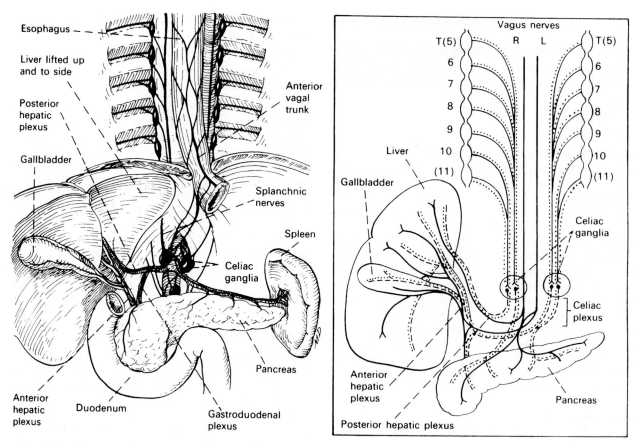

Figure 10-17 Connections of celiac ganglion and innervation of stomach. (From Kimmey MB, Silverstein FE. Diseases of the gastrointestinal tract. In: Bonica JJ, ed. *The Management of Pain*. Philadelphia, PA: Lea & Febiger, 1990:1189, with permission.)

Proximal duodenum
Liver
Gall bladder
Spleen
Portions of the pancreas

Superior Mesenteric Ganglia

This ganglion is found wrapped around the superior mesenteric artery. As mentioned above, it is often fused with the celiac ganglia. The superior mesenteric ganglia also receive preganglionic axons from the thoracic splanchnic nerves. Its distribution of postganglionic axons reaches the territory supplied by the superior mesenteric artery (Fig. 10.19):

Distal duodenum
Portions of the pancreas
Jejunum
Ileum
Ascending colon
Proximal two thirds of the transverse colon

Inferior Mesenteric Ganglia

The most ventral of the three prevertebral ganglia, the inferior mesenteric ganglia, surrounds the abdominal artery of the same name. It receives axons from the three lumbar splanchnic nerves

and supplies postganglionic axons to the vascular territory of the inferior mesenteric vessels, namely the (Fig. 10.18):

Distal third of the transverse colon
Descending colon
Sigmoid colon
Rectum

Postganglionic fibers from the prevertebral ganglia follow their specific blood supplies through the mesenteric ligaments to reach the specific organs. The termination of these noradrenergic fibers is primarily on the neurons in the enteric ganglia (91). Sympathetic fibers also terminate in the muscular coat of blood vessels, and an abundance of these fibers reaches the sphincter musculature of the enteric wall. Only scattered sympathetic fibers are present in the muscularis externa and submucosa of the gastrointestinal tract (92). There are almost no adrenergic cell bodies in the enteric plexus; therefore, most enteric adrenergic fibers are of external origin. In general, stimulation of the sympathetic fibers inhibits the activity of cholinergic neurons of the parasympathetic system and slows peristalsis and motility.

The parasympathetic innervation of the organs located below the thoracoabdominal diaphragm has a dual origin, which also segregates along vascular and embryologic divisions. The organs of the foregut and midgut, serviced by the celiac and superior mesenteric arteries, receive parasympathetic preganglionic fibers from the vagus nerve (Figs. 10.17–10.19). The vagus nerve follows the esophagus through the diaphragm to enter the abdominal cavity on

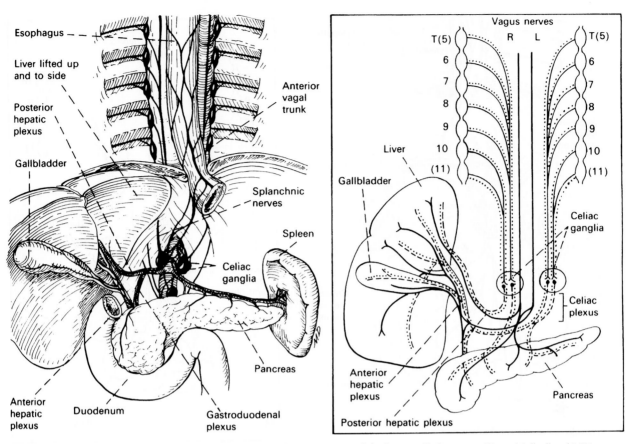

Figure 10-18 Connections of celiac ganglia and the innervation of the liver and biliary tree. (From Mulholland MW, Debas HT. Diseases of the liver, biliary system, and pancreas. In: Bonica JJ, ed. *The Management of Pain*. Philadelphia, PA: Lea & Febiger, 1990:1215, with permission.)

the walls of the stomach. The esophageal hiatus of the diaphragm is the last place the vagus can be identified as a distinct nerve. Vagal axons, however, continue into the abdominal cavity, joining those of the sympathetic system in the celiac and superior mesenteric ganglia and forming mixed nerves, which pass along celiac and superior mesenteric blood vessels eventually to reach the abdominal viscera. Vagal fibers are plentiful in the walls of the stomach and small bowel, and a few reach as far distally in the enteric plexus as the splenic flexure of the large colon. The preganglionic vagal axons terminate on neurons in enteric ganglia. Short postganglionic fibers from these neurons innervate the glands and course within the layers of smooth muscle of the alimentary canal. Cholinergic stimulation increases glandular secretions and peristaltic activity.

The organs of hindgut origin (transverse colon to anus) receive parasympathetic preganglionic innervation from the pelvic splanchnic nerves (Fig. 10.20). These nerves arise in the lateral horn of the S2-S3 spinal cord segments and exit the spinal canal with the sacral nerve roots. As the roots pass along the pelvic wall on their way to the greater sciatic foramen, the delicate pelvic splanchnic nerves are given off. These thin nerves course through the endopelvic fascia to reach the inferior hypogastric plexus surrounding the walls of the rectum. Once in the hypogastric plexus, these parasympathetic preganglionic fibers can ascend to the origin of the inferior mesenteric artery. By hitchhiking along the branches of this artery, they reach upward to the splenic flexure of the large colon. Not all parasympathetic axons from the pelvis follow this route to reach the inferior abdominal organs. Some preganglionic

fibers in the inferior hypogastric plexus gain access to the enteric plexus in the wall of the rectum and ascend along the colon to reach more proximal levels of the hindgut. The preganglionic axons of the pelvic splanchnic nerves eventually terminate on the neurons of the enteric nervous system. Stimulation of the parasympathetic fibers increases gut peristalsis and mobility.

The enteric ganglia and plexus within the walls of the gut form a highly complex and elaborate network, often referred to as the third division of the autonomic nervous system. It exerts a major influence over all activities in the gut (6,93). The enteric nervous system is estimated to possess as many neurons as are found in the entire spinal cord (94). The enteric system is divided into two layers: The external layer is the myenteric plexus (Auerbach's) controlling the muscularis externa, and the internal layer is the submucosal (Meissner's) controlling the glandular and immune components of the submucosal layers. A full understanding of these structures requires a knowledge of the gastrointestinal histology and is beyond the scope of this review (95,96).

Numerous neurotransmitters and neuromodulators are found within enteric neurons, for example:

Acetylcholine
Serotonin
Purines
Gamma-amino butyric acid
Histamine
There are also many peptides such as
Substance-P

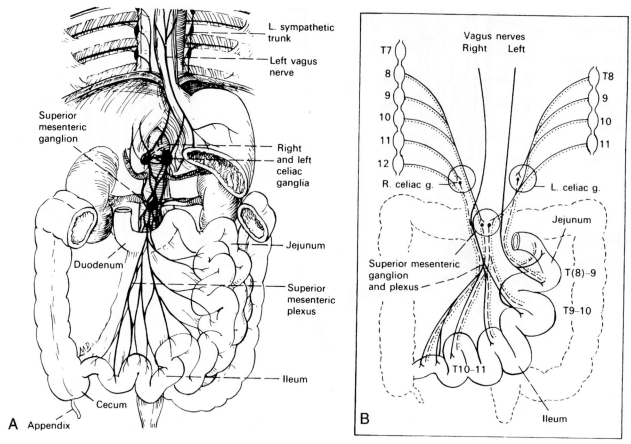

Figure 10-19 Connections of superior mesenteric ganglion and the innervation of the small bowel. (From Kimmey MB, Silverstein FE. Diseases of the gastrointestinal tract. In: Bonica JJ, ed. *The Management of Pain.* Philadelphia, PA: Lea & Febiger, 1990:1198, with permission.)

Somatostatin
Vasoactive intestinal polypeptide
Enkephalins

Recently, nitric oxide has been described as a significant noncholinergic, nonadrenergic mechanism of neurotransmission in the enteric nervous system as well as elsewhere (97,98). Nitric oxide is synthesized from the amino acid arginine by neurons in the myenteric plexus and is a potent smooth muscle relaxing factor. For this reason, it is postulated to be important in dilation of the alimentary canal.

Three levels of sensory information processing are necessary for the proper regulation of gastrointestinal tract function (6,87). The first level features afferent neurons that form a short loop interconnecting the gut mucosa, submucosa, or muscle to the enteric ganglia only. These neurons are responsible for local reflexes along the gut wall. The second level of sensory information processing involved is arranged in a longer loop involving afferent neurons from the mucosa that project to the prevertebral ganglia along the aorta. These sensory neurons participate in intra-abdominal reflex arcs coordinating various regions of the gastrointestinal system. Neither of these two sensory levels can reach consciousness; thus, we are generally unaware of the reflex control activity occurring in the gut wall. Finally, the third level of sensory feedback loops involves afferent neurons that project from the gut wall to the brainstem via the vagus nerve or to the spinal cord via the thoracic, lumbar, and pelvic splanchnic nerves. These visceral afferent neurons assist the CNS in integrating the activity of the alimentary canal with that

of external environmental conditions. Information in this third sensory level can, on occasion, reach consciousness.

There are significant differences in distribution, morphology, and neurochemistry between the visceral afferent fibers associated with sympathetic nerves and those coursing with the parasympathetic nerves. There are very few large, encapsulated nerve endings in the gut wall, most of which are related to axons from the parasympathetic vagus nerve. However, the majority of afferent terminals in the gut are small-caliber, naked nerve endings (87). In the vagus nerve, mechanoreceptive, chemoreceptive, and polymodal fibers have been described with their receptive fields in the mucosa and submucosa of the gut wall. At least in the stomach, very few of these vagal fibers contain calcitonin gene–related polypeptide, a neuropeptide typically related in nociceptive afferent fibers of the somatic tissue. However, some nociceptive information is carried in the vagus nerve because pain from a hiatal hernia can be referred to the face (99) via the vagus nerve. Little is known of nociceptive function in vagal fibers below the level of the diaphragm. The visceral afferent fibers that follow the sympathetic nerves to the spinal cord are mechanoreceptive and chemoreceptive, and they tend to be distributed to the mesenteries and peritoneal ligaments of the gut and along its vascular system. In contrast to the vagal fibers, those projecting to the spinal cord are mostly of small caliber and are rich in calcitonin gene–related polypeptide, suggesting that they have a role in nociception. Their endings are commonly distributed within the mesentery and supporting ligaments of the abdominal organs (88). These nerve endings are frequently present

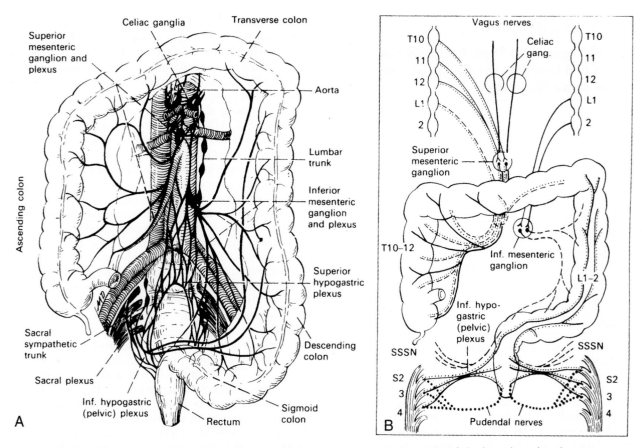

Figure 10-20 Connections of inferior mesenteric ganglion and the innervation of the large bowel and rectum. SSSN, sacral sympathetic splanchnic nerve. (From Kimmey MB, Silverstein FE. Diseases of the gastrointestinal tract. In: Bonica JJ, ed. *The Management of Pain.* Philadelphia, PA: Lea & Febiger, 1990:1199, with permission.)

near the branch points for the vasculature in the peritoneal lining. Few small-caliber nerve endings are present within the visceral organs themselves. (See additional comments concerning vagal activity in Chapter 8.)

Physiologic (68) and clinical studies support the general separation of regulatory information into the vagal system and nociceptive information into the spinal cord. Stimulating the greater thoracic splanchnic nerve at surgery elicits severe pain; however, blockade of the splanchnic nerve relieves pain (100). In addition, applying local anesthetic to the greater thoracic splanchnic nerve after abdominal surgery prevents the endocrine metabolic responses such as increased plasma cortisol and urinary adrenaline levels that are usually present in the early stages of recovery (101). The projection of the viscera afferent fibers through the sympathetic system creates a nociceptive map of the abdominopelvic organs on the dorsal horn of the spinal cord. This map has been demonstrated in humans by sectioning the white rami commicans during the surgical treatment of visceral pain [White and Sweet, as cited in Jänig and Morrison (88)]. A summary of the organotopic map of the human viscera is presented in Table 10.1. The position of a specific organ in the visceral afferent organotopic map of the spinal cord coincides approximately with the origin of the sympathetic efferent system to that specific organ. The nociceptive input to the spinal cord over these visceral afferent fibers is not precisely mapped; instead, input from any one organ overlaps considerably with that from surrounding organs (88).

Hepatobiliary Tree and Pancreas

The vasculature and parenchyma of the liver and pancreas, as well as their associated ducts, receive innervation from both divisions of the autonomic nervous system (Fig. 10.18). In addition, these organs have an abundant supply of visceral afferent fibers that course in the vagus and thoracic splanchnic nerves. Preganglionic sympathetic innervation to these organs arises in thoracic segments at approximately T6 to T9-T11 and approaches the abdomen through the thoracic splanchnic nerves. Sympathetic ganglionic neurons are located in the celiac ganglia. Their postganglionic axons reach the liver and pancreas by hitchhiking on the hepatic and pancreatic branches of the celiac trunk. Preganglionic parasympathetic axons, derived from the vagus nerve, pass through the fascia of the celiac region and follow the vasculature to the target organs. Little is known concerning the effects of autonomic nerve stimulation on liver function. However, in general, sympathetic activation drives the liver toward increasing the output of glucose (102).

A significant percentage of the axons in the vagus and thoracic splanchnic nerves traveling to the liver and pancreas are sensory in nature. Approximately 90 of the vagal axons and 50 of the splanchnic axons to the liver are visceral afferent fibers (103). These two afferent systems perform different functions (13). Those afferent axons traveling with the vagus nerve respond to such stimuli as plasma glucose concentration, portal venous blood osmotic pressure, and temperature changes. The visceral afferent fibers associated with the splanchnic nerves are high-threshold

TABLE 10.1

Visceral Organs and Their Approximate Spinal Cord Level for the Origin of Their Preganglionic Neurons[a]

Heart	T1-5	
Stomach	T5-9	
Liver and gall bladder	T6-9	
Pancreas	T5-11	
Small intestine	T9-11	
Colon and rectum	T8-L2	S2-4
Kidney and ureters	T10-L1	
Urinary bladder	T10-L1	S2-4
Ovary and fallopian tube	T9-10	
Testicle and epididymus	T9-10, L1-2	S2-4
Uterus	T10-L1	
Cervix		S2-4
Prostate	L1-2	

[a]These levels create a viscerotopic map in the lateral horns of the spinal cord.

mechanoreceptors and chemoreceptors located in the walls of the biliary system, among other places, and are responsive to stretch and bradykinin concentration. The evidence available to date suggests that all pain sensation from the liver and biliary tree is transmitted via the splanchnic nerves and not the vagus nerve.

Kidney and Urinary Tract
Kidney

Although the kidney is primarily controlled by endocrine mechanisms, it does receive significant innervation from the sympathetic adrenergic system that regulates, in part, the retention of sodium (Table 10.1) (104–107). Alterations in the neural activity in sympathetic fibers are involved in the generation of certain forms of hypertension (108). Very little vagal parasympathetic (cholinergic) input to the kidney has been reported. This organ does, however, receive neuropeptide-containing, primary afferent fibers that course along with the adrenergic fibers (Fig. 10.21).

The kidney receives most of its innervation from the thoracolumbar spinal cord. Preganglionic sympathetic neurons regulating the kidney are located in the lateral horn of the spinal cord extending approximately from segments T11 to L1. Their axons enter the abdominopelvic plexus over the lower thoracic and first lumbar splanchnic nerves (Table 10.1). The postganglionic sympathetic adrenergic fibers are derived from laterally positioned ganglia (sometimes called aorticorenal ganglia) in the celiac and superior mesenteric plexuses and course into the hilus of the kidney along the renal vasculature.

The adrenergic axons of the mammalian kidney terminate on the (109):

Afferent and efferent glomerular arterioles
Proximal and distal renal tubules
Ascending limb of Henle loop
Juxtaglomerular apparatus

All portions of the cortical tubular nephron are under neural influence. The relative density of adrenergic fibers is greatest around the ascending limb of the loop of Henle, followed in decreasing

relative density by the distal convoluted tubule and the proximal convoluted tubule (110,111). α-adrenoceptors have been located on the proximal convoluted tubule (112) as well as on the smooth muscle of the vasculature. Sympathetic innervation of the kidney is involved in the normal regulation of sodium retention, both by increasing the transport of sodium across the tubule walls and by directly increasing the release of renin from the juxtaglomerular apparatus (113,114). Studies have shown that there is increased activity in the renal sympathetic nervous system in essential hypertension in humans (108).

A dual sensory innervation of the kidney exists: afferent fibers follow the thoracic splanchnic nerves back to the spinal cord and the vagus nerve back to the brainstem. Within the kidney, peripheral endings of both mechanoreceptors and chemoreceptors are found in close association with ureteric blood vessels (arteries and veins) and in the walls of the pelvis of the ureter (115). Their cell bodies are in the dorsal root ganglia located mainly in segments at the thoracolumbar junction (T10-L3), and their central processes terminate in the dorsal horn of the spinal cord. These afferent axons are classified as A and C-fibers. Vagal afferent fibers, both mechanoreceptors and chemoreceptors, play a role in renorenal reflexes. The mechanoreceptors are also involved in modulating cardiovascular reflexes, thus regulating blood pressure (115). Pain is the only detectable sensory perception that can be elicited from the kidney (13). This modality is carried in the visceral afferent fibers of the thoracic splanchnic nerves to reach the spinal cord and the spinothalamic tracts. In a study of the sympathetic renal afferent fibers in the primate, all spinothalamic tract cells excited by renal afferent fibers were also excited by somatic afferent fibers, indicating a powerful somatovisceral convergence on these cells (116). This convergence has been suggested as a mechanism to explain the referral of pain from the kidney out to somatic structures such as the flank of the body. In addition, this relationship may explain the changes in the tone of muscle innervated by the segments T10-L1 that accompany renal infection or inflammation.

Ureter

The ureter is the conduit for urine from the kidney to the bladder. Its primary function of the ureter is the unidirectional flow of urine from the kidney to the urinary bladder. Although it is richly invested with nerves (117), peristalsis in the ureter is primarily myogenic in nature, driven by specialized pacemaker cells (118). The course of the ureter is retroperitoneal, lying along the posterior abdominal body wall and embedded in the transversalis fascia. The walls of the ureter consist of interlacing bundles of smooth muscle fibers woven into a theca muscularis. Individual smooth muscle cells interconnect via numerous gap junctions, making the muscularis a functional syncytium (119). Modified smooth muscle cells within the muscular layer serve as pacemakers, initiating peristaltic contractions (120). A plexus of efferent and afferent nerve fibers that are capable of regulating the pacemaker cells is wrapped around the muscularis (119).

The ureter receives its innervation in a segmental fashion. The upper portion is innervated by the lower thoracic and upper lumbar segments (T10-L1) and by the vagus nerve. The lower portion of the ureter is innervated by the upper lumbar segments (L1-L2) and the pelvic splanchnic nerves (Table 10.1). The sympathetic innervation reaches the upper ureter through the lesser thoracic and lumbar splanchnic nerves. Ganglionic neurons are located in the celiac and associated renal and gonadal (testicular or ovarian) ganglia. The lower ureter receives its sympathetic innervation from lumbar and sacral splanchnic nerves that contribute to ganglia located in the superior and inferior hypogastric plexus (121).

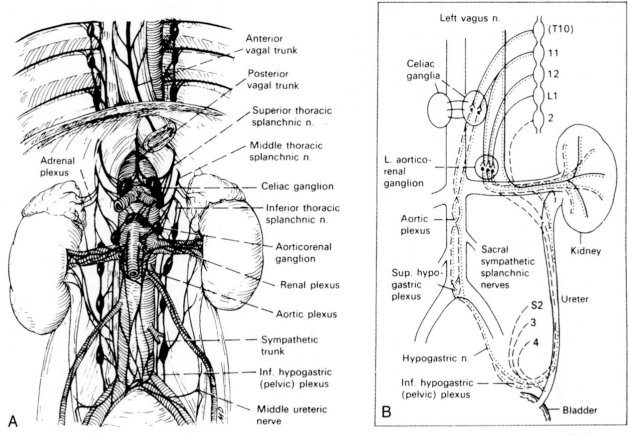

Figure 10-21 Innervation of the kidney. (From Ansell JS, Gee WF. Diseases of the kidney. In: Bonica JJ, ed. *The Management of Pain*. Philadelphia, PA: Lea & Febiger, 1990:1233, with permission.)

Fibers containing tyrosine hydroxylase and neuropeptide-Y, markers for sympathetic axons, are in the outer muscle layers and the surrounding adventitia of the human ureter (122–124). Activation of α-adrenergic receptors increases ureter peristalsis and elevates luminal pressures; whereas activation of β-adrenergic receptors decreases ureter peristaltic frequency and lowers intraureter pressures (125). The actual role of the noradrenergic system in human ureter peristalsis has been questioned, and it appears that control over the surrounding vascular system is the dominant theme for the ureteric nerves (118).

Parasympathetic innervation for the upper portion of the ureter arises in the vagus nerve and reaches the ureter through the celiac and superior mesenteric plexus. The lower portion receives its cholinergic innervation from spinal segments S2-S4. These pelvic splanchnic nerves communicate with the ureter via the inferior hypogastric plexus. Acetylcholine-containing neurons are present in the mural ganglia of the ureter, and fibers containing acetylcholine are present in the mammalian ureter. These fibers are of greatest density as the ureter enters the vesical wall. Stimulation of the ureter wall with acetylcholine results in an increased contractile activity and an increased basal tone of the mural smooth muscle (125,126). Acetylcholine also relaxes the ureter resistance arteries using a mechanism involving endothelium-derived nitric oxide (125).

Afferent fibers to the ureter are derived from dorsal root ganglia ranging from L2-L3 to S1-S2 (in guinea pigs) (127). Two classes of mechanoreceptors have been described in the ureter walls (128). One class has low thresholds and is responsive to peristaltic-type contractions of the ureteric smooth muscle. The other class of mechanoreceptor has higher thresholds of activation and is most likely related to nociception. Many of these primary afferent fibers contain neuropeptides such as substance-P and calcitonin gene–related polypeptide, thereby suggesting that they are involved in nociceptive activities.

Pain, presumably from these nociceptors, is the only sensory perception obtainable from the human ureter (13). In the thoracolumbar dorsal horn of the spinal cord, input from the ureter converges with somatic input from thoracolumbar spinal segments. Pain from distention of the ureter is often referred to the somatic body wall over a range of body segments. From the upper ureter, pain refers to the area from the anterior superior spine of the ileum anteriorly to the border of the rectus abdominis muscle (T11-T12). From the middle ureter, pain refers to the area from the inguinal ligament anteriorly to the rectus abdominis muscle (T12-L1). From the lower ureter, pain refers to the suprapubic area (L1) and below into the scrotum or labia (L2) (121). This descending segmental pattern of primary afferent fibers from the ureter is responsible for the descending movement of facilitated segments as any obstructing material moves through the ureteric lumen.

Urinary Bladder

The muscular components of the urinary bladder can be divided into two anatomical and functional parts: the body (or detrusor urinae muscle) and the base (or the trigone muscle). The detrusor urinae muscle is the larger of the two parts and is active during expulsion of urine from the bladder. The trigone muscle surrounds the openings of the ureter in the base and the opening of the urethra in the neck of the bladder. It acts as an internal sphincter and, when contracted, helps to prevent the flow of urine from the bladder. The detrusor and the trigone tend to oppose each other in activity. Both detrusor and trigone muscles comprise multiple layers of smooth muscle fibers and receive an efferent innervation from the large autonomic pelvic plexus. A third muscle related to bladder function is located inferior to the trigone in the layers of the perineum. It is the deep transverse perineal muscle; the portion of this muscle that surrounds the urethra is called the sphincter urethra. Unlike the detrusor and trigone, this component of the perineal diaphragm is composed of skeletal muscle and innervated by branches of the pudendal nerve, a somatic nerve (S2-S4).

The autonomic innervation of the urinary bladder is accomplished through the hypogastric plexus that is embedded in endopelvic fascia (Fig. 10.22). Parasympathetic preganglionic (cholinergic) fibers from the intermediolateral nucleus of spinal segments S2-S4 enter the hypogastric plexus via the pelvic splanchnic nerves. These axons continue anteriorly into the vesicle plexus to terminate on ganglionic neurons located in the walls of the bladder. Their postganglionic (cholinergic and purinergic) axons supply motor innervation to all portions of the bladder wall. Stimulation of the parasympathetic system, which occurs during voiding, is excitatory to the detrusor muscle and inhibitory to the trigone muscle (129).

Sympathetic preganglionic fibers arise in the intermediolateral nucleus of spinal segments T11-L2 (Fig. 10.22). They leave the sympathetic trunk coursing on lumbar and sacral splanchnic nerves to enter the inferior hypogastric plexus, eventually targeting prevertebral ganglia (130). Sympathetic postganglionic (adrenergic) axons pass anteriorly through the inferior hypogastric plexus and ultimately contribute to the vesicle plexus in the bladder adventitia. Their major target is the smooth muscle cells of the trigone muscle with a much smaller contribution to the smooth muscle of the detrusor urinae. Sympathetic tone facilitates contraction of the trigone muscles and relaxation of the detrusor urinae muscle, which is necessary to allow expansion of the bladder while it is filling (130).

The vesicle plexus contains many ganglionic neurons traditionally associated with the parasympathetic system. However, it is now clear that these neurons also receive input from adrenergic axons in the sympathetic system. Thus, the sympathetic system can influence the activity of the parasympathetic system by modulating the activity of the ganglion cells. The ganglion cells innervating the trigone muscle have α-adrenoceptors on their membranes and respond to sympathetic stimulation with contraction. Conversely, ganglion cells innervating the detrusor muscle have β-adrenoceptors on their membranes and respond to sympathetic stimulation with relaxation. It is through this differential distribution of adrenoceptors that the sympathetic nervous system is capable of increasing the tone in the trigone while simultaneously relaxing the detrusor urinae (130).

The sphincter urethrae muscle, or external urethral sphincter, at the base of the bladder, is skeletal muscle; it receives its innervation from the perineal branches of the pudendal nerve (Fig. 10.22). This is a somatic nerve containing axons from motoneurons located in the ventral horn of the spinal cord (S2-S4).

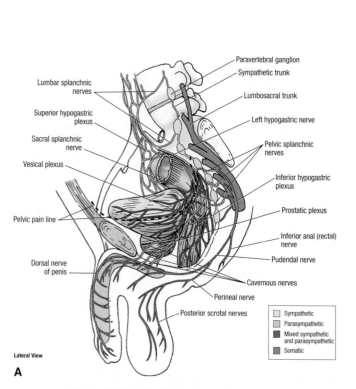

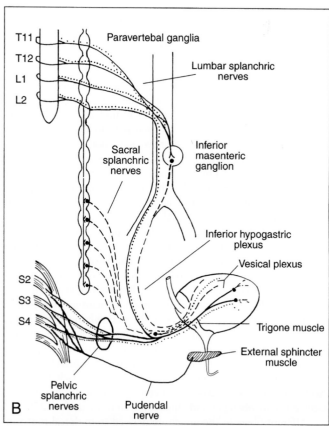

Figure10-22 The hypogastric plexus and the innervation of the male pelvic basin. **A.** This figure demonstrates the distribution of autonomic nerves to the pelvic and perineal organs. (Figure taken from A. M. Agur and A. F. Dalley. *Grant's Atlas of Anatomy.* Philadelphia, PA: Lippincott Williams & Wilkins, 2009.) **B.** This figure illustrates the origin of pelvic and perineal nerves in the male. (Figure taken from W. F. Gee and J. S. Ansell. Pelvic and perineal pain of urologic origin. In: J. J. Bonica, ed. *The Management of Pain.* Philadelphia, PA: Lea & Febiger, 1990:1368–1394.)

The release of urine from the bladder requires an integrated viscerosomatic reflex involving:

1. Excitation of the parasympathetic system to activate the detrusor urinae muscle.
2. Inhibition of the sympathetic system to relax the trigone and internal sphincteral muscles.
3. Subsequent inhibition of the pudendal nerve to relax the external sphincteral muscles.

Vesicle afferent fibers arise from mechanoreceptor endings in the connective tissue and epithelium of the vesicle mucosa and travel over the lumbar and pelvic splanchnic nerves as well as pudendal nerves to reach the cord at the L1-L2 and S2-S4 levels. Cell bodies for these nerves are present in the associated dorsal root ganglia. Many of these fibers contain neuropeptides such as those represented in the small-caliber, primary afferent fibers system (130). The afferent fibers reach only to the dorsal horn of the spinal cord near their segmental level of entry; however, a small number of these fibers enter the spinal cord and follow the ascending tracts rostrally to terminate in the lower regions of the medulla.

Sensory information from distension of the bladder initiates the reflexes involved in voiding. Initial filling of the bladder triggers low-level afferent volleys that increase the tone in the trigone muscle and external sphincter muscles and inhibit the tone in the detrusor urinae muscle, allowing the bladder to serve as a reservoir for urine. After a certain level of filling is reached, a higher intensity of afferent volleys from the bladder wall reverses these reflexes such that the detrusor urinae muscle tone is enhanced and the tone of the trigone and external sphincter is inhibited. This reversal of reflexes prepares the bladder for voiding. The last step, relaxation of the external sphincter, requires cooperation of the suprasegmental control of the bladder musculature, allowing volitional control of voiding (130).

Reproductive Tract

The pelvic and perineal organs of the male and female reproductive systems receive both sympathetic and parasympathetic innervation through the complex abdominopelvic plexus (Fig. 10.23). This innervation targets the glandular cells and smooth muscle of the vasculature as well as the mural smooth muscle present in the tubular portions of these organs. The origin of this innervation varies according to the embryonic origin of the specific organs. The testis and the ovary, which arise in the gonadal ridge of the posterior abdominal wall, receive their afferent and efferent supply

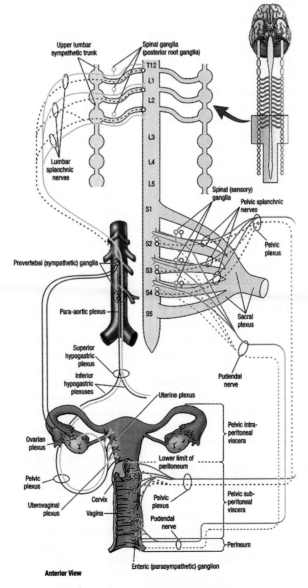

Figure 10-23 The origin and distribution of the hypogastric plexus in the female pelvic basin. (Figure taken from A. M. Agur and A. F. Dalley. *Grant's Atlas of Anatomy*. Philadelphia, PA: Lippincott Williams & Wilkins, 2009.)

from the abdominal portions of the abdominopelvic plexus. The remaining pelvic organs of reproduction are innervated from the pelvic portion of the plexus. Afferent fibers are present in each of these organs, and their input to the spinal cord is a key feature in the presentation of pelvic pain.

Testis and Ovary

Gonadal tissue receives sympathetic innervation from preganglionic neurons located in spinal segments T10 and T11. These preganglionic axons target neurons in the celiac and superior mesenteric ganglia. The gonadal (spermatic or ovarian) plexus of fibers arises from these ganglia and follows the course of the gonadal arteries. Additional sympathetic postganglionic axons join the gonadal plexus from the superior hypogastric plexus in the lower abdomen. In females, the gonadal (ovarian) plexus innervates the ovary and extends on to reach the uterine tubes. In males, the gonadal (spermatic) plexus joins the spermatic cord with the vas deferens and proceeds through the inguinal canal to reach the scrotum. Adrenergic fibers in the testis are present around blood vessels and interstitial cells of the seminiferous tubules and in the tubules of the epididymis (125). Stimulation of the sympathetic nervous system initiates strong peristaltic waves in the vas deferens, which is responsible for the propulsion of sperm. Parasympathetic innervation of the gonadal tissue is less dense than that of the sympathetic fibers. Cholinergic fibers arise from the vesical plexus and join the gonadal plexus as it passes through the pelvis. These fibers primarily target the vas deferens and the seminal vesicles.

Afferent fibers from the testis, epididymis, and vas deferens extend through the gonadal plexus to reach the thoracolumbar spinal cord. Fibers arising in the testis target segment T10, those from the epididymis enter the spinal cord at T11 and T12, although those from the vas deferens enter at T10-L1 (131). Afferent fibers from the ovary also ascend in the gonadal plexus to enter the spinal cord at the T10 level. The return of afferent axons from the gonadal tissue to the lower thoracic level of the spinal cord is responsible for the referral of pain to the thoracolumbar junction and the facilitation of segments in this area consequent to irritation of the gonadal tissue.

Uterus, Uterine Tube, Cervix, and Vagina

The distal portion of the abdominopelvic plexus bifurcates as it descends over the sacral promontory to enter the pelvic basin. The pelvic portion of this complex neural structure is called the inferior hypogastric or pelvic plexus. This network of ganglia and fibers sweeps laterally along the pelvic walls to surround the midline organs of the female pelvis. As this plexus crosses over the transverse cervical ligament, its fibrous network thickens to form the elaborate plexus of Frankenhuser (a regional subset of the inferior hypogastric plexus). From here, autonomic axons accompany the uterine vessels medially along the transverse cervical ligament to gain access to the uterus, cervix, and vagina. The remainder of the inferior hypogastric plexus extends anteriorly to surround the bladder (this collection of fibers is often referred to as the vesical plexus).

Sympathetic preganglionic neurons capable of influencing the uterus and cervix are located in the T10-L2 spinal segments (Fig. 10.23). Their axons target neurons in the celiac ganglia and other prevertebral ganglia. Postganglionic fibers from these ganglia descend into the pelvic basin coursing in the superior and inferior hypogastric plexus to eventually reach the uterus. For the most part, these adrenergic fibers end on the vasculature of the

uterus. Some axons terminate in the smooth muscle of the myometrium, particularly in the longitudinal layer (132) and among the glands of the endometrium. The parasympathetic input to the uterus and cervix arises in the intermediolateral nucleus of spinal segments S2-4. These axons target ganglia located in the plexus of Frankenhuser; whereas postganglionic (cholinergic) axons extend from this plexus into the uterus following the uterine artery. Most of the cholinergic input to the uterus is confined to the vascular supply with a small amount reaching the glands of the endometrium and a few fibers in the circular muscle layer of the myometrium (132). Beyond regulation of the vasculature, the function of this elaborate autonomic innervation of the uterus is not well known. Evidence suggests that stimulation of the adrenergic and cholinergic inputs can enhance the contraction of mammalian uterine myometrium (133). The number and size of adrenergic nerves appears to increase in the uterus during pregnancy (134), further suggesting a role for these fibers in the uterine contractions of labor and delivery.

The uterus, cervix, and vagina receive a complex afferent innervation that influences the referral of pain during parturition (135). Experimental studies in cats demonstrate that afferent fibers from the uterus and cervix enter the spinal cord over a range of levels (T12-S3) (136). The majority of fibers from the fallopian tubes have cell bodies in the dorsal root ganglia of the lumbar segments, whereas the majority of fibers from the cervix have cell bodies in the dorsal root ganglia of the sacral segments. Clinical studies suggest that the afferent fibers from the human uterus project to even higher levels of the spinal cord (T10) (135) and that the majority of pain fibers from the uterus enter the thoracolumbar spinal cord (137,138). Nociceptive fibers from the uterus pass upward through the superior hypogastric plexus and lumbar splanchnic nerves to enter the spinal cord over the white rami of the lower thoracic and lumbar segments. For this reason, the white ramus at L1 can be particularly large. The pathways handling sensory information from the female reproductive tract are split. Input from above the cervix ascends through the superior hypogastric plexus to the thoracolumbar junction, although afferent fibers from the cervix and below descend into the sacral spinal cord (68). This arrangement of primary afferent fibers is responsible, in part, for the presentation of low-back pain late in pregnancy as well as accompanying facilitation of spinal segments around the thoracolumbar junction.

Erectile Tissue of the Penis and Clitoris

The sympathetic innervation of the vasculature and erectile tissue in the penis and clitoris has its origin in the intermediolateral cell column of spinal cord segments T11-L2 (Fig. 10.23). At least two routes exist through which these fibers reach the penis. One route involves preganglionic axons that arise in the thoracolumbar spinal cord and synapse in the associated paravertebral ganglia. From these ganglia, adrenergic postganglionic fibers join the hypogastric plexus to pass into the pelvic basin, eventually entering the penis at its root on the perineal diaphragm. The second route comprises sympathetic preganglionic axons from thoracolumbar segments that pass by the paravertebral ganglia to terminate in pelvic ganglia located deep in the pelvic plexus. Postganglionic adrenergic axons from these ganglia reach the root of the penis or clitoris by following the associated perineal vasculature.

Parasympathetic innervation of the vasculature and erectile tissue arises in the sacral (S2-S4) spinal cord. Postganglionic axons from neurons in the scattered ganglia of the pelvic plexus join the sympathetic axons entering the penis or clitoris over its root. Nonadrenergic, noncholinergic axons, presumably from cells located in the pelvic ganglia, also innervate the erectile tissue. Somatic motor innervation of the clitoris and penis arises in Onuf's nucleus of the ventral horn of spinal cord segments S2-S4. Their axons travel the course of the pudendal to the perineum where they innervate the following structures, all of which are composed of skeletal muscle:

Bulbocavernosus muscles
Ischiocavernosus muscles
Superficial and deep perineal muscles
External urethral sphincters
Anal sphincters

The sex act requires coordinated viscerosomatic reflexes involving the organs and musculature of the pelvic and perineal region (130). Initially, somatic and/or emotional stimuli activate parasympathetic outflow from the sacral cord to the vasculature of the erectile tissue. The cholinergic fibers activate the release of nitric oxide from endothelial cells, which relaxes the vessel walls and results in increased perfusion of the tissue. Once the erectile tissue is engorged, additional stimuli initiate a sympathetic barrage from the thoracolumbar junction of the cord. This output results in contraction of smooth muscle in the vas deferens in the male and in the walls of the vagina in the female. Coordinated reflex activation of the perineal nerve subsequently results in contraction of the bulbospongiosus, ischiocavernosus, and transverse perineal muscles. The rhythmic contraction of these muscles assists in forcing the ejaculate along the urethra in the male and constricts the vestibule of the vagina in the female. Integration of these three efferent pathways (parasympathetic, sympathetic, and somatic) occurs in the circuitry of the sacral spinal cord segments and is necessary for successful completion of the sex act.

CONCLUSION

The autonomic nervous system is a major factor orchestrating the diverse functions of internal structures. Through an extensive network of connections, the autonomic nervous system helps maintain the normal rhythm of activity in the visceral organs as well as adjust their output to accommodate any external challenge. This conglomerate of interlocking systems, with its pervasive influence on our physiology and psychology, is called the neuroendocrine-immune network. This network is described in more detail in Chapter 8 and in Chapter 9 of the previous edition of this book (139).

REFERENCES

1. Clarke E, Jacyna LS. *Nineteenth-Century Origins of Neuroscientific Concepts.* Berkeley, CA: University of California Press, 1987.
2. McGeer PL, Eccles JC, McGeer EG. *Molecular Neurobiology of the Mammalian Brain.* New York, NY: Plenum Press, 1987.
3. Agnati LF, Bjelke B, Fuxe K. Volume transmission in the brain. *Am Sci* 1992;80:362–373.
4. Prechtl JC, Powley TL. B-afferents: A fundamental division of the nervous system mediating homeostasis? *Behav Brain Sci* 1990;13:289–331.
5. Wang FB, Holst MC, Powley TL. The ratio of pre- to postganglionic neurons and related issues in the autonomic nervous system. *Brain Res Brain Res Rev* 1995;21(1):93–115.
6. Goyal RK, Hirano I. The enteric nervous system. *N Engl J Med* 1996;334(17):1106–1115.
7. Renkin EM. Control of microcirculation and blood-tissue exchange. *Handbook of Physiology.* New York, NY: Oxford University Press, 1984; Sec. 2, Vol. IV:627–687.
8. Harati Y. Anatomy of the spinal and peripheral autonomic nervous system. In: Low PA, ed. *Clinical Autonomic Disorders.* Boston, MA: Little, Brown and Company, 1993:17–37.
9. Freire-Maia L, Azevedo AD. The autonomic nervous system is not a purely efferent system. *Med Hypotheses* 1990;32:91–99.
10. Dockray GJ, Sharkey KA. Neurochemistry of visceral afferent neurons. *Progress Brain Res* 1986;67:133–148.
11. Schott GD. Visceral afferents: their contribution to "sympathetic dependent" pain. *Brain* 1994;117:397–413.
12. Cervero F. Mechanisms of acute visceral pain. *Br Med Bull* 1991;47:549–560.
13. Cervero F. Sensory innervation of the viscera: peripheral basis of visceral pain. *Physiol Rev* 1994;74:95–138.
14. Vanhoutte PM, Shepherd JT. Autonomic nerves of the systemic blood vessels. In: Dyck PJ, Thomas PK, eds. *Peripheral Neuropathy.* Philadelphia, PA: W.B. Saunders, 1993:208–227.
15. Burnstock G. Cholinergic and purinergic regulation of blood vessels. *Handbook of Physiology.* New York, NY: Oxford University Press, 1980; Sec. 2; Vol. II.:567–612.
16. Joyner MJ, Halliwill JR. Sympathetic vasodilatation in human limbs. *J Physiol* 2000;526(3):471–480.
17. Bonica JJ. General considerations of pain in the head. In: Bonica JJ, ed. *The Management of Pain.* Philadelphia, PA: Lea & Febiger, 1990:651–675.
18. Mitchell GAG. The cranial extremities of the sympathetic trunks. *Acta Anat (Basel)* 1953;18:195–201.
19. Bevan JA, Bevan RD, Duckles SP. Adrenergic regulation of vascular smooth muscle. In: Bohr DF, Somlyo AP, Sparks HV, Geiger SR, eds. *Handbook of Physiology.* section 2, The Cardiovascular System: volume II, Vascular Smooth Muscle. Bethesda, MD: American Physiology Society, 1980:515–566.
20. Shepherd RFJ, Shepherd JT. Control of blood pressure and the circulation in man. In: Bannister R, Mathias CJ, eds. *Autonomic Failure.* Oxford, UK: Oxford Medical Publications, 1992:78–93.
21. Joyner MJ, Shepherd JT. Autonomic control of circulation. In: Low PA, ed. *Clinical Autonomic Disorders.* Boston, MA: Little, Brown and Company, 1993:55–67.
22. Kawarai M, Koss MC. Neurogenic cutaneous vasodilation in the cat forepaw. *J Auton Nerv Syst* 1992;37:39–46.
23. Jinkins JR, Whittemore AR, Bradley WG. The anatomic basis of vertebrogenic pain and the autonomic syndrome associated with lumbar disk extrusion. *Am J Roentgenol* 1989;152:1277–1289.
24. Yonehara N, Chen J-Q, Imai Y, et al. Involvement of substance P present in primary afferent neurons in modulation of cutaneous blood flow in the instep of the rat hind paw. *Br J Pharmacol* 1992;106:256–262.
25. Basbaum AI, Levine JD. The contributions of the nervous system to inflammation and inflammatory disease. *Can J Physiol Pharmacol* 1991;69:647–651.
26. Kidd BL, Gibson SJ, O'Higgins F, et al. A neurogenic mechanism for symmetrical arthritis. *Lancet* 1989;2:1128–1130.
27. Gonzales R, Sherbourne CD, Goldyne ME, et al. Noradrenaline-induced prostaglandin production by sympathetic postganglionic neurons is mediated by 2-adrenergic receptors. *J Neurochem* 1991;57: 1145–1150.
28. Levine JD, Fields HL, Basbaum AI. Peptides and the primary afferent nociceptor. *J Neurosci* 1993;13:2273–2286.
29. Keller JT, Marfurt CF, Dimlich RVW, et al. Sympathetic innervation of the supratentorial dura mater of the rat. *J Comp Neurol* 1989;290:310–321.
30. Keller JT, Marfurt CF. Peptidergic and serotonergic innervation of the rat dura mater. *J Comp Neurol* 1991;309:515–534.
31. Stead RH, Dixon MF, Bramwell NH, et al. Mast cells are closely apposed to nerves in the human gastrointestinal mucosa. *Gastroenterology* 1989;97:575–585.
32. Levine JD, Coderre TJ, Covinsky K, et al. Neural influences on synovial mast cell density in rat. *J Neurosci Res* 1990;26:301–307.
33. Levine JD, Dardick SJ, Roizen MF, et al. Contribution of sensory afferents and sympathetic efferents to joint injury in experimental arthritis. *J Neurosci* 1986;6:3423–3429.
34. Hardebo J-E. Activation of pain fibers to the internal carotid artery intercranially may cause the pain and local signs of reduced sympathetic and enhanced parasympathetic activity in cluster headache. *Headache* 1991;31:314–320.
35. Suzuki N, Hardebo J-E. The cerebrovascular parasympathetic innervation. *Cerebrovasc Brain Metab Rev* 1993;5(1):33–46.
36. Suzuki N, Hardebo J-E. Anatomical basis for a parasympathetic and sensory innervation of the intracranial segment of the internal carotid

artery in man. Possible implication for vascular headache. *J Neurol Sci* 1991;104(1):19–31.

37. Spalding JMK, Nelson E. The autonomic nervous system. In: Joynt RJ, ed. *Clinical Neurology*. Philadelphia, PA: JB Lippincott Co., 1986:1–58.

38. Williams PL. *Gray's Anatomy: The Anatomical Basis of Medicine and Surgery*. 38th ed. Edinburgh, Scotland: Churchill Livingstone, 1995.

39. Wilson-Pauwels L, Akesson E, Stewart P. Cranial Nerves: Anatomy and Clinical Comments. Toronto, Ontario, Canada: BC Decker Inc., 1988.

40. Haerer AF. *DeJong's The Neurologic Examination*. 5th Ed. Philadelphia, PA: JB Lippincott Co., 1992.

41. Grundy D. Speculations on the structure/function relationship for vagal and splanchnic afferent endings supplying the gastrointestinal tract. *J Auton Nerv Syst* 1988;22:175–180.

42. Lance JW. Current concepts of migraine. *Neurol India* 1993;43(suppl 3): S11–S15.

43. Ruskell GL. The orbital branches of the pterygopalatine ganglion and their relationship with internal carotid nerve branches in primates. *J Anat* 1970;106:323–339.

44. Suzuki N, Hardebo J-E, Skagerberg G, et al. Central origins of preganglionic fibers to the sphenopalatine ganglion in the rat. A fluorescent retrograde tracer study with special reference to its relation to central catecholaminergic systems. *J Auton Nerv Syst* 1990;30(2): 101–109.

45. Walters BB, Gillespie SA, Moskowitz MA. Cerebrovascular projections from the sphenopalatine and otic ganglia to the middle cerebral artery of the cat. *Stroke* 1986;17:488–494.

46. Hardebo J-E, Suzuki N, Ekblad E, et al. Vasoactive intestinal polypeptide and acetylcholine coexist with neuropeptide Y, dopamine-beta-hydroxylase, tyrosine hydroxylase, substance P or calcitonin gene–related peptide in neuronal subpopulations in cranial parasympathetic ganglia of rat. *Cell Tissue Res* 1992;267(2):291–300.

47. Suzuki N, Hardebo J-E, Owman C. Origins and pathways of cerebrovascular nerves storing substance P and calcitonin gene–related peptide in rat. *Neuroscience* 1989;31:427–438.

48. Moskowitz MA. The neurobiology of vascular head pain. *Ann Neurol* 1984;16:157–168.

49. Diamond S. Head pain. *Clin Symp* 1994;46(3):1–34.

50. Moskowitz MA. Basic mechanisms in vascular headache. *Neurol Clin* 1990;8(4):801–815.

51. Pick J. *The Autonomic Nervous System*. Philadelphia, PA: JB Lippincott Co., 1970.

52. Mitchell GAG. *Cardiovascular Innervation*. London, UK: E&S Livingstone, 1956.

53. Moore KL, Persaud TVN. *The Developing Human*. 6th Ed. Philadelphia, PA: WB Saunders, 1998.

54. Mizeres NJ. The cardiac plexus of nerves. *Am J Anat* 1963;112:141.

55. Standish A, Enquist LW, Schwaber JS. Innervation of the heart and its central medullary origin defined by viral tracing. *Science* 1994;263:232–234.

56. Standish A, Enquist LW, Escardo JA, et al. Central neuronal circuit innervating the rat heart defined by transneuronal transport of pseudorabies virus. *J Neurosci* 1995;15(3):1998–2012.

57. Levy M, Martin PJ. Neural control of the heart. *Handbook of Physiology*. section 2: The Nervous System vol. 1. New York, NY: Oxford University Press, 1979:581–620.

58. Talman WT. The central nervous system and cardiovascular control in health and disease. In: Low PA, ed. *Clinical Autonomic Disorders*. Boston, MA: Little, Brown and Company, 1993:39–53.

59. Baluk P, Gabella G. Some intrinsic neurons of the guinea-pig heart contain substance-P. *Neurosci Lett* 1989;104:269–273.

60. Quigg M, Elfvin L-G, Aldskogius H. Distribution of cardiac sympathetic afferent fibers in the guinea pig heart labeled by anterograde transport of wheat germ agglutinin-horseradish peroxidase. *J Auton Nerv Syst* 1988;25:107–118.

61. Quigg M. Distribution of vagal afferent fibers of the guinea pig heart labeled by anterograde transport of conjugated horseradish peroxidase. *J Auton Nerv Syst* 1991;36:13–24.

62. Hopkins DA, Armour JA. Ganglionic distribution of afferent neurons innervating the canine heart and cardiopulmonary nerves. *J Auton Nerv Syst* 1989;26:213–222.

63. Malliani A, Lombardi F, Pagni M. Sensory innervation of the heart. *Progress Brain Res* 1986;67:39–48.

64. Foreman RD, Blair RW, Ammons WS. Neural mechanisms of cardiac pain. *Progress Brain Res* 1986;67:227–243.

65. Bonica JJ. General considerations of pain in the chest. In: Bonica JJ, ed. *The Management of Pain*. Philadelphia, PA: Lea & Febiger, 1990:959–1000.

66. Ammons WS. Cardiopulmonary sympathetic afferent excitation of lower thoracic spinoreticular and spinothalmic neurons. *J Neurophysiol* 1990;64:1907–1916.

67. Beal MC. Viscerosomatic reflexes: a review. *J Am Osteopath Assoc* 1985;85:786–801.

68. Ruch TC. Pathophysiology of pain. In: Ruch TC, Patton HD, Woodbury JW, et al., eds. *Neurophysiology*. 2nd Ed. Philadelphia, PA: WB Saunders, 1965:345–363.

69. Thurlbeck WM, Miller RR. The respiratory system. In: Rubin E, Farber JL, eds. *Pathology*. Philadelphia, PA: JB Lippincott Co., 1988:542–627.

70. Barnes PJ, Baraniuk JN, Belvisi MG. Neuropeptides in the respiratory tract. Part II. *Am Rev Respir Dis* 1991;144:1187–1198.

71. Barnes PJ. Neurogenic inflammation in the airways. *Respir Physiol* 2001;125(1–2):145–154.

72. Drazen JM, Gaston B, Shore SA. Chemical regulation of pulmonary airway tone. *Annu Rev Physiol* 1995;57:151–170.

73. Bindoff LA, Heseltine D. Unilateral facial pain in patients with lung cancer: a referred pain via the vagus? *Lancet* 1988;1:812–815.

74. Morton DR, Klassen KP, Curtis GM. Clinical physiology of the human bronchi. I. Pain of tracheobronchial origin. *Surgery* 1950;28:669.

75. Sivarao DV, Goyal RK. Functional anatomy and physiology of the upper esophageal sphincter. *Am J Med* 2000;108(suppl 4a):27S–37S.

76. Richards WG, Sugarbaker DJ. Neuronal control of esophageal function. *Chest Surg Clin N Am* 1995;5(1):157–171.

77. Collman PI, Tremblay L, Diamant NE. The central vagal efferent supply to the esophagus and lower esophageal sphincter of the cat. *Gastroenterology* 1993;104(5):1430–1438.

78. Hightower NC. Applied anatomy and physiology of the esophagus. In: Bockus HL, ed. *Gastroenterology*. Philadelphia, PA: WB Saunders, 1974:127–142.

79. Goyal RK, Padmanabhan R, Sang Q. Neural circuits in swallowing and abdominal vagal afferent-mediated lower esophageal sphincter relaxation. *Am J Med* 2001;111(suppl 8A):95S–105S.

80. Collman PI, Tremblay L, Diamant NE. The distribution of spinal and vagal sensory neurons that innervate the esophagus of the cat. *Gastroenterology* 1992;103(3):817–822.

81. Pope CE. Heartburn, dysphagia, and chest pain of esophageal origin. In: Sleisenger MH, Fordtran JS, eds. *Gastrointestinal Disease: Pathophysiology, Diagnosis, Management*. Philadelphia, PA: WB Saunders, 1983:145–148.

82. Bennett J. ABC of the upper gastrointestinal tract: Oesophagus: Atypical chest pain and motility disorders. *Br Med J* 2001;323(7316): 791–794.

83. Bulloch K. Neuroanatomy of lymphoid tissue: a review. In: Guillemin R, Cohn M, Melnechuk T, eds. *Neural Modulation of Immunity*. New York, NY: Raven Press, 1985:111–141.

84. McHale NG. Innervation of the lymphatic circulation. In: Johnston MG, ed. *Experimental Biology of the Lymphatic Circulation*. Amsterdam, The Netherlands: Elsevier Science, 1985:121–140.

85. Benoit JN. Effects of alpha-adrenergic stimuli on mesenteric collecting lymphatics in the rat. *Am J Physiol* 1997;273(1 pt 2):R331–R336.

86. Elaut L. The surgical anatomy of the so called presacral nerve. *Surg Gynec Obst* 1932;55:581–589.

87. Mayer EA, Raybould HE. Role of visceral afferent mechanisms in functional bowel disorders. *Gastroenterology* 1990;99:1688–1704.

88. Jänig W, Morrison JFB. Functional properties of spinal visceral afferents supplying abdominal and pelvic organs, with special emphasis on visceral nociception. *Progress Brain Res* 1986;67:87–114.

89. Paintal AS. The visceral sensations—some basic mechanisms. *Progress Brain Res* 1986;67:3–19.

90. Cervero F, Tattersall JEH. Somatic and visceral sensory integration in the thoracic spinal cord. *Progress Brain Res* 1986;67:189–204.

91. Wood JD. Physiology of the enteric nervous system. In: Johnson LR, ed. *Physiology of the Gastrointestinal Tract*. vol. 1. New York, NY: Raven Press, 1981:1–37.

92. Gabella G. Structure of muscles and nerves in the gastrointestinal tract. In: Johnson LR, ed. *Physiology of the Gastrointestinal Tract.* vol. 1. New York, NY: Raven Press, 1981:197–241.

93. Goyal RK, Crist JR. Neurology of the gut. In: Sleisenger MH, Fordtran JS, eds. *Gastrointestinal Disease.* Philadelphia, PA: WB Saunders, 1989: 21–52.

94. Ottaway CA. Neuroimmunomodulation in the intestinal mucosa. *Gastroenterol Clin North Am* 1991;20:511–529.

95. Schofield GC. Anatomy of muscular and neural tissues in the alimentary canal. In: Code C, ed. *Handbook of Physiology.* Section 6, Alimentary Canal: volume IV, Motility. Bethesda, MD: American Physiology Society, 1968:1579–1627.

96. Fawcett D. *A Textbook of Histology.* 11th Ed. Philadelphia, PA: WB Saunders, 1986.

97. Stark ME, Szurszewski JH. Role of nitric oxide in gastrointestinal and hepatic function and disease. *Gastroenterology* 1992;103:1928–1949.

98. Sanders KM, Ward SM. Nitric oxide as a mediator of nonadrenergic noncholinergic neurotransmission. *Am J Physiol* 1992;262:G379–G392.

99. Blau JN, MacGregor EA. Migraine and the neck. *Headache* 1994;34(2): 88–90.

100. Cervero F. Neurophysiology of gastrointestinal pain. *Bailliere's Best Pract Res Clin Gastroenterol* 1988;2:183–199.

101. Shirasaka C, Tsuji H, Asoh T, et al. Role of the splanchnic nerves in the endocrine and metabolic response to abdominal surgery. *Br J Surg* 1986;73:142–145.

102. Nonogaki K, Iguchi A. Role of central neural mechanisms in the regulation of hepatic glucose metabolism. *Life Sci* 1997;60(11):797–807.

103. Mulholland MW, Debas HT. Diseases of the liver, biliary system, and pancreas. In: Bonica JJ, ed. *The Management of Pain.* Philadelphia, PA: Lea & Febiger, 1990:1214–1231.

104. Osborn JL. Relation between sodium intake, renal function, and the regulation of arterial pressure. *Hypertension* 1991;17(1 suppl):I91–I96.

105. DiBona GF, Wilcox CS. The kidney and the sympathetic nervous system. In: Bannister R, Mathias CJ, eds. *Autonomic Failure.* Oxford, UK: Oxford Medical Publications, 1992:178–196.

106. DiBona GF. Sympathetic neural control of the kidney in hypertension. *Hypertension* 1992;19(1 suppl):I28–I35.

107. DiBona GF, Jones SY. Analysis of renal sympathetic nerve responses to stress. *Hypertension* 1995;25(4 pt 1):531–538.

108. Hollenbreg NK. Renal vascular tone in essential and secondary hypertension. *Medicine* 1975;54:29–44.

109. DiBona GF. Neural control of renal function: cardiovascular implications. *Hypertension* 1989;13:539–548.

110. Barajas L, Powers K. Innervation of the renal proximal convoluted tubule of the rat. *Am J Anat* 1989;186:378–388.

111. Barajas L, Powers K, Wang P. Innervation of the renal cortical tubules: a quantitative study. *Am J Physiol* 1984;247:F50–F60.

112. Insel PA, Snavely MD, Healy D, et al. Radioligand binding and functional assays demonstrate postsynaptic alpha2-receptors on proximal tubules of rat and rabbit kidney. *J Cardiovasc Pharmacol* 1985;7:S9–S17.

113. DiBona GF, Kopp UC. Neural control of renal function. *Physiol Rev* 1997;77(1):75–197.

114. Gottschalk CW. Renal nerves and sodium excretion. *Annu Rev Physiol* 1979;41:229–240.

115. Ammons WS. Renal afferent inputs to the ascending spinal pathways. *Am J Physiol* 1992;262:R165–R176.

116. Ammons WS. Electrophysiological characteristics of primate spinothalamic neurons with renal and somatic inputs. *J Neurophysiol* 1989;61: 1121–1130.

117. Nemeth L, O'Briain DS, Puri P. Demonstration of neuronal networks in the human upper urinary tract using confocal laser scanning microscopy. *J Urol* 2001;166(1):255–258.

118. Santicioli P, Maggi CA. Myogenic and neurogenic factors in the control of pyeloureteral motility and ureteral peristalsis. *Pharmacol Rev* 1998;50(4):683–722.

119. Tahara H. The three-dimensional structure of the musculature and the nerve elements in the rabbit ureter. *J Anat* 1990;170:183–191.

120. Weiss RM. Physiology and pharmacology of the renal pelvis and ureter. In: Walsh PC, Gittes RF, Perlmutter AD, et al., eds. *Campbell's Urology.* Philadelphia, PA: WB Saunders, 1986:94–128.

121. Ansell JS, Gee WF. Diseases of the kidney and ureter. In: Bonica JJ, ed. *The Management of Pain.* Philadelphia, PA: Lea & Febiger, 1990: 1232–1249.

122. Edyvane KA, Smet PJ, Trussell DC, et al. Patterns of neuronal colocalization of tyrosine hydroxylase, neuropeptide Y, vasoactive intestinal polypeptide, calcitonin gene–related peptide and substance P in human ureter. *J Auton Nerv Syst* 1994;48(3):241–255.

123. Smet PJ, Edyvane KA, Jonavicius J, et al. Colocalization of nitric oxide synthase with vasoactive intestinal peptide, neuropeptide Y, and tyrosine hydroxylase in nerves supplying the human ureter. *J Urol* 1994;152(4):1292–1296.

124. Edyvane KA, Trussell DC, Jonavicius J, et al. Presence and regional variation in peptide-containing nerves in the human ureter. *J Auton Nerv Syst* 1992;39(2):127–137.

125. Stewart JD. Autonomic regulation of sexual function. In: Low PA, ed. *Clinical Autonomic Disorders.* Boston, MA: Little, Brown and Company, 1993:117–123.

126. Prieto D, Simonsen U, Martin J, et al. Histochemical and functional evidence for a cholinergic innervation of the equine ureter. *J Auton Nerv Syst* 1994;47(3):159–170.

127. Semenenko FM, Cervero F. Afferent fibres from the guinea-pig ureter: size and peptide content of the dorsal root ganglion cells of origin. *Neuroscience* 1992;47:197–201.

128. Cervero F, Sann H. Mechanically evoked responses of afferent fibres innervating the guinea-pig's ureter: an in vitro study. *J Physiol* 1989;412:245–266.

129. De Groat WC. Anatomy and physiology of the lower urinary tract. *Urol Clin North Am* 1993;20(3):383–401.

130. De Groat WC, Booth AM. Autonomic systems to the urinary bladder and sexual organs. In: Dyck PJ, Thomas PK, eds. *Peripheral Neuropathy.* Philadelphia, PA: WB Saunders, 1993:198–207.

131. Gee WF, Ansell JS. Pelvic and perineal pain of urologic origin. In: Bonica JJ, ed. *The Management of Pain.* Philadelphia, PA: Lea & Febiger, 1990:1368–1394.

132. Taneike T, Miyazaki H, Nakamura H, et al. Autonomic innervation of the circular and longitudinal layers in swine myometrium. *Biol Reprod* 1991;45:831–840.

133. Bulat R, Kannan MS, Garfield RE. Studies of the innervation of rabbit myometrium and cervix. *Can J Physiol Pharmacol* 1989;67:837–844.

134. Thilander G. Adrenergic and cholinergic nerve supply in the porcine myometrium and cervix. A histochemical investigation during pregnancy and parturition. *Zentralbl Veterinarmed A* 1989;36:585–595.

135. Bonica JJ. The nature of pain in parturition. *Clin Obstet Gynecol* 1975;2:499.

136. Kawatani M, Takeshige C, De Groat WC. Central distribution of afferent pathways from the uterus of the cat. *J Comp Neurol* 1990;302: 294–304.

137. Bonica JJ, McDonald JS. The pain of childbirth. In: Bonica JJ, ed. *The Management of Pain.* Philadelphia, PA: Lea & Febiger, 1990: 1313–1343.

138. Bonica JJ, Chadwick HS. Labor pain. In: Wall PD, Melzack R, eds. *Textbook of Pain.* Edinburgh, Scotland: Churchill Livingstone, 1989:482–499.

139. Willard FH, Mokler DJ, Morgane PJ. Neuroendocrine-immune system and homeostasis. In: Ward RC, ed. *Foundations for Osteopathic Medicine.* Baltimore, MD: Williams & Wilkins, 1997:107–135.

11

Physiological Rhythms/Oscillations

Complementary, Alternative, and Integrative Considerations of Biorhythms

THOMAS GLONEK, NICETTE SERGUEEF, AND KENNETH E. NELSON

KEY CONCEPTS

- An oscillation is any periodic vibration relative to an equilibrium position.
- Osteopathic Manipulative Technique (OMT) uses the laws of mechanical physics to generate effective therapeutic intervention.

"Vibration is an accepted fact in science. Solid bodies are composed of atoms which are vibrating at almost infinite velocities. One substance differs from another mainly in the modulus of vibritility, the different planes of substance representing the planes of gradually increasing vibratility. The higher vibratility governs and molds the lower, just as the sun centralizes the solar system. The most refined vibrations that mean life and light with all their accompaniments to the planets in the solar system. In man this vibritile characteristic also predominates, for within his organism he combines the higher and lower grades of vibratility in connection with mind, brain, bone, muscle, blood. So long as these combined vibratilities are in harmony the organism enjoys life and health" (1).

BIOLOGICAL CYCLES

Human physiology is dynamic. It is important to understand this point and keep it in mind when considering physiological phenomena. Everything in living things is changing with time—but not necessarily at the same rate. Keeping everything coordinated is paramount. Moreover, geology/physics impinges upon life processes; the more fit organisms are those that exploit the cycles of the solar system, from the oscillations of planets in their orbits to the vibrations of phospholipids in the cellular membrane.

Holistically, the totality of human physiology may be considered in the context of waves upon waves upon waves, wherein each rhythm or vibrational frequency, although independent, influences and is influenced by those frequencies above and below it. The authors have been working (Fig. 11.1) at physiological frequencies in the range of 0.002 to 0.500 Hz (Hertz, cycles/s), but the total picture is far grander than this.

Cellular Rhythms

A single-celled organism is completely surrounded by its external environment. As such, cellular physiology occurs in the context of that environment. Nutrients are withdrawn from the environment and waste materials are deposited into that same environment. These activities support cellular respiration: The cell exists autonomously. In the single-cell organism, the cell is either subject to the external movements of its environment or it must itself move within the environment in search of nutrients and to keep from being overwhelmed by its own waste products. This relationship between the cell and the environment becomes more complicated in the progression from single cell to multicellular organisms.

Multicellular organisms of higher phyla up to the level of Coelenterata (sponges) are organized in such a way that all of the constituent cells remain in direct contact with the external environment. Organisms of greater complexity contain individual cells that are, of necessity, not in direct contact with the external environment. This creates a new environment that is external to the cell but internal to the organism, thereby necessitating the need to regulate this resultant internal extracellular environment.

Cellular biochemistry demonstrates intrinsic rhythmic activity that creates a need to coordinate with the extracellular environment. The cell is absorbing nutrients and excreting waste products in harmony with its intrinsic biological rhythms. These rhythms dictate the need for similar rhythmicity of nutrient supply and waste transport in the extracellular environment. This can be accomplished by modulating the environment to provide for the needs of the cell or by modifying cellular activity to adjust to the provisions of the extracellular environment.

A component of this extracellular environment is other cells, cells that are nearby and carry out identical functions, and cells that are more distant but that act as integrated components of an organ. Such cells interact through processes of signal entrainment and signal modulation so that they perform as a regulated unit. For some organs, these regulated units exist as specific tissues having well-defined histology, for example the suprachiasmatic nucleus (SCN) in the brain, the atrioventricular node of the heart, the pancreatic ganglia (2). For other organs and systems, for example, smooth muscle, specific tissues have yet to be identified, yet physiological measurements indicate that they exist. Further, these internally regulated units communicate with other units within complex multiorgan systems and also with external signals from the environment; eating, for example, or activities such as singing and Tai Chi Chuan, all known collectively as zeitgebers. Because of this mutual dependency between the cell and the organism and its interaction with the environment, complex physiological rhythms and signaling have developed.

External Time Setters, Zeitgebers

Zeitgeber: Literally, "time-giver" [*zeit* "time" + *geber* "giver," coined by Jürgen Aschoff (3)]. A time cue capable of entraining circadian (and other) rhythms (3,4), it establishes the phase of an oscillating wave and can be used as a synchronizer for systems of waves.

When crowds of pedestrians started using London's Millennium (foot) Bridge, it began to sway from side to side. The pedestrians fell into step with the bridge's oscillations, which amplified them (5). The effect of pedestrian walking, a periodic mechanical cycle, was to entrain the bridge, which then began to entrain additional pedestrians. Later (6) it was determined that amplification of the swing was the result of the way people balance themselves while walking. The bridge had to be closed until it was strengthened with oscillation-damping reinforcements. This is an example of group entrainment of humans through an external mechanical motion. Humans are entrained by the bridge, which synchronizes the ambulatory rhythmic motion of the pedestrians, which in turn amplifies the oscillation of the bridge. [The bridge was modeled mathematically as a weakly damped and driven harmonic oscillator (5).] This is analogous to the amplification of the Traube-Hering wave in humans with incitant Osteopathic Manipulative Technique (OMT) (7,8) and the entrainment of this wave's frequency by baroreceptor outflow (9).

Everything must be synchronized in order that exchanges of energy take place. One must push the swing at exactly the right time to impart additional amplitude for the request "push me higher." The phenomenon is called resonance. This also is the principle behind incitant Osteopathic Manipulative Technique (OMT). This is why Osteopathic Manipulative Technique (OMT) works, because we are using the laws of mechanical physics to generate an effective therapeutic intervention. Cranial Osteopathic Manipulative Technique (OMT) is an exogenous zeitgeber.

Oscillations

An oscillation is any periodic vibration relative to an equilibrium position. As such, oscillations are characterized by:

Frequency: The number of complete oscillations occurring in a given unit of time.
Period: The time required for a complete oscillation or vibration.
Amplitude: The maximum displacement of a wave crest from its equilibrium position.

Period and frequency define the cycle, and amplitude defines the strength (the power).

Oscillating phenomena can regulate mechanical, chemical, physical, and physiological systems having interacting parts. They do so by continually sampling the system to determine the magnitude of an intervention that must be applied in order to maintain the system at equilibrium.

In the steady state, the position of equilibrium is subject to drift unless a corrective force (electrical, chemical, mechanical) is applied to oppose the drift. An oscillation is a dynamic phenomenon that is the result of forces acting upon the system and that provides a way to regulate the system by constantly returning it to the point of equilibrium. It is advantageous for a system to oscillate, because the oscillation provides a stable regulator, a reference point, if you will. Because of uncertainties in the universe, such as the motions of molecules caused by heat, chemical and physical systems lacking a reference will tend to drift and eventually become unstable. Oscillation is a mechanism for maintaining a system at its normative level of activity.

The body consists of multiple systems, each with their own equilibrium. Oscillation allows communication because waves can influence each other through the processes of entrainment, modulation, and phase coherence.

There are three components necessary for a system to oscillate. They are resonance, gain, and positive feedback, and all must be present. Resonance in this context is the ability of something to store energy at a certain frequency. Gain feeds energy into the oscillation at the resonant frequency to make up for inevitable losses. Positive feedback keeps the energy properly timed to reinforce the oscillation. If any one of them is missing or irregularly spread out (called dispersion), oscillation will not occur.

When visualized geometrically, oscillations in two dimensions appear as sinusoidal plots in three dimensions: Envision a train of footballs end to end. Physiological oscillations are usually combinations of sine waves, resulting in complicated looking waveforms (Fig. 11.5).

Rhythms

In rhythms, energy is provided regularly, but is delivered as a series of sharply focused impulses rather than as a smooth sinusoidal change. Usually the amplitudes of these rhythmic "spikes" are fairly uniform; think of the percussion section of an orchestra, or consider a train of neuronal impulses. (One way of looking at impulse trains is to consider them "digital" signals.) For digital signals, timing is everything because the energy is sharply focused. Further, we tend to think of rhythms in terms of slow periodic processes, such as the spinning of the Earth, even though the waveform may be quite sinusoidal, as in "circadian rhythms."

Chronobiology, Chronopharmacology, Chronotherapeutics

Most biological activities fluctuate throughout the day and contribute to a better adaptation to the organism's daily activity; they also are coordinated. During the last 30 years, chronobiology has aimed at studying these biological rhythms, explaining the operant biological mechanisms and (recently) identifying their methods of communication, their crosstalk. Moreover, the description of specific biological rhythm disorders and rhythm problems at the cellular and even the molecular level has prompted the emerging fields of chronopharmacology and chronotherapeutics.

It is all about timing. Where on the clock face are the hands pointing? Is the observed signal leading or trailing? Only when the timing is precisely matched will resonance occur and transfer of information take place.

In 1902, Littlejohn had this to say regarding biological oscillations: "The vital cycle depends upon vibration. Waves of vibration pass along the tissues, especially from the nerves and the brain to and along the muscle tissues. There is no function of the body that does not have peristaltic or rhythmic vibrations. . . . the power of osteopathic treatment occurs from its effect upon physiologic oscillations" (1).

Physiological Oscillations

The periodic physiological phenomena that exist in nature have been quantified, and there is a developing consensus that these rhythms are synchronized (10) from the level of the cell to that of swarms, and from periods of only millisecond duration (11) to rhythms spanning millennia (12). As preposterous as this may sound, it is, nevertheless, logically consistent with the evolution of the genome from its seminal progenitor, LUCA [last universal common ancestor (13)], and its requirement, like all machines, for a master time setter. Moreover, an evolutionary advantage will be imparted to those chromosomes that can time the activities of their organism to exploit the Earth's periods, hence the spur for development of a zeitgeber (3,4,14,15). At this moment, technology is providing the raw data, the objective measurements. From these, then, just as we gaze at a star and from its wiggles deduce the structure of a distant solar system (16), so in analogous fashion we can discern precisely how biological rhythms influence each other and how these rhythms synchronize biological systems (10).

Regarding the existence of a master oscillator intrinsic to all living systems, an important caveat to consider is that while there may be a specific discrete physical structure housing this oscillator, such a structure is not absolutely necessary. It is entirely possible that the mutual synchrony of an organism's oscillations may serve as the organismal reference clock [see "Jenna's clocks" (17)]. This is the concept of metastability in rhythm generation (18,19). The oscillation of electrically coupled pacemaker neurons has been, in fact, computationally modeled and compared successfully with tissue preparations (20).

Still, the idea of running a machine without a reference is uncomfortable. At this writing, the best candidate for a reference timer is the circadian clock residing in the SCN in man (21), yet this oscillator seems inappropriate as a reference, for example, for discerning (22) musical pitch. How do our brains tell us that the various instruments of the orchestra are in tune (23), when the fundamental frequency may be completely absent from the sound that reaches our ears (24)? And why are people all over the world comfortable with the pitch of A set to 440 Hz (25)? [Mozart's tuning fork oscillated at 421.6 Hz; however, Handel's oscillated at 422.5 Hz (26).] Moreover, there are pitch-sensitive neurons in marmoset monkeys that appear similar in pitch perception to humans (27). Could it be that all of life possesses a fundamental reference frequency without which it could not exist?

The circadian clock is referenced to the rotation of the Earth (the circadian zeitgeber), specifically the perception of light (28). The Earth is a good reference. It is stable by virtue of its size and its nearly perfectly circular orbit about the Sun. Successful life forms exploit the circadian cycle to gain evolutionary advantages over less well-adapted organisms.

An alternative reference is the oscillation of the cellular plasma membrane. The membrane is a good reference because all living things contain the same phospholipid components in their bilayer membranes. Further, the membrane oscillates at the high-frequency end of the biological rhythmic spectrum, a good position for a reference oscillator.

As mentioned above, a reference oscillator could result from the mutual synchronization of all oscillators in a living system. And there is another consideration; there apparently is a hierarchy (29) among oscillators in organisms having complex multiorgan systems (30–32). The SCN can entrain the peripheral clocks of the heart, kidney, liver, and pancreas, but, apparently, these peripheral clocks cannot entrain the SCN. "Thus, there may be tissue-specific differences in the molecular composition of the circadian clock, and clock components that have subtle effects on central clock function may play a more prominent role in the regulation of peripheral clocks and vice versa." (29). For a humanistic discourse concerning "who sets the clock and who keeps the time," see Ref. 33.

THE BIOLOGICAL RHYTHMIC SPECTRUM

The frequencies of biological rhythms can be considered in analogy to the electromagnetic spectrum of physics and chemistry, in that there exist frequency ranges where phenomena (and their measurement) occupy essentially nonoverlapping frequency bands that the research community has given convenient descriptive names (see Ref. 34, Table 1.1, p. 2). For example, the electromagnetic spectrum has been partitioned into bands for x-rays, visible light, infrared, and microwaves, among others. Between these bands discrete physical phenomena are fairly rare. These *gaps*, thus, provide convenient dividing points. Considering the biosphere and human physiology, one can devise analogous groupings.

(When a concept is in its infancy, investigators will describe their observations in terms familiar to themselves and usually in the language of their analytical methods. Thus, the electromagnetic spectrum has radio waves and gamma rays, which are studied by very different technologies. Considering periodic phenomena in the realm of biology, these phenomena also are described through a variety of terms that reflect the frames of reference and the analytical procedures of the individual investigators. This will lead to confusion when the same signal is referred to by different names, particularly when these names refer to different physiological functions. The problem is avoided when a specific signal is referred to by its frequency. A signal's frequency is its unequivocal name that does not depend upon the prejudices of investigators. Nomenclature problems are exacerbated, however, when the precision of measurement inadequately resolves adjacent signals. For this reason, there is often ambiguity as to the precise frequency of specific phenomena.)

The frequency range from annual through tenths of a second can be discussed in terms of frequency bands that more or less describe physiologic functions in mammals. Beginning with the low-frequency end, these may be described as follows: Annual/seasonal rhythms, for example, seasonal affective disorder (SAD); menstrual cycle; circadian rhythm, for example, sleep disorders; ultradian rhythms, for example, endocrine and digestive cycles; vasomotor phenomena, for example Traube-Hering waves; cardiac cycles, for example, RR variability, and finally, oscillations of the cellular membrane.

Biological rhythms, however, can be as long as millennia and as short as milliseconds. On the long end, signals are usually manifest as trains of spikes or pulses analogous to drum beat rhythms. On the short end, signals may appear as sinusoidal waves, such as Traube-Hering waves or electroencephalographic (EEG) waves, or as trains of spikes, such as nerve impulse trains or the electrocardiogram (ECG). Regardless of form, their common characteristic is that they are periodic phenomena that can be transformed into a spectrum of frequencies through the mathematical procedure of a Fourier transformation (FT) (Fig. 11.1). The FT converts the time-domain waveform, such as an EEG, into an *X-Y* frequency plot that displays the component signals of a wave along with their frequencies (how fast), their amplitudes (how strong), and their dispersion (how regular). Random oscillations, called noise, and incoherent signals simply produce another spectrum of noise that usually contains little to no useful periodic information.

Clinically, the physician will encounter conditions affecting periodic phenomena having frequencies from annual to fractions of a second. At the beginning of the 21st century, and particularly in the realm of medical science, these are the frequencies that have undergone the most intensive scrutiny.

Biological Rhythm Definitions

A number of terms describing frequency bands within the biological spectrum (defined below) have entered the biological rhythm/oscillation lexicon. Some terms are in common use and well understood as to precise meaning, for example, circadian. Individual research groups working in specific areas favor others, and there is overlap in meaning among investigators.

Geologic time: Pleistocene and Holocene to decades, periodic phenomena.

Annual, biannual, seasonal

Circatrigentan: About every 30 days (once a month).

Infradian (infradian < circadian): Relating to biological variations or rhythms occurring in cycles less frequent than every 24 hours (35).

Circadian: Relating to biological variations or rhythms with a cycle of about 24 hours (35). Circadian time (CT): A standardized 24-hour notation of the phase in a circadian cycle that represents an estimation of the organism's subjective time. CT 0 indicates the beginning of a subjective day, and CT 12 is the beginning of a subjective night. For example, for a nocturnal rodent, the beginning of a subjective night (i.e., CT 12) begins with the onset of activity, whereas for a diurnal species, CT 0 would be the beginning of activity. Bourdon suggested that the term circadian should be used only for endogenous rhythms.

Nyctohemeral: Both daily and nightly (35), restricted to rhythms other than endogenous rhythms.

Ultradian (ultradian > circadian.): Relating to biological variations or rhythms occurring in cycles more frequent than every 24 hours (35) but usually not applied to cardiovascular rhythms in the nominal range of 0.003 to 2.0 Hz, although these frequencies are ultradian.

Nanomechanical oscillatory motion: 1 to 10 kHz (11); cellular oscillations up to 10 kHz are possible (36).

Cycles from Millennia to Years

There is now hard evidence from speleothems (isotopic variations and organics present) for the regular waxing and waning of microorganism populations covering periods of millennia. At least three cycles from 20,000 to 10,000 year BP have been documented (12). Data from oxygen isotope ratios in stalagmites often vary in a cyclic fashion and correlate with marine oxygen isotope cycles and with other records of global climate change (the zeitgeber). At longer time scales, small mammal extinctions and turnover cycles, having periods in the range of 1 to 2.5 million years, correlate well with ice sheet expansions and cooling cycles that affect regional precipitation. It is inferred from more than 200 rodent assemblages from Central Spain that long-period astronomical climate forcing is a major determinant of species turnover [van Dam et al., their Fig. 0 (37)]. Imagine (if you can) what zeitgebers and what processes exist that are capable of regulating life over such gigantic periods of time?

In Illinois, we experience the periodic cicada (17-year locust) (38). Our population, brood XIII, is one of the more spectacular populations in North America in terms of numbers and the timing of their emergence. One of the authors has personally witnessed the ground beneath an old Forest Preserve District oak explode from a condition of no insects visible to no ground visible in less than 30 minutes, as if someone had fired a starting gun—a swarm, on cue, after 17 years, not unlike the synchronous spawning of corals (39). These phenomena are periodic, most certainly; however, their zeitgebers are not yet fully understood nor is their communication with life cycles of higher frequency, although surely such communication must exist.

Annual/Seasonal Cycles

Annual cycles abound. We have all witnessed migrating geese (their zeitgeber appears to be temperature) and migrating monarch butterflies. Bears and other animals hibernate or winter, usually with marked biochemical changes, as seen in frogs and toads (40,41), where the chemical signal for wintering may be phosphodiesters (42) derived from the phospholipids (43). Salmon populations migrate on an annual cycle (individual fish every 3 to 5 years), even when saltwater species have been translocated into fresh water lacking any of the fish's familiar chemical cues (44). Moreover, these Pacific Ocean species, when transplanted into (fresh water) Lake Michigan, migrate and spawn at the same time as their parent Pacific population (mid-September to mid-October). Leaves of deciduous trees fall from the trees. The zeitgeber here is the rapidly diminishing daylight at the autumnal equinox.

Higher vertebrates living outside the tropics compare changes in photoperiod (a daylight duration zeitgeber) with their circadian

clocks to adapt to seasonal changes in environment and to initiate reproductive activity. At the molecular level, light signals initiate coordinated gene-expression events in the brain, and the resultant increased thyrotrophin (TSH) in the pars tuberalis triggers long-day photoinduced seasonal breeding (45).

From the perspective of medicine, sudden cardiac death increases during winter months in both men and women, and the heart rate-corrected QT (QTc) interval exhibits a circadian variation. The question of a seasonal variation in QTc was answered through a retrospective analysis of 24,370 ECGs (46). It was found that the maximum monthly mean QTc interval for men (413 ± 18 ms; $N = 560$; $P < 0.05$) occurred in October, whereas the maximum for women (417 ± 16; $N = 350$; P, N.S.) occurred in March, but the variation for women was not significant. In a similar study of seasonal QT dispersion in 25 healthy subjects, again it was found that the winter dispersion was greatest (66 ± 21 ms) while the spring value was smallest (48 ± 18) (47). Thus, there exists a seasonal signal in heart rate QT interval.

For the human animal, SAD is an affective, or mood, disorder resulting in depressive symptoms in the winter or summer. (The summer condition is referred to as reverse SAD; both conditions mimic dysthymia.) SAD is (at least in part) a circadian rhythm sleep disorder that follows the seasonal darkening at high latitudes that shortens the light component of the circadian rhythm (48,49).

Garai et al. (50) observed seasonality in the occurrence of the first missed menstrual bleeding in perimenopausal women, indicating that human menstrual function is influenced by seasonally varying environmental factors. A similar process, although in the reverse direction, takes place at the start of the reproductive span (51). Seasonal variation in the timing of menarche also has been described, with increased rates during summer and early winter (52). In a historical sample of women born at the end of the 19th century, fecundability, which strongly depends on menstrual function, was higher during late spring and late autumn, and the strength of the variation depended on age.

Monthly Cycles (Circatrigentan Cycles)

The menstrual cycle in humans modulates, or is modulated by, body temperature variability (53). In normally cycling females, the body temperature varies in a predictable manner within the menstrual cycle. This menstrual cycle variation (see Ref. 54, Fig. 1) is well known within clinical medicine, unlike most other sources of temperature variation. It is often factored into temperature interpretations and has been used for fertility planning purposes (53). In the luteal phase of the menstrual cycle, there is a rise in mesor (mean temperature) and a decrease in the amplitude of the circadian temperature rhythm. It is believed, however, that these changes represent corrections over a 4- to 6-day time frame and are not immediate responses to ovulation, thus making them marginally useful for pinpointing ovulation (54). The menstrual cycle variation of a biological rhythm is known as a circamensal rhythm and has a period approximately equal to the length of one menstrual cycle.

Investigators have attributed circamensal rhythms to changes that occur in response to hormone levels during the menstrual cycle. For example, the menstrual cycle is modulated by a diurnal rhythm in free estradiol of four cycles per day (55). In addition, there is a circadian rhythm to serum estriol during late pregnancy (56). The circadian rhythm of body temperature also persists throughout the menstrual cycle. Thus, the menstrual cycle layers one rhythm on top of another existing rhythm (53). The result is a complex modulation of three waveforms.

In another example of a chemical entity acting as an entraining exogenous zeitgeber, this time between individuals, the existence of human pheromones was first suggested by the demonstration that women living together can develop synchronized menstrual cycles under specific conditions (57). The process (in rats) is mediated by two different pheromones (58). In a human study involving students and staff at The University of Chicago, odorless compounds from the axilla of women in the late follicular phase of their menstrual cycles accelerated the preovulatory surge of luteinizing hormone of recipient women and shortened their menstrual cycles. In a reciprocal action, compounds collected later in the cycle (at ovulation) had the opposite effect (59).

Regarding sleep-wake and rest-activity rhythms, the phase of circadian rest-activity rhythm may be modulated by the menstrual cycle; however, the sleep-wake cycle in normally cyclic healthy women does not appear to be affected (60).

Axoplasmic Flow (10 days)

Axoplasmic flow (macromolecules synthesized in hypoglossal nerve cell bodies and conveyed proximodistally in the axoplasm) oscillates with a period of 10 days (see Ref. 61, Fig. 5). This transport of neuronal protein was assessed using radioautography of incorporated tritiated leucine in the innervated muscle.

Circadian Rhythms (Frequency about 1 day, 24 hours)

The Earth's daily rotation about its axis has imposed potent selective pressures on organisms. The fundamental adaptation to the environmental day–night cycle is an endogenous 24-hour clock that regulates biological processes in the temporal domain. This clock coordinates physiological events around local (geophysical) time, optimizing the economy of biological systems and allowing for a predictive, rather than purely reactive, homeostatic control. Circadian clocks contribute to the regulation of sleep and reproductive rhythms, seasonal behaviors, and celestial navigation (62).

So what are the circadian rhythms? They are the external expression of an internal timing mechanism that measures daily time (63). (For light entrainment, see Ref. 28; for a review of light effects on humans, see Ref. 64.)

Circadian rhythms, such as locomotor activity, body temperature, and endocrine release, are regulated by a master pacemaker located in the SCN (65) that has a period of 24.18 hours (66). (For a perspective, see Ref. 67.) The circadian rhythm, which is regulated by the SCN clock, is reset by the environmental light–dark (LD) cycle (28), and this oscillation is called the light-entrainable oscillation (65). "The SCN imposes its rhythm on to the body via three different routes of communication: (a) The secretion of hormones; (b) The parasympathetic; and (c) The sympathetic. Imposed on these routes of communication are feedback loops" (68). The nature of these feedback loops is incompletely understood. They exist, however, as a myriad of dynamically counterbalancing entities, such that the whole reflects an integrated communications web.

The biological circadian clock was believed to be physically located exclusively in the SCN. However, cloning of the clock genes in the late '90s (for genetic and physical mapping, see Ref. 69) revealed that clock genes are expressed and oscillate with a circadian rhythm in each organ or cell, suggesting that each organ or cell has its own internal clock. These clock systems are called the peripheral clocks in comparison with the central clock in the SCN (70).

Concerning the timing of circadian clocks in tissues, fibroblasts from human skin biopsies were examined in culture following treatment with lentivirus containing a circadian promoter of the gene BMALL (71). This promoter directs the protein luciferase to be expressed. When the fibroblasts are infected with the lentivirus, they emit photons of light according to the circadian rhythm of their intrinsic clock. Surprisingly, the periods of the cultured fibroblasts did not depend on the time the biopsy was taken or on the site of the skin biopsy; it did depend on the individual who provided the biopsy [Brown and Schibler, Fig. 2 (71)]. Biopsies provided by all subjects exhibited a mean circadian period of 24.5 hours, however, which was similar to observations of others.

A number of clock genes, for example, Per1, Per2, Clock, Bmal1, Cry1, and Cry2, are expressed in the SCN of the hypothalamus (72,73). Moreover, these genes are expressed not only in the SCN, but also in other brain areas, as well as in peripheral organs (72,74–76). "The intracellular molecular clockwork of the SCN consists of interacting positive and negative transcriptional-/translational-feedback loops" (63). Maemura et al. (70) demonstrated that the CLOCK/BMAL heterodimer transcription factor upregulated 29 genes including transcription factors, growth factors, and membrane receptors and that these showed circadian oscillation.

"For orchestrated circadian timing, the collective SCN synchronizes the timing of slave oscillators, each of which is a multioscillatory entity. Synchronized slave oscillators in turn regulate local rhythms in physiology and behavior. A hierarchical multioscillatory system seems to confer precise phase control and stability on the widely distributed physiological systems it regulates" (77).

Rodents, which have been given an SCN lesion during a restricted-feeding schedule, however, are still able to anticipate mealtimes. This food-anticipatory activity appears to be mediated by the circadian oscillator because entrainment of this activity is limited to the circadian range (22 to 31 hours) (30,31). Thus, there are at least two types of biological clock oscillator: a light-entrainable oscillator, which is found in the SCN, and a feeding-entrainable oscillator the location of which was unknown to Damiola et al. in 2000 (32). Restricted feeding is an entraining signal for peripheral tissues (32,76,78), similar to light for the SCN. Peripheral clock entrainment by brain-driven fasting-feeding cycles allows peripheral tissues to anticipate daily fasting and daily feeding, potentially optimizing processes for food ingestion, metabolism, and energy storage and utilization (76). Such peripheral zeitgebers, however, *do not* entrain the SCN.

The circadian rhythm of mice is entrained by the LD cycle when food is plentiful; however, when access to food is restricted to the normal sleep cycle, mice shift many of their circadian rhythms to match food availability. A key transcription factor is BMAL1, which can be specifically disrupted (76). Restoration of BMAL1 within suprachiasmatic nuclei of the hypothalamus restores light-entrainable, but not food-entrainable, circadian rhythms. Restoration of this gene only in the dorsomedial hypothalamic nucleus, however, restores food entrainment but not light entrainment (79).

For opaque mammals, such as humans, light resets (28,80) the time of the central pacemaker in the SCM via ocular mechanisms, and the SCN clock then synchronizes peripheral oscillators via signal modulations, neuronal connections, or chemical signals. The peripheral clocks of semitransparent organisms, however, can be light entrained directly via nonocular mechanisms (81), as can the peripheral organ clocks of vertebrate tissues (82). Results from zebrafish heart and kidney tissue cultures indicate that the circadian system in vertebrates exists as a decentralized collection of peripheral clocks. Each tissue is capable of detecting light and using that signal as the zeitgeber to set the phase of the clocks they contain (82). Such a capability could impart a survival advantage to semitransparent fish embryos and fry.

Astronauts were examined during protracted space flight (83), where the circadian period (or absence thereof) is artificially established by the shorter orbital period of the space station. Systolic and diastolic blood pressures and heart rate were determined at 24-, 12-, and 8-hour intervals: (a) Systolic blood pressure during sleeping hours showed an unprecedented increase during space flight; (b) The approximately 24-hour circadian rhythms of blood pressure and heart rate shortened during the early stages of space flight, but after 6 months reverted to the established 24-hour flight activity cycle; and (c) Even during space flight, the periodic components of blood pressure and heart rate were preserved.

Regarding the diffusible gas neurotransmitter nitric oxide (NO), there is a circadian oscillation in urinary nitrate and cyclic GMP excretion rates, which are two marker molecules for systemic NO production in healthy humans. NO production is increased in the morning, concomitantly with the morning increase in blood pressure, indicating that NO may buffer blood pressure increase. In hypertension (HT), diurnal variation in these NO markers is absent, suggesting impaired NO formation in HT. The major change in peripheral arterial occlusive disease is an increased nitrate/cyclic GMP ratio, which points to increased oxidative inactivation of NO in this disease (84).

Regarding ocular tissues, there are circadian rhythms in axial elongation and choroidal thickness. Part of the underlying mechanism controlling the rhythm in elongation is the circadian rhythm in scleral proteoglycan synthesis (in isolated tissues) (85). Moreover, in the absence of temporal cues, a 24-hour rhythm in choroidal NO synthesis persists, indicating the presence of a circadian oscillator in the isolated tissue. Peak NO synthesis is coincidental with the peak in choroidal thickness in normal eyes, suggesting that NO might mediate the observed diurnal changes in choroidal thickness (86). [8-Nitro-guanosine 3′,5′-cyclic monophosphate is a new NO messenger that contains an NO_2 group on the purine ring system of (cyclic) GMP. This discovery further illuminates the downstream effects of NO that could be relevant to NO-linked biological responses and diseases (87).]

The Circadian Clock

The zeitgeber (3,4) for the circadian clock is light (28), although with man social zeitgebers also are important (88). The physiological circadian oscillator, however, resides within cells, and it can be relatively simple and remarkably regular. For example, three proteins, KaiA, KaiB, and KaiC [kai, Japanese for cycle; KaiC crystal structure at 2.8 Å resolution (89,90)] were identified as important for the daily activity of the cyanobacterium *Synechococcus elongates*. In a reconstituted system where these three proteins were mixed with adenosine 5′-triphosphate in a test tube, they spontaneously generated sustained oscillations in the phosphorylation state of one of the proteins (91,92).) Mutations in the KaiC protein changed the circadian rhythm in a manner identical to the results obtained in vivo. The oscillations arise from the slow, orderly addition and then subtraction of two phosphates from the KaiC protein. Phosphorylation-dephosphorylation is a well-established mechanism for regulating a protein's function. If the protein is part of a network of interacting factors, then its phosphorylation status may relay information that affects some cell behaviors.

Reversible phosphorylation usually occurs on a time scale of seconds or minutes and seems poorly suited for a clock ticking once a day; however, KaiC is phosphorylated at two sites and in a particular order: first on a threonine residue and then on a serine. Subsequently, the threonine and then the serine are dephosphorylated,

and the KaiC protein returns to the unphosphorylated state. The KaiA protein regulates these transitions by promoting autophosphorylation and inhibiting autodephosphorylation by KaiC.

It is known that phosphorylation-dephosphorylation by itself does not create an oscillator; however, in this zeitgeber system, the serine-phosphorylated form of KaiC (S-KaiC) binds stoichiometrically to both KaiA and KaiB. The formation of the three-protein complex prevents KaiA from activating KaiC phosphorylation. Thus, when the concentration of S-KaiC is high, KaiA is sequestered by S-KaiC and KaiB, and KaiC dephosphorylation predominates. When S-KaiC is low, KaiA is released and KaiC phosphorylation is activated. The rate that the clock ticks is, thus, regulated by the rate of a chemical reaction, which depends on the concentration of a key reactant—simple but elegant physical chemistry.

Although eukaryotic oscillators do not appear to operate the same way, and none have the three protein KaiA, KaiB, KaiC system, the design principles of the two oscillators are quite similar. Both circuits include double-negative-feedback loops that mitigate function as bistable triggers, and both include slow negative-feedback loops (63,77) for tunability and robustness (93). Robustness and tunability are essential elements of oscillatory systems, be they gene circuits or circadian clocks. We now have the ability to generate such oscillators in synthetic biological systems (94–96).

A feature of circadian clocks in both animals and plants is the incorporation of feedback loops. In plants, cyclic adenosine diphosphate ribose modulates the circadian oscillator's feedback loops and drives circadian oscillations of Ca^{++} release (97). In mice, phosphorylation by nutrient-responsive AMP-activated protein kinase enables the clock component cryptochrome to transduce nutrient signals to circadian clocks (98,99).

[Using DNA microarray technology, which is facile and rapid, temporal patterns of gene expression may be determined in whole organisms. Applied to the yeast cell cycle, Holter et al. (100) characterized the patterns of gene expression as consisting of two sinusoidal modes, each with a period of 2 hours, and about 30 minutes out of phase. Plotting the weights of these two functions for each gene monitored provides a graphical representation of the sequence that genes turn on and off. This clock mechanism operates at the level of gene expression; its action can be expected to modulate the activity of all other clock mechanisms by regulating the availability of clock proteins. The authors state, "…the complex 'music of the genes' is orchestrated through a few simple underlying patterns of gene expression change."]

The Redox State and Circadian Rhythms

"The concept that circadian rhythmicity and redox state are necessarily and intimately linked is widely accepted" (101). The relationships among cyclical melatonin production, oxidative stress, and circadian rhythms in a variety of organisms have been discussed at length (102).

The sirtuins, which are a highly conserved family of NAD^+ enzymatic silencing factors, have been connected to activities that encompass cellular stress resistance, genomic stability, tumorigenesis, and energy metabolism (103). SIRT1 (one family member) directly modifies core components of the circadian clock machinery, thus, for the first time, linking enzymatic genomic regulation with at least one established biorhythm (104,105).

Circadian Rhythms and Mental Health

A link between the circadian oscillation and Seasonal Affective Disorder (SAD) has been established, providing a proof of principle that circadian rhythms that are out of sync could underlie some mood disorders. Psychiatrists working with small patient groups have shown that correcting abnormal circadian rhythms can treat these disorders and also can benefit patients with neurodegenerative diseases, such as Alzheimer's. "The circadian model is clearly beginning to bear fruit," says David Avery, a psychiatrist at the University of Washington School of Medicine in Seattle. "It is logically getting extended beyond SAD and should lead to better treatments for a number of psychiatric disorders (48)."

Further, and logically, irregularities in higher frequency rhythms that are synchronized with the circadian rhythm, or that originate in the same neurological networks as the circadian rhythm, also may adversely impact mental health, and, conversely, treatment of such rhythmic irregularities may benefit mental well being. For example, humans can be classified as "larks," who are at their best in the morning, and "owls," who are more effective at night. In industrialized societies, it has been suggested that people suffer from "social jet lag" because their innate circadian rhythms or chronotypes are out of phase with their daily schedule (106).

Stem Cells

"Haematopoietic stem cell (HSC) release is regulated by circadian oscillations." (107) The number of HSC progenitors oscillated in synchrony with a steady-state, 12-hour light/12-hour dark cycle, peaking 5 hours after initiation of light (Zeitgeber time, ZT5) and reaching the nadir at ZT17 ($P = 0.005$). The number of HSCs in the circulation (mice) at ZT5 is twofold to threefold that at ZT17. "These results suggested that photic cues, processed in the central nervous system, could influence the trafficking of HSCs in unperturbed steady-state animals." HSC release is triggered by rhythmic expression of Cxcl12 in the bone marrow.

Ultradian Rhythms (Frequency Restricted Here to Higher Than 1/24 hours but Lower Than 1/minute

Definition: The Traube-Hering-Mayer (THM) oscillation, respiration, the cardiac rhythm, the pulse, the activity of neurons, the oscillation of the cellular membrane, and the angular velocity of molecular motors all exhibit ultradian rhythms. For the purpose of this work and in deference to current usage in the biomedical literature, we define the ultradian band to be that set of frequencies lying between the circadian band (once per 24 hours) and the low-frequency THM oscillation of hemodynamics (once per minute).

In analogy with the response of luteinizing hormone and follicle-stimulating hormone to pulsatile administration of gonadotropin-releasing hormone, an ultradian pulsatile secretory pattern has been described for all the classic fuel-regulatory hormones, including insulin, glucagon, growth hormone, cortisol, and epinephrine (see Ref. 108, for a review). The dominant signal for cortisol exhibited a period of one cycle per 80 to 90 minutes; a second signal with a power approximately 50% of the dominant signal occurred at a frequency of 240 min/cycle (see Fig. 2 of Ref. 108). Examining normal subjects, Sonnenberg et al. (109) found that the ultradian insulin secretion pulses with a periodicity of 75 to 115 minutes. In the in vivo canine pancreas, a nicotine-stimulated insulin release (period 7.6 ± 0.6) was blocked by the postsynaptic nicotinic receptor antagonist α-bungarotoxin, providing evidence that pancreatic ganglia may have a role in the generation of oscillatory hormone release (2). Insulin secretion has a common pacemaker (the hypothalamus) or a mutually entrained pacemaker with the cardiovascular, autonomic, and neuroendocrine systems (110).

The contractile lymphatic elements of the bat *Myotis lucifugus* can generate as high as 6 to 8 mm Hg pulsatile pressure at a rate of nine contractions per minute [0.15 Hz, measured in the wing by light microscopy at 640× (111)]. Lymph flow in the thoracic duct (anaesthetized and unanesthetized adult sheep) was determined by ultrasound transit time flow and found to be 5.2 ± 0.8 per minute. The prominent pulsatile signal has no relation to heart or respiratory rates (see Ref. 112, Fig. 2). The human leg generates pulses ranging from 1 to 9 per minute, with an average of 4 per minute. "Each pulse wave lasted for six to eight seconds—in most cases for six seconds" (113).

The nasal cycle [the phenomenon of relative nostril dominance (114)] exhibits a cycle that varies between 2 and 8 hours among subjects, with an average value of about 3 hours (115).

Skin-surface properties revealed, in addition to the circadian rhythm [forehead, forearm, shin (116,117)], ultradian (harmonic) cycles of 12 and 8 hours [face and forearm (117)]. Transepidermal water loss revealed a bimodal circadian rhythm with two peaks located at 08:00 and 16:00 along with the 12 and 8 hour harmonics. The 8-hour cycle also was detected for sebum excretion. The 12- and 8-hour signals were not detected for measurements of skin capacitance, pH, or temperature (117). Although not specifically reported by the authors, an 8-hour harmonic is apparent in the control record from the transmeridian (Chicago/Cologne) diurnal excretion pattern of 17-hydroxycorticosteroids [see Ref. (118), Fig. 1, top chart].

Autonomic Rhythms (Frequency Range 0.66/h to 30/min; 0.0004 to 0.5 Hz)

In 1942, using simultaneous pneumoplethysmographie of the tips of the fingers and toes and the posterosuperior portion of the pinna, Burch et al. (119) were able to differentiate five types of pressure waves (pulse wave, respiratory wave, and α, β, and γ waves) and obtain relative quantification of the contribution of each signal to that of the total waveform. In later work (120), these signals are attributed to the pulse, respiration, the 0.1 Hz oscillation [α, associated with the baroreflex and often referred to as the Mayer wave (121,122)], and a signal at about 0.02 Hz [β, associated with the thermoreflex (9,123)]. The γ wave varied in frequency from 1 to 8 per hour, with a mean value of 40 minutes (119); it has no assigned physiological function. (One half-cycle of this wave can be seen as the baseline slope in Figure 11.7.) Considering the plant Kingdom, the NADH oxidase activity of soybean plasma membranes oscillates with a temperature-compensated period of 24 minutes (124).

The 0.1 Hz oscillation exhibits the same frequency range as the cranial rhythmic impulse (CRI) and exhibits a characteristic sinusoidal waveform (Fig. 11.1) that may be determined through a wide range of instrumental methods: Plethysmography (119), photoelectric plethysmography (123), transcranial bioimpedance (125,126), NADH fluorescence and reflectance spectrophotometry (127,128), functional MRI (129,130), infrared (from acupuncture needles) (131), ultrasound (132,133), cranial bone movement (125,134), pulsatile (2 MHz) echo-encephalography (135), and including the sphygmometry of Louisa Burns (see Ref. 136, last figure, p. 59). Of particular importance among these studies are those involving brain cortical reflectance, where the oscillation was recorded in the absence of blood flow (127,128). Imaging of scattered and reflected light from the surface of neural structures can reveal the functional architecture within large populations of neurons. These techniques exploit, as one of the principal signal sources, reflectance changes produced by local variation in blood volume and oxygen saturation related to neural activity. It was found that a major source of variability in the captured light signal was a pervasive 0.1 Hz oscillation (137). Our work utilizing flowmetry to assess the signals in this band in the context of cranial osteopathy is presented below under the heading, "Osteopathic Manipulative Medicine and the Traube-Hering-Mayer Waveform."

With respect to the baroreflex in cardiac physiology, two mechanisms are invoked to explain rhythms of arterial pressure and RR interval occurring between 0.003 and 0.05 Hz (β signal, 0.18 to 3/min); the first of these is thermal regulation. This signal can be entrained by very-low-frequency thermal stimulation (such as alternating immersion of the arm in warm and cold water) (138). Based upon such data, Hyndman (138,139) suggested that they reflect thermoregulation, and Eckberg (140) agrees. There are no published data, however, to indicate whether human core temperature fluctuates spontaneously at these frequencies.

In a second proposed mechanism, RR interval rhythms are modulated by the renin-angiotensin-aldosterone system (141). Angiotensin-converting enzyme blockade augmented these RR rhythms in postinfarction patients (142); similar results were obtained using healthy volunteers (143). The incitant cranial manipulative procedure of bilateral temporal bone rocking specifically augments the low-frequency signal at 0.1 Hz (8). During the CV-4 procedure, the 0.1 Hz signal is suppressed until the still point is achieved. Upon release by the physician, this signal rebounds to levels significantly greater than that determined for the pre-treatment control (144). "This response to CV4 as measured by the laser-Doppler flowmeter was mirrored in the changes seen in heart rate variability" [from poster (145)]. Heart rate variability calculated from the ECG and the cardiac component of the flowmetry record demonstrated a correlation of 0.97 (P < 0.00, reflecting flowmetry's ability to detect RR interval with accuracy. The "Traube-Hering component of the laser-Doppler-flowmetry wave (0.08 to 0.15 Hz), when compared with the low-frequency component of ECG/heart-rate-variability (0.08 to 0.15 Hz), demonstrated a correlation of 0.712 (P = 0.00); this reflects simultaneous changes between the Traube-Hering component of the laser-Doppler-flowmetry wave and heart rate variability" (146). The RR interval also is entrained by the circadian rhythm (147), and is modulated by the liver (63,148) and kidney (63) peripheral clocks, blood pressure (83), and NO synthesis (84). (More under "Entrainment.")

Power spectral analysis of the RR interval in heart rate yields two prominent and well-characterized signals, the low-frequency domain signal (0.08 to 0.12 Hz) and the high-frequency domain signal (0.23 to 0.27 Hz). These signals provide an index of cardiac vagal activity (149). For example, after 15 days bed rest in a 6-degree head-down tilt position (N = 8 subjects), the spectral power of both signals was reduced approximately 50% (P = 0.012 and 0.017), with essentially no difference in the ratio of low- to high-frequency signals, which is an index indicative of cardiac sympathetic activity (P = 0.49) (150). The authors concluded that prolonged head-down-tilt bed rest reduced cardiac vagal activity, while changes in cardiac sympathetic activity were indistinguishable.

In a spectral power analysis involving systolic pressure, RR interval, and capillary blood flow, the prominent signal in this spectral band was found to lie in the region between 0.05 and about 0.2 Hz (3 to 12/min, centered at 0.1 Hz) in subjects having a resting breathing rate of 18/min (0.25 to 0.35 Hz). One hypothesis explains this signal as representing a simple cause-and-effect arterial baroreflex mechanism. A competing hypothesis attributes this signal to a "resonance," with the periodicity dictated by the time constants of norepinephrine release, vascular responses, and dissipation of vascular effects. The *frequency* of this signal does not appear to entrain with circadian or ultradian rhythms; however, the signal's *amplitude* does follow a circadian oscillation (147). Note that with borderline hypertensive subjects, the 0.1-Hz wave is shifted to lower frequencies (0.084 Hz/d) and displays a marked circadian frequency modulation (0.075 Hz, night). The lowered frequency observed with borderline hypertensive subjects is indicative of an increased risk for developing essential HT (151).

The influence of three types of breathing (spontaneous, frequency controlled [0.25 Hz], and hyperventilation with 100% oxygen) and apnea on RR interval, photoplethysmographic arterial pressure, and muscle sympathetic rhythms was determined (152). Coherence among the detected signals (0.05 to 0.5) varied as functions of both frequency and time. The mode of breathing did not influence these oscillations, and they persisted during apnea. The data document the independence of these rhythms from the respiratory activity and suggest that the close correlations that may exist among arterial pressures, RR intervals, and muscle sympathetic nerve activity at respiratory frequencies result from the influence of respiration on these measures rather than from arterial baroreflex physiology. The results indicated that correlations among autonomic and hemodynamic rhythms vary over time and frequency, and, thus, are facultative rather than fixed. We, however, do not agree with this interpretation but consider signal coherence a regulatory mechanism that if disrupted stimulates network components to create corrective responses.

Feedback loop mechanisms for generating the 0.1-Hz oscillation independent of zeitgeber regulation from the cerebral cortex fail to address the work of Dóra and Kovách (127). Their observed slowing of cortical oscillations (observed using fluorometric techniques directly assessing the cortex) by pentobarbital resembled the effects of barbiturates on cortical P_{O_2} and blood flow oscillations described by others (153,154). This suggests an underlying energy-dependent mechanism. The occasional absence of blood volume cycles during *persistent* cyt aa_3 redox fluctuations (in unanesthetized cats), and the complete postbarbiturate abolition of blood volume oscillations during *continued persistent* cortical cyt aa_3 oscillations, "strongly suggest that the cyclic increases in cortical oxidative metabolism represent the primary oscillatory process, followed by reflex hemodynamic changes." (128). Our prejudice is that there exists a 0.1-Hz oscillator and that it is located in the brain, perhaps in the SCN. Moreover, it is the amplitude of this signal and its dispersion that may be affected by cranial manipulation, but not its central frequency. Yet, although there is strong evidence for a central oscillator as the generator for the 0.1-Hz oscillation, there also is strong evidence supporting a resonance phenomenon (155,156) in the baroreceptor reflux loop (157). The matter, therefore, must be considered unresolved as of this writing.

Neurons, Impulse Trains (Frequencies up to 30 Hz)

The EEG record may be used to produces a plot of brain electrical activity, which in its simplest form is displayed as a time-domain plot of energy (voltage) as a function of time. The data also may be processed into two-dimensional brain plots or transformed via a FT procedure, into frequency-domain plots analogous to that presented in Figures 11.10 and 11.13. The raw EEG is usually described in terms of frequency bands: delta < 4 Hz; theta, 4 to 8 Hz; alpha, 8 to 12 Hz; beta, 12 to 36 Hz; and gamma >36 Hz. These bands, which represent the summed output of brain electrical activity at the position on the skull of the sensing electrode, can be used to assess the functional state of the brain and to document pathologies.

Employing the above EEG system of bands, Werntz et al. (158) demonstrated that relative changes of electrocortical activity have a direct correlation with changes in relative nostril dominance (the nasal cycle). In this cycle, the efficiency of breathing alternates predominantly through the right or the left nostril with a periodicity ranging from 25 to greater than 200 minutes. A relatively greater integrated EEG value in one hemisphere correlates ($P < 10^{-6}$) with predominant airflow in the contralateral nostril, establishing an interrelationship between cerebral dominance and peripheral autonomic nervous function.

Crosstalk between EEG bands, manifested as phase entrainment and amplitude modulation, has been documented (159). When low-frequency visual stimuli are presented at an appropriate rate, the low-delta band EEG oscillations of the cortex [~1.3 Hz (160)] entrain to the low-frequency stimulus, and the higher cortical frequencies (30 to 70 Hz gamma-band neuronal oscillations that appear integral to visual attention) are modulated in phase with the low-frequency band. A key functional property of these oscillations is the rhythmic shifting of excitability in local neuronal ensembles. It has been demonstrated (159) that when the stimuli are in a rhythmic stream, the delta-band oscillations in the primary visual cortex entrain to the rhythm of the stream, resulting in increased response gain for task-relevant events and decreased reaction times. Through hierarchical crossfrequency coupling, the delta phase also determines momentary power in higher-frequency activity. Consequently, cells become most excitable at the times when the stimulus is expected.

Regarding neuronal network processes, such as perception, attentional selection, and memory, gamma oscillations of the hippocampus split into distinct high- and low-frequency components that differentially couple to inputs from the medial entorhinal cortex, an area that provides information about an animal's current position, and a hippocampal subfield essential for storage of such information. These two types of gamma oscillation occur at different phases of the theta rhythm and mostly on different theta cycles. The results suggest routing of information as a possible function of gamma frequency variations in the brain and provide a mechanism for temporal segregation of information from different sources (161).

Thirteen examples of regular SCN cellular oscillations are shown by van den Pol and Dudek (162) in their treatise on communication within the SCN. Their Figure 3A illustrates a regular period of 100-ms pulses obtained from SCN slices. By contrast, calcium-induced oscillations in these same tissues exhibit a period of about 20 seconds, while glutamate induces calcium waves having a period of about 35 seconds.

Bendor and Wang (27) demonstrate the existence of neurons in the auditory cortex of marmoset monkeys that respond to both pure tones and missing fundamental harmonic complex sounds having the same fundamental pitch, providing a neural correlate for pitch constancy. These pitch-sensitive neurons are located in a low-frequency cortical region near the anterolateral border of the primary auditory cortex, and this finding is consistent with the location of a pitch-sensitive area identified in humans (163).

The Cellular Envelope (Frequency ≥1.6 kHz)

Cellular movements are generated at the molecular level by protein molecules that convert chemical energy into mechanical work (36). Prominent examples are the linear (164,165) and rotational motors (166) of eukaryotic cells. The linear motors are specialized to work by interacting with paired filaments of the cytoskeleton. Myosin motors generate motion along actin filaments, while kinesin and dynein motors move along microtubules (164,165). In certain situations, cells can generate oscillatory motion. The periodic motions of cilia and flagella are examples of such mechanical oscillation. The common structural feature of these cilia and flagella is the axoneme, a well-conserved machine composed of microtubule doublets organized in a cylindrical fashion. The activity of the dynein molecular motors coupled to the microtubules leads to periodic bending deformations and waves. Note that these waves are motions at the molecular level, very small relative to the macroscale of ordinary objects, so their frequencies can be expected to be very high.

The cellular wall of living *Saccharomyces cerevisiae* (baker's yeast), the only organism for which the vibration of the cellular envelope has been measured, oscillates at 1,600 Hz on the high end of its frequency range [range: 0.8 to 1.6 kHz (11)]. This is a fundamental oscillation at the level of a single cell; it is energy dependent and can be blocked by metabolic inhibitors. The magnitude of the forces observed suggests that concerted nanomechanical activity is operative in the cell. The authors believe "The observed motion may be part of a communication pathway or pumping mechanism by which the yeast cell supplements the passive diffusion of nutrients and/or drives transport of chemicals across the cell wall."

The plasma membrane of the animal cell ought to behave similarly, although its fundamental frequency could be considerably greater, since the animal cell in not constrained by a rigid cell wall. The spring constant of the animal membrane is approximately 0.002 N/m, that of the yeast 0.06 N/m, a difference of 30-fold, which conceivably could permit an oscillation as high as 54 kHz for the animal membrane, only 10-fold less than the commercial AM radio band. This cellular oscillation is an excellent candidate for an endogenous zeitgeber at the cellular level. It resides at the high end of the biological spectrum, which is an excellent position for a reference frequency, particularly if cellular membrane oscillations may be entrained, as in "brainwave synchronization," increasing net signal power. But that is another story (167).

The Integument as Antenna (Frequency Gigahertz)

Sweat ducts are capable of picking up 100-GHz radiation, the extremely high-frequency range lying between microwaves and terahertz radiation (168). This antenna behavior arises from the helical shape of the ducts. The ducts, which are filled with an electrolyte, act like coils of wire, that is, an inductance that resonates with radiation across the millimeter and submillimeter wavelength band. This helical antenna array makes skin a kind of biological metamaterial, in which the array's response to electromagnetic radiation is determined by physiological structure rather than composition. The spectral response has been correlated to physiological stress (see Ref. 168, Fig. 5).

ENTRAINMENT

Entrain: To mount a movement. Webster's: the process of carrying along or over (169). And what is carried along? Information is carried along.

Oscillations in Biological Communications

The scientist thinking about observations makes productive use of quiet time. In 1665, the Dutch physicist and inventor of the pendulum clock, Christiaan Huygens, was confined to his room by a minor illness. With nothing to do, he observed two of his clocks that were suspended by a common support and noted that they were locked in perfect synchrony and remained that way. Even if one was stopped and restarted out of phase with the other, synchrony would be regained shortly. Only if they were relocated to opposite sides of the room could the lockstep of their pendulums be disrupted. Thus was initiated a subbranch of mathematics: Theory of coupled oscillators. The Universe has ample examples of coupled oscillators: The realm of biology is particularly so (10). In the life sciences, in phenomena observed in medicine, oscillators appear to communicate through three basic modes: synchrony, commonly referred to as entrainment; modulation, our familiar AM and FM radio; and timing or phase.

Entrainment

Entrainment (synchrony) is what Huygens observed, oscillators in lockstep. The oscillators in this coupled system have the same frequency and the same phase. (They are each at the same point in their cycle. Imagine a wall full of identical clocks, each with its pendulum making the same angle with its clockwork, the wall, and the floor.) Groups of cells in local tissue clocks tick this way.

Should one cell fall off the pace, small corrective forces bring it back into synchrony at the mean frequency of the aggregate, the center-band output. How well the cellular aggregate does this is reflected in the amplitude and dispersion of the output signal at the mean frequency of the clock.

Amplitude (the power of the signal) is a measure of the strength of each component signal and the number of component signals in the aggregate. Further, it is a measure of signal dispersion, that is, how close is the frequency of each component oscillator to the mean frequency? And, additionally, how close is the phase of each oscillator to the mean phase of the aggregate? (They are at the same frequency, exactly, but have they fallen behind or are they running ahead, i.e., where on the circumference of a circle do they lie, and how close to the resultant vector do they lie?) The closer the component frequencies are matched AND the closer the component oscillator phases are matched, the greater will be the signal power at the center-band frequency and the narrower will be the signal width at half-height. [See the luminescent algae figure of Ref. 10, also digital entrainment with fireflies (170).] Regulation, that is, entrainment, is easy to observe in a power spectrum (120,141): A regulated signal rises well above the background noise, is narrow relative to the other signals in its band, and, at the apex of the signal, exhibits a well-defined frequency. Poorly regulated signals, by contrast, exhibit low signal to noise, are broad, sometimes to the point of being undetectable. Their center-band frequency may be difficult or impossible to locate or may exhibit multiple peaks (fine-structure). Such characteristics indicate loss of control, or decoupling of the coupled oscillators. These traits are exhibited by the respiratory (signal 3) and heart rate (signal 4) frequency peaks in Figure 11.1.

Coupled oscillators may exhibit continuous-wave (analog) properties, such as circadian cycles, digestive cycles, or low-frequency blood pressure (Traube-Hering) waves, or they may be pulsatile (fireflies, crickets chirping, neurons communicating via action potentials). Southeast Asian fireflies actually synchronize after individual flies begin flashing using a random-flash pattern. Subsequently, the male fireflies are entrained by their mutual light emissions to about three times every two seconds (170). Mathematically, continuous systems are easier to deal with than pulsatile systems; however, there now are mathematical tools for dealing with both systems (171).

Tissue Entrainment

A consensus is emerging that every living cell has a clock. This intrinsic clock times cellular events. Further, it can be entrained,

that is, reset, by a signal (physical, chemical, or electrical) external to the cell. Cells organized into tissues may mutually entrain themselves to generate an output signal of amplified power for the purpose of regulating an organ or set of organs. Such cells in the tissues of higher organisms may be entrained by the cellular milieu, which is external to individual component cells but internal to the organism. All cells can be entrained by the ecosystem in which they or their parent organism resides. The ecosystem signal may act directly on individual cells, for example, light through a transparent zebrafish juvenile, or indirectly through a signal transducing system, such as the photoreceptors and neurons of optical tissues in vertebrates. Moreover, bacteria have now been genetically engineered to coordinate their molecular timepieces (172). Cells in tissues also can be entrained by other signal generating tissues. Thus, our thermal regulating system and our blood pressure follow our circadian clock, and the RR interval in heart rate can be entrained by respiration.

Modulations, Mechanisms for Communication

An oscillating (periodic) wave can be varied in order to convey a message. For example, the sound of a trombone (the carrier wave form) may be varied in volume (amplitude), timing (rhythm, beat), and pitch to convey a musical message that is detected by our ears and processed by our brains. Ordinarily (but not necessarily always), a high-frequency sinusoid waveform, usually the highest frequency in any system, is used as a carrier signal. The three (key) signal parameters of amplitude ("volume"), phase ("timing"), and frequency ("pitch") are modified through interaction with a (usually) lower-frequency information signal to obtain the modulated signal. On the receiving side, a demodulator performs an inverse operation on the modulated signal to retrieve the original information. The information can be high or low frequency, coherent or incoherent in phase or not, and analog or digital in format.

In amplitude modulation, the frequency of the carrier waveform does not change but its strength varies with the modulating signal. Arterial pressure is modulated by the RR interval (140). In cranial treatment, manipulation amplifies the 0.1 to 0.2 Hz waveform in bloodflow velocity (8,144,173).

In frequency modulation, the strength of the carrier wave remains constant but the frequency of the carrier wave is changed. An identified 21% change of frequency of the 0.1 to 0.2 Hz waveform in bloodflow velocity (120,174) and heart rate variability (141) are examples of frequency modulation.

Phase modulation, which is modulation of the timing of the onset of a waveform with respect to a second waveform of the same amplitude and frequency, also is of considerable interest. The best example in biology is the phenomenon of jetlag, which involves resetting the phase of the circadian rhythm with respect to the destination's meridian following long-distance jet travel (175,176). The phase shifts of human biological rhythms observed in aircrews operating transoceanic routs are well documented (118,175–178); measurements have been recorded of sleep, fatigue, EEG, EMG, temperature, ECG, urine constituents, catecholamines, as well as outcomes records, including self-ratings, performance evaluations, sleep logs, and the Stanford Sleepiness Scale (179).

In digital modulation, a digital bit stream of either equal length signals or varying length signals modulates an analog carrier wave, and there are a multitude of digital modulation techniques. In a *hypothetical* scenario, nerve axon impulse trains could modulate the kHz signal of the cell membrane. We are not aware of any documented example of digital modulation in biology. The phenomenon, however, is possible, and, further, it would not be restricted to communication within a single organism, since the kHz frequencies of cell membranes are high enough for effective long-distance communication through empty space. Perhaps outliers like that reported in Michie and West (167) should be reconsidered with new experimentation.

Crosstalk Among Oscillators

Circadian rhythm is entrained externally by the daily LD cycle, a geological zeitgeber (3,4,28,80). Circadian rhythm in turn modulates ultradian rhythms, including the low-frequency rhythms of cardiovascular physiology. Normal cardiac sinus arrhythmia demonstrates circadian modulation as does digestive physiology involving liver, pancreas, and gastrointestinal rhythms. It is of interest to note that cellular level oscillations occur at, and are linked to, low-frequency vascular rhythms (127–129,180,181). Ultradian rhythms with similar frequencies entrain, and thereby amplify, one another. Low-frequency cardiovascular rhythms may be entrained by respiratory rate (122,182–184), including singing and chanting (185,186) and rhythmic postural change (9,187), including Tai Chi Chuan (188).

In vertebrates, the genesis of essential biological rhythms as widely separated in frequency as circadian and cardiac rhythms demand stability, yet the population of multiple local oscillators that generate these rhythms, the cells of an organ, for example, may be dispersed in intrinsic frequencies. This raises the question of how the constituent oscillators interact so that a stable population rhythm emerges. The evidence shows that, even outside the intrinsic frequency range of individual oscillators, a periodic input across a wide frequency range can produce a stable population rhythm. This feature arises from interactions at the single oscillator level, which with their intrinsic frequency spread confers the population with metastability for rhythm genesis (19).

In a study of 10 musically trained and untrained subjects where breathing was correlated to the rhythmic beat of a melodic line, the "data advance(d) the following hypothesis: musical rhythm can be a zeitgeber, with its ability to entrain respiration dependent on the strength of its signal relative to spurious signals from the higher neural centers that introduce noise into the central pattern generator. Tapping reinforces the zeitgeber, increasing its signal-to-noise ratio and thereby promoting entrainment" (185). (Also, see Ref. 189.)

A lower-frequency oscillation (*ca.* 0.02 Hz, 1.2 cpm) detected in arterial blood pressure also has been measured through skin-surface blood flowmetry (120) and photoelectric plethysmography (123). Kitney was able to entrain this signal (plethysmography of the right hand) through a hot-cold stimulus administered to the contralateral (left) hand (see Ref. 123, Fig. 2), thereby changing the signal's frequency and amplitude and also markedly reducing signal dispersion (signal spreading and multiple fine-structure). Entrainment could be accomplished only when the stimulus frequency lay within a short range of 0.02 Hz. In addition to demonstrating thermoentrainment (123), this experiment suggests that the natural signal at 0.02 Hz is linked with temperature regulation mechanisms, an interpretation that is consistent with previous work (190).

A Primary Reference Oscillator

It is known that circadian rhythm is linked closely to activity within the SCN (162,191,192). Visual stimulus, LD sensation, is transmitted from the retina to the SCN of the hypothalamus, to the upper thoracic intermediolateral cell column and from there through the superior cervical ganglion to the pineal (67). The daily LD cycle entrains the somewhat longer inherent circadian rhythm

(28), and at least one input pathway for light-entrainment proceeds through the p42/44-mitogen-activated protein kinase (MAPK) cascade of the SCN. The MAPK signal transduction pathway is a potent regulator of numerous classes of transcription factors and has been shown to play a role in neuronal plasticity (193).

The clock for low-frequency (0.1 to 0.2 Hz) cardiovascular oscillations appears to be located in the nucleus of the tractus solitarius linked to the baroreceptors innervated from the upper thoracic region. Whether these rhythms emanate from their respective zeitgebers or are the result of complex entrainment and modulations from multiple source signals is a subject of significant debate (19,120,127,128,154–157,194). Current thought appears to favor the complex multisource origin in a holistic matrix organized according to a hierarchical model in which neurons of the SCN of the hypothalamus may drive the central circadian clock and all the other somatic cells (195), thus linking everything from circadian (and probably even slower rhythms) to cellular level oscillations at least as high as that demonstrated from the yeast cell wall.

Individual cellular clocks in the SCN, the circadian center, are integrated into a stable and robust pacemaker with a period length of about 24 hours. The clock ticks via synchronization of clock gene transcription across hundreds of neurons (192). How the clock regulates cellular functions is being worked out. It is known that in the mouse, the core mechanism for the master circadian clock consists of interacting positive and negative transcription and translation feedback loops (196). In *Dorsophila*, despite the central role for the transcriptional regulator protein dTim, the relevance of another protein, mTim, remained equivocal; however, knockdown of mTim expression in the rat SCN disrupted SCN neuronal activity rhythms and altered levels of known core clock elements (197). Thus, the complete regulator consists of a zeitgeber and transmission proteins that carry the clock's timing signal to other elements in the cell's regulatory machinery. Moreover, the activity of these is further regulated through phosphorylation-dephosphorylation reactions (198) and the reduced or oxidized state of nicotinamide cofactors (199).

Circadian clocks produce output signals in order to impose their rhythms on organism behavior. These signals are controlled by the genetic machinery and have been identified as peptides or proteins. In *Drosophila*, the peptide PDF (for pigment-dispensing factor) was identified because of its resemblance to a peptide called pigment-dispensing hormone, which drives a daily rhythm of color changes in some crustaceans (200). Using mutant mice, Cheng et al. (191) showed that a cysteine-rich protein, prokineticin 2, secreted from the SCN, controls physiological and behavioral processes.

An early review by van den Pol and Dudek (162) provides background for research in the circadian zeitgeber and the means for intercellular communication in the SCN, including calcium spikes in presynaptic dendrites, ephaptic interaction, paracrine communication, glial mediation, and gap junctions; their Figure 3 is particularly valuable for showing the signals for intercellular communication and their relative time scales. For a review of the functional properties of the cellular circadian clocks of nonmammalian vertebrates, see Ref. 201.

As mentioned previously, the crystal structure of the central clock protein, KaiC, at the heart of the cyanobacterium clockwork has been determined as having a number of key residues involved in regulating KaiC phosphorylation status and circadian period (89). (For an overview, see Ref. 90.)

Multiple Oscillators

Entrainment (synchrony) of frequency occurs when two nonlinear oscillatory systems are coupled and operating at close but different frequencies (9,123,137,138); the coupling causes the two oscillators to lock into a common frequency. The THM oscillation has been entrained utilizing rhythmic alteration of body position (9), exposure to fluctuating temperature (123), and respiratory activity (9,122,182,183). Entrainment of THM has been accomplished using baroreceptors and vasomotor reflexes; the lower limit of the entrainment bandwidth is 0.0841 (SD 0.0030) cycles/s and the upper limit is 0.1176 (SD 0.0013) cycles/s (202). Entrainment of the THM by the respiratory rate specifically occurs over the same frequency range of 5 resp/min (0.083 cycles/s) to 7 resp/min (0.12 cycles/s) (184). Although cranial manipulation involves more complexity of intervention than merely modulating the primary (cellular) respiratory mechanism (PRM)/CRI, the concept of oscillatory entrainment offers an interesting explanation for this one aspect of treatment, as has been proposed by McPartland and Mein (203).

Breathing rate is modulated by musical tempo (204); no other aspect of music appears to be relevant. "Even short exposure to music can induce measurable and reproducible cardiovascular and respiratory effects, leading to a condition of arousal or focused attention that is proportional to the speed of the music and that may be induced or amplified by respiratory entrainment by the music's rhythm and speed" (204). The effect appears to be independent of preference, or repetition, or habituation, and is clearer when the rhythmic structure is simpler.

The gestalt of an orchestral performance, however, goes far beyond the musical demands of the score. "How interval, melody and harmony act on the emotions is central to our understanding of music." Moreover, there are data to suggest that affective and cognitive processing of music might involve different neural pathways (205). (See Ref. 189 for a comprehensive treatise on the subject of musicophilia.)

It really is a very odd business that all of us, to varying degrees, have music in our heads. If Arthur C. Clarke's Overlords were puzzled when they landed on Earth and observed how much energy our species puts into making and listening to music, they would have been stupefied when they realized that, even in the absence of external sources, most of are incessantly playing music in our heads (189).

In examining daily rhythms in sleep and waking performance, Dijk and Schantz (206) state, "in the absence of externally imposed LD and social cycles, sleep-wake cycles remain consolidated but desynchronize from the 24-hour day (external desynchrony). This loss of entrainment is accompanied by a dramatic change in the internal phase relationship between the sleep-wake cycle and the body temperature rhythm. The sleep-wake cycle shifts approximately 4 to 6 hours later, and most sleep initiations now occur at the body temperature nadir rather than before the temperature nadir. This change in the internal phase relationship suggests that separate oscillators drive the sleep-wake cycle and body temperature rhythm. The phenomenon of spontaneous internal desynchrony, during which the sleep-wake cycle oscillates with a period much longer or shorter than the rhythms of core body temperature, urine volume, and other physiological variables, provides stronger evidence for the existence of multiple oscillators."

Consider this musical relationship between rhythm and temperature. Birdsong has a precise, hierarchically organized structure that provides a look into the central control of motor neuron timing. A direct link between the clock of the premotor nucleus HVC (high vocal center) in zebra finch songbirds and the rhythm components of its song has been demonstrated by manipulating the biophysical dynamics in different regions of the forebrain (207). The clock signal may be slowed by cooling the HVC of the brain.

This cooling then slows the bird's song, thus linking temperature with rhythmic timing. Song tempo, syllable duration, and intervals between motif onsets are lengthened with cold; however, the stereotypical acoustic structure is not cold sensitive.

This idea of multiple oscillators is supported by a study of baroreceptor denervation (decerebrated cats), where sympathetic nerve discharge contains a prominent 10-Hz rhythmic component. The 10-Hz signal is ubiquitous to postganglionic sympathetic nerves with cardiovascular targets (e.g., heart, forelimb vasculature), and the 10-Hz discharges of these nerves are strongly correlated. It is has been proposed "that rather than arising from a single source, the 10-Hz rhythm is generated by a system of coupled brain stem oscillators, each targeting a different end organ." (208) The 10-Hz signal is interpreted as arising from an unrecognized form of phase walk in which the participating oscillators remain strongly coupled (208).

Other systems oscillate in a manner analogous to that of circadian systems but at different frequencies and for different purposes. In the nematode *Caenorhabditis elegans*, for example, proteins regulating the molting cycles of postembryonic development oscillate on a cycle of every 6 hours (209). In mice, cortical gamma oscillations (20 to 80 Hz) are generated by synchronous activity of fast-spiking inhibitory interneurons, with the resulting rhythmic inhibition producing neural ensemble synchrony (210).

Mathematical Models

Mathematical models describing mechanisms for intercellular communication have been developed. Li and Goldbeter (211) formulated a square-wave (pulsatile) model for intercellular communication and have analyzed the response to various types of stimulating systems (stochastic, chaotic), including the optimal periodic signal maximizing target cell responsiveness (34,212). In a hysteresis-based model, global transcription or translation rates have only small effects on the period; however, changes in these rates alter the signal amplitude (213).

Soto-Treviño et al. (20), using a model of the lobster pyloric pacemaker network, addressed the problem of coupling compartments that in isolation are capable of producing very different oscillations. At the neuronal network level, the model was used to explore the range of coupling strengths for which an intrinsically bursting neuron drives a tonic spiking neuron to burst synchronously with it. The model was tested and compared with the performance of isolated preparations of the stomatogastric nervous system of the spiny lobster *Panulirus interruptus*. The examples presented illustrate that neuromodulation can effectively modify neuronal network behavior.

Synthetic Genetic Oscillators

At the level of genes and proteins, positive and negative feedback loops of interacting molecular systems generate sustained oscillations, where it is possible to achieve a widely tunable frequency at near-constant signal amplitude (94). An engineered, synthetic tunable genetic oscillator in *Escherichia coli* has been created (95). The oscillator's modeled-network architecture contains linked positive and negative feedback loops. Oscillations in individual cells were monitored through repeated cycles using the fluorescence from incorporated yemGFP (monomeric yeast-enhanced green fluorescent protein) gene protein. The experiment demonstrated that the key design principle for constructing a robust genetic oscillator is a time delay in the negative feedback loop, which can mechanistically arise from the cascade of cellular processes involved in forming a functional transcription factor.

Apoptosis (Programmed Cell Death)

Apoptosis appears to be a universal feature of animal development, and abnormalities in it have been associated with an array of diseases, including certain cancers and neurodegenerative pathologies. In plants, it is essential for development and survival, including xylogenesis, reproduction, senescence, and pathogenesis (214). Employing two different sequential developmental stages, exponential growth and polynomial death, the process can be modeled by incorporating a parametric approach for exponential growth and a nonparametric approach based on the Legendre function (Legendre polynomial order 3) for polynomial death. The model was validated by a real example in rice (215) and should be universally applicable.

Cardiovascular-Respiratory Control/Congestive Heart Failure in Humans

A model of the cardiovascular-respiratory control system, incorporating constant state equation delays and the use of Legendre polynomials for feedback control, has been formulated (216). The model was used to study the transition from the awake state to stage 4 (NREM) sleep for normal individuals and for individuals suffering from congestive heart problems. The model steady states are consistent with observation both for the normal and the congestive heart state conditions. [Use of Legendre polynomials for feedback loop models (217,218) and for random regression modeling of longitudinal (time-dependent) data (219).]

Reviews

These literature citations refer to reviews focused on biorhythm frequency bands (10,34,36,38,110,138,156,162,169,201,220–223). Published mathematical models used to describe specific systems are given in these citations (20,34,36,80,123,137,138,171, 224,225). Osteopathic concepts clearly have a place here, particularly those treatments that incorporate oscillatory mechanisms (7,144,187,194,203).

Other Work Related to Biological Communication through Rhythms

Viewed as valuable by the authors of this chapter is the article on entrainment of the Earth's ice ages through frequency modulation of the Earth's orbital eccentricity (226). The documentation of this phenomenon demonstrates that frequency modulation represents a powerful regulatory mechanism, not only for radio transmissions, but also for the vast periods of geological time and most assuredly for all frequencies lying between these extremes.

The exceptional continuity that occurs among different cells, tissues, and organs when responding coherently to a set of stimuli as a function of self/species survival is appreciable. Coherent response alludes to a central rhythm that resonates throughout the cell and that is capable of synchronizing a diversity of physiological processes into a functional biological unity. It is probable that this rhythm exists for both prokaryotic and eukaryotic cells. Collectively, this resonance for the subphylum Vertebrata is hypothesized to emanate as the craniosacral respiration (227). Experimental data suggest that, at least, the circadian cycling of energy metabolism is mediated by an activator of gene expression (228).

It is this that lies at the basis of all mechanical systems of healing, the setting up of increase or the checking of the vibratile impulses, the correction in the distribution of the normal vibrations sent out from the brain center of control and distributed by co-ordination from the different planes of center activity—Littlejohn (1).

MAGNETORECEPTION

When considering the regulation of organisms through oscillating phenomena, one additional aspect of communication physics needs to be considered: There is a sixth sense, magnetoreception, and this sense also can be expected to give rise to oscillating (magnetic) fields. There are at least two different mechanisms for intracellular magnetic detection (229): (a) The biological compass composed of magnetite crystal chains (230) that are present in many species from microorganisms through vertebrates. (b) The radical-pair mechanism (231), which is based on the cryptochrome protein, an intracellular entity that produces two possible intermediate states depending upon its orientation to the ambient magnetic field. Because cryptochrome is located in the retina, it has been proposed that it feeds information to the brain through the optic nerves. Such a system is analogous to the light-entrainment system of the circadian clock (28).

So, what will studies of magnetoreception reveal? Magnetite crystals are aligned along cellular microtubules, a position where they could efficiently modulate cell membrane oscillations. Thus, from what is known today, a system of biomagneto-communication certainly is physically possible.

OSTEOPATHIC MANIPULATIVE MEDICINE AND THE TRAUBE-HERING-MAYER WAVEFORM

As was pointed out at the beginning of this chapter, Littlejohn observed over one hundred years ago that human physiology is dynamic (1). Everything in life is changing with time, but not necessarily at the same rate. Holistically, human physiology may be considered in the context of waves upon waves upon waves (Fig. 11.1, top, trace a), wherein each independent vibrational frequency influences and is influenced by those frequencies above and below it. Within the broad spectrum of physiologic rhythms, one area is of particular interest to practitioners of osteopathic manipulative medicine, the frequency range from 0.003 to 0.50 Hz (0.18 to 30 cpm). In cardiovascular physiology, this range is subdivided, by spectral peaks, into very-low-frequency (0.003 to 0.05 Hz, 0.18 to 3.0 cpm), low-frequency (0.10 to 0.20 Hz, 6.0 to 12 cpm), and higher-frequency (0.25 to 0.50 Hz, 15 to 30 cpm) components (140). The very-low-frequency peak reflects autonomic (parasympathetic) and renin-angiotensin interaction. The low-frequency spectral peak is predominantly the result of sympathetic, baroreflex, activity. The activity in the higher-frequency area, pulmonary respiration, impacts the cardiovascular system through the interaction of the autonomic (parasympathetic and sympathetic) nervous system (141).

In osteopathic manipulative medicine, the PRM (232) is often monitored by palpating the CRI (233–237). The rate of the CRI, first measured by Woods and Woods in 1961 (238), has since been measured repeatedly, with a reported range of 2 to 14 cpm (0.03 to 0.23 Hz) (125,131,173,226,238–246). This frequency range encompasses the low-frequency peak between 0.10 and 0.20 Hz in cardiovascular physiology.

In the mid-19th century, activity in the 0.10 and 0.20 Hz frequency range was observed in blood pressure, independent of pulmonary respiration (247,248). This low-frequency rhythm has since been identified as Traube-Hering waves (249–251), as Mayer waves (122) or as THM waves (120). To avoid confusion, rather than using eponyms in the discussion that follows, the oscillations will be identified by their frequencies.

Oscillations in the low-frequency range of 0.10 to 0.20 Hz have been identified throughout human physiology: blood pressure

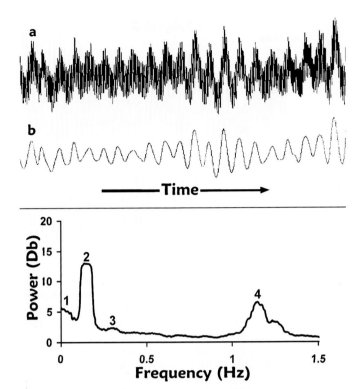

Figure 11-1   Top traces (a) and (b): (a) Waves upon waves upon waves; the time-domain record of a complete blood flow velocity record, demonstrating the heart rate waveform upon the low-frequency baroreflex waveform upon the very-low-frequency waveform. (b) Filtered record showing respiratory, low-, and very-low-frequency components only. **Bottom spectrum:** The FT, frequency-domain spectrum of waveform (a), demonstrating: (*1*) very-low-frequency signal component, (*2*) low-frequency signal component, (*3*) higher-frequency respiration signal, and (*4*) the heart rate spectral component.

(122,138,247,248), heart rate variability (122,252–254), pulmonary blood flow (250), peripheral blood flow (122,250,252,255,256), muscle sympathetic tone (254), cerebral blood flow and movement of the cerebrospinal fluid (126,148,251,255,257,258), and cerebral cortical cellular activity (128,129,180,181). Because these phenomena occupy the same frequency range as the CRI, it was decided to monitor that particular frequency in a known physiologic phenomenon to provide insight into cranial osteopathy.

Peripheral vascular manifestations of the low-frequency, 0.10 to 0.20 Hz, rhythm are readily measured by laser-Doppler flowmetry and may be recorded simultaneously with cranial osteopathic procedures. In the basic science protocols described below, where the low-frequency, 0.10 to 0.20 Hz, rhythm was monitored, a laser-Doppler perfusion monitor (Transonic Systems, Inc., Ithaca, NY) was employed to determine Doppler velocity of circulating blood that was then digitized for subsequent data reduction (WinDaq data acquisition and playback software).

This method provides time-domain records that may be obtained simultaneously with cranial diagnostic and therapeutic procedures. These records provide striking illustrations of what cranial practitioners have been describing for years. They lend themselves to the identification of the interaction between the practitioner and the subject and for determination of the rate of the CRI. The recorded bloodflow velocity record is the result of a very complex group of physiological processes with multiple contributing frequencies, resulting in waves upon waves upon

waves (Fig. 11.1, top, trace a). Because of this complexity, visually identifying where any given intervention actually has an effect is extremely difficult, if not impossible.

However, because these complex visual records are digital, the data may be converted mathematically through an FT (Fig. 11.1, bottom). This provides frequency-domain spectra that clearly identify the frequencies of individual spectral peaks (location on the *x*-axis), their power (height of any given spectral peak, *y*-axis) and dispersion, or irregularity, (width of a spectral peak measured at half-height) that result in the complex waves upon waves upon waves of the visual time-domain records. FT spectra may be filtered—spectral regions selected and then inverse FTs performed—to create time-domain records that focus upon the contribution of any spectral area to the observed time-domain record (Fig. 11.1, top, trace b). Frequency-domain records also may be analyzed comparatively to determine where in the complex waveform an intervention has had effect. This may be done by comparing the relative height of consecutive measurements of the same spectral peak. Or by subtracting one FT spectrum from another, and thereby calculating the changes that have occurred in frequency, power, and dispersion throughout the entire spectrum as a magnitude difference spectrum (Figs. 11.10 and 11.13).

These methods provide opportunities to study cranial osteopathy in the context of quantifiable aspects of human physiology through cutaneous bloodflow velocity. The following protocols were implemented by our group with able assistance, in the first protocol, from Celia M. Lipinski, D.O. and Arina R. Chapman, D.O. These studies, spanning a period from 1998 to the present, represent our attempt to quantify the CRI and demonstrate the effect of cranial manipulation upon the vibrations manifest in human bloodflow velocity.

The Research Protocols

Protocol 1: *Comparing low-frequency bloodflow velocity waves with cranial palpation* (120). First, it was appropriate to establish a correlation between the palpated CRI and the 0.10 to 0.20 Hz oscillation.

Twelve subjects participated in this study. With the laser-Doppler probe affixed to the subject's earlobe, they rested quietly on an Osteopathic Manipulative Technique (OMT) table. A baseline flowmetry record was then obtained. Next, an experienced examiner, blinded to the laser-Doppler record, monitored the CRI. As they palpated, they identified the CRI, saying "f" for flexion/external rotation and "e" for extension/internal rotation. At each verbal indication, an event mark (EM) was entered into the computer by the recording technician.

Figure 11.2 is the compressed laser-Doppler flowmetry time-domain records of two subjects. The palpation of the CRI is indicated by the vertical EMs on the right side of each record.

The flowmetry records for each subject were Fourier transformed and dissected, removing frequencies above 0.50 Hz. Inverse FT was performed on the remaining data, resulting in a time-domain record of frequencies below 0.50 Hz. This demonstrated that the dominant low-frequency wave phenomena apparent in the original flowmetry records represented the low-frequency, 0.10 to 0.20 Hz, wave and not harmonic aberrations from some other frequency (Figs. 11.3 and 11.4).

Of the 12 subjects, 11 provided data suitable for analysis. Six hundred thirteen low-frequency wave peaks (maxima) and troughs (minima) were visually identified. One hundred sixty-six flexion/external rotation events and 162 extension/internal rotation events

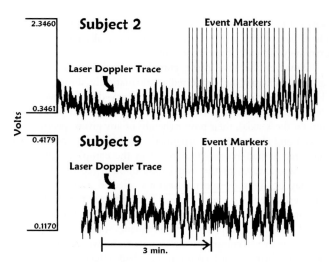

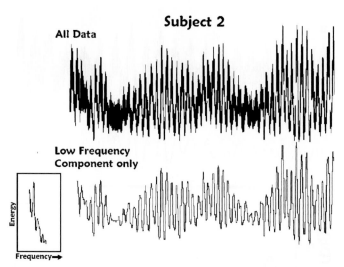

Figure 11-2 Compressed laser-Doppler-flowmeter bloodflow velocity (waveform) and flexion-extension records (vertical EMs) from two subjects.

(n = 328) were identified. These were associated equally between low-frequency maxima (n = 164) and minima (n = 164).

There was no correlation between palpation (flexion/external rotation, extension/internal rotation) and the low-frequency wave maximum or minimum in the flowmetry record (Pearson R value, –0.085; approximate significance, 0.123). In further analysis, the time of each palpation event was compared with the time recorded for the nearest maximum or minimum in the flowmetry record. The paired t-test, in this case, showed *no statistical difference* between the flowmetry low-frequency 0.10 to 0.20 Hz wave record and the palpated CRI. With 328 data pairs, both groups of time values were highly correlated (correlation, 1.000; significance, 0.000).

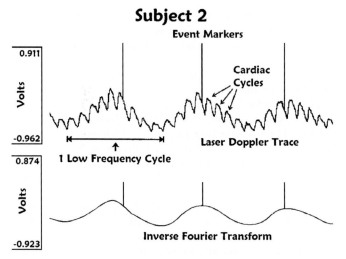

Figure 11-3 Expanded laser-Doppler-flowmeter relative-blood-velocity record of Subject 2: **Top**—Flowmeter trace, revealing cardiac cycle fine-structure. The double-headed arrow indicates the wavelength of one low-frequency cycle. **Bottom**—Low-frequency waveform component only of the top trace. The bottom waveform was created from the top waveform by filtering (removing) the high-frequency cardiac component, leaving only the very-low-frequency, low-frequency, and respiratory components. Inverse FT of this digitally filtered data generates the bottom trace. Both traces are in register with respect to time, and the event markers indicate the positions of the palpatory findings.

Figure 11-4 Inverse FT time-domain spectra from Subject 2: Top trace, all frequency-domain data used in the inverse computation; bottom spectrum, only the frequency component lying below 0.5 cycles/s (30 cycles/min) used. The bottom spectrum is the trace resulting from very-low-, low-, and respiratory frequency contributions. The insert box shows that portion of the FT frequency-domain spectrum used to compute the inverse very-low-, low-, and respiratory frequency spectrum.

Even though over the length of the recording the low-frequency, 0.10 to 0.20 Hz, waves demonstrated a frequency modulation of up to 20%, the palpation events precisely mirrored the oscillating flowmetry wave.

Discussion of Protocol 1: This study demonstrated that the CRI and the low-frequency, 0.10 to 0.20 Hz, bloodflow velocity waves are concomitant phenomena. The bloodflow velocity waves demonstrated a frequency modulation of up to 20% that was precisely mirrored by the palpation record. This frequency modulation also was reported by Lockwood and Degenhardt in their analysis of Frymann's 1971 data from instrumental measurement of the CRI (174,259).

The flowmetry records and FT of the data contained within them consistently demonstrate contribution from the very-low-frequency (0.003 to 0.05 Hz, 0.18 to 3.0 cpm) and low-frequency (0.10 to 0.20 Hz, 6.0 to 12 cpm) components. These frequencies in bloodflow velocity are remarkably consistent with the "slow tide" (six cycles in 10 minutes) and the "fast tide" (8 to 12 cpm) of the PRM as described by Becker (260) (Fig. 11.5).

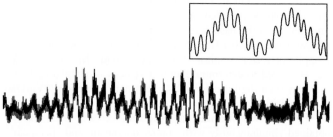

Figure 11-5 Waves upon waves, flowmetry record demonstrating the contribution from the very-low-frequency (0.003 to 0.05 Hz, 0.18 to 3.0 cpm) and low-frequency (0.10 to 0.20 Hz, 6.0 to 12 cpm) components. These frequencies in bloodflow velocity are remarkably consistent with the "slow tide" (6 cycles in 10 minutes) and the "fast tide" (8 to 12 cpm) of the PRM as described by Becker (260). Inset shows the low-frequency wave with the heartbeat upon it.

Additionally, it is of interest to note that the palpated CRI in this study was consistently palpated, such that ratio of the CRI to the low-frequency (0.10 to 0.20 Hz) oscillations was 1:2 (Fig. 11.2). This relationship was recognized retrospectively when additional flowmetry records were analyzed to measure the rate of the CRI (see *Protocol 5*) (Fig. 11.13).

Protocol 2: *Affecting low-frequency bloodflow velocity waves by cranial manipulation* (7). When the palpable CRI and low-frequency, 0.10 to 0.20 Hz, bloodflow velocity oscillations were demonstrated to be temporally concomitant, the question then arose: Does cranial manipulation exert an effect upon the low-frequency oscillations?

Twenty-three subjects were randomly divided into control (*n* = 13) and experiment (*n* = 10) groups. The laser-Doppler probe was affixed to the subject's earlobe. Subjects rested quietly on an Osteopathic Manipulative Technique (OMT) table. A baseline flowmetry record was obtained, followed by cranial manipulation (experimental group) or sham intervention (control group). The sham intervention consisted of 5 minutes of cranial palpation using a biparietal modification vault-hold. Subjects in the experimental group received an individually determined cranial treatment, applied until a therapeutic endpoint was achieved (5 to 10 minutes). Immediately following the sham or manipulative intervention, a 5-minute postintervention laser-Doppler recording was acquired. During the entire process the subjects, in both groups, remained on the treatment table; the laser-Doppler recording was continuous and the probe was undisturbed.

FT was performed upon the pre- and postintervention flowmetry records of each subject. Four major component signals from the flowmetry records were analyzed: very-low-frequency signal (0.003 to 0.05 Hz), low-frequency signal (0.10 to 0.20 Hz), higher-frequency, respiratory, signal (0.25 to 0.50 Hz), and the cardiac signal (1.0 to 1.5 Hz). Preintervention and postintervention data were compared for both the control and the experimental groups (Fig. 11.6).

For the control group, the very-low-frequency signal decreased to an almost significant degree ($P = 0.054$) while the low-frequency ($P = 0.805$), higher-frequency ($P = 0.715$) and cardiac ($P = 0.511$) signals showed no statistically significant changes. The experimental group showed a significant decrease of the very-low-frequency signal ($P = 0.001$) and an increase of the low-frequency signal ($P = 0.021$). The higher-frequency ($P = 0.747$) and cardiac ($P = 0.788$) signals showed no significant changes.

The effects of the cranial treatment seen in Figure 11.6, although visually exceptional, are consistent with changes induced in all of the subjects. Figure 11.7, a compressed continuous flowmetry record (~30 minute duration), demonstrates the progressive organization resulting from the increased low-frequency wave activity readily seen from the end of the treatment period through the posttreatment period.

Discussion of Protocol 2: This study demonstrated that cranial manipulation, specifically directed at cranial patterns of individual

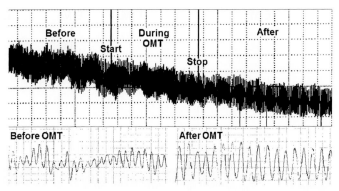

Figure 11-7 Continuous flowmetry record of approximately 30-minute duration. Although the record is greatly compressed to afford visualization of it in its entirety, the progressive organization resulting from the increased low-frequency wave activity can be readily seen from the end of the treatment period through the posttreatment period. The bottom tracings are the contributions to the flowmetry record from very-low-, low-, and respiratory frequencies before and after manipulation.

subjects, affected bloodflow velocity oscillations. The amplitude of the very-low-frequency (0.003 to 0.05 Hz) wave decreased and that of the low-frequency (0.10 to 0.20 Hz) wave increased. It is of interest to note here that cranial manipulation has been demonstrated to exert a comparable effect upon similar frequency oscillations (0.08 to 0.20 Hz) in intracranial fluid content as measured by transcranial bioimpedance (258).

Because the low-frequency wave in bloodflow velocity is mediated by sympathetic, baroreflex, activity (141), cranial manipulation can be inferred to affect the autonomic nervous system. Additionally, since the control palpation did not greatly affect bloodflow velocity oscillations, control palpation may be used as a sham treatment in future research.

Protocol 3: *Affecting low-frequency bloodflow velocity waves on demand* (8). Since individually determined cranial manipulation changed bloodflow velocity, it was decided to see if an affect could be obtained on demand, using palpation only, alternating with incitant bitemporal rocking. This alternating palpation and manipulation sequence was continued for a total of 35 minutes (maximum recording time for an uninterrupted laser-Doppler record). To eliminate the possibility that there might be an independent oscillation in bloodflow physiology, two different time sequences were decided on for the protocol. Five- and seven-minute intervals, both divisible into 35, were chosen. The timing of the treatment/nontreatment sequence was established for each subject before the initiation of the protocol.

Fifteen subjects participated. The laser-Doppler probe was placed in the midline on the subject's forehead. It was felt that the previously used ear site was too close to the temporomastoid region (area being manipulated) and could therefore be directly affected by the intervention.

The subjects rested upon the Osteopathic Manipulative Technique (OMT) table with their heads upon the practitioner's hands in position for the manipulative procedure. A baseline bloodflow velocity record was obtained. Following this, incitant bitemporal rocking was performed synchronous with the subject's CRI. The manipulation was stopped and, without changing hand placement, a period of cranial-palpation-only followed. This alternating sequence continued uninterrupted for the maximum laser-Doppler recording time.

Figure 11.8 shows the compressed, 35-minute long, flowmetry records for two subjects treated with cranial manipulation at

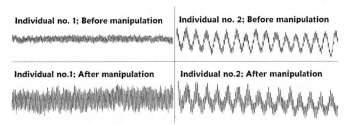

Figure 11-6   Laser Doppler blood flow recording of two individuals, before and after cranial manipulation.

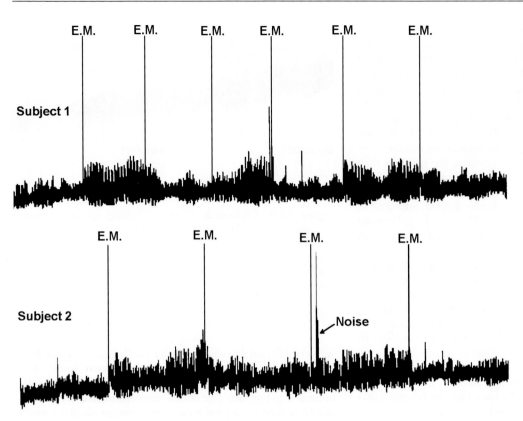

Figure 11-8 Compressed laser-Doppler-flowmetry, relative blood velocity waveforms, of two subjects treated by cranial manipulation at designated 5-minute (Subject 1) and 7-minute (Subject 2) intervals. EM indicate points in time when cranial manipulation started and stopped.

5-minute (Subject 1) and 7-minute (Subject 2) intervals. EMs identify where cranial manipulation was started and stopped. Expansion of the first and third nontreatment/treatment pairs of the flowmetry record for Subject 1 (Fig. 11.9) clearly shows the low-frequency (0.10 to 0.20 Hz) wave and the amplifying effect upon it resulting from incitant manipulation.

Using FT, the very-low-frequency, low-frequency, higher-frequency and cardiac rate, signals were identified to determine which changed. Signal intensities as a function of the respective component's frequency are plotted in Figure 11.10 for Subject 1: third nontreatment segment (top), third treatment segment (center).

Figure 11.10 (bottom) exhibits the difference spectrum obtained by subtracting the data in Figure 11.10 (top) from the data in Figure 11.10 (center). It demonstrates that the incitant cranial manipulation increased the very-low-frequency signal and greatly increased the low-frequency signal. Additionally, the heart rate can be seen, from the resultant sinusoidal shape for the cardiac signal, to have increased from approximately 70 to 82 beats per minute.

Discussion of Protocol 3: This study demonstrated that incitant cranial manipulation could, on demand, alter the physiologic parameters of bloodflow velocity. The low-frequency (0.10 to 0.20 Hz) component increased most markedly and the very-low-frequency component (0.003 to 0.05 Hz) increased to some degree. These effects occurred within a few seconds and, in this instance, the flowmetry record returned to near-baseline levels within fractions of a minute after the intervention was stopped. FT analysis, however, revealed that the flowmetry record does not return precisely to baseline following intervention, rather it exhibits a small residual effect with a considerably longer half-life. This persistent residual amplification may, in part, account for the therapeutic effect of some forms of cranial manipulation.

Protocol 4: *Affecting low-frequency bloodflow velocity waves by Compression of the Fourth Ventricle (CV-4)* (144). Because incitant cranial manipulation affected the amplitude of the low-frequency oscillations, it was decided to study the response to CV-4, a manipulative procedure that, during its application, is intended to dampen the CRI. CV-4 offers the advantage of having a specific starting point and a generally agreed upon physiologic end point, the still point. This endpoint is then reportedly followed by amplification of the CRI. This allowed us to measure the duration of time the CV-4 procedure was applied and any impact it had on bloodflow velocity.

Twenty-eight experienced cranial practitioners performed the CV-4, each with a different subject ($N = 26$; two subjects participated twice). One physician plus one subject at one treatment constituted one statistical case.

The physician sat at the head of an Osteopathic Manipulative Technique (OMT) table. The subject lying supine, with the laser-Doppler probe attached to the midline of their forehead, rested quietly for an equilibration period. A baseline record of 5 to 7 minutes, the Control (C) segment (Fig. 11.11, Control), was then obtained. During the Control segment period, no treatment was administered, but the subject's head rested upon the physician's hands in the appropriate position for palpatory diagnosis and treatment using CV-4. At the end of the Control segment, the physician was instructed to begin implementation of CV-4, and upon the treating physicians' indication that they had started, an EM was entered into the record by the technician (Fig. 11.11).

The Treatment (T) phase lasted until the physician indicated that they had obtained their therapeutic goal. At this point, a second EM was entered into the flowmetry record, indicating the end of the Treatment segment (Fig. 11.11, Treatment). The physicians removed their hands from contact with the subject's head, and the Response (R) to treatment was followed for an additional 5 to 7 minutes (Fig. 11.11, Response). Both treating physicians and subjects were blinded to operations at the computer console.

The duration of Treatment for the CV-4 procedure from the 28 individual records (Table 1) was computed by measuring the

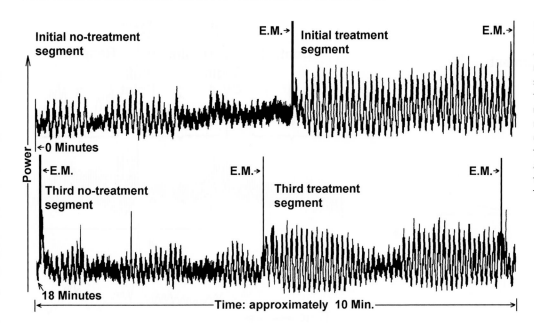

Figure 11-9 Expansion of the laser-Doppler flowmetry record of Subject 1 of Figure 8: The **top record** shows the initial resting segment followed by the first treatment segment; the **bottom record** shows the analogous segment pair beginning at 18 minutes, both records demonstrating that incitant cranial treatment amplifies the power of the low-frequency oscillation.

time elapsed on the flowmetry record between the first EM, when the physician started the procedure, and the EM indicating they had attained their therapeutic goal. The mean duration of Treatment was 4.43 minutes, range 8.65 minutes (minimum 1.42, maximum 10.07), a standard deviation ± 2.22 minutes, and a variance of 4.94. This duration is consistent with a published report of 3 to 7 minutes for CV-4 application (260).

The impact of the CV-4 procedure was then determined. Among the 28 CV-4 records obtained, high-frequency noise in 8 (29%) records made them unsatisfactory for data reductions and statistical analyses. The remaining 20 records, ranging from 15 to 24 minutes duration, were useable. Each of these records contained the three continuously linked segments (total waveform segments = 60) separated by the EMs. These segments (Fig. 11.11), the pretreatment resting period (Control), the CV-4 treatment period (Treatment), and the immediate response period (Response), were identified for intergroup comparisons. Within each segment, a 4- to 6-minute portion of the record was selected. The shortest of these segments, for each subject, was identified and its duration, to the nearest 0.01 second, noted. Portions of the remaining two segments, from that record, each of identical duration as the shortest segment, were extracted for FT.

FT spectra, for each of the segments, were then computed to generate 60 frequency-domain spectra (Fig. 11.12). Point-by-point subtraction, generating Control minus Treatment (C – T), Treatment minus Response (T – R), and Control minus Response (C – R) difference spectra, was then carried out (Fig. 11.13). The resulting difference spectra were plotted and then integrated to obtain spectral signal areas.

From these difference spectra, signal areas were computed from three signals in the low-frequency region. The 0.02 Hz signal represents physiological activity in the range of the very-low-frequency wave; the 0.10 Hz signal represents activity consistent with the low-frequency wave. A new minor signal, at 0.08 Hz, was resolved in flowmetry data but not reported in earlier work. Sufficient data at this point were accumulated verifying the existence of this minor resonance. Additionally, areas were computed from both the low- and the high-frequency halves of the cardiac signal (centered approximately at 1.10 Hz), and minimum and maximum frequency components of the cardiac signal were recorded.

To determine significance among the three groups (C – T, T – R, C – R) for each selected signal-area and frequency value analysis of variance was used. Seven scalar variables were considered: areas of the signals centered at 0.02, 0.08, and 0.10 Hz; areas of the lower-frequency and higher-frequency cardiac bands; and the frequencies at the maximum amplitude (either positive or negative) of both cardiac bands. Also evaluated were pair-wise comparisons between group pairs, using Scheffé, Bonferroni, Tukey, and Least-Significant Difference range tests (respectively, from most conservative).

Significant differences were identified for the minor signal at 0.08 Hz (sig. = 0.041) and the low-frequency signal at 0.10 Hz (sig. = 0.000). There was no significant difference for the very-low-frequency signal at 0.02 Hz or for any of the four cardiac signal variables. Using the Scheffé range test, significant differences were found only for the 0.10-Hz area variable at the alpha.05 level; however, the 0.08-Hz signal did exhibit parallel differences at the.072 level. Therefore, it is believed that both signals are affected together, and in the same sense, by the CV-4. The differences in significance between the two variables most likely reflect the much lower signal-to-noise ratio of the minor 0.08-Hz signal than fundamental differences in the behavior of each signal band with manipulation.

The variable that demonstrates the largest mean difference in response to CV-4 is the low-frequency area of the 0.10-Hz signal, where all three combinations, C – R, C – T, and T – R, are significantly different from each other.

Discussion of Protocol 4: This study demonstrated that the duration of the CV-4 was 4.43 ± 2.22 minutes, consistent with the previously published report of 3 to 7 minutes (260). During its application, bloodflow velocity was affected in a manner consistent with what would be expected from descriptions of the impact of CV-4 upon the CRI (234). As the occipital was held in extension to decrease the amplitude of the CRI, the low-frequency oscillation was damped and essentially eliminated when a still point was obtained (Figs. 11.11 and 11.13). The therapeutic impact of CV-4 is said to be increased amplitude of the CRI, which enhances the fluid motion of the PRM (234); following CV-4, the amplitude of the low-frequency wave in bloodflow velocity increases (Fig. 11.11).

Protocol 5: *The Rate of the CRI* (245). It is important to establish normative values when studying physiologic phenomena.

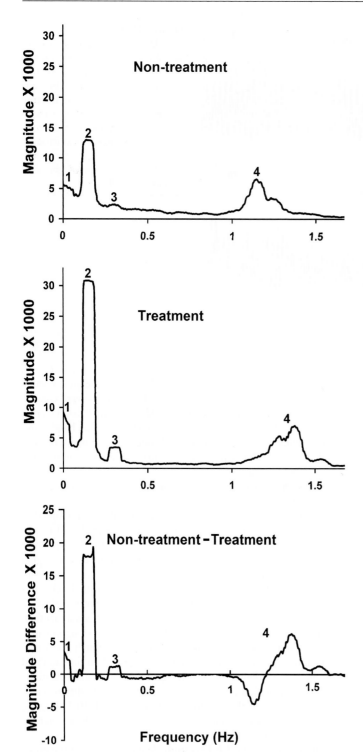

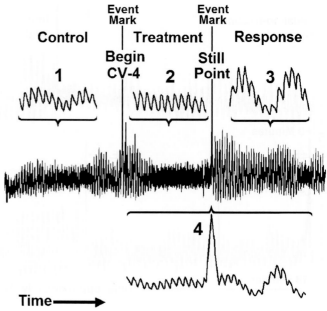

Figure 11-11 Real-time demonstration of the flowmetry record of a CV-4, consisting of a baseline bloodflow velocity record, the Control segment, the Treatment segment, and the posttreatment, Response segment. The EMs were entered into the record by the research technician upon verbal indication by the treating physician at the onset and culmination of treatment. The insets (*1*, *2*, and *3*) are representative segments (~2 minutes each) of the flowmetry record for each of the three segments of the procedure. Inset (*4*) is that portion of the record immediately before and following the still point.

Figure 11-10 FT magnitude spectra: Plotted is component intensity as a function of component frequency for Subject 1: Third nontreatment segment (**Top**) and third treatment segment (**Center**), with the (*1*) very-low-, (*2*) low-, (*3*) respiratory, and (*4*) cardiac frequencies identified. **Bottom:** Magnitude difference spectrum obtained by subtracting the nontreatment spectrum from the treatment spectrum: In this difference spectrum, the pronounced signal enhancement of the low-frequency, 0.10 Hz oscillation (*2*) stands out. Also, the heart rate (*4*) increased from approximately 70 to 82 beats/min during cranial manipulation.

Using laser-Doppler flowmetry in comparison to cranial palpation, we measured the palpated rate of the CRI. We further determined how clinicians palpate the CRI in comparison to the flowmetry record.

The CRI rate was determined from the records of 44 different examiners, each palpating a different subject. The examiners were experienced osteopathic physicians attending various professional meetings. Each palpated a different subject who was recruited randomly from attendees at the same meetings.

The laser-Doppler probe was placed onto one earlobe, and the subject then rested quietly on an Osteopathic Manipulative Technique (OMT) table. Examiners were seated at the head of the table. With a contact position of their preference, the examiners palpated their subject's CRI. As they palpated, they said, "f" indicating the perception of the flexion/external rotation and "e" indicating extension/internal rotation. At each verbal indication, an EM was entered into the computer by the recording technician. Continuous, unbroken records were recorded for each subject. The recording length, nominally of 5- to 15-minute duration, was determined by the examiner.

A portion of each record was selected for computation where the CRI was palpated consistently, without large "palpatory gaps." Calculating from 44 records acquired, the mean rate for the palpated CRI was 4.54 cpm, with a range of 7.26 (minimum 1.25, maximum 8.51). The standard deviation was 2.08, the standard error 0.313, and the variance 4.32.

The vast majority of examiners in this study palpated the CRI such that a flexion event was perceived coincident with one low-frequency oscillation and an extension event perceived coincident with the next low-frequency oscillation. This resulted in a ratio

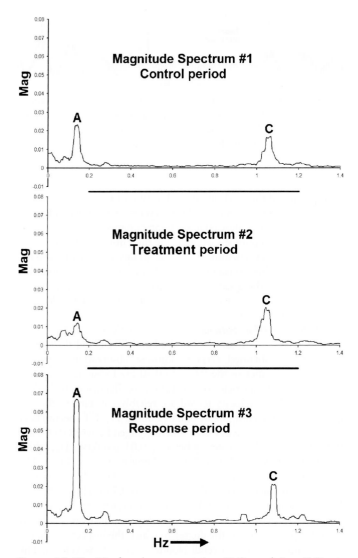

Figure 11-12 FT of each segment, (no. 1) Control, (no. 2) Treatment, and (no. 3) Response, of the CV-4 procedure, with the low-frequency (A) and cardiac (C) components indicated.

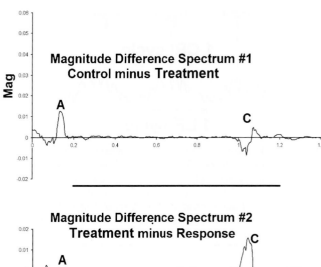

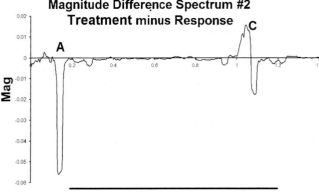

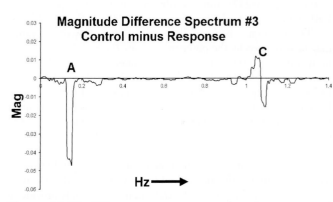

Figure 11-13 Difference spectra comparing the component parts (Control, Treatment, and Response) of the CV-4 procedure, with the low-frequency (A) and cardiac (C) components indicated: (no. 1) Control minus Treatment, (no. 2) Treatment minus Response, and (no. 3) Control minus Response.

of palpated CRI to recorded low-frequency (0.10 to 0.20 Hz) oscillations of 1:2. (Fig. 11.14). It is worthwhile to note that infrequently an examiner palpated the CRI at a 1:1 ratio to the low-frequency oscillation (Fig. 11.15).

During flowmetry recording, irregularities were observed resulting in gaps in both the palpatory and the flowmetry records. In some instances, these gaps were recognized and reported by the examiners as "still points" (Fig. 11.16) (261).

Discussion of Protocol 5: This study provides a normative rate for the CRI and insight into previously unexplained discrepancies in its reported rate. Also, by observing the relationship between the palpated CRI and bloodflow velocity, an explanation may be advanced for the difficulties encountered when sequentially comparing palpated rates for the CRI for the purpose of establishing interrater reliability.

The rate of the CRI, first reported as 10 to 14 cpm (238), has remained the accepted rate in the majority of osteopathic textbooks (233–237). Review of the literature, however, reveals an interesting paradox. Studies using palpation tend to report lower rates for the CRI (240–244) than those obtained by instrumentation (125,131,174,239,258) (Fig. 11.17). This occurs independent of

the type of instrumentation, such as plethysmography applied to the upper extremity (236), infrared light reflected from acupuncture needles implanted into the cranial bones of human subjects (131), retrospective analysis of data obtained by Frymann using a pressure transducer placed upon the head (173), and fluctuation of intracranial fluid content using transcranial electrical bioimpedance (125,258) (Fig. 11.17 and companion Table).

The palpated CRI rate in this study (4.54 ± 2.08 cpm, 0.04 to 0.11 Hz) is consistent with the lower rates obtained by palpation and reported by the majority of previous investigators (240–244) (Fig. 11.17 and companion Table 17). The inconsistency between palpation and instrumentation may be explained by the observation that the majority of examiners in the current study palpated such that a flexion event was perceived coincident with

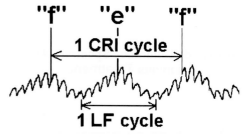

Figure 11-14 Palpation of the CRI compared to the laser-Doppler blood flow velocity record. The top trace shows the low-frequency (LF) oscillation (oscillating trace) and the CRI (palpation of "flexion/extension," vertical EMs) in a 2:1 ratio. Bottom trace: Compressed flowmetry record demonstrating the 2:1 ratio. This is the most frequently encountered LF oscillation to CRI ratio demonstrated by skilled examiners.

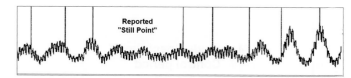

Figure 11-16 Pause in the palpation record coincidental with a decrease in low-frequency oscillation amplitude. Several examiners have commented on the perception of a "still point" at such times, although they were blinded to the flowmetry record.

one low-frequency oscillation and an extension event perceived coincident with the next low-frequency oscillation (Fig. 11.14). This resulted in a ratio of palpated CRI to recorded low-frequency (0.10 to 0.20 Hz) oscillations of 1:2. If instrumental measurement of the CRI tracks the dominant low-frequency oscillation, then the discrepancy between the palpated and instrumental measurements is explained.

There is, however, the issue of the higher palpated rate (10 to 14 cpm) consistent with the rates obtained by instrumentation, reported by Woods and Woods (238) and identified in osteopathic textbooks (233–237). Infrequently an examiner will palpate the CRI at a 1:1 ratio to the low-frequency oscillation (Fig. 11.15).

The difference between these palpation-to-flowmetry ratios may be explained by the observation from *Protocol 4* of the previously unreported 0.08 Hz (4.5 cpm) frequency wave in bloodflow velocity. The reported rate for the CRI in this study is 2.46 to 6.62 (4.54 ± 2.08) cpm, or 0.04 to 0.11 Hz. The low-frequency wave between 6 and 12 cpm (0.10 to 0.20 Hz) is twice as great. Thus, it may be concluded that the majority of individuals track the 0.04 to 0.11 Hz frequency while some individuals track the greater 0.10 to 0.20 Hz frequency.

It is worth noting here that an additional study (*Protocol 6*), using an entirely different method to measure the CRI rate, fully corroborates the findings of *Protocol 5* (246). This study provides a statistical *N* of 727 subjects, consisting of several smaller groups, from 16 to 86 individuals each, divided according to level of experience, that is, students with 1-year training, students with 2-year training and practitioners with 1 to 25 years of postgraduate experience. Participants palpated CRI rates on each other. Half of each group acted as examiners, while the other half were subjects. The examiners palpated the CRI using the classically described vault hold (233,234). They were not told how long they would be palpating, only to count the number of complete biphasic CRI cycles that they palpated during the acquisition period. The number of cycles each examiner reported was kept private so that no one was aware of the rates other participants reported. Following this, the pairs exchanged positions, and the protocol was repeated. The statistician

then computed the CRI rate in cycles/min for each recorded value by dividing the total number of CRI cycles counted per subject by the time in minutes allowed at each measurement session.

The mean reported CRI rate for the entire study (*N* = 727) was 6.88 ± 4.45 cycles/min. When the groups were subdivided and analyzed according to experience level, it is of interest to note that examiners with the greatest experience level palpated at a rate of 4.78 ± 2.57, a rate that is identical to the rate (4.54 ± 2.08 cpm) reported in *Protocol 5*.

Additional Observations: *Variability in the Flowmetry Record:* To date with more than one hundred and fifty blood flow velocity recordings obtained, certain additional observations regarding bloodflow velocities in the 0.003 to 0.50 Hz frequency range can be made. The frequencies of the various oscillatory contributions to the bloodflow velocity record are reliably constant in the frequencies that the component signals exhibit. The FT spectral peak of the very-low-frequency component (ranged between 0.003 and 0.05 Hz) is found consistently between 0.01 and 0.04 Hz, and the low-frequency spectral peak (ranged between 0.10 and 0.20 Hz) is found consistently between 0.10 and 0.17 Hz. The respiratory, or higher-frequency, spectral peak (0.25 to 0.50 Hz) is more variable, dependant upon the individual's respiratory rate. Despite this consistency, visibly distinctive variability occurs from record to record depending upon the degree to which the respective components contribute to the overall bloodflow velocity waveform. This results in visually recognizable patterns in the oscillations observed in the blood flow velocity record. Six flowmetry record subsets have been identified (Fig. 11.18) that are observed with reasonable frequency (264).

Three of these subsets exhibit a regular waveform that is easily recognized either in the original record or a record filtered using inverse FT. They differ in the amplitudes of the very-low-frequency and low-frequency signal components. In high-amplitude, strong-regular (sr) and intermediate-regular (ir) records, the regular waveform can be observed in the original record (Fig. 11.18, 1 and 2). In the weak-regular (wr) record, the regular waveform is masked by the high-frequency cardiac signal, which must be removed by filtering in order to observe the lower-frequency regular waveform (Fig. 11.18, 3) (262).

Flowmetry records in certain cases lack any visibly distinct low-frequency waves. CRI palpation of subjects exhibiting such a flowmetry record is often extremely difficult. Weak-irregular (wi) records are characterized by diminished very-low-frequency and low-frequency components (Fig. 11.18, 4). Often a relatively strong respiration signal also is present. Records with greatly diminished or undetectable low-frequency wave components are characterized as "low-baro" (lb) records (Fig. 11.18, 5) Excessive noise is the characteristic of high-noise (hn) records (Fig. 11.18, 6). This noise emanates from the subject. It is not an artifact of experimentation and cannot be removed by moving the probe to a new location (262).

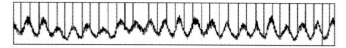

Figure 11-15 Bloodflow velocity record and CRI (palpation of "flexion/extension") in a 1:1 ratio.

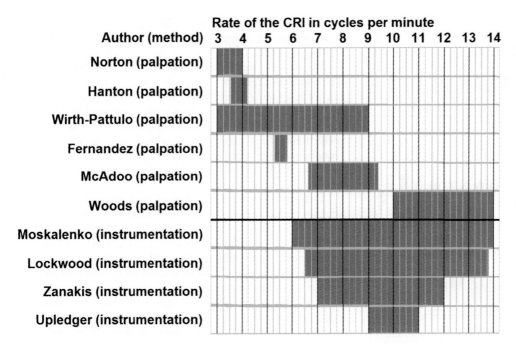

Rate of the CRI in cycles per minute

Author (method) — Norton (palpation), Hanton (palpation), Wirth-Pattulo (palpation), Fernandez (palpation), McAdoo (palpation), Woods (palpation), Moskalenko (instrumentation), Lockwood (instrumentation), Zanakis (instrumentation), Upledger (instrumentation)

Figure 11-17 A graphic representation of quantified rates for the CRI reported in the literature over the past 45 years. It is of interest to note that (with the exception of Woods, 10 to 14 cpm) when palpation is employed to obtain data, the reported rate tends to be lower (3 to 9 cpm), while if data are obtained by instrumentation, of any type, the reported rate tends to be higher (7 to 14 cpm).

Figure 11-17 Companion Table Caption. Comparison of palpated and instrumental CRI rates.

Interrater Reliability: During flowmetry recording, irregularities were observed resulting in gaps in both the palpatory and the flowmetry records. In some instances, these gaps were recognized and reported by the examiners as "still points" (Fig. 11.16) (261) When calculating the rate of the CRI (144), it was necessary that portions of each record be selected where the CRI was palpated consistently, without large "palpatory gaps." This was necessary because examiners often had difficulty consistently following the CRI. Additionally, it has now been noted, in two separate publications, that the CRI demonstrates a significant frequency modulation, which causes the rate to vary rhythmically approximately 20% (120,174).

Even if the issue of individual examiners palpating at 1:1 and 1:2 when comparing palpated CRI to the low-frequency oscillation in the flowmetry record is not given consideration, the irregularity of the palpatory records, the presence of still points, and the presence of a frequency modulation of 20% in the rate of the CRI will all contribute to such temporal variability in the sequential palpatory records of two individuals tracking the CRI that sequential interrater reliability becomes virtually impossible to establish. (This addresses the inability to demonstrate interrater reliability between sequential examiners but not between two examiners simultaneously palpating.)

Conclusions from the Above Six Protocols

From the protocols described, the following conclusions can be drawn:

1. Palpation of the CRI tracks identifiable frequencies in bloodflow velocity (*Protocol 1*).
2. The very-low-frequency (0.003 to 0.05 Hz, 0.18 to 3.0 cpm), low-frequency (0.10 to 0.20 Hz, 6.0 to 12 cpm) components of the flowmetry record, respectively, are remarkably consistent with the "slow tide" (six cycles in 10 minutes) and the "fast tide" (8 to 12 cpm) of the PRM as described by Becker (260) (*Protocol 1*).
3. Cranial palpation alone may be employed as sham treatment for research into the clinical impact of cranial manipulation (*Protocol 2*).

4. Cranial manipulation appears to exert effects upon baroreflex physiology (*Protocols 2 to 4*).
5. Cranial manipulation affects the low-frequency, 0.10 to 0.20, Hz signal, and to a lesser extent the very-low-frequency, 0.003 to 0.05 Hz, signal in bloodflow velocity and does so in a manner consistent with the type of manipulative procedure being employed (*Protocols 2 to4*).
6. A signal of frequency 0.08 Hz (0.04 to 0.11 Hz) has been identified in the flowmetry record that is closely related to the 0.10 to 0.20 Hz signal. Both are demonstrated to be affected by cranial manipulation, in this case CV-4 (*Protocol 4*).
7. Although not everyone appears to be palpating the CRI at the same frequency, everyone tracks the 0.10 to 0.20 Hz signal, with the majority tracking at 0.04 to 0.11 Hz or one CRI cycle to two low-frequency bloodflow velocity waves (*Protocol 5*).
8. The nearly identical palpated rates for the CRI of 4.54 ± 2.08 cpm (*Protocol 5*) and 4.78 ± 2.57 cpm (*Protocol 6*) appear to indicate that the majority of experienced practitioners are tracking the 0.08-Hz (4.5 cpm) minor signal (*Protocol 4*).
9. A new normative range for the CRI of 2 to 7 cpm, as palpated by experienced examiners, has been identified (*Protocols 5 and 6*).

Human physiology abounds with oscillating phenomena in the low-frequency (0.10 to 0.20 Hz) range. Many of these phenomena can be directly or indirectly linked to oscillations in the autonomic nervous system, particularly, but not limited to, the sympathetic nervous system. The CRI, with reported rates ranging from 2 to 14 cpm (0.04 to 0.23 Hz), shares the spectral frequency band with these physiologic phenomena. It is naïve, therefore, to draw the conclusion that these measurable phenomena are the PRM, or even the CRI. They are not. But they are certainly linked to one another and offer points of access through which the elusive aspects of cranial osteopathy may be studied.

The above protocols represent only the beginning of the work that needs to be done. They provide potential explanation for the physiology underlying the PRM. The conclusions offered, although controversial to some, cannot be denied. Although the oldest

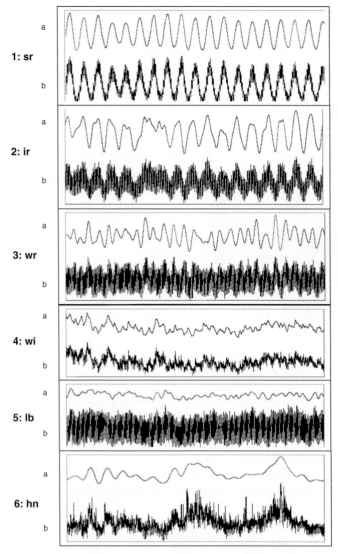

Figure 11-18 Observed flowmetry record subgroups: sr (47% of cases), ir (9%), wr (11%), wi (17%), low barrow (lb; 13%), and hn (3%). For each subgroup illustrated, the filtered trace (a), top, shows the oscillation created from only the very-low-, low-, and respiratory frequency components (below 0.5 Hz), and the bottom trace (b) shows the complete data record containing all component frequencies.

protocol involving flowmetry was published a decade ago, these studies have not, as yet, been replicated. It also must be acknowledged that these studies provide no clinical validation of cranial osteopathy. They address only basic science issues and offer no understanding as to how modulation of low-frequency physiological oscillations provides any therapeutic benefit. The door has been opened for further study.

CLOSING REMARKS

This chapter has looked at the entire frequency spectrum of oscillation that affects human beings, from milliseconds to millennia. Oscillation impacts all aspects of human life. The steady state, the position of equilibrium in any system, is subject to drift unless a corrective force is applied to oppose the drift. Oscillation is a process that regulates the drift of a system by constantly returning it to a point of equilibrium. Thus, it is advantageous for systems to oscillate. Oscillation provides a stable regulator, a reference point. It is a means for maintaining a system at its normative level of activity.

Oscillations are, in fact, energy. They are NOT matter. They are transmitted by matter, and in the process they transmit information. That information is a product of the frequency and power of the oscillation. It is further enhanced by the interaction of the specific oscillatory frequency with that of other oscillations. The strength of an oscillation may be augmented by entrainment with other oscillations of appropriate frequency. The resultant synchrony increases the power of the communicating frequency.

Frequency defines an oscillation's position within any given (frequency-domain) spectrum. It is a function of the rate of the regulated processes. Oscillation is a form of communication. The power of the communicating oscillation can be transferred to other frequencies through appropriate modification, that is, the various modes of modulation. Modulation is the result of communication among interacting frequencies.

The timing or phase of a given oscillation can enhance or negate another oscillation. To the degree that two oscillations are in phase, the power of the resultant oscillation will be augmented (or diminished).

A guitar string, in of itself, makes no sound until energy is provided by plucking the string. The string then oscillates at the frequency that its length, diameter, and tension dictate. This in turn excites the surrounding air that carries the waveform to your ear from where the information from the energy of the waveform is transmitted to your auditory cortex to be interpreted. The complexity of the message may be increased by simultaneously, plucking several strings to form a cord, and by sequentially playing cords to produce a tune. When several variations of that tune are provided by many musical instruments, a symphony results.

This simple example applies to all waveforms in all the ways that the laws physics permit their interaction. Oscillations all carry information and are subject to synchrony, modulation, and phase. They interact with other oscillations with resultant harmony or dissonance. Thus, it has been said, "The order of music is a bastion against chaos" (263). It may be an oversimplification, but health can be seen as harmony among physiological oscillations and disease as dissonance (264). As Littlejohn pointed out (1):

> It is this that lies at the basis of all mechanical systems of healing, the setting up of increase or the checking of the vibratile impulses, the correction in the distribution of the normal vibrations sent out from the brain center of control and distributed by co-ordination from the different planes of center activity.

Practitioners of manual therapeutics are aware of the significance placed upon oscillatory rhythms in several aspects of osteopathic theory and practice. Certainly, the low-frequency oscillation of the CRI immediately comes to mind (144). In this paradigm, the incitant procedure of temporal rocking and the intentional dampening of the rhythm with CV-4 are both examples of therapeutic control of a biological oscillation. Fulford's percussion hammer is another such example. This device vibrates in the range of the frequency of middle C on the piano (262 Hz) and is proposed to affect fascial dysfunction (265). (Middle C is the major sixth relative to A at 440 Hz.)

There are, however, many more examples that may not immediately spring to mind. Among the first therapeutic procedures taught to osteopathic students is the soft tissue stretching of the spinal paravertebral musculature. The student is taught to laterally stretch the paravertebral soft tissues, to gently release them, and then to repeat the process. The aware student quickly realizes that there is a comfortable rate with which this procedure can be applied. One may have had a similar experience when performing rib raising or the pedal fascial lymphatic pump of Dalrymple. As Dr. Littlejohn indicated, the body will respond optimally when therapeutic manual procedures are applied rhythmically and at the proper frequency. Not just in the case of the examples here listed, but for essentially all types of manipulative treatment from cranial and indirect functional to direct articulatory and even high-velocity low-amplitude procedures. Additionally, the application of vibratory forces may be employed diagnostically, like sonar, that in skilled hands can pinpoint a locus of dysfunctional restriction (266).

When performing an examination of any tissue, after having read this chapter, should clinicians take the time of day into consideration because of the presence of the circadian rhythm? Is the patient hungry and their ultradian rhythms no longer synchronized with their circadian rhythms? Is their heart rate variability damped and no longer responding to their circadian or ultradian signals?

Contemporary medicine considers homeostatic parameters and defines pathology as existing outside of those parameters. As such, therapies are commonly directed at lowering or raising the abnormal average. There may well be a better way! As Dr. Littlejohn indicated, the body will respond optimally when therapeutic procedures are applied rhythmically and at the proper frequency. He proposed that the therapeutic effect of osteopathic treatment is through the use of the physiological frequencies to affect the oscillations that share those frequencies. Thus, it is proposed that osteopathic treatment entrains physiological phenomena replacing dissonance with enhanced power and harmonic resonance (1,194,203).

REFERENCES

1. Littlejohn JM. The physiological basis of the therapeutic law. *J Am Osteopath Assoc* 1902;2:42–60.
2. Stagner JI, Samols E. Role of intrapancreatic ganglia in regulation of periodic insular secretions. *Am J Physiol* 1985;248:E552–E530.
3. Aschoff J. Zeitgeber der tierischen Tagesperiodik. *Naturwiss* 1954;41(3):49–56.
4. Aschoff J. Exogene und endogene Komponente der 24-Stunden-Periodik bei Tier und Mensch. *Naturwiss* 1955;42(21):569–575.
5. Strogatz SH, Abrams DM, McRobie A, et al. Crowd synchrony on the Millennium Bridge. *Nature* 2005;438:43–44.
6. Macdonald JHG. Lateral excitation of bridges by balancing pedestrians. *Proc R Soc A* doi:10.1098/rspa.2008.0367 19 pages (2008).
7. Sergueef N, Nelson KE, Glonek T. The effect of cranial manipulation on the Traube-Hering-Mayer oscillation as measured by laser-Doppler flowmetry. *Altern Ther Health Med* 2002;8(6):74–76.
8. Nelson KE, Sergueef N, Glonek T. Cranial manipulation induces sequential changes in blood flow velocity on demand. *Amer Acad Osteop J* 2004;14(3):15–17.
9. Nasimi SGAA, Harness JB, Marjanović DZ, et al. Periodic posture stimulation of the baroreceptors and the local vasomotor reflexes. *J Biomed Eng* 1992;14:308–312.
10. Strogatz SH, Stewart I. Coupled oscillators and biological synchronization. *Sci Am* 1993;269(6):102–109.
11. Pelling AE, Sehati S, Gralla EB, et al. Local mechanical motion of the cell wall of *Saccharomyces cerevisiae*. *Science* 2004;305(20 Aug):1147–1150.
12. Xie S, Huang J, Hu C, et al. Lipid distribution in a subtropical southern China stalagmite as a record of soil ecosystem response to paleoclimate change. *Quatern Res* 2003;60(3):340–347.
13. Boussau B, Blanquart S, Necsulea A, et al. Parallel adaptations to high temperatures in the Archaean eon. *Nature* 2008;456(7224):942–945.
14. Wever R. Zum Mechanismus der biologischen 24-Stunden-Periodik. *Biol Cybern* 1964;2(3):127–144.
15. Lubkin V, Beizai P, Sadun AA. The eye as metronome of the body. *Surv Ophthalmol* 2002;47(1):17–26.
16. Sasselov DD. Extrasolar planets. *Nature* 2008;451(7174):29–31.
17. Davenport TF. Jenna's clocks. *Nature* 2010;463:700-EOA, para. 15–16.
18. Piepoli M, Sleight P, Leuzzi S, et al. Origin of respiratory sinus arrhythmia in conscious humans. An important role for arterial carotid baroreceptors. *Circulation* 1997;95(7):1813–1821.
19. Chang H-S, Staras K, Gilbey MP. Multiple oscillators provide metastability in rhythm generation. *J Neurosci* 2000;20(13):5135–5143.
20. Soto-Treviño C, Rabbah P, Marder E, et al. Computational model of electrically coupled, intrinsically distinct pacemaker neurons. *J Neurophysiol* 2005;94:590–604.
21. Vitaterna MH, King DP, Chang A-M, et al. Mutagenesis and mapping of a mouse gene, *Clock*, essential for circadian behavior. *Science* 1994;264:719–725.
22. Schouten JF. The perception of subjective tones. *Proc Sect Sci* 1938;41:1086–1093.
23. Sacks OW. Papa blows his nose in G: absolute pitch. In: *Musicophilia: Tales of Music and the Brain*. New York, NY: Vintage Books (a division of Random House, Inc.) 2008:129–139; chap 9.
24. Zatorre RJ. Finding the missing fundamental. *Nature* 2005;436(7054):1093–1094.
25. International Conference, 1939, adopted by the International Organization for Standardization in 1955.
26. Swenson EE. The history of musical pitch in tuning the pianoforte. http://www.mozartpiano.com/articles/pitch.html. 2007. Pitches from Ellis AJ.
27. Bendor D, Wang X. The neuronal representation of pitch in primate auditory cortex. *Nature* 2005;436:1161–1165.
28. Wever R. Autonome circadiane Periodik des Menschen unter dem Einfluss verschiedener Beleuchtungs-Bedingungen. *Pflügers Arch* 1969;306(1):71–91.
29. Pando MP, Morse D, Cermakian N, et al. Phenotypic rescue of a peripheral clock genetic defect via SCN hierarchical dominance. *Cell* 2002;110(1):107–117.
30. Mistlberger RE. Circadian food-anticipatory activity: formal models and physiological mechanisms. *Neurosci Biobehav Rev* 1994;18(2):171–195.
31. Marchant EG, Mistlberger RE. Anticipation and entrainment to feeding time in intact and SCN-ablated C57BL/6j mice. *Brain Res* 1997;765:273–282.
32. Damiola F, Le Minh N, Preitner N, et al. Restricted feeding uncouples circadian oscillators in peripheral tissues from the central pacemaker in the suprachiasmatic nucleus. *Genes Dev* 2000;14:2950–2961.
33. Raffaelli D. Zeitgeber. *The Chicago Shimpo* 2008;5738(Nov. 21):4-EOA.
34. Goldbeter A. *Biochemical Oscillations and Cellular Rhythms*. Cambridge, UK: Cambridge University Press, 1997. Table 1.1, p. 2.
35. Bourdon L, Buguet A. Bases de la chronobiologie: les rythmes nycthéméraux. *J Fr Ophtalmol* 2004;2:2S5–2S10.
36. Jülicher F. Mechanical oscillations at the cellular scale. *C R Acad Sci (Paris) Ser IV* 2001;6:849–860
37. van Dam JA, Aziz HA, Sierra MÁÁ, et al. Long-period astronomical forcing of mammal turnover. *Nature* 2006;443(7111):687–691.
38. Kath WL, Ottino JM. Rhythm engineering. *Science* 2007;316:1857–1858.
39. Guest J. How reefs respond to mass coral spawning. *Science* 2008;320(5876):621–623.
40. Burt CT, Glonek T, Bárány M. Analysis of phosphate metabolites, the intracellular pH, and the state of adenosine triphosphate in intact muscle by phosphorus nuclear magnetic resonance. *J Biol Chem* 1976;251(9),2584–2591.
41. Glonek T. Applications of ^{31}P NMR to biological systems with emphasis on intact tissue determinations. In: Stec WJ, ed. *Phosphorus Chemistry Directed Towards Biology*. New York, NY: Pergamon Press, 1980:157–174.
42. Burt CT, Glonek T, Bárány M. ^{31}P nuclear magnetic resonance detection of unexpected phosphodiesters in muscle. *Biochemistry* 1976;15(22):4850–4853.

43. Glonek T, Merchant TE. ^{31}P NMR of phospholipid glycerol phosphodiester residues. *J Lipid Res* 1990;31:479–486.

44. Bardygula-Nonn LG, Black MB, Baranyai PS, et al. Naturally spawning chinook salmon (*Oncorhynchus tshawytscha*) from the effluent of a wastewater treatment plant. *J Freshwater Ecol* 1996;11:439–445.

45. Nakao N, Ono H, Yamamura T, et al. Thyrotrophin in the pars tuberalis triggers photoperiodic response. *Nature* 2008;452(7185):317–322.

46. Beyerbach DM, Kovacs RJ, Dmitrienko AA, et al. Heart rate-corrected QT interval in men increases during winter months. *Heart Rhythm* 2007;4(3):277–281.

47. Voon WC, Wu JC, Lai WT, et al. Seasonal variability of the QT dispersion in healthy subjects. *J Electrocardiol* 2001;34(4):285–288.

48. Avery DH, Eder DN, Bolte MA, et al. Dawn simulation and bright light in the treatment of SAD: a controlled study. *Biol Psychiatry* 2001;50(3):205–216.

49. Bhattacharjee Y. Is internal timing key to mental health? *Science* 2007;317:1488–1490.

50. Garai J, Világi S, Répásy I, et al. Short communication: seasonal onset of menopause? *Hum Reprod* 2004;19:1666–1667.

51. Smits LJ, Zielhuis GA, Jongbloet PH, et al. Seasonal variation in human fecundability. *Hum Reprod* 1998;13:3520–3524.

52. Brundtland GH, Liestöl K. Seasonal variations in menarche in Oslo. *Ann Hum Biol* 1982;9:35–43.

53. Kelly G. Body temperature variability (Part 1): a review of the history of body temperature and its variability due to site selection, biological rhythms, fitness, and aging. *Altern Med Rev* 2006;11(4):278–293.

54. Coyne MD, Kesick CM, Doherty TJ, et al. Circadian rhythm changes in core temperature over the menstrual cycle: method for noninvasive monitoring. *Am J Physiol Regul Integr Comp Physiol* 2000;279(4):R1316–R1320.

55. Bao A-M, Liu R-Y, van Someren EJW, et al. Diurnal rhythm of free estradiol during the menstrual cycle. *Eur J Endocrinol* 2003;148:227–232.

56. Goebel R, Kuss E. Circadian rhythm of serum unconjugated estriol in late pregnancy. *J Clin Endocrinol Metab* 1974;39:969–972.

57. McClintock MK. Menstrual synchrony and suppression. *Nature* 1971;229:244–245.

58. McClintock MK. Estrous synchrony: modulation of ovarian cycle length by female pheromones. *Physiol Behav* 1984;32:701–705.

59. Stern K, McClintock MK. Regulation of ovulation by human pheromones. *Nature* 1998;392:177–179.

60. Liu HY, Bao AM, Zhou JN, et al. Changes in circadian sleep-wake and rest-activity rhythms during different phases of menstrual cycle. *Sheng Li Xue Bao* 2005;57(3)389–394.

61. Korr IM, Appeltauer GSL. The time-course of axonal transport of neuronal proteins to muscle. *Exp Neurol* 1974;43(2):452–463.

62. Herzog ED, Schwartz WJ. Invited review: a neural clockwork for encoding circadian time. *J Appl Physiol* 2002;92:401–408.

63. Reppert SM, Weaver DR. Molecular analysis of mammalian circadian rhythms. *Annu Rev Physiol* 2001;63:647–676.

64. Wever RA. Light effects on human circadian rhythms: a review of recent andechs experiments. *J Biol Rhythms* 1989;4(2):161–185.

65. Inouye S-I T, Shibata S. Neurochemical organization of circadian rhythm in the suprachiasmatic nucleus. *Neurosci Res* 1994;20(2):109–130.

66. Czeisler CA, Duffy JF, Shanahan TL, et al. Stability, precision and near-24-hour period of the human circadian pacemaker. *Science* 1999;284:2177–2181.

67. Moore RY. A clock for the ages. *Science* 1999;248:2102–2103.

68. Buijs RM, Scheer FA, Kreier F, et al. Organization of circadian functions: interaction with the body. *Prog Brain Res* 2006;153:341–360.

69. King DP, Zhao Y, Sangoram AM, et al. Positional cloning of the mouse circadian *Clock* Gene. *Cell* 1997;89(4):641–653.

70. Maemura K, Takeda N, Nagai R. Circadian rhythms in the CNS and peripheral clock disorders: role of the biological clock in cardiovascular diseases. *J Pharmacol Sci* 2007;103:134–138.

71. Brown SA, Schibler U. La variance de la période circadienne chez l'homme, dans sa peau. *Med Sci (Paris)* 2006;22(5):474–475.

72. Dunlap JC. Molecular bases for circadian clocks. *Cell* 1999;96(2):271–290.

73. Hastings M, Maywood ES. Circadian clocks in the mammalian brain. *Bioessays* 2000;22(1):23–31.

74. Zylka MJ, Shearman LP, Weaver DR, et al. Three *period* homologs in mammals: differential light responses in the suprachiasmatic circadian clock and oscillating transcripts outside of brain. *Neuron* 1998;20:1103–1110.

75. Takumi T, Taguchi K, Miyake S, et al. A light-independent oscillatory gene mPer3 in mouse SCN and OVLT. *EMBO J* 1998;17(16):4753–4759.

76. Lamia KA, Storch K-F, Weitz CJ. Physiological significance of a peripheral tissue circadian clock. *Proc Natl Acad Sci USA* 2008;105(39):15172–15177.

77. Reppert SM, Weaver DR. Coordination of circadian timing in mammals. *Nature* 2002;418(6901):935–941.

78. Hara R, Wan K, Wakamatsu H, et al. Restricted feeding entrains liver clock without participation of the suprachiasmatic nucleus. *Genes Cells* 2001;6:269–278.

79. Fuller PM, Lu J, Saper CB. Differential rescue of light- and food-entrainable circadian rhythms. *Science* 2008;320(5879):1074–1077.

80. Wever R. Zum Mechanismus der biologischen 24-Stunden-Periodik. II. Der Einfluss des Gleichwertes auf die Eigenschaften selbsterregter Schwingungen. *Kybernetik* 1963;1:213–231.

81. Plautz JD, Kaneko M, Hall JC, et al. Independent photoreceptive circadian clocks throughout *Drosophila*. *Science* 1997;278:1632–1635.

82. Whitmore D, Foulkes NS, Sassone-Corsi P. Light acts directly on organs and cells in culture to set the vertebrate circadian clock. *Nature* 2000;404:87–91.

83. Shiraishi M, Kamo T, Kamegai M, et al. Periodic structures and diurnal variation in blood pressure and heart rate in relation to microgravity on space station MIR. *Biomed Pharmacother* 2004;58:S31–S34.

84. Bode-Böger SM, Böger RH, Kielstein JT, et al. Role of endogenous nitric oxide in circadian blood pressure regulation in healthy humans and in patients with hypertension or atherosclerosis. *J Investig Med* 2000;48:125–132.

85. Nickla DL, Rada JA, Wallman J. Isolated chick sclera shows a circadian rhythm in proteoglycan synthesis perhaps associated with the rhythm in ocular elongation. *J Comp Physiol A* 1999;185(1):81–90.

86. Yom SM, Nickla DL. There is a circadian rhythm in nitric oxide synthesis in isolated chick choroid. *Invest Ophthalmol Vis Sci* 2005;46:Abs. 1985–B754.

87. Sawa T, Zaki MH, Okamoto T, et al. *Nat Chem Biol* 2007;3(11):727–735.

88. Wever R. Zur Zeitgeber-Stärke eines Licht-Dunkel-Wechsels für die circadiane Periodik des Menschen. *Pflügers Arch* 1970;321:133–142.

89. Pattanayek R, Wang J, Mori T, et al. Visualizing a circadian clock protein: crystal structure of KaiC and functional insights. *Mol Cell* 2004;15(3):375–388.

90. Yarnell A. Cracking the biological clock. *Chem Eng News* 2004;2:40–41.

91. Nakajima M, Imai K, Ito H, et al. Reconstitution of circadian oscillation of cyanobacterial KaiC phosphorylation in vitro. *Science* 2005;308:414–415.

92. Poon AC, Ferrell Jr JE. A clock with a flip switch. *Science* 2007;318:757–758.

93. Gore J, van Oudenaarden A. The yin and yang of nature. *Nature* 2009;457(7227):271–273.

94. Tsai TY-C, Choi YS, Ma W, et al. Robust, tunable biological oscillations from interlinked positive and negative feedback loops. *Science* 2008;321(5885):126–129.

95. Stricker J, Cookson S, Bennett MR, et al. A fast, robust and tunable synthetic gene oscillator. *Nature* 2008;456(7221):516–519.

96. Tigges M, Marquez-Lago TT, Stelling J, et al. A tunable synthetic mammalian oscillator. *Nature* 2009;457(7227):309–312.

97. Dodd AN, Gardner MJ, Hotta CT, et al. The *Arabidopsis* circadian clock incorporates a cADPR-based feedback loop. *Science* 2007;318(5857):1789–1792.

98. Lamia KA, Sachdeva UM, DiTacchio L, et al. AMPK regulates the circadian clock by cryptochrome phosphorylation and degradation. *Science* 2009;236:437–440.

99. Suter DM, Schibler U. Feeding the clock. *Science* 2009;326:378–379.

100. Holter NS, Mitra M, Maritan A, et al. Fundamental patterns underlying gene expression profiles: simplicity from complexity. *Proc Natl Acad Sci USA* 2000;97(15):8409–8414.

101. Foyer CH. Review. *Ann Bot (Lond)* 2002;89:500–501.

102. Vanden Driessche T, Guisset J-L, Petiau-de Vries GM, eds. *The Redox State and Circadian Rhythms*. Dordrecht: Kluwer Academic Publishers, 2000.

103. Finkel T, Deng C-X, Mostoslavsky R. Recent progress in the biology and physiology of sirtuins. *Nature* 2008;460:587–591.

104. Asher G, Gatfield D, Stratmann M, et al. SIRT1 regulates circadian clock gene expression through PER2 deacetylation. *Cell* 2008;134:317–328.

105. Nakahata Y, Kaluzova M, Grimaldi B, et al. The NAD⁺-dependent deacetylase SIRT1 modulates CLOCK-mediated chromatin remodeling and circadian control. *Cell* 2008;134:329–340.

106. Phillips ML. Of owls, larks, and alarm clocks. *Nature* 2009;458(7235):142–144.

107. Méndez-Ferrer S, Lucas D, Battista M, et al. Haematopoietic stem cell release is regulated by circadian oscillations. *Nature* 2008;452(7186):442–447.

108. Weigle DS. Pulsatile secretion of fuel-regulatory hormones. *Diabetes* 1987;36(6):764–775.

109. Sonnenberg GE, Hoffmann RG, Johnson CP, et al. Low- and high-frequency insulin secretion impulses in normal subjects and pancreas transplant recipients: role of extrinsic innervation. *J Clin Invest* 1992;90:545–553.

110. Shannahoff-Khalsa DS, Kennedy B, Yates FE, et al. Low-frequency ultradian insulin rhythms are coupled to cardiovascular, autonomic, and neuroendocrine rhythms. *Am J Physiol* 1997;272:R962–R968.

111. Hogan RD. The initial lymphatics and interstitial fluid pressure. In: Hargens AR, ed, *Tissue Fluid Pressure and Composition*. Baltimore, MD: Williams & Wilkins; 1981:155–163.

112. Onizuka M, Flatebø T, Nicolaysen G. Lymph flow pattern in the intact thoracic duct in sheep. *J Physiol* 1997;503.1:223–234.

113. Olszewski WL, Engeset A. Lymphatic contractions. *N Engl J Med* 1979;300:316-EOA.

114. Kayser R. Die exacte Messung der Luftdurchgängigkeit der Nase. *Arch Laryngol Rhinol* 1895;3:101–120.

115. Keuning J. On the nasal cycle. *Inter Rhinol* 1968;6:99–136.

116. Yosipovitch G, Xiong GL, Haus E, et al. Time-dependent variations of the skin barrier function in humans: transepidermal water loss, stratum corneum hydration, skin surface pH, and skin temperature. *J Invest Dermatol* 1998;110(1):20–23.

117. Le Fur I, Reinberg A, Lopez S, et al. Analysis of circadian and ultradian rhythms of skin surface properties of face and forearm of healthy women. *J Invest Dermatol* 2001;117:718–724.

118. Wegmann HM, Brüner H, Jovy D, et al. Effects of transmeridian flights on the diurnal excretion pattern of 17-hydroxycorticosteroids. *Aerospace Med* 1970;41(9):1003–1005.

119. Burch GE, Cohn AE, Neumann C. A study by quantitative methods of the spontaneous variations in volume of the finger tip, toe tip, and postero-superior portion of the pinna of resting normal white adults. *Am J Physiol* 1942;136:433–447.

120. Nelson KE, Sergueef N, Lipinski CM, et al. Cranial rhythmic impulse related to the Traube-Hering-Mayer oscillation: comparing laser-Doppler flowmetry and palpation. *J Am Osteopath Assoc* 2001;101(3):163–173.

121. Mayer S. Über spontane Blutdruckschwankungen. *Sitzungb d k Akad d W math naturw* 1876;67:281–305.

122. Peňáz J. Mayer waves: history and methodology. *Automedica* 1978;2:135–141.

123. Kitney RI. An analysis of the nonlinear behaviour of the human thermal vasomotor control system. *J Theor Biol* 1975;52:231–248.

124. Morré DJ, Morré DM. NADH oxidase activity of soybean plasma membranes oscillates with a temperature compensated period of 24 min. *Plant J* 1998;16(3):277–284.

125. Moskalenko YE, Kravchenko TI, Gaidar BV, et al. Periodic mobility of cranial bones in humans. *Human Physiol* 1999;25(1):51–58, 62–70.

126. Moskalenko YE, Kravchenko TI, Vainshtein GB, et al. Slow-wave oscillations in the craniosacral space: a hemoliquorodynamic concept of origination. *Neurosci Behavioral Physiol* 2009;39(4):377–381.

127. Dóra E, Kovách AGB. Metabolic and vascular volume oscillations in the cat brain cortex. *Acta Physiol Hung* 1981;57(3):261–275.

128. Vern BA, Schuette WH, Leheta B, et al. Low-frequency oscillations of cortical oxidative metabolism in waking and sleep. *J Cerebral Blood Flow Metab* 1988;8(2):215–226.

129. Kiviniemi V. Spontaneous blood oxygen fluctuation in awake and sedated brain cortex—a BOLD fMRI study. Academic Dissertation. Oulu, HI: Oulu University Press, 2004. ISBN 951-42-7387-7 (nid.); ISBN 951-42-7388-5 (PDF) http://herkules.oulu.fi/isbn9514273885/; ISSN 0355-3221 http://herkules.oulu.fi.issn03553221/.

130. Schmidt SH. Bandwidth-specific functional connectivity of physiological low frequency oscillations in fMRI. Medizinische Fakultät Charité—Universitatsmedizin Berlin (Dissertation in English) 2009: 70 pp. http://www.diss.fu-berlin.de/diss/receive/FUDISS_thesis_000000008598.

131. Zanakis MF, Cebelenski RM, Dowling D, et al. The cranial kinetogram: objective quantification of cranial mobility in man. *J Am Osteopath Assoc* 1994;94(9):761-EOA.

132. Ueno T, Ballard RE, Shuer LM, et al. Noninvasive measurement of pulsatile intracranial pressure using ultrasound. *Acta Neurochir* 1998;71(suppl):66–69.

133. Ueno T, Ballard RE, Macias BR, et al. Cranial diameter pulsations measured by non-invasive ultrasound decrease with tilt. *Aviat Space Environ Med* 2003;74(8):882–885.

134. Retzlaff EW, Michael DK, Roppel RM. Cranial bone mobility. *J Am Osteopath Assoc* 1975;74:869–873.

135. Campbell JK, Clark JM, White DN, et al. Pulsatile echo-encephalography. *Acta Neurol Scand* 1970;46(suppl 45):6–57.

136. Burns L. Viscero-somatic and somato-visceral spinal reflexes. *J Am Osteopath Assoc* 1907;7(2):51–60; reprinted *J Am Osteopath Assoc* 2000;100(4):249–258.

137. Mayhew JEW, Askew S, Zheng Y, et al. Cerebral vasomotion: a 0.1 Hz oscillation in reflected light imaging of neural activity. *Neuroimage* 1996;4:183–193.

138. Hyndman BW. The role of rhythms in homeostasis. *Kybernetik* 1974;15:227–236.

139. Hyndman BW, Kitney RI, Sayers BMcA. Spontaneous rhythms in physiological control systems. *Nature* 1971;233:339–341.

140. Eckberg DL. Physiological basis for human autonomic rhythms. *Ann Med* 2000;32(5):341–349.

141. Akselrod S, Gordon D, Ubel FA, et al. Power spectrum analysis of heart rate fluctuation: a quantitative probe of beat-to-beat cardiovascular control. *Science* 1981;213:220–222.

142. Bonaduce D, Marciano F, Petretta M, et al. Effects of converting enzyme inhibition on heart period variability in patients with acute myocardial infarction. *Circulation* 1994;90:108–113.

143. Taylor JA, Carr DL, Myers CW, et al. Mechanisms underlying very-low-frequency RR-interval oscillations in humans. *Circulation* 1998;98:547–555.

144. Nelson KE, Sergueef N, Glonek T. The effect of an alternative medical procedure upon low-frequency oscillations in cutaneous blood flow velocity. *J Manip Physiol Thera* 2006;29(8):626–636.

145. Guinn KK, Rodriguez C, Bucheli D, et al. Reproducibility assessment of the response to CV4 as measured by the laser Doppler flowmeter and electrocardiogram. *J Am Osteopath Assoc* 2007;107(8; Abs. P7):332-EOA.

146. Guinn K, Seffinger MA, Ali H, et al. Validation of transcutaneous laser Doppler flowmeter in measuring autonomic balance. *J Am Osteopath Assoc* 2006;106(8):475–476.

147. Pagani M, Somers V, Furlan R, et al. Changes in autonomic regulation induced by physical training in mild hypertension. *Hypertension* 1988;12:600–610.

148. Hara K, Nakatani S, Ozaki K, et al. Detection of B waves in the oscillation of intracranial pressure by fast Fourier transform. *Med Inform* 1990;15(2):125–131.

149. Cevese A, Gulli G, Polati E, et al. Baroreflex and oscillation of heart period at 0.1 Hz studied by α-blockade and cross-spectral analysis in healthy humans. *J Physiol* 2001;531.1:235–244.

150. Crandall CG, Engelke KA, Pawelczyk JA, et al. Power spectral and time based analysis of heart rate variability following 15 days head-down bed rest. *Aviat, Space, and Environ Med* 1994;65:1105–1109.

151. Takalo R, Korhonen I, Majahalme S, et al. Circadian profile of low-frequency oscillations in blood pressure and heart rate in hypertension. *Am J Hypertens* 1999;12:874–881.

152. Badra LJ, Cooke WH, Hoag JB, et al. Respiratory modulation of human autonomic rhythms. *Am J Physiol Heart Circ Physiol* 2001;280:H2674–H2688.

153. Clark LC Jr, Misrahy G, Fox RP. Chronically implanted polarographic electrodes. *J Appl Physiol* 1958;13(1):85–91.

154. Moskalenko YE. Regional cerebral blood flow and its control at rest and during increased functional activity. In: Ingvar DH, Lassen NA, eds. *Brain Work, Alfred Benzon Symposium VIII.* Copenhagen: Munksgaard, 1975;343–352.

155. Guyton AC, Harris JW. Pressoreceptor-autonomic oscillation: a probable cause of vasomotor waves. *Am J Physiol* 1951;165:158–166.

156. Julien C. The enigma of Mayer waves: facts and models. *Cardiovasc Res* 2006;70:12:21.

157. Bertram D, Barrès C, Cuisinaud G, et al. The arterial baroreceptor reflex of the rat exhibits positive feedback properties at the frequency of Mayer waves. *J Physiol* 1998;513:251–261.

158. Werntz DA, Bickford RG, Bloom FE, et al. Alternating cerebral hemispheric activity and the lateralization of autonomic nervous function. *Human Neurobiol* 1983;2:39–43.

159. Lakatos P, Karmos G, Mehta AD, et al. Entrainment of neuronal oscillations as a mechanism of attentional selection. *Science* 2008;320(5872): 110–113.

160. Lakatos P, Chen C-M, O'Connell MN, et al. Neuronal oscillations and multisensory interaction in primary auditory cortex. *Neuron* 2007;53(2):279–292.

161. Colgin LL, Denninger T, Fyhn M, et al. Frequency of gamma oscillations routes flow of information in the hippocampus. *Nature* 2009;462(7271):353–357.

162. van den Pol AN, Dudek FE. Cellular communication in the circadian clock, the suprachiasmatic nucleus. *Neuroscience* 1993;56(4):793–811.

163. Penagos H, Melcher JR, Oxenham AJ. A neural representation of pitch salience in nonprimary human auditory cortex revealed with functional magnetic resonance imaging. *J Neurosci* 2004;24:6810–6815.

164. Rayment I, Rypniewski WR, Schmidt-Bäse K, et al. Three-dimensional structure of myosin subfragment-1: a molecular motor. *Science* 1993; 261:50–58.

165. Rayment I, Hazel M, Holden HM, et al. Structure of actin-myosin complex and its implications for muscle contractions. *Science* 1993;261: 58–65.

166. Noji H. The rotary enzyme of the cell: the rotation of F1-ATPase. *Science* 1998;282:1844–1845.

167. Michie D, West DJ. An experiment on 'telepathy' using television. *Nature* 1957;180:1402–1403.

168. Feldman Y, Puzenko A, Ben Ishai P, et al. Human skin as arrays of helical antennas in the millimeter and submillimeter wave range. *Phys Rev Lett* 2008;100(12):128102(4). (Ed. NOTE. This funny inclusive pagination is correct. The article page is 128102, and there are 4 pages to the article all numbered 128102.)

169. Gove PB, ed. *Webster's Third New International Dictionary of the English Language Unabridged.* Springfield, MA: G. & C. Merriam Co.; 1976.

170. Buck J, Buck E. Synchronous fireflies. *Sci Am* 1976;234(5):74–79, 82–85.

171. Mirollo RE, Strogatz SH. Synchronization of pulse-coupled biological oscillators. *SIAM J Appl Math* 1990;50(6):1645–1662.

172. Danino T, Mondragón-Palomino O, Tsimring L, et al. A synchronized quorum of genetic clocks. *Nature* 2010;463(7279):326–330.

173. Sergueef N, Nelson KE, Glonek T. Changes in the Traube-Hering wave following cranial manipulation. *Amer Acad Osteop J* 2001;11:17-EOA.

174. Lockwood MD, Degenhardt BF. Cycle-to-cycle variability attributed to the primary respiratory mechanism. *J Am Osteopath Assoc* 1998;98(1): 35–43.

175. Klein KE, Wegmann HM, Hunt BI. Desynchronization of body temperature and performance circadian rhythm as a result of outgoing and homegoing transmeridian flights. *Aerospace Med* 1972;43(2): 119–132.

176. Klein KE, Wegmann H-M. The resynchronization of human circadian rhythms after transmeridian flights as a result of flight direction and mode of activity. In: Scheving LE, Halberg F, Pauly JE, eds. *Chronogiology.* Tokyo: Igaku Shoin Ltd., 1974:564–570.

177. Klein KE, Brüner H, Holtmann H, et al. Circadian rhythm of pilots' efficiency and effects of multiple time zone travel. *Aerosp Med* 1970;41(2): 125–132.

178. Wever RA. Phase shifts of human circadian rhythms due to shifts of artificial zeitgebers. *Chronobiologia* 1980;7:303–327.

179. Wegmann HM, Gundel A, Naumann M, et al. Sleep, sleepiness, and circadian rhythmicity in aircrews operating on transatlantic routes. *Aviat Space Environ Med* 1986;57(12, suppl):B53–B64.

180. Vern BA, Leheta BJ, Vern JC, et al. Interhemispheric synchrony of slow oscillations of cortical blood volume and cytochrome aa$_3$ redox state in unanesthetized rabbits. *Brain Res* 1997;775:233–239.

181. Vern BA, Leheta BJ, Juel VC, et al. Slow oscillations of cytochrome oxidaseredox state and blood volume in unanesthetized cat and rabbit cortex. Intethemispheric synchrony. *Adv Exp Med* 1998;454:561–570.

182. Sayers BMcA. Analysis of heart rate variability. *Ergonomics* 1973;16(1): 17–32.

183. Barman SM, Gebber GL. Basis for synchronization of sympathetic and phrenic nerve discharges. *Am J Physiol* 1976;231:1601–1607.

184. Ahmed AK, Harness JB, Mearns AJ. Respiratory control of heart rate. *Eur J Appl Physiol Occup Physiol* 1982;50:95–104.

185. Haas F, Distenfeld S, Axen K. Effects of perceived musical rhythm on respiratory pattern. *J Appl Physiol* 1986;61(3):1185–1191.

186. Bernardi L, Sleight P, Bandinelli G, et al. Effect of rosary prayer and yoga mantras on autonomic cardiovascular rhythms: comparative study. *Brit Med J* 2001;323(7327):1446–1449.

187. Sergueef N, Nelson KE, Glonek T. The effect of light exercise upon blood flow velocity determined by laser-Doppler flowmetry. *J Med Eng Technol* 2004;28(4):143–150.

188. Kuo T, Huang G, Chen J, et al. Influence of Tai Chi Chuan on autonomic control of heart rate. 5th IOC World Congress on Sport Sciences (Sydney 31 Oct.–5 Nov., 1999, with the Annual Conference of Science and Medicine in Sport). Abs. 102b.

189. Sacks OW. *Musicophilia: Tales of Music and the Brain.* New York, NY: Vintage Books (a division of Random House, Inc.), 2008. (Quotation on p. 43).

190. Burton AC. The range and variability of the blood flow in the human fingers and the vasomotor regulation of body temperature. *Am J Physiol* 1939;127:437–453.

191. Cheng MY, Bullock CM, Li C, et al. Prokineticin 2 transmits the behavioural circadian rhythm of the suprachiasmatic nucleus. *Nature* 2002;417:405–410.

192. Yamaguchi S, Isejima H, Matsuo T, et al. Synchronization of cellular clocks in the suprachiasmatic nucleus. *Science* 2003;302:1408–1412.

193. Butcher GQ, Dziema H, Collamore M, et al. The p42/44 mitogen-activated protein kinase pathway couples photic input to circadian clock entrainment. *J Biol Chem* 2002;277(33):29519–29525.

194. Nelson KE. The primary respiratory mechanism. *Amer Acad Osteop J* 2002;12(4):25–34.

195. Pardini L, Kaeffer B. Feeding and circadian clocks. *Reprod Nutr Dev* 2006;46(5):463–480.

196. Shearman LP, Sriram S, Weaver DR, et al. Interacting molecular loops in the mammalian circadian clock. *Science* 2000;288:1013–1019.

197. Barnes JW, Tischkau SA, Barnes JA, et al. Requirement of mammalian *Timeless* for circadian rhythmicity. *Science* 2003;302:439–441.

198. Lin JM, Kilman VL, Keegan K, et al. A role for casein kinase 2α in the *Drosophila* circadian clock. *Nature* 2002;420:816–820.

199. Rutter J, Reick M, Wu LC, et al. Regulation of clock and NPAS2 DNA binding by the redox state of NAD cofactors. *Science* 2001;293: 510–514.

200. Renn SCP, Park JH, Rosbash M, et al. A *pdf* neuropeptide gene mutation and ablation of PDF neurons each cause severe abnormalities of behavioral circadian rhythms in *Drosophila*. *Cell* 1999;99(7):791–802.

201. Falcón J. Cellular circadian clocks in the pineal. *Prog Neurobiol* 1999;58:121–162.

202. McHale NG, Roddie IC, Thornbury KD. Nervous modulation of spontaneous contractions in bovine mesenteric lymphatics. *J Physiol* 1980;309:461–472.

203. McPartland JM, Mein EA. Entrainment and the cranial rhythmic impulse. *Altern Ther Health Med* 1997;3(1):40–45.

204. Bernardi L, Porta C, Sleight P. Cardiovascular, cerebrovascular, and respiratory changes induced by different types of music in musicians and non-musicians: the importance of silence. *Heart* 2006;92:445–452.

205. Ball P. Facing the music (1st of a 9-part essay series). *Nature* 2008;453(7192):160–162.
206. Dijk D-J, von Schantz M. Timing and Consolidation of human sleep, wakefulness, and performance by a symphony of oscillators. *J Biol Rhythms* 2005;20(4):279–290.
207. Long MA, Fee MS. Using temperature to analyse temporal dynamics in the songbird motor pathway. *Nature* 2008;456(7219):189–194. Doi: 10.1038/nature07448.
208. Gebber GL, Das M, Barman SM. An unusual form of phase walk in a system of coupled oscillators. *J Biol Rhythms* 2004;19(6):542–550.
209. Jeon M, Gardner HF, Miller EA, et al. Similarity of the C. elegans developmental timing protein LIN-42 to circadian rhythm proteins. *Science* 1999;286:1141–1146.
210. Cardin JA, Carlén M, Meletis K, et al. Driving fast-spiking cells induces gamma rhythm and controls sensory responses. *Nature* 2009;459(7247):663–667.
211. Li Y-X, Goldbeter A. Pulsatile signaling in intercellular communication. *Biophys J* 1992;61:161–171.
212. Goldbeter A. Periodic signaling as an optimal mode of intercellular communication. *News Physiol Sci* 1988;3:103–105.
213. Barkai N, Leibler S. Circadian clocks limited by noise. *Nature* 2000;403:267–268.
214. Greenberg JT. Programmed cell death: a way of life for plants. *Proc Natl Acad Sci USA* 1996;93:12094–12097.
215. Cui Y, Zhu J, Wu R. Functional mapping for genetic control of programmed cell death. *Physiol Genomics* 2006;25:458–469.
216. Batzel JJ, Kappel F, Timischl-Teschl S. A cardiovascular-respiratory control system model including state delay with application to congestive heart failure in humans. *J Math Biol* 2005;50:293–335.
217. Kappel F, Propst G. Approximation of feedback controls for delay systems using Legendre polynomials. *Conf Sem Mat Univ Bari* 1984;201:1–36. ISSN: 0374–2113.
218. Kappel F, Salamon D. Spline approximation for retarded systems and the Riccati equation. *Siam J Control Optim* 1987;25(4):1082–1117.
219. Kominakis A, Volanis M, Rogdakis E. Genetic modeling of test day records in dairy sheep using orthogonal Legendre polynomials. *Small Rum Res* 2001;39(3):209–217.
220. Rossi E, Lippincott B. The wave nature of being: ultradian rhythms and mind-body communication. In: Lloyd, D, Rossi E, eds. *Ultradian Rhythms in Life Processes: An Inquiry into Fundamental Principles of Chronobiology and Psychobiology.* New York, NY: Springer-Verlag, 1992:371–402.
221. Shannahoff-Khalsa DS, Kennedy B, Yates FE, et al. Ultradian rhythms of autonomic, cardiovascular, and neuroendocrine systems are related in humans. *Am J Physiol* 1996;270:R873–R887.
222. Glass L. Synchronization and rhythmic processes in physiology. *Nature* 2001;410:277–284.
223. Vitaterna MH, Takahashi JS, Turek FW. Overview of the circadian rhythms. *Alcohol Res Health* 2001;25(2):85–93.
224. Ottesen JT. Modelling of the baroreflex-feedback mechanism with time-delay. *J Math Biol* 1977;36:41–63.
225. Eyal S, Akselrod S. Bifurcation in a simple model of the cardiovascular system. *Method Inform Med* 2000;39(2):118–121.
226. Rial JA. Pacemaking the ice ages by frequency modulation of Earth's orbital eccentricity. *Science* 1999;285:564–568.
227. Crisera PN. The cytological implications of primary respiration. *Med Hypotheses* 2001;56(1):40–51.
228. Liu C, Li S, Liu T, et al. Transcriptional coactivator PGC-1α integrates the mammalian clock and energy metabolism. *Nature* 2007;447(5767):477–481.
229. Bohannon J. Seeking nature's inner compass. *Science* 2007;318:904–907.
230. Diebel CE, Proksch R, Green CR, et al. Magnetite defines a vertebrate magnetoreceptor. *Nature* 2000;406:299–302.
231. Ritz J, Thalau P, Phillips JB, et al. Resonance effects indicate a radical-pair mechanism for avian magnetic compass. *Nature* 2004;429:177–180.
232. Sutherland WG. *The Cranial Bowl.* Mankato, MN: Free Press Company, 1939, reprinted, 1986.
233. King HH, Lay E. Osteopathy in the cranial field. In: Ward RC, ed. *Foundations for Osteopathic Medicine.* 2nd Ed. Baltimore, MD: Lippincott Williams & Wilkins, 2003;985–1001.
234. Magoun HI. *Osteopathy in the Cranial Field.* 2nd Ed. Kirksville, MO: The Journal Printing Company, 1966.
235. Upledger JE, Vredevoogd JD. *Craniosacral Therapy.* Chicago, IL: Eastland Press, 1983.
236. Sergueef N. *Le B.A.BA du Crânien.* Paris: SPEK, 1986.
237. DiGiovanna E, Schiowitz S, ed. *An Osteopathic Approach to Diagnosis and Treatment.* 2nd Ed. Philadelphia, PA: J. B. Lippincott Raven Co., 1997.
238. Woods JM, Woods RH. A physical finding relating to psychiatric disorders. *J Am Osteopath Assoc* 1961;60:988–993.
239. Upledger JE, Karni Z. Strain plethysmography and the cranial rhythm. *Proc XII Internat Conf Med Biol Eng.* Jerusalem, Israel, Aug 19–24, 1979, Part IV, p. 69.5.
240. Fernandez D, Lecine A. L'enregistrement de l'onde de Traube-Hering et de la palpation cranienne simultanée. *Kinésithérapie Scientifique* 1990;292:33–40.
241. Norton JM, Sibley G, Broder-Oldach R. Characterization of the cranial rhythmic impulse in healthy human adults. *Amer Acad Osteop J* 1992;2(3):9–12,26.
242. Wirth-Pattullo V, Hayes KW. Interrater reliability of craniosacral rate measurements and their relationship with subjects' and examiners' heart and respiratory rate measurements. *Phys Ther* 1994;74(10):908–916.
243. McAdoo J, Kuchera ML. Reliability of cranial rhythmic impulse palpation. *J Am Osteopath Assoc* 1995;95(8):491-EOA.
244. Hanten WP, Dawson DD, Iwata M, et al. Craniosacral rhythm: reliability and relationships with cardiac and respiratory rates. *J Orthop Sports Phys Ther* 1998;27(3):213–218.
245. Nelson KE, Sergueef N, Glonek T. Recording the rate of the cranial rhythmic impulse. *J Am Osteopath Assoc* 2006;106(6):337–341.
246. Sergueef N, Greer MA, Nelson KE, et al. The palpated cranial rhythmic impulse (CRI): its normative rate and examiner experience. *Int J Osteopath Med* 2010. Under review.
247. Traube L. Ueber periodisdche Thätigkeits-Aeusserungen des vasomotorischen und Hemmungs-Nervencentrums. *Cbl Med Wiss* 1865;56:881–885.
248. Hering E. Über den Athembewegungen des Gefäßsystems. *Sitzungb d k Akad d W math naturw* 1869;60:829–856.
249. Hulett GD. Some fundamental considerations, subsection, the cell doctrine insufficient. *Principles of Osteopathy.* Kirksville, MO: The Journal Publishing Co., 1903:27–32; chap II.
250. Szidon JP, Cherniack NS, Fishman AP. Traube-Hering waves in the pulmonary circulation of the dog. *Science* 1969;164:75–76.
251. Jenkins CO, Campbell JK, White DN. Modulation resembling Traube-Hering waves recorded in the human brain. *Europ Neurol* 1971;5:1–6.
252. Akselrod S, Gordon D, Madwed JB, et al. Hemodynamic regulation: investigation by spectral analysis. *Am J Physiol* 1985;249:H867–H875.
253. Fuller BF. The effects of stress-anxiety and coping styles on heart rate variability. *Int J Psychophysiol* 1992;12:81–86.
254. Saul PJ, Rea RF, Eckberg DL, et al. Heart rate and muscle sympathetic nerve variability during reflex changes of autonomic activity. *Am J Physiol* 1990;258:H713–H721.
255. White DN. The early development of neurosonology: III. Pulsatile echoencephalography and Doppler techniques. *Ultrasound Med Biol* 1992;18:323–376.
256. Mevio E, Bernardi L. Phasic changes in human nasal and skin blood flow: relationship with autonomic tone. *Ann Otol Rhinol Laryngol* 1994;103(10):789–795.
257. Clarke MJ, Lin JC. Microwave sensing of increased intracranial water content. *Invest Radiol* 1983;18:245–248.
258. Moskalenko YE, Frymann V, Weinstein GB, et al. Slow rhythmic oscillations within the human cranium: phenomenology, origin and informational significance. *Human Physiol* 2001;27(2):171–178.
259. Frymann VM. A study of the rhythmic motions of the living cranium. *J Am Osteopath Assoc* 1971;70:928–945.
260. Becker RE. Life in Motion. In Brooks RE, ed. *The Cerebrospinal Fluid Tide.* Portland, OR: Rudra Press; 1997:p.107, Chapter 3.
261. Glossary Review Committee, Educational Council on Osteopathic Principles (ECOP) of the American Association of Colleges of Osteopathic Medicine (AACOM). Glossary of Osteopathic terminology. In: Ward RC,

ed. *Foundations for Osteopathic Medicine*, 2nd Ed. Baltimore, MD: Williams & Wilkins; 2003:1251.

262. Nelson KE, Sergueef N, Glonek T. Cranial osteopathy and the baroreflex, Traube-Hering (Mayer) oscillation. *Proceedings of the International Research Conference in Celebrating the 20ᵗʰ Anniversary of the Osteopathic Center for Children, Feb. 6–10, 2002, San Diego, California*, King HH, ed. Indianapolis, Indiana: American Academy of Osteopathic Medicine, 2005:39–51. ISBN: 0940668203; Library of Congress Catalog Number 20059222465.

263. Sacks OW. Said on Public Television, March, 2010.

264. Sacks OW. Keeping time: rhythm and movement. In: *Musicophilia: Tales of Music and the Brain*. New York, NY: Vintage Books (a division of Random House, Inc.), 2008:254–269; chap 19.

265. Fulford RC. *Dr. Fulford's Touch of Life*. New York, NY: Pocket Books, 1996.

266. Comeaux Z. *Harmonic Healing*. Berkeley, CA: North Atlantic Books, 2008.

12 Anatomy and Physiology of the Lymphatic System

HUGH ETTLINGER AND FRANK H. WILLARD

KEY CONCEPTS

- The lymphatic system removes fluid, particulates, and extravasated proteins from the interstitium, maintaining osmotic balance between the extracellular, intracellular, and intravascular fluids
- Inflammation is the generalized response of the body to injury or infection.
- Virtually all vascularized tissues have lymphatic capillaries that provide lymph drainage.

The extracellular fluid provides the environment in which cellular exchange of gases and nutrients takes place. Within these confines, intrinsic homeostatic mechanisms operate to maintain concentration gradients for cellular exchange. The lymphatic system plays an integral role in this process, removing fluid, particulates, and extravasated proteins from the interstitium, to maintain osmotic balance between the extracellular, intracellular, and intravascular fluids (Fig. 12.1). Overall, approximately 10% of intravascular protein and fluid volume "leak" out into the interstitial space each day and must be returned to the circulation via the lymphatics. Acute inflammation disrupts the homeostatic process in the interstitium and dramatically increases the burden on the lymphatic system. This chapter will review the anatomy and physiology of the lymphatic system, including the role it plays during inflammation and healing.

Inflammation is the generalized response of the body to injury or infection. It is a hallmark of most acute illness. Inflammation is perhaps most accurately viewed as part of a process by which the body defends against injury or infection and repairs the injured tissue. This process involves the vascular system, the immune system, and the nervous system, as well as the surrounding connective tissues. A wide variety of chemical mediators, produced locally and systemically, communicate between the cells of these systems, and control the progression of inflammation and healing. Continuous production and removal of these inflammatory mediators is essential for smooth and efficient progression and resolution of inflammation and healing. Delay in the removal of inflammatory mediators and exudates early in the process may result in prolonged inflammation with poor or delayed healing. Delayed removal of mediators later in the process may lead to a prolonged healing process, eventually leading to adhesions and/or fibrosis. The tissue drainage provided by the lymphatics offers an escape route for many of these mediators, as well as the inflammatory exudate, and plays a role in virtually every aspect of the inflammatory process. Understanding the factors influencing lymph formation and removal from tissue is critical to the Osteopathic diagnosis and treatment of any patient with an acute or chronic inflammatory process.

THE LYMPHATIC SYSTEM AND INFLAMMATION

Vasodilatation and increased capillary permeability occur early in the inflammatory process, and together are responsible for the tremendous influx of fluid and plasma protein into the interstitium of the inflamed tissue. This leaves a preponderance of red blood cells in the intravascular space, greatly increasing its viscosity, and potentially creating stasis of venules and capillary beds (Movat and Wasi, 1985). The lymphatic system, therefore, becomes responsible for virtually all fluid drainage from inflamed tissues. The rate of blood supply, and the delivery of antibodies, centrally produced mediators, medications, and the oxygen and nutrients necessary to fuel cellular activities will be limited, or even determined, by the rate of lymph flow.

Normal venous drainage will be restored when capillary permeability returns to normal and the osmotic gradient between the interstitium and the vascular system permits sufficient fluid return to reduce the viscosity of capillary blood. Capillary permeability is controlled by a variety of endogenous vasoactive mediators, including histamine, bradykinin, and prostaglandin E. Although these mediators can be inactivated locally, there is evidence that lymph drainage also provides a means by which they are removed and/or inactivated. Bradykinin has been shown to be inactivated systemically by plasma (Hurley, 1984). Histaminase, responsible for 30% of histamine breakdown, has been identified in high levels in the thoracic duct (Atkinson, 1994). Prostaglandin E has been identified in the lymph effluent draining from inflamed tissues (Movat and Wasi, 1985). The relative importance of tissue drainage and other mechanisms in the inactivation of these mediators has not been elucidated. The osmotic pressure in the interstitium will change when proteins and other osmotically active particles are removed. Extravasated protein and large particulates cannot return via the venous system, even when capillary permeability is maximally increased (Hurley, 1984), nor is there any evidence that protein is catabolized in the interstitium (Aukland and Reed, 1993). It is therefore evident that the removal of protein from tissue depends heavily on the lymphatic drainage of the tissues.

Inflammation generates both local and central immune responses. Locally, chemotactic mediators draw neutrophils and monocytes to the area. Neutrophils release lysosomal enzymes into the interstitium that can kill bacteria, but can also be destructive to local tissues. They are responsible for much of the tissue damage that accompanies acute and chronic inflammatory processes. The tissue damage created by neutrophilic lysosomes can be similar to that caused by pancreatic enzymes. However, a recent study has suggested that the macrophage in combination with the lymphatic system may serve to blunt the effect of the neutrophil in chronic inflammatory diseases. As the inflammation progresses, the polymorphonuclear leukocytes (also termed PMNs) undergo apoptosis and the remains are ingested by macrophages in a manner that does not release lysosomal enzymes or provoke proinflammatory responses (Lawrence and Gilroy, 2007). If the PMNs are not phagocytized, they eventually undergo secondary necrosis, releasing their damaging lysozymes into the tissue. The ingesting macrophages

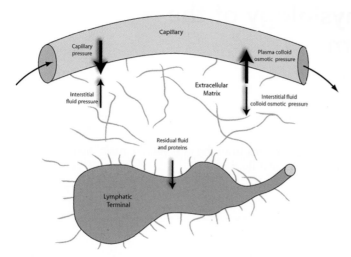

Figure 12-1 Tissue fluid homeostasis and the lymphatic system. Blood is passing from left to right in this capillary (small curved arrows). The high capillary pressure on the left side of the bed forces fluid and small proteins outward into the extracellular matrix (large downward arrow). Toward the right side of the bed, the oncotic pressure from concentrated proteins in the capillary blood draws fluid back into the capillary. Residual fluids and proteins are left in the extracellular matrix; these fluids pass into the terminal lymphatic vessels for reentry into the system circulation through the venous connections in the upper thorax.

must then be either removed from the tissue or themselves undergo apoptosis. Bellingan et al. (1996) have found most macrophages are removed via lymphatic drainage, implicating lymph drainage in another important aspect of resolving the inflammatory process.

Lymph drainage has been shown to dramatically reduce the tissue-damaging effects of pancreatic enzymes with obstruction of the main pancreatic duct in dogs (Witte and Witte, 1984). Neutrophilic lysosomes have been identified in lymph draining from inflamed tissues (Movat and Wasi, 1985). Drainage of these enzymes may be important in limiting their destructive effects on tissues.

Central immune responses involve stimulation of T-cells and B-cells by antigen in lymph nodes and other lymph organs. Delivery of antigen to these lymphoid organs occurs entirely by lymphatic drainage of antigen and antigen-containing macrophages from the site of injury. Weakening of antigenic stimulation has been demonstrated in chronic lymph stasis and lymphedema (Witte and Witte, 1984). Conversely, the B-cell response to immunization in medical students was increased by manipulating the rate of lymph drainage using the lymphatic pump technique (Measel, 1982).

Systemic responses to inflammation occur in the liver and brain. The proinflammatory cytokine interleukin-1 (IL-1) is involved in the stimulation of both of these organs. IL-1 stimulates the production of acute phase reactant proteins from the liver (Movat and Wasi, 1985). It has also been shown to reach circumventricular organs in the ventricular system of the brain, where it produces fever and stimulates the hypothalamic-pituitary axis (Dinarello, 1992). IL-1 is produced by monocytes and macrophages locally during an inflammatory process. Although there are systemic sources of IL-1 production, locally produced IL-1 has been shown to produce fever and stimulate acute phase protein production (Movat and Wasi, 1985). Locally produced IL-1 gains access to the systemic circulation via lymphatic drainage. Both prostaglandins and leukotrienes have been found in lymphatic drainage of inflamed tissues, and there is evidence that lymphatic drainage is involved

in the removal and inactivation of bradykinin and histamine. A variety of inflammatory mediators, including bradykinin, prostaglandins, leukotrienes, IL-1, and histamine, can stimulate primary afferent nociceptors (Levine et al., 1993), potentially resulting in hyperalgeasia of the surrounding tissue. As these mediators are dissipated, the rate of depolarization of the primary nociceptors will remit, and inflammatory pain will be reduced.

The repair of injured or infected tissue proceeds as the acute inflammatory process resolves. Fibroblasts, which lay down the matrix of the scar tissue, are stimulated by the inflammatory exudate, as well as several complementary factors and cytokines. As the balance between proinflammatory and profibroblast forces shifts, the inflammatory process shifts to the healing phase. By continually clearing the interstitium of exudate, including inflammatory mediators, the lymphatics can allow this shift to occur more rapidly and smoothly. Should proinflammatory mediators remain in the interstitium, acute inflammation will persist, and healing will be delayed. The healing process resolves when the inflammatory exudate is removed, and fibroblast activity decreases. Persistence of the inflammatory exudate in peripheral tissue will lead to excess local scarring and fibrosis. Plasma proteins, when trapped in the interstitium, attract monocytes. Platelets, extravasated into the tissue, release growth factors such as epidermal growth factor, platelet-derived growth factor, and transforming growth factor β (TGF-β). The latter, TGF-β, helps in the conversion of monocytes to macrophages. These latter cells also release numerous growth factors including Fibroblast Growth Factor (FGF) and TGF-β, which attract and stimulate fibroblasts, eventually leading to fibrogenesis, which can contribute to tissue repair in the acute state as well as fibrosis of tissue in the chronic state (Witte and Witte, 1984; also see chapter 7 on the fascial system in this volume). Repeated experimental injection of plasma into soft tissue produced both chronic inflammation and scar formation (Witte and Witte, 1984). The lymphatics are the predominant means by which the inflammatory exudate is removed, and so are intimately involved in the progression and resolution of the healing phase of the inflammatory process.

The process of inflammation and healing is the bodies' response to injury and infection. The lymphatics play a role in every aspect of this process. In essence, the lymphatic system is responsible for maintaining an interstitial environment conducive to the rapid, unimpaired progression and resolution of this complex process.

There are several categories of disease processes which warrant a focus on the lymphatic system:

1. Chronic inflammatory diseases: These range from smoldering, subclinical infections such as osteomyelitis to autoimmune and collagen vascular diseases such as rheumatoid arthritis. Although most chronic inflammatory diseases are attributed to persistent inflammatory stimuli, there are suggestions that reduced lymph drainage may play a role. Weak antigenic stimulation of regional lymphocytes was found in experimental lymphedema (Witte and Witte, 1984). This finding was implicated in the susceptibility to infection that often complicates lymphedema. Increased lymph drainage from the site of infection should improve immune response and local circulation.

Rheumatoid arthritis is thought to occur as a response to immune complexes. These complexes, and the inflammatory exudate they produce, are removed by lymphatic drainage. The inflammatory exudate is responsible for the pain and tissue destruction associated with this disease. Increased lymph production and drainage from rheumatoid ankles has been demonstrated in humans; in addition, this drainage contained elevated levels of proinflammatory cytokines (Olszewski et al., 2001).

2. Fibrotic diseases: Progressive interstitial fibrosis is a characteristic of chronic lymphedema. The pattern and time course of the fibrosis produced by experimental lymphedema is strikingly similar to a variety of diseases, including cirrhosis, interstitial lung diseases such as silicosis, regional ileitis, and even atherosclerosis (Witte and Witte, 1984). Each of these diseases involves repeated inflammatory events with a progressive build-up of protein rich tissue fluid, influx of leukocytes, release of proinflammatory cytokines, and fibroblast stimulation, eventually leading to fibrosis. Postoperative adhesions, common in abdominal surgeries with peritonitis, or other massive inflammatory processes, may result from inadequate drainage of the abdominal exudates. Similarly, surgeries involving lymph node dissections or disruption of lymphatics, such as a modified radical mastectomy, may result in lymphedema from fibrosis and adhesions. OMT to promote lymph drainage early in these diseases may help prevent the development of these long-term problems.

ANATOMY OF THE LYMPHATIC SYSTEM

General Aspects

Virtually all vascularized tissues have lymphatic capillaries that provide lymph drainage, the only exceptions being the central nervous system, bone and bone marrow, the maternal placenta, and the endomyceum surrounding muscle fibers. Cartilage, the lens and cornea of the eye, the epidermis, and the inner portion of the walls of large blood vessels are not vascularized and also have no lymph drainage. The lymph system begins in the interstitial space of tissues with initial lymphatics, also termed terminal lymphatics, or lymph capillaries (Fig. 12.1). These coalesce into collecting channels, which drain into progressively larger prenodal or afferent vessels (Fig. 12.2). All lymph then passes through one or more lymph nodes, which filter and alter the lymph in a variety of ways before draining into larger postnodal or efferent trunks. These trunks ultimately return lymph to the venous system either via the thoracic duct on the left or the right lymphatic duct. Lymph from the lower portion of the body, as well as the left thorax and part of the left lung, the left arm, and the left side of the head and neck return via the thoracic duct. Lymph from the heart, all of the right lung and the right arm, right side of the head and neck and diaphragm drain to the right lymphatic duct (Fig. 12.3).

ANATOMY OF THE LYMPH VESSELS

Initial Lymphatics—Lymphatic capillaries are blind-ended terminals that end in interstitial spaces (Fig. 12.2). They comprise endothelial cells in a single layer, which contain no tight junctions, and are therefore permeable to large particles and proteins. Although their morphology differs in different tissues, there are notable similarities in anatomic microstructure that are critical to the function of these capillaries in lymph formation. Initial lymphatics consist of overlapping endothelial cells lacking tight junctions but contain anchoring filaments. Anchoring filaments are collagenous bundles that attach to the external aspect of the lymphatic endothelium and imbed into the interstitial matrix (Figs. 12.1 and 12.2). Their form and function are described in a series of articles by Leak (Leak, 1976, 1987; Leak and Burke, 1966; Leak and Jamuar, 1983). During situations of edema, anchoring filaments prevent the collapse of the initial lymphatics as interstitial pressure rises. These filaments also cause the lymphatic vessel to change shape and volume in response to tissue movement (Fig. 12.4). The overlapping endothelial cells are theorized to act as a "primary

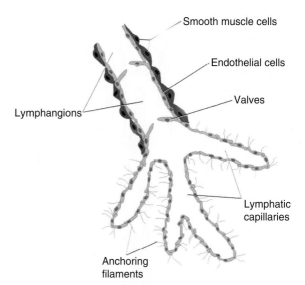

Figure 12-2 The cytoarchitecture of the terminal lymphatics. The terminal lymphatics or lymphatic capillaries are seen as endothelial-lined cul-de-sacs anchored into the surrounding extracellular matrix by small filaments. The endothelial cells overlap creating one-way valves allowing fluid in the ECM to leech into the terminal lymphatic but preventing back drainage. The terminal lymphatics lack smooth muscle walls. The collecting vessels begin at the first valve and have both smooth muscle walls and periodic valves derived from the endothelium. (Modified from L. N. Cueni and M. Detmar. The lymphatic system in health and disease. Lymphat.Res.Biol. 6 (3-4):109-122, 2008.)

valve system" that prevents reflux of fluid into the interstitium from the initial lymphatic (Mendoza and Schmid-Schonbein, 2003; Trzewik et al., 2001; Schmid-Schonbein, 2003). A recent study demonstrated the lack of adhesion molecules at the junction of the endothelial cells of the initial lymphatic, a structural feature necessary for this function (Murfee et al., 2007). In addition, the basement membrane of the terminal lymphatic is discontinuous, thereby facilitating the movement of fluid into the vessel (Witte et al., 2006). This arrangement provides for a one-way flow of lymphatic fluids from the extracellular space into the initial lymphatic vessels. It is important to note that these valves do not act as filters; thus, fluid moving into the lumen of the terminal lymphatic vessel has the approximate composition of extracellular fluid. Finally, lymphatic capillaries lack smooth muscle cells in their walls; thus, they are dependent on outside forces to both fill the terminal vessel and then expel lymph into the collecting vessels; this concept will be discussed further in the section on lymph formation. The discontinuous basement membrane, open interendothelial junctions, and the anchoring filaments all help to distinguish the terminal lymphatic from a capillary bed (Witte et al., 2006).

COLLECTING VESSELS

The initial lymphatic ends at the first bicuspid valve, which demarcates the beginning of the collecting vessel (Fig. 12.2). Collecting vessels develop a thin connective tissue layer to support the endothelium, and an increasing amount of smooth muscle, which is arranged in a woven mat surrounding the vessel and concentrated near the valves. The smooth muscle layer progressively thickens in a proximal direction and eventually the vessels develop a three-layer arrangement much like a small vein, with a tunica intima, media, and adventitia. Lymphatic vessels differ from veins in that they have far more valves in the vessels to prevent backflow. Lymphatic

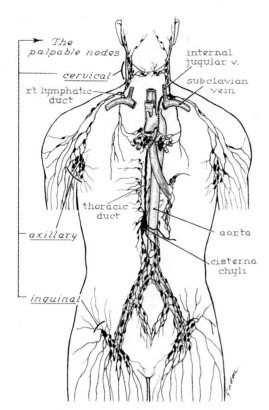

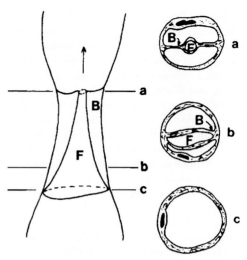

Figure 12-5 The collecting vessel valves. On the left is a longitudinal view of the valve in a collecting vessel. On the right are cross-sections taken through the valve at three separate levels indicated by the horizontal lines. The leaflets of the valve are fused to each other and to the wall of the vessel. As one progresses up the valve, the fusion of the leaflets moves closer to the midline making it impossible for the valve to invert and thus producing one-way flow. (Taken from Swartz MA. The physiology of the lymphatic system. *Adv Drug Deliv Rev* 50(1–2):3–20, 2001.)

Figure 12-3 The lymphatic system scheme. This diagram illustrates the overall distribution and flow patterns of the lymphatic system. (Taken from Basmajian JV. *Grant's Method of Anatomy*. Baltimore, MD:Williams & Wilkins Company, 1975.)

valves are bicuspid, collagenous, and attach so as to have their narrow end pointed in the direction of the lymph flow, that is toward the larger vessels (Fig. 12.5). They operate at low flow rates and, since the valve flaps are adherent to the vessel wall, are closed by retrograde fluid pressure. The vessel between the valves and the proximal valve constitute the "lymphangion."

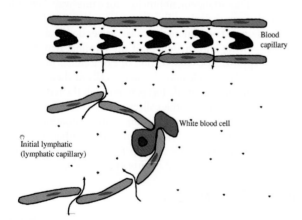

Figure 12-4 The mechanics of the terminal lymphatic vessel. An endothelial cell–lined blood vessel is seen above and a terminal lymphatic below. Fluid, particulates, and protein diffuse out of the vessel and into the extracellular matrix. From the matrix, these items can enter the terminal lymphatic vessel by passing through the small gaps in the endothelial lining. Due to the overlapping nature of these endothelial cells, back flow from the lymphatic into the matrix cannot occur. (Taken from Swartz MA. The physiology of the lymphatic system. *Adv Drug Deliv Rev* 50(1–2):3–20, 2001.)

Lymph is passed through nodes before draining into larger postnodal vessels. The collecting vessels prior to the lymph nodes are termed the afferent (prenodal) vessels, while those draining the node are termed the efferent (postnodal) vessel (Fig. 12.6). Lymph nodes are encapsulated and contain sinusoids that allow the lymph to "percolate" through a large surface area of cells and vessels. This filtration system is the means through which antigens in the lymphatic fluid are trapped and immune responses are generated. Foreign particles are also removed by nodal macrophages via this mechanism. The lymph sinusoids are permeable to fluid and small particles. This provides an area for exchange between the lymphatic and the venous systems. Free water may travel down a hydrostatic gradient from lymphatics to the venous system, effectively concentrating postnodal lymph (Adair et al., 1982). This can improve the overall efficiency of the lymphatic system since removal of protein from the extracellular space is considered the primary function of the lymphatic system (Adair and Guyton, 1985). Increased venous pressure or congestion in the area of the nodes will interfere with this process, thereby increasing the resistance to lymph flow (Adair and Guyton, 1983; Aukland and Reed, 1993). Osteopathic treatment to decongest areas around nodes, such as the popliteal spread or pectoral lift, may help maintain the downward hydrostatic gradient between the lymphatic and the venous systems.

Postnodal or efferent vessels follow fascial planes, progressively moving toward the midline of the body, where they enter the mediastinum in either the abdomen, thorax, or cervical region. Eventually, the postnodal vessels drain into the right lymphatic duct or left thoracic duct. These large lymphatic ducts, such as the thoracic duct, are organized histologically like a medium-sized vein, except for the greater amount of smooth muscle and valves. Spontaneous, peristaltic contractions have been consistently observed in the thoracic duct of various species; the rate of these spontaneous contractions can be modulated by the sympathetic nervous system (Reddy and Staub, 1981).

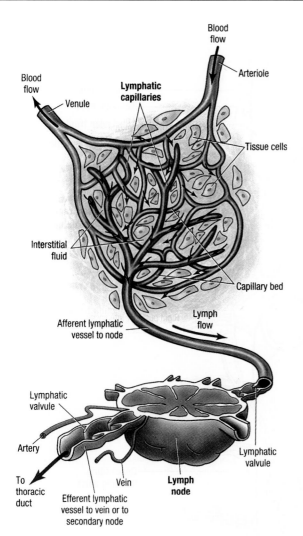

Figure 12-6 The lymphatic system. This figure illustrates the afferent lymphatic collecting vessels arising in the tissue between the arterial and venous system and extending to the lymph nodes. The efferent vessels arise in the capsule of the lymph node and progress toward the thoracic duct. (Taken from Agur AM, Dalley AF. *Grant's Atlas of Anatomy*, Philadelphia, PA: Lippincott Williams & Wilkins, 2009.)

INNERVATION OF LYMPHATIC VESSELS

The smooth muscle in the wall of the lymph vessel contains adrenergic, cholinergic purinergic, and peptidergic nerves (Alessandrini et al., 1981; Witte et al., 2006), although a sympathetic innervation has been more consistently observed (McHale, 1990). Chemical stimulation in vitro of the adrenergic receptors causes contraction of the lymphatic smooth muscle (Thornbury et al., 1989); the effect of cholinergic stimulation has been variable (McHale, 1990) and has been questioned by a more recent study (Thornbury et al., 1989). Beta adrenergic receptors have been identified that cause relaxation of lymphatic smooth muscle (Ikomi et al., 1997). Electrical stimulation of sympathetic nerves and/or ganglia also consistently increases the contractility of the smooth muscle, increasing stroke volume of the vessels (Benoit, 1997; McGeown et al., 1987; Thornbury et al., 1993). The innervation, like the presence of smooth muscle, is greatest in the larger vessels. The overall effect of sympathetic stimulation, which appears to be increasing lymph flow, is mediated via the alpha receptors. The role of

beta-receptors and cholinergic innervation has not yet been fully elucidated. Eliminating the effects of the sympathetic nervous system on the lymph vessels does not eliminate the peristaltic contractions but prevents field stimulation from increasing lymph flow (Hollywood and McHale, 1994), indicating the sympathetic nervous system does not initiate the peristaltic contractions, but is capable of modifying the intrinsic rate of contraction. This modification is most likely accomplished by varying the sensitivity of the autoregulatory mechanism in the lymphatic vessels to stretch (Witte et al., 2006). The finding of peptide containing fibers in the innervation of the lymph vessels suggests the possibility of sensory reflex modulation of lymph pumping, as well as an alternate means of modifying the pumping rate, as the lymphatic smooth muscle is responsive to substance P, which was identified in the peptidergic nerves (Hukkanen et al., 1992).

All lymph organs have been demonstrated to receive a sympathetic innervation; however, no consistent findings of parasympathetic innervation have been reported (Nance and Sanders, 2007). Sympathetic stimulation has been shown to modify lymphocyte activity (Felten et al., 1984), as well as cause contraction of the lymph node capsule, resulting in an increase in the output of lymphocytes from nodes (McGeown, 1993; McHale and Thornbury, 1990; Thornbury et al., 1990). It has been theorized that the primary role of the sympathetic innervation of the lymphatic system is to modify the immune response, rather that increase flow through the vessels (McHale, 1992).

REGIONAL LYMPH DRAINAGE

The movement of lymphatic fluids progresses from the peripheral tissues toward the midline of the body and, once on the midline, upward toward the cervicothoracic junction where these fluids are returned to systemic circulation through the jugular or subclavian veins. In general, lymph from the two lower extremities, pelvic basin, abdomen, left thorax, left upper extremity, and left side of the head targets the thoracic duct for return to the venous compartment. Lymphatic vessels draining the right thorax, upper extremity, and right side of the head flow into the right lymphatic duct before entering the venous compartment (Fig. 12.7).

There are slight variations in the structure and of initial lymphatics and collecting channels in various organs and tissues that offer insight into the physiology of lymph formation and propulsion. Some of those differences will be described here as well as the main pathways of drainage of the lymph system.

Peripheral Tissues

There is a superficial and deep drainage of the upper and lower extremities. The superficial drainage follows subcutaneous routes to proximal nodes at the axilla and inguinal areas. Deep drainage follows the neurovascular structures to the same ultimate endpoint and has various nodes at intermediary sites. The upper limb lymph exits the axilla via a somewhat vulnerable route through the thoracic outlet, exiting the limb beneath the pectoralis minor muscle, and entering the thorax through the costoclavicular space (Fig. 12.8). Here, the upper extremity lymph channels join with those from the anterior thoracic wall including the breast tissue in the female. The lower extremity drainage enters the abdomen through the femoral triangle, in close proximity to where the iliopsoas tendon crosses the hip joint (Fig. 12.9). The deep drainage of the foreleg passes into the popliteal space between the two heads of the gastrocnemius and exits the popliteal space between the heads of the hamstrings. The small, pliant lymph vessels are most vulnerable to tissue

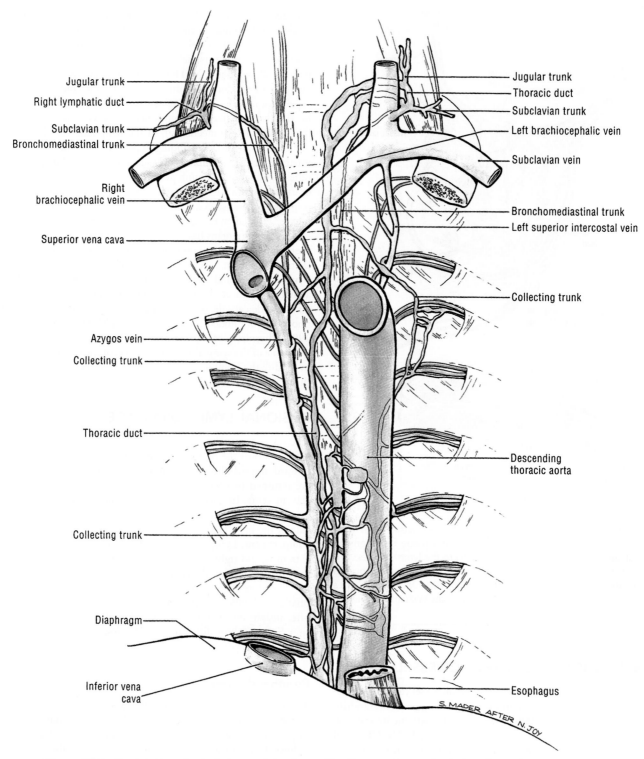

Figure 12-7   Regional lymphatic drainage of the thorax. The thoracic duct and right lymphatic duct are shown in green. (Taken from Agur AM, Dalley AF. *Grant's Atlas of Anatomy*, Philadelphia, PA: Lippincott Williams & Wilkins, 2009. Figure 1-73.)

tension as they pass through narrow spaces such as these. When sufficient tension is present, it may limit the lymphatic drainage of the respective extremity. Increasing outflow pressure has been shown to reduce lymph flow in vitro (Eisenhoffer et al., 1993).

The small collecting vessels draining skeletal muscle have been shown to have significantly less smooth muscle. In fact, the smooth muscle wall of the lymphatic vessels does not develop until the

vessel is relatively large in size, suggesting the effectiveness of the skeletal muscle contraction in propulsing the lymph through these small vessels (Schmid-Schonbein, 1990b).

The synovial fluid of large joints is drained via the lymphatic system. Radiolabeled tracer placed into the synovial space of the knee joint of a pig could be followed as it was removed through the lymphatic channels and entered the thoracic duct. The synovial

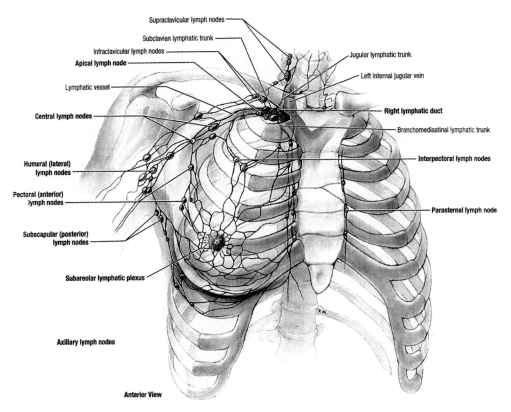

Figure 12-8 Regional lymphatic drainage of the upper extremity. The lymphatic drainage of the upper extremity is seen entering the axillary region where it merges with that of the anterior chest wall including the breast tissue in the female. (Taken from Agur AM, Dalley AF. *Grant's Atlas of Anatomy*. Philadelphia, PA: Lippincott Williams & Wilkins, 2009. Figure 1-8.)

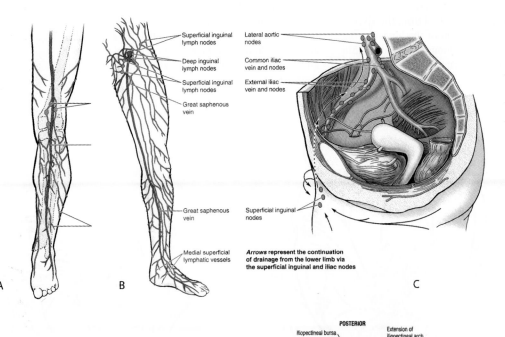

Figure 12-9 Regional lymphatic drainage of the lower extremity. Lymphatic drainage from the lower extremity is directed to the inguinal region, from which it passes along iliac nodes to reach the preaortic and aortic nodes. **A** and **B** are anterior and lateral views of the lymphatic drainage of the lower extremity, respectively. In **C** the drainage of the inguinal nodes in to the iliac nodes is illustrated. Illustration **D** is a cross-section through the femoral triangle illustrating the narrow region through which the lymphatic drainage must pass. This is a lateral. (Taken from Agur AM, Dalley AF. *Grant's Atlas of Anatomy*, Philadelphia, PA: Lippincott Williams & Wilkins, 2009. Figures 5-7 and 5-18.)

tracer was estimated to have a half-life of approximately 8.3 hours suggesting that synovial clearance via lymphatics is relatively quick from the large joints of the extremities (Jensen et al., 1993).

Head and Neck

The deep cervical vessels and nodes lie in the carotid sheath, and this is the terminal pathway for all drainage of the head and neck (Fig. 12.10). Superficial drainage will usually pass through superficial nodes before passing to deep nodes. Many of these nodes lie along the sternocliedomastoid muscle. Others lie in the supoccipital space, over the parotid gland, and under the mandible. Much of the deep drainage, including that of the ear, sinuses, pharynx, upper larynx, and upper teeth, drain via the upper nodes through the jugulodigastric node, which open into the deep chain in a narrow space between the mastoid process and the angle of the mandible. Drainage through this area may also be affected by local tissue tension.

Thorax

The heart has endocardial, myocardial, and epicardial lymph drainage (Fig. 12.11A). The vessels also have little smooth muscle and depend on myocardial activity for flow. The flow of drainage is from endocardial to myocardial to epicardial. The epicardial channels converge on the posterior aspect of the heart into a single, principal lymphatic trunk that drains to a pretracheal node and the cardiac lymph node. The drainage of the heart enters the right thoracic trunk (Fig. 12.11F). The pericardium drains into the thoracic duct and enters the left subclavian vein.

The lymphatics of the lung drain the pulmonary vasculature and also the bronchial airways (Fig. 12.11B). Lymph channels travel as far as the terminal bronchiole and are thought to be important in the drainage of particulates and fluid from the alveoli. Pulmonary lymph is formed by the expansion of the lungs during respiratory excursions, and drains out of the lungs at the hilum into the tracheobronchial nodes and into the right lymph trunk and thoracic duct (Fig. 12-11E & G).

Abdomen

There is lymphatic drainage of the gut tube, abdominal viscera, and mesenteries (Fig. 12.12A-D). The lymphatics of the intestines have lacteals for the unique purpose of absorbing fat (chyle) as part of the digestive process, giving abdominal lymph the characteristic milky color and consistency. The collecting lymphatics of the gut tube are similar to that of skeletal muscle, lacking smooth muscle for an unusually long distance, indicating the ability of peristalsis to propel lymph in this area (Schmid-Schonbein, 1990a,b). The lymphatic drainage of the mesenteries follows the vascular structures back through the roots, where they join the iliac and preaortic nodes on route to the cysterna chyle and thoracic duct. The preaortic and aortic nodes are clustered around the three large unpaired arteries on the anterior aspect of the aorta, the celiac, superior mesenteric, and inferior mesenteric arteries (Fig. 12.12A-D).

Peritoneal and Pleural Fluid

Diaphragmatic stomata have been discovered on the inferior, and to a lesser degree the superior surface of the diaphragm that are open to the peritoneal and pleural cavities, respectively (Negrini et al., 1991; Tsilibary and Wissig, 1977; Wang, 1975). These stomata are believed to act as "prelymphatics," connecting to the diaphragmatic lymphatic channels and represent a major pathway for the drainage of peritoneal and pleural fluid. Of radiolabeled tracer absorbed out of the abdomen of a sheep, 42% returned into circulation via the diaphragm and the remainder passed through other routes that include the organ walls and somatic body wall (Abernethy et al., 1991). In another study, Zakaria et al. (1996) found three routes for the removal of radiolabeled tracer from the peritoneum: 55% passed through the diaphragmatic, 30% through visceral lymphatics, and 10% to 15% through parietal lymphatics. Given these data, the diaphragm may be acting like a large sponge, absorbing fluid from the peritoneal and pleural cavities as it relaxes and pumping that fluid into the lymphatic collecting ducts on each contraction.

Figure 12-10 Regional lymphatic drainage from the head and neck. Lymphatic channels in the neuro- and visceral cranium converge on the carotid sheath, from which lymph passes downward to join the right lymphatic duct or the thoracic duct on the left.

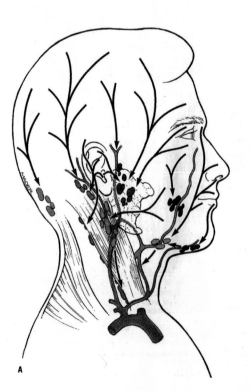

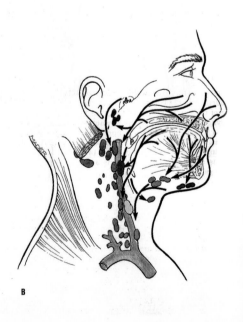

A

B

PHYSIOLOGY AND MECHANICS OF LYMPH FLOW

The movement of lymph is a fairly complex process involving several steps or stages. Fluid must first move from the interstitium into the initial lymphatic. It then travels through a series of progressively larger vessels until it drains into right lymph trunk or the thoracic ducts, which in turn drain into the subclavian veins. Lymph formation involves the movement of fluid across a permeable membrane.

Fluids move in the direction determined by the sum of the hydrostatic and osmotic gradients across the membrane (Fig. 12.1). Capillaries generally have a hydrostatic gradient that moves fluid out at their arterial end and an osmotic gradient that returns fluid to the capillary at the venous end. The search for similar hydrostatic and osmotic gradients across the lymphatic endothelium to account for the formation of lymph has been without success. Sampling of fluid from the initial and small collecting lymphatics has consistently shown a protein concentration identical to interstitial fluid (Benoit

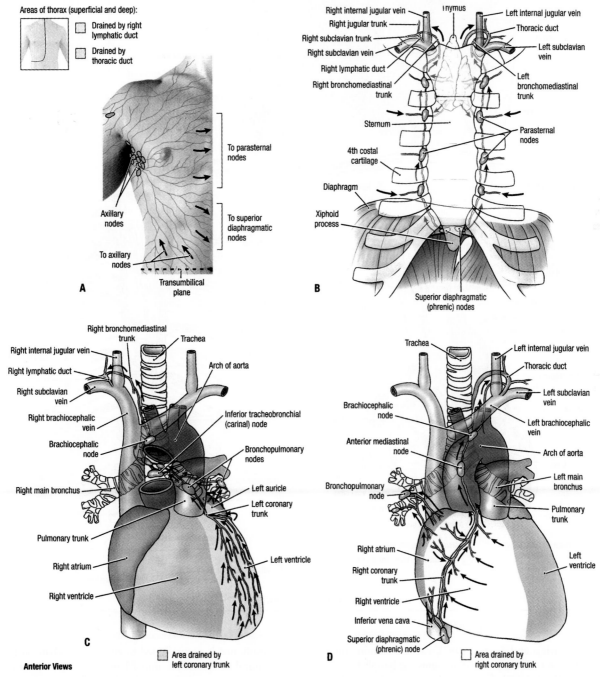

Figure 12-11   Regional lymphatic drainage from the thorax. **A.** The lines of superficial lymphatic drainage have been marked on the skin of the left thorax of a male. **B.** The substernal lymphatic drainage from the diaphragm to the superior thoracic inlet is illustrated. **C** and **D.** The lymphatic drainage of the myocardium along the anterior interventricular route (left anterior interventriclar artery, **C**) and the anterior atrioventricular route (right coronary artery, **D**) routes have been illustrated. **E.** The lymphatic drainage of the tracheobronchial and esophageal systems are illustrated. **F.** the lymphatic drainage routes of the posterior aspect of the heart is illustrated. **G.** The deep lymphatic drainage of the retroesophageal area is illustrated.

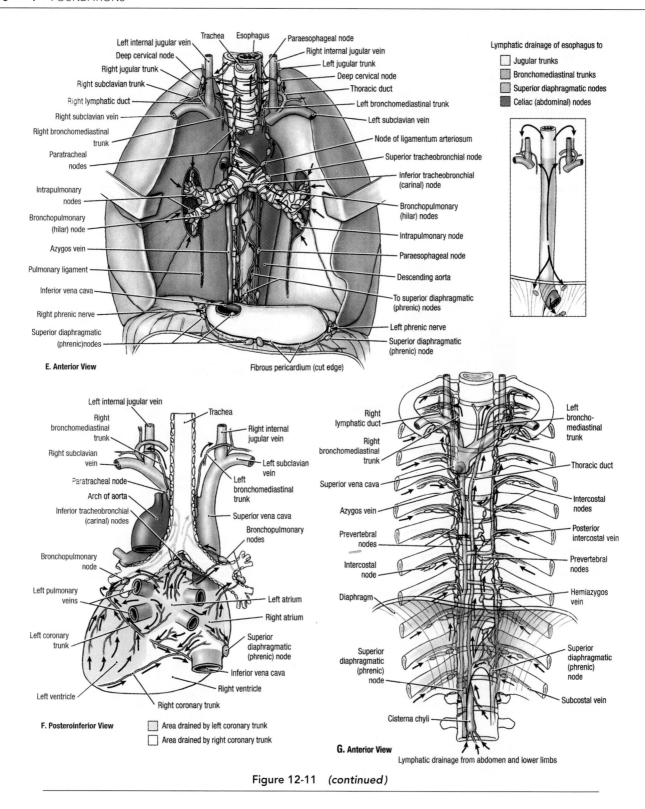

E. Anterior View

Trachea Esophagus
Left internal jugular vein
Deep cervical node
Right jugular trunk
Right subclavian trunk
Right lymphatic duct
Right subclavian vein
Right bronchomediastinal trunk
Paratracheal nodes
Intrapulmonary nodes
Bronchopulmonary (hilar) node
Azygos vein
Pulmonary ligament
Inferior vena cava
Right phrenic nerve
Superior diaphragmatic (phrenic)nodes

Paraesophageal node
Right internal jugular vein
Left jugular trunk
Deep cervical node
Thoracic duct
Left bronchomediastinal trunk
Left subclavian vein
Node of ligamentum arteriosum
Superior tracheobronchial node
Inferior tracheobronchial (carinal) node
Bronchopulmonary (hilar) nodes
Intrapulmonary node
Paraesophageal node
Descending aorta
To superior diaphragmatic (phrenic) nodes
Left phrenic nerve
Superior diaphragmatic (phrenic) node

Fibrous pericardium (cut edge)

Lymphatic drainage of esophagus to
☐ Jugular trunks
▨ Bronchomediastinal trunks
▨ Superior diaphragmatic nodes
■ Celiac (abdominal) nodes

F. Posteroinferior View

Left internal jugular vein
Right bronchomediastinal trunk
Right subclavian vein
Paratracheal node
Arch of aorta
Inferior tracheobronchial (carinal) nodes
Bronchopulmonary node
Left pulmonary veins
Left coronary trunk
Left ventricle
Right coronary trunk

Trachea
Right internal jugular vein
Left subclavian vein
Left bronchomediastinal trunk
Superior vena cava
Bronchopulmonary nodes
Left atrium
Right atrium
Superior diaphragmatic (phrenic) node
Inferior vena cava
Right ventricle

☐ Area drained by left coronary trunk
☐ Area drained by right coronary trunk

G. Anterior View
Lymphatic drainage from abdomen and lower limbs

Right lymphatic duct
Right bronchomediastinal trunk
Superior vena cava
Azygos vein
Prevertebral nodes
Intercostal node
Diaphragm
Superior diaphragmatic (phrenic) node
Cisterna chyli

Left broncho-mediastinal trunk
Thoracic duct
Intercostal nodes
Posterior intercostal vein
Prevertebral nodes
Hemiazygos vein
Superior diaphragmatic (phrenic) node
Subcostal vein

Figure 12-11 *(continued)*

et al., 1989; Zawieja and Barber, 1987), virtually eliminating the possibility that an osmotic gradient accounts for lymph formation (Aukland and Reed, 1993). Similarly, the discovery of a negative interstitial pressure in most tissues eliminates the possibility of a continuous hydrostatic gradient from the capillary to the initial lymphatic (Aukland and Reed, 1993; Guyton and Barber, 1980). Although a negative pressure has also been found in the initial lymphatic, there appears to be a small uphill gradient between the interstitium and the lymphatics (Aukland and Reed, 1993). Without a net osmotic or hydrostatic gradient to account for the formation

of lymph, one is naturally led to consider mechanical forces. The anatomical design of the initial lymphatic allows it to respond to a variety of forces in its environment. There are two anatomical features of initial lymphatics that are crucial in this regard.

The anchoring filaments that tether the outside of the lymphatic endothelial cells to the collagen of the interstitium cause the lymphatic to change shape and volume in response to tissue movement. Alternating movements create alternating volume changes in the initial lymphatic. These produce intermittent pressure gradients that move fluid into the initial lymphatic. In the lung, for example, movements of inhalation and exhalation alternately increase and decrease intralymphatic volume. The increased volume during inhalation lowers intralymphatic pressure and produces a gradient for the influx of fluid. During exhalation, the fluid is propelled forward into the collecting vessel. In the intestine, lymphatics lie between layers of muscle where they respond to peristalsis as well as the movement of the diaphragm during breathing. Interestingly, the resting position of the abdominal lymphatics appears to be an open position, that is, anchoring filaments hold the endothelial cells apart. This position is best suited for response to the compressive forces of peristalsis and the downward movement of the diaphragm (Schmid-Schonbein, 1990a,b). The situation appears reversed in the lungs, which allows the lymphatics to respond to expansion during exhalation. This suggests a structure/function relationship, where the lymphatic structure develops to best utilize the local forces available for lymph formation.

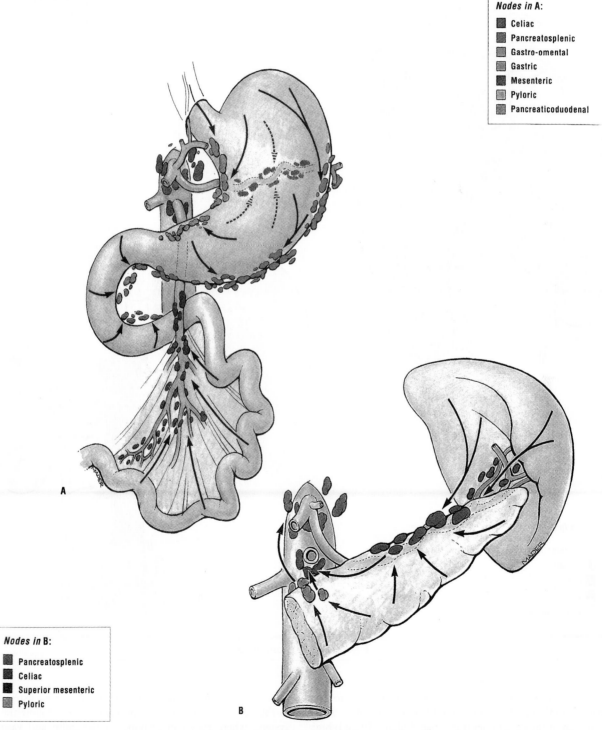

Nodes in A:

- Celiac
- Pancreatosplenic
- Gastro-omental
- Gastric
- Mesenteric
- Pyloric
- Pancreaticoduodenal

Nodes in B:

- Pancreatosplenic
- Celiac
- Superior mesenteric
- Pyloric

Figure 12-12 Lymphatic drainage of the abdominal organs: **A.** Regional lymphatic drainage of the stomach and proximal small bowel is illustrated. **B.** Regional lymphatic drainage of the spleen and pancreas is illustrated. **C.** the lymphatic drainage routes of the large bowels are illustrated. **D.** the lymphatic drainage routes of the liver and kidneys are illustrated.

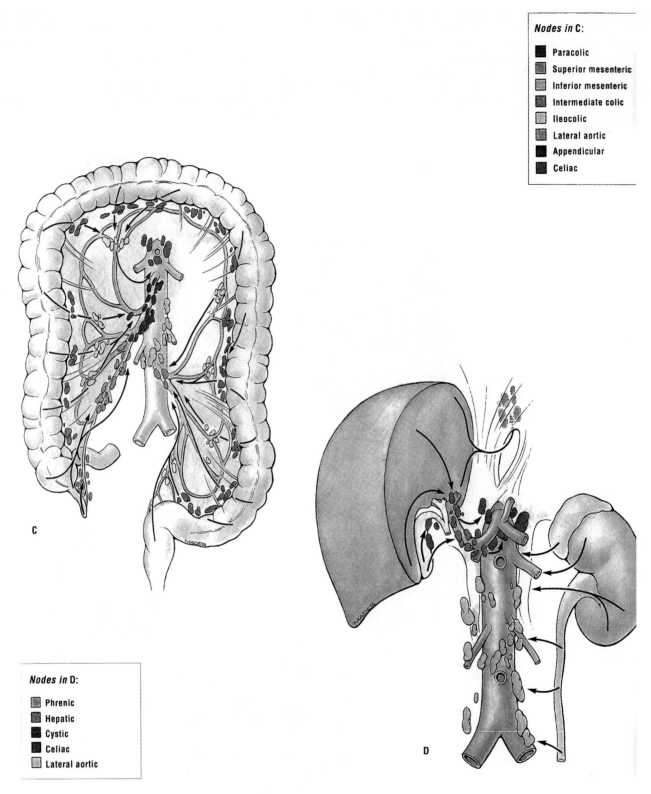

Nodes in C:

■ Paracolic
■ Superior mesenteric
■ Inferior mesenteric
■ Intermediate colic
□ Ileocolic
■ Lateral aortic
■ Appendicular
■ Celiac

Nodes in D:

■ Phrenic
■ Hepatic
■ Cystic
■ Celiac
■ Lateral aortic

Figure 12-12   (continued)

Lymphatics have been shown to respond to a variety of forces, including skeletal muscle contraction (Mazzoni et al., 1990), passive motion of the extremities (Gnepp and Sloop, 1978; Ikomi and Schmid-Schonbein, 1996; Ikomi et al., 1997), external tissue compression (McGeown et al., 1987), arterial pulse, and arteriolar vasomotion (Intaglietta and Gross, 1982). Lymphatics are oriented in tissue to maximize their exposure to the various external forces in their environment. Many lymphatics closely follow the arterial system, where they can respond to the pulse and vasomotion. Those in muscle are situated between layers, where they are effectively compressed. Although the forces that form lymph are varied, all involve movements that alternately expand and compress the initial lymphatics, creating oscillatory, dynamic pressure gradients between the interstitium and the initial lymphatic.

At the terminal lymphatic, passive motions could play an important role in loading the vessel with extracellular fluids (Witte et al., 2006). Alternating passive movements could not effectively form lymph if bidirectional flow across the lymphatic endothelium were possible. This is prevented by the overlapping endothelial cells in the initial lymphatic. These cells form a valve mechanism that allows the movement of fluid into the initial lymphatic, but prevents movement out (Schmid-Schonbein, 2003). Coupled with the anchoring filaments, this allows the lymphatic to utilize alternating tissue motion to create unidirectional movement of fluid from the interstitium into the lymph system. Additionally, this feature also allows the initial lymphatic to respond to fluctuations of fluid in the interstitium. A fluid pulse creates a pressure wave in the interstitial fluid. As the pulse approaches the lymphatic, a gradient is produced that opens the endothelial cells and permits fluid to enter. After the pulse crosses, the cells close preventing backflow out of the lymphatic. Arteriolar vasomotion appears to create a fluctuant displacement of interstitial fluid, which may influence lymph movement (Intaglietta and Gross, 1982). Fluid fluctuation may account for the movement and exchange of fluid within the interstitium. Capillary hydrostatic gradients dissipate quickly and do not account for the movement of fluid within the interstitial spaces (Aukland and Reed, 1993).

After moving into the initial lymphatic, fluid is propulsed through the collecting channels. These channels contain bicuspid valves that ensure unidirectional flow of lymph (Schmid-Schonbein, 1990b). An intrinsic myogenic pump has been identified that accounts for significant lymph propulsion. This pump consists of smooth muscle in the wall of the lymph vessel and the valves. Lymphatic smooth muscle exhibits spontaneous contractions that are peristaltic, traveling distal to proximal at a rate of 4 to 5 mm/s (Ohhashi et al., 1980). Evidence suggests that the contraction wave migrates retrogradely along the lymphatic vessels (Macdonald et al., 2008). A pacemaker initiates the spontaneous contractions (Beckett et al., 2007; Benoit, 1991; McHale and Meharg, 1992; Ohhashi et al., 1980; Van Helden, 1993; Van Helden et al., 2006). The pacemakers are situated in the wall of the lymphatic vessel between the endothelial cell layer and the surrounding smooth muscle; they begin just beyond the first valve (McCloskey et al., 2002; Ohhashi et al., 1980). The impulses are then coupled to the smooth muscle along the vessel in order to propagate a wave of contraction, producing a peristaltic action. Hogan proposed a mechanical coupling, based on the finding of stretch receptors in the lymphatic wall distal to the valve that initiated a smooth muscle contraction of the lymphangion (Hogan and Unthank, 1986). The initial pacemaker, located just proximal to the first valve near the initial lymphatic capillary, is also responsive to vessel distention and is stimulated by the distension created by lymph formation. The contraction of this distal segment propulses fluid beyond the valve where stretch receptors continue to stimulate smooth muscle contraction, and the peristaltic wave is propagated. In this model then, lymph propulsion is dependent on filling of the terminal lymphatic, or lymph formation.

More recent studies have demonstrated electrical coupling of smooth muscle cells (Crowe et al., 1997; Zawieja et al., 1993), likely mediated by calcium (Cotton et al., 1997). This, combined with a spontaneously contracting pacemaker, would allow a completely independent, electrically coupled peristaltic wave. Zawieja et al. (1993) found both upstream and downstream propagation of the contractions, supporting the idea of electrical coupling, since a volume-dependent mechanism should only propagate contraction centrally.

Crowe's study suggests that both electrical and mechanical coupling contribute to the propagation and coordination of

the intrinsic lymph pump (Crowe et al., 1997). They found that without a minimum amount of filling, no contractions occurred. They also found that more than half of the specimens studied, the contractions were preceded by a transient dilatation of the vessel, and that the propagation of the wave occurred relatively slowly, consistent with mechanical coupling. A minority of lymph specimens (9/22) demonstrated characteristics of electrical coupling, bidirectional propagation at a more rapid speed. Crowe's group also found that perfusion-induced contractile activity in most lymphangions, regardless of how the contraction was propagated, and that the contraction frequency was dependent on the rate of perfusion. Lymph formation then appears to be capable of initiating propulsion in some cases and significantly modifying it in others. Currently, there continues to be debate as to the relative importance of these two mechanisms in the functioning of the intrinsic lymph pump, but little debate about the relative importance of this pumping mechanism in the propulsion of lymph through the lymph vessel (Ohhashi et al., 2005; Witte et al., 2006). Ohhashi gives evidence of two separate pacemaker mechanism, one near the valve that responds to filling, and one near the middle of the lymphangion that responds to adrenergic stimulation, which may represent the source of the electrical pacemaker.

Lymph propulsion is also modified by a variety of other factors. Lymphatic smooth muscle responds to both adrenergic and humoral influences. Adrenergic stimulation has been shown to increase contractility and stroke volume of lymphatic smooth muscle (McHale, 1992). Humoral influences are important in lymph propulsion during inflammation. This area of study is in its early stages. An experimentally induced inflammatory process caused an increase in the stroke volume of the lymphatic vessels and an increase in lymph drainage (Benoit and Zawieja, 1992). Endotoxin, on the other hand, has a strong negative effect on lymph pumping and may explain some of the hemodynamic consequences of septic shock (Johnston et al., 1987). In vitro, IL-1 and prostaglandin E_1 reduced lymph contractile activity (Hanley et al., 1989), while bradykinin, PGH_2, and NO increased lymph contractility (Johnston and Gordon, 1981; Shirasawa et al., 2000; Yokoyama and Benoit, 1996), as did Substance P (Zawieja, 1996). Neurogenic and humeral influences appear less important in the myogenic pump than volumetric displacements (Aukland and Reed, 1993).

The effect of external forces of lymph propulsion is somewhat controversial. Lymphatic vessels lack anchoring filaments that would allow them to respond to the various forces that form lymph. On the other hand, the anatomical design of a thin-walled vessel with valves is consistent with propulsion from external compression. This is supported by the finding that lymphatics in the intestine and skeletal muscle have an absence of smooth muscle for a much greater distance from their origin than those from other tissues (Schmid-Schonbein, 1990b), presumably because compression from muscle contraction provides the necessary propulsive forces. Most studies on the effect of external forces on lymph flow do not distinguish the effect of these forces on lymph formation and propulsion. A study by McGeown et al. (1987) attempted to distinguish the effects of external compression on lymph formation versus propulsion. They created an inflammatory process on the hoof of a sheep, and then applied compressive forces to the hoof, directly over the area of lymph formation, and compared that to compression over the metatarsal area, where the larger collecting vessels are found. The study demonstrated a fourfold increase in flow when the forces were applied to the hoof, the area of lymph formation, and virtually no change when applied to the metatarsal area, where the collecting vessels were found. Although this study by itself does not exclude the possibility that external forces contribute to the propulsion of lymph, it provides compelling evidence that external forces are most effective in promoting formation of lymph. A further study demonstrated that the ability of external pressure to increase lymph flow was both rate and amplitude dependent (McGeown et al., 1988). This carries significant clinical implications for osteopathic approaches to lymph drainage, and should be considered in the design of Osteopathic treatment plans to promote lymph drainage, especially those using "lymphatic pump" techniques. Since lymph formation has been shown to initiate and/or strongly increase lymph propulsion, treatment to enhance lymph formation may increase lymph drainage in a number of important ways.

Postnodal lymph continues to move centrally, eventually draining into the right lymphatic duct or left thoracic duct before reentering the venous circulation at the subclavian vein. There have been numerous studies of the forces that move lymph through the thoracic duct (Browse et al., 1971; Browse et al., 1974; Dumont, 1975; Reddy and Staub, 1981; Schad et al., 1978). The smooth muscle in the thoracic duct exhibits spontaneous contractions similar to other lymphatic smooth muscle (Reddy and Staub, 1981). Respiration has been shown to have a consistent effect on the flow and pressures within the thoracic duct (Browse et al., 1971). Although these studies do not exclude the effect of respiration on the formation of lymph in the thorax and abdomen, and its contribution to thoracic duct flow, pressure changes associated with respiration are considered important in central lymph flow (Aukland and Reed, 1993).

Osteopathic treatment has been directed toward improving lymph drainage since the time of A.T. Still. Early writing by Millard focused on removing obstruction to the flow of lymph by treating somatic dysfunction along the course of fluid return (Millard, 1922). Although this concept has not been studied experimentally, it stands to reason that tissue strain in the area of lymph vessels will increase the resistance to lymph flow through those vessels. Earlier descriptions of lymph drainage pathways attempted to identify areas where compression might be likely. Experimentally increasing resistance to lymph flow has reduced lymph flow in distal lymphatics (Aukland and Reed, 1993).

J. Gordon Zinc discussed osteopathic treatment to improve the intrathoracic pressure gradients for their effect on central or terminal lymph drainage (Zinc, 1970, 1973). Treatment to improve thoracic excursion and increase negative intrathoracic pressure may not only increase thoracic duct flow, but it will also help stimulate lymph formation in the thorax and abdomen.

Lymph pump techniques, directed at actually moving lymph, have also been part of the Osteopathic approach to the lymphatics. McGeown's recent studies about the effects of external compression (McGeown et al., 1987, 1988), and the discovery of the intrinsic peristaltic contractions of lymphatic smooth muscle responsible for a considerable proportion of lymph propulsion, suggest that specific treatment to pump lymph should be directed toward lymph formation at the site of inflammation or lymphedema. Stimulation of the myogenic pacemaker by increasing lymph formation may also increase lymph propulsion.

REFERENCES

Abernethy NJ, Chin W, Hay JB, et al. Lymphatic removal of dialysate from the peritoneal cavity of anesthetized sheep. *Kidney Int* 1991;40(2): 174–181.

Adair TH, Guyton AC. Introduction to the lymphatic system. In: Johnston MG, ed. *Experimental Biology of Lymphatic Circulation.* Amsterdam, The Netherlands: Elsevier; 1985:1–12.

Adair TH, Guyton AC. Modification of lymph by lymph nodes. II. Effect of increased lymph node venous blood pressure. *Am J Physiol* 1983;245(4):H616–H622.

Adair TH, Moffatt DS, Paulsen AW, et al. Quantitation of changes in lymph protein concentration during lymph node transit. *Am J Physiol* 1982;243(3):H351–H359.

Alessandrini C, Gerli R, Sacchi G, et al. Cholinergic and adrenergic innervation of mesenterial lymph vessels in guinea pig. *Lymphology* 1981;14(1):1–6.

Atkinson TP, White MV, and Kaliner MA. Histamine and serotonin. In: Inflammation: Basic Principles and Clinical Correlations, edited by Gallin JI, Goldstein IM, and Snyderman R, New York NY:Raven Press, 1992, p. 193–209.

Aukland K, Reed RK. Interstitial-lymphatic mechanisms in the control of extracellular fluid volume. *Physiol Rev* 1993:73(1):1–78.

Beckett EA, Hollywood MA, Thornbury KD, et al. Spontaneous electrical activity in sheep mesenteric lymphatics. *Lymphat Res Biol* 2007;5(1):29–43.

Bellingan GJ, Caldwell H, Howie SE, et al. In vivo fate of the inflammatory macrophage during the resolution of inflammation: inflammatory macrophages do not die locally, but emigrate to the draining lymph nodes. *J Immunol* 1996;157(6):2577–2585.

Benoit JN. Relationships between lymphatic pump flow and total lymph flow in the small intestine. *Am J Physiol* 1991;261(6 pt 2):H1970–H1978.

Benoit JN. Effects of alpha-adrenergic stimuli on mesenteric collecting lymphatics in the rat. *Am J Physiol* 1997;273(1 pt 2):R331–R336.

Benoit JN, Zawieja DC. Effects of f-Met-Leu-Phe-induced inflammation on intestinal lymph flow and lymphatic pump behavior. *Am J Physiol* 1992;262 (2 pt 1):G199–G202.

Benoit JN, Zawieja DC, Goodman AH, et al. Characterization of intact mesenteric lymphatic pump and its responsiveness to acute edemagenic stress. *Am J Physiol* 1989;257(6 pt 2):H2059–H2069.

Browse NL, Lord RS, Taylor A. Pressure waves and gradients in the canine thoracic duct. *J Physiol* 1971;213(3):507–524.

Browse NL, Rutt DR, Sizeland D, et al. The velocity of lymph flow in the canine thoracic duct. *J Physiol* 1974;237(2):401–413.

Cotton KD, Hollywood MA, McHale NG, et al. Outward currents in smooth muscle cells isolated from sheep mesenteric lymphatics. *J Physiol (Lond)* 1997;503(pt 1):1–11.

Crowe MJ, von der Weid PY, Brock JA, et al. Co-ordination of contractile activity in guinea-pig mesenteric lymphatics. Physiol J.(Lond.) 500 (1):235–244, 1997.

Dinarello CA. Role of interleukin-i and tumor necrosis factor in systemic responses to infection and inflammation. In: Gallen JI, ed. *Inflammation: Basic Principles and Clinical Correlations.* New York, NY: Raven Press, 1992:211–232.

Dumont AE. The flow capacity of the thoracic duct-venous junction. *Am J Med Sci* 1975;269(3):292–301.

Eisenhoffer J, Elias RM, Johnston MG. Effect of outflow pressure on lymphatic pumping in vitro. *Am J Physiol* 1993;265(1 pt 2):R97–R102.

Felten DL, Livnat S, Felten SY, et al. Sympathetic innervation of lymph nodes in mice. *Brain Res Bull* 1984;13:693–699.

Gnepp DR, Sloop CH. The effect of passive motion on the flow and formation of lymph. *Lymphology* 1978;11(1):32–36.

Guyton AC, Barber BJ. The energetics of lymph formation. *Lymphology* 1980;13(4):173–176.

Hanley CA, Elias RM, Movat HZ, et al. Suppression of fluid pumping in isolated bovine mesenteric lymphatics by interleukin-1: interaction with prostaglandin E$_2$. *Microvasc Res* 1989;37(2):218–229.

Hogan RD, Unthank JL. Mechanical control of initial lymphatic contractile behavior in bat's wing. *Am J Physiol* 1986;251(2 pt 2):H357–H363.

Hollywood MA, McHale NG. Mediation of excitatory neurotransmission by the release of ATP and noradrenaline in sheep mesenteric lymphatic vessels. *J Physiol (Lond)* 1994;481(pt 2):415–423.

Hukkanen M, Konttinen YT, Terenghi G, et al. Peptide-containing innervation of rat femoral lymphatic vessels. *Microvasc Res* 1992;43(1):7–19.

Hurley JV. Inflammation. In: Staub NC, Taylor AE, eds. *Edema.* New York, NY: Raven Press, 1984:463–488.

Ikomi E, Zweifach BW, Schmid-Schonbein GW. Fluid pressures in the rabbit popliteal afferent lymphatics during passive tissue motion. *Lymphology* 1997;30(1):13–23.

Ikomi F, Schmid-Schonbein GW. Lymph pump mechanics in the rabbit hind leg. *Am J Physiol* 1996;271(1 pt 2):H173–H183.

Intaglietta M, Gross JF. Vasomotion, tissue fluid flow and the formation of lymph. *Int J Microcirc Clin Exp* 1982;1(1):55–65.

Jensen LT, Henriksen JH, Olesen HP, et al. Lymphatic clearance of synovial fluid in conscious pigs: the aminoterminal propeptide of type III procollagen. *Eur J Clin Invest* 1993;23(12):778–784.

Johnston MG, Gordon JL. Regulation of lymphatic contractility by arachidonate metabolites. *Nature* 1981;293(5830):294–297.

Johnston MG, Elias RM, Hayashi A, et al. Role of the lymphatic circulatory system in shock. *J Burn Care Rehabil* 1987;8(6):469–474.

Lawrence T, Gilroy DW. Chronic inflammation: a failure of resolution? *Int J Exp Pathol* 2007;88(2):85–94.

Leak LV. The structure of lymphatic capillaries in lymph formation. *Fed Proc* 1976;35(8):1863–1871.

Leak LV. Lymphatic endothelial-interstitial interface. *Lymphology* 1987;20(4):196–204.

Leak LV, Burke JF. Fine structure of the lymphatic capillary and the adjoining connective tissue area. *Am J Anat* 1966;118(3):785–809.

Leak LV, Jamuar MP. Ultrastructure of pulmonary lymphatic vessels. *Am Rev Respir Dis* 1983;128(2 pt 2):S59–S65.

Levine JD, Fields HL, Basbaum AI. Peptides and the primary afferent nociceptor. *J Neurosci* 1993;13:2273–2286.

Macdonald AJ, Arkill KP, Tabor GR, et al. Modeling flow in collecting lymphatic vessels: one-dimensional flow through a series of contractile elements. *Am J Physiol Heart Circ Physiol* 2008;295(1):H305–H313.

Mazzoni MC, Skalak TC, Schmid-Schonbein GW. Effects of skeletal muscle fiber deformation on lymphatic volumes. *Am J Physiol* 1990;259 (6 pt 2):H1860–H1868.

McCloskey KD, Hollywood MA, Thornbury KD, et al. Kit-like immunopositive cells in sheep mesenteric lymphatic vessels. *Cell Tissue Res* 2002;310(1):77–84.

McGeown JG, McHale NG, Thornbury KD. The role of external compression and movement in lymph propulsion in the sheep hind limb. *J Physiol (Lond)* 1987;387:83–93.

McGeown JG, McHale NG, Thornbury KD. Effects of varying patterns of external compression on lymph flow in the hindlimb of the anaesthetized sheep. *J Physiol (Lond)* 1988;397:449–457.

McGeown JG. Splanchnic nerve stimulation increases the lymphocyte output in mesenteric efferent lymph. *Pflugers Arch* 1993;422(6):558–563.

McHale NG. Lymphatic innervation. *Blood Vessels* 1990;27:127–136.

McHale NG. The lymphatic circulation. *Ir J Med Sci* 1992;161(8):483–486.

McHale NG, Meharg MK. Co-ordination of pumping in isolated bovine lymphatic vessels. *J Physiol (Lond)* 1992;450:503–512.

McHale NG, Thornbury KD. Sympathetic stimulation causes increased output of lymphocytes from the popliteal node in anaesthetized sheep. *Exp Physiol* 1990;75(6):847–850.

Measel JW Jr. The effect of the lymphatic pump on the immune response: I. Preliminary studies on the antibody response to pneumococcal polysaccharide assayed by bacterial agglutination and passive hemagglutination. *J Am Osteopath Assoc* 1982;82(1):28–31.

Mendoza E, Schmid-Schonbein GW. A model for mechanics of primary lymphatic valves. *J Biomech Eng* 2003;125(3):407–414.

Millard FP. Applied anatomy of the lymphatics. Kirksville, MO: The Journal Printing Company, 1922.

Movat HZ, Wasi S. Severe microvascular injury induced by lysosomal releasates of human polymorphonuclear leukocytes. Increase in vasopermeability, hemorrhage, and microthrombosis due to degradation of subendothelial and perivascular matrices. *Am J Pathol* 1985;121(3):404–417.

Murfee WL, Rappleye JW, Ceballos M, et al. Discontinuous expression of endothelial cell adhesion molecules along initial lymphatic vessels in mesentery: the primary valve structure. *Lymphat Res Biol* 2007;5(2): 81–89.

Nance DM, Sanders VM. Autonomic innervation and regulation of the immune system (1987–2007). *Brain Behav Immun* 2007;21(6):736–745.

Negrini D, Mukenge S, Del Fabbro M, et al. Distribution of diaphragmatic lymphatic stomata. *J Appl Physiol* 1991;70(4):1544–1549.

Ohhashi T, Azuma T, Sakaguchi M. Active and passive mechanical characteristics of bovine mesenteric lymphatics. *Am J Physiol* 1980;239(1): H88–H95.

Ohhashi T, Mizuno R, Ikomi F, et al. Current topics of physiology and pharmacology in the lymphatic system. *Pharmacol Ther* 2005;105(2):165–188.

Olszewski WL, Pazdur J, Kubasiewicz E, et al. Lymph draining from foot joints in rheumatoid arthritis provides insight into local cytokine and chemokine production and transport to lymph nodes. *Arthritis Rheum* 2001;44(3): 541–549.

Reddy NP, Staub NC. Intrinsic propulsive activity of thoracic duct perfused in anesthetized dogs. *Microvasc Res* 1981;21(2):183–192.

Schad H, Flowaczny H, Brechtelsbauer H, et al. 1978. The significance of respiration for thoracic duct flow in relation to other driving forces of lymph flow. *Pflugers Arch* 1975;378(2):121–125.

Schmid-Schonbein GW. Mechanisms causing initial lymphatics to expand and compress to promote lymph flow. *Arch Histol Cytol* 1990a;53(suppl):107–114.

Schmid-Schonbein GW. Microlymphatics and lymph flow. *Physiol Rev* 1990b;70(4):987–1028.

Schmid-Schonbein GW. The second valve system in lymphatics. *Lymphat Res Biol* 2003;1(1):25–29.

Shirasawa Y, Ikomi F, Ohhashi T. Physiological roles of endogenous nitric oxide in lymphatic pump activity of rat mesentery in vivo. *Am J Physiol Gastrointest Liver Physiol* 2000;278(4):G551–G556.

Thornbury KD, Harty HR, McGeown JG, et al. Mesenteric lymph flow responses to splanchnic nerve stimulation in sheep. *Am J Physiol* 1993;264 (2 pt 2):H604–H610.

Thornbury KD, McHale NG, Allen JM, et al. Nerve-mediated contractions of sheep mesenteric lymph node capsules. *J Physiol (Lond)* 1990;422:513–522.

Thornbury KD, McHale NG, McGeown JG. Alpha- and beta-components of the popliteal efferent lymph flow response to intra-arterial catecholamine infusions in the sheep. *Blood Vessels* 1989;26(2):107–118.

Trzewik J, Mallipattu SK, Artmann GM, et al. Evidence for a second valve system in lymphatics: endothelial microvalves. *FASEB J* 2001;15(10): 1711–1717.

Tsilibary EC, Wissig SL. Absorption from the peritoneal cavity: SEM study of the mesothelium covering the peritoneal surface of the muscular portion of the diaphragm. *Am J Anat* 1977;149(1):127–133.

Van Helden DF. Pacemaker potentials in lymphatic smooth muscle of the guinea-pig mesentery. *J Physiol* 1993;471:465–479.

Van Helden DF, Hosaka K, Imtiaz MS. Rhythmicity in the microcirculation. *Clin Hemorheol Microcirc* 2006;34(1–2):59–66.

Wang NS. The preformed stomas connecting the pleural cavity and the lymphatics in the parietal pleura. *Am Rev Respir Dis* 1975;111(1):12–20.

Witte CL, Witte MH. Lymphatics in the pathophysiology of edema. In: Johston MG, ed. *Experimental Biology of the Lymphatic Circulation*. New York, NY: Elsevier, 1984:167–188.

Witte MH, Jones K, Wilting J, et al. Structure function relationships in the lymphatic system and implications for cancer biology. *Cancer Metastasis Rev* 2006;25(2):159–184.

Yokoyama S, Benoit JN. Effects of bradykinin on lymphatic pumping in rat mesentery. *Am J Physiol* 1996;270(5 pt 1):G752–G756.

Zakaria ER, Simonsen O, Rippe A, et al. Transport of tracer albumin from peritoneum to plasma: role of diaphragmatic, visceral, and parietal lymphatics. *Am J Physiol* 1996;270(5 pt 2):H1549–H1556.

Zawieja DC. Lymphatic microcirculation. *Microcirculation* 1996;3(2):241–243.

Zawieja DC, Barber BJ. Lymph protein concentration in initial and collecting lymphatics of the rat. *Am J Physiol* 1987;252(5 pt 1):G602–G606.

Zawieja DC, Davis KL, Schuster R, et al. Distribution, propagation, and coordination of contractile activity in lymphatics. *Am J Physiol* 1993;264 (4 pt 2):H1283–H1291.

Zinc JG. The osteopathic holistic approach to homeostasis: 1969 Academy Lecture. American Academy of Osteopathic Medicine Yearbook, 1970:1–10.

Zinc JG. Applications of the osteopathic holistic approach to homeostasis. American Academy of Osteopathic Medicine Yearbook, 1973:37–47.

13

Mechanics of Respiration

FRANK H. WILLARD

KEY CONCEPTS

- The thoracoabdominal wall is a fibroelastic cylinder controlled by the respiratory muscles; fixation of the upper border of the ribs facilitates inhalation while fixation of the lower border of the ribs enhances exhalation.
- The thoracoabdominal diaphragm is a dome-shaped muscle, its function is greatly facilitated by its vertical component, termed the zone of apposition.
- The abdominal muscles play a role in fixing the lower border of the ribs as well as compressing the abdominal viscera and thereby expanding the zone of apposition to support the actions of the diaphragm.
- Structural changes in some respiratory muscles are seen at the molecular, cellular and gross structural levels in disease states such as COPD, kyphosis, and obesity, these changes decrease motion, ultimately decreasing the ability of the respiratory mechanism to supply adequate pumping activity.
- An emphasis is placed on having sufficient motion in the respiratory musculature to insure adequate ventilation of the tissue; an important role of the Osteopathic physician is to improve the range of motion in the respiratory mechanism.

INTRODUCTION

Definition of Respiratory Mechanics

The thorax is a flexible fibroelastic cylinder that is rhythmically distorted by the action of numerous respiratory muscles that are located both within the thorax and abdomen and extremities (Fig. 13.1). The changing shape of this cylinder creates the alternating inhalation and exhalation events necessary for perfusing the lung with air; these movements constitute the mechanics of breathing. Diseases that alter the shape of the thorax or its compliancy can have a substantial impact on the mechanics of respiration and, consequently, on the health of the individual.

Importance of Respiratory Mechanics in Osteopathic Manipulative Medicine

While alternating thoracoabdominal pressures are critical for the aeration of the pulmonary alveoli, this movement is also an important influence on the redistribution of fluid in the lymphatic system as well as the movement of blood in the venous network associated with the epidural venous plexus of Batson located in the spinal canal (See Chapter 12 on the lymphatic system). These facts emphasize the importance of striving for smooth continuous respiratory movements in the thoracoabdominal wall of the patient regardless of the etiology of their particular disease processes. This chapter will examine the anatomy and function of the muscles involved in respiration and the alteration of these movements in specific diseases involving structural changes in the thoracic wall as well as considering the influence of respiratory activity on the movement of fluids in the low pressure systems of the torso.

MUSCLES OF THE THORACIC CYLINDER

Intercostal, Scalene, and Abdominal Muscles

Anatomy of the Intercostal, Scalene, and Abdominal Muscles

The intercostal muscles form a distensible fibroelastic sheet surrounding the rib cage (Fig. 13.1). The sheet is divided into three incomplete layers. These layers are arranged in loose helical spirals (Fig. 13.2), each layer having a different pitch to the helix. Together, these layers act to both protect and alter the structural geometry of the thoracic wall and thus the volume of the pleural sacs. This fibromuscular tube is anchored from above by the scalene muscles that attach to the first and second ribs and below by the abdominal muscles that attach to the subcostal margin (Fig. 13.3).

The scalene muscles. Three scalene muscles—anterior, medius, and posterior—extend from the transverse processes of the cervical vertebrae (anterior C3-6, medius C1-7, and posterior C4-6) to reach the first rib and, to a lesser extent, the second rib (reviewed in O'Rahilly, 1986) (Figs. 13.2, 13.3 and 13.4). Occasionally, a scalenus minimus is found descending from the 6th and 7th transverse process to reach the inside of the 1st rib and the fascia of the apical pleural of the thoracic cavity (Sibson fascia). With the neck fixed in position by tonic contraction of the longus and paraspinal muscles, contraction of the scalene muscles elevates the first and second ribs, an important first step in inhalation. Activity in the scalene muscles is obligatory even in quiet respiratory movements (De Troyer and Estenne, 1988).

External intercostal muscle. This thin sheet of muscle arises from the costotransverse ligaments posteriorly at the level of the tubercle of the rib and tapers to become a membrane anteriorly at the level of the costochondrial junction. In the upright position, the orientation of the muscle fibers is close to vertical (Figs. 13.1-13.3, 13.5, and 13.6). Throughout its course in each interspace, the muscle is attached to the lower margin of the rib and costal cartilage above and to the upper margin of the rib and costal cartilage below (O'Rahilly, 1986). The external intercostal muscle is thickest and thinnest best developed in the superior posterior aspect of the thorax, thinnest inferior and medially (De Troyer et al., 2005). The pitch of its helical spiral is from superioposterior to inferioanterior (Fig. 13.2). Based on its geometry, thickness, and data from electromyography (EMG) studies, the external intercostal is a powerful muscle of inhalation in the human with the exception of its most anteromedial border, where the muscle is thinnest. This latter region, located in the anterior portions of spaces 6 to 8, appears to represent a weak muscle of exhalation (De Troyer et al., 2005).

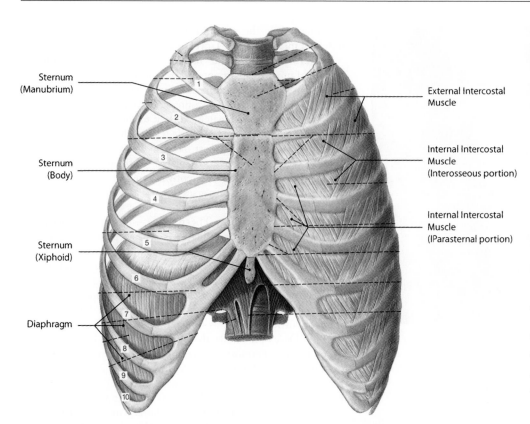

Sternum
(Manubrium)

Sternum
(Body)

Sternum
(Xiphoid)

Diaphragm

External Intercostal
Muscle

Internal Intercostal
Muscle
(Interosseous portion)

Internal Intercostal
Muscle
(IParasternal portion)

Figure 13-1 This figure illustrates the invasion of muscle fibers by proinflammatory cytokines such as interleukin-6 and tumor necrosis factor-α. Once in the muscle these cytokines can act through at least two routes to enhance muscle wasting. In (**A**) TNF-α works with interferon-g to suppress the ability of the nuclear transcription factor MyoD to stimulate production of myosin. Thus, less myosin heavy chain is produced in the myocyte. IL-6 is also capable of enhancing the production of ubiquitin and ubiquitin-ligase, two proteins used in labeling cellular protein for degradation by the proteosome as shown in (**B**). Thus, cachexia and muscle atrophy develops due to the blockage in myosin production and enhancement of its destruction. (Taken from C. D. Clemente. *Anatomy: A Regional Atlas of the Human Body.* Baltimore: Williams & Wilkins; 1997.)

Internal intercostal muscles. The internal intercostal muscles are found deep to the external intercostals (Fig. 13.1–13.3, 13.5–13.7). These thin muscles arise from the lateral border of the sternum and wrap around the ribs to eventually become a thin membrane in the posterior intercostal spaces (Fig. 13.1). Like the external intercostal muscles, the internal is attached to the lower margin of the rib and costal cartilage above and to the upper margin of these structures below. The muscle is thickest in the anterior

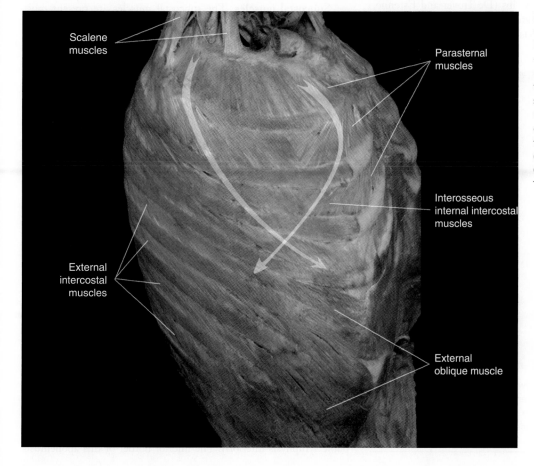

Scalene
muscles

External
intercostal
muscles

Parasternal
muscles

Interosseous
internal intercostal
muscles

External
oblique muscle

Figure 13-2 This is a lateral view of the thorax demonstrating the helical spirals established by the external and internal intercostal muscles. The arrow that starts on the left represents the pitch of the spiral of the external intercostal muscle while the arrow beginning on the right represents the same for the internal intercostal muscle. (Taken from the Willard/Carreiro Collection.)

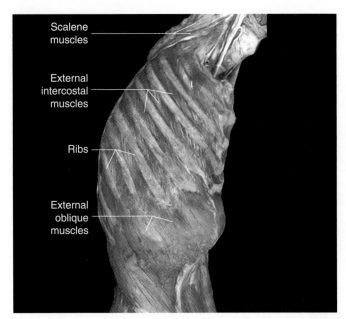

Figure 13-3   This is a lateral view of a male thorax and upper abdomen. The skin and superficial fascia have been removed to reveal the external intercostal and external oblique muscles. (Taken from the Willard/Carrerio Collection.)

and superior portions and tapers as it passes posteriorly (O'Rahilly, 1986). The resulting spiral pitch of its muscle fibers is oriented from superioanterior to inferioposterior. The muscle is divided into two functionally distinct components. The parasternal portion exists between the costal cartilages, while the interosseous intercostal muscle exists between the bony ribs (De Troyer and Estenne, 1988). Analysis of geometry, thickness, and EMG data supports the contention that the interosseous portion is strictly involved in

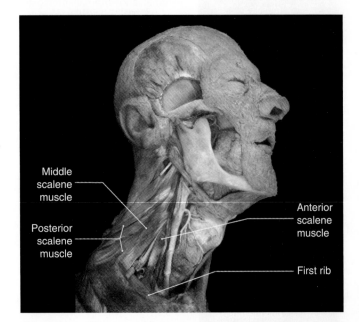

Figure 13-4   This is an oblique view of a male head and neck with the skin, superficial fascia, and upper extremity removed to display the three scalene muscles. A deep dissection was done into the temporal region for other purposes. (Taken from the Willard/ Carreiro Collection.)

exhalation while the parasternal portion represents a significant muscle of inhalation (De Troyer et al. 1998, 2005).

Innermost intercostal muscles. The innermost internal intercostal muscles are oriented orthogonal to the ribs (Fig. 13.7). These muscles are very thin and inconsistent in their presence. When present, the internal investing fascia of the innermost internal intercostal muscle is intimately adhered to the endothoracic fascia. Given this muscle's close geometric relationship with the rib, contraction of the muscle is most likely to assist in moving the ribs closer to each other. Functional analysis of the internal intercostal muscle by EMG analysis is currently lacking. The muscle is related embryologically to the transverses thoracic and transverses abdominus muscles.

Transversus thoracis. The transverses thoracis muscle, also termed sternocostalis or triangularis sternae muscle, arises from the inner surface of the lower sternum, xiphoid process, and lower costal cartilages (Fig. 13.7). It radiates outward to attach to the inner borders of the costal cartilages of ribs 2 through 6 (O'Rahilly, 1986). Only rarely is the muscle symmetric in disposition; often, additional slips of the muscle can be found scattered in the second through fourth interspace as seen in the specimen displayed in Figure 13.7. Developmentally, the muscle appears to be most closely related to the innermost internal intercostal group of muscles and the transverses abdominus muscle. In Figure 13.7, the transverses thoracis muscle is seen blending with the superior border of the transverses abdominus muscle; this is most apparent on the left side of the specimen. The transverses thoracis muscle is active typically on forced exhalation. Quiet, restful breathing in humans does not appear to use the muscle. However, exhalation below functional residual capacity (FRC) such as in speech and forceful exhalation such as in coughing, expectoration, and laughing utilize the power of this muscle (De Troyer et al. 1987, 2005).

Subcostal muscles. The subcostal muscles are present most often in the lower segments of the thorax. These muscles arise from the inner aspect of the rib near its angle and descend two to three ribs below to find an attachment to the upper margin of a rib (O'Rahilly, 1986). The subcostal muscles run in the same plane as the innermost intercostals and appear to be an embryological derivative of that layer. The subcostal muscles are most prominent in the inferior portion of the thorax and with the exception of the 12th rib and remain lateral to the angle to the rib at all levels. The common orientation of these muscles with the internal intercostal suggests a possible function in exhalation.

Levatores costarum. The levatores costarum are a group of small muscles located deep to the paraspinal muscles and attached to the ribs on their posterior aspect. These muscles arise from the transverse process at the level of the costotransverse joint and extend downward diagonally to attach to the rib or ribs below (Fig. 13.8). The short head (brevis) of the muscle attaches one rib below its origin while the long head (longus) attaches two ribs below. Given the position of these muscles on the rib, it is evident that they contribute to elevating the rib on inhalation (De Troyer et al. 2005) but have not received extensive physiological examination to date.

The external oblique muscle. The outermost abdominal muscle arises from the external and lower borders of the lower eight ribs. The attachment of this muscle interdigitates with the slips of the serratus anterior and latissimus dorsi, both extremity muscles, as well as fusing with the external intercostal muscle of the lower eight ribs (Fig. 13.9). The muscle fibers form a broad thin sheet passing anterior and inferior, similar to those of the external intercostals, to reach their attachment to a medially positioned aponeurosis, which extends from the xiphoid process superiorly to the pubic symphysis inferiorly. The inferior border of this aponeurosis

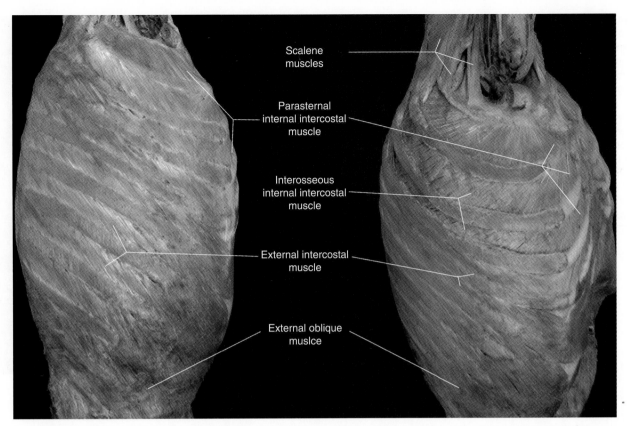

Figure 13-5 These are lateral views of the thorax to illustrate the distribution of the intercostal muscles. In the dissection on the left the external intercostal muscle id exposed. In the dissection of the right, the external intercostal muscle in the first 3 interspaces has been removed to expose the internal intercostal muscle. (Taken from the Willard/Carreiro Collection.)

participates in the formation of the inguinal ligament and its medial border contributes to the rectus sheath (O'Rahilly, 1986). The muscle fibers of the external oblique rarely extend below a line drawn between the umbilicus and the anterior superior iliac

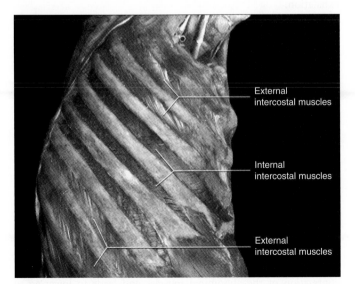

Figure 13-6 A lateral view of the thorax. IN this dissection, the skin, superficial fascia and upper extremity were removed. The external intercostal muscle is seen in the first two interspaces, This muscle was removed in the next three interspaces to reveal the internal intercostal muscles. The external intercostal is seen in the remaining interspaces. (Taken from the Willard/Carreiro Collection.)

spine, the remainder of the sheet being aponeurosis. Contraction of the external oblique muscle is capable of distorting the human rib cage (Mier et al., 1985). The external oblique is quiet during restful breathing but engaged during forceful exhalation (Epstein, 1994).

Internal oblique muscle. The internal oblique muscle has a radiate shape (Fig. 13.10), emanating from the region of the iliac crest and low back and attaching along a line from the pubic symphysis upward along the rectus sheath and posteriorly along the subcostal margin to reach the thoracolumbar fascia. Specifically, the broad sheet of muscle takes its origin from a curved line involving the upper portion of the inquinal ligament anteriorly, the iliac crest centrally, and the thoracolumbar fascia posteriorly. From this line, the fibers of the muscle radiate inferiorly to reach the conjoint tendon and pubic symphysis; in doing so, they help form the falx inquinalis under which the spermatic cord or round ligament will pass. Superiorly this muscle radiates toward the back were fibers attach to the inferior margin of the subcostal cartilage as well as interdigitate with the internal intercostal muscles. The middle fibers of the muscle pass anteriorly around the curve of the abdomen to join a medially positioned aponeurosis, which eventually splits to house the rectus abdominis muscle (O'Rahilly, 1986). Quiet respiration does not appear to engage the internal oblique muscle; however, it will become active on forced exhalation (Epstein, 1994).

Transversus abdominis muscle. Internal to the abdominal oblique lies a third muscle with a predominant horizontal fiber orientation (Fig. 13.11). The transverses abdominis arises from the lateral portion of the inguinal ligament, the iliac crest, the thoracolumbar fascia, and the inferior margin of the lower costal cartilages. On the posterior aspect of the anterior abdominal wall,

Figure 13-7 This is a posterior view of the anterior thoracic wall. The anterior wall was removed by sectioning the ribs laterally. The parietal pleural was removed from the right side of the wall but has been retained on the left side. The transversus thoracis muscle is seen radiating away from the inferior portion of the sternum. Note the asymmetry of this muscle. Slips of the innermost intercostal muscle can be seen in the upper interspaces. (Taken from the Willard/Carreiro Collection.)

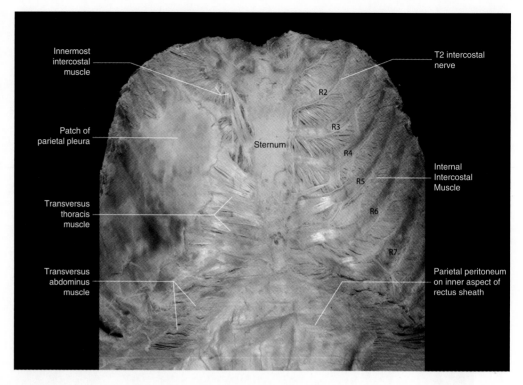

the transverses abdominis dovetails with slips of the diaphragm along the subcostal margin. Medially, the fibers of this broad, flat muscle attach to an aponeurosis that extends from the xiphoid process superiorly to the conjoint tendon inferiorly (O'Rahilly, 1986). All muscle fibers are horizontally oriented except for the most inferior border where the muscle bands turn downward dramatically to joint those of the internal oblique and form the conjoint tendon. The horizontal orientation of the muscle fibers allows this muscle to act as a retinaculum, pulling the rectus sheath toward the posterior body and increasing the intra-abdominal pressure. This mechanical action has the effect of raising the diaphragm in the thoracic cavity (De Troyer and Estenne, 1988). EMG studies have demonstrated that the transverses thoracis is an obligatory muscle of respiration and is active in both exhalation and inhalation, ceasing its activity only as it approaches the portion of maximum inhalation (De Troyer et al., 2005).

Rectus abdominis muscle. The rectus abdominis muscle forms a vertically oriented band of muscles extending from the pubic crest and symphysis to the xiphoid process and medial subcostal margin (Fig. 13.12). The muscle is typically divided into four plates by three tendinous horizontal bands. The rectus abdominis is housed in a dense fibrous connective tissue wrapping termed the rectus sheath. Essentially the sheath is composed of anterior and posterior plates derived from the splitting of the aponeurosis of the internal oblique. This sheath completely surrounds the muscle with the exception of the posterior wall inferior to the umbilicus; here, a defect in the posterior wall of the fibrous sheath transmits the rectus abdominis muscle. Inferior to this line, termed the arcuate line, the posterior wall is composed primarily of the transversalis fascia. Although a major function of the rectus abdominis is flexion of the torso and counter balancing the paraspinal muscle of the back, the rectus, when used in combination with the other abdominal muscle particularly the transverses abdominis, functions as a corset trussing the abdominal organs in place and pushing them upward to make a fulcrum (see section on the diaphragm) over which the

thoracoabdominal diaphragm is draped (De Troyer and Estenne, 1988).

Combined Function of the Intercostal, Scalene, and Abdominal Muscles

The various intercostal muscles have differing functions in respiratory movements. The external intercostal muscle and the parasternal muscle are key players in inhalation, while the interosseous portion of the internal intercostal muscle is involved in exhalation.

However, electrical stimulation of any isolated intercostal muscle will close the ribs regardless of its location, thus the factors differentiating the action of the external intercostal and parasternal muscle from the remainder of the internal intercostal muscle must reside outside the geometry of these muscles alone. The actions of the intercostal muscles are dependent on the resistance to motion at either end of the thoracic cylinder. This resistance is dependent on the state of contraction of the muscles attached to the cylinder ends. Fixation of the first rib supports inhalation and fixation of the subcostal margin facilitates exhalation. The function of the scalene muscles is to fix the position of the first rib and thus initiate inhalation. A function of the abdominal muscles is to fix the position of the lower ribs thereby initiating exhalation. The contraction of the intercostal muscles is coordinated with the activity of the scalene and abdominal muscles. As the scalene muscles contract, a wave of activity begins in the superior external intercostal and parasternal muscles sweeping sequentially down the thoracic wall from the first interspace. A reverse or ascending wave is seen following contraction of the abdominal muscles and leads to lowering of the ribs and exhalation (De Troyer and Estenne, 1988; De Troyer et al., 2005).

Control over the sequential contraction of the intercostal muscles has been shown to reside in the pattern of connectivity regulating ventral horn interneuron activity. These cells regulate the discharges of the ventral horn motor neurons, which in turn

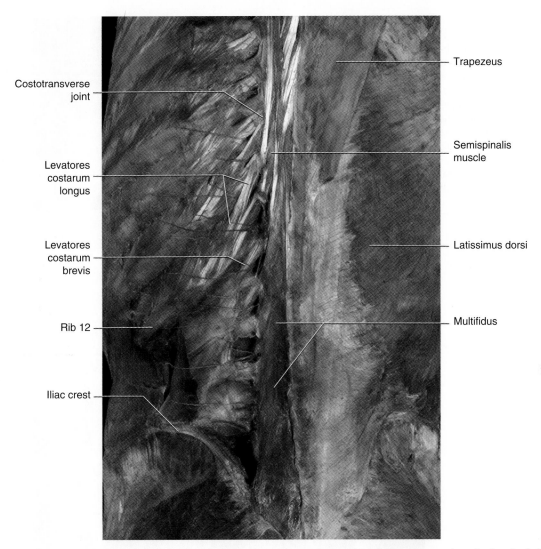

Costotransverse joint

Levatores costarum longus

Levatores costarum brevis

Rib 12

Iliac crest

Trapezeus

Semispinalis muscle

Latissimus dorsi

Multifidus

Figure 13-8 Posterior view of the back with the paraspinal muscles on the left side removed to display the levatores costarum muscles. Levatores costarum longus spans two segments while brevis spans one segment. (Taken from the Willard/Carreiro Collection.)

innervate the intercostal muscles. The spinal cord interneurons are modulated by input coming from both the medullary portion of the brainstem and peripheral input from muscle spindles. However, this combined input is relatively weak compared to that of the central respiratory drive potential present in the ventral horn, thus suggesting that the spinal interneurons of the ventral horn are the dominant force (De Troyer et al., 2005). Therefore, as with the control of individual muscle contractions in such repetitive actions as locomotion, there is a central pattern generator formed by the interneuronal pool in the ventral horn. This group of cells generates repetitive patterns of activity for the motor neurons to deliver to the appropriate skeletal muscles. These patterns can be influenced by both the descending activity from the medullary brainstem and the peripheral activity from the muscle afferent fibers; ultimate control however appears to reside in the spinal cord.

The Pumphead in the Thoracic Cylinder

The Thoracoabdominal Diaphragm

The diaphragm is often described as a dome-shaped structure composed of skeletal muscle and tendinous attachments that partially close the passage from thorax to abdomen (Fig. 13.13). However, if the diaphragm is removed from the body and spread on the flat surface, it takes on the shape resembling that of a large butterfly with the central tendon as the body and the leaflets resembling head, wings, and tail. Each of the diaphragm's leaflets is named by its attachments. The sternal leaflets (head of the butterfly) are small and attach to the posterior aspect of the xiphoid process; occasionally they are missing. The costal leaflets (wings of the butterfly) are the largest and attach to the lower six ribs where their muscle fibers interdigitate with muscular slips from the transverses abdominis. These two leaflets form the broad sheet of diaphragmatic muscle that courses vertically along the internal margin of the ribs. Finally, the lumbar leaflets (tail of the butterfly) extend from the medial borders of the central tendon inferiorly to form two aponeurotic arches, as well as the cura of the diaphragm.

The medial arcuate ligament of the diaphragm attaches to the body of L1 medially arches over the psoas muscle and the tip of the anterior surface of the L1 transverse process laterally. The lateral arcuate ligament attaches to the anterior aspect of the L1 transverse process medially and reaches over the quadratus lumborum muscle to anchor laterally to the tip of the 12th rib near its midpoint. The

Figure 13-9 Lateral view of the torso illustrating the external oblique muscle and its attachment to the rectus sheath and the inguinal ligament. Note the interdigitation of the external intercostal muscle with the finger-like attachments of the serratus anterior. In addition, the most inferior fibers of the pectoralis major also blend into the superior medial attachment of the external oblique. (Taken from the Willard/Carreiro Collection.)

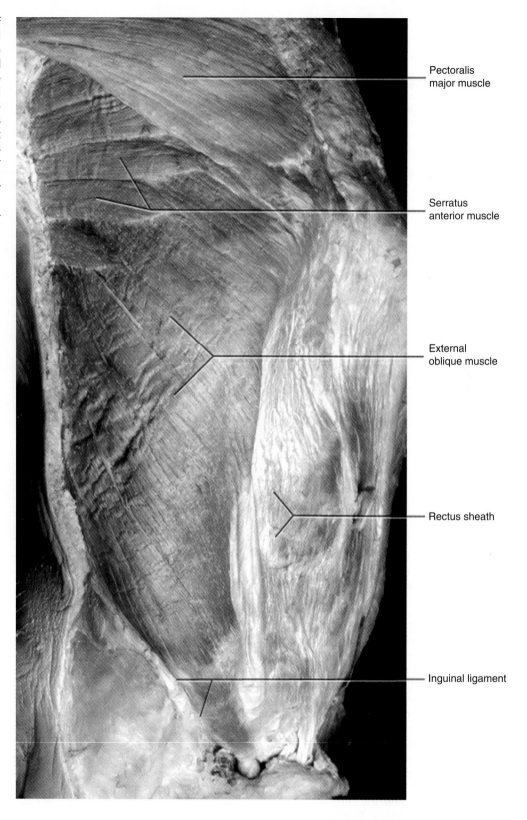

Pectoralis major muscle

Serratus anterior muscle

External oblique muscle

Rectus sheath

Inguinal ligament

midline portion of the lumbar leaflets forms the cura of the diaphragm. Both cura arise from the medial most portion of the central tendon and sweep downward, attaching to the anterior longitudinal ligament on the bodies of the upper three lumbar vertebrae. The right crus is larger than the left. The medialmost fibers of each crus unite on the midline to form the median arcuate ligament that surrounds aorta as it passes from thorax to abdomen.

Function of the Diaphragm

The dome shape of the diaphragm is created by a piston of viscera including the liver, stomach, and spleen, which is forced upward into the central tendon by the abdominal musculature (Fig. 13.14), particularly the transverses abdominis. Much of the costal leaflet passes vertically along the wall of the rib cage to reach the subcostal margin and their attachment. This dome-shaped arrangement

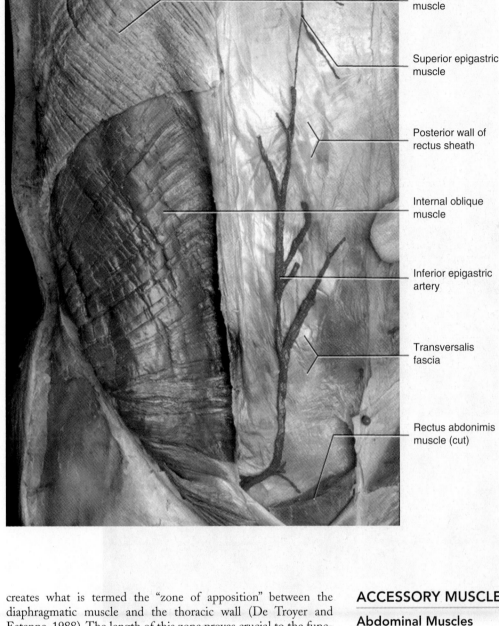

External oblique
muscle

Superior epigastric
muscle

Posterior wall of
rectus sheath

Internal oblique
muscle

Inferior epigastric
artery

Transversalis
fascia

Rectus abdonimis
muscle (cut)

Figure 13-10 The internal oblique muscle. This is an anterior view of the abdominal wall. The skin and superficial fascia have been removed. The external oblique muscle was cleaned and a window cut into the muscle to expose the internal oblique. This photograph demonstrates the middle fibers of the internal oblique as they arise from the iliac crest and attach to the rectus sheath. (Taken from the Willard/Carreiro Collection.)

creates what is termed the "zone of apposition" between the diaphragmatic muscle and the thoracic wall (De Troyer and Estenne, 1988). The length of this zone proves crucial to the function of the diaphragm. With the visceral piston placed in the full upright position, contraction of the costal leaflets will pull the subcostal margin upward while attempting to force the visceral piston downward. If the visceral piston is adequately buttressed by the abdominal musculature, the central tendon only descends a short distance, less than two segmental interspaces, and the subcostal margin of the ribs is elevated. Since the lower ribs are attached by movable joints anteriorly and posteriorly, the body of the rib rotates outward and upward (referred to as "bucket-handle" motion). Thus, the abdominal viscera can be considered to function to form a fulcrum over which the diaphragm is bent. The motion occurring across this visceral fulcrum greatly increases the volume of the thorax while minimizing the amount of descent required by the central tendon. It is important to realize that for the diaphragm to maximally lift the ribs during respiration it has to maintain its vertical zone of apposition along the costal wall. Structural changes that alter this arrangement can significantly impair the ventilatory mechanics of the diaphragm.

ACCESSORY MUSCLES OF RESPIRATION

Abdominal Muscles

External and Internal Oblique Muscles

Neither the external nor the internal oblique is active on quiet respiration. However, both muscles will become involved in respiratory movements during forced exhalation (reviewed in Epstein, 1994). These muscles exert a downward pull on the subcostal margin thus sliding the thoracic walls over the diaphragm and visceral organs, in essence seating the piston high in the cylinder. This gloving motion helps to decrease the volume of the pleural cavities in the thorax and thus facilitates exhalation. The gloving motion is also important in re-creating the large zone of apposition preceding the next respiratory cycle.

Limb Girdle Muscles

Seratus Anterior Muscle

The most powerful of the limb muscles capable of influencing the ribs is the seratus anterior. This thin, sheet-like muscle arises from the fleshy attachments to the anterior surface of the first eight or nine ribs (Fig. 13.15). Each band of the muscle wraps around the thorax

Figure 13-11 This is a lateral view of a male abdomen. The skin, superficial fascia and the external and internal oblique muscles have been removed to reveal the transversus abdominis muscle. The rectus sheath has also been removed. The whitish material is the transversalis fascia. Cotton has been placed in the abdominal cavity to expand the transversus abdominis muscle to is full extent. (Taken from the Willard/Carreiro Collection.)

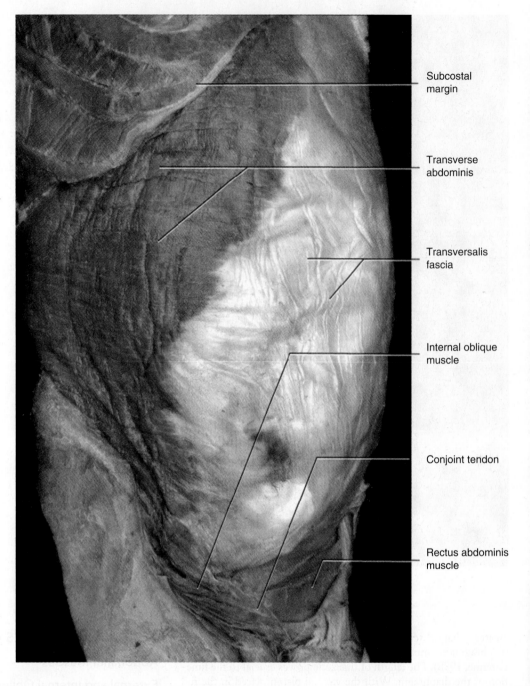

Subcostal margin

Transverse abdominis

Transversalis fascia

Internal oblique muscle

Conjoint tendon

Rectus abdominis muscle

passing between the posterolateral thoracic wall and the scapula to reach the medial border of this bone. The involvement of the seratus anterior with movement of the scapula is well detailed in numerous anatomy books and will not be covered here. If the upper extremity is fixed by grasping an external object, the seratus can assist in raising the ribs. Thus, the seratus anterior can become an accessory muscle of respiration in stressful situations. Use of this muscle to assist in respiration can be observed in cases involving hyperinflation of the chest such as chronic obstructive pulmonary disease (COPD). Here, the patient may grasp the bed rails, fixing the scapula, in an effort to recruit the seratus and assist in respiratory movements.

Oropharyngeal Muscles and Respiratory Movements

Protecting Airway Patency

The upper airway (the larynx and above) is a collapsible tubular structure. Compromise of the airway lumen can occur during inspiration and neonates are especially vulnerable to this event. Several

muscles act in concert to protect the patency of the air; these are the muscles of the tongue such as the genioglossus and those of the hyoid such as the geniohyoid, sternohyoid, stenothyroid, and thyrohyoid (Thach, 1992; reviewed in Lee et al., 2007). Bursts of activity in phase with inspiration have been recorded from these muscles (reviewed in Thach, 1992). In addition, an especially important muscle for opening the airway is the posterior cricoarytenoid muscle since it is the only abductor of the vocal folds. Although little is known concerning the respiratory-related activity of this muscle in humans, work in other species has confirmed an inspiratory rhythm in the muscle. Contraction of all of these upper airway muscles functions to increase airway rigidity and protect the patency of the lumen (Fig. 13.16). The neural pathways underlying the presence of a respiratory rhythm in the upper airway muscles have not been fully worked out. However, this activity may be in part due to pressure changes in the lumen of the airway detected by trigeminal afferent fibers and relayed to the hypoglossal nucleus through the trigeminal complex (Hwang et al., 1984).

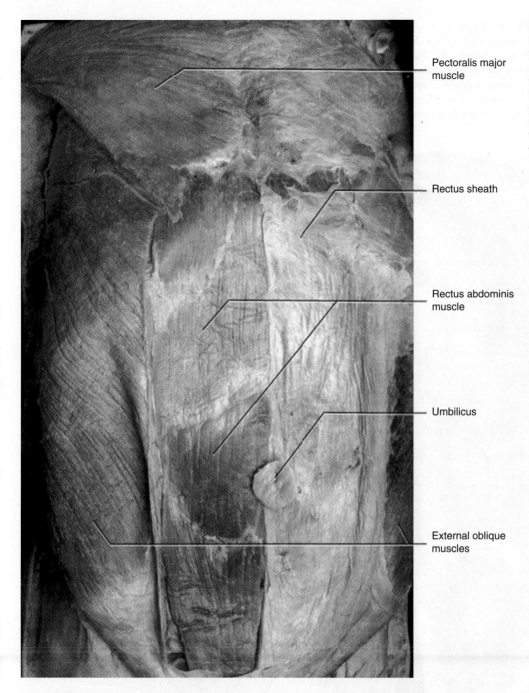

Figure 13-12 This is an anterior view of the anterior abdominal wall. The skin and superficial fascia have been removed to reveal the rectus sheath. The sheath has been removed on the right side of the individual to reveal the rectus abdominis muscle. (Taken from the Willard/Carreiro Collection.)

Pectoralis major muscle

Rectus sheath

Rectus abdominis muscle

Umbilicus

External oblique muscles

RESPIRATORY MUSCLE PATHOLOGY

Airway Diseases

Structural Changes in COPD

COPD currently is the fourth most common cause of death worldwide and has been estimated to rise to the third most common cause by 2020 (Barnes, 2004). It is most often related to smoking although it can be caused by exposure to any noxious gas including poorly ventilated cooking fumes.

Functionally COPD involves the increased resistance to airflow, typically expressed as a reduction in forced ventilation rate with air trapping in the lungs at end-stage exhalation. At a tissue level, COPD involves loss of alveolar architecture and narrowing of the small airways either through thickening of the wall from chronic inflammation or plugging with mucous secretions. Structurally, air trapping in the lungs at full exhalation results in hyperinflation with enlargement of the A-P dimension of the chest as is

typically seen on clinical and radiographic examination of the patient with COPD (Celli, 1995). The hyperinflation is due to either loss of static recoil in the parenchymal tissue or to dynamic hyperinflation, for example, the presence of residual air in the lung at the end point of exhalation (reviewed in Fitting, 2001). In essence, the narrowing of the distal end of airway allows air to be drawn into the alveoli but impedes movement of the air out of the lung. In hyperinflation, the diaphragm is typically lower in the thoracic cavity and shorter in length with a slightly increased radius of curvature.

Structurally the diaphragm in the COPD patient creates a straighter line between the subcostal margins at a lower level in the thorax, thereby significantly reducing the zone of apposition (Cassart et al., 1997) as well as the overall surface area of the muscle (Fig. 13.17). Normally the zone of apposition represents 60% of the muscle's length, but that can be reduced to 40% in COPD. This structural change significantly decreases the efficiency of the diaphragm as a muscle of inhalation (Cassart et al., 1997).

In addition, the reduced length of the muscle alters the length–tension relationship for the muscle fibers; this reduction in length–tension relationship further compromises the diaphragm's efficiency. In the physically lowered state, contraction of the diaphragm can, in fact, become an expiratory action in nature.

An example of this expiratory conversion of the diaphragm is seen when attempting deep inhalations from the flatten state with a marked reduction in the zone of apposition. The subcostal margin is drawn inward at the end stage as the flattened diaphragm pulls the ribs inward; this is a paradoxical motion termed Hoover sign (reviewed in De Troyer and Estenne, 1988). However, it appears that not all of the inward motion of the subcostal margin during attempted inhalation can be blamed on the loss of the zone of apposition. Additional inward force is most likely derived from the

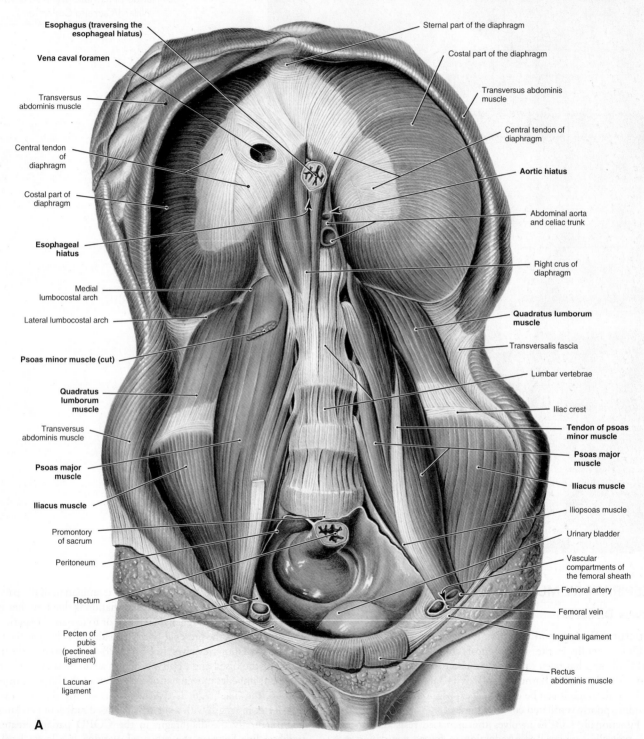

A

Figure 13-13   The inferior surface of the thoracoabdominal diaphragm. In **A.** the abdomen has been opened to reveal the inferior surface of the diaphragm. In **B.** a similar approach has been taken with a human dissection. Abbreviations are as follows: Aor, hiatus for the aorta; Eso, hiatus for the esophagus; IVC, hiatus for the inferior vena cava. ((**A**) is taken from Clemente CD. *Anatomy: A Regional Atlas of the Human Body.* Baltimore: Williams & Wilkins; 1997; (**B**) is taken from the Willard/Carreiro Collection.)

A significant change involves the fiber types present in the muscle of the diaphragm. Current estimates of respiratory muscle histological composition in the normal adult human diaphragm indicate that 55% of the fibers are of the slow type (type I fibers), 21% fast oxidative (type IIA fibers), and 24% fast glycolytic (type IIB and 2X fibers). Intercostal muscle histology finds greater than 60% are slow fibers (reviewed in Polla et al., 2004). This relatively high percentage of type I (slow twitch) fibers present normally is thought to represent an adaptation imparting the respiratory muscles a fatigue-resistant quality (Ottenheijm et al., 2008).

Interestingly, the diaphragm muscle of COPD patients demonstrated a further increase in the slow-twitch fibers with a shift to the slow isoforms of the myofibrillar proteins (Levine et al., 1997; reviewed in Polla et al., 2004). Stubbings et al. (2008) have shown a strong negative correlation between the forced expiratory volume in 1 second (FEV_1) and the percentage of type I fibers contained in the diaphragm. Thus, all COPD patients in their study had a higher percentage of type I fibers in the diaphragm and a lower FEV_1. In addition, there was a positive correlation between the FRC and the percentage of type I fibers in the diaphragm. Thus COPD individuals had a greater percentage of type I fibers and a greater residual of trapped air in the lung than the non-COPD controls.

The shift toward increasing type I fibers in the diaphragm muscle of COPD patients is suggestive of a further adaptive process to help minimize diaphragm muscle fatigue in these patients (Ottenheijm et al., 2008). It was also demonstrated that the amount of ATP consumption was proportional to the rate of the contraction. Since type IIA fibers contract faster than type I, then for a given contraction of equal length, type I fibers consume significantly less ATP than type IIA fibers. From this, it is clear that the shift to type I fibers with reduced consumption of ATP in the COPD patient helps to conserve energy.

The benefits of an increased percentage of type I fibers in the diaphragm may be partially offset by a decreased amount of myosin in each sarcomere. Since the contractile force of a muscle is related to the density of myosin per sarcomere, the muscle fibers of the COPD patient are weaker in nature (Balasubramanian and Varkey, 2006).

These structural changes in fiber type found in the diaphragm were not detectable in other respiratory muscles such as the intercostal muscles, nor have they been documented in other muscles of the body. In fact, evidence suggests that the extremity muscles suffer a reverse effect. Histological observation has demonstrated a shift from type I to type II fibers with a concordant reduction in the diameter of both type I and II fibers that is proportional to the severity of the of the COPD as measured by a reduction in FEV_1 (Gosker et al., 2003). Atrophy, fatty replacement, and fibrosis were enhanced in the extremity muscles of the COPD patients when compared to control subjects. Other metabolic and microstructural changes in extremity muscles of COPD patients have been reviewed recently (Balasubramanian and Varkey, 2006). All of these alterations in muscle anatomy and chemistry contribute to significantly increased weakness in COPD patients, a weakness and muscle mass loss that can be exacerbated by glucocorticoid therapy and reduced motion seen in a sedentary existence.

System Influences

COPD however is much more than a pulmonary system disorder; widespread systemic effects of the disease have been documented in patients with this disease. Systemic proinflammatory cytokines result in cardiovascular effects and generalized muscle wasting secondary to muscle and bone loss (reviewed in Balasubramanian and Varkey, 2006). The weight loss seen in COPD most likely is associated with cachexia secondary to elevated proinflammatory

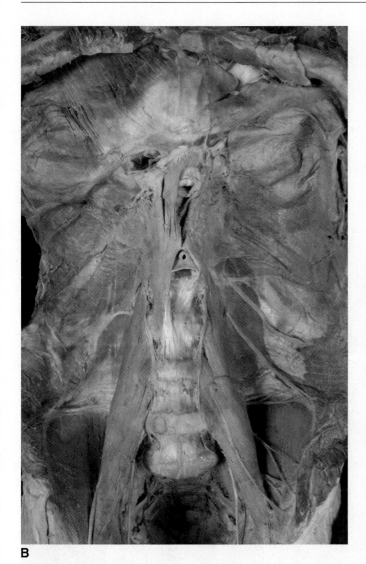

B

Figure 13-13 *(continued)*

large negative intrathoracic pressure against which the diaphragm is pulling in the COPD patient (Laghi and Tobin, 2003).

Biochemical Changes in Respiratory Muscles in COPD

Along with the structural changes seen in the diaphragm of patients with COPD, significant histological and biochemical changes result in adaptations aimed at increasing the efficiency of the muscle.

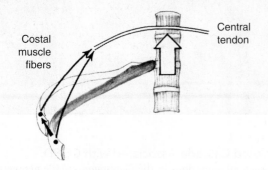

Figure 13-14 The abdominal viscera (*arrow*) act as the fulcrum of the diaphragm allowing it to elevate the ribs. (Taken from De Troyer A and Estenne M. Functional anatomy of the respiratory muscles. *Clin Chest Med N Am* 1988;9:175–193.)

Figure 13-15 The upper illustration is a lateral view of the serratus anterior in a specimen where the scapula has been freed from the body wall but sectioning the latissimus dorsi, trapezius and rhomboid muscles and cutting the clavicle. The scapula was then abducted as far laterally as possible to stretch the serratus to its full length. The lower illustration is an anterior view of a specimen prepared in a similar manner. The scapula has been fully abducted to expose the serratus anterior muscle. (Taken from the Willard/ Carreiro Collection.)

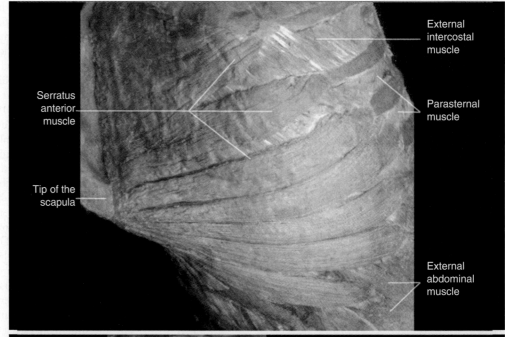

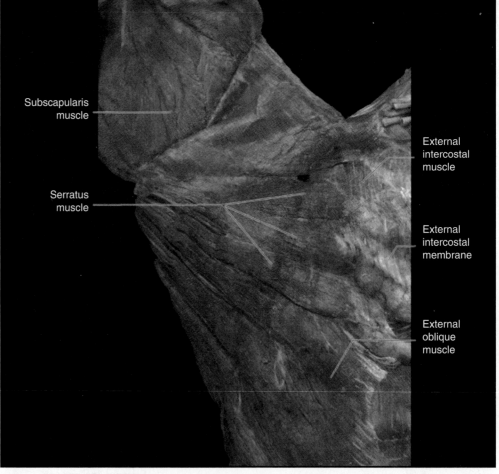

cytokines such as TNF-α in circulation. The weight loss problem is best termed cachexia—selective muscle loss and protein degradation—not malnutrition, which is more generalized (Debigare et al., 2001). In essence, in COPD, the body has entered a negative energy balance state. In addition to the musculoskeletal system, cardiovascular, renal, and nervous system dysfunctions have been documented in COPD (Agusti et al., 2003).

Downward Cascade Associated with COPD

The structural alterations in the diaphragm muscle geometry and fiber type make rapid breathing movements more difficult; thus, a sedentary lifestyle is common with COPD. It is well demonstrated that extremity muscle wasting is also a common feature of COPD associated with both a sedentary lifestyle and the systemic release of rhabdomyolytic proinflammatory cytokines (Gosker

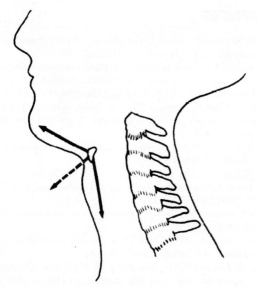

Figure 13-16 This is a schematic view of the muscles supporting the hyoid bone. Simultaneous contraction of these muscle pulls the hyoid anteriorly opening the airway. (Taken from van de Graaff WB, Gottfried SB, Mitra J et al. Respiratory function of hyoid muscles and hyoid arch. *J Appl Physiol* 1984;57(1):197–204.)

et al., 2003). Proinflammatory cytokines also have a stimulatory effect on the activity of osteoclasts, thereby enhancing the loss of bone. Principal areas of bony regression involve the proximal femur and the endplates of the vertebral bodies (reviewed in

Balasubramanian and Varkey, 2006). These changes increase the patient's susceptibility to femoral neck fractures and vertebral body collapse. Chronic hypoxemia, a condition that is ubiquitous in the later stages of COPD, will exacerbate many of the previously noted changes in musculoskeletal system. Diminished protein synthesis secondary to hypoxemia leads to diminished production of myosin in muscle sarcomeres and lower production of oxidative enzymes in mitochondria (reviewed in Balasubramanian and Varkey, 2006).

Thus in COPD, a downward spiral is established; compromised respiratory muscle function leads to reduced motion as well as hypoxia and inflammatory reactions. All of these results culminate in loss of muscle and bone mass with further reduction of motion in the patient. Lack of activity favors the stagnation of proinflammatory substances in the tissue further exacerbating the process. Although movement and exercise cannot restore the damage that has occurred in the lung, it can help arrest the downward spiral and improve the quality of life for the patient. The osteopathic approach to COPD should include consideration of the overall body structure and function in an effort to enhance the patient's ability to increase motion.

Obesity

Structural Changes

Abdominal obesity expands the subcostal margins of the rib cage without necessarily altering the superior margin. With

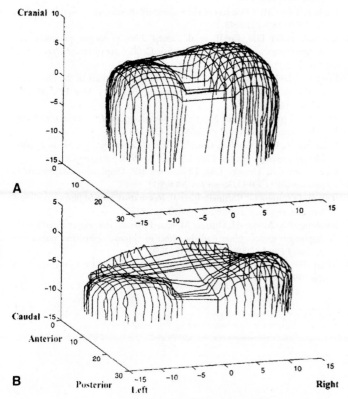

Figure 13-17 This figure illustrates a comparison of the shape of the diaphragm in a normal individual (**A**) and a patient with COPD (**B**). Tracings represent three-dimensional reconstructions derived from a spiral CT imaging study. (Illustration taken from Cassart M, Pettiaux N, Gevenois PA, et al. Effect of chronic hyperinflation on diaphragm length and surface area. *Am J Respir Crit Care Med* 1997;156(2 pt 1):504–508.)

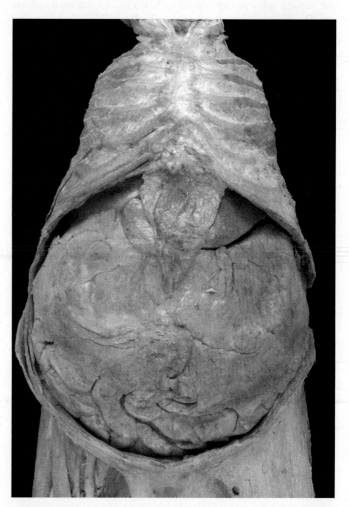

Figure 13-18 The torso of an obese female illustrating the flared, bell-shaped subcostal border. (Taken from the Willard/Carreiro Collection.)

the expanding subcostal margin, the rib cage takes on a more bell-shaped appearance (Fig. 13.18). When this occurs without raising the apex of the diaphragm, the entire muscle becomes more flattened in shape. In essence, the lateral margins are moving outward and upward getting closer to the level of the apex of the diaphragm and thereby reducing the zone of apposition. Attempted deep excursions of the diaphragm result in lower the apex closer to the level of the subcostal margin and can convert the diaphragm into a muscle of exhalation.

Influence on Systemic Disease

In an effort to maintain consistent minute volume of oxygen to the lung in the face of reduce amplitude of rib motion, the frequency has to rise; thus, a high-frequency, low-amplitude panting results. The hypoxia that associates with reduced respiratory muscle capacity, in a manner similar to that described for COPD, may be a partial cause of the systemic inflammatory response seen in morbidly obese patients.

Kyphosis

Structural Changes

Individuals with decreased bone density can suffer either acute or progressive loss of height in the anterior aspect of the vertebral bodies. In such cases, the vertebral column slumps anteriorly creating a kyphotic posture in the thorax with enhanced lordotic curvature of the cervical spine as compensation. The kyphotic curvature allows the ribs to move downward effectively diminishing, and in many cases completely eliminating, the intercostal spaces. Loss of the intercostal muscles prevents the upward and outward movement of the ribs on inhalation, thereby compromising the depth of the respiratory excursion and the efficacy of respiratory movements. Again a downward spiral of health ensues; compromised respiration yields hypoxia and reduced motion. Restricted movements lead to increased bone loss, furthering kyphosis and loss of thoracic motion.

SUMMARY

The anatomy of mandatory and selected accessory muscles of respiration has been reviewed. The structure of these muscles has been related to their specific functions in the respiratory movements. Dysfunction of these muscles occurs in a number of disorders such as COPD, obesity, and kyphosis. The implications of these structural changes on the respiratory movements have been examined and their resulting systemic effect considered. Each disorder leads to a vicious downward spiral involving motion restriction, hypoxia, inflammation, and further motion restriction. The role of the Osteopathic Physician is to help the patient restore homeostasis by facilitation motion in both the thorax and the extremities in an effort to arrest the vicious cycle.

REFERENCES

Agusti AG, Noguera A, Sauleda J, et al. Systemic effects of chronic obstructive pulmonary disease. *Eur Respir J* 2003;21(2):347–360.

Balasubramanian VP, Varkey B. Chronic obstructive pulmonary disease: effects beyond the lungs. *Curr Opin Pulm Med* 2006;12(2):106–112.

Barnes PJ. Small airways in COPD. *N Engl J Med* 2004;350(26):2635–2637.

Cassart M, Pettiaux N, Gevenois PA, et al. Effect of chronic hyperinflation on diaphragm length and surface area. *Am J Respir Crit Care Med* 1997; 156(2 pt 1):504–508.

Celli BR. Pathophysiology of chronic obstructive pulmonary disease. *Chest Surg Clin N Am* 1995;5(4):623–634.

Debigare R, Cote CH, Maltais F. Peripheral muscle wasting in chronic obstructive pulmonary disease. Clinical relevance and mechanisms. *Am J Respir Crit Care Med* 2001;164(9):1712–1717.

De Troyer A, Estenne M. Functional anatomy of the respiratory muscles. *Clin Chest Med N Am* 1988;9:175–193.

De Troyer A, Kirkwood PA, Wilson TA. Respiratory action of the intercostal muscles. *Physiol Rev* 2005;85(2):717–756.

De Troyer A, Legrand A, Gevenois PA, et al. Mechanical advantage of the human parasternal intercostal and triangularis sterni muscles. *J Physiol* 1998;513(pt 3):915–925.

De Troyer A, Ninane V, Gilmartin JJ, et al. Triangularis sterni muscle use in supine humans. *J Appl Physiol* 1987;62(3):919–925.

Epstein SK. An overview of respiratory muscle function. *Clin Chest Med N Am* 1994;15(4):619–639.

Fitting JW. Respiratory muscles in chronic obstructive pulmonary disease. *Swiss Med Wkly* 2001;131(33–34):483–486.

Gosker HR, Kubat B, Schaart G, et al. Myopathological features in skeletal muscle of patients with chronic obstructive pulmonary disease. *Eur Respir J* 2003;22(2):280–285.

Hwang JC, John WM, Bartlett D Jr. Afferent pathways for hypoglossal and phrenic responses to changes in upper airway pressure. *Respir Physiol* 1984;55(3):341–354.

Laghi F, Tobin MJ. Disorders of the respiratory muscles. *Am J Respir Crit Care Med* 2003;168(1):10–48.

Lee KZ, Fuller DD, Lu IJ, et al. Neural drive to tongue protrudor and retractor muscles following pulmonary C-fiber activation. *J Appl Physiol* 2007;102(1):434–444.

Levine S, Kaiser L, Leferovich J, et al. Cellular adaptations in the diaphragm in chronic obstructive pulmonary disease. *N Engl J Med* 1997;337(25): 1799–1806.

Mier A, Brophy C, Estenne M, et al. Action of abdominal muscles on rib cage in humans. *J Appl Physiol* 1985;58(5):1438–1443.

O'Rahilly R. 1986. *Gardner, Gray & O'Rahilly Anatomy: A Regional Study of Human Structure.* 5th Ed. Philadelphia, PA: W.B. Saunders Comp.

Ottenheijm CA, Heunks LM, Dekhuijzen RP. Diaphragm adaptations in patients with COPD. *Respir Res* 2008;9:12.

Polla B, D'Antona G, Bottinelli R, et al. Respiratory muscle fibres: specialisation and plasticity. *Thorax* 2004;59(9):808–817.

Stubbings AK, Moore AJ, Dusmet M, et al. Physiological properties of human diaphragm muscle fibres and the effect of chronic obstructive pulmonary disease. *J Physiol* 2008;586(10):2637–2650.

Thach BT. Neuromuscular control of upper airway patency. *Clin Perinatol N Am* 1992;19:773–788.

14 | Touch

FRANK H. WILLARD, JOHN A. JEROME, AND MITCHELL L. ELKISS

KEY CONCEPTS

- Our brain derives much of its perception of the world around us through the activity of our receptors in the skin and particularly from the skin over our hands.
- The communication developed through the touch of the physician in the physical and structural exam is the first step in helping the patient retrace his or her steps back to a healthy state of body and mind.
- Touch is a perception that is emergent from neural activity in a complex network that includes the somatic sensory cortex as well as numerous other regions of the cerebrum.

INTRODUCTION

Touch as a Primary Sensation

The sense of touch plays an important role in our awareness of the world around us. From the moment we awake in the morning, our hands contact the surrounding objects and communicate to us where we are and what we are doing. Throughout the day, touch provides a focal point for orientation and communication between us and the environment as well as between us and others in our lives. Our brain derives much of its perception of the world around us through the activity of our receptors in the skin and particularly from the skin over our hands. We make contact and explore surrounding objects and individuals using the somesthetic sense generated by touch with our hands. Texture, shape, weight, and size as well as friend, foe, harmless, or dangerous can all be determined, in part, through palpation. Our response to touch is filtered by the highly individualistic and personal emotional axes of our brain. Thus, whether the touch evokes kindness and trust or hatred and anger all depends on the context of the environment in which the touch occurs and the background of our daily lives. Finally, touch is a dynamic process, adapting to use or disuse, differing between sexes, changing with age and varying with culture.

Touch as a Primary Mechanism for Communicating with Patients

Touch can be a primary diagnostic tool. The physician touches the patient; the patient, in many ways, touches the physician. The dynamics of this contact between individuals are essential to the establishment of a trusting, respectful relationship (Fig. 14.1). The communication developed through the touch of the physician in the physical and structural exam is the first step in helping the patient retrace his or her steps back to a healthy state of body and mind. What begins as a palpatory examination quickly becomes a tactile conversation. The physician gains greater proprioceptive awareness of the structural impediments underlying physical as well as emotional and behavioral dysfunctions.

Significance of Touch to an Osteopathic Physician

Students begin to develop discriminative palpatory skills by touching other students, gradually transferring these abilities to the examination of patients. Through repeated practice, palpation progresses into deeper layers of the body—skin, fascia, muscle, bone, joint, and finally viscera—slowly unmasking the health of the tissue to the examiner. Palpation of tissue may tell the skilled physician much more about the state of the patient's health than the patient can put into words. Putting the patient at ease while the physician is diagnostically touching him or her includes an explanation of intention and nature of the touching, its purpose, and what the patient is likely to experience. This dialogue enhances confidence and trust. Skillful touching and communication forges a deep verbal and tactile relationship between the physician and the patient. Gradually, the skilled osteopathic physician develops tactile memories of tissue dysfunctions both within a patient and across multiple patients. With time, palpatory skills may be used to monitor the patient's progress in his or her return to a healthy state. Even with chronic illness where healing and cure are unlikely, there is a reestablished human connection based upon compassionate touch and careful attention to the dialogue. This is the osteopathic path to restored function and self-healing. This chapter explores the biophysical mechanisms involved when the contact between the skin of the examining physician and the skin of the patient is converted into touch in the minds of both individuals.

TOUCH: ANATOMY AND PHYSIOLOGY

Overview

We do not see with our eyes alone, we do not hear with our ears alone, nor do we touch with our hands alone; instead seeing, hearing, and touch are accomplished when our brain interacts with the information provided by receptor epithelia located in our eyes, ears, and hands. Thus, it is to this neural-based process that we must turn to understand our perception of touch. Touch is a perception that is emergent from neural activity in a complex network that includes the somatic sensory system as well as portions of many cortical regions in the cerebrum. This activity begins with the formation of a stimulus code in the peripheral process of primary afferent neurons distributed in the dermis and epidermis throughout the extremities, body, and head. The characteristic features encoded by these sensory neurons are stimulus quality, intensity, duration, and location on the surface of the body. The primary neurons bring this stimulus code to the dorsal aspect of the spinal cord. While some of this information is delivered to the dorsal horn of the spinal cord, a significant amount ascends the cord to reach the dorsal column nuclei in the caudal medulla. From these nuclei,

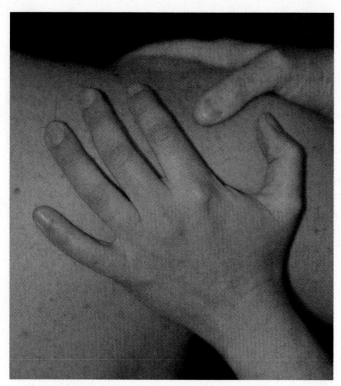

Figure 14-1 Touch in osteopathic medicine.

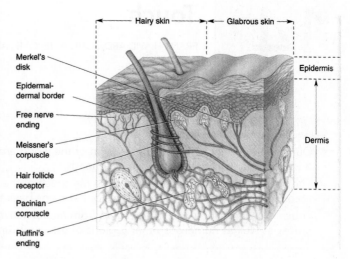

Figure 14-2 The sensory endings typically involved in tactile sensation. (Taken from Bear M, Connors BW, Paradiso MA. *Neuroscience: Exploring the Brain*. Philadelphia, PA: Lippincott, Williams & Wilkins, 2001, Figure 12-1.)

projections ascend through the brainstem to the posterior and ventral thalamus and are relayed on to the postcentral gyrus of the parietal cortex.

The entrance of primary axons into the spinal cord is done in an orderly fashion; thus, their addition to the spinal tracts creates a topographic map of the body—termed a somatotopic map. In essence, these maps, composed of nuclei and fiber tracts, contain information based on the segmentation pattern of the body. This orderly arrangement is preserved in the medulla, thalamus, and postcentral gyrus of the cerebrum. From the postcentral gyrus, the sensorineural code is mapped to several somatic sensory regions in the parietal cortex; these codes are modified and distributed across a large network of neural connection involving parietal, insular, occipital, temporal, and frontal lobes of the cerebral cortex. It is in this cortical network that the somesthetic input becomes integrated with that from our other senses, such as eyes and ears. Our perceptions of touch represent abstractions derived through extraction from the activity of these complex neural networks on the surface of our cerebrum. These perceptions are also colored by interaction with the pervasive emotional systems also present in the human forebrain.

CENTRAL PROCESSING: FROM PHYSICAL STIMULUS TO NEURAL CODE

The Primary Afferent Neurons Have Peripheral Processes in the Skin Deep Tissue and Central Processes in the Spinal Cord

Most of our sensation of touch arises from mechanical energy generated as an object makes contact with our skin. In the dermis underlying the epidermis, there are at least two major groups of primary afferent nerve endings: free endings that can give us a sensation of general contact with an object and encapsulated endings that purvey discriminative and localizable touch (Fig. 14.2). Free nerve endings are typically associated with unmyelinated or lightly myelinated axons and are discussed in Chapter 15. The peripheral processes of the encapsulated endings are illustrated in Figure 14.2; they include Merkel discs, Meissner corpuscles, pacinian corpuscles, and Ruffini endings typically found in glabrous skin. However, additional specialized receptors are found innervating the bases of follicles in hairy skin. Typically, the encapsulated endings are associated with well-myelinated (Group II) axons. The cell bodies for these fibers are invariably found in the dorsal root ganglia or the trigeminal ganglion. Central processes of these neurons course through the dorsal root to enter the spinal cord through the dorsal root entry zone (Fig. 14.3).

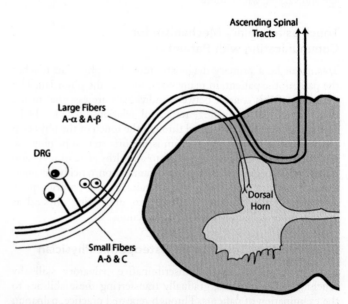

Figure 14-3 The dorsal root entry zone. The fibers of the dorsal root segregate prior to entering the dorsal horn of the spinal cord.

The Primary Afferent Neurons Detect Physical (Mechanical) Stimuli in the Peripheral Tissue, Develop a Sensorineural Code Based on the Stimulus, and Conduct This Information to the Spinal Cord and Brainstem

Primary afferent fibers detect various aspects of mechanical energy in the skin and encode this information into a series of discharge patterns that are conducted to the spinal cord (1). Four general patterns of activity have been cataloged based on the response properties and general position of each sensory neuron in the dermis. Two types of receptors have rapidly adapting endings and quickly change discharge patterns to a static stimulus; these are the Meissner and pacinian corpuscles, both with onion skin–like encapsulations. These rapidly adapting receptors are much better at recording a dynamic or moving stimulus than a static stimulus. The other two receptors, Merkel discs and Ruffini endings, demonstrate slowly adapting discharge patterns, much better designed to detect a static stimulus. Of these four types of receptors, the Meissner corpuscles and Merkel discs are located superficially at the epidermal-dermal junction, while the pacinian corpuscle and Ruffini ending are located in the deeper portion of the dermis. Each of these receptors is capable of encoding a specific characteristic of the physical stimulus presented to the skin; thus, for any given object touching the skin in any specific manner, a unique sensorineural code will be generated. This sensorineural code is conducted into the spinal cord by the central processes of the primary neurons.

The Position of the Sensory Axon in the Dorsal Root Entry Zone Is Related to Its Function

The dorsal root enters the spinal cord through the dorsal root entry zone; this zone is segregated based on fiber size. The small fibers move laterally in the root and enter directly into the dorsal horn. These fibers encode nociceptive stimuli and activate appropriate reflexes (see Chapter 15). Conversely, the large myelinated fibers shift medially, passing over the dorsal horn and gaining entrance to the more medially located dorsal columns of the spinal cord. As fibers add to the dorsal columns, they do so in an orderly manner, thus preserving the topography of the body. The dorsal columns ascend the full length of the spinal cord to reach the inferior aspect of the dorsal column nuclei located at the cervicomedullary junction.

Central Processing of Fine Tactile Information Begins in the Dorsal Column Nuclei

Neurons in the dorsal column nuclei receive the large myelinated, Group II afferent fibers in an orderly, somatotopic fashion. Within the dorsal column nuclei, each ascending axon synapses on a limited number of neurons, thereby maintaining the high fidelity of the information. These synapses are large and secure to ensure transmission of the information to the target neurons. In addition, the neurons of the dorsal column nuclei also receive the synaptic endings of corticonuclear fibers arising in the parietal cortex; thus, central processing of the sensorineural code really begins at this point.

The Chief Sensory Nucleus of the Trigeminal System Is Analogous to the Dorsal Column Nuclei

Primary afferent neurons innervating touch corpuscles in the face have their cell bodies in the trigeminal ganglion. Central projections from these ganglionic neurons reach the chief sensory nucleus in the trigeminal complex, which is located in the pontine portion of the brainstem (Fig. 14.3). The chief sensory nucleus is similar in function to the dorsal column nuclei; thus, the chief nucleus represents the first relay for discriminative information from the face. Projections from the chief sensory nucleus cross the midline and ascend to the contralateral thalamus.

The Posterior Thalamus Receives the Ascending Sensory Tracts from the Dorsal Column Nuclei and Trigeminal System

Axons from the dorsal column nuclei cross the midline and ascend to the posterior thalamus in a large, well-organized fiber tract termed the medial lemniscus. Above the pons, the medial lemniscus is joined in its course by the ascending trigeminal fibers from the chief sensory nucleus of the trigeminal system. These combined sensory pathways enter the posterior aspect of the thalamus to terminate in the ventroposterior nucleus (Fig. 14.3). Laterally, the ventroposterior thalamic nucleus (VPL) receives axons from the medial lemniscus in an orderly fashion, thus preserving the topographic map of the body (feet laterally positioned and arms more medially located). Medially, the ventroposterior thalamic nucleus (VPM) receives ascending axons from the chief sensory nucleus, representing discriminative sensory information from the face. Thus, the thalamus is the first region in the ascending sensory systems where the body and the face are represented in somatotopic register with each other.

The Thalamocortical Circuitry Functions as a Unit in the Processing of Sensory Information

Neurons in the ventroposterior thalamic nuclei project axons in an orderly fashion onto the postcentral gyrus of the parietal cortex—the primary region of the somatic sensory system. Precisely mapped reciprocal connections from primary somatic sensory cortex to ventroposterior thalamus mean that the thalamocortical circuitry acts as an interlocked functioning unit. The reciprocal connections between the thalamus and the overlying cortex establish a strong oscillating rhythm through which information is transferred to the cerebral cortex.

The Neocortex Is Partitioned into Functional Regions Based on Its Distinct Cytoarchitecture and Connectivity

Human cerebral neocortex is partitioned in several domains principally associated with motor or sensory functions; these domains are surrounded by significantly larger cortical regions, termed association cortex, which are given over to the integration of cortical information between multiple sensory and motor areas (Fig. 14.4). The primary somatic sensory cortex is located along the postcentral gyrus and is directly posterior to the somatic motor cortex located on the precentral gyrus (Figs. 14.5 and 14.6). Although these cortical areas were originally defined by their distinct cytoarchitecture, they have been confirmed and elaborated based on their connections and functions. Three distinct regions are present in the primary somatic sensory cortex—areas 3, 1, and 2—with area 3 further subdivided into 3a and 3b (Fig. 14.6). Although each of these areas is organized into a somatotopic map of the body including the hand, neurons in each of these areas receive a different type of input from the periphery. This map is arranged by body segments proceeding from the trigeminal nerve through the cervical segments located laterally on the convexity of the cortex and eventually extending medially to the sacral segments located on the medial aspect of the

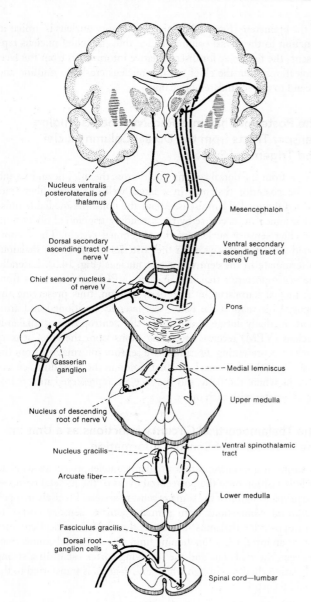

Nucleus ventralis posterolateralis of thalamus

Mesencephalon

Dorsal secondary ascending tract of nerve V

Ventral secondary ascending tract of nerve V

Chief sensory nucleus of nerve V

Pons

Gasserian ganglion

Medial lemniscus

Nucleus of descending root of nerve V

Upper medulla

Nucleus gracilis

Ventral spinothalamic tract

Arcuate fiber

Lower medulla

Fasciculus gracilis

Dorsal root ganglion cells

Spinal cord—lumbar

Figure 14-4 The spinal cord and brainstem pathways involved in tactile sensation. (From Campbell WW. *DeJong's The Neurologic Examination*. Philadelphia, PA: Lippincott Williams & Wilkins, 2005, Figure 32.4.)

cortex just above the corpus callosum. There is a disproportional representation of hands and mouth, which is reflective of increased density of sensory receptors; this disproportionate representation translates into increased sensitivity and sensory discrimination for the hand and oral regions of the body (Fig. 14.7).

Primary Somatic Sensory Cortex Receives High-Fidelity Sensory Information

Each region receives input from differing sources: Group I muscle afferent input coming from muscle spindles and Golgi tendon organs targets area 3a; area 3b receives input from Group II slowly adapting cutaneous receptors, while area 1 receives input from rapidly adapting receptors, although this differentiation is not complete. Finally, area 2 neurons are very complex; they receive input from joint receptors, periosteum, and deep fascias but respond more to movement than to individual stimuli (2). Unlike areas 3a, 3b, and 1

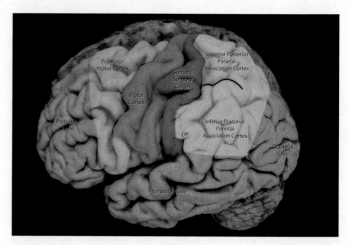

Figure 14-5 The location of the somatic sensory cortex on the convexity of the cerebral hemisphere. The primary somatic sensory cortex (areas 3, 1, and 2) is illustrated in blue; posterior to the primary somatic sensory area lies the large posterior parietal association cortex. It is divided into superior and inferior regions by the intraparietal sulcus (*black line*). (Used with permission from the Willard/Carreiro Collection, University of New England.)

where digit representation is relatively discrete, digit representation is overlapping in area 2, thus creating a more complex pattern of neural activity (3). Considering the areas posterior to the primary somatic sensory cortex, it is found that precise topography is lacking

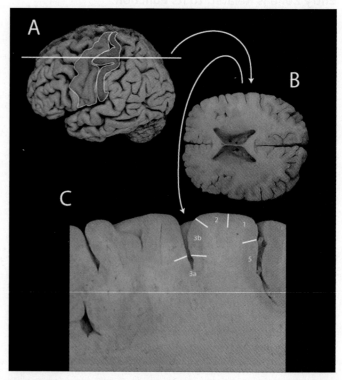

Figure 14-6 Primary somatic sensory cortex. **A.** A lateral view of the brain that demonstrates the primary somatic sensory cortex in blue and the primary motor cortex in red. The white line illustrates the plane of section for the cut demonstrated in **(B)**. **C.** Magnification of the postcentral gyrus illustrating the approximate locations of areas 3a, 3b, 1, and 2. (Used with permission from the Willard/Carreiro collection, University of New England.)

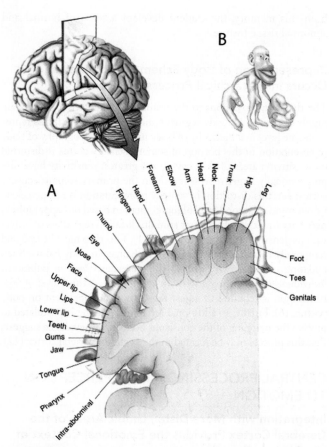

Figure 14-7 The somatotopic organization of the primary somatic sensory cortex. The upper left corner presents a lateral view of the brain with the primary somatic sensory cortex illustrated in green. **A.** A section parallel to the postcentral gyrus demonstrating the approximate location of the body map. **B.** A figurine demonstrating the distortion in the sensory map; areas of the body such as the hands and the mouth with increased density of sensory receptors received a disproportionally large representation in the cortical sensory map. (From Bear M, Connors BW, Paradiso MA. *Neuroscience: Exploring the Brain.* Philadelphia, PA: Lippincott, Williams & Wilkins, 2001.)

and neuronal response properties are very complex; this is in keeping with regions involved in higher cortical functions (3).

Representation of Body Schema on the Primary Somatic Sensory Cortical Surface Is Plastic and Can Be Influenced by the Environment

Often, the impression given by textbook descriptions of sensory maps is that these systems are relatively hardwired from birth; nothing could be further from the truth. Cortical mapping is very dynamic and can expand in response to exercise and contract in response to nonuse (4; reviewed in Refs. 5,6). Witness the expansion of the cortical maps for the digits seen in musicians such as a violinist; a similar expansion undoubtedly occurs in the cortex of a physician when training his or her hands in palpation. A similar expansion was seen in the digital representation of experimental subjects with sight who were taught to read Braille. Conversely, anesthesia, immobilization, or removal of a digit results in a rapid loss of the cortical area representing the missing digit, and the newly available territory is claimed by surrounding digit

representations. Such reallocation of territory occurs on a larger scale when an entire extremity is lost. Abuse of the somatic sensory system can also alter the cortical somatotopic maps. Studies that created chronic repetitive strain injury in primates have demonstrated a loss in precision of the somatic sensory cortical maps, suggesting that proper rehabilitation following such injury may involve reforming and refining these cerebral projection maps (7). These studies suggest that learning any type of manual skill will alter the cortical surface map; thus, as students hone their palpatory skills, their cortical somatic sensory map is most likely responding by allocating increased area for the representation of digits.

CENTRAL PROCESSING: FROM NEURAL CODE TO PERCEPTION

Primary Somatic Sensory Cortex Is Involved in a High-Speed Feedback Pathway for Primary Motor Cortex

The dorsal column–medial lemniscus pathway is a high-speed pathway carrying touch and proprioceptive sensory information to the primary somatic sensory cortex. Intracortical connections map these data onto the primary motor cortex where it can act as a feedback system regulating discrete movements of the hands and feet. Motor cortex can control the actions of individual muscles in the distal extremities through the corticospinal tracts and their connections in the ventral horn of the spinal cord. Using this system, we can regulate the force we apply during palpation of an object (1). The osteopathic physician utilizes this feedback system as he or she learns to adjust the depth of palpation accomplished by his or her fingers.

Integration with Surrounding Areas of Association Cortex Provides the Complexity of the Sensory Experience

The primary somatic sensory cortex has our tactile world mapped in a high-fidelity Cartesian system of intersecting body segments and receptor types as previously described. Yet, we know that we do not feel specific receptor types or specific segmental boundaries; instead, we feel objects, textures, and shades of firmness, often colored by emotions; clearly, this is not happening solely on primary somatic sensory cortex. Rather, data from the Cartesian map on primary somatic sensory cortex are projected outward to surrounding cortical regions termed association cortex; typically, these are located in the posterior parietal cortex, the parietal operculum, and the inferior temporal cortex. The association areas establish complex interconnections with numerous surrounding cortical regions as well as the primary somatic sensory areas. In addition, portions of these association areas also map to other major sensory systems such as the visual system and auditory system; thus, neurons in these areas are often polysensory in nature. What emerges is a complex neuronal network involving high-fidelity data representation in the primary cortex and numerous network activity nodes spread across the posterior association cortex of the brain. The sustainability of activity in these nodes depends on the power contained in the thalamocortical circuitry; each region of the node is mapped to a unique region in the thalamus. Repeated thalamocortical oscillations augment the intracortical connections and contribute to network sustainability. In addition to repetitive thalamic input, dense connections from the prefrontal cortex serve to augment and reenforce the activity on this network. It is currently believed that from the summated activity of this complex neuronal interaction emerge our sensations of feeling, sight, and audition.

Two Major Processing Streams Through the Cerebral Cortex Help Integrate Somatic Sensory Input with Other Sensory Systems to Render Our Complex Feelings of Touch

The dorsal visuospatial stream, or "where pathway," involves occipital cortex projections to the superior posterior parietal lobule (Fig. 14.8). This stream processes information involved with attention to the stimulus as well as location of the stimulus. Activity in this information stream helps in fitting the stimulus into a three-dimensional map of extrapersonal space. The ventral visuospatial stream or "what pathway" involves occipital cortex projections to the inferior temporal lobe. This stream provides information useful in recognizing, cataloging, and naming a stimulus. The somatic sensory parietal cortex has a dorsally directed projection that appears to participate in the "where pathway" and ventrally directed projections that contribute to the "what pathway" (8). This cortical organization affords us the ability to integrate visual and somesthetic senses into coherent images.

CENTRAL PROCESSING: FROM PERCEPTION TO COGNITION

The Prefrontal Cortex Is Involved in Reenforcing the Network Established in the Posterior Association Cortex Contributing to the Formation of Tactile Memories

Dorsolateral prefrontal cortex is strongly interconnected with the posterior parietal cortex and the inferior temporal cortex. These prefrontal cortex connections function to integrate information between the dorsal and the ventral information streams in the posterior association cortex (9). Through this integration of multiple distributed cortical networks, prefrontal cortex helps to create tactile memories. Thus, the prefrontal cortex uses the same information streams in parietal and temporal cortical areas that initially process tactile information to create our working memory of the experience (10). Tactile memory is used to compare tissue feelings;

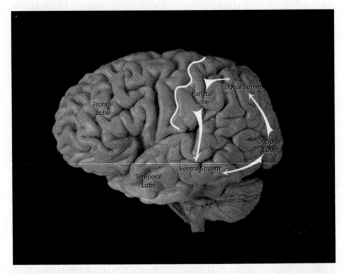

Figure 14-8 The information processing streams in the posterior association cortex. A dorsal stream arises from the visual and somatic sensory cortex termed the "where pathway." A ventral stream arises from the visual and somatic sensory cortex and is termed the "what pathway." (Used with permission from the Willard/Carreiro Collection, University of New England.)

from this memory, the student develops a sense of normal and abnormal tissue texture.

Representation of Body Schema Is Complex and Occurs in Hierarchical Process of Layers

The thalamic projections to the primary somatic sensory cortex are highly organized by body segment and by receptor type; this represents one level in a hierarchy of body maps. The topography of body representation in this portion of somatic sensory cortex is distorted by sensitivity; areas of skin having the greatest sensitivity have disproportionally larger representation in the primary somatic sensory cortex; yet, this distortion in sensory representation is not perceived by our mind. A second level of representation based on topography is necessary to accurately register stimulus location regardless of innervations density and tissue sensitivity (11). This map must be updated temporally to account for age-related changes in body habits. Such updating occurs slowly; witness the clumsiness seen in pubescent individuals experiencing a "growth spurt" (12). A third level of representation is required to adjust the body map dependent on body posture (6). Finally, an additional level of processing is postulated to involve the mapping of the conscious body image; evidence suggests that this process may be located in the posterior parietal cortex (12).

CENTRAL PROCESSING: FROM PERCEPTION TO EMOTION

Integration with More Distal, Limbic Areas of the Cerebral Cortex Provides the Emotional Context of the Sensory Experience

The somatic sensory pathways discussed so far in this chapter all involve input from well-myelinated systems with elaborate encapsulated sensory endings. An additional nonmyelinated sensory arising from fibers with naked nerve endings also provides input through the thalamus to the cerebral cortex. This latter system targets a portion of the insular cortex in a region that represents an extension of the somatic sensory cortex around the operculum into the lateral fissure. This small fiber input system is postulated to play a significant role in modulating our body's response to touch through its influence on the autonomic nervous system. This input also appears to influence our emotional state through its projections to the orbital prefrontal cortex and the anterior cingulate gyrus (13). These regions of the brain are associated with what many researchers have termed the limbic system—a loosely defined system that is believed to strongly regulate to our emotions (14). Activity in the orbital prefrontal cortex affects a strong reinforcement system, augmenting our positive or negative impressions of the particular tactile stimuli (15,16). Thus, tactile stimuli, using high-speed myelinated pathways, gain access to a discriminative and cognitive cortical system, allowing analytical evaluation of touch such as one might use in physical diagnosis; however, there is an additional component of the tactile information, which employs slower, less well myelinated systems that percolate through a strong cerebral emotional filter in and that play a large role in our final impression of touch (17).

This emotional aspect of touch gathers all of our past experiences—good or bad—to color our feelings and influence our decisions. To touch another is to be touched back, in essence tactility is bidirectional, intimate and reciprocal. The physician's and patient's boundaries are united with the intent to heal. The intangible emotions of physicians as they touch patients, encompassing all of their past experiences, may thus play a large role in the diagnosis that they pronounce and the treatment that they endorse.

REFERENCES

1. Kandel ER, Schwartz JH, Jessell TM. *Principles of Neural Sciences.* 4th Ed. New York, NY: Elsevier, 2000.
2. Iwamura Y, Tanaka M, Hikosaka O. Overlapping representation of fingers in the somatosensory cortex (area 2) of the conscious monkey. *Brain Res* 1980;197(2):516–520.
3. Young JP, Herath P, Eickhoff S, et al. Somatotopy and attentional modulation of the human parietal and opercular regions. *J Neurosci* 2004;24(23): 5391–5399.
4. Buonomano DV, Merzenich MM. Cortical plasticity: from synapses to maps. *Annu Rev Neurosci* 1998;21:149–186.
5. Tommerdahl M, Favorov OV, Whitsel BL. Dynamic representations of the somatosensory cortex. *Neurosci Biobehav Rev* 2010;34(2):160–170.
6. Medina J, Coslett HB. From maps to form to space: touch and the body schema. *Neuropsychologia* 2010;48(3):645–654.
7. Byl NN, Merzenich MM, Jenkins WM. A primate genesis model of focal dystonia and repetitive strain injury: I. Learning-induced dedifferentiation of the representation of the hand in the primary somatosensory cortex in adult monkeys. *Neurology* 1996;47(2):508–520.
8. Prather SC, Votaw JR, Sathian K. Task-specific recruitment of dorsal and ventral visual areas during tactile perception. *Neuropsychologia.* 2004; 42(8):1079–1087.
9. Rao SC, Rainer G, Miller EK. Integration of what and where in the primate prefrontal cortex. *Science* 1997;276(5313):821–824.
10. Gallace A, Spence C. The cognitive and neural correlates of tactile memory. *Psychol Bull* 2009;135(3):380–406.
11. Serino A, Haggard P. Touch and the body. *Neurosci Biobehav Rev* 2010;34(2):224–236.
12. Longo MR, Azanon E, Haggard P. More than skin deep: body representation beyond primary somatosensory cortex. *Neuropsychologia* 2010;48(3):655–668.
13. Olausson H, Lamarre Y, Backlund H, et al. Unmyelinated tactile afferents signal touch and project to insular cortex. *Nat Neurosci* 2002;5(9):900–904.
14. Morgane PJ, Mokler DJ. The limbic brain: continuing resolution. *Neurosci Biobehav Rev* 2006;30(2):119–125.
15. Rolls ET. The functions of the orbitofrontal cortex. *Brain Cogn* 2004; 55(1):11–29.
16. Rolls ET. *Emotion Explained.* Oxford: Oxford University Press, 2005.
17. Damasio AR. *Descartes' Error.* London: PaperMac, 1996.

Nociception and Pain: The Essence of Pain Lies Mainly in the Brain

FRANK H. WILLARD, JOHN A. JEROME, AND MITCHELL L. ELKISS

KEY CONCEPTS

- Tissue injury activates small primary afferent fibers in a process termed nociception.
- Nociceptive information from these afferent fibers passes through the dorsal horn of the spinal cord to reach the brainstem and thalamus.
- In the brainstem reflexes are initiated that can modify the individual's homeostatic mechanisms in a protective manner.
- From the thalamus, numerous cortical areas are engaged, creating a matrix of activity in the cerebrum contributing to the emergence of our feelings of pain.
- Based on this feeling of pain, protective physiological and psychological reflexes are initiated by the individual.
- Acute injury typically results in acute pain, a process which should resolve as the tissues heal.
- However, each level in the system is capable of sensitizing to the nociceptive activity and thereby enhancing our response both physiologically and psychologically to the noxious event.
- Excessive modification in the neural circuitry involved in processing nociception can lead to activity that out lasts the inciting event, thus entering the realm of chronic pain.
- In chronic pain patterns, protective physiological and psychological reflexes now become pathological, such dysfunction will affect the individual overall health and well being.
- Continued obsession with the pain further facilitates the involved forebrain circuitry creating a progressively worsening downward dysfunctional cycle carrying the individual into despair and depression.
- It is the role of the osteopathic physician to identify the physical (somatic and visceral) as well as behavioral factors contributing to these chronic dysfunctional patterns. It is the philosophy and practice of the osteopathic physician to assist the patient in seeking ameliorative and restorative strategies in the quest to regain health.

INTRODUCTION: THE NOCICEPTIVE SYSTEM AND PAIN

Every organism requires some form of protective system to detect and avoid potential external and internal environmental threats and to craft the behavioral expression of defensive behaviors. An ideal protective system would activate just before tissue damage is done and cease activation when the threat has remitted. In addition to protective reflexes, such a system should also trigger a strong learning experience that sensitizes the organism to future situations and helps foster avoidance behavior. Humans are endowed with just such a system; it is composed of small slowly conducting peripheral nerve fibers that can trigger rapid defensive responses at both spinal cord and brainstem levels as well as slower longer-lasting defensive changes involving neural, endocrine, and immune adaptations orchestrated from complex forebrain circuits. Accompanying these physiological and behavioral adaptations, there can also be a hard-to-define feeling of unpleasantness often simply termed "pain." The activity generated by a dangerous or potentially dangerous stimulus is not pain, it is best termed nociception, a mechanical and neurochemical process that is similar in physiology and intensity regardless of the individual concerned; pain is however the perception placed on this activity by the brain; pain is the learning experience. Thus pain arises, not from the small, primary afferent fibers in the periphery detecting a stimulus, but from the response of complex interacting systems contained in the forebrain, reacting to the barrage of nociceptive peripheral input. Along with the response to noxious stimulus, the "feeling of pain" also involves the integration of many previous situations as well as being set in the context of current emotional status of the individual; for this reason, painful

feelings may vary tremendously in intensity and quality from individual to individual as well as within an individual over time.

In this chapter, we will examine the small-fiber systems in the periphery that respond to potentially damaging stimuli and their initial short-loop reactions in the gray matter of the spinal cord. Next, a treatment of longer loop reflexes generated in the brainstem and forebrain will be developed. This will be followed by considering the integration of nociceptive input into the other defensive systems such as the endocrine response and the immune response to make an elaborate supersystem sculpting the organisms overall physiological and behavioral adaptations. Emphasis will be placed on the role of integrating the emotional circuitry of the brain into the defensive response in an effort to understand normal individual adaptations as well as the pathological responses associate with chronic pain scenarios. As with any physiological system, the central processes can regulate the peripheral systems; therefore, we will explore the descending neuronal and endocrine systems that influence the operation of the input systems both at the peripheral level and in the spinal cord and brainstem.

Finally, as with any complex system, failures can and do occur frequently. Complete loss of the small-fiber system, which can occur in certain familiar disorders, has catastrophic consequences for the individual concerned. Lack of a warning system allows self-mutilation to occur and the eventual demise of the musculoskeletal system (reviewed in Nagasako et al., 2003). From the study of such patients, it is clear that the normal activity of a nociceptive system is necessary for the maintenance of health in the individual. However, other seeds for destruction are contained in the very nature of the power in the system. The nociceptive system is a feed-forward system, explosive in activity and designed to mount a quick, effective, and powerful protective response. The mechanisms underlying this powerful response require strong inhibition if they are to be adequately controlled; loss of these controls leads to excessive responses, very similar to the development of seizures disorders expressed in the cerebral cortex. This excessive activity in the nociceptive pathways or in the target regions of the forebrain can generate the feelings of pain when no peripheral generator exists. Facilitation of this activity can lead to physical neuronal damage with a resulting deepening and hardening of the aberrant synaptic patterns such that eventually an indelible chronic pain circuit becomes ingrained in the patient. This chapter will discuss some of the mechanisms involved in establishing these chronic pain patterns and their effect on the general health of the individual.

DISTINCTION BETWEEN PAIN AND NOCICEPTION

When we injure ourselves, we activate small primary afferent fibers in that carry action potentials to the spinal cord capable of initiating protective reflexes. This is a mechanical and electrochemical process termed nociception, the activation of sensory fibers by noxious stimuli. However, this event allow does not necessarily result in a sensation of pain. The spinal cord can become facilitated and relay these nociceptive signals to the brainstem where other reflexes concerning the autonomic nervous system and endocrine system may be then be initiated; however, these events still do not necessarily result in a sensation of pain. In fact, all of these events can occur without conscious awareness of the situation. Projections from the spinal cord and trigeminal brainstem nuclei also reach the thalamus and activate thalamocortical circuitry generating a network of activity on the cerebral cortex. Regions of the cortex involved in localization, the autonomic nervous system, emotions and affectation are involved creating a large matrix of activity from which pain is an emergent feeling (Chapman, 2005). Thus the feeling of pain, which is defined as an unpleasant sensation, does not arise from any one region in the cerebrum but instead from a network which itself is colored by our past physical and emotional experiences.

Since nociception and pain are separate but related entities, they can be disassociated from each other. People can experience physical trauma and not feel pain and, conversely, patients can experience much pain but lack any physical evidence of ongoing nociception in peripheral tissue. Many of the patients that you will experience fall into this latter category. This chapter will focus on the mechanisms of nociception first and then consider the experience of pain and its impact on the patient's health.

DISTINCTION BETWEEN ACUTE AND CHRONIC PAIN

Fundamentally, pain can be divided into two major categories: that which is good for you (protective), termed eudynia, and that which is not (maladaptive), termed maldynia. Good pain is commonly designated as acute pain. It is an expected symptom of tissue damage; it is protective in nature and lessens in intensity as the tissue returns to normal. Chronically recurring or unremitting pain is not a normal experience; it is a pathology and as such is an indicator that something has gone seriously wrong with the nociceptive system. Either tissue is very abnormal in its composition (chronic inflammation) and thus a constant nociceptive signal is being generated, or the neural pathways of the spinal nociceptive system and the cerebral cortex have become facilitated and as such have suffered a significant change in organization and are malfunctioning. A combination of both peripheral tissue and central system dysregulation is also possible. Ultimately, this abnormal activity can result in the system overresponding

to noxious stimuli (hyperalgesia) or even nonnoxious stimuli (allodynia) or, in some cases, simply generating spontaneous activity that the brain then interprets as continuous pain. Chronic pain, that is pain which is persisting past a reasonable, acute period of time (2 to 4 months), is often associated with a wide array of biopsychosocial reactions (Gatchel et al., 1996) and is now a pathological state.

Both acute and chronic pain involve facilitation in the spinal dorsal horn or trigeminal system. Spinal facilitation is reasonably well understood and the mechanisms by which this initially protective state converts into a pathology are slowly becoming understood. This transition from acute to chronic pain states represents a breeching the body's inherent capacity to heal its self and has to be understood as such in order to achieve effective treatments in the clinic. A significant manifestation of chronic pain can be the presentation of altered function in the musculoskeletal and visceral systems of the body. Recognizing the signs and symptoms of spinal cord or trigeminal nuclear facilitation and its manifestation as chronic pain becomes critical to the differential diagnosis of its myriad of etiologies. A major feature of this chapter will be consideration of the conversion from an acute pain scenario to that of a chronic pain disease; to begin we will examine the peripheral nervous system and discuss its involvement in nociception and the perception of pain.

THE PERIPHERAL NERVOUS SYSTEM

Compartments of the Peripheral Nervous System

The peripheral nervous system of the body can be divided into three major compartments. The first is the somatic system that innervates the skin, dermis, fascias, and deep tissues such as muscle, bone, tendon, and enthesis as well as joint capsule. The second is the visceral system that provides sensory innervation to the organs of the body located the in the thoracic, abdominal, and pelvic cavities. Finally, a third category consists of vascular afferent fibers that course along the neurovascular bundles and provide innervation to the vascular system both in the somatic and the visceral locations.

Primary Afferent Neurons Innervate Peripheral Tissue

The sensory cells of the peripheral nervous system are termed primary afferent neurons. Their cell bodies are located in a dorsal root ganglion. The central processes of these cells terminate in the spinal cord or brainstem (Fig. 15.1). In general, these primary afferent neurons are divided into four fundamental types of fibers based on the size of their axon and the type of peripheral ending (Table 15.1). The four fiber types of the peripheral nervous system can be grouped into roughly two general categories: large-caliber myelinated fibers with encapsulated endings and small-caliber unmyelinated or lightly myelinated fibers with naked nerve endings. Although this division is not perfect, it is supported by evidence that suggests the cell bodies of the two types differ in size, the development of the two groups occurs on differing timetables, and their immunohistochemistry is differentiated (Prechtl and Powley, 1990; Fitzgerald, 2005).

The Large-fiber System Is Mainly Involved with Discrimination and Proprioception

The large-fiber sensory system is composed of heavily myelinated, rapidly conducting A-alpha and A-beta fibers. Of these, the A-alpha fibers are the largest and connect to muscle spindle and Golgi tendon organs at their distal endings, while the A-beta fibers are slightly smaller in diameter and are typically attached to cutaneous touch corpuscles or related endings located in deeper tissues such as joint capsules. Table 15.1 compares the properties of these two rapidly

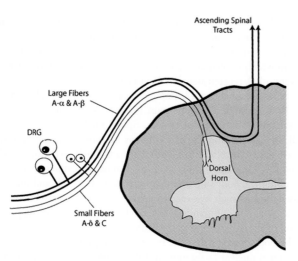

Figure 15-1 The termination of primary afferent fibers in the spinal cord. Large myelinated fibers with large cell bodies in the dorsal root ganglion (DRG) can be seen passing dorsal to the dorsal horn to enter the dorsal columns while small laterally positioned fibers with small cell bodies in the DRG are shown entering the dorsal horn laterally. (Used with permission from the Willard/Carreiro collection.)

conducting fiber systems. Typically, members of the largest fibers are easily activated, being sensitive to low levels of mechanical energy, and have the fastest conduction velocities. The ascending projections of the large-fiber system travel in the dorsal column–medial lemniscus system as well as the spinocerebellar systems to reach the thalamus from which they are relayed on to somatic sensory cortex (Fig. 15.2). This mapping is fairly precise and supports high-fidelity representation of the homunculus on the postcentral gyrus of the cerebral cortex (reviewed in Kandel et al., 2000). Collectively, the large-fiber system gives us the sensory modalities of vibratory sense, discriminative touch, and proprioception. Individual fibers of this system are said to be line labeled in so much as they represent a specific modality; varying the intensity of the stimulus for this fibers does not significantly alter the modality that they represent. Thus, an A-beta fiber associated with a Pacinian corpuscle, when activated, gives the individual a sense of vibration regardless of the intensity of the activation. This consistency in sensory perception contributes to the accuracy and precision of the system. An additional property, prominent in the large-fiber system, is ability of many of its endings to undergo adaptation to repetitive stimuli. In such fibers, repetitive

stimuli initially activate the fiber ending, which then adapts to the stimulus by altering its shape in such a way that it becomes nonresponsive to that particular stimulus. Adaptation of these fibers facilitates the detection of novel stimuli in the environment.

The Large-Fiber System is Active in Pain Control

Although the major target of A-beta fibers is the dorsal column nuclei of the brainstem, many of these fibers, as they enter the spinal cord, give collateral branches that invade the dorsal horn as well. These collateral branches, through an inhibitory mechanism, can modulate the transmission of information in the small-fiber system in the dorsal horn and thereby prevent nociceptive information from ascending in the spinal cord tracks. This mechanism has been termed the gate-control theory of pain modulation and appears to play a significant role in controlling the activity of the small-fiber system. (Melzack and Wall, 1965). Conversely, under situations of intense peripheral stimuli involving inflammation, some members of the large-fiber system have been observed to undergo a phenotypic change such that they can now activate dorsal horn neurons and produce a neuropeptide termed substance-P, a marker for the small-fiber system (Neumann et al., 1996). This alteration in fiber function would have profound effects on the amplification of signal in the dorsal horn and the patient's perception of pain.

THE SMALL-FIBER SYSTEM

The small-fiber sensory system is composed of A-delta and C-fibers; collectively these fibers have been referred to as primary afferent nociceptors (PANs). The A-delta fibers have a thin myelin sheath; whereas the C-fibers only have a thin wrapping derived from the Schwann cell but no myelin. A common feature of these fiber types is their termination as an exposed or naked axon ending, also termed free nerve ending, embedded in the extracellular matrix of the surrounding tissue. In general, many of these small-caliber fibers have high thresholds of activation, requiring tissue-damaging or potentially tissue-damaging levels of energy before generating action potentials. However, there are some A-delta fibers with thresholds of activation in the same range as the large-fiber systems previously described (Meyer et al., 2006); these low-threshold fibers will not be considered further.

The Small-Fiber System Targets The Dorsal Horn

The central process of the small-caliber fibers terminates in the ipsilateral dorsal horn of the spinal cord (Fig. 15.1) or if the fiber arises

TABLE 15.1

Classification of Fiber Types in the Peripheral Nervous System

Classification	Fiber Size and Velocity	Myelin	Origin	Receptor Organ	Effective Stimulus
Group Ia (Aα)	12–20 µm; 70–120 m/s	Yes	Muscle	Annulospiral	Stretch—low threshold
Group Ib (Aα)	2–20 µm; 70–120 m/s	Yes	Muscle	Golgi tendon organs	Active contraction of muscle
Group II (Aβ)	5–12 µm; 30–70 m/s	Yes	Muscle	Flower-spray	Stretch—low Threshold
		Yes	Skin	Touch corpusles	Mechanical deformation of skin
Group III (Aδ)	2–5 µm; 12–30 m/s	Yes	Muscle and skin	Nociception	Mechanical deformation of skin; heat; cold; chemical stimulation
Group IV (C-fibers)	0.5–1 µm; 0.5–2 m/s	No	Muscle and skin	Nociception	Mechanical deformation of the skin; heat; chemical stimulation

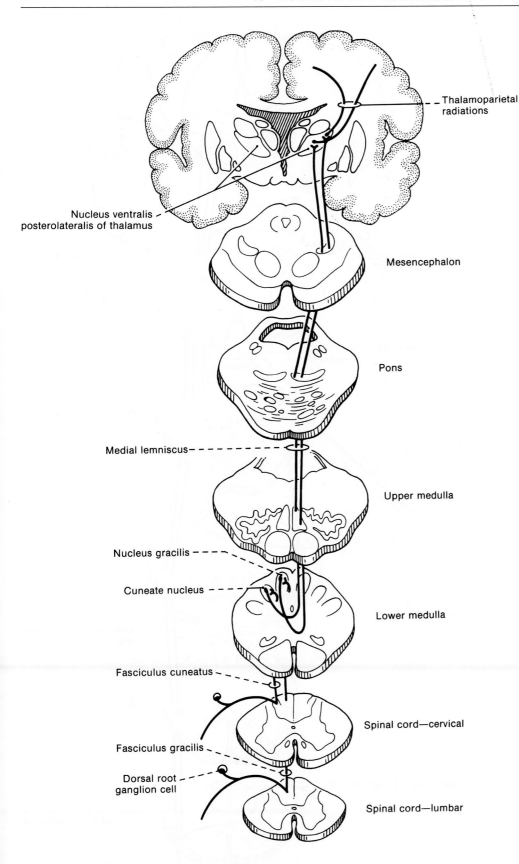

Figure 15-2 The dorsal column—medial lemniscal system. (From Campbell WW. *DeJong's the Neurologic Examination*, Philadelphia, PA: Lippincott Williams & Wilkins, 2005.)

Thalamoparietal radiations

Nucleus ventralis posterolateralis of thalamus

Mesencephalon

Pons

Medial lemniscus

Upper medulla

Nucleus gracilis

Cuneate nucleus

Lower medulla

Fasciculus cuneatus

Spinal cord—cervical

Fasciculus gracilis

Dorsal root ganglion cell

Spinal cord—lumbar

in the trigeminal territory of the face, its central process terminates in spinal trigeminal nucleus of the medullary brainstem. Specifically, these small-diameter afferent fibers reach laminae I, II, and V of the dorsal horn as well as the central portion of the gray matter around lamina X. Ascending projections from the dorsal horn neurons cross the midline in the anterior white commissure of the spinal cord and course upward in the anterolateral tract or system to reach the brainstem and thalamus (Fig. 15.3). Low-level activation of the small-fiber systems (most likely A-delta fibers) gives us the perception of touch without much localizing capability; however, increasing the activity of this system transforms the perception from that of touch to the sensation of pain. Thus, instead of being line labeled such

Figure 15-3 The Anterolateral or spinothalamic system. (From Campbell WW. *DeJong's the Neurologic Examination.* Philadelphia, PA: Lippincott Williams & Wilkins, 2005.)

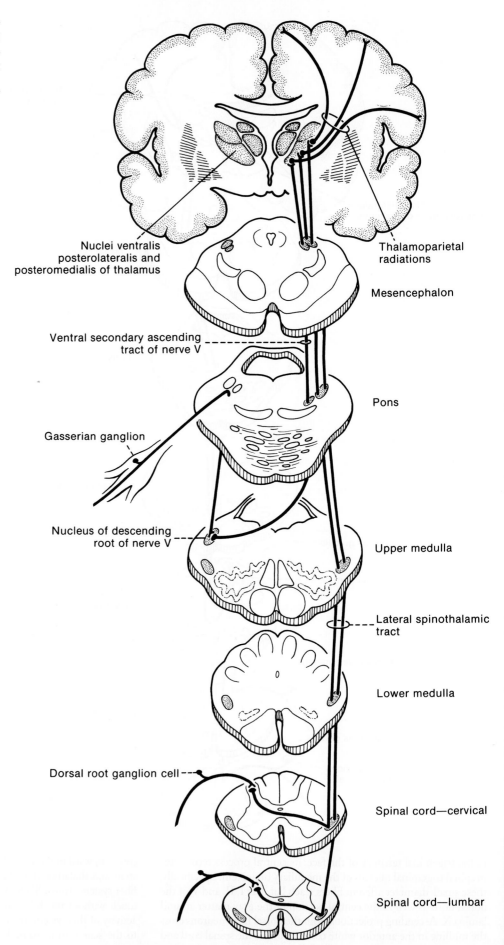

Nuclei ventralis posterolateralis and posteromedialis of thalamus

Thalamoparietal radiations

Mesencephalon

Ventral secondary ascending tract of nerve V

Pons

Gasserian ganglion

Nucleus of descending root of nerve V

Upper medulla

Lateral spinothalamic tract

Lower medulla

Dorsal root ganglion cell

Spinal cord—cervical

Spinal cord—lumbar

as the large-fiber system, some members of the small-fiber system appear to change their specificity with the intensity of activation.

The Output of the Small-Fiber System is Protective in Nature

In addition to warning signals (pain sensation), the small-caliber system activates a complex response from the brainstem termed by Hans Selye the general adaptive response (Selye, 1946). This response involves alterations in the autonomic nervous system and the hypothalamic-pituitary-adrenal axis, both reflexes which will contribute to the inherent ability of the body for self-regulation and the reestablishment of health. These concepts will be further discussed toward the end of the chapter.

An additional distinctive property of the small-caliber system is its ability to sensitize to repetitive stimuli. Unlike the large-fiber system, which tends to adapt to a stimulus, many of the components in the small-fiber system—either at the level of the peripheral neuron, spinal cord neurons, or even higher in the CNS—will increase their sensitivity to the stimulus. This enhanced activity secondary to sensitization has significant implications for the small-fiber system in the pathology of chronic pain (Ji et al., 2003).

SUMMARY

Both small- and large-fiber systems can play a role in the human perception of pain. However, typically, the small-caliber system has by far the greatest impact. In normal tissue, only small fibers transmit nociceptive information and only their activity is perceived as pain. In addition, the large-fiber system helps to gate the activity of the small-fiber system and control the amount of nociceptive information gaining access to the spinal cord neurons. However, in injured tissue, the situation changes dramatically. The large-fiber system can now become a key player involved in generating the perception of pain. The next section of this chapter will be focused on the anatomical organization and functional properties of the small fibers and their interaction with the large-fiber system in pathologic situations.

SMALL-FIBER LOCATION

PANs terminate with naked nerve endings in numerous tissues throughout the body. The specific locations in which these fibers terminate are important for understanding the patterns of pain that they develop.

Skin And Fascia

PANs are present in the dermis and underlying fascia throughout the body (Munger and Ide, 1988). Upon entering the dermis, much branching of these fibers occurs before their termination. A variety of molecular receptor types are present on cutaneous afferent fibers (Julius and Basbaum, 2001). The PANs in the deep fascia are mostly associated with blood vessels, while a few in the dermis can have small terminal branches that actually penetrate the epidermis to end embedded between cells of the squamous epithelium; these are termed intraepithelial endings. PANs also reach the specializations of the integument such as the nail beds, tympanic membrane, and cornea.

Muscle

Muscle nerves can be as much as 50% small fibers in composition (Mense and Simons, 2001). Within the muscle, PANs are seen to course in the connective tissue surrounding the vasculature. While PANs do not directly innervate myocytes, they do remain in the

surrounding connective tissue termed the perimycium and are thought to play a major role in regulating the vascular dynamics of the muscle. Many of these small fibers contain neuropeptides such as substance-P and calcitonin gene–related peptide consistent with their role as sensory fibers and neurosecretory fibers. Thresholds for activation muscle PANs are usually somewhat lower than that necessary actually to damage the surrounding muscle tissue. Distribution of the PANs is complex; many of these fibers have more than one receptive field in the peripheral tissue, and often the two fields are not contiguous. Muscle PANs appear to be sensitive to inflammatory substances and to the breakdown products resulting from intense muscle activity. Finally, muscle PANs are well noted for their ability to increase activity in the spinal cord, leading to sensitization of the dorsal horn neurons (Wall and Woolf, 1984).

Tendon

The PANs found in tendons are not very well characterized at this time. Mense describes small fibers in the peritendineum and in the enthesis but not in the body of the tendon (Mense and Simons, 2001). Alpantaki described nerve networks extending the length of the human bicep tendon and especially dense at the enthesis, but not in the tendon–muscle junction (Alpantaki et al., 2005). The small fibers in these neural networks contained several neuropeptides typically associated with sensory fibers such as PANs. Concentration of these fibers at the enthesis could be related to the notably painful presentation of enthesitis.

Blood Vessels

Somatic and visceral blood vessels receive small-caliber sensory fibers as well as a sympathetic innervation. PANs follow the sympathetic nervous system coursing in the tunica adventitia of these blood vessels. These small vascular fibers release vasodilatory neuropeptides and can act as a counter-regulatory force to the vasoconstrictive nature of the sympathetic system. This is especially interesting in light of the fact that the somatic peripheral vasculature does not receive a parasympathetic innervation; thus, the PANs could be providing some, if not most, of the external dilatory signals to the vasculature (Premkumar and Raisinghani, 2006).

Nerves

The connective tissue sheath surrounding nerves contains a PAN innervation (Bove and Light, 1995). Where studied, these fibers contain and release proinflammatory neuropeptides and have high thresholds of activation similar to nociceptors. It is possible that some of the pain arising from chronic injury of a nerve could be arising from the PANs in the connective sheath surrounding the nerve rather than from the discharge of axons contained within the nerve itself.

Joints

Joints typically receive multiple articular nerves. These nerves have been demonstrated to contain as much as 80% small-caliber (C-fiber range) axons; of these small fibers, there is approximately an even split between those of the sympathetic nervous system and PANs (Schaible and Grubb, 1993). Fibers of all calibers innervate the joint capsule, ligaments, menisci, and surrounding periosteum; however, only small-caliber, peptide-containing fibers are typically seen in the synovial membranes. Increased density of innervation is a feature in abnormal, osteoarthritic joints and suggests that the PAN system is plastic and dynamic and can respond to injury by proliferating into the damaged tissue along with the blood supply (Fortier and Nixon, 1997).

Viscera

The axons entering viscera are typically small in size, being in the Aδ- and C-fiber range (Bielefeldt and Gebhart, 2006). Afferent fibers enter the thoraco-abdomino-pelvic cavity either with the vagus nerve or the splanchnic nerves. These fibers are distributed via suspensory ligaments (mesenteries and mesocolons) to the hollow viscera. Sensory innervation can be found in the suspensory ligament as well as in the muscular wall and mucosa of the organ. Solid organs, such as the liver, are primarily innervated in the region of the fibrous capsule with very little projecting into the organ parenchyma. Many fibers are mechanoinsensitive, responding only to inflammatory compounds in the tissue. As such, they have been termed silent nociceptors to denote the lack of initial response to mechanical deformation (Cervero and Jänig, 1992), for example, during surgery. Although the total number of visceral afferent fibers is marginal compared to the somatic afferent system, the visceral system compensates for this by heavy branching and ramification of the central terminals in the spinal cord and brainstem (Cervero, 1991).

Meninges

Small-caliber fibers innervate the dura and extracerebral blood vessels surrounding the brain. These small fibers are components of the trigeminovascular system. Their cell bodies are located in the trigeminal ganglion and their peripheral processes follow the cerebrovascular system until it penetrates the brain. Inflammatory irritation of these fibers plays a crucial role in migraine and other vascular head pains (Sanchez del Rio and Moskowitz, 2000).

Annulus Fibrosis

PANs penetrate approximately one third of the way into the disc, reaching most of the annulus fibrosis but do not extend into the nucleus pulposis (Stilwell, 1956; Groen et al., 1990). These fibers are derived from the sinu vertebral nerve (recurrent meningeal) posteriorly and from the prevertebral plexus (somatosympathetic nerves) anteriorly (Jinkins et al., 1989). Many of these fibers contain neuropeptides typical of small-caliber primary afferent fibers and are involved in discogenic pain. In addition, PANs are found in the anterior and posterior longitudinal ligaments and in the facet joint capsules as well as in other ligaments of the vertebral column. This network of small-caliber fibers surrounding the vertebral column is involved in the axial pain syndromes (Willard, 1997).

SUMMARY

PANs have an almost universal distribution in the body; only a few areas have been demonstrated to be devoid of PANs. These regions include such regions as brain parenchyma, articular cartilage, the parenchyma of the liver, and lung and the nucleus pulposis. The density of small-fiber distribution is not uniform throughout the tissue of the body, being greatest in the dermis and more scattered in distribution through the visceral organs. There also appears to be some differential distribution of neupeptides within various regions of the body. The widespread and plentiful nature of these small-caliber primary afferent fibers is a testament to their important role in the maintenance of our health.

SMALL-FIBER ACTIVATION

Primary afferent nociceptors can respond to mechanical, heat, and chemical irritation. Several different forms of membrane-bound receptor mechanisms and ion channels are present and a variety of events can activate these fibers (Table 15.1). However, not all PANs have the same constellation of receptors. Mechanical distortion of tissue can open ion channels of some PANs and initiate

depolarization of the fiber. Thermal stimuli also open thermal-sensitive ion channels on some PAN fiber membranes. These heat-sensitive channels have been identified and were originally described as vanilloid receptors (V1) or, as more recently termed, "transient receptor potential channels" (TRPV1). However, the chemoreceptors are the more important of the receptor types related to chronic pain seen in the musculoskeletal. Substances released in the environment of the chemoreceptive PANs, during tissue injury or inflammation, activate receptors located on the exposed membrane of these fibers (Fig. 15.4). Many different substances (called alodynogens) can activate or sensitize PANs, either directly through their receptors or indirectly by stimulating the production of other compounds that in turn can activate their receptors; thus, chemoreceptive PANs are responsive to a wide range of modifications in the chemical milieu of the surrounding tissue (Levine et al., 1993). Receptors are of three general types: ion channels, G-protein-coupled receptors, and cytokine-type receptors (Table 15.2).

There is a growing list of alodynogens capable of activating PANs; some of the better known examples are listed in Table 15.3. Most of these substances are present either in a blocked form or sequestered in cells, to be unlocked or released in the face of tissue injury. Histamine is contained in the granules of mast cells, which is situated along neurovascular bundles in fascia. Injury disrupts the mast cell releasing the histamine into the tissue. Similarly, disruption of vascular endothelial cells releases prostaglandins into the surrounding tissue. Finally, bradykinin, a plasma protein produced in the liver, is present in blocked form termed preprobradykinin. Tissue damage activates enzymes similar to the clotting cascade that ultimately results in the release of bradykinin in the surrounding tissue.

Inflammation releases a cascade of chemicals, many of them capable of helping cleanse the tissue and stimulating wound repair in short-term exposure; however, most of these substances are also alodynogens. PANs have receptors for many of these chemicals and can record their release into the tissue by depolarization and action potential formation. Peripheral release of neuropeptide allodynogens from PANs can initiate or exacerbate an inflammatory response (Fig. 15.5). Some of these same substances are also used as neurotransmitters or neuromodulators, released from the central process of the PAN in the dorsal horn. PAN activation serves as a warning and initiates spinal cord and brainstem level reflexes to protect the injured area. In addition, exposure to some of these compounds activates G-protein-signaling cascades capable of sensitizing the PAN. In essence, the PANs are introceptors, sensitive to the quality of our tissue and can inform the central nervous system of our tissue health.

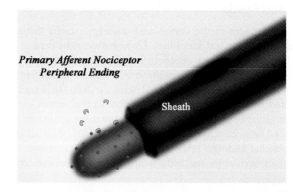

Figure 15-4 Primary afferent fiber ending. Primary afferent nociceptors are covered with a Schwann cell sheath containing little or no myelin. At the end of the fiber, the sheath terminates to expose the naked end of the axon. The membrane of the axon has receptors that can detect chemicals in the surrounding extracellular fluids. (Used with permission from the Willard/Carreiro collection.)

TABLE 15.2

PAN Receptors and Their Activating Substances

PAN Receptor Class	Activating Substances	Examples	Function
Ion-channels	Heat; mechanical force	Transient receptor potential channels (vanilloid receptors); proton-gated channels; sodium channels; potassium channels; calcium channels; serotonin (5-HT3) channels	Na^{++} and Ca^{++} influx into the axon
G-Proteins	Bradykinin, Prostaglandin; Ednocannabinnoids	BK-1, BK-2, DP, EP, FP, IP, TP	Initiate second messanger cascades in the axon
Cytokine receptors	Growth factors and cytokines	Trk-A, Trk-B, Trk-C, NT-4/5. NT-3, IL-1RI, sIL-6R, TNFR1	Modify surrounding ion channel activity

PANS CONTRIBUTE TO A FEED-FORWARD ALLOSTATIC PROCESS INVOLVED IN SOMATIC DYSFUNCTION AND TISSUE REPAIR

When activated, certain PANS can secrete potent, proinflammatory neuropeptides that enhance the release of histamine, prostaglandins, and cytokines. A feed-forward loop is established, with the PANs releasing substances that ultimately provoke additional activity from the same fiber. Importantly, this feedback loop has no established end point or set point. These types of reactions, rapidly fulminating, epitomize a process characterized by the term allostasis (Schulkin, 2003a). In allostatic processes, rapid change in the tissue chemistry is protective and contributes to the long-term survival of the individual. This is contrary to homeostasis, in which inhibitory feedback control establishes boundary parameters that oscillate around a defined set-point. Allostatic processes lack immediate boundaries or set-points; thus, this inflammatory process can potentially run out of control and become a chronic issue. Eventually, the increasing systemic levels of norepinephrine and glucocorticoids, due to long-loop inhibitory feedback systems, should aid in suppressing the inflammatory response. Acute exposure to an allostatic process can be very protective, creating an area of increased sensitivity to mechanical stimulation (allodynia), an increased response to a stimulus which is normally painful (hyperalgesia), and in initiating protective reflexes.

Most likely, the allostatic condition involving the release of alodynogens and the enhancement of the inflammatory soup of chemicals in the tissue environment resulting in sensitization of the PANs epitomizes the conditions found in somatic dysfunction. The potentiated PANs would generate a condition of hyperalgesia and the surrounding inflammatory cocktail would produce edema or a boggy, ropy texture to the tissues on palpation. Increased sensitivity to touch and tissue texture changes are two of the cardinal manifestations of somatic dysfunction (Denslow, 1975).

NERVE DAMAGE AND THE FEELINGS OF PAIN

Acute damage to a peripheral nerve fiber is usually relatively painless and, when done experimentally, rarely produces more than a few seconds of rapid axonal discharges. Acute damage to the dorsal root ganglion can produce long periods of excitation and rapid firing lasting 5 to 25 minutes; thus, the ganglion is the most sensitive part of the nerve to compressive injury. However, acute compression of a chronically injured, inflamed nerve represents a different situation and will produce several minutes of repetitive firing; it has been suggested that this long-duration rapid firing is the basis for radicular pain (Howe et al., 1977). Injury to a nerve can facilitate sprouting from the peripheral terminal of fibers within the nerve; this can be accompanied by the invasion of sympathetic axons into the dorsal root ganglion with inappropriate synapse formation and abnormal sprouting of axon terminals in the dorsal horn (McLachlan et al., 1993; Amir and Devor, 1996; Ramer and Bisby, 1997). All of these scenarios can contribute to the development of an intense chronic pain condition, termed neuropathic pain, which is pain initiated or caused by a primary lesion of dysfunction in the nervous system (Merskey and Bogduk, 1994).

THE SPINAL CORD AND PAIN

When PANs become active, they transmit a signal to the dorsal horn of the spinal cord via their central process (Fig. 15.5). Various cells, including both neurons and glia in the dorsal horn, are influenced by this sensory information. Interestingly, the response of the dorsal horn cells can outlast the activity of the PAN. The sustainability of this activity pattern among neurons in the dorsal horn represents central sensitization and is believed to be a major component of numerous pain syndromes. The interaction in the spinal cord of the central process of PANs from various regions in the body can substantially alter acute pain patterns (referral and association patterns), as well as states of chronic pain.

PANS TERMINATE IN THE DORSAL HORN OF THE SPINAL CORD

The central process of the PANs enters the spinal cord by coursing in the lateral aspect of the dorsal root entry zone, entering

TABLE 15.3

The Alodynogens and their Receptors

Alodynogen	Receptor	Origin
Bradykinin	BK1 and BK2	Plasma protein from liver
Histamine	H1	Mast cells
Serotonin	5-HT2A	Blood platelets
Prostaglandins	DP, EP, FP, IP, TP	Vascular endothelial cells
ATP	Purine	Local cell rupture
Protons	Vanilloid receptor (VR1)	Local cell rupture

Figure 15-5 Activation of a PAN and the release of proinflammatory compounds into the surrounding tissue. Tissue irritation results in the release of proinflammatory compounds from the distal ends of some primary afferent nociceptors. Interactions with compounds from immune cells, mast cells, and platelets result in an inflammatory soup that sensitizes the PAN leading to the increased release of neurotransmitters and neuromodulators in the dorsal horn of the spinal cord (used with permission from the Willard/Carreiro collection).

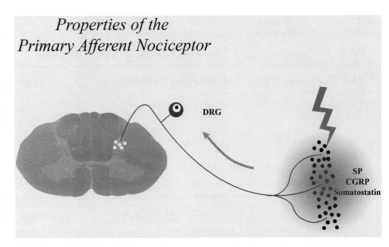

Properties of the Primary Afferent Nociceptor

the dorsal most aspect of the dorsal horn and extending inward to terminate generally in laminae I, II, and V. Conversely low-threshold, mechanoreceptive fibers tend to terminate deep in laminae III through VI. The organization of the PANs in the dorsal horn is orderly, forming a somatotropic body map extending roughly from medial to lateral across the dorsal horn (Wilson and Kitchener, 1996); however, much overlap in receptor territories exist allowing for referral of activity patterns to associated regions of the somatotropic map.

PANs represent a heterogeneous population of fibers; thus, not all PANs are the same in terms of anatomy and neurochemistry. Beyond the size difference seen between Aδ-fibers and C-fibers, the C-fibers divide into two groups: those that contain neuropeptides such as calcitonin gene–related peptide or substance-P and those that do not contain neuropeptides (Hunt and Rossi, 1985; Todd, 2006). The neuropeptide-containing fibers seem to terminate principally in laminae I, while the non–peptide-containing fibers terminate in laminae II. This dichotomy of fiber types and distributions suggests that differing aspects of nociception could be carried by specialized PANs; specifically, the peptidergic PANs terminating in lamina I are thought to be involved in localization, and the nonpeptidergic fibers in lamina II are more associated with the affective nature of the pain (Braz et al., 2005).

DORSAL HORN NEURONS AND PAN CENTRAL SYNAPSES

The three anatomical types of dorsal horn neurons are 1) projection cells, 2) interneurons, and 3) propriospinal cells. Projection cells, the best studied of the three types, send their axons upstream in the ascending tracts to reach brainstem and thalamus. Local circuit interneurons confine their projections to the segment that their cell body is located within, while propriospinal cells represent a combination of the first two types; their axons ramify in the spinal cord, interconnecting the various segments, but do not extend out of the spinal cord. Several different forms of projection cells exist in the spinal cord (Cervero, 2006); each form of these cells receives synaptic endings from the PANs. Projection cells in the superficial layer of the dorsal horn are relatively specific to PAN input and have been termed nociceptor-specific cells. The interaction of PANs with the superficial dorsal horn neurons is complicated and still not well understood (Graham et al., 2007). Projection cells located deep in the dorsal horn typically respond to a wide range of inputs, including Aβ–fibers, Aδ–fibers, and C-fibers, and have therefore been termed wide-dynamic-range (WDR) neurons (Mendell, 1966). Although gentle mechanical stimulation can activate a WDR neuron; maximal response from these cells can only be obtained from noxious stimuli (Willis, 1979). Evidence does support the concept that our affective perception of pain is related to the activity of the WDR neuron, while our perception of the pain location may be due to the activity of the nociceptor-specific cells (Mayer et al., 1975); however, these concepts remain a controversial area in perceptual neuroscience.

EXAMINATION OF A PAN CENTRAL SYNAPSE

Central Pan Synaptic Terminals Contain At Least Two Types of Neurotransmitters

The central process of the neuropeptide-containing PANs forms terminals on the dendrites of dorsal horn neurons. A closer look at the neurochemistry of these PAN synapses will help in understanding the central sensitization of dorsal horn neurons. Neuropeptide-containing PAN synaptic terminals produce excitatory amino acids, such as glutamate or aspartate, and neuropeptide neurotransmitters, such as substance-P or calcitonin gene–related peptide (Basbaum, 1999). These transmitters are coreleased from the terminal; however, while the amino acid is released during any sufficient depolarization of the ending, neuropeptide release requires more prolonged summation of depolarizations such as would occur during tonic discharges (Millan, 1999).

Excitatory Amino Acid

The most common excitatory amino acid (EAA) in the PAN central terminal is glutamate. Release of glutamate activates the alpha-amino-3-hydroxy-5-methyl-4-isoxazolepropionic acid (AMPA) receptors on the postsynaptic surface. AMPA receptors are ion channels that allow sodium to enter the cell when open, as such these channels can cause a rapid depolarization of the postsynaptic process when activated. This type of transmission is relatively quick, involving milliseconds at most, and has thus been termed fast transmission. Most neurons in the dorsal horn express AMPA receptors on their membranes.

Neuropeptide

A specific population of PAN central terminals contain neuropeptides as well as excitatory amino acids. Upon release, these peptides diffuse onto receptors located on the postsynaptic membrane, but not necessarily in the synaptic cleft. Tonic or repeated activation of the PAN is required to cause enough peptide release to activate the peptide receptors. Thus, the time required to obtain adequate volume of peptide release, and the longer diffusion route to a more distant receptor complex, combine to increase the time required for a response (Millan, 1999). When activated by attachment to the peptide, the peptide-receptor complex internalizes into the post-synaptic neuron through a process of endocytosis (Mantyh et al., 1995). Thus, the peptide is acting on the postsynaptic neuron in a way that is similar to some hormones in that it physically enters the postsynaptic cell to effect changes at the cytosolic and nuclear levels. Once across the cell membrane, the peptide-receptor complex can act as an enzyme and initiate second-messenger cascades leading to the phosphorylation of the AMPA receptor as well as surrounding NMDA receptors. Phosphorylation of EAA receptors allows calcium ions to enter, thereby facilitating the activity of the dorsal horn neuron. This type of transmission requires seconds to minutes and has thus been termed slow transmission. The result of this cascade of events is a potentiation of the responsiveness of dorsal horn cells that contributes to central sensitization that is the response properties of these dorsal horn neurons undergo a left-ward shift on the stimulus-response curve. Interestingly, excessive activation of the PANs can lead to the spread of neurons express-ing receptors for SP in the dorsal horn (Abbadie et al., 1997); this change would also facilitate the response of the dorsal horn neu-rons to afferent stimuli.

BEHAVIOR OF NOCICEPTIVE NEURONS IN THE DORSAL HORN

Transient Change in Dorsal Horn Circuitry—Activity-Dependent Plasticity

Neurons in the dorsal horn demonstrate a plasticity in their response properties that is directly related to the afferent activity to which they are exposed (Abbadie et al., 1997). This type of plas-ticity is characteristic of any biological system that is adaptive in nature. Through these plastic changes, afferent activity involving PANs can result in sensitization of the dorsal horn circuitry. These rapid changes in sensitivity represent a form of allostasis, similar to that already described in the periphery, and can be very protec-tive in the short term. Numerous cellular mechanisms contribute to the plasticity of the dorsal horn system (Ji et al., 2003). Initially, dorsal horn cells show a progressive increase in activity to a train of constant stimuli, an event termed wind-up, which will cease when the stimulus ceases. Prolonged exposure to the stimulus leads to the development of a classic form of central sensitization, where the heightened central neural response outlasts the end of the periph-eral stimulus by tens of minutes. High-frequency PAN stimulation of dorsal horn neurons can result in a much longer lasting response termed long-term potentiation (LTP); in fact, the duration of the response exceeds that of most experimental studies. Other events contributing to the sensitization of the dorsal horn neuron include the activation of protein kinase enzymes. Within the postsynaptic neurons, protein kinase activation with subsequent phosphoryla-tion events can lead to the induction of numerous genes; this form of sensitization is referred to as transcription dependent and can be very long lasting in nature. While the large projection neurons are undergoing an excitatory form of sensitization, their surround-ing inhibitory neurons can also be changing their activity. Long-term depression can occur in inhibitory interneurons located in the dorsal horn, resulting in reduced inhibition on the projection neu-rons and thus, more information traveling upstream to the brain-stem, thalamus, and cerebral cortex. Finally, two additional events can lead to a permanent form of sensitization: inhibitory cell loss (Scholz et al., 2005) and rearrangement of synaptic connections (Doubell et al., 1997; Abbadie et al., 1997).

Central Sensitization and Secondary Hyperalgesia

Sensitization of dorsal horn neurons can alter their response properties, typically shifting the response versus stimulus intensity curve to the left. An additional prominent feature of sensitization is the expansion of the neuron's receptive field. Expansion of the cell's receptive field outside the area of immediate injury will contrib-ute to the formation of secondary hyperalgesia (Cook et al., 1987; Laird and Cervero, 1989; Hylden et al., 1989; Grubb et al., 1993; Koerber and Mirnics, 1996). That is, noninjured tissue contiguous with the primary site of injury will develop increased sensitivity to mechanical stimuli. In addition to receptive field expansion, some dorsal horn neurons, particularly those driven by skeletal muscle afferent fibers, can develop new and, in some cases, noncontiguous receptive fields (Mense, 1991).

Irritation of the noncontiguous receptor fields results in the sensation of pain in the area of primary and secondary hyperalge-sia (Hoheisel et al., 1993; Mense and Simons, 2001). While the expansion of the receptive field contributes to the phenomena of secondary hyperalgesia, the development of new, noncontiguous receptive fields could contribute to the expression of either tender points or trigger points.

Central Sensitization and Glial Cell Activation

The classic notion is that a neuronal synaptic chain extends from periphery to cerebral cortex representing the pathways for process-ing nociception and generating the sensation of pain. However, recent evidence has forced a revisal of this concept to include other cells, such as glia, that can modify the information processing in the neuronal chain (Watkins et al., 2007). Glial cells form a matrix surrounding all dorsal horn neurons and central neurons in general. Multiple types of glia are present but the ones most associated with immune responses are the astrocytes and microglia. In the dorsal horn (and to date only in this region), these two glial cell types express receptors for substance-P. Interaction with SP can activate these two forms of glia. Activated glial cells release proinflamma-tory cytokines such as tumor necrosis factor-α and interleukins 1 and 6. Although it is not clear at this time how proinflammatory cytokines work in the dorsal horn, it is certain that they contribute to increasing spinal facilitation and hyperalgesia. Activated glia also increase the production of NO and PGE2 in the dorsal horn; both substances are known to increase spinal facilitation and the resulting hyperalgesia; interestingly, these glial cells also increase the release of SP from the central terminals of the PANs, thus creating another feed-forward loop in the interoceptive system pathways. Neurons in the dorsal horn have been demonstrated to express receptors for proinflammatory cytokines and IL-1 is known to increase the influx of calcium ions through the NMDA receptor, also increasing spinal facilitation. Thus, multiple factors occurring within the dorsal horn are combining to create plastic changes in the dorsal horn neurons. Finally, glial cell–neuron interaction can explain the formation of mirror-image pain, that is, pain that occurs contralateral to injured tissue (Wieseler-Frank et al., 2005). Spinal cord glial cells are inter-connected with each other by gap junctions, thereby constructing a large and complex syncytial matrix that extends across the mid-line in the spinal cord. Blocking the spread of information through these glial gap junctions prevents the development of mirror-image pain in experimental models. From all of this, it is clear that glia cell activity in the dorsal horn can modify the processing of nociceptive information and increase the sensation of pain. While protective in the short term, this response has the potential to fulminate and become part of a chronic problem.

Permanent Change in the Dorsal Horn Circuitry

All of the changes in dorsal horn circuitry discussed so far appear to be reversible; however, excessive PAN stimulation or peripheral nerve injury can also result in a permanent alteration in the dorsal horn. The smallest neurons in the dorsal horn, typically GABA-ergic neurons, appear to undergo an apoptotic cell death following excessive activation (Scholz et al., 2005). Loss of these neurons would diminish the inhibition in the spinal cord circuitry thus creating a more easily excited segment, possibly one that displays spontaneous activity. A second method of permanent change in the dorsal horn involves the sprouting of Aβ-afferent fibers following peripheral nerve injury (Neumann and Woolf, 1999). The normal distribution of the Aβ-afferent fibers is focused on the deeper layers of the dorsal horn. In animal models, following nerve injury, the terminals of the Aβ-afferent fibers can be seen in the superficial layers replacing sites occupied typically by PANs. Both of the above alterations in the dorsal horn circuitry would create permanent change and could contribute to chronic pain scenarios.

DORSAL HORN INVOLVEMENT IN MODIFIED PAIN PRESENTATION PATTERNS

Dorsal Horn Alteration in Chronic Pain States

Normal plasticity in the dorsal horn circuitry is necessary to insure adequate warning information and protective reflexes during the healing process. To be protective, these changes have to occur rapidly; they typically involve numerous feed-forward events without an immediate set-point, thus fitting the definition of an allostatic process (Schulkin, 2003a). However, excessive activation of the dorsal horn or inadequate control mechanisms (to be discussed below) can turn the normal plasticity into a pathologic response that leads to the development of a chronic pattern of abnormal neuronal activity, underlying the onset of chronic pain in the patient. Adaptive changes that can become pathologic include the spread of neurons expressing receptors for SP (Abbadie et al., 1997), expansion of dorsal horn neuron receptive fields, the loss of GABA-ergic inhibitory interneurons, and the sprouting of Aβ-fibers into the superficial layer of the dorsal horn. Thus, the chronic pain state can be considered as a failure of normal allostatic mechanisms leading to a pathological condition similar to other chronic stress-related diseases such as depression (Schulkin et al., 1994; McEwen, 2003), type 2 diabetes mellitus (Stumvoll et al., 2003), and cardiovascular disease (McEwen, 1998).

Clinical Expressions of Sensitization

Following the onset of central sensitization, the activity pattern of neurons in the dorsal horn is altered. Expanding receptive fields of dorsal horn neurons create a zone of increased sensitivity that surrounds the initial injury site, which is termed secondary hyperalgesia. Many dorsal horn neurons have projections or at least collateral axons that terminate in the ventral horn. Sensitization of dorsal horn neurons can then alter the activity patterns of the large ventral horn alpha motoneurons (Grigg et al., 1986; He et al., 1988). The ventral horn output can produce muscle spasms and, when prolonged, increased muscle tone and hyperreflexia akin to that seen in spasticity

Convergence of Visceral and Somatic Input in the Dorsal Horn

Visceral afferent fibers from thoracoabdominal and pelvic organs enter the spinal cord through the dorsal root and terminate in the lateral aspect of the deep dorsal horn (fig. 15.6; also see Chapter 9 on Somatic dysfunction, spinal fascilitation and viscerosomatic integration). Visceral PAN input overlaps with much of the somatic PAN input and many cells in the dorsal horn can be driven by both visceral and somatic input (Sato et al., 1983; Sato, 1995). Somatic input can sensitize dorsal horn neurons eliciting specific reflexes. Subsequent visceral input can activate the previously facilitated circuit, eliciting a similar pain pattern and some of the same reflexes. The reverse situation is also often seen clinically, as pointed out by Sir Henry Head many years ago (Head, 1920): that is, visceral input first sensitizes the dorsal horn circuitry and subsequent somatic injury elicits the previous visceral pain pattern and associated reflexes (Henry and Montuschi, 1978).

Influence of Primary Afferent Fibers Along the Spinal Cord

As PANs enter the spinal cord through the dorsal root entry zone, they undergo a trifurcation (Fig. 15.7). One branch enters the dorsal horn at that segment, one branch ascends, and one descends along the dorsal margin of the dorsal horn in a bundle of fibers termed Lissauer's tract (Carpenter and Sutin, 1983). Older diagrams of PAN termination clearly indicated this branching pattern (Ramon y Cajal, 1909), although it has been removed from most modern text for simplification. The division of the PAN is important since it can result in the spreading of information up and down the spinal cord to reach distant segmental levels. How far this information can spread is not clear, cutaneous PANs spread out

Figure 15-6 The convergence of PANs for cutaneous, deep somatic, and visceral sources on the WDR neurons in the dorsal horn of the spinal cord. Primary afferent fibers from visceral, deep somatic, and cutaneous sources are shown converging on a WDR neuron in the dorsal horn of the spinal cord (used with permission from the Willard/Carreiro collection).

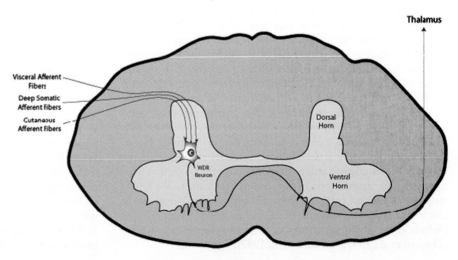

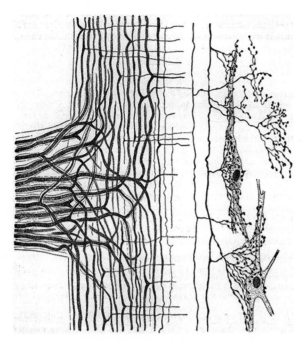

Figure 15-7 The trifurcation of primary afferent fibers as they enter the spinal cord. This is a longitudinal view of the spinal cord taken through the upper portion of the dorsal horn. Primary afferent fibers are seen entering the vertically oriented tract of Lissauer from the left. Upon entry into the tract, these fibers trifurcate giving a branch to the dorsal horn at the point of entry, an ascending branch to higher spinal levels, and a descending branch reaching lower spinal levels. (From Ranson SW and Clark SL. *The Anatomy of the Nervous System: Its Development and Function.* Philadelphia, PA: W.B. Saunders Comp., 1959; Figure 141.)

at least two to three segments, while visceral PANs have reported distributions involving greater than five segments (Sugiura et al., 1989); however, even greater distances are possible (Wall and Bennett, 1994).

The three-dimensional distribution of PAN information in the spinal cord allows for the interpretation of otherwise confusing pain patterns. For example, a patient could have an existing area of spinal facilitation in the midthoracic region consequent to an old process such as gall bladder disease. A recent revival of this old pain pattern, despite the prior removal of the gall bladder, could indicate the new onset of another disease process such as myocardial ischemia or gastric ulcer. The visceral PANs from the myocardium or the stomach enter the spinal cord in the upper thoracic region; early in the disease processes their input may be present in lower thoracic segments due to segmental spread of afferent input, but below the threshold of detection by the patient. However, spread of low-grade neural activity in the caudal direction could easily activate the portion of the spinal cord originally sensitized by the remote history of gall bladder disease. The patient perceives the gall-bladder-associated pain pattern, however this time the etiology of the nociception lies in the myocardium and not in the gall bladder. In general, the recent and otherwise unexplained revival of an old pain pattern should be considered the harbinger of new disease until proven otherwise.

The Dorsal Horn and Dorsal Root Reflexes

Normally, one thinks of the dorsal root as a strictly afferent system carrying action potentials from the peripheral tissue into the

spinal cord only; however, it is now known that under appropriate conditions, the dorsal root can act as an efferent pathway from the spinal cord; when this type of antidromic activity occurs in an intact sensory nerve it has been termed a dorsal root reflex (Rees et al., 1994). Centrifugally conducted activity on dorsal rootlets has been known since the late nineteenth century but was not really in detail examined until the middle of the 20th century (Willis, 1999). Dorsal root reflexes can are present in both large myelinated and in small myelinated and unmyelinated fibers (see Willis, 1999 for a discussion of the difficulties in recording DRRs from the smallest fibers); in this review, we will focus on those reflexes present in the small fibers such as PANs. To trigger these reflexes in PANs, the initial input stimulus to the spinal cord has to be in the range required to activate the PANs (C-fiber range). When such an afferent barrage reaches the dorsal horn, a wave of depolarization, termed primary afferent depolarization (PAD), occurs and is spread outward for several segments up and down the spinal cord. Interestingly, dorsal horn depolarization is facilitated by central sensitization of dorsal horn neurons; thus, past experience can influence the magnitude of this depolarization event. When an area of the dorsal horn depolarizes, the central terminals of other primary afferent fibers contained within this area also depolarize. This mechanism is most likely a spin-off event of presynaptic inhibition and is known to involve GABA-a receptors and GABA released by local interneurons as well as being influenced by serotonin receptors (Peng et al., 2001). Significant depolarization of the central terminals of primary afferent fibers can result in the generation of action potentials within these fibers that move antidromically (outward) to invade the peripheral terminals of this PAN. The resulting antidromic output from the dorsal horn can be recorded as a compound action potential, termed dorsal root potential (DRP) on adjacent dorsal rootlets that have been truncated. In the peripheral terminals of these PANs, the antidromic action potentials act similar to those involved in a classic axon reflex, that is they trigger the release of neuropeptides into the peripheral tissue (Fig. 15.8), thus either initiating or exacerbating an inflammatory reaction. Antidromic activity over dorsal roots can occur both ipsilateral and contralateral to the input root (Rees et al., 1996). DRR have been demonstrated to play a significant role in the spread of peripheral inflammation (Lin et al., 1999). Finally, recent studies have revealed that DRRs can be enhanced by stimulation of the periaqueductal gray region of the midbrain (Peng et al., 2001); this finding has significant implications with respect to the generation of diffuse pain patterns and will be reconsidered in the section on descending pain control mechanisms.

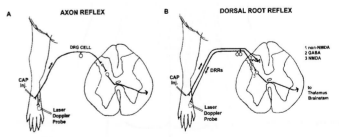

Figure 15-8 Comparison of an axon reflex to a dorsal root reflex. **A.** Diagram of an axon reflex. **B.** Diagram of a dorsal root reflex. Note that the dorsal root reflex simply involves the conduction of an action potential to the spinal cord, depolarization of surrounding fibers in the dorsal horn, and the conduction of an action potential out to the periphery on a depolarized sensory fiber. (From Willis WD. Dorsal root potentials and dorsal root reflexes: a double-edged sword. *Exp Brain Res* 1999;124:395–421.)

ASCENDING PATHWAYS FOR PAIN

The Anterolateral System in the Spinal Cord and Brainstem

Information from the neuronal activity in the dorsal horn is projected upstream to the brainstem and thalamus via dorsal horn neurons with long ascending axons (Fig. 15.9). These projection neurons arising mainly in laminae I, IV-V, and VII-VIII in the dorsal horn send their axons contralaterally to reach the anterior and lateral quadrant of the spinal cord (Dostrovsky and Craig, 2006). Most of these neurons represent either nociceptive-specific cells located in lamina I or wide-dynamic-range cells located in the deeper laminae of the dorsal horn. Axons from these neurons leave the dorsal horn to ascend diagonally, crossing the midline of the spinal cord in the anterior white commissure. The tract formed by these axons has been termed the anterolateral tract (ALS); within the ALS axons are arranged such that the cervical fibers are positioned most medially and the sacral fibers are most lateral. Also, anterior-lateral segregation of axons occurs within the tract such that the anterior portion of the ALS contains fibers activated by light touch and the lateral portions of the ALS contain more of the pain and temperature responsive fibers. Finally, based on target site, two basic components of the anterolateral tract can be identified: the spinoreticular and spinothalamic tracts.

Spinoreticular Tracts

The spinoreticular fibers arise from neurons located in the dorsal horn and terminate in nuclei of the medulla, pons, and midbrain. Specific sites targeted by the spinoreticular fibers include the

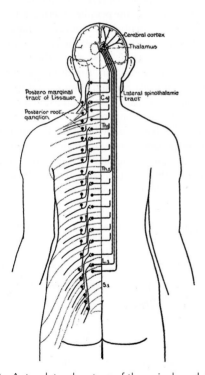

Figure 15-9 Anterolateral system of the spinal cord. The entry of spinal nerves is shown on the left with their synapse on a dorsal horn neuron. The spinothalamic axons arise in the dorsal horn, decussate over the midline, and ascend to the brainstem and thalamus in the anterolateral tract, also termed spinothalamic tract. (From Larsell O. *Anatomy of the Nervous System.* New York, NY: Appleton-Century Crofts, Inc., 1942. Figure 205.)

catecholamine cell groups (A1 to A7), subnucleus reticularis dorsalis, the ventrolateral medulla, the parabrachial nucleus, periaqueductal gray, and the anterior pretectal area (Westlund, 2005; Dostrovsky and Craig, 2006). Since these areas are thought to regulate much of the descending brainstem-spinal cord projections, they therefore could play a significant role in the modulation of pain. Of these two tracts in the anterolateral system, the spinoreticular appears to be the most important in regulating the arousal system of the brainstem.

Spinothalamic Tract

Axons from dorsal horn neurons that project to the thalamus form the spinothalamic tract; these axons are also embedded in the ALS system along with those projecting to the brainstem. In fact, many of the brainstem terminals can be collateral branches of the spinothalamic fibers. Spinothalamic axons located in the lateral most portion of the ALS tend to be most responsive to pain and thermal stimuli. At the rostral end of the spinothalamic tract a division occurs; the larger fibers in the tract remain laterally positioned to enter the thalamus, terminating in the vicinity of the ventroposterior and ventromedial nuclei, while the finer fibers in the tract segregate and enter the medial thalamus and terminate in the intralaminar nuclei. This arrangement creates medial and lateral pain systems in the thalamus. Many of the ascending fibers entering the medial thalamus appear to be of brainstem origin rather than spinal cord origin. In general, the lateral pain system is thought to be a phylogenetically newer system involved with localization of the noxious stimulus, while the medial system is an older system more likely involved in arousal and affectation of event.

Thalamic Representation of Pain

Until this point in the chapter, we have been describing a nociceptive system, a system that can generate a signal in response to tissue-damaging or potentially damaging energy. At the level of the thalamus a transition occurs, we are no longer describing a strictly nociceptive system but a system that can precipitate a feeling of pain and its associated emotions such as anxiety and depression. Neural activity below the thalamus can occur without perception resulting in reflexes as well as certain behaviors; however, the thalamus and cerebral cortex function as a unit and it is at the thalamocortical level that perception is initiated. While the spinal cord and brainstem can initiate primitive, withdrawal-type reflexes to nociceptive stimuli, the thalamocortical system is required to initiate more elaborate evasive movements as well as the complicated psychological responses to painful situations.

The thalamus is a major target for ascending information from the spinal cord and brainstem to the cerebral cortex. Two pain systems, medial and lateral, can be identified in the thalamus, separated from each other anatomically and having differing functions (Dostrovsky, 2006; also see Fig. 15.10). Functional imaging has demonstrated that the thalamus is the site where active is most expected in the acute pain state (May, 2007).

Lateral Pain System

The spinothalamic tract (often termed the neospinothalamic tract) innervates laterally and ventrally positioned nuclei of the thalamus including the ventroposterior lateral nucleus, ventromedial nucleus, portions of the posterior nuclear group, and portions of the ventrolateral nucleus (Fig. 15.10). These structures rapidly relay information to somatic sensory and insular cortex and play a role in

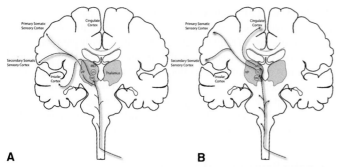

A   **B**

Figure 15-10   The ascending nociceptive systems in the thalamus. **A.** This figure demonstrates the projection of spinothalamic axons to the ventroposterior (ventral caudal) and ventromedial nuclei of the lateral thalamus and their relationship with primary and secondary somatic sensory cortex and in the insular cortex. **B.** Other spinothalamic and spinoreticulothalamic axons terminate in the central lateral and dorsomedial nuclei of the medial thalamus. Their cortical representation involves the cingulated cortex as well as the major somatic sensory areas.

the localizing qualities and intensity of the pain perception. In one published case of a patient with a lesion involving the postcentral gyrus of the cerebral cortex (a significant target of the lateral pain system of the thalamus), the individual lost the ability to accurately localize painful stimuli but retained the ability to experience the affective nature of the pain (Ploner et al., 1999).

Medial Pain System

The medial fibers of the spinothalamic tract (often termed the paleospinothalmic fibers) enter the thalamus medially (Fig. 15-10) to innervate the centromedian nucleus, centrolateral nucleus, dorsomedial nucleus, nucleus submedius, and the intralaminar nuclei (Dostrovsky, 2006). In the hypothalamus, this system innervates the paraventricular nucleus. Included in this ascending system would be projections from lower brainstem areas that have themselves been innervated by the spinoreticular axons. These connections form the medial pain system and primarily relay to the prefrontal cortex and anterior cingulate cortex, areas critical for the transformation of sensation to perception. The medial pain system is slower than its lateral counterpart and is more closely related to the affective and emotional nature of pain (Sewards and Sewards, 2002). Damage, typically from vascular accidents, involving the lateral and posterior thalamus appears to unmask spontaneous activity in the medial system. The unfortunate patient experiences an intense burning pain, usually in a limb, that is refractive to analgesics. This presentation is termed the thalamic pain syndrome or the syndrome of Dejerine-Roussy (Victor and Ropper, 2001).

The Cerebral Cortical Pain Matrix—From Sensation to Perception

Our understanding of the role of the forebrain in pain processing was limited to animal and electrophysiological studies until sophisticated human brain imaging methodologies were refined and complex meta-analysis of study results performed (Apkarian et al., 2005; Tracey and Mantyh, 2007). Appreciation of brain involvement in pain perception was also slowed by the state of physiology at the turn of the century (Head and Holmes, 1911), which questioned the participation of the cortex in human pain perception. In fact, Ronald Melzack in the 1970s at one point even proclaimed

that neuroscientists were "scooping out the brain" and ignoring the fact that a person could have, for example, a pain in their foot and not have a foot as illustrated with phantom limb pain (Melzack, 1991).

Fortunately, there has been a flood of refined scientific data driven by recent technologies such as a positron emission PET scan, functional MRI, single-photon computed tomography (SPECT), magnetoencephalography MEG), and electroencephalography (EEG) studies that have visualized the brain processing nociception (see Davis, 2005). These studies measure such factors as perfusion, metabolism, glucose, and oxygen utilization. We now have data to explain how a painful experience can occur in the forebrain without a concurrent primary nociceptive input in the peripheral nerve (Derbyshire et al., 2004; Eisenberger and Lieberman, 2004; Singer et al., 2004; Casey, 2004). The shift in mindset that considers pain that is unrelated to or out of proportion with the nociceptive stimulus as being a disease state rather than a symptom has accelerated treatment paradigms. When examining a patient with a chronic pain pattern it is now necessary to consider the whole person and their environment rather than just the presenting signs and symptoms; this is an approach that is quite consistent with the Osteopathic Philosophy.

With the brain now available for direct examination, there has been a virtual revolution in accessing the role of forebrain structures in the formulation of a neural matrix used in the perception of pain (Tracey, 2005a; Tracey, 2005b). These data have emphasized the concept that facilitation, long known to occur in the spinal cord secondary to tissue injury, can also occur in the forebrain profoundly influencing our perception (Apkarian et al., 2005). In addition, it is now clear that both bottom-up and top-down processing occurs in pain perception, with the forebrain structure responding to signals from the spinal cord as well as providing descending modulatory information that can influence many ascending signals, all of which creates the complex sensory experience termed pain.

MRI has been particularly useful in identifying pathways and brain regions involved in encoding various aspects of the pain matrix (Tracey and Mantyh, 2007), thereby linking nociception system to pain perception. The lateral-medial division seen in the thalamus is reflected in the organization of the cerebrum, with the lateral component of the nociceptive pathway involved in pain localization and recording pain intensity, while the medial system is encodes an emotional-motivational component. This later system is further tempered by powerful escape and avoidance behaviors (Price, 2000), sculpting the biopsychosocial modulation of pain. Pain is a conscious perception and an emergent property of a complex neuromatrix through which the brain transforms a nociceptive input into a disagreeable perception (Melzack, 1999; May, 2007). Based on functional imaging studies, the areas involved with the pain matrix include the somatic sensory cortex, insula, anterior cingular cortex, prefrontal cortex, and amygdala (Fig. 15.11).

Cortical level activity does appear to be related to pain perception. Coghill and coworkers found a significant correlation between the intensity of the patient's feelings of pain and the amount of cortical activity detectable with functional imaging (Coghill et al., 2003). Specifically, the neural activity was present in somatic sensory cortex, anterior cingulated cortex, and prefrontal cortex. A similar correlation was not found in the thalamus suggesting that cortical level processing is closely tied to our perception of pain.

No one portion of the cortex can entirely account for the perception of pain. Conversely, the perception emerges from simultaneous activity and the interaction of numerous cortical areas of this matrix (Chapman, 2005). Each of these areas will be discussed below. The behavioral responses elicited are shaped by previous

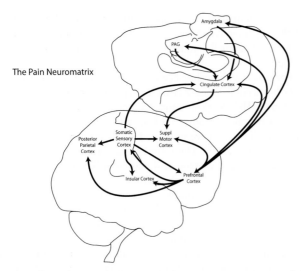

The Pain Neuromatrix

Figure 15-11 The pain Neuromatrix. Numerous regions of the cerebral cortex are interconnected and function to process nociceptive information. From this matrix emerges our complex feelings of pain. (Used with permission from the Willard/Carreiro collection.)

learning, stress levels, attention and arousal, memories, as well as cognitive, emotional, genetic, age-related, gender-related, and sociocultural factors. Pain is inherently unpleasant and associated with real or anticipated tissue damage; its presentation can be masked in a cloud of abnormal body function, chronic pain, and suffering. What has become very clear is that many factors influencing the pain experience are centrally mediated.

Recent studies raise the possibility that patients suffering from chronic pain scenarios may have undergone a significant alteration in the base mechanism of brain function. In 2001, Raichle proposed a Default Mode Network (DMN) as a means of understanding the baseline activity of the cerebrum (Raichle et al., 2001). The DMN represents the resting state of connected activity in representative cortical and subcortical structures. These structures show basal activity when the person is conscious and relaxed. The activity of the DMN is typically greatest at rest and decreases during cognitive processing. Using f-MRI, Blood Oxygen Level Dependent (BOLD) analysis and *functional connectivity* MRI (fc-MRI), signal fluctuations of various regions of interest and their temporal relationship are being explored.

DMN includes prominently the structures of posterior cingulate cortex (PCC) and ventral anterior cingulate cortex (ACC). In addition, the ventromedial prefrontal cortex (VMPFC) and the left inferior parietal cortex (LIPC) are involved. The ventral ACC is linked to limbic and subcortical structures of orbitofrontal cortex (OFC), nucleus accumbens, hypothalamus, and midbrain. These connections represent an emotional affective link in the brain. The PCC is mainly related to cortical structures suggesting a role in consciousness. These all show a decrease in activity on f-MRI, in healthy subjects, when they are asked to perform a simple task. At the same time, with task performance, attention, and cognition, there is an increase in activity in the ventrolateral prefrontal cortex (VLPFC) and in the dorsolateral prefrontal cortex (DLPFC). The lateral prefrontal regions include the OFC, left DLPFC, bilateral IPC, left inferolateral temporal cortex, and the left parahippocampal gyrus (PHG) (Greicius et al., 2003).

Chialvo has confirmed with f-MRI the DMN activity at rest in healthy subjects reveals an equilibrium that shows a decrease in activity when they are asked to pay attention or perform a task

(Baliki et al., 2008). However, in chronic back pain subjects, the DMN activity does not reduce when the subjects are asked to perform simple tasks (Baliki et al., 2008). Those with pain were able to perform the tasks as well as the healthy subjects, but they used their brains differently. This effect was greatest among the patients who had been in pain for the longest period of time. Though the study group was small, it suggests functional reorganization of the brain, altered patterns of brain activity and a possibly irreversibility of these patterns in patients with chronic pain.

Somatic Sensory Cortex (SCC)

The somatic sensory portion of the cerebral cortex is divided into two major regions—SI and SII (Fig. 15.12). SI is located on the post central gyrus and receives input from the ventroposterior thalamic nuclei, while SII is positioned at the base of the post-central gyrus wrapping over the operculum and reaching into the posterior insula lobe and receives input from the ventroposterior inferior nucleus, a small thalamic nucleus closely related to the VP complex (Friedman and Murray, 1986). SI has a high-fidelity representation of the contralateral body, while SII contains a less well-defined representation of the body bilaterally (Millan, 1999; Casey and Tran, 2006). Although considerable question has existed in the older literature as to how much if any nociception is represented in the somatic sensory cortex, recent function mapping studies have shed much light on this situation (reviewed in Aziz et al., 2000). SI appears to be involved in the localization-discrimination of a painful stimulus. At least one carefully documented case of a parietal stroke involving SI in a human diminished the patient's ability to localize a painful stimulus but left him with a strong unpleasant feel induced by the stimulus (Ploner et al., 1999).

Visceral sensory information is also represented on the surface of the parietal cortex. Visceral afferent fibers from the thoracic and upper lumbar spinal cord ascend in the dorsal columns to reach the ventral and medial thalamic nuclei, from which they are relayed to both SI and SII cortex. Although SI can be activated by some noxious visceral stimuli, SII appears to function as primary cortex for visceral information (Aziz et al., 2000). From SII, connections are established with the anterior cingulated cortex and the insular cortex. Ramping up the delivery of visceral noxious stimuli will result

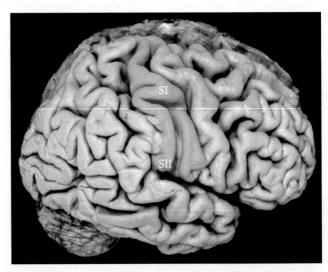

Figure 15-12 Areas I and II of the somatic sensory cortex. (Used with permission from the Willard/Carreiro collection.)

in the spread of the activation outward from SII into the region of the anterior cingulate and insular areas. Thus, SII has been depicted as a gateway into the paralimbic regions of cortex. The differential processing between visceral and somatic nociceptive stimuli at the cortical level may underlie the difference in feeling that characterizes visceral and somatic pains (Aziz et al., 2000).

Insular Cortex (IC)

Located in the depths of the lateral sulcus, between the frontoparietal cortex above and the temporal cortex below (Fig. 15.13), the insula is a major area in the pain cortical pain matrix (Hofbauer et al., 2001). This region of cortex receives thalamic projections from the ventromedial nucleus and posterior nuclei (Friedman and Murray, 1986), areas that are innervated by the spinothalamic tract (reviewed in Craig, 2002). The insula also receives cortical projections from adjacent somatic sensory areas. In primates, SI and SII project to the rostral and caudal portions of the insula (Friedman and Murray, 1986). The same regions of insular cortex that receive pain-related projections feed this information into the limbic forebrain, including such structures as the hypothalamus, amygdala, anterior cingulate cortex, and medial prefrontal cortex (Augustine, 1996; Jasmin et al., 2004). Finally, the insula also has descending projections to the brainstem through which it exerts control over the autonomic nervous system (Jasmin et al., 2004) as well as apparently regulating the descending pain control systems. The insular cortex activity is anatomically heterogeneous (M.-M. Mesulam and E. J. Mufson. Insula of the old world monkey. I: architectonics in the insulo- orbito-temporal component of the paralimbic brain. J.Comp.Neurol. 212:1-22, 1982.) and processing in its posterior portion may be more related to sensory aspects of pain. The anterior IC is anatomically more continuous with PFC and as a result it may be more important in emotional, cognitive, and memory-related aspects of pain perception. Recent studies have documented the presence of opioids such as dynorphin and enkephalin in the insular cortex and suggested a role for these opioid systems in the generation of cortically mediated analgesia (Evans et al., 2006)

One possible interpretation of this neurological arrangement is that the insula, working through the autonomic nervous system, helps to orchestrate physiological response to pain, including pain control or enhancement depending on the situation (Craig, 2002). Interestingly, disruption of the deep white matter at the caudal border of the insula can produce an intense central pain, similar

in quality to thalamic pain; an event termed pseudothalamic pain syndrome (Schmahmann and Leifer, 1992). Conversely, a tumor compressing the posterior aspect of the insula altered tactile perception and the perception of mechanical and thermal pain by raising pain thresholds (Greenspan and Winfield, 1992). Finally, damage to the insula or disconnection of the somatic sensory areas of parietal cortex from the insula has been proposed as the mechanism for the presentation of asymbolia for pain (Geschwind, 1965). In asymbolia, patients can localize the painful stimulus but do not experience the normal emotional or affective nature of the pain. In this state, it is proposed that the link between the somatic sensory system and the limbic system has been interrupted.

Besides interoceptive (somatic and visceral) input, the insula also is the target of olfactory, gustatory, and vestibular information (Shipley and Geinisman, 1984). Recent studies suggest that the anterior insular cortex plays a significant role in forming a short-term memory of an acute pain (Albanese et al., 2007) and possibly integrating the response into a balanced homeostatic mechanism. Thus, the insula could be pooling a wide range of information and passing it on to the limbic system as well as regulating autonomic response patterns (May, 2007).

Anterior Cingulate Cortex (ACC)

A common feature of almost all studies using functional imaging to examine the cerebral processing of pain is the engagement of anterior cingulated cortex. The ACC is traditionally considered part of the limbic system and, as such, is located on the medial aspect of the cerebral hemisphere, wrapped around the genu of the corpus callosum (Fig. 15.14). A major afferent contribution to the anterior cingulate cortex arises in the dorsomedial nucleus of the thalamus and constitutes a significant portion of the medial pain system. Other contributions arise in the intralaminar nuclei of the thalamus and, as such, also involve the medial thalamic pain system.

Activation of ACC has been repeatedly reported in PET studies of somatic or visceral pain and linked to the emotional response to pain (Rosen et al., 1994; Hsieh et al., 1996). Lesions of the ACC do not destroy the ability to perceive acute pain or reduce pain

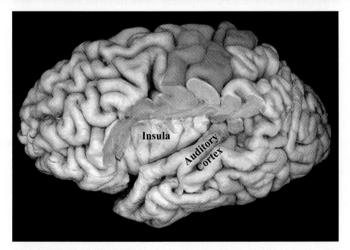

Figure 15-13 The insular cortex. (Used with permission from the Willard/Carreiro collection.)

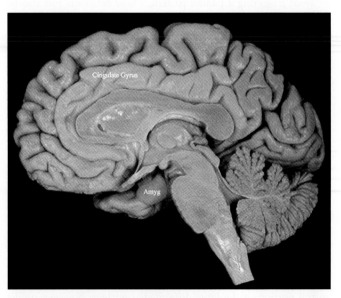

Figure 15-14 The cingulate cortex and the amygdale. (Used with permission from the Willard/Carreiro collection.)

related behaviors; however, they do blunt the affective nature of the pain (Rainville et al., 1997; Johansen et al., 2001; May, 2007).

The anterior cingulate cortex is also associated with the anticipatory emotional aspects of pain (Sewards and Sewards, 2002; Wager et al., 2004). Anticipation can be a particular problem for patients with chronic pain because such patients are already in varying degrees of distress. Researchers have used imaging techniques to characterize brain activation related to the intensity of expected pain and experienced pain, finding that pain-related brain activation overlapped partially with expectation-related activation in regions including anterior insula and the anterior cingulate cortex (Koyama et al., 2005). The ACC is not only involved in the actual perception of pain but also in imagined pain experience and in the (empathic) observation of another human receiving a painful stimulus (Devinsky et al., 1995). When expected pain decreased, activation in this portion of the cerebral cortex also diminished.

The relationship between activity in the ACC and our anticipation and expectation of pain feelings is very strong. Anticipation and expectation have a powerful influence on our eventual perception of pain. Directing attention away from a painful stimulus is known to reduce the perceived pain intensity and results in decreased activation of ACC subregions responsive to painful stimulation (Petrovic et al., 2000; Frankenstein et al., 2001). The placebo response in pain seems to be mediated, at least in part, by the ACC (Wager et al., 2004; Rainville and Duncan, 2006) as does the response to hypnosis (Faymonville et al., 2003; Derbyshire et al., 2004) and numerous other pain distracting techniques discussed in chapter 16.

Pain can be learned through the conditioned process of operant learning, possibly involving processing in the ACC. In some instances, for example, individuals might receive positive reinforcement for the expressions of pain. In studies of patients with chronic back pain who were given a painful electrical stimulation, those with a "solicitous" spouse present had an exacerbated pain response compared with those in the company of a nonsolicitous spouse. Imaging showed that the brain of patients with a solicitous spouse had increased activity in the ACC (Hampton, 2005).

Anticipation of pain can lead to the development of avoidance pain behaviors (Fordyce, 2009). These behavioral patterns represent powerful reflexive activity initiated in an attempt to minimize or avoid triggering a painful pattern. These behaviors can also be learned and are fairly automatic and not always in the patient's conscious awareness. The anticipation of pain can cause patients to avoid movement, tense the muscles, or move completely differently—disrupting mechanisms for posture and balance. These biomechanical imbalances may affect dynamic function, increase energy expenditure, alter proprioception, change joint structure, impede neurovascular function, and alter metabolism. Osteopathic manipulative techniques could be employed to not only restore posture and function but to also reduce fear of movement and the experience of anticipatory pain.

Prefrontal Cortex (PC)

It has been known since the early 1990s that pain is represented in multiple areas of the cerebral cortex and that these areas included portions of the prefrontal cortex (Talbot et al., 1991). In humans, the prefrontal cortex is formed by the very prominent rostral pole of the frontal lobe (Fig. 15.15). This region of cortex receives extensive afferent projections from the medial thalamus including the rostral portion of the large dorsomedial nucleus; however, unlike the other regions of the cortical pain matrix, the prefrontal cortex does not receive input from any portion of a thalamic nucleus

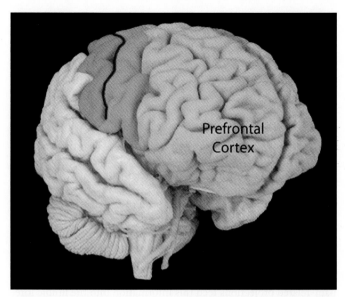

Figure 15-15 The prefrontal cortex. The darker red and blue stripes represent the precentral and postcentral gyri, respectively. (Artwork by Rachel Milner; used with permission from the Willard/Carreiro collection.)

known to receive ascending nociceptive information. Instead, the prefrontal cortex is activated in response to nociceptive stimuli via other regions in the cortical pain matrix such as the ACC (Bushnell and Apkarian, 2006; also see Fig. 15.11).

The prefrontal cortex can be divided into two major regions (Parent, 1996). The prefrontal cortex proper, usually termed dorsolateral prefrontal cortex (DLPFC) represents the convex surface of the frontal lobe. The second region is the orbitofrontal prefrontal cortex (OFC) involving the inferior or orbital surface and the medial (mesal) surface of the frontal lobe. In most functional MR imaging studies, the use of the term OFC also includes the anterior region of the cingulated cortex (ACC) as well.

The prefrontal cortex is activated in some but not all studies of brain representation of nociceptive events; in addition, when prefrontal cortex does demonstrate neuronal activity it is not necessarily proportional to the intensity of the painful stimulus (Coghill et al., 1999; reviewed in Bushnell and Apkarian, 2006). The dorsolateral portion of PFC is thought to be involved with executive functions and appears to play a significant role in the attentive and cognitive aspect of pain (Lorenz et al., 2003). The distinction in functional activity between the OFC and ACC is still not clear in the literature; however, it has been suggested that the strong affective-motivational character of pain develops from activity to this region (Treede et al., 1999) and that the ACC specifically is involved in the unpleasantness of some painful stimuli, while the orbitofrontal cortex, with its massive limbic system connections, may process some of the secondary effects of pain such as emotional feelings and suffering.

Although the precise role of the DLPFC in the forebrain pain matrix is not known at this time, there is a strong suggestion that it is intimately involved in regulating our perception of pain. Consistent with this concept is the observation that, in a paradigm using a thermal probe to sensitize skin, increased activity in the DLPFC correlated with suppression of activity in the medial thalamus and midbrain (Lorenz et al., 2003). This phenomenon suggests that given the proper conditions, the DLPFC can initiate a source of descending inhibition on the ascending nociceptive pathways.

A significant problem encountered when attempting to assign specific pain processing functions to anatomically defined regions of the prefrontal cortex relates to the alteration in cortical activity patterns with temporal sequence (acute vs. chronic). In a recent metastudy reviewing published functional imaging studies of acute and chronic pain patients, it was concluded that the thalamic-somatic sensory cortical pathways leading to activation of the insular cortex and ACC are strongly involved in acute pain patients, whereas in chronic pain patients these same pathways appeared somewhat reduced in activity; conversely in these latter patients, the DLPFC area imaged with increased activity (Apkarian et al., 2005). The shift in brain activity between acute and chronic pain states strongly suggests a plasticity exists in the forebrain processing and that the chronic pain state is a pathology representing uncontrolled or dysregulated activity in certain forebrain areas.

The role of the DLPFC in the pathology of long-term pain states is further suggested by the observation that a significant alteration in brain chemistry (Grachev et al., 2000) and an accompanying loss of neural tissue (Apkarian et al., 2004) occur in this region in patients suffering from various forms of chronic pain (Obermann et al., 2009). The loss in gray matter from the DLPFC was related to the duration of the chronic pain scenario, thereby suggesting some type of fulminating process. Since the loss of gray matter volume has been seen in numerous different forms of chronic pain (May, 2008), it therefore does not appear related to the origin of the pain, but rather to its chronicity.

Interestingly, since studies have shown that the DLPFC is not directly involved in recording the intensity, quality, or location of pain, it may play a more general role in our attending, or not attending to pain. This concept would fit well with the generally accepted role of the DLPFC in working memory, controlling our attention to stimuli, and weighting our decision on whether or not to act on neuronal information processed in other regions of cerebral cortex. Recent studies have pointed to the DLPFC as playing a significant role in our attention to painful stimuli (Lorenz et al., 2003). The amount of activity imaged in the midbrain and thalamus—representing ascending information—triggered by a noxious stimulus was inversely proportional to the activity imaged in the DLPFC. In essence, it is suggested that this region of the prefrontal cortex functions to modulate activity in the ascending pathways and therefore the amount of pain that we may feel. Thus, pathological mechanisms occurring in DLPFC could manifest as increased activity in cortical pain matrix even in the absence of noxious peripheral stimuli. In such a situation, a patient could be feeling significant amounts of pain even though there is no obvious peripheral source for the pain.

Like the dorsolateral PFC, the ventrolateral PFC does not receive direct input for regions of thalamus responding to spinothalamic tract activity. Therefore it also relies of activation to nociceptive stimuli via other cortical areas. Functional imaging studies have provided data linking the activity of VLPFC to descending pain modulation systems in the brainstem (reviewed in Wiech et al., 2008). Recent evidence has tied VLPFC to pain modulation consequent to specific religious beliefs. This context-dependent pain modulation specifically involved the right (nondominant) VLPFC and engaged the ventral midbrain suggesting the initiation of activity in the descending pain modulation systems to create increased tolerance to painful stimuli (Wiech et al., 2008).

All of these observations taken together strongly suggest that the PFC plays a major role in determining our attention to a painful stimulus as well as our ability to modulate the intensity of our feelings of pain. The importance of these observations in developing a sound strategy for pain management in chronic pain patients

and of getting the patient to accept the treatment strategy cannot be over stated. Total lack of confidence in the strategy and obsession over the pain state can initiate a downward spiral that results in pain management failure as well as magnification of the perceived pain on the part of the patient.

Amygdala

The amygdala is located on the medial aspect of the temporal lobe, forming a prominent enlargement termed the uncus, which is visible externally (Fig. 15.14). The amygdala receives numerous projections from most associative portions of the cerebral cortex—particularly the orbitofrontal cortex—as well as a set of subcortical projections from the parabrachial region of the pontomesencephalic border of the brainstem termed the spino-parabrachio-amygdaloid pathway (Jasmin et al., 2004). Intensely painful stimuli, acting through the spino-parabrachio-amygdaloid pathway, exert a strong drive on portions of the amygdala (Neugebauer and Li, 2002). This aspect of the medial temporal lobe is well known for its ability to facilitate (a form of central sensitization), and through this process to form memories of fear-provoking stimuli (Schafe and LeDoux, 2004). Efferent fibers from the amygdala provide a strong drive on hypothalamic and brainstem areas involved in control of the sympathetic-adrenal system. In this manner, the amygdala is capable of initiating a strong arousal response to a painful stimulus, or to the threat of a painful stimulus (Gauriau and Bernard, 2002).

Some of the input to the amygdala is subcortical in nature—that is, it passes from the posterior thalamus to the amygdala without cortical processing. This mechanism provides a possible explanation for patients who, having been exposed to a traumatic event at some earlier point in their life, later experience strong emotional arousal over seemingly inconsequential stimuli. This type of presentation would resemble that seen in posttraumatic stress disorder or PTSD. The initial traumatic event or events facilitated areas in the medial temporal lobe. Subsequently, innocuous stimuli that might only tangentially be related to the initial event can now evoke a major protective response from the amygdala. Given its plasticity, it is possible that the amygdala is a junction point between chronic pain states and those of depression and anxiety along (McEwen, 2005) with the concomitant physiological responses (Neugebauer et al., 2004).

Cerebellum and Basal Ganglia

Functional imaging of an individual exposed to various pain states has frequently demonstrated the involvement of the cerebellum and basal ganglia in the central processing nociceptive information (Bingel et al., 2004; Bushnell and Apkarian, 2006). The cerebellum arises mostly from the pontine portion of the brainstem. The cerebellum is often seen to contain neural activity in pain imaging studies of pain states (Saab and Willis, 2003). Nociceptive events have also been demonstrated to alter neuronal activity in the cerebellar vermis and portions of the hemispheres. Descending pathways from the deep cerebellar nuclei reach several brainstem locations that contribute to the control of nociceptive activity. Nociceptive-related cerebellar activity could relate to the coordination of motor programs necessary to control the individual's pain-related movements. The cerebellum is very clearly involved in learning and memory related to the motor system, and recent studies have suggested that the cerebellum can control large areas of the cerebral cortex, extending much beyond pure motor function (Fiez, 1996; Barinaga, 1996). Supporting this contention is the observation that patients suffering cerebellar damage can present with cognitive and behavioral deficits as well as the expected ataxic movements

(Schmahmann and Sherman, 1998; Schmahmann, 2004). Thus, it is possible that the cerebellar activity evoked by pain is involved in cognitive learning processes.

The basal ganglia are located in the deep white matter of the cerebrum and have well-described connections with much of the cerebral cortex (Parent, 1996). This collection of nuclei represents an integral part of a recurrent pathway linking various regions of the cerebral cortex. Like the cerebellum, the basal ganglia function to regulate the output of the cerebral cortex. A fairly consistent finding in most broad-based functional imaging studies is the involvement of the putamen, a portion of the basal ganglia, in the processing of nociceptive information. As a functional unit, the basal ganglia is known to exert inhibitory influences on the thalamocortical circuitry; thus in processing nociceptive input, the basal ganglia may be modulating the amount of activity in the medial thalamocortical circuits that are critical to the perception of pain (reviewed in Chudler and Dong, 1995). In support of this concept are the observations that diseases of the basal ganglia can interfere with pain thresholds and pain sensitivity.

The Pain Matrix

Our current understanding of supraspinal pain mechanisms based on recent neuroimaging studies and meta-analyses shows a nociceptive system, from primary afferents through the cerebral cortex, strongly modulated by the interactions of ascending and descending pathway (Head and Holmes, 1911; May, 2007). At the level of the forebrain, it has become apparent that no one region in the cerebrum is responsible for our feelings of pain, instead a complex network of reciprocally interconnected regions of the cerebrum respond to noxious stimuli. Our feelings and emotions related to pain are an emergent property of this distributed neural network, termed the pain matrix (Ingvar, 1999; Fig. 15.16). Three separate but interconnected systems for generating the emergent feelings of pain have been defined in this distributed network:

1. A sensory-discriminative system that codes pain location and intensity
2. An affective-motivational system that encodes the suffering associated with the feelings of pain.
3. A cognitive-behavioral system that encodes our conscious behavior to a painful stimulus or to an ongoing painful experience.

The somatosensory cortices on the postcentral gyrus are involved in encoding intensity, temporal and spatial aspects of nociception and thereby functions mainly in the sensory-discriminative zone. Conversely, the anterior cingulate cortex plays a role in the affective-emotional component, as well as in pain-related anxiety and attention. The insula, through its interaction with the autonomic nervous system, appears to be mediating both affective-motivational and sensory-discriminative aspects of pain perception. The prefrontal cortex,

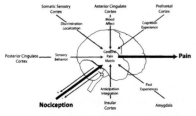

Figure 15-16 The pain neuromatrix takes nociceptive input from the spinal cord (or trigeminal system) and converts into a feeling associated with emotions. (Used with permission from the Willard/Carreiro collection.)

while not having intensity-coding properties, devotes significant amount of processing to the cognitive and emotional introspections and planning strategies underlying efforts to cope with the pain. Finally, the amygdala has emerged as the junction point for anxiety and depression, the negative aspects of pain, sensitizing to past pains and coloring out reception of future painful stimuli.

Pain perception is now clearly distinguished from nociception by the significant engagement of brain regions critical to sensory, affective, and evaluative assessments (Turk et al., 1993; Jerome, 1993). These areas involve:

1. Selectively reviewing all information at the onset of pain.
2. Retaining various aspects of the information to be analyzed and organized into meaningful patterns (i.e., "pain matrix").
3. Comparing this noxious stimulus information to pain information already catalogued in short- and long-term memory.
4. Transmitting recognized pain patterns to specific brain appraisal systems, including those responsible for attaching affect and meaning to the experience; and those responsible for translating the pain experience into behaviors, musculoskeletal reactions, and problem solving routines.
5. Selecting and executing various problem-solving strategies in an effort to adapt and cope with pain.

These pain strategies both influence and are influenced by the patient's neuromusculoskeletal environment.

The Endogenous Pain Control Systems

In response to injury, our body can suppress the transmission of nociceptive information through the spinal cord thus facilitating our ability to focus on escape and survival. Then, when safe to do so, reverse the situation by enhancing nociceptive transmission thereby facilitating protective guarding of the injured structure. To accomplish this control, our brain has the ability to modulate activity in the spinal cord, regulating the amount of information that is allowed to rise to consciousness. Descending pathways of brainstem origin and involving such neurotransmitters as serotonin and norepinephrine among others perform modulation of the dorsal horn and spinal trigeminal nucleus (Mayer and Price, 1976; Fields and Basbaum, 1978); as such these pathways form an endogenous and powerful antinociceptive system (Basbaum and Fields, 1978). Ascending nociceptive information reaches areas in the medulla, rostral pons, and midbrain; in turn these areas can initiate a complex descending pain control system capable of significantly modifying signal transmission in the dorsal horn. This descending system is named for its major nuclei in the brain stem: the periaqueductal gray-rostral medulla- dorsal horn (PAG-RM-DH) system.

This PAG-RM-DH system is under dynamic top-down modulation by brain mechanisms that are associated with anticipation and other cognitive and affective factors. When activated, the descending brainstem pain control systems can dampen pain sensation and inhibit behavior reactions typically evoked by nociception (Fields et al., 2006). This type of pain suppression can permit the use of an injured body part on an emergency basis. Such events are reported in combat situation as well as in competitive athletic events and other high-stakes crisis situations. In this way, the endogenous pain control system can represent a very adaptive behavior.

In addition to its descending control, the PAG-RM-DH system is also capable of enhancing our sensitivity to pain, an event that can also be protective in some situations (Fields et al., 2006). By promoting activities that limit aggravation of the painful area, through immobilization or other protective measures, these systems may have a positive effect on healing. Therefore, enhancing the neurotransmission of nociception and the associated perception of pain may serve an adaptive role. Unfortunately, an extended period of pain facilitation or diminished pain inhibition may no longer be serving an obvious adaptive function and infact creating excess suffering.

A second, descending pain control system has been identified (reviewed in Le Bars, 2002). Unlike the PAG-RM-DH system, when this second system is activated by primary afferent fiber discharge, it provides a diffuse blanket of inhibition over the entire spinal cord, with the exception of the segment that is stimulated. This second system is termed Diffuse Noxious Inhibitory Controls (DNIC). Once DNIC has been initiated, a second nociceptive stimulus at a distance in the body from the first is blunted in its affect on the spinal cord. The neural pathways utilized in DNIC are separate from those of the PAG-RM-DH and involve the subnucleus reticularis dorsalis in the medulla. However, like the PAG-RM-DH system, DNIC is modulated by multiple supraspinal mechanisms. DNIC has been demonstrated in humans and appears to have similar effects in males than females (France and Suchowiecki, 1999), despite the fact that men generally have a higher threshold for pain than women. In women, DNIC was demonstrated to vary somewhat during the menstrual cycle, being most effective during the ovulatory phase (Tousignant-Laflamme and Marchand, 2009).

The observation that at least some of the pain modulation system can facilitate nociceptive transmission as well as inhibit it at the spinal or trigeminal level, coupled with the knowledge that multiple forebrain areas, especially those long felt to be located in the limbic system, exert a strong regulation over these pathways, gives rise to some very intriguing possibilities. Complex supraspinal networks, influenced by emotions and hormones, could be responsible for enhancing as well as suppressing our feeling of pain from a noxious stimulus. Thus, the social and psychological context of the injury along with the degree of anticipation and anxiety as well as the individual's past experience with similar or related stimuli and their current body physiology may have a lot to do with that individual ultimate responds to a noxious stimulus.

Finally, it is important to note that what has been described as "descending endogenous pain control pathways" may be only a specific function of a much more broad-based system controlling numerous aspects of the spinal cord. It has been long known that areas in the brainstem, closely related to those involved in pain modulation, control the functions of the spinal components of the autonomic nervous system as well as the activity of motoneurons in the ventral horns (reviewed in Mason, 2005). Thus, the so-described pain control system may be an integral component of a larger brainstem system controlling spinal facilitation in general.

Pain Perception

There is a significant distinction between nociception and pain perception. Nociception occurs at the peripheral nerve, spinal cord, and brainstem level. It facilitates spinal cord and brainstem circuits, triggering reflexes and unconscious adaptive behavior. Conversely, pain perception begins with the activation of thalamocortical circuitry. The initial stages of pain perception most likely involve the primary and secondary somatic sensory cortical areas, but then rapidly spread outward on the pain matrix to engage numerous other regions such as the insula, anterior cingular, amygdale, and prefrontal cortex as previously described. The perception of pain is a construct (Chapman, 2005) that emerges

from the sum total of activity in this matrix and not a specific property of anyone region. The brain scans a pain threat or the potentially painful event for recognizable patterns in an effort to attach meaning and emotions and to generate strategies to problem solve. Each component of the cortical pain matrix provides aspects of the physiological, emotional, and cognitive response. The native activity in each of these cortical regions is strongly colored by the sum total of previous experience, such as past pains, emotional events—in essence—the baggage of life. It follows then that experience of a given pain and the subsequent emotional reactions that it generates may differ significantly between individuals.

At this point, it is important to distinguish between what is termed acute pain and the more ominous state termed chronic pain. Acute pain, also termed physiological pain or eudynia (good pain) occurs when a noxious stimulus is present. Peripheral nerve and central systems in the spinal cord, brainstem, and forebrain can sensitize and ramp-up activity, but acute pain will remit with the natural course of tissue repair. In contrast, chronic pain, also termed surgical pain or maldynia (bad pain) is pain that is still present 3 to 6 months following the expected natural healing of the injured tissue. In this way, chronic pain represents dysregulation in the normal sensitization systems either at a peripheral nerve, spinal cord, brainstem or forebrain level. From these observations, two significant conclusions can be made. First, chronic pain is a pathology representing altered neuronal activity—such as neuronal cell death—in multiple areas including possibly prefrontal cortex, more so than simply prolonged nociceptive activity triggered by peripheral generators. Second, the longer patients are exposed to chronic pain, the more sensitization mechanisms are stressed and falter leading to greater pain scenarios. Clinically, this means that the longer patients experience chronic pain patterns, they more intense these patterns will become and the harder it will be to ameliorate these pain syndromes.

Pain Behaviors and Problem-Solving Processes

Problem solving implies that humans have the capacity to identify and incorporate potentially useful stimuli, to translate and transform the information received from the stimuli into meaningful patterns, and to use these patterns in forming an optimal response. As the individual thinks about the factors surrounding a painful or damaging event, reasoning and learning are taking place. The individual quickly learns to anticipate damaging events and makes adjustments to optimize their chances for adaptation, new learning, and long-term survival (Sanders, 2002). Historically, the basic need to successfully anticipate and avoid potential tissue-damaging events has set the stage for considerable complex thinking and innovative problem solving. Humans have evolved to become quite good at anticipating, avoiding, or minimizing pain. When these skills are augmented with the ability to create symbols for communication, and to share language, reasoning, and abstract thinking, the result is the capacity for minimizing tissue damage and avoiding persistent pain and new learning.

Persistent pain, as has been documented, can lead to spinal cord excitability, brain reorganization, and self-perpetuating neuronal activity. The psychosocial consequences include anxiety, depression, and a reduction in quality of life (Melzack, 1993). The osteopathic physician often sees a patient who continually seeks medical attention in search of any treatment that will either interrupt the pain signal or help them manage the impact of the pain on their lifestyle. Without pain control, the patient suffers, and the suffering continues until the threat has passed. Pain and suffering form a dynamic-plastic system; dynamic in that the pain matrix continually responds to nociception, and plastic in that it also continually changes as a result of nociception. The constant resynthesis of pain information, coupled with the constant cognitive-emotional appraisals, positions the individuals to either suffer or learn and adapt (Jerome, 1993).

The philosophy of whole-person, health-oriented care that underwrites the Osteopathic profession provides a unique opportunity to help the patient suffering from chronic pain. Pain expression is closely tied to the condition of the musculoskeletal system and thereby acts as a bridge between the body and the mind. This bridge is a two-way street allowing the emergent activity in the mind to influence the physical condition of the musculoskeletal system as well.

Thoughts, Feeling, and Words

When nociception reaches the thalamocortical level and reaches consciousness as pain, thoughts, feelings and words are put to the event, conscious memories form, and behavior adaptations occur. Continuous nociception and activation of past pain memories encourage the assignment of words to pain experiences; lumping a large variety of pain experiences into pain beliefs that form the basis for future thoughts, feelings, behaviors and the problem-solving strategies employed in response to the pain experience. Emotional appraisals of the pain become highly charged when the pain is perceived as having a significant personal impact on function and quality of life. This becomes especially apparent when there is little or no understanding of the origin of the pain or of the future course of the pain.

The emotional appraisal process at the onset of pain begins with orienting and startle reflexes, and feelings of arousal, preparing the individual to engage in more focused attention. Further appraisal might determine that the noxious stimulus is not harming tissue but hurts, and this may cause some anxiety and irritability. If the appraisal concludes that some harm is also occurring, one may develop a feeling of fear about the impact and meaning of the pain. This process can lead to "catastrophizing" about horrible consequences coming from the pain situation (Sullivan et al., 2001; Turk and Monarch, 2002). Pain perception and cortical activity can vary with the patient's degree of vigilance or their perspective on pain, catastrophizing (Seminowicz and Davis, 2006).

In either case, there is generalized musculoskeletal tension, autonomic arousal, and visceral and motor responses, such as those that would be called on to fight or flee. If a person is unable to take any action, they may feel anger and want to fight or sadness from a sense of loss of control because they can't stop the pain or run from it. Over time, the loss of control and decline in personal mastery over the pain leads to depression.

If the pain extends beyond normal healing time, 3 to 6 months leading to the diagnosis of chronic pain (Merskey and Bogduk, 1994), the patient makes further more global appraisals in an effort to understand the overall biopsychosocial effect of their pain on function and quality of life. Emotions attached to this global appraisal include shame, fostered by a sense that one has failed to reach social cultural standards for mastering and living with chronic pain; or guilt, fostered by a sense that one has transgressed personal, family, and/or group member's expectations for adequately coping with pain. As a result of these ongoing cognitive-emotional appraisals, new behaviors are selected, more emotions are labeled and linked to painful musculoskeletal sensations, and the experience of pain and suffering reaches full expression, often through the musculoskeletal system.

Pain and Stress

The neural and endocrine linkage between the nociceptive system and the stress-response system is very strong (Schulkin, 2003a). Both systems operate on a feed-forward mechanism that is adaptive in nature. Neither the stress-response axis, nor the pain-response system has an established set-point around which it operates; thus, when activated, both are open-ended responses that meet the current definition for an allostatic event (Schulkin, 2003a). Both systems offer mechanisms that are protective in the short term or acute response. Acute pain and acute stress are symptoms of a problem that has occurred and that typically will resolve. Both systems can become pathologic (disease) when prolonged. Chronic pain and chronic stress represent diseases that no longer are responding to a triggering stimulus but have taken on a life of their own in the patient.

Both the pain response system and the stress response system have long-loop, slow feedback control system that attempt to reestablish the normal homeostatic rhythms of the body once the nociceptive event or the stressor remits. Destruction of these long-loop control systems through excitotoxic pathologic mechanisms is known to occur. This breakdown in control results in an inability to downregulate either the pain response or the stress response or both (Lee et al., 2002; Schulkin, 2003a; Schulkin, 2003b). In essence, both systems are stuck in the "on" position. In addition, long-term exposure to activity in either or both chronic pain and chronic stress system can result in the onset of depression. Indeed, there is strong crossover between each system. Patients with chronic pain chronically activate the stress response system, often resulting in the onset of depression, while those caught in a chronic stress response are more inclined to develop chronic pain as well (Magni et al., 1994).

Allostatic Mechanisms

Pain—and the stress it creates in the body and brain—is, in essence, an allostatic process influenced by a complex network (i.e., pain matrix) of cortical and subcortical brain structures. All levels of the nociceptive system are capable of an allostatic (feed-forward) response to noxious stimuli. At the level of PANs, peripheral sensitization can occur, in a feed-forward process, enhancing the activity of the fiber. In the spinal cord, central sensitization occurs, again in a feed-forward process, creating regions of segmental facilitation. Similar facilitation also occurs, again using feed-forward mechanisms, in the forebrain areas such as the amygdala. At this level, emotional experiences surrounding the painful event can facilitate amygdaloid activity, resulting in enhanced fear memories and increased drive on the neuroendocrine systems of the hypothalamus and midbrain. These systems increase the production and release of norepinephrine and cortisol resulting in an enhanced protective response to arousal-provoking stimuli such as pain. While such a response may be highly protective in the short-term situation, long-term exposure to allostatic mechanisms is known to be pathologic to numerous body systems thus predisposing one to physiological dysregulation (Chapman et al., 2008) as well as to such psychological states as depression and anxiety. Viewed in this light, chronic pain is the end product or disease that occurs in the nociceptive system when a normal allostatic response such as acute pain exceeds its control systems and becomes fixed in a pathologic state.

Keen understanding of pain from the peripheral generation of a nociceptive signal to its conversion into a painful feeling in the forebrain is necessary to provide a framework for managing somatic dysfunction. The person in pain is more than a biologic event; he or she is a thinking, feeling individual capable of sophisticated problem solving. Such a person, when confronted with chronic pain, actively seeks information, makes decisions, and attempts to put forth their best effort possible in adapting to the painful condition. Osteopathic treatment is aimed at taking the patient beyond the symptom of pain by exploring and treating factors in the patient's life that appropriately modified will facilitate recovery, prevent the reoccurrence of chronic pain, and improve their health and inherent recuperative and restorative powers.

REFERENCES

Abbadie C, Trafton J, Liu HT, et al. Inflammation increases the distribution of dorsal horn neurons that internalize the neurokinin-1 receptor in response to noxious and non-noxious stimulation. *J Neurosci* 1997;17(20):8049–8060.

Albanese MC, Duerden EG, Rainville P, et al. Memory traces of pain in human cortex. *J Neurosci* 2007;27(17):4612–4620.

Alpantaki K, McLaughlin D, Karagogeos D, et al. Sympathetic and sensory neural elements in the tendon of the long head of the biceps. *J Bone Joint Surg Am* 2005;87(7):1580–1583.

Amir R, Devor M. Chemically mediated cross-excitation in rat dorsal root ganglia. *J Neurosci* 1996;16(15):4733–4741.

Apkarian AV, Bushnell MC, Treede RD, et al. Human brain mechanisms of pain perception and regulation in health and disease. *Eur J Pain* 2005;9(4):463–484.

Apkarian AV, Sosa Y, Sonty S, et al. Chronic back pain is associated with decreased prefrontal and thalamic gray matter density. *J Neurosci* 2004;24(46):10410–10415.

Augustine JR. Circuitry and functional aspects of the insular lobe in primates including humans. *Brain Res Rev* 1996;22(3):229–244.

Aziz Q, Schnitzler A, Enck P. Functional neuroimaging of visceral sensation. *J Clin Neurophysiol* 2000;17(6):604–612.

Baliki MN, Geha PY, Apkarian AV, et al. Beyond feeling: chronic pain hurts the brain, disrupting the default-mode network dynamics. *J Neurosci* 2008;28(6):1398–1403.

Barinaga M. The cerebellum: movement coordinator or much more? *Science* 1996;272(5261):482–483.

Basbaum AI. Spinal mechanisms of acute and persistent pain. *Reg Anesth Pain Med* 1999;24(1):59–67.

Basbaum AI, Fields HL. Endogenous pain control mechanisms: review and hypothesis. *Ann Neurol* 1978;4:451–462.

Bielefeldt K, Gebhart GF. Visceral pain: basic mechanisms. In: McMahon SB, Koltzenburg M, eds. *Wall and Melzack's Textbook of Pain*. 5th Ed. Edinburg: Elsevier Churchill Livingston, 2006:721–736.

Bingel U, Glascher J, Weiller C, et al. Somatotropic representation of nociceptive information in the putamen: an event-related fMRI study. *Cereb Cortex* 2004;14(12):1340–1345.

Bove GM, Light AR. Calcitonin gene-related peptide and peripherin immunoreactivity in nerve sheaths. *Somatosens Mot Res* 1995;12(1):49–57.

Braz JM, Nassar MA, Wood JN, et al. Parallel "pain" pathways arise from subpopulations of primary afferent nociceptor. *Neuron* 2005;47(6):787–793.

Bushnell MC, Apkarian AV. Representation of pain in the brain. In: McMahon SB, Koltzenburg M, eds. *Wall and Melzack's Textbook of Pain*. 5th Ed. Philadelphia, PA: Elsevier Churchill Livingstone, 2006:107–124.

Carpenter MB, Sutin J. *Human Neuroanatomy*. 8th Ed. Baltimore, MD: Williams and Wilkins, 1983.

Casey KL. Central pain: distributed effects of focal lesions. *Pain* 2004;108(3):205–206.

Casey KL, Tran TD. Cortical mechanisms mediating acute and chronic pain in humans. In: *Handbook of Neurology*. Vol 81. 2006:159–177.

Cervero F. Mechanisms of acute visceral pain. *Br Med Bull* 1991;47:549–560.

Cervero F. Pain and the spinal cord. In: *Handbook of Clinical Neurology*. Vol 81 (3rd Series). 2006:77–92.

Cervero F, Jänig W. Visceral nociceptors: a new world order? *Trends Neurosci* 1992;15(10):374–378.

Chapman CR. Psychological aspects of pain: a consciousness studies perspective. In: Pappagallo M, ed. *The Neurological Basis of Pain*. New York, NY: McGraw-Hill, 2005:157–167.

Chudler EH, Dong WK. The role of the basal ganglia in nociception and pain. *Pain* 1995;60(1):3–38.

Coghill RC, McHaffie JG, Yen YF. Neural correlates of interindividual differences in the subjective experience of pain. *Proc Natl Acad Sci U S A* 2003;100(14):8538–8542.

Coghill RC, Sang CN, Maisog JM, et al. Pain intensity processing within the human brain: a bilateral, distributed mechanism. *J Neurophysiol* 1999;82(4):1934–1943.

Cook AJ, Woolf CJ, Wall PD, et al. Dynamic receptive field plasticity in rat spinal cord dorsal horn following C-primary afferent input. *Nature* 1987;325:151–153.

Craig AD. How do you feel? Introception: the sense of the physiological condition of the body. *Nat Rev Neurosci* 2002;3(8):655–666.

Davis K. Brain imaging of pain. In: Pappagallo M, ed. *The Neurological Basis of Pain*. New York, NY: McGraw-Hill, 2005:151–156.

Denslow JS. Pathophysiologic evidence for the osteopathic lesion: the known, unknown, and controversial. *J Am Osteopath Assoc* 1975;74:415–421.

Derbyshire SW, Whalley MG, Stenger VA, et al. Cerebral activation during hypnotically induced and imagined pain. *Neuroimage* 2004;23(1):392–401.

Devinsky O, Morrell MJ, Vogt BA. Contributions of anterior cingulate cortex to behaviour. *Brain* 1995;118:279–306.

Dostrovsky JO. Brainstem and thalamic relays. In: *Handbook of Clinical Neurology*. Vol 81(Chap 10). 2006:127–139.

Dostrovsky JO, Craig AD. Ascending projection systems. In: McMahon SB, Koltzenburg M, eds. *Wall and Melzack's Textbook of Pain*. 5th Ed. Edinburg: Elsevier Churchill Livingston, 2006:187–203.

Doubell TP, Mannion RJ, Woolf CJ. Intact sciatic myelinated primary afferent terminals collaterally sprout in the adult rat dorsal horn following section of a neighbouring peripheral nerve. *J Comp Neurol* 1997;380(1):95–104.

Eisenberger NI, Lieberman MD. Why rejection hurts: a common neural alarm system for physical and social pain. *Trends Cogn Sci* 2004;8(7):294–300.

Evans JM, Bey V, Burkey AR, et al. Organization of endogenous opioids in the rostral agranular insular cortex of the rat. *J Comp Neurol* 2006;500(3):530–541.

Faymonville ME, Roediger L, Del FG, et al. Increased cerebral functional connectivity underlying the antinociceptive effects of hypnosis. *Brain Res Cogn Brain Res* 2003;17(2):255–262.

Fields HL, Basbaum AI. Brainstem control of spinal pain-transmission neurons. *Ann Rev Physiol* 1978;40:217–248.

Fields HL, Basbaum AI, Heinricher MM. Central nervous system mechanisms of pain modulation. In: McMahon SB, Koltzenburg M, eds. *Wall and Melzack's Textbook of Pain*. 5th Ed. Edinburg: Elsevier Churchill Livingston, 2006:125–142.

Fiez JA. Cerebellar contributions to cognition. *Neuron* 1996;16(1):13–15.

Fitzgerald M. The development of nociceptive circuits. *Nat Rev Neurosci* 2005;6(7):507–520.

Fordyce W. Behavioral methods for chronic pain and illness. St. Louis, MO: Mosby, 2009.

Fortier LA, Nixon AJ. Distributional changes in substance P nociceptive fiber patterns in naturally osteoarthritic articulations. *J Rheumatol* 1997;24(3):524–530.

France CR, Suchowiecki S. A comparison of diffuse noxious inhibitory controls in men and women. *Pain* 1999;81(1–2):77–84.

Frankenstein UN, Richter W, McIntyre MC, et al. Distraction modulates anterior cingulate gyrus activations during the cold pressor test. *Neuroimage* 2001;14(4):827–836.

Friedman DP, Murray EA. Thalamic connectivity of the second somatosensory area and neighboring somatosensory fields of the lateral sulcus of the macaque. *J Comp Neurol* 1986;252(3):348–373.

Gatchel RJ, Garofalo JP, Ellis E, et al. Major psychological disorders in acute and chronic TMD: an initial examination. *J Am Dent Assoc* 1996;127(9):1365–1370, 1372, 1374.

Gauriau C, Bernard JF. Pain pathways and parabrachial circuits in the rat. *Exp Physiol* 2002;87(2):251–258.

Geschwind N. Disconnection syndrome in animals and man. Part I. *Brain* 1965;88:237–294.

Grachev ID, Fredrickson BE, Apkarian AV. Abnormal brain chemistry in chronic back pain: an in vivo proton magnetic resonance spectroscopy study. *Pain* 2000;89(1):7–18.

Graham BA, Brichta AM, Callister RJ. Moving from an averaged to specific view of spinal cord pain processing circuits. *J Neurophysiol* 2007;98(3):1057–1063.

Greenspan JD, Winfield JA. Reversible pain and tactile deficits associated with a cerebral tumor compressing the posterior insula and parietal operculum. *Pain* 1992;50(1):29–39.

Greicius MD, Krasnow B, Reiss AL, et al. Functional connectivity in the resting brain: a network analysis of the default mode hypothesis. *Proc Natl Acad Sci U S A* 2003;100(1):253–258.

Grigg P, Schaible HG, Schmidt RF. Mechanical sensitivity of group III and IV afferents from posterior articular nerve in normal and inflamed cat knee. *J Neurophysiol* 1986;55:635–643.

Groen GJ, Baljet B, Drukker J. Nerves and nerve plexuses of the human vertebral column. *Am J Anat* 1990;188:282–296.

Grubb BD, Stiller RU, Schaible HG. Dynamic changes in the receptive field properties of spinal cord neurons with ankle input in rats with chronic unilateral inflammation in the ankle region. *Exp Brain Res* 1993;92(3):441–452.

Hampton T. Pain and the brain: researchers focus on tackling pain memories. *JAMA* 2005;293(23):2845–2846.

He X, Proske U, Schaible HG, et al. Acute inflammation of the knee joint in the cat alters responses of flexor motoneurons to leg movements. *J Neurophysiol* 1988;59:326–340.

Head H. *Studies in Neurology.* Vol II. London: Henry Frowde and Hodder & Stoughton, Ltd, 1920.

Head H, Holmes G. Sensory disturbances from cerebral lesions. *Brain* 1911;34:102–254.

Henry JA, Montuschi E. Cardiac pain referred to site of previously experienced somatic pain. *Br Med J* 1978;2(6152):1605–1606.

Hofbauer RK, Rainville P, Duncan GH, et al. Cortical representation of the sensory dimension of pain. *J Neurophysiol* 2001;86(1):402–411.

Hoheisel U, Mense S, Simons DG, et al. Appearance of new receptive fields in rat dorsal horn neurons following noxious stimulation of skeletal muscle: a model for referral of muscle pain? *Neurosci Lett* 1993;153(1):9–12.

Howe JF, Loeser JD, Calvin WH. Mechanosensitivity of dorsal root ganglia and chronically injured axons: a physiological basis for the radicular pain of nerve root compression. *Pain* 1977;3(1):25–41.

Hsieh JC, Hannerz J, Ingvar M. Right-lateralised central processing for pain of nitroglycerin- induced cluster headache. *Pain* 1996;67(1):59–68.

Hunt SP, Rossi J. Peptide- and non-peptide-containing unmyelinated primary afferents: the parallel processing of nociceptive information. *Philos Trans R Soc Lond B Biol Sci* 1985;308(1136):283–289.

Hylden JLK, Nahin RL, Traub RJ, et al. Expansion of receptive fields of spinal lamina I projection neurons in rats with unilateral adjuvant-induced inflammation: the contribution of dorsal horn mechanisms. *Pain* 1989;37:229–243.

Ingvar M. Pain and functional imaging. *Philos Trans R Soc Lond B Biol Sci* 1999;354(1387):1347–1358.

Jasmin L, Burkey AR, Granato A, et al. Rostral agranular insular cortex and pain areas of the central nervous system: a tract-tracing study in the rat. *J Comp Neurol* 2004;468(3):425–440.

Jerome JA. Transmission or transformation? Information processing theory of chronic human pain. *Am Pain Soc J* 1993;2(3):160–171.

Ji RR, Kohno T, Moore KA, et al. Central sensitization and LTP: do pain and memory share similar mechanisms? *Trends Neurosci* 2003;26(12):696–705.

Jinkins JR, Whittermore AR, Bradley WG. The anatomic basis of vertebrogenic pain and the autonomic syndrome associated with lumbar disk extrusion. *Am J Roentgenol* 1989;152:1277–1289.

Johansen JP, Fields HL, Manning BH. The affective component of pain in rodents: direct evidence for a contribution of the anterior cingulate cortex. *Proc Natl Acad Sci U S A* 2001;98(14):8077–8082.

Julius D, Basbaum AI. Molecular mechanisms of nociception. *Nature* 2001;413(6852):203–210.

Kandel ER, Schwartz JH, Jessell TM. Principles of Neural Sciences. 4th Ed. New York, NY: Elsevier, 2000.

Koerber HR, Mirnics K. Plasticity of dorsal horn cell receptive fields after peripheral nerve regeneration. *J Neurophysiol* 1996;75(6):2255–2267.

Koyama T, McHaffie JG, Laurienti PJ, et al. The subjective experience of pain: where expectations become reality. *Proc Natl Acad Sci U S A* 2005;102(36):12950–1295.

Laird JM, Cervero F. A comparative study of the changes in receptive-field properties of multireceptive and nocireceptive rat dorsal horn neurons following noxious mechanical stimulation. *J Neurophysiol* 1989;62(4):854–863.

Le Bars D. The whole body receptive field of dorsal horn multireceptive neurones. *Brain Res Brain Res Rev* 2002;40(1–3):29–44.

Lee AL, Ogle WO, Sapolsky RM. Stress and depression: possible links to neuron death in the hippocampus. *Bipolar Disord* 2002;4(2):117–128.

Levine JD, Fields HL, Basbaum AI. Peptides and the primary afferent nociceptor. *J Neurosci* 1993;13:2273–2286.

Lin Q, Wu J, Willis WD. Dorsal root reflexes and cutaneous neurogenic inflammation after intradermal injection of capsaicin in rats. *J Neurophysiol* 1999;82(5):2602–2611.

Lorenz J, Minoshima S, Casey KL. Keeping pain out of mind: the role of the dorsolateral prefrontal cortex in pain modulation. *Brain* 2003;126(pt 5):1079–1091.

Magni G, Moreschi C, Rigatti-Luchini S, et al. Prospective study on the relationship between depressive symptoms and chronic musculoskeletal pain. *Pain* 1994;56:289–2897.

Mantyh PW, DeMaster E, Malhotra A, et al. Receptor endocytosis and dendrite reshaping in spinal neurons after somatosensory stimulation. *Science* 1995;268(5217):1629–1632.

Mason P. Deconstructing endogenous pain modulations. *J Neurophysiol* 2005;94(3):1659–1663.

May A. Neuroimaging: visualising the brain in pain. *Neurol Sci* 2007;28(suppl 2):S101–S107.

May A. Chronic pain may change the structure of the brain. *Pain* 2008;137(1):7–15.

Mayer DJ, Price DD. Central nervous system mechanisms of analgesia. *Pain* 1976;2(4):379–404.

Mayer DJ, Price DD, Becker DP. Neurophysiological characterization of the anterolateral spinal cord neurons contributing to pain perception in man. *Pain* 1975;1(1):51–58.

McEwen BS. Protective and damaging effects of stress mediators. *N Engl J Med* 1998;338(3):171–179.

McEwen BS. Mood disorders and allostatic load. *Biol Psychiatry* 2003;54(3):200–207.

McEwen BS. Glucocorticoids, depression, and mood disorders: structural remodeling in the brain. *Metabolism* 2005;54(5 suppl 1):20–23.

McLachlan EM, Jänig W, Devor M, et al. Peripheral nerve injury triggers noradrenergic sprouting within dorsal root ganglia. *Nature* 1993;363(6429):543–546.

Melzack R. The gate control theory 25 years later: new prospectives on phantom limb pain. In: Bond MR, ed. New York, NY: Elsevier, 1991.

Melzack R. Pain and the brain. *APS Journal* 1993;2(3):172.

Melzack R. From the gate to the neuromatrix. *Pain* 1999;(suppl 6):S121–S126.

Melzack R, Wall PD. Pain mechanisms: a new theory. *Science* 1965;150(3699):971–979.

Mendell LM. Physiological properties of unmyelinated fiber projection to the spinal cord. *Exp Neurol* 1966;16(3):316–332.

Mense S. Physiology of nociception in muscles. *J Manual Med* 1991;6:24–33.

Mense S, Simons DG. Muscle pain: understanding its nature, diagnosis, and treatment. Philadelphia, PA: Lippincott, Williams & Wilkins, 2001.

Merskey H, Bogduk N. Classification of chronic pain: descriptions of chronic pain syndromes and definitions of pain terms. 2nd Ed. Seattle, WA: International Association for the Study of Pain Press, 1994.

Meyer RA, Ringkamp M, Campbell JN, et al. Peripheral mechanisms of cutaneous nociception. In: McMahon SB, Koltzenburg M, eds. *Wall and Melzack's Textbook of Pain.* 5th Ed. Edinburg: Elsevier Churchill Livingston, 2006:3–34.

Millan MJ. The induction of pain: an integrative review. *Prog Neurobiol* 1999;57(1):1–164.

Munger BL, Ide C. The structure and function of cutaneous sensory receptors. *Arch Histol Cytol* 1988;51(1):1–34.

Nagasako EM, Oaklander AL, Dworkin RH. Congenital insensitivity to pain: an update. *Pain* 2003;101(3):213–219.

Neugebauer V, Li W. Processing of nociceptive mechanical and thermal information in central amygdala neurons with knee-joint input. *J Neurophysiol* 2002;87(1):103–112.

Neugebauer V, Li W, Bird GC, et al. The amygdala and persistent pain. *Neuroscientist* 2004;10(3):221–234.

Neumann S, Doubell TP, Leslie T, et al. Inflammatory pain hypersensitivity mediated by phenotypic switch in myelinated primary sensory neurons. *Nature* 1996;384(6607):360–364.

Neumann S, Woolf CJ. Regeneration of dorsal column fibers into and beyond the lesion site following adult spinal cord injury. *Neuron* 1999;23(1):83–91.

Obermann M, Nebel K, Schumann C, et al. Gray matter changes related to chronic posttraumatic headache. *Neurology* 2009;73(12):978–983.

Parent A. *Carpenter's Human Anatomy*. 9th Ed. Baltimore, MD: Williams & Wilkins, 1996.

Peng YB, Wu J, Willis WD, et al. GABA(A) and 5-HT(3) receptors are involved in dorsal root reflexes: possible role in periaqueductal gray descending inhibition. *J Neurophysiol* 2001;86(1):49–58.

Petrovic P, Petersson KM, Ghatan PH, et al. Pain-related cerebral activation is altered by a distracting cognitive task. *Pain* 2000;85(1–2):19–30.

Ploner M, Freund HJ, Schnitzler A. Pain affect without pain sensation in a patient with a postcentral lesion. *Pain* 1999;81(1–2):211–214.

Prechtl JC, Powley TL. B-afferents: a fundamental division of the nervous system mediating homeostasis? *Behav Brain Sci* 1990;13:289–331.

Premkumar LS, Raisinghani M. Nociceptors in cardiovascular functions: complex interplay as a result of cyclooxygenase inhibition. *Mol Pain* 2006;2:26.

Price DD. Psychological and neural mechanisms of the affective dimension of pain. *Science* 2000;288(5472):1769–1772.

Raichle ME, Macleod AM, Snyder AZ, et al. A default mode of brain function. *Proc Natl Acad Sci U S A* 2001;98(2):676–682.

Rainville P, Duncan GH. Functional brain imaging of placebo analgesia: methodological challenges and recommendations. *Pain* 2006;121(3):177–180.

Rainville P, Duncan GH, Price DD, et al. Pain affect encoded in human anterior cingulate but not somatosensory cortex. *Science* 1997;277(5328):968–971.

Ramer MS, Bisby MA. Rapid sprouting of sympathetic axons in dorsal root ganglia of rats with a chronic constriction injury. *Pain* 1997;70(2–3):237–244.

Ramon y Cajal S. *Histologie du Systeme Nerveux de l'Homme et des Vertebres*. L. Azoulay, trans. Madrid (1952–1955): Instituto Ramon y Cajal del C.S.I.C., 1909.

Rees H, Sluka KA, Lu Y, et al. Dorsal root reflexes in articular afferents occur bilaterally in a chronic model of arthritis in rats. *J Neurophysiol* 1996;76(6):4190–4193.

Rees H, Sluka KA, Westlund KN, et al. Do dorsal root reflexes augment peripheral inflammation? *Neuroreport* 1994;5(7):821–824.

Rosen SD, Paulesu E, Frith CD, et al. Central nervous pathways mediating angina pectoris. *Lancet* 1994;344(8916):147–150.

Saab CY, Willis WD. The cerebellum: organization, functions and its role in nociception. *Brain Res Brain Res Rev* 2003;42(1):85–95.

Sanchez del Rio M, Moskowitz MA. The trigeminal system. In: Olesen J, Tfelt-Hansen P, Welch KMA, eds. *The Headaches*. 2nd Ed. Baltimore, MD: Lippincott, Williams and Wilkins, 141–15, 2000.

Sanders SH. Operant conditioning with chronic pain: back to basics. In: *Psychological approaches to the Management of Pain: A Practitioner's Handbook*. New York, NY: Guilford Press, 2002:128–137.

Sato A. Somatovisceral reflexes. *J Manipulative Physiol Ther* 1995;18(9):597–602.

Sato A, Sato Y, Schmidt RF, et al. Somato-vesical reflexes in chronic spinal cats. *J Auton Nerv Syst* 1983;7:351–362.

Schafe GE, LeDoux JE. The neural basis of fear. In: Gazzaniga MS, ed. *The Cognitive Neurosciences*. 3rd Ed. Cambridge, MA: A Bradford Book, MIT Press, 2004:987–1003.

Schaible HG, Grubb BD. Afferent and spinal mechanisms of joint pain. *Pain* 1993;55:5–54.

Schmahmann JD. Disorders of the cerebellum: ataxia, dysmetria of thought, and the cerebellar cognitive affective syndrome. *J Neuropsychiatry Clin Neurosci* 2004;16(3):367–378.

Schmahmann JD, Leifer D. Parietal pseudothalamic pain syndrome. Clinical features and anatomic correlates. *Arch Neurol* 1992;49(10):1032–1037.

Schmahmann JD, Sherman JC. The cerebellar cognitive affective syndrome. *Brain* 1998;121 (pt 4):561–579.

Scholz J, Broom DC, Youn DH, et al. Blocking caspase activity prevents trans-synaptic neuronal apoptosis and the loss of inhibition in lamina II of the dorsal horn after peripheral nerve injury. *J Neurosci* 2005;25(32):7317–7323.

Schulkin J. *Rethinking Homeostasis*. Cambridge, MA: The MIT Press, 2003a.

Schulkin J. Allostasis: a neural behavioral perspective. *Horm Behav* 43(1):21–27, 2003b.

Schulkin J, McEwen BS, Gold PW. Allostasis, amygdala, and anticipatory angst. *Neurosci Biobehav Rev* 1994;18(3):385–396.

Selye H. The general adaptive syndrome and the diseases of adaptation. *J Clin Endocrinol* 1946;6:117–173.

Seminowicz DA, Davis KD. Cortical responses to pain in healthy individuals depends on pain catastrophizing. *Pain* 2006;120(3):297–306.

Sewards TV, Sewards MA. The medial pain system: neural representations of the motivational aspect of pain. *Brain Res Bull* 2002;59(3):163–180.

Shipley MT, Geinisman Y. Anatomical evidence for convergence of olfactory, gustatory, and visceral afferent pathways in mouse cerebral cortex. *Brain Res Bull* 1984;12:221–226.

Singer T, Seymour B, O'Doherty J, et al. Empathy for pain involves the affective but not sensory components of pain. *Science* 2004;303(5661):1157–1162.

Skinner EA, Edge K, Altman J, et al. Searching for the structure of coping: a review and critique of category systems for classifying ways of coping. *Psychol Bull* 2003;129(2):216–269.

Stilwell DL. The nerve supply of the vertebral column and its associated structures in the monkey. *Anat Rec* 1956;125:139–169.

Stumvoll M, Tataranni PA, Stefan N, et al. Glucose Allostasis. *Diabetes* 2003;52(4):903.

Sugiura Y, Terui N, Hosoya Y. Difference in distribution of central terminals between visceral and somatic unmyelinated (C) primary afferent fibers. *J Neurophysiol* 1989;62:834–840.

Sullivan MJ, Thorn B, Haythornthwaite JA, et al. Theoretical perspectives on the relation between catastrophizing and pain. *Clin J Pain* 2001;17(1):52–64.

Talbot J, Marrett S, Evans A, et al. Multiple representations of pain in human cerebral cortex. *Science* 1991;251:1355–1358.

Todd AJ. Anatomy and neurochemistry of the dorsal horn. In: *Handbook of Neurology* 2006; 81(3rd Series):61–76.

Tousignant-Laflamme Y, Marchand S. Excitatory and inhibitory pain mechanisms during the menstrual cycle in healthy women. *Pain* 2009;146 (1–2):47–55.

Tracey I. Functional connectivity and pain: how effectively connected is your brain? *Pain* 2005a;116(3):173–174.

Tracey I. Nociceptive processing in the human brain. *Curr Opin Neurobiol* 2005b;15(4):478–487.

Tracey I, Mantyh PW. The cerebral signature for pain perception and its modulation. *Neuron* 2007;55(3):377–391.

Treede RD, Kenshalo DR, Gracely RH, et al. The cortical representation of pain. *Pain* 1999;79(2–3):105–111.

Turk DC, Melchenbaum D, Genest M. *Pain and Behavior Medicine: A Cognitive Behavioral perspective*. New York, NY: Guilford Press, 1993.

Turk DC, Monarch ES. Biopsychosocial perspective on chronic pain. In: *Psychological Approaches to the Management of Pain: A Practitioner's Handbook*. New York, NY: Guilford Press, 2002:128–137.

Victor M, Ropper AH. *Principles of Neurology*. 7th Ed. New York, NY: McGraw-Hill Health Professions Division, 2001.

Wager TD, Rilling JK, Smith EE, et al. Placebo-induced changes in FMRI in the anticipation and experience of pain. *Science* 2004;303(5661):1162–1167.

Wall PD, Bennett DL. Postsynaptic effects of long-range afferents in distant segments caudal to their entry point in rat spinal cord under the influence of picrotoxin or strychnine. *J Neurophysiol* 1994;72(6):2703–2713.

Wall PD, Woolf CJ. Muscle but not cutaneous C-afferent input produces prolonged increases in the excitability of the flexion reflex in the rat. *J Physiol (Lond)* 1984;356:453–458.

Watkins LR, Wieseler-Frank J, Hutchinson MR, et al. Neuroimmune interactions and pain: the role of immune and glial cells. In: Ader R, ed. *Psychoneuroimmunology*. Vol 1, 4th Ed. Amsterdam The Netherlands: Elsevier Academic Press, 2007:393–414.

Westlund KN. Neurophysiology of pain. In: Pappagallo M, ed. *The Neurological Basis of Pain*. New York, NY: McGraw-Hill, 2005:3–19.

Wiech K, Farias M, Kahane G, et al. An fMRI study measuring analgesia enhanced by religion as a belief system. *Pain* 2008;139(2):467–476.

Wieseler-Frank J, Maier SF, Watkins LR. Immune-to-brain communication dynamically modulates pain: physiological and pathological consequences. *Brain Behav Immun* 2005;19(2):104–111.

Willard FH. The muscular, ligamentous and neural structure of the low back and its relation to back pain. In: Vleeming A, Mooney V, Snijder CJ, Dorman T, Stoeckart R, eds. *Movement, Stability and Low Back Pain*. Edinburgh: Churchill Livingstone, 1997:3–35.

Willis WD. Physiology of dorsal horn and spinal cord pathways related to pain. In: Beers RF, Bassett EG, eds. *Mechanisms of Pain and Analgesic Compounds*. New York, NY: Raaven Press, 1979:143–156.

Willis WD. Dorsal root potentials and dorsal root reflexes: a double-edged sword. *Exp Brain Res* 1999;124(4):395–421.

Wilson P, Kitchener PD. Plasticity of cutaneous primary afferent projections to the spinal dorsal horn. *Prog Neurobiol* 1996;48(2):105–113.

Chronic Pain Management

MITCHELL L. ELKISS AND JOHN A. JEROME

KEY CONCEPTS

- Pain is an unpleasant sensory and emotional experience. Acute pain is a symptom; chronic pain is a disease.
- The pain neuromatrix is nested in the central nervous system, where modulation, transmission, and transduction of noxious stimulation occur.
- The musculoskeletal, immune, neurologic, and endocrine (MINE) systems interact as one "supersystem" in response to nociception.
- Body unity and structure/function interrelationships guide osteopathic thinking regarding chronic pain management.
- Stress dysregulates the MINE supersystem, predisposing one to chronic pain.
- Chronic pain results from a sustained loss of a system's ability to function normally with regard to its own self-regulation and/or its normal regulatory role interacting with other systems.
- Osteopathic assessment of chronic pain is dynamic, patient focused, and comprehensive.
- Osteopathic pain management integrates the five models as the standard of care for pain management.

INTRODUCTION

The National Institute of Health describes pain as a leading public health problem affecting more than 75 million Americans, more than the number of people with diabetes, heart disease, and cancer combined (1). This translates into 70 million health care visits a year, making pain a leading cause for health care utilization (2). In a large study of primary care practices, 50% of patients regularly reported experiencing pain and associated dysfunction. Health care utilization for chronic pain patients is *five times* that of those without chronic pain (3).

In the evaluation and management of patients with chronic pain, osteopathic medicine offers a particularly illustrative example of its unique diagnostic and therapeutic potential. The principles that have defined osteopathic philosophy and practices can be readily recognized as central to the process of diagnosis and treatment of patients with chronic pain.

In osteopathic medicine, the emphasis is placed on evaluating, not just the painful region of the patient, but the "person who is in pain"; taking into consideration the general health of their body, their relations with family and close associates, as well as their cultural background. In this manner, the pain syndrome is seen as nested in ever-expanding circles of influence. Each element in this nested array represents a diagnostic vector capable of affecting other elements, at every other level (Fig. 16.1).

Chronic pain management has been formally studied only since the late 20th century. In that time, we have come to understand profound influence that noxious peripheral stimuli can have on the musculoskeletal, immune, and endocrine systems as well as the central nervous system (CNS). In the spinal cord, brainstem and forebrain regions, synaptic organization and function can change rapidly, in response to acute nociceptive input (4). Such changes can range from the molecular, to the gross, structural levels, involving alterations in gene expression and protein synthesis. These immediate responses can be transient or long term, and, unfortunately, given the right circumstances, can become permanent. Certainly, one of the most profound findings in the recent research on pain is the dynamic or plastic nature of this beast and its pervasive influence on body physiology and behavior (5).

Therefore, it is important to keep in mind, when evaluating a patient in pain, that the process is dynamic and may rapidly evolve in catastrophic directions.

Detailed and repeated examinations are required to monitor the situation. Treatment protocols must have both a strong evidence-based grounding and the confidence of the patient in order to succeed (6). Finally, the irony involved in evaluating a patient in pain is that for the patient this is a first-person subjective experience, strongly colored by prior experience, that the physician is attempting to convert into a third-person investigation, for the purpose of diagnosis and the design of an appropriate treatment and management regimen.

Pain is an unpleasant sensory and emotional experience. In 1982, the subcommittee on Taxonomy of the International Association for the Study of Pain (IASP) redefined pain by integrating both physiological and psychological components. This definition was published in *Pain* (IASP) (7) as well as in the *Proceedings of the 3rd World Congress on Pain* (8).

Pain: An unpleasant sensory and emotional experience associated with actual or potential tissue damage, or described in terms of such damage.

> Note: Pain is always subjective. Each individual learns the application of the word through experiences related to injury in early life. Pain is the experience that we associate with actual or potential tissue damage. It is always unpleasant and therefore an emotional experience. Many people report pain in the absence of tissue damage or any pathophysiological cause; usually, this happens for psychological reasons. This definition avoids tying pain to the stimulus. Activity induced in the nociceptor and nociceptive pathways by noxious stimulus is not pain, which is always a psychological state.

The following policy statement on pain was adopted by the American Osteopathic Association's House of Delegates in 1997 and reviewed in 2002 and 2005. Chronic pain means "a pain state in which the cause of the pain cannot be removed or otherwise definitively treated and which in the generally accepted course of

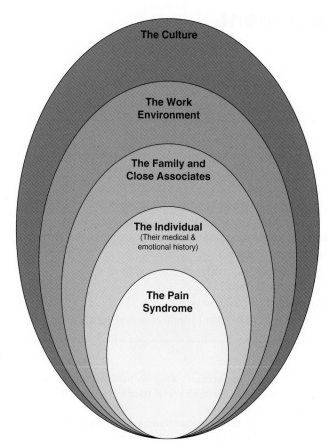

Figure 16-1   The nested spheres of influence on the pain syndrome.

medical practice, no relief or cure of the cause of the pain is possible or none has been found after reasonable efforts" (9,10). Osteopathic physicians recognize a duty and a responsibility to treat patients suffering from chronic pain. Certainly, the differences between acute pain and chronic pain represent qualitatively different experiences for both patient and clinician.

In this chapter, we learned that nociception is related to the process of detecting real or potential tissue damage. Specialized A-delta and C fibers (nociceptors) respond to a variety of noxious stimuli. They convert the chemical, mechanical, or thermal stimuli into altered neuronal activity. This is largely transmitted to the dorsal horn in segment derived, organized, receptive patterns. The nociceptor responses themselves are affected by local chemical and neural activity. In their normal state, they respond to energies capable of damaging cells. In abnormal states, they can demonstrate altered response characteristics associated with hyperalgesia and painful responses to noninjurious stimuli, known as allodynia. Nociception can be disrupted or enhanced by descending modulation from the brain and brainstem. In chronic pain, there is a bias toward greater nociceptive facilitation and less inhibition.

Pain is the response to nociception. When the system is healthy, it represents nociceptor-driven activity in the spinal cord and brain. When the system is not healthy, it may represent impaired function of the peripheral nervous system (PNS) or CNS. Pain may be experienced even when there is no noxious stimulus (i.e., phantom limb pain) (11).

Therefore, pain is a perception. This perception is part of a greater pain experience.

Suffering is a negative affective experience and response to pain. It is seen in association with pain and other psychic states (i.e., "a broken bone can cause pain... while the suffering of a broken

heart may often be inconsolable"). Suffering is associated with activity in specific brain regions. It, too, is under the influence of ascending and descending influences. It is a feeling. This feeling is part of a greater pain experience. It frequently leads to pain behaviors. Often, it is this suffering that is the primary concern driving a patient to seek health care.

Acute pain is a symptom. Acute pain is usually associated with a well-defined biological cause and a rapid onset that alerts you to the possibility of tissue damage. It usually vanishes as healing occurs. Acute pain follows an injury to the body and implies a natural healing process of short duration. It is only expected to persist as long as the tissue pathology itself. Acute pain is often, but not always, associated with objective physical signs of:

- Increased cardiac rate
- Increased systolic and diastolic blood pressure
- Increased pupil diameter
- Striated muscle tension
- Decreased gut motility
- Decreased salivary flow
- Decreased superficial capillary flow
- Fear and/or anxiety
- Releases of glycogen, adrenaline, and noradrenaline

These are collectively understood as the alarm response and the secondary stages of resistance/healing that can lead to recovery. These changes in nociceptive activity have been assumed to be roughly proportional to the intensity of a noxious stimulus. The enormous biologic value of acute pain is to promote a rapid orientation to the noxious stimulus, and, to promote reactions to minimize or escape the damage being done by the noxious stimulus. Some pain fosters rest, protection, and care of the injured area during healing, thereby promoting recuperation. In other situations, acute pain can be suppressed temporarily in the service of a greater circumstance. These examples can be seen on the battlefield, the athletic field, and in emergency, crisis situations as anyone might experience (11).

The overall behavioral signs of acute pain are agitation and the emerging flight-or-fight reaction. Patients with acute pain are anxious about the pain's intensity, meaning, and impact on themselves and their lifestyles (12). This is rapidly followed by the resistance phase during which the organism resists a compromise of homeostasis. Through allostatic actions of the integrated musculoskeletal (M), immune (I), neural (N), and endocrine (E) systems, the person is led toward recovery.

Unfortunately, and rather often, pain persists after initial healing. It may persist after all conventional medical treatments and drugs have been tried to little or no avail. A constant barrage of erratic nociceptive impulses into the brain provides no new or useful information, but the adverse signal continues to reach consciousness. As an example, a patient with a failed back surgery 2 years postoperatively does not need to experience pain every time he moves his spine to remind him that he has scar tissue, adhesions, and functional changes in the structure of his back. Since he is no longer in the acute healing phase, the information provided by this type of repetitive noxious stimulation may lead to central sensitization, with musculoskeletal, immunologic, neurologic, endocrinologic disturbances, and abnormalities of regional cerebral blood flow (13) and metabolism.

Chronic pain is a disease that can affect both the structure and the function of the CNS (14). Pain patients imaged with functional magnetic resonance imaging (f-MRI), positron emission tomography (PET), single-photon emission computed tomography (SPECT), and magnetoencephalography (MEG) have revealed changes in neural processing that differentiates chronic pain from acute pain (15–17).

In patients with irritable bowel syndrome (18) with chronic pain, there is cortical thinning, and cell loss in the anterior cingulate cortex and anterior insula. Similar changes are also seen in chronic tension headache (22) and chronic back pain (4). In addition, effects are seen on thalamic and prefrontal gray matter density, as well as on ascending and descending pain-modulating pathways (19). In the fibromyalgia syndrome, there is an altered sensitivity to stimulation, with sensitization in pain-related neural activity (20). In migraine sufferers, there has been a reported thickening of the somatosensory cortex (21).

It is also reasonable to consider that a person's inherent structural/functional neural capacity may predispose them to the development of chronic pain. Genetically determined or acquired disturbances in the neural circuitry affecting neurotransmitter production and metabolism, receptor morphology and function, ion channel structure and function, disturbances of the neurons, their cell bodies and metabolism, their axons, their transmission properties, their structure and function, the tracts in which they run, the nuclei that they form, and their neuronal/glial interactions, all help create a pain neuromatrix.

The pain neuromatrix is nested in the CNS, where modulation, transmission, and transduction of noxious stimulation occur. At the basic biochemical level, when noxious stimulation of muscle afferent C fibers is prolonged and persistent, excitatory amino acid and neurotransmitters are released in greater amounts and for longer periods (23), the resulting activation of *N*-methyl-D-aspartate (NMDA) receptors and the release of substance P, both centrally and peripherally, lead to hyperexcitability of PNS and CNS neurons with expansion of the size of the painful area beyond the original site of damage. This peripheral and central sensitization, the enlargement of peripheral pain receptor fields (24), allows noxious sensations to be experienced as more painful (hyperalgesia) (25) and even non-noxious sensations as painful (allodynia).

Primary hyperalgesia occurs at the site of tissue damage as an increased sensitivity to heat or mechanical stimulation. This primary hyperalgesia is due to peripheral sensitization (26). That is one way in which a healthy peripheral nerve can be chronically activated at its periphery. For heat, it has been linked to sensitization of the peripheral terminals of the primary pain afferents (27). The primary afferent can also be sensitized by descending noradrenergic and serotonergic systems that work directly, in the spinal cord, on the primary afferent's central terminals (presynaptic) and on the segmental interneurons to increase their sensitivity in chronic pain states. *Secondary hyperalgesia* occurs around the site of tissue damage, manifesting as an increased sensitivity to mechanical stimulation only. This secondary hyperalgesia is due to central sensitization. It is in this enlarged receptive field that mechanical stimulation elicits abnormally increased responses from second-order afferents in the spinal cord to normal afferent input. It is, in part, NMDA receptor mediated. It appears to be related to increased synaptic efficacy, which is molecularly similar to long-term potentiation (LTP). This represents a form of intercellular learning. It, too, is subject to descending modulation of both inhibitory and excitatory influences.

The lateral system ascends to the lateral thalamus, synapses, and projects to the primary and secondary somatosensory cortex and the insular cortex. The insular cortex and claustrum appear to represent a site of major sensory modality convergence. It is largely associated with the discriminative aspects of stimulus quality, intensity, location, and duration.

The medial system projects to the brainstem and ultimately to the medial thalamus. It sends projections to the anterior cingulate cortex. The insular and anterior cingulate cortex project to the amygdala and then to the brainstem. From the brainstem, projections can be ascending and descending. The descending projections can inhibit and disinhibit the activities in the spinal cord and lower brain stem and in this way contribute to primary and secondary hyperalgesia.

The medial nociceptive system has been associated with general arousal, emotional, autonomic, motor responses, leading the drive to end the painful problem. Here, then, afferent sensory information is linked to efferent autonomic and gross motor actions of defense and avoidance. This activity may be studied with objective measures of chemical levels, neural activity, and gross behaviors.

The cognitive evaluation occurs in view of past experience, memory, and expectation and is cortically and subcortically mediated. The way a person feels and thinks about their pain condition actually can affect the way they process and cope with pain. Cognitive elements promote modulation of the medial and lateral ascending nociceptive systems and provide a connection to the conscious experience.

The endogenous opioid system is richly represented at all levels of the neuraxis involved in pain processing. It is part of the parallel distributed and integrated endogenous system for relieving pain. It is part of the medicine chest to which A.T. Still referred. It, however, can be inadequate in states of chronic pain. Ironically, the long-term use of exogenous opioids, usually from the doctor, can inhibit the body's capacity to respond to pain. The chronicity of pain is associated with structural and functional changes at multiple levels of the neuraxis (4). It can involve changes in excitability, lowered thresholds and higher gain in the system, changes in receptors, channel-mediated changes, and second messenger effects, transduction and translational effects at the cellular level, and changes in synaptic efficacy (14). This form of LTP is part of the neural basis for learning, known as *plasticity*. Plasticity means that the nervous system has the capacity to change its structure in response to environmental demands (28,29). Maladaptive plasticity (4,30) at several levels of the nervous system is the biology behind the continuation of pain long after the original offending event has passed, depriving pain of its functional role of protection, withdrawal, adaptation, and functional recovery (4,31,32). Plasticity can also be influenced by and can certainly influence the development of depression and anxiety (27,39).

When pain results in the activation of peripheral nociceptive afferents, there is tremendous activity in the brain. It is clear that pain perception requires a brain. "No brain, no pain." Proceeding from the peripheral receptive fields associated with the pain, there is an activation of limbic, autonomic, brainstem, and spinal cord networks of modulation (33–36).

Parallel neural networks of processing pain information are responsible for the pain behaviors resulting from the peripheral activation of nociceptors (12,38). These parallel networks are always represented in some ratio to each other. The ratio varies as the *symptoms* of acute pain become the *disease* of chronic pain (37).

Finally, it is important for the osteopathic physician to recognize that a systems network understanding of chronic pain would not be complete without consideration of the structural/functional *interactions* of the musculoskeletal, immune, neurologic, and endocrine (MINE) systems in response to nociception. *The MINE systems interact as one "supersystem" in response to nociception.*

Chapman talks about a system of "reciprocal, neural, endocrine, and immune interactions" (36) in the human response to pain and stress. In this, he posits a coherent model of interacting systems with global and local features. From there, complex pain behaviors emerge as immune (I), neurologic (N), and endocrine (E) interactions (i.e., INE system). Chapman's comprehensive, systematic review of the immune-neural-endocrine systems as they respond to pain and stress is a clear elaboration of principles, which are characteristic of osteopathic medical thinking. This, then, joins the works of Denslow and Korr, as further demonstration of the underlying biologic, anatomic, and physiologic substrata of human functioning. When Chapman describes his INE system, he calls it a "nested system." It provides a nest for the INE systems and is itself nested in a larger, more complex system. That is, it is nested, nurtured and nurturing, defended and defending a greater system. This greater system is the neuromusculoskeletal system whose activity is crucial to our survival. The neuromusculoskeletal system "enables us to respond to, interact with, and even alter, the external environment. Through its activity, our needs are expressed and met. It is through the use of our neuromusculoskeletal system by which we define our niche as a unique species on the planet" (ECOP, 2000).

The reciprocal interactions of these four systems—musculoskeletal (M), immune (I), neurologic (N), and endocrine (E)—as they interact in response to nociception form a *MINE system* that is continually adjusting to incoming information from both internal and external environments.

Many of the behavioral responses of the MINE system can be observed and measured. The behaviors occur at levels of scale, from the molecular to the cellular, to the whole human level. The responses represent both incoming information about the outer world and outward directed responses designed to meet and satisfy the needs and drives of that person to decrease their pain. The four individual systems that comprise the MINE system demonstrate feedback effects that can be both facilitating and inhibiting. They show connection, through their common shared receptors and their associated ligands. Neurotransmitters, peptides, hormones, cytokines, and endocannabinoids are the biochemical messengers, responsible for some of the interactive crosstalk between these four systems.

The final pain effects of the MINE system interactions vary depending on where, when, and how they are expressed and reinforced by the environment. Pain inhibitory or excitatory systems and MINE feedback and feed-forward mechanisms are all at work. Though elements within each individual MINE system can be reduced to relatively simple observable physical/chemical activity, their coordinated interactive efforts create a more complex system of observable pain behaviors.

Figure 16-2 MINE supersystem in response to noniceptive input.

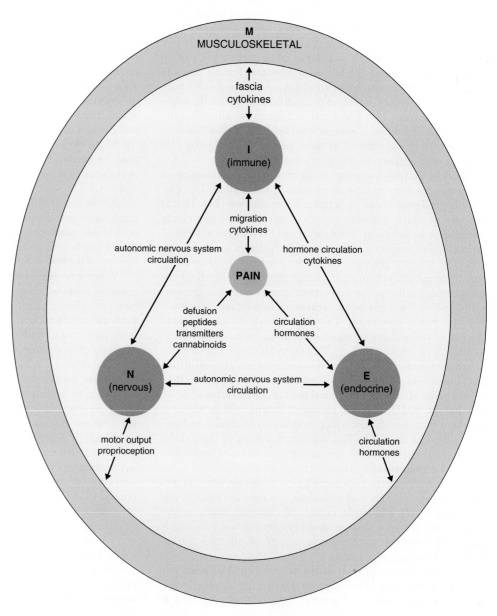

For example, measurements can be made of afferent nociceptive activity in primary afferent neurons, ascending secondary afferents, brainstem, subcortical and cortical neurons; hormone levels and endocrine activity; and immune system expression of cytokines. These are the simple activities. The fight or flight response, the endocrine aspect of stress response, and the inflammatory reaction are examples of more complex pain behavior. Even more complex is the individual's ability to recognize danger and avoid it and run or fight as needed. The ability to fight off infection, the ability to recover from abuse or trauma, or the capacity to suffer are representative behaviors of even greater complexity. These coordinated complex whole-body behaviors are based upon simple principles occurring at every level of the system.

Dysregulation within the MINE system also has individual components that can be measured, modeled, and understood. The multitude of possible states and phases, for each of the four systems, from the level of the atomic, to the whole human, represent all the possibilities for healing or obstruction. "Remove all obstruction; and when it's intelligently done, nature will kindly do the rest." (A.T. Still)

The human pain system is thus characterized as dynamic. The dynamics of these systems are very sensitive to initial nociceptive conditions. That is, even though many parameters can be measured and monitored, in the face of apparent deterministic anatomic, physiologic, and pathophysiologic principles, there is still an inherent unpredictability. Because there is such sensitivity to nociception, one must be able to account for and manage every circumstance at every scale, at every moment. This is obviously not possible with chronic pain. Furthermore, slight variations or perturbations in one or another system can result in exponential expression or change from that perturbation. Therefore, with nociception, there is unpredictability. Pain behaviors in the patient often appear random, nonlinear, or chaotic; yet these behaviors are characteristic for dynamic systems. Complexity and emergence of chronic pain behaviors, in this complex pain system, is natural. *Body unity and structure/function interrelationships guide osteopathic thinking regarding chronic pain management.*

Each of the MINE subsidiary systems has an inherent capacity for self-regulation, self-learning, and health maintenance. Any of these subsidiary systems can also break down. Chronic pain, therefore, is likely an effect or consequence of system breakdowns or dysregulation.

Sometimes it is easy to understand why a patient might be hurting and other times it is less easy to explain how a particular set of circumstances might result in a patient's unique pain expression and experience. Understanding this dynamic pain system's extreme sensitivity to initial and/or prolonged nociceptive conditions makes it understandable that some people will become chronically painful (36).

The idea of holistic, interactive, nested systems, such as the MINE supersystem, is an idea consistent with osteopathic philosophy. The MINE system has properties greater than the sum of its individual subsidiary systems. The MINE system explains how individuals are able to live and adapt, respond to, and survive stressful pain situations and how they can mount a defensive response to a stressor/pain crisis, recover from that response, survive, and maintain health. The four systems themselves are interdependent, show reciprocity of structure and function, demonstrate self-regulation, and produce and maintain the necessary biologic products to sustain their own continued existence. *Homeostasis serves to regulate* the internal resources ready to be called upon when stressed by pain. From a system's analysis, homeostasis exists as an attractor, or basin of attraction within which the body maintains its internal milieu.

Allostasis is the set of adaptive reactions that help the individual maintain homeostasis in the face of any number of stressors. Pain, trauma, illness, aging, excess or deficiency can all call forth a stress response. This is a mobilization of internal resources to meet stressor challenges. First, there is an alarm response, which is accompanied by both immediate stressor resistance and a slower forming recovery response. In fact, a critical part of the recovery response is its ability to down-regulate the pain defensive response when the threat is over. This avoids overactivity of the defensive catabolic responses of active resistance and permits self-mediated recovery and return to anabolic conditions. The defensive response turns itself on, and then turns itself off, when it is appropriate. If the stressor prevails, exhaustion results. If the individual prevails, recovery occurs. The range of an individual's collective biopsychosocial responses, as well as their ability to tolerate pain intrusion and still maintain homeostasis, helps to define their level of health.

Failure to self-manage pain symptoms might occur if the defensive response is inadequate or excessive. An inadequate or excessive recovery response is associated with clinical symptoms as seen in chronic pain, especially in the musculoskeletal system. *The musculoskeletal system is ultimately involved in all pain processes and management.*

One thing essential to understanding the MINE system is an appreciation of the musculoskeletal (M) system. The musculoskeletal system is particularly available for observation and palpatory evaluation. It is the system within which the INE systems are nested. It executes the flight or the fight, and maneuvers in the external world to secure the necessary objects of sustenance, food, drink, breath, and through movement it allows seeking behaviors, interpersonal behaviors, and collectively communal behaviors. It, too, is built upon basic behaviors reiterated at cellular, tissue, and organism levels. This system, too, shows feedback, and feedforward mechanisms. The musculoskeletal system is interactive with the other systems, not only through a common chemical language but also through a system of mechanical linkages that can be shown to have transduction, transmission, and response capability in effecting pain coping behaviors (39).

Mechanical transducers include muscle, tendon, ligament, bone, fascia, and fibroblast. The transmission occurs along planes of physical connection. The patterns of connection can be described as mechanical, anatomical, neurological, or biomolecular. The effects may include skeletal muscle behavior, whether segmental, regional, or global. They may be seen in coordinated and patterned motor system responses. They may be seen in the transformation of fibroblasts to myofibroblasts when they are under mechanical stress (39). Similarly, the behavior of bone in response to stress loading is a dynamic process. Certainly, the musculoskeletal system is body wide in its presence and in its purpose. From the cytoskeleton to the integrins to the intercellular connective tissues, from the osteon to the bones, from the myofibril to the muscle groups, from the local fascia to the entire body of fascia, there is reiteration in every scale. There is complexity and there is predictability in the musculoskeletal system. It is a part of the body's essential response to pain and stress. The musculoskeletal system interacts with the immune system, nervous system, and the endocrine system, not to mention, the respiratory, circulatory, digestive, and eliminative systems.

Stress dysregulates the MINE, predisposing one to chronic pain—dysregulation in the MINE system's ability to respond to stress, at any of its component sites, or its numerous interfaces compromises one's overall ability to heal or recover from pain/stress. Whether from extraordinary stress, compounding comorbidities, confounding social stressors, or intrinsic system vulnerability, nociception can create dysregulation and become chronic pain.

The musculoskeletal system responds to pain/stress. It is the active agent of fight and flight, and why muscles tense, contract with a purpose, and relax, when the stress has passed. The musculoskeletal system affects the nervous system through the proprioceptive stream of information that complements the flow of nociceptive afferent information. The musculoskeletal system affects the endocrine system through its complex relationship with the SMA and hypothalamic-pituitary-adrenal (HPA) systems. The musculoskeletal system affects the immune system particularly by enabling the movement of cells and their products, along the fascial networks, which are responsible for mounting immune responses.

The immune system responds to pain/stress with an inflammatory response. The combined effects of cytokines, lymphoid tissue, and immune active cells are to focus attention on internal directed vigilance. Tissue trauma elicits an elaboration of immune active molecules at the site of trauma and systemically, to trigger both the acute, inflammatory, phase reaction at the site of injury, and a more global acute phase reaction, which has been dubbed, the "sickness response" (i.e., see Chapter 10: Somatic Dysfunction). Proinflammatory cytokines and immune cell (lymphocytes, granulocytes, neutrophils, and macrophages) are "circulated" through blood vessels, lymphatics, and along fascial networks.

The immune system interacts with the nervous system. Nociceptor activation causes release of substance P and neurokinase A at the site of the disturbance. These are immune stimulating neuropeptides. The neurogenic inflammation is a part of the initiating mechanism and propagation of the immune defensive response. This inflammatory response is sensitive to sympathetic enhancement from primary nociceptor activation. The immune system interfaces with the endocrine system. This is accomplished largely by cytokines, such as interleukins 1 and 6, and their receptors that are found throughout the HPA and the sympathetic-adrenal-medullary (SAM). The immune system affects the musculoskeletal system via the structure and function of tissues that are responding to potential invasion. These are local, mechanical, anatomic, and neurologic, in their pattern of organized, coordinated involvement. Features of tissue texture abnormalities, both acute and chronic, can be associated with the primary pain response of reactive nervous, immune, and endocrine systems.

The nervous system responds to pain/stress. In a bidirectional manner, tissue trauma, anticipated or perceived, elicits transduction of the threat into an information signal, transmission of that information, and effecting of a response, adaptive in nature. When wounds occur and primary afferent nociceptors (PAN's) are aroused, their signal activity increases, and they contribute to their own peripheral responsivity, by producing peripheral neurogenic inflammation in concert with the immune system. These nociceptors and immune system elements show connectivity in the periphery, where they participate in the acute inflammatory reaction, a part of the acute phase reaction. Peripheral sensitization is the result, with additional neural contribution from the sympathetic mediated peripheral effects.

Dorsal horn (central) sensitization refers to the lowered threshold and increased responsiveness, which occurs in secondary afferents from severe or protracted nociceptive stimulation. It occurs by glutamate and NMDA receptor mechanisms. There are inhibitory and excitatory influences from segmental, polysegmental, and descending mechanisms, which help determine the afferent sensitivity of ascending transmission. Central connections in the thalamus, hypothalamus, locus coeruleus (LC), solitary nucleus (visceral and somatic convergence), amygdala, periacqueductal gray (PAG), and the cerebellum are the sites of relay and response of the ascending neural message. Further projection to the insula and anterior cingulate cortex appears to represent convergent sites for affective (amygdala), motivational (LC), and primary sensory processing. Multiple sensory modalities are integrated and coordinated. Of course, the somatosensory cortex is activated. Descending influences may be inhibitory or excitatory. The presence of inadequate inhibition or excessive excitation can explain a circumstance in which chronic pain may develop.

In the alarm response, a stage of defensive arousal, the hypothalamus, amygdala (affective intensity), and PAG (pain modulation) are engaged. They coordinate sensory input with emotional content and cognitive meaning with the goal of driving behaviors that favor survival. They are connected with higher-order cortical structures and lower-order brainstem and subcortical elements to foster learning and ultimate mastery.

The nervous system's alarm response affects the endocrine system via the HPA axis and the SAM axis. The nervous system also affects the immune system. The vagus nerve has an afferent role and an efferent role in mediating inflammatory responses by modulating cytokine levels. The nervous system affects the musculoskeletal system. Acutely, in stress it shunts blood to the skeletal muscles and away from the viscera (sympathetic). In recovery, it shifts to a resting state, decreasing skeletal muscle shunting, and becomes more supportive of visceral, vegetative processes (parasympathetic).

The endocrine system is seen to respond to stress in fast defensive arousal and in the slower process of recovery. Hormone variably affects the nervous system. At the level of the LC, noradrenergic engagement occurs. Through the HPA, the hypothalamic periventricular nucleus and the pituitary, adrenal effects are reinforced or restrained. Corticotrophin-releasing hormone (CRH), proopiomelanocortin, as a precursor for adrenocorticotrophic hormone, and glucocorticoids, are involved in a feedback-dependent response system. This affects adrenocortical behavior through glucocorticoid (cortisol) release. The LC, noradrenergic axis, affects adrenomedullary behavior through release of epinephrine, norepinephrine, and neuropeptide Y. Through the effects of CRH and its receptors CRH-1 and CRH-2, the endocrine system initiates defensive arousal and recovery, respectively. It affects the immune system through its effects on cytokines. HPA axis activation affects the cytokines differentially at times encouraging inflammation, other times encouraging recovery and resolution of inflammation. It affects the musculoskeletal system. Through an activated sympathetic state of arousal, there is shunting of blood to the necessary fight or flight participants. This is the musculoskeletal system.

Other nested systems responding to stress include the visceral, arterial, venous lymphatic, and respiratory/circulatory systems. These nested systems are also intra-active and interactive. The majority of their communication is via the holistic musculoskeletal, circulatory, and nervous systems. They share many of the same properties and demonstrate similar feedback and feed-forward modulation. The feed-forward aspect allows the ability to mount a rapidly accelerating and amplified response when needed. The feedback aspect is part of a process of deceleration that helps control the acute defensive reactions and prevent their excesses. Excesses or deficiencies, in positive and negative feedback, create the potential for dysregulation. These dysregulatory mechanisms can also be related to the problem of chronic pain. This can occur when the fast immediate arousal state does not yield to the slow response recovery phase, or when the response to the stressor fails to readjust to the normal level after the stress has passed. Hypervigilance and hyperreactivity continue as the system, using McEwen's metaphor, fails to hear the all-clear signal (28) and back off. It can occur when the classic changes in cortisol and HPA axis regulation fail to occur. Disturbances in the coordination of the elements involved in the MINE system can result in circumstances predisposing to chronic pain.

Chronic pain results from a sustained loss of a system's ability to function normally with regards to its own self-regulation and/or its normal regulatory role interacting with other systems.

Impaired connectivity of the neuromusculoskeletal system, the autonomic nervous system, the LC, the endocrine, HPA and SMA axes, and the immune cytokines can lead to pain system dysregulation. Coordination of the MINE system is disrupted when the mechanisms of interaction are impaired. This can lead to an inadequate recovery. In this same vein, the system and its set points can be altered by experience such as seen in both posttraumatic stress disorder (PTSD) (40,41) and in chronic pain.

Autonomic dysregulation is first manifested by loss of inter r-wave intervals on ECG. This electrophysiologic variable typically fluctuates in association with inhalation and exhalation. Its variability is modulated by vagal nerve activity and reflects the balance of sympathetic and parasympathetic activity. Its presence is a sign of health and stress-managing capacity. Its absence is a sign of autonomic dysregulation and portends a lesser capacity to respond and recover from stress.

Sensory dysregulation can lead to chronic pain. Excessive facilitation, as in the phenomenon of wind-up, can lead to a sensitized state and chronic pain. Deficient inhibition at any level of the neuraxis can lead to a chronic pain predisposition.

The Default Mode Network (DMN dysregulation) of Raichle shows changes of function and structural distribution of brain activity in patients with chronic pain compared to healthy controls (42). The neuroendocrine and biochemical systems, and their set point changes, contribute to the suffering and misery associated with chronic pain. It is as though these patients continue to experience the memory of pain and are unable to stop.

Endocrine dysregulations, as it affects the HPA axis and cortisol release, can be measured and correlated with diurnal fluctuations and in the response to dexamethasone suppression and/or corticotrophin stimulation. This informs the clinician as regards the inherent endocrine capacity to respond to stress. When disturbed, as in depression, it can lead to an increased incidence of dysregulation and chronic pain.

Immune system dysregulation is exemplified in the complex relation of Th1, proinflammatory, and Th2, anti-inflammatory cytokines. Th1/Th2 ratios can be measured and can be quantified as a sign of dysregulation. Glucocorticoids and catecholamines can locally stimulate Th1 changes, but globally have a Th2 effect. This suggests that they can promote local inflammation while maintaining generalized, opposing, anti-inflammatory effects. An inadequacy of Th1 response, as seen in the chronically stressed, may reflect a compromised ability to respond to stress.

A pattern of objective clinical signs (115) also emerges with dysregulation as the patient in chronic pain now reports:

- Sleep disturbance
- Decreased libido
- Irritability
- Depression
- Decreased activity level
- Deterioration in interpersonal relationships
- Change in work status
- Increased preoccupation with health and physical function

Over time, patients in chronic pain become hypervigilant to all incoming stimuli, their behavior regresses, and they demand pain control from the medical community at any cost. The environment around the patient in chronic pain also often reinforces these ongoing pain behaviors. The pain behaviors are expressed through the musculoskeletal system and are integrated into the patient's lifestyle.

> Every aspect of human life is acted out by the body's muscles and joints…These are the body parts that act together to transmit and modify force and motion…Everything man does to express his aspirations and convictions can be perceived by others only through his bearing and demeanor and utterances, and these are composites of myriads of finely controlled motions.
> —L.M. Korr

The end result is that chronic pain becomes the focal point of the individual's life. This leads to demoralization and suffering. The outcome of dysregulation is the refractory, enduring pain experience commonly referred to as the "chronic pain syndrome."

The person in pain expresses structural changes and functional disturbances, associated with their unique thoughts, feelings, and pain behaviors, through the musculoskeletal and visceral systems. Immunologic, neurologic, and endocrine systems are also continually responding to the moment-by-moment changes of the musculoskeletal system, in response to prolonged pain. With this rich afferent input of the musculoskeletal system into the CNS, it is inevitable that continuous redundant pain has profound consequences on the patient's mind, body, and spirit.

An osteopathic model of pain goes beyond the biological level of sensory modalities and neurological transmissions to include dynamic interactions among and within the mind, body, spirit, and social environment to describe each patient's unique pain presentation (131). For the osteopathically trained physician, pain is more than sensation and perception (Fig. 16.3).

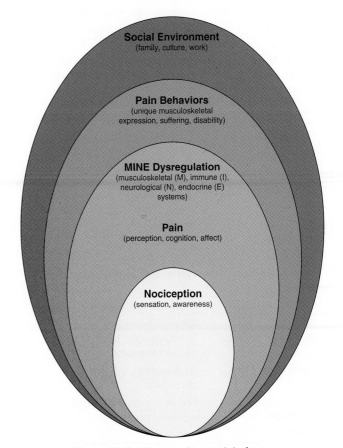

Figure 16-3 Osteopathic model of pain.

It is fundamentally recognized that nociception sets in motion a conscious awareness of discomfort, thoughts, emotions, and dysregulation of the MINE systems, which are displayed throughout the musculoskeletal system. Over time, the social environment (i.e., family, culture, work, etc.) responds to the pain, suffering, and system dysregulation to further shape and reinforce each unique and highly individualized aspect of the pain presentation (132,133). This model, which builds on the biopsychosocial model (134) and Loesers conceptual model of pain (135), emphasizes the critical role of system dysregulation (Chapman, 2008). And also more importantly, it recognizes the central role of the neuromusculoskeletal system that "is ultimately involved in all pathophysiological processes, regardless of where or how they originate." (ECOP, 2000).

Osteopathic assessment of chronic pain is dynamic, patient focused, and comprehensive.

Osteopathic evaluation includes a complete biopsychosocial history, physical examination, osteopathic structural examination, and follow-up visits for both reassessment of the pain management plan and review of the patients' pain scores and functional capacities (43) (see also Table 16.1).

TABLE 16.1

Investigations to Support History and Physical Examination

Categories of Tests	Examples of Tests
Psychometric testing	Formal neuropsychologic evaluation, McGill Pain Questionnaire (MPQ)
Diagnostic imaging	X-ray, computerized tomography (CT), MRI
Functional diagnostic imaging	Isotope scan, PET, blood oxygen level dependent-MRI (BOLD-MRI), fluoro-deoxyglucose-PET (FDG-PET), O2-PET, ultrasound (US)
Neurophysiologic testing	Electroencephalography (EEG), MEG, electromyography (EMG), nerve conduction velocity (NCV), evoked potentials (EP), quantitative sensory testing, vibration threshold
Fluid testing (serology)	Blood, urine, feces, cerebrospinal fluid (CSF)
Tissue testing (histology)	Nerve biopsy, tissue biopsy
Cellular testing (cytology)	Morphology, function, energy, transformation
Molecular testing	Immunologic, hormonal, neurotransmitters
Genetic testing	HLA testing, inherited disorders
Diagnostic anesthetic blockade	Nerve blocks, facet blocks, epidural blocks

Patients and their individualized pain management programs are routinely evaluated for benefits and side effects of treatment, and impact on activities of daily living (ADL). These are regularly queried and appropriately documented. The physician interprets these data through their medical knowledge and formulates a description of the patient in biopsychosocial terms, that is an integrated biological, psychological, and social diagnosis (44,45).

The osteopathic physician recognizes that the palpatory examination provides clues to the underlying pain generators. Pain generators may be confirmed by an effective therapeutic response, even temporarily, to manual correction (OMT). "Somatic dysfunction may be causative, reflective, reactive or perpetuating, or a combination (43)." In summary, osteopathic thinking requires more than assessing somatic dysfunction and relying on pain intensity scores. Comprehensive osteopathic care for chronic pain takes into account patient's moods, beliefs about pain, coping efforts, resources, response of the family members, and the impact of pain on the patient's functional quality of life (QOL). The patient reporting the pain must be evaluated, not just the pain (46).

The general medical history holds many keys to understanding chronic pain. The past medical history includes a childhood and early life history, a history of previous or current medical conditions and trauma (41). Of particular importance is a history of dysregulations of the musculoskeletal system, immunologic system, nervous system, and endocrine system (i.e., MINE system).

Active listening is essential for both understanding pain and developing trust. Chronic pain management begins with careful listening and observations, is followed by the physician-guided examination, and is completed with the review of historical record. The patient is seen as a whole person affected by many spheres of influence. They have sought your help because their health and sense of well-being is challenged. They hurt. What they have tried on their own for pain has failed. They often fear the worst, or they fear you'll find nothing wrong and tell them the pain is in their "head."

The simple message is "I know you have pain. I believe that your pain is real. I want to know all about you and the pain you are experiencing. I will treat your pain in parallel with the necessary investigations to exclude serious underlying pathology. The goal is to identify the reasons for the pain to restore function and to reduce your pain to the lowest possible level."

A common mnemonic of PQRST (pain, quality, radiation, severity, temporal) is a good starting point for the focused pain history.

Pain: Most frequently used pain assessments are single-item Verbal Rating Scales with 0 being "no pain" and 10 being "unbearable pain." These assessments rely on patients' self-reported experience of pain intensity or unpleasantness. A great deal of information is available about the psychometric qualities and properties of these single-item numeric rating scales. A systematic review of clinical and randomized controlled clinical trials shows them to be reliable and valid (46).

In addition to pain scores' intensity, multidimensional measurements of affective response, coping, function, and QOL and analgesic use allow a more comprehensive approach to measuring pain and function (46). These measures are designed to assess ability to engage in functional activities such as walking, sitting, lifting, performing ADL, and an overall sense of satisfaction and QOL.

Quality: One of the most frequently used pain assessment instruments is the McGill Pain Questionnaire (MPQ) (70–72). This instrument has three parts including a descriptive scale (pain intensity), a front and back of a drawing of a human figure on which patients indicate the location of their pain, and a pain-rating index based on patient selection of adjectives from 20 categories of words reflecting sensory, affective, and cognitive components of pain. The MPQ provides a great deal of information in less than 5 minutes (Fig. 16.4) with good test/retest reliability (66–69).

Radiation: where is the pain, and to where does it travel or refer? (see pain drawing on MPQ). Look for dermatome patterns, peripheral nerve distribution patterns, or CNS patterns.

Severity (*intensity*): how bad it is; sometimes the pain intensity score and behavioral observations can be corroborating or contradicting, (i.e., 10/10 but the patient looks comfortable. or 2/10 and they look dreadful).

Temporal (*intensity and duration*): Another useful clinical parameter of pain assessment is a pain, intensity—time curve. These can be graphed. Basically, over a 24-hour period of time, how does the pain wax and wane? This line of questioning can be valuable. For example, a subarachnoid hemorrhage is likely to produce severe pain rapidly; meningitis may take hours or days to reach maximum intensity, while a muscle tension headache patient may describe maximal pain continuously.

The graph can include the temporal characteristic of pain resolution. Over what period of time does the pain diminish and to what degree? The pain of trigeminal neuralgia comes like a lightning bolt and typically goes away in a matter of seconds to minutes. Cluster headache crescendos rapidly and while severe is usually gone within 1 to 3 hours.

Pain of neuropathy is commonly constant, reported as worse when the patient is trying to relax or sleep, yet gets better when distracted. It is important to know how the pain returns and with what temporal characteristics. The peristaltic rhythm of colonic pain, the morning stiffness of osteoarthritis, or pain associated with menses are examples of temporal aspects.

It is useful to understand and classify pain by its intensity and persistence over time. This can lead to differential diagnoses based on differential anatomy, physiology, and pathology (Table 16.2).

The patient is queried regarding the *impact on their affective state*. What is their mood? Are they depressed, worried, angry, or fearful and what is the history of these feelings? To what degree and in what ways is the patient suffering? What is the *impact on their cognitive state*? (Use Pain Coping Skills) What is their self-image and, how has it been affected by pain? What is the *impact on the patient's ADL*? Are they able to eat, dress, wash, and toilet? Can they do the shopping, cooking, and cleaning? Are they able to work? Are they completely unable to work, do they have a limited ability to work, are they on disability? Are they seeking disability? Has there been an effect on their mobility? Can they walk, bend, stand, sit, or lie without pain? Can they exercise? What do they do for exercise and has it changed because of their pain? Has this affected how they view themselves or how they feel? How has this affected their nutrition? Have they lost their appetite, are they not eating adequately, has it affected the availability of healthy food choices, or are there physical impediments to eating? *Lifestyle changes* and *high-risk choices* such as increased alcohol use, drug use, lack of exercise, and comfort eating are other important factors (see Chapter 32: Health Promotion).

How is their *sleep*? Do they have trouble falling asleep, staying asleep, staying awake, or getting enough sleep? Do they feel refreshed after sleeping?

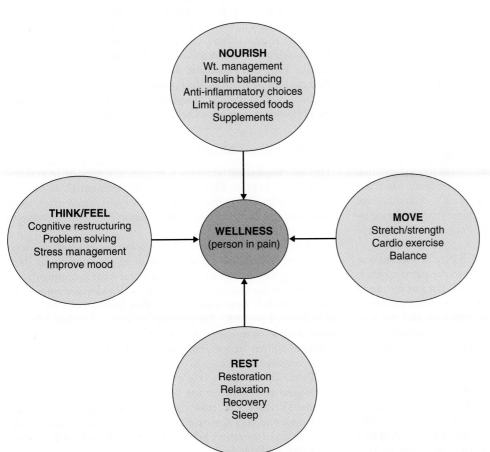

Figure 16-4 Wellness is appreciated through multiple interacting systems.

TABLE 16.2

Assessment/Diagnosis: Temporally Defined

Temporal Character	Clinical Examples
Acute	Trauma, illness
Acute, recurring	Migraine
Subacute	Longer-lasting insult or time to resolution
Chronic	Low back pain, neck pain, daily headache, fibromyalgia, irritable bowel syndrome
Chronic, progressive	Malignancy, degenerative, inflammatory
Chronic with acute recurrences	Spondylosis

TABLE 16.3

Assessment/Diagnosis: Location Defined

Anatomic Location	Clinical Examples
Visceral	Liver, lung
Vascular	Large vessel, small vessel
Muscular	Muscle, myofascial pain syndrome
Skeletal	Bone, joint, capsule, ligament, tendon
Nervous system	Cortical, thalamic, brain stem, spinal cord, peripheral nerve, autonomic nervous system
Other	Skin, eyes, ears, nose, mouth

What is the impact on their *family* life? How have the family dynamics and interpersonal relationships been affected? Is there a family history that is relevant? Are there family members with migraine, degenerative disc disease, connective tissue disease, substance abuse, or other abuses? Who are the caregivers? What is the impact on the *community*? Has there been a change in the patient's role in the community? Do they derive care giving from the community? What is the cultural stigma or stereotype associated with admitting, showing, or seeking treatment for pain? What are the *economic implications* of their pain? Are they missing work, losing wages, receiving or seeking disability payments? What is their degree of health care utilization? Are they seeking *medicolegal* redress?

What are the *environmental stressors*? Is there poverty, malnutrition, dysfunctional living circumstances, toxic exposure, substance abuse, high-risk behaviors?

Ultimately, the behavioral model assesses the pain and its impact on the patient's *QOL*.

The osteopathic physician is uniquely trained to evaluate the musculoskeletal system. Through observation, palpation, and motion testing, key information is gathered. The neurological/musculoskeletal system is known as reflector and effector of the entire organism and all its systems. The combination of this information with the general physical exam and appropriate evidence-based test results provides the osteopathic physician with a comprehensive data set. This allows for a most complete biopsychosocial evaluation of pain, physical functioning, system dysregulations, and adaptive response patterns.

The osteopathic physical examination is patient focused and solution oriented. It can allow a connection to the patient, otherwise unavailable. The musculoskeletal system is not just for securing a diagnosis. It provides an avenue for treatment that can target the nociceptors, the pain experience, the suffering, and the pain behaviors. Armed with the knowledge of anatomy, physiology, and pathologic physiology, a dynamic, interactive, systems analysis can be made. Specific diagnostic considerations include ongoing tissue injury, effects of neurologic processing, presence and degree of suffering, cognitive and affective disruptions, musculoskeletal manifestations, as well as premorbid, and subsequent, adaptive responses. The diagnostic systems analysis will typically describe multiple axes of dysfunction. This leads directly to an integrated diagnostic assessment and an active treatment plan (Table 16.3).

The formal biomechanical/musculoskeletal examination is integral to osteopathic medicine.

Besides the obvious orthopedic aspects of the examination, the characteristic evaluation for static asymmetry, tissue texture abnormalities, and restriction of motion has become an integral part of the osteopathic examination. Static asymmetry looks at posture, spinal curvature, and limb asymmetry. Tissue texture abnormalities and motion restrictions can be examined for in local, regional, and even global fashion. The important thing is to be doing this part of the examination mindful of what the patient's major pain complaints might be. Be sure to examine where it hurts. How does it look, how does it feel, how does it move? Knowing exactly where it hurts also suggests any number of associated mechanical, anatomical, and neurological associations, visceral and somatic, that can augment the biomechanical examination and its contribution to a comprehensive diagnosis. Patients in pain are sometimes not touched by their doctors. Sometimes, their painful areas are not directly examined and, as a result, their complaints are not fully understood, and the physician's formulations believed (Table 16.4).

The Neurologic Model

The neurological examination is particularly relevant in evaluating patients in pain. This is designed to ferret out those patients with irritation of a previously healthy nervous system from those with disorders of the nervous system that might be predisposing to painful states.

Always when evaluating the holistic nervous system, both peripheral and central, the questions to be answered are, is there something wrong, where is it localized, and what is causing it?

It begins with an evaluation of the patient's level of arousal and content of their consciousness. Are they bright and alert, or are they dull and sluggish? Are they making sense? Are they delirious, demented, or encephalopathic? Have they taken too much medication or do they have encephalitis? Are they mood appropriate to their complaints?

Particular attention to the cranial nerves is obviously appropriate in pain complaints of the head, face, and the special sensory organs. The eyes, ears, nose, and mouth are known to be richly innervated and very sensitive. Smell, sight, eye movements, facial strength, facial sensation, hearing, taste, speech, and swallowing are all evaluable (Table 16.5).

TABLE 16.4

Assessment/Diagnosis: Pathophysiology Defined

Pathologic Process	Clinical Examples
Malignant	Primary, metastatic, para-neoplastic
Degenerative	Trauma, wear and tear, apoptotic
Inflammatory	Immune mediated, organ effects
Immunologic	Antibodies, interleukins, tumor necrosis factor, etc.
Respiratory, circulatory	Local, regional, global
Energy, metabolic	Local, regional, global
Endocrine	Hormones, releasing factors
Infection	Local, regional, global
Somatic dysfunction	Local, regional, global
Trauma	Severity, complexity
Neurogenic	Neoplasm, infarction, demyelination, trauma, infection, degenerative, migraine
Psychogenic	Somatoform, depression, anxiety, hypervigilance, personality disorder, malingering, catastrophizing

TABLE 16.5

Management of Nociceptive Activity

Type of Intervention	Clinical Examples
OMT	Direct, indirect
Anesthesia	Local, regional, sympathetic
Medication, systemic	NSAID, opiates, pregabilin, gabapentin, lamotrigine, acetaminophen
Medication, local	Lidocaine, NSAID, OTC topical
Surgery	Removal, repair, restoration, ablation, stimulation
Biofeedback	EMG, temperature, galvanic skin response (GSR), EEG
Physical therapy	Heat, cold, laser, ultrasound, electrical stimulation, traction, exercise, balance
Acupuncture	With or without electrical stimulation, local, systemic

Sensory Examination

Sensory testing is designed to evaluate the peripheral nerves, which lead to spinothalamic and dorsal column pathways, from their peripheral elements to their central pathways and connections. Further testing is aimed at evaluating cortical and subcortical components of sensory processing. Obviously, in pain conditions, sensory processing is hugely relevant. An attempt to recognize a pattern of sensory dysfunction is sought. Is there altered sensation in the territory of a peripheral nerve or is it the territory of a nerve root with dermatomal features? Do the small fibers that respond to pinprick and temperature react differently than the larger fibers that respond to touch, vibration, and proprioception? Sometimes, this can point to a disorder of the peripheral nerves such as a small fiber neuropathy. These conditions are known to have association with peripheral neuropathic pain. Is there a sensory level suggestive of a spinal cord etiology? Is there a hemisomatic distribution of sensory changes suggesting a central source? Are their dissociations of sensory deficits? For example, is there loss of pain and temperature with preservation of touch as in syringomyelia? Is there loss of pain and temperature on one side of the body with loss of touch on the other as in hemisection lesions of the spinal cord? Are there deficits in touch and proprioception with sparing of pinprick sensation, as in dorsal column disorders such as vitamin B_{12} deficiency or multiple sclerosis? Does the sensory loss include the face on one side and the arm and leg on the other side suggestive of brainstem pathology? Or, does the sensory loss involve the face, arm, and leg on the same side suggesting a disorder at the level of the thalamus or sensory cortex? These central lesions have long been known to be cause for central pain syndromes, such as thalamic pain syndrome, or parietal pain syndrome. Whether from cerebral infarction, neoplasm, trauma, or demyelinating disease, they can represent vexing conditions to manage.

Armed with a pin, tuning fork, and wisp of cotton, the sensory evaluation is pursued. Not just patterned disturbances are relevant. Sometimes, the patients response themselves are illuminating. Do they have allodynia, hyperpathia, or hyperalgesia indicating unusual sensitivity to stimuli? Or, do they have sensory loss in areas that are reported as painful, so-called, anesthesia dolorosa? Do they complain of pain in parts they no longer have, as in phantom pain syndrome? Do they have dissociations between their ability to feel and localize painful stimuli and their ability to manifest appropriate affect or cognitive correlates? This can be seen in some of the cerebral hemispheric disorders.

It is particularly important to assess the sensory status in the area or areas of complaint. Is it normal or abnormal? If abnormal, is it more or less sensitive? Is there indifference? If the sensory exam is abnormal, do the sensory findings correlate with the pain in some way? Is there a pattern of sensory loss suggesting a neurological localization?

Motor Examination

The motor examination begins with the casual examination while the patient walks into your office, moves about your examination room, describes their pain problem, participates in the examination process, passively and actively. Because pain is at least part of the problem, a particular eye toward the patient's signs of protective behaviors, such as limping or hobbling, is made. Looking for and documenting signs of suffering, such as grimacing, moaning, or crying, is done. Sad, anxious, angry affective behaviors are part of the casual motor examination, as are observations of the cognitive behavioral manifestations, like resigned, slumpedshouldered, head drooped, slow moving postural adjustments. This, by the way, is an important opportunity to broaden your osteopathic impressions

TABLE 16.6

Management of Pain Perception

Type of Intervention	Clinical Examples
OMT	Direct, indirect
Education	Information about pain and self-management
Exercise	Stretch, balance, strengthen
Medication	Opiates, TCA, NSRI, cannabinoids
Cognitive and behavioral therapies	Insight, hypnosis, relaxation training Operant and respondent conditioning

TABLE 16.7

Management of Suffering

Type of Intervention	Clinical Examples
OMT	Direct, indirect
Cognitive and behavioral therapy	Psychotherapy, cognitive restructuring, hypnosis, imagery, relaxation
Relaxation	Biofeedback, progressive relaxation
Breathing exercise	Yoga, tai chi, diaphragmatic breathing
Medication	Opiates, antidepressants, anticonvulsants
Surgery	Ablation, deep brain stimulation

regarding the entirety of the burden that has befallen the patient (Table 16.6).

The formal testing of the motor system includes passive tests of motor tone looking for flaccidity, spasticity, or rigidity, as well as atrophy, or fasciculations. In patients with pain, there may be guarding, which must be considered. Likewise, in active testing of strength, pain may limit effort or willingness to exert a particular action or many different actions. This is best recorded as pain limited strength testing. Testing for strength can be done both regionally and locally. So, while testing general arm and leg raising, grip and toe wiggle, may be enough for a screening exam, sometimes a meticulous muscle-by-muscle, limb-by-limb, and trunk exam must be conducted, particularly, if there are pain complaints, associated with symptoms of weakness, cramping, spasms that can be localized. In those cases, the more thorough version of motor examination is mandated (Table 16.7).

Furthering the motor examination requires tests of the reflexive properties of the body. These include the segmental, monosynaptic myotatic reflexes. These tendon reflexes can be obtained from most myotendinous junctions, but are usually tested at elbow, wrist, hand, knee, and ankle. Their hypo- or hyper-reactivity must be ascertained. Is there a pattern to the reflex and motor findings?

Is there a problem in the muscles generally with proximal weakness and normal reflexes? Do they have distal weakness and reflex loss due to neuropathy? Do they have weakness of one side of the body involving the leg, arm, and face with hyperactive reflexes on that same side suggesting a CNS disorder?

Some reflexes are usually not present in adults and are considered pathologic when present.

Plantar responses that are extensor, thumbs that flex with middle finger flicking are signs of upper motor neuron deficiency.

Palms that grasp when stroked, chins that twitch when the palm is stroked, loss of extinction to glabellar tapping, rooting and sucking signs are generally hemispheric deficiency signs.

Somewhere, you are also collating this information with what you have already obtained in the mental, cranial nerve, and sensory exams.

Cerebellar/Motor Examination

The cerebellar testing includes an assessment of gait and posture, coordination, and balance. The cerebellum has great capacity for learning and remembering and mostly what it learns is how to balance and move. In general, signs of imbalance are just that. They are signs of imbalance in the body proper. Balance is what we seek, when we seek health.

The patient stands, walks, eyes open, eyes closed, along an imaginary tight rope. They stand on one leg; they touch their finger to their nose and their heel to their shin. Rapidly alternating motions can be tested, including finger and foot tapping. The qualities of their speech and eye movements are assessed.

Fifty percent of the neurons of the CNS are in the cerebellum, which occupies only 10% of its volume. It has a prominent role in the nervous system's contribution to health or disease. Its activities are, for the most part, not consciously appreciated. It is becoming clear that the cerebellum is involved in all manner of dysfunctions, including pain and somatic dysfunction.

Autonomic Model

Autonomic testing has largely been performed earlier in the examination. The heart rate, respiratory rate, blood pressure, state of the pupils, tears and saliva, color and temperature of the limbs, associated sudomotor activity, sweaty and clammy features have likely been noticed by now. The presence of goose flesh due to piloerection or skin mottling has already been observed during the general physical but here is reformulated in the context of overall autonomic behavior. Is the pattern sympathetic driven, sympathetic exhausted, or parasympathetic in nature? Is it generalized or regional?

The evaluation of the skin provides the most external opportunity for evaluation and can lead to important observations about regional, dermatomal, or local problems. The tuft of hair over the midline lower back may overlie a neural tube closure defect like a spina bifida. The blistered rash over a single dermatome can be the presentation of Herpes zoster or shingles. It is noteworthy that for the skin to be evaluated, in fact for an adequate examination to be performed, the patient must be disrobed. With modesty and respect, patients should be undressed, gowned, and examined.

The fascial system, another of the body's holistic systems, is an organizing tissue like no other. It is continuous from top to bottom, front to back, inside to outside. It invests every tissue type, from its outer most coverings to its deepest cellular structures. In its investments, it is found to be continuous. Current research has now revealed intracellular and intercellular linkage through this same fascial system. Connective tissue, collagen, integrins, cytoskeletons are the levels of scale in which the reiterated properties of mesodermal derivatives serve as a principal organizer for the multitude of the body's structures and functions. As a mechanical force transducer, a mechanical force transmitter, and an effector tissue, the fascial system impacts immunologic, neurologic, and endocrinologic, and, of course, musculoskeletal functions and structures. Its many functions will be discussed elsewhere, but its evaluation in patients suffering pain can be uniquely rewarding. It can reveal biomechanical linkages between internal and external structures as well as information regarding the patient's unique constellation of painful parts.

The Respiratory/Circulatory Model

The respiratory/circulatory testing demands a thorough examination of both the cellular and the whole-body adequacy of oxygen, blood, lymph, interstitial fluid, and cerebrospinal fluid dynamics. Good health requires the maintenance of adequate arterial, venous, lymphatic, cerebrospinal, and interstitial fluid dynamics. The cardiovascular exam evaluates the very essence of circulatory function, from the pump to the pipes. Every region must be considered for the adequacy of its blood supply and the health of its components. Is there leg pain from claudication? Is it due to peripheral vascular disease? Is it due to neurogenic claudication, as a result of spinal stenosis?

Is their head pain associated with an indurated, tender superficial temporal artery? Is their acute low back pain (LBP) associated with an abdominal bruit and loss of pedal pulses? This is one of the holistic systems of the body that reaches every single cell and influences every single function. The "rule of the artery" must always be considered.

In some texts, the respiratory system is considered as part of a cardiorespiratory system. But it merits its own consideration as another of the holistic systems of the body. The adequacy of breath, the dependence on adequate oxygenation, again, can be seen to affect every organ, every system, every cell and cellular function. The examination considers the patient's color, their respiratory effort and capacity, as well as its adequacy. Signs of chronic insufficiency like clubbing of the fingers raise concerns for more widespread problems. Ultimately, the adequacy of the cardiorespiratory system is vital to the essential well being of the individual. In managing pain, optimization of respiratory and circulatory structure and function is critical. Of course, this involves auscultation, palpation, and observation of the thoracic space. Examination of the heart, lungs, lymphatic structures, great and small vessels, diaphragm, and thoracic inlet comprise the test.

There are palpable reactions of the musculoskeletal system to stress/pain (see Chapter 14 The Physiology of Touch). Touching the patient's pain is more than a euphemism. It is an experience for doctor and patient alike. It is an opportunity to validate a patient-centered subjective experience with more objective physical data. As a clinician, you will always feel more confident in diagnosis when you have been able to reproduce the patient's symptoms. This is not always possible even with a meticulous and comprehensive examination. Sometimes, the examination process is straightforward; other times, it remains elusive. Patients themselves feel better understood when they are examined and touched in ways that inform the examiner regarding the nature of their pain. Understanding the generators and mechanisms of a painful process enhances the therapeutic options. Therefore, understanding what actions exacerbate or initiate the pain is essential. Ask the patient to demonstrate the behaviors, positions, movements, and activities that influence their pain. Pay attention to what worsens and what improves the symptoms.

At some point in the examination, if it has not already occurred, provocative testing is pursued. This means attempting to reproduce or aggravate the pain. If the clinical scenario suggests nerve root compression, then intervertebral foraminal compression with vertebral side ending and extension may exacerbate the nerve root symptoms. Straight leg raising that causes pain to radiate down the leg suggests nerve/nerve root entrapment that is affected by neurofascial stretch. Compression or traction on peripheral nerves that reproduces symptoms can be diagnostic of conditions like thoracic outlet syndrome, carpal tunnel syndrome, cubital tunnel syndrome, tarsal tunnel syndrome, or piriformis syndrome. Skeletal percussion can help identify a bony source of pain, as in fracture or metastasis. Visceral palpation can identify a visceral source of pain.

Palpation of the myofascial system, systematically seeking tender points, can reveal the trigger points of myofascial pain syndrome, Chapman's points of neurolymphatic dysfunction, the muscles, tendons, ligaments, skeletal, and connective tissue generators of pain.

At times, the relationship between the tender points and the pain complaint is obvious. They sprain their ankle and their talofibular ligament is tender. Other times it is less obvious; their appendix is inflamed and their abdominal wall is tender. The relationship of the tender places and the pain complaints is usually related to their segmental, autonomic, and central relations.

The pattern of tenderness may reveal patterns of musculoskeletal involvement that involve multiple structures. This pattern can be analyzed to reveal whole-body patterns of strain and trauma. This is an example of forensic Osteopathy. This provides an opportunity to correlate the patterns of dysfunction with the biomechanical/musculoskeletal behaviors of origin. This can reveal the traumatic vectors of strain.

Even more important than the attempts to increase pain are the efforts to reduce pain. Besides asking the patient to demonstrate what helps, maneuvers such as distraction or compression are performed. Attention to the functional anatomy and neurology of the maneuvers can reveal keys to diagnosis as well as treatment. OMT, as will be described in greater detail in this text, is a uniquely osteopathic approach to this process. For example, the confirmation of a cervical origin to a headache by relieving it using manual cervical distraction provides useful diagnostic information. In addition, it provides critical understanding that can be translated into therapeutic strategy (Table 16.8).

Behavioral Model

The psychological examination has been ongoing and largely done by now. Has the patient been anxious, tense, fearful, angry, worried, or depressed? Are they catastrophizing (50–53) about their pain? Is their belief in their pain so firmly maintained as to disagree with logic or rational argument? Do they fear pain (54–56), or movement (i.e., kinesiophobia) (57–59) and avoid activity? Patients who catastrophically (mis)interpret their pain are prone to become fearful and consequently engage in protection (e.g., escape/avoidance) behaviors, such as guarding and resting. Paradoxically, these behaviors may increase pain and pain disability rather than reducing them (60). There are a large number of patients with musculoskeletal pain who avoid physical activities unnecessarily because of the fear that movement can be harmful. As a result of inactivity and withdrawing, they feel helpless, have little initiative to comply, and find themselves depressed (39). *Pain sets in a still joint. Depression sets in a still person.* "Motion is a basic function of life" (ECOP). In fact, prolonged bed rest is no longer recommended for the management of LBP; it is ineffective and may even delay recovery. Recent guidelines encourage the patient to continue to stay active, continue

TABLE 16.8

Pain-Related Behavior Management

Type of Intervention	Clinical Examples
OMT	Direct, indirect
Meditation	Mindfulness meditation, self-hypnosis
Visual imagery	Guided, self-guided. Distraction and visualization training
Behavioral therapies	Functional recovery programs (Fordyce), operant conditioning, interdisciplinary pain programs
Exercise	Healthy activity, prescribed stretch, strengthening, endurance, balance training

TABLE 16.9

Behavioral Indication of Pain

Anatomic Location	Clinical Examples
Vocalizations	Sighs, moans, crying, pleading
Facial expressions	
• Brow bulge	• Bulging, creasing and/or vertical furrows above and between eyebrows
• Eye squeeze • Nasolabial furrow	• Lowering and drawing together of the eyebrows (squeezing and bulging of eyelids)
• Horizontal mouth	• Pulling upward and deepening • A distinct horizontal stretch/pull at the corners of the mouth
Motor activity	Slow movement Avoidance of activity for fear of pain
Disposition	Irritable, withdrawn, sad, aggressive
Body postures, gesturing	Limping or distorted gait Rubbing or supporting the affected area Frequent position changes Rigid posture, guarded movement
Behaviors to avoid pain	Inactivity and rest to avoid pain Excessive use of medication/health care system Social withdrawal/reduction of ADLs Outward symbols of distress (self-prescribed collars, canes, braces) Addictions

Adapted from Turk (133). Psychological Approaches to Pain Management: *A Practitioners Handbook*. 2nd. Ed. New York: Guilford; 2002.

ordinary activities, and work as normal, and this leads to faster recovery and lower risk of chronic pain and disability (61,62).

The osteopathic physician remembers that pain is a complex, subjective perceptual phenomenon with intensity, quality, time course, personal impact, and meaning—"That you assess the person, not just see the pain" (63). Persons experiencing nociception display a large range of reactions that are indicative of pain, distress, fear, anger, depression and/or suffering. Their autonomic arousal, muscle tension, endocrine, immune, and neurologic reactions add to the pain behaviors (Table 16.9). The pain behaviors further develop and change through learning and are molded by past painful experiences (64,65).

It is important not to mistake these pain behaviors as being synonymous with malingering. Malingering is a conscious purposeful effort to defraud and fake symptoms of pain for financial and/or emotional gain. In many cases, chronic pain behaviors do not automatically correlate with conscious deception, but rather they are behaviors that are unintended and result either from unrelieved pain or environmental reinforcement. Most patients who display pain behaviors are not aware of them nor are they consciously motivated to obtain reinforcements from others. There is little support for the contention of outright faking of pain or that the process of malingering is widespread (63).

Formulation and Execution of Osteopathic Pain Management

It has been our contention that proper therapy depends upon a proper diagnosis. That is why in a chapter titled Chronic Pain Management, so much emphasis and time has been devoted to assessment. We have learned that the diagnostic process is multivariate and it is reasonable to conclude that therapeutic plans are best conceived as offering benefit at multiple levels. Our diagnosis must include relevant medical diagnoses, including medical, affective, cognitive, and behavioral comorbidities. It must include an understanding of the involved nociceptive mechanisms, peripheral and central. Finally, our diagnosis must include an understanding of the biopsychosocial impact on the patients' function and QOL. Our targets, therefore, are the peripheral, spinal, and forebrain structures and their functions. They include

the MINE systems. Additional targets include comorbidities, psychiatric, social, behavioral, and medical. In all patients, with or without chronic pain, general advice is offered regarding proper nutrition, levels of activity and exercise, on sleep and rest, as well as the importance of creating and maintaining thoughts of wellness (122).

The Osteopathic Pain Management Plan is Evidence Based and Comprehensive

Osteopathic treatment decisions are based on systematic reviews and evidence-based considerations. (For current reviews, see The American Pain Society [APS] and the American College of

Physicians systematic reviews, utilizing both the Oxman criteria and the Cochrane Database [In *Ann Intern Med* 2007;147(7):492–504]). Their therapeutic prescription, after reviewing all the evidence on nonpharmacologic therapies for chronic pain (>4 weeks duration) when compared to placebo, sham, or no treatment found *good evidence* for spinal manipulation, exercise, cognitive-behavioral therapy, and interdisciplinary rehabilitation. The only nonpharmacological therapies with *fair-to-good evidence* of efficacy for acute pain (<4 weeks duration) are superficial heat and spinal manipulation. The choice and sequencing of these therapies and the methods of tailoring therapy to the unique individual patient is the true art of osteopathic care.

The therapeutic plan is aimed at removing noxious influences, at any level or location. Concurrently, efforts at optimizing structure and function are the objective goals for moving toward health. The inherent vitality and capacity for wellness of the patient is the focus for therapy. From the molecular, cellular, systemic, and regional perspectives, therapeutic strategies are conceived. They are often stratified. First, we will try treatment A and if not successful will change to treatment B. They are typically multifaceted. Sometimes, they are additive and even synergistic. In this way, they represent a microcosmic, multidisciplinary, therapeutic plan. Of course, in some situations, multiple different health care providers are involved in delivering and coordinating the plan. This represents the macrocosmic interdisciplinary therapeutic team.

In some cases, there is clear synergy of therapies. The total amount of therapeutic efficacy is greater than the sum of the individual therapeutic efforts. Likewise, the idea that interdisciplinary management can offer synergistic therapeutic opportunities has led to the creation of interdisciplinary pain management centers treating both pain and disability.

The osteopathic mission through both OMT and the doctor–patient relationship is to restore postural and mechanical alignments, manage fascial strain, and tissue texture changes to encourage the patient's innate ability to heal (116,117). Osteopathic thinking has long considered pain as a symptom closely linked to somatic dysfunction. In addition to neuromuscular factors *triggering nociception* and the initial report of pain, biopsychosocial factors often *worsen and perpetuate* pain. Osteopathic physicians need to approach patients in chronic pain with support and empathy while drawing heavily from the expertise of their pain specialist colleagues. Caring for chronic pain often warrants an interdisciplinary approach blending osteopathic thinking and the best evidence-based knowledge about biopsychosocial treatments (73,74). The goal is to assist the patients internal healing and their ability to mount a homeostatic response. Each therapeutic prescription needs to be individualized.

Biopsychosocial Interventions Decrease Suffering

Much of the disabling nature of chronic pain thus stems from cognitive and affective factors and cannot be explained by objective physical measures alone (75,76). Osteopathic interventions are biopsychosocial and they target nociception in an attempt to decrease distress and increase functioning (77,78). Four systematic reviews (79–82) and a recent meta-analysis (83) of random controlled trials (RCTs) of specific measurement domains such as pain expression, functional activity level, health-related QOL, and depression substantiates the efficacy of treating the psychological factors of chronic pain.

Specifically, these RCTs showed cognitive behavioral treatments (Table 16.10) were *moderately superior* to no treatment, placebo, and wait-list controls. Positive effects of psychological

TABLE 16.10
Common Components of Cognitive Behavioral Treatment of Chronic Pain

Strategy	Focus of Treatment
Cognitive restructuring	Self-statement reanalysis to change pain, distressing thoughts, and decrease anxiety
Challenging irrational beliefs	Catastrophizing, all or none thinking, negative predicting, selectively focusing on pain, over generalizations, jumping to conclusions, fatalistic viewpoints
Motivating patients	Reduce social isolation, improve communication and problem-solving skills and outcome expectancy
Desensitize patients	Pacing activities, goal setting, muscular relaxation training
Reinforce activity	Operant and respondent conditioning
Teach self-management	Breathing techniques, bio-feedback, imagery training, distraction techniques
Educate on mind/body/spirit	To understand body unity and our inherent capacity for self-regulation, self-learning, and the importance of healthy lifestyle choices
Relapse prevention	Pain coping skills, support groups, family interventions, caregiver support/education, breakthrough pain rescue planning

interventions when compared to these various control groups were noted for pain intensity, pain-related interference, health-related QOL, and depression. Both cognitive and behavioral and self-regulatory treatments were specifically found to be efficacious in decreasing suffering (83).

The robust nature of these studies should encourage confidence in the osteopathic physician as they advise and counsel the chronic pain patient in the areas of pain catastrophizing (84), fear avoidance (85), managing psychiatric comorbidities (76), reinforcing pain relevant conversations (86), and the promotion of pain self-management and self-healing (87). *The strength of osteopathic medicine in managing chronic pain comes through talk and touch. Nothing can be more powerful.*

Exercise is Treatment for Chronic Pain

The body is made to move. At every stage of life and health, there is a range of activity that can be realized. There is a minimum, and there is a maximum. Within this window of physicality is the domain of exercise and conditioning. Outside of this window is the realm of atrophy and injury.

In 2003, the Center for Disease Control (CDC) presented information on over 200,000 individuals in the United States and found less than half engage in activities that fulfill the CDC's minimal recommendations for exercise (88). Females were significantly less active than males, and their activity levels were also found to be progressively lower with age (89).

Exercise significantly enhances physical and psychological health (90–91), contributes to antidepressant and anxiolytic effects (92–97), and benefits sleep (69,90). Prescriptive exercises can begin to teach the patient to think about health-oriented behaviors. Exercise affects posture, balance, flexibility, strength, and coordinates movement to promote the optimal structure and function. Over time, exercise promotes lessening of tension and stress as the patient learns to support their own health. This has impact on the Respiratory/Circulatory, and Metabolic/Energy systems.

Metaregression analysis found the best outcomes for exercise incorporating the following elements (98):

- Individualized regimens
- Supervision
- Stretching
- Strengthening

When exercise included these features, compared to no treatment, pain scores went down nearly 20% and functions scores improved by 60%! The standard exercise course includes educating the patient, clearly defined goals, a program of 30 minutes performed twice daily and beginning with low-stress activities (walking, aquatic exercise, stationary bike with rest breaks), and encouraging self-management. (99).

Relaxation exercises can also be taught along with exercise when anxiety, fear of movement or pain, and chronic muscle tension interfere with performances (100–102).

OMT can provide further solace and comfort while the patient is in your hands (102,104). It is likely that maladaptive pain states can be partially characterized by excessive suffering (105). To this end, making the patients calm allows the intrinsic systems to function more optimally.

Suffering can be relieved, at least temporarily. The reduction of suffering is part of the process of altering pathologic activity in the limbic and autonomic domain. Once the lack of value of suffering has been realized, like getting the attention of those around, including caregivers and health professionals, its value quickly diminishes.

Osteopathic medicine is at its most essential level a mechanism for changing pain-related behaviors (116,117). From the OMT effects on segmental, regional, and global neuromusculoskeletal activity, to its calming limbic and autonomic effects, it is attempting to change behaviors. At the whole-person level, OMT affords the patient an opportunity to feel better. Even if only transient, OMT permits the patient a glimpse of their capacity for having less pain.

Educating the patient to gain understanding and self-manage pain is therapeutic. Enabling the patient to understand their pain generators and pain management strategies allows a patient to self-manage their symptoms. The patient is empowered by accurately understanding the causes, treatments, and prognoses relative their pain. This is education.

Active listening skills (see Part II: Approach to Patient) and sound advice can help the patient maintain a reality-based expectation for course and outcome. Patient education can be conducted one on one, but is typically carried out in small group sessions (eight to ten patients). Clinical trials show this group model helping to increase activity levels and effectively applying pain self-management skills (106). In addition, pain support groups are an extremely powerful and low-cost strategy for educating large numbers of patients with chronic pain (107). The goal is to help patients cope with and adjust to their pain and condition. In support groups, patients reconceptualize the meaning of their pain, their cognitive and emotional appraisals, and problem-solving strategies (108). They review how their pain impacts themselves and their lifestyle and identify the events in the environment that reinforce their pain behaviors and musculoskeletal reactions. If not taught in a group therapy model, the following concepts form at least an outline for teaching coping strategies within the doctor–patient relationship. These concepts are also the foundational ideas for the advice given to the pain patient on how to think about and manage their pain (37). Patients who have to "live with their pain" are taught to hold the following ideas as true:

1. My pain is real. It occurs in my body, I have a reaction to it in my head.
2. I accept that I may need, outside help to control my pain, and I refuse to quit or give in to the pain and the deterioration it causes.
3. At times my pain has had an overwhelming influence on my life, but I believe that I can choose how I react to it.
4. My best efforts and those of the medical community have not stopped my pain. This is not necessarily a fault of mine or a shortcoming of medicine. I will no longer fight with myself about this or blame medicine. No fight, no blame.
5. I will recognize some aspects of my coping with pain that I am doing well, and will also admit to myself mistakes that I have made.
6. I will forgive myself unconditionally for my past mistakes and forgive others whom I perceive are responsible for my pain and troubles.
7. I will fix any mistakes I've made struggling to live with the pain.
8. I will go forward with hope that the pain will someday pass or be relieved; and, at the same time, recognize that I have to cope with the pain that I have.
9. I will strive for higher goals, making pain a side issue, to be managed as necessary.
10. I now recognize there is more to my life than struggling with pain.
11. With this knowledge, I will separate myself from my pain management program or doctor, with the complete understanding that I may return at any time.
12. I understand that I have more important goals in my life than coping with pain and I will strive toward them as my mission.

Remembering that "Pain runs in front of the skillful surgeon's scalpel or anesthesiologist's needle;" a laudable goal, if possible, is to find and block nociception.

To control acute pain, anesthetic blockade of neural transmission to virtually any part of the body can temporarily be achieved by direct application of local anesthetics (nerve blocks), such as procaine, lidocaine, tetracaine, or bupivacaine. In some severe cases, substances that destroy neural tissue can be injected (neurolytic block) in an effort to permanently obliterate the neural transmission mechanisms.

Diagnostically, nerve blocks determine specific pathways of involvement that aid in the differential diagnosis, of the site or transmission mechanisms, of a given pain. Prognostically, they partially predict the probable effectiveness of neurolytic or neurosurgical procedures. Interestingly, the pain-relieving effects of local anesthetics can often exceed the duration of the chemical blockade of neural transmission. The reason for this is not completely understood. It might be a result of decreasing sympathetic reflexes and skeletal muscle tension. Perhaps it results from the creation of pain-free time during which the patient can restructure their cognitive and emotional processing routines or learn new behavior patterns that help in coping with pain. The treatment of acute pain adequately may help prevent some cases of chronic pain. For example, the use of topical anesthesia before starting an IV, the use of adequate local anesthesia before an invasive procedure, the use of nitrous oxide with dental procedures, all represent ways of preventing the unnecessary experience of pain.

Treating the symptom (nociception) alone rarely leads to lasting results. Dysregulation in the MINE systems, and pain-induced changes in thinking, feelings, and behaviors must be addressed, often in an interdisciplinary team approach.

In some cases, chronic pain medication can be seen as a helpful measure. Chronic pain requires chronic care. Medications for chronic pain involve three main categories:

1. Nonopioid analgesics: aspirin, salicylate salts, acetaminophen, and nonsteroidal anti-inflammatory drugs (NSAIDs)
2. Opioid analgesics
3. Analgesic adjuvants

These drugs are prescribed according to the World Health Organization's analgesic ladder (108). It involves choosing among these three groups based primarily on pain intensity. Many mild-to-moderate acute pains readily respond to nonopioid analgesics alone; they are the obvious first choice. Some moderate-to-severe pains may require combining the nonopioid analgesics with a low-dose opioid preparation, the second step in the analgesic ladder. The third step is the addition of a *time-released* opioid preparation to the nonopioid analgesics. At any of these three steps, analgesic adjuvants might also be useful.

The APS and the IASP outline a number of important concepts to remember when choosing drugs to manage chronic pain:

1. Analgesia should be integrated into a comprehensive patient evaluation and management plan.
2. The emotional and cognitive aspects of pain must be recognized and treated.
3. Individualize route, dosage, and schedule.
4. Administer analgesics on a regularly predetermined time schedule.
5. Recognize and treat side effects.
6. Do not use placebos to assess nature of pain.
7. Watch for development of tolerance.
8. Use analgesic adjuvants.
9. Block pain transmission whenever possible.
10. Consider a multimodality approach that applies both pharmacologic and nonpharmacologic therapies.

These organizations are a constant source of updated information on the rapidly changing pharmacologic knowledge base regarding pain control with drugs. (See the section "Resources" at the end of this chapter for contact information.)

It is important to remember, that for chronic pain, management with medication "as needed" is often insufficient. Adequate management of ongoing pain is better accomplished using time-contingent, long-acting medications with adequate medication for breakthrough pain (118). This also frees the patient from constantly thinking about how much pain they have and wondering if and when they should be medicating. This therefore is another example of the potential use of preventive pain management principles.

When narcotics are a part of the medication regimen especially at the end-of-life care (119,120), special communication and contracting between physician and patient also becomes necessary. Monitoring benefits, side effects, and possible inappropriate drug use becomes a part of the standard osteopathic pain management (121). Finally, one must remember that opioids can also activate pronociceptive mechanisms creating *opioid-induced hyperalgesia* (129) through distinct cellular mechanisms such as spinal dynorphin, glutamatergic activity, and descending facilitation (125,126). Diminished opioid analgesic efficacy may be opioid tolerance, increased nociception, and/or opioid-induced pain sensitivity (127). These complex pain management patients may require opioid rotation, adding adjunctive medications, combining an NMDA-receptor antagonist, or a trial of opioid tapering (126–129).

Interdisciplinary rehabilitation is the osteopathic standard of care for complex chronic pain management. The APS and the American College of Physicians recently released the clinical practice guidelines for treating back pain, and recommended *interdisciplinary rehabilitation* and exercise therapy for chronic LBP patients (99). The advantages and benefits of an interdisciplinary approach to managing pain, especially when it is chronic, are well documented (81). Treatment in interdisciplinary pain rehabilitation programs is considered the premier treatment for chronic pain (82,106,124). As reported by Flor et al. (73), behavioral outcomes, including return to work, were significantly better, for interdisciplinary, compared with unimodal treatments. Their analyses extend these findings by demonstrating that interdisciplinary treatments were superior to other treatments at improving work-related outcomes at both short-term and long-term follow-up. Using local treatments to reduce noxious stimulation can be multidimensional. Physical measures such as heat and cold, topical agents, local injections of anesthetics, acupuncture, and electrical stimulation (TENS) all can be seen as affecting nociception locally. Systemic medications that have local effects include NSAIDs, narcotics, channel and receptor blockade (sodium, calcium, glutamate), and the expanding list of anti-inflammatory agents targeting recently discovered elements of the inflammatory cascade (tumor necrosis factor, leukotrienes, interleukins, etc.) As the nociceptive signal is processed rostrally, additional sites of intervention become available.

OMT throughout the stages of treatment, as a strategy, can address primary causes and secondary manifestations, and in so doing, can enhance healing capacity. It fosters an individualization of treatment designed to influence health restoration, recovery, and disease prevention. Using palpatory, diagnostics, and therapeutics, the customized therapeutic program can be furthered.

Special considerations arise when there is damage to the peripheral or CNS. The traditional treatments may be less effective as the nature of the pathophysiology is different. Peripheral blockade with local anesthetics, affecting sodium channels, anticonvulsants with effects on glutamate and NMDA transmission, SNRI antidepressants, affecting NE and 5-HT, opiates, and all the rest are possibly well-timed, coordinated options in an evolving interdisciplinary treatment plan.

In this interdisciplinary model, the patient, as leader, in partnership with the physician creates a health care team. Through the use of appropriate consultants and caregivers, coordinated pain management can be delivered. Consulting physicians in pain management, anesthesiology, psychiatry, osteopathic manipulative medicine, physiatry, orthopedics, neurosurgery, general surgery, gynecology, oncology, EENT, neurology, internal medicine, endocrinology, immunology, pharmacology, addictionology, behavioral medicine, sleep medicine, or any other subspecialty required is part of the process of team building. Coordinated nursing services are also appropriate when medical acuity or complexity requires a protracted need for health services. This includes patients hospitalized in pain centers, outpatient pain management centers, primary care–based pain management programs, and medical appliance–related health care (intrathecal or epidural pumps, implanted brain and spinal cord stimulators, etc.).

The fact that anything ever heals is a reminder of the miracle of life.

From a simple paper cut that heals without much thought to a pelvic fracture that requires surgery and thoughtful rehabilitation, there is represented a spectrum of the ongoing manifestation of one of Osteopathy's guiding principles. A broken bone is likely to heal relatively quickly in a healthy person. A sprained ankle might take longer to heal if the patient is misbehaving or suffers with comorbidities that interfere with healing. A more serious injury, with greater tissue injury, or with more systems or sites of involvement is likely to take longer to rehabilitate, even in a healthy person. Most healing is less than perfect, leaving its mark, a scar, a memory on the mind, on the body and on the spirit.

By integrating the five models, the osteopathic perspective seeks to restore optimal structural and functional relations. A comprehensive palpatory examination and a review of psychological factors is required for chronic pain management (43). We know the neuromusculoskeletal system is the primary source of a number of neck, low back, spinal, and extremity pain problems. Here, again, is a setting where OMT can be of particular therapeutic value.

Recently, the APS and the American College of Physicians clinical practice guidelines recommend heat, spinal manipulation, and time to allow the natural healing processes to occur (83), as mainstays for treatment of LBP. Neck and low back syndromes are often related to disturbances of muscle, tendon, ligament, joint capsule, joint, or disc. Appropriate use of OMT can encourage healing and health maintenance. Other examples exist (see Part III: Problem-Based Osteopathic Patient Management). By optimizing structure and function the patient course can be positively affected.

In chronic pain states, whether primary or secondary, there are always manifestations of somatic dysfunction, compensatory structural adaptations, and altered sense of self-confidence for healing. OMT, at this level, is useful by promoting afferent reduction through direct and indirect techniques, muscle relaxation, and improved mobility. This includes attempts at balancing muscle tension and identifying and treating pain generating compensatory musculoskeletal processes. For example, a patient with a limp, from a musculoskeletal or neurologic pathology, may secondarily develop LBP. Treating the back pain helps treat the compensatory process and may suggest preventive strategies. This treats aspects of the pain arising remotely.

When there is ongoing tissue damage or inflammation, efforts to reduce the destructive or inflammatory process is a first step in pain management. This might include OMT, medications, systemic and topical, physical modalities like, heat, cold, traction, compression, TENS, acupuncture, biofeedback, rest, and positioning for comfort. This leads to general recommendations regarding behaviors best suited to recuperation. This can include specific exercises and restrictions, both for daily life and work. It would include advice about sleep and rest requirements. It might invoke a conversation about nutritional optimization as it relates to wellness. This includes a discussion of supplements, foods, herbs, and medications.

Medications have a role in helping the body manage its nociceptive load. Anti-inflammatory agents, immunosuppressants, glutamate antagonists and NMDA receptor antagonists, opiates, NSRI antidepressants, topical anesthetics and anti-inflammatory agents, even intrathecal and intraventricular administration of medication may be useful depending on the circumstance.

There are times when surgical intervention, removing the inflamed gallbladder, decompressing the nerve root, etc., is the clear and best option. Anesthesiologic interventions like trigger point injections, nerve blocks, sympathetic blocks, even spinal cord stimulators can be of selective utility. Now, we also have deep brain stimulation as an extreme option for extreme circumstances. Surgical procedures can influence the suffering aspect of pain and leave the pain experience otherwise intact. Through ablation and deep brain stimulation of structures like the thalamus, hypothalamus, and amygdala, this can be accomplished. Due to its invasive nature, it is usually reserved for patients with malignant clinical courses. Still it is the patient who must be up to the healing process (Table 16.11) to fully benefit. (For an excellent review of presurgical psychological screening and pain outcome (109)).

The ultimate goal of chronic pain management is, "Wellness," fostered by self-regulation, self-healing, and health maintenance. This notion of wellness refers to the balance and recuperative capacity of an individual (Fig. 16.5). It takes into effect inherited constitution, acquired conditions through illness, injury, and abuse, as well as the restorative and healthful aspects of an individual. Their nutrition, exercise regimen, sleep habits, state of mind, support system, and willingness to enter into health-oriented partnerships with doctors and others help determine their reservoir for health (123). This includes their ability to recover from or successfully live with a variety of chronic conditions. It reflects the vulnerability of any given individual to develop pathology in response to a variety of stressors. These pathologies can manifest as organ pathology, musculoskeletal dysfunction, and/or system dysregulation.

Osteopathic chronic pain management is a true art and true science. Chronic pain, like so many other conditions, cannot be cured. Patients can learn to live successfully in spite of chronic pain. This requires the patient and practitioner forming a therapeutic alliance; a partnership for health. In this context, medical investigations can be conducted, psychologic and sociologic information can be

---

TABLE 16.11

Psychological Factors that Interfere with Pain Relief

Number of failed surgeries

Length of pain duration
History of smoking/alcohol overuse/medication failures
Job dissatisfaction/disability payments
Unhealthy food choices/obesity
Stress, anxiety, fear or panic associated with pain
Personality disorders, hypervigilance, somatization
Catastrophic misinterpretations of bodily sensations
Fear of movement, lack of exercise
History of physical, emotional, sexual abuse
Insomnia, nonrestorative sleep

McGILL PAIN QUESTIONNAIRE

PATIENT'S NAME

DATE   TIME   AM/PM

PRI: S   A   E   M   PRI(T)   PPI
(1-10) (11-15) (16) (17-20) (1-20)

1 FLICKERING ___ QUIVERING ___ PULSING ___ THROBBING ___ BEATING ___ POUNDING ___	11 TIRING ___ EXHAUSTING ___
2 JUMPING ___ FLASHING ___ SHOOTING ___	12 SICKENING ___ SUFFOCATING ___
3 PRICKING ___ BORING ___ DRILLING ___ STABBING ___ LANCINATING ___	13 FEARFUL ___ FRIGHTFUL ___ TERRIFYING ___
	14 PUNISHING ___ GRUELLING ___ CRUEL ___ VISCIOUS ___ KILLING ___
4 SHARP ___ CUTTING ___ LACERATING ___	15 WRETCHED ___ BLINDING ___
5 PINCHING ___ PRESSING ___ GNAWING ___ CRAMPING ___ CRUSHING ___	16 ANNOYING ___ TROUBLESOME ___ MISERABLE ___ INTENSE ___ UNBEARABLE ___
6 TUGGING ___ PULLING ___ WRENCHING ___	17 SPREADING ___ RADIATING ___ PENETRATING ___ PIERCING ___
7 HOT ___ BURNING ___ SCALDING ___ SEARING ___	18 TIGHT ___ NUMB ___ DRAWING ___ SQUEEZING ___ TEARING ___
8 TINGLING ___ ITCHY ___ SMARTING ___ STINGING ___	19 COOL ___ COLD ___ FREEZING ___
9 DULL ___ SORE ___ HURTING ___ ACHING ___ HEAVY ___	20 NAGGING ___ NAUSEATING ___ AGONIZING ___ DREADFUL ___ TORTURING ___
10 TENDER ___ TAUT ___ RASPING ___ SPLITTING ___	PPI 0 NO PAIN ___ 1 MILD ___ 2 DISCOMFORTING ___ 3 DISTRESSING ___ 4 HORRIBLE ___ 5 EXCRUCIATING ___

BRIEF ___ MOMENTARY ___ TRANSIENT ___	RHYTHMIC ___ PERIODIC ___ INTERMITTENT ___	CONTINUOUS ___ STEADY ___ CONSTANT ___

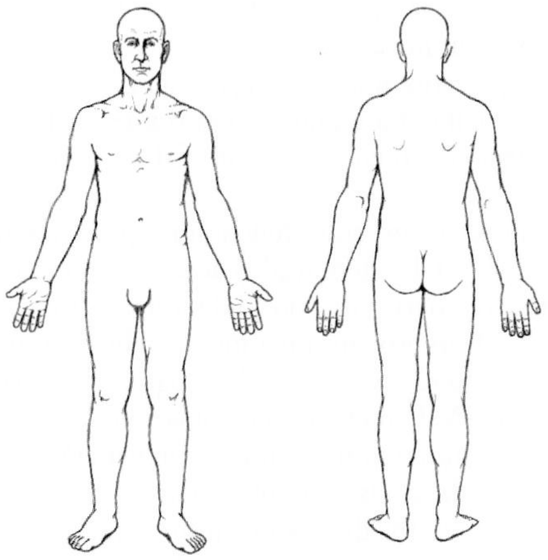

E = EXTERNAL
I = INTERNAL

COMMENTS:

The descriptors fall into four major groups: sensory, 1 to 10; affective, 11 to 15; evaluative, 16; and miscellaneous, 17 to 20. The rank value for each descriptor is based on its position in the word set. The sum of the rank values is the pain rating index (PRI). The present pain intensity (PPI) is based on a scale of 0 to 5. Copyright © 1970 Ronald Melzack.

Figure 16-5 McGill Pain Questionnaire.

gathered, all in an effort to educate the patient and the practitioner. Treating begins by educating the patient about their unique constitutional predisposition, heredity, effects of trauma and illness, and lingering learned behavioral/neurophysiologic traits on how they contribute to their burden of pain. Then, in healing fashion, this information is slowly reformulated into a workbook of health-restoring activities. This workbook includes counsel on nutrition, exercise, rest and sleep, and mental attitude. This advice is included with recommendations regarding traditional medical care, traditional osteopathic manipulative medical care, and whatever care of the future whose evidence-based value is yet to be proved.

With our growing knowledge of the MINE correlates of chronic pain experience and behavior, we can offer a more comprehensive, individualized program for traveling toward wellness. Whether it is nanobot delivery/repair systems or new biochemically targeted molecules, we are prepared to critically evaluate biomedical research of the future, as well as the past and present. Utilizing the osteopathic precepts of *self-healing* and a *self-contained medicine chest*, we and our patient are drawn toward interventions that encourage the expansion and enhancement of these inherent capacities.

Recognizing the primacy of structure/function reciprocity and having the neuromusculoskeletal system readily accessible for evaluation enable osteopathic physicians to enjoy unique access to biologically relevant physical diagnostic information, thereby creating a more complete patient-centered evaluation. As a logical corollary, it also allows an avenue of OMT intervention that is uniquely well tailored and therapeutically useful to the chronic pain patient.

Pain management tests the skills of all physicians. Whether it is the symptom of acute pain or the disease of chronic pain, proper management is dependent on proper assessment. The more multifactorial and biopsychosocial the evaluation can be and the more comprehensive and patient focused the treatment plan, the greater the decrease in reported pain scores and the better the QOL at 2-year follow-up (81–85). Being comprehensive and incorporating the five models (see Chapters 1 and 5) assures the patient feels heard and thoroughly understood. At many levels, the patient feels "touched" by the osteopathic physician.

As an important aside, this collaborative doctor–patient relationship allows the osteopathic *physician* to participate in the patients' healing process and in so doing to help to heal themselves. Physicians are certainly not immune to the problems of chronic pain. In this way, the focus of caring for one's self is encouraged, which is generally not well supported at the professional or institutional level.

In summary, the physician's goal is to restore both physical functioning and adaptive musculoskeletal responses through the simultaneous use of physiological and psychological interventions (110). When managing chronic pain, it is routine to use osteopathic manipulative techniques (104), exercise, sleep, nutritional, and psychological counseling. Combining the five models into a comprehensive treatment approach increases the chances of a successful outcome (103,111). A treatment plan that simultaneously addresses the biological, psychological, and social factors of chronic pain is more likely to succeed and decreases chronic pain perception and behavior (111–114).

Pain is the most common element in the symptoms presented to physicians. But as so eloquently stated by John Loeser (105):

> It is *suffering*, not pain, that brings patients into doctor's offices in hopes of finding relief. Astounding developments in our understanding of the mechanisms of nociception should not cause us to lose sight of our patients' goals. Chronic pain is far more than a sensory process. We must maintain the biopsychosocial model of chronic pain if we are to provide effective health care to our patients. Understanding the components of pain facilitates this goal. Suffering is an emergent property of the human brain and is dependent upon consciousness. It too is worthy of study by scientists and of concern to clinicians.

Successful management of chronic pain depends on much more than knowledge. Knowledge must be teamed with keen observation, patience, and compassion. Many physicians have come to believe that treating chronic pain and suffering, with all its biopsychosocial elements, reflects both the true art and the true science of osteopathic medicine.

This is truly a labor of body, mind, and spirit.

REFERENCES

1. Health, United States. *With Chartbook on Trends in the Health of Americans.* Hyattsville, MD: National Center for Health Statistics; 2006 Centers for Disease Control and Prevention. *National Diabetes Fact Sheet. General Information and National Estimates on Diabetes in the United States,* 2005. *Morbidity and Mortality Weekly: Prevalence of Heart Disease: 2007. Morbidity and Mortality Weekly: Prevalence of Stroke,* 2007.
2. Litcher-Kelley L, Martino SA, Broderick JE, et al. A systematic review of measures used to assess chronic musculoskeletal pain in clinical and randomized controlled Clinical trials. *J Pain* 2007;8(12):906–913.
3. Kerns RD, Otis J, Rosenberg R, et al. Veterans' reports of pain and associations with ratings of health, health-risk behaviors, affective distress, and use of the healthcare system. *J Rehabil Res Dev* 2003;40(5):371–379.
4. May A. Chronic pain may change the structure of the brain. *Pain* 2008;137(1):7–15.
5. Gatchel RJ, Robinson RC, Peng YB, et al. Pain and the brain. *Pract Pain Manage.* 2008;8(5):28–40.
6. Marcus D. Treatment of non-malignant chronic pain. *Am Acad Fam Physicians* 2003;61(5):1331–1346.
7. International Association for the Study of Pain. Pain terms: a list with definitions and notes on usage. *Pain* 1982;14:205.
8. Mersky H. Development of a universal language of pain syndromes. In: Bonica JJ, Lindblom U, Iggo A, eds. *Advances in Pain Research and Therapy.* New York, NY: Raven Press; 1983:37–52.
9. D'Alonzo GE, Bgorkman-Stipp K. AOA adopts policies on treatment of patients in pain: an overview. *JAOA* 2005;105(5):29–31.
10. Licciardone VC. The unique role of osteopathic physicians in treating patients with low back pain. *J Am Osteopathic Assoc* 2004;104(suppl 8):13–18.
11. Melzack R. The gate control theory 25 years later. New prospectives on phantom limb pain. In: Bond MR, ed. *Proceedings of the 6th World Congress on Pain.* New York, NY: Elsevier; 1991.
12. Jerome JA. Transmission of transformation? Information processing theory of chronic human pain. *Am Pain Society J* 1993;2(3):160–171.
13. Raichle ME, MacLeod AM, Snyder AZ, et al. *Proc Natl Acad Sci USA* 2001;98:676–682.
14. Apkarian AV, Sosa Y, Sonty S, et al. Chronic back pain is associated with decreased prefrontal and thalamic gray matter density. *J Neurosci* 2004;24:10410–10415.
15. Apkarian AV, Bushnell MC, Treede RD, et al. Human brain mechanisms of pain perception and regulation in health and disease. *Eur J Pain* 2005;9:463–484.
16. Baliki MN, Chialva DR, Geha PY, et al. Chronic pain and the emotional brain: Specific brain activity associated with spontaneous fluctuations of intensity of back pain. *J Neuroscience* 2006;26:12165–12173.
17. Craig AD. Interoception: the sense of physiological condition of the body. *Curr Opin Neurobiol* 2003;13:500–505.
18. Davis KD, Pope G, Chen J, et al. Cortical thinning in IBS: Implications for Homeostatic, Attention, and Pain Processing. *Neurology* 2008;70:153–155.
19. Schmidt-Wilcke T, Leinisch E, Straube A, et al. Gray matter decreases in patients with chronic tension type headache. *Neurology* 2005;65:1483–1486.

20. Vierck CJ Jr. Mechanisms underlying development of spatially distributed chronic pain (fibromyalgia). *Pain* 2006;124:242–263.

21. Alexandre FM, Granzlera C, Snyder J, et al. Thickening in the somatosensory cortex of patients with migraine. *Neurology* 2007;69:1990–1995.

22. Couch JR, Lipton RB, Stewart WF, et al. Head or Neck Injury increases the risk of chronic daily headache. *Neurology* 2007;69:1169–1177.

23. Urban MB, Gebbart GF. Central mechanisms in pain. *Med Clin North Am* 1999;83(3):585–596.

24. Allemer SR, Bradley LA, Crofford LJ, et al. The neuroscience and endocrinology of fibromyalgia. *Arthritis Rheum* 1997;40(11):1928–1939.

25. Bennett RM. Emerging concepts in the neurobiology of chronic pain: evidence abnormal sensory processing in fibromyalgia. *Mayo Clin Proc* 1999;74(4):385–398.

26. Treede RD. Pain and hyperalgesia: definitions and theories. In: Cervero F, Jensen TS, eds. *Handbook of Clinical Neurology*. New York: Elsevier B.V. *Pain* 2006;81(3rd ser):3–10.

27. Johnstone T, vanReekum CM, Urry HL, et al. Failure to regulate: counterproductive recruitment of top-down prefrontal-subcortical circuitry in major depression. *J Neurosci* 2007;27(33):8877–8884.

28. May A, Hajak G, Ganbbauer S, et al. Structural brain alterations following 5 days of interventions: dynamic aspects of neuroplasticity. *Cereb Cortex* 2007;17:205–210.

29. Draganski B, Gaser C, Volker B, et al. Neuroplasicity: changes in grey matter induced by training. *Nature* 2004;427:311–312.

30. Flor H, Nikolajsen L, Staehelin Jensen T. Phantom limb pain: a case of maladaptive CNS plasticity? *Nat Rev Neurosci* 2006;7:873–881.

31. Woolf CJ, Salter MW. Neuronal plasticity: increasing the gain in pain. *Science* 2000;288:1765–1769.

32. Flor H. Cortical reorganization and chronic pain: implications for rehabilitation. *J Rehabil Med*. Vol. number is (suppl.41) 2003:66–72.

33. Julius D, Basbaum AI. Molecular mechanisms of nociception. *Nature* 2001;413:203–210.

34. Marchand F, Perretti M, McMahon SB. Role of the immune system in chronic pain. *Nat Rev Neurosci* 2005;6:521–532.

35. Scholz J, Woolf CJ. The neuropathic pain triad: neurons, immune cells and glia. *Nat Neurosci* 2007;10:1361–1368.

36. Chapman CR, Tuckett RP, Song CW. Pain and stress in a systems perspective: reciprocal neural, endocrine, and immune interactions. *J Pain* 2008;9(2):122–145.

37. Loeser JD. Pain as a disease. In: Cervero F, Jensen TS, eds. *Handbook of Clinical Neurology*. New York: Elsevier B.V. *Pain*. 2006;81(3rd ser): 11–20.

38. Jerome JA. Information processing theory of chronic pain [bulletin]. *Am Pain Soc J* 1992;1:7–10.

39. Langevin HM. Connective tissue: a body-wide signaling network? *Med Hypotheses* 2006;66(6):1074–1077.

40. Bedi US, Arora R. Cardiovascular manifestation of post-traumatic stress disorder. *J Natl Med Assoc* 2007;99:642–649.

41. Roth RS, Geisser ME, Bates R. The relationship of post-traumatic stress symptoms to depression and pain in patients with accident related chronic pain. *J Pain* 2008.

42. Chialvo D. *J Neurosci* 2008;28:1398–1403.

43. Kuchera ML. Osteopathic manipulation medicine consideration in patient with chronic pain. *JAVA* 2005;105(4):29–36.

44. Smith RC. *Patient-Centered Interviewing: An Evidence-Based Method*. Philadelphia, PA: Lippincott Williams & Wilkins; 2002.

45. Wells-Federman C, Arnstein P, Caudill M. Nurse-led pain management program: effect on self-efficacy, pain intensity, pain related disability, and depressive symptoms in chronic pain patients. *Pain Manag Nurs* 2002;3:131–140.

46. Turk DC, Melzack R. *Handbook of Pain Assessments*. 2nd Ed. New York, NY: The Gilford Press; 2001.

47. Kelso JAS. *Dynamic Patterns: The Self Organization of Brain and Behavior*. Cambridge, MA: MIT Press; 1995.

48. Paice JA, Cohen FL. Validity of a verbally administered numeric scale to measure cancer pain intensity. *Cancer Nurs* 1997;20:88–93.

49. Wilke D, Lovejoy N, Dodd M, et al. Cancer pain intensity measurements: concurrent validity of three tools—finger dynamometer, pain intensity number scale, visual analogue scale. *Hospice J* 1990;6:1–13.

50. Sullivan MJ, Bishop SR, Pivik J. The pain: catastrophizing scale development and validation. *Psychol Asses* 1995;7:524–532.

51. Sullivan MJ, Thorn B, Haythornthwaite JA, et al. Theoretical perspectives on the relation between catastrophizing and pain. *Clin J Pain* 2001;17: 52–64.

52. VanDamme S, Crombez G, Bijttebier P, et al. A confirmatory factor analysis of the Pain Catastrophizing Scale: invariant factor structure across clinical and non-clinical populations. *Pain* 2002;96:319–324.

53. D'Eon JL, Harris CA, Ellis JA. Testing factorial validity and gender invariance of the pain catastrophizing scale. *J Behav Med* 2004;27:361–372.

54. McNeil DW, Rainater AJ. Development of the fear of pain questionnaire—iii. *J Behav Med* 1998;21:389–410.

55. Osman A, Breitenstein JL, Barrios FX, et al. the fear of pain questionnaire—iii: further reliability and validity with nonclinical samples. *J Behav Med* 2002;25:155–173.

56. Albaret MC, MunozSastre MT, Cottencin A, et al. The fear of pain questionnaire: factor structure in samples of young, middle-aged and elderly European people. *Eur J Pain* 2004;8:273–281.

57. Goubert L, Crombez G, VanDamme S, et al. Confirmatory factor analysis of the tampa scale for Kinesiophobia: invariant two-factor model across low back pain patients and fibromyalgia patients. *Clin J Pain* 2004;20: 103–110.

58. Roelofs J, Goubert L, Peters ML, et al. The Tampa Scale for Kinesiophoboa: further examination of psychometric properties in patients with chronic low back pain and fibromyalgia. *Eur J Pain* 2004;8:495–592.

59. Woby SR, Roach NK, Urmston M, et al. Psychometric properties of the TSK-11: a shortened version of the Tampa Scale for Kinesiophobia. *Pain* 2005;117:137–144.

60. Vlaeyen JW, Linton SJ. Fear avoidance and its consequences in chronic musculoskeletal pain: a state of the art. *Pain* 2000;85:317–332.

61. European Commission, Research Directorate General. *COST ACTION B13: Low Back Pain: Guidelines for its Management*. Brussels: European Commission, Research Directorate General; 2004.

62. Royal College of General Practitioners. *Clinical Guidelines for the Management of Acute Low Back Pain*. London: Royal College of General Practitioners; 1999.

63. Turk DC. Pain clinical updates. *Int Assoc Study Pain* 1993;1(3):1–4.

64. Fordyce WE. *Behavioral Methods for Chronic Pain and Illness*. St. Louis, MO: Mosby; 1976.

65. Fordyce WE. Environmental factors in the genesis of low back pain. In: Bonica JJ, Liebeskind JE, Albe-Fessard DG, Eds. *Advances in Pain Research and Therapy*. Vol 3. New York: Raven Press; 1979:659–666.

66. Reading AE, Everitt BS, Sledmere CM. the McGill Pain Questionnaire: a replication of its construction. *Br J Clin Psychol* 1982;21:339–349.

67. Love A, Leboeuf DC, Crisp TC. Chiropractic chronic low back pain sufferers and self-report assessment methods: Part 1. A reliability study of the visual analogue scale, the pain drawing and the McGill Pain Questionnaire. *J Manipulative Physiol Ther* 1998;12:21–25.

68. Holroyd KA, Holm JE, Keefe FJ, et al. A multi-center evaluation of the McGill Pain Questionnaire: results from more than 1700 chronic pain patients. *Pain* 1992;48:310–311.

69. Turk DC, Rudy TE, Salovey P. The McGill Pain Questionnaire reconsidered: confirming the factor structures and examining appropriate uses. *Pain* 1985;21:385–397.

70. Melzack R. The McGill Questionnaire: major properties and scoring methods. *Pain* 1975;1:277–299.

71. Melzack R, Ed. *Pain Measurement and Assessment*. New York: Raven Press; 1983.

72. Melzack R. The short-form McGill Pain Questionnaire. *Pain* 1987;30: 191–197.

73. Flor H, Fydrich T, Turk D. Efficacy of multidisciplinary pain treatment center: a meta-analytic review. *Pain* 1992;49(2):221–230.

74. Gatchel R, Okifuji A. Evidence based scientific data documenting the treatment and cost effectiveness of comprehensive pain programs for chronic nonmalignant pain. *J Pain* 2006;7(11):779–793.

75. Waddell G. A new clinical model for the treatment of low back pain. *Spine* 1987;12:632–644.

76. Banks SM, Kerns RD. Explaining high rates of depression in chronic pain: a diathesis-stress framework. *Psychol Bull* 1996;119:95–110.

77. Nielson WR, Weir R. Biopsychosocial approaches to the treatment of chronic pain. *Clin J Pain* 2001;17(suppl 4):S114–S127.

78. Smith B, Gribbin M. Introduction. *Clin J Pain* 2002;14(supp 4):S1–S4.

79. Guzman J, Esmail R, Karjalainen K, et al. Multidisciplinary rehabilitation for chronic low back pain: systematic review. *Br Med J* 2001;322:1511–1516.

80. Morley S, Eccleston C, Williams A. Systematic review and meta-analysis of randomized controlled trials of cognitive behavior therapy for chronic pain in adults, excluding headache. *Pain* 1999;80:1–13.

81. vanTulder MW, Ostelo R, Vlaeyen JWS, et al. Behavioral treatment for chronic low back pain: a systematic review within the framework of the Cochrane Back Review Group. *Spine* 2001;26:270–281.

82. vanTulder MW, Koes BW, Bouter LM. Conservative treatment of acute and chronic nonspecific low back pain: a systematic review of randomized controlled trials of the most common interventions. *Spine* 1997;22:2128–2156.

83. Hoffman BM, Papsa RK, et al. Mata-analysis of psychological interventions for chronic low back pain. *Health Psychol* 2007;26(1):1–9.

84. Sullivan MJ, Thorn B, Rodgers W, et al. Path model of psychological antecedents to pain experience: Experimental and clinical findings. *Clin J Pain* 2004;20:164–173.

85. Vlaeyen JW, Linton SJ. Fear-avoidance and its consequences in chronic musculoskeletal pain: a state of the art. *Pain* 2000;85:317–332.

86. Kerns RD, Haythornthwaite J, Southwick S, et al. The role of marital interaction in chronic pain and depressive symptom severity. *J Psychosom Res* 1990;34:401–408.

87. Kerns RD, Habib S. A critical review of the pain readiness to change mode. *J Pain* 2004;5:357–367.

88. Centers for Disease Control and Prevention. *Morb Mortal Wkly Rep* 2004;53(2):25–28.

89. King AC, Kiernan M. Physical activity and women's health: issues and future directions. In: Gallant S, Keita G, Royak-Schaler R, Eds. *Health Care for Women: Psychological, Social, and Behavioral Influence*. Washington, DC: American Psychological Association; 1997:133–146.

90. Blair SN, Horton E, Leon AS, et al. Physical activity, nutrition, and chronic disease. *Med Sci Sports Exerc* 1996;28:335–349.

91. Bouchard C, Shepherd RJ, Stephens T, eds. *Physical Activity, Fitness, and Health: International Proceedings and Consensus Statement*. Champaign, IL: Human Kinetics; 1994.

92. Dimeo F, Bauer M, Varahram I, et al. Benefits from aerobic exercise in patients with major depression: a pilot study. *Br J Sports Med* 2001;35(2):114–117.

93. Dunn A, Trivedi M, Kampert J, et al. Exercise treatment for depression: efficacy and dose response. *Am J Prev Med* 2005;28(1):1–8.

94. Fox K. The influence of physical activity on mental well-being. *Public Health Nutr* 1999;2(3A):411–418.

95. Paluska S, Schwenk T. Physical activity and mental health: current concepts. *Sports Med* 2000;29(3):167–180.

96. Salmon P. Effects of physical exercise on anxiety, depression, and sensitivity to stress: a unifying theory. *Clin Psychol Rev* 2001;21(1):33–61.

97. Strohle A, Feller C, Onken M, et al. The acute antipanic activity of aerobic exercise. *Am J Psychiatry* 2005;162:2376–2378.

98. Hayden JA, vanTulder MW, Tomlinson G. Systematic review: strategies for using exercise therapy to improve outcomes in chronic low back pain. *Ann Intern Med* 2005;142:776.

99. Headley B. Posture correction—begin with motor control re-training. *Phys Ther Forum* 1993;3:9.

100. Holroyd KA, Penzien DB, Hursey KG, et al. Change mechanisms in EMG biofeedback training: Cognitive changes underlying improvements in tension headache. *J Consult Clin Psychol* 1984;52:1039–1053.

101. Arena JG, Blanchard EB. Biofeedback and relaxation therapy for chronic pain disorders. In: Gatchel RJ, Turk DC, eds. *Chronic Pain; Psychological Perspectives on Treatment*. New York NY: Guilford Press 2002: 179–230.

102. Arena JG, Blanchard EB. Biofeedback therapy for chronic pain disorders. In: Loeser JD, Butler SD, Chapman CR, Turk DC, Eds. *Bonica's Management of Pain*. 3rd Ed. Baltimore, MD: Williams & Wilkins; 1990: 1755–1763.

103. Seaman DR, Cleveland C. Spinal pain syndromes: nociceptive, neuropathic, and psychologic mechanisms. *J Manipulative Physiol Ther* 1999;(7):458–472.

104. Anderson GB, Lucente T, Davis AM, et al. A comparison of osteopathic spinal manipulation with standard care for patients with low back pain. *N Engl J Med* 1999;341(19):1426–1431.

105. Loeser JD. Pain and suffering. *Clin J Pain* 2000;16(suppl 2):S2–S6.

106. Turk DC, McCarberg B. Non-pharmacological treatments for chronic pain: A disease management contest. *Dis Manage Health Outcomes* 2005;13(1):19–30.

107. Leo RJ. *Concise Guide to Pain Management for Psychiatrists*. Arlington, VA: American Psychiatric Publishing, Inc.; 2003.

108. Turk DC. A cognitive-behavioral perspective on treatment of chronic pain patients. In: Turk DC, Gatchel RJ, Eds. *Psychological Approaches to Pain Management*. New York: Guilford Press; 2002:138–158.

109. Robinson ME, Riley JL. Presurgical psychological screening. In: Turk DC, Melzack R, Eds. *Handbook of Pain Assessments*. Vol 20. New York, London: The Guilford Press; 2001:385–399.

110. Aranoff GM. *Pain Centers—A Revolution in Health Care*. New York, NY: Raven Press; 1988.

111. Friedrich M, Gittler G, Arendasy M, et al. Long term effect of a combined exercise and motivational program on the level of disability of patients with chronic low back pain. *Spine* 2005;30:995–1000.

112. Chou R, Qaseem A, Snow V, et al. Diagnosis and treatment of low back pain: a clinical practice from the American College of Physicians and the American Pain Society. *Ann Intern Med* 2007;147:478–491.

113. Sullivan MJ, Stanish WD. Psychologically based occupational rehabilitation: the Pain-Disability Prevention Program. *Clin J Pain* 2003;19:97–104.

114. Berry PH, Chapman CR, Covington EC, et al. *Pain. Current Understanding of Assessment Management and Treatments*. Reston, VA: National Pharmaceutical Council and the Joint Commission of Accreditation of Healthcare Organizations; December 2001.

115. Carr DE, Ed. Pain in depression—depression in pain. *Int Assoc Study Pain*. 2003;11(5):2–6.

116. Licciardone JC, Brimhall A, King L. Osteopathic manipulative treatment for low back pain: a systematic review and meta-analysis of randomized controlled trials. Data reviewed at the Osteopathic Research Council Meeting OCCYIC VI: "Hot Topics in Osteopathic Manipulative Research". April 7–8, 2005, Fort Worth, TX.

117. Stanton DF, Dutes JC. Chronic pain and the chronic pain syndrome: the usefulness of manipulation and behavioral interventions. *Phys Med Rehabil Clin N Am* 1996;7:863–875.

118. Rasor JR, Harris G. Opioid use for moderate to severe pain. *JAOA* 2005;5(6):2–7.

119. AOA position statement on end-of-life care. House of Delegates of AOA, July 2005. Available at: http://www.jasa.org/cqi/reprint/105/3-suppl/25.

120. American Osteopathic Association. End-of-Life Committee. AOA's position against use of placebo's for pain management at end-of-life. *JAOA* 105(suppl);2005:2–5.

121. Galluzzi KE. Management of neuropathic pain. *JAOA* 2005;105(suppl-4):12–19.

122. Oken BS. Complementary and alternative medicine: overview and definitions. In: Oken BS, Ed. *Complimentary Therapies in Neurology: An Evidence Based Approach*. New York, NY: The Parthenon Publishing Group; 2004:1–7.

123. Morris DB. In: Jensen TS, Wilson PR, Rice AS, Eds. *The Challenges of Pain and Suffering in Clinical Pain Management: Chronic Pain*. London: Arnold; 2003.

124. Loeser J, Turk DC. Multidisciplinary pain management. In: Loeser JD, Butler SD, Chapman CR, Turk DC, Eds. *Bonica's Management of Pain*. 3rd Ed. Baltimore, MD: Williams & Wilkins; 1990:2069–2079.

125. Vanderah TW, Ossipov MH, Lai J, et al. Mechanisms of opioid-induced pain and antinociceptive tolerance: descending facilitation and spinal dynorphin. *Pain* 2002;92:5–9.

126. Mao, J. Opioid-induced abnormal pain sensitivity: implications in clinical opioid therapy. *Pain* 2002;100:213–217.

127. Angst MS, Clark JD. Opioid-induced hyperalgesia: a qualitative systematic review. *Anesthesiology* 2006;104:570–587.

128. Baron MJ, McDonald PW. Significant pain reduction in chronic pain patients after detoxification from high-dose opioids. *J Opioid Manag* 2006;2:277–282.

129. Visser E, Schug SA. The role of ketamine in pain management. *Biomed Pharmacother* 2006;60:341–348.

130. Mao J. Opioid-induced hyperalgesia. Pain Clinical Updates. In: *Association for the Study of Pain.* Vol XVI, Issue 2, Elsevier; February 2008.

131. Gatchel RJ, Maddrey AM. The biopsychosocial perspective of pain. In: Raczynski J, Leviton L, Eds. *Healthcare Psychology Handbook.* Vol II. Washington, DC: American Psychological Association Press; 2004.

132. Gatchel RJ. *Clinical Essentials of Pain Management.* Washington, DC: American Psychological Association; 2005.

133. Turk DC, Monarch ES. Biopsychosocial perspective on pain. In: Turk DC, Gatchel RJ, Eds. *Psychological Approaches to Pain Management: A Practitioners Handbook.* 2nd Ed. New York: Guilford; 2002.

134. Engel GL. The need for a new medical model: a challenge for biomedicine. *Science* 1977;196(4286):129–136.

135. Loeser JD. Concepts of pain. In: Stanton-Hicks J, Boaz R, Eds. *Chronic Low Back Pain.* New York: Raven Press; 1982.

136. Ecop. Core Curriculam for Osteopathic Principles Education Chicago: American Association of Osteopathic Medicine (AACOM); February 4, 1983.

17 Psychoneuroimmunology—Basic Mechanisms

DAVID A. BARON, ROSE J. JULIUS, AND FRANK H. WILLARD

KEY CONCEPTS

- Psychoneuroimmunology (PNI) is the study of the interaction between psychological processes, the nervous system, and the immune system of the human body.
- While clinical observations have noted the dynamic interplay between the nervous, endocrine, and immune systems in homeostasis regulation and stress adaptation, it was not until the 20th century that research has formally investigated these mechanisms.
- Osteopathic philosophy and principles emphasize the unity between the structure and the function of multiple body systems. The osteopathic physician is best suited to appreciate and study the interplay between the different systems of the body and behavior, health, and disease.
- Understanding the basic functions and mechanisms of the HPA axis, the central and peripheral nervous systems, is key to elucidating the processes through which the PNI systems integrate to affect health and disease.
- Stress impacts the body's endocrine, immune, central, and peripheral nervous systems, with direct influences on individuals' health and disease susceptibility. Furthermore, stress reduction can improve overall health and well-being.
- Depression and anxiety symptoms are commonly comorbid with many chronic physical diseases. These psychiatric symptoms can complicate the physical illnesses and increase morbidity and mortality. The osteopathic physician should maintain a low threshold for treatment of depressive and anxiety symptoms.
- Many somatic illnesses have behavioral and psychological manifestations. The osteopathic physician should be aware of these in order to properly diagnose and treat patients.

INTRODUCTION

Psychoneuroimmunology (PNI) conceptualizes the brain, endocrine, and immune functioning as an interactive supersystem. As Rubinow first pointed out (new ref), the immune, neuroendocrine, and central nervous systems (CNSs) are all stimulus-response systems that are similar in the functions they subserve and tightly integrated in their actions. The reciprocal regulatory effects of these systems provide a basis (but not proof) for the belief that brain-behavior-endocrine-immune interactions are clinically relevant and not reducible to characteristics of component systems.

At the core of PNI research is a demonstration of the interconnectedness of the body, mind, and behavior, and its impact on health and disease. Basic PNI principles stress the hardwiring of emotions to the body's physiologic functions. The CNS, autonomics, the endocrine, and the immune system all contribute to the body's inherent work in regulating and trying to maintain homeostasis. Pert et al. (2) first suggest that the intimate integration of these three systems warrants their consideration as a single system. All three systems can function as sensory and effector organs, recognizing foreign antigen and other incoming physiologic signals. All three also transmit signals as part of their basic function. The immune response can be modulated by input from nervous and neuroendocrine systems. The high degree of similarity and integration between these systems is sensible due to the fact that their common task is to preserve homeostasis and assure consistency and integrity of body cells and tissues, for which integration and regulatory redundancy is an obligation (1). The more research elucidates the mechanisms through which these complex systems interact, the further advances can be made in the diagnosis and treatment of disease and in the promotion of health.

HISTORY OF PSYCHONEUROIMMUNOLOGY RESEARCH

Despite centuries of interest, clinical observation, and anecdotal reports, research on the complex interactions between the CNS, the endocrine, and the immune system has only taken place in modern medicine. This in part is due to the lack of an understanding of the complexities of immune functioning and limited availability of biologic probes to observe and measure the impact of one system on another. Walter Cannon, a physiology professor at Harvard University, coined the term *homeostasis* to reflect the need of the organism for regulation and balance of all its systems. He conducted research with animals, noting that affective states such as psychological distress, anxiety, and rage were associated with cessation of the movements of the stomach. His findings were published in 1911 in a book titled *The Mechanical Factors of Digestion*. Hans Seyle would continue to expand on Cannon's early work, studying the physiologic adaptation of animals to stress. Through his research, he ultimately developed a clinical model for adaptation to stress, consisting of three stages: a brief alarm reaction, prolonged resistance, and a terminal stage of exhaustion and death (3).

George F. Solomon (4), M.D. ultimately coined the term *psychoneuroimmunology* in 1964, in his paper, "Emotions, Immunity, and Disease: A Speculative Integration." In this paper, Solomon offers a theoretical explanation of how emotional states can diminish immunocompetence, ultimately resulting in physical disease. These speculations were of significant interest to the mental health community. However, they did not enjoy a similar level of acceptance by the medical community as a whole and especially not by immunologists. Without data derived from well-controlled research studies, the consensus was that something as imprecise and variable as emotion could not impact on a seemingly hard-wired physiologic process like immune function. No reasonable explanation existed for how these systems could communicate with each other.

Despite repeated reports of illness following a significant stressor, nothing more substantial than observation and anecdotal reports existed to convince the nonbelievers. Ader (5) made an accidental finding that immunosuppression could be classically conditioned in mice, by pairing taste aversion (saccharine) with an immunosuppressive medication (cyclophosphamide). He conditioned rats by using saccharine combined with cyclophosphamide. When given to the rats, the elixir induced nausea and suppressed the rats' immunity. Ultimately, Ader gave the rats saccharine alone, and this neurologic signaling via taste was able to stimulate immune suppression. These findings ignited research interest in PNI. For the first time, direct evidence demonstrated the potential for external manipulation of the immune system. Intriguing questions followed. If immunologic response could be behaviorally conditioned to turn off, could it be conditioned to turn on? Could this help explain why the patient, who shortly after giving up the will to live, dies or conversely why some patients refuse to succumb and ultimately defy the odds to survive life-threatening illness? These and related questions stimulated PNI research.

In addition to stress-induced immune suppression, altered immune functioning has been reported in patients with mood disorders and other psychiatric syndromes. The Greek physician, Galen, reported the relationship between clinical depression and physical illness in the second century C.E. He observed that melancholic (depressed) women were especially susceptible to breast cancer. In an effort to replicate and further explain this observation, Levy et al. (6) measured natural killer (NK) cell activity (a measure of immune function) and psychological stress in women with breast cancer. They found NK activity to be a reliable and valid predictor of the patient's prognosis relative to their lymph node status. In a separate study, these same authors reported that 51% of baseline NK activity changes could be accounted for by assessing a patient's adjustment to diagnoses, depressive symptoms, and perceived lack of social support. They concluded, based on multiple clinical trials, that differences in NK cell activity and overall prognosis could be predictably determined by assessing baseline stress, as measured by emotional adjustment, depression or fatigue, and lack of social supports.

Alterations in immune function were demonstrated in patients with psychotic illnesses as early as the 1940s (7). Early studies in the 1970s also reported an increase in the prevalence of herpes simplex virus in patients with psychotic depression when compared with age-matched nondepressed controls. Unfortunately, these early studies did not monitor any specific immune parameters. This research and findings would be replicated in a similar fashion in future PNI research as it applies to stress, mood disorders, and clinical outcomes.

OSTEOPATHIC PHILOSOPHY AND PSYCHONEUROIMMUNOLOGY

The concept of PNI was the central theme of A.T. Still's original theories that formed the basis of the Osteopathic philosophy. Still was ahead of his time in postulating that the body communicated with itself and that the CNS was integral to the somato-visceral, visceral-somatic response. Still opened the first Osteopathic psychiatric hospital, the Still-Hildreth Clinic in Missouri in 1916. Although not yet recognized as an area of clinical investigation at that time, core PNI concepts were prominent in the proposed etiology and treatment of the patients treated at the clinic. Essentially, a broad-based appreciation of inextricable structural and functional relationships between somatic dysfunction, hormonal systems, central and peripheral nervous system, and resultant mood and behavior formed the rationale for explaining symptom onset and treatment interventions. The idea that the brain could be the target organ of hormonal fluctuation occurring in other parts of the body would later be described as hormonal neuromodulation.

PSYCHONEUROIMMUNOLOGY MECHANISMS

PNI mechanisms are founded on some core clinical observations and research findings:

- The autonomic nervous system, particularly the sympathetic nervous system (SNS), directly innervates lymph organs and tissues. The SNS can change blood flow/supply to lymphoid tissue.
- Immune cells have receptors for neurotransmitters such as norepinephrine, which is released from sympathetic nerve terminals. This allows the SNS to directly affect immune functioning.
- Immune cells also have receptors for hormones.
- As elucidated by Pert, neuropeptides are present on the cells walls in the CNS as well as in the immune system (2).
- Cytokines made by immune cells, such as macrophages, can directly act on the nervous system.
- Cytokine receptors are expressed in the CNS as well as in the periphery.
- Stress impacts the immune, nervous, and endocrine systems.

These clinical observations generate support for the idea that nervous, endocrine, and immune systems can interact, in part, through neuropeptides and neurotransmitters and more generally that psychological effects and physical health are intricately linked.

The structure and function of the HPA axis is thought to be central to the physiologic response of the body to stress, as its activation occurs in response to stress. Part of the HPA axis response to stimuli involves the release of cortisol, ACTH, and corticotropin-releasing hormone (CRH). The stimulation and release of these mediators has CNS effects on arousal, sensory processing, stimulus habituation, pain, sleep, and memory, and depends on whether the stressor is acute or chronic. Chronic increases in cortisol can also have multiple physiologic effects, including hyperglycemia, increased visceral adipose, increased blood pressure, decreased bone density, and increased lipids. The response of the HPA axis is also modulated by the autonomic nervous system, which works to maintain homeostasis through the sympathetic branch, regulating arousal, and parasympathetic branch, regulating relaxation. Often when the HPA axis is stimulated together with the SNS during a stressor, the result is a diminished immune response (8). Reactions of the HPA axis and the nervous system in response to stress have been demonstrated as risk factors for diseases such as viral infection and autoimmune diseases (9).

The HPA axis is also stimulated in the process of inflammation. Macrophages generate numerous proinflammatory cytokines, such as interleukin (IL)-2, IL-6, IL-1, IL-10, tumor necrosis factor-α and interferon-gamma (INF-γ), in response to stress. These cytokines in turn stimulate ACTH and cortisol secretion. These same cytokines are active in the brain and the periphery. When cytokines are released in response to stress and inflammation, the effect on the body is weakness, malaise, sleep and appetite disturbances, and difficulties with memory and concentration. Proinflammatory cytokines also cause serotonin levels to be decreased within the CNS, by increasing its enzymatic turnover (10).

The HPA axis, the nervous system, and the interaction of the two are disturbed in disorders of chronic inflammation, such as rheumatoid arthritis and systemic lupus erythematosus (SLE) (11). Persistent inflammation is linked with a multitude of diseases, including heart disease, arthritis, renal and pulmonary disease, diabetes, infection, and cancer. Cytokines and IL-6 stimulate the production of C-reactive protein (CRP), an important risk factor in heart disease (12). In fact, Ridker et al. (12) found a 2.6 increase in risk of death among individuals with high CRP and IL-6 levels. IL-6 and other inflammatory cytokines have also been implicated in muscle wasting, osteoporosis, and arthritis. INF-α has been shown to increase anxiety-like behaviors in rhesus monkeys and to induce ACTH and cortisol (13).

CRH has been studied as another key mediator between the central nervous, endocrine, and immune systems. It is a major regulator of the HPA axis, the autonomic nervous system, and the immune system and is widely distributed in the brain and the periphery of the body. CRH dosed in the CNS has been shown to cause decreases in immune responses in numerous studies, including immunoglobulin M (IgM) and IgG levels (14–16). CRH receptors in the amygdala are associated with immune response (17).

In collaboration with the immune and endocrine systems, the nervous system is known to mediate the body's response to stress in a multitude of ways. First, as mentioned above, autonomic nerves directly innervate lymphoid tissue, including the spleen. Second, lymphoid cells have B-adrenergic specific receptors. The SNS stimulates and potentiates immune responses to inflammation and infection through β_2 adrenergic receptors and neuropeptides, such as neuropeptide Y (18). Cole et al. (19) demonstrated that activation of the SNS accelerates HIV replication and progression. Wilder (20) demonstrated that sympathetic activity exacerbates arthritis in rats. Kuis (21) found that evidence for disturbed sympathetic activity in response to stress has a negative impact on juvenile idiopathic arthritis.

THE EFFECTS OF STRESS ON HEALTH AND DISEASE

The arrival of a good circus consisting of clowns is a greater benefit upon the health of a town than that of twenty Asses laden with drugs.
—Dr. Thomas Sydenham

Throughout history, medical researchers and clinicians have observed and reported the effect of stress on health and disease. Stress impacts multiple body systems, the behaviors and the health of the individual, with implications for morbidity and mortality. Despite the general acceptance of this concept by health care providers, it is difficult to define stress and its impact on health and disease. Early concepts focused on stress being a force of universality, acting on a passive body, with all organisms reacting in a similar way to the disruption. More modern concepts emphasize stress not as a universally experienced phenomenon, but rather that experienced uniquely by every individual. Research to date has shown that an individual's reaction to stress is dependent on a myriad of factors, including the type of stress, chronicity of the stress, genetic predisposition, health status, psychological factors, coping strategies, and the interplay between all these variables.

The role of stress, the stress response, and health is a central concept in PNI research. The idea that emotional stress is a biologic phenomenon that has a modulatory effect on immune functioning, and ultimately health, has historically not been fully accepted by the medical community. Over the last few decades, significant discoveries and clinically meaningful advances have been made by

PNI investigators. Researchers at Temple University's Center for Substance Abuse Research have reported provocative findings suggesting chemokines function as neurotransmitters within the CNS (22,23). These findings further demonstrate how emotional stress, which impacts the immune response system including chemokines, may directly affect central neuronal functioning via synaptic transmission modulation. As this area of investigation continues to progress and the extant literature grows, a critical question is the direct impact of emotional stress on physical health. When does a down-regulation of immunocompetency result in the actual onset, of exacerbation, of disease? How much of an immune alteration is required before susceptibility to physical illness is more likely to occur? Translational research in this area has yet to answer these highly relevant clinical questions. The answer is most assuredly as complex as the interaction between stress and immunomodulation. The intricate nature of this interaction is further complicated by epigenomic phenomena and the concept of context dependency. In addition, recent preclinical investigations have demonstrated that stress resilience is biologically mediated, but can be altered through nonbiological interventions. This was highlighted by Meili and colleagues who discovered stress resilience in rat pups could be altered as a result of maternal overgrooming. The overgroomed pups not only increased their stress resistance but also bred more stress-resistant pups themselves compared to genetically similar siblings.

Psychological distress arises when a person perceives that imposed demands have exceeded their ability to cope with them. There is a significant physiologic response to stress, and this response further impacts the ability to cope both physically and psychologically with the stressor. The response also directly impacts an individual's objective physical and mental health, with effects on disease incidence, morbidity, and mortality. Early PNI research using animal models linked stress with acute infections and inflammation. Rasmussen et al. (24) and others found that mice subjected to psychological stress were at increased risk of developing herpes simplex virus infections. Amkraut et al. (25) and others also demonstrated that psychologically stressed rats were more susceptible to developing adjuvant-induced arthritis.

Specific immunologic mechanisms have been demonstrated to mediate the body's immune response to stress. In the early 1980s, Kiecolt-Glaser published a series of prospective studies examining the effects of emotional stress on the function of the immune system. Kiecolt-Glaser et al. (26) measured NK cell activity, γ-interferon (INF-γ) production by lymphocytes, stimulated with concanavalin A and mitogen responses in medical students prior to important examinations. Medical students stressed by examinations had poorer immunity and were thus susceptible to active herpesvirus infection (27). The results of these studies demonstrated that emotional stress did in fact have a measurable negative effect on the immune system. NK cell activity has been further studied by many as a key factor in the body's response to stress and infection. A robust response should be seen in NK cell activity when pathogens and/or non–self-entities are recognized by the body. Numerous studies have demonstrated a decrease in NK cell activity in response to severe life stress (28).

Would the results from research in acute infections and stress be similar in studies of patients with chronic illness? Castes et al. (29) conducted a prospective study of 35 asthmatic children to evaluate the impact of a psychosocial intervention on immune function. The immune measures studied were NK cell number and activity, IL-2 (30), and leukocyte affinity for IgE receptors (an important marker related to asthma attacks). Clinical outcomes assessed included the number of asthma attacks, use of bronchodilators, and overall pulmonary improvement in pulmonary functioning during the psychosocial interventions, as compared to the six months before entry into the study. In fact, surface markers for IgE in the children receiving the psychosocial interventions became similar to nonasthmatic children. Smyth et al. (31) report similar findings in adults with asthma and rheumatoid arthritis. These well-designed clinical trials offer preliminary data supporting the hypothesis that psychosocial stress can and does affect immune functioning and ultimately wellness.

A more recent view of the relationship between PNI and cancer by Kiecolt-Glaser (32) reports "substantial evidence from both healthy populations under stress as well as individuals with cancer associated psychological stress for immune deregulation and that stress may also enhance carcinogenesis and through alterations in DNA repair and or apoptosis." The study concludes that psychological and behavioral factors could influence the incidence and progression of cancer through psychosocial influences on immune function. Decreased NK cell activity has been recognized in patients with cancer under stress (33), and a reduced NK cell activity has been linked to diminished capacity to resist tumor suppression in animals.

Severity of the stressor is an important variable in terms of the body's reaction to the stimulus. Loss of a spouse or other significant other is considered one of the most severe psychological stressors. Research has demonstrated decreases in immune function, specifically mitogen-induced lymphocyte proliferation among individuals who have lost spouses (34,35).

Just as type of stressor is important to the overall response of the neuroendocrine system on the body, so too does the individual's perception of and reaction to the stressor work in mediating the body's response. Irwin et al. (36) demonstrated that the severity of affective symptoms in response to psychologic stressors correlates with the NK cell activity, that is, those with a greater severity of affective symptoms such as depression have greater decreases in NK cell activity. Greater levels of perceived stress and depressive symptoms have been shown to predict susceptibility to infection with viruses such as the rhinovirus (37) as well as delays in wound healing (11).

Chronicity of the stressor is also relevant to understanding the different physiologic responses on the body. One study showed that while an initial response to a stressor (in this study foot shock) is immune suppression, repeat exposure to the stressor elicited immune enhancement, and this process was mediated by central CRH (38). Other research demonstrates activation of the immune system in response to acute stress and an inhibition of immune responses under exposure to chronic stress. Chronic stress of caring for a loved one with Alzheimer dementia is associated with delays in wound healing and in long-term immune changes.

Since it is established that stress significantly influences immunity, an important next research question is *Can stress-reduction mediate the body's immune response?* In one important study, students who were taught relaxation training had a significant increase in NK cell activity compared to students who had not received stress-reduction training. This was the first well-controlled clinical human study that demonstrated evidence of immune enhancement resulting from a psychological intervention (39). Not only did stress reduction improve immune response, but students who were not taught stress-reduction techniques self-reported an increase in infectious illness symptoms around exam time (24). These provocative experiments clearly demonstrated an effect in otherwise healthy subjects. Another study showed that relaxation interventions decreased inflammatory response (40). Additionally, research in cancer patients has demonstrated longer survival time and improved immune function among patients enrolled in support and psychoeducation groups (41,42).

MOOD DISORDERS AND IMMUNE FUNCTION

A merry heart doeth good like a medicine but a broken spirit dries the bones.
   —Galen

Immunologic alterations have been reported in a number of psychiatric disorders. Schleifer et al. (43) demonstrated that depressed patients have a decreased number of peripheral T cells compared with those of nondepressed control subjects. Their data suggest that the functional activity of lymphocytes, as well as the number of circulating immunocompetent cells, is reduced in patients with clinical depression. They also speculate that the altered immune functioning in patients with depression might be related to the severity of their depressive symptoms. Indeed, patients with depression have also been found to have decreases in NK cell activity in several studies (44,45). Affective symptoms such as depression and anxiety appear to stimulate proinflammatory cytokines such as IL-6 (46).

Depression is a common comorbidity in many physical illnesses. Research has documented prevalence rates of depression among patients with a variety of chronic medical conditions, often higher than in the general population. Table 17.1 highlights these prevalence rates. Not only are many diseases associated with an onset of clinical depression and anxiety, but depression and anxiety symptoms themselves can be significant risk factors for the progression of many diseases, with effects on morbidity and mortality (47). Depressive symptoms are associated with lower immune responses, such as lower T lymphocyte counts, along with higher

TABLE 17.1

Prevalence of Depression in Patients with Comorbid Medical Illness

Comorbid Medical Illness	Prevalence Rate (%)
Cardiac disease	17–27
Cerebrovascular disease	14–19
Alzheimer disease	30–50
Parkinson disease	4–75
Epilepsy	
Recurrent	20–55
Controlled	3–9
Diabetes	
Self-reported	26
Diagnostic interview	9
Cancer	22–29
HIV/AIDS	5–20
Pain	30–54
Obesity	20–30
General population	10.3

Source: Reproduced from Evans, DL, Charney, DS, Lewis L, et al. Mood disorders in the medically ill: scientific review and recommendations. *Biol Psychiatry* 2005;58:175–189, with permission.

rates of infection (9). La Via et al. (48) demonstrated that among patients with generalized anxiety, symptom severity was correlated with immune suppression and increased disability from upper respiratory infection. Severity of anxiety symptoms has also been associated with decreased NK cell activity (46).

Depression as a clinical syndrome, as well as depressive symptoms, has been shown to impact morbidity and mortality related to cardiovascular health. Cardiovascular disease risk is increased significantly among patients with depression (47). Also, the prevalence of depression among patients with cerebrovascular and cardiac disease is higher than that in the general population. As Evans et al. (47) point out, the prevalence of depression may be even higher, as many patients with cardiovascular disease have symptoms that may not meet criteria for a diagnosis of major depression, but that are clinically significant. These subsyndromal symptoms still may impact morbidity and mortality in these patients. Frasure-Smith et al. (49) conducted a large prospective study of patients' status post acute coronary syndrome and monitored them for depressive symptoms as well as inflammatory markers. Findings demonstrated that depressive symptoms were risk factors for further cardiac morbidity, and that a higher level of CRP was also a risk factor. In another longitudinal prospective study of over 5,000 elderly men and women, Arbelaez et al. (50) found that greater depressive symptoms were associated with an increased risk of ischemic stroke. Depression is postulated to exert its physiologic effects on cardiovascular health by influencing inflammation of vessels, increasing platelet activation, promoting hypercoagulability, changing autonomic function (decreased heart rate variability and increased QT), and increasing in plasma cortisol (47).

Given the documented association between depression and cardiovascular morbidity and mortality, one might consider a low threshold for treatment of depressive and anxiety symptoms in this context. The trial, Enhancing Recovery In Coronary Heart Disease Patients (ENRICHD), demonstrated safety for SSRI treatment in the context of cardiac disease. Future research will focus on potential cardioprotective benefits SSRI may have, hypothesized to be beneficial due to their assumed inherent antiplatelet activity.

Depression is also an associated risk factor for diabetes morbidity and mortality (47). Depressed patients may be less adherent to medications, placing them at risk for higher blood glucose levels and associated progression of the disease (51). Additionally, depression, through its effects on the HPA axis, can promote insulin resistance and inflammation.

Much research has investigated the association between depression and cancer. In addition to having possible depression as a result of coping with the psychological and physical aspects of their diagnosis and treatments, studies have suggested that affective symptoms may decrease survival time (52) and increase mortality (53). There is even some suggestion that stress may lead to an increased risk of cancer (47).

Lowering the threshold for treatment of comorbid depression is warranted given the association between depression, its symptoms, and many other physical illnesses. To date, research has attempted to document the safety and efficacy of using antidepressants in the context of many physical comorbid conditions.

SOMATIC CONDITIONS WITH BEHAVIORAL AND PSYCHIATRIC MANIFESTATIONS

Many somatic illnesses have behavioral and psychological manifestations. While not all the mechanisms are clearly understood, the presentation and associations of somatic conditions with behavioral and psychiatric manifestations highlight the interconnectedness between physical and mental health, and relate strongly to PNI

concepts. For example, Stein (54) reports behavioral pathology and neuropsychiatric impairment of patients with autoimmune and viral conditions associated with SLE and multiple sclerosis (MS). In turn, stress can also aggravate the symptoms associated with many of these and other conditions. Stress has been shown to predict CD4 cell loss in HIV. Table 17.2 highlights some somatic pathology with psychiatric manifestations. It is important for the osteopathic physician to be especially mindful of these conditions in the assessment and diagnosis of patients.

HEALTH BEHAVIORS

Health behaviors clearly influence the physical responses of the body, with implications for health and disease. Behaviors such as tobacco smoking, drug dependence, and sleep deprivation have been shown to further decrease the body's immunity independent of other factors such as depressive symptoms, and that many of these behaviors interact synergistically with depression to cause greater decreases in immunity than either factor alone (18). Chronic sleep deprivation may stimulate the SNS and the HPA axis (55). As well, partial sleep deprivation during a single night was demonstrated by Irwin et al. (56) to produce a reduction in NK activity. Kripke et al. (57) demonstrated increased mortality associated with poor sleep.

RELEVANCE OF PSYCHONEUROIMMUNOLOGY TO MEDICAL PRACTICE

Why is PNI an important topic for study? The implications of research in this area are paramount for the diagnosis and treatment of patients with a myriad of chief complaints and diagnoses. Particularly, mental health issues are often ignored or viewed as unimportant for treating physically ill patients. Most of medical education focuses on the diagnosis and treatment of so-called organic pathologic conditions. Yet, PNI research underscores that all illness, regardless of whether its manifestation is physical or mental, is organic. Psychosocial issues, while often seen as separate

TABLE 17.2
Medical Conditions with Psychiatric Manifestations
Delirium
Epilepsy
Dementia
CVA
Structural brain abnormalities
Nutritional deficiencies (B_{12}, A, D, zinc)
Endocrinopathies (thyroid anomalies, hypoglycemia, Addison's, Cushing's)
Infections (HSV, syphilis, HIV, TB, prion disease, encephalitis)
MS
Huntington's
Wilson disease
Parkinson disease
SLE
Neoplastic disease

and distinct from biologic concerns, directly influence multiple body systems and impact the health and disease of the individual. To put in context the need to understand this interplay, consider the following facts:

- Emotionally distressed patients visit their doctors more than nondistressed patients.
- Emotionally distressed patients are hospitalized more often than nondistressed patients.
- Emotionally distressed patients have greater morbidity and mortality than nondistressed patients and generally poorer health outcomes for many physical diagnoses.
- People with emotional distress commonly visit their doctors with physical symptoms and complaints, never reporting psychological symptoms.
- Emotional distress and other psychological issues directly impact patient adherence to medications and other biologic treatments.
- Nearly two thirds of all physician visits fail to confirm a biologic diagnosis.
- Numerous biologic diseases can manifest themselves with psychiatric symptoms.
- Medical illness can precipitate emotional distress, which complicates medical treatment and increases medical costs.
- Emotional distress often goes unrecognized and untreated in medical encounters.
- Appropriate mental health treatment reduces emotional distress, medical utilization, and costs.
- Savings from reduced medical costs can offset the cost of providing mental health treatment and stress-reduction training, which may result in lower overall health care costs.

In everyday medical practice, both in inpatient and outpatient settings, these facts are often ignored, leading to a striking mismatch between the true needs of patients and the health care services delivered. The result is less effective care, frustration for both patient and physician, and the waste of ever-shrinking health care resources. Worse, it can lead to dangerous misdiagnosis of patients, with disastrous health consequences, including disability and death. If nothing else, PNI research underscores the need to assess patients' emotional distress. Osteopathic physicians in particular are likely to encounter patients with musculoskeletal complaints with a component of stress contributing to their illness. Eliciting information from patients on their stressors, their perception of their stress level (see Chapter 19) along with their current mood and mental state, making appropriate referrals and recommending appropriate stress-management techniques, will positively impact their overall health, improving disease and disability. For patients suffering from ongoing illness, identifying and addressing these issues may improve their response to other somatic treatments.

CASE VIGNETTES

Case 1

A 47-year-old woman presents to your office complaining of frequent low back pain, headaches, poor sleep, and a cold she "just cannot kick." The patient has been in your practice for 12 years and has enjoyed good health. She lives a healthy lifestyle, watches her diet, exercises regularly, does not smoke or drink in excess, and comes in yearly for a physical. Her routine labs are normal. Her physical exam reveals musculoskeletal tension in her lumbar, midthoracic, and cervical regions. The remainder of her physical exam is unremarkable, except for mild congestion in her lungs and a nonproductive cough. She appears more stressed than usual, and when questioned admits to ongoing marital discord and trouble with her teenage son. She also reports failing health in the parents and concerns over their ability to care for themselves much longer. She reports feeling tired most of the time and rarely gets a restful night's sleep. It takes her up to three hours to fall asleep due to worrying about her life circumstances. She does not meet diagnostic criteria for depression or generalized anxiety disorder.

Discussion

This patient's physical complaints are real and likely related to the chronic emotional stress she is experiencing. Although immunologic measures were not attained, an appropriate treatment strategy would include OMT for her musculoskeletal complaints, conservative symptomatic treatment of her pulmonary symptoms, analgesics as needed for her headache (if not relieved by cervical OMT), and a stress-reduction strategy focusing on coping skills to deal with her stressful life issues (marriage, son, and parents). Special attention should be paid to normalizing her sleep. Chronic initial insomnia (difficulty falling asleep) is commonly associated with life stress and often responds to effective stress management. Disruptive and diminished sleep can play an important role in contributing to physical pain and susceptibility to organic pathology.

Case 2

A 58-year-old man, who has been your patient for the past 6 years, suffers an acute myocardial infarction. He survives the event and is being stabilized in the coronary care unit (CCU). You have treated the patient for depression in the past with antidepressant medication and referred him for psychotherapy. Although he was compliant with his medications, he never followed up on referrals for therapy. When you visit him in the CCU, his is very depressed and convinced he is going to die. He is hopeless, helpless, and expresses guilt over not being a good husband or father. Your attempts to cheer him up are unsuccessful. You inform his cardiologist of his history of Major Depression and restart his antidepressant medication and arrange for a psychiatry consult while in the CCU.

Discussion

It is critically important to address the patient's depression. Major depression is a major, independent risk factor for mortality in patients with cardiac disease. The precise mechanism for the increased morbidity and mortality is not fully known. However, the extant literature is robust and well replicated in confirming this clinical association. All physicians treating patient with cardiac disease should routinely screen for depression.

PATIENT EDUCATION

...I can trust the principles that I believe are found in the human body. I find what is necessary for the health, comfort, happiness of man, the passions, and all else. Nothing is needed but plain, ordinary diet and exercise.
—A.T. Still

The physician should emphasize the importance of lifestyle alterations such as cutting down on caffeine, maintaining a healthy diet, quitting smoking, and exercising regularly. Other stress-reduction strategies can be tailored to the patient's lifestyle and can be a key component to disease prevention. It is the responsibility of physicians to educate their patients about the importance of maintaining a healthy lifestyle. Make patients aware of target organs and areas particularly vulnerable to stress, such as the heart, kidney, gastrointestinal tract, and musculoskeletal system. Some patients with chronic medical conditions should be educated on the potential associated psychological consequences of their condition and the physician should be regularly screening for these. Patient counseling should also include protecting patients from claims of miracle cures or unsound, potentially dangerous interventions, such as unproven megavitamin therapies.

Virtually all adult patients have some awareness of the noxious effects of chronic stress on overall health. The lay media and press are replete with stories on the importance of stress reduction, and the ill effects of the stressful times we live in. As physicians, it is important to teach patients to first identify emotional stress, particularly chronic low-grade stress that often goes unidentified. By the time a patient acknowledges their inability to manage their life stress, adverse health consequences have already been set in motion. Stress may be self-medicated with alcohol or drugs, which results in additional health problems. It is important for physicians to give patients the "permission" to discuss stress, as they may be reluctant to address these issues as not having medical relevance.

Osteopathic philosophy highlights the importance of treating the whole patient, not just diseased or dysfunctional organs. Every physical complaint should be evaluated as context dependent, that is, how does the current life setting impact on the symptom presentation? The field of PNI demonstrates the need to evaluate stress as an important factor in the etiology and treatment of disease.

CONCLUSIONS

Our understanding of the intricate complexity of the body, its individual systems, and their interconnectedness, is rapidly expanding. Since the first edition of this text in 1997, significant advances have been made in understanding the basic mechanisms of PNI. Early clinical observation is rapidly becoming scientifically proven fact. As with other core osteopathic concepts, the key to continued acceptance in the medical community, and ultimately to the enhancement of health of patients, is the study of and adherence to the principles of methodologically sound scientific research. PNI research has demonstrated that the CNS is in direct and constant bidirectional communication with the immune and endocrine systems. The goal of future research is to better understand their "language" and how to identify and manipulate it to promote health and treat disease. The challenge of the next generation of osteopathic researchers and clinicians is to continue to investigate and to expand on the work of this exciting and important field.

REFERENCES

1. Rubinow DR. Brain, behavior and immunity: an interactive system. *J Natl Cancer Inst* 1990;(monograph no. 10):7982.
2. Pert CB, Ruff MR, Weber RJ, et al. Neuropeptides and their receptors: a psychosomatic network. *J Immunol* 1985;135:820–826.
3. Neylan TC. Hans Selye and the field of stress research. *J Neuropsychiatry Clin Neurosci* 1998;10:230.
4. Solomon GF, Moos RH. Emotions, immunity and disease. *Arch Gen Psychiatry* 1964;11:657–674.
5. Ader R, Cohen N. Behaviorally conditioned immunosuppression. *Psychosom Med* 1975;37:333–340.
6. Levy SR, Lippman M, d'Angelo T. Correlation of stress factors with sustained depression of natural killer cell activity and predicted prognosis in patients with breast cancer. *J Clin Oncol* 1987;5:348–353.
7. Freeman H, Elmadjuan F. The relationship between blood sugar and lymphocyte levels in normal and psychotic subjects. *Psychosom Med* 1947;9: 364–371.
8. Glaser, R, Kennedy, S, Lafuse W, et al. Psychological stress-induced modulation of IL-2 receptor gene expression and IL-2 production in peripheral blood leukocytes. *Arch Gen Psychiatry* 1990;47:707–715.
9. Kemeny M, Cohen F, Zegens L. Psychological and immunological predictors of genital herpes recurrence. *Psychosom Med* 1989;51:195–208.
10. Muller N, Schwarz MJ. The immune-mediated alteration of serotonin and glutamate: towards an integrated view of depression. *Mol Psychiatry* 2007;1–13.
11. Kemeny ME, Schedlowski M. Understanding the interaction between psychosocial stress and immune-related diseases: a stepwise progression. *Brain Behav Immun* 2007;21:1009–1018.
12. Ridker PM, Cushman M, Stampfer MJ, et al. Inflammation, aspirin, and the risk of cardiovascular disease in apparently healthy men. *N Engl J Med* 1997;336:973–979.
13. Felger JC, Alagbe O, Hu F, et al. Effects on interferon alpha on rhesus monkeys: a nonhuman primate model of cytokine induced depression. *Biol Psychiatry* 2007;62:1324–1333.
14. Irwin MR, Vale W, Britton KT. Central corticotropin-releasing factor suppresses natural killer cytotoxicity. *Brain Behav Immun* 1987;1:81–87.
15. Irwin M, Jones L, Britton K, et al. Central corticotropin-releasing factor reduced natural cytotoxicity: time course of action. *Neuropsychopharmacology* 1989;2:281–284.
16. Strausbaugh H, Irwin M. Central corticotropin releasing hormone reduced cellular immunity. *Brain Behav Immun* 1992;6:11–17.
17. Hauger RL, Irwin M, Lorang M, et al. Chronic pulsatile administration of corticotropin releasing hormone into the central nervous system downregulates amygdala CRH receptors and desensitizes splenic natural killer cell responses. *Brain Res* 1993;616:283–292.
18. Irwin MR. Human psychoneuroimmunology: 20 years of discovery. *Brain Behav Immun* 2008;22:129–139.
19. Cole SW, Kemeny ME, Fahey JL, et al. Psychological risk factors for HIV pathogenesis: mediation by the autonomic nervous system. *Biol Psychiatry* 2003;54(12):1444–1456.
20. Wilder RL. Neuroendocrine-immune system interactions and autoimmunity. *Annu Rev Immunol* 1995;13:307–338.
21. Kuis W, de Jong-de Vos van Steenwijk C, Sinnema G, et al. The autonomic nervous system and the immune system in juvenile rheumatoid arthritis. *Brain Behav Immun* 1996;10:387–398.
22. Adler MW, Rogers TJ. Are chemokines the third major system in the brain? *J Leukoc Biol* 2005;78:1204–1209.
23. Adler MW, Geller EB, Chen XH, et al. Viewing chemokines as a third major system of communication in the brain. *AAPS J* 2006;7:E865–E870.
24. Rasmussen AFJ, Marsh JT, Brill NQ. Increased susceptibility to avoidance-learning stress or restraint. *Proc Soc Exp Biol Med* 1957;96:183–189.
25. Amkraut AA, Solomon, GF, Kraemer HC. Stress, early experience and adjuvant-induced arthritis in the rat. *Psychosom Med* 1971;33(3):203–214.
26. Kiecolt-Glaser JR, Garner W, Speicher C, et al. Psychosocial modifiers of immunocompetence in medical students. *Psychsom Med* 1984;46:714.
27. Glaser R, Rice J, Sheridan J, et al. Stress-related immune suppression: health implications. *Brain Behav Immun* 1987;1:7–20.
28. Irwin MR, Miller AH. Depressive disorders and Immunity: 20 years of progress and discovery. *Brain Behav Immun* 1997;21(4): 374–383.
29. Castes M, Hagel I, Palenque M, et al. Immunological changes associated with clinical improvement of asthmatic children subjected to psychosocial intervention. *Brain Behav Immun* 1999;13:1–13.
30. Glaser R. Stress-associated immune dysregulation and its importance for human health: a personal history if psychoneuroimmunology. *Brain Behav Immun* 2005;17:321–328.
31. Smyth M, Stone, A, Hurwitz A, et al. Effects of writing about stressful experiences on symptom reduction with asthma or rheumatoid arthritis, a randomized trial. *JAMA* 1999;281:1304–1309.
32. Keicolt-Glaser J, Glaser R. Psychoneuroimmunology and cancer: fact or fiction? *Eur J Cancer* 1999;35:1603–1607.

33. Lutgendorf Sk, Sood AK, Anderson B, et al. Social support, psychological distress, and natural killer cell activity in ovarian cancer. *J Clin Oncol* 2005;23:7105–7113.

34. Bartrop RW, Lazarus L, Luckhurst E, et al. Depressed lymphocyte function after bereavement. *Lancet* 1977;16:834–836.

35. Schleifer SJ, Keller SE, Camerino M, et al. Suppression of lymphocyte stimulation following bereavement. *JAMA* 1983;250(3):374–377.

36. Irwin M, Daniels M, Smith TL, et al. Impaired natural killer cell activity during bereavement. *Brain Behav Immun* 1987;1:98–104.

37. Cohen S, Tyrrel DAG, Smith AP. Psychological stress and susceptibility to the common cold. *N Eng J Med* 1991;325:606–612.

38. Irwin M, Vale W, Rivier C. Central corticotropin-releasing factor mediates the suppressive effect of stress on natural killer cytotoxicity. *Endocrinology* 1990;126:2837–2844.

39. Kiecolt-Glaser, JR. Stress, personal relationships, and immune function: health implications. *Brain Behavior Immun* 1999;13:61–77.

40. Lutgendorf SK, Logan H, Kirchner L, et al. Effects of relaxation and stress on the capsaicin-induced local inflammatory response. *Psychosom Med* 2000;62:524–534.

41. Spiegel D. Bloom JR. Kraemer HC, et al. Effect of psychosocial treatment on survival of patients with metastatic breast cancer. *Lancet* 1989;2:888–891.

42. Fawzy FI, Fawzy NW, Hyun CS, et al. Malignant melanoma: effects of early structured psychiatric intervention, coping and affective state on recurrence and survival 6 years later. *Arch Gen Psychiatry* 1993;50:681–689.

43. Schleifer SJ, Keller SE, Siris SG, et al. Depression and immunity. *Arch Gen Psychiatry* 1985;42:129–133.

44. Irwin M, Patterson T, Smith TL, et al. Reduction in immune function in life stress and depression. *Biol Psychiatry* 1990;27:22–30.

45. Irwin M, Lacher U, Caldwell C. Depression and reduced natural killer cytotoxicity: a longitudinal study of depressed patients and control subjects. *Psychol Med* 1992;22:1045–1050.

46. Kiecolt-Glaser JK, McGuire L, Robles BS, et al. Psychoneuroimmunology and Psychosomatic Medicine: back to the future. *Psychosom Med* 2002;64:15–28.

47. Evans DL, Charney DS, Lewis L, et al. Mood disorders in the medically ill: scientific review and recommendations. *Biol Psychiatry* 2005;58:175–189.

48. La Via MF, Munno I, Lydiard RB, et al. The influence of stress intrusion on immunodepression in generalized anxiety disorder patients and controls. *Psychosom Med* 1996;58:138–142.

49. Frasure-Smith N, Lesperance F, Irwin MR, et al. Depression, C-reactive protein and two-year major adverse cardiac events in men after acute coronary syndromes. *Biol Psychiatry* 2007;62(4):302–308.

50. Arbelaez JJ, Ariyo AA, Crum RM, et al. Depressive symptoms, inflammation and ischemic stroke in older adults: a prospective analysis in the cardiovascular health study. *J Am Geriatr Soc* 2007;55:1825–1830.

51. De Groot M, Anderson R, Freedland KE, et al. Association of depression and diabetes complications: a meta-analysis. *Psychosom Med* 2001;63:619–630.

52. Brown KW, Levy AR, Rosberger Z, et al. Psychological distress and cancer survival: a follow-up 10 years after diagnosis. *Psychosom Med* 2003;65:636–643.

53. Stommel, M, Given BA, Given CW. Depression and functional status as predictors of death among cancer patients. *Cancer* 2002;94:2719–2727.

54. Stein M. Future directions for brain, behavior and the immune system. *Bull NY Acad Med* 1992;68(3):390–410.

55. Redwine L, Haufer RL, Gillin JC, et al. Effects of sleep and sleep deprivation on interleukin-6, growth hormone, cortisol and melatonin levels in humans. *J Clin Endocrinol Metab* 2000;85(10):3597–3603.

56. Irwin M, Mascovich A, Gillin JC, et al. Partial sleep deprivation reduces natural killer cell activity in humans. *Psychosom Med* 1994;56:493–498.

57. Kripke DF, Garfinkel L, Wingard DL, et al. Mortality associated with sleep duration and insomnia. *Arch Gen Psychiatry* 2002;59(2);131–136.

Psychoneuroimmunology— Stress Management

JOHN A. JEROME AND GERALD G. OSBORN

KEY CONCEPTS

- Empathy for stress-related problems and their many manifestations
- Stress and related somatic complaints, including those related to somatic dysfunction
- Signs and symptoms of depression
- Signs and symptoms of anxiety
- Signs and symptoms of alcohol abuse
- Signs and symptoms of insomnia
- Adaptive methods for coping with stress
- Overview of treatment techniques
- Impact of the doctor/patient relationship

DEFINITION OF STRESS

Stress is a condition experienced when the physical, mental, emotional, or social environment makes unwanted inescapable demands. These demands exceed resources and create a sense of powerlessness and inability to control the stressor or effect change.

The person under stress responds as a unit (i.e., mind, body, and spirit) and coordinates an adaptive response to the stressor. The main physiological components of the stress system response are activation of the hypothalamic—pituitary—adrenal (HPA) axis, autonomic nervous system arousal, and adrenalin secretion in the "fight or flight" response. Being aroused by stress provides a biologic advantage that enables the individual to rapidly respond to danger. Historically, the stress system response enhanced survival and adaptive responses. We ignored a pain, fought back, ran to safety on broken bones, and scrambled to the top of the food chain.

Osteopathic philosophy teaches us that damaging stress levels are reached when perceived threats or dangers upset the biopsychosocial balance. Prolonged hypersympathetic activity can be deleterious to health and can facilitate disease. Thoughts, emotions, and behaviors in response to stressors are in a blended and complex relationship that can affect both anatomy (structure) and physiology (function).

Seyle (1) first described these interdependent processes of responding to stress as the general adaptation syndrome. Seyle believed that our response to stress was a specific syndrome following certain patterns and affecting specific organs. Stress itself could be induced by a variety of internal or external stimuli.

When patients are continually stressed, they move through three response stages. First, there is a startle response and orientating reflex as the patient becomes aware of the stress and is biologically alarmed. Adrenal, cardiovascular, respiratory, and musculoskeletal functions increase.

Next is an attempt to cope and problem-solve biologically, psychologically, and socially. The patient mobilizes all resources to meet and resist the stressor. If the patient is successful, mastery and learning occur. If the patient fails, he or she becomes exhausted physically, mentally, and emotionally.

The third stage, exhaustion, is what the osteopathic physician sees clinically as a variety of dysfunctional signs and symptoms affecting any and all organ systems. As coping responses fail, the exhaustion depletes adaptive reserves and resistance disappears. Patients then experience somatic dysfunction and present themselves to the primary physician requesting treatment for symptoms of stress-related problems.

In primary care, stress-induced somatic complaints are the mechanisms underlying the symptoms for 20% to 35% of all patients seeking treatment from physicians (2,3). In the United States, more than 33% of the population is susceptible to acute or chronic stress and the physical and psychological disorders caused by stress (4). Studies in several populations have also found that 10% of patients account for about 30% of primary care visits (5,6). These high utilizers of medical services represent a group of patients who have physical disease *as well* as concomitant distress (7).

The onset of stress-related illness is a complex phenomenon that incorporates the tissue pathology (musculoskeletal abnormalities), psychosocial and behavioral response to that physical insult, and the environmental factors that maintain or reinforce that disability (even after the initial cause has been resolved). A significant portion of the variance in an individual response to any disease outcome is accounted for by the manner of behavior and emotional response to the stress of the illness (8). In fact, the majority of today's health woes—obesity, cancer, and anxiety disorders to heart disease, hypertension, and adult-onset diabetes—are actually relatively new "diseases of civilization" brought on by our behavioral choices and mind-body interactions.

Our current understanding of stress-induced illnesses suggests that these processes are a complex interplay between genetic physiologic, environmental, and behavioral factors that influence health and disease. Behavioral mechanisms can alter the nervous system, endocrine system, and immune system, directly influencing health. Diet, exercise, drugs, alcohol, and tobacco use, along with a variety of other behaviors, also modify disease progression and/or disease risk (see Chapter 32). Finally, behaviors directly related to seeking or avoiding medical care also have important consequences on prevention, early detection, and adherence with medical regimens.

This chapter presents a framework for understanding and clinical management of stress-related illness. It includes guidelines for the cognitive/behavioral management of the effects of stress related to:

Anxiety
Depression
Alcohol abuse
Insomnia

CONCEPTUALIZING STRESS

No life is without stress. There are, however, adaptive and maladaptive manners of coping, even under the most stressful circumstances. Although there are many events that can happen in our lives that are completely unexpected, many of life's difficulties can be anticipated and managed effectively. Many people accept high levels of stress in their lives but do not appreciate the high price they pay. Medical research has shown that a life lived in chronic stress can trigger and activate psychophysiologic disorders such as hypertension, peptic ulcer disease, and coronary artery disease (9). In essence, a feed-forward loop is established where each added consequence of stress becomes a factor in raising the levels of stress.

More recent research in psychoneuroimmunology shows a relationship between stress and attenuation of immune responses (see Chapter 17). Mental health researchers have long known that stress plays a strong role in various forms of anxiety and depressive disorders, as well as in many forms of substance use and abuse.

Most recently, stress has been conceptualized as an organism's nonspecific response in an attempt to adapt to demands. Those demands can cover the spectrum of psychological, social, and physiological functioning. Even ordinary day-to-day events, whether seen as positive or negative, involve adoption to change. The concept of adoption to change now dominates current thinking about stress. In 1967, Holmes and Rahe verified the stress of adaptation (10). They developed a scale and assigned points to 43 common life events to develop a stable and objective point of reference. They were not concerned with how people interpreted or felt about these events but merely with whether they happened. They demonstrated that the greater number of points a person scored over a 1-year period, the greater the probability of illness occurring within the next 2 years. Later research determined that if the person assessed the event as a negative life experience, the impact was more severe (11). Based on these findings, the preventive implications are clear. Although a number of stress scales are now available, the Holmes & Rahe Social Readjustment Scale remains one of the most highly validated and widely used (Table 18.1). This scale can be easily incorporated into medical practice and used liberally to help patients assess their judgments and vulnerabilities based both on the stressful event and their perception (positive or negative) of the event and develop increasingly effective anticipatory coping strategies.

TABLE 18.1

Social Readjustment Scale

	Life Events	Holmes Points
1	Death of spouse	100
2	Divorce	73
3	Marital Separation	65
4	Jail term	63
5	Death of close family member	63
6	Personal injury of illness	53
7	Marriage	50
8	Fired from job	47
9	Marital reconciliation	45
10	Retirement	45
11	Change in health of family member	44
12	Pregnancy	40
13	Sex difficulties	39
14	Having a baby	39
15	Business readjustment	39
16	Change in financial state	38
17	Death of a close friend	37
18	Change to different line of work	36
19	Change in number of arguments with spouse	35
20	Mortgage large in relationship to income	31
21	Foreclosure of mortgage or loan	30
22	Change in responsibilities in work	29
23	Son or daughter leaving home	29
24	Trouble with in-laws	29
25	Outstanding personal achievement	28
26	Spouse begins or stops work	26
27	Begin or end school	26
28	Change in living conditions	25
29	Change in personal habits	24
30	Trouble with boss	23
31	Change in work hours or conditions	20
32	Change in residence	20
33	Change in schools	20
34	Change in church activities	19
35	Change in recreation	19
36	Change in social activities	18
37	Small mortgage in relation to income	17
38	Change in sleeping habits	16
39	Change in number of family get-togethers	15
40	Change in eating habits	13
41	Vacation	13
42	Christmas	12
43	Minor violations of the law	11

Source: Reprinted from Holmes TH, Rahe RH. The social readjustment rating scale. *J Psychosom Res* 1967;7:17–20, with permission.

Stress can also be self-generated. The "type A personality" first described by Friedman and Rosenman has now become a household word (12). Although it has been argued excessively as to whether the "type A personality" is a feature of coronary artery disease, the adaptive style of a person with type A characteristics can hardly be envied. Research beyond Friedman & Rosenman's seminal work indicates that competitiveness, impatience, and difficulty dealing with anger and hostility are the core characteristics of people prone to coronary artery disease. It might be difficult to completely alter these maladaptive styles, but counseling and education can modify them to the point where a patient's risks are significantly lowered (13).

Change the Stressor

Before seeking medical treatment, the patient probably has already tried to change the stressor without much success. In this situation, casual advice usually doesn't work, even when coming from a physician. Compliance with physician advice is low, particularly in the current climate of health care delivery where the pace is hectic and often impersonal. As patients shift between physicians and insurance plans in a managed care environment, the personal relationships once forged between physician and patient disappear. Trusting relationships are difficult to establish under these circumstances, increasing the likelihood that professional advice will go unheeded.

Many patients who come to a primary care setting are looking for help with stress-related symptoms. A primary care, osteopathically oriented approach assesses all the disturbing psychosocial and organic problems, including the neuromusculoskeletal elements, so that a long-term treatment strategy can be developed. In such cases, after a detailed history is taken and complete physical examination, the treatment strategy incorporates all elements of the osteopathic philosophy. It includes:

Palpatory diagnosis
Manipulative treatment
Exercise, diet, smoking, alcohol, drug cessation
Appropriate medication
Coping strategy education

There is a palpable reaction of the musculoskeletal system to stress whether from inside the body or from environmental or social influences. When hands-on procedures are used to identify stress-induced somatic dysfunction, the experienced osteopathic practitioner can determine whether the observed pattern of somatic dysfunction is associated with primary neuromusculoskeletal dysfunction, contribution from somatovisceral or viscerosomatic components, or a more complex behavioral dysfunction. Designing all aspects of treatment to include modification of the biopsychosocial causes and maladaptive responses to stress is important. The primary care physician must constantly be aware that clinically evident stress reflects two realities:

1. A patient's response to stress-inducing events produces biopsychosocial consequences.
2. A patient's long-term stress management style is an important factor determining health or disease and an area in which the physician must intervene for long-term adaptive change.

Change Response to Stress

Significant stress-related conditions are often found in primary care outpatients (14–16). By changing the patient's response to stress, one immediately treats some of the autonomic components of stress-related somatic dysfunction and their antecedents, which can be so impactful on the patient's general health. Success is more likely when physicians educate patients, guide and mentor their adaptation, and teach them coping and stress-mastery skills. In a primary care practice, diagnosis begins by accurately reviewing four of the most common behavioral consequences of stress:

Depression
Anxiety
Substance abuse
Insomnia

When the exact diagnosis is made, carefully inform the patient and then guide him or her through a process of problem identification and problem solving designed to either relieve or cope with the stress. The remainder of this chapter reviews these four stress-induced problem areas from a cognitive behavioral standpoint. Emphasis is on rapid techniques for diagnosis and on specific strategies to be employed within the doctor-patient relationship.

DEPRESSION

Feeling "down" is a universal experience. Being sad or "blue" accompanies disappointments, setbacks, or losses in life. The depressed mood usually lasts a short time and passes. For some people, however, the sadness becomes intense and long lasting, coloring every aspect of their existence. The future seems hopeless. They see the world as an overwhelming place in which they are unable to concentrate, sleep, or solve the routine problems of life.

In the United States, the problem of clinical depression is monumental. Clinical depression results in the hospitalization of 6% of all women and 3% of all men, with 15% of all who are severely clinically depressed eventually committing suicide (17,18). There is emerging evidence that depressed patients have a significant loss of cells in the prefrontal cortex, a brain area important in discerning reward verses punishment, in shifting mood from one state to the other, and in exerting cortical restraint on the amygdala fear system through the HPA axis and the sympathetic nervous system. An increase in cortisol and norepinephrine secretion represents a highly adverse biochemical environment, a condition that is likely to contribute to many different adverse outcomes, including increased visceral fat, insulin resistance, increased inflammation, enhanced blood coagulation, deficient fibrinolysis, decreased bone formation, and increased bone resorption.

The *Diagnostic and Statistical Manual of Mental Disorders*, Fourth Edition (*DSM-IV*) (19) and the *Guidelines for Detection and Diagnosis in Primary Care* categorize mental health diagnoses. The word "depression" refers to a syndrome in which a variety of signs and symptoms occur. Typically, there is a change from previous adequate emotional functioning to a depressed mood and a loss of pleasure in life's usual activities. The depressed person feels sad or empty most of the time and often experiences impairment in interpersonal, social, or occupational functioning. Conceptually, these symptoms may be grouped as disturbances in:

- Emotions (depressed mood, loss of interests/pleasure, worthlessness or guilt).
- Ideation (worthlessness/guilt, death/suicide).
- Neurovegetative or somatic symptoms (sleep, appetite/weight, psychomotor, energy, concentration).

If five or more of these symptoms are present for more than 2 weeks, a diagnosis of *major depressive disorder* is considered. The diagnosis

TABLE 18.2

Structured Interview Questions for Depression[a]

For the last 2 weeks, have you had any of the following problems nearly every day?

1. Trouble falling or staying asleep, or sleeping too much?	YES	NO
2. Feeling tired or having little energy?	YES	NO
3. Poor appetite or overeating?	YES	NO
4. Little interest or pleasure in doing things?	YES	NO
5. Feeling down, depressed, or hopeless?	YES	NO
6. Feeling bad about yourself, or that you are a failure or have let yourself or your family down?	YES	NO
7. Trouble concentrating on things, such as reading the newspaper or watching television?	YES	NO
8. Being so fidgety or restless that you were moving around a lot more than usual? If No: What about the opposite—moving or speaking so slowly that other people could have noticed?	YES	NO
9. In the last 2 weeks, have you had thoughts that you would be better off dead or of hurting yourself in some way? (Tell me about it.)	YES	NO

SCORING: If five or more of Nos. 1 to 9 are yes, one of which is No. 4 or 5, then consider *major depressive disorder.* If the condition has persisted over the last 2 *years* and the patient reports that it was hard to do their work, take care of things at home, or get along with other people, then consider *dysthymia.*

[a]Primary care evaluation for mental disorders (Prime-MD).
Source: From Spitzer RL, Williams JB. *PRIME-MD Clinical Evaluation Guide.* New York, NY: Biometrics Research, New York State Psychiatric Institute, 1994, with permission.

becomes *dysthymia* if over the last 2 years the patient reports having felt these symptoms and says that for more than half of that time it was hard to work, take care of simple things at home, or get along with people. These symptoms (all but depressed mood) may be more readily recalled using the mnemonic "SIG: E CAPS" (i.e., "prescribe energy capsules"): Sleep, Interest, Guilt, Energy, Concentration, Appetite, Psychomotor, and Suicide.

Measurement of Depression

The diagnosis and management of depression in a patient can be facilitated through numerous self-administered inventories, such as the Zung Depression Scale (20,21), the Beck Depression Inventories (22,23), and the MMPI Depression Scale (24,25). These inventories provide reliable and valid measures of the severity of depression. The patient can initially be tested for a baseline measure and then repeatedly tested with the same instrument to measure progress. More recently developed structured interviews such as the PHQ-9 (26,27) allow one to quickly (i.e., in 8.4 minutes) determine the presence of pivotal signs and symptoms (Table 18.2). The PHQ-9 is a 9-item self-report instrument assessing the nine symptoms of DSM-IV major depression, which is feasible to use, reliable, and valid in primary care settings (28). The PHQ-9 establishes the clinical diagnosis of depression and does not require further confirmation. This allows the clinician more time to be spent on patient education and negotiation of the treatment plan. The PHQ-9 sum score can also be used to track the severity of patient symptoms over time (29).

Medical disorders with intrusive symptoms of depression must also be ruled out (Table 18.3). Unfortunately, there is no evidence to support routine laboratory testing in the diagnosis of depression. Complete blood count (CBC), a basic chemistry profile, liver function tests, TSH, Rapid plasma reagin (RPR), B$_{12}$, and folate levels are only helpful when underlying medical conditions are suspected. This situation is made more complex by the fact that depression

has also been reported as a serious adverse effect of more than 100 commonly prescribed drugs (Table 18.4).

Tricyclic antidepressants and serotonin reuptake inhibitors are the gold standards for initiating management of many serious, possibly organic, depressions (30,31). Recoveries are often dramatic as the patient reverts to predepression levels of functioning. Given the distribution of depression in the population and the long-term treatment protocols used in management, primary care physicians are exposed to a tremendous amount of publicity and marketing from pharmaceutical companies to manage the symptoms of depression with their various products.

Cognitive Behavioral Factors in Depression

Depression in response to stress can be well understood within the framework of learning theory (32). Deficits in social skills can set the stage for unrewarding social, vocational, and personal relationships causing subsequent feelings of depression. Studies with animals and humans exposed over time to inescapable stress have shown that the subjects failed to demonstrate simple behaviors to escape or avoid the stress and subsequent punishment (33,34). In a laboratory setting, when exposed to inescapable electric shock, dogs and humans felt helpless and both suffered from naturally occurring depression. Human and animal groups showed similar response patterns of passivity, slowed learning, impaired problem solving, and loss of appetite. Their inability to stop the stressor or to escape from the stressor initiates cognitive processes that lead to a sense of powerlessness. Victims of inescapable stress lower their future expectations for control over stress and have measurably lower self-esteem and lower motivation.

Beck (23,32,35) describes negative schemas as a learned maladaptive thinking process that often leads to depression. When faced with stressful events, some patients routinely employ negative views of themselves and their abilities (i.e., negative schemas) and are dominated by themes of failure and personal inadequacies.

TABLE 18.3

Medical Illnesses and Conditions with Intrinsic Symptoms of Depression

Parkinson disease

Normal pressure hydrocephalus

Multiple sclerosis/stroke

Brain tumors (temporal lobe)

Adrenal insufficiency syndrome

Hyperparathyroidism

Vitamin B_{12} or iron deficiency

Serum sodium or potassium reductions

Hypercalcemia

Cancer

Metal (thallium, mercury) intoxication

Chronic pain and disease (i.e., fibromyalgia, diabetes mellitus)

A common symptom in geriatric populations

20%–24% of medical inpatients

Neurologic disorders (i.e., related to abnormal catecholamines or indoleamine metabolism)

Cardiac disease

Serious medical injury (i.e., spinal cord, end-stage renal disease)

Dementia, head trauma, seizure disorders

Source: From Derogatis LR, Wise TN. *Anxiety and Depressive Disorders in the Medical Patient. Clinical Practice No. 4.* Washington, DC: American Psychiatric Press, 1989:121, with permission.

TABLE 18.4

Drugs with Known Propensity to Induce Clinical Depression

Antihypertensives

Reserpine

  α-methyldopa

  Guanethidine

  Clonidine

  Propranolol

  Hydralazine

Hormones

  Corticosteroids

  Progesterone

  Estrogen

Central nervous system depressants

  Benzodiazepines

  Barbiturates

  Alcohol

Neuroleptics

  Haloperidol

  Fluphenazine

Cardiovascular agents

  Digitalis

  Procainamide

Antiparkinsonian drugs

  L-Dopa

  Amantadine

Antimicrobials

  Cycloserine

  Gram-negative agents

  Sulfonamides

Source: From Derogatis LR, Wise TN. *Anxiety and Depressive Disorders in the Medical Patient. Clinical Practice, No. 4.* Washington, DC: American Psychiatric Press, 1989:125, with permission.

They have learned to expect their performance to be worse than that of others, and view the world as an overwhelming place, laden with burdens, and filled with excessive demands and daily defeats.

Over time, negative depression themes become stable, long-standing thought patterns creating downward cognitive spirals. Once the pattern begins, the patient will organize new experiences as depressing and selectively direct attention to the negative aspects of current and future stressors. Thus, these depression-prone patients perceive the present as depressing, remember the past the same way, and respond to the future in a fixed, negative manner, independent of what occurs in their environments.

There are six basic cognitive errors in logic that a patient learns over time (Table 18.5). Insight into these faulty reasoning patterns is helpful for some depressed patients. Patients who respond positively to cognitive therapy by changing their patterns of thought, appear to have sustained benefits; the risk of relapse over one year was lower than that of patients who had responded to medications and were then switched to placebo (36). Osteopathically trained physicians routinely work with their patients' cognitive stress coping styles in addition to pharmacologically managing their depressive symptomatology. Drug therapy and cognitive behavioral treatments augment and complement one another in patients diagnosed with major clinical depression; administering these strategies simultaneously yields a superior result (37–40).

ANXIETY

Chronic anxiety is a generalized state of apprehension in response to stress. The chronically threatened individual will eventually begin to experience *distress* in everyday situations that would not normally have elicited such reactions in the past. An anxious reaction is a basic, genetically programmed human response to a real or imagined threatening stressor. The biologic changes elicited by an anxious reaction have specific adaptive survival value in their acute state. They represent alertness and arousal responses for better behavioral and biologic focusing and coping with the threat. It is when feelings of anxiety becomes dysregulated and a constant part of the patient's life that a state of pathology occurs.

An anxious reaction represents one of several built-in stress programs that patients can use to adapt to and cope with new

TABLE 18.5

Faulty Reasoning Patterns Noted in Depression-prone Patients

Arbitrary inference—drawing a specific conclusion in the absence of evidence to support the conclusion.

Selective abstraction—drawing a conclusion based on a detail taken out of context.

Overgeneralization—drawing a broad, global conclusion on the basis of one or more isolated pieces of information.

Magnification and minimization—exaggerating the significance of negative events and minimizing the significance of positive events.

Personalization—relating external events to oneself when there is no realistic basis for making such a connection.

Absolutistic, dichotomous thinking—placing all experiences in one of two opposite categories.

Source: From Beck, AT, Rush AJ, Shaw BF, Emery G. *Cognitive Therapy of Depression: A Treatment Manual.* New York, NY: Guilford, 1979, with permission.

TABLE 18.6

Medical Disorders and Conditions Associated with Disproportionately High Amounts of Anxiety

Hyperthyroidism

Cardiac disease (e.g., arrhythmias, paroxysmal tachycardias)

Mitral valve prolapse

Pernicious anemia

Respiratory disease

Endocrine disorders (e.g., hypoglycemia)

Porphyria

Depressive illness

Presenile or senile dementias

Effects of drug or alcohol use/withdrawal

Caffeine/tobacco use

Hypoglycemia

Pheochromocytoma

Epilepsy

---

threats in their environment. Physically, anxiety is a state of fear with especially strong manifestations in the hypothalamic, sympathetic, autonomic, adrenal, and reticular neuroendocrine networks orchestrated from such forebrain limbic structures as the amygdala. Chronic anxiety is a maladaptive response to a stressful stimuli primarily involving the neurotransmitters norepinephrine, serotonin, and gamma-aminobutyric acid (GABA). Research has also focused upon possible HPA axis abnormalities and the potential role of cholecystokinin (41). Imaging studies in patients with GAD have shown differences in regional brain activity. As an example, one report using positron emission topography measurements found high relative metabolic rates in parts of the occipital, temporal, and frontal lobes, and cerebellum, during a passive viewing task in patients with anxiety relative to normal control subjects (42). Experienced osteopathic physicians soon learn that chronic exposure to anxiety-inducing stress without adequate coping strategies often involve irrational cognitive appraisals of threats that, in turn, can lead to further and commonly excessive anticipatory anxiety.

Lifetime prevalence rates for anxiety based on DSM IV criteria are estimated at 4.1% (43). The prevalence is estimated to be 8% in the primary-care setting (44). The number of office visits with a recorded anxiety disorder diagnosis increased from 9.5 million in 1985 to 11.2 million per year in 1994 and 12.3 million per year in 1998 (16). Twice as many women as men have the disorder (43,45).

Anxiolytic benzodiazepines are among the most commonly prescribed medications in the United States, and primary care physicians write 85% of these prescriptions. Unfortunately, the diagnosis of anxiety is complicated by the fact that anxiety is often not the patient's chief complaint. Rather, patients experiencing anxiety generally complain of physical problems (46). Primary care physicians often focus exclusively on these physical symptoms, failing to note that the patient's complaints are really created by unreported

or unrecognized anxiety and chronic autonomic arousal including disturbed sleep-wake cycles.

Further complicating the situation is the fact that some medical problems magnify the state of anxiety. Table 18.6 lists medical disorders and conditions associated with high amounts of anxiety. Laboratory studies to consider include a CBC, chemistry panel, serum thyrotropin (TSH) (47), urinalysis, electrocardiogram (in patients over 40 with chest pain or palpitations), and any other specific studies required to diagnose a suspected medical cause of anxiety. Urine or serum toxicology measurements of drug levels can be obtained for drugs or medications suspected in the etiology of anxiety.

Measurement of Anxiety

Anxiety inventories such as the state-trait anxiety inventory (48) and anxiety subscales of the MMPI-2 (24,25) measure individual differences in anxiety susceptibility and the patient's tendency to perceive a wide range of situations as threatening. The inventories also measure the patient's reported response to these situations with associated activation and arousal of the autonomic nervous system, an important index of the anxiety state.

These measurements can also be routinely collected in the primary care setting. A seven-item anxiety questionnaire (GAD-7) has been developed and validated in a primary care setting (Table 18.7) (49). GAD-7 is a patient self-assessment tool that can facilitate screening. It is important that positive results from the test (a score of 8 or higher) should be followed by clinician interview to establish the diagnosis of generalized anxiety disorder (GAD). The GAD-7 tool has been validated to screen for generalized anxiety, as well as for other types of anxiety (panic disorder, social anxiety disorder, and posttraumatic stress disorder [44]). Additionally, a shorter version of the GAD-7 (referred to as the GAD-2), using only its first two items of the original test and employing a cutoff score of 3 or more to initiate further evaluation, may be equally sensitive to the GAD-7 (44).

TABLE 18.7

Structured Interview Questions for Generalized Anxiety Disorder (GAD-7)

1. Have you felt nervous, anxious, or on edge on more than half the days in the last month?	YES	NO

In the last month, have you *often* been bothered by any of these problems?

2. Feeling restless so that it is hard to sit still?	4. Muscle tension, aches, or soreness?	6. Trouble concentrating on things, such as reading a book or watching TV?
3. Getting tired very easily?	5. Trouble falling asleep or staying asleep?	7. Becoming easily annoyed or irritated?

8. Are three or more of Nos. 2–7 checked?	YES	NO
9. In the last month, have these problems made it hard for you to do your work, take care of things at home, or get along with other people?	YES	NO
10. In the last 6 months, have you been worrying *a great deal* about *different things, and has this* been on more than half the days in the last 6 months? (Count as yes only if yes to both.)	YES	NO
11. When you are worrying this way, do you find that you can't stop?	YES	NO
12. These current anxiety symptoms *are not* due to the biologic effects of a physical disorder, medication, or other drug?	YES	NO

SCORING: Yes to 1, 8, 9, 10, 11, and 12 constitutes a probable diagnosis of *generalized anxiety disorder.*

Source: From Spitzer RL, Williams JB. *PRIME-MD Clinical Evaluation Guide.* New York, NY: Biometrics Research, New York State Psychiatric Institute, 1994, with permission.

Anxiety Treatments

An osteopathically oriented approach for managing anxiety involves treating both the physical symptoms of chronic fear and the mechanisms of learned and reinforced maladaptive arousal in response to prolonged stress. Benzodiazepines can be prescribed to reduce the paralyzing anxiety associated with a clear external stressor. These are most effective if prescribed on a *temporary* emergency basis with the goal of preventing dependence and iatrogenic withdrawal anxiety when medications are stopped. Thus, one should avoid chronic use of these pharmaceuticals. Physical symptoms can also be controlled by muscular relaxation training, controlled diaphragmatic breathing, and biofeedback (50,51). Structural examination and manipulative treatment should be used to assure appropriate function of the respiratory muscles. Supportive therapy and cognitive behavioral therapy (CBT) are frequently recommended as first-line psychological treatment for GAD. A meta-analysis found CBT to be effective in reducing symptoms in patients with GAD (22). CBT in primary care settings that have integrated mental health resources are particularly effective (52). Osteopathic care attempts to reduce anxiety by enhancing coping abilities, providing interpersonal support, and training the patient to reduce learned anxiety associated with stress while also establishing and maintaining normalized function of the somatic system.

Also, general measures to improve coping ability such as a healthy diet, moderate exercise, weight control, and mobilizing a support system of family and friends can set the stage for effective long-term anxiety management. Positive outcomes of the proposed treatment will result when the primary care physician enters collaborative management relationships with anxious patients. The goal of these relationships is to alleviate overly aroused patients' fears as they learn new coping styles.

ALCOHOL USE AND DEPENDENCE

The use of alcohol as a coping strategy is uniquely human. As our society becomes more complex and ambiguous, more patients use alcohol to manage stress. Medical care for alcohol abuse has become routine work in primary care practice (53–55). The reported use and abuse of intoxicating chemicals that alter the physiology of the body and the central nervous system dates back to the ancient Egyptian papyri and the Greek amphitheater at Delphi. Alcohol abuse and dependency have become a self-medication strategy for stress that is socially tolerated and modeled for our children. Approximately 10% of Americans (10 million people) abuse alcohol (56). A survey of mental health and substance abuse disorders in nearly 20,000 American adults found a 13.5% lifetime prevalence rate for alcohol abuse or dependence (57,58). Alcohol abuse and dependence runs in families (59). First-degree relatives have a three- to fourfold higher prevalence compared with the general population; this number is twofold higher in identical twins of alcohol-dependent individuals (60,61).

Alcohol as Response to Stress

The excessive use of alcohol accounts for a wide spectrum of health and social problems. Alcohol plays a casual or a contributing role in deaths resulting from accidents, homicides, and suicides, as well as diseases such as cirrhosis and cancer. Beyond the negative effects on individuals with alcoholism, the disorder also has been estimated to negatively affect the lives and health of many other people. Alcohol abuse is implicated in 50% of all divorces, in 45% to 68% of spouse abuse cases, and in up to 38% of child abuse cases. Alcohol abuse is especially harmful during pregnancy. Fetuses can be seriously harmed by alcohol. Fetal alcohol syndrome is now one of the three leading causes of prenatal mental retardation in the United States, and it is completely preventable.

In low concentrations, alcohol depresses the brain's neuronal and synaptic transmission systems, including inhibitory center. These depressant effects create three self-reinforcing psychological and behavioral patterns:

Euphoria effects
Disinhibiting effects
Anxiety-relieving effects

Initial euphoria effects reflect central nervous system sedation, temporarily increasing self-esteem, courage, and confidence. To the alcoholic, these disinhibiting and anxiety-relieving effects seem almost magical.

As dependence and abuse develop, biologically, alcohol acts as an antagonist at N-methyl-D-aspartate receptors and as a facilitator at GABA receptors. It also interacts with multiple other neurotransmitter systems in the brain such as the endogenous opioid, serotonin, and ultimately dopamine systems (62,63). Corticotropin-releasing factor, which is involved in stress responses, may play a role in mediating alcohol enhancement of GABA neurotransmission and thus could be involved in the relationship between stress and alcohol abuse (64).

The National Council on Alcoholism and Drug Dependence and The American Society of Addiction Medicine define alcoholism as a primary chronic disease with genetic, psychosocial, and environmental factors influencing its development and manifestations (65). The disease is often progressive and fatal. It is characterized by impaired control over drinking, preoccupation with the drug alcohol, use of alcohol despite adverse consequences, and distortion of thinking, most notably denial. Each of these symptoms may be continuous or periodic.

A person who abuses alcohol rarely changes these maladaptive behaviors without strong, consistent, systematic, and long-term treatment. The first step involves accurate diagnosis so that the appropriate treatment can follow. A number of useful examiner and self-administered questionnaires are available, but the most useful diagnostic screen consists of four simple questions. The screen's acronym, CAGE, comes from the critical word in each question (66):

1. Have you ever tried to *Cut* down on your drinking?
2. Are you *Angry or Annoyed* when people ask you about your drinking?
3. Do you ever feel *Guilty* about your drinking?
4. Do you ever take a morning *Eye* opener?

One positive response suggests the possibility of alcoholism and merits further exploration. Two positive answers make the likelihood of alcoholism extremely high. Three positive responses to questions 1 through 3, or a single positive response to question 4, is most likely diagnostic for the condition. The helpful features of these questions are their simplicity, sensitivity, and efficiency. These questions take under two minutes to ask and they should be included in every initial ambulatory and hospital admission workup.

Alcohol abuse often is a symptom of psychiatric illness, most commonly anxiety and mood disorders. The ubiquity, social acceptance, and relative low cost of alcoholic beverages make drinking an effective short-term and maladaptive long-term manner of self-medication. If the alcohol problem is a primary disorder (alcohol-related disorder, *Diagnostic and Statistical Manual of Mental Disorders*, Fourth Edition [*DSM-IV*]) (67), substance abuse treatment alone suffices. If the alcohol problem is secondary to a psychiatric disorder (dual diagnosis), specific attention to the underlying illness must be addressed simultaneously with the substance abuse disorder. The most useful recent method to diagnose psychiatric disorders efficiently and accurately in an ambulatory care setting is the Prime-MD (Primary Care Evaluation of Mental Disorders) (68). Prime-MD is a well-validated and highly reliable questionnaire that screens for psychiatric disorders (see Table 18.8). Patients fill out a questionnaire and the physician then discusses with the patient any positively endorsed symptoms. The questionnaire is specific for most of the common psychiatric disorders presenting to primary care practice, including mood, anxiety, somatoform concerns, and alcohol-related problems.

If a psychiatric disorder is coexistent with alcoholism, referral for psychiatric consultation and comanagement is strongly recommended. Compulsory inpatient treatment followed by close monitoring for incipient relapse yields the best results (69).

Alcohol as Cause of Further Stress

Once alcohol use becomes a primary stress management strategy, a cascade of further physical and psychosocial stressors will follow (Table 18.9). Evidence of brain plasticity and atrophy (shrinkage) has also been documented in various imaging studies of addicts with results indicating that frontal lobes, limbic system, and cerebellum are particularly vulnerable to damage and dysfunction. Atrophy of the brain contributes to transient or persistent loss of memory, diminished cognitive ability, and compromised reasoning and decision making, depending upon which brain areas are affected and severity and duration of chronic substance abuse (64,70,71). With abstinence, maintained for more than 6 months, partial function may return, but studies have shown that full recovery of these compromised structures is usually not attained.

Alcohol might have been initially used to manage stress, but disruption in work, personal, and social relationships, and isolation are the final consequences. The urgent need to drink concentrates the patient's remaining energies on securing and ingesting alcohol. Denial, minimization, and self-deception are used to explain the alcoholic's deterioration, especially when discussing alcohol use with the primary care physician. When the patient's self-esteem or prominence in the community is at risk, lying, evasion, and other manipulative behaviors emerge as strategies to avoid admitting the problem to the primary care physician and to others. At the point of threatened or actual loss of job, family, home, or health, the physician may intervene and encourage the patient to enter an alcohol treatment program.

Primary care physicians normally refer patients with recurrent alcoholism who need active motivational counseling that treats the biopsychosocial components of addiction (see Table 18.10). Alcohol abuse is a chronic, relapsing disease, and these patients often require consistent interventions by the primary care physicians. The recent research has shown that 5 to 15 minutes of motivational counseling can reduce heavy drinking by 25% (72,73). The recovering alcoholic will need a physician's guidance (Table 18.11) and family support to learn to face life's stressors without the use of intoxicants. With support from the physician, the family, and a peer support group, the patient can change his or her maladaptive stress management style and abstain from alcohol (55,74).

TABLE 18.8

Structured Interview to Elicit Information on Probable Alcohol Abuse/Dependence

Opening Inquiries:

Have … you thought you should cut down on your drinking? Why?		
Has … someone complained about your drinking? Who? Why?		
Do … you feel guilty or upset about your drinking? Why?		
Have … you had five or more drinks in a single day in the past month?		
How often have you had that much to drink in the past 6 months?		
Has that caused any problems?		
1. Has a doctor ever suggested that you stop drinking because of a problem with your health? (Count as yes if patient has continued to drink in the last 6 months after doctor suggested stopping.)	YES	NO
Have any of the following happened to you *more than one time* in the last 6 months?		
2. Were you drinking, high from alcohol, or hung over while you were working, going to school, or taking care of other responsibilities?	YES	NO
3. What about missing or being late for work, school, or other responsibilities because you were drinking or hung over?	YES	NO
4. What about having a problem getting along with other people while you were drinking?	YES	NO
5. What about driving a car after having several drinks or after drinking too much?	YES	NO
SCORING: Yes to most questions. (Consider responses to opening inquiries and other information known about the patient, such as information obtained from a family member.)		

Source: From Spitzer RL, Williams JB. *PRIME-MD Clinical Evaluation Guide.* New York, NY: Biometrics Research, New York State Psychiatric Institute; 1994, with permission.

OSTEOPATHIC MANIPULATIVE TREATMENT

Osteopathic Manipulative Therapy

The musculoskeletal components of the stress response are important when considering manipulation as a modality for stress management. The musculoskeletal system is the physical expression of emotions and feelings (ECOP, 2000). In patients with prolonged depression, anxiety, or fear, those parts of the body that are used to express these emotions tend to have increased tone, altered biomechanics, and lack efficient postural mechanics. Conversely, in the face of altered connective tissues of the parts of the body involved with the expression of a particular emotion, there is often inability of the patient to adequately express or communicate that emotion. While applying OMT, many physicians have encountered emotional releases as the connective tissues begin to regain their functions (ECOP, 2000).

The physician may also encounter lifestyle choices, attitudes, and habits that directly affect the musculoskeletal system. They include poor sleeping habits and chemical dependency (i.e., alcohol abuse causing fatty degeneration and atrophy of the muscle), and the physician may learn about high-risk behaviors, sociocultural values, and views of health and disease that interfere with or

---

TABLE 18.9

Alcohol-related Stress-induced Factors Affecting Somatic Dysfunction

Increased central nervous system excitability
Associated vitamin and nutritional deficiencies
Cirrhosis
Wernicke-Korsakoff syndrome
Alcoholic dementias
Functional gastrointestinal changes with and without gastrointestinal bleeding
Pancreatitis
Esophageal varices
Blackouts; brief amnesic periods
Ataxia and poor coordination

TABLE 18.10

Biobehavioral Components of Addiction-Management Models

1. A public declaration
2. Attend to withdrawal syndrome
3. Aerobic exercise
4. Attacking learned behaviors
5. A supportive group
6. Diary of progress
7. Track economic rewards
8. Track interpersonal rewards

TABLE 18.11
Physician Tasks
The tasks of the physician are to
Develop a strong relationship built on trust
Make the diagnosis of alcoholism compassionately
Elicit the support of family and friends
Refer the alcoholic to a recognized recovery program
Reinforce the stress management techniques

facilitate the adaptive response to stressors. Counseling, problem solving, and education are at the core of complete and comprehensive osteopathic stress management.

Cognitive Behavioral Counseling

Systematic review of English-language studies listed in Medline (through November 2006) and the Cochrane Database of Systematic Reviews (2006, issue 4) identified ample evidence supporting the use of cognitive-behavioral counseling (75) for relief of both the stress of chronic pain and depression (76–79). Cognitive therapy assumes that a patient's misconceptions and attitudes about the world and themselves precede and produce symptoms such as anxiety and depression. Therapy identifies habitual ways in which patients distort information (e.g., automatic thoughts) and teaches patients to identify, evaluate, and respond to their dysfunctional thoughts

and beliefs, using a variety of techniques to change thinking, mood, and behavior (See Chapter 16; Table 16.10). Cognitive therapy is a structured, goal-oriented, problem-focused, and time-limited intervention. This active approach involving principles of learning, help the patient develop new and adaptive ways of behaving. Treatment also attempts to alter behavior by systematically changing the environment that produces the behavior; such behavioral changes are believed to lead to changes in thoughts and emotions.

The osteopathic physician employs all their interpersonal skills (see Part II, Approach to the Patient), to elicit information on the patients perceptions of stressors but more importantly, the thoughts, feelings, and behaviors that contribute to lifestyle choices and stress-related symptoms (Fig. 18.1). As a clinician, on average you will perform 200,000 patient interviews during your career (80). The goal is to elicit personal and symptom data, and through an osteopathic health oriented approach, formulate a description of the patients stress-related symptoms and the biopsychosocial factors involved (81,82). The next step is to interpret and synthesize this information along with laboratory and physical/palpatory assessments to formulate the biopsychosocial description, a diagnosis and recommendations for treatment (83,84).

Problem Solving

Many patients need to construct understandable and easy-to-explain models of the complex interaction of stressful factors in their environment to effectively cope with stress. The physician must provide the patient with simplified models of how the world works and which steps must be taken to problem solve stress. Many patients like to use simple models to increase their understanding of health problems and the subtle and complex factors surrounding

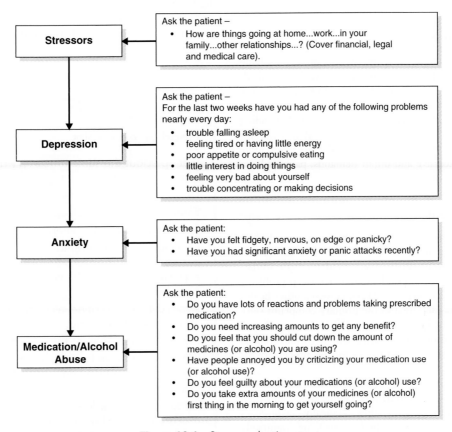

Figure 18-1   Stress evaluation steps.

the risks posed by a stressor. Setting the stage for decreased anxiety and adaptive coping is as easy as taking a moment to listen to the patient's conceptual model of the stressors in his or her life. From there, the physician in a collaborative relationship can offer concrete explanations of the stressors and the risks imposed sharing expert knowledge with the patient (85). One example is telling a patient with back pain that he or she has degenerative disc disease and osteoarthritis. Stated as such this can sound intimidating and hopeless; however, to help the patient understand the diagnosis, the physician can describe the condition from the patient's perspective. Thus, in this example, the patient's diagnosis could be described as "an aging back with stiffness that can be treated in many ways."

Patient Education

Knowledge gives a sense of control and can powerfully mitigate stress (83,84). Education provides patients with information about their diagnosis, its treatment, how to recognize signs of relapse, relapse prevention, and strategies to cope with the reality of prolonged stress. Patients can be given a sense that they can cope by learning to anticipate a potential stressor. The perception that a stressor can be accurately anticipated or stopped increases one's range of problem-solving possibilities and consequent feelings of control. By giving a patient information about stressors before the patient's exposure to them, researchers have reduced the threatening appraisals made when the stressor is experienced. Studies have determined that the stress of surgery or of common medical procedures can be reduced by giving patients accurate expectations, particularly in terms of pain and recovery time. In essence, through adequate patient education and the development of appropriate coping skills, the inescapable stress becomes escapable, the unmanageable stress becomes manageable, and the patient regains control over their life.

Assertiveness Training

The physician often teaches assertiveness and problem-solving techniques. These techniques are most effective with individuals who experience stress as a result of difficulties in self-expression. A lack of appropriate interpersonal skills exacerbates stress-related physical symptoms. For example, an overwhelmingly demanding boss or spouse may be a common cause of stress-related symptoms seen in a primary care setting. By teaching verbal strategies to more effectively deal with excessive and unfair demands, patients learn new and more effective coping behaviors.

Insomnia Management

In the United States, approximately 10 million people consult their health care provider annually for sleep disorders, with half receiving prescriptions for sleeping medications. Epidemiologic studies suggest that 20% to 35% of respondents describe sleep problems as severe or constant for as long as 14 years; however, other health problems are commonly identified as the primary complaint (86). Persistent insomnia is not life threatening. When compared with good sleepers, however, insomniacs experience more (87,88) somatic complaints, anxiety, depression, and have a greater propensity for alcohol and other substance abuse.

An inability to remain asleep is most common initial presentation; this is soon followed by difficulty falling asleep and then by abnormal early morning awakening. Typically, insomniacs are chronically aroused autonomically (anxious), or cognitively distressed and unable to stop thinking and worrying at bed time.

They worry about not getting to sleep and then are too aroused at bedtime to sleep. This worrying leads to fears that they will have poor daytime performance if they cannot make themselves sleep. This initiate a viscous downward cycle, insomnia begets more insomnia and leads to poor learned sleep habits and routines that further exacerbate the insomnia. When insomnia lasts more than 3 weeks, it becomes ingrained and requires specific behavioral strategies to counteract the learned aspects of the insomnia. Current strategies that can mitigate the insomnia include such things as relaxation therapies, stimulus control, distraction techniques, and sleep hygiene education. Evidence from clinical trials and meta-analysis suggests that these sleep habit strategies for insomnia are as effective as sedative hypnotics for acute treatment and more effective for long-term therapy (89,90). CBT for insomnia typically involves visits over six to eight weeks and can be administered in group format (91). Effectiveness has even been shown for patients with insomnia associated with medical and psychiatric disorders (93), and for older patients and chronic hypnotic users (93). A review of evidence-based treatments for insomnia found that 70% to 80% of patients with chronic insomnia showed benefit from sleep habit strategies (94).

Insomnia can be managed effectively by teaching sleep hygiene techniques that employ a variety of sleep habit strategies (Table 18.12). These techniques form the foundation for the guidance that the osteopathically trained physician gives to the patient. When sleep is restored, the patient feels more alert, and there are fewer stress-related somatic complaints. Patients practicing good sleep habits also report improved concentration, better problem solving, and more effective management of their stress.

Augmenting sleep habit strategies with medication for sleep during short intervals is another method used to manage insomnia. A prescription for exercise and a muscular relaxation training tape to be used in the evening hours will also promote better sleep. All this, coupled with encouragement by the osteopathic physician who functions both as educator and guide, will alleviate insomnia.

TABLE 18.12

Good Sleep Habits

Get up about the same time every day, regardless of when you go to bed.
Go to bed only when sleepy.
Establish relaxing presleep rituals.
Exercise regularly and keep active.
Organize your day around regular times for eating and outdoor activities with regular exposure to bright light, which synchronizes circadian cycles.
Avoid caffeine, nicotine, alcohol, excessive warmth, and hunger at bed time.
If you nap, try to nap at the same time every day.
When laying down to sleep, relax all your muscles, particularly your face and jaw, and breath slowly and evenly.
If you do not fall asleep in 20 minutes, get back up and return to bed when sleepy.

Muscular Relaxation

Progressive relaxation is based on the premise that muscle tension is closely related to anxiety. Individuals feel a significant reduction in experienced anxiety as their tense muscles are taught to relax. The teaching of progressive muscular relaxation skills follows a standard procedure. The individual practices muscle relaxation after he or she decides which muscle groups are tense. For example, the individual is instructed to tighten his or her jaw and notice a pattern of feeling strain in these muscles. After maintaining the tension for approximately 10 seconds, the subject is instructed to let the muscle group completely relax, and then to notice a difference in sensation as the places that were previously tense and strained relax. After a few minutes of relaxation, repeat the sequence. The main goal of the training program is to teach individuals what it feels like to relax each muscle group and to provide practice in achieving greater relaxation. Once the individual can discriminate the pattern of tension in a particular muscle group, omit the instruction to tense before relaxing. Instead, the individual must relax the muscle from the present level of tension. The original relaxation procedure required months of training with hundreds of trained muscle sites. Clinical practice employs a much more abbreviated form of training and is easy to teach to the patient in a primary care setting.

Biofeedback

In biofeedback paradigms, the individual is taught to use physiologic monitoring equipment to perceive physiologic processes. Once the physiological process is perceptible, the individual is taught to monitor the process. By receiving auditory or visual feedback, one learns about the close relationship between mind and body. The availability of sensitive recording devices for home use has made it possible to work on these skills in a more organized and regular manner. There are a number of systematic and well-controlled outcome studies that show the clinical effectiveness of Electomyographic Biofeedback (95–97). Temperature biofeedback, which is also receiving positive support in the literature, has been shown to control Raynaud phenomena and migraine headaches. From an osteopathic perspective, biofeedback makes it possible to extend voluntary control over some elements of somatic dysfunction by decreasing arousal responses affecting somatic and viscerosomatic reflex activities. Learning to master these responses helps develop a sense of control and improves confidence in one's self-healing abilities.

Social Support

One of the major factors attenuating stress is an effective system of psychosocial support. The physician should conceptualize a patient's support system as a network of expanding concentric circles with the patient's closest confidant at the center. This social network gives a person the feeling that he or she is valued and cared about. The idea that people need to be surrounded by groups of people who provide love and a sense of belonging is not new. The patient needs help to identify mentors and significant others in his or her environment whom he or she can trust and with whom he or she can share feelings. The importance of having person(s) in whom we can confide cannot be overemphasized in buffering the effects of life stress. Most times, this central confidant is a spouse or best friend, or it could be anyone who demonstrates care, concern, and respect for feelings and opinions. This confidant serves the preventive role of ensuring that all burdens and troubles can be shared. A system of support ranges from the confidence of having

trusted advice available when planning a predicted transition to the comfort and nurturing of friends, neighbors, and community during an unforeseen tragedy. Confidants also help professionals, such as the clergy or physicians, to provide assistance. The osteopathic physician assumes an important role by providing this help and counseling the stressed patient. Referrals to self-help groups in the community such as Alanon and Recovery, Inc. can help to reduce the patient's self-absorption. Participation in these groups also leads to the development of outside interests that are compatible with a lifestyle free of addictions. Last, but certainly not least, religious faith provides the opportunity for a spiritual confidant. Patients for whom a spiritual dimension to life is important derive great comfort and benefit from their belief in power and meaning beyond what can be known in life in the world. Physicians should not underestimate the positive healing power of spiritual belief systems.

Spiritual Support

For patients undergoing elective open heart surgery for coronary artery disease, those experiencing strength or comfort from their spiritual feelings are three times more likely to survive than are those without spiritual support. Those who participate in social and community groups (such as local school programs, senior centers, historical societies, etc.) also have three times the survival rate of those who do not take part in social activity. A 1995 study (98) involving 232 patients over age 55 found that seniors who had both "protective factors," that is, spiritual and social support, enjoyed a 10-fold increase in survival. The amount or type of spiritual or social activity did not matter as much as the *participation, comfort, and support derived from the activity* (98). Why and how spiritual feelings and social support extend life after open heart surgery is not understood. There are many studies corroborating this health-enhancing, life-prolonging effect in a variety of circumstances and population groups. It is well documented, for example, that Mormons (both clergy and devout members) have extremely long life expectancies. The physiologic mechanisms behind longevity, health, and social support are not well understood, however (see Chapter 30, "Integration of Mind/Spirit").

Group Support

Encourage your patient to become involved in settings and groups of people who are coping with stress. This can lead to new patterns of coping behaviors. For example, patients with intractable pain fear physical movement. Having them attend a group aquatic exercise program lets them observe others, perhaps older or in poorer health than themselves, moving without damage or injury. This vicarious learning lessens the patient's apprehension when the painful area is moved. In managed care population studies, group sessions for identified high utilizing distressed patients, including education, social support, and coping skills, as well as an opportunity to individually interact with a physician after the session, improved patient satisfaction and led to lower costs for hospitalization, as well as fewer emergency department visits and subspecialty referrals (7,99).

CONCLUSIONS

The osteopathically trained physician has many available tools to employ a broad approach to stress-related problems, including varieties of somatic dysfunction. Anxiety, depression, insomnia, and drug and alcohol abuse are common symptoms seen in primary care offices. Osteopathic management can be practiced in three ways:

1. By treating symptoms as they are reported and observed.
2. By giving advice on managing stressors.
3. By guiding and mentoring stress-related responses toward positive coping behaviors and strategies (the most rewarding).

Successful diagnosis depends on the understanding the interaction of the biopsychosocial factors that lead to stress-induced problems. Successful treatment depends on giving clear explanations so that the patient understands the mechanisms that perpetuate his or her distress. The long-term goal to assist the patient toward self-mastery and self-healing through a collaborative doctor—patient relationship based on treating the whole person—mind, body, and spirit.

REFERENCES

1. Seyle H. *The Stress of Life*. Rev. Ed. New York, NY: McGraw Hill, 1976.
2. Centers for Disease Control. *Ten Leading Causes of Death in the United States*. Washington, DC: Government Publishing Office, 1980.
3. Surgeon General's Office. *Healthy People*. Washington, DC: Government Printing Office, 1979.
4. Surgeon General's Office. *Report on Nutrition and Health*. Washington, DC: Government Printing Office, 1988.
5. Katon W, Von Korff M, Lin E, et al. Distressed high utilizers of medical care. DSM-III-R diagnoses and treatment needs. *Gen Hosp Psychiatry* 1990;12:355.
6. Gill D, Dharpe M. frequent consulters in general practice: a systematic review of studies of prevalence, associations and outcome. *J Psychosom Res* 1999;47:115.
7. Gatchel RJ, Oordt MS. *Clinical Psychology and Primary Care*. Washington, DC: American Psychological Association, 2003.
8. Spiegel D. Healing words: emotional expression and disease outcome. *JAMA* 1999;281:1328–1329.
9. Cohen S, Tyrell DAJ, Smith AP. Psychological stress and susceptibility to the common cold. *N Engl J Med* 1991;325:606–612.
10. Holmes TH, Rahe RH. The social readjustment rating scale. *J Psychological Res* 1967;7:17–20.
11. Sarason IG, Johnson JH, Siegel JM. Assessing the impact of life changes: development of the life experiences survey. *J Consult Clin Psychol* 1978;46(5):932–946.
12. Friedman M, Rosenman RH. *Type-A Behavior and Your Heart*. New York, NY: Knopf, 1984.
13. Freidman M, Ulmer, D. *Treating Type-A Behavior and Your Health*, New York, NY: Knopf, 1984.
14. Anderson SM, Harthorn BH. The recognition, diagnosis and treatment of mental disorders by primary care physicians. *Med Care* 1989;27;869–886.
15. Toft T, Fink P, Christiansen K, et al. Mental disorders in primary care: prevalence and co-morbidity among disorders. results from the functional illness in primary care (FIP) study. *Psychol Med* 2005;35(8):1175–1184.
16. Barrett JE, Barrett JA, Oxman RE, et al. The prevalence of psychiatric disorders in a primary care practice. *Arch Gen Psychiatry* 1988;45:1100–1106.
17. Copas JB, Robin A. Suicide in psychiatric patients. *Br J Psychiatry* 1982;141:503–511.
18. Kessler RC, Chiu WT, Demier O, et al. Prevalence, severity, and comorbidity of 12-month DSM-IV disorders in the National Comorbidity Survey Replication. *Arch Gen Psychiatry* 2005;62:617.
19. American Psychiatric Association. *Diagnostic and Statistical Manual of Mental Disorders*. Rev. 4th Ed. Washington, DC: American Psychiatric Association, 1994.
20. Zung WWK. A self-rating depression scale. *Arch Gen Psychiatry* 1965; 12:6370.
21. Zung WWK. A rating instrument for anxiety disorders. *Psychosomatics* 1971; 12:164–167.
22. Beck AT. *Depression: Clinical, Experimental and Theoretical Aspects*. New York, NY: Harper & Row, 1967.
23. Beck AT. *Cognitive Theory and the Emotional Disorders*. New York, NY: International Universities Press, 1976.
24. Hathaway SR, McKinley JC. *MMPI Manual*. Minneapolis, MN: Psychological Corp., 1943.
25. Dahlstrom WG, Welsh GS. *An MMPI Handbook*. Minneapolis, MN: University of Minnesota Press, 1972.
26. Spitzer RL, Williams JB, et al. *PRIME-MD Clinical Evaluation Guide*. New York, NY: New York State Psychiatric Institute, Biometrics Research Dept., 1994.
27. Spitzer RL, Williams JB. Utility of a new procedure for diagnosing mental disorders in primary care. *JAMA* 1994;272(22):1749–1756.
28. Kroenke K, Spitzer RL, Williams JB. The PHQ-9: validity of a brief depression severity measure. *J Gen Intern Med* 2001;16:606.
29. Lowe B, Unutzer J, Callahan CM, et al. Monitoring depression treatment outcomes with the patient health questionnaire-9. *Med Care* 2004;42:1194.
30. Cameron OG. *Presentations of Depression*. New York, NY: John Wiley and Sons, 1987.
31. Nezu AM, Nezu CM. *Problem-Solving Therapy for Depression*. New York, NY: John Wiley and Sons, 1989.
32. Beck AT, Rush AJ, Shaw BF, et al. *Cognitive Therapy of Depression: A Treatment Manual*. New York, NY: Guilford, 1979.
33. Overmier JB, Seligman MEP. Effects of inescapable shock upon subsequent escape and avoidance learning. *J Comp Psychol* 1967;64:2333.
34. Seligman MEP, Maier SF. Failure to escape traumatic shock. *J Exp Psychol* 1967;74:19.
35. Beck, AT. How an anomalous finding lead to a new system of psychotherapy. *Nat Med* 2006;12:1139.
36. Hollon SD, DeRubeis RJ, Shelton RC, et al. Prevention of relapse following cognitive therapy vs medications in moderate to severe depression. *Arch Gen Psychiatry* 2005;62:417.
37. DeRubels RJ, Hollon SD, Amsterdam JD, et al. Cognitive therapy vs medications in the treatment of moderate to severe depression. *Arch Gen Psychiatry* 2005;62:409.
38. Chilvers C, Dewey M, Fielding K, et al. Antidepressant drugs and generic counseling for treatment of major depression in primary care: randomized trial with patient preference arms. *BMJ* 2001;322:772.
39. Dimidjian S, Hollon SD, Dobson KS, et al. Randomized trial of behavioral activation, cognitive therapy and antidepressant medication in the acute treatment of adults with major depression. *J Consult Clin Psychol* 2006;74:658.
40. Otto, MW, Smits, JAJ, Reese, HE. Combined psychotherapy and pharmacotherapy for mood and anxiety disorders in adults: review and analysis. *Clin Psychol: Sci Pract* 2005;12:72.
41. Brawman-Mintzer O, Lydiard RB. Biological basis of generalized anxiety disorder. *J Clin Psychiatry* 1997;58(suppl 3):16.
42. Wu JC, Buchsbaum MS, Hershey TG, et al. PET in generalized anxiety disorder. *Biol Psychiatry* 1991;29:1181.
43. Grant BF, Hasin DS, Stinson FS, et al. Prevalence, correlates, co-morbidity, and comparative disability of DSM-IV generalized anxiety disorder in the USA: results from the National Epidemiologic Survey on Alcohol and Related Conditions. *Psychol Med* 2005;35:1747.
44. Kroenke K, Spitzer RL, Williams JB, et al. Anxiety disorders in primary care: prevalence, impairment, comorbidity, and detection. *Ann Intern Med* 2007;146:317.
45. Harman JS, Rollman BL, Hanusa BH, et al. Physician office visits of adults for anxiety disorders in the United States, 1985–1998. *J Gen Med* 2002;17:165.
46. Katon W, Vitalliano PP, Russo J, et al. Oanic disorder: spectrum of severity and somatization. *J Nerv Ment Dis* 1987;175:12.
47. Fricchione, G. Clinical practice. Generalized anxiety disorder. *N Engl J Med* 2004;351:675.
48. Spielberger CD, Gorsuch RC, Lushene RE. *Manual for the State-trait Anxiety Inventory*. Palo Alto, CA: Consulting Psychologists, 1970.
49. Spitzer RL, Kroenke K, Williams JB, et al. A brief measure for assessing generalized anxiety disorder: the GAD-7. *Arch Intern Med* 2006;166:1092.
50. Keabie D. *The Management of Anxiety*. New York, NY: Churchill Livingstone, 1989.
51. Kennerley H. *Managing Anxiety*. Oxford, UK: Oxford University Press, 1990.

52. Rollman BL, Belnap BH, Mazumdar S, et al. A randomized trial to improve the quality of treatment for panic and generalized anxiety disorders in primary care. *Arch Gen Psychiatry* 2005;62:1332.

53. Whitlock EP, Polen MR, Green CA, et al. Behavioral counseling interventions in primary care to reduce risky/harmful alcohol use by adults: a summary of the evidence for the U.S. Preventive Services Task Force. *Ann Intern Med* 2004;140:557.

54. Substance Abuse and Mental Health Services Administration. National Household Survey on Drug Abuse (NHSDA); population estimates 2001. Rockville, MD: U.S. Department of Health and Human Services, Substance Abuse and Mental Health Administration (SAMHSA), 2001.

55. Whitclock EP, Green CA, Polen MR. Behavioral Counseling Interventions in Primary Care to Reduce Risky/Harmful Alcohol Use. Systematic Evidence Review. No. 30 (Prepared by the Oregon Healthcare Research and Quality, April 2004 (Available at www.ahrq/gov/clinic/serfiles.htm.).

56. Saltz R. Clinical practice. Unhealthy alcohol use. *N Engl J Med* 2005;352:596.

57. Kendler KS, Walters EE, Neale MC, et al. The structure of the genetic and environmental risk factors for six major psychiatric disorders in women. Phobia, generalized anxiety disorder, panic disorder, bulimia, major depression, and alcoholism. *Arch Gen Psychiatry* 1995;52:374.

58. Regier DA, Farmer ME, Rae DS, et al. Comorbidity of mental disorders with alcohol and other drug abuse. Results from the Epidemiologic Catchment Area (ECA) Study. *JAMA* 1990;264:2511.

59. Gordis E. Genes and the environment in complex diseases: a focus on alcoholism. *Mol Psychiatry* 1997;2:282.

60. Prescot CA, Kendler KS. Genetic and environmental contributions to alcohol abuse and dependence in a population-based sample of male twins. *Am J Psychiatry* 1999;156:34.

61. Heath AC, Bucholz KK, Madden PA, et al. Genetic and environmental contributions to alcohol dependence risk in a national twin sample: consistency of findings in women and men. *Psychol Med* 1997;27:1381.

62. Sass H, Soyka M, Mann K, Zieglgansberger W. Relapse prevention by acamprosate. Results from a placebo-controlled study on alcohol dependence. *Arch Gen Psychiatry* 1996;53:673.

63. Wise RA. Drug-activation of brain reward pathways. *Drug Alcohol Depend* 1998;51:13.

64. Nie Z, Schweltzer P, Roberts AJ, et al. Ethanol augments GABAergic transmission in the central amygdala via CRF1 receptors. *Science* 2004;303:1512.

65. Morse RM, Flavin DK; for the Joint Committee of the National Council of Alcoholism and Drug Dependence and the American Society of Addiction Medicine to Study the Definition and Criteria for the Diagnosis of Alcoholism. The definition of alcoholism. *JAMA* 1992;268:1012.

66. Ewing JA. Detecting alcoholism, the CAGE Questionnaire. *JAMA* 1984;252:1905–1907.

67. American Psychiatric Association. Alcohol-related disorders. In: *Diagnostic and Statistical Manual of Mental Disorders*. 4th Ed. Washington, DC: American Psychiatric Association, 1994:116–118.

68. Spitzer RL Williams JBW, et al. Utility of new procedure for diagnosing mental disorders in primary care. *JAMA* 1994;272(22):1749–1756. (PRIME-MD materials are available from Dr. Robet Spitzer, Biometrics Research Department, New York State Psychiatric Institute, New York, NY.)

69. Walsh DC, Higson RW, et al. A randomized trial of treatment options for alcohol abusing workers. *N Engl J Med* 1991;325:775–782.

70. Gordis, E. The neurobiology of alcohol abuse and alcoholism: building knowledge, creating hope. *Drug Alcohol Depend* 1998;51:9.

71. Di Chiara G, Imperato A. Drugs abused by humans preferentially increase synaptic dopamine concentrations in the mesolimbic system of freely moving rats. *Proc Natl Acad Sci U S A* 1988;85:5274.

72. Estee S, Lee N, He L. *Substance Use Outcomes: Six-Month follow-up survey of WASBIRT clients April 2004-January 2005*. Olympia, Washington: Department of Social and Health Services, Research and Data Analysis Division, 2006.

73. Fleming MR, Mundt MP, French MT, et al. Brief physician advice for problem drinkers: long-term efficacy and benefit-cost analysis. *Alcohol Clin Exp Res* 2002;26:36–43.

74. U.S. Department of Health and Human Services. Healthy people 2010: With understanding and improving health and objectives for improving health. November 2020. www.healthypeople.gov/hp2020.

75. Chou R, Huffman LH; American Pain Society; American College of Physicians. Nonpharmacologic therapies for acute and chronic low back pain; a review of the evidence for an American Pain Society/American College of Physicians clinical practice guideline. *Ann Intern Med* 2007;147(7):145.

76. Dobson KS. A meta-analysis of the efficacy of cognitive therapy for depression. 3 consult *Clin Psychol* 1989;57:414.

77. Elkin I, Shea MT, Watkins JT, et al. National Institute of Mental Health Treatment of Depression Collaborative Research Program. General effectiveness of treatments. *Arch Gen Psychiatry* 1989;46:971.

78. Craigheadm WE, Craighead LW, Illardi SS. Psychological treatments for major depressive disorder. In: Nathan PE, Gorman JM, eds. *A Guide to Treatments that Work*. New York, NY: Oxford University Press, 1998;226.

79. Jacobson NS, Dobson KS, Truax PA, et al. A component of cognitive-behavioral treatment for depression. *J Consult Clin Psychol* 1996;64:295.

80. Davidoff F, Deutsch S, Egan KL, et al. Who *Has Seen A Blood Sugar?—Reflections On Medical Education*. Philadelphia, PA: American College of Physicians, 1996.

81. Smith RC. *Patient-Centered Interviewing: An Evidence-Based Method*. Philadelphia, PA: Lippincott Williams & Wilkins, 2002.

82. Smith RC. Evidence-Based Interviewing: (Tape 1) Patient-Centered Interviewing & (Tape 2) Doctor-Centered Interviewing (February 2001)—Produced by Michigan State University Broadcasting Services, Eric Schultz, Producer—Available from Marketing Division, Instructional Media Center, Michigan State University via any of the following: PO Box 710, East Lansing, MI 48824; 2) 517–353–9229; 3) 517–432–2650; 4) www.msuvmall.msu.edu/imc (Accessed 3/7/05).

83. Brody H. *The Healing Power*. New Haven, CT: Yale University Press, 1992.

84. Brody H. The biopsychosocial model, patient-centered care, and culturally sensitive practice. *J Fam Prac* 1999;48:585.

85. Taal E, Rasker JJ, Wiegman O. Patient education and self-management in the rheumatic diseases: a self-efficacy approach. *Arthritis Care Res* 1996;9:229–238.

86. Rosekind MR. The epidemiology and occurrence of insomnia. *J Clin Psychiatry*. 1992;53(suppl 6):46.

87. Lesch DR, Spire J-P. Clinical electroencephalography. In: Thorpy MJ, ed. *Handbook of Sleep Disorders*. New York, NY: Marcel Dekker Inc., 1990:1331.

88. Buysse DJ, Reynolds CF III. Insomnia. In: Thorpy MJ, ed. *Handbook of Sleep Disorders*. New York, NY: Marcel Dekker Inc., 1990:375–433.

89. Perlis ML, Junquist C, Smith MT, et al. *Cognitive Behavioral Treatment of Insomnia: A Session-by-Session guide*. New York, NY: Springer Science and Business Media, Inc., 2005.

90. Siversten B, Omvik S, Pallesen S, et al. cognitive behavioral therapy vs zopiclone for treatment of chronic primary insomnia in older adults: a randomized controlled trial. *JAMA* 2006;295:2851.

91. Verbeek IH, Konings GM, Aldenkamp AP, et al. Cognitive behavioral treatment in clinically referred chronic insomniacs: group versus individual treatment. *Behav Sleep Med* 2006;4:135.

92. Morin CM, Bootzin RR, Buysse DJ, et al. Psychological and behavioral treatment of Insomnia: update of the recent evidence (1998–2004). *Sleep* 2006;29:1398.

93. Morganthaler T, Kramer M, Alessi C, et al. Practice parameters for the psychological and behavioral treatment of insomnia: an update. An American academy of sleep medicine report. *Sleep* 2006;29:1415.

94. Cognitive Behavioral therapy for Insomnia, by Charles Morin, available at: http://therapyadvisor.com/taTreatment.aspx?disID=38&trID=21. Accessed on October 2 2008.

95. Drexler AR, Mur EJ, Gunther VC. Efficacy of an EMG-biofeedback therapy in fibromyalgia patients. A comparative study of patients with and without abnormality in MMPI psychological scales. *Clin Exp Rheumatol* 2002;20:677–682.

96. Ferraccioli G, Ghirekki L, Scita F, et al. EMG-biofeedback training in fibromyalgia syndrome. *J Rheumatol* 1987;14:820–825.

97. Mur E, Drexler A, Gruber J, et al. Electomyography biofeedback therapy in fibromyalgia. *Wiener Medizinische Wochenschrift* 1999;149:561–563.

98. Oxman TE. Lack of social participation or religious strength and comfort as risk factors for death after cardiac surgery in the elderly. *Psychosom Med* 1995;57:681–689.

99. Scott J, Gade G, McKenzie M, et al. Cooperative health care clinics: a group approach to individual care. *Geriatrics* 1998;53:68.

Life Stages—Basic Mechanisms

JED MAGEN, ALYSE LEY, DEBRA WAGENAAR, AND STEVE SCHEINTHAL

KEY CONCEPTS

- Human development involves the complex interaction of biological influences and environmental effects.
- Infants come equipped with preprogrammed capabilities that have evolved to maximize survivability.
- Adolescence marks a time of profound biobehavioral shifts with reorganization of cognitive, emotional, and biologic functioning.
- The definition of adulthood and the transition to geriatric status is fluid.
- While we often tend to view elderly individuals as a homogeneous group, there are actually tremendous variations in the physical and emotional aspects of aging.
- The definition of "older adult" depends upon the context in which it is given. Age-related changes begin by the third or fourth decade of life.
- The major focus of geriatric care is optimizing function, avoiding institutionalization, and maintaining the older adult in the community.
- A mental status examination is a part of thorough geriatric evaluation.

Human development involves the complex interaction of biological influences and environmental effects. From the time of conception through death, the individual continuously develops. The process of development and the phases of development, however, follow a paradigm that is discontinuous. Transitions from one phase of development to another are characterized by "biobehavioral shifts" (1). These times of transition involve relatively abrupt reorganizations of biologic, cognitive, affective, and social characteristics resulting in more complex behaviors and abilities by the organism (2). Recent studies have demonstrated that the dramatic physiologic and "psychological competencies" that occur in early development, especially during the first two years of life, are temporally correlated with the anatomic, biochemical, and physiologic changes occurring in the brain (3).

The timing and genesis of a biobehavioral shift is mediated by and dependent upon the expression, repression, and depression of genes that are themselves both environmentally and biologically influenced. Phenotype is the observable physical or biochemical characteristics of an organism as determined by both genetic makeup and environmental influences. Cells can modulate functions in response to internal and environmental factors. The theory of "phenotypic plasticity" explains the ability of a specific environmental stressor to alter the phenotypic expression of a gene (4). Defects in plasticity alter genes and stem cell processes leading to many forms of cancer (5,6). From an evolutionary perspective, organisms continuously attempt to manipulate their environment in ways that are beneficial to them. An abnormality in development resulting in a disorder or disease process may be an adaptive response to an environmental stressor. The influence of genes in early development may also result in a disease process in later development. For example, gene and prenatal environmental interactions are correlated with adult health, including the risk of coronary artery disease and type 2 diabetes (7). Genes not only impact physiologic mechanisms resulting in disease, they also shape psychological developmental outcomes. Serotonin transporter promoter polymorphism, or the variation in serotonin transporter genes, is linked to temperament, antisocial behavior, and substance abuse disorders among adolescents (8).

The move from childhood to adolescence is a particularly cogent example of a "biobehavioral shift." Puberty is associated with an upsurge in sexuality with very different behaviors toward the opposite sex, for example, an increase in aggression and striking physical changes and cognitive changes (9). Relationships during adolescence transform from a family-centered focus to a peer relations focus. Adolescence also marks a change in the epidemiology of various disorders. Illustrating this change, the sex ratio for depression changes from 1:1 to a larger predominance in females.

PRENATAL PERIOD

Rapid development during the prenatal period is influenced by multiple factors. Embryogenesis is affected by the complex interactions between genes and the intrauterine environment. Genetic predispositions are determined by maternal and paternal gene composition prior to conception. The association between maternal age and the increased risk of chromosomal abnormalities such as trisomy 21 has long been established. Paternal age also appears to contribute to the etiology of birth defects, including heart, gastrointestinal, and musculoskeletal defects, as well as chromosomal abnormalities (10).

In utero environmental factors, such as exposure to alcohol, drugs, maternal malnutrition, and maternal stress, influence prenatal growth and development. Cigarette smoking and malnutrition are associated with decreased fetal growth and low birth weight. Alcohol exposure can result in fetal alcohol syndrome, which occurs in 1 in 500 to 1,000 live births, and includes characteristic facial features, mental retardation, behavioral abnormalities, and language delays (11). There is now evidence that fetal alcohol exposure should be considered in the pathogenesis of some cases of attention deficit hyperactivity disorder (ADHD), depressive disorder, oppositional defiant disorder, conduct disorder, and specific phobia (12). Maternal wellbeing is essential to fetal growth and development. Multiple studies have demonstrated the influence of maternal psychopathological symptoms and the impact on the developing fetus. Untreated depression during pregnancy has been linked to preeclampsia, spontaneous abortion, early labor, bleeding during gestation, small fetal size, low birth weight, preterm delivery, increased neonatal care unit admissions, and elevated cortisol levels in the neonate (13). Prenatal exposure has also been linked to early childhood behavior disorders. Children born to mothers who endured intimate partner violence during pregnancy have significantly more behavioral disorders than their counterparts (14). Prenatal stress has been implicated as an important factor in the neurodevelopment of cognitive abilities and fearfulness during infancy (15).

Attachment begins prior to infancy. As the embryo completes its transition into a fetus and the fetus develops into the neonate, mothers and other family members undergo an emotional transformation. In preparation for childbirth and caring for the infant, mothers often become preoccupied with herself and the pregnancy. This phenomenon is especially pronounced after fetal movement is detected. Fathers may initially experience attachment when viewing their fetus through sonographic examination or when they can feel fetal movement through the mother's abdomen. Complications such as preterm delivery can adversely affect the infant and the developing relationship with parents. The complex measures used to sustain premature infants oftentimes make it difficult for parents to develop attachments to their infant. Parents may not perceive the infant responding to them as a term infant would. This lack of reciprocal interaction can begin to shape the infant-parent interaction and add to complications in growth and development, sometimes leading to later behavioral difficulties. The neonatal care unit is not an atmosphere that fosters the parent child dyad. Parents of preterm children are often unable to feed or care for their infant in the usual ways. Preterm infants are at risk for severe neurological and physical disabilities as well as eating disorders, ADHD, learning disabilities, visual-motor disorders, and language impairment. The stress of preterm delivery and adjustment to caring for a medically ill child places the mother-infant relationship in jeopardy. Early family support and intervention while the infant is in the hospital and during the transition home help to decrease stress and the risk of maternal depression, thereby increasing positive mother-child interactions (16,17).

INFANCY

On the 18th day of gestation, the nervous system begins to develop (114). Brain growth and development in the fetus proceeds in a predictable manner from the brainstem to the cerebral cortex (18). At birth, the gross anatomical structure of the brain is nearly identical to the adult brain, but the complex neural connections and pathways will continue to develop until adulthood. The limited capacity of the female pelvis to accommodate the fetal head forces brain growth to continue outside the uterus. Given this limit on brain size, infants are equipped with only those capabilities needed for survival. The brainstem is almost fully functional in the newborn but the forebrain and limbic structures are immature by comparison (19). Infants come equipped with preprogrammed capabilities that have evolved to maximize survivability. Adaptive reflexes including rooting, sucking, grasping, and Moro allow the infant to feed and maintain close contact with the caregiver. Less overt capabilities are also present in the infant at birth. Newborns engage in complex visual activities. They scan patterns by means of eye movements going back and forth across edges (20). At birth, infants discriminate their mother's voice from the voice of others. Between one and four months of age, infants gain the ability to discriminate speech sounds (21). These and other abilities allow infants to participate in the dyadic interaction with the primary caregiver known as attachment. These innate preprogrammed behaviors and capabilities are critical in the attachment process. Attachment can be defined as "an enduring emotional bond uniting one person with another" (22). Preprogrammed behaviors and predispositions of the infant serve to help develop a secure attachment between the infant and care giver, allowing optimal psychosocial development to take place. Instinctive caregiver behaviors also contribute to the attachment process. Caregivers tend to hold infants at a distance maximizing face-to-face contact, engage in exaggerated greeting behaviors, and imitate infants' facial and vocal expressions. All these behaviors promote attachment (24). Newborns reciprocate by making eye contact and vocalizing. The temporal relationship that exists between the neurobiological development of the brain and the emergence of more complex behaviors is evident in the acquisition of developmental milestones that allow the infant to participate in more complex interactions with caregivers and their environment. The appearance of a social smile by eight weeks helps to engage the caregiver, thereby promoting the reciprocal relationship. By 2 to 3 months, preprogrammed neonatal reflexes begin to disappear allowing the emergence of more complex abilities. Cortical inhibition of the brainstem causes the palmer reflex to recede and spontaneous crying becomes less prominent. Simultaneously, the hippocampus and surrounding structures develop the sophistication to permit the beginnings of recognition memory, allowing the infant for the first time to store events from the immediate past, thereby promoting the infant caregiver relationship. Working memory, the ability to compare past and present, emerges in the form of stranger and separation anxiety develops at approximately 7 to 10 months of age and coincides with the maturation of the prefrontal cortex, hippocampus, limbic system and the integration of the hypothalamic-pituitary axis (25).

New behaviors that elicit stimulation from caretakers conversely contribute to brain growth and development in infants. The brain grows most rapidly during the first year of life. Glucose use in the cerebral cortex rises from birth to 4 years; at age 4 it is twice that of the adult. During the first two years of life, there is tremendous growth and proliferation of neurons, axons, dendrites, and synapses. As time passes, these complex networks are pruned in part based upon how actively they are used (26). This "use it or lose it" phenomenon partly accounts for the smaller brain growth seen in cases of deprivation. Failure to thrive is typified by infants who do not demonstrate appropriate growth or achievement of developmental milestones. This diagnosis can be divided into two categories based on whether the etiology is organic or environmental. The earliest sign of failure to thrive is often the lack of a social smile. This is the direct result of the inability to achieve a relationship with the caretaker that involves handling and positive interaction. There is experimental evidence that touch, in part, operates as a soothing mechanism in animals by activating brain opiates (27). This mechanism may be operative in the therapeutic effects of osteopathic manipulative medicine.

The importance of closeness and touch is well documented in the literature on breast feeding and developmental outcomes. Breast milk provides multiple health, nutritional, and immunologic benefits as well as the perfect natural setting for bonding and attachment to take place. Breast feeding has also been implicated in the earlier development of language and motor skills (28). A growing body of research indicates that breast feeding is associated with increased cognitive abilities and later academic achievement (29). The long-chain polyunsaturated fatty acids, docosahexaenoic acid and arachidonic acid, found in human milk are essential in the growth and development of the central nervous system (CNS). Many studies suggest that the fatty acids found in breast milk confer long-term benefits as well. Early infancy and childhood nutrition are linked to diabetes and atherosclerosis in adulthood (30,31).

Infancy is a critical time for attachment and bonding. Decreases in the normal expected quantity or quality of stimulation as seen in post partum depression may have profound effects on the development of the infant. Infants of depressed mothers exhibit dysregulated neurobiological rhythms including elevated norepinephrine and cortisol levels, decreased vagal tone, and right frontal EEG activation. They show lower scores on the Bayley Scale for infant development and growth delays up to 12 months ?(32). Maternal impairment during infancy may have lasting effects throughout childhood. Post partum depression has been linked to emotional, cognitive, and behavioral disorders in infants and children (33). An analysis of the literature on child behavior demonstrates the

negative effect of post partum depression on "later distractibility, antisocial and neurotic behavior" that may continue until age 5. The degree of cognitive and behavioral effects on the child is directly correlated to the severity and duration of the depressive episode in the mother (34).

Adaptability, the ability to modulate and change behaviors in conjunction with the environment, is an important attribute in both infants and caregivers. For example, a parent who is unable to remain calm and soothe an irritable, cranky infant is likely to have an infant who is in fact irritable and crying most of the time. The situation, sometimes labeled as colic, may be the result of a mismatch between what the parent is able to provide and what the child needs. Competent caregivers are able to modulate their infant's arousal caused by displeasure, fear, or frustration by calming the infant and returning him or her to a tolerable emotional state. Given at least average parenting, most infants are able to obtain the stimulation and nurturance needed from the environment to progress developmentally (35,36).

Age	Gross Motor	Fine Motor	Language	Social
1 month	Elevates head momentarily from prone position	Tight fist grasp	Responds to sounds	Prefers the human face
3 months	Steadily holds head up in midline	Hands held open at rest, reaches for objects	Coos	Anticipates feeding
4–5 months	Rolls over	Hand-to-hand transfer	Laughs	Visually explores environment
6 months	Sits up	Raking grasp	Babbles	Stranger recognition
9 months	Crawls, pulls self to standing position	Immature pincer grasp, holds bottle	Waves bye-bye, understands "no"	Plays games "pat a cake"
12 months	Walks	Mature pincer grasp	Uses single words	Begins to imitate actions
18 months	Runs	Scribbles, three block tower	Combines two words	Copies parent tasks
24 months	Walks up/down steps	Draws a line, removes shoes and pants, seven block tower	Follows two-step commands, uses two-word sentences	Parallel play
3 years	Rides tricycle	Draws circle, undresses self completely	Vocabulary at least 250 words, uses three word sentences	Gender identity, full name and age
4 years	Jumps, hops on one foot, alternates feet going up and down stairs	Draws square or plus sign, dresses self completely	Knows songs, poems, and colors	Plays cooperatively with others
5 years	Skips, jumps over object	Draws triangle	Writes name, some letters, and numbers	Plays games and understands rules

AGE 1 TO 5

Prominent language, motor, social, and emotional changes develop between the ages of one and five. The abundant number of synapses and continued growth and proliferation of neural connections in the first 2 years is demonstrated in the rapid acquisition of developmental skills and milestones. Expressive language becomes evident by the end of the first year. Receptive language exceeds expressive language until approximately the age of 4 to 5. The child's language progresses from cooing (3 to 6 months) and babbling (6 to 18 months) to single words (12 months). The appearance

of single words between the age of 8 and 18 months marks a transition after which time there is rapid acquisition of words (37). At this age, children also begin to walk allowing them to explore their environment more independently. A sense of one's own body also begins to emerge in a coherent way. Gender identity appears to be set by age two and a half (38). As the children gain motor and language skills, a sense of self and independence develops. With increasing self-reliance and a developing ability to understand and evaluate social situations comes the appearance of behavior that differs from those desired by the parents. The suddenly-less-than-compliant

2- to 3-year-old has entered the "terrible twos," a period often marked by a strong need for autonomy that often leads to oppositionality. Consistent and calm limit setting often helps parents navigate through this sometimes challenging time.

Children in the United States become interested in toilet training between age 2½ and 4. Most children in the United States are trained by age 3. Readiness for toilet training is based upon social-emotional skills, the acquisition of motor skills and sphincter control. Intensive toilet training prior to 27 months of age is not associated with earlier completion of training and is likely to take significantly longer to master (39). It is important not to develop a battle of will around toileting issues. Healthy children with complicated toilet training more often are found to have constipation and difficult temperaments (40).

The toddler and preschool years are often complicated by the introduction of a new sibling. Many children will feel displaced by this intruder. It is not unusual for children to oscillate between excitement and anger. Children often displace anger onto inanimate objects such as toys. Regressive behaviors including bedwetting, thumb sucking, or oppositionality may be observed. Opportunities to be alone with parents, to engage in pleasurable activities, and to safely displace anger are essential.

Parenting is crucial in the growth and development of children. Children who are exposed to adverse events during early childhood may be impacted for life. Child Protective Services investigated 3.5 million cases (5% of all children in the United States) of child abuse or neglect in 2004. The majority of abuse cases and deaths from child maltreatment occur in children under the age of 4 (41). Children who are abused or neglected in early life suffer enduring behavioral and neurobiological consequences. At a minimum, they appear to have increased vulnerability for psychiatric disorders (42). Abuse is correlated with a host of maladaptive behaviors and psychiatric difficulties in young children, including personal and academic difficulties, aggression, suicidal behavior, risk taking, and diagnosable psychiatric disorders (43). Recent literature suggests that exposure to early childhood abuse and/or neglect may alter brain structure and function. Exposure to abuse is associated with EEG abnormalities, alterations in the corpus callosum, and decreased synapse density and volume in the hippocampus. There appear to be critical periods during early childhood when discrete brain regions are most sensitive to stress and likely to be altered (44). Early maltreatment has a dramatic impact on the developing hypothalamic-pituitary axis. Child abuse has long-term consequences on basal cortisol levels and the ability of the Hypothalamic Pituitary Adrenal (HPA) axis to respond to stress (45).

SCHOOL AGE CHILD

Generally, children from school age to puberty are considered to be school age or latency age children. The major tasks of this period are cognitive development and socialization. Central experiences for children during this period are the family and school. Attendance at preschool or public school may be a child's first experience with adults other than parents. A premium is placed in this setting on the ability to interact in socially appropriate ways with other children and adults. Rapid advances in interactional abilities take place. Children begin to learn strategies for continuing interactions and for reengaging after rejection and failure in groups. Self-concept and internalization of self-identity is heavily dependent on these early experiences in school. Cognitively, Jean Piaget noted that young school age children are dominated by "centrition." They tend to view events as happening to them or in some way being affected by them. For example, children in this age group who experience parental divorce usually think that they, in some way,

caused the divorce. It is not unusual to see increases in depression, oppositional, and angry behaviors and declines in school grades as a result. Objects also tend to be measured and defined by only a few of several possible dimensions and may be classified in idiosyncratic ways. Children may measure the volume of a column of water exclusively by its height or width without taking into account changes in both parameters (46). Piaget termed this preoperational thinking. Children who learn how to recognize constant qualities or quantities of material even when the material changes shape or color are said to have achieved the concrete operational level.

This is also a time period when personality is rapidly developing and changing. A 6 year old is very different cognitively, socially, and emotionally from a 10 year old. There is always debate about what the major influences on personality are. Table 19.1 lists those thought to be most important. We have discussed temperament in an earlier section of this chapter. Basic components of parenting include consistency and limit setting. The importance of parenting is reflected in the numbers of programs developed to help parents with these kinds of skills. Most do not have any experimental verification. One well-known model that seems to have empirical validity has been used in schools and by mental health professionals for over 30 years. The Love and Logic model (Charles Fey, Ph.D.) (http://www.loveandlogic.com/) postulates that (1) children learn the best lessons when they're given a task and allowed to make their own choices (and fail) when the cost of failure is still small; and (2) that the children's failures must be coupled with love and empathy from their parents and teachers. The California Evidence-Based Clearinghouse for Child Welfare reports no research studies that document efficacy. Expressed emotion (EE) is a concept that, in contrast, is well studied in many different populations. EE consists of parental critical comments, hostility, and overcontrol. High levels of criticism especially have been correlated with poorer outcomes in children with physical disabilities and psychopathology (47,48). School quality seems to be related to both academic achievement and to healthy personality development. The way children relate to peers is important in overall adjustment. Students who had good relationships with teachers and peers did better in terms of engaging in school emotionally and behaviorally (49). There is good evidence that on balance, birth order affects intellectual performance (50) and personality characteristics within the family constellation, but perhaps not outside the family (51). It has been pointed out that the protests of the 1960s resulted in a cohort of individuals who are less likely to listen to authority and to follow social conventions (52).

TABLE 19.1
Major Influences on Personality Development in Children
1. inherited physiologic patterns known as temperament
2. parental practices and personality
3. quality of schools attended
4. relationships with peers
5. ordinal position within the family
6. historical era in which late childhood and early adolescence are spent

Source: From Kagen J. The role of parents in children's psychological develoment. *Pediatrics* 1999;104(1 Suppl): 164–167.

TABLE 19.2

Common Psychiatric Disorders in School Age Children

Separation anxiety disorder

Attention deficit hyperactivity disorder

Learning disorders

Oppositional defiant disorder

Psychiatric disorders as listed in Table 19.2 commonly begin in this age group. Depressive disorders are present but are less common. Children date the onset of internalizing disorders like depression earlier than their parents so that when identified, depression and anxiety disorders have likely been present for a longer time. On the other hand, parents and children agree about the timing of onset of externalizing disorders like oppositional defiant disorder (53).

It appears that childhood behavioral disorders are fairly stable into adolescence, so that the presence of a behavior disorder in childhood is predictive of disorder into adolescence (54). Importantly for adults, it appears that most lifetime psychiatric disorders first appear in childhood (53). This makes identification of psychiatric disorders in children critically important for treatment and prevention. In one survey of 1,060 pediatric practices, approximately 16% of patients were identified with psychiatric disorders and 55% of parents who reported a psychiatric disorder did not report discussing it with their pediatrician (55). Rates of use of mental health services for children are lower than indicated based on rates of disorder (56). Based on this and other data, identification and referral for children and adolescents with psychiatric disorders is a problem. Primary care practitioners can improve identification by using parent-and patient-completed standardized questionnaires they can then review (57). Table 19.3 lists some of these questionnaires.

ADOLESCENCE

Adolescence marks a time of profound biobehavioral shifts with reorganization of cognitive, emotional, and biologic functioning. Adolescence generally coincides with the onset of puberty. In females, breast budding precedes menarche by about 1 year (58). In males, the onset of puberty is marked by pubic hair and penile growth (58).

TABLE 19.3

Standardized Questionnaires for use in Identifying Psychiatric Disorder in Children and Adolescents

Pediatric symptom checklist-17

Beck depression inventory (age 16 and older)

Child depression inventory

Child behavior checklist

Strengths and difficulties questionnaire

The initiation and onset of puberty illustrates the complex interplay of genes and environment. The initiation of puberty is under control of multiple genes (59), and it is estimated that genes account for about 75% of the variation in time of onset of puberty (60). Consider, however, that female athletes tend to have delayed menarche based on body fat levels determined by diet and exercise. This illustrates the complex interplay of genetic and environmental factors.

Cognitive and social-emotional factors are extremely important during this time period. Cognitively, adolescents move from the state of concrete operations to formal operational processes (47). They begin to grasp highly abstract concepts and manipulate them. They develop the ability to use deductive and inductive reasoning to solve problems.

Development of these executive functions is related to marked changes in brain growth and organization that occur in adolescence. There may be a critical period for brain growth and development during this time. The prefrontal cortex and limbic systems undergo extensive reorganization. Dopaminergic and serotonergic inputs increase to frontal lobes, and there is an increase in gray matter volume resulting, in part, in greater frustration tolerance and better ability to delay impulses. There appears to be overproduction of neurons and synapses early in adolescence and pruning later on. As in earlier childhood, the amount, types, and quality of interaction and stimulation probably heavily influence this remodeling/production/pruning process (61). For example, tasks of selective attention, working memory, and problem solving improve consistently during this period and correlate with frontal cortical synaptic pruning and myelination (62). Drugs or injuries related to sensation seeking can cause profound behavioral and neurobiological distortions affecting the rest of life. Some studies show that in animals, adolescent brains are uniquely sensitive to alcohol (63).

Perhaps the hallmark of adolescence is the process of separation-individuation (64). Adolescents develop a relatively stable adult personality structure that tends to endure and as part of the process, they gradually separate from their family. Many factors contribute to and interact with this critical developmental process. Cognitively, adolescents can now conceive of a larger world and others outside their family as being relevant and important. Their peer group begins to be more important than parents regarding matters like dress, opinion, and in numerous other ways. They are overwhelmingly concerned with relationships with the same and opposite sex. This is not accidental or only determined by cultural norms. Adolescents use these new relationship abilities and their newly developed ability to think independently in order to separate from their family, build an increasingly independent lifestyle, and develop a character structure capable of self-regulation and independent action. Most adolescents have some conflict with their parents around at least a few things, and this may even enhance the process. However, viewing this time as a developmental period of turbulence does not seem to be true for a substantial number of adolescents. Offer and colleagues (65) documented a large group of male adolescents who seemed to go through this period of time in a "continuous growth" mode. They found little evidence of conflict or turmoil with family members, and this group was able to integrate various experiences of adolescence and to accept cultural and societal norms without conflict.

Some adolescents separate in maladaptive ways. Individuals who engage in delinquent acts are in part choosing an alternative path of separation from the family. There is also good evidence for gene-environment interactions related to some maladaptive behaviors. For example, Nilsson and colleagues report that individuals with the short variant of the MAO-A gene and who had been maltreated or abused or who came from families with poor relationships showed the highest scores on alcohol-related problems (66). Another group reported in 2007 that in a sample of males referred for forensic assessment, high adversity in child impacted later life violence only if the short form of the serotonin transporter gene was present (67). These studies demonstrate that one has to have both the gene and the environmental insult to develop the maladaptive behaviors described.

Individuals with chronic diseases may need more care and may not be able to become as independent as quickly as peers. In reaction, they may become neglectful of diets or insulin injections or other care needs. Adolescent diabetics with frequent ketoacidotic episodes might be engaging in a maneuver to express independence in the only way easily available. The opposite also occurs. Some adolescents never really separate and remain childish and enmeshed with parents. College and professional education can extend adolescent-like dependency into the 20s and 30s with continuing financial dependence on parents. This pattern may be particularly pertinent to medical students.

Other patterns of progression through adolescence occur. That which we consider normative is, in part, culture bound. In some cultures, preadolescent and early adolescent male homosexuality in normative and does not seem to result in large numbers of homosexual adults. In a number of cultures, there is a sharp demarcation between adolescence and adulthood with rites of passage.

Hamburg (68) comments that the fundamental requirements for healthy adolescent development are:

1. finding a valued place in a constructive group
2. learning how to form close, durable human relationships
3. feeling a sense of worth as in individual
4. achieving a reliable basis for making informed choices
5. knowing how to use the support systems available to them
6. expressing constructive curiosity and exploratory behavior
7. believing in a promising future with real opportunities
8. finding ways to be useful to others
9. learning to live respectfully with others in circumstances democratic pluralism
10. cultivating the inquiring and problem-solving skills that serve lifelong learning and adaptability

Practitioners seeing adolescents should be supportive of normal developmental processes. Seeing adolescents alone for at least a part of the medical visit is important and supports the process of separation-individuation.[52]

ADULT DEVELOPMENT

The definition of adulthood and the transition to geriatric status is fluid. For instance, medical students often have a prolonged period of dependency on others due to the length of training without opportunity to be employed. One is earning money while in residency, but is still in many ways a trainee. The transition to independent wage earner is gradual. Meanwhile, medical students and residents are often establishing families, having children, and acquiring all the other traditional trappings of independent adult life.

Furthermore, individuals progress through life stages at different rates. A 35-year-old woman may be a new mother, or in some settings, a new grandmother.

Personality is generally quite stable in adulthood. This should not be taken to mean that here are no changes. An individual at age 30 is certainly going to be different from the same individual at 40 or 50. However, change is much more gradual than in younger age groups. A sudden personality change is grounds for suspecting CNS disease. For instance, a patient who presents with the development of depression at age 52 with no history of psychiatric disorder, or a patient who begins to make impulsive decisions and sexually inappropriate comments needs to be worked up medically for space-occupying lesions as well as neurodegenerative disorders.

Eric Erickson's psychosocial stages of development in adulthood include:

1. Intimacy versus Isolation: Developing a cooperative, close, and supportive relationship with a spouse or significant other, often leading to starting a family, is a major task. Negotiating between parents around who does what at home and who takes care of the children at what times are major issues in a society where often both spouses work. Nontraditional family settings with a single parent or two parents of the same sex are more and more common and present their own challenges related to intimacy, childcare, and support.
2. Generativity versus Stagnation: A concern for and active involvement in guiding the next generation is a characteristic of individuals who achieve generativity. People who are generative also have fulfilling work and relationships. Contrast this lifestyle and values to persons who are without intimate relationships and who dislike their work and are waiting to retire.
3. Integrity or Ego Integrity versus Despair: This stage is discussed under geriatrics below.

One of the few studies to look at long-term aging followed several groups of men and women over a 60-year period. George Vaillant describes six factors in middle age (50) that have seem to be correlated with getting to age 80:

- Having a warm marriage
- Possessing adaptive coping strategies
- Not smoking heavily
- Not abusing alcohol
- Getting ample exercise
- Not being overweight

These people are more likely going to be the "happy well," people "who subjectively enjoy their lives and are objectively healthy" (69). Physicians see these people less often in their offices than the worried well or those who have debilitating chronic illnesses.

GERIATRICS

Introduction

Aging is a diverse, complex phenomenon that requires the physician become aware of both normal and pathological changes associated with it. The osteopathic physician's holistic perspective is especially advantageous in helping geriatric patients with complex medical, psychosocial, and end-of-life issues. While we often tend to view elderly individuals as a homogeneous group, there are actually tremendous variations in the physical and emotional aspects of aging. To this end, physicians must be aware of the normal and pathological changes linked to late-life development. Osteopathic physicians bring a comprehensive patient view and manual medicine skills that are tremendously valuable when treating chronic diseases and associated musculoskeletal disorders that are so often seen in elderly individuals.

The definition of "older adult" depends upon the context in which it is given. The establishment of Medicare in 1965 provided the cut off at age 65, an age at which individuals could receive full Medicare and Social Security benefits. Gerontologists have used a broader definition, considering age 60 the beginning of late life. In contrast, some cultures equate the term "old" with what the western world would consider middle age, that is, age 45. However, more recently geriatricians have divided late life into young old (age 65 to 75), older-old (age 75 to 85) and old-old (age 85+) (70).

The 2000 U.S. Census reports that 12.4% of the U.S. population is over age 65. Among the older population, those "old-old" age 85 years plus showed the highest percentage increase, moving from 3.1 million to 4.2 million adults nationally. In 2000, there were over 50,000 centenarians living in the United States, suggesting increasing longevity for our oldest citizens (71). Centenarians are expected to exceed 1 million by 2040. Of note, by 2030, the older population is expected to double from 2000 census figures, increasing to 71.5 million people (72). The oldest living adult was Jeanne Calment, who died in 1997 at age 122 in France (73).

Cellular Changes Associated with Aging

There are a number of possible explanations for why cells decline resulting in aging of the organism. Although no single theory is generally accepted, researchers currently view the impact of environment upon genetic substrate as a possible reason for such variability in the aging process.

Hayflick limit purports that genes do not drive the aging process, but the general loss of molecular fidelity does. There are a finite number of cell divisions possible. This theory explains that aging is the result of changes that occur in molecules that have existed at one time with no age changes. Aging is considered a molecular disorder with an escalating loss of molecular fidelity that ultimately exceeds repair and turnover capacity and increases vulnerability to pathology or age-associated disease (74).

Telomere shortening is another theory of cellular aging. Telomeres serve to camouflage chromosome ends from the DNA damage response machinery. Telomerase activity is required to maintain telomeres. One consequence of telomere dysfunction is cellular senescence, a permanent growth arrest state. The introduction of telomerase is proposed as a method to combat ageing via cell therapy and a possible method to regenerate tissue (75).

The free radical theory of aging by Harman proposes that reactive oxygen species are a cause of aging. Chronic states of oxidative stress exist in cells even under normal conditions. However, an imbalance leads to a steady-state accumulation of oxidative damage in a variety of macromolecules that increases during aging, resulting in a progressive loss in the functional efficiency of various cellular processes (76).

Genes may also impact the aging process. Developmental genetics theorists propose that aging is genetically programmed and controlled by influences in the second half of life. Both oxidative stress and DNA methylation are possible regulators of gene expression. Examples of genetic influences in aging are Apolipoprotein (ApoE-4) in the development of Alzheimer disease and coronary heart disease and longevity (77).

Inflammation may be linked to cellular aging. A large number of studies have documented changes in Zinc metabolism in experimental animal models of acute and chronic inflammation and in human chronic inflammatory diseases. In particular, modification of zinc plasma concentration as well as intracellular disturbance of antioxidant intracellular pathways have been found associated to age-related inflammatory diseases, like atherosclerosis. Zinc deficiency in individuals genetically predisposed to a dysregulation of inflammation response may play a crucial role in causing adverse events and in reducing the probability of successful aging (78).

Other aging theories focus on inflammation and evolution. Chronic inflammatory conditions (as demonstrated by increased homocysteine and plasma cholesterol levels) may shorten the lifespan by causing cellular damage and diverting resources (79). Evolutionary theories include the notion that genes that are adaptive in early life may be harmful later in life when natural selection is not operative.

Physical Changes Associated with Aging

Age-related changes begin by the third or the fourth decade of life. Physical changes appear to happen earlier and more dramatically than do psychological changes. Although previously considered a constant phenomenon, genetic research offers another explanation, namely that individual genes impact the rate of aging decline (80).

Body Composition Changes

Throughout life, there are three specific periods in which there is notable increase in fat mass, specifically early in life, during pregnancy and lactation, and with aging. The increase in body fat and decrease in lean body mass and body water seen in aging may be protective from an evolutionary standpoint, providing body calorie reserves to withstand periods of illness (81). Total and central body fat increase with aging.

Because of these changes in total body fat, drugs that are lipid soluble may have prolonged half-lives in the elderly. This alternation in pharmacokinetics with aging must be accounted for when prescribing or evaluating treatment regimes in this population. For example, while diazepam (Valium) has a half-life of 20 hours in a 20-year old, due to increased fat storage the half-life in an 80 year old may be 80 to 100 hours (82).

Skin Changes

Skin changes are well-known markers of aging. The skin loses its elasticity and sagging appears. Wrinkles increase significantly during the second half of life. Other changes include the loss of subcutaneous fat, sweat glands, and increased capillary fragility. Chronic inflammation also appears strongly linked to many preventable and treatable skin diseases and conditions such as visible skin aging. Mucocutaneous inflammation may be the final common pathway of many systemic and mucocutaneous diseases (83). Sex steroids modulate epidermal and dermal thickness as well as immune system function, and changes in these hormonal levels with aging and/or disease processes alter skin surface pH, quality of wound healing, and propensity to develop autoimmune disease, thereby significantly influencing potential for infection and other disease states (84).

Skin issues become increasingly important in the elderly. These include bruising, skin tears, changes in body temperature regulation, and pressure sores (85). Adequate nutrition and mineral supplementation, management of shear forces, body positioning, and physical health are a few of the many critical components of good skin care management in late life.

Sensory Changes

Hearing and vision decline with normal aging. Ophthalmic changes include loss of elasticity of the lens resulting in presbyopia. Many older adults experience a variety of visual perceptual problems resulting from aging-related changes in the optics of the eye and degeneration of the visual neural pathways. These problems consist of impairments in visual acuity, contrast sensitivity, color discrimination, temporal sensitivity, motion perception, peripheral visual field sensitivity, and visual processing speed (86). Visual changes can make it more difficult to read, encouraging older adults to use back lighting as well as large print materials to accommodate to these changes.

Hearing diminishes with well-documented loss of auditory neurons and cochlear hairs (87). The resulting presbycusis (a decreased ability to hear high-pitched sounds) can also lead to misunderstanding of information and conversations. It becomes increasingly difficult to hear conversation with background ambient noise, making conversation in a crowd quite difficult. Paranoia may result from misunderstanding and sensory loss. An older adult may withdraw from social situations as a way to deal with hearing loss or ensuing paranoia. Accepting the need for hearing aids can be a slow process for some older adults who experience denial of their problem.

Taste and smell change with aging. In general, both young and elderly confuse salty and sour much more than they confuse sweet and sour (88). Changes in taste can impact diet and nutrition, causing decreased food intake and enjoyment in eating. The sense of smell is more impaired by aging than is the sense of taste (89). As with taste, if smell is impaired the older adult may be less likely to enjoy the smell of food and the impact of smell on digestion and appetite.

Brain Changes
Age-related neuronal dysfunction, which must underlie observed decline in cognitive function, probably involves a host of other subtle changes within the cortex that could include alterations in receptors, loss of dendrites, and spines and myelin dystrophy, as well as the alterations in synaptic transmission (90). Loss of brain weight with cerebral atrophy has been demonstrated on MRI. Both whole brain metabolism and frontal lobe metabolism decrease significantly with age (38% and 42%, respectively), whereas cerebellar metabolism does not show a significant decline with age (91). Many elderly individuals demonstrate increased time to recall memories. On the whole, it is important to know that memory loss and dementia are never normal parts of the aging process.

Musculoskeletal Changes
Age-related changes to the musculoskeletal system have tremendous impact on the older adult. Muscles achieve peak force in women in their 40s and then force trends downward for those in their 50s and 60s, with significant reductions by the 70s. Tactile acuity, vibration sensitivity, and joint position sense for a non–weight-bearing toe-matching task were significantly reduced by the 40s or 50s, with further reductions by either the 60s or 70s (92). In addition, decreased muscle mass and demineralization contribute to falls and to fractures as well as spontaneous compression and stress fractures. Decreased mobility and the pain of osteoarthritis can lead to social isolation and the inability to complete activities of daily living (ADLs). The osteopathic physician's holistic philosophy and manipulative therapy skills are well suited for addressing musculoskeletal issues.

Cardiopulmonary Changes
Calcification and sclerosis of arteries and heart valves can affect blood pressure and hemodynamic response to exertion. The main changes in the cardiovascular system include loss of large artery compliance, dysfunction of some of the systems modulating resistance vessel tone, increased activity of the sympathetic nervous system, and reduced hemodynamic responses to inotropic agents (93). These changes may contribute to fatigue, decreased endurance and depression.

The structural changes associated with the pulmonary system and aging include chest wall and thoracic spine deformities that impair total respiratory system compliance leading to increase work of breathing. The lung parenchyma loses its supporting structure causing dilation of air spaces: "senile emphysema." Respiratory muscle strength decreases with age and can impair effective cough, which is important for airway clearance. The lung matures by age 20 to 25 years, and thereafter aging is associated with progressive decline in lung function. The alveolar dead space increases with age, affecting arterial oxygen without impairing carbon dioxide elimination (94). There is a decline in alveolar surface area, a decrease in vital capacity, and a decrease in the partial pressure of arterial oxygen. These changes may contribute to the experience of shortness of breath, a significant cause for the new onset of anxiety in the older patient.

Liver Changes
Several age-related changes in the liver have been documented, including (a) a decline in liver volume, (b) an increase in the hepatic dense body compartment (lipofuscin), (c) moderate declines in the Phase I metabolism of certain drugs, (d) shifts in the expression of a variety of proteins, and (e) diminished hepatobiliary functions. Other more subtle changes (e.g., muted responses to oxidative stress, reduced expression of growth regulatory genes, diminished rates of DNA repair, telomere shortening) may contribute to reduced hepatic regenerative capacity, shorter post–liver transplant survival, and increased susceptibility to certain liver diseases in the elderly (95). Overall liver mass decreases. As liver function decreases with decreasing drug clearance, older adults are increasingly at risk for delirium and increased drug-drug interactions. The osteopathic physician working with an older adult should be aware of decreased liver clearance with many drugs and anticipate the CNS effects of prescribed medications.

Renal Changes
The function of the kidney as well as its morphology changes markedly with age. The glomerular filtration rate falls progressively, independent of overt pathology. Glomerular, vascular, and accompanying parenchymal changes occur (96). The number of nephrons is reduced and creatinine clearance declines. This impacts the kidney's ability to clear drugs. Care must be taken when prescribing drugs that are cleared through the kidney as drug toxicity may result quite rapidly. In addition, as chronic kidney disease is quite prevalent in late life, special care should be taken with drug prescribing and dosing to avoid kidney-related drug toxicity.

Immunologic Changes
With increasing age, the competence of the immune system to fight infections and tumors declines. Age-dependent changes have been mostly described for human CD8 T cells (97). Antibody production decreases and autoantibodies increase with age. These changes may account for the higher rate of infection, autoimmune disease, and perhaps malignancy with age.

Psychological Changes Associated with Aging

Late life has been described as a season of change and loss. Older adults are faced with a variety of predictable losses including retirement, reduction in income, loss of spouse, death of friends and peers, loss of health, and change of living environment. The elder may experience a shift from an internal locus of control to an external one, as many life changes occur outside of one's control.

A number of developmental theorists have addressed the psychological issues associated with aging. Erickson identified the last stage of aging as "integrity vs. despair." In this stage, the older adult is faced with looking back on their life and determining meaning and value in their history. Regrets for mistakes, losses and life events left undone can create bitterness and frustration. Erickson believes that successful resolution of this stage results in wisdom.

High levels of extraversion and low levels of neuroticism are associated with reduced risk of mortality in old age and that these associations are mediated in part by personality-related patterns of cognitive, social, and physical activity (98). Older adults who are more outgoing may be able to weather the changes associated with late life more flexibly than those who are more introverted. Anxiety also appears to play a role in survival in that elders with low levels of anxiety appear to survive longer than those with high levels of anxiety.

Comprehensive Geriatric Assessment

The major focus of geriatric care is optimizing function, avoiding institutionalization, and maintaining the older adult in the community. The geriatric multidisciplinary assessment is defined as a multidimensional interdisciplinary process focused on determining a frail elderly person's medical, psychological, and functional capacity in order to develop a coordinated and integrated plan for treatment and long-term follow-up (99). Team members may include a geriatrician, nurse practitioner, social worker, dietician, pharmacist, psychiatrist, physical therapists, and other medical specialties. The domains addressed in a comprehensive geriatric assessment include competency and communication, functional status, physical status, nutrition, mobility, symptoms and distress, psychological/social status, spiritual issues, care services, and quality of life (100).

Components of the Medical Assessment

Geriatric patients need a thorough medical assessment as in no other age group is the interface of physical, behavioral, and social issues so great. The presentation of a variety of disorders may be different in a young versus older population; physicians should be mindful of these differences. Examples include abdominal pain from a ruptured diverticuli that presents as often with less pain and less inflammation in an older adult when compared to a younger person. Depression may present as memory changes for an older adult, less likely in a younger person. Drug interactions can be more serious for older adults, both because of the multiple medications many older adults take as well as the drug interactions that may occur.

Older adults may under report symptoms, perhaps due to embarrassment or misconceptions about normal aging. Before beginning the history, physicians should determine if there are any significant deficits of vision, hearing, or cognition that may impact the patient's ability to relate their story. Physicians often have to spend more time with patients because of cognitive slowing and a lengthy life history. Other informants such as children or care providers should be interviewed since they may be able to provide another perspective on patient functioning or problems. Informants should be encouraged to bring an accurate list of the patient's medications as medication adherence/confusion may prove to be a key element of the comprehensive geriatric assessment.

Table 19.4 outlines those issues that should be a component of the geriatric assessment. Unlike other age groups, the geriatric patient should be assessed for ADLs such as dressing, toileting, bathing, continence, feeding, and transferring. Independent activities of daily living should also be assessed including housekeeping, laundry, finances, cooking, medication management, transportation,

---

TABLE 19.4

Components of the History in a Geriatric Assessment

- Dentition/dentures
- Feeding difficulties
- Hearing status
- Vision status
- Bowel and bladder control
- Nutrition
- Infections
- Osteoporosis
- Status of feed/gait
- Fall risk
- Osteoporosis
- Decubitus ulcers
- Mood/affect
- Thought process and memory
- Advanced directives
- Abuse
- Medications and polypharmacy issues

---

and telephone use. The elder's ability to complete these is essential information needed to help determine the level of care that is needed from independent living to residential care.

A number of assessment instruments can be helpful in obtaining history from the patient. For falls and gait issues, the "Get-up and go" test (101) can be a helpful assessment of balance and ambulation issues (Table 19.5).

The geriatric patient should have a physical exam as part of their geriatric assessment. The components of the physical exam are not unlike those of a younger adult with special attention being focused on issues associated with aging. The osteopathic physician should be mindful of modesty issues with older adults and sensitively examine in a warm comfortable environment. Table 19.6 outlines issues to focus on with respect to each area of the physical exam.

A mental status examination is a part of thorough geriatric evaluation. Appearance can inform the clinician about self-neglect and

---

TABLE 19.5

The Get-up and Go Test

Initial check:

All older persons who report a single fall should be observed as they:

- From a sitting position, stand without using their arms for support
- Walk several paces, turn and return to the chair
- Sit back in the chair without using their arms for support

Note: Individuals who have difficulty or demonstrate unsteadiness performing this test require further assessment.

TABLE 19.6

Key Components of the Geriatric Physical Examination

Vital signs

- Assess for orthostatic hypotension (Blood pressure sitting and standing)
- Assess temperature
- Monitor weight with each visit

Skin

- Evaluate for common skin lesions in aging including lentigo, senile keratosis, senile purpura, pressure sores, or evidence of falls

Head

- Assess vision and eye movements, evidence for cataracts
- Assess hearing
- Evaluate skull for trauma with a history of falls
- Examine patient for cerumen impacting ear canal
- Auscultate for carotid bruits

Cardiopulmonary system

- Evaluate for systolic ejection murmurs (common secondary to aortic valve changes associated with aging)
- Presence of peripheral pulses
- Assessment for leg edema
- Auscultate for bibasilar rales and possible atelectasis secondary to immobility

Abdomen

- Assess hernias
- Deep palpation for aortic size
- Palpate for enlarged bladder
- Rectal examination and assessment for stool in blood
- Prostate exam in men

Musculoskeletal

- Evaluate gait
- Assess posture
- Range of motion of upper and lower extremities
- Feet evaluation for ulcers and nail care
- Osteopathic structural evaluation of muscle and joint for somatic dysfunction

Neurological exam

- Evaluate vibration (may be normal in older adults)
- Reflexes (ankle reflex may be absent in normal older adult)
- Observe for asymmetrical test results (could be suggestive of stroke)
- Mini-Mental State Exam to evaluate cognition (Table 19.4)

TABLE 19.7

The Geriatric Depression Scale

Scoring system: Answers indicating depression are highlighted. Each bold faced answer counts as one (1) point.

1.	Are you basically satisfied with your life?	yes/**no**
2.	Have you dropped any of your activities and interests?	**yes**/no
3.	Do you feel that your life is empty?	**yes**/no
4.	Do you often get bored?	**yes**/no
5.	Are you in good spirits most of the time?	yes/**no**
6.	Are you afraid that something bad is going to happen to you?	**yes**/no
7.	Do you feel happy most of the time?	yes/**no**
8.	Do you often feel helpless?	**yes**/no
9.	Do you prefer to stay in your room rather than going out?	**yes**/no
10.	Do you feel you have more problems with memory than most?	**yes**/no
11.	Do you think it is wonderful to be alive?	yes/**no**
12.	DO you feel worthless the way you are now?	**yes**/no
13.	Do you feel full of energy?	yes/**no**
14.	Do you feel that your situation is hopeless?	**yes**/no
15.	Do you think that most people are better off than you?	**yes**/no

Score > 5 = Probable Depression Score_____.

dementia issues. Orientation and short-term memory assessment are invaluable tools to understand whether a patient will be able to live independently and comply with complex medical treatments. Mood assessment is critical to evaluate for any level of depression that may impair functioning or quality of life. The Geriatric Depression Scale (102) (Table 19.7) can be used for older adults without cognitive impairment. For patients with cognitive decline in which one suspects dementia, the Cornell Scale for Depression in Dementia (103) may be used to assess the cognitively impaired patient for depression (Table 19.8).

Likewise, evaluating the patient for thought disorder is vital to help understand the clarity of thinking process and the patient's ability to participate in their care. The neurological exam should periodically include a standardized cognitive assessment (Table 19.9). The Mini-mental state exam (MMSE) (104) is one such cognitive exam frequently used both as a baseline and an outcomes measure of cognitive decline.

Pathologic Changes Associated with Aging

Humans are social animals. Late life is fraught with losses and changes to the social support network. Social networks work as buffers for stresses and moderate losses. Older adults who lose their social networks due to death, changes in location or illness tend to not do

TABLE 19.8

The Cornell Scale for Depression in Dementia

a	0	1	2	**A. Mood-related signs**
				1. Anxiety: anxious expression, rumination, worrying
				2. Sadness: sad expression, sad voice, tearfulness
				3. Lack of reaction to present events
				4. Irritability: annoyed, short tempered
a	0	1	2	**B. Behavioral disturbance**
				5. Agitation: restlessness, hand wringing, hair pulling
				6. Retardation: slow movements, slow speech, slow reactions
				7. Multiple physical complains (score 0 if gastrointestinal symptoms only)
				8. Loss of interest: less involved in usual activities (score only if change occurred acutely, i.e., in <1 month)
a	0	1	2	**C. Physical signs**
				9. Appetite loss: eating less than usual
				10. Weight loss (score 2 if >5 lb in 1 month)
				11. Lack of energy: fatigues easily, unable to sustain activities
a	0	1	2	**D. Cyclic functions**
				12. Diurnal variation of mood: symptoms worse in the morning
				13. Difficulty falling asleep: Later than usual for this individual
				14. Multiple awakenings during sleep
				15. Early morning awakening: earlier than usual for this individual
a	0	1	2	**E. Ideational disturbance**
				16. Suicidal: feels life is not worth living
				17. Poor self-esteem: self-blame, self-deprecation, feelings of failure
				18. Pessimism: anticipation of the worst
				19. Mood congruent delusions: delusions of poverty, illness, or loss

Score_____ score > 12 = Probable Depression Score.

Ratings should be based on symptoms and signs occurring during the week before interview. No score should be given if symptoms result from physical disability or illness

Scoring system: a, unable to evaluate; 0, absent; 1, mild to intermittent; and 2, severe.

as well physically or psychologically as those adults whose lives are more stable. Assessing the older adult's social network is critical to understanding the nature and scope of support around them as this may impact their ability to function. The osteopathic physician will want to understand other components of support including financial and physical status. This is critical to help the patient access appropriate services as well as to guide treatment and therapy decisions. A team approach is likely to be helpful in collecting this information and providing more interventions than any single health professional may be. Even with a strong social and financial support system in place, the older adult may be more vulnerable to a number of issues including depression, anxiety, dementia, and psychosis.

Depression

Depression is prevalent in late life. Although many older adults present with subsyndromal depressive symptoms that may not meet DSM-IV-TR criteria for major depression, depression continues to impact functioning significantly in late life. Increased somatic symptoms may be present for some older adults, leading to somatization and a focus on bodily functions. Eight to twenty percent of older adults in the community and up to 37% in primary

care settings suffer from depressive symptoms (105). Table 19.10 describes the symptoms associated with major and minor depression (106) in the elderly.

Suicide risk is also high. Being male as well as having mental illness (particularly depression), physical illness, and interpersonal discord are all risk factors for suicide in the elderly (107). To this end, a thorough evaluation of mood and suicidal ideation should be done with the older patient including the use of a thorough psychiatric examination to obtain information about the patient's current presentation, history, diagnosis, and to recognize suicide risk factors therein; the necessity of asking very specific questions about suicidal ideation, intent, plans, and attempts; the process of making an estimation of the patient's level of suicide risk is explained; and the use of modifiable risk and protective factors as the basis for treatment planning (108).

When older adults consider suicide, they choose the most lethal means and do not tell their physician prior to their attempts. Older patients may not realize or acknowledge that they are depressed. In fact, many patients will deny that they are depressed yet admit to symptoms of hopelessness, decreased energy, anhedonia, sleep changes, and changes in appetite. Other etiologies must also be considered including iatrogenic causes for depression, recent loss (spouse, children, friends, and pets) and advancing medical illnesses.

TABLE 19.9

Mini-Mental State Exam

Orientation	Maximum Score
1. What is the (year) (season) (date)(day)(month)?	5
2. Where are we? (state)(country)(town)(hospital)(floor)	5

Registration	
As the patient if you may test his memory. Then say the names of three unrelated objects, clearly and slowly. After you have said all three, ask him to repeat. This first repetition determines the score (0–3) but keep saying them until he can repeat all three, up to six trials.	3

Attention and calculation	
Ask the patient to begin with 100 and count backward by 7, stop after 5 subtractions (93,86,79,72,65). If the patient cannot do serial 7s, ask him to spell the word WORLD backwards.	5

Recall	3
Ask the patient to recall the three items repeated above.	

Language	2
Naming: Show the patient a wristwatch and pencil and ask the name.	
Repetition: Repeat the phrase "No ifs, ands, or buts" after you.	1
3-Stage Command: Give the patient a blank paper and ask him to take the paper in his right hand, fold it in half, and put it on the floor. One point for each part correctly executed.	3
Reading: On a blank page of paper print "CLOSE YOUR EYES." Ask the patient to do what it says.	1
Writing: Give the patient a blank piece of paper and ask him to write a sentence that must contain a subject and a verb.	1
Copying: Ask the patient to copy the figure of intersecting pentagons. All 10 angles must be present and 2 must intersect to form a four-sided figure.	1

SCORING:

MAXIMUM 30

Mild impairment MMSE >21; Moderate MMSE 10–20; Severe MMSE <9.

Depression is treatable in late life and should not be considered merely a normal reaction to loss. Antidepressants may be helpful for the neurovegetative signs of depression such as sleep disturbance, weight changes, and depressed mood. However, because of decreased renal and liver clearance, antidepressant dosages used should be one half to one third of a younger adult's dosage to eliminate the possibility of toxicity. A variety of selective serotonin reuptake inhibitors or noradrenergic-serotonergic reuptake inhibitors may be used safely in the elderly. Frequent visits with the physician to both monitor for side effects and provide encouragement in waiting for antidepressant response (which may take 6 to 12 weeks) is encouraged.

Psychotherapy is helpful in managing depression as old age is fraught with a number of losses. Cognitive behavioral, interpersonal, and supportive therapies are helpful for the older adult (109). Used in combination with antidepressant medication, psychotherapy can provide additional help in dealing with the adjustment to life changes as well as problem solving.

Anxiety

There is significant overlap between depression and anxiety in late life. Anxiety may manifest itself as panic, generalized anxiety, or simple phobias of theft or loss. Feeling nervous or restless may be signs of anxiety, but in the older patient anxiety is very closely tied to medical illness. Pulmonary disorders such as chronic obstructive pulmonary disease can create hypoxia and mimic the signs and symptoms of anxiety. Cardiac disease has also been associated with anxiety in older adults (110).

Although often used, benzodiazepines can be highly problematic for older individuals. This class of drug is associated with falls, delirium, and even depression. A better choice to manage anxiety is the use of a selective serotonin reuptake inhibitor. Benzodiazepine use should be short term and of low potency in order to reduce risks associated with these medications.

Cognitive behavioral therapy has been demonstrated to be highly effective for the management of anxiety (111). Learning to deal with irrational thoughts, developing strategies for replacing negative thoughts with positive ones, and helping a patient find solutions for overwhelming worries are all practical functions of psychotherapy.

Dementia

Dementia is a syndrome of brain deterioration characterized by short-term memory loss, disorientation, word-finding difficulties,

TABLE 19.10

Symptoms Associated with Major and Minor Depression

Major depressive disorder

- Depressed or irritable mood for >2 weeks
- Five or more of the following symptoms >2 weeks that impair social, occupational or other important areas of functioning:
  - a. diminished interest or pleasure
  - b. significant weight change
  - c. insomnia or hypersomnia
  - d. psychomotor agitation or retardation
  - e. fatigue
  - f. feelings of worthlessness or guilt
  - g. diminished ability to concentrate
  - h. recurrent thoughts of death

Minor depression

Presence of 2–5 symptoms of major depressive disorder. In addition, these symptoms may also be associated with minor depression:

- Increased somatic preoccupation
- Anergic, anhedonia
- Isolation
- Pessimistic attitude
- Fatigue
- Increased emotional sensitivity
- Increased mood reactivity

apraxia, and agnosia with significant functional decline. It is estimated that currently around 24 million people have dementia in the world, with the number being projected to double every 20 years, and that 60% of dementia patients live in developing countries, with the proportion being raised to more than 70% by 2040 (112). Patients with dementia require increased caregiving supervision and care because of their memory loss.

A number of behavioral issues can arise with dementia. These include psychosis, depression, agitation, and physical aggression. Personality changes may also result making docile individuals premorbidly aggressive or paranoid. These behavioral issues can be particularly troublesome to caregivers and are the place where the osteopathic physician, considering the impact of mind-body-environment, can help provide psychoeducation, behavioral strategies to minimize excessive stimulation, and support for the family caregivers (113).

Pharmacological treatment for the management of dementia currently includes acetylcholinesterase and glutamate inhibitors (114). Antidepressants can be helpful in the management of depression in dementia. Atypical antipsychotics have been used in the management of agitation and psychosis in dementia; however, they have recently come under scrutiny for increased risk of cerebrovascular risk and sudden death (115).

Delirium

Delirium is characterized by an acute confusional state, usually fairly sudden in nature, in which the patient has fluctuating sensorium, attentional deficits, waxing and waning levels of alertness, and intermittent psychosis. Delirium is common in the elderly and its manifestation may be frightening for family members witnessing an abrupt change in the patient. Delirium may result from many sources including medications (anesthetics, pain medications), infection, electrolyte imbalance, hypoxia, and sensory loss.

Systematic detection and intervention programs and special nursing care appeared to add large benefits to traditional medical care in young and old surgical patients and modest benefits in elderly medical patients (116). Special attention to sensory loss such as hearing or vision may help target interventions (hearing aids, glasses) that can reduce the risk for the development of delirium (117). Osteopathic physicians should work to identify those medical and environmental causes for delirium. Providing psychoeducation to caregivers and family is also an important component in trying to aggressively anticipate the problem of delirium in the older adult.

Psychosis

Older schizophrenics have more multiple medical problems as a result of chronic illnesses due to poor lifestyle choices as well as lack of health care. Often, these individuals are frail and may be suffering from cardiac or pulmonary diseases. These illnesses may hamper the pharmacokinetics of antipsychotic medications they are using to manage their psychosis. Elderly patients may be at greater risk for tardive dyskinesia and parkinsonian side effects of antipsychotic medications (118).

Psychosis may result from schizophrenia, mood disorders, or organic etiologies. Since new onset psychosis in older individuals is much more likely to be related to an organic etiology, it requires a thorough medical workup. Schizophrenics may also develop dementia. In addition, older adults with premorbid schizoid or schizotypal personality disorders may develop late-life schizophrenia.

REFERENCES

1. Zeanhan CH, Anders TF, Seifer R, et al. Implications of research on infant development for psychodynamic theory and practice. *J Am Acad Child Adolesc Psychiatry* 1989;28(5):657–668.
2. Emde RN, Easterbrooks MA. Assessing emotional availability in early development. In: Frakenbert WK, Emde RN, Sullivan JW, eds. *Early Identification of Children at Risk.* New York, NY: Plenum Publishing, 1985.
3. Herschkowitz N, Kagan J, Zilles K. Neurobiological bases of behavioral development in the first year. *Neuropediatrics* 1997;28(6):296–306.
4. Reser J. Schizophrenia and phenotypic plasticity: schizophrenia may represent a predictive, adaptive response to severe environmental adversity that allows both bioenergetic thrift and a defensive behavioral strategy. *Med Hypotheses* 2007;69(2):383–394.
5. Feinberg AP. Phenotypic plasticity and the epigenetics of human diseases. *Nature* 2007;447(7143):433–440.
6. Weidman JR, Dolinoy DC, Murphy SK, et al. Cancer susceptibility: epigenetic manifestation of environmental exposures. *Cancer J* 2007;13(1):9–16.
7. Eriksson JG. Epidemiology, genes and the environment: lessons learned from the Helsinki Birth Cohort Study. *J Intern Med* 2007;261(5):418–425.
8. Gerra G, Garofano L, Castaldini L, et al. Serotonin transporter promoter polymorphism genotypes is associated with temperament, personality traits and illegal drug use among adolescents. *J Neural Transm* 2005;112(10):1397–1410.
9. Rutter M. Continuities and discontinuities in socio-emotional development: Empirical and conceptual perspectives. In: Emde RN, Harmon RJ, eds. *Continuities and Discontinuities in Development.* New York, NY: Plenum Publishing, 1984:41–68.
10. Yang Q, Wen SW, Lader A, et al. Paternal age and birth defects: how strong is the association? *Hum Reprod* 2007;22(3):696–701.

11. McMillan JA, DeAngelis CD, Feigin RD, et al. *Oski's Pediatrics: Principals and Practice.* 3rd ed. Philadelphia, PA: Lippincott, Williams & Wilkins, 1999:2228.

12. Fryer SL, McGee CL, et al. Evaluation of psychopathological conditions in children with heavy prenatal alcohol exposure. *Pediatrics* 2007;119(3): 733–741.

13. Bonari L, Pinto N, et al. Perinatal risks of untreated depression during pregnancy. *Can J Psychiatry* 2004;49(11):726–735.

14. McFarland JM, Groff JY, O'Brien JA, et al. Behaviors of children who are exposed and not exposed to intimate partner violence: an analysis of 330 black, white, and Hispanic children. *Pediatrics* 2003;112(3):202–207.

15. Berman K, Sarkar P and O'Connor TG, et al. Maternal stress during pregnancy predicts cognitive ability and fearfulness in infancy. *J Am Acad Adolesc Psychiatry* 2007;46(11):1454–1463.

16. Forcada-Guex M, Pierrehumbert B, Borghini A, et al. Early dyadic patterns of mother-infant interactions and outcomes of prematurity at 18 months. *Pediatrics* 2006;118(1):e107–e114.

17. Salt A, Redshaw M. Neurodevelopmental follow-up after preterm birth:follow up after two years. *Early Hum Dev* 2006;8(3):185–197.

18. Nelson A, Bloom E. Child development and neuroscience. *Child Dev* 1997;68:970–987.

19. Joseph R. Environmental influences on neural plasticity, the limbic system, emotional development, and attachment; a review. *Child Psychiatry Hum Dev* 1999;29(3)189–208.

20. Haith MM. *Rules that Babies Look By.* Hillsdale, NJ: Erlbaum, 1980.

21. Eimas PD, Siqueland ER, Josczyk P, et al. Speech perception in infants. *Science* 1971;171;303–306.

22. Thompson RA. Attachment theory and research. In: Lewis M, ed. *Child and Adolescent Psychiatry: A Comprehensive Textbook.* Baltimore, MD: Williams & Wilkins, 1991:100–108.

23. Kraemer GW. Psychobiology of early social attachment in rhesus monkeys. *Ann NY Acad Sci* 1997;807:401–408.

24. Emde RN. Development terminable and interminable:innate and motivational factors from infancy. *Int J Psychoanal* 1988;69:23–42.

25. Herschkowitz N, Kagan J, Zilles K. Neurobiological bases of behavioral development in the first year. *Neuropediatrics* 1997;28(6):296–306.

26. Singer W. Development and plasticity of cortical processing architectures. *Science* 1995;270;758–764.

27. Kuhn CM, Schanberg SM. Responses to maternal separation: mechanisms and mediators. *Int J Dev Neurosci* 1998;16(3–4):261–270.

28. Dee DL, Ruowei L, Li-Ching L, et al. Association between breastfeeding practices and young children's language and motor skill development. *Pediatrics* 2007;119;S92–8.

29. Horwood JL, Fergusson DM. Breastfeeding and later cognitive and academic outcomes. *Pediatrics* 1998;101(1):1–7.

30. Heird WC, Lipillonne A. The role of fatty acids in development. *Annu Rev Nutr* 2005;25:549–571.

31. Lanting CI, Boersma ER. Lipids in infant nutrition and their impact on later development. *Curr Opin Lipidol* 1996;7(1):43–47.

32. Van der Kolk B, Fisler R. Childhood abuse and neglect and loss of self regulation. *Bull Menninger Clin* 1994;58:145–168.

33. Payne JL. Antidepressant Use in the postpartum period: practical considerations. *Am J Psychiatry* 2007;164(9):1329–1332.

34. Grace SL, Evindar A, Stewart DE. The effect of postpartum depression on child cognitive development and behavior: a review and critical analysis of the literature. *Arch Women's Ment Health* 2001;6:263–274.

35. Winnecott DW. *Primitive Emotional Development.* New York, NY: Basic Books, 1945.

36. Siberry GK, Iannone R. *The Harriet Lane Handbook.* 15th ed. St. Louis, MO: Mosby, 2000:193–195.

37. Baker L, Cantwell DP. The development of speech and language. In: Lewis M, ed. *Child and Adolescent Psychiatry: A Comprehensive Textbook.* Baltimore, MD: Williams & Wilkins, 1991:100–108.

38. Money J, Hampson JL. An examination of some basic sexual concepts: the evidence of human hermaphroditism. *Johns Hopkins Hosp Bull* 1995;97: 301–319.

39. Blum NJ, Taubman B, Nemeth N. Relationship between age at initiation of toilet training and duration of toilet training. *Pediatrics.* 2003;111: 810–814.

40. Schonwald A, Sherritt L, Stadtler A, et al. Factors associated with difficult toilet training. *Pediatrics* 2004;113:1753–1757.

41. U.S. Department of Health and Human Services, Administration on Children, Youth and Families. Child Maltreatment 2008; Washington, DC: U.S. Government Printing Office, 2010. Available at: http//www.acf.hhs.gov

42. Glaser D. Child Abuse and neglect and the brain-a review. *J Child Psychol Psychiatry* 2004;41(1):97–116.

43. Kaplan SJ, Pelcovitz D, Labruna V. Child and adolescent abuse and neglect research: a review of the past 10 years. Part 1. Physical and emotional abuse and neglect. *J Am Acad Child Adolesc Psychiatry* 1999;38(10): 1214–1222.

44. Teicher MH, Tomoda A, Andersen SL, Neurobiological consequences of early stress and childhood maltreatment: are results from human and animal studies comparable? *Ann NY Acad Sci* 2006;1071;313–323.

45. Trolls AR, Gunnar MR. Child Maltreatment and the developing HPA axis. *Horm Behav* 2006;50(4):632–639.

46. Combrinck-Graham L. Development of school age children. In: Lewis M, ed. *Child and Adolescent Psychiatry: A Comprehensive Textbook.* Baltimore, MD: Williams & Wilkins, 1991:100–108.

47. Maniati M, Tzikas D, Hibbs ED, et al. Maternal expressed emotion and metabolic control of children and adolescents with diabetes mellitus. *Psychother Psychosom* 2001;70:78–85.

48. McCarty CA, Lau AS, Valeri SM, et al. Parent-child interactions in relation to critical and emotionally overinvolved expressed emotion (EE): is EE a proxy for behavior? *J Abnorm Child Psychol* 2004;32(1):83–93.

49. Furrer C, Skinner EA. Sense of relatedness as a factor in children's academic engagement and performance, *J Educ Psychol* 2003;95:148–162.

50. Sulloway FJ. Birth order and intelligence. *Science* 2007;316(5823):1711–1712.

51. Harris JR. Context-specific learning, personality, and birth order. *Current Dir Psycholog Sci* 2000;9(5):174–177.

52. Kagen J. The role of parents in children's psychological development. *Pediatrics* 1999;104(1 suppl):164–167.

53. Costello EJ, Egger H, Angold A. 10 year research update review: The epidemiology of child and adolescent psychiatric disorders: I Methods and public health burden. *J Am Acad Child Adolesc Psychiatry* 2005;44(10): 972–986.

54. Sourander A. Childhood predictors of externalizing and internalizing problems in adolescence-a prospective follow-up study from age 8 to 16. *European Child and Adolesc Psychiatry* 2005;14(8):415–423.

55. Briggs-Gowan MJ, Horwitz SM, Schwab-Stone ME, et al. Mental health in pediatric settings: Distribution of disorders and factors related to service use. *J Am Acad Child Adolesc Psychiatry* 2000; 39(7):841–849.

56. Better Health for Our Children: A National Strategy. The Report of the Select Panel for the promotion of Child Health. United States Congress and the Secretary of Health and Human Services. Vol IV: Background Papers. Ed.198956.

57. Gardner W, Kelleher KJ, Pajer KA. Multidimensional adaptive testing for mental health problems in primary care. *Med Care* 2002;40(9):812–823.

58. Brook GG. Endocrinological control of growth at puberty. *Br Med Bull* 1981;37:281–285.

59. Ojeda SR, Lomniczi A, Mastronardi C, et al. Minireview: the neuroendocrine regulation of puberty: Is it the time ripe for a systems biology approach? *Endocrinology* 2006;147(3):1166–1174.

60. Hughes IA, Kumanan M. A wider perspective on puberty. *Mol Cell Endocrinol* 2006;254:1–7.

61. Crews F, He J, Hodge C. Adolescent cortical development: A critical period of vulnerability for addiction. *Pharmacol Biochem Behav* 2007;86(2):189–199.

62. Blakemore SJ, Choudhury S. Development of the adolescent brain: implications for executive function and social cognition. *J Child Psychol Psychiatry* 2006;47:296–312.

63. Crews FT, Mdzinarishvili A, Kim D, et al. Neurogenesis in adolescent brain is potently inhibited by ethanol. *Neuroscience* 2006;137:437–445.

64. Erickson H. Elements of a psychoanalytic theory of psychosocial development. In: Greenspan SI, Pollock GH, eds. *The Course of Life: Psychoanalytic Contributions Toward Understanding Personality Development, II Later Adolescence, and Youth.* Washington, DO: National Institute of Mental Health: 1987;357–372.

65. Offer D. Adolescent development: a normative perspective. In: Greenspan SI, Pollock GH. eds. *The Course of Life: Psychoanalytic Contributions Toward*

Understanding Personality Development, II Later Adolescence, and Youth. Washington, DO: National Institute of Mental Health 1991; 357–372.

66. Nilsson KW, Sjoberg RL, Wargelius HL, et al. The monoamine oxidase A (MAO-A) gene, family function and maltreatment as predictors of aggressive behavior during male adolescent alcohol consumption. *Addiction* 2007;102(3):389–398.

67. Reif A, Rosler M, Freitag CM. Nature and nurture predispose to violent behavior: Serotonergic genes and adverse childhood environment. *Neuropsychopharmology* 2007;32(11):2375–2383.

68. Hamburg D. Toward a strategy for healthy adolescent development. *Am J Psychiatry.* 1997;154;6–12.

69. Vaillant G. *Aging Well. Surprising Guideposts to a Happier Life from the Landmark Harvard Study of Adult Development.* Boston, MA: Little Brown and Company, 2002:373.

70. Craik FIM, Salthouse TA, eds. *The Handbook of Aging and Cognition.* 3rd Ed. New York, NY: Psychology Press and Taylor and Francis Group, 2008.

71. Census Bureau. Census 2000 Brief. US Dept of Commerce; Economics and Statistics Administration, October 2001.

72. Humes K. The population 65 years and older: aging in America; The Book of the States 2005; US Census Bureau. US Dept of Commerce, Economics and Statistics Administration; pp. 464–468.

73. Harman D. Aging: Phenomena and theories. *Ann NY Acad Sci.* 1998 Nov 20;854:1–7

74. Hayflick L. Biological Aging is no longer an unsolved problem. *Ann NY Acad Sci* 2007;1100:1–13.

75. Shawi M, Autexier C. Telomerase, senesescence and ageing. *Mech Ageing Dev* 2008;129(1–2):3–10.

76. Muller Fl, Lustgarten MS, Jang Y, et al. Trends in oxidative aging theories. *Free Radic Biol Med* 2007;43:477–503.

77. Hamet P, Tremblay J. Genes of aging. *Metabolism* 2003;52(10):5–9.

78. Vasto S, Mocchegiani E, Candore G, et al. Inflammation, genes and zinc in aging and age related diseases. *Biogerontology* 2006;7(5–6):315–327.

79. Mattson MP. Gene-diet interactions in brain aging and neurodegenerative disorders. *Ann Intern Med* 2003;139(5 pt 2):441–444.

80. Austad SN. What science is discovering about the body's journey through life. New York, NY: Wiley, 1997:220–244.

81. Zafon C. Oscillations in total body fat content through life: an evolutionary perspective. *Obes Rev* 2007;8(6):525–530.

82. Murry JB. Effects of valium and Librium on human psychomotor and cognitive functions. *Genet Psychol Monogr* 1984;109(2D Half):167–197.

83. Thornfeldt CR. Chronic inflammation is etiology of extrinsic aging. *Cosmet Dermatol* 2008;7(1):78–82.

84, Dao H Jr, Kazin RA. Gender differences in skin: a review of the literature. *Gend Med* 2007;4(4):308–328.

85. Inouye SK, Studenski S, Tinetti ME, et al. Geriatric syndromes: clinical, research, and policy implications of a core geriatric concept. *J Am Geriatr Soc* 2007;55(5):780–791.

86. Jackson GR, Owsley C. Visual dysfunction, neurodegenerative diseases, and aging. *Neurol Clin* 2003;21(3):709–728.

87. Frisina RD, Walton JP. Age-related structural and functional changes in the cochlear nucleus. *Hear Res* 2006;216:216–223.

88. Stevens JC, Cain WS. Changes in taste and flavor in aging. *Crit Rev Food Sci Nutr* 1993;33(1):27–37.

89. Winkler S, Garg AK, Mekayarajjananonth T, et al. Depressed taste and smell in geriatric patients. *J Am Dent Assoc* 1999;130(12):1759–1765.

90. Dickstein DL, Kaboso D, Rocher AB, et al. Changes in the structural complexity of the aged brain. *Aging Cell* 2007;6(3):275–284.

91. Tumeh PC, Alavi A, Housenia M, et al. Structural and functional imaging correlates for age-related changes in the brain. *Semin Nucl Med* 2007; 37(2):69–87.

92. Low Choy NL, Brauer SG, Nitz JC. Age-related changes in strength and somatosensation during midlife: rationale for targeted preventative intervention programs. *Ann NY Acad Sci* 2007;1114:180–193.

93. Moore A, Mangoni AA, Lyons D, et al. The cardiovascular system. *Br J Clin Pharmacol* 2003;56(3):254–260.

94. Sharma G, Goodwin J. Effect of aging on respiratory system physiology and immunology. *Clin Interv Aging* 2006;1(3):254–260.

95. Floreani A. Liver diseases in the elderly: an update. *Dig Dis* 2007; 25(2):138–143.

96. Martgin JE, Sheaff MT. Renal ageing. *J Pathol* 2007;211(2):198–205.

97. Czesnikiewicz-Guzik M, Lee WW, Cui D, et al. T cell subset-specific susceptibility to aging. *Clin Immunol* 2008;127(1):107–118.

98. Steunenberg B, Beekman AT, Deeg DJ, et al. Personality and the onset of depression in late life. *J Affect Disord* 2006;92(2–3):243–251.

99. Langhorne P. Comprehensive geriatric assessment for older hospital patients. *Br Med Bull* 2005;71:45–50.

100. Arseven A, Chang Chih-Hung, Arseven OK, et al. Assessment instruments. *Clin Geriatr Med* 2005;21:121–146.

101. Mathias S, Nayuak US, Isaccs B. Balance in elderly patients: the "get-up and go" test. *Arch Phys Med Rehabil* 1986;67(6):387–389.

102. Yesavage JA. Geriatric depression scale. *Psychopharmacol Bull* 1988; 24(4):709–711.

103. Alexopoulos GS, Abrams RC, Young RC, et al. Cornell scale for depression in dementia. *Biol Psychiatry* 1988;23(3):271–284.

104. Folstein MF, Whitehouse PJ, Cognitive impairment of Alzheimer disease. *Neurobehav Toxicol Teratol* 1983;5(6):387–389.

105. Callahan CM, Hendrie HC, Nienaber NA, et al. Suicidal ideation among older primary care patients. *J Am Geriatr Soc* 1996b;44:1205–1209.

106. Rapaport MH, Judd LL, Schettler PJ, et al. A descriptive analysis of minor depression. *Am J Psychiatry* 2002;159:637–643.

107. Grek A. Clinical management of suicidality in the elderly: an opportunity for involvement in the lives of older patients. *Can J Psychiatry* 2007; 52(6 suppl 1):47S–57S.

108. Jacobs DG, Brewer ML. Application of the APA practice guidelines on suicide to clinical practice. *CNS Spectr* 2006;11(6):447–454.

109. Miller MD. Using interpersonal therapy (IPT) with older adults today and tomorrow: a review of the literature and new developments. *Curr Psychiatry Rep* 2008;10(1):16–22.

110. Kloner RA. Natural and unnatural triggers of myocardial infarction. *Prog Cardiovasc Dis* 2006;48(4):285–300.

111. Gorenstein EE, Papp LA. Cognitive-behavioral therapy for anxiety in the elderly. *Curr Psychiatry Rep* 2007;9(1):20–25.

112. Oiu C, DeRonchi D, Fratiglioni L. The epidemiology of the dementias: an update. *Curr Opin Psychiatry* 2007;20(4):380–385.

113. Ouldred E, Bryant C. Dementia care: Part 2: understanding and managing behavioural challenges. *Br J Nurs* 2008;17(4):242–247.

114. van Marum RJ. Current and future therapy in Alzheimer's disease. *Fundam Clin Pharmacol* 2008;22(3):265–274.

115. Schneider LS, Dagerman K, Insel PS. Efficacy and adverse effects of atypical antipsychotics for dementia: meta-analysis of randomized, placebo-controlled trials. *Am J Geriatr Psychiatry* 2006;14(3): 191–210.

116. Cole MG, Primeau FJ, Elie LM. Delirium: prevention, treatment and outcome studies. *J Geriatr Psychiatry Neurol* 1998;11(3):126–137.

117. Nouye SK, Leo-Summers L, Zhang Y, et al. A chart-based method for identification of delirium: Validation compared with reviewer ratings using the confusion assessment method. *J Am Geriatr Soc* 2005;53(2):312–318.

118. Correll CU, Schenk EM. Tardive dyskinesia and new antipsychotics. *Curr Opin Psychiatry* 2008;21(2):151–156.

The Patient Encounter

The Initial Encounter

FELIX J. ROGERS

INTRODUCTION

The first encounter with a patient is the culmination of medical training and the fulfillment of clinical practice. As J. Willis Hurst (1) explains, the purpose of the initial history and physical evaluation is to gain information and, just as importantly, to establish a bond between the patient and the physician (1).

With the increasing availability of sophisticated, accurate, and expensive diagnostic tests, physicians in training typically devote a large amount of time to learn about these studies. As a consequence, an emphasis on the approach to the patient at the bedside has been diminished. Physicians who train to perform surgical or other interventional procedures recognize that a certain minimum number are required for proficiency. In the same way, a minimum number of bedside examinations are necessary for proficiency.

The information to be gathered on each patient is appropriate for the context of that evaluation. For a new patient visit in a primary care office or a patient hospitalized in a general medical or surgical ward, the standard patient history and physical examination is appropriate. The subspecialty evaluation, such as the presentation to an ophthalmologist, urologic surgeon, or specialist in sports medicine, may be much more focused.

KEY ASPECTS OF PATIENT EVALUATION

Because there are many fine references on bedside patient evaluation, this section of the textbook does not attempt to recreate that content; rather, it will emphasize unheralded aspects of the patient evaluation that warrant more attention. These include the evaluation of the musculoskeletal system in the context of the public health perspective of clinical problems in this area (Chapter 21: Public Health Aspects: screening and prevention and Chapter 22: The Musculoskeletal Component), an assessment of the influences of the environment (Chapter 23: Environmental Issues), and an evaluation of the patient in the context of complementary and alternative medicine and nonosteopathic forms of manual medicine (Chapter 24: Interface of Osteopathic Medicine with Complementary and Manual Medicine Practitioners).

Presently, members of the Educational Council on Osteopathic Principles promote the use of five models to be used in patient assessment and treatment, including the biomechanical, respiratory/circulatory, neurologic, metabolic-energy, and behavioral or biopsychosocial models. These form the organizing principles for the basic science and clinical chapters of this textbook.

Regardless of the presenting complaint of the patient and irrespective of the specialty interest of the health care provider, all physicians have some inherent obligations. For example, some clinical problems occur with such a magnitude that all physicians need to be involved. Examples include hypertension, which affects an estimated 42 million Americans; hypercholesterolemia, affecting 100 million Americans; and obesity and overweight, which affect two third of all Americans. Likewise, diabetes and cancer are such prevalent public health problems that physicians need to be vigilant for manifestations of these disorders. Some problems, such as vaccinations for influenza for the elderly, require that every encounter with the patient become an opportunity for intervention (Chapter 30: Life Cycles—Health Promotion). This is the basis for hospital-based initiatives to provide influenza and pneumococcal vaccinations for all appropriate patients admitted to the hospital.

PATIENT RAPPORT

The information that is gathered as part of the initial patient evaluation is considered in the context of establishing osteopathic medical care. Consider the influence of context in the following four examples of patients with chest pain:

- A 38-year-old man who is in danger of losing his home to foreclosure begins to experience chest pain after he is laid off from his job.
- A 67-year-old man has experienced typical effort angina at progressively lower levels of exertion over the past 4 weeks; he is awakened from his sleep with chest pain at 2 AM.
- A 67-year-old woman indulged in an unusually opulent feast with lots of fatty food and alcohol; she is awakened from her sleep with chest pain at 2 AM.
- An 84-year-old woman with lung cancer metastatic to bone, brain, and adrenal glands comes to the hospital with chest pain.

It should be obvious that the context of the patient presentation means that we cannot take a "one-size-fits-all" approach to chest pain, since the above patients have chest pain related, respectively, to stress/anxiety, unstable angina, gastroesophageal reflux, and chest pain that may be cardiac in the setting of end-stage lung cancer.

More often, the context of the patient evaluation involves subtleties that can only be discerned after careful evaluation. The development of rapport with the patient is critical to this approach, as are the principles for patient care (2) that identify the patient as the focus for care. There are tools that can be used to assist physicians in developing rapport; perhaps the most important of these is professionalism, which seeks to raise the standard of physician behavior, while enhancing that individual's sensitivity to cultural, socioeconomic, and religious differences (Chapter 26: Professionalism). In addition, the awareness of the importance of the mind-body relationship can open new avenues to understanding the patient's presenting complaint and provide insight into working collaboratively with the patient to resolve health problems (Chapter 27: Mind-Body Medicine). The role of spirit in health care is discussed much more widely than it is understood. This section explores that consideration and offers a few concrete points to assist in expansion of patient care into this arena (Chapter 28: Spirituality and Health Care).

DECISION MAKING AND EVIDENCE

After collection of information on a patient and with the establishment of appropriate rapport, the physician is then ready to embark on medical decision making. As with any other aspect of health care, decision making (also called clinical problem solving) is based on principles that have been validated and can be taught to newcomers to the field. A portion of this section of the textbook is devoted to an explication of medical decision making (Chapter 25: Clinical Decision Making).

Implementation of the patient care plan is multifaceted. The goal is to base that care plan on clinical evidence derived from well-designed and well-conducted research trials (Chapter 32: Evidence-Based Medicine). In one sense, clinical evidence is like a net. When used properly, it is a safety net that sustains the physician and his/her practice and supports him/her in terms of the many pressures that confront physicians in medical care. However, it can also be a net that holds one down. Physicians are expected to meet the standard of evidence-based medicine, and failure to do so is constraining and increases the potential for malpractice liability.

Finally, evidence-based medicine presents a challenge in terms of keeping the focus on the individual patient. Scientific evidence must be based on sufficient numbers of patients to generate meaningful information. At the moment of the patient encounter, however, there is just one person who matters: the patient. There is often a significant challenge of discernment, to define the manner in which your decision making is properly formed by the research literature.

PATIENT-CENTERED CARE

The issue of patient-centered care touches on a core osteopathic premise. To focus on the patient is more difficult than it might appear at first glance. Frequently, it is not considered as part of the approach to the patient interview or to medical decision making. Physicians, by nature, are goal oriented. To stop and assess the patient's values may appear to disrupt the flow of information gathering and development of the patient care plan. A chapter in this section (Chapter 29: Patient-Centered Model) offers both

Seven Aphorisms for the Successful Physician

1. *Distinguish between a* goal *and a* guideline. A goal is a guiding principle that we may or may not attain, similar to the North Star, which can lead us, but we may never get there. An example of a goal in osteopathic medicine is "treatment of the whole person." The individual person presenting for health care is far too complex for any one physician to fully understand every aspect of that individual. Still, we do our best to maintain a holistic approach. In contrast, a practice guideline is a statement developed by an expert group based on the best available medical evidence. Physicians are expected to adhere to guidelines and to fulfill those requirements.

2. *Maintain a focus.* Sometimes you will hear a physician say that he or she performed a "comprehensive" history and physical examination. Even if a truly comprehensive exam existed, it would often be inappropriate. A physician should be capable of a general evaluation of the patient. Then, as specific concerns arise, a detailed, complete assessment can be made in that one area. For example, a full assessment of each of the cranial nerves is unnecessary in the assessment of a patient complaining of chest pain, but some basic evaluation of the neurologic status is necessary in all patients.

3. *The patient is the hero.* Many physicians gladly accept the expressions of praise and gratitude offered by patients and their family members. Some even accept the description of "heroic." But the reality is that the patient is the hero. Frequently, they come to the health care system with life-threatening medical problems or with the fear that they have these problems. Patients who have advanced heart disease, unrelenting gastrointestinal problems, or cancer are expected to arrive for their appointments on time, be polite, respond respectfully, tolerate physicians who are late, and maintain good cheer in the face of crippling health care costs. The fact that many of them still have time to bring in home-cooked pies or cookies and to send thank-you notes is really remarkable.

4. *Poor historians are outnumbered by poor history takers.* Patients often come to the health care encounter in a frightened state, and typically they don't know what information the physician needs. Because of this, their answers can be vague and even misleading. It is the physician's job to provide leadership during the interview process. Clearly, there is a delicate balance between providing direction and also giving plenty of opportunity for thoughtful, careful listening.

5. *Be brief.* It's big world out there. There is a lot to learn, and there is a lot to do. Use your time well. Learn to distinguish what is important and what is urgent.

6. *In medicine, there is no finish line.* Although there are many mileposts in the practice of medicine, there is really no stopping point. In terms of physician education, milestones can be the basic science and clinical science aspects of medical school, postgraduate training, and then specialty programs. Because the world of medicine and science advances so rapidly, physician education must be an active, continuous process. Likewise, a patient is seen on day one, and their clinical course develops by the time the patient is seen in follow up. Each patient encounter represents the opportunity to integrate developments in the patient's clinical course with new information that

(continued)

> is available. Even when a patient dies, the finish line is not clear cut: there are still issues to handle in terms of providing consolation and solace for the family.
>
> 7. *Our patients have much to teach us.* How did the great clinicians become so? One has to suspect that they did not go through life committing the same mistakes time again. Instead, they were present in each moment, taking the opportunity to adjust their medical practice to the changing circumstances of their patients and to new developments in medical science.

philosophical and practical points to address this topic. Patient-centered care also becomes especially clear when decision making must be conducted in the context of end-of-life decisions (Chapter 31: End of Life Care).

Finally, there is the issue of documentation. One institution puts this in a grand context: "In God We Trust. All others must document." Behind this glib statement is the recognition that, if events are not documented, there may be no evidence that they happened. Younger members of the medical profession frequently spend a good deal of time documenting information that is not needed and failing to document information that becomes the foundation of the conclusions and care plans that they propose. Several tools are available to assist the physician, including the time-tested problem list and, more recently, the electronic health record. Box 20.1 presents useful aphorisms for this purpose.

The patient encounter is the most fulfilling aspect of being a doctor. It might be considered to be the litmus test of who we are. This includes the position as a physician, a professional, and as a person. It gives us the chance to live every day from a new perspective, since all of us change every day: the patient, the field of medicine, and, of course, each of us. Try to savor the experience!

REFERENCES

1. Hurst JW, Morris DC. The history: symptoms and past events related to cardiovascular disease. in Schlant RC, Alexander RW, eds. *The Heart, Arteries, and Veins.* 8th Ed. New York, NY: McGraw-Hill, 1994:205.
2. Rogers FJ, Glover J, D'Alonzo GE, et al. Proposed Tenets of Osteopathic Medicine and Principles for Patient Care, *J Am Osteopath Assoc* 2002; 102:63–65.

21 Public Health Aspects

MARGARET AGUWA

KEY CONCEPTS

- A host of factors impact the development, incidence, and prevalence of disease and illness among the population.
- We, as a society, must act collectively to assure the conditions in which people can be healthy.
- Public health functions include assessment and monitoring of health, formulation of public policies, and ensuring access to appropriate and cost-effective care.
- Advocation of concepts of public health with utilization of the principles of osteopathic medicine will further our ability to enhance the health and well-being of all patients.
- The desirable results of efforts of public health and osteopathic medical practice include longevity with health and the elimination of health disparities.

INTRODUCTION

There is sometimes a perception that a discipline like osteopathic medicine, which prides itself on its holistic approach to health care, thrives on its own merit. Evidence, however, shows that without the strides made through public health concepts and practices, all medical fields would not exist as we know them today. In the later 19th century, Andrew Taylor Still, the founder of osteopathic medicine, established four basic principles as the basis for the profession's philosophy and practice. More recently, in 2002, a multidisciplinary ad hoc committee of osteopathic clinicians and researchers proposed an updated set for these tenets of osteopathic medicine and associated principles of patient care that are to reflect the relevance of scientific approach to care. These proposed tenets and principles found by Rogers et al. are:

Tenets:

1. A person is the product of dynamic interaction between body, mind, and spirit.
2. An inherent property of this dynamic interaction is the capacity of the individual for the maintenance of health and recovery from disease.
3. Many forces, both intrinsic and extrinsic to the person, can challenge this inherent capacity and contribute to the onset of illness.
4. The musculoskeletal system significantly influences the individual's ability to restore this inherent capacity and therefore to resist disease processes.

Principles:

1. The patient is the focus for health care.
2. The patient has the primary responsibility for his or her health.
3. An effective treatment program for patient care is founded on these tenets.

These tenets and principles form the overarching ideology and the basis for the use of structural diagnosis and osteopathic manipulative medicine.

Through education rooted in these principles, evidence-based practice, and diligent doctor-patient partnerships, osteopathic physicians, particularly primary care specialists, provide exceptional and holistic care to their patients. In the early 1800s, medical practice became centered on various developments achieved through public and community health efforts. Since the early 14th century, simple acts such as hand washing and proper management of human waste have produced significant impacts on the health of individuals as well as reducing the adverse effects that communicable diseases have on the population at large. Today, although public health efforts seem to be relegated to the background of medical practice, they have remained important facets in managing the health of global communities.

Recognized as a leading figure in the early development of public health in America, Winslow (1920) described public health as "the science and art of preventing disease, prolonging life and promoting physical health and efficiency through organized community efforts for the sanitation of the environment, the control of community infections, the education of the individual in principles of personal hygiene, the organization of medical and nursing science for the early diagnosis and preventive treatment of disease, and the development of the social machinery which will ensure to every individual in the community a standard of living adequately for the maintenance of health" (Winslow, 1920). Over the years, components such as research for diseases, injury prevention, and promotion of healthier lifestyles were added to encompass the totality of the field. In 1988, the Institute of Medicine published a landmark report titled "The Future of Public Health in the 21st Century" and defined public health as "What we, as a society, do collectively to assure the conditions in which people can be healthy." Therefore, activities that include organized community efforts to identify, prevent, and counter threats to the health of the public and improve the health and well-being of people can be categorized as public health.

CORE FUNCTIONS OF PUBLIC HEALTH

The three core functions of public health include:

1. Assessing and monitoring the health of communities and populations at risk to identify health problems and priorities
2. Formulating public policies designed to solve identified local and national health problems and priorities
3. Ensuring that all populations have access to appropriate and cost-effective care, including health promotion and disease prevention services, and evaluating the effectiveness of that care

Many of the dramatic achievements of public health in the 20th century have contributed to the improvement of the quality of life of people globally and resulted in increased life expectancy, reduction in infant and child mortality, and elimination of many communicable and infectious diseases in many industrialized nations.

While doctors usually treat individual patients one-on-one for a specific disease or injury, public health practice requires that professionals monitor and diagnose the health concerns of entire communities and promote healthy behavior and practices to ensure that populations stay healthy.

However, the prevalence of certain chronic diseases, such as diabetes, hypertension, and cardiovascular disorders, as well as the recent occurrences of certain communicable illnesses like SARS, Ebola Fever, HIV/AIDS, and methicillin-resistant staphylococcus aureus, Norovirus and the H1N1 influenza infections, signal the need for a paradigm shift in the overall evaluation and management of many patients especially on a community basis.

TRENDS IN POPULATION MEDICINE

The recent trends in population medicine today show that in America:

- There is increasing racial and ethnic diversity.
- Life expectancy of the population continues to increase.
- People are getting more involved in their own health care and seeking alternative ways to manage their health while demanding more from their physicians.
- More people today are living with some form of chronic disease such as hypertension, diabetes, heart disease, cancer, Chronic Obstructive Pulmonary Disease, or chronic pain.
- There are increasing numbers of people without health insurance coverage.
- There are increasing concerns about real or perceived threats associated with natural disasters, massive biohazard accidents, and terrorist acts that could have a significant impact on the health of the community.

These trends should motivate physicians to become more aware and more involved in disease prevention, health maintenance, promotion of healthy lifestyles, and emergency preparedness for their patients. In 2006, a report by the U.S. Centers for Disease Control and Prevention (CDC) indicated the alarming rise in the numbers of Americans suffering with chronic diseases such as diabetes type 2, a disease that remains the leading cause of adult blindness, lower-limb amputation, kidney disease, blindness, and nerve damage, thereby contributing significantly to health policy issues and public health concerns. The CDC also reports that a majority of the top ten causes of mortality in the United States are due to preventable illnesses. The study, "Measuring the health of Nations" conducted by the London School of Hygiene and Tropical Medicine, ranks the United States the nation with the highest in the rate of preventable deaths among 19 most industrialized nations when comparing matters about health status and morbidity (Nolte and McKee, 2008). According to this study, more than 100,000 Americans die each year from lack of timely and effective medical care. The study focused on how a variety of conditions including diet, lifestyle, and various preventable and treatable chronic diseases and risk factors contribute to mortality rates. Of the 19 nations studied, the United States is the only one without universal health care coverage yet spends significantly more money in health care services than any of the other countries. Other studies have shown similar findings and conclusions (Danaei et al., 2009).

The results of this study raise an important question regarding what this nation and the health care system can do not only to improve these statistics but also to energize the health of the population in general. Health care reform, modifications in clinical practice, and fostering positive lifestyle changes may be necessary to achieve this goal.

A critical look at the osteopathic medicine reveals significant similarities of prevention, holism, and community inclusion between its tenets and the philosophical approach to public health. The basic principle of osteopathic medicine recognizes the important connections and the inseparable link between the physical, mental, emotional, and spiritual factors in the maintenance of optimal functioning in the context of the individual, family, and society.

In addition to their medical education, skills, and talents, there exists a wide range of resources and tools that help osteopathic physicians to successfully integrate and apply various procedures, including osteopathic manual medicine, in their practices in order to foster health promotion, disease prevention, early diagnosis, timely treatment, and standard of care that are based on clinical evidence.

To become fully conversant with these methods, physicians, particularly those who provide general medical care in the primary care of their patients, may have to make some changes in the methodologies of their practices. Osteopathic medical students will need to learn and think differently regarding the way health care services are delivered as well.

THE PATIENT ENCOUNTER

Currently, the patient encounter consists of the individual patient-centered approach: an approach to providing health care and occasional comprehensive primary care for people of all ages and medical conditions. It is a way for a physician-led medical practice, chosen by the patient or insurer, to integrate health care services for that patient. Frequently, the patient confronts episodic sporadic care within a complex and confusing health care system associated with referrals, insurance rejections, copay requirements among other regulations.

The Healthy People 2010 concept challenges individuals, communities, and professionals to take specific steps to ensure that good health, as well as long life, is enjoyed by all. The two overarching goals of the Healthy People 2010 are:

- **Goal 1: Increase Quality and Years of Healthy Life:** designed to help individuals of all ages increase life expectancy *and* improve their quality of life.
- **Goal 2: Eliminate Health Disparities:** designed to foster the elimination of health disparities among different segments of the population thereby improving community health and health for all.

While the Healthy People proposes the improvement of health for all, it targets two primary concerns: (a) specific chronic illnesses and (b) the health of vulnerable populations that focus on specific health indicators to be used in measuring the health of the nation over the 10-year span of its existence (2000–2010). The ten specific health indicators, listed below, are termed The Leading Health Indicators and reflect the major health concerns in the United States at the beginning of the 21st century. These indicators were selected on the basis of their ability to motivate action, the availability of data to measure progress, their contribution to disease process, morbidity and mortality, and their longitudinal importance as public health issues.

The leading health indicators are:

- Physical activity
- Overweight and obesity
- Tobacco use
- Substance abuse
- Responsible sexual behavior
- Mental health
- Injury and violence
- Environmental quality
- Immunization
- Access to health care

Physicians are encouraged to review the needs of individual patients they see, as well as those of the populations in the communities they serve to determine which specific health recommendations to implement in their practices. While each patient is unique, there are certain basic examination and screening procedures that should be performed for each patient as a part of the overall health care service.

What to do for Each Adult Patient at Every Visit

The management of a patient at each visit can determine the potential of early diagnosis of disease and thereby contribute significant to health care outcomes. These recommendations are provided partly to help establish standard of patient care and also to provide guidance in record keeping in order to monitor changes and further take corrective clinical action. While these recommendations assist physicians in making clinical decisions regarding the care of their patients, they cannot be substituted for the individual judgment brought to each clinical situation by the physician based on his/her knowledge, expertise, and experience. As with all clinical matters, they reflect the best understanding of the science of medicine in the regular management of patients and in the provision of care that are valuable in health maintenance, early diagnosis of disease, or considerations in health status changes. These recommendations are to be carried out regardless of the specialty of the physician. Variations on recommendations relating to pediatric patients are not discussed in this chapter.

The following health indices should be recorded at each visit:

- **Vitals**: BP, pulse, temperature, respiration, weight;
- **Presenting complaint(s)**: medical history as relates to the complaint(s), past occurrences, quality, differences and similarities of symptoms, and any management thereof;
- **Medications/and changes**: prescribed, over-the-counter, herbs, vitamins, and other supplements—compliance with recommendations, appropriate use, abuse, and misuse;
- **Functional Status**: ability to perform activities of daily living, including emotional and physical aspects;
- **Review of Lifestyle Behaviors and Activities**: smoking, regular exercise, nutritional factors, rest, meditation, job, family life;
- **Other Changes**: including consultations with other health care providers for secondary or tertiary care.

What to do for Adult Patients Annually

Despite lack of evidence to support annual physical exams for asymptomatic adults, patients report considerable enthusiasm for such exams. While many physicians may consider this an essential aspect of health maintenance for their patients, research has shown that only specific patients, particularly those with manageable chronic illnesses, should receive yearly medical check-ups. Healthy individuals with minimal or no risk factors, and those with documented healthy lifestyles can be monitored less frequently.

Effective monitoring of all patients requires the implementation of evidence-based clinical medicine. Pediatric procedures should be followed accordingly.

Items for the Annual Patient Screening and Evaluation include:

- Review of vaccinations and immunizations
- Healthy lifestyles evaluation
- Motor vehicle safety
- Safe workplaces

REVIEW OF VACCINATIONS AND IMMUNIZATIONS

Each patient's yearly evaluation should include a review of their vaccination/immunization status to determine the needs of the patient for protection against communicable diseases and potentially preventable epidemics. Appropriately timed adult and childhood immunizations can reduce or prevent morbidity and mortality related to illnesses such as influenza, pneumococcal infection, hepatitis B, diphtheria, tetanus, measles, mumps, and rubella. Vaccination of adults at risk for various communicable and infectious diseases can reduce the expenses associated with preventable causes of adult morbidity and mortality. While diphtheria, tetanus, measles, mumps, and rubella affect children at a higher rate than adults, the wide scope of positive results of childhood immunizations has shown that morbidity and mortality attributable to these preventable illnesses can also be substantially reduced by selective immunization of at-risk adults.

HEALTHY LIFESTYLES EVALUATION

Items to consider in the Healthy LifeStyles Evaluation include tobacco use, alcohol abuse and misuse, exercise, coping with stress, and diet and weight maintenance.

TOBACCO USE STATUS

The use of tobacco products—cigarettes, cigars, and chewing tobacco—should be monitored and recorded in the patient's chart and reviewed annually. Since the recognition of the health hazards of tobacco use, U.S. surgeon generals as far back as 1957 have given reports on the health risks associated with tobacco and further emphasized the causal relationship between smoking and lung cancer. In 2004, the U.S. Department of Health and Human Services reported an increase in averted deaths due to the multiple factors of government policy on smoking, public health focused attention on smoking cessation, and the decreased use of tobacco in all its forms, which improved the understanding of the health hazards associated with smoking and the use of tobacco products.

ALCOHOL ABUSE AND MISUSE

While the use of alcohol in moderation has been found to have beneficial effects on cognition and the cardiovascular system (Mayo Clinic.com); (Galanis et al., 2000) excessive drinking can lead to serious health problems and even sudden death. Therefore, obtaining information about the drinking habits of the patient is useful in determining the need for intervention if abuse or misuse of alcohol is suspected.

EXERCISE

It is well known in the medicine that part of a healthy lifestyle includes regular physical activities. There are known merits of exercise such as preventing chronic health conditions, boosting confidence and self-esteem, improving the immune system, enhancing overall well-being maintaining weight and supporting the body structure, and many others. According to a Mayo Clinic report, these benefits exist regardless of age, gender, or physical ability. The report further maintains that exercise has positive influence on almost every body function and subsequently can reduce the incidence and prevalence of diseases that result in significant morbidity and mortality.

COPING WITH STRESS

Stress has both positive and negative effects on the body. The body's reaction to stress, particularly in the long term, can trigger the development of serious illnesses or even make an existing physical or mental condition worse. Some researchers such as Astin et al. (2003) and Pelletier (2004) support these assertions and further recommend evidence-based mind-body intervention modalities for patients. The chapter on Mind–Body Interactions is a good follow-up reading.

DIET AND WEIGHT MAINTENANCE

Recent studies by Avenell et al. (2004) and O'Brien et al. (2004) have shown that obesity is a major public health problem in adults and a significant growing issue in children. In light of the current obesity crisis, prevention of weight gain and better weight maintenance are critical. Therefore, inquiring and reviewing diet, weight management and maintenance are important facets of the regular patient encounter.

MOTOR VEHICLE SAFETY

Improvements in motor vehicle safety have contributed to large reductions in motor vehicle–related deaths (Harfst and Marshaw, 1990). While these improvements include engineering efforts to make both vehicles and highways safer, additional successful efforts of personal behaviors regarding use of safety belts, child safety seats, and increased use of motorcycle helmets, designated driver, and reduced speed limits have had positive impacts on injuries and deaths related to vehicular use.

SAFE WORKPLACES

Common work-related health injuries and illnesses such as coal workers' pneumoconiosis (black lung), and asbestosis, and repetitive stress injuries have been significantly reduced since the emergence of the policies for safer workplaces, use of ergonomically structured work stations, and the monitoring of work hours and the work environment. It is, however, necessary to review the patient's work environment and any potential hazards that might contribute to occupational-related injuries.

RECOMMENDATIONS FOR PREVENTIVE SERVICES

In view of the constantly changing and challenging bulk of medical literature on patient care and management, the U.S. Preventive Services Task Force (USPSTF) (1996) recently provided a guide on which clinical judgment can be made regarding intervention and treatment protocols.

Recommendation Categories

These recommendations were developed with consideration of overall costs, patient preferences, and the quality of the overall evidence for a service on a three-point scale of good, fair, and poor (Table 21.1).

TABLE 21.1

U.S. Preventive Services Task Force Recommendation Categories

Category	Description
SR/A	Strongly recommend: Good quality evidence exists hich demonstrates substantial net benefit over harm; the intervention is perceived to be cost-effective and acceptable to nearly all patients.
R/B	Recommend: Although evidence exists which demonstrates net benefit, either the benefit is only moderate in magnitude or the evidence supporting a substantial benefit is only fair. The intervention is perceived to be cost-effective and acceptable to most patients.
NR/C	No recommendation either for or against: Either good or fair evidence exist of at least a small net benefit. Cost-effectiveness may not be known or patients may be divided about acceptability of the intervention.
RA/D	Recommend against: Good or fair evidence which demonstrates no net benefit over harm.
I	Insufficient evidence to recommend either for or against: No evidence of even fair quality exists or the existing evidence is conflicting.

Strength of Recommendations

The USPSTF grades its recommendations according to one of five classifications (A, B, C, D, and I) reflecting the strength of evidence and magnitude of net benefit (benefits minus harms). These classifications represent gradation of the strongest evidence (A) to (I) where research has shown insufficient evidence of any derivable benefits. In addition, the USPSTF provides a 3-point scale (good, fair, and poor) for determining the quality of evidence to support the above recommendations.

A new approach to patient care, the "Medical Home" system was proposed several years ago by physicians who were looking for different and better ways to deliver health services, improve quality of care, and also receive appropriate remuneration. The new paradigm asserts that with burgeoning health care costs, increasing number of the uninsured, and the health care burden associated with retirees and the "baby boomers," there is dissatisfaction among patients, physicians, insurers, and the public in general about the way the current health care systems function. Initially suggested by the American Academy of Pediatrics in 1992, "Medical Home" recommends a major fundamental shift from the patient-centered care to the family-centered care that fosters an accessible, multidisciplinary, culturally effective, compassionate, continuous, coordinated, and comprehensive method of care delivery with the concept of relationship building. In early 2007, several medical groups, including the American Osteopathic Association, the American Academy of Family Practice, and the American College of Physicians, joined in endorsing this system. The Medical Home guidelines consist of six index domains: Organizational Capacity, Chronic Condition Management, Care Coordination, Community Outreach, Data management, and Quality Improvement. While some physicians especially those in solo medical practices may find it challenging to systematically apply the Medical Home concept, its principles reflect the philosophical approaches found in both osteopathic medicine and public health. Some modifications and flexibility within this system might make it appealing to more physicians.

The Doctor's Role

In addition to having the expertise to provide standard of care, the doctor will also need to be a communicator of information in succinct and clear ways, a facilitator and coordinator of the gamut of services that the patient requires, and further act as an advocate and coach inspiring the patient to work toward achieving better health. Physicians need to understand that patients expect to be treated promptly, courteously, and correctly. They expect their care to be personalized and communicated to them in terms they understand. These practices can reflect positive and effective relationships between the patients and their doctors.

The Patient's Role

As the U.S. health care system continues to evolve and change, patients and their families seem to be taking more active roles in their own health care. It is becoming more and more essential that patients actively partner with their physicians and also take more responsibility for understanding their care, proactively advocate for themselves, engage in open dialogue and communication with their doctor, and become knowledgeable in their own health profiles. Given these circumstances, the patient becomes an active participant in his/her own health care and by extension in the health care of those that depend on them. The patient's role thereby complements and supports the role of the physician. As research reminds us (Steinbrook, 2006a,b), the concept of personal responsibility in health care is that by following healthy lifestyles (exercising, maintaining a healthy weight, and not smoking) and complying with good judgment (keeping appointments, heeding physicians' advice, and using a hospital emergency department only for emergencies), people can enjoy better health, improved quality of life, and greater longevity at a more reasonable cost.

Society's Role

There are many examples of initiatives that are meant to promote personal responsibility. The World Health Organization no longer hires persons who smoke, suck, chew, or snuff any tobacco product, although it will still recruit people "who do not have a healthy lifestyle." In several US states and local communities, laws have been enacted to restrict smoking in public areas such as restaurants, hospitals, and schools. Airlines no longer permit smoking during flight, initially due the efforts of the flight attendants who wanted to minimize their exposure to cigarette fumes and finally by public regulations that ratified the ban.

SUMMARY

The key to successful preventative and curative treatment of patients is to first understand that a host of factors impact the development, incidence, and prevalence of disease and illness among the population. How we, as physicians, interact with the patient is essential to good clinical management and the outcomes. The application of

established preventive measures as advocated through the concepts of public health coupled with the utilization of the principles of osteopathic medicine will further our ability to enhance the health and well-being of all patients. It is in this way that the tenets of osteopathic medicine can be sustained.

REFERENCES

American College of Physicians Task Force on Adult Immunization/Infectious Diseases Society of America; *Guide for Adult Immunization*. 3rd Ed. Philadelphia, PA: American College of Physicians, 1994.

Astin JA, Shapiro SL, Eisenberg DM, et al. Mind-body medicine: state of the science, implications for practice. *J Am Board Fam Pract* 2003;16(2):131–147.

Avenell A, Broom J, Brown TJ, et al. Systematic review of the long-term effects and economic consequences of treatments for obesity and implications for health improvement. *Health Technol Assess* 2004;8(21):iii–iv, 1–182.

Danaei G, Ding EL, Mozaffarian D, et al. The preventable causes of death in the United States: comparative risk assessment of dietary, lifestyle, and metabolic risk factors. *PloS Med* 2009;6(4).

Editorial. A role for public health history. *Am J Public Health* 2004;94(11):1851–1853.

Galanis DJ, et al. A longitudinal study of drinking and cognitive performance in elderly Japanese American men: The Honolulu-Asia Aging Study. *Am J Public Health* 2000;90:1254–1259.

Harfst DL, Mashaw JL. *The Struggle for Auto Safety*. Cambridge, MA: Harvard University Press, 1990.

Joint principles of a patient-centered medical home released by organizations representing more than 300,000 physicians; an AAFP White Paper, February 2007; American Academy of Family Physicians 2007; www.aafp.org

Mayo Clinic.com; Alcohol Use, Why Moderation is Key. Mayo Clinic Reports: http://www.mayoclinic.com/health/exercise

National Library of Medicine: Images of the Public Health Services; U.S. Department of Health and Human Services; Public Health Service Institute of Medicine; The Future of Public Health in the 21st Century. 1988.

Nolte E, McKee CM. Measuring the health of nations: updating an earlier analysis. *Health Aff* 2008;27(1):58–71 (Millwood) http://www.ncbi.nlm.nih.gov/entrez/query.fcgi?linkbar=plain&db=journals&term=1544–5208

O'Brien SH, Holubkov R, Reis EC. Identification, evaluation, and management of obesity in an academic primary care center. *Pediatrics* 2004;114(2):e154–e159.

Pelletier KB. Mind-body medicine in ambulatory care: an evidence-based assessment. *J Ambul Care Manage* 2004;27(1):25–42.

Rogers FJ, D'Alonzo GE, Glover JC, et al. Proposed tenets of osteopathic medicine and principles for patient care. *JAOA* 102(2): 63–65.

Starfield B, Shi L. The medical home, access to care, and insurance: a review of the evidence. *Pediatrics* 2004;113:1493–1498.

Steinbrook R. Imposing personal responsibility for health. *N Engl J Med* 2006a.

Steinbrook R. Imposing personal responsibility for health. *NEJM* 2006b;355(8):753–756.

Schwenk TL. Physicians enthused about annual "Check-Ups". *Arch Intern Med* 2005.

U.S. Centers for Disease Control; Update on adult immunization: recommendations of the Immunization Practices Advisory Committee (ACIP). MMWR 1991:40(RR-12):1–94.

U.S. Department of Health and Human Services, Office of Disease Prevention and Health Promotion. Available at: http://www.healthypeople2010.gov

U.S. Department of Health and Human Services; *The Health Consequences of Involuntary Exposure to Tobacco Smoke: A Report of the Surgeon General*. U.S. Department of Health and Human Services, Centers for Disease Control and Prevention, National Center for Chronic Disease Prevention and Health Promotion, Office on Smoking and Health, 2006.

U.S. Preventive Services Task Force: Guide to clinical preventive services. 2nd Ed. Alexandria, Virginia: International Medical Publishing; 1996.

Wikipedia, "What is Public Health". Available at: http://www.whatispublic health.org

Winslow CEA. The untilled fields of public health. *Mod Med* 1920;2:183–191.

22

Musculoskeletal Component

WOLFGANG G. GILLIAR

KEY CONCEPTS

- Juxtaposing the viewpoints of public health and individual patient care with the musculoskeletal system and its varied disorders demonstrates their impact and burden on the health care system.
- A recent shift from static structural diagnosis to a dynamic patient concept is the guide for assessment of the "three fundamental pillars" of health care.
- Appreciation of the primary role of the musculoskeletal system in health and disease is fundamental to the philosophy and approach to the patient of the osteopathic system of care.
- Central tools of osteopathic management approaches include the use of refined functional examinations and the application of specific osteopathic manipulative interventions.
- Recent public health initiatives and prevention strategies have targeted chronic disorders having significant musculoskeletal consequences of major functional loss.
- Physiologic mechanisms viewed from the perspective of somatic dysfunction facilitate osteopathic management within an integrated musculoskeletal approach.

INTRODUCTION

The musculoskeletal system continues to play a central role in the osteopathic paradigm of patient care ever since its inception at the end of the nineteenth century. As osteopathic medicine has grown from a virtually purely "hands-on" profession of healers to a present-day system much akin to the orthodox allopathic model of disease and pathology, its uniqueness and distinctiveness have been challenged in most recent years. According to the World Health Organization (2003), "...although the diseases that kill attract much of the public's attention, musculoskeletal or rheumatic diseases are the major cause of morbidity throughout the world, having a substantial influence on health and quality of life, and inflicting an enormous burden of cost on health systems ..." With many assumptions remaining about the profession and its practitioners, we want to take a closer look at the osteopathic approach to the individual patient from a musculoskeletal perspective, while viewing it as one that is embedded in and guided by the greater challenges of public health and health policy at the same time.

Musculoskeletal Function and Burden: Perspectives of Public Health and Medical Care

Musculoskeletal or rheumatic conditions include over 150 diseases, disorders, or syndromes. These are progressive and painful conditions that present as a leading cause of morbidity and disability, giving rise to enormous health care expenditures and loss of work (2). Musculoskeletal conditions account for more disability and more costs to the U.S. health care system than any other condition (3). The musculoskeletal conditions with greatest impact on society include rheumatoid arthritis, osteoarthritis, osteoporosis, spinal disorders, and severe limb trauma (2).

Low back pain is the most prevalent of the spinal disorder group and is treated most commonly in the primary health care setting (4). This condition presents with significant disability among young adults, leading to not only considerable personal challenges but also to a large societal burden in all developed. Low back pain is thought of primarily as a self-limiting problem with a spontaneous recovery in those who experience their first activity-related episode. Nonetheless, about 40% of patients with low back pain have recurrences within 6 months, and up to 60% have recurrences within 1 year (5). Furthermore, with the increasing age of the population, this burden will not only increase but is expected to become a major challenge to society at large. In addition, when coupled to the shift in lifestyle toward greater activity in the very same population, there is greater risk of injury, abuse, and overuse.

The Shift from Structure to Function

The central focus in musculoskeletal care in recent years has prominently shifted away from a symptom- or a disease-based description of disability *toward* the concept of *function*. This change is innately reflected in the adoption of the current operative term of "musculoskeletal system," as it goes beyond one specific physician's specialty of care, say orthopedics, neurology, or rheumatology, for instance. The new emphasis in the musculoskeletal system is *away* from a static structural description toward an understanding of abilities and health rather than disability. Thus, medicine has been moving away from "linear" or purely anatomic disease classifications, typically utilized in the orthodox medical model to a dynamic, interactive system. This reflects the desire to integrate human functioning within a larger context, based on the biopsychosocial model (6). This system, in which activity is the center of consideration, is represented in Figure 22.1 and Table 22.1.

For the purposes of this chapter, it is helpful to recall that a particular disorder or set of disorders can be approached vis-à-vis two fundamental perspectives:

1. the Public Health Domain
2. the Health Care Domain

The mission of public health is to promote physical and mental health, prevent disease, injury, and disability, and to protect the public from environmental hazards (7). The public health domain is distinct from health care in that public health focuses on the

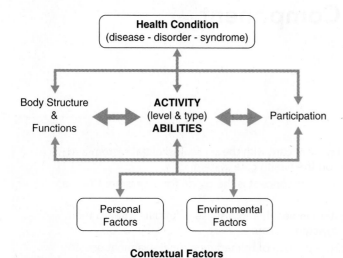

Contextual Factors

Figure 22-1   Activity level and type are the center of a functional approach to the patient, where structure and function interact on one level, while at the same time, personal and environmental factors play into the entire patient situation as well as the disease process itself. (Modified from Public Health Functions Steering Committee, "Public Health in America," U. S. Department of Health and Human Services, June 1995, accessed August 28, 2008. Available at: http://www.health.gov/phfunctions/public.htm.; WHO [2002].)

prevention of disease within populations, while health care focuses on the treatment of disease in individuals (8). With a common vision of ensuring good health and often pursuing overlapping strategies to achieve this vision, there exists no consensus on the precise boundaries between the two disciplines (8). This is a point worth remembering, especially when considering the three fundamental axes making up the *health policy equation* that guide the entire health system, namely, access, quality, and cost (Fig. 22.2).

PUBLIC HEALTH ASPECTS OF MUSCULOSKELETAL DISORDERS

Currently in the United States, more than 30% of the entire population is affected by musculoskeletal problems that require medical care. This figure alone represents an increase by more than two percentage points over the past decade (9), indicative of a prevalence of more than 11.5 million people. While musculoskeletal diseases rarely are a cause of death and do not have the high visibility of conditions such as heart problems, respiratory problems, and cancer, they are nonetheless much more prevalent and are a major cause of pain and reduced quality of life (10). In 2005 alone, 107.7 million adults, that is one in two aged 18 and over, reported suffering from a musculoskeletal condition lasting three months or longer during the prior year. This is nearly twice the number who reported any other medical condition (9). In addition, nearly 15% of the adults aged 18 and older are reported to be unable to perform at least one common activity, such as self-care, walking, or rising from a chair, on a regular basis due to their musculoskeletal condition (9). Table 22.2 compares the diseases with high mortality with those that lead to significant disability (self-reported), with the latter having a significant impact on disability and function, and thus contributing in the USA to significant health care expenses.

The annual direct and indirect costs of nearly US$ 850 billion for musculoskeletal care represent 7.7% of the gross domestic product (GDP) of the United States (9), corresponding to nearly half of the entire health care costs in the United States. These figures are particularly impressive when realizing that the future health expenditures will dramatically rise even more as a result of factors that are *directly linked* to the musculoskeletal system. These factors include *intensity of care* (longer life span, greater prevalence of chronic disease) and aging of the population, especially when the baby boomer generation (persons born between 1946 and 1964) enters the Medicare program in 2011, shifting a significant burden to the public sector (9).

TABLE 22.1

Functional Approach to the Patient

Health Condition	Intervention/Medical Care	Prevention/Public Health
Health Condition (disease, disorder, or syndrome)	Medical treatment/care Medication(s)	Health Promotion Nutrition Immunization Exercise
Impairment	Medical treatment/care Manual medicine approaches/manipulation Medication(s) Surgery	Prevention of further functional deterioration or development of further activity limitations
Activity limitation	Assistive devices Personal assistance Rehabilitative intervention/treatment	Preventive rehabilitation Prevention of the development of participation restrictions
Participation restriction	Accommodation Public education Antidiscrimination laws Universal design	Environmental change Employment strategies Accessible services Universal design Lobbying for change

Source: Modified from WHO (2002). Definitions used in the bio-psycho-social function model and indicating how the different levels of disability are linked to the different levels of approaches: intervention (e.g., medical care) and prevention (e.g., public health sector).

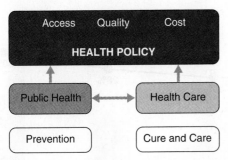

Figure 22-2 Health Policy as shaped by the three "pillars" of access, quality, and cost of health care issues. The public health sector deals primarily with prevention, and the individualized patient health care sector (e.g., hospitals, clinics, doctors' offices, etc.) deals with the care and cure of disease or disorders. However, the borders between the two often overlap and may be blurry.

Musculoskeletal health care utilization and the economic costs of musculoskeletal diseases are the focus of a recent comprehensive monograph published by the American Academy of Orthopaedic Surgery (9). The report highlights and substantiates the growing impact and burden musculoskeletal problems will have on both the health care industry and on the individual patient. A brief review of the reported findings will be presented here to address some of the major considerations such as (a) musculoskeletal disease prevalence, (b) musculoskeletal health care utilization, (c) musculoskeletal medical care expenditures, and (d) impact of musculoskeletal diseases on the U.S. economy.

Prevalence

Between nearly 90 million people and 108 million people reported musculoskeletal conditions as a primary health concern during the 2002–2005 period (9). When including people in whom the musculoskeletal disease is a byproduct of another condition, nearly 50% (46.6%) of the population reported some musculoskeletal disease (135.6 million people) (9). Figure 22.3 shows prevalence of musculoskeletal diseases and percentage of total population, United States, 1996–2004.

Utilization

Persons with musculoskeletal conditions account for a rather large share of health care utilization. Since 1999 to 2001, utilization has been increasing steadily, especially that associated with the consumption of prescription medication, which is twice the amount in the 2002–2004 as compared with the 1996–1998 interval.

Expenditures

Overall, the total average *individual* expenditure rose by 23% from $4,751 in the 1996–1998 interval to $5,824 (9). The aggregate total expenditures increased by nearly $150 billion from 361.0 billion to a total of $ 510.0 billion during this time frame, corresponding to a more than 40% increase. Within a 6-year period, it is noteworthy that the percentage of the GDP represented by expenses associated with MSK disease has risen from 4.4% (1996–1998 aggregates) to 4.6% (2002–2004 aggregate numbers).

TABLE 22.2

Causes of Death and Disability in the United States (2006)

Most Common Causes of Death in the United States* (2006)	Main Causes of Disability Among U.S. Adults Over 18 Years of Age**
Disease of the heart (28.5% of total)	**Arthritis or rheumatism (19% of total)**
Cancer/malignancy (22.8% of total)	**Back or spine problems (16.8% of total)**
Stroke/cerebrovascular accident (6.7% of total)	Circulatory/heart trouble (6.6% of total)
Chronic lower respiratory diseases (5.1% of total)	Lung or respiratory trouble (4.9% of total)
Accidents (nonintentional injuries) (4.4% of total)	Mental or emotional problems (4.9% of total)
Diabetes Mellitus (3.0% of total)	Diabetes (4.5% of total)
Alzheimer disease (2.7% of total)	Deafness/hearing problems (4.2% of total)
Influenza and Pneumonia (2.4% of total)	**Stiffness of deformity of limbs/extremities (3.6% of total)**
Nephritis/kidney diseases (1.7% of total)	Blindness or vision problems (3.2% of total)
Septicemia (1.4% of total)	Stroke (2.4% of total)
Intentional self-harm/suicide (1.3% of total)	Cancer (2.2% of total)
Chronic liver disease (1.1% of total)	**Broken bone/fracture (2.1% of total)**
Primary hypertension/hypertensive renal disease (0.8% of total)	High blood pressure (1.9% of total)
Parkinson disease (0.7% of total)	Mental retardation (1.5% of total)
Homicide (0.7% of total)	Senility/Dementia/Alzheimer disease (1.1% of total)

Note: The table compares the most common causes of death in the United States in descending order and the main causes of self-reported disability of adults older than 18 years of age in the United States.

Sources: Mortality figures (left column): http://www.cdc.gov.nchs/data/nvsr/nvsr57/nvsr57_14.pdf and for disability figures (right column): http://www.cdc.gov/mmwr/preview/mmwrhtm/mm5816a2.htm#tab1

Figure 22-3 Prevalence of musculoskeletal diseases and percentage of total population, United States, 1996–2004. While the 2% increase in prevalence between the 1996–1998 and 2002–2004 time intervals appears rather modest, it reflects an increase of nearly 12 million people in the same time frame. (Modified after reference WHO Technical Report Series. The burden of musculoskeletal conditions at the start of the new millennium. Available at: http://whqlibdoc.who.int/trs/WHO_TRS_919.pdf, accessed August 24, 2009.)

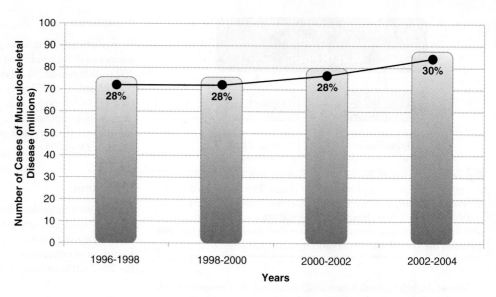

Economic Impact

The direct total costs for all four conditions studied (e.g., gout, osteoarthritis, rheumatoid arthritis, spine disorders) including earning losses are highest for those associated with disorders of the spine, followed by those associated with osteoarthritis and allied disorders, gout, and rheumatoid arthritis (9). When further including with spine disorders, the total costs for spine care amounted to $120 billion US$, which is nearly three times that used for treatment of osteoarthritis and allied disorders, and nearly four times that used for treatment of gout or rheumatoid disease each (9).

PUBLIC HEALTH INITIATIVES AND PREVENTION STRATEGIES

The monumental impact of musculoskeletal conditions worldwide is now recognized by the United Nations, the World Health Organization, World Bank, and numerous governments throughout the world through support of the Bone and Joint Decade 2000 to 2010 initiative (9,11).

Realization of the impact from bone and joint disorders on society, the health care system, and on the individual, combined with the awareness that resources need to be more efficiently used, culminated in the proposal for the "Decade of the Bone and Joint from 2000 to 2010" (12). The Bone and Joint Decade 2000–2010 aims to improve the health-related quality of life for persons with musculoskeletal disorders by working in partnership with all stakeholders to raise awareness, identify needs, empower patients, promote cost-effective prevention and treatment, and advance understanding through education and research to improve prevention and treatment (13). The major areas of focus are osteoporosis, rheumatoid arthritis, back pain, and musculoskeletal trauma (13).

Drawing on a number of major documents produced by various national and international groups over the last few years, an international task force of the Bone and Joint Decade came together to develop standards for the care of acute and chronic musculoskeletal pain (14). The group's document is a product of the World Health Organization Collaborative Centre for Evidence-Based Health Care in Musculoskeletal Disorders (15) that has set forth the following three goals:

1. To identify barriers and facilitators that affect successful implementation of health strategies for better musculoskeletal health
2. To identify the costs of musculoskeletal conditions and develop economic models for cost-effectiveness

3. To monitor for ongoing activities relating to musculoskeletal conditions etiology, prevention, and treatment

Another recent example of successful international collaborative efforts is reflected in a series of publications on the topic of neck pain and its burden on the health care sector as published in the journal *Spine* (16). The authors who made up the working group actually developed a new conceptual model for the evaluation and treatment of neck pain and then presented a new classification system based on a "domain approach" to neck pain by using "axes" of diagnostic categorization similar to a system used in the psychiatry/psychology literature (16).

With respect to manipulative and exercise therapy for neck pain, the group's best evidence synthesis suggests that such therapies are more effective than alternative strategies for patients with neck pain. Their recommendations for future efforts include studies of noninvasive interventions for patients with radicular symptoms and on the design and evaluation of neck pain prevention strategies (17).

THE OSTEOPATHIC PERSPECTIVE—APPROACH: REAL AND PERCEIVED BENEFITS

In the United States, Osteopathic Medicine is described as a complete system of medical care with the philosophy of treating the whole person, not just symptoms (28). Currently, there are more than 60,000 osteopathic physicians (D.O.—Doctor of Osteopathic Medicine) reflecting a significant growth in numbers in the recent years (18).

DOs may use all accepted methods of treatment, including drugs and surgery, while they place special emphasis on the body's musculoskeletal system, preventive medicine, and holistic patient care (19). With about half of DOs practicing in general or family medicine, general internal medicine, or general pediatrics, they are most likely to be primary care specialists although they can be found in all specialties (19).

It would seem plausible to hypothesize that osteopathic medicine, by virtue of its medical education and philosophical underpinnings, is uniquely positioned to provide a comprehensive medical and manipulative perspective to a variety of medical disorders in general, and musculoskeletal problems in particular. The remainder of this chapter will take a closer look at the current supportive evidence of such claims. Of interest in the discussion will be the concept of the "art of osteopathic medicine," which provides satisfactory patient care even in situations where there is no "published evidence."

According to Cypress (1983), low back pain was the most common reason for office visits to osteopathic physicians based on the 1977–1978 National Ambulatory Medical Care Surveys (NAMCS) (20).

Subsequently, based on the NAMCS of nearly 40,000 ambulatory care visits to osteopathic physicians, Koch and McLemore report in 1987 (21) that "although office-based DOs gave ample evidence of their prominent concern with the musculoskeletal system, this concern did not appear to dominate their office practice." The closest counterpart to osteopathic office care was found in the care provided in the offices of MDs in general or family practice. Most DOs in office practice were best characterized as generalists who brought the added dimension of a specialized philosophy and training to the conduct of their professional tasks. With respect to musculoskeletal disease, the same authors found that DOs were more focally involved with injuries and musculoskeletal disease, conditions which, according to prior NAMCS studies, were among the most likely to be associated with symptomatic pain (22,23).

This allowed Koch and McLemore to further conclude that apparently, the use of manipulative therapy "reduced the perceived need for pain medication, albeit to an unknown extent" (20). The following patient and physician characteristics were specifically reported: "The DO's special concern for the musculoskeletal system is evident in the finding that back symptoms were the major reason for a patient visit. Back and neck symptoms alone motivated about 1 of every 10 visits to the osteopathic physician."

More recently, Licciardone and Herron (23) report that a majority of those patients who visit an osteopathic physician receive treatment for musculoskeletal disorders. Furthermore, based on a national telephone survey, Licciardone further reports in 2003 (25), that a majority of those patients who visit a DO also receive spinal manipulation. Among those persons who reported being life time users (16% of the respondents), 84% received primary care, while 52% reported receiving osteopathic manipulative treatment (OMT) and 25% received specialty care.

Musculoskeletal Disorders, Health Care Access, Cost, and Quality

The Osteopathic Survey of Health Care in America (OSTEO-SURV II), a national random telephone survey, confirmed that most patients visiting osteopathic physicians (52% in the 1998 and 2000 administrations) continue to seek treatment for musculoskeletal conditions (25).

In the United States, osteopathic physicians, allopathic general and family physicians, chiropractors, orthopedic surgeons, and other medical specialists are the main providers of low back pain care. Millions of office visits per year are attributed to low back pain, and almost half of the visits may involve spinal manipulation provided by osteopathic physicians or chiropractors (25).

With respect to the quality component of the health care equation, it is noted that unlike treatment modalities offered by many allopathic physicians, including orthopedic surgeons and neurosurgeons, and spinal manipulation provided by chiropractors, OMT can be readily integrated with other primary health care services when patients visit osteopathic physicians (26).

Considering that the majority of low back pain is mechanical, consideration should be given to the nonspecific low back pain as a multifactorial problem, yet all the while considering the "sprain/strain" model to be more reflective of somatic/segmental dysfunction (27).

Osteopathic Structural Examination

The primary goal in the osteopathic management of a patient with a particular condition, especially with a musculoskeletal component (as the presenting or the associated phenomenon), is to view the influences of posture, regional, and segmental dysfunctions upon the entire organism or specific body regions. The goal of the osteopathic structural examination (OSE), which searches for functional aberrations within the musculoskeletal system, is to determine the presence of one or multiple segmentally related somatic dysfunction(s) and its/their relevance within the overall clinical presentation. Perhaps the greatest contribution from the osteopathic manipulative approach and integrative thought is the evaluation of a diagnostic and therapeutic framework defining the various dysfunctions that affect the musculoskeletal system, with a goal of restoring maximal function within postural balance (28).

The OSE has as the primary goal the determination and specification of the entity known as somatic dysfunction (ICD 9:739). The examination routine builds upon and is integrated into the standard neuro-orthopedic and medical examination routine. By using the OSE, the physician is able to obtain information about the tissues and body regions otherwise not available through the standard medical exam or diagnostic imaging or laboratory studies.

The OSE takes on special consideration in the musculoskeletal system and also is important when dealing with nonmusculoskeletal issues, especially when mediated through viscerosomatic reflexes.

A Rational Approach to the Patient

In order to maximize the individual person's functional capacity, osteopathic medicine's philosophical and practical approach has always emphasized the individual's capacity for self-healing when appropriately guided and fostered, including the use of manual medicine approaches. Thus, so it appears, osteopathic medicine has inherently "practiced" medicine using the biopsychosocial model throughout. More research is needed that will look at such factors as cost-effectiveness, impact, outcomes, and expediency of care as provided by medical providers, and osteopathic physicians, in particular. The "standard" research methods, however, may not suffice. New tools or approaches to the study of functional abilities as well as impairments and disabilities are needed in order to fully "catch" the multilayered effects a fully integrated hands-on approach has within the medical setting (29).

With the growing international collaborative efforts, it is becoming evident that what should guide patient management is a comprehensive and patient-centered approach based on the best available evidence. In addition to recommending specific evidence-based practices for neck pain, the members of the *Bone and Joint Decade 2000–2010 Task Force on Neck Pain and Its Associated Disorders* performed an analysis of their own group's activities and "internal workings" in a "Self-Study of Values, Beliefs, and Conflict of Interest," which led to a set of "Guiding Principles" (30). From this, it is apparent that such guiding principles are helpful, if not necessary, in advancing sound consensus.

Musculoskeletal Issues and Medical Diagnoses

Of growing recent interest to clinicians and basic science researchers alike are the often surprising interrelationships that have been observed to exist between many nonmusculoskeletal and musculoskeletal conditions as well as particular medical issues related to various musculoskeletal problems.

When a patient enters the osteopathic physician's office, the musculoskeletal component assumes a central role for either of the two following reasons or a combination of both:

1. The presenting complaint is related to the musculoskeletal system.
2. The presenting complaint is a medical issue that is accompanied by musculoskeletal issues.

The physician skilled in both aspects, that is one having achieved a well-educated understanding of both the full spectrum of medical care *and* the musculoskeletal system, is best situated to determine the most appropriate patient-specific approach.

Organic Versus Musculoskeletal Pain

AN INTERESTING CASE

A woman in her early 60s was referred for osteopathic manipulation by her internist because of unresolved upper and midback pain of several weeks' duration. Laboratory and radiographic studies had been unremarkable. The history revealed a "strain" after the patient had picked up her granddaughter. Initial osteopathic evaluation revealed no localizing neurologic deficits or other "red flags" but found both chronic and acute tissue changes in the midthoracic region. The patient received myofascial trigger point injections with Lidocaine and OMT in the first visit.

In her follow-up visit one week later, the patient reported that the presenting pain had completely disappeared after the initial treatment, only to return "like gang-busters" 2 to 3 hours after the injection. Follow-up examination revealed more acute soft-tissue changes and somatic dysfunctions, prompting the contact of the patient's internist to rule out viscerosomatic disease.

The MRI of the spine revealed a space-occupying lesion in the thorax, which by biopsy turned out to be a mesothelioma. The patient succumbed approximately 6 months later.

Organic pain may mimic musculoskeletal pain. The more common organ-system related pain syndromes that present as either pseudospine pain or pain referred to various regions of the axial skeleton and/or the extremities include the following (29):

- *Cancer and the entire body system*—85% of patients who have bone cancer report pain; 50% of patients who have breast cancer report pain; and approximately 40% of patients who have lung or gastrointestinal cancer report pain.
- *Cardiovascular disease* that may present with pain mimicking musculoskeletal disease include abdominal aortic aneurysm, angina, myocardial infarction, pericarditis, and mitral valve prolapse.
- *Lung diseases* include such entities as a pulmonary embolus, pneumonia, and tracheobronchial pain.
- *Gastrointestinal diseases* include cholecystitis, duodenal ulcer, irritable bowel syndrome, and pancreatitis, among others.
- Symptoms/signs related to the *genitourinary system* include sources such as cystitis, nephrolithiasis, and prostatitis.
- *Gynecologic* considerations include endometriosis, pelvic inflammatory disease, and ectopic pregnancy, as well as cancer.

Recent research advances in the basic and clinical sciences have shown in the care of the patient with diabetes, for instance, that the skeleton is more than the support and biomechanical "connector organ" of the body, as it is "actually an endocrine organ," which produces hormones that act outside of bone (31). The spine is now believed to influence the body's insulin and glucose levels. For instance, Osteocalcin, a hormone released by bone cells, is reported to direct the pancreas to produce more insulin: all the while it is thought to signal fat cells to increase their sensitivity to insulin (31).

The Patient Visit: Cardinal Questions

From a direct and practical medical management standpoint, in the evaluation of a patient with a musculoskeletal issue, there are four cardinal questions that need to be answered in each clinical situation, especially when associated with apparent or true medical emergencies involving complaints of pain, stiffness, or swelling affecting the spine and joints of the extremities.

1. **Is there a systemic organic disease that could explain the symptoms?**

This question would lead to the appropriately targeted medical evaluation of the patient ruling out the prominent "red flags." The osteopathic physician's medical education allows her/him to easily integrate the "red flag thinking" into the standard medical examination. The OSE may provide immediate clues for diagnosis (e.g., presence of viscerosomatic reflexes) and osteopathic treatment may provide information about prognosis in response to manipulative treatment that may be provided as an adjunct or primary treatment intervention for a particular situation.

2. **Are the symptoms due to neurologic deficits that are becoming progressively worse (e.g., low back pain, with worsening leg pain and loss of bowel and/or bladder control, for instance, in cauda equina syndrome)?**

   In this case, surgical referral is then most likely indicated.

3. **Are there social or psychological stress factors that influence or worsen the patient's pain perception (e.g., impending job loss, family discord, prolonged disability, loss of function), both vocationally and avocationally that may have precipitated psychological issues?**

4. **Is there a history of major trauma—even if remote?**

This question includes trauma that may have required hospitalization in the past, for instance. Of significance is any report in which the patient volunteers the information that the "wind has been knocked" out of him/her. If there is such a history, it may imply longstanding adaptive or compensatory changes in the entire musculoskeletal system such that areas of "stress" are created throughout the body, which may cause symptoms "away" (centripetal from) the location of original injury. For instance, a patient with shoulder pain may present with a pelvic dysfunction that had never been detected, and vice versa, leading to all sorts of muscle, fascial, articular, and capsular changes that may create an "individualized" pain presentation.

Integrated Osteopathic Evaluation and Management

The aim of individual patient management is to comprehensively address both the patient's pain and his/her functional deficits and, using best medical practice, to work toward goals that are determined in partnership between patient and physician (32). Both the patient's vocational and avocational interests must be taken into account when developing a management plan. Furthermore, it is prudent to build projections of time frames according to which one would expect certain improvements to occur in order to allow monitoring patient progress. It should be remembered that even when best care is rendered, patient expectations and preferences may affect outcome (33).

Manual medicine treatment may assume an integral role in the management of the various musculoskeletal disorders or particular presentations. This is especially true when the approach to the individual patient is appropriately coordinated within the entire patient medical management process; from obtaining a meaningful history to integrating a structural/functional musculoskeletal examination, and implementing a comprehensive treatment plan with appropriate follow-up, all the while determining specific medical and functionally meaningful end points.

As shown in Table 22.3, the OSE thus builds upon and refines findings elicited in the standard neuro-orthopedic examination by using specific manual medicine approaches (56), by:

1. Paying specific attention to findings of asymmetry in posture, regional, and segmental regions

2. Determining both the degree and the quality of motion abnormalities/restrictions or hypermobility
3. Eliciting abnormal soft-tissue findings in muscle and fascial structures
4. Eliciting specific findings through controlled provocative testing

---

TABLE 22.3

The OSE Embedded in the Standard Patient Visit Routine Based on the Problem-oriented SOAP-format Approach

	Patient's Chief Complaint **Pain—Loss of Function—Lifestyle Changes**	**Physician Activity/Task**
Subjective		

	1. History of present illness
	2. Detailed pain history and medical history
	3. Functional history/loss of function
	4. Is there sinister organic pathology ("red flags")
	   a. nonmusculoskeletal related history
	   b. musculoskeletal related history
	5. Any history of trauma? Recent vs. remote
	6. Review of systems, social, family history, medication use, allergies, prior interventions/studies, etc.
		Standard Medical Interview and questions (including stress and stressors)
		Osteopathic considerations
		a. trauma, even if remote
		b. work habits (vocational)
		c. avocational components (hobbies, etc.)
		d. stress and stressors (unit/function/outcome)
		e. any "mechanical issues" that could contribute or exacerbate an underlying/associated medical issue
		f. patient goals and why he/she came to the visit

Objective	**Standard Neuro-Orthopedic Exam**	**Physician Activity/Task**

	1. "LOOK": General Inspection
	          Gait—posture—deformities—skin
	2. "FEEL": Palpation of gross structures
	3. "MOVE": Range of motion (quantity)
	4. Neuro exam: Sensory-motor examination
	5. Special tests: Provocative tests
	6. Adjunct studies: Laboratory/Imaging/
	          Neurodiagnostics
		Appropriate
		Exams/evaluation
		Standard medical exams
		Osteopathic
		Integration using the structural
		examination routine—to be correlated with the other findings
		KEY element: Integration of structural OMM exam into the entire clinical scenario (contextual)

	Osteopathic Structural Exam **Screen—Scan—Segmental Exam**	

	1. "LOOK": Specific joints, spine and tissues
	         after general exam
	2. "FEEL": Detailed tissue/joint palpation
	3. "Move": Segmental/joint specific motion
	         testing; quality and quantity
	4. Function: Muscles and Fasciae/"Points"
	5. Specific tests: Provocative testing of specific
	         joints/regions	

Assessment	**Diagnosis—Assessment—Clinical Impression**	**Physician Activity/Task**
	1. Structural level: "organic" 2. Functional level: "dysfunction" 3. Pain perception level: pain and behavior	1. RATIONALE for which studies are essential/helpful — and which might be "superfluous" 2. RATIONALE for the correlation of osteopathic diagnostic findings to the clinical presentation 3. RATIONALE as to what techniques are indicated and contraindicated 4. RATIONALE as to what patient goals and physician goals would need to be prioritized and what outcome is expected in what time frame 5. Provides the framework of what additional information is essential to have and how to obtain it
Plan	**Treatment—Planning—Management**	
	1. Comprehensive, patient-specific planning and time projections 2. Setting meaningful functional goals 3. Periodic reevaluation with appropriate parameters to monitor progress or lack thereof	

5. Helping select the appropriate additional diagnostic studies as indicated by the patient's presentation and specifically defined patient and physician goals with specific outcomes and time frames in mind

The key is that the presenting complaints and findings per each visit's assessment should be reviewed anew and monitored on an ongoing basis and compared with the initially set patient-physician goal so as to allow meaningful monitoring of the progress or lack thereof. The patient's pain should be assessed within the greater context of patient expectations and elicited goals. Patients may be "ok to live with some pain," as long as they can do what they want or need to do.

SUMMARY

The incidence of musculoskeletal problem in the general population is so high that a typical patient is likely to have MSK problems in addition to the other medical issues. Neck and back pain are among the leading source for cost generation in the United States, and there is no change for the better predicted given the aging of the population. The cost associated with the diagnostic and therapeutic management of chronic musculoskeletal diseases or disorders is expected to continue to rise. Musculoskeletal disorders have a profound effect on aging and lifestyle and vice versa. Consideration of the role that somatic dysfunction plays in the musculoskeletal system may provide improvement in quality, cost, and access to care. The osteopathic physician is able to positively influence the (a) access, (b) quality, and (c) cost dimensions *directly*. Osteopathic physicians are well prepared to take on the challenge of muscle and bone disorders, especially when considering the duality of either (A) medical issues that are accompanied by musculoskeletal issues or (B) musculoskeletal issues that are accompanied by medical problems. The ability of treating both simultaneously should enhance access, quality, and cost through a best-practice approach.

REFERENCES

1. Rogers FJ, D'Alonzo GE Jr, Glover JC, et al. Proposed tenets of osteopathic medicine and principles for patient care. *J Am Osteopath Assoc* 2002;102:63–65. www.who.int/chp/topics/rheumatic/en/index.html, accessed April 17 2008.
2. Haralson R, Zuckerman JD. Prevalence, health care expenditures, and orthopedic surgery workforce for musculoskeletal conditions. *JAMA* 2009;302(14):1586–1587.
3. Koes BW, vanTulder MW, Thomras S. Diagnosis and treatment of low back pain. *BMJ* 2006;332:1430–1434.
4. Frymoyer JW. Back pain and sciatica. *N Engl J Med* 1988;318:291–300.
5. *Towards a Common Language for Functioning, Disability and Health.* Geneva, Switzerland: ICF The International Classification of Functioning, Disability and Health, World Health Organization publication, 2002.
6. Public Health Functions Steering Committee, "Public Health in America," U. S. Department of Health and Human Services, June 1995, accessed August 28, 2008. Available at: http://www.health.gov/phfunctions/public.htm.
7. Salinsky E, Public Health Emergency Preparedness: Fundamentals of the "System" NHPF Background Paper April 3, 2002, available at: www.nhpf.org/pdfs_bp/BP_Public_Health_4-02.pdf, accessed August 29, 2008.
8. *The Burden of Musculoskeletal Diseases: Chapter 9–United States Bone and Joint Decade.* Rosemont, IL: American Academy of Orthopaedic Surgeons, 2008.
9. WHO Technical Report Series. The burden of musculoskeletal conditions at the start of the new millennium. Available at: http://whqlibdoc.who.int/trs/WHO_TRS_919.pdf, accessed August 24, 2009.
10. Woolf AD, Zeidler H, Haglung U, et al. Musculoskeletal pain in Europe: its impact and a comparison of population and medical perceptions of treatment in eight European countries. *Ann Rheum Dis* 2004;63:342–347.
11. Walsh NE, Brooks P, Hazes JM, et al. Bone and joint decade task force for standards of care for acute and chronic musculoskeletal pain. Standards of care for acute and chronic musculoskeletal pain: the Bone and Joint Decade (2000–2010). *Arch Phys Med Rehabil* 2008;89(9):1830–1845.
12. http://www.boneandjointdecade.org/default.aspx?contId=229, accessed February 24, 2009.
13. Brooks PM. Impact of osteoarthritis on individuals and society: how much disability? Social consequences and health economic implications. *Curr Opin Rheumatol* 2002;14(5):573–577, 2002 Sep).
14. World Health Organization: Collaborating Centre for Evidence-Based Health Care in Musculoskeletal Disorders. Available at: www.who.int/whocc/Detail.aspx?cc_ref=SWE-60&cc_city=lund&cc_code=swe&, accessed 10/28/2008
15. Guzman J, Haldeman S, Carroll LJ, et al. Clinical practice implications of the Bone and Joint Decade 2000–2010 Task Force on neck pain and its associated disorders: from concepts and findings to recommendations *Spine* 2008;33(4 suppl):S199–S213.
16. Hurwitz EL, Carragee EJ, van der Velde G, et al. Bone and Joint Decade 2000–2010 Task Force on neck pain and its associated disorders. Treatment of neck pain: noninvasive interventions: results of the Bone and Joint Decade 2000–2010 Task Force on neck pain and its associated disorders. *Spine* 2008;33(4 suppl):S123–S52.
17. http://www.osteopathic.org/index.cfm?PageID=aoa_ompreport_profession#dos, accessed October 23, 2008.
18. www.bls.gov/oco/ocos074.htm, accessed October 22, 2008.
19. Cypress BK. Characteristics of physician visits for back symptoms: a national perspective. *Am J Public Health* 1983;73:389–395.
20. Koch H, McLemore T. National Center for Health Statistics: Highlights of osteopathic office practice, National Ambulatory Medical Care Survey, 1985. *Advance Data From Vital/ and Health Statistics. No.* 138. DHHS Pub. No. (PHS) 87–1250. Hyatsville, MD: Public Health Service, September 18, 1987.
21. Knapp D, Koch H. National Center for Health Statistics, The Management of New Pain in Office-based Ambulatory Care, National Ambulatory Medical Care Survey. *Advance Data From Vital and Health Statistics. No. 97.* DHHS Pub. No. (PHS) 84–1250. Hyattsville, MD: Public Health Service, June 13, 1984. National Center for Health Statistics.
22. Koch H. The Management of Chronic Pain in Office-based Ambulatory Care, National Ambulatory Care Survey. Advance Data From Vital Health Statistics. No. 123. DHHS Pub. No. (PHS) 86–1250. Public Health Statistics. Hyattsville, MD: Public Health Service, August 29, 1986.
23. Licciardone JC, Herron KM. Characteristics, satisfaction, and perceptions of patients receiving ambulatory healthcare from osteopathic physicians: a comparative national survey. *J Am Osteopath Assoc* 2001;101:374–385.
24. Licciardone JC. Awareness and use of osteopathic physicians in the United States: results of the Second Osteopathic Survey of Health Care in America (OSTEOSURV-II). *J Am Osteopath Assoc* 2003;103:281–289.
25. Licciardone JC. A comparison of patient visits to osteopathic and allopathic general and family medicine physicians: results from the National Ambulatory Medical Care Survey, 2003–2004 *Osteopath Med Prim Care* 2007;1:2.
26. Licciardone J. The unique role of osteopathic physicians in treating patients with low back pain. *J Am Osteopath Assoc* 2004;104(11 suppl):13–18.
27. Dvorak J, Dvorak V, Gilliar W, et al. *Musculoskeletal Manual Medicine— Diagnosis and Treatment.* New York, NY/Stuttgart, Germany: Thieme Publishers, 2008;3:135–144.
28. Dvorak J, Dvorak V, Gilliar W, et al. *Musculoskeletal Manual Medicine— Diagnosis and Treatment.* New York, NY/Stuttgart, Germany: Thieme Publishers, 2008;3:238–239.
29. Reardon R, Haldeman S. Self-study of values, beliefs, and conflict of interest: the Bone and Joint Decade 2000–2010 Task Force on neck pain and its associated disorders. *Spine* 2008;33(4S suppl):S24–S32.
30. SCHAFFER Amanda: *The New York Times*, October 16, 2007: In Diabetes, a Complex of Causes.
31. Gilliar S. Clinical disorders and syndromes of the upper limb. In: Dvorak J, Dvorak V, Gilliar W, eds. *Musculoskeletal Manual Medicine.* Stuttgart, Germany/New York NY: Thieme Verlag, 2008:252–255.
32. Van der Windt, DAWM, Bouter LM. Physiotherapy or corticosteroid injection for shoulder pain? *Ann Rheum Dis* 2003;62:385–387.

Environmental Issues

NATALIE A. NEVINS

INTRODUCTION

Our environment is made up of all the things around us. It can be broken down into our natural world such as air, water, and earth, and our man-made world such as our homes, buildings related to work, pollution, and chemicals. Our environment includes the foods we eat, the clothes we wear, and even our socioeconomic status. As human beings, we have an intimate relationship with our environment. We cannot be separated from the food and water we eat and drink, or the environment in which we live. Too often, we take environmental issues for granted and dismiss them as a factor in health. As a physician, it is vitally important to remember these aspects when evaluating patients. An environmental history is a key component to obtaining an accurate picture of your patient's complete health status. You are your environment.

THE INTERACTION OF GENETICS AND ENVIRONMENT

Some liken the role of genetics in your overall health as a loaded gun, and the environment as the actual trigger. Patients often ask themselves the "why me" question. How is it possible for one person to smoke like a chimney for years and never develop lung cancer, and another individual who smokes significantly less yet develops lung cancer? Current research is leading scientists to believe that factors in our environment, such as pollution and man-made chemicals, as well as naturally occurring gases and radiation may be setting us up for disease (1). The National Academy of Science has reported that as much as 25% of developmental disabilities may be caused by environmental factors.

A study in 2006 evaluated the effects of polychlorinated biphenyls (PCBs) on the cognitive function of adolescents. The study found that there were "significant correlations between serum PCB concentrations and three subtest scores: delayed recall index (p = 0.019), long-term retrieval (p = 0.004), and comprehension knowledge (p = 0.043). These subtle negative effects provide a warning that more serious effects could occur from greater exposure to environmental PCBs" (2). PCBs were banned in the 1970s, but they are classified as persistent organic pollutants that bioaccumulate in mammals. They were used in many everyday items such as wood flooring, adhesives, and paints to name just a few. Thus, many homes and buildings that were built with the use of PCB-contaminated items continue to be a health threat, especially to those of lower socioeconomic status (3). If we do not ask our patients about their environment, we will miss important epidemiological information that will help us diagnosis, treat, and, more importantly, prevent disease.

ENVIRONMENT AS THE TRIGGER FOR DISEASE DEVELOPMENT

Several common environmental factors can impact health (4–7), as shown in Table 23.1.

Examples of work-related environmental diseases include:

- Carpal tunnel syndrome
- Hearing loss
- Vibrational trauma
- Musculoskeletal pain
- Asbestosis/pleural plaques

Examples of environmental diseases related to chemical/biological/radiation sources include:

- Birth defects
- Cancer
- Dermatitis
- Emphysema
- Fertility problems
- Lead/mercury poisoning
- Nervous system disorders
- Vision problems
- Waterborne diseases
- Kidney/liver disease
- Asthma
- Allergies

PATIENT HISTORY

When taking a social history of your patient, it is imperative to include an environmental history that includes both occupational and nonoccupational information. Specific questions will give you the detailed information you need to properly evaluate and care for your patients.

Keep in mind that chemicals leave residue behind even outdoors. Children and pets crawl on floors and play outside, and young children place almost everything in their mouths. We tend to have close contact with our pets and they often sleep with us; thus, a pet could contaminate our indoor living spaces. Most patients are not aware of what kinds of chemicals are in their home-cleaning products or pesticides, or the chemicals used where they work. All employers are mandated by the government to maintain a Material Safety Data Sheet (MSDS) that is accessible to all employees giving a complete list of all chemicals used in the workplace. Patients should be encouraged to maintain a file with a copy of the MSDS from all of their jobs (8).

TABLE 23.1

Examples of Environmental Health Factors

Natural world	Air	Water	Soil	Chemical	Biological	Social
Examples						
Dust	Radon gas	Mercury	Arsenic	Mold	Fungi	Pollen
Man-made world	Structures: home and work	Schools	Farms	Factories	Community buildings	Roads
	Transportation: public and private	Land	Waste management	Pollution	Chemicals	
Examples						
Organophosphates	Pharmaceuticals	Latex	Asbestos	Epoxy resins	Cigarette smoke	Carbon monoxide
Lead paint	PCBs	Noise	Pesticides	Ozone		

NONOCCUPATIONAL AND OCCUPATIONAL ENVIRONMENTAL HEALTH HISTORY

Begin asking questions systematically. The questions apply to pediatric, adult, and geriatric patients. You need to ask specific questions as most patients are unlikely to realize that environmental information could be pertinent to their problem. Box 23.1 provides a sample of some of the key questions to ask your patients. It is not intended to be a comprehensive list of all possible questions. Your general history should have the majority of your open-ended questions. An environmental history should be focused on the details; be a detective.

Key Questions in an Environmental Health History

- Is the problem acute or chronic?
- Are the symptoms worse when at home or work?
- What chemicals are used in and outside the home (e.g., pesticides, paints, solvents, glue, cleaners, etc.)?
- Do any of the chemicals have a warning label (such as "Do not use around small children or pets")?
- Is the home near any manufacturing companies? If so, what kind?
- Does a family member work around chemicals? If so, what are the chemicals?
- Are any of the household pets sick?
- Does anyone else in the home or neighborhood have the same symptoms?
- Is there peeling paint around the home or in the neighborhood? Are there abandoned buildings accessible to the children?
- Is there new construction in or around the home?
- Are medications and chemicals out of reach of children?
- Has there been any recent water leakage in the home? Is there black mold growing on walls?
- What protective equipment is used when handling chemicals in and outside the home? Are these chemicals used around pets or children's toys?

- Have there been visitors to the home from another country? Has there been travel outside the country?
- Has the home been tested for carbon monoxide or radon gas?
- Does anyone smoke in or around the home?
- Do you use well water?
- Is the patient eating a strict vegan diet?

Focused Occupational History Questions

- Type of work: current and past 10 years
- Chemical or radiological exposures
- If there are chemicals in the workplace, does the patient have a copy of the MSDS?
- If working with or around chemicals, what protective gear does the patient use?
- If working with or around chemicals, does the patient shower at work and change clothes before going home?
- Does the patient work in manufacturing? If so, what kind?
- Does the patient work outside? If so, in what capacity?
- Is any machinery used (e.g., heavy, loud, grinding vibrational, etc.)?
- If working with or around machinery, what kind of protective equipment is used?
- Does the patient work with animals? If so, what kind?

CASE VIGNETTE: ENVIRONMENTAL ILLNESS

Mary is a 40-year-old health care worker who is in good health with a medical history of only reactive airway disease (RAD). She reports to the clinic with chief complaints of new-onset shortness of breath, nonproductive cough, and wheezing that started 3 weeks ago. She denies any other symptoms. She states that she has not had a flare-up of her RAD for over 5 years. Her RAD is known to be triggered by dust mites, mold, and dog dander. She admits to trying allergy medication and an albuterol inhaler without significant improvement in her symptoms. The patient reports that she moved into a new house 3 weeks ago, that is a new construction home. It has been professionally cleaned three times, but her symptoms seem to

(continued)

be getting worse. She reports that she has attempted to "dust proof" her new house (hardwood floors, no drapes, dust mite covers on her pillows and mattress, air purifier in her bedroom). She has a cat that does not go outside.

Physical examination reveals normal vital signs. The remainder of the exam was normal except for; head exam revealed dark circles (allergic shiners) under each eye. Nasal and throat exam revealed boggy and pale nasal mucosa with clear drainage and cobblestoning of the posterior pharynx. On pulmonary evaluation, the patient had both inspiratory and expiratory wheezing. The remainder of the lung exam was normal.

Investigation of the patient's new home revealed an access panel in her bedroom closet that connected to the room for the washer and dryer. When the panel was removed black mold (stachybotyris) was found covering all of the inner drywall in the access space. A professional mold removal company was hired to eradicate the mold. The patient's symptoms completely resolved after the space was cleaned.

Resources Box

There are many resources to assist the practicing clinician with understanding the impact of environmental issues on health. The Toxicity and Exposure Assessment for Children's Health (TEACH), is a Web site run by the EPA that contains summaries of scientific literature and U.S. Regulations regarding children's environmental health currently focusing on 18 known chemicals of health concern (www.epa.gov/teach/). Many information portals can be accessed through the EPA Web site. Other useful sites are The National Center for Environmental Assessment (NCEA), www.cfpub.epa.gov/ncea/, The National Institute for Occupational Safety and Health (NIOSH), www.cdc.gov/niosh/, National Institute of Environmental Health Sciences (NIEHS) www.niehs.nih.gov/, and The Centers for Disease Control and Prevention, www.cdc.gov/Environmental/.

Patient Education: Easy Steps to Personal Environmental Health

As a physician, your job is not only to diagnose and treat medical problems, but also to educate patients on how to prevent health problems in the first place. Below you will find some important tips to help you educate patients on how to maintain good health.

1. Read labels on house and garden chemicals. Crosscontamination is common and can lead to accidental self-poisonings. Patients should carefully follow instructions on the handling of chemicals especially around children and pets. Use gloves, masks, and eye protection when recommended. When possible use nontoxic, biodegradable products in and around the home.
2. Turn down the volume. Noise pollution is real and can cause permanent hearing damage. Use ear plugs when working with loud equipment and when attending loud concerts (9).
3. Use a carbon monoxide detector in your home. Carbon monoxide can leak from faulty heaters and is produced from the exhaust of cars. Detectors are inexpensive and easy to install.
4. Know the hazards of your job. All businesses are required to have an MSDS file of the known chemicals used on a job site. Encourage patients to ask their employer for a copy of this information to include with their chart.
5. Immediately deal with any water leakage in the home. Look for any signs of mold (commonly found in wet areas around washing machines, windows, and bathrooms). Remove all mold from your home (10).
6. Keep chemicals and medications out of reach of children. Use child-proof locks on all accessible cabinets that contain household cleaners/chemicals.
7. Don't smoke/don't allow others to smoke around you. There are over 4,000 known chemicals in tobacco smoke, and it is a known carcinogen.
8. Allergy sufferers and asthmatics should consider using an air purifier in their homes. Use dust mite covers on pillows and bedding. Avoid being outside, and exercising outside

when air pollution levels are rated as high; this is especially important for young children with asthma (11–15).
9. Wash your hands. Many diseases such as the common cold, flu, and diarrheal diseases are passed passively by people touching bacteria- or virus-laden objects, and then introducing those pathogens into their own system, or contaminating venues affecting many people, such as a food buffet. Hand washing after using the bathroom or changing an infant's diaper is common knowledge, but reminding your patients can be helpful. Alcohol-based hand sanitizers and plain soap and water will kill the majority of these pathogens.
10. Be careful with the use of pesticides around and in your home. Extreme caution should be used when applying insect repellents to children. They should never be applied over open wounds, or directly to the face or hands. Use the smallest amount possible, and never under clothing.
11. Use sun block. Apply according to instructions and repeat the application if remaining outdoors for an extended period of time or after getting wet. Even waterproof sunscreens need to be reapplied after prolonged time in the water. Use age-appropriate sun block.
12. Eat a healthy balanced diet with plenty of fresh fruits and vegetables. If a patient is eating a strict vegan diet, supplements may be needed to get all the basic nutrients required, especially for young children. Vegetable protein can be less bioavailable than animal protein sources. The average adult should be getting approximately 0.9 g of protein per day per kilogram of weight, and the protein sources used should be able to provide all of the essential amino acids needed.
13. Use caution when visiting the beach. It can pose serious health threats to the young, old, and those with a compromised immune system from contaminated water. Patients should always pay attention to signs for beach closures due to pollution and bacterial contamination (16).
14. Grow plants. Plants have been shown to help reduce toxins in the environment, and they make and release oxygen into the air.

SUMMARY

Every individual on this planet is impacted by their environment. Sometimes that impact moves us toward health, and sometimes toward illness. A complete patient history, taking into account the potential environmental impact, along with a thorough physical exam will give you the information you need to come up with a functional differential diagnosis. Every patient encounter is an opportunity to counsel patients on how to improve their quality of life. Always include "Patient Education" on environmental issues; it will go a long way toward helping your patients have the happy healthy life they deserve.

REFERENCES

1. Wright L. Looking deep, deep into your genes: discoveries about the impact of the environment on our DNA could revolutionize our concept of illness. *Onearth* 2007; 29(2):32–35.
2. Newman J, Aucompaugh AG, Schell LM, et al. PCBs and cognitive functioning of Mohawk adolescents. *Neurotoxicol Teratol* 2006;28:439–445.
3. Lin CM, Li CY, Mao IF. Increased risks of term low-birth-weight infants in a petrochemical industrial city with high air pollution levels. *Arch Environ Health* 2004;59(12):663–668.
4. Daly G. Hundreds of man-made chemicals—in our air, our water, and our food—could be damaging the most basic building blocks of human development. *Onearth* 2006;27(4):20–27.
5. George CM, Smith AH, Kalman DA, et al. Reverse osmosis filter use and high arsenic levels in private well water. *Arch Environ Occup Health* 2006;61(4):171–175.
6. Yeoh B, Woolfenden S, Wheeler D, et al. Household interventions for prevention of domestic lead exposure in children (Protocol). *Cochrane Database System Rev* 2006;(2):CD006047. Doi: 10.1002/14651858.CD006047.
7. Aas RW, Holte KA, Moller A. Worksite intervention for neck and back disorders in workers (Protocol). *Cochrane Database System Rev* 2005;(4):CD005498. Doi: 10.1002/14651858.CD005498.
8. Guidotti TL. Environmental and occupational health: a "critical science" [Editorial]. *Arch Environ Occup Health* 2005;60(2):59–60.
9. Kateman E, Verbeek J, Morata T, et al. Interventions to prevent occupational noise induced hearing loss (Protocol). *Cochrane Database Syst Rev* 2007;(1):CD006396. DOI: 10.1002/14651858.CD006396.
10. Cummings KJ, Van Sickle D, Rao CY, et al. Knowledge, attitudes, and practices related to mold exposure among residents and remediation workers in posthurricane New Orleans. *Arch Environ Occup Health* 2006;61(3):101–108.
11. Sheikh A, Hurwitz B, Shehata Y. House dust mite avoidance measures for perennial allergic rhinitis. *Cochrane Database Syst Rev* 2007;(1):CD001563. DOI: 10.1002/14651858.CD001563.pub2.
12. Lee JT, Son JY, Kim H, et al. Effect of air pollution on asthma-related hospital admissions for children by socioeconomic status associated with area of residence. *Arch Environ Occup Health* 2006;61(3):123–130.
13. Cakmak S, Dales RE, Judek S. Respiratory health effects of air pollution gases: modification by education and income. *Arch Environ Occup Health* 2006;61(1):5–10.
14. Eiswerth ME, Douglass Shaw W, Yen ST. Impacts of ozone on the activities of asthmatics: Revisiting the data. *J Environ Manage* 2005;77(1): 56–63.
15. Millstein J, Gilliland F, Berhane K, et al. Effects of ambient air pollutants on asthma medication use and wheezing among fourth-grade school children from 12 Southern California Communities Enrolled in The Children's Health Study. *Arch Environ Health* 2004;59(10): 505–514.
16. Dwight, RH, Fernandez LM, Baker DB, et al. Estimating the economic burden from illnesses associated with recreational coastal water pollution—a case study in Orange County, California. *J Environ Manage* 2005;76(2):95–103.
17. NIH Publication #02–5081 Health. The National Institute of Environmental Health Sciences (NIEHS). NIEHS is one of the National Institutes of Health departments within the U.S. Department of Health and Human Services.
18. Clarke CC, Mowat FS, Kelsh MA, et al. Pleural plaques: a review of diagnostic issues and possible nonasbestos factors. *Arch Environ Occup Health* 2006;61(4):183–192.
19. Wu T, Bhanegaonkar AJ, Flowers JW. Blood concentrations of selected volatile organic compounds and neurobehavioral performance in a population-based sample. *Arch Environ Occup Health* 2006;61(1): 17–25.

24 Osteopathic Medicine within the Spectrum of Allopathic Medicine and Alternative Therapies

JOHN M. MCPARTLAND

KEY CONCEPTS

- The primary care physician (PCP) works with an interdisciplinary health team that includes allied health professionals (e.g., nurses, dentists, physical therapists, etc.) as well as practitioners of complementary and alternative medicine (CAM), such as acupuncturists, naturopaths, and massage therapists.
- Osteopathic physicians are uniquely poised to integrate osteopathic principles and practices with the care provided by allopathic physicians and CAM practitioners, creating a system of integrative medicine.
- Sources of reliable information regarding the risks and benefits (safety and efficacy) of CAM therapies are available. The physician should develop guidelines for choosing local CAM practitioners and formulate a referral strategy.

INTRODUCTION

Treating the person as a whole includes the whole of the patient's "health care team." Interacting with other providers becomes imperative when the osteopathic physician serves as the primary care physician (PCP). Since the majority of osteopathic physicians serve as PCPs, this chapter comes from the PCP perspective. The patient's interdisciplinary health team includes physicians (osteopathic and allopathic) and allied health professionals such as nurses, dentists, podiatrists, physical therapists, occupational therapists, psychologists, social workers, counselors, and registered home health aides. Patients frequently employ complementary and alternative medicine (CAM) practitioners, such as chiropractors, naturopaths, acupuncturists, homeopaths, midwives, and massage therapists. Lastly, patients may self-prescribe Over The Counter (OTC) drugs, dietary supplements, and medicinal herb preparations. The physician must obtain a history of the patient's CAM practitioners and self-prescribed CAM modalities, and document that history. Patients frequently fail to disclose CAM use, so the physician should make specific queries regarding CAM. The patient's attitudes toward other practitioners can be gauged by verbal and nonverbal clues (e.g., tone of voice, body posture, eye contact). Ask the patient or a family member to bring in all pharmaceuticals and nutraceuticals for review.

Osteopathic physicians are uniquely poised to integrate osteopathic principles and practices (OPP) with the care provided by allopathic physicians and CAM practitioners, creating a system of *integrative medicine*. This chapter describes the interactions between osteopathic physicians, allopathic practitioners, and CAM health care providers, delivered within a historical context. For a book-length description of these interactions, see Gevitz (2004).

Allopathic Medicine

Allopaths were initially forbidden to associate with osteopaths or accept patient referrals from osteopaths. Finally in 1961, the AMA Judicial Council deemed it ethical for MDs to work with DOs. After the AMA quit attacking osteopathy, it tried co-opting the profession by assimilation. This danger loomed in the California merger debacle during the 1960s. Another act of integration by the AMA—the sanctioning of mixed-staff hospitals—contributed to the decline of osteopathic hospitals. Of the 127 osteopathic hospitals accredited by the American Osteopathic Association (AOA) in 1974, only 59 remained in 1999 (Gevitz, 2004). A new assimilation threat began in 1968 when the AMA opened its residency programs to DOs. Thus, association and assimilation have posed a double-edged sword. Will the integration of OPP with allopathic medicine endanger our unique osteopathic identity? Dr. Still was wary of integration, "Medicine and osteopathy as therapeutic agencies have nothing in common either theoretically or practically, and only an inconsistent physician will attempt to practice both" (Still, 1903).

Nevertheless, within Dr. Still's lifetime, osteopathic physicians began integrating OPP with allopathic approaches. Arguably, some allopathic approaches may inform and reinforce OPP. Certainly, the integration of reductionist allopathic research methods by J. Stedman Denslow, D.O., led to breakthroughs in understanding the "osteopathic lesion" or somatic dysfunction. These advances, in turn, sped innovations in osteopathic manipulative treatment (OMT), such as the development of muscle energy technique (MET), functional and counterstrain techniques, and even (at least in part) osteopathy in the cranial field. The allopathically derived philosophy of "evidence-based medicine" has been embraced by many osteopathic physicians (see Chapter 32).

In contrast, J. Martin Littlejohn exported Dr. Still's staunch antiallopathic paradigm to England. He established the British School of Osteopathy (BSO) in 1915. One may speculate that "carrying the torch of osteopathy" by spurning allopathic-flavored advancements hampered osteopathic evolution in England. Indeed, when this author introduced MET into the curriculum at the New Zealand osteopathic school in 2001, former BSO faculty in New Zealand were unfamiliar with many MET concepts. The former BSO personnel taught articulatory techniques and were inexperienced in counterstrain, myofascial release, and many cranial concepts.

As American DOs have integrated allopathic approaches, some American allopaths have adopted OPP approaches. Holistic medicine has become an allopathic specialty! The American Board of Holistic Medicine was established in 1996 and currently seeks affiliation with the American Board of Medical Specialties. Allopathic physicians have long employed manipulative treatment as a procedure. In 1955, an AMA committee that investigated osteopathic education had reported, "The use of manipulative therapy is decreasing in colleges of osteopathy and is increasing in the orthopedic and physiatry departments of medical schools" (Cline, 1955). Ironically, many osteopathic physicians use OMT-style techniques developed by allopaths, such as Travell and Simons' approaches to myofascial triggerpoints (Kuchera and McPartland, 2002). *Principles of Manual Medicine*, 3rd ed., by Philip Greenman, a well-regarded osteopathic text, highlights proprioceptive rehabilitation developed by Vladimir Janda, M.D. (to whom that book is dedicated).

COMPLEMENTARY AND ALTERNATIVE MEDICINE

Widespread American use of CAM promoted federal funding of the Office of Alternative Medicine (OAM) in 1991, which soon enlarged into the National Center for CAM (NCCAM). NCCAM defines CAM as a group of diverse medical and health care systems, practices, and products that are not presently considered to be part of conventional medicine. The list of what is considered to be CAM changes continually, as therapies that are proven to be safe and effective become adopted into conventional health care and as new approaches to health care emerge (NCCAM, 2007). Many CAM practices employ manipulative and body-based techniques (McPartland and Miller, 1999).

Is osteopathic medicine alternative? This debate has raged in the *Journal of the American Medical Association* (*JAMA*) and the *Journal of the American Osteopathic Association* (*JAOA*) (McPartland, 1999a,b). After the AMA dropped osteopathy from its list of medical cults in 1961, DOs lost their "alternative" identity in many people's minds. One of the first comprehensive reference works on alternative medicine did not mention osteopathic medicine in its otherwise encyclopedic coverage of CAM modalities (Bauman et al., 1978). To show how osteopathic medicine straddles the divide between allopathic medicine and CAM, the NCCAM classifies osteopathic physicians as "conventional medical providers," while it designates OMT as a CAM technique (NCCAM, 2007).

The AOA initially distanced itself from the OAM and NCCAM. In 1995, the First International Congress on Alternative and Complementary Medicine featured an "osteopathy workshop" led by an allopathic physician, Peter Bower, M.D. The AOA changed its position in 2001, and the Bureau of Osteopathic Clinical Education and Research facilitated research collaborations with NCCAM. NCCAM has awarded multiple grants to the Osteopathic Research Center.

RELATIONS WITH CHIROPRACTORS

The AMA waged a fierce war against chiropractic, the largest CAM profession. The chiropractic profession eventually countered with a federal antitrust suit, which the AMA lost in 1990 and paid damages. Early osteopaths distrusted chiropractors, calling them plagiarists. The AOA teamed with the AMA to defeat the initial chiropractic-licensing bills (Norman, 1912). The DOs softened their stance, however, and by the 1980s DOs were granting hospital privileges to chiropractors at Doctors Hospital in Detroit and the Seattle Osteopathic Hospital (Wardwell, 1992). Research collaborations between osteopathic colleges and chiropractic schools began in 1993 (McPartland et al., 1997). In 2005, the AOA officially recognized that chiropractors, naturopaths, acupuncturists, homeopaths, and numerous other nonphysician clinicians have unique and valid roles in health care (AOA, 2007). The very existence of this chapter you are reading attests to the acceptance of CAM by AOA leadership.

REFERRAL PATTERNS

Interactions between providers, in the form of referrals and consultations, necessitate effective communication. Residency programs provide training in the physician-to-physician referral process. Web-accessible primers are available (e.g., Harris, 1998). The consultation letter from an osteopathic specialist to an allopathic PCP calls for particular attention; referring physicians may be hypersensitive to perceived arrogance by a consultant (Greene et al., 2006). OMT specialists have a special opportunity to provide evidence-based education in their consultation letters. Consultation letters can be improved by including problem lists, patient-centered assessments, prognostic statements, contingency plans, and the clear enunciation of consultants' reasoning behind further tests and changes to current management (Scott et al., 2004). Use of structured letter templates may facilitate the consistent inclusion of key information to referring physicians.

Increasing use of CAM makes it crucial that the physician formulate a referral strategy both clinically sound and ethically appropriate. The physician's first step is with the patient, fostering open communication and a nonthreatening environment, enabling the patient to enlist the physician as an ally. Choosing a CAM modality requires a balance between the patient's preferences and evidence to the contrary. A framework for choosing a CAM modality was developed by Adams et al. (2002). The major relevant issues included the severity and acuteness of illness; the curability of the illness by conventional forms of treatment; the associated side effects of the conventional treatment; the evidence of efficacy and safety of the desired CAM treatment; the level of understanding of risks and benefits of the CAM treatment combined with the patient's knowing and voluntary acceptance of those risks; and the patient's persistence of intention to use CAM therapies.

Once a specific CAM modality has been chosen, the next step is finding the right practitioner. Considerations include patient recommendations, advice from colleagues, and verification of the CAM practitioner's licensure. In the absence of licensure requirements, the PCP should open a dialog with the practitioner and ask about duration of training, CAM certification, and membership in professional societies (Frenkel and Borkan, 2003). Collaborating with CAM practitioners in a professional manner will be in the patient's best interests. The PCP who refers a patient to a CAM practitioner is responsible for ensuring the practitioner's competency and safety. With time, the PCP will develop a list of trusted CAM practitioners in the community. The PCP should monitor the results of the referral and schedule periodic reviews with the patient. Additional guidelines for choosing CAM practitioners are available (see the NCCAM and Rosenthal Center Web sites cited below). Fully integrated clinics and hospitals need to establish policies governing CAM practitioners' credentialing and hiring, scope of practice, informed consent, and malpractice liability (Cohen et al., 2005).

The final consideration is cost. CAM therapies are rarely reimbursed by third-party payors. Few CAM modalities are included in the *Resource-Based Relative Value Scale* (*RBRVS*), which Medicare and Health Maintenance Organization (HMOs) use to determine provider reimbursement schedules. And listing in the *RBRVS* does not guarantee reimbursement; OMT gained inclusion in 1998, but OMT specialists still struggle with some private insurers and managed care entities. Most third-party payors accept claims from chiropractors. The FDA stopped classifying acupuncture needles as "experimental devices," thus facilitating reimbursement. Homeopathy and herbal medicine consultations may be reimbursed if the practitioner is licensed as a physician or holding another license allowing the prescription of drugs.

EVALUATING CAM USE

Your patient may have already seen a CAM practitioner, or taken herbal compounds, or ask for advice regarding information gleaned from the Internet. Providing advice regarding CAM practitioners follows the steps described above and further behooves the osteopathic physician to become acquainted with CAM practitioners in the area. Recommending source material regarding herbal medicines and other CAM modalities can be more problematic. Books become outdated and Web sites are ephemeral. Some of the best-known references written by CAM "authorities" are frighteningly biased (McPartland, 1998).

Herbal remedies and dietary supplements may be the most important CAM modalities to understand, because they act pharmacologically and may interact with conventional medications. In contrast, homeopathic remedies employ an "energetic" activating force, rather than a pharmacologic one, and will not crossreact with medications (albeit indirectly, if they ill-advisedly replace allopathic medications). Attitudes toward herbal remedies are often polarized into two extremes: some people believe that herbs are simultaneously *dangerous* and *clinically ineffective* (in other words, all side effect and no benefit). Other people naïvely believe that herbs are *always curative* and *incapable of causing harm* (all benefit and no side effects). Of course, neither extreme is true. Perhaps the best evidence-based text for busy physicians is *The 5-Minute Herb & Dietary Supplement Consult* (Fugh-Berman, 2003).

Although Web sites can be ephemeral things, reliable online sources of information regarding CAM modalities include:

- NCCAM (http://nccam.nih.gov/),
- Cochrane Collaboration (www.cochranelibrary.com/clibhome/clib.htm),
- Bandolier (www.medicine.ox.ac.uk/bandolier/),
- Clinical Evidence (www.clinicalevidence.com/ceweb/conditions/index.jsp),
- TRIP Database (www.tripdatabase.com/),
- Rosenthal Center (www.rosenthal.hs.columbia.edu/),
- PubMed (www.ncbi.nlm.nih.gov/sites/entrez).

Several of these sources are proprietary and require subscription fees, so access may be an issue. PubMed may be insufficient as a standalone search engine for retrieval of CAM information; McPartland and Pruitt (2000) showed that PubMed yielded only a third of published clinical trials regarding saw palmetto that were located in an expanded literature search. Nevertheless, using PubMed as a search engine may be preferable to general search engine portals (e.g., Google), which typically access low-level pages that are not peer reviewed. The Internet is saturated with both good and bad health information, and studies have shown that consumers are not good judges of quality (Greenberg et al., 2004). Judging the accuracy of CAM information is uniquely challenging because CAM is generally not supported by biomedical literature. Some Internet sites clearly state they have instituted peer review processes, and these sites are preferable.

SUMMARY

In *Medical Economics*, a physician with both MD and DC degrees proclaimed, "The most valuable degree is one I don't have: the DO… They have it all: pharmacology, surgery, and manipulation" (Gilley, 1989). Osteopathic medicine has grown in recognition and prestige, especially within the past 30 years. Osteopathic practitioners now find themselves where several worlds collide. One world, allopathic medicine, holds sway with its pharmaceutical- and government-funded dominance. Yet at the same time, allopathic practitioners are losing the confidence of the American public. Another world, CAM, generates little gravitational force within the "medical-industrial complex," but a rising number of Americans trust and support CAM practitioners. Osteopathic physicians are uniquely prepared to integrate allopathic medicine and CAM within our unique OPP art and science.

REFERENCES

Adams KE, Cohen MH, Eisenberg D, et al. Ethical considerations of complementary and alternative medical therapies in conventional medical settings. *Ann Intern Med* 2002;137(8):660–664. Available at: www.annals.org/cgi/reprint/137/8/660.pdf.

American Osteopathic Association. Position paper: non-physician clinicians, 2007. Available at: https://www.do-online.org/index.cfm?PageID=aoa_position.

Bauman E, Brint A, Piper L, et al., eds. *The Holistic Health Handbook*. Berkeley, CA: And/Or Press, 1978.

Cline JW. Report of the committee for the study of relations between osteopathy and medicine. *JAMA* 1955;158:736–742.

Cohen MH, Hrbek A, Davis RB, et al. Emerging credentialing practices, malpractice liability policies, and guidelines governing complementary and alternative medical practices and dietary supplement recommendations: a descriptive study of 19 integrative health care centers in the United States. *Arch Intern Med* 2005;165(3):289–295. Available at: http://archinte.ama-assn.org/cgi/content/full/165/3/289

Frenkel MA, Borkan JM. An approach for integrating complementary-alternative medicine into primary care. *Fam Pract* 2003;20(3):324–332. Review. Available at: http://fampra.oxfordjournals.org/cgi/reprint/20/3/324

Fugh-Berman A. *The 5-Minute Herb & Dietary Supplement Consult.* Philadelphia, PA: Lippincott Williams & Wilkins, 2003.

Gevitz N. *The DOs: Osteopathic Medicine in America.* 2nd Ed. Baltimore, MD: Johns Hopkins University Press, 2004.

Gilley LD. An MD-DC tells what you can learn from chiropractic. *Med Econ* 1989;66:136–143.

Greenberg L, D'Andrea G, Lorence D. Setting the public agenda for online health search: a white paper and action agenda. *J Med Internet Res* 2004;6(2):e18.

Greene BR, Smith M, Allareddy V, et al. Referral patterns and attitudes of primary care physicians towards chiropractors. *BMC Complement Altern Med* 2006;6:5. Available at: www.biomedcentral.com/1472-6882/6/5

Harris ED. Learnable skills: guidelines for referring physicians and consulting physicians. Stanford University Medical Staff Update, 1998. Web site: http://med.stanford.edu/shs/update/archives/feb98/harris.htm

Kuchera ML, McPartland JM. Myofascial trigger points as somatic dysfunction, pp. 1034–1050 In: Ward R, Ed. *Foundations for Osteopathic Medicine.* 2nd Ed. Baltimore, MD: Lippincott Williams & Wilkins, 2002:1472 pp.

McPartland JM. Book review: the alternative medicine handbook. *JAMA* 1998;280:1635–1636.

McPartland JM. Is osteopathic medicine "alternative"? *JAMA* 1999a;281:1893.

McPartland JM. Is osteopathy "holistic"? *J Am Osteopath Assoc* 1999b;99:239–240.

McPartland JM, Brodeur R, Hallgren RC. Chronic neck pain, standing balance, and suboccipital muscle atrophy. *J Manipulative Physiolog Ther* 1997;21(1):24–29.

McPartland JM, Miller B. Bodywork therapy: a review of system. *Phys Med Rehabil Clin N Am* 1999;10:583–602.

McPartland JM, Pruitt PL. Benign prostatic hyperplasia treated with saw palmetto: a literature search and an experimental case study. *J Am Osteopath Assoc* 2000;100:89–96.

National Center for Complementary and Alternative Medicine, 2007. What is CAM? Web site: http://nccam.nih.gov/health/whatiscam/

Norman PK. Chiro bill vetoed. *JAOA* 1912;12:429.

Scott IA, Mitchell CA, Logan E. Audit of consultant physicians' reply letters for referrals to clinics in a tertiary teaching hospital. *Intern Med J* 2004;34(1–2):31–37.

Still AT. What will become of the MD DO? *J Osteopathy* 1903;10:366.

Clinical Decision Making

ROBERT A. CAIN

KEY CONCEPTS

- The former "art" of practicing medicine has given way to the more modern "clinical decision making."
- This transition represents a comprehensive process of evaluation, testing, resource utilization, and demonstration of treatment effectiveness.
- The extensive evaluation and treatment options of today were not available to our predecessors.
- The physician impact on the health care system requires knowledge of and attention to the reimbursement process.
- Physicians are increasingly asked to demonstrate improvement and outcomes in practice and within the health care system.

INTRODUCTION

Let us begin with a few questions that we will attempt to answer as this chapter progresses. Is clinical decision making the same as making a diagnosis? If not, then what is clinical decision making? How is clinical decision making today different from the past? How do the daily activities of a physician impact clinical decision making?

Probably no aspect of a practicing physician's day is more important than decision making, yet it is perhaps least studied by members of the profession. Although an increasingly important part of medical practice, few physicians have any type of formal training in the decision-making process (1). Despite this, reality is that our daily choices as physicians drive outcomes related to quality, safety, and cost.

TEACHING DECISION MAKING

It can be difficult to teach decision making in a way that makes for an interesting classroom experience. This should not come as a surprise given the topic is not "the stuff" that makes medicine or surgery interesting. For most trainees, a practical approach emerges during residency, as few individuals have an interest in regularly applying rigorous methods to or mastering the conceptual theories behind clinical decision making.

There is little evidence to support that practicing physicians read about or take courses on decision making. In fact, few continuing medical education courses teach critical thinking skills. Experience alone appears to account for the improvement in decision making by individual physicians that occurs over time. A three-question survey was recently conducted of thirty career emergency medicine physicians who work in a setting where decision-making complexity and level of uncertainty are potentially the highest in medicine (1). The survey asked about the last time they read a journal article or book explicitly on decision making, if they read the *Journal of Medical Decision Making*, and how important they thought decision making was in their practice. The results are found in Box 25.1.

Clinical decision making is the effective use of information to implement an effective plan of care. Quite simply, it is the "critical thinking" or processing of information that comes after a stimulus (the patient presentation) and before a response (the testing and/or treatment). This is shown in Figure 25.1, along with what is likely the most common question asked by a physician, "What is happening with this patient?" The information gained from the time-honored completion of a proper history and physical examination is combined with what is learned from other forms of testing and evaluation to guide the development of a final plan of care based upon available forms of treatment. Indeed, clinical decision making encompasses the "art" of making a diagnosis and beyond that it considers the effective use of resources and implementation of the right treatment.

Consider for a moment the expansion of medical and surgical capabilities over the last century. Sir William Osler has been quoted as saying that a patient's history alone can solve many problems encountered in medicine, and this was likely true at the time. In the late nineteenth century, the "art" of making a diagnosis was essentially limited to information elicited from a patient's history and findings gathered during a physical examination. Few reliable tests existed and effective therapies were virtually nonexistent for most conditions.

The practice of medicine has changed dramatically since the days of Dr. Osler, and concerns exist about inadequacies in the training process that has changed far less during the same time period (2). Today, there are at least 26 major specialties in medicine and surgery with a vast number of sub-specialty areas recognized or under development. As a result, methods developed to teach clinical decision making must to some degree be applicable across specialties, requiring us to identify elements common to each.

The potential exists for every physician encountering a patient to have a different perspective on how best to approach clinical decision making. Consider for a moment the story of the six blind men and the elephant (Fig. 25.2). There are many versions of this tale, but the essence is that a group of blind men are asked to describe an elephant using only their sense of touch. Although each man describes well the specific part of the animal he touches, the final picture when the descriptions are combined looks little if anything like an elephant. This old story suggests that reality may be viewed differently depending upon one's perspective.

How often is this true when practicing medicine? It is easy to become focused upon a problem from only one perspective, yours. Such focus limits your ability to solve problems. Perhaps this fact alone supports osteopathic belief regarding the need for a more holistic approach to health care.

Results of Physician Survey Regarding Decision Making

- Question 1—when was the last time you read a journal article or book explicitly on decision making?
    - within the last 6 months: 0%
    - within the last year: 0%
    - within the last 5 years: 20%
    - not since residency training: 80%
- Question 2—do you read the journal *Medical Decision Making*?
    - yes   3%
    - no   97%
- Question 3—how important is decision making to your practice?
    - not very important   0%
    - moderately important   0%
    - very important   100%

There appear to be three critical questions involved with the clinical decision-making process that impact all physicians regardless of their specialty. What is the nature of the problem—acute or chronic? What is the severity of the problem? What information is or is not necessary to appropriately diagnose and treat the problem?

Attempts have been made to loosely describe levels of decision making in medicine (Table 25.1). Such attempts are based upon the complexity of the presenting problem with consideration to the required knowledge and involved skills. Consider for a moment the emergency physician faced with decision making that typically occurs in an acute setting. He or she will likely have limited information and significant time constraints when making a diagnosis. This is a direct contrast to the office-based rheumatologist who will most likely make decisions about subacute or chronic processes. Such a physician will usually have more extensive information at hand and the potential luxury of multiple visits to arrive at a diagnosis and treatment plan. The severity of the problem may be equal for both patients, but the path taken to problem solve will be quite different. A physician whose practice tends to deal with patients described by levels five and six may prefer or be required to use a different method of decision making than one whose patients tend to be described by level two or three.

This suggests that a single method of clinical decision making does not exist. The situation and degree of uncertainty will drive the approach taken by the physician (1). The problem will in general be seen by the treating physician from his or her perspective dependent upon training and experience.

In order to be effective, physicians must be aware of how different forms of decision making impact their specific type of practice, the types of errors commonly seen with each form, and the methods to improve their decision-making skills. It is however not enough to teach physicians what to do as part of some methodical process; we must also teach them what not to do and what to avoid.

The medical education process is undergoing its first major change in almost 100 years (2). Work-hour limitations have recently been placed upon trainees in the United States and abroad. It remains unclear how such changes will impact the resident training process and clinical decision making in the future. The time spent in the operating room has been reduced as a result of the 80-hour work week rule, replaced in many cases by other nonclinical activities (3). The requirements for internal medicine training have changed as well, reflecting decreased inpatient continuity from the limited work hours. Residency training program changes include increased time for ambulatory training, enhanced didactics, and developing skills lab experiences. A decrease in the amount of time spent providing actual patient care may require that we develop new ways to teach decision making. Traditionally, we have relied upon immersion learning within a time-served apprenticeship as the primary method for resident development (3). This is being replaced in almost all teaching facilities by a more formal, structured, competency-based training program.

The work hour limitation reflects a perceived need to protect the public from error as a result of faulty decision making. Quality indicators do exist for some specialties to suggest that workloads exist above which error is more likely to occur. Specifically, such a threshold has been identified in the specialty of radiology with regard to the number of abdominal CT cases interpreted by a physician per day (4). Because of these types of examples, Pat Croskerry, M.D., Ph.D., an expert in the field of decision making, has suggested that the successful decision maker may become the well-rested physician working in an optimized workplace, who is not driven by a pressure to perform, is aware of the most common forms of error and bias, and is able to blend intuition and analysis to the task at hand.

OSTEOPATHIC THOUGHT

What is osteopathic thought and how does it impact clinical decision making?

One of the early concepts taught to osteopathic medical students is the need to avoid focusing on the obvious problem before you as a clinician, and to instead focus on what is often not so

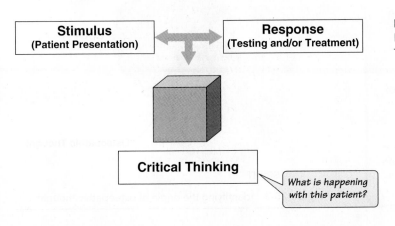

Figure 25-1 Clinical decision making, based upon Stephen R. Covey's *The 7 Habits of Highly Effective People*, 1989.

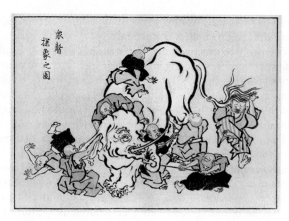

Figure 25-2   The parable of the Six Blind Men and the Elephant.

obvious. This might be stated as, "don't treat the symptom, find and treat the cause."

Our founder Andrew Taylor Still expressed this in another way when he said, "The object of the physician is to find health, anyone can find disease." A conscious choice to make clinical decisions in a manner that promotes and maintains health requires a different thought process than one focused upon treating symptoms and the effect of disease.

It is critical we remember this perspective when developing the patient–physician relationship. The complaint bringing a patient to us may be far different from an unspoken problem actually troubling them. The need to investigate further (and actually doing so) provides us with an opportunity to identify and treat

---

TABLE 25.1

Levels of Decision Making in Medicine

Level	
1	self-evident problem with clear-cut treatment
2	self-evident problem with limited thought about treatment
3	simple problem, requires linear thought with essentially clear-cut decision making
4	narrow differential diagnosis to presenting problem requiring limited medical knowledge and use of testing
5	broad differential diagnosis to presenting problem requiring moderate medical knowledge and more extensive use of testing
6	very broad differential diagnosis to presenting problem requiring complex medical knowledge and extensive use of testing
7	life-threatening problem + any of the above levels

Source: Adapted from Rosen P, et al. *Emergency Medical Concepts and Clinical Practice.* St. Louis, MO: Mosby Year-book, Inc., 1998.

---

something that might otherwise have been missed. There are however a variety of threats to the patient–physician relationship in this current health care environment, including managed care, litigation, decreasing resources, and loss of privacy (5). All of these (and undoubtedly more) have the potential to shift our perspective away from the goal of making good clinical decisions designed to assist our patients with maintenance of their own health. Our decisions and behaviors often send a hidden message that we are treating a disease, offsetting the effects of illness or overcoming bad behaviors, when indeed we should be providing the tools necessary to achieve and maintain an optimum state of health. As an example, consider what a patient imagines an inhaler containing a medication to treat COPD to do when prescribed. Do they believe the inhaler provides them a way to offset the effects of smoking and that the medication is in fact a cure for their problem? In such a case, our message must be clear that the medication is only a bandage covering up the problem by limiting symptoms. The real intervention is the lifestyle change leading to smoking cessation.

Three distinct components are often used to identify the domains within which an osteopathic physician operates. These domains are mind, body, and spirit. Their intersection likely represents what is termed osteopathic thought (Fig 25.3).

It has been suggested that an osteopathic physician should build upon the proposed new tenets of osteopathic medicine when developing an effective plan of care. Simultaneously while doing so, he/she should incorporate evidence-based medicine (EBM), optimize the patient's natural healing capacity, address the primary cause of disease and emphasize health maintenance and disease prevention (5).

It is tempting in the need to be efficient with our time to focus only upon the needs of the body, but research clearly shows that a failure to address underlying mental illness, such as depression, in a patient with chronic disease results in a less-than-optimal outcome (6,7). Such patients are often less compliant and present with varied and less common symptoms, complicating the decision-making process. Although it may be argued by some that treating within the domain of the mind is not their responsibility, it is just as easily argued that professional behavior dictates proper referral and follow-up on subsequent visits as critical to achieving best outcomes. Consultation with another physician for management of mental illness may indeed help to control the primary disease, although arguments can be made about division of care among specialists being less optimal than primary care by one physician.

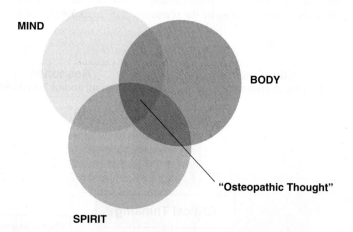

Figure 25-3   Identifying the origin of osteopathic thought.

With regard to the domain of the human spirit, failure to identify the underlying beliefs of a patient may mean a lost opportunity to recognize the critical support systems they are missing or may make it difficult to understand their decisions about testing, procedures or treatment. The end result is that our ability to make effective clinical decisions can be compromised without adequate information.

At least one small study has suggested that communication differences exist between osteopathic and allopathic physicians (8). It is possible these communication differences represent one effect of osteopathic thought. The major differences identified in the *Journal of the American Osteopathic Association* study were associated with psychosocial aspects of patient care. Addressing these critical areas during a patient encounter may help to provide a more complete "picture" as we begin the process of clinical decision making. In fact, the simple act of asking questions or addressing issues of a psychosocial nature may result in an opportunity to provide more complete and comprehensive health care through the development of a stronger patient-physician relationship. Proper research may demonstrate that "osteopathic thought" results in more effective resource utilization for our health care system and improved outcomes for our patients.

The osteopathic approach to patient care is a more complete one if we maintain an ongoing awareness of this mind-body-spirit connection. The primary difference appears to be the amount and type of information gained by thinking within the osteopathic paradigm. Simply put, osteopathic thought creates a different perspective from which our critical thinking takes place.

DEVELOPMENT OF CLINICAL DECISION MAKING

Use your five senses…learn to see, learn to hear, learn to feel, learn to smell and know that by practice alone you can become expert.
—Sir William Osler

For those who argue the practice of medicine can be reduced to branching algorithms, making it pure science to be practiced by an individual using a handheld computer, others note that clinical decision making is an art, blending and balancing science with physician senses.

It is virtually impossible to write about or teach a single method of decision making and expect that it can be applied by every physician and in all types of clinical encounters. Each of the recognized processes has some kind of limitation dependent upon the clinical situation. It is more likely that at any given time a physician may need to call upon one or more of these different processes to deal with an individual patient. However, all too often as a result of constraints placed upon us by a busy practice, shortcuts in decision making become a significant part of physician behavior.

A balancing of physician senses is an important part of the clinical decision-making process. These senses are developed over time and represent tools that are always with us during a patient encounter. The three most important senses are sound, sight, and touch. The first two are critical to the rapid analysis often required of physicians in determining whether a given patient is "sick or not sick" (9). Such an analysis will often guide what kind of a search must follow to elicit additional information and arrive at a treatment plan.

Consider for a moment how hearing can be a critical part of the patient encounter and decision-making process. Is their voice weak? Do they speak rapidly? Does their speech pattern suggest an inability to form cohesive thoughts? From such information we begin to formulate our first thoughts about what is wrong with the patient. The habitual use of empathic listening skills is likely to affect our thinking process as well and as a result provide a better understanding of the patient before us.

Sight is important to identify any number of patient characteristics. Does the patient appear to be in pain? Do they appear anxious? How are they dressed? What is their breathing pattern? Do they engage your gaze or do they look away? Visual sense is a basic part of the physical exam. It contributes to our documentation about the general appearance of the patient and our subsequent decisions.

Although sound and sight can provide us with a significant amount of information about a patient, touch provides a unique opportunity to expand our perspective on diagnosis and to develop the patient–physician relationship. Like our ears and eyes, our hands are readily available to help provide information about a patient. Palpation as a skill is learned early in medical school and is employed in a variety of ways including joint evaluation, point of maximal cardiac impulse, and establishing the presence or the absence of organ enlargement. These are common components of the basic physical examination, but we cannot as osteopathic physicians forget the role of the structural evaluation, perhaps identifying an otherwise unrecognized viscero-somatic reflex. In an effort to save time, the structural exam is often limited or even worse overlooked, an act that may limit our ability to fully integrate osteopathic thought into patient care.

The development of clinical decision-making skills is a continuously evolving process with at least three defined stages—the medical student, the resident, and the experienced clinician (Fig. 25.4).

The student focuses heavily upon what has been termed the hypotheticodeductive method. A very structured pattern is learned and applied to obtaining the history, completing the physical examination, ordering tests, and arriving at a decision (10). Each step guides the next. Early in residency this same pattern is used, but as experience is gained another form of decision making emerges parallel with the hypotheticodeductive method. It is known as pattern recognition or template matching. This form of thinking seems to represent simultaneous information gathering and decision making. It is as if the physician chooses a likely diagnosis based upon expanded use of the senses already described. With the exception of complex cases, pattern recognition often becomes the dominant form of decision making for the experienced physician.

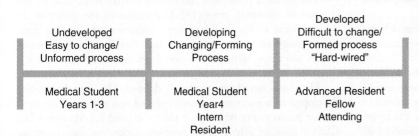

Figure 25-4 Development of the decision-making process.

Undeveloped Easy to change/ Unformed process	Developing Changing/Forming Process	Developed Difficult to change/ Formed process "Hard-wired"
Medical Student Years 1-3	Medical Student Year4 Intern Resident	Advanced Resident Fellow Attending

Effective decision making requires us to be flexible and avoid becoming locked into pattern recognition alone. An over-reliance upon pattern recognition may result in misdiagnosis. It is associated with certain types of errors the clinician should be aware of when making decisions. Unfortunately, the time constraints of practice often force pattern recognition to become dominant. Oddly, this happens at the same time it is demanded we use resource wisely and make choices to limit risk of litigation from malpractice. The "well-calibrated" physician therefore needs to balance their thinking process with task uncertainty (1). Ultimately, the chosen approach must optimize quality and safety for the patient.

It is also important to note that there may be additional methods of decision making across the various medical specialties. Surgical decision making may be somewhat different as a result of the environment within which a surgeon functions. A skilled (developed) surgeon must have situation awareness and be able to rapidly choose appropriate courses of action (3).

It is unlikely that an experienced physician will make a significant shift in his or her decision-making process without some force motivating the behavior change. This directly reflects that a "hard-wiring" of behavior takes place over time and reduces the likelihood that meaningful change will occur. The practicing physician is also faced with other constraints that limit the possibility of change, time being among the most obvious. An understanding of how experienced physicians think combined with the appropriate use of incentives and application of cognitive forcing strategies might help with the development of continuing medical education designed to improve their decision-making process (11). Such an effort is completely different than that required to promote the development of good decision-making skills among medical students, who are yet to become "hard-wired."

COMMUNICATION SKILLS

Clinical decision-making and physician communication skills are closely linked. In fact, good decision making is aided by a strong doctor–patient relationship. The astute clinician readily recognizes that each visit is a new opportunity to question, listen and observe (10).

Attention to the interpersonal component of human communication extends our interaction during a patient encounter to include an understanding of the involved emotions. Such an approach directly reflects what has previously been described as "osteopathic thought" and its attendant association with the psychosocial aspects of patient care. It is necessary that awareness exists of both the emotions of the patient and the physician. A patient detecting a disinterested physician is likely to limit the information provided or may alter their responses in order to answer what they perceive the physician wants to hear (10).

The development and utilization of empathic listening is critical, as a good history still remains the backbone of the decision-making process. Tests should never be substituted for this basic component of patient care hoping that the results will provide the answer. Such an approach is potentially harmful to the patient and wasteful to the health care system (10).

Listening must follow a proper line of questioning. Open-ended questions are far more likely to result in patient-centered answers and are less likely to be leading (10). Permitting the patient an adequate amount of time to tell their story is critical. Some sources have demonstrated that on average physicians stop listening to a patient within eighteen seconds after they have started to speak (12). Limiting the patient as a primary resource for information can easily result in error from misuse of "availability" or the tendency to judge the likelihood of an event by the ease with which relevant examples come to mind (10,13). By way of example, a physician might rapidly decide without adequate information that a patient with cough and fever has influenza, determining this because he has seen four other similar cases throughout the day. This is an example of a heuristic. Heuristics, what otherwise might be thought of as rules of thumb, intuitions, abbreviations, simple judgments and short cuts, are often part of dynamic decision making and represent a form of pattern recognition or template matching (1).

There is growing recommendation to involve the patient in his or her own treatment plan by including them more actively in the decision-making process. This is thought to be important to optimize outcomes and has come to be known as patient-centered care. It requires that we undertake an effort to understand what the patient wants or desires in addition to helping them understand what we are proposing. A patient may view very differently their participation with the decision-making process from that desired by physicians; thus, their involvement should be delineated as the patient–physician relationship is established (14).

There is one other important aspect of communication skills to be considered as it may affect the decision-making process. Physicians must often interact with each other in order to gain additional information that is needed to make a diagnosis and develop a plan of care. This requires an ability to listen and question in a manner that promotes cooperative patient care. When considering collaborative decision making among physicians, there are two factors that can influence the process. These are prediscussion knowledge of the patient and problem and an awareness of each other's knowledge and talents (15).

ERROR AND CLINICAL DECISION MAKING

Despite public perception from legal advertising, errors in diagnosis (misdiagnosis) actually happen in only a minority of cases. Based upon autopsy data, this has been estimated at 15% by A.S. Elstein (10,16). Keep in mind that misdiagnosis is something different from medical mistakes, which are primarily errors of action (10). The majority of errors in diagnosis are due to flaws in physician thinking.

Significant performance variability has been demonstrated among physicians as a whole and within a given specialty. At least one study of radiologists conducted by E. James Potchen, M.D., at Michigan State University demonstrated a variability in agreement of 20% between physicians interpreting a series of sixty chest x-rays (10,17). A 5% to 10% variability was noted when the same radiologist was compared using his or her own interpretation on two separate occasions. The potential "miss rate" was substantially higher depending upon whether the radiologist was asked to "rule-in" or "rule-out" a diagnosis. It might be assumed that the variability represents a difference in the decision-making process associated with a request to find versus to exclude an abnormality. This once again reminds us that perspective affects decision making.

The medical profession has been less than responsive to the concept of admitting error (18). Unfortunately, the ability to do so is critical to successful process improvement. Dealing proactively with error may help us to understand and avoid certain pitfalls associated with time-honored practices used to establish a diagnosis.

Heuristics have been previously defined. The use of heuristics developed as a necessity in medicine and was the approach used by our predecessors when no evidence existed for treatment (1). Clinical problem solving at the time was dependent upon expertise and the needs of the patient. It is only since the advent of rigorous scientific research, especially the development of randomized controlled trials (RCTs), that evidence supporting decision making has emerged. Unfortunately, many variables exist that impact our ability to make good decisions despite the presence of strong evidence supporting any given treatment plan (1).

The term "cognitive disposition to respond" (CDR) has been proposed as an alternative to words with negative connotations such as error, bias, sanction, and fallacy (1). A CDR represents those actions or behaviors likely to have an impact upon the decision-making process, and over 30 types have been identified (1). Examples of these are found in Box 25.2, demonstrating the somewhat whimsical names that have in some cases been applied. Explanations of these are available in work by Croskerry (1) or in the AHRQ glossary (19).

Many of these CDRs are derived from three metaheuristics: representativeness, availability, and anchoring (1). Availability has been previously defined. Representativeness occurs when physician thinking is overly influenced by what is typically true, failing to consider possibilities that contradict their mental template of a disease and attributing symptoms to the wrong cause (19). Anchoring occurs when physicians allow first impressions to exert excessive influence upon the diagnostic process. Although we are taught in training to "trust our first impressions," the bias occurs if we continue to maintain a diagnosis as accurate even when there is evidence to the contrary (19).

The duration of medical practice, gender of the physician, and the type of specialty under consideration may all be associated with certain types of CDR and differences in approach to decision making. Knowledge-based, skill-based, and rule-based errors occur with greater or lesser frequency at different points in a physician's career (1). It has already been stated that emotions can affect our decisions, but what about known personality types? The various medical specialties are associated with personality differences (1). Surgeons have been shown to make decisions about undertaking surgery even when information to the contrary is provided to them (1,20). Certain CDRs have been shown to occur more frequently among women than men suggesting that gender contributes to the decision-making process as well (1,21).

CDRs That May Influence Clinical Decision Making

- Aggregate bias
- Gambler's fallacy
- Premature closure
- Anchoring
- Gender bias
- Psych-out error
- Anticipated regret
- Hindsight bias
- Representativeness restraint
- Ascertainment bias
- Ignoring negative evidence
- Search satisfying
- Availability
- Multiple alternatives bias
- Sutton's slip
- Base-rate neglect

- Omission bias
- Triage cueing
- Commission bias
- Order effects
- Unpacking principle
- Confirmation bias
- Outcome bias
- Vertical line failure
- Diagnosis momentum
- Overconfidence bias
- Visceral bias
- Ego bias
- Playing the odds
- Ying-Yang out
- Fundamental attribution error
- Posterior probability error
- Zebra retreat

It is quite possible that certain CDRs are already hard-wired in the development phase of decision making (1). If so, cognitive forcing strategies might be developed to heighten the awareness of medical students and physicians, potentially teaching ways to avoid predictable problems. Simulation and rehearsal are evolving activities at all levels of medical education that may help us with this process. Simulation and rehearsal programming typically includes a debriefing session that is used to review and learn from performance. The "debrief" session is critical to promote behavior change and accelerate learning. During such sessions, it is possible to focus upon observed CDRs.

HYPOTHETICODEDUCTIVE REASONING

This form of reasoning might be looked upon as a "paper" form of problem solving. Because this method can be time consuming, it is most useful in the classroom for training purposes, but under the right conditions, it also has its place in clinical practice (9).

The most likely situation for this method of decision making to be employed is a nonurgent consultation where a complex diagnosis presents itself. Unfortunately, the health care environment we exist in today discourages long visits with patients (both due to patient volume and financial constraints) and limits practical use of this approach in daily clinical practice. Decision making involving the development of hypotheses is best employed when there is more time or less risk involved allowing for the development of several responses or options (1).

Hypotheticodeductive reasoning represents linear thinking during which a diagnosis is established as part of a progressive exercise in logic. When compared to pattern recognition, this form of clinical decision making begins by asking the question, "What might this be" instead of making the statement, "I know what this is."

This method is commonly employed by trainees where a high degree of uncertainty exists about a diagnosis. The linear thought process allows the trainee to investigate the case and break it into manageable pieces. It is also employed by experienced consultants when the complexity of a case is high. This is especially true if the consultant desires to avoid diagnosis momentum (22). Diagnosis momentum is the tendency to assume that the diagnosis made by previous physicians is correct and then building upon their decisions, potentially propagating established errors.

This form of reasoning integrates Bayes' theorem within the context of the clinical decision-making process. It requires that we have a sense of probability as to the diagnosis under consideration and as to the proper interpretation of test results. Each diagnosis has its own initial probability based on its prevalence. Understanding the concept of prevalence is crucial, because common diseases automatically have a greater initial likelihood than uncommon diseases (23). At least some understanding of sensitivity/specificity and positive and negative predictive values is required in order that test be used appropriately. Such simple biostatistics help to guide steps in the decision-making process by collecting information in a purposeful and logical sequence.

By using Bayes' theorem, hypotheticodeductive reasoning takes relevant information and estimates the probabilities for a wide range of diagnoses (23). It does this repetitively and sequentially as new information is added, eventually leading to the development of what is commonly termed the "differential diagnosis." The process often begins even before the patient is seen, driven by available history, documented chart information, and support staff comments (23).

Consider the following example. A 60-year-old male presents with blue lips and fingers. A series of questions begins to arrive at a diagnosis and develop a treatment plan. The response to each question or result of each test guides the next step. The physician might begin by trying to determine if the finding represents a life-threatening condition. He may ask the patient if he is short of breath, suspecting that a breathing disorder is causing cyanosis to be present. This might be followed by a question to determine if he smokes. A negative response may change the line of questioning, asking next if he has chest pain. While this historical information is obtained, pulse oximetry is found to be normal, prompting the physician to ask how the patient long his lips and fingers have been blue. When the patient responds, "Only since preparing the blueberry pie I just gave to your staff," the line of questioning changes and the importance of good staff communication becomes obvious.

TEMPLATE MATCHING

Template matching represents a "real-time" process with regard to physician decision making. It is most useful at the bedside and especially in urgent situations. It is often visual in nature, although historical information contributes to the decision as well (10). Essentially, the physician is asking, "What does the picture presented by this patient best fit?"

Template or pattern matching is nonlinear reasoning in that "thinking" about the diagnosis begins from the start of the patient encounter (10). The physician is likely to exclaim an almost immediate, "I know what this is" (even if not spoken) instead of undertaking a deeper inquiry to ask, "What might this be?" As such, this is a form of forward reasoning or arriving at a decision even before all information has been gathered (9).

This process relies heavily upon use of shortcuts or what has been previously described as "heuristics." It is acquired rather than taught, meaning that some degree of clinical expertise must be present to incorporate intuition as part of the process (23). The result frames a patient within a certain clinical context. This "pre-establishing" of a diagnosis may lead to certain kinds of errors and less than desirable outcomes in more complex cases.

As an example, think again about the 60-year-old male presenting with blue lips and fingers. If the evaluating physician reacts using minimal critical thinking, suspecting profound hypoxemia as a cause of the cyanosis, a completely different pathway might be followed. The patient might immediately be placed on oxygen and testing undertaken before all the necessary information is accumulated, in this case learning that the effect is the result of having made a fresh blueberry pie. The "preestablishing" of a diagnosis delays identifying the real cause of the patient's presentation, adds cost to the system, and places the patient at risk from unnecessary testing.

Pattern recognition as a form of decision making may lead to a higher rate of error. Such errors can be primary or secondary in nature (22). A primary framing error results from a physician's own flawed decision making from excessive use of shortcuts. A secondary framing error results from a physician accepting and carrying forward an existing diagnosis based upon the decision making of a colleague.

ALGORITHMS

Algorithms have been suggested by quality improvement experts as a means to overcome weaknesses in the health care system as a result of studies suggesting that educational efforts alone do not change physician practice behavior (24,25). The algorithms serve as a form of reminder, helping to guide the clinical decision-making process.

Until recently, these algorithms were added to the practicing physicians approach to patient care as a means to improve outcomes for a variety of inpatient and outpatient conditions.

Now some medical schools have chosen to incorporate a curriculum that focuses upon the use of algorithms to develop in-depth clinical decision-making skills in medical students. The most common presenting signs and symptoms are used as a starting point for patient evaluation.

At least one osteopathic medical school has elected to teach from a curriculum based upon the 120 most common presenting signs and symptoms (26). This clinical presentation model, originally developed in Canada, is now being used by ATSU's School of Osteopathic Medicine in Arizona (27). Each clinical presentation is associated with an algorithm developed to assist the learner toward a diagnosis. Such an approach does create a methodical thought process if followed without shortcuts.

Algorithms use decision trees, typically branching pathways of yes/no and present/absent, to guide the physician through the evaluation process. "Real-time" and "paper" decision making are combined when using algorithms, and it is quite easy to develop computer assistance for this type of process. Both forward and backward reasoning may be included, concurrently recognizing patterns and developing hypotheses.

This type of decision making is commonly promoted by third-party payers believing that it improves outcomes and reduces waste by decreasing over-utilization.

EVIDENCE-BASED MEDICINE IN CLINICAL DECISION-MAKING

> *Weigh evidence and [do] not go beyond it.*
> —Sir William Osler

The development and promotion of EBM principles has introduced yet another approach to clinical decision making. Unfortunately, many physicians in practice appear to misunderstand the potential power of this form of problem solving as they have been exposed to a somewhat skewed version of EBM often promoted by third-party payers. EBM is more than just the identification and use of best evidence. EBM in fact provides a framework for identifying best practices by finding and using best evidence, considering clinical experience and circumstance, and incorporating patient interests when undertaking decision making (28).

Perhaps for the physician, these elements of EBM can be thought of as the legs of a stool (Fig. 25.5). The role of the clinician is to balance these legs in a manner that promotes a best practice. Clinical expertise represents individual experience and recall of collective outcomes. Distant events tend to be less remembered while recent events tend to be more remembered, and bad events are more likely to be remembered versus routine good outcomes. Few

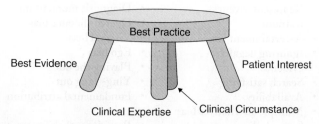

Figure 25-5 Best practice as represented by a level stool with four equal legs.

physicians can objectively ask and assess themselves with regard to the question—how am I performing? (2). This is likely because our selective memory skews the impact of clinical expertise.

Best evidence represents primarily the physician's fund of medical knowledge. This means that best evidence tends to be limited by our individual cognitive abilities and by the always and fast changing world of medical research. While patient interests may seem easiest to understand, we must be aware that strong communication skills are required to obtain information, then adequately educate and inform them about choices and options.

Clinical context or situation is unique for every case and can alter our decision-making process. Best practice can also be defined by the intersection of the four major aspects of EBM (Fig. 25.6). No one aspect alone is capable of defining a best practice.

Evidence as derived from a variety of research sources represents probability (29). Higher levels of evidence as based upon predetermined grading systems can be considered to have greater validity in the decision-making process. Those with the highest levels should in fact stimulate a physician to change practice habits when identified. In general, best evidence utilizes specific information about populations and generalizes it to the individual patient.

Evidence stands in direct contrast to the inference or logic that must be applied when considering clinical context in the decision-making process (29). This is especially true in the practice of surgery, where an individual case may require unexpected and immediate consideration of best practices, expertise and patient interest if an intraoperative emergency arises. Rigorous data from RCTs or other forms of research are often unavailable in such circumstances (29). There is no good method associated with teaching this process. It requires the application of general knowledge to a specific situation.

Clinical experience calls upon the progressive development of a personal reference source for measuring when and how to apply specific evidence, while patient interest may ultimately determine whether or not our decision-making process is applicable to a given situation.

Consider the following example with regard to these four elements of the EBM decision-making process:

An 88-year-old male presents with acute blood loss from a lower GI bleed. The patient has a history of coronary artery disease and complains of anginal chest discomfort. His hemoglobin is 6.0 gm/dL. Best evidence supports the use of blood products to increase oxygen carrying capacity, and clinical experience tells us that use of blood products in this case will likely be of benefit. When you request permission to administer packed red blood cells, the patient informs you he is a Jehovah Witness and unwilling to accept blood products as part of his treatment. Based upon his religious beliefs it is unlikely you will convince him otherwise; thus, in this clinical situation an alternative decision will be required. This results in a return to "point A" of the process. It will require the development of a new clinical question and a new search for best evidence to support another approach to treatment. Since this new treatment may be unfamiliar to you (meaning that you have little clinical experience), patient interest becomes critical in the decision-making process as a result of the specific clinical situation.

Patient safety and quality outcomes are driving forces behind the practice of EBM.

IMPACT OF TECHNOLOGY AND RESOURCE UTILIZATION

Perhaps no area of medicine has been impacted more by technology and the third-party payer system than the physician-patient relationship. The strength and nature of this relationship greatly impacts our approach to clinical decision making, yet it is being challenged on several fronts.

Resource utilization is a new concept faced by practitioners when making decisions about patient care. It requires that we attune ourselves to the value of information gained from a given procedure and treatment while considering the demands placed upon the overall health care system. The greater the intensity of the problem and the longer its duration the greater are the demands upon the health care system.

The most basic approach to patient care and clinical decision making begins with a simple timeline. This timeline has only two points—the beginning of the problem (disease development) and the end of the problem (disease resolution). The duration of the problem (length of the timeline) and other critical points between the beginning and the end (such as onset of symptoms) is unique for each patient and disease process. However, this simple linear model of patient care no longer exists, requiring an expansion of our thinking process in order to be highly successful as a practitioner today. In the current health care environment, clinical decision

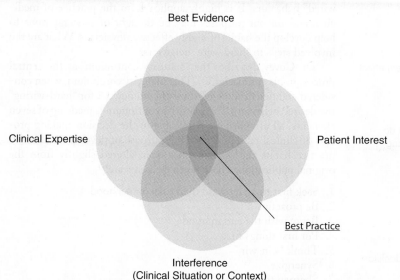

Best Evidence

Clinical Expertise

Patient Interest

Best Practice

Interference
(Clinical Situation or Context)

Figure 25-6 Identifying the components of best practice for optimal decision making.

making is impacted by at least three major elements of resource utilization and these are:

1. Overall outcome for the patient
2. Timing of intervention or treatment
3. Effects upon the health care system

Each of these elements represents a different axis of the decision-making process, potentially creating a three-dimensional framework in which a physician must learn to operate (Fig. 25.7). As described by this framework, there are only two optimum pathways to follow in clinical decision making. These are:

■ Doing something that results in a good outcome and a positive system effect
■ Not doing something that results in a good outcome and a positive system effect

This three-dimensional thinking is radically different from the decision-making process of physicians trained prior to the advent of managed care and pay for performance. Although we cannot lose sight of the dictum, "first do no harm," there are clearly other factors that become important when making decisions about patient care in today's health care environment.

We have progressed from linear thought to this complex arrangement in a relatively short period of time. Initially, our primary interest as physicians relied upon clinical expertise and patient interest. To these have been added best evidence and system interests as well. Although decision making resulting in a good outcome for the patient should still be our primary goal, it is quite possible to be censured for failing to recognize our impact upon the system. In fact, this awareness of our impact upon the "system" is the basis of the systems-based practice competency domain described by the ACGME and AOA as something to be mastered by a resident prior to graduation. Hopefully, this demand will better prepare future graduates to function effectively in practice.

Clinical decision support systems (CDSSs) are interactive computer programs designed to assist physicians with decision-making tasks. The concept is not new, going back to the 1950s before the right technology existed. Based upon a definition proposed by Dr. Robert Hayward of the Centre for Health Evidence, CDSSs link health observations with health knowledge to influence health choices by clinicians for improved care. Such systems can assist with decisions about when we should or should not do something over the course of patient evaluation and care.

Although CDSS may help to limit the adverse impact of our decisions upon the health care system, they should not be a replacement for physician judgment and should not override the primary importance of our role to assist patients to find a state of optimum health.

One other aspect of technology to impact our decision-making process is the sheer volume of information available to us today as a result of the internet and electronic publishing methods. Keep in mind that more information is not always better information. A significant amount of material published is of little use to the average practitioner and a large portion of it is not what we would call "evidence-based," thus raising questions about its usefulness in daily practice.

It is important that we learn to access information from highly valid sources, hopefully filtering relevant from irrelevant in the process. Point-of-care resources are under development that will eventually make possible the almost immediate access to useful filtered information that can impact the decision-making process in a real-time manner.

CLINICAL REASONING FOR OSTEOPATHIC PHYSICIANS

Clinical reasoning for osteopathic physicians (CROPs) is a modern and unique approach to decision making. It was created using various aspects of existing approaches to problem solving with the goal of assisting physicians with decision making in the current health care environment.

CROP requires that certain good habits become "hard-wired" into physician behaviors for life. These behaviors represent the AOA domains of competency and are based upon the model of patient care promoted by the new tenets of osteopathic medicine. It is here that "osteopathic thought" can be used to create a unique approach to decision making for osteopathic physicians, thus setting them apart from their allopathic counterparts.

What is different about CROP? It accepts that there is no one right way to make clinical decisions, yet provides in itself a structured framework for decision making. Its basis is found in the work of Stephen R. Covey, Ph.D. In his highly acclaimed work, *The Seven Habits of Highly Effective People*, Dr. Covey published what has become an internationally recognized approach to effecting change on a personal level (30). This change focuses upon the development of good habits or what we might think of as "hard-wired" behaviors. It is highly applicable to the practice of medicine, and for our purposes may be thought of as suggestions to help develop the habits of highly effective physicians. What are the involved steps to "hard-wire" behaviors?

Dr. Covey describes the "maturity continuum" as the central process in his approach (30). This maturity continuum, when considered and practiced regularly, is the framework for "hard-wiring" the desired behaviors. The maturity continuum is made up of seven elements, all of which are applicable to the decision-making process of clinical reasoning. For the purpose of developing effective practice habits the sequence has been altered slightly from the original publication. These seven elements are:

1. Seek first to understand then to be understood
2. Be proactive
3. Begin with the end in mind
4. Put first things first
5. Think "win-win"
6. Synergize
7. Sharpen the saw

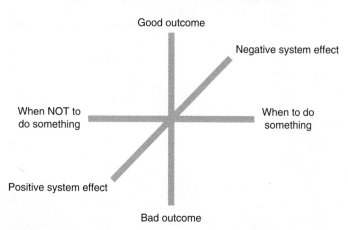

Figure 25-7 Resource utilization elements impacting decision making.

"Seek first to understand then to be understood" occupies the position of central importance in CROP as it is felt to represent the need to develop a strong patient–physician relationship. As previously expressed, this relationship is considered to be critical to the decision-making process. This is the point where empathic listening and speaking become important, as well as the need to be aware of the emotions involved during the patient encounter (the physician's and the patient's). This is the foundation for all of the elements that follow. The component of EBM reflecting patient interest is identified while developing this element during first and subsequent encounters. It is based upon a mastery of the competency domains of professionalism and communication/interpersonal skills.

To "be proactive" represents the critical need to maintain and apply current medical knowledge. It requires not only that physicians maintain a commitment to lifelong learning and incorporate evolving technology or treatments into their practices, but also that they not lose focus upon the osteopathic principles we believe are important to maintaining health. To "be proactive" infers that we make decisions in a methodical manner and work to avoid reactive practices that waste resources and potentially result in less-than-optimal outcomes for our patients. This requires an awareness of best evidence within the context of practicing EBM. It is based upon a mastery of the competency domains of medical knowledge and practice-based learning.

"Begin with the end in mind" represents the needs to understand and communicate the anticipated outcomes and endpoints of any planned treatment. As physicians, we should always understand the desired effect of selected treatments. One way of doing this is to become comfortable with the basic statistical concepts of number needed to treat/harm and positive/negative predictive values. Understanding these values and incorporating them into our clinical decision-making process expands the communication possibilities with our patients. This element is based upon a mastery of the competency domains of medical knowledge and communication/interpersonal skills.

To "Put first things first" represents the need to develop a linear or sequential plan of care. No plan can foresee every need of the individual patient, but population-based studies describe for us the behavior of most acute and chronic problems. Understanding that these often follow a similar path can help us to determine the points at which testing and treatment are best undertaken. This requires the development of clinical expertise within the context of practicing EBM. This element is based upon a mastery of the competency domains of medical knowledge and practice-based learning.

Think "win-win" represents a consideration of the impact our decisions have upon the patient, the practice, and the health care system as a whole. Although it is important to remember that the needs of our patient at the moment must always come first, today it is also important to consider how our decisions affect the patient and the system over time. Such consideration to the rationale use of health care services may help to prevent rationing in the future and in fact may provide physicians with the means to maintain greater autonomy over decision making. This "win-win" paradigm should be considered across the spectrum of decision making from the most basic (whether or not to use an antibiotic) to the most complex (whether or not to start dialysis in a dying patient) choices. This element is based upon a mastery of the competency domain of systems-based practice.

"Synergize" represents the need to view decision making within the context of a team, calling effectively upon other physicians and professionals who contribute to positive outcomes for patients.

The concept of synergy helps us to understand the strengths of the evolving health care team that provides care for patients. It is quite important that physicians (especially the primary physician) maintain a central role as members of this team. All team members should understand that a "project" requires a manager (the physician) to be successful. The idea of patient care viewed as a "project" while initially foreign is actually quite accurate. Project management is defined by cost, time, features, and quality. Indeed, effective clinical decision making requires an awareness of these same components. The function of the physician on the team is critical to balancing a desired outcome (quality and features) with effective use of resources (cost and time). This element is based upon a mastery of the competency domain of systems-based practice.

"Sharpen the saw" is the last element of the maturity continuum. It represents the need for us to maintain our own health if we are to provide proper care to our patients. We are all aware that rapid changes are taking place in the health care environment. For example, the demand upon radiologists has been particularly disturbing as the number of images they view per day rises dramatically, possibly creating a less-than-safe working environment in some facilities (31,32). As previously noted, Croskerry has suggested that the successful decision maker of the future may be one who has an optimized workplace, is well rested, and is not driven by pressure to perform. This element is based upon a mastery of the competency domain of professionalism.

Each of the elements of the maturity continuum represents strong professional behaviors that if practiced habitually can augment the decision-making process. The elements are summarized in Table 25.2. They provide a "hard-wired" template to follow whether dealing with the easiest or the most difficult of cases. The first four elements represent our independent growth as physicians. The remaining three elements recognize that we as physicians are a small part of a greater whole, promoting the concept of interdependence in order to improve patient care. In this manner of thinking, effective patient care as a competency domain results from the mastery and application of all the other domains.

The practice of these habits is critical to the next component of CROP. Physicians must be aware of certain "root activities" where repetitive clinical decision making is prominent. In order to be effective, a physician must also "hard-wire" his or her approach to each of these "root activities" including:

- Admitting a patient
- Caring for a patient
- Discharging a patient
- Dealing with unexpected outcomes
- Communicating with patients, families, and colleagues
- Accessing and using information

Applying a "hard-wired" template to each of these "root activities" provides the greatest opportunity for a successful clinical practice, including a positive impact upon patient safety and quality outcomes.

Once these behaviors and templates are in place, certain primary elements of medical knowledge are required to support good decision making within the context of the CROP concept. These elements should drive our learning process both in medical school and subsequently as practicing physicians. The capable physician should possess a knowledge base that includes the elements listed in Box 25.3.

A strong understanding of disease behavior, especially chronic disease, is essential. This means an awareness of what happens from the point of disease development to the final outcome. The natural history of chronic disease has been previously described and assists

TABLE 25.2

Association of the Covey "Habits," Desirable Decision-Making Behaviors, and the Seven AOA Competency Domains

Covey Habit to be "Hard-wired"	Desirable Impact on Decision-Making Behavior
	Associated AOA Competency Domain
Seek first to understand, then to be understood	Creates strong physician–patient and physician–physician relationships based upon "osteopathic thought"
	Communication and interpersonal skills, professionalism, patient care
Be proactive	Encourages use of current best practices and incorporation of recommended treatment guidelines
	Medical knowledge, practice-based learning and improvement, professionalism, patient care
Begin with the end in mind	Undertakes testing or treatment with clear goals and defines expected outcomes for patients
	Medical knowledge, communication and interpersonal skills, practice-based learning and improvement, patient care
Put first things first	Develops and sequentially carries out well-defined treatment plans
	Medical knowledge, practice-based learning and improvement, patient care
Think win-win	Understands and becomes a part of the health care system by solving problems for patients, physicians, and the community
	Systems-based practice
Synergize	Draws upon the strength of fellow physicians and diverse support staff to create a safe environment providing quality patient care
	Systems-based practice
Sharpen the saw	Recognizes the need to take care of "self" and others by being well rested, optimizing the workplace, and avoiding excessive pressure to perform
	Professionalism

us with this process (Fig. 25.8). Understand that the divisions listed are artificial, but they do provide a generalization of the expected changes over time (23). Appropriate questions must be asked during the clinical decision-making process to recognize where the patient is at any given time with regard to the various stages. Such "thinking" is easily done within the context of timelines and with consideration to several questions:

- How is this disease or problem expected to behave?
- How is treatment expected to work?
- How much improvement do I expect?
- What variations have I seen previously?
- How do outcomes compare to expectations?

Elements of a Capable Physician's Knowledge Base

- Recognizing signs and symptoms or at-risk populations
- Utilizing available screening or diagnostics
- Understanding the course of illness/complaint or natural history of disease
- Adapting therapeutic guidelines
- Undertaking the right procedure or treatment at the right time
- Identifying desired outcomes and endpoints

As osteopathic physicians, our approach to patient care should also include proper attention to psychosocial issues that impact illness and decision making. Maintaining an awareness of the mind-body-spirit connection defines a central core for the successful practice of osteopathic medicine.

The final critical component of CROP is the development of the differential diagnosis. The list of possible diagnoses for any patient may be very limited or it may be very extensive. If we are

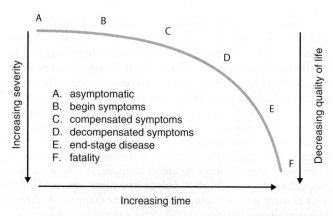

Figure 25-8 Natural history of chronic disease. (Adapted from Rosen P, et al. *Emergency Medicine Concepts and Clinical Practice.* St. Louis, MO: MosbyYearBook, Inc., 1998.)

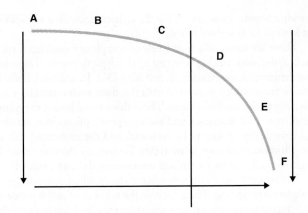

Figure 25-9   Natural history of chronic disease. (Adapted from Rosen P, et al. *Emergency Medicine Concepts and Clinical Practice.* St. Louis, MO: MosbyYearBook, Inc., 1998.)

Differential Diagnosis Descriptors

- **Rule out Dx**—this is the most important diagnostic possibility and represents the greatest potential risk to the patient
- **Probable Dx**—this is the most likely alternative to the primary diagnosis under consideration
- **Possible DX**—this is a closely related alternative, but even less likely based upon presenting information
- **Consider Dx**—this is a possible mimic of the apparent diagnosis and represents variable risk dependent upon many factors; the ability to recognize that it is not the likely diagnosis expands our thought process and our understanding of the patient we are evaluating

not careful, this important step in the "thinking" process can overutilize pattern recognition, resulting in a limited list of possible diagnoses.

Certain descriptors (Box 25.4) are useful for trainees during the previously described "development phase" of clinical decision making to assist with the construction of a differential diagnosis. These same descriptors can also be used to expand the practicing physician's list of possible diagnoses after clinical decision-making practices have been "hard-wired." As such, they can be applied as a cognitive forcing strategy to drive change in the "developed" clinician when performance is less than optimal.

It has been said that the physician of the future will not be successful because of what he or she knows, but rather he or she will be successful because of how they access and use information (33). As we have previously commented, the use of CDSSs and algorithms can successfully replace certain tasks that have traditionally been under the control of the physician. Our place as decision makers will rely upon an ability to problem solve using methods that cannot be replaced by a microprocessor.

CROP is a means to accomplish this role in a successful fashion because of the way it expands our view of decision making. CROP permits us to merge advanced forms of evaluation and technology into a basic process that has little cost, is easy to learn, and has been shown under other conditions (business, leadership, and education) to be reproducible in a variety of settings (30). The "hard-wired" behaviors are with us at all times, unlike CDSSs that are expensive and may not always be available.

In summary, CROP consists of five very specific components that if considered regularly provide a strong basis for effective decision making beyond the simple desire to reach a diagnosis. These five steps include:

1. The physician should develop a "hard-wired" template for thinking comprehensively about decision making (the effective physician habits)
2. The physician should develop a "hard-wired" template to approach the repetitive activities of practice (the "root activities")
3. The physician should develop the primary elements of medical knowledge to better understand disease states, using this as a foundation to be built upon through lifelong learning (the "capability concept")
4. The physician should develop a strong understanding of expected disease behavior (awareness of the natural history of disease)
5. The physician should utilize cognitive forcing strategies to expand the differential diagnosis for a problem under evaluation (the use of differential diagnosis descriptors)

Perhaps if we are able to utilize this approach habitually in our decision-making process we will one day find that our health care system becomes less reactive to medical problems and instead approaches evaluation and treatment in a proactive manner. Such an approach is consistent with both primary care and osteopathic principles. Several studies have shown differences in resource utilization and patient outcomes in areas of the country where such practices are emphasized (34). This suggests that the goals of high-quality patient care and optimal resource utilization are not incompatible. Reactive care is in general costly and offered under crisis situations that well-planned decision making carried out in a longitudinal and methodical fashion might help to avoid (Fig. 25.9).

DOCUMENTATION

One final topic remains to be discussed that is closely related to clinical decision making. It directly impacts our ability to be reimbursed as physicians and is critical to the practice of medicine in the present health care system. The topic is medical decision-making as defined by the third-party payer, specifically the Centers for Medicare and Medicaid Services (CMS) under guidelines produced during the 1990s.

The process of clinical decision-making that we have outlined in this chapter requires translation from our minds to paper in order to create a billable situation for our practices and a permanent record of our actions. The "thought" associated with clinical decision making can be extensive and the associated documentation can easily become overwhelming. It is therefore important to have at least some understanding of the current documentation guidelines as they pertain to medical decision making. This short section is not meant to substitute for extensive works on this topic, but rather to provide a summary of how documentation should be undertaken to express the "thinking" process physicians utilize during a patient encounter.

To begin, it is important to point out that many authorities consider documentation of medical decision making to be the true test for determining the evaluation and management (E/M) level associated with a specific patient encounter. The content of an H&P can be easily upcoded, especially since the development of electronic medical record systems. Complexity of the medical decision-making process and the nature of the presenting medical problem therefore become the most heavily weighted factors determining the E/M service (35). It is important then that we provide adequate evidence within the written document to support the level of E/M service billed.

There are essentially four levels of complexity associated with medical decision making accepted by third-party payers. These are straightforward, low, moderate, and high (36). In addition, there is specific terminology associated with the three main variables contributing to the level of a claim. These three variables are the number of potential diagnoses and management options, the amount and complexity of data to be reviewed, and the associated risk of complication, morbidity, or mortality. To simplify these variables, it might be said that they represent uncertainty, data, and risk (35).

Uncertainty represents a number of things when converting our thoughts into writing. These include the number of problems dealt with during an encounter, how uncertain the physician is about the diagnosis, the number of options for managing the diagnoses, and how uncertain the physician is about which management option to choose (35).

The spectrum of diagnostic uncertainty can be expressed as:

- An already diagnosed problem that is improved or resolved/resolving
- An already diagnosed problem that is inadequately controlled, worsening, or failing to change
- An identified but undiagnosed problem for which the H&P is adequate to establish a diagnosis
- An identified but undiagnosed problem for which additional information is needed

Since documentation of uncertainty relies upon diagnostic possibilities it is important to consider this spectrum, as the level of complexity for billing purposes shifts from straightforward to high based upon these descriptions (35). A single diagnosis involving a stable condition cannot be considered as more than "minimal" based upon the aforementioned spectrum, whereas a new complaint requiring further evaluation significantly elevates the level of uncertainty.

It is best that physicians document what was done to acquire needed information. This should be obvious from the written plan, and at the very least a minimal comment should be added to describe why any testing was ordered (35). Documentation should also be present that addresses the initiation of or any change in treatment (35).

Data as a variable represent a review of information other than that gained from the H&P. This includes test results ordered during the evaluation that you will have to interpret, old records or history from another source (such as family), any discussion with other treating physicians, and personal review of available test data (such as looking at imaging studies).

Risk represents danger posed to the patient resulting from their interaction with the health care system. It does not reflect malpractice risk or risk to the physician and staff. It includes risk associated with the presenting problem(s), any diagnostic procedures requested and management options chosen (35). When developing the risk variable of medical decision making, you should always consider and document co-morbidities and the urgency of the problem. Specific documentation should be included about any planned surgical or invasive procedures. In general, risk is related to the episode being documented and not the long-term risk associated with a diagnosis (35). Risk determination should be based upon what may happen during and immediately following any treatment or testing. Of interest in the stratification process, any visit involving a prescription drug represents at least moderate risk.

How do we use this information in a meaningful fashion?

The problem-oriented medical system described by Lawrence Weed, M.D., nearly 50 years ago is an excellent method for documentation (9). Although the system as a whole has failed to be adopted for a variety of reasons, one component, the SOAP note (an acronym standing for subjective, objective, assessment, and plan) provides a meaningful way to record the patient encounter. Following detailed documentation of the history and physical using accepted CMS guidelines, the documentation of assessment (including a differential diagnosis) and plan easily provides what is needed to meet the requirements of the third-party payers. The assessment should outline the diagnostic possibilities, while the plan should reflect data review (completed or to be accomplished) and risk (based upon the documented testing or treatment). While some physicians choose to separate their assessment and plan others choose to document their plan immediately following each element of the assessment.

Conversion of our thoughts into written words is critical not only to the reimbursement process but also for successful communication between health care professionals. The record of our decision-making process when clear and understandable assists staff and other consultants, enhances transfer of care, reduces inefficiencies in the system, and may help to prevent error.

SUMMARY

We began this chapter by asking a few questions about clinical decision making and then attempting to provide answers to those questions within the various sections. Modern clinical decision making expands greatly upon what has previously been called the "art of making a diagnosis." It is a comprehensive process reflecting not only evaluation and testing, but also resource utilization and treatment effectiveness. One primary difference in clinical decision making today is the extensive evaluation and treatment options that were not available to our predecessors. Of particular note, clinical decision making now requires that we pay attention to the reimbursement process (pay-for-performance) and the impact we have upon the health care system.

Physicians are progressively being asked to show how they are undertaking methods to improve their practice behavior and outcomes (practice-based learning) and how to perform optimally within the health care system (systems-based practice). These two domains of competency directly impact clinical decision making. The development of Good Medical Practice-USA by the National Alliance for Physician Competence has caused the Federation of State Medical Boards to suggest reform of the physician licensure/relicensure process (37). Such changes will hopefully encourage continuing medical education by physicians to better understand how the decision-making process impacts them, their patients, and the health care system as a whole.

In conclusion, probably no other part of a physician's day is more important than the process of clinical decision making. A reasonable attempt by physicians to understand the most common methods of decision making and the errors associated with each can have an impact upon misdiagnosis (safety) and outcomes (quality).

REFERENCES

1. Croskerry P. The theory and practice of clinical decision-making. *Can J Anesth* 2005;52:R1. Available at: http://www.cja-jca.org/cgi/content/full/52/suppl_1/R1. Accessed January 21, 2008.
2. Initiative to transform medical education-recommendations for change in the system of medical education. *Am Med Assoc* June 2007.
3. Flin R, Youngson G, Yule S. How do surgeons make intraoperative decisions? *Qual Safe Health Care* 2007;16:235–239.

4. Fitzgerald R. Error in radiology. *Clin Radiol* 2001;56:938–946.
5. Proposed tenets of osteopathic medicine and principles for patient care. *JAOA* 2002;102:63–65.
6. Katon WJ. The depressed patient with comorbid illness. Program and abstracts of the 154th Annual Meeting of the American Psychiatric Association; May 5–10, 2001; New Orleans, LA. Industry Symposium, Part 2, 43B.
7. Wells KB, Stewart A, Hats RD, et al. The functioning and well-being of depressed patients: results from the outcomes study. *JAMA* 1989;262:914–919.
8. Carey CS, Motyka TM, Garret JM, et al. Do osteopathic physicians differ in patient interaction from allopathic physicians? An empirically derived approach. *J Am Osteopath Assoc* 2003;103(7):313–318.
9. Sprafka SA. *Foundations for Osteopathic Medicine*. 2nd Ed. Philadelphia, PA: Lippincott Williams & Wilkins, 2003.
10. Groopman J. *How Doctors Think*. New York, NY: Houghton Mifflin Company, 2007.
11. Croskerry P. Cognitive forcing strategies in clinical decision making. *Ann Emerg Med* 2003;41:110–112.
12. Communication patterns of primary care physicians. *JAMA* 1997;277:350–356.
13. Tversky A, Kahneman D. *Cognit Psychol* 1973;5:207–232.
14. Fraenkel L, McGraw S. Participation in medical decision making: the patient's perspective. *Med Decis Making* 2007;27:533–538.
15. Christensen C, Larsen J. Collaborative medical decision making. *Med Decis Making*. 1993;13:339–346.
16. Higgs J, Jones MA. *Clinical Reasoning in Health Professions*. Woburn, MA: Butterworth-Heinemann, 1995.
17. *J Am Coll Radiol*. 2006;3:423–432.
18. Kaldjian LC. Disclosing medical errors to patients: attitudes and practices of physicians and trainees. *Online J Gen Intern Med*. Available at: http://www.springerlink.com/content/th831725521204p43/fulltext.html. Accessed February 23, 2008.
19. Agency for Healthcare Research and Quality, M&M Rounds on the Web, Glossary of terms available at: http://www.ahrq.gov/qual/hcq.gloss.pdf. Accessed February 19, 2008.
20. Gaba D, Howard SK, Jump BA. Production pressures in the work environment. California anesthesiologist' attitude and experiences. *Anesthesiology* 1994;81:488–500.
21. Byrnes JP, Miller DC, Schafer WD. Gender differences in risk-taking: a meta-analysis. *Psychol Bull*. 1999;125:367–83.
22. Croskerry P. Achieving quality in clinical decision making: Cognitive strategies and detection bias. *Acad Emerg Med* 2002;9(11):1184–1204.
23. Rosen P, et al. *Emergency Medicine Concepts and Clinical Practice*. St. Louis, MO: Mosby Year-book, Inc., 1998.
24. Smith W. Evidence for the effectiveness of techniques to change physician behavior. *Chest* 2000;118:8S–17S.
25. Millenson ML. *Demanding Medical Excellence*. Chicago, IL: The University of Chicago Press, 1999.
26. ATSU School of Osteopathic Medicine of Arizona, Clinical Presentation Model, SOMA Web site. Available at: http://wwwatsu.edu/soma/medschool_future/curriculum.htm. Accessed February 23, 2008.
27. Mandin H, Harasym PH, Eagle C, et al. Developing a "clinical presentation" curriculum at the University of Calgary. *Acad Med* 1995;70:186–193.
28. Straus, SE. *Evidence-based Medicine: How to Practice and Teach EBM*. 3rd Ed. Philadelphia, PA: Elsevier Churchill Livingstone, 2005.
29. Marshall JC. Surgical decision making: integrating evidence, inference, and experience. *Surg Clin North Am* 2006;86(1):201–215.
30. Covey SR. *The Seven Habits of Highly Effective People*. New York, NY: Fireside, 1989.
31. Sunshine JH, Cypel YS, Schepps B. Diagnostic radiologists in 2000: basic characteristics, practices, ad issues related to the radiologist shortage. *Radiology* 2002;178(2):291–301.
32. Bhargavan M, Sunchine JH. Workload of radiologists in the United States in 1998–1999 and trends since 1995–1996. *Radiology* 2002;179(5):1123–1128.
33. Shaughnessay AF, Slawson, DC. Are we providing doctors with the training and tools for lifelong learning? *Br Med J* 1999;319:1280.
34. Starfield B, Shi L, Macinko J. Contributions of primary care to health systems and health. *Milibank Q* 2005;83(3):457–502.
35. Edsall R, Moore K. Thinking on paper: guidelines for documenting medical decision making. Available at: http://www.aafp.org/online/en/home/publications/journals. Accessed January 21, 2008.
36. Centers for Medicare & Medicaid Services, 1997 Guidelines, Documentation Web site. Available at: http://www.cms.hhs.gov/MLNProduct/Downloads/MASTER1.pdf. Accessed February 24, 2008.
37. Good Medical Practice-USA, National Alliance for Physician Competence, 2007. Available at: https://gmpusa.org/Docs/Good%20-%20Medical%20Practice%20-%20USA%20version%200.1%20final.pdf. Accessed February 24, 2008.

26 Professionalism

KARI HORTOS AND SUZANNE GUIMOND WILSON

KEY CONCEPTS

- As a group, physicians are granted status, autonomy, and the ability to self-regulate.
- A traditional societal contract expects the application of knowledge and skills to benefit individuals and society.
- Additional challenges to professionalism have arisen in the digital age: internet applications, electronic mail, and social networking Web sites.
- Andrew Taylor still taught that each person should be treated as a unique individual, not as a disease entity. Osteopathic physicians have consistently maintained this thought as the core of their professionalism.
- Professionalism is a personal journey for each osteopathic phys
- ician's understanding of how to demonstrate attributes of knowledge, skill, altruism, and duty.

INTRODUCTION

Osteopathic physicians have valued professionalism since the days of A.T. Still. Some authors have suggested that medical professionalism is the cornerstone of the societal contract between the physicians and the public (Whitcomb, 2007). As a group, physicians are granted a status, ability to self-regulate, and to be autonomous in exchange for an expectation that they will use their knowledge and skills to benefit individuals and society. Although there is consensus about the importance of professionalism, descriptions of it vary widely. Each author or organization tends to have a slightly different notion of how professionalism should be defined and the characteristics that comprise it.

To add to the complexity, expectations for professional behavior tend to evolve over the professional life cycle of an osteopathic physician, and recent research is providing greater insight into how subtle differences in demonstrations of professionalism impact patient relationships and outcomes. Additional challenges to professionalism have arisen in the digital age as internet applications, electronic mail, and social networking Web sites have become increasingly popular among physicians (Farnan et al., 2008). For all of these reasons, this is an opportune time to take a systematic look at professionalism as it relates to osteopathic physicians.

Professionalism and Osteopathic Philosophy

Although many of the foundations for osteopathic medicine defined by Still were mechanical in nature, he also taught that each person should be treated as a unique individual, not as a disease entity (Seffinger et al., 2003). A pioneer of holistic health, he developed the four key principles of osteopathic philosophy, one of which being that the person is a unity of body, mind, and spirit. The importance for the osteopathic physician to be mindful of the uniqueness of individual patient needs and the need to maintain a humble attitude when approaching the application of medicine is summarized in Still's basic premise: "It is the patient who gets well, and not the practitioner or the treatment that makes them well" (Seffinger et al., 2003).

The Osteopathic Oath (modified from the Hippocratic Oath in 1938), shown in Box 26.1, also places the health and needs of the patient as the central focus of care; as well as the importance of maintaining the general welfare of the community.

In 2002, the *Journal of the American Osteopathic Association* published a set of principles for patient care to accompany the proposed tenets of osteopathic medicine. These tenets and principles were developed by a multidisciplinary ad hoc committee under the leadership of Felix Rogers, D.O. (Rogers et al., 2002).

The principles of patient care are:

1. The patient is the focus for health care.
2. The patient has the primary responsibility for his or her health.
3. An effective treatment program for patient care is founded on the tenets of osteopathic medicine and
   - incorporates evidence-based guidelines,
   - optimizes the patient's natural healing capacity,
   - addresses the primary cause of disease, and
   - emphasizes health maintenance and disease prevention.

These recently defined principles of patient care further enhance the osteopathic physician's understanding of how to demonstrate the professional attributes of knowledge, skill, altruism, and duty.

Professionalism in the Preclinical Years

At time of matriculation, most osteopathic medical students are typically given some type of document that outlines student rights and responsibilities and communicated expectations about professionalism. For example, at Michigan State University, COM students are "expected to demonstrate academic professionalism and honesty, and to maintain the highest standards of integrity according to a code of honor that embodies a spirit of mutual trust and intellectual honesty" (Michigan State University College of Osteopathic Medicine website, n.d.). Though such guidance is an important beginning, it must be recognized as being unique to the values and culture of the organization that authored them. These early forms of guidance also tend to make a medical student's initial glimpse at professionalism relatively narrow because it relates specifically to one's role as a student and focuses upon academic honesty.

The guidance offered by medical schools on professionalism has been recently expanded as more schools are broadening their institutional policies to specifically address what students should and should not post online (Chretien et al., 2009).

In 2001, the Accreditation Council for Graduate Medical Education ("ACGME") began the "Outcome Project," a long-term

The Osteopathic Oath

"I do hereby affirm my loyalty to the profession I am about to enter.

I will be mindful always of my great responsibility to preserve the health and the life of my patients, to retain their confidence and respect both as a physician and a friend who will guard their secrets with scrupulous honor and fidelity, to perform faithfully my professional duties, to employ only those recognized methods of treatment consistent with good judgment and with my skill and ability, keeping in mind always nature's laws and the body's inherent capacity for recovery.

I will be ever vigilant in aiding in the general welfare of the community, sustaining its laws and institutions, not engaging in those practices which will in any way bring shame or discredit upon myself or my profession.

I will give no drugs for deadly purposes to any person, though it may be asked of me.

I will endeavor to work in accord with my colleagues in a spirit of progressive cooperation and never by word or by act cast imputations upon them or their rightful practices.

I will look with respect and esteem upon all those who have taught me my art.

To my college I will be loyal and strive always for its best interests and for the interests of the students who will come after me.

I will be ever alert to further the application of basic biologic truths to the healing arts and to develop the principles of osteopathy which were first enunciated by Andrew Taylor Still"

(American Osteopathic Association Web site, n.d.).

initiative with increasing emphasis on educational outcomes. Professionalism is one of the general competencies outlined in the Outcome Project described as "a commitment to carrying out professional responsibilities, adherence to ethical principles, and sensitivity to a diverse patient population." They have developed excellent educational resources to aid residency programs and physicians in teaching and assessing professionalism (ACGME Outcome Project Website, n.d.).

The American Osteopathic Association (AOA) quickly followed suit in adopting core competencies. In the AOA version, the six competency areas were accompanied by an additional one: OPP. The AOA also provided more detailed guidance on the core competency of professionalism, adding several required elements to assist in understanding (Box 26.2).

In this guidance from AOA, professionalism encompasses patient advocacy, ethics, collaborative relationships with colleagues; ongoing learning; sensitivity to diverse patient populations; self-health; honesty; confidentiality; and compassion among other things.

Along with graduate medical education, osteopathic medical schools have been required to incorporate the core competencies. Consequently, as medical school progresses, each COM is obligated to teach and evaluate professionalism along with all the other seven required core competency areas. As this occurs, additional descriptors are brought to bear in an effort to accurately capture professionalism so that it can be effectively taught, reviewed, and evaluated. Accrediting bodies and specialty groups contribute additional information by offering their own interpretations and professionalism becomes larger, encompassing a variety of areas beyond the purely academic.

The taxonomy lists for professionalism are abundant and daunting. As shown in Table 26.1, there are many different descriptors

Core Competency of Professionalism

Competency 5: PROFESSIONALISM

DEFINITION

Residents are expected to uphold the Osteopathic Oath in the conduct of their professional activities that promote advocacy of patient welfare, adherence to ethical principles, collaboration with health professionals, life-long learning, and sensitivity to a diverse patient population. Residents should be cognizant of their own physical and mental health in order to effectively care for patients.

REQUIRED ELEMENTS

1. Demonstrate respect for patients and families and advocate for the primacy of patient's welfare and autonomy.

Suggested methodology to achieve compliance:

   a. Present an honest representation of a patient's medical status and the implications of informed consent to medical treatment plans.

   b. Maintain a patient's confidentiality and demonstrate proper fulfillment of the physician's role in the doctor–patient relationship.

   c. Commitment to an appropriate and nonexploitive relationship with patients.

   d. Inform patients accurately of the risks associated with medical research projects, the potential consequences of treatment plans, and the realities of medical errors in medicine.

   e. Treat the terminally ill with compassion in the management of pain, palliative care, and preparation for death.

   f. Participate in course/program (compliance and end of life). Workshops, lectures, bedside, and clinic/office teaching

   g. Role modeling behavior

AOA Report of the Core Competency Task Force (2003)

TABLE 26.1				

Professionalism Descriptors

	AAMC	ACGME	American Board of Internal Medicine, American College of Physicians-XXX (ACP-SIM), European Federation of Internal Medicine	GMC
Accountability		+		
Advocacy/Primacy of patient welfare	+			+
Altruism	+	+		
Appropriate relationships			+	+
Avoidance of conflict of interest	+		+	
Clinical skills/Professional competence	+		+	+
Commitment to excellence/ Quality improvement		+	+	
Communication/Listening	+			+
Compassion	+	+		
Condition managing	+			
Ethical probity/Sound ethics	+	+		
Honesty/Honesty with patients	+		+	+
Improving access to care			+	
Integrity/Trustworthiness		+		+
Knowledge/Scientific knowledge	+		+	+
Patient autonomy			+	+
Professional responsibilities			+	+
Pt. Confidentiality/Patient privacy			+	+
Reasoning	+			
Respect/Treat every patient politely and considerately	+	+		+
Responsiveness to patient needs		+		+
Sensitivity to (patient diversity)		+		+
Social contract			+	
Social justice/Just distribution of finite resources			+	
Work with colleagues to serve patients' interests				+

Source: Inui, T. A Flag in the Wind: Educating for Professionalism in Medicine. Washington, DC: Association of American Medical Colleges, 2003.

of professionalism such as honesty, trust, fairness, respect, personal accountability, altruism, competence, skill, integrity, commitment to excellence (Inui, 2003). Some of these descriptors are objective and amenable to measurement; however, some of them are arguably subjective, difficult to quantify, and open to varied interpretation.

Although we all agree "good physicians" should embody these virtues, the challenge arises with how we should educate, apply, and measure such traits when professionalism (like beauty) is in the eye of the beholder. It is much like trying to teach and quantify love. We as humans agree that love exists, but we have yet been able to establish a tool with which to measure it. Certainly, many attributes of professionalism such as knowledge, academic honesty, and accountability can be identified and measured during the

preclinical years in the academic "course work" setting. However, the true labor of professionalism becomes apparent with the onset of clerkship training and continues to unfold for the duration of the osteopathic physician's clinical career.

Professionalism in the Clerkship and Residency Years

Multiple organizations have offered differing definitions of professionalism. In his landmark publication on professionalism "A Flag in the Wind: Educating for Professionalism in Medicine," Thomas Inui, MD, has condensed the work from the Association of American Medical Colleges (AAMCs) Medical School Objective Project defining the "attributes of the good physician as falling into four large domains—being knowledgeable, skillful, altruistic and dutiful" (2003). The expanded description for each attribute is summarized below:

- Knowledgeable (scientific method, biomedicine)
- Skillful (clinical skills, reasoning, condition managing, communication)
- Altruistic (respect, compassion, ethical probity, honesty, avoidance of conflicts of interest)
- Dutiful (population health, advocacy, and outreach to improve nonbiologic determinants of health, prevention, information management, health systems management) (Inui, 2003)

Medical schools and professional organizations have striven to develop meaningful curricula and evaluation tools to help physicians produce clinicians who will understand and fulfill such societal expectations.

Yet, it must be recognized that the early clinical experiences that medical students encounter in clerkships can be disquieting. They may find themselves thrust into situations where decision making is driven more by insurance restrictions than doing what is best for the patient. When this occurs, they will witness the frustration of their mentors and role models. Quickly, medical students realize that although they are taught that professionalism is important and highly valued, embodying it consistently in clinical situations is not simple or easy at all. Some authors have reported that such early clinical experiences may actually contribute to a decline in empathy (Newton et al., 2008) and moral development during the medical school years (Patenaude et al., 2003). Based on such findings, some authors have voiced concern that more should be done to prevent deterioration during the clinical years in medical school (Branch, 2000; Self et al., 1998).

In a recent article published in Academic Medicine 2007, medical students who are "immersed in learning professionalism, observe that most of the professionalism literature missed the mark" (Brainard and Brislen, 2007). These authors indicate that there is a "hidden curriculum" in the actual practice of medicine that places such issues as efficiency, productivity, or academic hierarchy ahead of the patient's needs. The accompanying cynicism and despair many medical students and physicians describe in response to the "hidden curriculum" are reflections of a grieving process.

The increased use social networking among the technically savvy medical students can also be problematic. "Medical students may not be aware of how online posting can reflect negatively on medical professionalism or jeopardize their careers." (Chretien et al., 2009) The authors suggested including a digital media component in the formal professionalism curriculum to help the student manage their "digital footprint." (Chretien et al., 2009; Gorindo and Groves, 2008).

All of this information should be a serious wake-up call for physicians. It is imperative that we examine the expectations we place on medical students, the impact of their clinical experiences, and what we might do differently to lessen or reverse these negative influences as much as possible.

Professionalism and the Staff Physician

Once a physician has completed residency, obtained certification, and become established in practice, professionalism becomes codified in daily activities. Epstein (2002) wrote "Professional competence is the habitual and judicious use of communication, knowledge, technical skills, clinical reasoning, emotions, values and reflection in daily practice for the benefit of the individual and the community being served." This expansive description captures the multifaceted demands of professionalism in daily practice

and the intention that such activities will enable the physician to benefit society through his or her work. Although all of these aspects are important to professionalism, much has recently been learned in the areas of communication and physician self-awareness, and these areas are summarized below.

Communication Skills

Communication is one of the primary skills for an osteopathic physician's effectiveness in the "art" of medicine. These skills help to elicit a patient's story, promote rapport, influence patients' understanding, compliance, and emotional well-being (Novack et al., 1992). Historically, communication skills were considered to be a "soft" science, something physicians developed "at patients' bedsides, in their rounds as residents, and as students at the elbows of master clinicians" (Traveline et al., 2005). Currently, it is appreciated that many of these skills can be taught and, consequently, this is a focus of learning early in medical school so that baseline skills are present prior to contact with actual patients.

Published literature has long shown the value of effective physician-patient communication on improving health outcomes of common clinical conditions such as headache, hypertension, diabetes, and anxiety (Stewart, 1995). Research has affirmed the importance of communication skills and their effect on health care outcomes for racial and ethnic groups (Ashton et al., 2003); gays and lesbians (Harrison, 1996); and the functionally illiterate (Williams, 2002). Low patient satisfaction scores for hospitalists and emergency department physicians have been documented when communication skills are deficient. Some work has been done on developing targeted sets of communication skills expressly to assist physicians and when implemented, there are indications that this does improve those satisfaction scores (Keller et al., 2002).

Empathy has been measured as a neurobiological response in studies using positron emission tomography. This chapter suggests that "the physicians' use of empathy warrants consideration as a clinical procedure" because of the features of having "a medical indication; a skilled interpersonal performance requiring emotional labor; and an attempted improvement in the patient's psychobiology" (Adler, 2007). Adler (2007) indicates further that the benefits of affective attunement help the patient to feel understood, but also benefit the physician for they foster a deeper understanding of the patient's unique situation and clinical presentation.

As technology has advanced, electronic mail has become readily available as a potential tool for communication between the patient and physician, but ethical, legal, and clinical concerns have been raised about the use of e-mail (Luo et al., 2009) Guidelines for clinical use of e-mail are now available through several organizations such as the American Medical Association.

However important communication may be for special situations, a case could be made that in our current practice environment, improved communication skills are important for all physicians—now more than ever before. In busy practices, physicians face emotionally charged situations, crisis decision making, family contacts, conflicting interests, and much more on a daily basis. Improved listening and communication skills can be a tremendous benefit to an individual physician in addressing such issues, in boundary setting, and in clarifying expectations.

Physician Personal Awareness

Because physicians use themselves as instruments of diagnosis and therapy, it can be extremely valuable for a physician to have an insight into how his or her personality, life experiences, and feelings can impact interactions with patients, families, and other professionals (Novack et al., 1992). In Novack et al.'s (1992) article "Calibrating the Physician," a number of studies are discussed which evaluate factors impacting doctor-patient communication such as the physician's core beliefs, family of origin, gender issues, and sociocultural influences.

In addition, studies have documented a general drop in physician satisfaction most prominent in areas with a high penetration of managed care (Gallagher and Levinson, 2004). In one longitudinal observational study, Murphy et al. (2001) reported a decline in the patient rating of their doctor's communication and interpersonal skills over a 3-year period of time. The authors suggested that possible factors driving this decline might include the distractions of organizational restructuring, mergers, and pressures to increase productivity without compromising standards of care. All of these examples are commonplace in health care environment today.

Consequences of Lack of Professionalism

Just as outstanding physicians are recognized by their continuous professionalism, the absence of professional behaviors can be a signal that an individual practitioner is at risk for problems.

Papadakis et al. (2005) have published a number of studies extrapolating behavior patterns observed in medical students and their associated risks for future disciplinary actions by medical boards. The three types of unprofessional behavior categories that were significantly associated with disciplinary actions were (a) irresponsibility, (b) diminished capacity for self-improvement, and (c) poor initiative (Teherani et al., 2005). Examples of unprofessional conduct included observed behaviors such as unreliable attendance at clinic, lack of follow-up on activities related to patient care, argumentativeness, failure to accept constructive criticism, lack of motivation, and poor attitude. A list of the most frequent subsequent violations that lead to disciplinary action on the part of state medical boards included use of drugs or alcohol, incompetence, negligence, conviction for a crime, and also unprofessional conduct (Teherani et al., 2005).

A case-controlled descriptive design study was published that established a relationship between psychological indices as measured by the California Psychological Inventory ("CPI") with measures of professionalism during medical school (Hodgson et al., 2007). The CPI was administered at time of matriculation. The authors indicated that those physicians who demonstrated unprofessional behavior in medical school tended to score significantly lower on four CPI scales. Low scores on the four CPI scales indicated the following patterns of behavioral deficits: responsibility (self-indulgent, lack of discipline), communality (unconventional, changeable, and moody), well
-being (perceived unfair treatment, health, or personal problems), and rule respecting (rebellious, cynical). Finally, it has been recognized that physicians who receive a disproportionate number of patient complaints and subsequent malpractice claims often struggle with interpersonal behaviors such as establishing rapport, expectation management, and communication effectiveness (Hickson et al., 2002).

Professionalism—A Lifelong Personal Commitment

There are an abundance of suggestions for enhancing education for professionalism from medical schools and professional organizations. The remainder of this chapter will be devoted to providing practical resources for individual physicians to incorporate into their lifelong implementation plan for professionalism. The suggestions below are organized according to the attributes of professionalism provided in Table 26.1.

Knowledge and Skills

The continuing medical education requirements of licensing agencies and certifying boards provide the structure for maintaining some form of lifelong learning. Current clinical knowledge status is also regularly assessed through periodic specialty certification boards. Participating and receiving feedback from hospital quality assurance programs also promotes the ongoing outcome measurement of clinical skills application. Many hospitals have opportunities for participation in peer review, M&M conferences, grand rounds, and other activities that enable the practicing physician to keep abreast of knowledge and skills in his/her clinical specialty area.

Individual practitioners can become more self-aware of their personality and communication preferences by taking the Myers-Briggs Type Indicator personality questionnaire, a process that provides many helpful insights. Keirsey (1998) and Meyers (1980) have expanded on the concepts of personality preferences in their books. Deborah Tannen, Ph.D., is a professor in linguistics and has published a number of useful books and journal articles on gender communication patterns (Tannen, 1990).

Increased understanding of religious and cultural differences may be obtained from attending local college classes, community programs, and/or online resources. Volunteering to help patients and families with understanding medical information in the context of their own cultural and religious issues may also be a very valuable source of personal learning.

Altruism and Duty

In his article "Professionalism and Humanism beyond the Academic Health Center," Swick (2007) suggests using the humanities to show our own personal humanity. Swick's article includes a list of selected works by physician authors that he believes convey the values of humanism and professionalism. Inui (2003) emphasizes the link between personal and professional growth and development that can be further enhanced through such mechanisms as ethics training and social medicine courses—history, medicine, health, and society.

There are two established professional development small groups to consider; Balint groups and "Literature & Medicine: Humanities at the Heart of Health Care." The aim of a Balint group is to help the doctors with the psychological aspect of their patients' problems—and their problems with their patients. The focus of the work is on the doctor–patient relationship. Additional information about Balint groups and workshops can be found on their Web site.

Literature and Medicine: Humanities at the Heart of Health Care was created by the Maine Humanities Council and is a workplace program that gives people involved in the delivery of health care an opportunity to come together and reflect on their roles as health care providers through the medium of literature. Detailed information of the program is available on their Web site.

Confront the Facts

In addition to all of the efforts medical schools make to include the elements of Professionalism in their curriculum, we must add one more—"Confront the Brutal Facts." In his book *Good to Great*, Jim Collins (2001) devoted an entire chapter titled "Confront the brutal facts, yet never lose faith". Based on the author's extensive research, one of the elements that enables companies to become great is their ability to confront the most brutal facts of reality while maintaining faith that they will prevail regardless of difficulties. Based on Collin's guidance, the osteopathic profession needs to foster a "climate where the truth is heard." We must help our students and ourselves move through their grief process to find acceptance (Kübler-Ross, 2003); and to be forthright about the fact that the daily application of professionalism is a continuous struggle. The majority of physicians are high academic achievers striving for the "A" in all areas of medicine, including professionalism. The brutal truth about professionalism is that it is composed of a number of important elements that must be done the best that we can in the face of resource limitations and at times, conflicting priorities.

As a case in point, let's take compassion and medical knowledge, two fundamental qualities of professionalism. While a student might achieve an "A" in compassion by spending an extra 30 minutes with an upset family member; he/she sacrificed an obligation to pursue medical knowledge by missing noon lecture. Although this is admittedly a simplistic example, the message is absolutely crucial for creating an environment where the truth is heard. We must encourage acceptance of the struggle involved in balancing conflicting demands while attempting to embody the multiple elements of professionalism. We must also affirm that fact that in spite of the difficulties we face each day, on balance, professionalism prevails because of our devotion to it and our steadfast determination to keep trying to do the very best that we can at it.

Authenticity is the Heart of Professionalism

Professionalism comprises a set of expected behaviors. Institutions select the behaviors of professionalism that will be measured to determine competency (Cohen, 2007). There is another important element of professionalism—caring—which is harder to quantify. Caring, also described by Cohen as humanism, denotes an intrinsic set of "deep-seated convictions about one's obligations toward others." It is possible for physicians to "go through the motions" of professional behavior without actually believing in the virtues that support them (Cohen, 2007). The bond between the *behaviors* of professionalism and the *attribute* of caring is critical to the delivery of meaningful health care and is sustained by the osteopathic physician's ability to be authentic. "All humans have authenticity detectors…that psychic mechanism by which we can recognize the ring of truth that helps us determine if that person is trustworthy" (Spence, 1995). We fuel our authenticity by telling the truth about ourselves which in turn strengthens the trust in our relationships. For example, physicians are often reluctant to admit that "they don't know," concerned that this disclosure would undermine the patient's confidence in their care. However, the act of fabricating a diagnosis when the physician is unsure is readily picked up by the patient and could actually undermine the patient's trust and confidence in that physician. When we dare to tell the truth, all the elements of communications, physical and verbal, automatically come together to deepen our authenticity.

Professionalism is a Journey

The osteopathic physician does not become a professional but rather chooses to be professional daily. The truth about our days is that even when they are carefully planned with our very best "time-management" skills, circumstances will arise that are unplanned, competing, and all worthy of our full attention. What do we do? Employing the concept developed by the Covey team of "integrity in the moment of choice" is one approach (Covey et al., 1994). Covey writes that we increase our ability to act with integrity when we "pause; ask with intent, listen without excuse and act with courage," it includes asking questions such as "What's the best use of my time right now?" It is important to avoid rationalizing your choices and to choose your actions based on enduring principles (Covey et al., 1994). Professionalism is processed based, and it demands daily effort and regular self-examination.

SUMMARY

Professionalism has been a cherished ideal since the foundation of osteopathic medicine. Although much has been done in recent years to better delineate the traits and behaviors associated with professionalism, it still remains a personal journey for each physician.

REFERENCES

ACGME Outcome Project. (n.d.). Retrieved January 10, 2008 from web site, http://www.acgme.org/outcome/comp/compMin.asp.

Adler H. Toward a biopsychosocial understanding of the patient-physician relationship: an emerging dialogue. *J Gen Intern Med* 2007;22:280–285.

American Osteopathic Association. (n.d.) *The Osteopathic Oath.* Available at: http://www.osteopathic.org/index.cfm?PageID=ado_oath. Retrieved January 8, 2008.

Ashton C, Haldet P, Paterniti D, et al. Racial and ethnic disparities in the use of health services: bias, preferences or poor communication? *J Gen Intern Med* 2003;18:146–152.

Brainard A, Brislen H. Learning professionalism: a view from the trenches. *Acad Med* 2007;82(11):1010–1014.

Branch W. Supporting the moral development of medical students. *J Gen Intern Med* 2000;15:503–508.

Chretien K, Greysen S, Chretien J, et al. Online posting of unprofessional content by medical students. *J Am Med Assoc* 2009;302(12):1309–1315.

Cohen J. Linking professionalism to humanism: what it means, why it matters. *Acad Med* 2007;82(11):1029–1028.

Collins J. *Good to Great.* New York, NY: Harper Collins Publishers, 2001.

Covey S, Merrill A, Merrill R. *First Things First.* New York, NY: Simon & Schuster, 1994.

Epstein R, Hundert E. Defining and assessing professional competence. *J Am Med Assoc,* 2002;287(2):226–235.

Epstein R. Mindful practice. *J Am Med Assoc* 2008;282(9):833–839.

Farnan J, et al. The YouTube generation: implications for medical professionalism. *Perspect in Biol Med* 2008;51(4):517–524.

Gallagher M, Cummings M, Gilman D, et al. Report of the core competency task force. 2003. Available at: http://scs.msu.edu/cc/docs/AOATaskForce Report.pdf. Retrieved May 6, 2008.

Gallagher T, Levinson W. A prescription for protecting the doctor-patient relationship. *Am J Manage Care* 2004;10(2):61–68.

Gorindo T, Groves J. Web searching for information about physicians. *J Am Med Assoc* 2008;300(2):213–215.

Harrison A. Primary care of lesbian and gay patients: educating ourselves and our students. *Fam Med* 1996;28:10–23.

Hickson G, Federspiel C, Pichert J, et al. Patient complaints and malpractice risk. *J Am Med Assoc* 2002;287(22):2951–2957.

Hodgson C, Teherani A, Gough H, et al. The relationship between measures of unprofessional behavior during medical school and indices on the California psychological inventory. *Acad Med* 2007;82(10 suppl):S4–S7.

Inui T. *A Flag in the Wind: Educating for Professionalism in Medicine.* Washington, DC: Association of American Medical Colleges, 2003.

Keller V, Goldstein M, Runkle C. Strangers in crisis: communication skills for the emergency department clinician and the hospitalist. *J Clin Outcomes Manage* 2002;9(8), 439–444.

Kübler-Ross E. *On Death and Dying—What the Dying have to Teach Doctors, Nurses, Clergy and their own Families.* New York, NY: Scribner, 2003.

Luo J, et al. Cyberdermatoethics I: ethical, legal, technologic and clinical aspects of patient-physician e-mail. *Clin Dermatol* 2009;27:359–366.

Michigan State University College of Osteopathic Medicine Statement of Professionalism (n.d.). Available at: http://www.com.msu.edu/aa/professionalism.php. Retrieved November 12, 2009.

Murphy J, Chang H, Montgomery J, et al. The quality of physician-patient relationships [Electronic Version]. *J Fam Pract* 2001;50(2):1–9.

Newton B, Barber L, Clardy J, et al. Is there hardening of the heart during medical school? *Acad Med* 2008;83(3):244–249.

Novack D, Suchman A, Clark W, et al. Calibrating the physician, personal awareness and effective patient care. *J Am Med Assoc* 1992;278(6):502–509.

Papadakis M, Teherani A, Banach M, et al. Disciplinary action by medical boards and prior behavior in medical school. *N Engl J Med* 2005;353(25):2673–2682.

Patenaude J, Niyonsenga T, Fafard D. Changes in students' moral development during medical school: A cohort study. *Can Med Assoc J* 2003;168(7):840–844.

Rogers F, D'Alonzo G, Glover J, et al. Proposed tenets of osteopathic medicine and principles for patient care. *J Am Osteopath Assoc* 2002;102(2):63–65.

Seffinger M, King H, Ward R, et al. Osteopathic philosophy. In: Ward R. ed. *Foundations for Osteopathic Medicine.* 2nd Ed. Philadelphia, PA: Lippincott, Williams & Wilkins, 2003:3–18.

Self D, Olivarez S, Baldwin D. The amount of small-group case-study discussion needed to improve moral reasoning skills of medical students. *Acad Med* 1998;73(5):521–523.

Spence G. *How to Argue and Win Every Time.* New York, NY: St. Martin's Press, 1995.

Stewart, M. (1995). Effective physician-patient communication and health outcomes: a review. *Can Med Assoc J* 1995;152(9):1423–1433.

Swick H. (2007). Professionalism and humanism beyond the academic health center. *Academic Medicine, 82*(11), 1022–1028.

Tannen D. *You Just Don't Understand.* New York, NY: Ballentine Books, 1990.

Teherani A, Hodgson S, Banach M, et al. Domains of unprofessional behavior during medical school associated with future disciplinary action by a state medical board. *Acad Med* 2005;80(10 suppl):S17–S20.

Traveline J, Ruchinskas R, DeAlonzo G. Patient-physician communication: why and how. *J Am Osteopath Assoc* 2005;105(1):13–18.

Whitcomb M. Professionalism in medicine. *Acad Med* 2007;82(11):1009.

Williams M. Recognizing and overcoming inadequate health literacy, a barrier to care. *Cleve Clin J Med* 2002;69(5):415–418.

27

Mind-Body Medicine

HOWARD SCHUBINER

> ## KEY CONCEPTS
>
> ■ The experience of illness has a powerful effect on individuals, perhaps the determining factor in the eventual outcome.
>
> ■ Personality factors have been shown to affect the development of certain illnesses.
>
> ■ The biopsychosocial model of patient care correctly conceptualizes components of disorders, but may not differentiate the degree to which these factors are present in particular disorders.
>
> ■ Disorders affecting relatively young, healthy people with little evidence of attendant increased mortality can be effectively treated using a purely psychological or "mind-body" approach.
>
> ■ The unconscious mind can perpetuate physical symptoms that begin with a clear physical cause.

INTRODUCTION

As George Engel (1) pointed out in 1977, all patients with an illness have physical, psychological, and social components that interact in complex relationships to impact the onset, course, and outcome of their illness. The experience of illness has a powerful effect on individuals and, for some patients, may become the determining factor in the eventual outcome. In addition, factors such as social support, stable living situations, and personality factors have been shown to play important roles in health outcomes (2).

For example, the Canadian Health Study found that an individual's perception of health was more highly correlated with longevity than were other more objective measures of health, such as the number of chronic diagnoses (3). The Alameda longitudinal study found that individuals with higher levels of social support (defined as being married, being involved in religious or social groups, or having close friends) had 50% lower mortality over the course of 9 years (4). Conversely, depression is associated with increased mortality after a myocardial infarction (5).

Personality factors have also been shown to affect the development of certain illnesses. The longitudinal study of physicians and attorneys from the University of North Carolina showed that those who reported higher levels of hostility and anger during graduate school were more likely to develop myocardial infarctions and had higher mortality rates later in life (6). Hostility also appears to predict cardiovascular mortality among middle-aged men (7). Stress and emotional reactions to stress have been shown to alter a variety of markers that are associated with poor health outcomes, such as tissue necrosis factor, interleukin 6, and C-reactive protein (2,8).

When the biopsychosocial model of patient care was proposed, it provided physicians with a way to conceptualize illness and the relationship between the patient and the illness. In this model, there is an interaction between the physical disease process (pathologic changes in the body), the psychologic makeup of the individual, and the social milieu of the patient. A generation of physicians and psychologists has used this model in research and patient care to elucidate complex relationships between illness and disease. Although this model correctly points out that all disorders have components of biologic, psychologic, and social determinants, it may not differentiate the degree to which these factors are present in particular disorders.

Cancer and cardiovascular diseases comprise the major causes of mortality in the United States and have a clear age-related prevalence. Although there is significant literature documenting relationships between these diseases and psychological factors, there is little evidence that psychosocial interventions affect the course of the pathological disorder and virtually no evidence that these disorders can be cured by psychosocial treatments (9,10). It may be inferred that psychosocial treatments are best characterized as helping to cope with the effects of these primarily biologic processes.

A second group of disorders can be considered to have more equal balance between biologic and psychosocial factors. Disorders such as asthma, rheumatoid arthritis, and inflammatory bowel disease cause clear pathologic changes, but they also occur in younger individuals and can follow a course that is mild, moderate, or severe. There is some literature to suggest that psychosocial interventions can improve the symptoms in these disorders, but true cures appear to be less likely (11). Psychosocial interventions can be considered for these disorders to attempt to decrease exacerbations of the underlying process.

A third group of disorders is the subject of this chapter: disorders affecting relatively young, healthy people with little evidence of true pathologic changes in the body, nor evidence of increased mortality due to the disorders. These disorders comprise a wide range of syndromes but can be grouped into pain syndromes (including headaches, migraine, back pain, neck pain, whiplash, fibromyalgia, temporomandibular joint syndrome, and chronic abdominal and pelvic pain syndromes), autonomic nervous system (ANS)–related disorders (including irritable bowel syndrome, interstitial cystitis, postural orthostatic tachycardia syndrome, reflex sympathetic dystrophy, and functional dyspepsia), and neurologic-psychologic syndromes (including insomnia, fatigue, paresthesias, and tinnitus). These disorders are not generally considered to be psychosomatic disorders; however, there is ample evidence that these disorders are primarily caused by physiologic, rather than pathologic conditions within the body and that they can be effectively treated using a purely psychological or "mind body" approach (12,13).

Table 27.1 outlines the differences between these three categories of illness vis-à-vis psychological processes.

TABLE 27.1

Physical, Psychological, and Social Interactions

Group	Examples	Epidemiology	Role of Psychological Factors	Treatment Aim Biomedical/Psychological
1	Cancer CAD	Increases with age; mortality common	Associated but not causative	Rx disease/cope with stress
2	Asthma IBD RA	Young to middle age; morbidity common	May cause exacerbations	Rx disease/prevent exacerbations
3	HA, LBP, Fibromyalgia Whiplash	Young to middle age; no mortality; no tissue destruction	Causative of symptoms	Rx symptoms/control or cure

CAD, coronary artery disease; IBD, inflammatory bowel disease; RA, rheumatoid arthritis; HA, headaches; and LBP, low back pain.

HISTORICAL BACKGROUND

In 1934, Harriman reported a case of a former nun who secretly got married but suddenly developed paralysis of her right arm at the very moment at which she was going to convey this news to her family in a letter (14). This is an example of a conversion reaction caused by great conflict in the unconscious mind of this patient. In the 1600s and 1700s, common consequences of stressful events and strong unconscious emotions were so-called hysterical paralysis and hysterical seizures (15).

Changes in society and advances in medicine (e.g., discovery of deep tendon reflexes, which could quickly distinguish organic from psychogenic paralysis) caused these syndromes to greatly diminish in occurrence. When a medical condition is clearly viewed as being psychogenic by a culture (and by the medical profession), the unconscious mind will be less likely to produce that syndrome. However, humans continue to experience great stresses and strong emotions and these emotions are commonly manifest as physical (and psychological) symptom complexes. Therefore, paralysis and seizures have been replaced in the 21st century with chronic back pain, fibromyalgia, fatigue. irritable bowel syndrome, and other similar disorders (15).

In 1950, Hans Selye described the General Adaptation Syndrome in rats who had been subjected to stress in the laboratory. These rats showed signs of immune dysfunction (shrunken thymus glands) and ANS overactivity (peptic ulcers and enlarged adrenal glands) (16). Building on the prior work of Walter Cannon, who described the fight or flight response (17), this ushered in the era of understanding that stress and emotional disturbances could cause physical changes in the body. In 1975, Robert Ader found that rats given cyclophosphamide in bowls of saccharine (with its characteristic taste) developed immune suppression that was reproducible when they were later exposed simply to saccharine (18). These findings (which have been reproduced in humans) (19) confirmed that the mind can cause physical disorders via the sympathetic nervous system and that these pathways can be conditioned by classic behavioral techniques.

In the 1970s, Dr. John Sarno, a rehabilitation physician in New York City began to question the conventional wisdom of ascribing most chronic back and neck pain to musculoskeletal derangements in the spine (20). He noted that radiological imaging studies were often predictive of neither the level of pain or neurologic symptoms, nor the course of the illness. Since then, several studies have documented that MRI findings have little correlation with low back pain (LBP). For example, in those without LBP, 64% were found to have disc bulging, protrusion, or extrusion (21). In follow-up studies, the development or persistence of back pain shows no correlation with MRI findings (22,23). Despite increased spending for surgery, injection therapies, and other modalities, disability for back pain has risen in the last decade (24). Noting the lack of efficacy for these therapies, Deyo and colleagues have suggested that invasive treatments be curtailed (25).

Dr. Sarno explored the theory that stressful situations, the response to stressful situations, and both conscious and unconscious emotions were the actual cause of the physical symptoms seen in many of his patients. He developed a psychoeducational approach for these patients and has found success in curing patients with chronic musculoskeletal symptoms. In addition, he has found that many patients had concomitant symptoms in other systems (such as GI and GU systems) and psychiatric symptoms (such as anxiety, depression, insomnia, fatigue) improved along with the musculoskeletal symptoms when some of the underlying psychological issues were identified and addressed. The key component of this approach however is not in the psychological treatment modalities, but in the recognition that while the physical symptoms are real, these symptoms are not due to a pathologic derangement in the body, but that they are caused by mental processes and therefore they can be cured with a purely psychological approach (26).

NEUROPSYCHOPHYSIOLOGIC MECHANISMS OF MIND-BODY SYNDROMES

The mechanisms for psychophysiological dysfunction producing psychosomatic syndromes have begun to surface in recent years. There are two distinct pathways involving the CNS, by which musculoskeletal pain can be amplified and/or reduced. The current prevailing paradigm for physiological pain modulation—the gate-control theory—acknowledges that an individual's emotional state can modulate the perception of pain (27).

An area of the brain known as the "rostral anterior cingulate cortex" (rACC; sometimes referred to as the "medial prefrontal cortex" is known to modulate the intensity of pain that an individual perceives (28,29).

The psychological function of the rACC has been described as generating the emotional response to a perceived error (30).

In contrast to the rACC, the dorsolateral prefrontal cortex (DLPFC) is able to decrease the perceived intensity of pain, in part by inhibiting the rACC (31). The role of the DLPFC in reducing perceived pain intensity is further supported by studies that show atrophy or neurodegeneration of this brain region in patients with persistent LBP, compared to controls (32–34). Among the many psychological functions of the DLPFC, the most pertinent to our discussion is its role in the interaction between cognitive and emotional processing. The DLPFC has been shown to be activated by praise and feelings of positive self-worth (35).

In addition to the above mechanisms, researchers have shown that stress causes increases not only in cortisol but also in inflammatory cytokines such as tissue necrosis factor-α and nuclear factor kappa-B (NF-κB) which induces expression of proinflammatory cytokines such as TNF-α, interleukin-6, and interleukin-1β (36). All of these cytokines are known to cause sensitization of peripheral nociceptors which lead to increased pain (37,38).

Figure 27.1 describes a hypothesis of the mechanisms that underlie psychosomatic syndromes. The process may start with an injury or significant conscious or unconscious stressors, but the syndrome may become perpetuated by sensitization of afferent nerve fibers, amplification of signals by the amygdala and the anterior cingulate cortex, and reinforcement of efferent signals in the ANS. These processes all occur in the unconscious part of the brain. Conscious and willful activity in the DLPFC can attenuate these processes as shown (39,40).

PSYCHOLOGICAL ISSUES

Numerous studies document the role of the unconscious mind in determining human behavior. For example, being presented with words such as old, wise, retired, and gray in a word experiment caused those participants to walk slower than a control group (41). People who were shown subliminal words related to assertiveness later were more likely to interrupt the investigator than those who were shown subliminal words related to politeness (42). People who briefly held an iced coffee drink in their hand rated a stranger as being less friendly than did people who held a warm cup of coffee (43). It is estimated that approximately 95% of our thoughts and feelings reside in the unconscious mind and while a human brain can take in about 11 million bits of information each second, the conscious brain can only process about 40 bits of information in a second and that the vast majority of our thoughts and emotions occur in the unconscious mind (44).

The unconscious mind can perpetuate physical symptoms that begin with a clear physical cause, such as a car accident or an injury. In these cases, the mind may "use" the opportunity of the accident in order to develop pain that serves a function for the individual, such as relieve them from a difficult work situation. A study that created a sham (or placebo) car accident showed that 10% of the participants had neck pain 4 weeks after the "accident," even though their necks did not move during the sham accident. Those who were most likely to develop neck pain were those who were under the most stress and emotional distress at the time of the accident (45). In contrast, demolition car drivers who have an average of over 150 crashes per race rarely develop chronic neck pain (46). And a study of people involved in motor vehicle accidents in Lithuania showed no difference in neck pain or headaches compared to a group of people who had not been in car accidents, suggesting that whiplash is potentially a "culture-bound syndrome" (47).

The unconscious mind is also more likely to produce symptoms that run in the family, for example, headaches and abdominal pain, or symptoms that are discussed in magazines and television shows or advertisements. Another mechanism for the "choice" of a particular symptom complex is due to prior learning. For example, someone who had an injury to a certain area is more likely to develop psychogenic pain in that area since the neurological pattern of pain and nerve sensitization has been produced in the past and is remembered by the brain.

Finally, some symptoms are symbolically representative of a clear psychological process, such as a man who develops groin pain after an extramarital affair. It appears that the unconscious mind is likely to produce physical symptoms at times of severe stress as an outlet or an escape mechanism for the buildup of unacceptable emotions that have no outlet. It is also possible that the unconscious mind is alerting the individual to what it perceives to be dangerous situations through the development of pain. For example, a woman who migrated to the United States from India developed

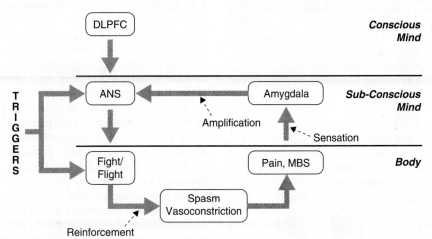

Figure 27-1 This figure represents the theorized pathways that produce and perpetuate the mind-body syndrome. These pathways can begin due to an injury or stressful events that produce strong unconscious emotions in the amygdala. Afferent sensory nerves develop sensitization over time and send signals to the amygdala. Signals in the brain get amplified by emotions and the ANS activates the fight or flight mechanisms, which produces muscle spasm, and vasoconstriction, which worsens the physical symptoms in the body. These pathways get reinforced over time and this creates a vicious cycle of pain and increased emotional responses. A variety of triggers (such as certain positions, places, weather changes, foods, or situations) can act as conditioned responses and add to the neurologic pathways that perpetuate pain. In the conscious portion of the brain, the DLPFC area can act to attenuate and break the cycle at the level of the ANS.

fibromyalgia at a time in her life when she was beginning to think of doing some more things for herself such as taking classes at a local college. However, her husband took an extra job, she had three adolescent children who required a great deal of attention, and then both her mother-in-law and her brother moved into the home. Being a dutiful person who was obligated to others before her own desires, she put aside her own desires and she sublimated her feelings of resentment. Her body reacted to this set of stressors and repressed emotion with a widespread painful process, which responded to the psychological intervention mentioned below.

Another example is that of a firefighter who developed neck pain after a fall in a burning building and was on disability from work due to severe neck pain. Although he had similar injuries in the past and had bounced back from them, this fire was different because it caused the death of one of his friends. Following the fire, in his conscious mind of course, he wanted to improve and return to work; however, his unconscious mind would not let him and found a way to create pain, which prevented him from returning to active duty. Once he understood that there was no significant pathological process in his neck and that the underlying cause of his pain was due to emotions triggering a pattern of nerve pathways creating pain, he completed the psychological interventions described below and had a dramatic resolution of his symptoms allowing him to return to work. Table 27.2 outlines conditions for which a psychosomatic etiology is common.

MANAGEMENT OF MIND-BODY SYNDROMES

Current treatment approaches to patients with these unexplained symptom complexes consist of pain medications, modulators of pain perception, such as pregabalin and gabapentin, exercise, osteopathic manipulation, and physical therapy. These modalities are all successful in many patients; however, certain patients do not respond and

appear to require alternative approaches. Psychological approaches typically consist of cognitive behavioral therapy and stress reduction. Studies using mindfulness meditation have shown a reduction in pain for patients with chronic musculoskeletal pain (48) and fibromyalgia (49,50). Cognitive-behavioral therapy, which works in part by reducing psychosocial stress, has also been shown to be effective in chronic musculoskeletal pain (51–54). Finally, studies using therapeutic writing techniques in fibromyalgia have shown reductions in pain comparable to standard pharmacological therapy (55,56).

A model for treatment of these "mind-body syndromes" consists of the following steps. First, each patient is asked to read *The Mindbody Prescription* by Dr. Sarno (26). This gives the patient a basic understanding of how physical symptoms, which are real, located in the body and often severe, can be caused by conscious and unconscious emotional turmoil.

Second, each patient has a 60 to 90 minute office visit to rule out any physical disorders that require conventional medical attention and to search for patterns of psychosomatic symptoms across their life span beginning in childhood. It is important to listen carefully to the patient's life story and to help them uncover particular stressors and emotional reactions that have triggered such psychosomatic symptoms. It is useful to attempt to help the patient understand the role of conditioned responses that serve as stimuli triggering the neurologic pathways that have developed over time (e.g., certain positions, activities, weather changes, foods, locations).

It is necessary to explain the physiologic pathways between the emotional centers of the brain (amygdala) and the ANS, which creates the physiologic substrates of pain and other symptoms (e.g., sensitized nerve pathways) in order to help them understand the role of the unconscious mind in producing emotions that can produce significant physical symptoms despite being suppressed.

It is critical to normalize and destigmatize psychosomatic disorders and accept them as a part of being "human," and to explain how simple psychological techniques can alter the vicious cycle of pain and offer hope that their symptoms are curable.

An important step in the treatment process is patient participation in a 4-week seminar. Participants receive a workbook and instructions for performing specific therapeutic writing exercises to help them express emotions and better cope with prior and current stressors, specific meditative exercises based on mindfulness meditation developed for this purpose, specific declarative and affirmative sentences that are spoken to oneself as a method for disrupting patterns of neurologic connections that promote symptoms, and exercises to develop and carry out activities that previously caused symptoms or are pleasurable and desirable.

Finally, follow-up is conducted to plan for the future depending on the response obtained to this program. Patients may require individual psychotherapy as an adjunct to the program. The program is also available on the internet (57) and in a self-help book (58).

In 1976, Ivan Illich warned of the potential iatrogenic consequences of a classification of disease that labels patients (59). When patients with psychosomatic disorders are labeled as having degenerative disc disease on the basis of an MRI or as having fibromyalgia on the basis of an arbitrary classification system, the stage is set for a vicious cycle of exacerbation of symptoms and of psychologic status. Eugene Carragee also warned of this process occurring in patients with back pain, "ill-considered attempts to make a diagnosis on the basis of imaging studies may reinforce the suspicion of serious disease, magnify the importance of nonspecific findings, and label patients with spurious diagnoses" (60).

The tremendous advances in biomedical technology over the past several decades have led to an overemphasis on the biologic, while ignoring the psychologic and the social causes of common symptoms.

TABLE 27.2	
Conditions for Which a Psychosomatic Etiology is Common	
Types of Disorders	**Clinical Conditions**
Chronic pain syndromes	Tension headaches Migraine headaches LBP Neck pain Whiplash Fibromyalgia Temporomandibular joint syndrome Chronic abdominal and pelvic pain syndromes Chronic pain syndromes
ANS-related disorders	Irritable bowel syndrome, Interstitial cystitis, postural orthostatic tachycardia syndrome, reflex sympathetic dystrophy, functional dyspepsia
Neurologic syndromes	Insomnia Chronic fatigue Paresthesias Tinnitus

In addition, there has been a surge in expenditures for complementary and alternative treatments. An alternative nosology of disease has been created by this movement and includes labels such as chronic yeast infection, chronic food allergies and deficiencies of natural hormones, gastric acid or various nutritional supplements. Such "diagnoses" can have similar effects to medical labeling, that is, turning a person with functional symptoms due to stressors into a patient with a "disease."

APPLICATION TO PATIENT CARE

Therefore, in the course of routine patient care, it is critical for physicians to be aware of the probability that psychosomatic disorders will occur in most people during the course of their lifetime. A careful history and physical examination should include investigation into the potential for both organic and functional disorders; that is, examining not only for signs of nerve root compression, tumor, or infection, but determining the psychological and social factors that may have led to this set of symptoms at this point in a person's life.

The most important question to ask is "What was happening in your life at the time these symptoms began?" For patients who present with the new onset of headaches, bowel or bladder symptoms, or painful conditions that are not determined to have a clear pathologic basis, some amount of probing regarding stressors and underlying emotions may be required to uncover feelings of guilt, fear, resentment, or anger. Careful listening is important to validate the suffering of the patient and to reassure the patient that you take their condition seriously. Listening for and probing to obtain the psychosocial context of this point in a patient's life will allow the physician to understand the potential contribution of psychosocial factors in the illness and will serve as starting point for understanding and potentially curing those ailments that are purely functional.

It is critical to inform the patient with a psychosomatic illness that they are "not crazy," but that these conditions commonly occur in most people. If the patient feels they are being told, "It's all in your head," they will be less likely to improve. It is better to tell patients that all symptoms have a cause and we have to get to the root cause of the symptoms in order to cure them. A careful psychosocial history with emphasis on their childhood stressors as well as their adult stressors is necessary in order to uncover potential root causes. Looking carefully for temporal relationships between stressors (even mild stressors can precipitate significant symptoms if they trigger an emotional response connected to childhood stressors) is important to confirm a psychosomatic etiology.

Once a psychosomatic condition is diagnosed, the management should consist of the following:

Avoid excessive rest and disability. Encourage routine activities and exercise as tolerated.

Reassure about the lack of serious disease and inform the patient that they do have a condition. One useful term is "mind-body syndrome." Emphasize that mind-body syndrome is real and that their symptoms are very real, but they are curable.

Avoid excessive testing and excessive referral to specialists who may be likely to reinforce the suspicion of serious disease. Explain the results of nonspecific test findings (such as degenerative disc changes) as findings that are within the range of normal.

Explain how the mind-body syndrome causes real symptoms and how physiologic mechanisms in the brain and body create this vicious cycle (see Fig. 27.1).

Consider a referral to a physician or psychologist who specializes in this condition or to a counselor who can help the patient understand and cope with their childhood and adult stressors.

Give them resources, such as books by Dr. John Sarno or web sites such as www.tarpityoga.com or www.unlearnyourpain.com.

A tremendous amount of money is spent on the diagnosis and treatment of psychosomatic disorders. The majority of people will have physical and psychological symptoms at some time in their life due to psychological states. If psychosomatic disorders were widely recognized by the lay public and medical professionals (both traditional and alternative), there would be increased potential for alleviation of common symptoms, decrease in medical costs, and prevention of chronic symptom complexes. The treatment of these disorders requires a careful history, judicious use of diagnostic tests to rule out serious pathologic processes, attention to past and current psychosocial stressors and reactions to these stressors, validation of the real nature of the symptoms ("It's not all in your head"), explanation of the psychophysiologic basis of functional symptoms, and brief educational and psychologic interventions. In this way, patients are empowered to gain control over their symptoms, understand themselves better, and obtain tools to improve their psychological states.

REFERENCES

1. Engel GL. The need for a new medical model: a challenge for biomedicine. *Science* 1977;196(4286):129–136.
2. Kiecolt-Glaser JK, McGuire L, Robles TF, et al. Psychoneuroimmunology: psychological influences on immune function and health. *J Consult Clin Psychol* 2002;70(3):537–547.
3. Mossey JM, Shapiro E. Self-rated health: a predictor of mortality among the elderly. *Am J Public Health* 1982;72:800–808.
4. Berkman LF, Syme SL. Social networks, host resistance, and mortality: a nine-year follow-up study of Alameda County residents. *Am J Epidemiol* 1979;109:186–204.
5. Carney RM, et al. Depressions and five year survival following acute myocardial infarction: a prospective study. *J Affect Disord* 2008; epub.
6. Barefoot JC, Dahlstrom WG, Williams RB. Hostility as a predictor of survival in patients with coronary artery disease. *Psychosom Med* 1983;45:59–63.
7. Matthews KA, et al. Hostile behaviors predict cardiovascular mortality among men enrolled in the MRFIT trial. *Circulation* 2004;109(1):66–70.
8. Steptoe A, et al. Acute mental stress elicits delayed increases in circulating inflammatory cytokine levels. *Clin Sci (London)* 2001;101(2):185–192.
9. Stephen JE, Rahn M, Verhoef M, et al. What is the state of the evidence on the mind-cancer survival question, and where do we go from here? *Support Care Cancer* 2007;15(8):923–930.
10. Linden W, Stossel C, Maurice J. Psychosocial interventions for patients with coronary artery disease: a meta-analysis. *Arch Intern Med* 1996;156(7):745–752.
11. Smyth JM, Stone AA, Hurewitz A, et al. Effects of writing about stressful experiences on symptom reduction in patients with asthma or rheumatoid arthritis: a randomized trial. *JAMA* 1999;281(14):1304–1309.
12. Schechter D, Smith AP, Beck J, et al. Outcomes of a mind-body treatment program for chronic back pain with no distinct structural pathology—a case series of patients diagnosed and treated as tension myositis syndrome. *Altern Ther Health Med* 2007;13(5):26–35.
13. Schubiner H, Hsu M. The psychodynamic treatment of chronic musculoskeletal pain unresponsive to conventional medical care: a report of five illustrative cases (submitted).
14. Harriman PL. A case of hysterical paralysis. *J Abnorm Psychol.* 1934–1935;29:455–456.
15. Shorter E. *From Paralysis to Fatigue: A History of Psychosomatic Illness in the Modern Era.* New York, NY: The Free Press, a division of Simon and Schuster Inc., 1992.
16. Selye H. *The Physiology and Pathology of Exposure to Stress: A Treatise Based on the Concepts of the General Adaptation Syndrome and the Diseases of Adaptation.* Montreal, AR: Acta Incorporated Medical Publishers, 1950.

17. Cannon WB. *Bodily Changes in Pain, Hunger, Fear and Rage: An Account of Recent Researches into the Function of Emotional Excitement.* New York, NY: D. Appleton, 1929.

18. Ader R, Cohen N. Behaviorally conditioned immunosuppression. *Psychosom Med* 1975;37(4):333–340.

19. Goebel MU, et al. Behavioral conditioning of immunosuppression is possible in humans. *FASEB J* 2002;16(14):1869–1873.

20. Sarno J. *Mind Over Back Pain.* New York, NY: Harper Collins, 1984.

21. Jensen MC, Brant-Zawadzki MN, Obuchowski N, et al. Magnetic resonance imaging of the lumbar spine in people without back pain. *N Engl J Med* 1994;331(2):69–73.

22. Borenstein DG, O'Mara JW Jr, Boden SD, et al. The value of magnetic resonance imaging of the lumbar spine to predict low-back pain in asymptomatic subjects: a seven-year follow-up study. *J Bone Joint Surg Am* 2001;83-A(9):1306–1311.

23. Savage RA, Whitehouse GH, Roberts N. The relationship between the magnetic resonance imaging appearance of the lumbar spine and low back pain, age and occupation in males. *Eur Spine J* 1997;6(2):106–114.

24. Martin BI, Deyo RA, et al. Expenditures and health status among adults with back and neck problems. *JAMA* 2008;299:656–664.

25. Deyo RA, Mirza SK, Turner JA, et al. Overtreating chronic back pain: time to back off? *J Am Board Fam Med* 2009;22:62–68.

26. Sarno JE. *The Mindbody Prescription: Healing the Body, Healing the Pain.* New York, NY: Warner Books, 1998.

27. Melzack R, Wall PD. Pain mechanisms: a new theory. *Science* 1965;150(699):171–179.

28. Baliki MN, Chialvo DR, Geha PY, et al. Chronic pain and the emotional brain: specific brain activity associated with spontaneous fluctuations of intensity of chronic back pain. *J Neurosci* 2006;26:12165–12173.

29. deCharms RC, Maeda F, Glover GH, et al. Control over brain activation and pain learned by using real-time functional MRI. *Proc Natl Acad Sci U S A* 2005;102:18626–18631.

30. Fitzgerald KD, Welsh RC, Gehring WJ, et al. Error-related hyperactivity of the anterior cingulate cortex in obsessive-compulsive disorder. *Biol Psychiatry* 2005;57:287–294.

31. Schmahl C, Bohus M, Esposito F, et al. Neural correlates of antinociception in borderline personality disorder. *Arch Gen Psychiatry* 2006;63:659–667.

32. Apkarian AV, Sosa Y, Sonty S, et al. Chronic back pain is associated with decreased prefrontal and thalamic gray matter density. *J Neurosci* 2004;24:10410–10415.

33. Schmidt-Wilcke T, Leinisch E, Gansssbauer S, et al. Affective components and intensity of pain correlate with structural differences in gray matter in chronic back pain patients. *Pain* 2006;125:89–97.

34. Grachev ID, Ramachandran TS, Thomas PS, et al. Association between dorsolateral prefrontal N-acetyl aspartate and depression in chronic back pain: an in vivo proton magnetic resonance spectroscopy study. *J Neural Transm* 2003;110:287–312.

35. Hooley JM, Gruber SA, Scott LA, et al. Activation in dorsolateral prefrontal cortex in response to maternal criticism and praise in recovered depressed and healthy control participants. *Biol Psychiatry* 2005;57:809–812.

36. Zingarellli B. Nuclear factor kappa B. *Crit Care Med* 2005;33(12 suppl):S414–S416

37. DeRijk R, Michelson D, Karp B, et al. Exercise and circadian rhythm-induced variations in plasma cortisol differentially regulate interleukin-1 beta (IL-1 beta), IL-6, and tumor necrosis factor-alpha (TNF alpha) production in humans: high sensitivity of TNF alpha and resistance of IL-6. *J Clin Endocrinol Metab* 1997;82:2182–2191.

38. Cunha TM, Verri WA Jr, Silva JS, et al. A cascade of cytokines mediates mechanical inflammatory hypernociception in mice. *Proc Natl Acad Sci U S A* 2005;102:1755–1760.

39. Kong J, Kaptchuk TJ, Polich G, et al. Placebo analgesia: findings from brain imaging studies and emerging hypotheses. *Rev Neurosci* 2007;18(3–4):173–190.

40. Wiech K, Kalisch R, Weiskopf N, et al. Anterolateral prefrontal cortex mediates the analgesic effect of expected and perceived control over pain. *J Neurosci* 2006;26(44):11501–11509.

41. Bargh JA, Chen M, Burrows L. Automaticity of social behavior: direct effects of trait construct and stereotype activation on action. *J Pers Soc Psychol* 1996;71:230–244.

42. Bargh JA. Auto-motives: preconscious determinants of social interaction. In: Higgins T, Sorrentino RM, eds. *Handbook of Motivation and Cognition.* New York, NY: Guilford Press, 1990;93–130.

43. Willliams LE, Bargh JA. Experiencing physical warmth promotes interpersonal warmth. *Science* 2008;322:606–607.

44. Wilson TD. *Strangers to Ourselves: Discovering the Adaptive Unconscious.* Cambridge, MA: Belknap Press of Harvard University, 2002.

45. Castro, WHM, et al. No stress—no whiplash? Prevalence of "whiplash" symptoms following exposure to a placebo rear-end collision. *Int J Legal Med* 2001;114:316–322.

46. Simotas A, Shen T. Neck pain in demolition derby drivers. *Arch Phys Med Rehabil* 2005;86(4):693–696.

47. Schrader H. Headache after whiplash: a historical cohort study outside the medico-legal context. *Lancet* 1996;347:1207–1211.

48. Plews-Ogan M, Owens JE, Goodman M, et al. A pilot study evaluating mindfulness-based stress reduction and massage for the management of chronic pain. *J Gen Intern Med* 2005;20:1136–1138.

49. Kaplan KH, Goldenberg DL, Galvin-Nadeau M. The impact of a meditation-based stress reduction program on fibromyalgia. *Gen Hosp Psychiatry* 1993;15:284–289.

50. Astin JA, Berman BM, Bausell B, et al. The efficacy of mindfulness meditation plus Qigong movement therapy in the treatment of fibromyalgia: a randomized controlled trial. *J Rheumatol* 2003;30:2257–2262.

51. Kole-Snijders AM, Vlaeyen JW, Goossens ME, et al. Chronic low-back pain: what does cognitive coping skills training add to operant behavioral treatment? Results of a randomized clinical trial. *J Consult Clin Psychol* 1999;67:931–944.

52. McCarberg B, Wolf J. Chronic pain management in a health maintenance organization. *Clin J Pain* 1999;15:50–57.

53. Johansson C, Dahl J, Jannert M, et al. Effects of a cognitive-behavioral pain-management program. *Behav Res Ther* 1998;36:915–930.

54. Haugli L, Steen E, Laerum E, et al. Learning to have less pain—is it possible? A one-year follow-up study of the effects of a personal construct group learning programme on patients with chronic musculoskeletal pain. *Patient Educ Couns* 2001;45(2):111.

55. Broderick JE, Junghaenel DU, Schwartz JE. Written emotional expression produces health benefits in fibromyalgia patients. *Psychosom Med* 2005;67:326–334.

56. Gillis ME, Lumley MA, Mosley-Williams A, et al. The health effects of at-home written emotional disclosure in fibromyalgia: a randomized trial. *Ann Behav Med* 2006;32:135–146

57. Schubiner H. *Mind Body Syndrome.* www.unlearnyourpain.com

58. Schubiner H. *Unlearn Your Pain.* Ann Arbor, MI: Sheridan Books, Inc., 2009.

59. Illich I. *Medical Nemesis: The Expropriation of Health.* New York, NY: Pantheon, 1976.

60. Carragee EJ. Persistent low back pain. *NEJM*, 2005;352:1891–1898.

28 Spirituality and Health Care

FELIX J. ROGERS

KEY CONCEPTS

- Spirit defined as an "animating or vital principle" can be viewed from a broad range of perspectives. For the physician, the patient represents the primary focus.
- Many people seek to discern the degree to which their own lives are aligned with this animating principle. For the astute clinician, individual patients are often the best guides.
- The role of the physician is to enhance the patient in her/his quest, and not to promote the physician's personal value system.
- The nature of the human condition is such that illness and disease do occur. Physicians can do much to promote understanding and provide comfort.

INTRODUCTION

The starting point and the first stumbling block to treating a person in terms of body-mind-spirit is to understand what is meant by each of these terms. In osteopathic medicine, we feel they have come to represent a comprehensive approach to an individual. Elsewhere, body-mind-spirit has become such an increasingly popular term that it has been applied as a catchphrase, a means to promote a product. Interested readers who would like to verify the extent to which this term has become a marketing slogan are invited to do an Internet search. Ironically, a match for "osteopathic medicine" does not emerge. Chapter 27 has addressed the topic of mind–body interactions. This chapter will address the spirit component.

DEFINING SPIRIT

Teresa of Avila (1515–82), mystic and founder of the reformed Carmelites, stated, "I can't understand what the mind is, or how it differs from soul or spirit. They all seem the same to me." (1) Tenzin Gyatso, the 14th Dalai Lama, citing the Buddhist principle of emptiness, remarks that Buddhism does not recognize spirit as an independent part of a person:

> … if we examine our own conception of selfhood, we will find that we tend to believe in the presence of an essential core to our being, which characterizes our individuality and identity as a discreet ego, independent of the physical and mental elements that constitute our existence. The philosophy of emptiness reveals that this is not only a fundamental error but also the basis for attachment, clinging, and the development of our numerous prejudices (2).

Hazrat Inayat Khan, who introduced Sufism, the mystical component of Islam, to the western world, writes: "… If we define spirit, it cannot be spirit; the spirit that can be defined cannot be spirit. The best definition of spirit is 'that which is not matter'" (3).

Given that the religious community itself has difficulty in defining a term that at least by appearances belongs in that domain, let's turn to historical and secular approaches. In the tradition of the Abrahamic faiths, spirit, *ruah* has an original meaning of breath, wind. A similar semantic development is found in the Greek *pneuma*. The English word "spirit" is derived from the Latin *spiritus* but contains the basic meaning of "breath," "blow" (4). In one dictionary, spirit is described as an animating or vital principle in man (and animals); that which give life to the physical organism, in contrast to it purely material elements; the breath of life (5). Spirituality, in a narrow sense, concerns itself with matters of the spirit, which is closely tied to religious belief and faith. Especially in modern America, many are concerned that a distinction be drawn between spirituality and religion. Here's one useful formulation: "Spirituality is the way you find meaning, hope, comfort and inner peace in your life. Many people find spirituality through religion. Some find it through music, art or a connection with nature. Others find it in their values and principles" (6).

Andrew Taylor Still had strong spiritual feelings that were intertwined with his osteopathic philosophy. He stated "God is the Father of osteopathy and I am not ashamed of the child that is of his mind" (7). On the other hand, throughout *Osteopathy, Research and Practice*, Still described the osteopathic physician as a mechanic (8). He reasoned that the good osteopathic physician should know the cause of the problem, but he was not to waste time on the reason for the cause. Of the tenets of osteopathic medicine, published in Kirksville in 1953 (9), the first was equally blunt: the body is a unit. It was expanded with the publication of the first edition of *Foundations of Osteopathic Medicine* (10):

The body is a unit; the person is a unit of body, mind and spirit.

In that textbook, Irvin M. Korr, Ph.D., develops further this expansion of the concept of unity:

> Important and valid as is the concept of body unity, it is incomplete in that it is, by implication, limited to the physical realm. Physicians minister not to bodies but to individuals, each of whom is unique by virtue of his or her genetic endowment, personal history, and the variety of environments in which that history has been lived. The person, obviously, is more than a body, for the person has a mind, also the product of heredity and biography. Separation of body and mind, whether conceptually or in practice, is an anachronistic remnant of such dualistic thinking as that of the 17th century philosopher-scientist, René Descartes. It was his belief that body and mind are separate domains, one publicly visible and palpable, the other invisible, impalpable, and private. This

dualistic concept is anachronistic because, while it is almost universally rejected as a concept, it is still acted out in much of clinical practice and in biomedical research. Clinical and biomedical research (as well as everyday experience) has irrefutably shown that body and mind are so inseparable, so pervasive to each other, that they can be regarded and treated as a single entity. It is now widely recognized (whether or not it is demonstrated in practice) that what goes on (or goes wrong) in either body or mind has repercussions in the other. It is for reasons such as these that I prefer unity of the person to unity of the body, conveying totally integrated humanity and individuality (11).

SCIENCE AND RELIGION

Judging from what we know of present-day primitive cultures, religion, magic, and medical treatment were seen in prehistory as inseparable from each other. Primitive man apparently often distinguished between ordinary conditions (such as old age, cough, cold, and fatigue) and illnesses caused by spirits and evil forces that required the special services of a medicine man, shaman, or witch doctor (12).

Plato (circa 429–347 BCE), a contemporary of Hippocrates, a student of Socrates, and the teacher of Aristotle, was one of the most influential thinkers in the history of the western world. His interests were mainly in the nature of the soul and matter. His medical speculations were logical but without direct experimentation. Physicians who supported his doctrine, especially in the third century BCE and thereafter, were called dogmatists. For them, reasoning superseded observation.

Aristotle (384–322 BCE) was the son of a physician. He, along with Hippocrates before him, and Galen afterward, were the principal authorities of pagan, Christian, and Muslim medical thought until the Middle Ages.

During the Middle Ages, in Judaic thought, disease was equated with punishment for sin or with divine disfavor. Early Christian churches did little to change this popular viewpoint. In some respects, the attitude of the Islam toward the origin of disease was similar to the Judeo-Christian idea, in that Allah caused illness as punishment for a person's sins, or for reasons beyond human comprehension, but sickness was usually borne without moral stigma. While one might hope for miracles through prayer, one could also seek divine help through the agency of a physician (13).

In the 17th century, the Age of Reason represented a major turning point in the history of science. Instead of asking *why* things occur, scientists turned to *how* things happened. This represented a shift in emphasis from speculation to experimentation. Interpretations became mechanistic and the language of science became mathematical (14) René Descartes (1596–1650) promoted ideas that would become a transition between the earlier influences of Aristotle and Galen and the Age of Reason. The scientific approach gained momentum during the Industrial Revolution.

The medical profession stands at the door between science and religion, at times taking the role of arbitrator, and offering scientific explanation when the *how* clashed with religions interpretation of the *meaning* of the event. Remarkable advances of science in the last few decades have led to discoveries that were formerly in the exclusive realm of religion. This difference in perspective can be highlighted by the example of a sunrise. Gerard Manley Hopkins (1844–1889), English poet and Jesuit, practiced pantheism; that is, he saw God in everything. His famous poem *God's Grandeur* concludes with this description of a sunrise.

Oh, morning, at the brown brink eastward, springs—
Because the Holy Ghost over the bent
World broods with warm breast and with ah! bright wings.

In contrast, a scientist might point out that visible red light has a wavelength of about 650 nm. At sunrise and sunset, red or orange colors are present because the wave lengths associated with these colors are less efficiently scattered by the atmosphere than the shorter wave lengths of the colors blue and purple. If the blue and violet light has been removed as a result of scattering, red and orange are more readily seen. In this example, the sunrise is measurable, and a personal perspective determines the attribution of God's hand, or explanation by scientific facts. Much of what we deal with in medicine involves issues for which nothing can be measured, such as hope, faith, and out of body experiences, which engenders lively debate.

With the development of functional magnetic resonance imaging, diverse pharmacologic agents, improved understanding about epilepsy, and deep brain stimulation treatments, discreet brain regions are now identified that have been associated with language, art, and religion. At one end of the spectrum, Francis Collins, head of the Human Genome Project, states that molecular biology and brain function argue for the existence of a personal God (15). At the other end, British neurologist Michael Trimble proposes that some of the greatest religious figures in history had what were probably complex partial seizures (16).

Some individuals who have survived cardiac arrest report out-of-body experiences during the time of their resuscitation. Sometimes, this is reported by patients following surgery with general anesthetic. Experimentally, out-of-body experiences in the brain can be repeatedly elicited during stimulation of the posterior part of the superior temporal gyrus on the right side using electrodes that have been implanted to suppress tinnitus (17). Out-of-body experiences may also be reported by sufferers of migraine headaches or epilepsy. Recently, neuroscientists have developed methods to induce an out-of-body experience in healthy volunteers using head-mounted video displays that give people a different perspective on their own bodies. The sense of touch was used to enhance the illusion (18,19). So, when a person describes an out-of-body experience, did it actually happen, or did this just seem to happen, and can it be explained by firing of a few neurons? If you are taking care of the patient for whom this occurred, does it matter?

Francis Collins offers a conciliatory statement to resolve the battle between science and religion. "Science is the only reliable way to understand the natural world and its tools when properly utilized can generate profound insights into material existence. But science is powerless to answer questions such as "Why did the Universe come into being?" "What is the meaning of human existence?" "What happens after we die?" One of the strongest motivations of humankind is to seek answers to profound questions and we need to bring all of the power of both the scientific and spiritual perspectives to bear on understanding what is both seen and unseen" (20).

PRAYER, HEALING, AND MIRACLES

Prayer has long been used as a coping mechanism for illness. A survey of more than 31,000 adults indicated that 36% of U.S. adults use some form of alternative remedies. When prayer is included in the definition of complementary and alternative medicine (CAM), the number of U.S. adults using CAM rose to 62% (21).

Prospective randomized trials can be evaluated in terms of spirituality, worship service attendance, frequency of prayer/meditation, and intercessory prayer. In a study of 503 patients with acute myocardial infarction who had depression or low social support, there was no evidence that self-reported spirituality, frequency of church attendance, or frequency of prayer is associated with cardiac morbidity or all-cause mortality (22). Although measurable outcomes in terms of mortality or morbidity do not occur, prayer has been demonstrated to provide a coping mechanism for cardiac surgery patients, likely mediated through optimism (23). Jantos and Kiat (24) suggest four plausible mechanisms whereby there may be a benefit: (a) a relaxation response, (b) placebo, (c) expression of positive emotions, and (d) a channel for supernatural intervention. These authors conclude that spirituality has an impact on the health and well-being of individuals, and this needs to be reflected in patient care. Patients consider prayer and spiritual issues to be important, and they yearn for open dialogue with their caregivers concerning important spiritual beliefs and practices. Such information may be relevant to understand a patient's resources for coping with illness.

Intercessory prayer has been the subject of sufficient study that large-scale, multicenter randomized controlled trials are available now to assess intercessory prayer with other noetic interventions (healing practices that are not mediated by tangible elements).

The STEP study was a randomized controlled trial of 1,802 patients undergoing coronary artery bypass surgery at six U.S. medical centers (25). Two third of the patients were told they might receive prayer on their behalf; one half of these patients received intercessory prayer and half did not receive prayer. A third of the patients received prayer after being told they would receive it. Prayers were performed by members of three religious groups remote from the hospital. At 30-day follow-up, 1,201 patients did not know whether they had received prayer. Fifty-two percent of the people who actually received prayers suffered surgical complications. Fifty-one percent of the patients who did not receive prayer suffered complications. Six hundred and one patients knew they received prayers, and 59% of them suffered complications (relative risk 1.14, 95% CI: 0.02–1.28).

The MANTRA II study was a randomized trial of 748 patients undergoing percutaneous coronary intervention or catheterization at nine USA medical centers (26). Three hundred seventy one patients were assigned prayer and 377 patients no prayer. Three hundred seventy four were assigned music, imagery, and touch therapy (MIT) and 374 did not receive MIT. There were four study groups: (a) standard care only, (b) prayer only, (c) MIT only, and (d) prayer plus MIT. There were no differences in the primary composite end point of in-hospital major adverse cardiovascular events, 6-month readmission, or death. However, mortality at 6 months was lower in the MIT therapy than the group with no MIT therapy (hazard ratio: 0.35, 95% CI: 0.15–0.82, $p = 0.016$). Patients who received MIT also had a significant decrease in anxiety and emotional distress prior to the catheterization. MIT therapy was administered by practitioners certified in level 1 Healing Touch (27).

The outcomes for intercessory prayer were summarized in two systematic reviews. The Cochrane database summarized 10 studies ($N = 1,646$) (28). Individual studies did find some effects. Most data were equivocal. Evidence presented prompted the authors to say it was interesting enough to suggest that further study is warranted into the human aspects of the effects of prayer. The review concluded that it is impossible to improve or disprove in trials any supposed benefit that derives from God's response to prayer. The results of the review and meta-analysis of prayer and health by Masters and Spielmans (29) are presented in Figure 28.1.

Forest plots and confidence intervals for 15 trials are summarized. When the studies are combined, the effect does not reach statistical significance. In addition to evaluating distant intercessory prayer, they also considered the frequency of prayer, content of prayer, and prayer as a coping strategy. In these categories, not all evidence regarding prayer is positive. The authors conclude that a highly developed model of prayer as coping would include integration of other aspects of the individual's personality, cognitive abilities, physical skills, and socioenvironmental context.

The large-scale review by Jonas and Crawford, *Healing, Intention and Energy Medicine* (30) goes beyond intercessory prayer and healing prayer to include mind–matter interactions, qigong, and the therapeutic effects of music. No well-designed, well-conducted

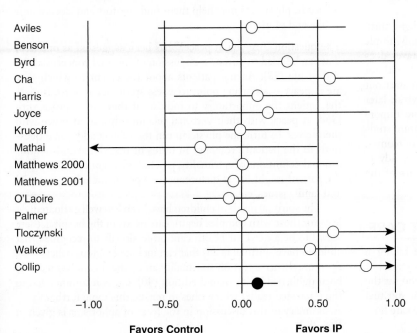

Figure 28-1 The effects of distant intercessory prayer summarized for 15 individual studies. The effect size and confidence intervals for each individual study is shown. Open circles to the right of the zero identity line represent effect sizes that favor intercessory prayer, while those to the left favor control patients. The overall combined effect is shown in the solid circle at the bottom of the figure. From Masters and Spielmans (28).

randomized controlled trials demonstrated statistically significant beneficial effects of any of these interventions.

A PARADIGM SHIFT?

Readers are cautioned against drawing the conclusion that this discussion of science and religion lays out a simple conflict. Because science is expressed by humans, its implementation may reflect some unscientific behavior. One example demonstrates bias. Years ago, a delegation from Jehovah's Witness, a religious group that does not permit its members to receive blood transfusions, made a presentation to a hospital staff, indicating that the staff performed too many blood transfusions. The initial response from the staff was negative: all transfusions seemed appropriate and met standard scientific guidelines. The transfusion committee agreed. In turn, Jehovah's Witness representatives pointed out that preoperative preparation and intraoperative techniques, including use of cell savers, could eliminate many transfusions. In the end, everyone won. The staff adopted the recommendations, and surgery became safer for Jehovah's Witness patients, and other patients were spared unnecessary transfusions.

A more daunting example of how science may be reported to us comes from observations reported over the past few years from the National Institutes of Health, the Center for Disease Control, and other institutions that receive funding from the federal government. Recently, scientists have reported unprecedented pressure from governmental bodies to reconfigure scientific reports to conform to political viewpoints. Over the past decade, several national and international medical publications reported another troublesome problem: information presented as scientific fact may not be so, since drug companies concealed the degree to which information was selectively presented.

Religion may employ some values beneficial to science. Although science is morally neutral, the inventions of science, such as weapons of mass destruction and stem cell research, challenge our society because of the threat they pose without alignment to some moral or ethical context, which may be supplied by religion. At the same time, many religions would be well served by an attitude expressed by the Dalai Lama, "…certainly some specific aspects of Buddhist thought will have to be modified in the light of new scientific insights" (31).

The scientific study of prayer may lead to a paradigm shift, one that is likely to be more obvious to the nonbeliever. Multiple randomized, controlled trials show that intercessory prayer does not have measurable benefit in clinical outcomes. This should not be a challenge to religious faith. Research studies often start out with "hard" endpoints, such as death or length of survival; later they move to "soft" outcomes, some of which are more important to patients, such as quality of life. In this regard, future studies of noetic interventions might assess nonclinical outcomes, such as happiness, hope, and acceptance, in the face of adversity, at least some of which have been described as fruits of the spirit (32).

APPROACH TO SPIRITUALITY IN PATIENT CARE

Although health professionals may be uncomfortable taking a spiritual history and assessment of a patient, patients expect it and others may welcome it. Further, the Joint Commission for the Accreditation of Healthcare Organizations requires that spiritual assessment be made for each patient admitted to an acute care hospital or nursing home, or seen by a home health agency.

Spiritual assessment should, at a minimum, determine the patient's denomination, beliefs, and what spiritual practices are important to the patient. This information would assist in determining the impact of spirituality, if any, on the care/services being provided and will identify if any further assessment is needed. The standards require organizations to define the content and scope of spiritual and other assessments and the qualifications of the individual(s) performing the assessment (33).

The World Health Organization has established a quality of life instrument to assess facets of spirituality, religion, and personal beliefs (34).

Surveys of patients in an ambulatory setting indicate that many but not all patients welcome a carefully worded inquiry about their spiritual or religious belief in the event that they become gravely ill (35). As a general statement, patients who were more interested having their physician address this topic had a serious or life-threatening illness, and were in general not interested in this at a routine office visit (36). Writing on behalf of the Working Group on Religious and Spiritual Issues at the End of Life, Bernard Lo, M.D., et al. (37) offered a practical guide for physicians to discuss religious and spiritual issues at the end of life. They address four topics:

1. Some patients may explicitly base decisions about life-sustaining interventions on their spiritual or religious beliefs. Physicians need to explore those beliefs to help patients think through their preferences regarding specific interventions.
2. Other patients may not bring up spiritual or religious concerns but are troubled by them. Physicians should identify such concerns and listen to them empathetically, without trying to alleviate the patient's spiritual suffering by offering premature reassurance.
3. Some patients or families may have religious reasons for insisting on life-sustaining interventions that physicians advise against. The physician should listen and try to understand the patient's viewpoint. Listening respectfully does not require the physician to agree with the patient or misrepresent his or her own views.
4. By responding to patient's spiritual and religious concerns and needs, physicians may help them find comfort and closure near the end of life.

The question "Are you at peace?" has been suggested as one item that can be used to initiate a discussion of spiritual concerns at the end of life (38). Asking patients about the extent to which they are at peace is a starting point to assess spiritual concerns. It gives the patient the opportunity to indicate if they are at peace with God, at peace with their personal relationships, or at peace with themselves. In turn, the physician can then direct additional questions to the patient's response in terms of traditional and nontraditional definitions of spirituality, psychological concerns, or topics the patient might list as disturbances of peace, including financial and family issues, etc.

The spiritual needs of children have been less well evaluated. At least for those with complex health care needs in the hospital, there seems to be a need for health care professionals to recognize that children have spiritual needs that can include religious beliefs (39). A comprehensive text on spirituality and patient care has recently been published in its second edition (40) and is recommended to the interested reader who wishes to pursue this topic further. A summary of this discussion in the form of aphorisms is given in Box 28.1.

Aphorisms for Spirituality in Patient Care

1. Ask open-ended questions to initiate a discussion.
2. Ask the patient to say more.
3. Acknowledge and normalize the patient's concerns.
4. Use empathetic comments.
5. Ask about the patient's emotions.
6. The profound issues of spirituality offer a prime opportunity for patient-centered care.
7. The issue of spirituality may center on the *meaning* of the challenging illness. Avoid the temptation to supply that meaning to patients, especially to a locus external to the person who is living that meaning. (e.g., "This has meaning in God's plan for you" or, "Future patients will benefit from your battle with this disease.")
8. Spiritual issues at the end of life are a challenge for authenticity.
9. Live your life in such a manner that you develop the courage to be happy; take that happiness to the bedside for your patients.
10. Allow goodness, kindness, and love to be expressed.

The first five points are modified from Lo, et al. ref 37. The author is indebted to William A. Russell, M.D., for providing the last four points from his perspective as a pediatrician.

SUMMARY

A definition of spirit as "an animating or vital principle" is useful because it can be productively viewed from a broad range of perspectives. The scientist, the atheist, the existentialist, and the religious person can all use this as a starting point. While the physician will have his or her own perspective, the patient will represent a primary focus.

Many people choose to take an intentional or mindful approach to the life journey incorporating to some degree what Plato called "the examined life." They establish a process of discerning the degree to which their own life is aligned with this animating principle. A survey of poetry, art, music, religion, philosophy, and even "the school of hard knocks" makes clear the rich human experience in the pursuit of this path. For young people, preoccupied with the development of the ego, their question may be "Who am I?" Halfway through life, some people awake one day with the question "Is this all there is?" This characteristic of the midlife crisis may be approached in terms of alignment with the animating principle, or with renewed efforts in the materialistic quest (red sports car, floozy romantic love interest), in which case a second midlife crisis may later appear!

No matter what the person's age, serious, potentially fatal illness represents a threat to this animating principle that may call forth powerful personal responses: "What does it all mean?" "Will I ever get better?" "Has my life been worthwhile?" "What happens after I die?" Appropriately, many patients change their orientation in order to enhance this animating force, according to their understanding and the nature of their illness. For example, some will seek any and all forms of treatment that might extend their life, whether or not it is of proven value. Others, for example the young man or woman who has survived his or her first heart attack, may finally adopt the heart-healthy lifestyle they have been hearing so much about. Another may choose at this time to decline chemotherapy or dialysis and spend the rest of her or his time with family and friends.

The effective physician is likely to be one who spends some time focusing on these issues; personal growth is a component of professionalism. (See Chapter 26, Professionalism.) The astute clinician is likely to be a keen observer of how other people have pursued this basic question. Of the many examples extant (heroes, saints, parent figures), individual patients may be some of the best guides. Physicians should always be aware that their role is to enhance the patient in his or her quest and not to promote their own value system.

Many of the issues raised by patients represent profound questions, and our answers are not much better now than when they were first raised thousands of years ago. We can help with two of them. When the patient asks if they will get better or be cured, it is helpful to understand our role in healing and our contribution to health and wholeness. The nature of the human condition is such that illness and disease do occur. Physicians can do much to help patients move toward the understanding of wholeness and recognition that health includes our adaptation to the presence of some illness, whether it is a consequence of aging, or a disease process.

When the patient asks what happens when he or she dies, we cannot address what occurs after their death. We can speak to what happens *while* they die. And, there, we can always provide comfort. No physician should use the term "I have nothing more to offer." When patients reach the final stages in their life, the world of medicine has a wealth of resources to alleviate pain and provide psychological and emotional support. These include hospice care, hospital or outpatient spiritual support services, and pastoral care by clergy and laity (see Chapter 31).

REFERENCES

1. May GG. *The Dark Night of the Soul*. SanFranciso, CA, New York, NY: Harper, 2004:124–125.
2. Gyatso T. His Holiness the Fourteenth Dalai Lama. *The Universe in a Single Atom. The Convergence of Science and Spirituality*. New York, NY: Broadway Books, 2005:46.
3. Khan HI. *The Heart of Sufism*. Boston, MA: Shambala Publications, 1999:93.
4. Gehman HS, ed. *The New Westminster Dictionary of the Bible*. Philadelphia, PA: Westminster Press, 1970:901.
5. *Shorter Oxford English Dictionary*. Oxford, England: CT Onions Ed., 1964.
6. familydoctor.org editorial staff. Spirituality and Health. Available at: www.familydoctor.org. Accessed April 25, 2008.
7. Still AT. *Osteopathy: Research and Practice*. Kirksville, MO: privately published by the author, 1910. Quoted in Adler P, and Northup GW. *100 Years of Osteopathic Medicine*. Northville, IL: Monograph. Medical Communications, Inc., 1978:21.
8. Still AT. *Osteopathy: Research and Practice*. Kirksville, MO: privately published by the author, 1910. Quoted in Adler P, and Northup GW. *100 Years of Osteopathic Medicine*. Northville, IL: Monograph. Medical Communications, Inc., 1978:23.
9. Special Committee on Osteopathic Principles and Osteopathic Technic. Kirksville College of Osteopathy and Surgery. An interpretation of the osteopathic concept. Tentative formulation of a teaching guide for faculty, hospital staff and student body. *J Osteopath* 1953;60(10):7–10.
10. Ward RC, ed. *Foundations of Osteopathic Medicine*. Baltimore, MD: Williams & Wilkins, 1997:4.
11. Ward RC, ed. *Foundations of Osteopathic Medicine*. Baltimore, MD: Williams & Wilkins, 1997:8.
12. Lyons AS, Petrucelli RJ. *Medicine: An Illustrated History*. New York, NY: Henry N. Abrams, 1978:31.
13. Lyons AS, Petrucelli RJ. *Medicine: An Illustrated History*. New York, NY: Henry N. Abrams, 1978:298.
14. Lyons AS, Petrucelli RJ. *Medicine: An Illustrated History*. New York, NY: Henry N. Abrams, 1978:427.
15. Collins FS. *The Language of God: The Scientist Presents Evidence for Belief*. New York, NY: Free Press, 2007:197–211.

16. Trimble MR. *The Soul and the Brain: the Cerebral Basis of Language, Art and Belief.* Baltimore, MD: John Hopkins University Press, 2007:137–141.

17. DeRidder D, Van Laere K, Dupont P, et al. Visualizing out-of-body experience in the brain. *New Engl J Med* 2007;357:1829–1833.

18. Ehrson HH. The experimental induction of out-of-body experiences. *Science* 2007;317:1048.

19. Lennggenhager B, Tadi T, Metzinger T, et al. Video ergo sum: manipulating body self-consciousness. *Science* 2007;317:1096–1099.

20. Op cit. 14, page 6.

21. Barnes PM, Powell-Griner E, McFann K, et al. Complementary and alternative medicine use among adults: United States, 2002. *CDC Advance Data Report No. 343.2004.* Available at: http://nccam.nih.gov/news/report. Pdf on April 18, 2008.

22. Blumenthal JA, Babyak MA, Ironson G, et al. Spirituality, religion and clinical outcomes in patients recovering from an acute myocardial infarction. *Psychosom Med* 2007;69:501–508.

23. Ai AL, Pederson C, Tice TN, et al. The influence of prayer coping on mental health and cardiac surgery patients. The role of optimism and acute distress. *J Health Psychol* 2007;12(4):580–596.

24. Jantos M, Kiat H. Prayer as medicine: how much have we learned? *Med J Aust* 2007;186:S51–S53.

25. Benson H, Dusek JA, Sherwood JB, et al. Study of the therapeutic effects of intercessory prayer (STEP) in cardiac bypass patients: a multicenter randomized trial of uncertainty and certainty of receiving intercessory prayer. *Am Heart J* 2006;151(4):934–942.

26. Krucoff MW, Crater SW, Gallup D, et al. Music, imagery, touch and prayer as adjuncts to interventional cardiac care: the monitoring and actualization of noetic training (MANTRA) II randomised study. *Lancet* 2005;366:211–217.

27. Hover-Krane, Mentgen D. *Healing Touch: A Resource for Healthcare Professionals.* Delmar, NY: Albany, 1996.

28. Roberts L, Ahmed I, Hall S. Intercessory prayer for the alleviation of ill health. *Cochrane Database Syst Rev* 2008;1.

29. Masters KS, Spielmans GI. Prayer and health: review, meta-analysis and research agenda. *J Behave Med* 2007;30:329–338.

30. Jonas WB, Crawford CC. *Healing, Intention and Energy Medicine. Science Research Methods and Clinical Implications.* London: Churchill Livingstone, 2003.

31. Paul of Tarsus. *Galatians* 5:22–23

32. Op cit Gyatso, T. p.5

33. Spiritual Assessment. Oakbrooke Terrance, Illinois: Joint Commission on Accreditation of Healthcare Organizations: Last revised January 2004. Available at: http://www.jointcommission.org/AccreditationPrograms/Hospitals/Standards/FAQs/Provision+of+Care/Assessment/Spiritual_Assessment.htm. Accessed April 25, 2008.

34. WHOQOL SRPB Group. A cross-cultural study of spirituality, religion and personal beliefs as components of quality of life. *Soc Sci Med* 2006;62:1486–1497.

35. Ehman TW, Ott B, Schwart TH, et al. Do patients want physicians to inquire about their spiritual or religious beliefs if they become gravely ill? *Arch Int Med* 299;159(15):1803–1806.

36. McCord G, Gilcrest VJ, Grossman SD et al. Discussing spirituality with patients. A rationale and ethical approach. *Ann Family Med* 2004;2(4):356–361.

37. Lo B, Ruston D, Kales LW, et al.; For the Working Group on Religious and Spiritual Issues at the End of Life. Discussing religious and spiritual issues at the end of life: a practical guide for physicians. *JAMA* 2002;287:749–754.

38. Steinhauser KE, Voyls CI, Clipp EC, et al. "Are You At Peace?" One item to probe spiritual concerns at the end of life. *Arch Intern Med* 2006;166:101–105.

39. Bull A, Gillies M. Spiritual needs of children with complex healthcare needs in hospital. *Paediatr Nurs* 2002;19(9):34–38.

40. Koenig HG. *Spirituality in Patient Care: Why, How, When and What.* West Conshohocken, PA: Templeton Foundation Press, 2007.

29

Patient-Centered Model

RICHARD BUTLER

KEY CONCEPTS

- Osteopathic principles and philosophy call for a patient-centered approach to the medical encounter.
- Patient-centered care is more than a set of definable communication skills; it is a value that endorses the importance of providing information and facilitating patient involvement.
- Medical encounters often fail to provide patient-centered care.
- Patient-centered skills can be learned; however, the influence of improving patient-centered communication on health outcomes is less clear.
- Patient perception that they have found common ground with their physician appears to be an essential aspect of the patient-centered method.

INTRODUCTION

Proposed tenets of osteopathic medicine and principles for patient care (Rogers et al., 2002) have put forth that "a person is the product of a dynamic interaction between body, mind and spirit," and that "the patient is the focus for healthcare." These tenets direct osteopathic students and practitioners to provide care to patients that may be described as "whole patient" care or "patient-centered care."

The purpose of this chapter is to guide the student through a definition of patient-centered care from multiple perspectives and to review the evidence identifying the efficacy of such an approach. We will also review the striking evidence that it is common for patients in today's health care system to experience care that is not patient centered. The clinical skills and system changes needed to ensure the delivery of a more patient-centered approach to care will also be discussed.

PATIENT-CENTERED CARE IN THE CONTEXT OF THE MEDICAL ENCOUNTER

Patient-centered care within the context of the medical encounter has been defined and described by many. Perhaps the earliest proponent of an expanded model of medical care in the United States was George Engel (1977, 1980). Dr. Engel articulated the limitations of applying a strict biomedical conceptualization to patients presenting with medical illness. He developed an approach to care that he defined as the biopsychosocial model. The application of this model to the medical encounter has been described as patient-centered care (Stewart, 2003, p. 123) or relationship-centered care (Tresolini and the Pew-Fetzer Task Force, 1994).

In its essence, patient-centered care may be viewed as a core value implemented through a set of clinical skills. Information and involvement are at the heart of the patient-centered model. Patients are encouraged to express their values and preferences prior to the implementation of diagnostic or therapeutic interventions. The physician uses a cluster of communication skills with the specific intent of (a) identifying and responding to patients' ideas and emotions regarding their illness and (b) reaching common ground about the illness, its treatment, and the roles that the physician and the patient will assume (Epstein, 2000). This is consistent with the practice and application of evidence-based medicine, one component of which is the assessment of patient values. (Sackett et al., 2000, p. 1)

Patient-centered care is in contrast to a more prevalent model in health care that may be best described as benevolent paternalism: an approach to care where the well-meaning physician determines what is best for the patient and applies diagnostic and therapeutic interventions with little or no dialogue between the patient and physician (Braddock et al., 1999; Coulter, 1999). Benevolent paternalism is recognized when clinicians make statements to patients such as, "It is time for your mammogram," or "You need to have a colonoscopy," or "Your hemoglobin A1C should be below 7.5%." These statements represent possible choices that patients can make in their care, each with its own potential for benefit and harm. A patient-centered approach would engage patients in the evaluation of these choices, identifying the opportunity for benefit and risk juxtaposed against the relative value or importance of the choice given the overall state of the patient's life at the time (Austoker, 1999). Although difficult for many physicians to grasp, now is not always the right time for a patient to quit smoking, reduce their drinking, start a diet, begin exercising, start a new blood pressure medication, engage in screening, or practice stress reduction techniques (Rollnick et al., 1999, pp. 34–36).

The patient-centered approach encourages physicians to cultivate healing relationships based on who the patient is rather than who the physician would have him be (Epstein, 2000). This method, however, is not a simple passive acceptance of each patient, but a skilled and directive approach to the doctor–patient relationship based on respect, empathy, and a shift toward power sharing with the goal of enhancing and optimizing patient health.

Stewart (2003) has described six interactive components of the patient-centered method:

1. Exploring both the disease and the illness experience
2. Understanding the whole person
3. Finding common ground
4. Incorporating prevention and health promotion
5. Enhancing the patient–doctor relationship
6. Being realistic

Specific communication skills are utilized to facilitate the implementation of these components.

PATIENT-CENTERED CARE IN THE BROADER CONTEXT OF SYSTEMS OF CARE

There is increasing concern that our current system of health care fails to deliver consistently safe and effective patient-centered care. Perhaps the most visible light focused on this problem came with the publication of Institute of Medicine's (IOM) report, *To Err Is Human* (Kohn et al., 2000). This report described a dysfunctional and disintegrated health care system where the risk for harm to patients is real and often not appropriately addressed. In the follow-up publication, *Crossing the Quality Chasm: A New Health System for the 21st Century*, the IOM called for reform to ensure safe, effective, patient-centered, timely, efficient, and equitable health care delivery. Patient-centered care was defined as, "providing care that is respectful of and responsive to individual patient preferences, needs, and values and ensuring that patient values guide all clinical decisions" (Committee on Quality Health Care in America, Institute of Medicine, 2001, pp. 39–40).

Other national organizations have joined in the call for a more patient-centered health care system. The Institute for Healthcare Improvement has defined "ten simple rules" to guide reform (Institute for Health Care Improvement, 2008). The first four of these rules identify components that are recognized as the foundations of a patient-centered model of medical care: (1) care is based on continuous healing relationships, (2) care is customized according to the patient needs and values, (3) the patient is the source of control, and (4) knowledge is shared and information flows freely.

The American Osteopathic Organization, in collaboration with other professional societies, is calling for the development of new model of primary care delivery known as The Patient-Centered Medical Home (PC-MH) (American Academy of Family Physicians, American academy of Pediatrics, American College of Physicians, and American Osteopathic Association, 2007). The PC-MH is based on seven guiding principles, one of which is a "whole person orientation." In this model, the primary care physician is placed at the center of a system designed to provide coordinated and integrated comprehensive care for patients of all ages.

Other proposed changes to enhance patient-centered care at a system level include allowing patients to schedule their own appointments and providing open access to their electronic medical record. New models for chronic disease management that include group visits and coaching patients to become more engaged and active in the medical encounter are also being implemented (Bergeson and Dean, 2006).

THE CURRENT STATE OF DOCTOR-PATIENT COMMUNICATION

When one begins to look inside the medical encounter for evidence of patient-centered communication, a concerning picture starts to arise. For example, investigators have studied how well physicians assess the reasons why patients present for medical care in different clinical settings. This task, which should occur early in a medical encounter, is known as assessing the patient's agenda and is a basic component of patient-centered care.

Agenda setting in primary care visits was assessed by Marvel et al. (1999). The investigators evaluated 264 medical encounters performed by 29 board-certified family physicians. The physicians in this sample failed to elicit the patient's initial statement concern in 25% of the encounters. In the 75% of encounters where the agenda was assessed, physicians allowed patients to complete their initial statement of concern only 28% of the time, with the remaining patients being interrupted and redirected after a mean of

23.1 seconds. The patients in the sample who were allowed to complete their initial statement of concern took an average of only 6 more seconds to do so. In addition, interrupting patients increased the risk of late arising concerns by more than twofold (the patient who at the end of a visit states, "Doctor, did I tell you that I am also having chest pains?"), resulting in an inefficient and potentially dissatisfying encounter for both the patient and the physician.

Agenda setting and other communication skills were evaluated in emergency room encounters by Rhodes et al. (2004). These investigators analyzed 93 emergency department encounters performed by 24 emergency medicine residents and 8 nurses. The physicians in this sample failed to introduce themselves in one third of the encounters and indicated their level of training in only 8%. Only 20% of patients were allowed to complete their presenting complaint without interruption; the remaining 80% patients were interrupted in a mean of 12 seconds. Discharge instructions, an important component of emergent and urgent medical encounters, lasted 76 seconds on average (7 to 202 seconds). Only 16% of patients were asked if they had any further questions and clinicians never confirmed patient understanding.

The exploration of the emotional aspects of illness, known as empathic communicationis another important component of the patient-centered method. Suchman et al. (1997) evaluated empathic communication in 23 encounters performed by generalist physicians in outpatient settings. The investigators found that patients rarely expressed emotions directly, but tended to offer indirect clues to the emotional impact of their illness. Physicians commonly ignored the emotional content offered by patients, often diverting the conversation back to the exploration of the biomedical aspects of the encounter. Physician failure to acknowledge emotional content frequently resulted in patients engaging in repeated attempts at emotional expression, often with increasing intensity, placing efficiency and satisfaction within the encounter at risk.

In a similar study, Levinson et al. (2000) found that physician failure to respond to emotional clues presented by patients in primary care and surgical settings resulted in encounters that tended to last longer compared to encounters where emotional expression was acknowledged and facilitated. Taken together, these observations suggest that the expression of emotion appears to be an important and perhaps essential aspect of the medical encounter for many patients. These results should challenge the common assumption that allowing patients to express emotions will cause physicians to lose control of the direction and duration of the medical encounter.

Involving patients in medical decision making is another communication element at the heart of the patient-centered approach. Braddock et al. (1999) evaluated the nature and completeness of informed decision making in 1,057 routine medical encounters with 59 primary care physicians (family practice and general internal medicine) and 65 general and orthopedic surgeons. The investigators developed a taxonomy of decision making, recognizing that medical decisions vary in terms of complexity and uncertainty. Seven elements of informed decision making were identified. Through a consensus process, the authors determined which of these elements should be included for decisions of varying complexity. A medical decision was defined as "complete" if all of the required elements were present. Basic decisions, such as checking a TSH level in patients on thyroid replacement therapy or electrolytes in patients on antihypertensive therapy, were considered complete if only two of the seven elements were present: discussing the nature of the decision and asking the patient to voice a preference. Complex decisions, such as prostate cancer screening or genetic testing for breast cancer risk, should include all seven of the elements.

The 1,057 encounters included 3,552 decisions, 1,857 of which were basic, 1,478 were intermediate, and 217 were complex. About one in five (17.2%) of the "basic decisions" contained the two required elements for completeness and only one of the "complex decisions" in the entire sample contained the required seven elements.

In a type of secondary analysis, the investigators asked how often the two essential elements required for basic decisions were present in any decision, regardless of complexity. For this analysis, any decision making was defined as complete if the physician simply discussed the nature of the decision and asked the patient to voice a preference. An example of complete decision making at the most basic level might be, "Because of your age, we should probably check a PSA level. Is that OK with you?" Although two component basic decision making could be viewed as the moral minimum for any decision, only one in five decisions (20.4%) in the entire cohort, regardless of the level of complexity, met this very basic level of completeness. Surgeons tended to outperform primary care physicians (21.8% vs. 18.9% complete, respectively), but results for both groups were shockingly low. If patient-centered care is performed on a platform of information and involvement, this evidence suggests that current medical care frequently falls short of the ideal.

On perhaps a more positive note, some evidence suggests that osteopathic physicians might be more patient-centered compared to our allopathic counterparts. Carey et al. (2003) evaluated audiotapes of 54 medical encounters with 11 osteopathic and 7 allopathic physicians to determine if osteopathic and allopathic primary care physicians differed in a communication style. In a blinded analysis, osteopathic physicians were more likely to discuss preventive measures, health issues in relation to family life and social activities, and the patient's emotional state compared to allopathic physicians. These results suggest that osteopathic principles and training are congruent with the patient-centered approach.

EVALUATING THE EFFECT OF PATIENT-CENTERED COMMUNICATION ON MEDICAL AND HEALTH OUTCOMES

Although it is clear that communication problems in the medical encounter are common, it may be less clear if educational interventions can improve physician communication behavior or if improved communication will result in improved health outcomes. Before one can suggest wide-ranging changes in the structure of the doctor-patient encounter, some evidence of feasibility and benefit should exist.

Rao et al. (2007) performed a systematic review to evaluate the effectiveness of communication interventions on subsequent communication behaviors in the medical encounter. The authors identified 36 randomized controlled trials that met their inclusion criteria. Educational interventions varied and focused on physicians only, patients only, or a combination of both and may have utilized one or more educational strategies of varying intensity. In general, physicians exposed to the various interventions tended to exhibit more patient-centered behaviors and receive higher global ratings of their communication. When patients were the target of the interventions, they tended to be more involved during the encounter and obtain more information compared to control patients. However, the investigators noted that many of the effective interventions required fairly intense educational efforts and recognized that easy integration into a busy practice setting may not be feasible.

Perhaps the most important and effective educational approaches will be achieved through the integration of comprehensive communication curriculum into medical school curriculum when students are still forming their professional identity (Kalet et al., 2004; Yedidia et al., 2003). Indeed, most if not all medical schools have formal communication skills curriculum and methods to assess the acquisition of these skills. Whether these skills can be maintained when students are placed into the "real world" of clinical medicine is not entirely clear.

Although it is apparent that educational interventions are able to change physician and patient communication in the medical encounter, it remains less clear if these changes actually result in measurable differences in medical outcomes. In an attempt to answer this question, Griffin et al. (2004) conducted a systematic review of randomized controlled trials evaluating the impact of communication interventions on changes in measurable health outcomes or satisfaction. Communication interventions were directed at patients, practitioners, or both. Measurements of changes in the communication process evaluated either patient participation in the encounter, such as question asking or information seeking, or changes in physician communication style, such as addressing psychosocial issues or attending to patient emotion. A range of outcome measures were evaluated with some studies including more than one assessment. Changes in health outcomes included the evaluation of objective measures of disease processes such as change in blood pressure or glucose control, or changes in subjective measures of illness experiences such as self-reported symptoms of anxiety, depression, functional status, well-being, and quality of life. Other health-related outcome measures included changes in cost, patient knowledge, and adherence to treatment. Changes in satisfaction usually involved measurements of patient satisfaction with the process and outcomes of care.

The authors screened more than 21,200 reports and performed a full assessment of 148 of these to identify 35 trials that met their inclusion criteria. The quality of the reviewed and included trials varied considerably and rigorous outcome measurements were lacking in many of the studies. Most of the trials occurred in primary care settings and included patients with common chronic medical problems. Median follow-up time was only 4 weeks. Only four of the trials that utilized objective measures of health outcomes met all of the prespecified quality criteria.

Communication process improved to a significant degree in 22 of 30 (73%) of the trials that evaluated these measures. However, in six trials, at least one measurement of communication process deteriorated. Objective measures of health outcomes, including HBA1c levels, blood pressure control, and cholesterol levels, favored the intervention group in five of six trials (83%). Subjective measures of health outcomes, including pain ratings, functional status, well-being, and other psychological symptoms such as depression and anxiety, favored the intervention group in 21 of 25 trials (84%). Neither of the two studies that measured medication adherence favored the intervention group. Patient satisfaction with the process of care was higher in the intervention group in 17 of the 27 (63%) trials that assessed this outcome. In contrast, satisfaction increased in control group in 7 of the 27 trials (23%).

The authors concluded that although there is significant evidence to support the concept that interventions directed at changing the process of communication between doctors and patients can lead to a more patient-centered style, the influence of these changes on health-related outcomes is variable and less certain. It is clear from this review that there remains a significant need for more and higher quality research before one can state with a degree of certainty that patient-centered communication will consistently lead to improved health outcomes.

Our understanding of what constitutes the essential components of the patient-centered method was deepened by a well-designed observational cohort study performed by Stewart et al. (2000). Medical encounters between 39 family physicians and 319 of their patients were evaluated to determine the influence of both objective measures of physician-patient communication and subjective measures of patient perception of patient centeredness on health-related outcomes and the subsequent utilization of medical resources. Audiotapes of the medical encounters were scored for the degree of patient-centered communication in the following three domains: physician exploration of the disease and illness experience, understanding the illness in the context of the whole person, and finding common ground. Immediate postencounter interviews were conducted with the patients to determine their perception of the patient centeredness of the visit. The investigators developed a total patient-centeredness score and two subscores rating the exploration of the disease and illness, and the finding of common ground. The utilization of medical care resources during the subsequent 2-month period was assessed by determining the use of diagnostic testing and referrals related to the main complaint of the visit and the number of return visits to the physician. Health outcomes included patient ratings of symptom severity and level of concern immediately postvisit and in telephone interviews conducted 2 months later.

In a somewhat surprising finding, objective ratings of patient-centered communication from audiotape analysis failed to correlate with either subsequent resource utilization or patient-reported health outcomes. However, subjective measures of the patient's perception of patient centeredness were associated with decreased postvisit levels of discomfort and concern about symptoms and improved mental health scores at two months. Subsequent health care utilization was also influenced by the perception of patient centeredness. Patients who perceived the encounter to be more patient centered were 40% less likely to receive diagnostic tests and 50% less likely to be referred. This relationship was even stronger for the subscore of reaching common ground where there was an 80% reduction in diagnostic testing and 60% reduction in referrals.

This study seems to indicate that patient perception may be far more important than objective counts of the occurrence of specific communication skills. It appears that the physician striving to improve health outcomes through a more patient-centered approach should continually ask themselves and the patient, "Are we achieving common ground in this encounter?"

IMPROVING THE PATIENT-CENTERED APPROACH

There are several well-accepted models designed to help students and physicians conceptualize and learn the essential communication tasks and skills of a more patient-centered medical encounter. Most medical schools have identified one of the accepted models and have developed structured curriculum based on essential texts and readings. It is beyond the scope of this chapter to discuss these models in depth; rather, each medical student must engage in the curriculum at his or her school. The following suggestions have been derived from the synthesis of several models, as well as clinical experience.

The first step in any encounter, for new or return patients, and regardless of the setting, is to invest in the beginning. This is accomplished by assessing the patient's agenda early with the use of open-ended questions. An example for a new patient might be (after you have introduced yourself to the patient), "How were you hoping that I can help you?" Facilitative comments are used to ensure that the patient has given you a complete statement of their concerns. For example, a patient may be presenting with a complaint of headaches. After you have heard a bit about the nature of the initial problem, it is important to stop the patient and check for additional concerns. The physician might say, "So it sounds like the main reason for your visit today is headaches. Before I learn more about them, it's helpful for me to know if there are other concerns that you may have. What else is on your mind?" For return appointments, it is appropriate to acknowledge that you may have requested the follow-up visit, while still being sure to assess the patient's agenda for new concerns or complaints. An example might be, "The reason I asked you to come back was to see how you were doing with the adjustment in your insulin dose. But before we start, how about you, what do you want to be sure we accomplish in today's visit?" Or, "In addition to checking on your diabetes, what other issues are on your mind that we may need to talk about today?" I also find it helpful to check with the patient later in the encounter to be sure we are meeting our mutual agenda. "So, if we accomplish these three things today, will that meet your needs?"

Even when the reason for the visit is quite clear and focused, such as in an emergency department, it may still be appropriate to initiate the encounter with an open-ended question. An example might be, "The nurse tells me that you have a pretty bad injury to your hand. Before I take a look, how are you holding up?" The question, "How are you holding up?" is particularly useful in emergency room settings because it actively encourages patients to disclose emotional aspects of their illness and will create opportunities for the physician to offer brief moments of support and empathy in what is often an emotionally charged environment of care. While examining the laceration, the physician can efficiently assess the patient's complete agenda by stating, "It's clear this laceration is the main reason you came in. However, it's helpful for me to know if there are any other concerns that you may want to tell me about while we get you fixed up. What else is going on?"

As the studies described earlier point out, patients often fail to directly verbalize the emotional content of their illness. It is therefore important to be alert to and acknowledge nonverbal expressions of emotion and create opportunities for patients to talk about their feelings. These conversations do not need to be long or dominate the discussion of medical topics. Brief comments like, "you seem uncomfortable" or "you have been suffering a lot with these headaches" gives the patient permission to describe the more complicated and frightening aspects of their illness. As mentioned earlier, failure to acknowledge the emotional domains of illness may prolong the encounter and harm satisfaction. Remember, there is a human relationship embedded within every doctor–patient relationship.

Education and the involvement of patients in medical decision making is another essential and moderately complex task. An in-depth discussion of this area is beyond the scope of this chapter. However, a few comments may be helpful. As physicians offer diagnostic and therapeutic options and advice to patients, it is important to recognize that it is perhaps the norm for patients to feel some degree of ambivalence about many of these decisions, particularly more complex decisions. Simply reflecting this ambivalence can be very helpful to patients. An example might be, "On the one hand you can see your blood pressure is remaining elevated and that is concerning to you. You worry about having a stroke like your father and you would like to keep that from happening to you. And yet on the other hand you do not really like taking medication.

It's expensive and it seems that it makes you feel tired and not like yourself. You don't like the thought of adding a new pill to the two that you are already taking. Do I have that right?" You can then ask patients. "What do you see as your options?" or "How can I help you with this decision?"

It can also be helpful to present a menu of choices while creating space for the patient to decide. An example might be, "I see three options for your blood pressure that all seem reasonable and safe in the short run, and maybe there are some that I haven't thought about. The first would be to keep things the same and watch what happens to your blood pressure readings. A second approach might be to work a bit harder on diet and exercise and to really be sure that you are taking all of your pills as prescribed. A third would be to add a new pill. What are your thoughts? Do any of these options sound reasonable, or do you see others we may not have talked about?"

An approach that may be helpful and efficient when discussing higher complexity decisions, such as the acceptance of screening, is to talk to patients about groups of people and then ask the patient to decide which, if any, group they see themselves most likely to fit into. An example might be, "There are some patients who value doing all they can to lower their risk of dying from a cancer like colon cancer. These patients see the benefits of screening and are willing to undergo these tests even in the face of some uncertainty about the benefits and acknowledging the small, but real potential for harm. They, for the most part, choose to undergo screening. And then there are other patients who do not feel so strongly. They tend to be more concerned about the potential risks for harm and tend to want to avoid undergoing tests and medical procedures. They are willing to accept the small but real risk that some day they may develop a cancer that might have been helped or even cured by screening. These patients, for the most part, choose not to undergo screening. How about you? What group do you see yourself fitting into? And is there more information that you might need to help you decide?"

All medical encounters should conclude with some review of what has transpired and the plans for ongoing and follow-up care. It may be helpful to have patients summarize their understanding prior to leaving. At a minimum, it is clearly helpful to check with patients by asking, "Does today's plan make sense?" followed by the more open-ended question, "What other questions do you have?" Asking the patient about any concerns regarding the treatment plan can be very enlightening. It actively pulls for the emotional content of the patient's illness and may provide insight to important issues that could hinder compliance. It will again offer brief opportunities to provide empathy and support to patients.

And lastly, the task of understanding the whole person in the context of a medical encounter is greatly facilitated by asking the simple question, "What would you like me to know about you as a person?" This question appears to be best asked early in the encounter after the patient's initial agenda has been assessed. I will often structure the question in the following manner: "So it seems that the main issues that bring you here today are your blood pressure, your diabetes, and the back pain that has been troubling you. Do I have that right? Before we explore these medical topics in more depth, I am wondering if I could learn a bit about you as a person. What would you like me to know about you?" This question can be both refreshing to patients and at times unsettling. Patients who have never been asked such a question by a physician may respond with some defensiveness by asking, "What do you mean? What do you want to know?" I gently stay with the question by reflecting, "Anything. Anything you would like me to know?" Sometimes I ask patients, "What do you love to do?" These discussions do not need to last long, but the simple process of a doctor actually being curious about a patient beyond their symptoms and illness can facilitate patient engagement in the encounter and the perception of being on common ground. It is this kind of information that allows a doctor to really know their patient.

SUMMARY

The time-pressured world of modern medical practice, defined by product lines, revenue generated per case, physician relative value units, corporate pressures on throughput, decreasing physician reimbursement, and the application of clinical guidelines to patients with little or no dialogue conspire against a more collaborative approach to the medical encounter. It is clear that with appropriate effort patient-centered communication skills can be defined and learned. However, the effect of these changes on measurable outcomes is less certain. There are many factors that influence health outcomes, only one of which is communication within the context of a medical encounter. Social economic status, job stress, social isolation, education status, and mental health factors are just a few of the known determinates of health that are not easily influenced within the confines of a professional medical encounter.

Patient-centered care appears to be more than a set of skills to be learned and applied; it is, perhaps, a way of being with patients. A patient-centered approach will require that physicians affirm a deep personal value that believes in the capacity of each patient to be a meaningful partner in their own health care, capable of making choices that fit with their values and broader life circumstances. It will also require a commitment to finding common ground with patients in the medical encounter. As Stewart et al. (2000, p. 800) state, "Physicians may learn to go through the motions of patient-centered interviewing without understanding what it means to be a truly attentive and responsive listener" (Stewart et al., 2000, p. 800). Our presence and how patients perceive us matters. Perhaps for no other reason, efforts to improve patient centeredness may be justifiable on moral and ethical grounds alone. After all, is this not the care that you hope one day to receive from your physician?

REFERENCES

American Academy of Family Physicians, American Academy of Pediatrics, American College of Physicians, and the American Osteopathic Association. *Joint Principles of the Patient-centered Medical Home*. 2007. Retrieved February 4, 2008, from the World Wide Web: http://www.aafp.org/online/etc/medialib/aafp_org/documents/policy/fed/jointprinciplespcmh0207.Par.0001.File.dat/022107medicalhome.pdf

Austoker J. Gaining informed consent for screening. *Br Med J* 1999;319:722–723.

Bergeson SC, Dean JD. A systems approach to patient-centered care. *JAMA* 2006;296(23):2848–2851.

Braddock CH, Edwards KA, Hasenberg NM, et al. Informed decision making in outpatient practice: time to get back to basics. *JAMA* 1999;282:2313–2320.

Carey TS, Motyka TM, Garrett JM, et al. Do osteopathic physicians differ in patient interaction from allopathic physicians? An empirically derived approach. *J Am Osteopath Assoc* 2003;103(7):313–318.

Committee on Quality Health Care in America, Institute of Medicine. *Crossing the quality chasm: a new health system for the 21st century*. Washington, DC: National Academy Press, 2001.

Coulter A. Paternalism or partnership? *Br Med J* 1999;319:719–720.

Engel GL. The need for a new medical model: a challenge for biomedicine. *Science* 1977;196:129–136.

Engel GL. The clinical application of the biopsychosocial model. *Am J Psychiatry* 1980;137:535–544.

Epstein RM. The science of patient-centered care. *J Fam Pract* 2000;49(9):805–807.

Griffin SJ, Kinmonth A-L, Veltman MWM, et al. Effect on health-related outcomes of interventions to alter the interaction between patients and practitioners: a systematic review of trials. *Ann Fam Med* 2004;2(6):595–608.

Institute for Healthcare Improvement. Quality rules: how far have we come. 2008 progress report. 2008. Retrieved February 4, 2008, from the World Wide Web: http://www.ihi.org/NR/rdonlyres/741D90B6–753B-4058-A1A2-FF0FB35595E5/0/2008ProgressReportFinal.pdf

Kalet A, Pugnaire MP, Cole-Kelly K, et al. Teaching communication in clinical clerkships:models from the Macy Initiative in Health Communications. *Acad Med* 2004;79(6):511–520.

Kohn LT, Corrigan JM, Donaldson MS, eds. *To Err Is Human: Building a Safer Health System*. Washington, DC: National Academy Press, 2000.

Levinson W, Gorawara-Bhat R, Lamb J. A study of patient clues and physician responses in primary care and surgical settings. *JAMA* 2000;284(8):1021–1027.

Marvel MK, Epstein RM, Flowers K, et al. Soliciting the patient's agenda: have we improved? *JAMA* 1999;281(3):283–287.

Rao JK, Anderson LA, Inui TS, et al. Communication interventions make a difference in conversations between physicians and patients: a systematic review. *Med Care* 2007;45(4), 340–349.

Rhodes KV, Vieth T, He T, et al. Resuscitating the physician-patient relationship: emergency department communication in an academic medical center. *Ann Emerg Med* 2004;44(3), 262–267.

Rollnick S, Mason P, Butler C, eds. *Health Behavior Change: A Guide for Practitioners*. London: Churchill Livingstone, 1999.

Rogers FJ, D'Alonzo GE, Glover JC, et al. Proposed tenets of osteopathic medicine and principles for patient care. *J Am Osteopath Assoc* 2002;102 (2):63–65.

Sackett DL, Straus SE, Richardson WS, et al., eds. *Evidence-based Medicine: How to Practice and Teach EBM*. London: Churchill Livingstone, 2000.

Stewart M. Evidence for the patient-centered clinical method as a means of implementing the biopsychosocial approach. In: Frankel RM, Quil TE, McDaniel SH, eds. *The Biopsychosocial Approach: Past, Present, Future*. Rochester, NY: University of Rochester Press, 2003.

Stewart M, Brown JB, Conner A, et al. The impact of patient-centered care on outcomes. *J Fam Pract* 2000;49(9):796–804.

Suchman AL, Markakis K, Beckman HB, et al. A model of emphatic communication in the medical interview. *JAMA* 1997;277(8):678–682.

Tresolini CP and the Pew-Fetzer Task Force. Health professions education and relationship-centered care: report of the Pew-Fetzer Task Force on Advancing Psychosocial Education. San Francisco, CA: Pew Health Professions Commission, 1994.

Yedidia MJ, Gillespie CC, Kachur E, et al. Effect of communications training on medical student performance. *JAMA* 2003;290(9):1157–1165.

30

Health Promotion and Maintenance

GERALD G. OSBORN AND JOHN A. JEROME

KEY CONCEPTS

- Decrease of overall mortality is due to effective public health measures for disease prevention aimed at large populations.
- Many of the most common noncommunicable diseases are strongly linked to lifestyle and behavior.
- Research into human nutrition continues to identify significant problems in the "western diet," with significant overlap in consensus of the constitution of a healthy diet.
- Physical activity is inversely correlated with morbidity as well as mortality.
- Tobacco and alcohol are readily available, relatively inexpensive, and legal substances that cause more human misery than all illegal substances combined.
- Ill health, disability, and death from unhealthy sexual practices are almost completely preventable.

INTRODUCTION

Historians of medicine and public health have described in detail the dramatic changes that have taken place in medical education, practice, and research in the 20th century. Most of these changes are the result of more effective and expansive technology that has enabled us to trade short-term mortality for long-term morbidity. Disability and death, especially from acute infectious disease, have been increasingly replaced by the chronic illnesses that make their appearance in middle age and late life.

In 1900, the average life expectancy at birth was 46.3 years for men and 48.3 for women. By 2005, however, life expectancy dramatically increased to 75.2 years for men and 80.4 years for women (1). The sweeping epidemiology study, *The Global Burden of Disease* (*GBD*), based upon more sophisticated analyses and egalitarian principles, sets life expectancy standards at birth to be 80 years for men and 82.5 years for women (2). These increases are mostly attributable to the decrease in infant mortality.

Overall mortality has decreased more due to research and technology developed toward more effective public health measures for disease prevention aimed at large populations than medical procedures aimed at individuals. These fundamental strides include the increasing promotion of clean air and water standards; high-quality, safe, affordable food; and safer living and work environments. This increased survival expectancy also includes a generally well-regulated pharmaceutical industry providing immunizations to prevent most common acute infectious diseases occurring early in life and effective antimicrobials to treat infectious diseases we fail to prevent.

These positive strides are now facing serious challenges due to increasing social and lifestyle changes, especially in Western societies. Further advancements in improving the long-term health of our patients depend, for the foreseeable future, upon our understanding the major impact of behavior on health and illness. This involves continuously educating our patients, encouraging their active participation in and cooperation with health maintenance, and motivating them to make choices that will promote the healthiest, most enriched, vigorously productive, and enjoyable lives possible. Growing old remains inevitable but fortunately for most, ill health is not.

Assisting our patients to live long and live well certainly does not mean emphasizing prevention and health maintenance to the neglect of research into increasingly effective technological interventions. New technologies will always be a vital component of the continuum of health care. The promise of effective genetic therapies is especially exciting and represents our most probable next revolution in eradicating chronic as well as acute illnesses (3). In the interim, however, preventive research in the form of improved screening, health maintenance, and positive health-related behavioral changes must be given at least equal emphasis. New strategies to promote positive behavioral change in our patients must be an enduring and vital component of osteopathic medical education, practice, and research if the profession is to make a significant improvement in the overall health of the population.

ADDRESSING THE BURDEN OF DISEASE

The *GBD* continues to represent the most current and profound ongoing study surveying health, injury, and illness worldwide. This investigation, which is a collaborative effort by the Harvard School of Public Health (HSPH), the World Health Organization (WHO), and the World Bank, has changed our understanding of the emerging patterns of illness and provided new methods to calculate its impact on the individual and society.

Looking at mortality is important but an incomplete method of measuring the impact of disease. The level of illness morbidity is increasing and is the more difficult health problem to measure. The *GBD* has assisted health policy planners and medical educators by developing and elaborating the concept of "Disability Adjusted Life Years" (DALY). This method is a means to more accurately determine and quantify the manner in which illnesses rob people of fulfilling and productive lives.

The *GBD* continues to confirm a number of startling shifts in the patterns of disease in countries with developed market economies and developing countries. Since the *GBD*'s data sets begin in 1990 and project out to 2020, and since its most recent data are so accurate, it provides a virtual road map to the changing face of global illness. One of the clearest trends continues to show that the disease patterns of developing nations are beginning to approximate those of the developed ones today. Noncommunicable diseases such as depressive disorders and heart disease are eclipsing the threats of the past, like infectious disease and malnutrition.

The use of the DALY method also continues to demonstrate the formerly drastically underestimated burden of mental illness.

Even in the original 1990 data, the **GBD** indicated that unipolar depressive disorder, bipolar disorder, schizophrenia, obsessive compulsive disorder, and alcoholism accounted for five of the top 10 leading causes of disability worldwide. The burden of psychiatric disorders is highest in the developed nations and this trend continues in an alarming direction. If osteopathic medicine is to make any significant strides in reversing this trend, the profession must pay much more attention to screening, early diagnosis, and expeditious interventions.

The **GBD** also highlights the striking and complex interlocking nature of behavioral risk factors and illness. The most common behaviors most closely associated with disease and ill health include tobacco use, alcohol abuse, and unsafe sexual practices. Given present behavioral trends, tobacco use alone will outweigh the burden of any single illness by 2020. Western nations have instituted preventive measures to lower tobacco use, but the developing countries are becoming the new emerging tobacco market, much to their detriment. Complicating things further is the manner in which some diseases aggravate and predispose to others causing further disability (e.g., hypertension and diabetes increase the risk for heart disease, stroke, and peripheral vascular disease) (4).

Many of the most common noncommunicable diseases are strongly linked to lifestyle and behavior. Osteopathic physicians committed to the most effective comprehensive care simply must place more emphasis upon promoting positive behavioral changes for their patients. We should remain excited about emerging "procedure-oriented" technological interventions but must immediately place more focus upon "the basic building blocks" of health to improve the care we provide. Attention to increasingly customizing comprehensive care in every patient encounter will heighten the efficacy of our treatment and most likely decrease health care costs. Awareness of the leading causes of death, as shown in Table 30.1, certainly emphasizes the value of comprehensive osteopathic care.

TABLE 30.1

Leading Causes of Death in the United States

Causes of Death	Number of Deaths in Thousands
1. Heart disease	652
2. Cancer	559
3. Stroke	144
4. Chronic respiratory disease	131
5. Accidents	118
6. Diabetes mellitus	75
7. Alzheimer's disease	72
8. Pneumonia and influenza	63
9. Inflammatory kidney disease	44
10. Suicide	33

Source: National Center for Chronic Disease Prevention and Health Promotion. Dept. of Health and Human Services (www.cdc.gov/nccdphp/). Last modified November 20, 2008.

IMPACT OF ILLNESS ON THE INDIVIDUAL AND SOCIETY

Nutrition

Nutritional sciences continue to reaffirm the aphorism by Oscar Wilde: "You are what you eat." Research into human nutrition has continued to identify significant problems in the "Western Diet," with the United States being the most striking example. Nutritionists acknowledge significant overlap in the general consensus of what constitutes a healthy diet. Within the past 7 years, however, the controversies about specific foods and especially the proportions of those foods have begun to escalate.

Pick Your Pyramid

More than a decade ago, the United States Department of Agriculture (USDA) created the "Food Guide Pyramid" as a useful model to illustrate to the general public what constitutes a healthy diet. In its first iteration, it received almost universal approval from nutritionists who agreed it was a major positive step. Disagreement was limited to "arguing around the margins" about types of foods and proportions, but the discourse was more relevant to research than practice. The USDA Pyramid has since been revised twice with the last major revision being in 2005 (Fig. 30.1). Since collection and review of nutritional research is ongoing, it is anticipated that the next revision might occur in 2010.

Controversy began after the second revision when nutritional researchers, especially those within the HSPH, openly questioned the influence of food industry on the final product. Because the USDA Guidelines determines the standards for all federal food programs, including school lunch programs, and influences the food shopping choices of many of the general public, even minor recommendations could affect sections of the food industry. The HSPH argued that the revision was not based solely upon the best nutritional science but reflected undue influence by lobbying efforts. The controversy spilled over from the scientific literature to health-related literature for the general public.

The HSPH responded with its own "Healthy Eating Pyramid" (HEP) within the next year and it was been updated in 2008. The Harvard Guidelines stress their version is based only on the best-available science and is easier for the general public to grasp. One major difference includes the HEP suggesting eating more protein from fish, especially those species containing high levels of omega 3 fatty acids and significantly limiting red meat. The HEP also stresses less dairy products and the use of a daily multivitamin, calcium, and vitamin D supplementation. It also emphasizes limiting salt, refined grains, and sugary drinks and, optionally, alcohol in moderation (5,6).

Increasing numbers of people, for reasons of health, spiritual faith, and/or concerns about the moral treatment of animals, are becoming strict vegetarians. For those people, both the USDA and the Harvard Pyramids are only partially useful. To ensure that these people get sufficient protein and vitamin coverage, the "Vegan Food Pyramid" was created (7) (Fig. 30.2).

All three pyramids are featured as charts for use in discussing and customizing prescriptive nutritional advice for patients. Simple readjustments tailored for the individual patient offer significant protection from developing some of the most disabling chronic problems including cardiovascular disease, stroke, hypertension, obesity, osteoporosis, and certain forms of neoplastic disease (8,9).

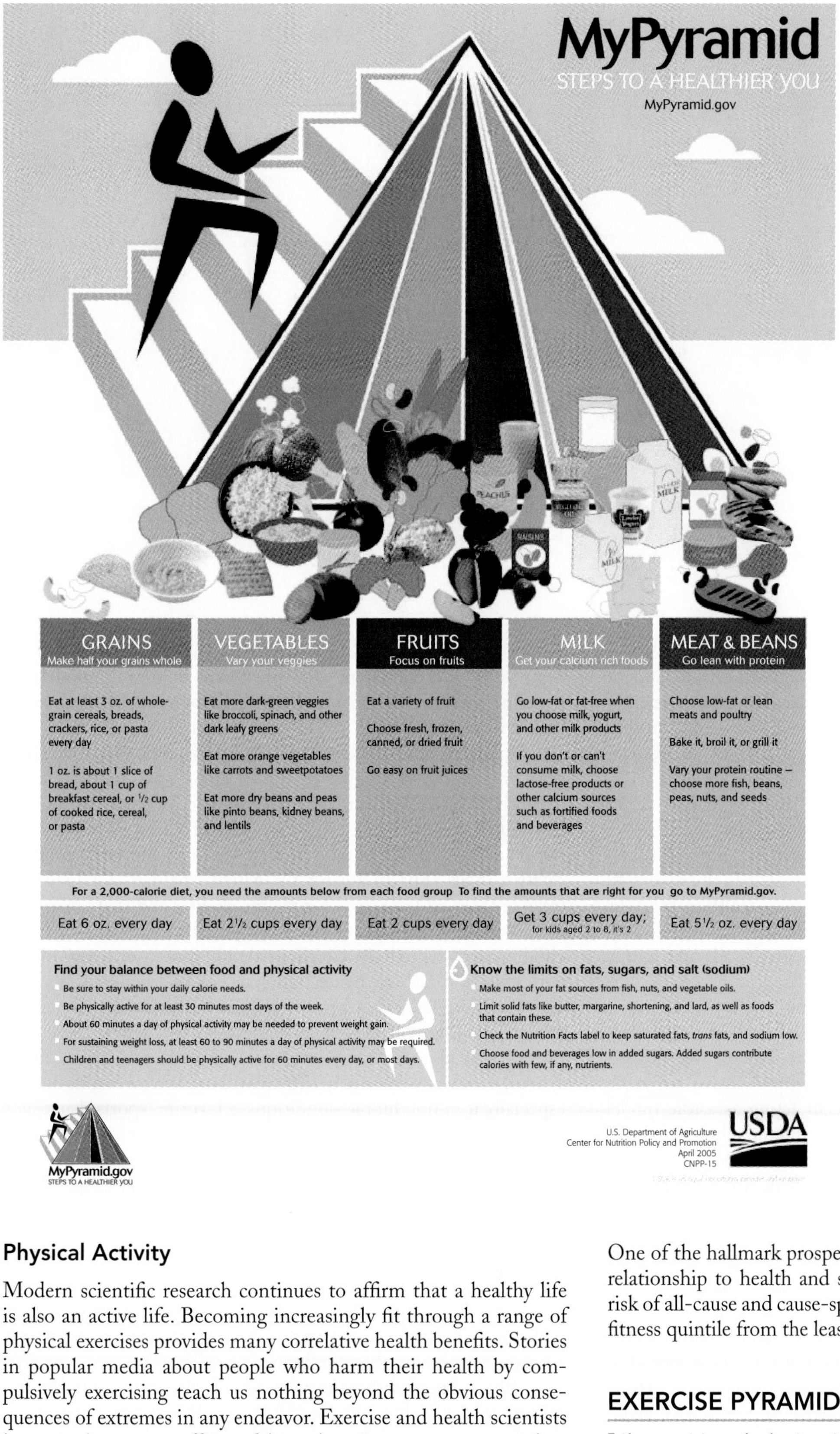

Figure 30-1 The USDA MyPyramid.

MyPyramid
STEPS TO A HEALTHIER YOU
MyPyramid.gov

GRAINS	VEGETABLES	FRUITS	MILK	MEAT & BEANS
Make half your grains whole	Vary your veggies	Focus on fruits	Get your calcium rich foods	Go lean with protein
Eat at least 3 oz. of whole-grain cereals, breads, crackers, rice, or pasta every day 1 oz. is about 1 slice of bread, about 1 cup of breakfast cereal, or ½ cup of cooked rice, cereal, or pasta	Eat more dark-green veggies like broccoli, spinach, and other dark leafy greens Eat more orange vegetables like carrots and sweetpotatoes Eat more dry beans and peas like pinto beans, kidney beans, and lentils	Eat a variety of fruit Choose fresh, frozen, canned, or dried fruit Go easy on fruit juices	Go low-fat or fat-free when you choose milk, yogurt, and other milk products If you don't or can't consume milk, choose lactose-free products or other calcium sources such as fortified foods and beverages	Choose low-fat or lean meats and poultry Bake it, broil it, or grill it Vary your protein routine — choose more fish, beans, peas, nuts, and seeds

For a 2,000-calorie diet, you need the amounts below from each food group To find the amounts that are right for you go to MyPyramid.gov.

Eat 6 oz. every day	Eat 2½ cups every day	Eat 2 cups every day	Get 3 cups every day; for kids aged 2 to 8, it's 2	Eat 5½ oz. every day

Find your balance between food and physical activity
- Be sure to stay within your daily calorie needs.
- Be physically active for at least 30 minutes most days of the week.
- About 60 minutes a day of physical activity may be needed to prevent weight gain.
- For sustaining weight loss, at least 60 to 90 minutes a day of physical activity may be required.
- Children and teenagers should be physically active for 60 minutes every day, or most days.

Know the limits on fats, sugars, and salt (sodium)
- Make most of your fat sources from fish, nuts, and vegetable oils.
- Limit solid fats like butter, margarine, shortening, and lard, as well as foods that contain these.
- Check the Nutrition Facts label to keep saturated fats, trans fats, and sodium low.
- Choose food and beverages low in added sugars. Added sugars contribute calories with few, if any, nutrients.

MyPyramid.gov
STEPS TO A HEALTHIER YOU

U.S. Department of Agriculture
Center for Nutrition Policy and Promotion
April 2005
CNPP-15

USDA

Physical Activity

Modern scientific research continues to affirm that a healthy life is also an active life. Becoming increasingly fit through a range of physical exercises provides many correlative health benefits. Stories in popular media about people who harm their health by compulsively exercising teach us nothing beyond the obvious consequences of extremes in any endeavor. Exercise and health scientists have much more to offer, and here there is more agreement than controversy in the benefits of increasing levels of physical fitness.

Nearly all systematic studies show that high levels of physical activity delay all-cause mortality but mostly due to lower rates of cardiovascular disease. These studies show also that physical activity is inversely correlated with morbidity as well as mortality.

One of the hallmark prospective studies of physical activity and its relationship to health and specific illnesses demonstrates that the risk of all-cause and cause-specific mortality declines across physical fitness quintile from the least fit to the most fit in both sexes (10).

EXERCISE PYRAMIDS

Like nutrition, the basic principles of exercise are fairly straightforward and easy to understand for most people. A number of research exercise programs, however, have taken their cues from nutritional science research and have developed their own "Exercise Pyramids." Also like eating a healthier diet, increasing levels of fitness offer additional protection from developing many diseases, including

Figure 30-2 *Vegan Food Pyramid (Courtesy of Joshua Wold and VeganFoodPyramid.com).*

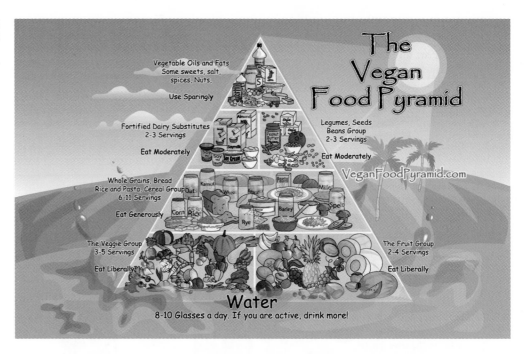

cardiovascular disease, stroke, obesity, non–insulin-dependent diabetes, and osteoporosis. Moreover, a regular comprehensive exercise program has benefits of better emotional and mental health, especially a reduction in feelings of anxiety and depression. Exercise has also been demonstrated to improve immune responses (11,12).

Exercise Pyramids have been created to assist with discussions about prescriptive exercise with patients; these models stress being active in ways that emphasize fun and enjoyment. The extent to which physical activity is paired with enjoyment is the extent to which it will probably be incorporated into a healthier lifestyle. Most people find exercise much more enjoyable when paired with a social activity. Physical activities shared with friends and family (including the four-legged kind) are more likely to become a life-enriching and ordinary activity of daily living.

Extremely important and most often left out of discussions about promoting health by physicians is the issue of role modeling. Osteopathic medicine embraces a comprehensive approach to health, and this includes the physician acting as a role model for vitality and fitness. Patients are much more likely to hear and accept prescriptive advice about health from a physician whose lifestyle exemplifies the behaviors being suggested. Almost regardless of prior levels of fitness, patients can be motivated to begin by first taking steps to increase their levels of activity in their daily lives.

The Exercise Pyramids give examples of this at their bases. Total fitness involves a balanced program consisting of preferably daily aerobic exercise, resistance exercise, and gentle stretching. Aerobics develop stamina, resistance training develops strength, and stretching increases flexibility and helps prevent injury. Patients should be encouraged to begin slowly, consistent with age and current fitness, and gradually increase their level of exercise to prescriptive goals. The levels of fitness they ultimately attain will involve many factors, especially their improved health status and the enjoyment and pride they derive from their efforts. Special attention must be taken with patients for whom exercise represents risk. For these patients, consultation with physical medicine and rehabilitation and/or physical therapy will greatly assist with the therapeutic effects of an exercise program (13). Development of an active lifestyle should begin early and consistent with physicians being role models for patients; parents can become the most important role models for their children to develop good health habits early.

Americans now spend over $12 billion yearly on health-related activities, mostly belonging to health clubs, spas, and/or buying expensive exercise equipment and clothing. While these amenities might add to the social enjoyment of exercise, fitness need not be expensive. Most important expenses should be to promote safety. (Shoes appropriate for the activity, helmets for bicycling, wrist braces and knee pads for in-line skating and skate boarding, etc.) Attention to proper clothing is especially important for young children and the elderly. Clothing should attend to function first with style and fashion being optional. For the increasingly active and fun lifestyles, other protective gear and measures should be taken including sun glasses and adequate sun screen. Adequate hydration is also extremely important. For exercise lasting under 1 hour, cool water is usually sufficient. For exercise lasting longer, especially if in hot, humid conditions, a favorite "sports drink" will provide additional glucose and electrolyte replacement, preventing excess fatigue, dehydration, and speed postexercise recovery. The old coach's advice is still valid: "Take frequent small drinks, if you wait until you feel thirsty, it's already too late."

Obesity

It is ironic that with both the current emphasis by many on health and fitness and the near-universal Western stigma toward people who are overweight, that obesity is now epidemic.

The good news is that the prevalence of obesity in adults has stabilized since 2003 but remains still at 34%. Worse news, however, is that the prevalence of obesity in children has continued to rise from 4.5% in 1970 to 16.3% in 2006. Researchers continue to debate the health risks of being mildly or even moderately overweight. They are in near complete agreement however about the health risks as body mass index (BMI) exceeds 30. The most recent list of health problems associated with obesity is listed for adults and children in Box 30-1, from the Centers for Disease Control (14).

Health Risks Associated With Obesity

- Coronary heart disease
- Type II diabetes
- Cancers (endometrial, breast, and colon)
- Hypertension (high blood pressure)
- Dyslipidemia (e.g., high total cholesterol or high levels of triglycerides)
- Stroke
- Liver and gallbladder disease
- Sleep apnea and respiratory problems
- Osteoarthritis (a degeneration of cartilage and its underlying bone within a joint)
- Gynecological problems (abnormal menses, infertility)

Health promotion researchers have conclusively demonstrated that simple caloric restriction alone does not produce long-term positive results for people who are overweight or obese. Moreover, unsupervised very-low-calorie-diets involve serious health risks (15). For most patients, de-emphasizing weight and emphasizing fitness is the best place to start. Educating, encouraging, and motivating patients to follow the recommendations of the Food and Exercise Pyramids can improve outcomes for both adults and children.

The best guides to monitor progress include the BMI and waist circumference at the navel. The measurement of waist circumference adds an important parameter because the presence of circumferential fat has been demonstrated to pose additional health risks. The ideal trajectory is a gradual weight loss of between 1 and 2 lb per week until the patients' goals are reached. The maintenance of health and fitness requires life-long attention. If former habits of unhealthy eating and sedentary lifestyle return, health risks will predictably again rise. Comprehensive management also requires confronting social pressures and misinformation about weight and the variation among somatotypes. The fashion and advertising industries create completely unrealistic standards of beauty. Even the photographs of fashion models are computer retouched to the point where the finished product represents an aesthetic ideal that does not exist in the natural world. Exciting research into the genetic control of hunger, satiety, and metabolism continues, but these treatments are still far into the future.

For some patients, the course of their weight problem has progressed to a point to where they are at imminent risk. It is here where more vigorous and even invasive surgical procedures are life saving. Medications and bariatric surgery are indicated in these circumstances, and these treatments are beginning to show increasing success. Patients still need to be educated beforehand that decreased health risks, even after successful acute treatment, require life-long behavioral changes. Literature written by physicians and exercise scientists for the lay public are many times very helpful and can easily be incorporated as a component of patients' overall fitness plans (16).

Substance Use and Abuse

Illegal substance abuse continues to be an ongoing social scourge and a significant public health problem. It is ironic however that the two substances that cause more human misery than all illegal substances combined are readily available, relatively inexpensive, and legal. Focusing upon the hazards of these legal substances to our patients is essential to the practice of osteopathic medicine.

Tobacco

Since the release of the first "Surgeon General's Report on Smoking" in 1964, the United States has made impressive strides in lowering the prevalence of smoking. Tobacco companies have been rightfully taken to task for the damage to public health for which they are responsible. As stated earlier though, these companies have merely shifted their markets outside the United States especially targeting developing countries. The strong statement from the *GBD* merits repeating here: "By 2020 tobacco is expected to kill more people than any single disease, surpassing even the HIV epidemic." The most recent Surgeon General's Report, while indicating clear successes, continues to stress that we have still much more room for improvement. The report expands the list of diseases that are directly related to smoking including acute myeloid leukemia, cataracts, abdominal aortic aneurysm, periodontitis, and cancers of the cervix, kidney, pancreas, and stomach (17,18). Most shocking is the more current report on the health consequences of second-hand smoke. Public health research now demonstrates clearly that involuntary exposure to tobacco smoke poses more serious health risks than expected, especially for infants and children. The report does not equivocate: "There is no risk-free level of exposure to second hand smoke." The evidence is now conclusive that second-hand smoke increases the risk for nonsmokers for heart disease, lung cancer, sudden infant death syndrome, respiratory infections, and asthma. The total costs of smoking are estimated at over $100 billion today. The negative effects of smoking on productivity are likewise staggering. The Office of Technology Assessment estimates the costs of lost productivity to be over $47 billion for smokers and lost productivity to second-hand smoke at over $8.6 billion. The message to our patients needs to be loud, firm, clear, and persistent: "If you don't smoke, don't ever start and if you do smoke, quit!"

Smoking cessation literature continues to show that most people who do smoke would prefer to quit and have made efforts to do so. Many smokers are able to quit on their own, but many go to their family physicians for help. The following are some very useful methods physicians can suggest that will increase the likelihood of success:

- Publicly declare a date to stop. Compose a written statement that includes a request of support from family, friends, and co-workers. Some programs even recommend announcing the intent to stop smoking in the local paper.
- Prepare by making efforts to minimize stress, eat a healthier diet, and begin a program of physical fitness.
- Attend to nicotine withdrawal by gradually smoking fewer cigarettes each day.
- Get rid of the "stash" and begin to buy cigarettes one pack at a time.
- Break up learned patterns of smoking by waiting at least 10 minutes before lighting up when craving begins. Smoke with the cigarette in the nondominant hand. Smoke only while standing. Any strategy that makes smoking more inconvenient will help.
- Maintain a positive attitude as the cessation date approaches. A helpful "cognitive restructuring" approach is to de-emphasize the idea of "giving something up," replacing it with a list of all that will be gained fro m your efforts.

On the quitting date and thereafter:

- Make sure all cigarettes are gone.
- Prepare for times of craving by substituting healthy alternatives: fresh fruit, carrot or celery sticks, xylitol chewing gum.

Many report brushing your teeth at times of craving to be a very helpful strategy:

- Increase fluid intake, especially drink water.
- Record progress in a diary or calendar.
- Financially reward yourself. Open an exclusive savings account and regularly deposit the money formerly spent on cigarettes. Be fair to yourself and also bank the spin-off savings from smoking damage to clothing, furniture, automobile interior, etc. Also save the cost of at least one visit to the doctor's office. Enjoy watching your savings grow!

Even with physician advice and coaching, some patients will have increased success with over-the-counter or prescription medications. Nicotine replacement products in all their delivery forms will attenuate withdrawal symptoms. Low-dose antidepressant medications have been demonstrated to be helpful, especially doxepin and bupropion. Also, low-dose clonidine has been shown in the literature to be helpful. Finally, a new medication for smoking cessation (varenicline) has been marketed so successfully that patients will request it by its brand name.

Forms of alternative/complementary medicine may have a place in a comprehensive smoking cessation program depending upon the knowledge base of the physician and the level of acceptance of the patient. One of the most common complementary treatment methods is acupuncture, but the clinical literature about its efficacy is quite mixed (19). When provided by a qualified therapist, acupuncture has demonstrated such a mild side effect profile that it could be included as adjunctive treatment.

An analysis of the literature on smoking cessation reveals the most successful smoking cessation programs use multimodal approaches sharing the commonalities of education, positive motivational encouragement by physicians and other health care professionals, face-to-face contact with a therapist, group therapy emphasizing mutual support, the offer of traditional and complementary treatment, and long-term follow-up (20,21).

Finally, patients who continue to experience relapse should be strongly encouraged to "never quit trying to quit." Helping patients to stop smoking may just be the physician's single most effective preventive effort. WAKE UP CALL: According to the WHO, 45 more people have died worldwide from smoking-related illnesses in the time it has taken you to read this section on tobacco (22).

Alcohol

Although the benefits of moderated alcohol intake have received increasing attention in the medical and popular literature, the abuse of alcohol accounts for a wide spectrum of health and social problems. Alcohol abuse plays a causal or contributing role in injury and deaths from accidents, homicides, and suicides.

Personal Safety

Attending to personal and family safety is a major component of a preventive health program. Educating patients by providing the best and most current information is key. Addressing personal safety issues can be incorporated into new patient screening and provided for current patients in the form of pamphlets. Some safety videos are also available.

AUTOMOBILES

Approximately 50,000 people in the United States die every year in automobile accidents. The automotive industry has made significant strides in making cars safer with the advent of air bags and antilock brakes. Laws that make the use of seat belts mandatory and call for infants and small children to be secured in the rear seats in protective seating have also helped reduce deaths from automobile accidents. Physicians can help patients better understand automobile safety issues by encouraging patients to:

- Purchase vehicles with the latest safety devices (i.e., air bags, antilock brakes)
- Keep automobiles safer through proper maintenance, especially of brakes and tires
- Obey speed limits and all traffic regulations
- Follow all regulations when operating recreational vehicles
- Wear an approved helmet and protective clothing when operating a bicycle, moped, or motorcycle
- Avoid driving while taking sedative medications
- *Never* drink alcohol before driving

HOME

Provide patients with information on how to maintain a safe environment in their home. The following list is not inclusive of all issues; rather it represents significant areas where simple attention can make a major difference in household safety. The general nature of these recommendations does not minimize their importance for the health of patients:

- Keep medicines, harmful chemicals, and cleaning products secure and especially out of reach of children.
- Prevent fires by judicious use of auxiliary home heating devices and by proper use of electrical appliances and outlets.
- If fire should occur, minimize danger and damage by the use of smoke detectors and fire extinguishers.
- Develop and practice an escape plan from the home in the event of fire or other disaster (i.e., earthquake, hurricane, tornado). Most local fire departments and electric companies will inspect your home and make safety recommendations at little or no cost.
- Patients who choose to own guns should keep them in a secure place, unloaded, with appropriate locking mechanisms on the triggers. Likewise, ammunition should be kept in a secure place, separate from the weapons.
- Keep power tools and lawn care equipment in good repair, especially their safety guards, and wear safety glasses and ear plus during their operation.
- Falls are a major cause of injury to older adults. Keep bathrooms and stairways free of obstacles and install appropriate lighting, handles, and banisters. Secure the edges of throw rugs to minimize trips and falls.
- In winter, keep sidewalks and outdoor stairs clear of snow and ice. This can be a component of a family's fitness plan.

SEXUALITY

Sexual behavior is a central component of healthy human functioning and a source of pleasure, comfort, and intimacy. Unfortunately, lack of knowledge about human sexuality can result in more than an unwanted pregnancy; it can result in illness and death. As well as providing the best possible counsel and information about contraception and family planning, physicians must also inform sexually active patients about safe-sex practices. Female patients suffer far more than male patients in the area of sexually transmitted diseases (STDs) due to their more complicated and lengthy reproductive roles. Again, ironically, ill health, disability, and death from unhealthy sexual practices are almost completely preventable. High-risk practices should immediately be curtailed. These include:

- Sex with an intravenous substance abuser
- Sex with a prostitute, stranger, or person whose sexual history is unknown
- Sex without the use of a condom
- Sex with any person who engages in any of the above behaviors

Further, patients should be advised that abstinence or maintaining a mutually monogamous relationship with one partner is the best method for preventing all types of STDs. For many people, however, this advice is not acceptable. In such cases, the physician should instruct patients to minimize high-risk behaviors. Although not 100% effective, consistent, and correct, use of condoms and other barrier contraceptives decrease risk of pregnancy and STDs and should be encouraged. Studies reveal that using contraceptives containing the spermicide nonoxynol-9 with condoms offers further projection if the barrier should fail.

FAMILY AND WORK

A healthy family life has long been known to be a source of comfort, joy, and inspiration. The family is the basic unit of society and needs the support of all. Fragmented, blended, or single-parent families need even more support. Families experiencing problems or who are in turmoil should be encouraged to seek help, whether it be support from caring relatives and friends, support groups, or professional family therapy. The primary care osteopathic physician should engage patients in constructive discussions about family health. Five general qualities shared by healthy families include:

- A clear understanding of each member's role and responsibilities
- An equitable distribution of power
- Support and encouragement
- Effective communication
- A shared system of values or beliefs

It should become routine in osteopathic, family-oriented health care to inquire about these characteristics in medical history taking and to promote them at every therapeutic opportunity (23,24).

Doing work that one finds meaningful is a source of pride and personal fulfillment. The most tragic work situation is for one to feel trapped in a work circumstance one despises. Many people, however, fail to take the steps necessary to make their work more meaningful or to prepare themselves to change jobs or careers. If patients find that, despite their best efforts, they are unhappy in their work, they should be encouraged to survey their situation and develop a plan of change. Opportunities for alternative education and training are more abundant and accessible now than ever before. Even in the most difficult economic circumstances, education is the best investment a person can make.

Many people unhappy with their work never take full advantage of what the situation offers. Most large employers have tuition-reimbursement plans for educational courses that go unused by employees. Patients should also be encouraged to cultivate friendships at work. If a workplace does not provide activities, patients can become agents of change who organize and develop work-related social or sports activities. Work need not be daily tedium and loathing, and even planning for a change can be the activity that lifts a patient's spirits and gives them hope and comfort. Work should not be a constant endeavor of joyless striving but rather an undertaking that provides meaning and satisfaction.

DOCTOR–PATIENT RELATIONSHIP

The doctor–patient relationship remains the single most powerful healing tool of the physician. Technology is obviously important, but the power of the doctor–patient relationship allows "high-tech" medicine to be used most wisely and to the greatest benefit. Primary and secondary prevention are two of the most important goals of the osteopathic physician, especially those in primary care practice. Physicians can do the most to encourage patients to become partners in their health care by using the power inherent in the doctor–patient relationship.

Most physicians agree that counseling is one of their most important tasks; paradoxically, most feel ineffective in this role. Many physicians feel generally pessimistic about their ability to motivate patients toward positive change. This pessimism exists partly due to a lack of effective training about behavioral change during medical school and in postgraduate medical education. Physicians generally underestimate the difficulty in changing behavior, even their own. Most wrongly believe their only duty is to provide information and end up preaching to or lecturing their patients, rather than informing them. Because this approach alone usually fails, physicians can become discouraged and stop trying to change patient behavior or begin to provide information in a cursory manner, never really expecting patients to cooperate.

Behavioral scientists investigating change as a process have proposed both general and specific approaches that are realistic, practical, and broadly applicable in health care settings. One of the most helpful models is that proposed by Prochaska and DiClemente (25,26). This model divides the process of change into stages. The duty of osteopathic physicians is then to assist their patients to identify the stage they are in and to move successfully into the next. This approach is useful in three important ways because it:

1. Acknowledges that change is difficult and requires planning.
2. Minimizes discouragement on the part of patient and physician.
3. Continually encourages positive work toward lasting or permanent change.

The stages of change include:

1. *Precontemplation*: In this first stage, patients are unaware of or perhaps deny the negative consequences of their behavior. This can include, for example, rationalizations like "I know lots of people who smoke who are healthy." The task of the physician in this stage is to make patients aware of the fallacy of such rationalizations by providing good information and/or by introducing therapeutic tension into the patient's belief systems.
2. *Contemplation*: At this stage, patients spend variable lengths of time reflecting on their behaviors and assessing both negative consequences of continuing a behavior and the probable benefits of positive change.
3. *Preparation*: Patients acknowledge that change is desirable. The physician's task is to negotiate a plan aimed at the higher likelihood of success.
4. *Action*: The patient and physician implement the plan for behavioral change with clear outcome measures to monitor progress.
5. *Maintenance*: Patients have experienced the reinforcing effects of their action plan to the point where the change becomes an ordinary part of their life.

The Prochaska/DiClemente model allows for the possibility and probability of relapse, especially with difficult changes like smoking cessation. If or when relapse occurs, rather than abandoning the process, the physician and patient move back to a prior stage to troubleshoot the problem before moving ahead again. Continuous attention and incremental improvement are far superior in the long run to giving up in frustration or demoralization.

A review of doctor–patient relationship literature proposes four specific sequential strategies for motivating patient cooperation and encouraging patients to take more personal responsibility for their health. These strategies are grounded in the patient compliance literature and have been expanded and integrated to include relevant social influences and psychotherapy research. A major contribution of this research has been the identification of the patient's health beliefs as a powerful predictor of cooperation with treatment. The review focuses on the critical importance of the doctor–patient relationship and interaction and then expands to the patient's relationship with the entire integrated primary care health team.

Patients who are not clear about what they are expected to do are unlikely to follow recommendations. A number of studies show major patient dissatisfaction with not receiving enough information from physicians. Dissatisfied patients are less likely to cooperate and may not ever return.

STRATEGY 1: INFORMING THE PATIENT

The physician should never make assumptions about a patient's knowledge and understanding, regardless of socioeconomic class or level of education. A confident level of baseline knowledge should first be established. The physician can implement this by allowing the patient time to explain their understanding of health problems and then identify any incorrect or idiosyncratic perceptions. The cultural belief system of patients should also be explored. Verbal instructions should be clear and can be supplemented with pictures and printed materials if necessary. The physician should avoid jargon whenever possible. The physician can check the patient's level of understanding by asking the patient to repeat instructions or demonstrate how they might share the instructions with a third party. This area of the doctor–patient relationship has been receiving more recent attention than any other aspect (27,28).

STRATEGY 2: OBTAINING COMMITMENT FROM THE PATIENT

This strategy involves the use of referent power, social power bestowed on a significant figure whose acceptance and approval are highly regarded and desired. The use of this referent power involves making direct and clear statements about a desired behavior change and eliciting the patient's commitment to cooperate. Using the example of smoking, this would involve stating in a nonjudgmental but direct and authoritative manner the detrimental effects of smoking, and then asking the patient directly for a commitment to stop. Physicians' success in eliciting this commitment is revealed in higher patient smoking cessation rates.

STRATEGY 3: NEGOTIATING AND TAILORING A REGIMEN

All treatment recommendations require a change from the patient's ordinary lifestyle (Box 30-2). The more complex the changes recommended, the more difficult it is for the patient to cooperate. The goal of negotiation is to arrive at an agreement. Through negotiation

---

History Taking and Behavior Change

1. Standard Osteopathic Examination
2. Review of five osteopathic domains (see Chapter 1)
3. Behavioral lifestyle choices
   (a) nutrition, body weight
   (b) physical activity
   (c) tobacco and alcohol use
   (d) personal safety, high-risk behaviors
   (e) sexual behaviors
   (f) family and work stress
4. Treatment recommendations
5. Health Promotion Counseling and strategies for behavioral change
6. Relapse Prevention Counseling and follow-up planning
7. Continuous reinforcement of self-management and patient responsibility throughout the examination and treatment

---

and exploration of lifestyle and belief system issues, a regimen can be tailored to the individual life circumstance of each patient. When the negotiated agreement is written up as a mutually binding contract, it is more likely to be kept. A verbal agreement may also suffice.

STRATEGY 4: ATTENDING TO THE PATIENT'S EMOTIONAL RESPONSES

The quality of the doctor–patient relationship is crucial at this point. Patients often complain, even bitterly so, about not being listened to or not having the opportunity to tell their story. Stories abound about technically competent but cold and aloof physicians. Research into doctor–patient relationships has shown that patients' judgments about physicians are made on the basis of the physician's ability to recognize and respond to emotional concerns. Positive behavior change occurs more often in the presence of a high-quality doctor–patient relationship. Patients in distress and suffering anxiety are not in the best condition to attend to the cognitive components of their instructions. When physicians attend to a patient's emotions and set the patient at ease, they facilitate routine history taking understanding and cooperation.

Physicians also need to communicate their interest and concern for their patients nonverbally. Several tactics communicate care and interest including smiling, sitting down, using appropriate eye contact, and not appearing to be rushed.

The osteopathic physician in the patient encounter has a distinct advantage over other health care professionals through the medium of touch and "the laying on of hands." Through the integrated verbal and nonverbal communication of care, trust is promoted, cooperation is maximized, and the doctor–patient relationship is further strengthened.

The use of the integrated primary care team in this process is summarized in Table 30.2. The primary care team encounter is *individualized* with active patient participation. Treatment is customized, flexible, and based on both physical examination and ongoing biopsychosocial findings. It is a collaborative, cooperative alliance between the health care team and the patient with the goal of facilitating the patient's own capacity to restore health and maintain optimal function of mind, body, and spirit. This is the true art and science of osteopathic care.

TABLE 30.2

Primary Care–Based Patient Encounter

Activity	Outcome	Agent	Adjunct
Screening	Identification of risky behavior	Physician Nurses Other staff	Questionnaires Interactive Computer
Informing	Knowledge	Physician Nurse Health educator	Written materials Video station
Counseling	Commitment to behavior change	Physician	Written contract
Training/education	Skills to make short-term behavior change	Physician Nurses Other staff Health educator Nutritionists	Written materials
Emotional support	Motivation	Entire PHCO team	Telephone calls/letters
Plan adjustment/motivation	Long term	Entire PHCO team	Telephone calls/letters Biologic measurement

Source: Reprinted with permission from Stoffelmayr B, Hoppe RB, Weber N. Facilitating patient participation: the doctor–patient encounter. *Prim Care* 1989;16:265–278.

SUMMARY

During the last century, the leading causes of death were diseases such as influenza, tuberculosis, pneumonia, diphtheria, and gastrointestinal infections. "Since then, the yearly death rate from these diseases per 100,000 people has been reduced from 580 to 30!" (1). Today, the major causes of premature death and disability result from behavioral factors, such as accidents and violence, or long-standing habits, such as smoking, high-fat diets, lack of routine exercise, stress, and alcohol abuse (2). Both the WHO and the HSPH predict that by 2020, in the developing countries where four fifths of our planet's people will live, seven out of ten deaths will be traced to lifestyle factors setting the stage for ischemic heart disease, depression, and chronic obstructive pulmonary diseases. In fact, by 2020, tobacco alone is expected to cause more premature death and disability than any single disease (22). Future improvements in health will come from managing the effects of unhealthy behaviors.

Most of the task of providing the highest quality, cost-effective care involves teaching and motivating patients. The place to begin in creating the desired behavior we wish to see in our patients is to make them clearly reflected in our own. Many physicians have been successful in altering their personal health behavior habits for the better, but there is always room for improvement. Doctor means teacher, and the old maxim remains sound: "Example isn't the best way to teach, ultimately it is the only way to teach."

REFERENCES

1. National Center for Health Statistics. *United States Health & Prevention Profile.* Hyattsville, MD: U.S. Department of Health & Human Services, 2005. Public Health Service. (All statistics cited in this chapter are taken from this source unless otherwise indicated.)
2. Murray CJL, Lopez AD. *The Global Burden of Disease: A Comprehensive Assessment of Mortality and Disability from Diseases, Injuries, and Risk Factors in 1990 and Projected to 2020.* Cambridge, MA: Harvard University Press, 2000.
3. Dimos JT, Rodolfa KT, et al. Induced pluripotent stem cells generated from patients with ALS can be differentiated into motor neurons. *Science* 2008;218–1221.
4. Kung HC, Hoyert DL, et al. Deaths: final data for 2005. *National Vital Statistics Reports; CDC* 2008;56(10):1–2.
5. McCullough ML, Feskanich D, Stampfer MJ, et al. Diet quality and major chronic disease risk in men and women: moving toward improved dietary guidance. *Am J Clin Nutr* 2002;76:261–271.
6. Harvard School of Public Health: Food Pyramids: What should you really eat? Website: www.the nutrition source,org, 2008.
7. The Vegan Food Pyramid: Website: www.veganfoodpsyramid.com, 2008.
8. Willett WC. Diet & cancer. *Oncologist* 2000;5(50):393–404.
9. Joint National Committee on Prevention, Detection, Evaluation and Treatment of High Blood Pressure and the National High Blood Pressure Education Program Coordination Committee. *Arch Intern Med* 1997;157:2413–2446.
10. Blair SN, Kohl WH III, Paffengarger RC Jr. Physical fitness and all-cause mortality. *JAMA* 1989;262:2395–2401.
11. Shin KS, et al. Aging, exercise training, and the immune system. *Immunol Rev* 1997;3:68–95.
12. Pyne DB, et al. Training strategies to maintain immunocompetence in athletes. *Int J Sports Med* 2000;(suppl 1):551–560.
13. Kisner C, Colby LA. *Therapeutic Exercise: Foundations and Techniques.* 5th Ed. Philadelphia, PA: F.A., Davis Co., 2007.
14. Obesity and Overweight: Health Consequences. Website: www.cdc.gov/nccdphp/dnpa/obesity/consequences.htm, 2008.
15. Very Low-Calorie Diets: Weight Control Information Network: USDHHS/NIH. National Institute of Diabetes and Digestive and Kidney Disease: Website: www.niddk,nih,gov/low_claorie.htm, 2008.
16. Roizen MF, Oz MO. *You: On a Diet, You: The Owner's Manual, You: Staying Young.* New York, London, Toronto, Sydney: Free Press, Simon & Schuster, 2007.
17. Surgeon General's Report on Smoking: Expanded List of Diseases Caused by Smoking. USDHHS, May 2004.
18. MacKenzie TD, Bartecchi CE, Schrier RW. The human costs of tobacco use. *NEJM* 1994;330:975–980.

19. Smoking Cessation: Alternative Medicine. Peace Health Website: www. healthwise.net. 2008. (Contains and extensive and well-researched bibliography.)

20. Kottke TE, Battista RN, et al. Attributes of successful smoking cessation interventions in medical practice. a meta-analysis of 39 controlled trials. *JAMA* 1988;259(19):2883–2889.

21. Coleman T. Smoking cessation: integrating recent advances into clinical practice. *Thorax* 2001;56:579–582.

22. World Health Organization: Statistics on Smoking, Fact Sheet: 2002.

23. Silliman B. *Resilient Families: Qualities of Families Who Survive and Thrive.* Laramie, WY: University of Wyoming Extension Service, Publication B-1018, June 1995.

24. First Things First: Building Healthy Families. Website: www.firstthings. org, 2008.

25. Prochaska JO, DiClemente CC, Norcross JC. In search of how people change: applications to addictive behaviors. *Am Psychol* 1992;47:1102–1104.

26. Prochaska JO, DiClemente CC. Stages of change in the modification of problem behaviors. In: Hersen M, Eisler RM, Miller PM, Eds. *Progress in Behavior Modification.* Sycamore, IL: Sycamore, 1994:183–218.

27. *Health Literacy.* Institute of Medicine of the National Academies. Website: www.iom.edu, 2008.

28. *Healthy People 2010, Health Communication Terminology.* USDHHS/ HRSA. Website: www.hrsa.gov/health literacy, 2008.

29. Ewing JA. Detecting alcoholism: the CAGE questionnaire. *JAMA* 1984;252:1905–1907.

30. To SE. Alcoholism and pathways to recovery: new survey results on views and treatment options. Medscape Website: CME January 2006. www. medscape.com. (Outstanding overview and well-referenced.)

31. Snipes GE. Accidents in the elderly. *Am Fam Physician* 1982;26:117–122.

32. Website: www.medicalalertreviews.com. 2008. (Excellent patient information resource.)

33. Holmes TH, Rahe RH. The social readjustment scale. *J Psychosom Res* 1967;7:17–20.

34. Friedman M, Rosenman RH. *Type A Behavior and Your Heart.* New York, NY: Knopf, 1973.

35. Friedman M, Ulmer D. *Treating Type A Behavior and Your Health.* New York, NY: Knopf, 1984.

36. Stoffelmayr B, Hoppe RB, Weber N. Facilitating patient participation: the doctor-patient encounter. *Prim Care* 1989;16:265–278.

31

End of Life Care

KAREN J. NICHOLS

KEY CONCEPTS

- The challenges of patient care at end of life are daunting.
- A significant opportunity is presented for offering each patient the most complete expression of osteopathic medicine's philosophy and practice.
- Physicians must respect and accommodate patient needs in communicating prognosis.
- Physicians must also respect family members' needs in order to understand the dying process and process grief.
- Student–physician interaction with the dying may be the ideal training ground for young doctors.

INTRODUCTION

The opportunity and ability to employ all the facets of being an osteopathic physician is never more needed than at the end of a patient's life. When there is no more surgical intervention possible or advisable, when there are no more tests and studies to conduct, when there is no more medication that can turn the tide of the inevitable decline, then the physician moves fully into utilizing her and his most important tool, the physician–patient relationship for psychological support.

End-of-life care is filled with demands and challenges that all physicians must deal with at some point. No discipline in medicine—except perhaps pathology—escapes the issues of end-of-life care. Ironically and unfortunately for their patients, physicians in those disciplines that are perceived as relatively immune to routinely dealing with end-of-life issues find themselves least prepared when these issues inevitably arise. Further, a very interesting phenomenon that occurs not infrequently is that the student physician who has taken the time to establish a rapport through caring may be the first physician the patient will turn to with questions and concerns at end of life. The wise medical student will learn the principles of end-of-life care to be able to assist all patients.

PRINCIPLES OF END-OF-LIFE CARE

To clarify the requirements for proper care, The Milbank Memorial Fund published a set of "Principles for Care of Patients at the End of Life: An Emerging Consensus among the Specialties of Medicine." (1) The American Osteopathic Association End-Of-Life Care Advisory Council prepared an osteopathic version of these principles, which were approved by the American Osteopathic Association (AOA) House of Delegates in 2000 (2,6).

RESEARCH INTO END-OF-LIFE CARE

The landmark study—"A controlled trial to improve care for seriously ill hospitalized patients: The study to understand prognoses and preferences for outcomes and risks of treatments (SUPPORT)"—gave the first clear understanding of how patients and families viewed their end-of-life care experiences (3). The phase I observation stage documented shortcomings in communication, frequency of aggressive treatment, and the characteristics of hospital death. It documented a strong indictment of the medical care system discovering that only 47% of physicians knew when

their patients preferred to avoid cardiopulmonary resuscitation, 46% of do-not-resuscitate (DNR) orders were written within 2 days of death, 38% of patients who died spent at least 10 days in an intensive care unit, and for 50% of conscious patients who died in the hospital, family members reported moderate-to-severe pain at least half of the time. Unfortunately, the Phase II intervention part of the study did not demonstrate any improvement in care or patient outcomes. The study's conclusions recommended greater individual and society commitment and more proactive and forceful measures to fill the gaps identified (3).

Many subsequent studies have sought to study the quality of end-of-life care and to understand the perception of both physicians and patients/families about expectations and knowledge of end-of-life care issues. The persistent lack of patients' knowledge of options at the end of life was studied by Silveira et al. (4). Of the 1,000 patients surveyed, there were 728 respondents. Only 23% to 46% of those responding demonstrated an appropriate awareness of four areas relevant to end-of-life care (4). All research points to the importance of more education of physicians and patients about end-of-life care issues.

GOALS OF CARE

The most important issue that needs to be addressed in dealing with patients at end of life is to determine their goals of care. What does the patient perceive as appropriate care at the end of his or her life? How does the patient wish to see himself or herself living out their final days? What does the patient see as the acceptable limits of his or her existence given the constraints of the current medical condition? These questions take the emphasis from "which procedure to perform" and move it to "how do you want to spend your final days?" The patient who states that he or she wants every measure employed to keep himself or herself alive every possible minute regardless of being aware of the surroundings leads the physician to create a very different care plan than one for the patient who states that he or she wants to spend the final days at home out of pain surrounded by loved ones. End-of-life decisions should be the result of the collaboration and mutual informing of the patient, the patient's family and the physicians, each sharing his or her own expertise to help the patient make the best possible decision, often in the worst possible circumstances.

Patients and families also need to understand that the goals of care can and should change as the disease progresses. "Initially, patients might hope that the cancer responds to chemotherapy or surgery. When disease control is no longer possible, patients might hope to live pain free, achieve closure on personal issues or die surrounded by friends and family" (5).

Adults with decision-making capacity should be informed of their choices, and they have the legal and ethical right to make their own decisions about their life, including the right to refuse recommended life-sustaining medical treatment. This position honors the patient's autonomy and liberty as guaranteed in the U.S. Constitution. This right exists even when the physician disagrees with the patient's decision (6).

Patients without decision-making capacity can have their choices adhered to by physicians who follow a previously executed advance directive described below. The principle of "best interests" (what would the reasonable and informed patient select) is invoked if the individual's wishes are not known. Quality of life should be viewed from the patient's perspective in all these decisions because quality of life can only be self-determined. Extreme caution must be exercised when trying to determine what constitutes quality of life for another person as research has shown that patients consistently assess their quality of life to be better than their caregivers think their patients do (6).

The over-riding issue is not what the family or friends want for the patient at end of life, but rather what would the patient want for him/herself. If the noncognitive patient were to awaken for only 15 minutes and be able to fully understand the circumstances, what decisions would the patient make? If the answer is unclear, society should err on the side of life. If the answer is clear, then refusal to follow the patient's wishes is unethical and illegal (6).

ADVANCE CARE PLANNING

Ideally, every person who comes to the hospital or care setting would have completed some type of document that falls under the category of "advance care planning." This approach was the impetus for the "Patient Self-determination Act of 1991," which requires that every person entering a facility that receives Medicare/Medicaid funding must be asked whether they have executed such a document or wish to do so. Provision of care is not predicated upon existence or absence of such a document, the only requirement is that the patient or family is aware that such information is available and that such a document could be created. Advance care planning documents generally include living wills or durable medical powers of attorney for health care affairs (proxy designation for health care affairs) and can be self-executed with or without the aid of an attorney. This medical power of attorney is separate and distinct from the legal power of attorney and neither one implies the presence or intent of the other. Such documents are available from many organizations and are also online. These documents carry the weight of law but can be superseded by the patient at any time. Living wills document the desired treatments but leave much room for interpretation when the situation doesn't match the directives, so a combination of a living will and a durable medical power of attorney may be best. When the physician, patient, and family have had these conversations earlier and are in agreement, there is little need for such documentation. However, when that is not the case, these documents can assist in settling disagreements. Ultimately, if agreement cannot be reached, the hospital ethics committee can also be called upon to assist these deliberations.

Sample living wills and durable medical powers of attorney can be downloaded from several Internet sites, search term: living will form.

WHOLE PATIENT ASSESSMENT

Nowhere is the principle of assessing the whole patient more important than at end of life. However, whole patient assessment does not imply that the physician will be employing futile treatment. Whole patient assessment implies that the patient at end of life is to be accorded the same well thought out evaluation and care as any other patient. A fever in a patient dying from heart failure is not caused by the heart failure and may be an indication of an easily treatable problem. Pedal edema in a patient with respiratory failure without cor pulmonale cannot be assumed to be due to the respiratory failure. More than one patient at end of life has had incorrect assumptions made about symptoms and has been denied simple and appropriate care just because he or she is "dying anyway." A proper patient assessment does not have to be painful, costly, onerous, or futile. It just has to be thoughtful and appropriate.

SYMPTOM MANAGEMENT

Closely tied to the approach of whole patient assessment is the requirement to provide proper symptom management. When whole patient assessment does not reveal a treatable cause for a specific symptom, there are appropriate interventions for those symptoms. The types of symptoms most frequently encountered as part of the end-of-life process that may not be indicative of another medical cause include dyspnea, nausea, vomiting, constipation, diarrhea, anorexia, cachexia, fatigue, weakness, fluid balance problems, edema, skin integrity, decubitus ulcers, odors, and insomnia. The physician caring for the patient with such symptoms at end of life is referred to the American College of Physician (ACP) Clinical Practice Guidelines (11) and Education for Physicians on End of Life Care (EPEC) (7) www.EPEC.org and to the Osteopathic EPEC (12) for best practices. www.osteopathic.org (search term "palliative care")

PAIN MANAGEMENT

Another aspect of patient care at end of life, which bears special mention, is that of proper pain management. The key concept about how much medication to provide to control pain is "it takes as much as it takes." All the restrictions and guidelines about dosing of pain medication do not apply at end of life for anyone other than the narcotic-naive patient. The principle of "go low and go slow" applies to every patient until the appropriate level of pain relief has been achieved. The other key concept of pain management is that pain medication should never be administered on a "prn" basis but as a continuous infusion to maintain a baseline of pain control. This level of control may have to be supplemented at times of unavoidable painful processes, or if the level of pain steadily escalates, but the patient should never be allowed to experience unrelieved pain. There is no need to fear addiction at end of life, although medication tolerance may be seen, expected, and properly managed with increased dosing. The proper usage of narcotics at the end of life in a person who is or was addicted to narcotics prior to acquiring the terminal illness requires more thoughtful planning, but no such person should ever be denied narcotics for the purposes of providing adequate pain relief.

DOUBLE EFFECT OR SECONDARY EFFECT AND TERMINATION SEDATION

Subtopics under pain management are the related principles of double effect or secondary effect and the issue of terminal sedation.

It is possible that a patient can be in so much pain at end of life, particularly with such diagnoses such as bone metastasis after the patient has passed the limits of radiation, that the patient's pain may be uncontrolled by any current measure. At that point, it is appropriate to present the option of controlling that pain by medicating the patient into a coma. This is called "terminal sedation." The patient is kept comfortable even though not cognizant of the surroundings. The appropriate level of pain medication dosing is determined by monitoring the patient's native blood pressure, respiratory rate, and heart rate to see the response of the body to the effects of the pain medication. Another natural response to uncontrolled pain that can be helpful in this assessment is grimacing. Monitoring how the body naturally responds to the relief of pain allows for appropriate adjustments in dosage, increasing to control the pain, and decreasing the dosage if the current medication level appears to be too strong for the body's present pain level. Such a required level of pain medication may result in the patient dying sooner than without that level of pain medication. The sheer anxiety of unrelieved pain can trigger the counter-regulatory hormones that can act to prolong life. Relief of that level of pain may decrease those same counter-regulatory hormones to the level that the life processes are no longer stimulated and the patient may die. The concept of double effect or secondary effect indicates that the primary and intended effect was to ease pain, and not to kill the patient. A well-designed study in a hospice population found no association between percentage of change in dose of opioids and time until death (13). The primacy of the intent of maintaining pain control is evident by the proper monitoring as described above.

HOSPICE AND PALLIATIVE CARE

The hospice concept of providing comfort when cure is no longer possible was initiated in England and quickly spread to the United States beginning in the 1970s. Although the number of patients who die while being cared for by hospice has been rising slowly, patients generally do not spend enough time in these programs to experience all the potential benefits. Such benefits include provision of medications and durable medical equipment, a major focus on aggressive pain management, counseling services both before and up to a year following death for the family, out patient medical support and in patient care for extremely demanding situations. More recently, palliative care programs have been developing across the United States to provide the expertise and standards of practice developed by hospice to patients who have needs for symptom control and supportive care earlier in their illness. All hospice programs fall under the umbrella of palliative care; however, palliative care is indicated beyond the specific time limits of and criteria for hospice, generally anticipated to apply to the specific diagnoses and limited to the last six months of life. The focus of hospice is to work toward death with dignity employing an entire team of professionals bringing the needed expertise to the entire galaxy of end of life. According to anecdotal experience, while designed to improve the quality of patients' lives as they fight their disease, good palliative care may help to increase life expectancy in certain diagnoses (7).

TRANSITIONS OF LIFE

There exists another aspect of assisting patients as they move toward the end of their lives that may be one of the most challenging, as Thomas Finucane, M.D., eloquently points out in an editorial in the November 3, 1999 issue of *JAMA* (8). It is the process of "moving through the transition from gravely ill and fighting death to terminally ill and seeking peace, shifting the goals of treatment from cure or longer survival to preservation of comfort and dignity."

Two conflicting issues clash here. The dying patient desperately wants to live as long as possible, as healthy as possible, able to enjoy life and people, without pain. When this is no longer possible, the patient also wants death to come swiftly, peacefully, and painlessly at the last possible minute. The physician also wants this scenario for every patient. The problem is medicine does not have the ability to predict the future and give patients a precise, reliable date and time when death will come. Ironically, many chronically ill patients never experience a time during which they are clearly dying of their disease; "the sickest patients are not necessarily the ones who die first" (8).

The result is the patient chooses to accept a less and less "ideal" quality of life, adjusting to more and more incapacitation and pain in exchange for one more day, and yearning for this day not to be the last. Some patients seem to accept death's coming easily, accepting the future, even choosing not to eat and drink. For many others, however, hope (no matter how faint) persists so strongly that surrender to the inevitable end of life is more excruciating than the pain and the struggle. Openly discussing this struggle to shift goals may be the only way to avoid a time where "do everything you can, doctor," in life becomes "why did this have to drag on so long?" after death (8).

This point is confirmed by a significant study of prognosis from George Washington University and the Department of Veterans Affairs published in *JAMA* (9). The study looked at seriously ill hospitalized patients with advanced chronic obstructive pulmonary disease, congestive heart failure, or end-stage liver disease. It found that the recommended clinical prediction criteria are not effective in identifying a population with a prognosis for survival of 6 months or less (9).

While we may not be able to predict the exact day of demise, we can predict that all indications point to the fact that the time is so short that hospice and palliative care is the best way to proceed, even though the patient and family may not be eager to hear that recommendation. The following words from the attending physician may be useful in the discussion: "Do you think it is time to consider a different type of treatment that focuses on your symptoms? I'll be here with you no matter what you decide." Another approach might be "I want to provide intense, coordinated care with a team of professionals who will treat your symptoms and help you stay comfortable" (5).

LEGAL MYTHS AND REALITIES

A significant barrier to proper care is lack of understanding on the part of the physician about legal issues at the end of life. Many physicians are not aware of the underlying principles vis-à-vis actual legal concerns. The body of law known as right-to-die cases extends ordinary treatment refusal doctrine to end-of-life decisions. The courts have affirmed a right to refuse life-sustaining treatment. Making a distinction between what treatment is life sustaining and what is not, is the difficulty. Meisel, Snyder, and Quill published a well-written set of "Seven legal barriers to end-of-life care: myths, realities and grains of truth," for the ACP—American Society of Internal Medicine End-of-Life Care Consensus Panel (10).

COMMUNICATING BAD NEWS

One of the major challenges at end of life is that of telling a patient that he/she is at the end of life. Every physician has to communicate uncomfortable information or to give the family/patient bad news at some time in the process of providing medical care. It is important to develop the skill of delivering this type of information. Most people want to know such information and delivering it well actually strengthens the patient–physician relationship. The patient/family not only learns the information but also learns that the physician who doesn't shy away from the hard issues can be trusted to tell the truth. Delivering such information thoughtfully fosters collaboration between the physician and the patient/family as they then have time to plan and cope.

COMMUNICATION PROTOCOL

There is a seven-step protocol that has been developed as part of the program "Education for Physicians on End of Life Care (EPEC)" that is recommended as an effective approach to communicating bad news (7). All these steps may need to be modified by the urgency of the situation. The emergency department setting with an elderly demented patient quickly approaching his or her final minutes dictates a different pace than in the office setting talking to an alert patient who needs to be advised of a condition with a long prognosis:

1. Know yourself. Whether they know it or not, physicians communicate their own emotional responses in the most subtle ways, so it is important to be aware of your own responses.
2. Create a plan. Allot adequate time without interruption. Plan what to say after confirming the medical facts. Don't delegate this job. Create an environment that is conducive to conversation.
3. Establish what the patient already knows. The patient may already have suspected the worst.
4. How much does the patient want to know? There can be various patient preferences, either declining to know the details or choosing to designate someone else to communicate on his or her behalf. This varies with race, ethnicity, culture, religion, socioeconomic status, age, and developmental level.
5. Say the information and stop to allow the patient/family time to process. Avoid a monologue, jargon, and euphemisms, and pause frequently.
6. Be prepared for emotions. Some may respond with tears, anger, and anxiety, and others may experience denial, blame, guilt, fear, and shame.
7. Plan for the next steps in the process of the disease and approach.

FAMILY REQUESTS TO WITHHOLD INFORMATION

If the family anticipates the worst and requests that information not be told to the patient, the physician still has a legal obligation to tell the patient. The family needs to discuss the reason for their fears of the information being shared. It is always the physician's responsibility to tell the truth to the patient, but it may be necessary to assist the family in working through their issues so that they see the importance of telling the truth and understand why it is not fair to the patient not to have this information. It may be appropriate to talk to the family and the patient at the same time.

LANGUAGE BARRIERS

When language is a barrier, the best approach is to obtain a translator as the family members who may be able to translate may have difficulty with the medical terms and concepts or may feel compelled to modify the news to protect the patient. A family translator may also not want to be the one to actually be the first to have to utter the words that will bring such dismay.

COMMUNICATING PROGNOSIS

When the physician is asked about prognosis and timing of death, it is helpful to find out why the patient wants to know. There may be a specific event coming up that the patient wishes to plan for, or the reasons for asking may be very ill-defined. The "planner" patient will want more details. Avoiding precise answers is appropriate indicating that the prognosis is either in hours instead of days, days instead of weeks, weeks instead of month, or in months instead of years. Precise answers can be perceived as a guarantee that no physician is able to provide.

THE TIME TO WITHDRAW INTERVENTIONS

Another aspect of communication that can be unexpectedly challenging is when the time comes for the invoking of the patient's wishes to withdraw interventions. It is unkind and unwise to ask the family "do you want us to take your family member off the ventilator now?" This approach puts the family member in the position of having to "make the decision to let Mom die," and actually having to say those words, when in reality that decision was already made by the patient some time ago. The better approach is to tell the family, "as we have discussed repeatedly, your mother indicated in her living will that when we got to this point she did not want life support continued, so we think it is time to take her off the ventilator, which we can do at 6 P.M. tomorrow." Allowing plenty of time for that information to sink in and for the family to respond, guides the rest of the treatment plan and timing.

WITHHOLDING AND WITHDRAWING TREATMENT

As was indicated in the "legal myths and realities" section, there is much misinformation about the difference between withholding and withdrawing treatment. In my experience in seminar after seminar that I have personally presented on end-of-life care topics, when I have polled physicians about which choice seems to be "harder" for the physician to perform, the results always indicate that physicians feel that choosing to withdraw treatment is more difficult to handle psychologically than withholding treatment. Nevertheless, all sources agree that there is no difference legally, morally, or ethically as the end result is the same, death of the patient (7). If the treatment is initially withheld, there is no possibility of determining whether or not it may have been successful.

On the other hand, if the specific treatment is instituted and is determined not to be successful, there is often significant reluctance to remove that treatment. In my opinion, this reluctance is based upon the fact that when the treatment is removed, the patient will likely die sooner than if the treatment had been continued, so the appearance is created that removing the treatment was the event that killed the patient. On the contrary, the disease process kills the patient. The treatment was shown to be ineffective in reversing the disease process and therefore was futile. The best approach to this difficult situation is to explain prospectively that a specific treatment will be instituted as a time-limited trial, with the time specified. At the appointed time, depending upon the natural course of the disease process and the chosen treatment, the issue is then revisited. Either the treatment is successful and is no longer needed, or the treatment is achieving desired results and a new time-limited plan is created, or the treatment is unsuccessful with no reason to continue and a plan to remove the treatment is created. The time-limited trial combines the advantages and avoids as much as possible the disadvantages of these two approaches to patient treatment.

ARTIFICIAL NUTRITION AND HYDRATION

Providing such support at end of life may at times be beneficial; however, sometimes this intervention may be excessively burdensome and may actually prolong the dying process. The use of artificial nutrition and hydration involves a medical procedure with potential side effects and complications. That fact is also the reason that the proper terminology is to use the technical medical phrase "artificial nutrition and hydration," not "providing food and water." A decision to not provide or to discontinue this intervention may pose some significant challenges particularly to families. Physicians need to assist patients and families to understand the role of artificial nutrition and hydration at the end of life, which is to provide temporary support to allow time for other interventions to have a chance to work. Families also need to understand that as body processes shut down, loss of the sensations of hunger and thirst are part of the dying process. Research has shown that discontinuing such support doesn't contribute to suffering, but those concerns may persist (6).

DO NOT (ATTEMPT) RESUSCITATE STATUS

This status is indicated for most patients when it is anticipated that there is only a short length of life remaining. It means that the physician continues to provide all comfort care and when the patient slips into the final minutes of life, nothing is done to stop that process. Sometimes physicians who have been reluctant to write an actual DNR order will indicate that any code procedure should be "slow" (when full resuscitative efforts are not expended with the pretense that they are). This is not appropriate as it represents an attempt to deceive, which is an ethical violation (6). Even in optimal circumstances, code procedures are not successful in the majority of patients, so any "restricted" code order (chemical code, do not intubate, no compressions) is even less likely to be successful, therefore seldom indicated.

Obtaining patient/family permission for a DNR status order can be very challenging. Following the principles in the paragraph "communicating bad news" will be helpful. A suggested sequence of discussion can be:

1. Gently introduce the topic of end of life, such as "it looks like your disease isn't really responding to treatment."
2. Let the patient/family respond about their thoughts, feelings, and impressions.
3. Introduce the next statement such as "we have all been working to meet your needs and want to be sure we follow your wishes in the event your time is near."
4. Again, let the patient/family respond.
5. Ask the question, "have you thought about what is most important to you in how you want to spend your final hours?"
6. If there is no clear direction from the patient/family, another question could be "in the event your heart stops, do you want to be kept alive on machines?"
7. It is always best to focus on the patient's goals of care. Having the patient explain his or her last-hour wishes can also lead to the question, "so it sounds like you want your last hours to be quiet and peaceful and free of pain, with no machines to prolong the inevitable?"
8. The best approach is to be osteopathic and focus on the whole person, letting the dialogue flow from your human-to-human relationship. It is important never to take away hope and also to

acknowledge that if the clinical situation improves, a change in DNR status can be made.

Families have specific needs at this time, as well as the patient (i.e.,) the need to understand the dying process, the need to have cultural and religious differences understood and honored, the need to process grief. The osteopathic physician understands the important contribution of the family to the patient's overall well-being.

SUDDEN ILLNESS

A particularly difficult aspect of end-of-life care arises when the terminal illness/trauma has occurred suddenly without warning and especially in an otherwise healthy and/or young person. All the principles of good communication apply. The physician must be aware that the level of understanding about the terminal illness including the options and pathway ahead will likely be minimal. Determining the approach to care will be a delayed "process" and may be much more contentious as the terminal nature of the illness is complicated by the unexpected nature of the situation. The grief and anger that result from the sudden and unplanned nature of the illness are almost inevitable. Frequently, the physician has never met that new patient and/or family until this event; so this fact further complicates patient care as there is no basis for trust in the physician–patient relationship. The best approach is always to be as open as possible, provide as much information as possible, and never withhold partial information waiting for more definitive testing. It is also appropriate to err on the side of life to allow families time to process the grief. The assistance of social workers and other support staff as well as any of the patient's or family's personal trusted advisors, especially including spiritual advisors, is never more valuable than in this situation.

MEDICAL FUTILITY

A further aspect of sudden illness but also of other terminal illnesses is the issue of medical futility. Present-day medical care has not been well served by the media where every illness is solved at the conclusion of the movie or the TV show. There is a very high expectation by the American public that with sufficient consultations, testing, and interventions, every patient can be saved, for the present day. Also, the lack of medical knowledge in the general population complicates this issue, as there is often little understanding of basic anatomic and physiologic principles. The physician is often faced with a demand/expectation that a particular intervention should be instituted, when there is no possibility that the intervention is appropriate or indicated for the diagnosis. An excellent example is that of the individual who has suffered a severe crush injury to the chest in a motor vehicle accident, which has created a diminished cardiac output that has prevented adequate perfusion of the kidneys resulting in kidney failure. The demand for a kidney transplant in this situation is a request for a medically futile procedure. While technically feasible, a kidney transplanted into this setting of inadequate perfusion is also doomed to fail. The best approach is a thorough explanation, assistance from social workers, and a willingness to understand, acknowledge, and tolerate the frustration of the person requesting the futile intervention.

PHYSICIAN-ASSISTED SUICIDE AND PHYSICIAN-ASSISTED DEATH

Currently in flux is the issue of physician-assisted suicide (PAS). While Oregon is the only state that currently allows the full legal provision of PAS, other state legislatures are also addressing this issue in various forms. The general provisions of the Oregon law require verification of terminal status without depression, a waiting period between a repeated request for PAS, and the ability to swallow the specified prescribed barbiturate in liquid form.

The U.S. attorney general filed a law suit against the state of Oregon opposing PAS and lost the case. In an interesting turn of events, although both the AOA and the American Medical Association officially oppose PAS, both organizations opposed the attorney general's lawsuit. This opposition was based on the premise of the lawsuit, which was that physicians should not be allowed to prescribe medication for an off-label use. Therefore, the implication was that since no medication is approved by the Food and Drug Administration for assisting a patient to commit suicide, that practice would have been judged illegal if the lawsuit had prevailed. Taking this outcome to the next step runs afoul of the fact that included in most state medical licensure statutes is the prerogative of physicians to use best judgment to prescribe medication for off-label purposes, so if this lawsuit had been successful, the unintended consequence would have set a chilling precedent leading to restriction of the lawful practice of medicine in every setting.

The AOA opposes the practice of PAS. Such a practice puts the physician in the position of making a determination as to whether to be on the side of working to save a patient or on the side of working to kill a patient. No physician should have to make that decision and no patient should wonder if the physician is weighing that option. In a survey of 988 terminally ill patients by Emanuel and associates in 2000, identified factors associated with a patient being less likely to consider euthanasia or PAS which were "feeling appreciated, being aged 65 years or older, and being African American." Factors associated with being more likely to consider euthanasia or PAS were "depressive symptoms, substantial care giving needs, and pain"(14). Foley (15) makes the strong point that competent care for the dying can relieve the concern of those patients considering PAS, and this approach should be advocated in preference to PAS.

There is also a move to change the descriptive title of this practice from PAS to physician-assisted death. This proposed change would appear to be an attempt to camouflage the fact that when the patient takes the prescribed medication for its intended purpose, the patient is committing suicide and the physician assisted that suicide by providing the means. PAS (where the physician provides the means and the patient acts) is also clearly differentiated from euthanasia (where the physician provides the means and completes the act for the patient).

There is no question this is a highly emotionally charged issue with no lack of strength of opinions on both sides. The perspective of proponents of physician-assisted suicide is PAS is the best alternative to other methods of ending one's life when the burdens of that life have become untenable from the patient's perspective. Only a small percentage of those patients in Oregon who have invoked the provision of this law, have actually consummated this method of ending their life, indicating that making this request was as much to provide the option for control of the dying process as to actually use that option.

STUDENTS AND END-OF-LIFE CARE

To what degree should students be involved in this process? Should students restrict participation to information gathering? If so, are there key elements to determine? How do they record their findings (this information doesn't exactly fit in the SOAP note)? Should students ever introduce discussion in this area? If so, are there limits to how they advance the information that they gain? Who is the recipient of the information they gather: attending,

case worker, hospital chaplain, or potential hospice person? This is a most provocative series of questions to which the answer is yes, no, maybe, sometimes, and even "I don't know." After learning how to diagnose and treat disease, the student on clinical rotation starts to experience the biggest challenge to being a physician, how to translate all that knowledge into real patient care. The patient who can't understand, refuses to listen, chooses not to follow the instructions, or hides the true problem out of fear is still the patient who needs care. The physician has to learn that he or she is frequently part of the trigger or reason the patient acts and responds in the way he or she does. The physician–patient relationship is ultimately the strongest tool the physician has to help the patient. The student physician cannot wait to learn to work in this relationship until after completion of residency.

On the other hand, the student physician is still a student working under the attending physician's license. The best guidance I can provide is to include the following question in every history and physical, "have you made anyone aware of your wishes for the end of your life through some tool like a living will?" The answer is to be precisely documented as stated by the patient, in the notes section of the chart in the appropriate manner with the rest of the history and physical information such as "last tetanus shot, last mammogram, last colonoscopy, etc." This simple question opens the door for the patient to walk through if desired. If the patient is not ready to discuss this topic, the answer will indicate it is time to move to the next topic. The student is not expected to probe any further, to answer questions, or to counsel the patient. The student is expected to bring to the attention of the attending physician (or designee such as a resident) if the patient requests further discussion or information. The student should function like a conduit to carry information and concerns from the patient to the attending physician who can assess the situation and decide what orders are appropriate, including a possible DNR status. The patient will set the tone, indicate the depth and length of the conversation, indicate whether further questions are appropriate, or whether the patient just wants a willing listener. Many times, the patient has been waiting for a physician to broach this topic. Two leaders in end-of-life care, Dr. Susan Block and Dr. J. Andrew Billings, have studied the student–physician interaction with the dying and suggest that end-of-life care may be the ideal training ground for young doctors (16).

SUMMARY

Although the challenges of patient care at end of life are daunting, it is a truly rewarding time to care for patients. Every one of our patients and each of us will pass through this experience. It can be handled well or be given short shrift. It may be the only opportunity to bring to bear all the best that osteopathic medicine has to offer, honoring the patient as a whole person and calling upon each osteopathic physician to create the milieu for the use of everything we have learned. To share this time with a patient and make his or her last days comfortable and meaningful is a true gift, a reciprocal gift that the patient and physician give each other. The physician who welcomes and embraces the interaction at end of life is touched in ways that won't be forgotten by the patient, the family, or the physician.

REFERENCES

1. Cassel CK, Foley KM. *Principles for Care of Patients at the End of Life: An Emerging Consensus among the Specialties of Medicine.* New York, NY: Milbank Memorial Fund, 1999.

2. Nichols KJ. Approach to optimal care at end of life. *JAOA* 2001;101: 586–593.

3. The SUPPORT Principal Investigators. A controlled trial to improve care for seriously ill hospitalized patients. The study to understand prognoses and preferences for outcomes and risks of treatments (SUPPORT). *JAMA* 1995;274:1591–1598.

4. Silveira MJ, DePiero A, Gerrity MS, et al. Patients' knowledge of options at the end of life: ignorance in the face of death. *JAMA* 2000;284:2483–2488.

5. Ngo-Metzger Q, August K, Srinivasan M, et al. End-of-life care: guidelines for patient-centered communication. *Am Fam Physician* 2008;77(2): 167–174.

6. The American Osteopathic Association End of Life Care Advisory Committee. End of Life Care Policy, approved by the American Osteopathic Association House of Delegates, 2004. Available at: www.osteopathic.org, accessed January 27, 2008.

7. *Education for Physicians on End-of-Life Care (EPEC) Trainers' Manual.* Princeton, NJ: The Robert Wood Johnson Foundation, 1999.

8. Finucane TE. How gravely ill becomes dying. A key to end-of-life care (editorial). *JAMA* 1999;282:1670–1672.

9. Fox E, Landrum-McNiff K, Zong Z, et al. Evaluation of prognostic criteria for determining hospice eligibility in patients with advanced lung, heart, or liver disease. SUPPORT Investigators. Study to Understand Prognoses and Preferences for Outcomes and Risks of Treatment. *JAMA* 1999;282:1638–1645.

10. Meisel A, Snyder L, Quill T. Seven legal barriers to end-of-life care: myths, realities, and grains of truth. *JAMA* 2000;284:2495–2501

11. Qaseem A, Snow V, Shekelle P, et al. Evidence-based interventions to improve the palliative care of pain, dyspnea, and depression at the end of life: a clinical practice guideline from the American College of Physicians. *Ann Intern Med* 2008;148:141–146.

12. Osteopathic education for physicians on end-of-life care (O-EPEC). Available at: www.osteopathic.org, accessed January 27, 2008

13. Portenoy RK, Sibirceva U, Smout R, et al. Opioid use and survival at the end of life: a survey of a hospice population. *J Pain Symptom Manage* 2006;32:532–540.

14. Emanuel EJ, Fairclough DL, Emanuel LL. Attitudes and desires related to euthanasia and physician-assisted suicide among terminally ill patients and their caregivers. *JAMA* 2000:284:2460–2468.

15. Foley KM, Competent care for the dying instead of physician-assisted suicide. *N Engl J Med* 1997;336:54–58.

16. Billings JA, Block S. Nurturing humanism through teaching palliative care. *Acad Med* 199873(7):763–765.

32

Evidence-Based Medicine

ROBERT CARDARELLI AND BRENT W. SANDERLIN

KEY CONCEPTS

- Evidence-based medicine (EBM) builds upon a framework of valid patient-oriented information dispensed within the time constraints of a typical practice.
- The EBM approach of today is, in effect, an elaboration of osteopathic medicine's break away from the harmful effects of 19th century medical treatments in pharmacotherapy and surgery.
- In the practice of EBM, an easily grasped series of steps allows physicians to utilize the best-available research in caring for their patients.
- The focus of EBM is the appraising of individual research studies of therapy, diagnosis, harm, and prognosis.
- EBM functions as a tool for the practicing physician. Repetition and practice are the key to becoming comfortable and efficient with the concepts and steps, allowing physicians to stay informed and to properly inform the patient.

INTRODUCTION

Physicians of today are confronted with an insurmountable amount of medical information from a variety of sources (1,2), much of which has the potential to change the way we practice medicine and care for our patients. Many medications or treatment modalities, which were formerly considered to be the standard of care, have now been shown to either be of questionable benefit or even to cause harm to our patients. Thousands of health care research articles are published each month (3)—far beyond the capacity of any physician to read. This knowledge explosion is primarily a result of electronic resources such as the Internet and has forced physicians to be selective in what they use to stay updated, thus making valid information, and the ability to assess for validity, more important than ever.

The concept of **Evidence-Based Medicine (EBM)** evolved in 1992 by the Evidence-Based Medicine Working Group (4). EBM is intended to provide a method for practicing physicians to efficiently utilize published research to improve the care they provide in their clinical practice. EBM builds upon a framework that allows physicians to provide the most valid patient-oriented information to patients within the time constraints of a typical practice (5).

Why is EBM important to osteopathic physicians? Andrew Taylor Still originally broke from traditional medicine as a result of his observation that the allopathic medicine of the time was often more harmful to the patient than no treatment at all, violating one of the key tenets of modern medicine—"first do no harm" (6). Osteopathic medicine was founded upon an ideology that the body can heal itself and that the physician's role was to assist it in this process. As scientifically valid treatments became available in pharmacotherapy and surgery, Still and other osteopathic physicians began to embrace and utilize them. For today's osteopathic physicians, it is important to use scientifically valid methods of treatment and diagnosis to care for our patients. EBM provides us with a framework to do this.

STEPS IN PRACTICING EVIDENCE-BASED MEDICINE

The practice of EBM is based upon a series of steps that allows physicians to utilize the best available research in caring for their patients (5). These **fundamental steps** are:

1. Ask an answerable question.
2. Search the available evidence.
3. Critically appraise the evidence for its validity, impact, and applicability.
4. Integrate this critical appraisal with the physician's clinical expertise and the patient's unique biology, values, and circumstances.
5. Evaluate and improve how one performed the first four steps.

Step 1: Ask an Answerable Question

There are two types of questions that one can ask: background questions and foreground questions. Background questions are those that ask for general knowledge or background about a certain condition, illness, or some aspect of health status and are commonly asked by learners early in their career. Foreground questions ask for specific information in order to perform clinical decisions or actions (5). Foreground questions have four components, also known as the "**PICO**" format: (a) patient and/or problem; (b) intervention or exposure; (c) comparison (if relevant); and (d) clinical outcome (including time if relevant) (5). An example of a foreground question is "In adults with diabetes mellitus, would the use of metformin lower the risk of having a cardiovascular event compared to taking a sulfonylurea?" Well-formulated questions create a basis for a well-defined literature search and appraisal process.

Step 2: Search the Available Evidence

Once an answerable question is formulated, the next step is to search the available evidence for an appropriate answer. It is important to realize that not all evidence is of equal value. Systematic reviews, randomized controlled trials, observational studies, and secondary publications are resources of evidence of varying degrees of reliability. The most reliable information comes from homogeneous systematic reviews (with or without meta-analyses) comprising multiple randomized controlled trials. The next most reliable information comes from individual randomized controlled trials followed by observational studies. Although this list represents a hierarchy, caution is advised since the best study design is determined by the study question. Moreover, a systematic review is only as good as the individual studies that are summarized in the review. Clinical guidelines are a source of evidence that must also be critically appraised since the development of a guideline may be based on expert opinion (low quality) or independent well-designed trials (high quality). Another valuable source of evidence for practicing physicians is secondary publications, such as *Journal of Evidence-Based Medicine*, which is a collection of articles from various journals that are already appraised for the reader with summary recommendations.

Step 3: Assess the Evidence for Validity, Impact, and Applicability

Physicians spend a considerable amount of time making therapeutic decisions, performing and ordering diagnostic tests, understanding the potential risks of their and the patients' actions, and assessing potential long-term outcomes of medical decisions. Hence, the focus of this introductory EBM chapter is on appraising individual research studies of therapy, diagnosis, harm, and prognosis. It should be noted that there are methods to appraise other types of articles such as decision prediction rules, cost-effective analyses, clinical guidelines, and so on. However, these are beyond the scope of this chapter and readers are encouraged to seek other valuable resources on these topics.

Shared Concepts Impacting a Study's Validity

When assessing the validity of therapeutic, diagnostic, harm, and prognostic articles, there are some core concepts that they all share. These concepts include blinding, accounting for all study participants at the end of the study, treating each study participant equally throughout the study, and ensuring the participants are similar to some extent. These concepts are discussed in more detail below and then followed by additional validity questions that are specific to the article type.

Blinding

In therapeutic and harm studies, study participants, clinicians, and investigators should not know who is allocated to the intervention group or control group. Unblinded studies have the potential to introduce significant bias into the study since participants, and researchers alike, may respond differently or intentionally (or unintentionally) alter the study's protocol. **Double-blinding** refers to keeping the participants and investigators (including clinicians) blinded to avoid conscious or unconscious actions that may jeopardize the integrity of the study.

In diagnostic studies, the test of interest is normally compared to a reference standard. Comparing a rapid streptococcal test to a throat culture is such an example. The testers should be blinded to the diagnostic test results (i.e., rapid streptococcal test) when performing and interpreting the reference standard test (i.e., throat culture).

Accounting for all Study Participants

All patients who started the study must be accounted for at the end of the study since a large loss of participants to follow-up may lead

to biased results. For example, if very sick patients do not complete a study or drop out of the study early because of death or unacceptable side effects, the outcome may appear falsely favorable if they are not accounted for. Furthermore, study participants should be analyzed in their original group assignment. This principle is called "**intention-to-treat analysis**" (7). A crude "**5 and 20 rule**" can guide readers in determining the completeness of the study (8). If less than 5% of the study population is lost to follow-up, one can be reassured that the loss to follow-up minimally impacts the results. However, if more than 20% of the study population is lost to follow-up, caution is advised. One must weigh the strengths and weakness of the study itself, such as the study's sample size and the length of the study, when there is a 5% to 19% loss to follow-up.

Treating all Participants Equally

Keeping study groups blinded would prove to be difficult if the intervention and the control groups were treated differently. For example, if study participants in the intervention group had more frequent follow-up visits or if the study pill looked and tasted differently than the placebo pill, participants may develop the suspicion that they were receiving the intervention or the placebo.

Ensuring Study Groups are Similar

The description of a study population is usually found in the first table of an article. Since there are always some established risk factors that may affect the outcome, it is important to determine whether these factors are equally balanced between study groups. Another important consideration is that the study's population should be relatively similar to the physician's practice population. This increases the likelihood that the study's results can be **generalized** to a specific patient population.

Additional Validity Criteria for Therapeutic Studies

Randomization is the most important factor that impacts the validity of a therapeutic study (9). It ensures that each person has the same probability of being chosen and assigned to a specific study group. Nonrandomized studies may consciously or unconsciously cause an imbalance of important factors that can potentially impact the study's final results.

Additional Validity Criteria for Diagnostic Test Studies

Both the diagnostic test and the **reference standard** test must be performed and compared to one another. This should not be an issue if the study is truly blinded. The reference standard establishes whether the disease of interest is present or not (10), allowing the diagnostic test's characteristics to be calculated (i.e., sensitivity, specificity, etc.).

Additional Validity Criteria for Harm Studies

The follow-up period in a valid harm study should be sufficiently long since short follow-up periods may allow too little time for the disease (outcome) to manifest. The length of the study is determined by the study question, intervention, outcomes of interest, and limiting circumstances (i.e., funding). Phase IV clinical trials represent the study period in which participants are followed over extended periods of time. Recent FDA actions, such as pulling certain medications off the market, highlight the importance of having sufficiently long follow-up periods to monitor potential adverse events.

Additional Validity Criteria for Prognostic Studies

Prognostic studies usually stratify the study group into cohorts based on comorbid conditions or factors that influence the outcome (11).

TABLE 32.1

Hypothetical Example for Calculating EER and CER

Study Plan	Received Beta-blocker	Received Placebo
Number of patients in each group	100	100
Died within 2 y since initial myocardial infarction	5	15

EER = 5/100 = 0.05 = 5%
CER = 15/100 = 0.15 = 15%
RRR = 0.15 − 0.05/0.15 = 0.67 or 67%
ARR = 0.15 − 0.05 = 0.10 or 10%
NNT = 1/0.10 = 10

These factors can include the stage of disease or other diseases that may impact the outcome of interest. Demographic factors (i.e., age, sex) and environmental risk factors must also be considered. These potential "**confounding**" factors can be addressed using statistical techniques or participants can be matched (i.e., paired up) at the start of the study.

Assessing the Importance of Studies

Once the validity of a specific article is established, the next step is to assess the magnitude of its treatment effects.

The Magnitude of Effects of Therapeutic Studies

Most studies report their outcome in a dichotomous fashion. For example, one may evaluate whether or not daily use of a beta-blocker prolongs life after an initial myocardial infarction (Table 32.1). One can then compare the event of interest (i.e., death rates) among those who received a beta-blocker and those who received nothing (or placebo). The proportion of those who died in the placebo group is the "**control event rate**" (CER), also considered the baseline risk.

The proportion of those who died in the intervention group (received beta-blocker) is called the "**experimental event rate**" (EER). The **relative risk reduction** (RRR; RRR = CER − EER/CER) is common term that is used to explain the magnitude of a treatment effect. However, the RRR conveys limited information to the clinician because it does not take the baseline risk into account, not giving the clinician the ability to discriminate large treatment effects from small ones. The **absolute risk reduction** (ARR; ARR = CER − EER) takes the baseline risk into account (12). By taking the reciprocal of the ARR, the **number needed to treat** (NNT; NNT = 1/ARR) can be calculated (5). The NNT corresponds to the number of patients who need to take the therapy (i.e., beta-blocker) to prevent one outcome (i.e., death) over a certain period of time.

The Magnitude of Diagnostic Test Characteristics

The characteristics of a diagnostic test can be calculated by using a **2 × 2 table**, as depicted in Table 32.2. The columns often refer to the presence or absence of the disease of interest as determined by a standard reference. The rows of the table are the "positive" or "negative" results of the diagnostic test of interest.

Based on Table 32.2, the **prevalence** of the disease (i.e., congestive heart failure) in the study population is 10.7%. A patient's **pretest probability** (the probability that a patient has the disease before the diagnostic test is performed) can be estimated by the prevalence if the patient is relatively similar to the study population. The **positive predictive value** is the probability that a patient has the disease if the diagnostic test is positive, whereas the **negative predictive value** is the probability that they do not have the disease if the test result is negative. **Sensitivity** is another characteristic of a diagnostic test that is commonly reported, which is defined as probability of a positive test given that the target disease is present. **Specificity** is defined as the probability of a negative result given that the target disease is not present. These parameters are then used to calculate the **positive (LR+) and negative (LR−) likelihood ratios** of diagnostic tests. The LR+ is the ratio of the true-positive rate to the false-positive rate. In the example in Table 32.2, a positive test result would be 9.77 times as likely in someone with

TABLE 32.2

Example of a 2 × 2 Table

Diagnostic test result		Target Disorder CHF	Target Disorder No CHF	Totals
	BNP ≥ 100	138 (a)	118 (b)	256 (a + b)
	BNP < 100	19 (c)	1196 (d)	1215 (c + d)
Totals		157 (a + c)	1,314 (b + d)	1,471 (a + b + c + d)

Prevalence = (a + c)/(a + b + c + d) = 157/1,471 = 10.7%
Positive predictive-value = a/(a + b) = 138/256 = 53.9%
Negative predictive-value = d/(c + d) = 1,196/1,215 = 98.4%
Sensitivity = a/(a + c) = 138/157 = 87.9%
Specificity = d/(b + d) = 1,196/1,314 = 91.0%
LR+ = sensitivity/(1 − specificity) = 0.879/1 − 0.91 = 9.77
LR− = (1 − sensitivity)/specificity = 0.25/0.88 = 0.28 (1 − 0.879)/0.91 = 0.13
BNP, B-type natriuretic peptide; CHF, congestive heart failure.

the disease as in someone without the disease. Likewise, the LR is defined as the ratio of the false-negative rate to true-negative rate. There are two mnemonics that are used in remembering the clinical applicability of specificity and sensitivity: (a) for a test with a high *Sp*ecificity, a *P*ositive result rules-*in* the diagnosis (**SpPin**) (5) and (b) for a test with a high *Se*nsitivity, a *N*egative result rules-*out* the diagnosis (**SnNout**) (5).

The Magnitude of Effects from Harm Studies

The magnitude of association in retrospective studies is reported as an **odds ratio** where a value of less than one confers a protective effect of the intervention and a value of greater than one confers a detrimental effect of the intervention. A sample calculation is shown in Table 32.3.

Prospective studies (i.e., clinical trials and cohort studies) report the magnitude of an association by using a "**Relative risk**" which is defined as "the ratio of the risk in the treated group (EER) to the risk in the control group (CER)" (5,13). Interpretation of the relative risk is the same as the odds ratio and a sample of a relative risk calculation is also shown in Table 32.3. The odds ratio and the relative risk are difficult to conceptualize for patients and physicians, and thus can be reported as the **Number needed to harm** (NNH). The NNH is defined as the number of patients who need to be exposed to the causative agent to produce one additional harmful event over a specified period of time (5,14). The calculation is shown in Table 32.3 but can only be utilized for clinical trials and cohort studies.

The Magnitude of Prognostic Study Results

The outcome of prognostic studies provides information about survival over time. A **survival curve** is one of the most common ways prognostic data are presented. It provides the proportion of individuals who are alive (i.e., have not had the outcome, such as death) at any given time point. Prognostic information can also be presented as the probability of being alive at a particular point in time, usually at 1- or 5-year time points. In addition, **median survival** is used to describe the amount of time in which 50% of patients have died. At times, all three measures are required to be fully informed about the prognosis of certain diseases.

Step 4: Applying the Evidence to the Patient

One of the strongest links between osteopathic medicine and EBM practice is the need to consider the whole patient in terms of cultural, economic, religious, and other special circumstances that impact the applicability of evidence to the specific patient. In fact, many physicians, especially osteopathic physicians, start the application of EBM at this step. A physician should take into account the patient's beliefs and wishes, such as lifestyle modification over taking a medication. Although the physician should be knowledgeable of the current guidelines and evidence, patient-centered decision making should be at the core of the patient–physician relationship (15). Social and economic factors regularly impact what the patient is willing to do regardless of what the evidence shows. High medication costs and copayments are common reasons why patients fail to take prescribed medications (16). These barriers must be considered at the clinical encounter in order to keep the best interest of the patients in mind. Patient-centered care involves offering and discussing alternative options for the patient to consider. Moreover, it involves listening, assessing, assimilating, and delivering a shared treatment plan with the individual patient. Without this, EBM truly becomes "textbook medicine."

As discussed earlier in the chapter, one can only apply the evidence of a study to a patient if the study population is similar to that patient. This applies to the demographic characteristics of the study population and also the factors that may have impacted the study's results. For example, a study assessing a medication's efficacy on heart failure symptomatology may have excluded diabetics or patients with a history of a myocardial infarction. The question becomes, "Can these results be applied to a patient who is a diabetic and had two previous myocardial infarctions?"

Step 5: Evaluate and Improve on Performance of Steps 1 to 4

This chapter is the first of many steps to becoming proficient in practicing EBM. This chapter outlined some of the basic EBM principles to allow physicians, residents, and medical students to begin understanding its importance. Repetition and practice are the key to becoming comfortable and efficient with the concepts and steps required to appraise different articles. EBM functions as a tool for the practicing physician, allowing them to stay informed and able to properly inform the patient. The systematic approach to appraising articles is only one part of EBM mastery. Failing to utilize personal expertise and consider patient values and expectations gives credit to those who criticize EBM as "textbook medicine." So what's next? Continue reading articles on EBM, attend sessions at conferences, and start appraising one article a week. As a guide to appraising articles, PowerPoint presentations and worksheets are available at no cost at http://www.hsc.unt.edu/depart ments/cebm/lectures.htm.

TABLE 32.3

Calculating an Odds Ratio (OR) and Relative Risk (RR)

	Adverse Outcome	No Adverse Outcome
Exposure to treatment	(a)	(b)
No exposure to treatment	(c)	(d)

Calculations:
OR = (a) × (d)/(b) × (c)
RR = [a/a + b]/[c/c + d]
EER = a/(a + b)
CER = c/(c + d)
Absolute risk increase (ARI): EER − CER
NNH = 1/ARI

REFERENCES

1. Osheroff JA, Forsythe DE, Buchanan BG, et al. Physicians' information needs: analysis of questions posed during clinical teaching. *Ann Intern Med* 1991;114:576–581.
2. Covell DG, Uman GC, Manning PR. Information needs in office practice: are they being met? *Ann Intern Med* 1985;103:596–599.
3. Virgilio RF, Chiapa AL, Palmarozzi EA. Evidence-based medicine, part 1. An introduction to creating an answerable question and searching the evidence. *J Am Osteopath Assoc* 2007;107:295–297.
4. Evidence-Based Medicine Working Group. Evidence-based medicine: a new approach to teaching the practice of medicine. *JAMA* 1992;268: 2420–2425.
5. Straus SE, Richardson WS, Glasziou P, et al. *Evidence-Based Medicine: How to Practice and Teach EBM.* 3rd Ed. St. Louis, MO: Elsevier, 2005.

6. Orenstein R. Andrew Taylor Still and the Mayo Brothers: convergence and collaboration in the 21st century osteopathic practice. *J Am Osteopath Assoc* 2005;105:251–254.

7. Hollis S, Campbell F. What is meant by intention to treat analysis? Survey of published randomized controlled trials. *Br Med J* 1999;319: 670–674.

8. Cardarelli R, Oberdorfer JR. Evidence-based medicine, part 5. An introduction to critical appraisal of articles on prognosis. *J Am Osteopath Assoc* 2007;107:315–319.

9. Guyatt GH, Sackett DL, Cook DJ. How to use an article about therapy or prevention: are the results of the study valid? (Users' guide to the Medical Literature, part 2A) *JAMA* 1993;270:2598–2602.

10. Mayer D. *Essential Evidence Based Medicine*. Cambridge University Press, 2004.

11. Hemingway H. Prognosis research: Why is Dr. Lydgate still waiting? *J Clin Epidemiol* 2006;59(12):1229–1238.

12. Guyatt GH, Sackett DL, Cook DJ. How to use an article about therapy or prevention: what were the results and will they help me in caring for my patients? (Users' guide to the Medical Literature, part 2B) *JAMA* 1994;271:59–64.

13. Rosner B. *Fundamentals of Biostatistics*. 6th Ed. Belmont, CA: Thomson Brooks/Cole, 2006.

14. Levine M, Walter S, Lee H, et al. How to use an article about harm. *JAMA* 1994;271(20):1615–1619.

15. Stewart M, Brown JB, Donner A, et al. The impact of patient-centred care on outcomes. *J Fam Pract* 2000;49(9):805–807.

16. Gottlieb H. Medication nonadherence: finding solutions to a costly medical problem. *Drug Benefit Trends* 2000;12(6):57–62.

Approach to the Somatic Component

33

Palpatory Examination

WALTER C. EHRENFEUCHTER AND ROBERT E. KAPPLER

KEY CONCEPTS

- No known device has been developed that exceeds the tactile sensitivity of the human hand.
- The development of palpation can be accomplished through various exercises.
- Familiarization with determination of layers of the body is the outcome of progressive developmental exercises.
- The learning process for the physician never stops.
- The development of a high level of palpatory skill is ongoing, requiring patience and practice.

INTRODUCTION

The scanning evaluation is carried out in all body regions indicated by abnormalities found in the screening exam. Therefore, findings of asymmetry, spinal curve abnormalities and abnormalities of body posturing, combined with regional range of motion testing, guide the physician in choosing the location(s) to perform layer-by-layer palpation. In the case of more than one area of abnormality being identified, typically it is the region of greatest motion loss that is evaluated first, that is where the key lesion is most likely located.

PALPATION DEFINED

The *Glossary of Osteopathic Terminology* defines palpation as the application of variable manual pressure to the surface of the body for the purpose of determining the shape, size, consistency, position, inherent motility, and health of the tissues beneath (1). Another definition is Palpation is the lightly placing of hands or fingers on the patient's body to discover changes from the normal condition of soft tissues, bones or organs beneath the surface of the skin, as well as the skin itself (2). The reality is that there has been no device developed that comes close to mimicking, let alone exceeding the tactile sensitivity of the human hand.

When performing palpation in a given region of the body, it is best to apply a layer-by-layer approach. This consists of:

- Observation
- Temperature
- Skin topography and texture
- Superficial fascia
- Muscle
- Tendons
- Ligaments
- Bone
- Erythema friction rub

Palpation always includes notation of any areas of tenderness, which is defined medically as the presence of pain elicited by palpation. How hard does one need to press to accomplish these various layers? Light surface palpation requires only a few grams of pressure. Deep bony palpation requires about 1,500 g of pressure or about 3.33 lb (8).

OBSERVATION

Visual observation of the skin surface must precede any palpatory examination (Fig. 33.1). Observation is made of the skin color, and any adnexal changes such as the presence of pimples, dry or scaly skin, folliculitis, and pigmentary changes. The spinal segments or body surface associated with any findings are noted for further review during the examination. These reflect local sympathetic nervous system changes and neural trophism that can be segmentally associated with somatic dysfunction.

TEMPERATURE

Skin temperature has been observed since the time of Hippocrates. He observed the patient for hot spots by having an assistant smear the patient with a thin layer of mud. Areas that dried first were warmer than those that did not.

Today the osteopathic physician evaluates the skin temperature by using the volar aspect of the wrist, or the dorsal surface of the hypothenar eminence of the hand. The physician does this by placing the wrists or hands a few centimeters above the area to be tested and using both hands to evaluate the paraspinal areas bilaterally simultaneously, searches for areas of thermal asymmetry (Fig. 33.2).

Heat radiation may be palpated in many other areas of the body (e.g., the abdomen or extremities). If the physician is unable to discern a temperature difference while off the skin surface, then he or she may at this point make very light contact with area to be examined. The hands are then lifted off, not dragged along the surface, and then replaced gently on the next levels to be examined. Again, the spinal segments or body regions of abnormality are noted.

Changes in temperature reflect a change in local blood flow that may be due to inflammation, or to the changes in sympathetic tone associated with segmental somatic dysfunction.

SKIN TOPOGRAPHY AND TEXTURE

A very light touch is used. Generally, the palmar surface of the fingertips is used for this type of palpation. This pressure will permit the finger pads to glide smoothly over the skin surface without excessive friction.

The skin is evaluated for sweat gland activity, greasiness (sebaceous gland activity), thickening, or roughness. The spinal segments or body regions of abnormality are noted. Gently pressing the fingers into the skin surface will allow the physician to evaluate for

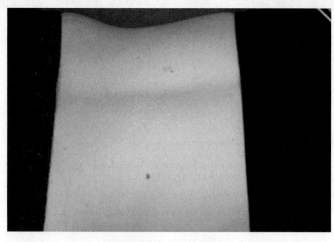

Figure 33-1 Observation.

changes in skin turgor and tension. These changes reflect a change in local sympathetic nervous system activity associated with segmental somatic dysfunction.

SUPERFICIAL FASCIA

The physician now makes a broader contact with the skin surface and presses gently with the palm of the hand to engage the fascia. The amount of pressure necessary typically causes slight reddening of the physician's nail beds (Fig. 33.3). The physician gently moves the hands cephalad and caudad, side to side, and clockwise and counterclockwise to elicit motion tensions and directions of ease and bind in the superficial fascia.

Gradually applying more pressure will allow the physician to evaluate deeper and deeper layers of fascia right down to the muscular investing fascia. The segmental levels or body regions associated with asymmetric bind of the fascias are noted, as well as the depth of penetration necessary to elicit that alteration. Any areas of tenderness are likewise noted.

MUSCLE

Deep palpation is defined as pressure sufficient to contact the periaxial tissues of the spinal column. Muscle is the next layer of tissue to be palpated, and additional pressure is required to feel through the superficial tissues to get to the musculature. The amount of pressure varies from patient to patient depending on the thickness of the subcutaneous fat layers. The thicker the fat, the more difficult it is to palpate changes in the deeper tissues.

Typically, the pads of the fingers are aligned perpendicular to the direction of the muscle fibers and firmly pressed into the muscle then rolled across the fiber bundles (Fig. 33.4). Sufficient pressure is

typically necessary to blanch the physician's nail beds. An irritable muscle will twitch in response to this "plucking" of the muscle.

The physician evaluates muscle turgor, tension, thickness, shape, and irritability. Many terms are used to describe the changes that are felt in abnormal musculature: ropiness, stringiness, fibrotic, dense, and so on. The segmental location of any of these changes is noted as well as the character of the muscle tissue at that location. While muscle hypertonicity may extend for a number of levels (e.g., T4-9 left paraspinal), the physician also notes the level of peak muscular change (T6 left PVM). The location of any tenderness elicited or trigger points discovered is also noted.

TENDONS

Although tendons are not readily palpable in the paraspinal tissues, in the periphery tendons should be traced to their bony attachments as well as their continuity with the muscle. Any fibrous thickening, change in elasticity, or tenderness should be noted. Tenderness at the muscle attachment to bone is termed an enthesopathy. Trigger points are commonly located in the myotendinous junction.

LIGAMENTS

The ligaments accessible to palpation vary with location in the spine. Palpation of the ligaments should include a search for the presence of the ligament (absence indicating a traumatic rupture or congenital absence), tension in the ligament (normal, excessive, or lax), and elicited tenderness.

BONE

Even deeper pressure will allow the physician to palpate the bony structures beneath the musculature. The bone is palpated for evaluation of normal contour, tenderness, and for motion.

ERYTHEMA FRICTION RUB

In erythema friction rub, the pads of the physician's second and third fingers are placed paraspinally and then in two or three quick strokes drawn cephalad to caudad down the spine (Fig. 33.5). The normal tissue response is initial blanching followed by reddening of the skin surface, followed by a slow fading of the redness back to normal skin color.

Any deviation from this by tissues remaining pale, remaining red, or becoming red initially instead of pale, is abnormal and the spinal levels and laterality of the findings are noted.

Most of us use fine palpation on a daily basis without realizing it. We do such things as picking coins out of a pocket or purse by touch. We readily differentiate between dimes, nickels, pennies, and quarters, based on the known characteristics of each coin (10).

Figure 33-2 Temperature.

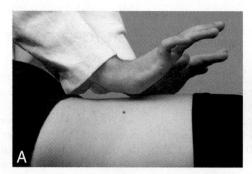

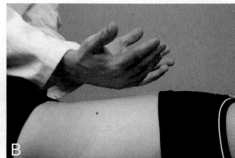

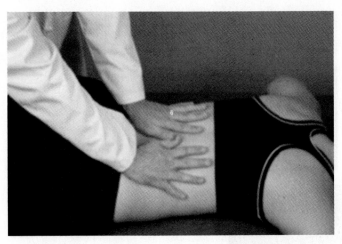

Figure 33-3 Palpating fascia.

There is no substitute for experience. Inexperienced examiners have been shown to be able to palpate motions as small as 1 mm in excursion. Experienced examiners have been shown to palpate motion as small as 0.0846 mm (3/100").

The diagnosis of somatic dysfunction requires at least two of the following:

- Tenderness
- Asymmetry
- Range of motion changes
- Tissue texture changes

The scanning examination, applied to areas of previously discovered screening abnormalities, provides further information on asymmetry, tenderness, and tissue texture changes associated with the somatic dysfunction. It also provides an opportunity for segmental localization.

There are three basic phases to kinesthetic observation (palpation):

1. Detection
2. Internal amplification and magnification (eyes closed)
3. Combining Nos. 1 and 2 with the physician's three-dimensional knowledge of anatomy yields analysis and interpretation (4).

What remains now is for the physician to interpret the results of the palpatory examination on a level-by-level basis. Table 33.1

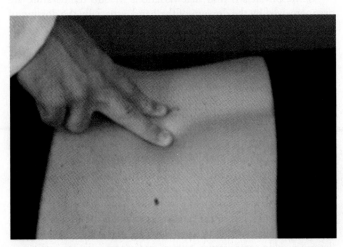

Figure 33-4 Palpating muscle.

outlines the changes one would expect in the presence of either acute or chronic somatic dysfunction. This would allow an examiner to ascertain whether a somatic dysfunction is new (acute) or old (chronic) or perhaps a combination of the two (acute exacerbation of a chronic condition). This determination is critical in choosing the correct manipulative techniques to apply to a given individual.

PALPATORY EXERCISES

Learning Palpatory Technique

To accomplish this task, it is necessary to teach the fingers to feel, think, see, and know. One feels through the palpating fingers on the patient; one sees the structures under the palpating fingers through a visual image based on knowledge of anatomy; one thinks what is normal or abnormal; and one knows with a confidence acquired by practice that what is felt is real and accurate.

Through complex peripheral and central processing, the smallest sensory perception can be amplified to the point of conscious recognition and analysis.

Exercise 1: Palpating Inanimate Objects

Purpose

To perceive slight tactile differences of tissue texture and motion. Exercises on inanimate objects serve to sharpen tactile concentration and attention. Concentration is essential. Close the eyes to eliminate extraneous stimuli. Pay attention to kinesthetic sensations received through the fingers.

Procedure

1. Put a mixture of coins in a pocket or purse. By touch, distinguish between heads and tails, and between pennies, dimes, nickels, and quarters. Identify date lines on the coins.
2. Locate a hair that has been placed under a sheet of paper; attempt to estimate its length. Add sheets of paper until you can no longer palpate the hair.
3. Palpate several types of human bones. Identify the bones and their component parts, envisioning the tissue that normally surrounds them.
4. Palpate a human bone and a solid plastic imitation of the same bone. Identify the characteristics of the human bone that distinguish it from the replica.

Mitchell (3) calls palpation a two-way communication system in which the patient's tissues react to the presence of the palpator's hand. This is more likely to occur when palpation has been practiced over a period of time.

Three steps define the process. The first is detection, the second is internal amplification or magnification, and the third is analysis and interpretation. This last step translates palpatory findings into meaningful anatomic, physiologic, or pathologic states (V. Frymann. Syllabus for workshop on palpation, 1990). Familiarity with osteopathic terminology permits description of palpatory findings in consistent terms.

Effective palpatory technique cannot be learned by observation. Watching another physician palpate a patient indicates where the hands are placed but gives little or no indication of the feel of tissues being palpated.

Many individuals have a dominant hand with which they prefer to palpate or motion test. This may or may not be the hand with which they write. Recognition of a dominant hand will allow the individual to develop a compensatory mechanism to obtain accurate information when using both hands.

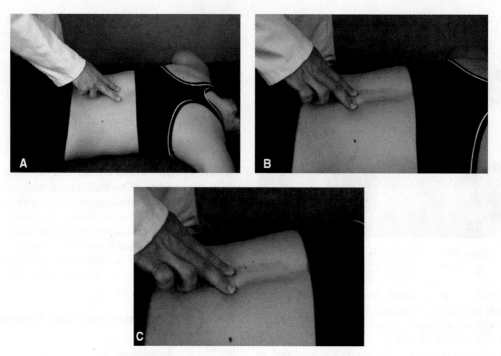

Figure 33-5   Demonstration of erythema friction rub.

Exercise 2: The Dominant Hand

Purpose

The purpose of this exercise is to determine the dominant hand. It is believed that when a person does not consciously think about it, he or she will put his or her dominant hand on top when the hands are clasped.

Position

This exercise can be done in a standing or sitting position.

Procedure

Without consciously thinking about it, clasp your hand together in front of you, with one hand on top of the other.

Results

The hand that *is* on top will most likely be your dominant hand. It is also believed that palpatory results are more consistent if the examiner has the dominant eye over the area that is being palpated.

For example, if one hand is stronger than the other, practice in applying equal pressure over equivalent structures can result in accurate interpretation of such manual information.

Interpretation of dominant and nondominant proprioceptive feedback from each hand is also a response that the individual can adjust.

Exercise 3: The Dominant Eye

Purpose

The purpose of this exercise is to determine the dominant eye. Some believe that palpation and the interpretation of palpatory findings are more accurate if palpation is performed with the dominant eye over the area being palpated.

Position

This exercise can be performed standing or sitting with a distant clock or visible object to look at.

Procedure

1. Look at the distant object with both eyes open (Fig. 33.6).
2. Extend your dominant hand and make a circle with your thumb and index finger that encircles your view of the distant object.
3. Now, close one eye, then open it and close the other eye.

Result

The eye that saw the object encircled with the fingers of your dominant hand is generally your dominant eye (6). Recognition of dominance, if it exists, and development of a compensatory mechanism is the main issue here; in time, apparent palpatory ambidexterity may result.

There are more touch (kinesthetic) nerve endings in the pads of the fingers than elsewhere in the hand. It is generally agreed that the thumb and/or the first two finger pads, rather than the fingertips, are the most sensitive part of the hand to train and use for palpation (V. Frymann. Syllabus for workshop on palpation, 1990).

Some physicians find that variations in skin temperature are best perceived by the dorsum of the hand, especially the dorsum of the middle phalanges of fingers two, three, and four; others use the palmar surface. Try both and see which is more effective for you. The coordinated use of the palms and the fingers around an object is best suited for obtaining a stereognostic sense of contour (4).

Flexibility of the joints of the elbows, wrists, hands, and fingers is important. Relaxation is also important to eliminate any muscle tension that would block perception. Strength of hands and fingers can be increased by using a finger exerciser, squeezing a ball, or playing a musical instrument that requires fingering. Because the hands are so important to a physician, they should be carefully protected and cared for. They are sensitive diagnostic instruments.

Light touch is thought by many persons experienced in palpation to be the most useful and easy to use. Very light touch, or light touch, consists of laying the hands passively on the skin or moving the hands lightly over the skin. Such light touch can be used to determine skin temperature, texture, moistness, oiliness, resistance, tone, and elasticity. It may be possible to determine skin temperature

TABLE 33.1

Palpatory Signs of Acute or Chronic Somatic Dysfunction

Signs	Manifestations
Pain	
Acute	Severe, cutting, or sharp
Chronic	Dull, achy with paresthesias.
Skin changes	
Acute	Warm, moist, red, inflamed
Chronic	Cool, pale
Vasculature	
Acute	Vessel injury with resultant release of endogenous peptides, chemical vasodilation, inflammation, and edema
Chronic	Vessels constricted due to increased sympathetic tone
Sympathetic activity	
Acute	Systemically increased sympathetic activity, but the local effect of this increased activity is overpowered by bradykinins released, so there is local vasodilation due to chemical effect
Chronic	Local vasoconstriction due to hypersympathetic tone; systemic tone has returned toward normal.
Musculature	
Acute	Locally increased muscle tonus, muscle contraction, spasm, ropiness, mediated via the muscle spindle. Minimal somatosomatic reflex effects.
Chronic	Decreased muscle tone, flaccid, mushy, limited range of motion likely due to fascial contracture. Common somatosomatic reflex effects.
Mobility	
Acute	Range of motion is often normal, but the quality is sluggish.
Chronic	Range of motion is diminished, but quality of remaining motion is normal.
Soft tissues	
Acute	Boggy edema, acute congestion, fluids from vascular leakage, and chemical reactions in the tissues.
Chronic	Congestion, doughy, stringy, fibrotic, thickened, exhibits increased resistance to penetration, contracted, contractured.
Adnexa	
Acute	Moist skin, no trophic changes
Chronic	Scaly, dry skin, pimples, folliculitis altered pigmentation (trophic changes).
Visceral	
Acute	Minimal somatovisceral reflex effects.
Chronic	Common somatovisceral reflex effects (5).

Paresthesias—crawling, tingling, itching, burning, or gnawing sensations (10).

sensation by passing the hand just above the skin. Firmer pressure communicates with the deeper cutaneous layers and fascial sheaths. It explores superficial muscles to determine their tone and mobility. Firm pressure and compression explore deeper muscle, fascia, and bony relationships.

Exercise 4: Layer Palpation

Purpose

The goal of this exercise is to palpate your own tissues and concentrate and perceive various layers and structures of the body by varying the pressure of palpation.

Position

The position for this exercise is seated comfortably beside a table with your nondominant arm resting on the table.

Procedure

1. Close your eyes and relax. Concentrate your attention through the palpating fingers of your dominant hand.
2. Lightly palpate the dorsum of the nondominant hand using the fingers of your dominant hand. Scarcely touching the surface, feel the contour of the hand.
3. Test palpation with the dorsal and palmar aspects of the palpating fingers to determine which is most sensitive to temperature.

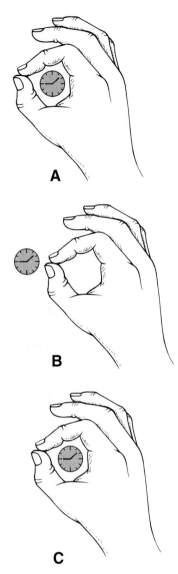

Figure 33-6   Right eye dominance. **A.** Both eyes open. **B.** Right eye closed; left eye open. **C.** Left eye closed; right eye open. (Modified from WA Kuchera, with permission.)

4. Using very light touch, palpate and describe skin texture, moisture, and thickness.
5. Gently pinch the skin on the back of the hand. Elevate it and release it. How long did it take for the skin to resume its normal configuration?
6. Evaluate skin drag on both the palm and dorsum of the hand. Skin drag is the estimation of the amount of resistance experienced when the pads of the fingers are lightly applied and moved (dragged) over the skin surface. On which aspect of the hand do the palpating fingers move most easily? Why? Describe any increase in skin drag that is due to excessive dryness, slight perspiration, or edema. Describe any decrease in drag resulting from excessive perspiration, oiliness, or atrophy.
7. Locate the veins and note their size and texture. Make a fist several times to engorge the veins and then describe the differences observed.
8. Locate the radial artery and describe the differences between it and a vein.

9. Increase the contact between your palpating fingers and the skin of your hand so that you create a shearing stress in the subcutaneous tissues. Shearing in this context refers to movement of tissues between layers. Note that with this palpation one can shear only so far before the palpating fingers slide on the skin. Shear across the hand in various directions describing what you feel. Does the skin move equally and easily in all directions?
10. Palpate the extensor tendon of the ring finger. Place two fingers along the length of the tendon; flex the ring finger, and palpate the sense of the linear movement along the tendon.
11. Palpate the tendon of the biceps at the elbow. How does it feel? It should be ropelike, smooth, and firm.
12. Place the thumb and index finger of the palpating hand on either side of the mid-phalangeal articulation of a finger on the opposite hand. Note the quality and range of various elements during flexion and extension. Now lighten your touch while performing the same movements. Notice how little contact is needed to distinguish flexion and extension.
13. Place your palpating fingers on the anterior surface of the proximal third of your other forearm. Using slightly more pressure than that used for skin, palpate the muscles used to flex the fingers. Now maintain palpatory contact during flexion of the middle finger. Describe the feel of these flexor muscles and fascia during the maneuver.

When you are examining a patient, tell the patient in general terms about the procedure as it goes along. This is especially important if significant tenderness might be elicited during deep palpation. Take the necessary time, moving gently and deliberately. Initially it is common to apply too much pressure in an attempt to feel the tissue. Avoid poking, prodding, tickling, or stirring the tissue. These actions can cause reflex irritation (4).

Louisa Burns, a noted early osteopathic researcher, made the following suggestions to those beginning to develop palpatory skills:

■ Palpate the objects with the lightest possible touch, scarcely touching the surface.
■ Be aware of surface elevations and temperature differences.
■ Using slightly more contact, palpate the surface.
■ Try to ascertain the qualities or characteristics of the substance of the object.
■ Describe perceptions as accurately as possible.

Exercise 5: Palpate Your Partner's Forearm

Purpose
The goal of this exercise is to determine the characteristics of different structures in the forearm of another person.

Position
You are seated comfortably, facing your partner, who is seated, facing you from across a narrow table.

Procedure
1. Grasp your partner's left forearm with your nondominant hand.
2. Lightly place the palm and fingers of your dominant hand over the dorsal forearm of your partner, just distal to the elbow. Close your eyes, relax, and concentrate your attention through the palmar surface of your fingers.
3. Without moving your hand, think skin. Try to perceive and describe skin temperature, texture, thickness, and moisture.

4. Next, compare the dorsal and palmar aspects of the forearm, and describe the differences. Which aspect is smoother? Thicker? Warmer? Drier?

5. Now, with a slightly firmer touch, concentrate on the second layer, the subcutaneous fascia. Gently move the skin of the forearm longitudinally and horizontally. How thick is it? How loose? Many of the tissue texture changes associated with somatic dysfunction are within this layer.

6. Gently and slowly increase the depth of touch until you feel the deep fascial layer that forms a sheath around the underlying structures. Think deep fascia. Is it smooth? Continuous? Firm?

7. While palpating the deep fascial layer; slowly move the hand horizontally across the forearm to identify areas of thickening that form fascial compartments between bundles of muscles. Identifying enveloping layers of deep fascia is often helpful in separating one muscle from another; use it to work with even deeper structures.

8. Palpating through the deep fascia, concentrate on the underlying muscle. Is it soft and compliant? How is its elasticity? Pay attention to individual muscle fibers and the directions in which they run.

9. Have your partner slowly open and close his or her hand as you note the quality and range of movement created by the contracting and relaxing muscle. Describe the difference. Palpate the forearm muscles as the hand is clenched. This sensation simulates the feel of the most common tissue texture abnormality (TTA) at the level of muscle or in areas of somatic dysfunction.

10. Still palpating at the level of muscle, move your hand slowly down your partner's forearm until you feel the musculotendinous junction, an area or region where the muscle is vulnerable to injury.

11. Move past the musculotendinous junction toward the wrist. Note the transition from muscle to musculotendinous junction to the smooth, round, firm feel of tendons.

12. Follow the tendons distally until you feel a structure that binds them at the wrist. This is the transverse carpal ligament (flexor retinaculum) and palmar carpal ligament (a thickening of the deeper anterolateral fascia). Note fiber direction, thickness, and firmness. How does it feel in comparison with the tendon? Compare the palpatory sensation over this area with that over tendons that are more superficially located.

13. Now place your index finger over the proximal radiohumeral joint at the dimple of the elbow. Place your thumb opposite your index finger, on the ventral side over the lateral side of the humeroulnar attachments. You should now be palpating the head of the radius. Describe the characteristics. Compare the feel of this living bone with a plastic model or with your memory of bone from a cadaver.

14. Move your thumb and index finger proximally until you locate the joint space. Your finger and thumb fall into it. You should not be able to feel the joint capsule. The joint capsule is not palpable because palpable joint capsules signal pathologic changes.

Palpatory skill involves more than a mechanism for finely tuned sensory perception. A more significant component is to be able to focus on the mass of information being perceived, paying close attention to those qualities associated with TTA, and bypassing many of the other palpatory clues not relevant at the time. These skills might be enhanced by trying to palpate a hair through several pages of a telephone directory.

Exercise 6: Palpatory Sensitivity

Purpose
The goal of this exercise is to determine and improve your sensory awareness.

Position
For this exercise, sit comfortably in front of a table with a phone book and objects of various thicknesses, including a human hair.

Procedure

1. Starting with the thickest object, place them, one at a time, under a page in the phone book and see if you can palpate their edges and dimensions.

2. Then add pages and palpate until you can no longer determine the objects' dimensions. How many pages were between your fingers and each object before you could no longer palpate it? Can you palpate the human hair through a single page from the phone book?

Palpatory sensitivity involves a process of developing mental filters. Consider an analogy in music, where the orchestra conductor focuses on the violins. The conductor is aware of the entire orchestra playing, but is diverting attention to a specific portion of sound that he or she perceives. The brain cannot process everything at once. By concentrating only on the portion you want, it becomes easy and fast to detect areas of significant TTA. In a comparison of student musculoskeletal examinations with experienced examiners, Kappler et al. (5) observed that the experienced examiners recorded fewer findings than student examiners, but the experienced examiner's findings were more significant. This shows that experienced physicians apply a filtering process to their palpatory data, rejecting insignificant findings without being consciously aware that they are doing this. The student is overwhelmed with the mass of palpatory data and has not yet developed this filtering process to reduce the data to a manageable component.

MOTION PERCEPTION

If any motion is present, describe the sensations transmitted through the fingers. Also, estimate the weight of objects, the amount of pressure needed to move them, and the resistance or force exerted against your pressure.

Perception of motion is an essential component of palpation. A major difference in palpation of living tissue is this sensed motion. Motion of the body is described as passive, active, and inherent (6).

Passive motion is brought about by the physician; it is movement done to the subject. Active motion is performed by the subject; it is deliberate, conscious muscular activity. Inherent motion is activity unconsciously generated within the body (J. Goodridge. Michigan State University College of Osteopathic Medicine. Biomechanics syllabus, 1986), such as respiratory motion or peristalsis. Inherent motion is postulated to occur in any of several ways:

- Biochemically, at the cellular or subcellular level
- As part of multiple electrical patterns
- As a combination of a number of circulatory and electrical patterns
- As some periodic pattern not yet understood

Experts agree that individuals can perceive tissue movement as minute as 1 mm (6). With practice and patience, inherent motion may be palpated.

By varying the palpation pressure, successive layers of tissue can be palpated. In palpating superficial tissue, use the lightest effective touch. To palpate successively deeper layers, apply only as much additional pressure as necessary. As a general rule, this means palpating to the depth of the tissue or structure to be examined, that is, down to but not through the structure being examined. The use of various depths of touch differs from physician to physician, usually depending on the model of diagnosis and treatment chosen.

Exercise 7: Palpating Spinal Motion and Paravertebral Tissues

Purpose
The goals of this exercise are to learn how to palpate living tissue in the classroom situation with an instructor available to demonstrate and interpret as needed and to be able to palpate the thoracic and lumbar spinal areas, testing for and finding any regions with relative resistance of the vertebrae and their spinous processes when passive flexion is introduced.

Position
Your partner sits on the table and you stand behind your partner.

Procedure

1. Using your finger pads, place the first three fingers of your dominant hand between the spinous processes of T1 and T2, T2 and T3, and T3 and T4. Remember to use the pads of your fingers. Place your other hand on the top of your partner's head.
2. Locate the spinous processes and interspinous ligaments, noting how they feel. Compare differences between the feel of the bone and the feel of the ligament.
3. Passively flex the head and neck while sensing for increasing tension of the interspinous ligaments. Note: One spinous process may move more easily than another (Fig. 33.7).
4. Using the fingers of both hands, palpate for temperature differences along the paravertebral thoracic and lumbar spine. Use either the palmar or dorsal surface of your fingers, depending on which you find to be more sensitive.
5. Using both hands simultaneously, stroke the back from C7 to L5. Which areas are warmer? Try to find a segment within the thoracic area that is either warmer or cooler than another segment. Compare left with right sides, and superior with inferior.

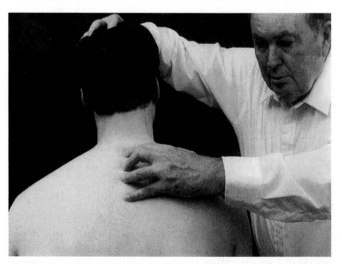

Figure 33-7 Palpating upper thoracic flexion-extension.

Stroking of this type is useful in identifying changes in contour, as well as identifying areas of edema and increased tissue tension.
6. Palpate for moisture differences, noting stickiness, dryness, wetness, waxiness, and slipperiness.
7. Proceeding from T2 to L5, lightly compress the paravertebral soft tissues. Then use deeper pressure, but less pressure than that required to palpate bone. You may notice that in some areas, tissues compress more easily; while in others, there is more resistance. Significant resistance indicates an area of TTA (1), which bears further investigation.
8. Lightly palpate the skin and subcutaneous tissue over the resistant site. This helps you identify the outer limits of tissue texture involved.

Developing Advanced Skills in Palpation of Tissue Texture Abnormality

Advanced palpatory skills require practice and experience. We try to define or describe what the tissues feel like. The important factor is an imprint in the brain of the sensation that is perceived. Attempting to translate this sensation into words is inadequate. It must be perceived. Comparing an area of tissue texture abnormally with an adjacent area without this tissue texture is essential. Experiences that involve **COMPARISON** are far more valuable than experiences palpating an abstract area.

Think of evaluating hot or cold water. If a hand is in warm water (e.g., 90°F) and this hand is used to evaluate a test beaker of water at 70°F, this beaker will seem cold. Now the hand is placed in water at 50°F, and then evaluate the temperature of 70°F water. The water in the test beaker will seem warm. Perceiving difference between water temperature or difference between tissue texture is best achieved by comparing one against the other.

A skilled osteopathic physician has developed a store of information in the brain about what tissues feel like, and especially the tissue texture change of somatic dysfunction. When the skilled examiner palpates an area, he or she can compare the current palpatory sensation with the store of information in the brain. This is a different type of comparison. To the novice, it appears to be evaluating the abstract but it is really a matter of comparing what is perceived with the palpation with prior experiences stored in the brain.

Once the osteopathic has developed this advanced skill in palpating, the skill is never lost. The author has experienced older osteopathic physicians who were almost frail, yet when they laid their hands on a patient, they immediately detected areas of tissue texture change.

The author's theory about this type of learning is that this is cerebellar learning. Cerebral learning is subject to the curve of forgetting. Cerebellar learning is never forgotten.

SUMMARY

Position your dominant eye over the structure being palpated. Place thumbs or finger pads over the area to be palpated. To ensure greater accuracy, mentally transfer your thoughts to the interface of your hand with the patient's body. Realize that resiliency or resistance to motion can be sensed in the initial movement during motion testing. You can miss these subtle findings and get hung up on gross motion restrictions, for example, how far a vertebral joint or tissue moves rather than the quality of the movement. Avoid the following common errors in palpation:

- Lack of concentration
- Too much pressure
- Excessive movement

These palpatory skills provide a method of obtaining practical experience in developing the art of palpation. There are many other exercises. Initially, palpation is practiced on a partner in the skills laboratory. During clinical clerkships, one gains additional experience by examining attending physicians' patients. Ultimately, palpatory experience is gained from palpatory examination of the physician's own patients. The physician continues to learn and never stops gaining experience. The preceding section shows how to get started in the process of obtaining palpatory data from the patient.

Remember that development of a high level of palpatory skill is an ongoing process, requiring patience and practice. "Osteopathy cannot be imparted by books. Neither can it be taught to a person intelligently who does not fully understand anatomy" A T Still (7).

REFERENCES

1. The Glossary Review Committee of the Educational Council on Osteopathic Principles. Glossary of osteopathic terminology. In: D'Alonzo GE, Jr, ed. *AOA Yearbook and Directory of Osteopathic Physicians*. Chicago, IL: American Osteopathic Association, 2000, Palpation;1242.

2. DiGiovanna, Schiowitz, Dowling. *An Osteopathic Approach to Diagnosis and Treatment*. 3rd Ed. Baltimore, MD: 2005.

3. Mitchell F, Jr. The training and measurement of sensory literacy in relation to osteopathic structural and palpatory diagnosis. *J Am Osteopath Assoc* 1976;75:881.

4. Kuchera WA, Kuchera ML. Palpation of soft tissue. In: *Osteopathic Principles in Practice*. 2nd Ed. Columbus, OH: Greyden Press, 1994:25, 112.

5. Kappler RE, Larson NJ, Kelso AF. A comparison of osteopathic findings on hospitalized patients obtained by trained student examiners and experienced osteopathic physicians. *J Am Osteopath Assoc* 1971;70(10):1091–1092.

6. Van Allen P, Stinson J. The development of palpation. *J Am Osteopath Assoc* 1941;40(5):207, 208.

7. Greenman PE. *Principles of Manual Medicine*. 2nd Ed. Baltimore, MD: Williams & Wilkins, 1996.

8. Patterson, et al. Determination of pressures used in osteopathic palpatory diagnosis. *JAOA* 103:382.

9. Kappler R. Chicago College of Osteopathic Medicine, 1971.

10. Nicholas & Nicholas. *Atlas of Osteopathic Techniques*. 1st Ed. Baltimore, MD: Lippincott, Williams & Wilkins, 2008:31–33.

11. Dorland's Illustrated Medical Dictionary.

12. Still AT. *Autobiography*, 192–193.

Screening Osteopathic Structural Examination

WALTER C. EHRENFEUCHTER

INTRODUCTION

The screening examination is designed to determine rapidly where in the body the most significant somatic dysfunctions reside. It is designed simultaneously to find larger orthopedic structural abnormalities that may be responsible for generating these dysfunctions.

The nature of the screening examination is that it is sensitive to the discovery of the presence of dysfunction, but not specific as to the spinal segments or structures involved, or for the tissues responsible for creating and maintaining the dysfunction.

The screen consists of two portions, a static postural examination and a dynamic part, which includes regional range-of-motion testing and observation of gait (1).

Static Postural Examination

Observation

The patient should be undressed enough to be able to accurately observe the overall configuration of the body without it being obscured by clothing. This also allows you to observe the patient for evidence of other serious diseases. One common finding is the presence of pigmented nevi with the possibility of malignant melanoma. The reality is that people do not get to see their backs. Skin tumors can grow quite large here prior to discovery. Patients sustain burns from heating pads, develop erythema ab igne from chronic heating pad use and develop discoloration of the skin, abrasions, and even ulceration in skin overlying points of chronic pressure.

Body Symmetry

Assessment of body symmetry constitutes the first portion of the overall structural examination. Some minor asymmetry is present in virtually all human beings. The goal of the examination is to determine what abnormal asymmetries are present in a given individual. Figure 34.1 shows examination for symmetry of posterior landmarks of the body. The posterior landmarks commonly used in the screening structural examination are in **bold** type in the following discussion.

Ankles and Feet

Arches—Observe the height of the arches on each foot. Most important is the fact that they are symmetric, not whether they are both flat or not.

Achilles Tendons—Observe the medial and lateral surfaces of the tendon. The curve of the tendon should be symmetric. Flattening of the normal curve on the medial side of the Achilles tendon indicates the likely presence of a valgus hindfoot deformity. The valgus hindfoot accompanies longitudinal arch collapse in the foot. Again, asymmetry becomes the most significant finding.

Significance—Unilateral arch collapse with valgus hindfoot can occur to assist the body in compensating for an anatomically long leg on the ipsilateral side, and dysfunctions of the pelvis that create a functionally long leg on the ipsilateral side (anterior rotation of the innominate, inferior innominate shear, etc.)

Legs

Observe the size and symmetry of the gastrocsoleus muscles. If asymmetric try to determine if one is enlarged, or if one is smaller. A large calf can be due to deep venous insufficiency in the ipsilateral leg, a small calf may indicate muscle atrophy due to chronic entrapment of the S1 or S2 nerve roots, or even the sciatic nerve itself.

Knees

Observe the popliteal creases. If unlevel in the presence of normal ankles and feet, they indicate the presence of a short tibia and fibula on the ipsilateral side.

Observe the shape of the popliteal fossa. If flattened or exhibiting a genu recurvatum, it indicates hyperextension of the knee and the presence of laxity of the posterior cruciate ligament. Again, if unilateral, it may represent a compensatory change for an anatomic or a functional long leg on the ipsilateral side.

Observe any medial or lateral deviation of the leg at the knee (genu valgus (knock kneed) or genu varus (bow legged). Typically, these are congenital or developmental deformities, although they can occur with advanced unilateral compartment arthritis of the knee. The presence of a unilateral varus or valgus deformity may shorten the ipsilateral leg and affect the rest of the body above. If bilateral, asymmetry may indicate a worsening of the condition again as a result of an anatomic or functional long leg.

Thigh

Observe the posterior thigh muscle mass. If enlarged, it may be due to venous insufficiency or thrombosis, or there is also the possibility of an underlying tumor. This author has personally had a patient present with low back pain and asymptomatic enlargement of one thigh. Further examination, imaging, and ultimately surgery resulted in the removal of a football-sized liposarcoma from the patient's thigh. Again, decreased size of the muscle mass unilaterally may indicate a chronic entrapment of the L5, S1, or S2 nerve roots, or the sciatic nerve's tibial division.

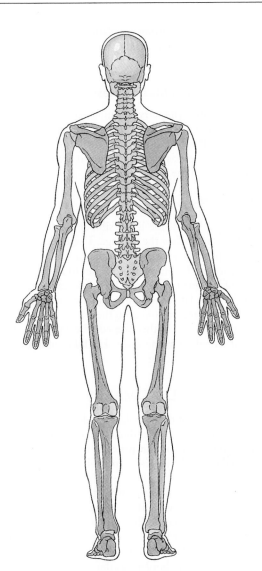

On examination note:
- Midgravitational line
- Achilles tendon: straight, curved?
- Position of feet
- Relation of spine to midline (curves, etc.)
- Prominence of sacrospinalis muscle mass
- Symmetry of calves
- Symmetry of thighs (including any folds)
- Symmetry of buttocks
- Lateral body lines
- Levelness of greater trochanters
- Prominence of posterior superior iliac spines
- Levelness of posterior superior iliac spines
- Levelness of iliac crests (supine, prone, sitting, standing)
- Fullness over iliac crests
- Prominence of scapula
- Position of scapula and its parts
- Levelness and relation of fingertips to body
- Arms (relations)
- Levelness of shoulder
- Neck-shoulder angles
- Level earlobes
- Level of mastoid processes
- Position of body relative to a straight vertical line through the midspinal line
- Posterior cervical muscle mass (more prominent, equal, etc.)
- Head position: lateral inclination

Figure 34-1 Examination for symmetry of posterior landmarks of the body. (From Nicholas & Nicholas. *Atlas of Osteopathic Technique.* Philadelphia, PA: Lippincott Williams & Wilkins; Figure 2.8.)

Gluteal Region

The gluteal folds should be symmetric; again, asymmetry may indicate a leg-length inequality. The **greater trochanters** should be palpated and assessed for levelness, again as a check for leg-length inequality. The gluteal muscle mass should be assessed for asymmetry. Enlargement may indicate the presence of a buttock tumor (lipoma is the most common), whereas atrophy may indicate chronic entrapment of the S1 nerve root or entrapment of the superior and inferior gluteal nerves in the greater sciatic foramen due to hypertrophy of the piriformis muscle.

Iliac Crests

The iliac crests should be assessed for symmetric height over their lateral aspect. Asymmetry could indicate the presence of an anatomic or functional leg-length inequality. If the legs have been symmetric all the way up to the gluteal folds and greater trochanters, asymmetry of the iliac crest height can indicate the presence of a short hemipelvis.

POSTERIOR SUPERIOR ILIAC SPINES

Again, the assessment is for symmetric localization relative to vertical displacement and anterior-posterior displacement. A low

posterior superior iliac spines (PSIS) can be caused by an anatomic or functional leg-length inequality, a short hemipelvis, and by innominate somatic dysfunction. Low PSIS results from posteriorly rotated innominate, or inferior innominate shear. High PSIS can result from anteriorly rotated innominate, or superior innominate shear. A posterior displacement of the PSIS indicates the possible presence of a posteriorly rotated innominate, anterior displacement an anteriorly rotated innominate. Posterior rotation or superior shear of the innominate is a common compensatory mechanism for an anatomic long leg.

Thoracic and Lumbar Spine

The spinous processes should all be in a vertical straight line. Large side-to-side deviations indicate the presence of a scoliosis. If there is leg-length inequality present, observe the scoliosis for its "fit" with the unlevel sacral base. This is done to determine whether the scoliosis is due to the leg-length inequality, or the patient has two separate conditions (2). Figure 34.2 shows lumbar scoliosis due to a 2-inch sacral base unleveling from an anatomic short left leg.

Mild scoliosis may be produced by segmental or group somatic dysfunction. The direction of the curve gives a general indication

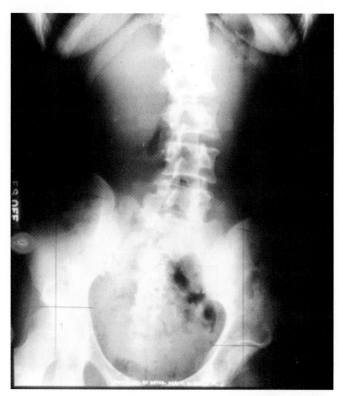

Figure 34-2 Lumbar Scoliosis due to 2-in sacral base unleveling from an anatomic short left leg. (Original photograph: Walter C. Ehrenfeuchter, D.O., F.A.A.O., with permission.)

of the sidebending component of the segmental dysfunctions. If the curve is due to a single segmental dysfunction, the dysfunction may be located at the bottom of the curve, the top of the curve, or right in the middle. If there is a group of dysfunctional segments, they are likely all sidebending and rotating in opposite directions.

The presence of a thoracic scoliosis can indicate a primary thoracic curvature, a secondary thoracic curvature compensating for a primary lumbar curve, or a secondary thoracic curvature compensating for an unleveling of the cranial base. The unlevel cranial base may be due to cervical spine abnormalities (e.g., Klippel Feil Syndrome), a head tilt due to asymmetric cervical muscle tone (Torticollis), or even somatic dysfunction of the cranial base.

Excessive prominence of a spinous process may indicate the presence of an angulate Kyphosis, which can be due to a congenital anomaly of the vertebral body, or possibly compression fracture.

Exaggeration of the kyphotic thoracic curve can occur due to flexed segmental dysfunctions, flattening of the kyphotic curve from extended segmental dysfunction. Exaggeration of the thoracic Kyphosis can occur in some conditions of the spine such as Scheuermann disease or diffuse idiopathic skeletal hyperostosis (DISH). DISH occurs more frequently in patients with type II diabetes mellitus.

Exaggeration of the lumbar lordotic curve can be due to an extended segmental dysfunction or a flexed or anteriorly rotated sacrum. Flattening of the lumbar lordotic curve can be due to a flexed segmental dysfunction or an extended or posteriorly rotated sacrum. It can also be flattened by muscle spasm or the presence of ankylosing spondylitis.

Observe the lumbosacral junction for the presence of skin anomalies including a hairy patch, pigmented nevus, port-wine stain, pilonidal sinus, pilonidal cyst, or lipoma. The presence of a

skin lesion has a strong correlation with presence of an underlying congenital bony abnormality including many forms of occult spinal dysraphism.

Paravertebral Muscle Mass

Observe for symmetry. Prominence of the paravertebral muscle mass can indicate the presence of vertebral rotation to the ipsilateral side. It may also represent hypertrophy or hypertonicity of the larger muscle mass. Uncommonly, it can be the result of a tumor or an abscess in the musculature.

Lateral Body Line

The lateral body line is the silhouette of the contour of the sides of the trunk below the rib cage. These become especially useful in obese patients where the condition of the lumbar vertebrae and the paravertebral muscles is harder to assess. For example, flattening of the left lateral body line and exaggeration of the curvature of the right lateral body line suggest the presence of a scoliosis in the lumbar region convex to the left. In the severely obese, the left lateral body line in this case could exhibit two skin folds, and the right lateral body line three skin folds, indicating the presence of the same sidebending curve.

SCAPULAR LANDMARKS

The position of the scapulas is under numerous muscular and postural influences. The landmarks that are of the greatest importance here are the **acromion process, the inferior angle**, **spine of the scapula,** and the medial scapular border.

A line across the shoulders should be perpendicular to the spinal column, regardless of what the spinal column is doing in the upper thoracic region. If the spinal column is vertical, the shoulders should be symmetrically horizontal. If a scoliosis has the spinal column sidebent right in this region, the right scapular landmarks will be lower than the left.

The medial border of the scapula should roughly parallel the spine, regardless of the position of the spine at this site. Forward carriage of one shoulder will result in the medial scapular border being farther from the spinous processes than its normal mate. Normally, the medial scapular border is approximately 2 to 3 inches. Rotation of the scapula due to shoulder muscle imbalances will result in a loss of the parallel relationship between the spine and the medial border of the scapula.

If the spine is vertically straight, and the scapulas are unlevel, it indicates a problem with the shoulder girdle. Typically, the spine of the scapula is even with the spinous process of T3, whereas the inferior angle of the scapula is even with the spinous process of T7 (transverse processes of T8). If one scapula is higher than this in position, scapula alta, it implies the presence of hypertonic or contractured musculature involving the shoulder elevators (upper trapezius, the rhomboids, and levator scapulae). If sufficiently high and present from birth, it represents a congenital Sprengel deformity. On the other hand, a scapula positioned lower than normal, scapula infra, can represent weakness of the shoulder elevators vs. hypertonicity of the shoulder depressors (latissimus dorsi, lower trapezius, lower serratus anterior).

Arm Position and Length

Viewing the position of the arms in relation to the trunk can give you further insight into dysfunctions of the shoulder girdle musculature by revealing rotations of the entire extremity. The distance of the arms from the torso also informs you as to the possibility of scoliosis decompensation or pelvic side shift. The length of the arms from acromion to fingertip should be observed. Just as you can have a patient with a short leg, you can also have a patient with a short arm. This becomes significant for work and sport activities involving the upper extremities.

Slope of the Shoulder

Observe the slope of the shoulder where it meets the neck. These two surfaces should be symmetric. They should meet the vertical muscle mass of the cervical spine in the mid-cervical region. Asymmetry must be interpreted in light of all the preceding data regarding scapular position. If a fold of skin attaches to the neck higher than the mid-cervical region, this constitutes a web neck, or pterygium colli. It may even attach as high as the mastoid process. This is associated with congenital disorders such as Klippel-Feil syndrome or Turner syndrome.

Cervical Spine

The cervical spinous processes should be vertically oriented. Slight deviations from this are the norm, since the mid-cervical spinous processes are bifid and it is not unusual for one fid to be longer than the other, giving one the impression that a cervical vertebra is out of line with the rest of the neck. This is a normal finding.

The paravertebral muscle masses should be symmetric. Prominence of a muscle mass unilaterally may indicate the presence of unilateral facet dislocation with overriding, enlarged facet joints due to arthritic changes, local muscle hypertonicity, or a hematoma within the musculature.

Head

The head should sit level on top of the cervical spine. A tilt of the head atop the neck indicates the presence of either asymmetric suboccipital muscle tone or the presence of hypertonicity or spasm of one of the larger muscles that attach to the cranium (torticollis). It can also represent the sidebending component of an occipitoatlantal somatic dysfunction. In rare cases, it represents head positioning to reduce the impact of some forms of diplopia.

The **mastoid processes** should be level and the inion positioned in the midline. Asymmetry of the mastoid processes in the presence of a head positioned symmetrically atop the neck should lead you to think of the possibility of cranial somatic dysfunction with involvement of the temporal bones. Likewise, the position of the pinnae of the ears should be observed. Asymmetry again suggests the presence of cranial somatic dysfunction involving the temporal bones.

Patient Seated

The same landmarks of the torso, shoulders, neck, and head are again examined with the patient in the seated position (Fig. 34.3). Any changes in pattern from what was previously observed indicate a strong influence from problems in the lower extremity from the hip joints and hip girdle musculature (including the psoas muscles) down to the feet. These problems would need to be identified and addressed before any clear conclusions can be made regarding the presence of somatic dysfunction from the pelvis on up.

Some structural and postural abnormalities of the body are more obvious when viewed from the anterior perspective.

Feet

Apparent in-toeing (pigeon toed) and out-toeing (duck footed) positions of the feet can be due to local foot deformities like metatarsus adductus, lower leg abnormalities like tibial torsion, of femoral abnormalities such as anteversion or retroversion of the femoral neck. They may also represent the position of the entire lower extremity under the influence of a shortened piriformis muscle (out-toeing) or iliopsoas muscle (in-toeing).

Knees

Observe again for varus, valgus, and recurvatum or flexion contracture deformities of the knees. Observe the tibial tuberosities for prominence as this may represent a case of Osgood-Schlatter disease.

Observe the height of the patellas relative to the tibial tuberosities. Search for the presence of patella alta (high-riding patella) or patella baja (low-riding patella).

Thighs

Observe the symmetry of the thigh muscle mass. Atrophy of the these muscles can occur as a result of long-standing knee disorders such as osteoarthritis, or from entrapment of the femoral nerve or L2, L3, or L4 nerve roots.

Pelvis

Observe the position of the anterior superior iliac spines (ASIS) and pubic bones. They are supposed to reside in the same anterior coronal plane. If not, it tells you there is either an anterior or a posterior pelvic tilt that can cause changes in the lumbar lordotic curve (anterior tilt—increased lordosis; posterior tilt—flattening of lordosis). Likewise, changes in the lumbar curve can force changes in the tilt of the pelvis. Pelvic tilt is also under the influence of the hip girdle musculature. Anterior tilt may be caused by hypertonic or contracted iliopsoas muscles, posterior tilt by hypertonic or contracted hamstrings.

Pelvic rotation about a vertical axis is also readily viewed from the anterior aspect, with shifting of the ASIS anteriorly or posteriorly in response to positioning of the entire pelvis.

Observe the pelvis for evidence of pelvic side shift. This can again be compensation for a leg-length discrepancy, or it can be due to a leg-length discrepancy depending on the individual. Side shift will increase the prominence of the greater trochanter on the side to which the pelvis has shifted and will increase the tension in the iliotibial band.

The symmetry of the ASIS may also be altered by the presence of virtually any of the innominate dysfunctions.

Abdomen

The prominence of the abdomen is often in response to the shape of the lumbar lordosis. If the lordosis is flattened, it will tend to flatten the abdomen. If the lordosis in increased, it will make the abdomen more protuberant. This author has seen a case of lordosis due to paralytic polio that was so severe that the anterior portion of the lumbar spine could be seen pressing against the abdominal wall and the vertebrae and anterior discs readily palpable just beneath.

Protuberance of the lower abdomen is common in the presence of an increased Kyphosis or from flattening of the diaphragm due to respiratory conditions such as emphysema or asthma.

Figure 34-3 Examination for symmetry of anterior landmarks of the body. (From Nicholas & Nicholas. *Atlas of Osteopathic Technique.* Philadelphia, PA: Lippincott Williams & Wilkins; Figure 2.7.)

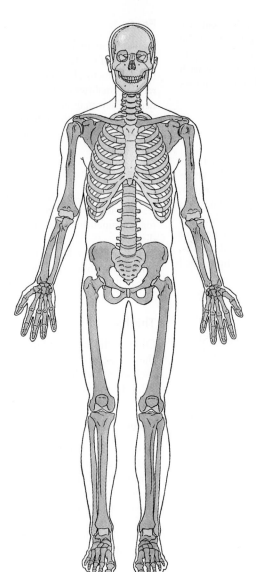

On examination note:
- Midgravitational line
- Lateral body line
- Position of feet
  - Pronation
  - Supination
  - Levelness of tibial tuberosities
- Levelness of patellae
- Anterior superior iliac spines
  - Level?
  - Anteroposterior: rotational prominence
- Prominence of hips
- Iliac crests, levelness
- Fullness over iliac crest
- Relation of forearms to iliac crests
  - One longer
  - Anteroposterior relation
  - Nearness to body
- Prominence of costal arches
- Thoracic symmetry or asymmetry
- Prominence of sternal angle
- Position of shoulders
  - Level or unlevel
  - Anteroposterior relations
- Prominence of sternal end of clavicle
- Prominence of sternocleidomastoid muscles
- Direction of symphysis menti
- Symmetry of face (any scoliosis capitis)
- Nasal deviation
- Angles of mouth
- Level of eyes
- Level of supraciliary arches (eyebrows)
- Head position relative to shoulders and body

If the spinal curves are normal and no respiratory condition exists, the protuberant abdomen provides evidence of visceroptosis and the patient should be evaluated for the same.

Normally, there is about three or four finger-breadths of space between the top of the iliac crest and the lower costal margin. This can be decreased by the presence of scoliosis. In severe or decompensated scoliosis, one side of the costal cage can literally be sitting on top of the iliac crest. At times, this can shift far enough laterally to put pressure on the liver or the upper left abdominal viscera. Elevation of liver or pancreatic enzymes can be the result.

Rib Cage

The prominence of the xiphoid process should be noted. It is not uncommon for the xiphoid to become more prominent as one ages. Then. due to clothing pressure or sleeping prone, it becomes tender to touch and the patient presents with "midepigastric pain" with the resultant unnecessary work-up. Palpation of the xiphoid will reproduce the patient's pain and render a diagnosis of xiphalgia.

Observe the patient for any deformities of the sternum. The pectus excavatum (funnel breast) is the most common (Fig. 34.4), pectus carinatum (pigeon breast) less so. Any deformity of the sternum should prompt an examination for occult congenital heart defects. While not a 100% correlation, heart defects are more common in patients with sternal abnormalities than in the general population.

Observe the prominence or lack thereof of the two halves of the rib cage. An anterior prominence of the rib cage on one side of the spine is frequently due to the rotational component of scoliosis. It is the analogue of the rib hump on the posterior side of the body.

Observe the costal cartilages for any deformity or swelling. Congenital abnormalities in the structure of the lower 4 or 5 costal cartilages are quite common. The normal rib cage is shaped something like an apple. A common abnormality is the presence of an outflaring of the lower rib cage. The resultant lateral sulci formed are called Harrison Grooves. These are most often familial, but can come about from any condition (such as very young pregnancy, large Wilms tumors) that bows out the growing costal cartilages. After skeletal maturity, the position of the cartilages is relatively fixed.

A visible or palpable ridge at one or more costochondral joints can indicate the presence of a "separated rib." When deformity is present at the time of injury, the articulation will often heal with

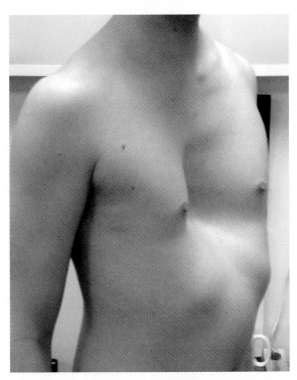

Figure 34-4 Pectus excavatum. (Original photograph Walter C. Ehrenfeuchter, D.O., F.A.A.O., with permission.)

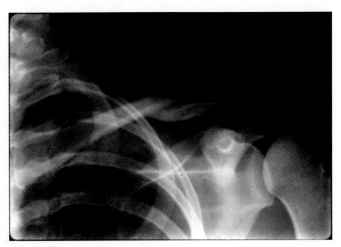

Figure 34-5 Deformed clavicle due to old fracture with malunion. (Original photograph Walter C. Ehrenfeuchter, D.O., F.A.A.O., with permission.)

a slight anteroposterior deformity. This is not amenable to correction after this injury has already healed.

Swelling of one or more costal cartilages (typically the second or the third) indicates the likelihood of Tietze syndrome, believed to be a viral infection of costal cartilage. This must be differentiated from the more common costochondritis that does not cause swelling of the cartilage, just tenderness.

Shoulders

Observe and palpate the clavicles for symmetry. Rarely will you see cases of congenital absence of the clavicles. A clavicle can be misshapen due to congenital anomaly, fracture during birth, or subsequent fracture at a later date. The length of the clavicle from sternum to acromion in part determines the position of the entire shoulder. The clavicle is the upper extremity's only bony connection to the axial skeleton. A shortened clavicle often causes anterior shoulder carriage, pulling the scapula farther away from the spinal column than its mate on the uninjured side. Figure 34.5 shows a deformed clavicle due to old fracture with malunion.

Cervical Region

Observe the patient for prominence of the sternocleidomastoid muscles and scalene muscles. Hypertonicity, contracture, and hematoma will shorten all of these commonly injured muscles. This will in turn alter neck and head carriage in response.

Head

Observe the carriage of the head atop the neck. Some dysfunctions in this region will be more obvious from an anterior view than the posterior.

Observe the position of the symphysis menti relative to the midline of the body and to the midline of the face. Observe the jaw for symmetry relative to the rest of the head. Lateral deviation of the jaw can signify a shortened portion of the mandible, with resultant dental abnormalities and the potential for temporomandibular dysfunction syndrome and pain. Asymmetry of the jaw can also be generated by somatic dysfunction of the temporal bones.

Observe the face for symmetry. Facial asymmetry can occur due to congenital malformation of the skull, as a result of birth trauma to the sphenobasilar synchondrosis, or acquired sphenobasilar somatic dysfunction as a result of head trauma or dental work. It can also occur as a result of facial bone somatic dysfunction as a result of trauma to the face. Facial asymmetry is often most evident in the shape of the orbits or entire face. Often, a visual determination of the cranial dysfunctions present can be made before palpating the motion of the head.

Figure 34.6 is a lateral view of normal posture with midgravitational line.

Knees

This may be the easiest way to observe genu recurvatum or flexion contracture of the knee. Again, symmetry may be more important than the mere presence of one deformity or the other.

Thighs

The lateral thigh surface should be smooth. If a deep groove is present running from the greater trochanter of the femur to the knee, it suggests shortening and contracture of the iliotibial band.

Pelvis

Anterior or posterior pelvic tilt is readily seen from the lateral aspect.

Lumbar Lordosis

Observe for a normal lumbar lordotic curve.

Figure 34-6 Lateral view of normal posture with midgravitational line. (From Nicholas & Nicholas. *Atlas of Osteopathic Technique.* Philadephia, PA: Lippincott Williams & Wilkins; Figure 2.9.)

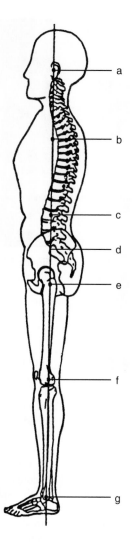

On examination note:
- Lateral midgravitational line
  - a   External auditory canal
  - b   Lateral head of the humerus
  - c   Third lumbar vertebra
  - d   Anterior third of the sacrum
  - e   Greater trochanter of the femur
  - f   Lateral condyle of the knee
  - g   Lateral malleolus
- Anterior and posterior body line
- Feet: degree of arching or flatness
- Knees: degree of flexion or extension
- Spinal curves: increase, decreased, or normal
  - Cervical lordosis: posterior concavity
  - Thoracic kyphosis: posterior convexity
  - Lumbar lordosis: posterior concavity
  - Sacrum, lumbosacral angle
- Arms: position relative to body
- Abdomen: prominence or flatness
- Sternal angle
- Thorax: prominence or flatness
- Head: relation to shoulder and body

Thoracic Kyphosis

Observe for a normal thoracic kyphotic curve.

Cervical Lordosis

Observe for a normal cervical lordotic curve.

Shoulders

Anterior shoulder carriage is readily apparent from the lateral view as is posterior carriage or a military-type posture. Anterior shoulder carriage with the scapula shifting superiorly and laterally will cause the acromion process to impinge upon the supraspinatus tendon. This can result in subacromial bursitis, rotator cuff tendonitis, frozen shoulder (fibrous adhesive capsulitis), and partial or total rupture of the supraspinatus portion of the rotator cuff.

Head Carriage

Note the position of the head relative to the rest of the trunk.

MID-GRAVITY LINES

Components of the posterior mid-gravity, anterior mid-gravity, and lateral mid-gravity lines are shown in Table 34.1.

Posterior Mid-Gravity Line

The posterior mid-gravity line (see Fig. 34.1) begins at a mid heel point, passes directly through the gluteal crease; the spinous processes of the sacral, lumbar, thoracic and cervical vertebrae; and the inion.

Assessment of body symmetry about this line makes readily apparent any pelvic side shift, any minor scoliotic curves, and head tilt.

If the line is reversed and begun at the inion passing down through the spine, other information can be gathered. In the presence of a scoliosis, no matter how severe, if it is a compensated curve, this plumb line will fall through the spinous process of S1. If decompensated, the plumb line will fall laterally to one side or the other.

If the body as a whole has compensated for a decompensated or traumatic spinal curve, even when the plumb line does not fall mid-sacrum, it may still fall normally at the mid heel point.

If the body is unable to compensate for any deformity above the feet, the plumb line will fall off of the mid heel point to one side or the other.

Posturing, which relieves or minimizes pain in any part of the body, can also shift this plumb line off of the mid heel point.

Anterior Mid-Gravity Line

The anterior mid-gravity line (see Fig. 34.3) again originates at the mid heel point, passes upward through the pubic symphysis, the

TABLE 34.1

Mid-Gravity Lines and Their Components

Mid-Gravity Line	Components
Posterior	• mid heel point • gluteal crease • spinous processes of the sacral, lumbar, thoracic, and cervical vertebrae • inion
Anterior	• mid heel point • pubic symphysis • umbilicus • xiphoid process • midsternum • episternal notch • symphysis menti • glabella
Lateral	• lateral malleolus • patella • greater trochanter of the femur • sacral promontory • midbody of L3 • greater tuberosity of the humerus • odontoid process of C2 • external auditory meatus

umbilicus, xiphoid process, midsternum, episternal notch, symphysis menti, and glabella.

Again, some truncal asymmetries and deformities are most visible from an anterior perspective, especially those involving the rib cage, jaw, and face.

A plumb line hung from the glabella can be used in much the same way that a plumb line from the inion is used.

Lateral Mid-Gravity Line

The normal lateral mid-gravity line (see Fig. 34.6) passes just anterior to the lateral malleolus, just posterior to the patella, through the greater trochanter of the femur, the sacral promontory, the midbody of L3, the greater tuberosity of the humerus, the odontoid process of C2, and the external auditory meatus.

Most of the anteroposterior deformities that can occur will cause pain in one part of the body or another and become a pathologic state in their own right.

An extreme abnormality of this weight bearing line is the situation where only the lateral malleolus is on the line. The rest of the points are anterior to this plane. Patients appear to be on the verge of falling forward and are in fact contracting every posterior truncal muscle they have to fight this gravitational tendency. Often, such patients have had their sense of normal posture disrupted by some trauma and have come to accept this distorted posture as correct. In addition to manipulative treatment, this type of patient will frequently require postural reeducation.

If the lateral malleolus is on the line as is the greater trochanter, but the knee is not, it demonstrates the presence of knee flexion contracture or genu recurvatum.

An increased lumbar lordosis will carry the points on L3 and the sacral promontory forward, but leave all other points on the line. This is often due to a bilaterally flexed sacrum or other anterior going sacral dysfunctions, or an extended dysfunction of the one or more of the lower lumbar vertebrae. It can also be due to weak lower abdominal musculature.

The "sway back" posture places the malleolar point on the mid-gravity line, but the only other point typically on the line is the greater tuberosity of the humerus. All other points fall anterior to the line. This posture commonly results from pregnancy. After the birth of the child, the body maintains this posture as it has learned this to be the normal. Abdominal strengthening exercises, osteopathic manipulative treatment, and postural re-education can all be used to correct this postural deformity.

Increased thoracic kyphosis tends to shift all points below the shoulder posterior to the weight bearing line except the malleolar reference point. Often, the head is carried anterior to the line for balance.

To a lesser degree, this is the same posture assumed by students while studying in a seated position. For every inch that the external auditory meatus is shifted anterior to the ideal mid-gravity line, an additional ten pounds of load is placed on the posterior cervical musculature. The solution is to relearn to sit upright. This can be assisted by raising the materials being read and propping them on something akin to a music stand. There are commercial devices that will do this. Artists and draftsmen have long used tilt top tables that take the strain off the neck and shoulders and allow the person to sit upright. So, put those heavy text books to good use and make them into a support for the notes you are studying from.

Some authorities prefer to reference the lateral mid-gravity line to the external auditory meatus, rather than the lateral malleolus. This changes the relative position of the landmarks for all the conditions listed above; it does not change the diagnoses (3–5).

REGIONAL RANGE-OF-MOTION TESTING

Regional range-of-motion testing is the last part of the screening structural examination. There are three things of note when performing these tests. First, any region with diminished range of motion is abnormal. Second, any region with increased range of motion is abnormal and may be compensating for an adjacent area that is hypomobile. Third, for the paired motions of sidebending and rotation, any left-to-right asymmetry is abnormal, even if the overall range of motion is normal.

The following screening range-of-motion exam will not pick every possible somatic dysfunction, but most will be discovered through it. In addition to measuring the ranges of motion, when possible, regional motion will be examined both actively and passively. The loss of active range of motion has many causes; the loss of the additional passive range of motion is most commonly associated with somatic dysfunction. The quality of that motion will also be assessed, as will any associated special tests.

Screening Ranges of Motion

Cervical Region

The normal range of motion for flexion is 45 to 90 degrees, and for extension is 45 to 90 degrees. The procedure for screening range of motion in the cervical region is:

1. The physician palpates between the spinous processes of C7 and T1 (Fig. 34.7).

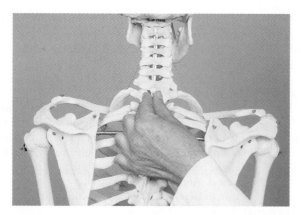

Figure 34-7 The physician palpates between the spinous processes of C7 and T1. (From Nicholas & Nicholas. *Atlas of Osteopathic Technique.* Philadelphia, PA: Lippincott Williams & Wilkins; Figure 3.1.)

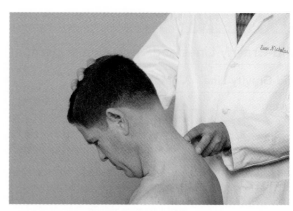

Figure 34-9 Passive forward bending. (From Nicholas & Nicholas. *Atlas of Osteopathic Technique.* Philadelphia, PA: Lippincott Williams & Wilkins; Figure 3.9.)

2. Instruct the patient to bend the head forward as far as he or she can go without pain. Normal range of motion is 45 to 90 degrees (Fig. 34.8).
3. After the patient has reached full active flexion, passively carry the head farther forward until motion is palpated at C7/T1 (Fig. 34.9).
4. Instruct the patient to return to the neutral position (Fig. 34.10).
5. Instruct the patient to bend the head backward as far as he or she can go without pain (Fig. 34.11).
6. Once the end of the active range of motion has been reached, the physician passively carries the head into further extension until motion is again palpated. (Fig. 34.12).

For sidebending, the normal range of motion is 30 to 45 degrees. The procedure for screening sidebending in the cervical region is:

1. The physician palpates over the Intertransverse spaces bilaterally between C7 and T1 (Fig. 34.13).
2. The patient is instructed to actively sidebend the head to the right to the pain-free limit of motion. Normal is 30 to 45 degrees (Fig. 34.14).

3. At the end of active right sidebending, the physician passively sidebends the patient's neck to the right while palpating for motion at C7/T1 (Fig. 34.15).
4. The patient is instructed to return his or her head to the neutral position (Fig. 34.16).
5. The patient is instructed to actively sidebend the head to the left as far as it will go without pain (Fig. 34.17).
6. At the end of the range of motion, the physician passively moves the patient's head into further left sidebending while palpating for motion at C7/T1 (Fig. 34.18).

The normal range for rotation in the cervical region is 70 to 90 degrees. The procedure for screening is:

1. The physician palpates over the Intertransverse space between C7 and T1 (Fig. 34.19).
2. The patient is instructed to actively turn his or her head to the right as far as it will go without pain. Normal range is 70 to 90 degrees (Fig. 34.20).
3. At the end of active right rotation, the physician passively turns the head farther while palpating for motion at C7/T1 (Fig. 34.21).

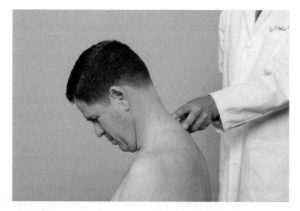

Figure 34-8 Instruct the patient to bend the head forward as far as he or she can go without pain. (From Nicholas & Nicholas. *Atlas of Osteopathic Technique.* Philadelphia, PA: Lippincott Williams & Wilkins; Figure 3.4.)

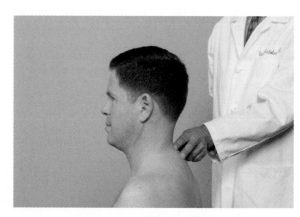

Figure 34-10 Neutral position. From Nicholas & Nicholas. *Atlas of Osteopathic Technique.* Philadephia, PA: Lippincott Williams & Wilkins; Figure 3.3.)

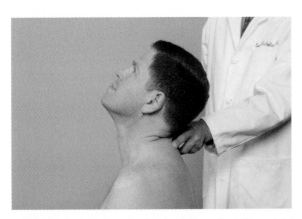

Figure 34-11   Active extension (backward bending). (From Nicholas & Nicholas. *Atlas of Osteopathic Technique*. Philadelphia, PA: Lippincott Williams & Wilkins; Figure 3.5.)

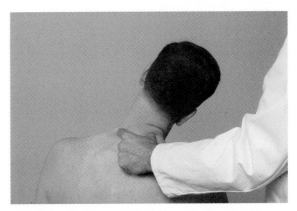

Figure 34-14   Active sidebending—right. (From Nicholas & Nicholas. *Atlas of Osteopathic Technique*. Philadelphia, PA: Lippincott Williams & Wilkins; Figure 3.12.)

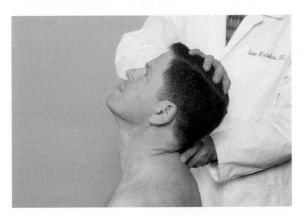

Figure 34-12   Passive extension (backward bending). (From Nicholas & Nicholas. *Atlas of Osteopathic Technique*. Philadelphia, PA: Lippincott Williams & Wilkins; Figure 3.10.)

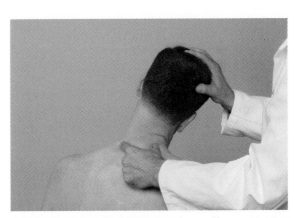

Figure 34-15   Passive sidebending—right. (From Nicholas & Nicholas. *Atlas of Osteopathic Technique*. Philadelphia, PA: Lippincott Williams & Wilkins; Figure 3.14.)

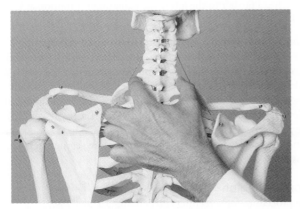

Figure 34-13   The physician palpates over the Intertransverse spaces bilaterally between C7 and T1. (From Nicholas & Nicholas. *Atlas of Osteopathic Technique*. Philadelphia, PA: Lippincott Williams & Wilkins; Figure 3.11.)

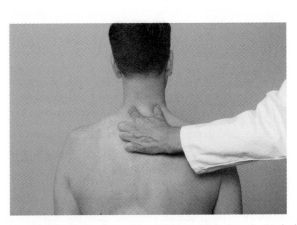

Figure 34-16   Neutral position. (From Nicholas & Nicholas. *Atlas of Osteopathic Technique*. Philadelphia, PA: Lippincott Williams & Wilkins; Figure 3.16.)

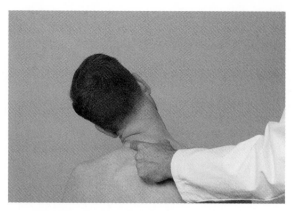

Figure 34-17 Active sidebending—left. (From Nicholas & Nicholas. *Atlas of Osteopathic Technique*. Philadelphia, PA: Lippincott Williams & Wilkins; Figure 3.13.)

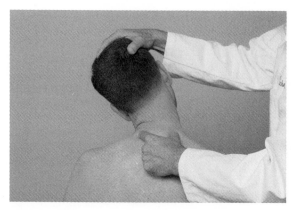

Figure 34-18 Passive sidebending—left. (From Nicholas & Nicholas. *Atlas of Osteopathic Technique*. Philadelphia, PA: Lippincott Williams & Wilkins; Figure 3.15.)

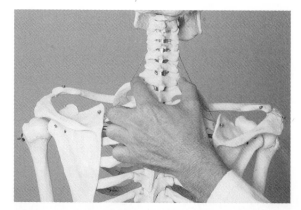

Figure 34-19 The physician palpates over the Intertransverse space between C7 and T1. (From Nicholas & Nicholas. *Atlas of Osteopathic Technique*. Philadelphia, PA: Lippincott Williams & Wilkins; Figure 3.11.)

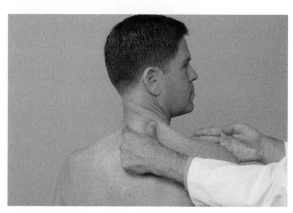

Figure 34-20 Active rotation—right. (From Nicholas & Nicholas. *Atlas of Osteopathic Technique*. Philadelphia, PA: Lippincott Williams & Wilkins; Figure 3.17.)

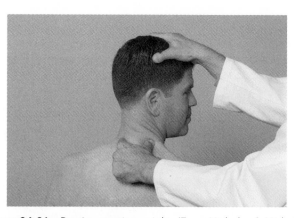

Figure 34-21 Passive rotation—right. (From Nicholas & Nicholas. *Atlas of Osteopathic Technique*. Philadelphia, PA: Lippincott Williams & Wilkins; Figure 3.19.)

4. The patient is instructed to return his or her head to the neutral position (Fig. 34.22).
5. The patient is instructed to actively turn the head to the left as far as it will go without pain (Fig. 34.23).
6. At the end of active left rotation, the physician passively turns the head farther to the left while palpating for motion at C7/T1 (Fig. 34.24).

A loss of approximately 50% of rotation in the cervical spine can have several types of dysfunction associated with it. First, since approximately 50% of cervical rotation occurs at C1 on C2, it could indicate a dysfunction at this level. It could also indicate the presence of hypertonicity of spasm of a long restrictor muscle such as levator scapulae or sternocleidomastoid. Lastly, it could indicate a group dysfunction of everything from C2 to C7. Less severe motion losses are typically due to one or more segmental dysfunctions from C2 to C7.

Thoracic Region

The procedure for screening sidebending T1 to T4 is:

1. The patient is seated on the side of the treatment table. The physician stands behind and at the side of the patient on the side to be tested. The physician palpates of the transverse processes of T4 (Fig. 34.25).

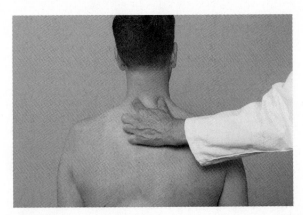

Figure 34-22   Neutral. (From Nicholas & Nicholas. *Atlas of Osteopathic Technique*. Philadelphia, PA: Lippincott Williams & Wilkins; Figure 3.16.)

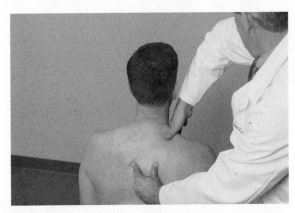

Figure 34-25   The physician palpates over the transverse processes of T4. (From Nicholas & Nicholas. *Atlas of Osteopathic Technique*. Philadelphia, PA: Lippincott Williams & Wilkins; Figure 3.21.)

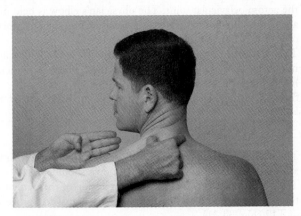

Figure 34-23   Active rotation—left. (From Nicholas & Nicholas. *Atlas of Osteopathic Technique*. Philadelphia, PA: Lippincott Williams & Wilkins; Figure 3.18.)

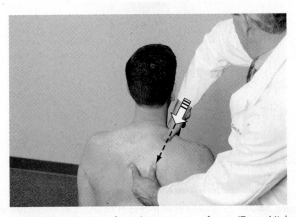

Figure 34-26   Palpating first rib—springing force. (From Nicholas & Nicholas. *Atlas of Osteopathic Technique*. Philadelphia, PA: Lippincott Williams & Wilkins; Figure 3.22.)

2. The physician places his first metacarpal-phalangeal joint over the first rib at the base of the neck. The physician's elbow is held high above the shoulder to deliver a springing force toward the spinous process of T4 (Fig. 34.26).
3. This produces passive sidebending of T1 to T4. Normal range of motion is 5 to 25 degrees. There is no active motion test for this range.
4. Steps 1 to 3 are repeated on the opposite side of the body.

The procedure for screening sidebending T5 to T8 is:

1. The patient is seated on the side of the treatment table. The physician stands behind and to the side of the patient on the side to be tested.
2. The physician palpates over the transverse processes of T8 (Fig. 34.27).
3. The physician places his first metacarpal-phalangeal joint over the midpoint of the shoulder. The physician's elbow is held high above the shoulder to deliver a springing force toward the spinous process of T8 (Fig. 34.28).
4. This produces passive sidebending of the thoracic spine from T5 to T8. Normal range of motion is 10 to 30 degrees. There is no active motion test for this range.
5. Steps one through four are repeated for the opposite side.

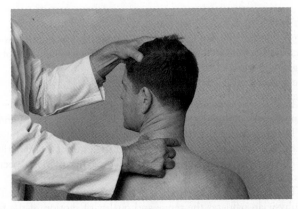

Figure 34-24   Passive rotation—left. (From Nicholas & Nicholas. *Atlas of Osteopathic Technique*. Philadelphia, PA: Lippincott Williams & Wilkins; Figure 3.20.)

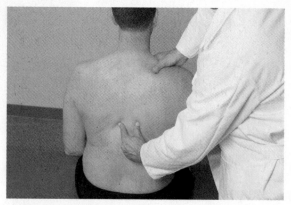

Figure 34-27 The physician palpates over the transverse processes of T8. (From Nicholas & Nicholas. *Atlas of Osteopathic Technique*. Philadelphia, PA: Lippincott Williams & Wilkins; Figure 3.25.)

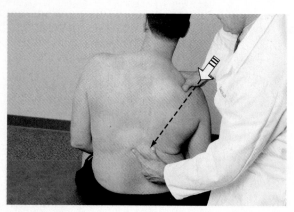

Figure 34-30 Springing over the acromioclavicular joint. (From Nicholas & Nicholas. *Atlas of Osteopathic Technique*. Philadelphia, PA: Lippincott Williams & Wilkins; Figure 3.30.)

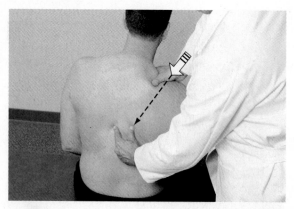

Figure 34-28 Springing over midpoint of shoulder. (From Nicholas & Nicholas. *Atlas of Osteopathic Technique*. Philadelphia, PA: Lippincott Williams & Wilkins; Figure 3.26.)

2. The physician places his first metacarpal-phalangeal joint over the acromioclavicular joint. The physician's elbow is held high above the shoulder to deliver a force toward the spinous process of T12 (Fig. 34.30).
3. This produces passive sidebending from T9 to T12. The normal range of motion is 20 to 40 degrees. There is no active motion test for this region.
4. Steps 1 through 3 are repeated for the opposite side of the body.

The procedure for screening rotation T9-12 is:

1. The patient is seated on the side of the treatment table with the arms crossed, holding on to his or her own shoulders.
2. The physician stands behind and to the side of the patient on the side to be tested and palpates over the transverse processes of T12 (Fig. 34.31).
3. The patient is instructed to turn his or her body as far as possible to the ipsilateral side. This is the active range of motion. Normal is 70 to 90 degrees (Fig. 34.32).
4. Once this has been accomplished, the physician grasps the patient's contralateral arm and attempts to rotate them farther in the same direction. This is the passive range of motion (Fig. 34.33).
5. Steps 1 to 4 are repeated for the opposite side of the body.

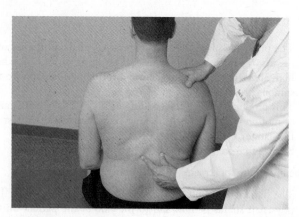

Figure 34-29 The physician palpates over the transverse processes of T12. (From Nicholas & Nicholas. *Atlas of Osteopathic Technique*. Philadelphia, PA: Lippincott Williams & Wilkins; Figure 3.29.)

Rib Motion

Screening for rib motion involves palpating for pump handle motion (Fig. 34.34) in the upper ribs and for bucket handle motion (Fig. 34.35) in the lower ribs.

The procedure for screening ribs 1 and 2 is:

1. The patient is supine on the treatment table. The physician is positioned at the head of the table and palpates over ribs 1 and 2. The thumbs are placed on the angles of rib 1. The index fingers are placed posterior to the clavicle over the anterior aspect of rib 1. The middle or ring fingers are placed over the anterior aspect of rib 2 (Fig. 34.36).
2. The patient is instructed to inhale and exhale deeply. The physician palpates the range and quality of motion of the first two ribs noting any asymmetry that may exist. The principal motion in this location is designated as pump handle. There is no passive motion test for this range (Fig. 34.37).

The procedure for screening sidebending T9-12 is:

1. The patient is seated on the side of the table. The physician stands behind and to the side of the patient on the side to be tested. The physician palpates over the transverse processes of T12 (Fig. 34.29).

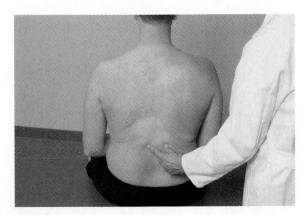

Figure 34-31 The physician palpates over the transverse processes of T12. (From Nicholas & Nicholas. *Atlas of Osteopathic Technique.* Philadelphia, PA: Lippincott Williams & Wilkins; Figure 3.33.)

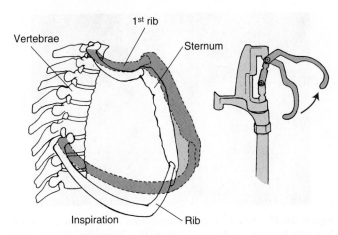

Figure 34-34 Pump handle motion. (From Nicholas & Nicholas. *Atlas of Osteopathic Technique.* Philadelphia, PA: Lippincott Williams & Wilkins; Figure 5.60.)

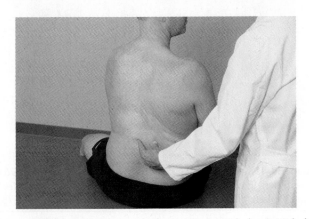

Figure 34-32 Active range of motion. (From Nicholas & Nicholas. *Atlas of Osteopathic Technique.* Philadelphia, PA: Lippincott Williams & Wilkins; Figure 3.34.)

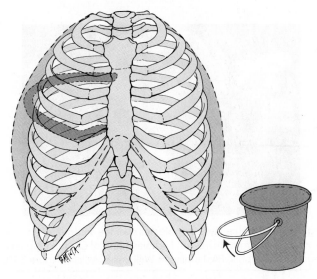

Figure 34-35 Bucket handle motion. (From Nicholas & Nicholas. *Atlas of Osteopathic Technique.* Philadelphia, PA: Lippincott Williams & Wilkins; Figure 5.61.)

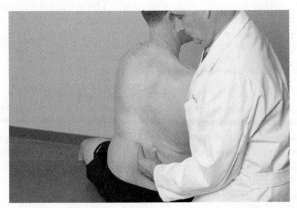

Figure 34-33 Passive range of motion. (From Nicholas & Nicholas. *Atlas of Osteopathic Technique.* Philadelphia, PA: Lippincott Williams & Wilkins; Figure 3.36.)

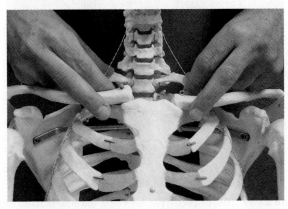

Figure 34-36 Palpating over anterior ribs 1 and 2. (From Nicholas & Nicholas. *Atlas of Osteopathic Technique.* Philadelphia, PA: Lippincott Williams & Wilkins; Figure 5.62.)

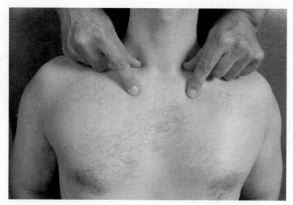

Figure 34-37   Palpating over anterior ribs 1 and 2—on skin. (From Nicholas & Nicholas. *Atlas of Osteopathic Technique*. Philadelphia, PA: Lippincott Williams & Wilkins; Figure 5.63.)

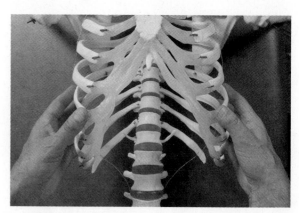

Figure 34-40   The physician palpates the lateral aspects of ribs 6 to 10. (From Nicholas & Nicholas. *Atlas of Osteopathic Technique*. Philadelphia, PA: Lippincott Williams & Wilkins; Figure 5.74.)

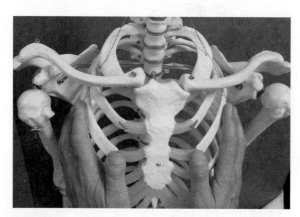

Figure 34-38   The physician palpates over the anterolateral aspect of ribs 3 to 5. (From Nicholas & Nicholas. *Atlas of Osteopathic Technique*. Philadelphia, PA: Lippincott Williams & Wilkins; Figure 5.70.)

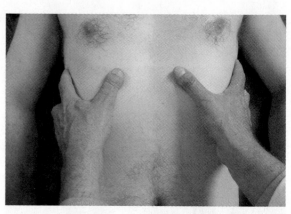

Figure 34-41   The physician palpates the lateral aspects of ribs 6 to 10—on skin. (From Nicholas & Nicholas. *Atlas of Osteopathic Technique*. Philadelphia, PA: Lippincott Williams & Wilkins; Figure 5.75.)

The procedure for screening ribs 3 through 5 is:

1. The patient is supine on the treatment table. The physician palpates over the anterolateral aspect of ribs 3 to 5. This is done with the physician standing at about the level of the patient's waist (Fig. 34.38).
2. The patient is instructed to inhale and exhale deeply. The physician palpates the range and quality of motion of ribs 3 through 5 noting any asymmetry that exists. The principal motion in this location is described as combined pump handle and bucket handle. There is no passive motion test for this range (Fig. 34.39).

The procedure for screening ribs 6 to 10 is:

1. The patient lies supine. The physician stands at the side of the patient at the level of the patient's pelvis. The physician palpates the lateral aspects of ribs 6 to 10 (Fig. 34.40).
2. The patient is instructed to inhale and exhale deeply. The physician palpates the range and quality of motion of ribs 6 through 10 noting any asymmetry that exists. The principal motion at this location is described as bucket handle. There is no passive motion test for this range (Fig. 34.41).

The procedure for screening ribs 11 and 12 is:

1. The patient is prone. The physician stands at the side of the table and palpates ribs 11 and 12. The thumbs go on the

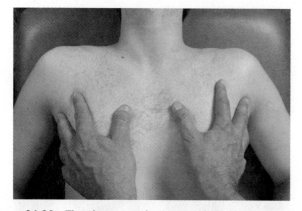

Figure 34-39   The physician palpates over the anterolateral aspect of ribs 3 to 5—on skin. (From Nicholas & Nicholas. *Atlas of Osteopathic Technique*. Philadelphia, PA: Lippincott Williams & Wilkins; Figure 5.71.)

inferior aspect of rib 12 with fingers over the tips of rib 11 (Fig. 34.42).

2. The patient is instructed to inhale and exhale deeply. The physician palpates the range and quality of motion of ribs 11 and 12 noting any asymmetry that exists. The typical motion for these ribs is described as caliper motion. There is no passive motion test for this range (Fig. 34.43).

Restriction of motion and motion direction of these lower ribs is under the strong influence of the quadratus lumborum muscle. Any restriction must be interpreted in light of this influence.

Lumbar Region

The procedure for screening flexion in the lumbar region is:

1. The angle created by lumbar flexion is formed using lines joining the lateral malleolus to the greater trochanter and the greater trochanter to the acromion process (Fig. 34.44).
2. The patient is instructed to slowly bend forward as if he or she is going to touch the toes. They should bend forward as far as possible. The normal range of active motion here is 70 to 90 degrees (Fig. 34.45).
3. Note to see that there is a normal reversal of the lumbar lordosis. Persistence of the lordosis indicates immobility of the

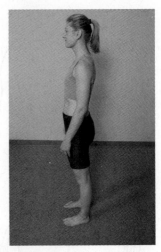

Figure 34-44   Patient in sagittal plane. (From Nicholas & Nicholas. *Atlas of Osteopathic Technique.* Philadelphia, PA: Lippincott Williams & Wilkins; Figure 3.34.)

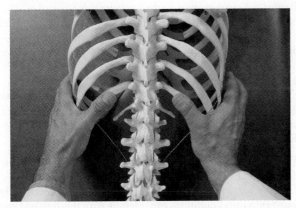

Figure 34-42   The physician palpates ribs 11 and 12. (From Nicholas & Nicholas. *Atlas of Osteopathic Technique.* Philadelphia, PA: Lippincott Williams & Wilkins; Figure 5.78.)

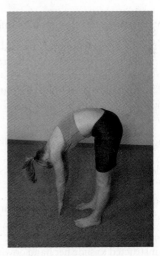

Figure 34-45   Active forward bending. (From Nicholas & Nicholas. *Atlas of Osteopathic Technique.* Philadelphia, PA: Lippincott Williams & Wilkins; Figure 3.39.)

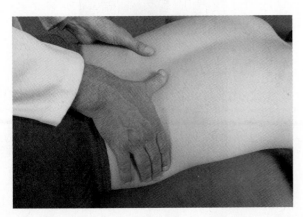

Figure 34-43   The physician palpates ribs 11 and 12—on skin. (From Nicholas & Nicholas. *Atlas of Osteopathic Technique.* Philadelphia, PA: Lippincott Williams & Wilkins; Figure 5.79.)

spine despite hypermobile hip joints and a normal range of motion.

4. If it is uncertain whether normal lumbar motion is occurring or not, the modified Shober test is used.

In this test, a mark is made on the skin midway between the PSIS. Measure down 5 cm and make another mark. Measure up 10 cm from the initial point and make another mark. The total distance in the erect position should measure 15 cm. With the trunk flexed, this distance should stretch to 20 cm. Less than this indicates a significant restriction of lumbar motion (Fig. 34.46).

Note: When Shober first described this test, he made only two marks, one midway between the PSIS and another 10 cm above. Early efforts to confirm the validity of this test with x-rays discovered that a significant number of times, the first mark was above the L5/S1 motion segment, so it was modified to include the downward measurement of 5 cm. Radiographic validation of the test came in the 1960s using metallic skin markers and lumbar x-rays (6–8).

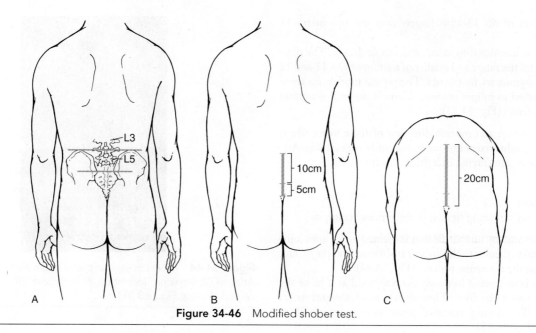

Figure 34-46 Modified shober test.

The procedure for screening extension in the lumbar region is:

1. The angle created by lumbar flexion is formed using lines joining the lateral malleolus to the greater trochanter and the greater trochanter to the acromion process (see Fig. 34.44).
2. The patient is instructed to place the arms out in front for balance and then bend backward as far as possible while keeping the knees straight.

The normal range for lumbar extension is 30 to 45 degrees (Fig. 34.47).

To screen sidebending/active range of motion in the lumbar region:

1. The posterior landmarks used for this measurement are a line from the mid heel point to the spinous process of S-1, and from S-1 to the spinous process of T1 (Fig. 34.48).
2. The patient is instructed to slide her hand down the lateral thigh toward the knee reaching as far as she can go (Fig. 34.49).

3. Note where the sidebending occurs. Is the arc of motion smooth or does the back "hinge" at a certain level?
4. Repeat the same motion to the opposite side.
5. Note any asymmetry in both the quantity and the quality of motion. Normal range of motion for this range is 25 to 30 degrees (9–11).

The Hip Drop Test

The hip drop test is performed to screen for sidebending/passive range of motion in the lumbar region. This test is interpreted as passive motion as the lumbar spine spontaneously responds to an artificially produced sacral base declination:

1. The patient is instructed to flex one knee, allowing the pelvis to drop on that side of the body. (Fig. 34.50).
2. Observe for symmetry of range and quality of motion. Many lower extremity conditions can interfere with this test: bad knees, tight iliotibial band, inability to dorsiflex the ankle, etc. (12).

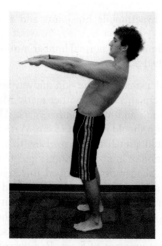

Figure 34-47 Lumbar extension (backward bending). (Original photograph: Walter C. Ehrenfeuchter, D.O., F.A.A.O., with permission.)

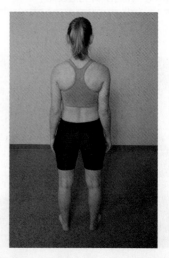

Figure 34-48 Posterior landmarks. (From Nicholas & Nicholas. *Atlas of Osteopathic Technique.* Philadelphia, PA: Lippincott Williams & Wilkins; Figure 3.41.)

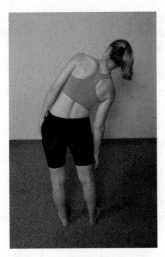

Figure 34-49   Active lumbar sidebending right. (From Nicholas & Nicholas. *Atlas of Osteopathic Technique*. Philadelphia, PA: Lippincott Williams & Wilkins; Figure 3.42.)

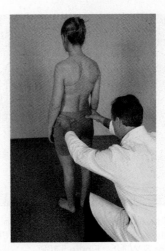

Figure 34-51   Standing flexion test—step 3. (From Nicholas & Nicholas. *Atlas of Osteopathic Technique*. Philadelphia, PA: Lippincott Williams & Wilkins; Figure 5.106.)

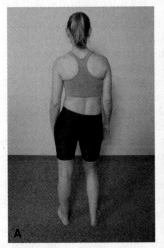

Figure 34-50   Hip drop test. (From Nicholas & Nicholas. *Atlas of Osteopathic Technique*. Philadelphia, PA: Lippincott Williams & Wilkins; Figures 3.45 and 3.46.)

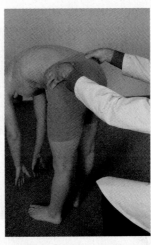

Figure 34-52   Negative standing flexion test. (From Nicholas & Nicholas. *Atlas of Osteopathic Technique*. Philadelphia, PA: Lippincott Williams & Wilkins; Figure 5.107.).

Iliosacral Motion

The screening test for innominate dysfunction is the standing flexion test:

1. The patient stands erect with the feet a shoulder width apart.
2. The physician stands or kneels behind the patient with his eyes at the level of the PSIS.
3. The physician's thumbs are placed on the inferior slope of the patient's PSISs. The physician maintains a firm pressure on the PSISs to ride with the bony landmarks, not shift due to skin or fascial drag (Fig. 34.51).
4. The patient is instructed to actively bend forward and try to touch her toes (Fig. 34.52).
5. The test is positive when asymmetry of the thumbs occurs. The side of a positive test is the one where the thumb on the PSIS moves at least one thumb breadth more cephalad at the end range of motion. (Fig. 34.53).
6. A positive standing flexion test indicates the side of likely iliosacral dysfunction. A false-positive test can be created by a leg-length discrepancy >½ in, contralateral tight hamstring,

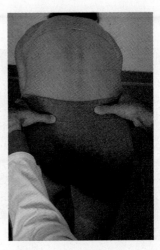

Figure 34-53   Positive standing flexion test—right. (From Nicholas & Nicholas. *Atlas of Osteopathic Technique*. Philadelphia, PA: Lippincott Williams & Wilkins; Figure 5.108.)

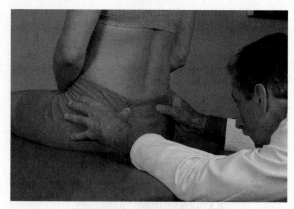

Figure 34-54 Seated flexion test—start position. (From Nicholas & Nicholas. *Atlas of Osteopathic Technique.* Philadelphia, PA: Lippincott Williams & Wilkins; Figure 5.109).

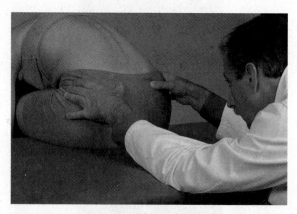

Figure 34-55 Negative seated flexion test. (From Nicholas & Nicholas. *Atlas of Osteopathic Technique.* Philadelphia, PA: Lippincott Williams & Wilkins; Figure 5.110.)

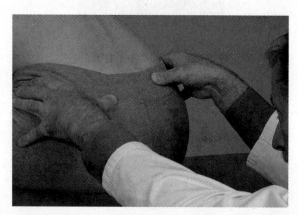

Figure 34-56 Positive seated flexion test—right. (From Nicholas & Nicholas. *Atlas of Osteopathic Technique.* Philadelphia, PA: Lippincott Williams & Wilkins; Figure 5.111.)

contralateral tight iliopsoas muscle, or the presence of a unilateral sacral dysfunction. If this test is negative, the presence of an iliosacral dysfunction is highly unlikely (13).

Sacroiliac Motion

The screening test for unilateral sacral dysfunction is the seated flexion test:

1. The patient is seated on a low stool or side of a treatment table with the feet touching the floor.
2. The physician stands or kneels behind the patient with his eyes at the level of the patient's PSISs.
3. The physician's thumbs are positioned on the inferior slopes of the PSISs (Fig. 34.54).
4. The patient is instructed to bend forward as far as possible (Fig. 34.55).
5. A positive test is one where the PSIS moves more cephalad by at least one thumb breadth at the end of the range of motion (Fig. 34.56).
6. Potential dysfunctions here include anterior and posterior torsions, and unilateral flexed and extended sacra (14).

An additional test for sacroiliac motion is the pelvic side shift test:

1. The patient stands erect with the feet shoulder width apart.
2. The physician stands behind the patient with one of the physician's hands contacting the patient's iliac crest and the other on the opposite deltoid/shoulder area.
3. The physician gently pushes the iliac crest/pelvis laterally (translates) to the opposite side utilizing the hand on the deltoid/shoulder to stabilize the thoracic spinal segments. The ease and amount of motion is noted.
4. The physician next switches hand positions and introduces motion to the opposite direction. Motion in each direction is now compared.
5. A positive pelvic side shift reveals freer translation to the side of the side shift and named for that direction. A positive pelvic side shift means that the sacrum (base of support) is positioned on the side of the freer motion and may indicate a possible long leg to the side of and/or a tight psoas muscle to the opposite side of the pelvic side shift.

Sacral Motion

The screening test for bilateral sacral dysfunction is the sacral rock test:

1. The patient is prone on the treatment table.
2. The physician stands at the side of the treatment table at the level of the patient's pelvis.
3. The physician places his cephalad hand on the sacrum with the heel of the hand at the sacral base, fingers pointing toward the coccyx (Fig. 34.57).
4. The physician's caudad hand reinforces the cephalad hand with the thumb and the index finger creating a space for the cephalad hand's wrist (Fig. 34.58).
5. The physician presses straight down into the sacrum so that any body movement is imparted to the sacrum.
6. The physician attempts to rock the sacrum through flexion (Fig. 34.59) and extension (Fig. 34.60). Bilateral sacral dysfunction feels exceptionally rigid—a so-called concrete pelvis (15).

Symptom Exacerbation or Remission

One of the important accompaniments of range-of-motion testing is the exacerbation or remission of patient symptoms. Table 34.2 includes a partial list of structures and conditions that would be

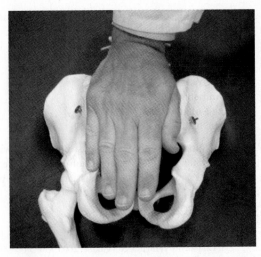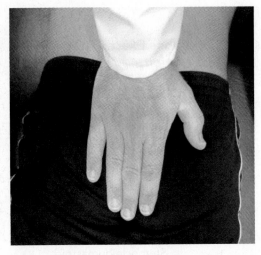

Figure 34-57   Sacral rock test—step 3. (Original photos: Walter C. Ehrenfeuchter, D.O., F.A.A.O., with permission.)

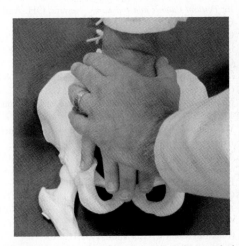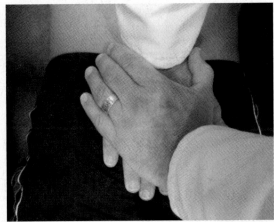

Figure 34-58   Sacral rock test—step 4. (Original photos: Walter C. Ehrenfeuchter, D.O., F.A.A.O., with permission.)

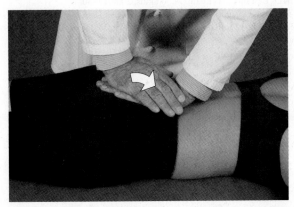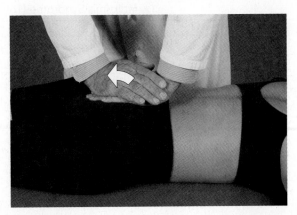

Figure 34-59   Sacral flexion. (From Nicholas & Nicholas. *Atlas of Osteopathic Technique.* Philadelphia, PA: Lippincott Williams & Wilkins; Figure 15.29).

Figure 34-60   Sacral extension. (From Nicholas & Nicholas. *Atlas of Osteopathic Technique.* Philadelphia, PA: Lippincott Williams & Wilkins; Figure 15.28).

TABLE 34.2

Structures and Conditions Exacerbated by Spinal Range of Motion

Structure	Motion	Condition
Cervical Spine	Flexion	Disc Herniation
		Posterior Muscles
	Extension	Facet Joint Disease
		Anterior Muscle
	Sidebending	Trapezius muscle
		Levator Scapulae muscle
	Rotation	Splenius capitis and cervicis muscles
		Sternocleidomastoid muscle
Thoracic Spine	Flexion	Paraspinal muscles
		Posterior shoulder girdle muscles
		Disc Herniation
	Extension	Facet Joint Disease
	Sidebending	Intercostal muscles
		Serratus Anterior muscle
	Rotation	Abdominal Oblique muscles
Lumbar Spine	Flexion	Disc Herniation
		Lumbar Paravertebral muscles
		Lumbosacral Ligaments
	Extension	Spondylolisthesis
		Facet Syndrome
		Spinal Stenosis
		Psoas Spasm
	Sidebending	Lateral Abdominal Wall muscles
		Iliotibial Band Syndrome
	Rotation	Abdominal oblique muscles
		Iliolumbar ligaments
		Piriformis Syndrome (16)

exacerbated by spinal range of motion. Listed muscle pains apply to both injury and muscle hypertonicity or spasm.

The diagnosis of somatic dysfunction requires at least two of the following:

- Tenderness
- Asymmetry
- Range-of-motion changes
- Tissue texture changes

The screening evaluation will at least provide you with regional data as to asymmetry and range-of-motion changes. "We know that if we are ever to know the whole, we must first know the parts." A.T. Still.

REFERENCES

1. Ward RC, Ed. *Foundations for Osteopathic Medicine*. 2nd Ed. Philadelphia, PA: Lippincott Williams & Wilkins, 2003:348–349.
2. Kappler RE. Postural balance and motion patterns. In: *Postural Balance and Imbalance*. Newark, OH. American Academy of Osteopathy, 1983:6–12.
3. Cathie AG. The applied anatomy of some postural changes (1945). In: *Postural Balance and Imbalance*. Newark, OH. American Academy of Osteopathy, 1983:44–46.
4. Cathie AG. Soft tissue changes that may follow postural defects (1949). In: *Postural Balance and Imbalance*. Newark, OH. American Academy of Osteopathy, 1983:47–49.
5. Cathie AG. The influence of the lower extremities upon the structural integrity of the body (1950). In: *Postural Balance and Imbalance*. Newark, OH. American Academy of Osteopathy, 1983:50–53.
6. Moll JMH, Wright V. Normal range of spinal mobility—an objective clinical study. *Ann Rheum Dis* 1971;30:341.
7. Macrae IF, Wright V. Measurement of back motion. *Ann Rheum Dis* 1969;28:584.
8. Von Schober P. Lendenwirbelsaule und kreuzschmerzen. *Munch Med Wochenschr* 1937;9:336.
9. Mitchell F, Jr, Moran PS, Pruzzo NA. *A General Osteopathic Postural/Structural Screening Examination: The Ten Step Screening Examination*. 1st Ed. Mitchell, *Moran & Pruzzo Associates, 1985*.
10. Cathie AG. *Regional Ranges of Passive Spinal Motion. 1974 Year Book of the American Academy of Osteopathy*, Colorado Springs, CO. 68–72.
11. Doege T, Ed. *Guides to the Evaluation of Permanent Impairment*. 4th Ed. American Medical Association, 1995:112–130.
12. Greenman PE. *Principles of Manual Medicine*. 2nd Ed. Baltimore, MD: Williams & Wilkins, 1996:18–35.
13. Mitchell FL Jr. *The Muscle Energy Manual-Volume I*. E. Lansing, MI. MET Press, 1995:100.
14. Mitchell FL Jr. *The Muscle Energy Manual-Volume I*. MET Press, 1995:110.
15. Nicholas & Nicholas. *Atlas of Osteopathic Techniques*. 1st Ed. Baltimore, MD: Lippincott Williams & Wilkins, 2008:17–30.
16. Simons DG, Janet G. et al. *Myofascial Pain and Dysfunction: The Trigger Point Manual*. 2nd Ed. Baltimore, MD: Lippincott Williams & Wilkins, 1999.

Segmental Motion Testing

WALTER C. EHRENFEUCHTER

INTRODUCTION

The final portion of the osteopathic structural examination is segmental definition. This is carried out guided by the findings in the screening examination and the scanning evaluation (layer-by-layer palpation). If there are no findings on the scanning exam for a given segment, it is unlikely that any significant somatic dysfunction exists at that segment and segmental definition is unnecessary.

VERTEBRAL UNIT

The vertebral unit is defined as two adjacent vertebrae with their associated intervertebral disc, arthrodial, ligamentous, muscular, vascular, neural, and lymphatic elements (Fig. 35.1).

Conventionally, when referring to motion of a single vertebra, we are in fact referring to that segment's vertebral unit. For example, when referring to the motion of L3, we are in reality referring to the motion of L3 in reference to L4.

Potential Segmental Motions

Using a Cartesian coordinate system, the position or motion of any vertebra can be described in space as a combination of rotation about any of the three axes and translation along any of the three axes. This system, while useful for biomechanical research purposes, is clinically cumbersome. For simplicity, the movements of the individual vertebrae are broken down into three components: flexion or extension, rotation, and sidebending (Table 35.1).

When referencing the position or motion of a vertebra, the position of a point on the superior endplate at the anterior most part of that endplate is used (Fig. 35.2).

Conventionally, the diagnosis of a segmental dysfunction may be described in one of two ways:

1. That vertebra's position relative to the vertebra below.
2. The directions of motion restriction of that vertebra relative to the vertebra below.

For example:

- Positional diagnosis—L5 flexed, sidebent right, rotated right
- Motion restriction diagnosis—L5 restricted in extension, left sidebending, and left rotation.

The two examples describe exactly the same segment, just from two different points of view.

In positional language, words end in -ed and -ent, as in flexed, extended, rotated, and sidebent. In motion restriction language, words end in -ing and -ion, as in flexion, extension, rotation, and sidebending.

When diagnosing somatic dysfunction, the positional diagnosis is determined and named for what the vertebra does most easily. In other words, the direction of freest motion, the direction of ease, is identified.

Physiologic Laws of Spinal Motion: Fryette's Principles

Fryette's principles regarding the physiologic laws of spinal motion include:

I—In the neutral range, sidebending and rotation are coupled in opposite directions

II—In sufficient flexion or extension, sidebending and rotation are coupled in the same direction (4)

III—Initiating movement of a vertebral segment in any plane of motion will modify the movement of that segment in other planes of motion.

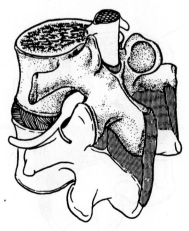

Figure 35-1 The vertebral unit.

TABLE 35.1

Vertebral Movements

Movement	Definition
Rotation	Movement in a transverse plane about a vertical axis
Sidebending	Movement in a coronal plane about an anterior-posterior axis
Flexion	Anterior movement in a sagittal plane about a transverse axis
Extension	Posterior movement in a sagittal plane about a transverse axis.

Laws I and II apply to thoracic and lumbar motion only. Sidebending and rotation are considered coupled motions (i.e., you cannot have one without the other). They were described by Harrison H. Fryette, D.O., in 1918. All of his observations regarding vertebral mechanics were made without benefit of x-rays; he used palpation only. Law III was described by C. R. Nelson, D.O., in 1948.

Neutral is a Range

Neutral in the world of spinal mechanics is not a single point, but rather a range in which the weight of the trunk is borne on the vertebral bodies and discs, and the facets are "idling" (3) (Fig. 35.3).

In this range, Law I applies. That is, when one or the other is introduced, sidebending and rotation will be coupled in opposite directions; the motion segment will sidebend right and rotate left or it can sidebend left and rotate right. This is referred to as Type I mechanics (Fig. 35.4). A dysfunctional segment held in this position is referred to as a Type I dysfunction.

NonNeutral Mechanics

In the thoracic and lumbar spine when sufficient flexion or extension beyond the neutral range occurs, sidebending and rotation will be coupled to the same side. The segment is flexed or extended and sidebent right, rotated right or sidebent left, rotated left. This is referred to as Type II mechanics (Fig. 35.5). A dysfunctional segment held in this position is referred to as a Type II dysfunction.

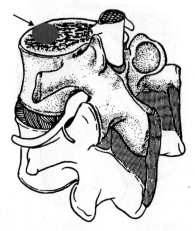

Figure 35-2   Point of reference for vertebral motion.

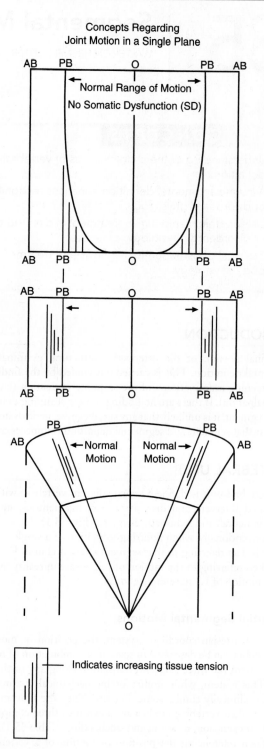

Figure 35-3   Neutral range. (From the *Kimberly Manual Outline of Osteopathic Manipulative Procedures*. Marceline, MO: Walsworth Publishing Company, 2000:10.)

Law III has been interpreted to mean that if motion is restricted in any one direction (e.g., rotation), then motion will also be restricted in sidebending and flexion/extension. If motion is improved in any one direction (e.g., flexion/extension), it will be found to have improved in rotation and sidebending as well.

Due to the cumbersomeness of the longhand descriptions of vertebral position, shorthand abbreviations and notations have been developed, as shown in Box 35.1.

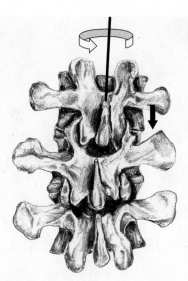

Figure 35-4 Fryette Type I mechanics. (Courtesy of Adam Ehrenfeuchter, San Francisco, CA.)

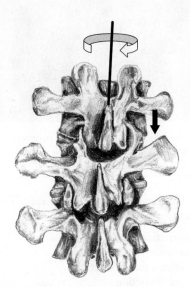

Figure 35-5 Fryette Type II mechanics.

Characteristics of Type I Dysfunctions

Type I dysfunctions tend to occur in groups (7), for example, T1-7 NR_RS_L. This constitutes typical scoliosis mechanics. This does not preclude their occurring singly, for example, T5 NR_RS_L.

Groups of Type I dysfunctions tend to compensate for a single Type II dysfunction. When present, the Type II dysfunction is typically at the apex of the group dysfunction, or at either end of the group.

Characteristics of Type II Dysfunctions

Type II dysfunctions tend to occur singly, although you may have two Type II dysfunctions adjacent to each other (7). More than that is rare. Extended Type II dysfunctions are frequently the product of the segmental muscle contraction that results from a viscerosomatic reflex and should prompt the search for visceral disease and dysfunction.

> ## Shorthand Abbreviations and Notations for Segmental Dysfunctions
>
> *Abbreviations*
>
> N—Neutral
> F—Flexed
> E—Extended
> L—Left
> R—Rotated
> R—Right
> S—Sidebent
>
> *Notations*
>
> Type I dysfunction:
>   L5 Neutral, rotated left, sidebent right
>   Or L5 NR_LS_R
>   Or L5 R_LS_R
> Type II dysfunction:
>   L5 flexed, rotated right, sidebent right
>   Or L5 FR_RS_R
>   Or L5 FRS_R

Classic Spinal Mechanics

Classic Fryette mechanics is exhibited by the typical thoracic and lumbar vertebrae. The motion pattern in these regions is determined by patterns of force generated by the discs, ligaments, and musculature. Motion patterns in the cervical spine are largely determined by the shape of the facet joints, independent of the discs, ligaments, and musculature.

Motion in the cervical region is often described in terms of Fryette "Like" mechanics. It is not Fryette mechanics in that it is independent of sagittal plane position.

The occiput on C-1 always follows Type I **Like** mechanics in that sidebending and rotation are always coupled to opposite sides, whether the occiput is flexed, extended, or neutral (6).

C1 on C2 is considered to only rotate, even though considerable (20 degrees) sagittal plane motion is possible. That is because dysfunctions typically are discovered only in the rotational component of C-1 motion (6).

C2-6 always follow Type II **Like** mechanics in that sidebending and rotation are always coupled to the same side, whether these segments are flexed, extended, or neutral (6).

C7 has inferior facet joints that are more thoracic in configuration and thus tends to follow classical Fryette mechanics (2,5).

Exceptions to the Laws of Spinal Mechanics

Single plane dysfunctions are quite possible and involve restriction of motion on both facet joints, for example, T10 flexed or L5 extended.

Compressive Dysfunctions are also possible and also involve restriction of motion of both facet joints, for example, Occiput compressed on C1.

Trauma to the supporting ligaments and/or discs can generate segmental instability and any direction of dysfunction is possible. These dysfunctions do not occur as a result of exaggerated physiologic motion of the spine, but are caused by external traumatic forces.

Advanced degenerative disc disease and degenerative facet joint disease lead to segmental instability and, again, any direction of dysfunction is possible. This can also lead to neural entrapment due to a phenomenon called dynamic lateral stenosis. Figure 35.6 shows a detailed view of lumbar vertebral column showing large osteophytes.

Congenital anomalies of the vertebrae or facet joints will also alter the motion characteristics of those segments. Facet tropism, a turning of the facet joints from their usual orientation, can dramatically alter the motion characteristics of a segment and may present with bony asymmetry and thus congenital asymmetric vertebral motion. Figure 35.7 shows a transitional lumbosacral segment causing atypical lumbosacral mechanics.

Categorizing Somatic Dysfunction

Somatic Dysfunction can be categorized by the tissue or structure most responsible for the motion restriction at that segment (8). Most dysfunctions are a combination of types, but it is helpful for the purpose of technique selection to consider searching

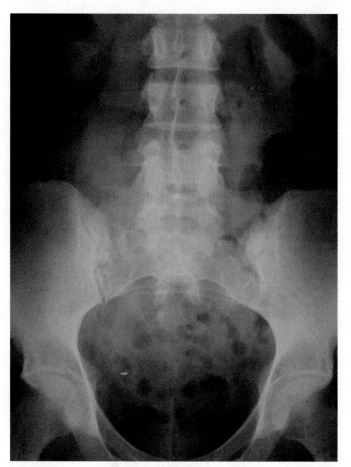

Figure 35-7 Transitional Lumbosacral Segment causing atypical lumbosacral mechanics. (Photograph courtesy of Walter C. Ehrenfeuchter, D.O., FAAO.)

for the reason for segmental restriction to exist. Types of somatic dysfunction include:

- Arthrodial restriction
- Muscular restriction
- Fascial and ligamentous restriction
- Edema-causing restriction

ARTHRODIAL RESTRICTION

This type of somatic dysfunction is maintained by the facet joint structure itself. The articular restriction is often accompanied by a reflex muscle guarding response that will not relax until the articular "lock" is released. When acquired by acute injury, these dysfunctions can be quite painful. Despite the level of pain and guarding, the patients often derive instantaneous relief when these dysfunctions are properly treated.

Articular restrictions may be generated by acute trauma, sustained muscle hypertonicity, repetitive motion injuries (microtrauma), fascial or ligamentous contracture, or poor posture.

The articular restrictions are maintained by a combination of thin layer adherence and muscle guarding response. If the dysfunction becomes chronic, it will lead to fascial contracture and desiccation of the facet joint.

Thin layer adherence is a process where two congruent surfaces are "glued" together by a typically lubricating substance when the said substance is spread thinly enough. For thin layer adherence to occur, one needs to have congruent surfaces and a lubricating substance.

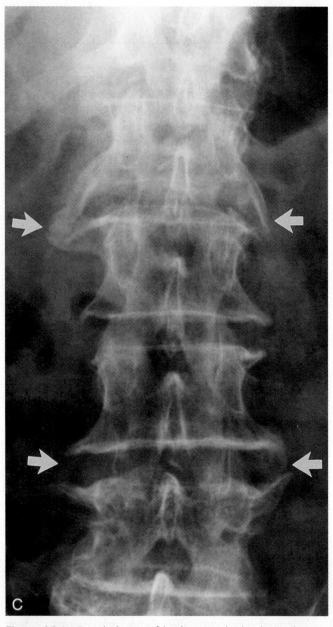

Figure 35-6 • Detailed view of lumbar vertebral column showing large osteophytes.

In a congruent joint, all joint surfaces are in complete contact with each other in the anatomic position. The spinal facet joints are congruent joints.

Synovial fluid when present in normal amounts is an exceptionally effective lubricant. It has been estimated that it makes the joint surfaces 10 times slipperier than ice on ice. It is very viscous and possesses a high surface tension (a single drop of normal synovial fluid can be strung out to a length of several feet without breaking).

So if you combine the congruent facet surfaces with the viscous synovial fluid and add a force that compresses the facet surfaces together, you get thin layer adherence and an articular dysfunction.

In the acute, traumatically induced articular dysfunction, where does the synovial fluid go? Some is squeezed out of the joint space and distends the capsule, one source of the pain. Over time, the synovial fluid is both adsorbed into the surface of the cartilage and removed from the capsule and surrounding tissues by the lymphatics.

MUSCULAR RESTRICTION

One very common cause of asymmetric and restricted segmental motion is the attached musculature. A detailed analysis of the influence of all the various muscles which attach to axial skeleton is beyond the scope of this book; however, some broad generalizations may be made.

Short restrictor muscles are those muscles that only cross one vertebral segment or cross one joint in the peripheral skeleton. When hypertonic, they will alter the positional and motion characteristics of just a single vertebral segment. Long restrictor muscles are those muscles that cross more than one vertebral segment on more than one joint in the peripheral skeleton. When hypertonic, they will alter the positional and motion characteristics of groups of vertebrae.

Deep Segmental Spinal Muscles

These muscles run only a segment or two adjacent to the spinal column and rib cage, and include such muscles as Rotatores Brevis, Levator Costorum Brevis, Interspinalis, Lateral Intertransverse, Rectus Capitis Posterior Minor, and a number of others. These muscles are short restrictors. They are also totally involuntary in their action. One cannot consciously think, "I want to sidebend L4 on L5, let me just contract the Lateral Intertransverse muscle at that segment." Nothing will happen. These muscles serve to balance the spinal column in response to larger movements of the trunk and long restrictor muscles. More importantly, they respond rapidly and in predictable patterns to facilitation of spinal cord segmental influences. They are believed to be the muscles that produce and maintain the extended Fryette Type II dysfunctions in response to viscerosomatic and somatosomatic reflexes. Their actions as a group in truncal posturing and locomotion are so complex that very little is known about how they function together.

Intermediate Spinal Muscles

These muscles run parallel to the spinal column and cross anywhere from two to eight or more segments and include such muscles as Multifidus, Semispinalis, Longissimus, Iliocostalis, Quadratus Lumborum, and Psoas Major to name but a few. These muscles are long restrictors. They are voluntary, motor muscles that move the trunk under the direction of volitional thought. They also function unconsciously in large truncal movements like those necessary to maintain balance and propulsion in the gait cycle. When these muscles are hypertonic, they produce sidebending of the spinal column and group curves usually composed of vertebrae engaged in Fryette Type I mechanics.

Superficial Back Muscles

These are muscles that are incidentally involved in spinal motion owing to their attachment to the spinal column or ribs. They are actually used to brace or move the extremities. These muscles include Trapezius, Latissimus Dorsi, Rhomboideus Major and Minor, Serratus Anterior, Pectoralis Minor, and more.

When hypertonic, they influence both motion of an extremity, but also spinal motion as well. An example of this would be hypertonicity of the Rhomboid Minor m. This would tend to draw the scapula medially and superiorly. If the Scapula is anchored by its other attached musculature, its attachment to the spinous processes of C7 and T1 would tend to rotate these vertebrae away from the side of the hypertonic Rhomboid (remember the reference point for vertebral rotation is on the front of the vertebra).

When these muscles go into a true spasm, they produce significant pain and will grossly distort the normal curves of the spine and body posturing. Additionally, this produces a host of adaptational responses that can be body wide in scope.

FASCIAL AND LIGAMENTOUS RESTRICTION

The ligaments of the spine can shorten due to fibrosis resulting from trauma, or due to inflammatory diseases of the spine. Which ligaments shorten or lose elasticity the most will determine which directions a vertebral segment can and cannot move.

Likewise, the fascial envelope in which the contractile elements of the muscles reside can shorten due to a host of causes (congenital, developmental, disuse, injury, inflammatory diseases of muscle). Again when shortened, they produce patterns of restriction that are identical to those that would occur if that same muscle were hypertonic. However, even with the contractile elements of the musculature relaxed, the more static investing fascia of the muscle remains shortened.

EDEMA-CAUSING RESTRICTION

The presence of fluid in the interstices of any region of the body will create motion restriction. Part of this is due to the presence of pain from fascial stretching and compartmental distention. Part of this is due to the actual presence of the fluid itself, distending fascial compartments, stretching tissues and thus taking some of the "slack" out of the fascia or joint capsules themselves. While no set pattern of dysfunction has been ascribed to segmental or regional edema, its importance has long been acknowledged by the Osteopathic profession.

END FEEL

The concept of end feel is one in which the characteristics of how the tissue feels at the end of range of motion testing for large joint motions, or for segmental motion testing has significant implications for the Osteopathic physician. The quality of the end feel is used to determine the most likely etiology of the motion restriction (articular, muscular, fascial, edema). Once this is determined, it is used by the physician to guide in the selection of which Osteopathic manipulative technique would be most useful in addressing that particular region or dysfunction.

Each etiologic agent of somatic dysfunction produces its one distinct end feel. Edema tends to produce a mushy or fluid-filled sponge kind of end feel. Muscle hypertonicity has a somewhat stretchy or rubbery end feel. Articular dysfunctions tend to have a more solid end feel with loss of the elasticity usually palpated in muscular of edematous restrictions. Ligamentous and fascial restrictions often have a very hard, abrupt end feel with near total loss of tissue elasticity.

It is not uncommon for a patient to exhibit several types of restriction in a single dysfunction, especially when these dysfunctions are chronic in nature. So one could apply a muscle energy technique to a segmental dysfunction and, on retesting, discover that now that the contractile elements of the muscle have relaxed, that the segment now exhibits a more fascial restriction type of end feel calling for the application of a direct myofascial release technique. Another example would be where edema is present, and after applying indirect myofascial release, or lymphatic approaches, the end-feel changes to one of articular restriction calling for an articulatory or high-velocity, low-amplitude thrust technique. Likewise, the failure of a technique to work for a given dysfunction may arise from a misinterpretation of the end feel by the inexperienced physician, not a poor application of a given technique. The technique may be applied perfectly, but if applied for the wrong tissue etiology of the restriction, it would be unsuccessful.

Primary and Secondary Somatic Dysfunction

A primary dysfunction is one that is caused by a trauma, or repetitive microtrauma. It serves as the initiating event for the generation of a variety of symptoms and events such as local pain, somatosensory referred pain, local muscle guarding responses, initiation of somatosomatic and somatovisceral reflexes, and creation of secondary somatic dysfunctions (10).

Secondary somatic dysfunction can arise secondary to a variety of other conditions. The following list of causes is not exhaustive, but contains many of the more common causes:

- Local diseases of the spine such as degenerative disc disease or facet joint osteoarthritis
- Mechanical effects of larger deformities such as Kyphosis or scoliosis
- Compensatory for primary or other secondary somatic dysfunctions
  - Viscero-somatic reflex–generated dysfunctions
  - Somato-somatic reflex–generated dysfunctions (11)

The Key Lesion

The key lesion is defined as that somatic dysfunction that causes and maintains a whole pattern of dysfunction including secondary somatic dysfunctions.

The key lesion frequently represents, on a percentage basis, the *most* restricted structure in a patient's body. A great deal of time and effort is often expended searching for the key lesion, as it is this dysfunction, that when corrected, will result in the greatest change for the better in the patient's overall body physiology (9).

SUMMARY

So what is it that the overall osteopathic structural exam is searching for? It is searching for larger deformities that give rise to secondary somatic dysfunctions. It is searching for evidence of musculoskeletal diseases that give rise to somatic dysfunction. It is searching for somatic dysfunctions that may be responsible for the patient's symptomatology or dysfunctional physiology. It is searching for the location of the key lesion. It is searching for the tissue responsible for maintaining the key lesion. It is searching for normal tissue behaving badly. It is in short the search for a 100% reversible entity. It is the search for somatic dysfunction. "When you know the difference between normal and abnormal you have learned the all absorbing first question……you must take your abnormal case to the normal, lay it down, and be satisfied to leave it" (1).

REFERENCES

1. American Academy of Osteopathy; Indianapolis, IN: *Autobiography* by A T Still, 228.
2. Nicholas & Nicholas. In: Intersegmental Motion Testing. *Atlas of Osteopathic Techniques.* Baltimore, MD: Lippincott, Williams & Wilkins, 2008; chap 5.
3. Fryette H.H. *Principles of Osteopathic Technic.* Carmel, CA: Academy of Applied Osteopathy, 1954:19.
4. Fryette H.H. *Principles of Osteopathic Technic.* Carmel, CA: Academy of Applied Osteopathy, 1954:22–26.
5. Fryette H.H. *Principles of Osteopathic Technic.* Carmel, CA: Academy of Applied Osteopathy, 1954:34.
6. Fryette H.H. *Principles of Osteopathic Technic.* Carmel, CA: Academy of Applied Osteopathy, 1954:30–31
7. Kimberly P.E. *Outline of Osteopathic Manipulative Procedures* (*The Kimberly Manual*)., Marceline, MO: Walsworth Publishing Company, 2000:11–12.
8. Greenman P.E. *Principles of Manual Medicine.* 2nd Ed. Baltimore, MD: Williams & Wilkins, 1996:36–37
9. *Glossary of Osteopathic Terminology.* April 2002.
10. *Glossary of Osteopathic Terminology.* April 2002.
11. *Glossary of Osteopathic Terminology.* April 2002.

36 Postural Considerations in Osteopathic Diagnosis and Treatment

MICHAEL L. KUCHERA

KEY CONCEPTS

- Alteration of postural alignment and recurrent somatic dysfunction are key manifestations of gravitational strain.
- Postural compensation is best understood as an integrated homeostatic process.
- Postural decompensation is associated with various pathophysiological states of gravitational strain.
- Patient education is a primary source of initiating the means to a successful management plan for issues of gravitational strain.
- The osteopathic medical profession has contributed many strategies to address issues of gravitational strain.

INTRODUCTION

The osteopathic postural-biomechanical model provides one of five major approaches to structuring osteopathic manipulative care. Viewing clinical findings through the "lens" of this model and interpreting those findings with the benefit of the growing evidence base can provide remarkable insights into multiple systems, structures, and functions.

The osteopathic postural assessment evaluates more than upright symmetry; it considers the homeostatic capability of integrated components of the neuromusculoskeletal system to resist constant gravitational stress and to adapt to ever-changing situations. In the incorporation of "body unity" principles, the osteopathic postural model interprets the physical body as a *tensegrity system* within which even minor changes in one body region may affect significant biomechanical, tensile, and ergonomic changes elsewhere. This interpretation expands an osteopathic practitioner's understanding of both etiology and treatment intervention. It also accepts that postural patterns are capable of providing a cogent glimpse of that patient's unique interrelationship of body, mind, and spirit. Carefully exploring the specific pattern of the "body unit's" homeostatic response provides clues to both the function and the dysfunction of key anatomical, physiological, and psychological structures.

Applying this model, the osteopathic physician seeks to achieve each patient's maximum function and to prepare that patient's neuromusculoskeletal system to respond optimally to postural realignment. To achieve this requires accessing and sometimes "reeducating" peripheral and central interactions that are biomechanically, physiologically, and psychologically linked. Conservative modalities available to the osteopathic physician for this purpose include osteopathic manipulative treatment (OMT), functional orthotics and orthopedic braces, exercise protocols, and patient education. These treatment modalities typically precede or accompany less conservative options ranging from prolotherapy to surgery.

The discussion in this chapter will make the case for considering the postural gravitational strain model whenever evaluating the health status of a patient. It will further describe how to implement the osteopathic postural care model in planning effective treatment strategies whenever a postural pattern for group spinal curves or recurrent skeletal, arthrodial, or myofascial dysfunction is diagnosed.

Nearly 2,500 years ago, Hippocrates said, "*The regimen I adopt will be for the benefit of my patients according to my abilities and judgment.*" The guidelines in this chapter lay out principles intended to enhance your ability to understand postural mechanisms as dynamic processes affecting interrelated structures throughout the body. With understanding and practice, your judgment in prescribing individualized postural treatment regimens will evolve and improve.

History and Unique Postural Contributions by the Osteopathic Profession

Neither the clinical observation of postural imbalance nor the use of radiographic assessment is unique to the osteopathic profession. However, osteopathic physicians integrated the two almost ninety years ago to better study structure and function.

In 1895, the discovery of the roentgen ray permitted visualization of structures inside the body. By 1898, the American School of Osteopathy in Kirksville, Missouri, had acquired the second machine west of the Mississippi and was producing the earliest roentgenologic studies of circulation (1). Hoskins and Schwab (2) introduced the standing postural x-ray series in 1921, opening the field for clinical interpretation and integration. Martin Beilke in 1936 acknowledged the value of the technique by observing, "The osteopathic profession can lay claim to these contributions as being strictly original and especially applicable to our approach in finding etiological factors in a given pathological process and in applying corrective measures" (3).

For many years, lack of standardization for postural radiographic procedures prevented the profession from combining important multicenter data needed to develop a common set of guidelines to interpret postural studies and formulate care. J. Stedman Denslow and his coworkers called for standardization in 1955 (4), although even today relatively few academic healthcare institutions outside of the osteopathic profession have adopted that recommendation.

Standard protocols provided measurable, accurate, and reproducible data to correlate with the osteopathic palpatory structural examinations. Published for decades thereafter in osteopathic literature, the profession documented the natural history of postural changes and also the consistency of radiographic postural findings (5,6). A compilation of many of the classic osteopathic articles discussing diagnosis, clinical impact, and treatment of postural subjects can be found in the *1983 Yearbook of the American Academy of Osteopathy, Postural Balance and Imbalance* (5). This compilation and a 1983 research study published in *Spine* (7) (itself based upon the osteopathic contribution to the importance of postural imbalance) would spark a second renaissance of osteopathic postural research that lasted nearly 2 decades.

Definitions and Basic Postural Principles

> If we regard posture as the result of the dynamic interaction of two groups of forces—the environmental force of gravity on one hand, and the strength of the individual on the other—then posture is but the formal expression of the balance of power existing at any time between these two groups of forces. Thus, any deterioration of posture indicates that the individual is losing ground in his contest with the environmental force of gravity (8).

Analysis of a patient's posture provides an enormous amount of information about that individual. If and how the patient compensates or decompensates under gravity's continuous stress speaks volumes about that patient's homeostatic reserves. The pattern and degree of antigravity (postural) muscle dysfunction, the presence and type of group spinal curves, and the locations of the resultant postural spinal crossovers offer clinically relevant insight into physical structure-function relationships. Observation of posture may also offer the clinician the first clues to the underlying emotional, spiritual, and psychological elements of a patient. Conversely, it may also suggest a source of physical pain and energy depletion that precipitates or perpetuates nonphysical dysfunctions within that individual.

The postural model encompasses a range of treatment strategies designed to impact general health status or to treat the underlying cause of specific problems. Such strategies play a central role in the management of certain spinal conditions such as scoliosis or spondylolisthesis that are associated with postural decompensation. In addition, such strategies may significantly improve symptoms associated with a wide range of neuromusculoskeletal conditions. Postural improvement can reduce and potentially eliminate gravity strain's constant precipitation and perpetuation of myofascial trigger points and other recurrent somatic dysfunction. Amelioration of gravity strain has been postulated to support homeostatic mechanisms by reducing nociception and segmental facilitation and by supporting the clinical goals defined by the osteopathic respiratory-circulatory model.

Base of Support and Center of Gravity

Posture is defined as the distribution of body mass in relation to gravity over a base of support. As an adult shifts from a standing to seated posture, this *base of support* shifts from the feet alone to a base that includes the pelvis. Theoretically, a center of mass for the entire body could be mathematically approximated using force plates or computer-assisted summation of horizontal cross-sectional measurements for any given posture. By definition, however, in the living human, the *center of gravity* must remain a *theoretical* point representing the weight center of the body for the given posture; the point about which the body balances in every direction moment to moment. For simplicity, osteopathic practitioners accept that the generic clinical center of gravity in an adult's passive upright standard posture lies approximately in the middle of the third lumbar vertebral body (9).

Balancing against gravity over a base of support is not a passive process. For example while standing, moving your arms from your sides to a horizontal position in front of your body shifts your body mass and, therefore, the center of gravity anteriorly. To keep from falling forward, dynamic homeostatic mechanisms are activated to alter total body posture from the toes to the head. The resulting posture will often be observed to increase regional spinal curves and requires energy from multiple muscles to maintain it.

Functional postural demands will also alter structure, usually first at the sites where structural anatomy changes. For example,

consider the compensatory response to gravity that begins as soon as an infant attempts to assume an upright position and continues throughout life (Fig. 36.1). In order to stand upright with the least amount of effort, the infant learns to balance the center of gravity by positioning various segments of the spine over the base of support formed by the region of anatomy immediately underneath. The "toddler" learning to walk then exercises postural control to adjust for falling forward as the mass of a lower extremity is moved forward.

These evolving regional changes typically take place at the so-called anatomical transition zones where anatomical "blocks" interface with anatomical spinal "rods." The transitional zones include the:

- *Lumbopelvic region* where the pelvis joins the lumbar spine
- *Thoracolumbar region* (or inferior thoracic outlet) where the lumbar spine joins the thoracic cage
- *Cervicothoracic region* (or superior thoracic inlet) where the thoracic cage joins the cervical spine
- *Craniocervical region* where the cervical spine joins the head

In this fashion, two secondary lordotic group curves normally develop in the cervical and lumbar regions to counterbalance the primary thoracic curve present at birth. These three spinal curves together will resist gravity much better than one single sagittal plane curve. They allow a person to function in an upright position; however, they result in human specific problems that affect both structure and function. These problems are characterized by coordinated compensation occurring in multiple regions and planes.

Optimal Posture

Postural homeostatic mechanisms automatically integrate a number of systems whose goal is to provide balance and stability during activities of daily living in the most energy-efficient manner possible. The musculoskeletal system contributes innately to postural homeostasis as a *tensegrity system* and is discussed later in this

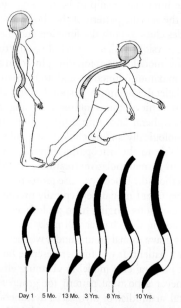

Figure 36-1 Changes in sagittal plane spinal curves from day 1 through age 10 years. (From Kapandji IA. *The Physiology of the Joints.* Vol 3. New York, NY: Churchill-Livingstone, 1974:17, with permission.)

chapter. (In architecture, tensegrity is defined as "the property of skeletal structures that employ continuous tension members and discontinuous compression members in such a way that each member operates with the maximum efficiency and economy.") (10) The neurological system contributes through its antigravity and balance functions to insure the body's "best attempt" at an upright position and orientation; it involves multisensory pathways to provide the visual, vestibular, and somatosensory data from proprioceptor and cutaneous receptors required to optimize these functions (11) The central nervous system (CNS) then integrates this sensory information to create an internal frame of reference that regulates the center of gravity and creates the optimal posture for that individual.

This best attempt by the body is *an optimal posture* for a given individual; a balanced configuration of the body with respect to gravity. Optimal standing postural alignment involves the total body and depends, in part, on balancing regional structures including cervical, lumbar, and thoracic curves under gravity's influence; it depends also on normal arches of the feet, vertical alignment of the ankles, and horizontal orientation (in the coronal plane) of the sacral base. The presence of *the* optimal or *ideal posture* suggests that there is a perfect distribution of the body mass around the center of gravity; the compressive force on spinal disks is balanced by ligamentous tension; and there is minimal energy expenditure from postural muscles (12,13). Structural or functional factors, however, frequently prevent achievement and maintenance of optimal or ideal posture. When this occurs, homeostatic mechanisms manifest compensatory patterns in an effort to provide maximum postural function within the existing structure of the individual. *Compensation* is the counterbalancing of any defect of structure or function (14).

An optimally balanced standing postural alignment in the coronal plane normally divides the body into two equal parts (Fig. 36.2A and B). The center of gravity line, or "weight-bearing

line," runs midway between the feet, through the pubic symphysis, along the midline of the vertebral column, and bisects the center of the suprasternal notch and glabella. Ideally, there would be no rotation in the horizontal plane of any body region (Fig. 36.2C) and no coronal plane side-bending asymmetry.

Optimal postural alignment in the sagittal plane (Fig. 36.2D) has been characterized by a weight-bearing line that passes through the lateral malleolus, midknee, femoral head, anterior third of the sacral base, middle of the body of the L3 vertebra, humeral head, and external auditory meatus.

Failure of the body to align optimally with respect to its center of gravity functionally stresses pain-sensitive soft tissues and joint facets that were not adapted for direct, sustained weight-bearing function. Thus, structural change, increased energy demands, and pain are the results of postural decompensation (15).

Common Postural Clinical Conditions
Postural Types: Body Unity Issues

Clearly, posture is not just a stack of spinal curves with musculoligamentous connectors. Posture is influenced by the patient's triune emotional, spiritual, and psychological sense of self and by their inner energy reserves. It has been astutely observed that posture, to a large degree, can be a somatic depiction of one's inner emotions; what has been termed a *somatization of the psyche* (16). In emotionally depressed patients, for example, the somatic posture is also often termed *depressed*. Sagittal plane curves are typically accentuated and patients seemingly hang from their soft tissues without the apparent energy to stand tall. (See Table 36.1 for other postural types associated with the psyche.) In some chronic conditions where both physical and psychoemotional dysfunction exist, it is often difficult to know whether the psychoemotional state or the posture is the primary factor maintaining the cycle.

Sometimes, the primary psychological issue does not directly manifest in the posture; instead, for example, it may lead to fluctuations in weight, such as obesity. Such changes may, in turn, cause secondary changes in posture by requiring a redistribution of body mass or the use of medications that affect postural homeostatic mechanisms. Some health professionals generalize certain body types (endomorphic, mesomorphic, or ectomorphic) as being "linked" to a corresponding personality; regardless, there are mass and distribution of mass issues that affect both posture and the energy demands required to implement postural change.

Even when body unity issues do not directly impact the manifestation of posture, they can subvert a well-planned treatment program. In particular, compliance, vanity, and patient education are body unity issues that must be addressed in a complete postural treatment regimen. Patients' philosophies toward illness, their way of life, their appearance, their education, and the environment in which they function all can affect their compliance, which in turn affects the outcome of the treatment program.

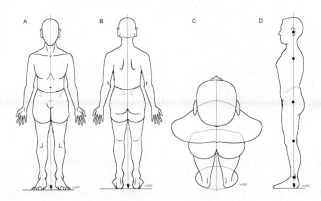

Figure 36-2 An optimally balanced standing postural alignment in the coronal plane (**A,B**) normally divides the body into two equal parts. The center of gravity line, or "weight-bearing line," runs midway between the feet, through the pubic symphysis, along the midline of the vertebral column, and bisects the center of the suprasternal notch and glabella. Ideally, there would be no rotation in the horizontal plane of any body region (**C**) and no coronal plane side-bending asymmetry. Optimal postural alignment in the sagittal plane (**D**) has been characterized by a weight-bearing line that passes through the lateral malleolus, midknee, femoral head, anterior third of the sacral base, middle of the body of the L3 vertebra, humeral head, and external auditory meatus. (Courtesy of William Kuchera, D.O., F.A.A.O.)

Spinal Biomechanics

"Biomechanics from the osteopathic perspective has evolved into a dual study of the adaptive responses of the body to gravitational force and the effects of alterations in joint mechanics that result from injury or impaired function" (17).

Spinal joints are designed to provide the motion in our activities of daily living and to permit the body unit to adopt the optimal dynamic posture in order to remain upright while doing so. Most ordinary and compensatory spinal motions involve a group of vertebral segments. In thoracic and lumbar group curves, such spinal motions follow Fryette's first principle of physiological motion and are necessary to allow for positional changes of the body. This

TABLE 36.1

Examples of Relationships Between Psyche and Posture

Psychological Tendency or Psyche	Posture	Implications
Healthy individuals who are open and ready internally to meet all external environment has to offer	Gentle, firm back curves; flexible body, pelvis-hips-knees	Capable of adaptation and homeostasis; maximal function within triune body
Depression; defeated individuals; downcast attitude; Those who feel, "I can't"	Posture is also "depressed." Head droops forward Trunk bends downward Shoulders project forward "Limp posture" resembles a very tired person	Tendency toward cervical and lumbar lordosis coupled with thoracic kyphosis. Posture leads to an abnormal stretch of ligaments and to pain. Bioenergically a fatiguing posture, as keeping this position causes overload on the extensor muscles. Posture adds physiological tiredness to the preexisting psychological feeling. Decreases depth of inhalation and compromises the respiratory-circulatory model.
Hyperkinetic individuals; aggressive individuals; anxiety; anger	Postural position very unbalanced Shoulders are carried anteriorly Pelvis is flexed Muscles are in a constant state of supported contraction	Postural muscles especially psoas prone to triggerpoints. Muscles of jaw, posterior neck, and shoulders especially tight
Individuals ashamed of body maturity (common in some girls reaching growth spurt earlier than boys of same age; development of breast tissue)	Posture is slumped with shoulders rolled inward	Prone for thoracic outlet symptoms from increased lordosis in neck and trigger points in pectoralis muscles
Proud, outgoing	Chest leads ("throw chest out")	Often a hard, rigid back
Threatened; fearful individual	Forward neck; prominent buttocks; protruding collapsed abdomen	Tightened buttocks, hamstrings and sphincters Tight thoracoabdominopelvic diaphragms
Shame, sorrow, sadness	Head hangs ("hang your head in shame")	
Obstinate or determined	Chin leads ("stick your neck out")	

Source: Some thoughts extracted from "psycho-orthopedics" by Sypher FF. Pain in the back: a general theory. *J Int College Surgeons*, 1960;33:6 and reported in Irvine WG. New concepts in the body expression of stress. *Can Fam Physician* 1973;38–42.

means that when the spine is in its neutral position (an absence of marked flexion or extension) and side bending is introduced, the vertebrae rotate into the produced convexity (18). (Rotation is to the opposite side of side bending.)

These types of dynamic spinal curves may be produced in the coronal plane by unilateral muscle contraction. Tension originating from this muscle creates a concavity, which results in a lateral curve. The involved thoracic and lumbar vertebrae rotate into the convexity. These Type I curves disappear when the muscle relaxes. Type I curves become a biomechanical problem when restriction occurs and the spine no longer straightens.

The total somatic body reaction that manifested as postural changes in response to less than ideal conditions is better understood by applying knowledge of spinal biomechanics. For example, the *bottom-up* spinal response to unleveling the sacral base in the coronal plane or an anatomically short lower extremity is guided by spinal biomechanical principles. To keep the eyes level at the opposite end of the body, the lumbar vertebrae located above the sacrum start to side bend away from the low sacral base thereby creating a scoliotic curve. As this Type I lumbar group curve forms, all other spinal regions capable of adjusting their alignment attempt to accommodate the new postural balance. Similarly, spinal biomechanics largely direct the postural response in a *top-down* spinal response to certain craniocervical dysfunctions or deformations.

Early postural compensation is associated with the development of a longer single lumbar or lumbothoracic scoliotic curve—convex on the side of the low sacral base. In this *C-shaped scoliotic curve*, the horizontal cephalad planes are typically depressed on the side opposite the depressed pelvic horizontal plane. Later, the compensatory mechanisms redistribute postural responsibilities resulting in the formation of several lateral curves. In this more *chronic* postural compensation (an *S-shaped scoliotic curve*), the shoulders and the greater trochanteric planes are typically depressed on the same side as the depressed sacral base. (The typical biomechanical response to sacral base unleveling is shown in Fig. 36.3.)

Postural patterns can be classified according to their capacity to be lessened by employing specific functional maneuvers that are appropriate for the regions' spinal biomechanics. If some spinal motion such as side bending can reduce a lateral curve, it is known as a *functional* or *secondary* curve. If it is unable to be reduced, it is known as a *structural, fixed,* or *primary* curve. A functional scoliotic, for example, is reversible; a structural scoliotic curve is nonreversible. Because structure and function are interrelated, many scoliotic curves are a mixture of these two classifications. This phenomenon is also seen with postural patterns in other planes.

Postures Seen in Pathology

Rational, conservative management of the postural components of patients with certain orthopedic disorders or structural pathology presupposes early and accurate diagnosis and a thorough understanding of the biomechanics involved. While the underlying cause is important for prognosis, knowing the static and dynamic effects of the pathology on spinal mechanics and on the homeostatic reserve required for compensation is central to the treatment design. For example and as discussed later in this chapter, management of patients with spondylolisthesis typically emphasizes sagittal plane strategies; management of scoliosis patients typically emphasizes coronal plane strategies. Table 36.2 lists examples of other pathological conditions in which the application of the osteopathic postural model is useful.

Postural Compensation: An Integrated Homeostatic Process

Genetic, traumatic, and habitual processes that require compensation accumulate and create an environment where few patients have ideal posture. Compensated postures are not ideal postures; they are, however, the result of several integrated homeostatic mechanisms working through the entire body unit to maximize

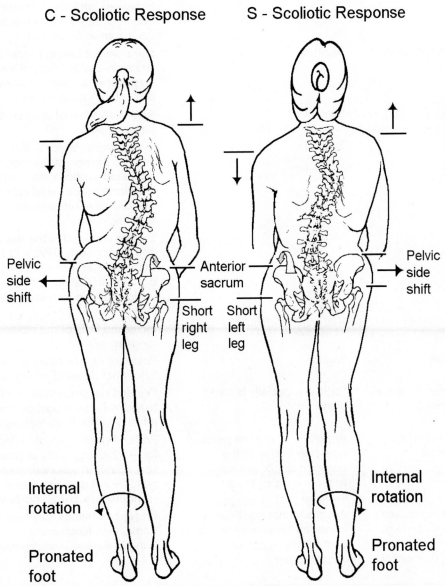

Figure 36-3 Typical postural compensation for short-leg syndrome. (Courtesy of William Kuchera, D.O., F.A.A.O.)

TABLE 36.2

Examples of Pathology and Posture

Pathology	Primary Plane(s) of Postural Involvement	Postural Effect
Cervical disk disease	Coronal and sagittal	Aggravating radiculopathy; Side bending toward can compromise nerve root; Decreased lordosis can move disk material posteriorly
Cervical osteoarthritis	Sagittal and coronal	Aggravating radiculopathy; Increased lordosis can close foraminal opening; Side bending toward can compromise nerve root
Lumbar disk disease	Horizontal, coronal and sagittal	Rotational stresses poorly tolerated by lumbar disks; flattened lordosis can move disk material posteriorly; side bending towards can compromise nerve root
Lumbar osteoarthritis	Sagittal and coronal	Aggravating radiculopathy; Increased lordosis can close foraminal opening; Side bending toward can compromise nerve root
Lumbar L5-S1 spondylolisthesis	Sagittal	Shifts weight bearing anteriorly to increase strain on posterior spinal elements; may aggravate back pain or nerve roots; increased iliolumbar ligament strain
Visceroptosis	Sagittal	Aggravates fascial drag on abdominal and pelvic organs
Osteoporosis	Sagittal	Osteoporosis typically first affects the anterior portion of the thoracic spine; increased kyphosis may increase pressure on anterior thoracic vertebral bodies; thoracic compression fractures may increase thoracic kyphotic curves
Uterine prolapse	Sagittal	Studies reported in the *Am J of Obstetrics and Gynecology* (1996 and 2000) demonstrated correlation of increased uterine prolapse in women with loss of lumbar lordosis and in increased thoracic kyphosis (risk increased 3.2×)
DJD of the hip	Coronal	Increased DJD of the hip seen on the long-leg side
Lumbar facet arthritis	Sagittal	Posterior weight-bearing mechanics transfer functional demand to lumbar facets
Any pathology where there is a congestive component	Sagittal especially but any plane	Postural decompensation affects the respiratory-circulatory model by decreasing the efficacy of the thoracoabdominopelvic pump
Any pathology worsened by hypersympathetic tone	Any plane where the postural crossover occurs at the common site of autonomics to the organs or tissues involved	Postural decompensation increases segmental facilitation (especially at crossover sites and secondarily at apices of postural curves); this typically will decrease blood flow, alter glandular functions, and/or increase pain
Any pathology that significantly compromises energy use (e.g., congestive heart failure or severe chronic obstructive pulmonary disease)	Any plane that significantly increases the energy demands of maintaining posture or effecting gait	Postural demands may take energy needed to maintain functional activities of daily living in severely compromised individuals

function. If not overly stressed, many compensated postures will remain relatively asymptomatic.

Postural compensation is coordinated by the CNS with continuous feedback provided by visual information, vestibular information from the semicircular canals, and kinesthetic/proprioceptive information from tendons and muscles (19). The resultant posture is manifested throughout the entire body to minimize energy requirements and to distribute and balance somatic stress, while keeping the eyes and semicircular canals as level as possible.

Postural homeostatic lessons are gradually "learned" by the evolving peripheral-CNS interrelationship. Influences begin with forces *in utero;* then from birth, throughout the growth process, and into senescence, soft tissue structures and functions both influence, and are influenced by, the cumulative functional demand placed upon them by postural compensation. As a result:

- Each person will progressively compensate in a different way depending, in part, on his or her unique intrinsic and extrinsic risk factors
- Postural preferences and patterns will conform within the resultant connective tissue structure
- Neuromusculoskeletal structures will remodel to reflect the functional demands placed upon them
- Functional capability will be limited by less than ideal structure.

These progressive and interactive neuromusculoskeletal compensatory processes impact postural diagnostic and treatment protocols. With regard to diagnosis, an osteopathic examination of selective soft tissue tensions and dynamic posture and segmental motion testing should be added to static postural alignment in the upright weight-bearing position. This combination illuminates structure-function interrelationships and provides clinical clues about the inherent capability of the patient's neuromusculoskeletal system to balance and maintain biomechanical alignment. Radiographic analysis of bony postural relationships (discussed later) adds further insight. With regard to therapeutics, recognition of the long-term nature of postural compensation suggests that a reversal toward ideal posture should be equally progressive and consistent if it is to succeed.

Potential Impact

Postural mechanisms acting from moment to moment may have only a transient negative impact on an individual. Persistent demands however lead to adaptations; in certain individuals, intrinsic or extrinsic factors may overtax one or more of the homeostatic processes that could lead to the manifestation of symptoms and eventually to postural decompensation.

Understanding how either postural compensation with adaptation or postural decompensation might negatively impact health requires a closer look at how each impacts tensegrity, group curves, and spinal mechanics. In this fashion, it becomes possible to predict and/or assess whether an individual's posture is contributing to negative functional or structural conditions.

Tensegrity

The *tensegrity model* plays a significant role in understanding the effects of postural stress, compensation, adaptation, or decompensation. Introduced by architect Buckminster Fuller in 1929 from the terms *tension* and *integrity*, tensegrity modeling has been successfully applied to biological systems. The model helps explain how most of the integrated structure-function arrangements in living systems require such little energy for their maintenance (*postural integrity*). The way in which bony tension elements are held together by connecting elastic elements (ligaments and antigravity muscles) helps create/maintain the balance between stability and

strength; it also explains how forces are dispersed through the body diffusely. The tensegrity model helps explain the predictable total structural response to tension change anywhere in the body.

In this model, it is recognized that:

- Areas of hypomobile somatic dysfunction may cause compensatory hypermobility elsewhere
- Hypermobility in one or more regions may affect compensatory hypomobility elsewhere
- Fascial patterning and musculoligamentous tensions take on primary importance as the model's connecting elements

It also helps to explain why certain global or local host factors adversely affect the capability of some individuals to successfully resist the effect of gravity strain or why injury to local sites (e.g., a foot or knee) may lead to secondary symptoms like back pain or headaches. For these reasons, a number of clinical models including osteopathic and orthopedic medicine cite tensegrity principles (16,20,21) when discussing the importance of postural balance and treatment.

Group Curves

Postural terminology applied to group curves is apparent in some situations and requires a thorough understanding of clinical medicine for others. Normal postural curves in the sagittal plane for example are termed *kyphotic* (forward bending) or *lordotic* (backward bending) *curves;* when they are pathological they are termed *kyphosis* and *lordosis*, respectively. Similarly, when pathological, coronal side bending (or *scoliotic* curves) of more than 5 degrees is termed *scoliosis*. Scoliosis is sometimes referred to as *rotoscoliosis* because rotation and side bending are inseparably linked. The pathology may be called a *kyphorotoscoliosis* if all three planes are significantly involved.

The terminology reflects the presence of an underlying continuum of responses to dynamic postural processes. Examples of this include the spine that is initially in a curved position to compensate for an anatomic short leg or certain structural deformities, postural balance adaptation, or even long-term positional change (such as may be required for a certain occupation) that becomes a pattern. In response to functional demands, the tissues associated with this curve change. Tissue texture changes become palpable and over time, tissues on the convex side become lengthened; those on the concave side become shortened. Bony remodeling in response to stress within the scoliotic group curve takes place, and the result is structural deformation of the vertebral body with lateral wedging and scoliosis (22). Longstanding curves with this type of anatomical adaptation resist change. Eventually, the curved position becomes the neutral position and is readily apparent in the analysis of standardized static postures.

In the process of postural compensation and adaptation, group curves in a given plane typically assume certain patterns. The most common patterns have group curves occurring in one direction in one region and in the opposite direction in the adjacent spinal regions, alternating so that the body can maintain some type of postural balance. Most commonly, these changes occur within the so-called transitional regions—areas where anatomic structure changes create the potential for the greatest functional change (Fig. 36.4).

Describing the pattern (23–25) of the group curves in various patient populations along with the location and direction of the major group curve provides a convenient way of summarizing common postural prototypes. Postural patterns or *patterning*, therefore, refers to useful and classifiable combinations of regional compensatory changes:

- Naming the anatomical locations of the postural *crossover* site provides clinical clues to potential somatovisceral sequelae or to sites at risk of arthritic change. Crossover sites are named

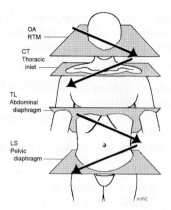

Figure 36-4 Compensation in the horizontal planes: Alternating pattern of rotation at transition zones. (Courtesy of William Kuchera, D.O., F.A.A.O.)

for the vertebral level where group curves change direction and crossover the ideal gravity line.

■ Naming the apices of group curves is also clinically helpful.

■ By international convention, group curves in scoliotic patterns are named for their convex side. For example, rotoscoliosis right means a postural curve that is convex to the right by being side bent to the left by more than 5 degrees.

Mechanics and Patterning

The biomechanical principles in postural compensation lead to fairly predictable response patterns to disturbances in one or more regional postural curve.

The systemic fascial or regional compensatory pattern will consist of an alternating directional pattern in one or multiple planes occurring at the transitional regions of the body (25) (Fig. 36.5A or its less common mirror image). (See the discussion of compensated fascial patterns in Chapter 51 and recognize the relationship this pattern has relative to the Postural and Respiratory-Circulatory models as a consequence):

■ In group postural curves, spinal side bending and rotation are biomechanically linked with each other (18) with the thoracic

and lumbar regions for example, typically manifesting curves that side bend in one direction and rotate in the opposite direction.

■ In sagittal plane postural curves, the degree of flexion or extension may manifest alone or in conjunction with all three cardinal planes.

With respect to the spinal mechanical compensatory pattern, gravity-induced changes in each plane of motion in the lumbopelvic region are particularly predictable because of this region's proximity to the L3 vertebral center of gravity.

■ In the sagittal plane, gravity encourages the sacral base to rotate anteriorly and encourages innominates to rotate posteriorly (Fig. 36.6) (26,27). This occurs because the L3 weight-bearing gravitational line falls anterior to the middle transverse sacral axis and behind the femoral axis. Homeostatic mechanisms that resist this counter-rotation are provided by muscular tone and by pelvic and lumbosacral ligaments (28). The anterior rotation of the sacrum in turn tends to increase all lordotic and kyphotic curves.

■ Compensatory changes in the coronal plane (as occurs with leg-length inequality) can also be generalized. As shown in Figure 36.3, the lumbar spine side bends away from and rotates toward the low sacral base. The pelvis as a unit typically side shifts and rotates around a vertical axis toward the long leg side. The innominate may attempt to compensate for the "short leg" by rotating anteriorly on the short leg side. This functionally lengthens that extremity. The innominate on the side of the apparent long leg may rotate posteriorly to functionally shorten that extremity. Often, on the long leg side, the foot assumes a pronated position, and the lower extremity internally rotates. The lumbosacral angle (LSA) increases 2 to 3 degrees. The increased LSA and pelvic rotation often mask the presence of an unlevel sacral base (29). The vertebrae of the most caudal scoliotic curve usually side bend away from and rotate toward the side of the apparent short leg.

■ Pelvic rotation in the horizontal plane occurs concomitantly with biomechanical stresses in the coronal plane (such as the short-leg syndrome) (30). This can present a therapeutic

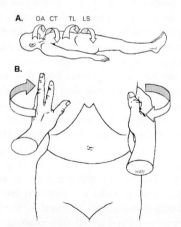

Figure 36-5 The systemic fascial or regional compensatory pattern will consist of an alternating directional pattern in one or multiple planes occurring at the transitional regions of the body. (Courtesy of William Kuchera, D.O., F.A.A.O.)

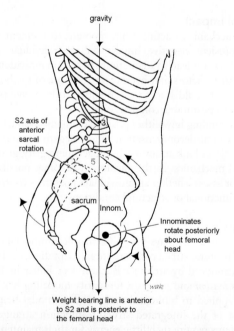

Figure 36-6 In the sagittal plane, gravity encourages the sacral base to rotate anteriorly and encourages innominates to rotate posteriorly. (Courtesy of William Kuchera, D.O., F.A.A.O.)

challenge when prescribing foot orthotics in an attempt to treat leg length or to level the sacral base. Strategies helpful in addressing this clinical challenge are described later in this chapter.

Relationship to Somatic Dysfunction

The consequences of postural compensation are most commonly asymptomatic; however, they may predispose an individual to prolonged or recurrent positions or adaptations that are less than ideal. As such, the postural element becomes a precipitator or perpetuator of certain somatic dysfunctions that may elicit symptoms. For example, it is widely quoted that posture is the most common precipitating and perpetuating factor for Travell myofascial trigger points (31). It contributes in the same fashion to recurrent dysfunctional muscle imbalance between the antigravity postural muscles and their antagonists.

In the thoracic and lumbar spine, somatic dysfunction secondary to postural compensation typically carries the freedom pattern of the neutral Type I spinal group curve mechanics that predominate in that patient; the restriction being in the opposite direction. If and when symptoms occur from Type I somatic dysfunctions, any pain or segmental facilitation generated is likely to be focused at the postural crossover sites where the most "work" is allowed or at the apices of the curves where the most restriction often exists. Should postural compensation in the sagittal plane predispose for somatic dysfunction that remains either flexed or extended outside the neutral range, the most symptomatic area may also be a single segment at the center of the sagittal postural curve. That segment is almost always symptomatic and may demonstrate somatic dysfunction that is either uniplanar (flexion or extension) or triplanar (Type II dysfunction).

Postural compensation or adaptation may also predispose and perpetuate fascial dysfunction at all four transitional zones. The directional pattern of compensatory regional fascial function and dysfunction is also an alternating one.

Postural compensation requires the work of muscles and, even prior to postural decompensation (discussed later), may predispose an individual to patterns of muscular somatic dysfunction. This is particularly true in patients who complain that their symptoms began after a particularly "long day on their feet." In these patients, look for muscular somatic dysfunction in their over-worked antigravity muscles and, if identified, in those of the same myotatic unit (muscles sharing the same function). Such muscular dysfunction symptomatology may range from achiness and hyperirritability to local crampy pain to the distantly referred pain and entrapments resulting from the development of myofascial trigger points. Antigravity/postural muscles are discussed further in this chapter.

Characteristically for this etiological cause, even after successful initial treatment of the individual arthrodial or myofascial somatic dysfunctions, the same pattern initially seen will often gradually recur until the primary postural element is addressed. Such recurrence should therefore trigger suspicion that postural compensation mechanisms underlay this diagnosis. It is important here to point out that the locations of somatic dysfunction in a primary postural pattern may be significantly different from a primary viscerosomatic pattern even though in both a pattern of recurrence is seen.

Some osteopathic physicians question the value of treating secondary group curve and regional fascial somatic dysfunctions; in treating posturally related somatic dysfunction they might focus only on any nonneutral Type II single segmental dysfunctions present. Others emphasize the importance of treating group curves when they are symptomatic or when the dysfunction might interfere with the success of implementing one of the osteopathic models of care. The correct answer to the question (of whether to treat or not) probably depends on asking another question about the patient involved.

"What is the functional significance of a group curve for the patient?" If the group curve contributes to dysfunction of the patient or prevents success in applying another treatment, then it should be treated.

Gravitational Strain Pathophysiology and Postural Decompensation

Gravitational force is universal, a systemic stressor, and an often underestimated and potentially progressive disruptor of postural homeostasis. Although it exerts a constant force on all structures, some individuals appear to be less capable of resisting gravitational effects than others. Possessing certain intrinsic (host) or extrinsic risk factors, these individuals may have weakened support mechanisms, increased functional demand on postural structures, and/or biomechanical disadvantages that challenge their ability to compensate for gravity's effect on their body systems (15,32–35). Considered in this fashion, posture is a secondary finding.

Of the many signature manifestations of pathophysiology resulting from the individual's chronic attempt to stave off the effects of gravity (15), altered postural alignment and recurrent somatic dysfunction are the most prominent. Other signs and symptoms indicative of *gravitational strain pathophysiology* (GSP) include low back pain, pain referred to the extremities, headache, somatovisceral manifestations, fatigue, and weakness will escalate in frequency and severity as key host compensatory mechanisms are progressively taxed.

Postural decompensation occurs when an individual's functional homeostatic mechanisms are overwhelmed (36) or when the degree of pathological change becomes structurally incapable of resisting gravitational force.

Predisposing Factors

The presence of a number of anatomic, congenital, and acquired conditions can stress postural compensatory mechanisms or accelerate the signs and symptoms of GSP and postural decompensation. In return, chronic postural functional demands will initiate and accelerate structural changes. This is a classic example of the reciprocity of structure-function interrelationships.

Patients with predisposing intrinsic or extrinsic factors will be at the highest risk of postural decompensation. Identifying these predisposing factors with an appropriate history and physical examination is an important diagnostic goal in the osteopathic postural model.

Intrinsic Factors

A number of host (intrinsic) factors decrease the ability to adequately resist gravity and create a predisposition towards postural decompensation. Examples include:

- Age (intrinsic factors related to muscle weakness, fascial elasticity, bone mass, etc.)
- Altered integrity or response from antigravity soft tissues (systemic hypermobility syndrome, various connective tissue disorders, muscular dystrophy, etc.)
- Incompetent bony antigravity structures (spondylolysis or spondylolisthesis, etc.)
- Poor tissue health (related to poor nutrition, inactivity with subsequent deconditioning, metabolic diseases, etc.)

Examples of host factors that increase asymmetry within the body and thereby magnify demands on postural compensatory mechanisms include:

- Altered base of support (unilateral pes planus [flat foot]), wearing shoes with high or worn heels, dysfunctional gait following ankle sprains or strains, anatomically short leg, etc.)

- Changes of body habitus (pregnancy, obesity, etc.)
- Congenital bony asymmetries (small hemipelvis, wedge vertebrae, etc.)
- Ergonomic factors associated with poor sitting or standing habits
- Strenuous posturing required by certain work environments or recreational activities such as gymnastics or carrying heavy rucksacks.

This chapter has already discussed a number of disorders which have known postural changes often due to each compromising one or more postural homeostatic mechanisms that result in a less efficient or defective host response (see pathologies or body unit issues related to posture).

Extrinsic Factors

Traumatic postural decompensation occurs when macrotrauma or recurrent microtraumas disrupt muscular, ligamentous, or bony stability of the spine. Such decompensation may occur more frequently in patients with a history of automobile accidents or surgical laminectomies (macrotraumas); or of carrying heavy loads for significant distances or certain high-level sport activities, as exist in gymnastics, weight-lifting, golf, or football (35) (microtrauma). Fractures of the spine, pelvis, or lower extremity may produce sacral base unleveling or the need for other compensatory changes above the area of the trauma. In addition, a few occupations actually increase extrinsic gravitational stress, for example, certain military pilots who experience multiple G-forces.

Responses of Tissues
Skeletal-Arthrodial Response

According to Wolff Law, bone remodels over time in response to the stress placed upon it (37). In this fashion, the vertebrae of patients with exaggerated or lateral postural curves will develop wedging of the vertebral body and exostoses (spurs). Posterior weight-bearing mechanics transfers weight onto the spinal facets, which results in modified function, increased calcium deposition that may appear on radiographs, and pain.

Degenerative change in spinal and other major weight-bearing joints (such as the hip) also occurs when there is accentuated functional demand and asymmetry. Degenerative arthritis of the hip joint that is accompanied by tenderness over the greater trochanter often develops on the long leg side (38).

One third of the sample population studied in a long-term radiographic postural study documented a chronic, progressive postural decline with spinal postural patterns which continued to evolve with age (6). The likelihood of several lateral curves evolving is higher when the leg-length inequality is >10 mm (39). The stereotypic posture of the geriatric patient depicts a decrease in total height as their kyphotic and lordotic curves are accentuated. In addition, the radiographic measurements of such patients show a height diminution (an increased pelvic index [PI] ratio) within the pelvis (32,40).

Regional (Transition Zone) Fascial Response

Postural patterning influences and is influenced by the fascias and related structures. J. Gordon Zink described patterns (25) that are clinically relevant to the diagnosis and treatment of fascial compensation and decompensation. Based on the palpatory fascial preference to motion, these fascial patterns may be classified as *ideal, compensated, or uncompensated* (Fig. 36.5A is one of two compensated—meaning directionally alternating—regional patterns). The postural influence on *fascial patterning* is important for understanding the effect that postural management has in improving the respiratory-circulatory model (41). Conversely, fascial preference

influences tissues and skeletal structures of each region and produces the dynamic postural characteristics of that body region.

Muscular Response

Gravitational stress placed on musculoligamentous structures is constant and is amplified in patients with less than ideal postural alignment. When the viscoelastic deformation properties of a muscle are unable to resist an imposed stress, predictable pathophysiological changes occur (15). These changes are both functional and structural. The *elastic* component represents the transient functional change in connective tissue length occurring in response to stress. The viscous component, on the other hand, is responsible for the more permanent (*plastic*) deformation of connective tissue that occurs with static postural change.

Stressed myofascial structures undergo sustained changes in length and deleterious change is most pronounced in shortened muscles (42). New collagen, with a half-life of 10 to 12 months, realigns the connective tissues in response to vectors of stress, perpetuating postural problems and maintaining the biomechanical amplification of gravitational stress. Postural patterns that are compensated are more likely to decompensate.

The structure of the muscle and its function are related; both playing a major role in the muscle patterns commonly seen in posture-initiated pain and dysfunction. In GSP, stressed antigravity muscles develop chronic, recurrent trigger points (43), consistent myotomal and sclerotomal pain patterns (44), and predictable functional changes. While postural (antigravity) muscles are structurally adapted to resist fatigue and function in the presence of prolonged gravitational exposure, when their capacity to resist stress is overwhelmed, they become irritable, tight, and shortened (45). Many muscles that are antagonists of these postural muscles, react when stressed by becoming weak or pseudoparetic (45). Therefore, GSP manifests as dysfunction in a *postural pattern* of tight and weak muscles or of myofascial trigger points (Fig. 36.7) (45–47). Recognizing such predictable patterns involving multiple muscles (Tables 36.3 and 36.4) should suggest GSP as a possible underlying

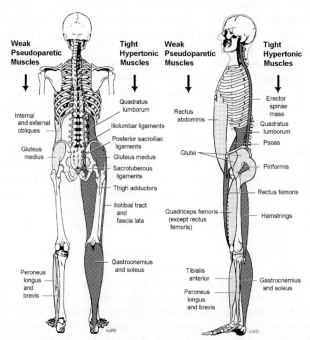

Figure 36-7 A postural pattern of tight and weak muscles or of myofascial trigger points. (Courtesy of William Kuchera, D.O., F.A.A.O.)

TABLE 36.3

Examples of Postural (Hypertonic-Prone) Muscles and Symptoms

Lower Body Muscle(s)	Symptoms
Iliopsoas	Inability to stand straight (psoas posturing); knees flexed; recurrent L1 or L2 NN somatic dysfunction; pain referred to back and anterior groin; positive Thomas test; may falsely increase PI measurements and decrease LS angle unless treated
Quadratus lumborum	Low back pain referred to the groin and hip; may be misdiagnosed as gr. trochanteric bursal disorder; exhalation 12th rib somatic dysfunction; diaphragm restriction
Thoracolumbar erector spinae	Low back pain; recurrent thoracolumbar somatic dysfunction; segmental facilitation
Hamstrings	Pain sitting or walking; pain disturbs sleep; pain referred to posterior thigh; straight leg raising limited mechanically; the combination of tight hamstrings on one side and tight rectus femoris on the other usually suggests postural strain seen with pelvic rotation in the horizontal plane; may cause false positive straight leg raising test
Rectus femoris	Pain deep inside the knee; the combination of tight hamstrings on one side and tight rectus femoris on the other usually suggests postural strain seen with pelvic rotation in the horizontal plane
Piriformis	Pain down posterior thigh; may entrap peroneal portion of sciatic nerve; perpetuated by(and perpetuates) sacroiliac dysfunction; associated with pelvic floor dysfunction, dyspareunia or prostatodynia
Thigh adductor (short)	Pain referral to the inguinal ligament, inner thigh, and upper medial knee
Gastroc-Soleus complex	Nocturnal leg cramps; pain referral to upper posterior calf, instep, and heel

The *"Lower Cross Syndrome"* (or *"Pelvic Cross Syndrome"*) reflects the *pattern* of lower body postural-phasic muscles in Tables 36.3 and 36.4 affecting the lower kinetic chain (lumbopelvic hip complex, knee, and ankle). The patient usually presents with anterior pelvic tilt, increased lumbar lordosis (swayback), and weak abdominals; they usually experience chronic low back pain, piriformis syndrome and anterior knee pain. This syndrome was popularized by Czech neurologists and manual medicine specialists, Vladimir Janda, M.D. and Karel Lewit, M.D.

Upper Body Muscles	Symptoms
Upper trapezius	Most likely muscle in body to develop TrPs; headache pain refers to occiput and/or to side of head near temple
Sternocleidomastoid	The SCM clavicular head is rich in proprioceptors (informs CNS where head is with respect to body), so dysfunction leads to postural instability & spatial disorientation; may veer off to one side while walking; refers pain to forehead bilaterally and ear. Sternal head may cause visual and ANS symptoms
Levator scapulae	Stiff neck (especially with rotation); pain to base of neck, vertebral border of the scapula and posterior shoulder
Pectoralis major (upper)	May cause chest wall pain with radiation down arm in anginal pattern (if on left) and intense nipple hypersensitivity
Pectoralis minor	Prominent in slumped postures with rolled in shoulders, increased kyphosis, and anterior neck carriage; May entrap brachial nerve and/or axillary artery leading to radial sided dysesthesias and possible loss of the radial pulse
Cervical erector spinae	Headache and neck pain; recurrent cervical somatic dysfunction
Scalenes	The entrappers—may entrap neurovascular bundle (esp lower trunk of the brachial plexus and/or subclavian vein) with dysesthesias to 5th digit and/or puffy hands; may also reflexly limit thoracic duct return leading to upper extremity swelling; TrPs may cause dysesthesia into thumb and index finger side of hand. May lead to recurrent elevated rib 1–2 somatic dysfunction

Janda's and Lewit's *"Upper Cross Syndrome"* reflects the *pattern* of lower body postural-phasic muscles in Tables 36.3 and 36.4 affecting the upper kinetic chain (neck, shoulder, upper chest). The patient usually presents with headaches, upper thoracic pain, and various Thoracic Outlet Syndrome signs and/or symptoms.

TABLE 36.4

Examples of Phasic (Pseudoparesis-Prone) Muscles and Symptoms

Lower Body Muscle(s)	Symptoms
Gluteus minimus	Pain characteristic when arising from chair; pain referral to buttock, lateral and posterior thigh; "pseudosciatica"; antalgic gait; positive Trendelenburg test
Gluteus medius	Pain aggravated by walking; pain referral to posterior iliac crest and sacroiliac joint; positive Trendelenburg test
Gluteus maximus	Restlessness; pain sitting or walking up hill; antalgic gait
Three Vasti (but *not* rectus femoris)	Buckling knee syndrome; weakness going up stairs; thigh and knee pain; patellar tracking imbalance; chondromalacia patellae
Rectus abdominis	Increased lordosis; constipation
Tibialis anterior	Pain referred to great toe and anteromedial ankle; may drag foot or trip when tired

Upper Body Muscle(s)	Symptoms
Mid/lower trapezius	Refers pain and tenderness to the region of the upper trapezius
Latissimus dorsi	Causes chronic midthoracic back pain but with the slack muscle, no particular position offers relief
Rhomboids	Ache between shoulder blades; cracking or scrunching sounds when move shoulder
Deep cervical flexors	Longus coli and longus capitus muscles leading to recurrent cervical somatic dysfunction; loss of neck stability

cause. In these patients, treatment of the dysfunctional postural alignment yields more lasting results than treatment of the secondary recurrent myofascial trigger points or muscle imbalances in isolation.

Finally, GSP and postural decompensation may also involve a loss of energy because of the increased active muscle contraction (48) needed to counteract gravity or to ambulate.

Ligamentous Response

Stabilizing ligaments are stressed in individuals with postural imbalance or diminished homeostatic abilities to resist gravity—in particular, the iliolumbar, sacrotuberous (ST), and long dorsal (posterior) sacroiliac ligaments; each having its own predictable sclerotomal pain pattern.

The iliolumbar ligaments (ILL) are critical for stabilizing the lumbar vertebrae with respect to the pelvis (28). They are usually the first structures to be involved with GSP and are also affected by both sacral and innominate rotations (Fig. 36.8). The attachments of these ligaments become tender to palpation when stressed—unilaterally in coronal plane postural strain and bilaterally in sagittal plane strain conditions. ILL calcification may occur with long-standing postural strain because calcium is laid down along lines of stress (Wolff law) (37). Functional changes include tenderness, edema, and pain referred to the lower extremity (Fig. 36.9); these findings disappear with treatment.

ST ligament and long dorsal sacroiliac (LDSI) ligaments resist anterior and posterior rotation of the sacrum respectively (Fig. 36.10) (49). The LDSI ligament connects the sacrum and the posterior superior iliac spine (PSIS), whereas the main part of the ST ligament connects the sacrum and ischial tuberosity.

Postural stress involves a more complex biomechanical interaction than is depicted in Figures 36.8 and 36.10. It involves interaction between these ligaments, the sacroiliac joint, the thoracolumbar fascia, and a variety of muscles including the multifidi, biceps femoris, and glutei (49). The pelvic girdle as a foundation for function and support must therefore be interpreted in its relationship to other areas of the spine and all four extremities.

Response of Related Neural, Vascular, Lymphatic, and Visceral Elements

The postural model overlaps with the respiratory-circulatory and neurological models of patient assessment and treatment. Each of these models looks to transition zones as key areas for identifying and treating somatic dysfunction.

The transition zones are closely linked to transverse diaphragms; dysfunction in these areas often results in reduction of venous and lymphatic return. Reduction of postural decompensation frequently improves respiratory homeostasis and reduces circulatory impediment. Additional symptoms originate at the individual's postural crossover sites, where the spinal curve crosses from side to side or anterior to posterior across the weight-bearing line (Fig. 36.11) and may secondarily occur at postural curve apical sites. These sites often manifest local subjective joint and myofascial tissue symptoms. The resultant nociception frequently links the postural model to the autonomic model through resultant facilitated segments (50,51) producing inappropriate increases in sympathetic activity. Posturally mediated facilitation, in turn, results in dysfunction of segmentally related vascular and lymphatic structures, somatovisceral reflex change, and subsequent related organ dysfunction.

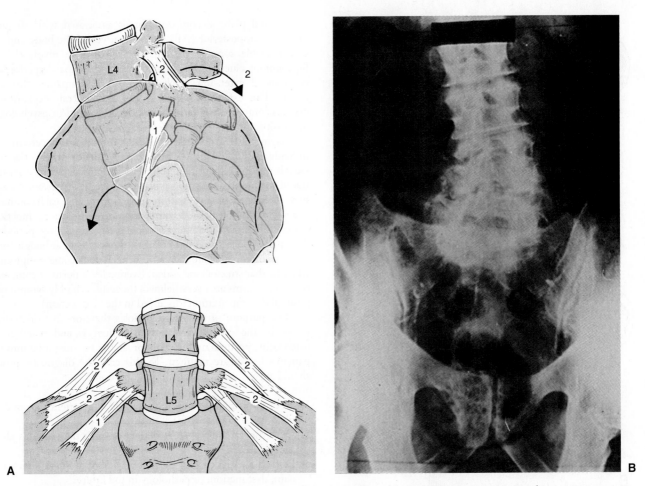

Figure 36-8   A. Anterior rotation of sacrum bilaterally stresses fibers labeled *1*. Posterior rotation of innominates bilaterally stress fibers labeled *2*. **B.** Calcification of iliolumbar ligament is an excellent example of structural change resulting from excess functional demand. (Radiograph from the Institute for Gravitational Strain Pathology Inc., with permission.)

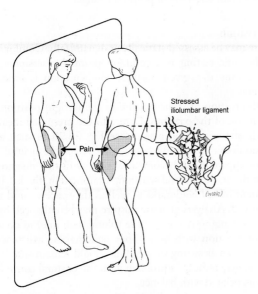

Figure 36-9   Iliolumbar ligament pain pattern from postural imbalance. (Courtesy of William Kuchera, D.O., F.A.A.O.)

Furthermore, in the coexistent presence of intervertebral foraminal compromise by cervical or lumbar degenerative disease (figure-of-eight deformities), increasing postural curves may further reduce homeostatic abilities to counter irritation or swelling in the area, resulting in altered axoplasmic flow, so-called double-crush phenomena, or radicular symptoms neurological model); each of these can also result in secondary myofascial trigger points (52–54).

In considering the postural model then, related neural, vascular, lymphatic, and visceral information should always be sought and an attempt should be made to correlate the site of GSP with local, visceral, or referred symptoms.

General Diagnostic Considerations

Observation and palpation of postural muscles, their antagonists, and regional or group spinal curves should be performed if possible with the patient in an upright, weight-bearing position. In this upright position, the patient is asked to move into various positions to determine whether any observed thoracic or lumbar rotoscoliotic group curve asymmetry can be functionally reduced or eliminated. The structural component in the coronal and horizontal planes is represented by the spinal asymmetry that is not modified by active or passive motion.

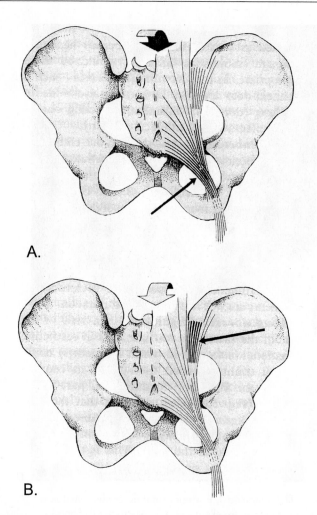

A.

B.

Figure 36-10   A. Sacrum rotating anteriorly winds up ST ligament. **B.** Sacrum rotating posteriorly winds up the LDSI ligament. (From Vleeming A, Snijders CJ, Stoeckart R, et al. The role of the sacroiliac joints in coupling between the spine, pelvis, legs, and arms. In: Vleeming A, Mooney V, Dorman T, et al., eds. *Movement, Stability, and Low Back Pain: The Essential Role of the Pelvis.* New York, NY: Churchill-Livingstone, 1997, with permission.)

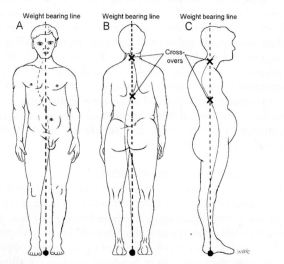

Figure 36-11   Postural crossover sites. (Courtesy of William Kuchera, D.O., F.A.A.O.)

Sagittal plane decompensation is associated with alteration of the anteroposterior (AP) regional curves of the body and specific palpable somatic patterns. In addition to myofascial and ligamentous clues, anterior sacral base and lumbar hyperlordosis, craniosacral extension mechanics often accompanies this condition. The extension phase of the craniosacral mechanism is often accompanied by fatigue, loss of energy, and/or psychological depression.

Asymptomatic postural compensation is of no concern in many individuals but constitutes a degree of risk for others. For individuals seeking patient care, recurrent symptoms may be eventually traced to the predisposition toward somatic dysfunction, nociception, facilitation, or stress within the tensegrity unit; each commonly engendered by postural decompensation. Furthermore, functional demands imposed by maintaining posture over long periods of time may induce structural changes; those which, although sometimes asymptomatic, are increasingly likely to become symptomatic when further stressors are added. Eventually, if postural compensation mechanisms are overwhelmed, the result is highly symptomatic postural decompensation (discussed in the next section).

The purpose of postural diagnosis therefore is to determine where in the continuum a given patient is and whether the osteopathic postural model could or should be integrated into that patient's healthcare regimen. To this end, the diagnostic process should answer at least four specific questions:

1. Does the patient's posture play a role in a patient's given complaint?
2. Does the patient's posture detract or limit the patient's ability for self-healing?
3. Does the patient's posture present a significant risk factor for pain, dysfunction, or pathology in the future?
4. Is the patient able to respond positively to a postural treatment regimen in a time- and cost-effective manner?

The postural diagnostic approach to answering these questions relies heavily on observation and palpation. It attempts to correlate other findings from the patient's history and physical examination in order to determine if any pertinent signs or symptoms exist. It may also bring in radiological or biomechanical tests to help quantify the extent and type of postural change.

Observation

Posture may be assessed statically or dynamically. Combining static and dynamic testing is a common postural assessment strategy to determine if a given postural compensation is functional or structural.

Observation of static posture in the upright position permits comparison of the patient's posture to the presumed ideal posture in each of the cardinal planes (see Fig. 36.2). In such a screening examination, postural curves that affect the neutral position become apparent and become the focus of further diagnostic testing. In the static postural screening examination, the levelness and alignment of key landmarks as well as the space around the body is observed. Analysis of static posture may be enhanced by using a grid or a hanging reference wire (plumb bob line) to obtain valuable information with or without radiographic assistance. Static postures such as sitting or standing should remain still; if they do not, this may indicate a problem with the postural control mechanisms associated with balance.

Suspicious regions identified in static testing may be further screened using dynamic positioning to determine if the postural curve is *functional* (with flexibility) or *structural* (with no change permitted with motion), or *mixed* (with some combination of both). Dynamic postural testing not only adds insight into the flexibility of obvious spinal curves that were apparent in static screening, it may also uncover minor or overlooked functional curves. Dynamic postural testing frequently provides information on the spinal biomechanics of the region being tested and can uncover areas of somatic dysfunction. Dynamic postural analysis looks at how postural elements react to particular motions and can be quantified using manual or electronic goniometers to measure the magnitude and symmetry of total or regional motion in the three cardinal planes.

Coronal and Horizontal Plane Observations

Coronal and horizontal plane postural disorders are anticipated with certain combinations of static and dynamic observations. To diagnose coronal plane problems, first stand behind the upright patient and observe (using simultaneous palpatory assistance) to assess the following key static anatomical landmarks (Fig. 36.12) for asymmetry from the horizontal plane:

- Mastoid processes
- Acromioclavicular joints
- Inferior scapula

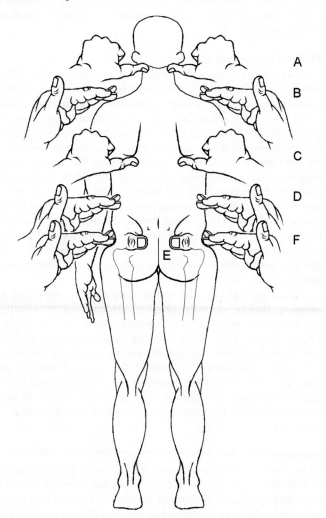

Figure 36-12 Levelness of horizontal planes. **A.** Occipital plane. **B.** Shoulder plane. **C.** Scapular plane. (inferior) **D.** Iliac crest plane. **E.** PSIS plane. **F.** Greater trochanteric plane. (Courtesy of William Kuchera, D.O., F.A.A.O.)

- Fingertips
- Iliac crests
- PSIS
- Greater trochanters
- Knee creases

In addition, observe the coronal plane for evidence of scoliotic curves and note the spinal level at which point the curve crosses an imagined midline (crossover sites). Sometimes, asymmetry due to shoulder muscle bulk arising from a *handedness pattern* may mislead the physician to think there is a scoliotic curve; in these cases, it may be helpful to observe the patient from the front as well. Lateral spinal curves in the back are often reflected in the front and are particularly easy to see in the chest hair pattern of some men. Look at the space around the body; is the space between one arm and the body greater on one side than the other?

Observation from the front of the body can also alert the doctor to horizontal plane problems. In the static postural diagnosis of this plane, an imaginary or actual plumb-bob line should equally bisect the body. Observations should include:

- Are midline structures like the nose and xiphoid process centered or not?
- Is the face turned with one ear more visible than the other?
- Is one humeral head, costal margin, or anterior superior iliac spine (ASIS) anterior to the other?

After static observation, add one or more dynamic tests. Two commonly used observational test combinations in postural analysis examples are shown in the adjacent Figure 36.13.

- Interpretation of the shape of the lumbar curve during a dynamic hip drop test in a patient with a lumbar Type I side-bending curve (Fig. 36.13A)
- Interpretation of static and dynamic postures in a patient with thoracic Type I double balanced side-bending curve (Fig. 36.13B and C)

The Adams forward-bending test is the most commonly used dynamic screening test for rotoscoliosis. It works because side bending and rotation in group curves are normally coupled Fryette Type I motions. The test involves standing behind the patient and observing for a "rib hump" as the patient slowly bends forward. Any

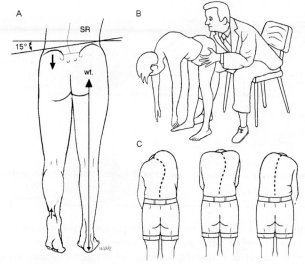

Figure 36-13 Assessment of structural or functional scoliosis. (Courtesy of William Kuchera, D.O., F.A.A.O.)

costal asymmetry should then be analyzed by having the patient (still flexed to the site of the asymmetry) try to side bend toward the high rib to see if levelness can be restored (Fig. 36.13C). Performed with care, this method should allow detection of scoliotic curves measuring as small as 10 degrees; when performed without focused attention, physicians have been documented to miss curves as large as 35 degrees. The forward-bending test has a sensitivity of only about 84% (less than Moire topography or scoliometer) but a specificity greater than both of those; it is most effective in thoracic scoliosis but has a high false-negative rate in the lumbar spine (55).

Sagittal Plane Observations

Viewing the static posture of patients from the side, the osteopathic physician should look for exaggerated or flattened kyphotic or lordotic curves. The clinician should also assess whether key anatomical landmarks are aligned from bottom to top along an imaginary ideal (Fig. 36.2D) or actual plumb bob line:

- Just anterior part to the lateral malleolus
- Just behind the midknee
- Femoral head
- Anterior one third of sacral base (radiographic observation only)
- Middle of the body of L3 (radiographic observation only)
- Humeral head
- External auditory meatus

Dynamic testing can be done while standing with the patient flexing and extending to determine the relative flexibility of the sagittal plane curves. Alternatively, in a functional lumbar lordosis, having the patient supine with bent knees as shown (Fig. 36.14) should permit the spinal curve to flatten onto the table (or floor). Inability to flatten this curve either actively or passively represents a sagittal plane structural component or pathology. When evaluating this element, be sure to simultaneously "observe with palpation" the lumbar spine as excessive or hypertrophied soft tissues in the adjacent flanks may mask the lordotic curve.

Palpatory Tissue Assessment

Musculoligamentous and fascial structures are affected early in patients with postural stress and somatic dysfunction here can be easily recognized with palpation.

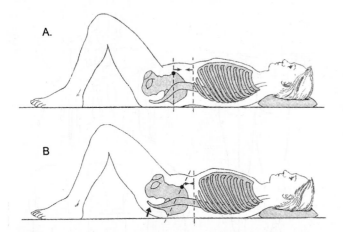

Figure 36-14   Lumbar lordosis, with patient actively attempting to flatten spine to table. **A.** Structural component (no reduction of lordotic curve). **B.** Flattening indicative of functional lordotic curve. (From Simon DG, Travell JG, Simons LS. *Myofascial Pain and Dysfunction: The Trigger Point Manual.* Vol I. Baltimore, MD: Williams & Wilkins, 1999, with permission.)

The symptoms arising from the resultant pathophysiological condition have associated palpable *tissue texture changes* that include the following:

- Muscle spasm in postural (antigravity) muscles
- Subtle weakness to muscle testing in postural antagonist (phasic) muscles
- Tenderness over ligamentous and osseotendonous attachments involved in postural stability
- Myofascial trigger points
- Edema or bogginess

Palpation identifies structural *asymmetries* of key landmarks and gathers information about the functional characteristics of the body unit. It is also the best tool for uncovering patterns of *restricted motion, tenderness*, pain, strain, or adaptations characteristic of postural disorders. Palpation of the postural response to certain movements helps to differentiate the degree to which a given postural curve is structural or functional (i.e., does it stay the same or increase or does it reduce or disappear?).

It is important not to miss these palpable changes or postural pattern clues, which are relatively early signs that postural compensation mechanisms are starting to be overwhelmed. If not recognized and addressed upon discovery, it is possible that the last step in the continuum of man's battle against gravity will be postural decompensation.

Postural Radiographic Series

As mentioned, posture and postural diagnoses involve the understanding of both static (structural) and dynamic (functional) characteristics; x-ray images primarily visualize the static or structural aspect of posture. Therefore, postural radiographs are typically performed after first using OMT to correct concomitant somatic dys*function*—especially preradiographic goals include normalizing lumbopelvic mechanics (56), and treating the larger postural muscles affecting the lower extremities and pelvis such as the quadratus lumborum (57), and iliopsoas (46) that are known to particularly distort static postural interpretation. Performed in this manner, an osteopathic postural series will document "repeatable findings when the state of the patient is unchanged and provide valid information concerning improvements or regressions in skeletal structure which are associated with changes in the patient's condition" (4).

These radiographs also contain information pertinent to assessing skeletal maturity (Fig. 36.15) and aid in identifying congenital anomalies and other structural deficiencies (see Fig. 36.16 and Table 36.5) that can enhance the potential for gravitational and other functional strain to overwhelm the body's homeostatic mechanisms or prevent their reversal through the employment of certain treatment strategies. Finally, postural radiographs may be used to quantify static postural distortion or decompensation from the ideal and to document improvement with treatment.

Protocol

While many radiologists are not trained to do postural studies specifically for osteopathic analysis, most will conduct them for referring physicians if informed of the protocol and necessary materials needed (such as is depicted in Fig. 36.17A and B) (58). The protocol involves two postural views, AP and lateral, which are captured in order to assess coronal, horizontal, and sagittal plane static postures (Figs. 36.18 and 36.19). These AP and lateral films are typically performed with the patient's shoes off to determine intrinsic postural discrepancies. At times, films may also be obtained with

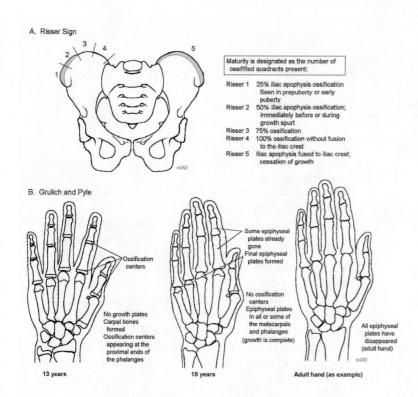

A. Risser Sign

Maturity is designated as the number of ossified quadrants present:

Risser 1   25% iliac apophysis ossification Seen in prepuberty or early puberty
Risser 2   50% iliac apophysis ossification; immediately before or during growth spurt
Risser 3   75% ossification
Risser 4   100% ossification without fusion to the iliac crest
Risser 5   Iliac apophysis fused to iliac crest; cessation of growth

B. Grulich and Pyle

Ossification centers

Some epiphyseal plates already gone
Final epiphyseal plates formed

No ossification centers
Epiphyseal plates in all or some of the metacarpals and phalanges (growth is complete)

No growth plates
Carpal bones formed
Ossification centers appearing at the proximal ends of the phalanges

All epiphyseal plates have disappeared (adult hand)

13 years   18 years   Adult hand (as example)

the patient wearing their shoes, with a therapeutic lift or orthotic in place, to determine the amount of sacral base unleveling that still remains to be corrected (i.e.). The exposure of the patient to ionizing radiation in this study is minimal. For example, this protocol is calculated to expose the patient to 0.12 rad for the AP postural view but could be reduced even further with only 0.011 rad to the gonads using a lead gonadal shield (57). Known pregnancy would nonetheless be a contraindication to performing a postural radiographic series.

Postural x-ray views taken according to a standardized protocol (with precise foot placement, locked knees, and consistent arm positions) can be accurately and consistently measured for static postural information by radiologists or attending nonradiologist physicians (59). Such a protocol is amenable to rapid adjustment and placement, making it practical even in busy radiology departments. Each time the patient is positioned in a reproducible weight-bearing posture and recorded with an independent vertical reference line (RL) on the film. The RL is unrelated to the position of the cassette, yet it is perpendicular to the line of the horizon. Measurements taken from the edge of the film may be inaccurate because of the variable position of the film within the cassette and therefore would produce misleading or nonreproducible results (57).

Lack of a standard protocol would render many measurements meaningless for the purposes of postural diagnosis, patient follow-up, or research. However, using standard protocols for taking and marking the films for postural measurements have been

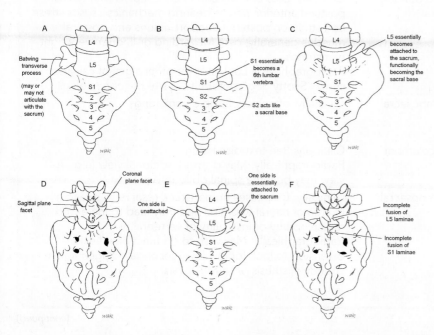

Figure 36-16 Common lumbosacral abnormalities: **A.** Batwing transverse processes of L5. **B.** Lumbarization of S1. **C.** Sacralization of L5. **D.** Facet asymmetry (zygopophyseal tropism) of L4. **E.** Partial sacralization of L5 (Bertolotti). **F.** Spina bifida occulta of both L_5 and of S. (Courtesy of William Kuchera, D.O., F.A.A.O.)

TABLE 36.5

Radiological Findings on Postural Films

Radiological Finding and Appearance	Best X-ray View	Implications/Comments
Congenital		
Bat-wing deformity	A-P lumbosacral	Clinically: May alter joint mechanics, pain and inflammation possible if rudimentary L5-iliac joint, alters sacral base level Radiographically: May be unable to accurately measure sacral base unleveling
Sacralization of L5 Partial Sacralization = Bertolotti syndrome	A-P and lateral lumbosacral (both help)	Clinically: Short lumbar curve (n = 4) leading to more functional demand per segment and increased likelihood of developing degenerative L4 spondylolisthesis Radiographically: Unable to measure PI or lumbosacral lordotic angle
Lumbarization of S1	A-P and lateral lumbosacral (both help)	Clinically: Long lumbar lever arm (n = 6) leading to less stability and increased incidence of low back pain Radiographically: Unable to measure PI
Spina bifida occulta	A-P lumbosacral	Clinically: May not mean anything however may be harbinger of other posterior spinal congenital anomalies; muscles may attach and therefore function differently; often externally small tuft of hair at vertebral site
Facet tropism	A-P and lateral lumbosacral (both help visualize)	So common that most radiologists do not even report its presence ("most commonly occurring congenital spinal anomaly"); asymmetric function; may
Horizontal L5-S1 facets with— listhesis (see Table 36.7, Type I)	Lateral lumbosacral	Clinically: Drop-off sign is at level lower than isthmic type because spine remains attached to
Small hemipelvis	A-P pelvis	Clinically: May be associated with smaller extremity and/ or face on same side; may lead to functional scoliosis in seated position (and similar symptoms)
Wedge vertebrae	A-P thoracolumbar	Radiographically: Impact on Cobb Angle process
Acquired		
Spondylolysis	Oblique lumbosacral	Clinically: May be asymptomatic but usually associated with increased sagittal plane stress and decompensation; called *prespondylolisthesis*
L5-S1 isthmic spondylolisthesis (see Table 36.7, Type IIA-B)	Lateral and oblique lumbosacral	Clinically: Loss of bony continuity coupled with typical postural anterior weight-bearing mechanics causes stress and strain on posterior support tissues and postural muscles generally; over Meyerding gr II, often very tight hamstrings Radiographically: Look also for other signs of calcified show "Scotty dog" deformity at site of spondylolysis
L4–5 degenerative spondylolisthesis (see Table 36.7, Type III)	Lateral lumbosacral	Clinically: often very flexible hamstrings
(Roto)scoliosis	A-P thoracolumbar	Clinically: See text discussion Radiographically: May distort traditional view (e.g., A-P view may become spinal oblique view)
Disk thinning	Lateral lumbosacral	Clinically: Decreases homeostatic reserve to swelling in area of neural foramina and may lead to increased radiculopathy or instability of vertebral unit Radiographically: May wish to do functional flexion-extension to look for low level secondary degenerative spondylolisthesis or retrolisthesis

(continued)

TABLE 36.5   *(Continued)*

Facet arthritis	AP and lateral	Seen in especially in posterior weight-bearing mechanics
Unlevel sacral base	A-P lumbosacral	Often a cause of functional scoliotic change above; coronal changes often linked to visual rotational change as well
DJD spurs, figure-of-eight vertebral foraminal changes; calcification of ligaments (e.g., iliolumbar)	Oblique as well as other views	Clinically: Structural signs of long-term functional demand (Wolff law) but themselves may be totally asymptomatic Radiographically: Should raise suspicion of postural stress warranting postural measurements
Fracture(s)	Multiple views; oblique view for optimal view of the pars interarticularis	Clinically: May cause reflect straightening of the spinal curve due to muscle spasm Radiographically: May not be able to accurately assess underlying lordotic angles due to straightening

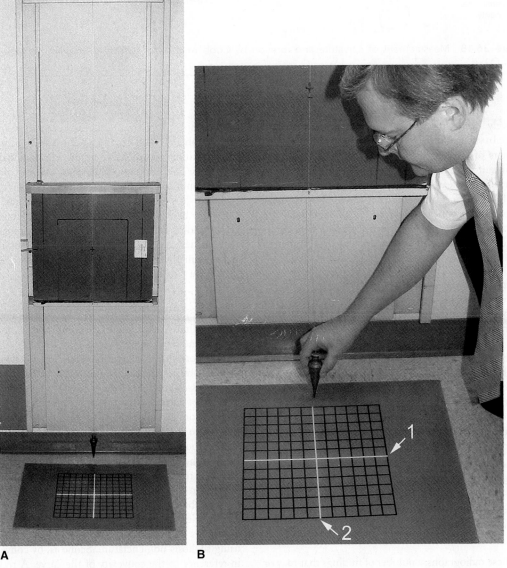

A   **B**

Figure 36-17   X-ray set-up. **A.** Vertical Bucky diaphragm and piano wire reference. **B.** Rectangular metal base plate with RLs. *1*, posterior line; *2*, midheel line.

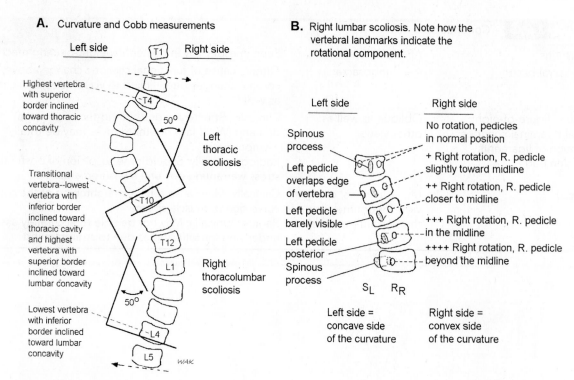

A. Curvature and Cobb measurements

Left side   T1   Right side

Highest vertebra with superior border inclined toward thoracic concavity

T4
50°

Left thoracic scoliosis

Transitional vertebra--lowest vertebra with inferior border inclined toward thoracic cavity and highest vertebra with superior border inclined toward lumbar concavity

T10

T12

L1   Right thoracolumbar scoliosis

50°

Lowest vertebra with inferior border inclined toward lumbar concavity

L4

L5   WAK

B. Right lumbar scoliosis. Note how the vertebral landmarks indicate the rotational component.

Left side   Right side

Spinous process

Left pedicle overlaps edge of vertebra

Left pedicle barely visible

Left pedicle posterior Spinous process

S_L R_R

No rotation, pedicles in normal position

+ Right rotation, R. pedicle slightly toward midline

++ Right rotation, R. pedicle closer to midline

+++ Right rotation, R. pedicle in the midline

++++ Right rotation, R. pedicle beyond the midline

Left side = concave side of the curvature

Right side = convex side of the curvature

Figure 36-18 Measurement of curvature and rotation by Cobb method. (Courtesy of William Kuchera, D.O., F.A.A.O.)

studied extensively for reproducibility, validity, and clinical relevance (60,61). In such studies (Fig. 36.20), interexaminer standard measurements of error are acceptably small and have been remarkably consistent in multiple studies (7,62,63). These might best be summarized as a mean error of <1.0 mm and a maximum error of 2.0 mm for linear measures and 2 degrees for angular measures. These were also the conclusions obtained when manual and computer-assisted measurements by different practitioners (radiologist, primary care physicians, and osteopathic medical students) (59) were compared.

General interpretation of postural radiographs

Postural measurements obtained in this way can be interpreted using the osteopathic postural model. This model presumes that static findings from postural radiographs will be correlated with various dynamic aspects of the clinical examination, including palpation, and can be used to uncover relevant structure-function and postural-biomechanical insights. To maximize the interpretation of the static information provided by postural x-rays, the osteopathic postural model also presumes that somatic dysfunction is corrected as much as possible *prior* to sending the patient for a postural radiographic series (56). The somatic dysfunctions that are most likely to create significant transient postural asymmetry on these films are:

- Sacral shear (unilateral sacral flexion)
- Innominate shear (e.g., superior or up-slipped innominate)
- Iliopsoas muscle spasm (46)
- Quadratus lumborum spasm (57)
- Innominate rotation

In interpreting these radiographs, a number of findings that may or may not be clinically relevant, including those listed in Table 36.5, are considered.

Examples of common lumbosacral anomalies appearing radiographically and having potentially significant impact when implementing the postural model are depicted in Figure 36.16 and Table 36.5. Several of these anomalies complicate the selection of landmarks used in postural measurements or in the interpretation of postural radiographic data. A few are recognized to cause low back pain or instability in a percentage of patients; others are widely believed to be incidental insignificant anomalies, but may be viewed as "risk factors," others potentially complicate the findings in those patients who are diagnosed as having regional instability.

Interpreting AP thoracolumbar postural radiographs

The standing AP film of the thoracic and lumbar regions contains both qualitative and quantitative information about posture in the coronal and horizontal planes.

By noting the relative positions of the two pedicles and the spinous process, thoracic or lumbar vertebral rotation can be qualitatively assessed in AP radiographic views (see Fig. 36.18B). In the absence of vertebral rotation, the spinous process is located equidistant from each pedicle. With right vertebral rotation (named in relation to the direction of movement of a reference point on the anterior portion of the vertebral body), the spinous process visualized on the x-ray film appears closer to the left pedicle. With left vertebral rotation, the spinous process appears closer to the right pedicle on the x-ray film.

Vertebral side bending is easily observed on the AP radiographic view and can be qualitatively reported. Quantitative measurements of group curves are often more formally reported by using scoliosis nomenclature. Scoliosis, by convention, is reported in reference to the convexity of the curve. A right scoliosis is side bent left (convex right). The Cobb method is commonly used to measure scoliotic curves (see Fig. 36.18A) and with care is accurate

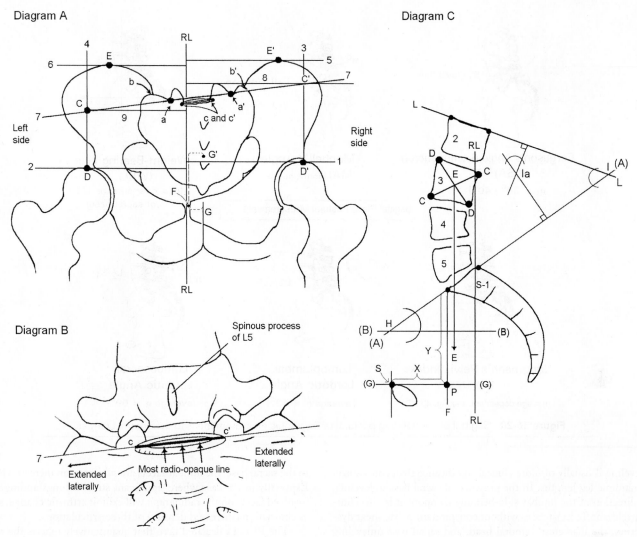

Figure 36-19 Measurements for a postural x-ray view. **A.** AP postural measurements. **B.** Landmark options for measuring sacral base unleveling. **C.** Lateral postural measurements. (Figs. 36.19A and C adapted from Kuchera WA, Kuchera ML. *Osteopathic Principles and Practice*. 2nd Ed. Rev. Columbus, OH: Greyden Press, 1994:63. Fig 36.19B adapted from Irvin RE, Suboptimal posture: the origin of the majority of idiopathic pain of the musculoskeletal system. In: Vleeming A, Mooney V, Dorman T, et al., eds. *Movement, Stability, and Low Back Pain: The Essential Role of the Pelvis*. New York, NY: Churchill-Livingstone, 1997:133–155.)

to within 3 degrees (64). Lines are constructed across the top of the superior vertebral segment and across the bottom of the inferior vertebral segment of a spinal scoliotic curve. Perpendicular lines are then constructed from these lines that intersect to form an angle—the Cobb angle measurement.

Interpreting AP lumbopelvic postural radiographs
The standing AP radiograph of the pelvis contains coronal and horizontal plane postural data. This film is especially important in evaluating the degree of sacral base unleveling, structural leg lengths, and pelvic rotation with the patient in a weight-bearing position; measures that are the central values influencing lift therapy in the osteopathic postural model. Roughening of the iliac crest where the iliolumbar ligament attaches or calcification of the iliolumbar ligament (see Fig. 36.8) (65) should be noted, as these are markers for postural stress.

Common measurements associated with coronal plane posture include the relatively straightforward iliac crest and femoral head

lines; horizontal lines quantifying any height asymmetry to these landmarks. The sacral base line used to report sacral base unleveling is determined in a less intuitive manner (see Fig. 36.19A and B). For clinically relevant reasons, this line is extended to the vertical lines extending from the femoral heads (4,59). The amount of sacral base unleveling is reported as the measured height difference of a line drawn across the top of the sacral base as extrapolated to its intersection with the femoral head lines. The margin of error in measuring sacral base unleveling, using this radiographic protocol, has been reported to be ±0.75 mm (57). Measurements using the different choices for landmarks (line of eburnation [see Fig. 36.19B] or the juncture of the sacral ala with either the iliac crests or the articular pillars) for identifying the sacral base are reported to have a variability of up to 2 mm (59,57). Therefore, the alternative selected should be that which has the least ambiguity or in which the set of reference points are most easily and accurately identified (34,56,66).

Because the osteopathic physician is more interested in leveling the sacral base than making the leg lengths equal, the sacral base

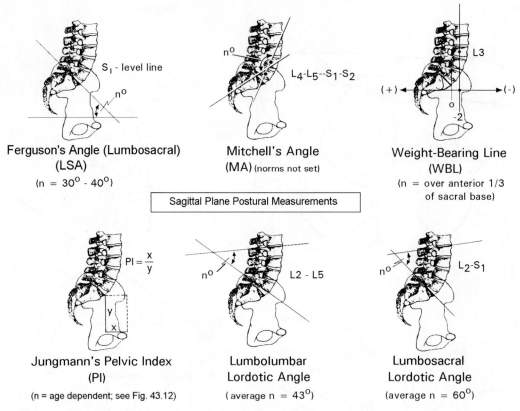

Figure 36-20 Sagittal plane standing postural radiographic measurements and their normal ranges.

unleveling is usually of more clinical significance than comparison of anatomic leg lengths. In the presence of sacral base unleveling, the direction of the lumbar side-bending component is also clinically relevant. In most cases without concomitant pelvic shear dysfunction, the iliac crest, femoral head, and sacral base unleveling measurements will be roughly equal. In larger discrepancies, however, it would appear that intrapelvic homeostatic adaptations are inadequate or overwhelmed leading to sacral base height unleveling that surpasses the difference in the femoral head heights (67).

Pelvic rotation is recognized qualitatively by observing asymmetry of the obturator foramina. It can be quantified by measuring the distance between the pubic symphysis and either the dark line representing the air in the gluteal crease or the median sacral crest (36). The pelvis is denoted to rotate in the direction in which the anterior portion of the pelvis (pubic symphysis) moves. In Fig. 36.19A, the pelvis is rotated to the left.

Interpreting lateral lumbopelvic postural radiographs

The standing lateral film of the pelvis provides a means for determining several sagittal plane postural measurements. (see Figs. 36.19C and 36.20) These include the angle of the sacral base (Ferguson angle), the weight-bearing line (WBL) from L3 relative to the sacral base, lumbar lordotic angles, and the PI. Normal values for these objective measures are summarized in Figure 36.20.

The ideal line of weight bearing (see Fig. 36.2D), previously described as running just anterior to the lateral malleolus, will be represented by a radiolucent line produced by the image of the metallic reference wire on the x-ray film. This *RL* can also be used to evaluate the approximate position of the center of gravity (body of L3) relative to the lateral malleolus of the ankle, the sacral base, and the femoral heads. The L3 WBL should ideally fall through the anterior one third of the sacral base. If this line falls posterior

to the sacral base, the lumbar facets are subject to an increased load. Especially in the case where significant stress is longstanding, the involved facets on the radiograph will exhibit arthritic change, seen as eburnation (increased density) of these articulations.

The PI is a calculated ratio that quantitatively reflects the relative position of the innominates to the sacrum (Fig. 36.21). Normal PI values are age related (40) and are typically less than 1.00. As the patient ages, this postural intrapelvic ratio approaches (or, in the same conditions, may exceed) the value of 1.00. PI has been documented to be increased in some patient populations, including athletes with high functional demand in the sagittal plane (35), patients with chronic low back pain (40), and those with L5-S1 isthmic spondylolisthesis (46). In the latter group, patients with an extremely high PI for their age should be examined for spondylolysis or spondylolisthesis. Conversely, PI has been shown to be very low for age in patient populations with L4-5 degenerative spondylolisthesis (68).

Lordotic angles are objective measurements of lumbar lordosis (Fig. 36.22) (69). The observation of hyperlordosis is significant in the evaluation of patients with sagittal plane postural problems. Some of these measurements may eventually prove to be relevant, whereas others may never add any clinical relevance. Radiographically, lumbar lordosis is often only qualitatively assessed as normal, increased, or decreased. It can be quantified however by measuring the angle created by lines along the top of L2 and S1 (*lumbosacral lordotic angle*), or the top of L2 and the bottom of L5 (*lumbolumbar lordotic angle*) (69). These angles average 60 and 43 degrees, respectively (70). A modification of the Cobb method can also be used to quantify other sagittal plane curves.

Postural radiographic summary

Abnormal static postural measurements can be viewed as being biomechanical (or functional) risk factors for a patient. Using the

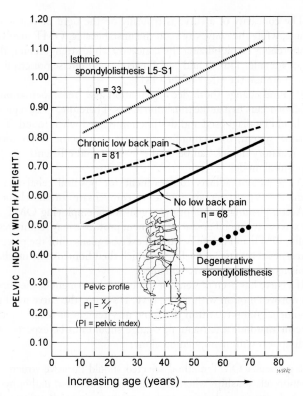

Figure 36-21 Pelvic index. (Courtesy of William Kuchera, D.O., F.A.A.O.)

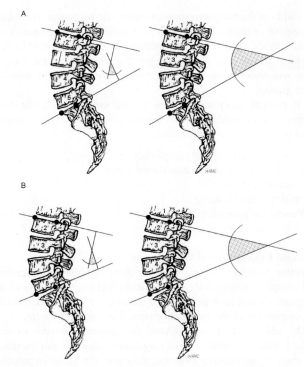

Figure 36-22 Lordotic angles of the lumbar A-P curve. **A.** Lumbosacral lordotic angle using L2 and S1 (average 60 degrees. **B.** Lumbolumbar lordotic angle using L2 and the bottom of L5 (average 43 degrees). (Courtesy of William Kuchera, D.O., F.A.A.O.)

standard radiographic protocol summarized in this chapter (58), measurements outside the normative range suggest a biomechanical disadvantage that increases functional demand. As the number of biomechanical risk factors increases, homeostatic maintenance of posture is more likely to fail. These factors not only strain musculoligamentous structures but also predispose the patient to the development of scoliosis, spondylolysis, or spondylolisthesis (71), or other postural diagnoses.

Balance Plates and Other Functional Postural Measures

Balance plates, computerized calculations of changing centers of mass during a particular activity, or even dynamic imaging procedures may also be additional quantitative measures used to understand the postural impact on structure and function. Some of these instruments can measure intersegmental as well as regional motions and are used to reinforce the palpatory determination of areas requiring manipulative treatment (hypomobile areas) and those that need strengthening exercise, prolotherapy, or extrinsic stabilization (hypermobile areas).

Correlation of static-dynamic diagnostic information within the structural-functional continuum will play a significant role in postural treatment regimens and in providing patient education concerning prognosis. Observation and palpation form the cornerstones of postural evaluation. Radiographic and computerized range-of-motion analyses provide additional or supportive information.

General Treatment Strategies

Properly designed postural care for patients with signs of GSP is often effective in ameliorating recurrent, predictable patterns of pain and dysfunction as well as relieving a wide range of secondary complaints (46,72). This is true for GSP with or without postural decompensation, and principles used to prescribe individualized treatment plans do not vary significantly regardless of which plane of posture is primarily involved.

Treating a patient with postural decompensation clearly requires appropriate diagnosis of postural structures and their functional capabilities, and the treatment plan benefits from an estimate of overall homeostatic reserves. Knowing the duration of any functional imbalance or adaptation and the amount of any postural decompensation influences both the scope of the treatment regimen and prognostic expectations. Identifying significant muscle imbalance or joint somatic dysfunction in the absence of structural group curves may prompt corresponding "functional" treatment goals that promote freer motion within an optimally balanced posture. Such imbalance and dysfunction in the presence of significant structural group curve involvement suggests adopting "structural" treatment approaches. In both cases, improved results are more likely when cumulative strategies decrease functional demand on postural structures, modify biomechanical risk factors, and allow postural homeostatic mechanisms to operate under more optimal conditions.

The prognosis for many functional care regimens is likely to be a significant reversal or resolution of signs and symptoms. Expectations for structural care, in some cases, may need to be limited to maximization of function within existing structural constraints. Likewise, realistic goals should involve attempting to slow or halt further postural decompensation in advancing curves.

Recalcitrant dysfunctions, or those that only respond transiently to traditional postural strategies, might require adjunctive treatment modalities to accomplish the goals set for care. These additional adjuncts are particularly indicated for patients who have reduced intrinsic homeostatic compensatory mechanisms; structural change due to GSP and postural decompensation (reducing the ability of the body to respond to otherwise successful treatment strategies); or those chronic back pain patients whose histories of failed surgical or medical management of concomitant arthritic, spondylolytic or disc disease suggest that their structural conditions will make it more difficult for the patient to functionally resist gravity.

If compensatory mechanisms remain overwhelmed, the following adjuncts could be combined with other conservative treatment of postural decompensation:

1. Postural education and compliance
2. OMT generally and to transitional zones
3. Postural exercise
4. Static postural bracing
5. Functional postural orthotics
6. Other miscellaneous approaches.

Postural Education and Compliance

Effective postural treatment regimens should emphasize education and compliance, especially in the initial phases of the reeducation program. Compliance is enhanced when the patient understands all components of the treatment protocol and their rationale.

In addition to other protocol components, provide to the patient sound *biomechanical and ergonomic education* emphasizing the choice of appropriate footwear, reduction of high heels, promotion of functional arches, and correction of pronation. Other useful education includes proper lifting technique and, when necessary to accomplish appropriate weight distribution, dietary counseling.

Counseling may also be helpful in modifying patients' *self-images* regarding their bodies or the choices they make affecting compliance. This is often required for successful treatment of the myofascial system. Teenage girls, for example, may slump severely because they are embarrassed about the development of their breasts. They may also not want to look taller than teenage boys who chronologically mature later. The personal attitude many teenage girls have toward their body must be changed through education about normal growth and development. Other patients need treatment of their primary psychological depression that results in a secondary postural slump. Proper postural education for the work site and other activities of daily living is also beneficial.

OMT Generally and to Transitional Zones

OMT is an integral part of care when applying the osteopathic postural model. It addresses predictable patterns of somatic dysfunction that consistently and recurrently accompany postural problems. It helps prepare the soma (muscles, joints, ligaments, and other supportive soft tissue) to better accept the positive postural change sought by postural care regimens. It addresses tensegrity issues by reducing tension and hypomobility that, if left alone, may prevent reversal of functional group curves physically or create pain in these sites (73).

In managing group curves affected by GSP or postural decompensation, several considerations exist concerning treatment of somatic dysfunction with OMT:

- The physician needs to identify and treat the cause of the curve. If the cause is functional, OMT might be used to remove that cause. Leveling the base of support by treating a unilateral pronated foot or a sacral shear somatic dysfunction in such a case would decrease the curve. If focal muscle hypertonicity has produced a curve, the muscle hypertonicity that produces the curve must be found. Causes of muscle hypertonicity are varied but if discovered and removed, the curve disappears.

- The concavity of a curve is typically on the tight or restricted side, while the convexity is on the unstable side. OMT involves stretching or mobilizing the concavity while strengthening the convex side. This should be followed by an exercise prescription to maintain the effect of the OMT.

- Postural change (both decompensation and "recompensation") often occurs first at the transition zones. Therefore, these regions should be diagnosed and dysfunction treated when found. The same system, to accomplish the first step in the respiratory-circulatory model, can be used effectively and efficiently in the postural model.

- As a patient adjusts to treatment for postural rebalancing, the spine must remain mobile to compensate for the change. Accomplishing such a primary goal while employing OMT or exercise in general postural treatment protocols may require regular OMT and carefully titrated exercise plans until the patient reaches that stage of healing in which their homeostatic mechanisms are no longer overwhelmed.

- If a curve has been present for some time, treatment of the curve improves motion within the curve. However, the curve itself or some asymmetry within the spine may remain or recur. Long-term anatomical (structural) change should not be expected to disappear with manipulation alone.

The particular OMT method selected should improve structure-function relationships where there is posture-induced pathophysiological change and do so with a minimum of side effects. In hypermobile areas, indirect method OMT is particularly useful for treating somatic dysfunction. It should be recognized that hypermobile areas may represent either primary traumatized tissue or regions of secondary compensation for other regions of restricted motion. In regions of longstanding hypomobility, direct methods, physical modalities, and stretching exercises are particularly useful. The percussion hammer technique (Fig. 36.23), as was taught by Robert Fulford, D.O., is clinically helpful in the treatment of

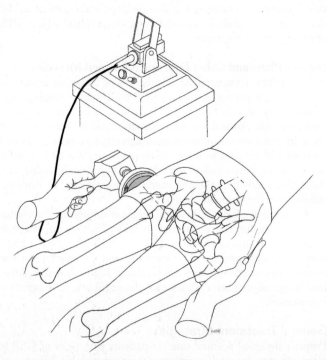

Figure 36-23 Percussion hammer technique. (Courtesy of William Kuchera, D.O., F.A.A.O.)

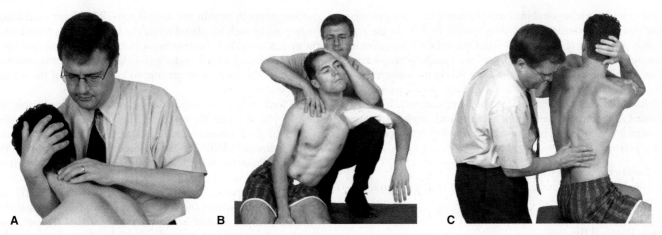

Figure 36-24   Seated OMT for postural transitional zones. (Courtesy of William Kuchera, D.O., F.A.A.O.)

some chronic postural problems (74). Examples of focused postural OMT to the transition zones are provided in Fig. 36.24 (seated) and Chapter 74 (supine).

Postural Exercise

Exercise is an often misunderstood and misused activity. The patient needs to be given a precise and realistic prescription for the goal, the dose, the frequency, and the duration of physical activities. In this manner, an exercise prescription can help the patient achieve rest, flexibility, strength, and endurance, depending on the desired goal. Specific *exercise* in postural decompensation cases should be designed first to rest, then to functionally enhance ineffective soft tissue structures, and finally to reintegrate the peripheral structures with their CNS controls.

Always consider the present status of the muscles and their ability to respond to a desired goal. In general, a person with decompensated posture requires a period of rest before exercise and compensation are effective; overly or continuously stressed or strained muscles cannot effectively be exercised until they have first

recovered (75). Thus, rest, medication, indirect OMT, and certain physical modalities may be necessary before beginning an individually designed exercise program; the appropriate exercise prescription for a patient with postural decompensation may be to *decrease* activities of daily living.

The bioenergetic cycle (76) (Fig. 36.25) describes the requirement of resting the body until it is physiologically capable of resuming its postural fight against gravity. Energy expenditure throughout each day is cyclical; sequencing is important for the efficacy of the process. Postural strain increases the expenditure in the early stages of the cycle and delays or even subverts later stages. When a person whose homeostatic reserves have been exceeded first lies down at night, it may take 30 minutes (or more) before the erector spinae and quadratus lumborum muscles relax and allow comfort in the supine position. These muscles, therefore, need to be monitored. Furthermore, reduction in both iliolumbar ligament tenderness and edema is an indicator that active postural exercises may then be effectively introduced to achieve strength, stability, and proprioceptive reeducation.

When the muscles are sufficiently recovered, certain exercise regimens are helpful for certain postural conditions. Pelvic coil exercises (77) are often beneficial for sagittal plane postural problems (Fig. 36.26). In patients with coronal plane postural decompensation, the exercises used in Konstantin, Poland, were shown to significantly improve postural alignment, but exercise in the United States was often deemed ineffective. More recently, many protocols for

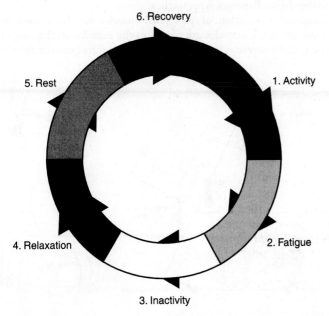

Figure 36-25   Bioenergetic model. (Modified from Jungmann M. *The Jungmann Concept and Technique of Antigravity Leverage.* Rangely, ME: Institute for Gravitational Strain Pathology, Inc., 1982. Courtesy of William Kuchera, D.O., F.A.A.O.)

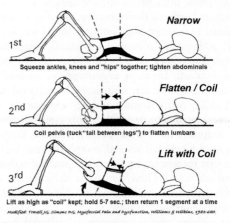

Figure 36-26   Pelvic narrow and coil exercises. (Courtesy of William Kuchera, D.O., F.A.A.O.)

trunk-specific exercises combined with correcting behavioral patterns have shown the benefits of including specific exercise in the regimens of all degrees of scoliosis (78–81). Optimally, effective postural exercise protocols include the goal of proprioceptive reeducation. Promotion of flexibility for realignment and selective strengthening for stability in hypomobile areas are goals for postural exercise.

As noted, exercise prescriptions should promote the healing of strained and injured tissues before striving to accomplish any other postural goal. Two basic rules of exercise are thereby advocated for these patients (82):

1. Avoid exercising to the point of fatigue.
2. Discontinue any exercise that causes pain until a reason for the pain is discovered.

Static Postural Bracing

Nonfunctional *braces* or *corsets* may be used as adjuncts to short-term treatment. Under certain conditions, they may be used for longer periods.

Static structural bracing has both positive and negative aspects. On the positive side, static braces promote rest and healing in a region of acute strain; they support the structure and initially reduce ligamentous and muscular functional stress. On the negative side, the muscles soon become dependent on the support provided. The longer the brace is worn, the weaker the patient's own muscles become. Static braces are therefore better for providing rest in an acute condition rather than for treating a chronic postural one.

Use of static bracing in chronic situations requires both care designed to prevent muscle atrophy and the patient's dependence on the static brace. It is therefore imperative that the physician links the patient's brace treatment with an ongoing exercise program. Ideally, to prevent weakness and physical dependency, a physician should rarely introduce a static brace without having a plan to replace it (83).

Functional Postural Orthotics

Functional postural *orthotics* are more appropriate choices than static braces for patients with chronic GSP and postural decompensation. Such devices serve to direct, guide, and/or reeducate the body, as opposed to directly taking over support. They are capable of influencing physiological parameters and reducing associated low back pain. With respect to postural realignment, this class of treatment modalities includes several specific orthotics. Functional postural orthotics discussed in this chapter include over-the-counter flexible foot supports, graduated incremental heel or sole lifts, and a custom-fitted pelvic orthotic device.

A functional orthotic device may be added to a patient's treatment regimen to enhance homeostatic postural mechanisms, prevent GSP, or increase efficacy of a postural treatment regimen. It is indicated for those patients exhibiting chronic or recurrent conditions resulting from, or aggravated by, postural strain or decompensation. Its use can realistically be expected to improve the body's ability to resist strain and decompensation by altering biomechanical alignment or assisting soft tissue structures. Concomitant symptoms such as back pain, headache, fatigue, muscle imbalance, and functional visceral complaints may be relieved in a program that incorporates a functional postural orthotic, OMT, and patient education. These symptoms alone (in the absence of the underlying postural cause) are not a sufficient indication for the use of adjunctive orthotic devices.

A foot orthotic that incorporates a unilateral heel lift adds length to one of the two lower extremities thereby leveling that base of support. This shifts the balance from side to side and affects posture primarily within the *coronal plane*. The direct mechanical impact of any such lift placed under the foot or heel is measured at the midcalcaneal line. In some ways, placing a unilateral shoe lift is similar to placing a shim under a table leg to balance the structure above it; in this case, in an attempt to level the top of the sacrum as a base of support.

A foot orthotic incorporating a unilateral anterior sole lift (usually placed under the metatarsal heads) will maximally affect posture in the *horizontal plane*. Located biomechanically anterior to the individual's WBL, an anterior sole lift will typically tip the structures above the feet backward. In this fashion, such a lift on the right will rotate the pelvis to the right.

A pelvic orthotic device, such as the Levitor (Fig. 36.27), has its greatest effect within the sagittal plane. This pelvic orthotic has been used in the United States since 1939 and is the only prescription, custom-fitted device for the pelvic base of support that is available for long-term use with chronic GSP or postural decompensation in the sagittal plane. It weighs 6 oz and is made of a high-test aluminum alloy that transfers pressure to cushioned pads; one over the superior portion of the pubic symphysis and the other on the posterior part of the sacral apex below the S2 middle transverse axis. This orthotic device was specifically designed to resist the counter-rotation of the sacrum and innominates that occur under the influence of the strain of gravity. It aids but does not replace the function of postural muscles, thereby avoiding the dependency caused by the prolonged use of static bracing.

While the mechanical design of each orthotic primarily affects one plane of motion, linked musculoskeletal biomechanics insure that all three of these examples affect postural change in all cardinal planes simultaneously (29). Treatment outcomes include improved balance mechanisms as demonstrated by changing graphic center-of-gravity plots and the reduction or reversal of lordosis, kyphosis, and scoliosis on postural radiographs (46). They also decrease low back pain, other musculoskeletal symptoms, energy demands, segmental dysfunction, and they appear to improve respiratory-circulatory functions.

Other Miscellaneous Approaches

Electrical stimulation of paraspinal muscles has been used in some centers. Electrodes are placed in the muscles on the side of the spinal convexity and are connected to a direct current from a

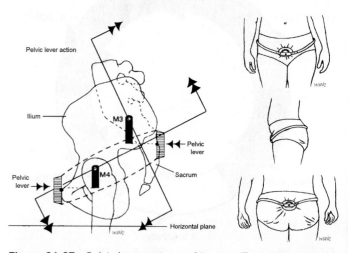

Figure 36-27 Pelvic lever action and Levitor. (From Jungmann M *The Jungmann Concept and Technique of Antigravity Leverage.* Rangely, ME: Institute for Gravitational Strain Pathology, Inc., 1982; with permission. Courtesy of William Kuchera, D.O., F.A.A.O.)

control box. An electrical current causes contraction of the muscles on the side of the convexity and is postulated to help reduce scoliotic curvature. Research suggests that, used alone, this modality is not effective in reversing scoliosis; but it is recommended by some centers as part of a unified treatment regimen to assist in muscle strengthening or pain relief.

Injection techniques using proliferative medication (*prolotherapy*) for ligamentous laxity may be employed if other conservative modalities alone fail to restore stability. Prolotherapy (sclerotherapy) consists of proliferant solution injected at a ligamentous attachment (44). When postural strain biomechanically overwhelms structural integrity, ligamentous laxity can result. Injection of a proliferant solution (such as 50% glucose) into the ligament at its fibro-osseous insertion can increase stability. Combined with exercise, OMT, and postural realignment to prevent return of musculoligamentous strain, this protocol can be an effective and conservative approach to hypermobility and ligamentous laxity (84).

When an insurmountable problem is primarily a structural one, so too is its treatment. In unstable situations, or in situations that have not responded to conservative care, surgery is a viable option to consider. In the case of severe scoliosis or highly symptomatic spondylolisthesis, this could consist of fusing vertebrae. Surgical implantation of orthopedic rods or other stabilizing apparatuses may also be required. Surgical techniques have even been successfully used to lengthen anatomically short legs.

In summary, numerous modalities are used to assist the body's postural response to gravity. An individually designed conservative program includes a carefully selected combination of patient education, OMT, exercise, and functional orthotics. All of these are aimed at modifying the structure-function relationship and enhancing the body's ability to self-heal. Therefore, postural balancing requires an understanding of the biomechanical nature and functional anatomy of each patient and a full understanding of osteopathic philosophy.

3-PLANAR POSTURAL CONSIDERATIONS: INTEGRATED POSTURAL TREATMENT OF SPECIFIC CLINICAL CONDITIONS

Coronal Plane Decompensation

Unleveling of the sacral base or a deformed vertebra resulting from a fracture or congenital deformation often leads to a compensation or adaptation that most predominantly affects the coronal plane curvatures of the spine. Motion (or lack thereof) in the coronal plane, however, is physiologically linked to that in the horizontal plane and lordosis (sagittal plane) has been specifically implicated as a destabilizing factor in the development and progression of scoliosis (85).

Occasionally, an unlevel sacral base is observed in a postural x-ray image with a straight spine above it. This requires muscular effort, resulting in spinal musculoligamentous strain that may manifest as back pain or headache. As the person grows older and the muscular compensation becomes inadequate, functional scoliosis manifests and structural scoliosis eventually develops (22).

Adaptation or decompensation in the coronal plane as measured in postural radiographic series also correlates with degenerative osteoarthritis of the hip (38), lumbar osteophytes (22,86), lumbar vertebral wedging (22), scoliotic patterns (especially where sacral base unleveling measures >10 mm) (67), and a variety of somatovisceral symptoms (34,87). This chapter will discuss the so-called short-leg syndrome as an example of a coronal plane

predominant functional condition and scoliosis as a predominantly structural condition.

Functional Considerations: "Short-Leg Syndrome"

References that attest to the existence of leg-length inequality in approximately 90% of the population have appeared in the medical literature since the latter half of the 1800s (88–90). John Hilton specifically mentioned lift therapy as a treatment for this problem in 1863: *Thus I have seen many patients wearing spinal supports, in order to correct a lateral curvature when the deformity might have and has been subsequently, corrected by placing within the shoe or boot a piece of cork thick enough to compensate for the shortness of the less well developed limb* (91).

Within the osteopathic profession, the term *short-leg syndrome* is a recognized misnomer. This text, however, will continue to refer to short-leg syndrome because of historical precedence. Regardless of the name, the cause of the condition may not be related to the actual length of the legs at all. It is called a syndrome because it is associated with a variety of related biomechanical findings and symptoms.

In the osteopathic postural model, an unlevel sacral base is the clinically relevant element in this syndrome even when the actual cause might extend all the way down to the arch of the foot or up to the cranium. Because a structural or a functional short lower extremity usually results in an unlevel sacral base, the spine that sits on that base compensates by changing its spinal curvatures. Subsequently, the person must often stand or walk differently. If the sacral base is unlevel for any reason, the innominates often rotate to compensate. This creates the appearance of a functionally short lower extremity. In either case, the most common spinal response is the development of a rotoscoliosis in which side bending of the most caudal curve is away from the side of the low sacral base, and usually on the side of the short leg. An atypical pattern in which the low sacral base is opposite the side of the low femoral head rarely does occur (67), however, and is clinically challenging to manage (Fig. 36.28).

Clinical Presentation

Compensatory measures are sometimes so good that any single landmark measurement may fail to provide a true and accurate

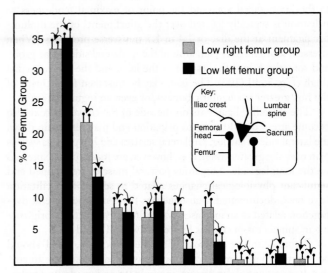

Figure 36-28 Frequency distribution of lumbosacral relationships to unlevel femoral head heights. N = 738. (From Kirksville College of Osteopathic Medicine, Kirksville, MO, with permission.)

diagnosis. Neither the alignment of spinous processes nor the level of the iliac crests (92) is a good single indicator of sacral base unleveling or short-leg syndrome. ASIS or hip-to-ankle measurements using a tape measure are also inaccurate (57,93–95). Comparison of the levels of the medial malleoli in the supine position is similarly inaccurate and potentially misleading (96,97). The greater trochanters in the standing position are somewhat more helpful clinically but can be in error when unilateral coxa varus or coxa valgus is present (98). Prevalence data and radiographic measurements definitely correlate much better than any of these clinical estimates of postural asymmetry. In one study of standing patients with known radiographic leg-length inequality, the wrong extremity was identified as being short in 13% of the clinical observations; more than half of the 196 clinical estimates of leg length were incorrect by more than 3/16 of an inch (97).

Recurrent patterns of somatic dysfunction of the pelvis, spine, cranium, or myofascial structures may also be a clue that the sacral base is unlevel or that a short leg is present. Soft tissue involvement with respect to the compensation occurring in the short-leg syndrome is particularly common throughout the entire body (tensegrity) and is a cause of many patient complaints. Tissues on the concavity shorten and demonstrate increased electromyographic activity (99,48). Tissues on the convex side lengthen. Patients with coronal plane postural imbalance develop tight abductors on one side of the pelvic sideshift and tight thigh adductors on the contralateral side. Associated horizontal plane imbalance often results in tight hamstrings on one side and tight rectus femoris muscle on the other thigh.

Coronal plane postural disorders are expected with certain combinations of static and dynamic findings such as constellations of asymmetry, recurrent somatic dysfunction, and tissue texture change. When this diagnosis is the result of leg length inequality, the standing trochanteric plane, the plane of the PSIS, and the iliac crests are usually depressed on the side of the depressed sacral base. Usually the more horizontal cephalad planes (shoulders, occipital) are also depressed to compensate for the unlevelness of the sacral base (39). The number of curvatures between the pelvis and the upper body will determine on which side the more horizontal cephalad planes are depressed in relation to the sacral base.

The iliolumbar ligament on the side of the convexity of the lumbopelvic curve is often the first structure to react to added stress in the lumbosacral area and the point of maximal tenderness to palpation is typically located over the attachments of the iliolumbar ligament at the iliac or L4 or L5 transverse processes. When stressed, it often refers pain around the ipsilateral side to the groin, and sometimes into the testicle or the labia and the upper medial thigh (Fig. 36.9) (100). The pain may be mistaken for arthritis of the hip, greater trochanteric bursitis, or even an inguinal hernia.

The sacroiliac ligaments on the side of the convexity may also become stressed and tender to palpation and may refer pain down the lateral side of the leg. Unilateral sciatica and hip pain, as well as pain over the greater trochanter, however, are more often expressed on the long leg side. Numerous postural muscles are strained and significant physiological changes related to segmental facilitation have been documented. Subsequently, there may be visceral dysfunction related to an increased sympathetic hyperactivity originating in spinal crossover areas located between T1 and L2.

Before definitive diagnosis of a patient's posture, OMT should be directed to all somatic dysfunction with particular care to correct dysfunctions of the sacrum, innominate, and quadratus lumborum. After OMT, the demonstration of a positive standing flexion test coexisting with a negative seated flexion test should raise the suspicion that lower extremity influences, such as a short lower extremity, are affecting the function of the sacroiliac joint and the patient's posture (101).

In problematic cases, it may be helpful to obtain a standard standing postural x-ray series. After first removing the patient's somatic dysfunction, this x-ray series primarily portrays structural data associated with the best homeostatic compensation possible by the patient at the time. These standardized standing postural x-ray images can then be used to measure coronal plane values accurately, including the heights of the iliac crest, femoral heads, and sacral base as extrapolated over the femoral heads. The radiographic series will also provide quantitative measures of the degree, location, and type of scoliotic compensatory curvatures as well as any congenital or acquired bony anomalies.

When reading the x-ray image (Fig. 36.29) obtained by standard methods, remember that there is still potentially a 2-mm human error in measurement. This can occur even with flawless technique by the radiologic technician and perfect patient cooperation. The further from the exposed radiographic film, the greater the x-ray diversion meaning there can be up to a 25% bony magnification (distortion) for structures furthest away from the film (39,102). Nonetheless, repeat studies on leg length inequality of 108 subjects found 85% with less than a 1.5-mm difference in measurement and 10% with less than a 3-mm difference; in only three subjects did the repeat study differ as much as 5 mm (38).

Compensatory changes such as innominate rotations, pelvic rotation, and changes in the LSA might alter the x-ray appearance, which can misrepresent the extent of the patient's actual problem. For these reasons, a leg length difference of <5 mm might not be treated unless the patient has other clinically relevant complaints and risk factors. Conversely, the desire to attain "peak physical performance" or to prevent long-term sequelae such as osteoarthritis of the hip (107) might be an indication to treat a patient in this case. Patterns of imbalance recorded along the spine may be caused by as little as a 1/16 of an inch (1.5 mm) difference in leg length. Clinical symptoms can occur in these cases, including low back pain (103,104).

Treatment Considerations

Typically, treatment of the so-called short-leg syndrome involves lifting the heel of the leg on the side of the depressed sacral base. This is especially true if there is a compensatory curvature that side bends to the side opposite the short leg. In the rare situation where the curve has its concavity toward the side of the short leg, it may be necessary to begin by lifting the side of the long leg. This first effects a change in the lumbar scoliosis and also relieves some of the pelvic and lumbar strain (105). The lift on the long leg side is later reduced to begin lifting the depressed side of the unlevel sacral base.

Heel lift treatment using the osteopathic postural model is always combined with OMT and is usually not attempted until after an appropriate OMT trial. The rationale for both was clearly implied by Harrison Fryette: *In the average case I do not attempt a correction until I have mobilized the lumbar joints and established rotation in them; furthermore, if this region cannot be rotated toward the midline, the lift will not do what it is intended of it, for the correction will not take place in the lumbar region—the spine higher up will compensate by increasing its curve and only more trouble will result* (106).

OMT may alleviate a functional condition that manifests as an apparent short-leg syndrome. In the situation in which lift therapy is indicated, OMT prepares the somatic tissues to accept the realignment needed to respond to the newly established sacral base level.

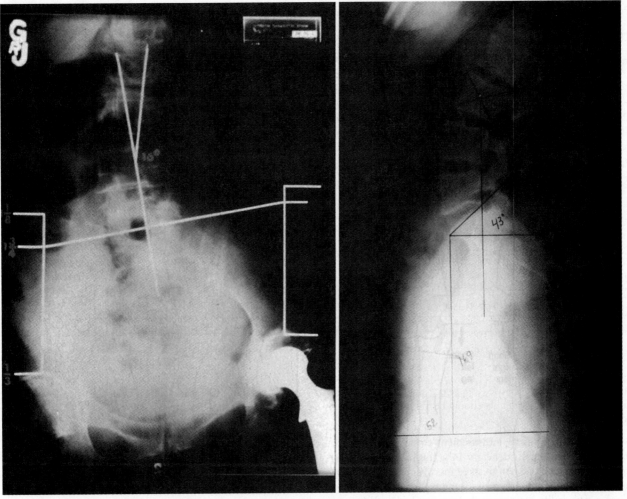

Figure 36-29 X-ray image marked for coronal **(A)** and horizontal **(B)** plane measurements. Ideal values would be no side-to-side unleveling of any of these landmarks and no pelvic rotation.

Whenever lift therapy is initiated, consider the implications of postural realignment and reeducation that must take place throughout the entire body. For many reasons, the initial amount of lift selected is rarely the full amount needed. In most cases, compensation, adaptation, and decompensation have occurred over a period of time, leading to shortening and fibrosis of soft tissues, bony remodeling, and regional somatic dysfunction. The easiest but least sensitive guideline used by clinicians is to select an initial lift that is one third to one half of the measured sacral base difference.

Attempts to formulate specific guidelines to better quantify the amount of lift are best appreciated by studying the writings of David Heilig, D.O., F.A.A.O. (107). Heilig found that one third to one half of the measured sacral base unleveling was too much initial lift in selected clinical situations. He developed a formula (Table 36.6) that considered the amount of lift to be directly proportional to the measured sacral base unleveling and inversely proportional to host factors such as the age, duration of the condition, and amount of compensation or adaptation acquired by the body. Heilig offered examples of patients who all had a 1/2-in sacral base unleveling but who, based on the formula, would receive different initial lifts.

One of the safest protocols taught at many of the colleges of osteopathic medicine is less complicated than the Heilig formula

yet sensitive to individual host factors. It employs a conservative "rule of thumb" that can later be modified by clinical experience and judgment. This protocol is designed to avoid any unexpected flare-ups of pain or somatic dysfunction that can occur if lift therapy is introduced too rapidly or if it exceeds the capability of the body to realign in response to the changes occurring in the sacral base level.

The following are only guidelines for the application of conservative lift treatment and must be adapted to each patient according to their individual evaluation and response (108):

- If lift therapy is required and if the patient is considered to be a "fragile" patient (arthritic, osteoporotic, elderly, having significant acute pain, etc.), begin with a 1/16-in lift and lift no faster than 1/16 of an inch every 2 weeks.
- If the spine is flexible and no more than mild-to-moderate strain is noted in the myofascial system, begin with a 1/8-in lift and lift at a rate no faster than 1/16 of an inch per week, or 1/8 of an inch every 2 weeks.
- If there was a recent and sudden loss of leg length on one side, as might occur following fracture or a recent hip prosthesis, and the patient had a level sacral base before the fracture or surgery, lift the full amount that was lost.

TABLE 36.6

The Heilig Formula and Patients with Same Sacral Base Leveling but Receiving Different Lifts

The Heilig formula suggests that the initial lift can be calculated as follows:

$L < [SBU]/[D + C]$

L, lift required; SBU, sacral base unleveling; D, duration; C, compensation.

Duration allotted as: (D = 1), 0–10 y; (D = 2), 10–30 y; (D = 3), 30+ y. Compensation allotted as: (C = 0), none observed; (C = 1), rotation of lumbar vertebrae into convexity of compensatory side bending; (C = 2), wedging of the vertebrae, altered size of facets, horizontal osseous developments from endplates, and/or spurring.

Patients With Same Sacral Base Leveling But Receiving Different Lifts

Case 1: Following fracture, minimal duration, no compensatory changes

$L = [SBU]/[D + C] = 1/2''/[0 + 1] = 1/2''$

Case 2: Patient age 35, injured in early youth, minimal compensation

$L = [SBU]/[D + C] = 1/2''/[2 + 1] = 1/2''/3 = 1/6''$

Case 3: Patient age 75, injured in youth, spurring, horizontal endplate development, rotation is marked

$L = [SBU]/[D + C] = 1/2''/[3 + 2] = 1/2''/5 = 1/10''$

Case 4: Patient age 26, polio affecting right leg in youth, minimal compensatory change

$L = [SBU]/[D + C] = 1/2''/[2 + 0] = 1/2''/2 = 1/4''$

Regardless of the method used to select the amount of the initial lift, certain other guidelines should be followed for optimum clinical results:

■ Because of magnification, measurement error, and compensatory changes, the final lift height in a chronic short-leg syndrome may only be one half to three fourths of the shortness in that leg measured by the standard standing x-ray method.

■ When a proper lift has eventually been reached and there are no pelvic or lower extremity somatic dysfunctions, the former positive standing flexion test should become negative. If a repeat x-ray image is desired, it should be taken using the same radiographic protocol and parameters that were used in the initial x-ray series, but with the shoes on and the lift in place.

Guidelines used in lift treatment are not absolute rules. One aspect of the art of medicine is an appreciation of the concerns that patients have about cost, cosmetic appearance, and convenience. Ideally, the shoe is rebuilt with every increment of lift to prevent alteration of foot mechanics and introduction of unwanted pelvic rotation. Few patients, however, would agree with this approach. The following guidelines, which emphasize clinical tolerances, can be pragmatically used in lift treatment. If problems arise, reducing the tolerances or insisting on continuing to the ideal lift may be necessary:

■ The true height of a lift is measured from the bottom of the lift to a point where the calcaneal bone strikes the lift; it is not measured at the posterior edge of the lift.

■ Up to and including 1/4-in of replaceable lift can be used inside of the shoe before the shoe no longer fits well.

■ Up to and including a total of a 1/2-in lift can be placed between the heel of the patient's foot and the floor before foot mechanics are significantly disturbed.

■ As a heel is progressively lifted, there is an increased tendency toward pelvic rotation, muscle imbalance, and alteration of foot mechanics.

Application of these principles to change the relative leg length by 1/2 in may result in:

■ 1/4-in lift being placed inside the shoe and 1/4 in added to the heel of that shoe

■ 1/2 in added to the heel of one shoe

■ 1/4 in added to one sole and 1/4 in removed from the opposite sole (108,109).

Many other combinations exist within these general guidelines, permitting the osteopathic practitioner the latitude to balance nonphysical factors (such as vanity and cost) with those related to posture.

Any increase in height beyond the 1/2-inch heel lift must be added to the heel and also to the anterior half-sole of the shoe (Fig. 36.30). This principle preserves the relationship of the heel to the forefoot by maintaining a certain normal angle.

Studies (34,104) indicate that an 80% reduction in subjective pain and other posture-related symptoms (including the degree of functional scoliosis) could be expected as a result of properly balancing the sacral base with lift therapy to within 1 mm of levelness.

Balancing the weight of both shoes might by desirable, especially if large lifts are required. If a big lift is needed, placing cork material between the shoe and the heel might be necessary to reduce the weight being added to one side. In some cases, small lead weights might be added to the other shoe to help maintain balance.

OMT helps the patient's spine to adapt to the functional changes required by the new postures as seen in progressive lift therapy for a short leg.

Compressive force makes bone grow faster. A lift under a growing child's foot may be expected to stimulate faster growth in the epiphyseal plates of that lower extremity. The physician must therefore closely monitor leg lengths when using lift therapy for a child. The height of the lift must be adjusted according to clinical responses and the results observed on follow-up x-ray studies.

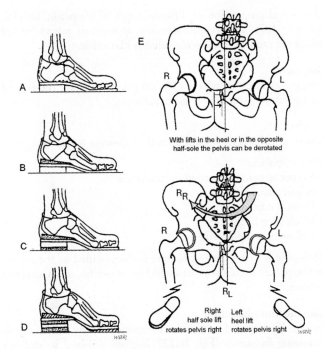

Figure 36-30 Principles of lift therapy. Heel lift measurements made at midcalcaneal line. **A.** Foot in a typical shoe. **B.** Heel lift in place. Maximum lift in shoe is 1/4 in. **C.** If more lift is needed, add to outside heel. **D.** If more than 1/2 in is required, or to create minimal disturbance of foot mechanics, the entire sole can be lifted. (Courtesy of William Kuchera, D.O, F.A.A.O.)

With lifts in the heel or in the opposite half-sole the pelvis can be derotated

Right half sole lift rotates pelvis right   Left heel lift rotates pelvis right

In growing athletes, alternating lower extremity growth parameters have been reported (107), and have prompted the clinical recommendation to check the pelvic and extremity levels at regular intervals. Fryette even remarked: "*In the last 15 years I have added lifts to the short side in many cases under the age of fourteen and in every case that I have kept under my observation for some time I have been astonished to find that the legs grew to the same length*" (110).

Structural/Pathological Considerations: Scoliosis

Scoliosis and rotoscoliosis are postural diagnoses with origins dating back to ancient Greece. Today, ten in every 200 children (10:200) develop scoliosis by the age of 10 to 15 years; 1 in every 200 (1:200) has clinical symptoms related to the curvatures. Boys and girls are equally affected, but the curvatures in girls are three to five times more likely to progress and produce subjective symptoms.

Curvatures are more likely to progress during times of rapid bone growth. Therefore, most cases (75% to 90%) of scoliosis in children are discovered—in part because of widespread screening programs—between the ages of 10 and 15 years.

Clinical Presentation

Scoliosis primarily affects the coronal plane. It is officially named according to the direction of the convexity of its curve. A curve that is side bent to the left is called a *right scoliosis* because the convexity of the curve is toward the right.

Symptoms and Screening

Children and adolescents with scoliosis are often asymptomatic and their scoliosis can go undiscovered. They, or a parent, may have only noticed that clothing does not fit properly. Therefore, school children and teens should be routinely screened for scoliosis between the ages of 10 to 15 years when they are experiencing rapid bone growth.

As the person gets older, several symptoms may bring the scoliotic patient to the physician. These include:

- Arthritic symptoms
- Backaches
- Chest pains
- Neck aches
- Headaches
- Symptoms of organ dysfunction

Physicians only casually looking for scoliosis may miss a curve of up to 35 degrees; careful screening with a physical examination alone however should pick up the majority of scoliosis more than 10 degrees.

As previously described, in the standing position, the space around the patient's body is analyzed, especially in the arm and waist area. Observe whether one hand hangs lower than the other or whether one hangs by the side while the other hand lies on or over the thigh. Look at the levelness of the occipital, shoulder, iliac crest, PSIS, and trochanteric planes (see Fig. 36.12). Run your fingers along the spinous processes from top to bottom. Have the patient forward bend and observe for an asymmetric "hump" along the horizon of vision. Its presence would indicate rotoscoliotic deformity with rotation to that side and side bending of the spine to the side opposite the hump.

If spinal curvature is found, have the patient bend over to that area of the spine and determine if the asymmetry goes away with side bending toward the side of the rib hump (see Fig. 36.13). Check the patient for conditions that could give the appearance of a short leg, such as sacral shear somatic dysfunction on that side. If you find somatic dysfunction, it can be corrected with manipulation. Recheck following OMT for lower extremity induced postural problems.

If the scoliotic curve remains, provide OMT until there is an adequate mobilization of the spine and then obtain a standardized standing postural x-ray image. The x-ray image provides the quantitative data to determine:

- Bony pathology
- Type and severity of spinal curvatures
- Amount of sacral base unleveling
- Femoral head and iliac crest levelness

Scoliosis may be classified by its reversibility, severity, cause, or location.

Classification: Reversibility

Scoliosis can be functional or structural. A simple physical examination technique used to assess the proportion of functional to structural scoliosis can be accomplished by standing behind a patient (Fig. 36.13B). The patient bends forward until maximal rib hump appears on horizon. With that much of the body forward bending, the patient swings the upper body, first left and then right, while the clinician observes the functional ability of the rib hump to lessen in degree. The amount of rib hump remaining during this maneuver indicates the associated structural scoliotic component. Functional scoliotic curves go away with side bending, rotation, or forward bending. If functional curves remain in the body too long, they may become structural (111). Structural scoliotic curves are fixed curves that do not reduce with side bending, rotation, or lift therapy.

Classification: Severity

Scoliotic curvatures are commonly and accurately measured from postural radiographs using the Cobb method (64) (see Fig. 36.18). The same vertebrae used to define the top and the bottom of the curve are used for future Cobb measurements to see if the curve is progressing. Scoliosis often increases rapidly during the growth spurt of adolescence. Take an x-ray image of the hands, iliac crests, or other epiphyses and obtain a bone age for those patients who have significant scoliotic progression. For females, the scoliosis is more likely to undergo a rapid progression. Significant progression of the curve is considered to be occurring if, on a second standardized postural x-ray taken within 5 months of the first one, there is a 5-degree or greater increase in the curvature.

The Cobb method is used to classify scoliosis as mild, modest, or severe (Fig. 36.31). The normal case shows no scoliosis. A curve of 5 to 15 degrees is assigned a mild severity classification. Moderate scoliosis curves measure 20 to 45 degrees. Severe scoliosis has a curve of more than 50 degrees and can be expected to affect both structure and systemic function. A thoracic curve of more than 50 degrees significantly compromises respiratory function; more than 75 degrees seriously compromises cardiovascular function. The effect on these two systems is inversely proportional to the degree of scoliosis and even mild curves impact exercise capacity (80).

Classification: Etiology

The following causes are listed according to decreasing frequency.

Idiopathic

This diagnosis accounts for 70% to 90% of scoliotic curves. By definition, the term *idiopathic* implies that there is no known reason for this type of scoliosis to occur. Osteopathic physicians believe that some of these may be explained as being compensatory curves that manifest as a response to an unlevel sacral (105) or cranial base (106). In cases where a biomechanical basis exists for the development of scoliosis, a diagnosis of an idiopathic scoliosis is erroneous. Other clinicians have implicated sagittal plane biomechanics in the genesis and progression of different types of idiopathic scoliotic patterns (107). Better understanding of scoliosis might further reduce the number of cases classified as idiopathic.

Congenital

Congenital cases, of which 75% are progressive, are the second most common associated cause of scoliosis.

Acquired

Acquired scoliosis may result from the following conditions:

- Osteomalacia
- Response to inflammation or irradiation
- Sciatic irritability
- Psoas syndrome
- Healed leg fracture
- Following a hip prosthesis

Obviously, if a short-leg syndrome is documented as the reason for the patient's scoliosis, this should be reclassified as an acquired scoliosis.

Classification: Location

Various locations of scoliosis are reported below according to decreasing frequency (Fig. 36.32). Regions involved in scoliosis may be balanced or unbalanced. Unbalanced curves are more likely to decompensate, while balanced curves are subject to degeneration at crossovers.

Double major scoliosis

These are balanced curves but they are subject to degeneration at the crossover regions of the spine (see Glossary at the end of the textbook). This is the most common scoliosis, with a thoracic and lumbar combination being the most frequent.

Single thoracic scoliosis

Cosmetically, this curve is rather noticeable. It is usually side bent right and rotated left, producing a left paraspinal rib hump.

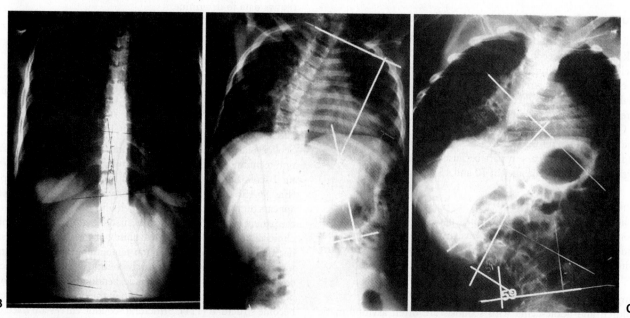

A,B   C

Figure 36-31 Curve patterns in idiopathic scoliosis. **A.** Mild (14 and 15 degrees). **B.** Moderate (38 degrees). **C.** Severe (59 and 85 degrees). Assessment of scoliotic severity defined by Cobb angle measurements for each portion of coronal plane curve. Classification system quoted allows a 5-degree gray zone between severity classes.

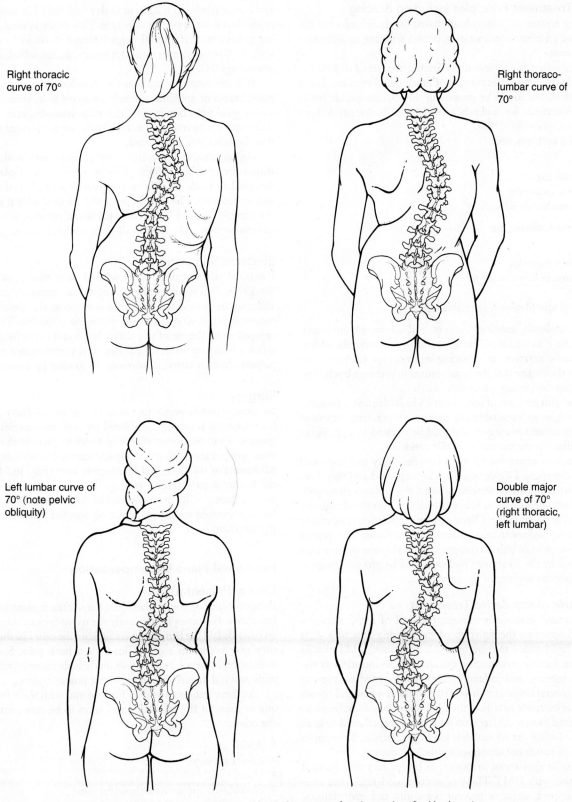

Right thoracic
curve of 70°

Right thoraco-
lumbar curve of
70°

Left lumbar curve of
70° (note pelvic
obliquity)

Double major
curve of 70°
(right thoracic,
left lumbar)

Figure 36-32 Curve patterns in idiopathic types of scoliosis classified by location.

If this type of curve should progress, it could compromise the function of the heart or lungs. It is the second most common scoliosis.

Single lumbar scoliosis
This curve is associated with arthritic change. It is the third most common scoliosis.

Junctional thoracolumbar scoliosis
This single curve scoliosis often results in structural (arthritic) change because it tends to be a longer curve that functionally overstresses the spine. It is not a common scoliosis.

Junctional cervicothoracic scoliosis
This scoliosis is very uncommon.

General Treatment Principles Including Bracing

Appropriate treatment protocols are based on classification of the scoliosis and take into consideration factors affecting an individual's compliance.

While a systematic review of the limited number of clinical trials concludes that the "effectiveness of bracing and exercises is not yet established, but might be promising" (112), osteopathic treatment considerations for scoliosis according to its severity follows these general guidelines (108).

For **mild scoliosis**, use:

- OMT
- Konstantin exercises
- Functional orthotics
- Patient and family education

For **moderate scoliosis**, use:

- OMT
- Konstantin exercises
- Patient and family education
- Bracing
- (Electrical stimulation—debatable efficacy)

For **severe scoliosis**, consider surgery and adjunctive measures, including those listed for moderate scoliosis. Adjunctively adding patient-specific exercises to a bracing regimen, for example, may help reduce the degree that the spine returns to prebrace levels after discontinuing the bracing procedure (113).

Anyone with scoliosis of more than 15 to 20 degrees, a progressive curvature, or an intractable low back pain that is irresponsive of conservative treatment measures, should be referred to a physician who specializes in the treatment of this condition.

The goals of treatment are to obtain flexibility and improved balance of the spine. Decide what can be improved and then correct the primary cause or at least prevent the scoliosis from progressing. Postpone fusions as long as possible without endangering function or the patient's life. Osteopathic manipulation is a definite part of the management of a patient with scoliosis. The person with scoliosis must be able to compensate for the new posture that is introduced by the treatment methods used to prevent progression or reduce the severity of the curvatures.

Osteopathic Manipulative Treatment

When structural scoliosis is present, the goal of direct manipulation is to optimize the function of the existing structure. It is not primarily intended to straighten the curvatures. OMT should remove joint somatic dysfunction but should also include soft tissue, fascial releases, and indirect treatments designed to improve the body's general range of motion. Stretch the lumbosacral tissues and institute exercises to reduce the LSA and strengthen the psoas and abdominal muscles. After structural strains are allowed to heal, introduce a formal set of scoliosis exercises (such as Konstantin [64]) and self-treatment strategies for the soft tissues.

Orthopedic appliances, orthotics, or braces may also be used in conjunction with OMT. These adjunctive modalities were conceived to support, align, or prevent deformity and may stabilize function of a hypermobile part of the body. Braces are more effective if the scoliosis is moderate, if the spine is mobile, and if the spine still has not fully matured.

Braces

The Milwaukee brace (Fig. 36.33A) was introduced in 1945 and has been the standard for scoliosis bracing for many years. It is individually fitted and easy to prescribe, but it is also hard to wear and is costly. It is worn 23 hours a day with only 1 hour allowed out of the brace for applying skin care. This brace is used in a growing patient with 20- to 40-degree curves. It works to control the scoliotic (lateral) curves until the spine matures, which is generally around age 21.

It is necessary to exercise the muscles that are supported by static braces or appliances. Studies suggest that, even for patients with a good reduction in the Cobb measurements, after a few years their curves return to approximately the extent present at the time that the brace was introduced.

An alternative brace for some patients with scoliosis is the Boston brace (Fig. 36.33B). This brace is made of plastic and is designed to work on deformities such as lordosis and rotation as well as scoliosis. The Boston brace can be used only if the apex of the curve is below T10. In these particular patients, it is helpful in addressing postural curves in all three cardinal planes.

Electrical Stimulation

Electrical stimulation was introduced as a treatment option in the 1970s. It was originally applied to the convexity of the curve and may be considered when the curve is in the thoracic region, measures 10 to 40 degrees, and the spine is flexible. This concept enjoyed some degree of popularity but is not often used today; its efficacy being up for debate. If electrical stimulation is applied to a patient's lumbar curve, it increases the lumbar lordosis.

Surgery

Surgical fusion is performed only in one out of every 1,000 scoliosis cases. It is usually considered for scoliosis patients with progressive 45 to 50 degree curves in order to prevent the heart and lung complications that accompany curvatures >50 degrees. The placement of stainless steel Harrington rods (Fig. 36.34) and spinal fusion is an extensive surgery. The mechanical power of the body is dramatically demonstrated by the propensity of the rods to become stressed and break, requiring another extensive surgery to replace them.

Horizontal Plane Decompensation

Clinical Presentation

Patients with horizontal plane problems often present with muscle imbalance. For example, frequently the rectus femoris muscle is tight on one side and the hamstrings are tight on the other. In this situation, they may complain more of knee than back pain. Such muscle imbalance, however, leads to a similarly wide range of symptoms as with postural disturbance in any other postural plane.

As these patients stand in front of you with their feet aligned, one or more of the following may seem to be more anterior than the other:

- ASIS
- Lower rib cage
- Hand
- Shoulder at the acromioclavicular joint
- Mastoid process

In compensated patients, the anterior component will alternate in sequential transition zones. Those with decompensation are more likely to be symptomatic because as they walk they are less capable of positioning one region of the body in line with the region above or below.

Posture in the horizontal plane is linked directly to that in the coronal plane. Interestingly, in use of orthotic devices to modify the

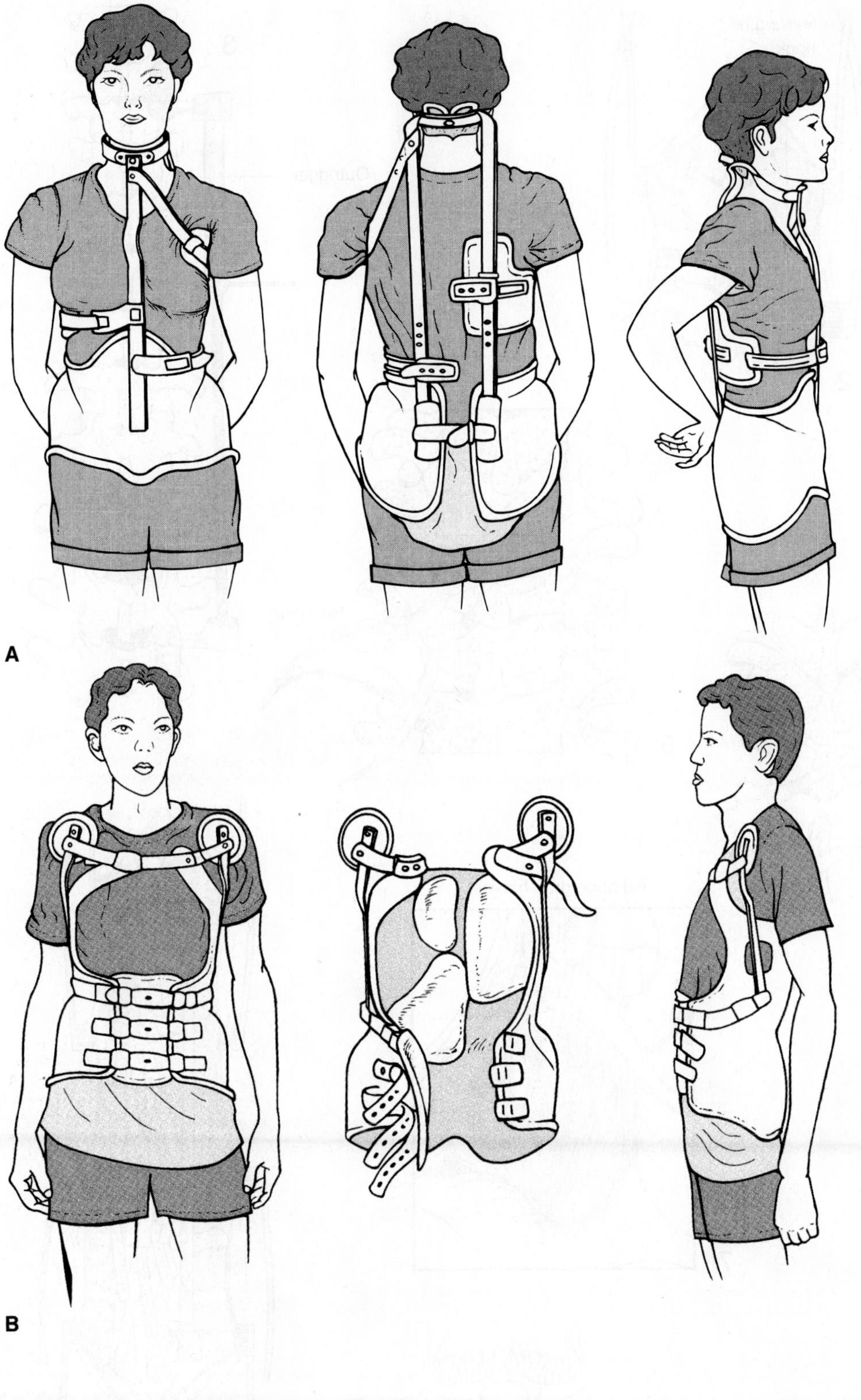

Figure 36-33 A. Milwaukee brace.
B. Boston brace.

other cardinal planes, the horizontal plane seems to be the second most affected. For example:

- Heel lift effects: coronal → horizontal → sagittal
- Levitor effects: sagittal → horizontal → coronal

Treatment Considerations—Functional Conditions

The functional orthotic best suited to modify posture in the horizontal plane is the anterior sole lift. The clinical use of anterior sole lifts (in distinction from heel lifts) or the combination of an anterior lift in one shoe and/or a heel lift in the opposite shoe to affect posture in the horizontal plane has largely been explored by osteopathic physicians, Ross Pope and James Carlson (114). An increase in the sole height of a shoe encourages rotation of the pelvis toward that same side. A unilateral heel lift rotates the pelvis to a lesser degree and rotates it away from the lifted side (108). Because this method is relatively new, few clinical trials have been performed. The predominance of clinical experience, however,

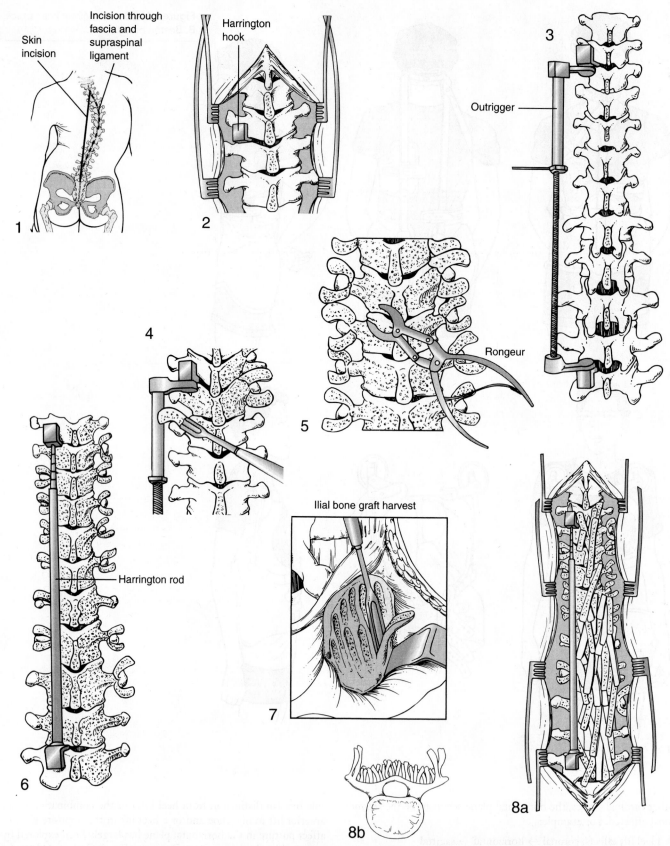

Figure 36-34   Surgical fusion with Harrington rod implantation. This extensive surgery is reserved for patients with curves >45 degrees. A major clinical goal is to stop structural progression of a curve before it seriously compromises cardiopulmonary function.

suggests the following guidelines, which are adapted to each individual patient's evaluation and response.

Anterior lift therapy rotates the pelvis toward the same side; heel lifts may rotate the pelvis away from the lift side. Treatment of both planes simultaneously is often warranted, as side bending and rotation are biomechanically linked motions. A heel lift pushes that side of the pelvis anteriorly in the horizontal plane because the lift is behind the axis of motion (i.e., rotates the pelvis away from the side of the heel lift). Anterior sole lifts create their effect anterior to the axis causing that side of the pelvis to rotate posteriorly in the horizontal plane (i.e., rotate the pelvis toward the side of the sole lift) (see Fig. 36.30).

In the treatment of pelvic rotation assuming coexistent sacral base unleveling, follow these principles:

For pelvic rotation <5 mm: Usually it is not necessary to treat a pelvic rotation <5 mm. However, if the sacral base unleveling is treated with heel lifts, this should be done according to the principles outlined for coronal plane postural balancing. Recheck to determine if any unwanted pelvic rotation occurs secondary to the heel lift therapy.

For pelvic rotation of 5 to 10 mm: For pelvic rotation of 5 to 10 mm, both sacral base (coronal plane) and rotational (horizontal plane) components are treated simultaneously. Begin with appropriate 1/8-inch anterior and heel lifts, progressively increasing in 1/8-in increments every 2 weeks.

For pelvic rotation > 10 mm: Pelvic rotations more than 10 mm should first be treated with an anterior (sole) lift of 1/4 in, and the postural study then rechecked before attempting heel lifts. Thereafter, sacral base unleveling and pelvic rotation are treated simultaneously with 1/8-in incremental changes in anterior (sole) and heel lifts every 2 weeks.

Treatment Considerations—Structural/ Pathological Conditions

Rotoscoliosis: See coronal plane structural conditions mentioned earlier.

Sagittal Plane Decompensation

Functional Considerations: Kyphotic/Lordotic Curves

In 1934 Ferguson noted, *Our spines were developed for the four-footed position and are not yet adapted to the erect, so mechanical weakness at the lumbosacral area is usual rather than exceptional. We must consider the lumbosacral area, not as normal or abnormal, but as mechanically sound or mechanically unsound* (115).

Clinical Presentation

Posture-related disorders in the sagittal plane include those defined by the degree of their lordotic and kyphotic curves; those defined by their distinctive pattern of somatic dysfunctions including muscle imbalance and trigger points; and those with related structural or pathological change such as lordosis, kyphosis, or isthmic L5-S1 spondylolisthesis.

Decompensation in predisposed individuals can occur simply by changing the height of the heels in the shoes worn daily or the number of hours spent on a certain type of flooring. Pregnancy, with progressive shifts in regional centers-of-gravity combined with circulating hormonal change (including relaxin), may lead to self-limited sagittal plane decompensation that reverses postpartum, or a more permanent postural condition can be traced back historically to that event.

As with any spectrum ranging from functional to structural disorders, there can be a great deal of overlap in diagnostic findings and treatment strategies. Each relies upon the biomechanical principles discussed in the earlier sections of this chapter. Often, treatment focuses on modifying the underlying functional disorders that aggravated or precipitated the eventual structural changes that define the structural, codable diagnosis.

Often, patients with exaggerated sagittal plane postural decompensation will present with bilaterally tender ILL and a history of recurrent psoas syndrome. They frequently have Barbor's so-called theatre-cocktail party syndrome (116) and, when asked, will tell you that their backs take a significant amount of time to relax after they lie down to rest. They may give a history of recurrent or chronic low back pain, headaches, and other bilateral signs and symptoms of GSP.

Treatment Considerations

Treatment for functional sagittal plane disorders incorporates the same general postural principles as in the other cardinal planes. There are specific recommendations however for the certain aspects of patient education, exercise, and manipulative components.

Patients with increased sagittal plane curves need to be told to avoid heels that exceed more than 1/2 in on their shoes; they may even benefit from a reverse heel. Sleeping on their stomach should be discouraged; sleeping on their sides with a pillow between their knees helps to reduce and relax overused quadratus lumborum muscles. It is particularly useful to advise this group of patients to sit upright with both feet on the floor directly below their knees. A normal lordotic curve should also be maintained at all times; slumping in an easy chair with prolonged bilateral shortening of the psoas muscles should be avoided. When standing in one spot for a prolonged period of time, a small step placed underneath one foot often provides stress relief on the low back.

An ideal exercise for patients with functional or structural sagittal plane problems is the *pelvic narrow-and-coil exercise.* (See Fig. 36.26). Alternatively, the patient can be encouraged to tilt their pelvis in the upright position against a door jamb.

A variety of OMT strategies are appropriate in addressing individuals who have sagittal plane postural decompensation. In addition to treatment of the transitional areas that is a part of every postural model treatment, specific sagittal plane care in the lumbosacral region includes techniques such as the "frog" mobilization for sacral nutation or lumbar hyperlordosis (Fig. 36.35).

Structural/Pathological Conditions: Kyphosis, Lordosis, and Spondylolisthesis

The treatment of pathologic change in the sagittal plane, including lordosis, kyphosis, and isthmic and dysplastic spondylolisthesis builds upon the treatment used for functional sagittal plane problems.

Dysplastic and Isthmic Spondylolistheses

Spondylolisthesis, which is often mistaken to be solely a congenital abnormality, is frequently and incorrectly treated as a single entity; rather, it is a structural outcome of several different processes, each with their own biomechanical and pathophysiological risks (see Table 36.7). Postural care is most beneficial in the case of the dysplastic and isthmic types and the remainder of this chapter will focus on isthmic L5-S1 spondylolisthesis as a bony structural change often initiated by stress occurring predominantly in the sagittal plane (46). This functional stress progresses through the previously described chronic, progression of compensation,

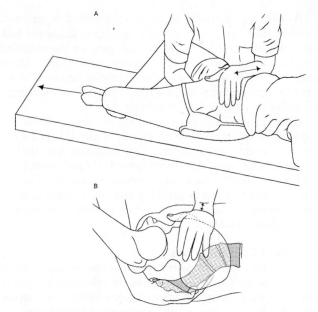

Figure 36-35 Treatment of pelvis. (Courtesy of William Kuchera, D.O., F.A.A.O.)

adaptation, decompensation leading to pathological spondylo*lysis*, and finally spondylolisthesis. In the osteopathic postural model, treatment is directed less to these acquired bony structural changes than to reducing functional demands placed on musculoligamentous structures ill-equipped to resist continued postural stresses in the region.

Background

The biomechanical principles of diagnosis and treatment of patients with sagittal plane postural problems can be directly applied to the management of patients with spondylolisthesis. The generic term *spondylolisthesis* is derived from the Greek roots roughly meaning *vertebra sliding down a slippery path*. It describes the common finding of a group of spinal disorders in which there is a forward displacement of one vertebra over another, usually the fifth lumbar over the body of the first sacral segment.

With the advent of modern radiology, the study of spondylolisthesis began, including its true incidence, location, classification, and significance. The classification of spondylolisthesis subsequently evolved into the currently accepted causal categories delineated by Wiltse et al. (117) shown in Table 36.7.

Regardless of specific hereditary and developmental factors, spondylolisthesis refers to a group of disorders having a particular common mechanical consequence. Applying the mechanical perspective permits better understanding of the general symptom complex. Applying mechanical treatment protocols provides the rational basis for osteopathic conservative management of patients diagnosed as having spondylolisthesis.

Causes: Hereditary Predisposition

Two observations argue against a person having a direct inheritance of spondylolisthesis. First, although there is an increased incidence of spondylolisthesis within family groups (118,119), a significant number of these family members exhibit different types of spondylolisthesis. Second, infants are rarely reported to have spondylolysis (also known as *prespondylolisthesis*). The incidence increases after children assume an active upright position and continues up until age 20, when it matches the 5% incidence of the general population (120).

The genetic link appears to be more likely involved in those factors that predispose the region to instability. Posterior defects such as spina bifida occulta and open sacrum are almost invariably inherited in dysplastic spondylolisthesis and in a third of patients with the isthmic type (120). This lack of posterior support may concentrate postural weight-bearing forces in the area, resulting in forward subluxation of the entire L5 unit in dysplastic spondylolisthesis. In this fashion and under certain biomechanical stressors, genetics could predispose a patient to stress fracture of the pars interarticularis which, in isthmic spondylolisthesis at the most commonly involved level, potentiates forward sliding of the anterior elements of L5 on S1 (119).

Conversely, degenerative spondylolisthesis (formally called *pseudospondylolisthesis*) occurs two to three times more frequently in African Americans, who are also known to have greater L5-S1 stability (121). In general, patients with degenerative spondylolisthesis have a low PI for age (68) (see Fig. 36.21) and higher incidences of sacralization of L5 or block-shaped L5 vertebrae. They also have a much lower incidence of posterior defects (121) than seen in the general population. The increased stability at L5 encourages instability higher in the lumbar spine.

Causes: Developmental Factors

Certain developmental factors have been statistically or logically implicated in spondylolisthesis. Foremost among these factors are posture and microtrauma (122–127).

Posture is strongly implicated in the development of spondylolisthesis and spondylolysis (prespondylolisthesis). Spondylo-"lysis" does not develop prior to the assumption of the standing posture. In one study, out of 125 institutionalized patients who had never assumed a standing position, none demonstrated a pars defect (123). No other primate has fully adopted human upright posture, nor does any other primate develop a lytic type of spondylolisthesis.

Postural decompensation as measured by the Jungmann PI is substantially higher in patients with L5-S1 spondylolisthesis (122) than in the general population. Increasing PI and increasing lumbosacral instability may, in part, address Wiltse's observation (117) that many patients develop lesions in the pars at approximately age 6 and then have no problems with it until their mid-30s.

Hyperlordosis, in particular, has been the postural fault most implicated in isthmic spondylolysis and spondylolisthesis (125,127,128). Increased lordosis transfers weight bearing from the vertebral bodies onto the articular facets in joint capsules (82). These structures are ill-adapted to continuously carry the body's weight. An anterior weight-bearing line is also known to create similar mechanics and should be looked for and evaluated. Certain activities, such as gymnastics, further increase backward bending demands in the lumbar spine. Subsequently, many young gymnasts permanently adopt an exaggerated lordotic posture. Not surprisingly, many female gymnasts demonstrate spondylolysis; having an incidence four times that of the general female population (129).

Other groups are specifically subject to increased stress in the lumbopelvic area and each has been shown to have an increased incidence of spondylolysis. These subpopulations included weight lifters, soldiers carrying backpacks, and college football linemen. Repetitive lumbosacral motion is a common characteristic in all types of spondylolisthesis except in those due to trauma. Therefore, frequent stress in posturally or congenitally unstable areas is implicated, especially during the adolescent growth spurt, in the development of fatigue fractures, the proposed basic lesion in isthmic spondylolisthesis (119).

TABLE 36.7

Classification of Spondylolisthesis

Diagnosis	Type	Percent	Criteria	Comments
Type I Dysplastic spondylolisthesis 	Dysplastic	21	Congenital deficiency of neural arch of L5 or upper sacrum. Insufficiency of superior sacral facets.	Two girls: one boy is the ratio; almost exclusively L5; lumbosacral facets also approach horizontal

Type IIA
Isthmic spondylolisthesis
 	
Type IIB
 	
	Isthmic
	Subtype A
	Subtype B
	Subtype C
		51	Pars interarticularis defect
			  A. Lytic-fatigue fracture of pars
			  B. Elongated but intact pars
			  C. Acutely fractured pars
				Almost exclusively L5
				  A. Most common type below age 50 y
				  B. Probably due to repeated microfractures healing elongated fashion as slippage occurs
				  C. History of severe trauma may heal with immobilization

Type III Degenerative spondylolisthesis 	Degenerative	25	Degenerative changes at apophyseal joints due to longstanding intersegmental instability	Four female: one male; three black: one white; six to nine times more common at L4; sacralization 4× general population; not seen before age 40; rare between 40 and 50; slippage 30% maximum
Type IV Traumatic spondylolisthesis 	Traumatic	1	Due to fractures in other areas of the bony hook than the pars	Heals with immobilization
Type V	Pathologic	2	Generalized or localized bone disease	Neoplasm, osteogenesis imperfecta, Paget disease, arthrogryposis, iatrogenic postlumbar fusion; Kuskokwim disease

Source: Reprinted with permission from Kuchera WQ, Kuchera ML. *Osteopathic Principles in Practice.* Columbus, OH: Greyden Press, 1994.

Diagnosis

Of the estimated 5% of the population with spondylolisthesis, approximately half are asymptomatic (130). Those who become symptomatic commonly do so after the age of 20. Preventive care depends on early and accurate diagnosis.

Diagnostic testing should include the following:

- Radiography
- PI measurement
- History
- Physical examination
- Spinal palpation
- Neurologic testing

Radiographic analysis

Radiology has greatly enhanced our ability to diagnose spondylolisthesis even in totally asymptomatic patients; it is a modality that provides prognostic data (122,131). It must be realized that there are significant differences between the measurements obtained from weight-bearing and non–weight-bearing x-ray films (131,132). From a pragmatic point of view, the standardized postural standing film series offers reproducible, functional, and postural data that are preferred.

Radiographically, gross spondylolisthesis can be seen and quantified on a lateral x-ray view. However, 45-degree oblique films may be necessary to see a subtle or unilateral spondylolysis (Fig. 36.36). In this view, the pars interarticularis in isthmic Type II-B spondylolisthesis has been described as the Greyhound of Hensinger because of the "long neck" rather than the "collar" on the "Scotty dog" (133).

Meyerding (134) provided the simplest system of grading (Fig. 36.37A). Spondylolisthesis is assigned the classification of I, II, III, or IV, respectively, for each one fourth of the vertebral body that the upper vertebra is displaced forward on the vertebra below. The more precise displacement measurement of Taillard (135) (Fig. 36.37B) can detect minor progression but it is rarely needed clinically. The Meyerding system is more commonly used, more quickly applied, and is clinically relevant.

The fastest progression of isthmic spondylolisthesis is seen between ages 9 and 15. Rarely is there progression in the Meyerding grading over the age of 20, especially in patients having a sclerotic buttress on the anterior lip of the sacrum (123,136).

Other signs of instability or its effects in the area can be seen with radiographic analysis (27,40,128,137,138) including:

- Angle of slip
- Osteophytes
- Calcified ligaments (especially iliolumbar)
- Increased PI
- Anterior weight-bearing mechanics
- Increased lordosis or LSA
- Disc narrowing

Whenever possible, radiographic typing of the spondylolisthesis should be performed because it might affect treatment or prognosis.

Clinical Presentation

The age of the symptomatic patient determines the clinical presentation. While spondylolisthesis is perhaps the most common cause of persistent low back pain and sciatica in children and adolescents (139), most children with spondylolisthesis in this age group do not have pain. These individuals are often identified when a school official or parent notes a change in gait or posture. If any pain is expressed, it is usually described as a dull ache in the buttock or posterior thigh; symptoms are rarely expressed below the knee (133).

Tight hamstrings (131,140) are found in 80% of young people with symptomatic spondylolysis or spondylolisthesis and to a lesser extent in asymptomatic patients. This finding probably results from postural stress and an attempt to stabilize the unstable lumbosacral junction (and is not from root impingement). Inability to bend over and touch one's toes reveals this deficit. It can also be used to uncover the nonfixed scoliosis (123,141) that exists in approximately 30% of these patients secondary to lumbar irritation and paraspinal spasm. Furthermore, as a result of having tight hamstrings, those patients having spondylolisthesis rated greater than grade II have a pathognomonic stiff-legged, short stride, waddling gait (142,143), in which the pelvis rotates with each step.

Distortion of the pelvis and trunk appears in patients having a Meyerding grade II or III. They have flared ilia in the back and an abdomen that is thrust forward. These young people have a short waist, a transverse abdominal crease at the level of the umbilicus, and flattened heart-shaped buttocks. Only 2% of young people demonstrate any objective neurologic change (82) requiring extensive electromyographic or myelographic workup.

One of the most consistent physical findings associated with patients younger than 30 years of age and with dysplastic or isthmic spondylolisthesis is tight hamstrings that restrict forward flexion of the trunk. In contrast, the most constant physical finding in patients older than 50 years of age with degenerative spondylolisthesis is the ease with which they are able to touch their toes without bending their knees or obliterating their lumbar lordosis.

The flexibility of a patient with degenerative spondylolisthesis is thought to result from laxity of the pelvicotrochanteric and hamstring muscle groups. The unstable spondylolisthetic joint at the L4-5 level predisposes the patient to manifest L5 root neurologic symptoms. The patient is more likely to have somatovisceral

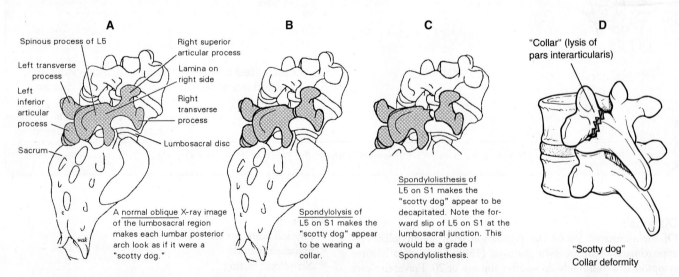

Figure 36-36 **A.** Normal 45-degree oblique radiographic view best visualizes pars interarticularis. **B.** Spondylolysis. **C.** Spondylolisthesis. **D.** Lysis pars interarticularis appearance as a collar. (From Roy S, Irvin R. *Sports Medicine: Prevention, Evaluation, Management, and Rehabilitation.* Englewood Cliffs, NJ: Prentice Hall, 1983:280, with permission.)

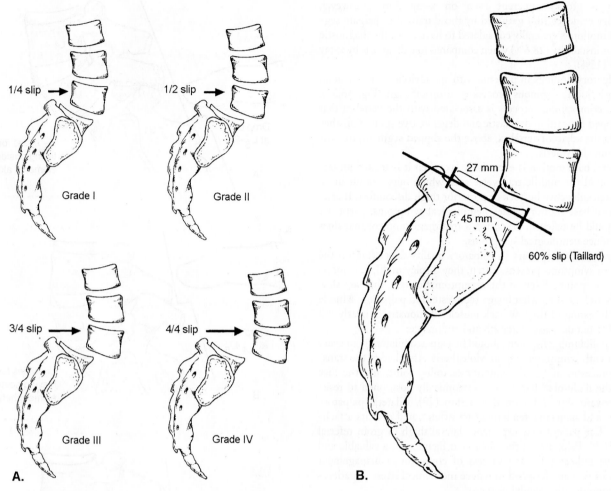

Figure 36-37   A. Classification of spondylolisthesis using the Meyerding system. **B.** Taillard method of classifying spondylolisthesis.

complaints of a hypersympathetic nature including constipation or irregular menses (72). Symptoms of pelvic congestion and vague lower extremity complaints are also common in adults with spondylolisthesis. These result from the hyperlordosis, visceroptosis, and poor thoracic abdominal diaphragmatic function that accompany spondylolisthesis (25,72,144,145).

Adult patients are more likely to complain of pain. Their pain is usually aggravated by moderate activity or prolonged standing and relieved by rest or limited activity. Because of chronic overt instability of the lumbosacral region, these patients have poorly responsive soft tissues (83), somatic dysfunction, and multiple myofascial points that, when stressed, react out of proportion to the initiating event and produce palpable spasm and low back pain. Pain can thus be caused by several structures in the area other than the spondylolisthetic segment. These structures are also subject to the instability of the region and the mechanical disadvantage that is localized there. It is, therefore, difficult to sort out when the pain is caused by spondylolisthesis, when it is the result of somatic dysfunction of muscular, ligamentous, or joint structures, or when it is of discogenic origin.

In patients older than 20 years of age with spondylolisthesis of <33%, pain is probably caused by one of three mechanisms (123):

- Disc degeneration at the level of the defect
- Root impingement by fibrocartilaginous build-up
- Referral from stressed posterior ligaments and soft tissues

In our clinical experience, pain in these patients is most commonly referred from trigger points in the quadratus lumborum, glutei, and piriformis muscles, and from iliolumbar and posterior sacroiliac ligaments. This best supports the third mechanism above.

The cauda equina becomes physically involved in isthmic spondylolisthesis patients with more than a 50% slip (more than a grade II). In these patients, low back pain is attributed directly to the spondylolisthesis itself. Because the dysplastic type carries the posterior arch forward, no more than 25% slippage is necessary to manifest a cauda equina syndrome (119). Degenerative spondylolisthesis, by nature of its mechanism, does not progress beyond a 30% slip (119,123,128). The instability of this joint (usually L4-5), coupled with physical continuity with the posterior arch, usually results in L5 root impingement. Myelograms performed on these patients generally show hourglass constriction (128) at that level. Therefore, the differential and accurate diagnosis of the primary cause of back pain in a patient with spondylolisthesis requires careful palpatory and neurologic physical examination and diagnosis in addition to the radiographic and historical findings just outlined.

Palpatory Findings

Increased intersegmental motion in the lumbosacral region is usually a sign of instability and severe degeneration. This increased motion is grossly apparent even on x-ray films. However, palpatory evidence (83) gathered by those trained to palpate segmental motion is generally considered to have twice the diagnostic yield for instability (28.6%) when compared to a diagnosis by x-ray studies (15%).

Palpatory findings in patients with spondylolisthesis reveal an anteriorly located spinous process or drop-off sign (Fig. 36.38). The anterior spinous process is associated with the vertebra that has slipped forward in dysplastic and degenerative spondylolisthesis. It is the adjacent vertebra, above the slipped segment, in isthmic spondylolisthesis.

Sacral base motion is excessively lax when it is rocked anteriorly around the middle transverse axis, which might result in an associated subjective buttock or posterior thigh discomfort. If testing sacral base motion causes neurological symptoms, particular care should be taken in designing a treatment protocol that does not produce neurological symptoms.

Paraspinal tissues vary in palpatory quality depending on the degree of symptoms present. Often, they display multiple myofascial tender points. Even in the asymptomatic state, they are slow to relax and are somewhat boggy (congested) to palpation. Muscle strength testing of the low back muscles demonstrates nearly full flexibility but decreased strength and endurance.

The iliolumbar ligament should be palpated bilaterally in every patient with symptomatic spondylolisthesis. Attached to the transverse processes of L5, the anterior sacroiliac joint, and the iliac crest, the iliolumbar ligament is anatomically positioned to resist any forward slip of L5 on the sacrum (28). Bilateral palpatory tension and subjective tenderness are often noted over its attachments. The patient may experience lateral thigh or groin referral (Fig. 36.9). Palpation of the iliolumbar ligament is a valuable and sensitive indicator for the success of conservative management programs that are designed to reduce mechanical stress in patients with symptomatic spondylolisthesis.

Neurological Findings

The physical examination of each patient should include a neurological evaluation including deep tendon reflexes, muscle strength testing, and straight leg raising. Electromyographic testing or imaging studies are indicated if radicular symptoms are present. It is especially important to assess the condition of the L4 disc (123) if surgical fusion is contemplated.

General Treatment Principles

Conservative management is 85% to 90% successful in degenerative spondylolisthesis (123,128). In the minority of children who are symptomatic, only 50% are successfully managed with conservative care (123,133). For immature patients with Meyerding grade III or IV spondylolisthesis, those with progressive subluxation, or a spondylolisthesis that is secondary to an acute fracture, conservative management is probably not indicated without extensive bracing or surgical fusion. The acute fracture group (Table 36.7) responds best to immediate immobilization (123).

For those patients requiring surgery (or bracing), conservative management should be added afterward because the conditions that led to the instability preoperatively are still present postoperatively. In all cases, conservative management should attempt to maximize structure-function relationships.

Patient Education

Education is a key component in the conservative management (130,146,147) of patients with either asymptomatic or symptomatic spondylolisthesis. Goals should center on decreasing

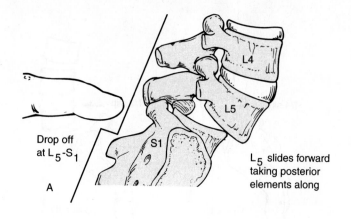

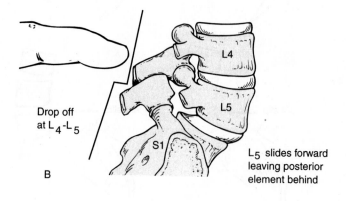

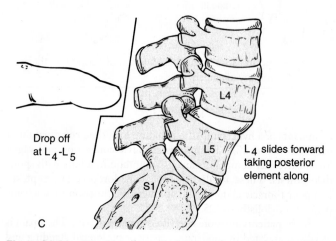

Figure 36-38 Location of anteriorly located spinous process (drop-off sign) depends on underlying mechanism of spondylolisthesis. **A.** In dysplastic spondylolisthesis, L5-S1 horizontal facets allow entire spine to glide forward creating drop-off between L5 and S1. **B.** In isthmic spondylolisthesis, pars defect between L5 and S1 allows anterior elements of L5 to slide forward along with the rest of the spine. Posterior elements of L5 remain behind with the sacrum, creating drop-off between L4 and L5. **C.** Degenerative spondylolisthesis at L4-5 does not affect anterior and posterior elements of the vertebral unit and therefore the drop-off sign is located between L4 and L5. (Courtesy of William Kuchera, D.O., F.A.A.O.)

stress in the unstable lumbosacral region through application of back mechanics, proper exercise and nutrition, and postural improvement techniques. Back schools that offer 36 hours of instruction in teaching back mechanics and appropriate choices for optimum back care are also effective (146). These approaches immensely increase patient compliance. In the absence of a back school, the individual practitioner should use a minimum of one patient visit (more if necessary) to explain lumbosacral mechanics. Patients are taught to lift properly and to avoid improper lifting, especially over the head, as this increases lumbar lordosis.

The osteopathic physician should advocate proper footwear; high heels in particular increase lumbar lordosis (82). Patients should be advised on correct sleeping, sitting, and standing postures; they should also be counseled on weight loss if necessary. This minimal investment of time reduces the frequency of reinjury or the failure of an otherwise well-conceived conservative program.

Pregnancy significantly affects posture by shifting the weight-bearing line anteriorly and accentuating the lumbar lordotic curve. Unfortunately, this postural stress occurs at a time when the hormonal changes of pregnancy also act to reduce soft tissue stabilization. Women with spondylolisthesis who are contemplating pregnancy should, if possible, prepare their posture and muscle tone in advance. They should also strictly adhere to their obstetrician's weight gain limits. Often, the addition of a Levitor is extremely beneficial, even if it is only for the duration of the pregnancy.

For young, asymptomatic individuals with less than a Meyerding grade I spondylolisthesis, avoid creating a back cripple with excessive restrictions. It is wise to direct these individuals toward a vocation not requiring heavy lifting or strenuous activity (148). In young, asymptomatic people with more than grade I spondylolisthesis, the same vocational goals are upheld but these individuals should also avoid contact sports. Inform young patients and their parents of the concerns and uncertainties involved; stress the need for close follow-up.

Exercise

The response to exercise does not depend on the type of spondylolisthesis (I, II, or III) (147). The goals of exercise are to eventually stabilize the lumbosacral region and diminish the lumbar lordosis (144,147). Weight loss for an overweight patient can also be facilitated by exercise.

Exercise should be of a flexion-type only, rather than flexion-extension combination programs (141). Gramse has reported excellent results with the flexion program (147). The variables examined included relief of pain, need for back supports, return to work status, and recovery. Combination flexion-extension exercise significantly reduced the effectiveness in all of these variables. Pelvic narrow and coil exercise (149–152) with the knees bent in the supine position is extremely effective (Fig. 36.26), although flattening the back against the wall while standing or bringing the chest to the thigh while sitting in a chair can also be beneficial.

The patient must be able to demonstrate their ability to maintain a reduced lordosis before abdominal strengthening exercises such as bent-knee sit-ups are considered. Good abdominal strength adjunctively supports weight-bearing and unloads the spine. Gymnastics, diving, and contact sports are not encouraged. Swimming, however, is considered an excellent activity to cultivate.

Osteopathic Manipulative Treatment

Several authors report a benefit (27,46,72,81,153) from the manipulative management of patients with spondylolisthesis. Manipulative treatment of the patient with spondylolisthesis is extremely helpful in attempting to redress some of the postural decompensation that has occurred over time and to alleviate segmental limitation of motion, which is known to upset the forces resisting spondylolisthesis (128).

The goals (27,46,72,82,154) are reduction of lumbar lordosis and somatic dysfunction. This transfers weight bearing from the posterior elements and tissues back to the vertebral bodies. It specifically relaxes strained, irritable lumbar paraspinal tissues, permitting them to better resist the stresses imposed by the activities of daily living. It also reduces the patient's somatic pain and somatovisceral symptomatology. These goals seek a gradual reestablishment of fascial and muscular balance in order to promote maximal functional weight-bearing posture.

The manipulative program is not simply directed to the lordosis and specific somatic dysfunctions; it also addresses biomechanical support structures. Because of the instability and injury in the lumbosacral junction, high-velocity techniques should be avoided in that area.

In correcting lordosis and recurrent lumbopelvic clinical conditions, the first concern is often balancing the pelvis horizontally (29,82,7). An undiagnosed or uncorrected unilateral, sacral shear somatic dysfunction thwarts the most expert manipulator in achieving this goal and renders functional orthoses such as the Levitor ineffective. This and other nonphysiological somatic dysfunctions can be treated promptly and effectively with OMT.

An unlevel sacral base needs gradual heel lift orthotics before instability and recurrent somatic dysfunction can be effectively addressed. A minimal heel lift, when indicated, can reduce the LSA by 2 to 4 degrees (29) and may move an anterior weight-bearing line as much as an inch posterior (155). Correction of a short leg is also extremely helpful in reducing long-term strain on the iliolumbar ligament. It eliminates somatosomatic referral of groin pain from this structure as well as reducing low back pain and instability in the lumbosacral junction (154,156). A heel lift may also be helpful to the one third of spondylolisthetic young people who have concomitant scoliotic change and the long-term somatovisceral changes resulting from it.

Any intrapelvic somatic dysfunction should be removed; the sacroiliac articulations should be freely mobile. Tight hamstring muscles are gently stretched with isometric muscle energy technique. The use of a vapocoolant spray and stretch over the hamstrings to achieve this goal is often helpful. Fascial unwinding of the lower extremities is well received by patients and eliminates many of the general congestive complaints in this area (J.G. Zink, *personal communication*, 1978).

The thoracic spine and thoracolumbar junction are addressed next. Schwab (153) reported improvement of compensatory lumbar lordotic stresses with mobilization of increased thoracic kyphosis. Fryette (82) emphasized that somatic dysfunction in this area must be corrected before any effective changes could be maintained in the lower lumbosacral junction. Additional consideration of the diaphragm and quadratus lumborum has proven particularly successful in helping to promote lymphatic drainage (25). The quadratus lumborum and the iliolumbar ligament are functionally and structurally related (156) and both should be treated.

Lastly, the lower lumbar region should be approached in a general manner with soft tissue, counterstrain, myofascial release, and fascial unwinding techniques. Address any specific somatic dysfunction with indirect technique. A clinically useful end point is achieved when the intrinsic rhythm of the craniosacral mechanism is easily palpated between the hands as they are monitoring both the thoracolumbar junction and sacrum.

Orthotics, Braces, and Casts

Orthotics play a significant role in the conservative management of patients with spondylolisthesis. The benefits of a heel lift orthotic in helping to lend stability to the lumbosacral region have already been discussed, and the heel lift orthotic is potentially a permanent part of the patient's treatment program. A corset-like lumbosacral support, conversely, should only be considered for short-term stability (83,130) Grieve (83), however, writes that a support should never be supplied without a plan to eliminate it. Most lumbosacral supports worn for prolonged periods weaken the patient's own supportive mechanisms (130), thereby increasing long-range instability and promoting dependence on the support. For short-term management of lumbar strain, however, these supports can be invaluable in reducing pain and preparing the tissues for a subsequent exercise program.

Types of immobilization, ranging from knee-to-nipple casting to ordinary body casts and corsets, have been studied for their use by patients with spondylolisthesis resulting from an acute fracture (133). The latter two types of immobilization suppress the extremes of bending but do a poor job of diminishing lumbosacral motion with walking (136).

The Levitor functional pelvic orthotic has proven to be extremely effective as an adjunct in the long-term management of symptomatic isthmic spondylolisthesis (27,71,72). Exerting pressure between the pubic symphysis and the base of the sacrum (Fig. 36.27), the Levitor effectively (157) aids in decreasing postural decompensation as measured by PI, in reducing the LSA, and in transferring weight bearing off the posterior tissues and forward to the vertebral bodies. By reducing the chronic strain on these tissues, symptomatic relief from low back pain is accomplished in days to weeks, and implementation of an exercise program can begin shortly thereafter.

Medication

Anti-inflammatory medication, analgesics, muscle relaxants, and bowel softeners all have a limited role in the symptomatic relief of various common symptoms experienced by patients with spondylolisthesis. Because spondylolisthesis is a chronic problem, narcotics have no place in symptom management of these patients. Vapocoolant spray-and-stretch technique and trigger point injection with local anesthetics may be helpful in relieving the secondary myofascial points that occur (152). Injections of proliferative agents are also useful for cases of ligamentous laxity uncorrected by conservative means (158).

Clinical Outcomes

Adjunctive use of the Levitor, for example, has been demonstrated to improve measurable sagittal plane risk factors and to reduce posture-related low back pain (157,159). In a 1985 study involving 109 patients with recalcitrant chronic low back pain, 30% of patients were found to improve with manipulation and postural exercise alone. When a functional orthosis (Levitor) was added to this program, 76% improved.

Degenerative Spondylolisthesis

Acquired degenerative spondylolisthesis has a different etiology and affects a different and more senior patient population. Patients with this pathology typically possess highly flexible hamstrings with very stable L5-S1 junction is in contradistinction with the very tight hamstrings and unstable L5-S1 of isthmic and dysplastic types of spondylolisthesis (see comparative Table 36.7). For this reason, postural care is only indicated in those patients who independently demonstrate the clinical findings to warrant the same.

SUMMARY

The postural-biomechanical model is one of several osteopathic approaches to patient care. It has several overlapping considerations with the neurological-autonomic model and the respiratory-circulatory model. Therefore, understanding this model is essential for the osteopathic physician.

REFERENCES

1. Smith W. Skiagraphy and the circulation. *J Osteopath* 1899;3:356–378.
2. Schwab WA. Principles of manipulative treatment: II. Low back problem. *J Am Osteopath Assoc* 1932;31:216–220.
3. Beilke M. Roentgenological spinal analysis and the technic for taking standing x-ray plates. *J Am Osteopath Assoc* 1936;35:414–418.
4. Denslow JS, Chace JA, Gutensohn OR, et al. Methods in taking and interpreting weight-bearing films. *J Am Osteopath Assoc.* 1955;54:663–670.
5. Peterson B, ed. *Postural Balance and Imbalance (1983 AAO Yearbook)*. Newark, OH: American Academy of Osteopathy, 1983.
6. Hagen DP. A continuing roentgenographic study of rural school children over a 15 year period. *J Am Osteopath Assoc* 1964;63:546–557.
7. Friberg O. Clinical symptoms and biomechanics of lumbar spine and hip joint in leg length inequality. *Spine* 1983;8(6):643–651.
8. Jungmann M, McClure CW. Backaches, postural decline, aging and gravity-strain. Abstract delivered at the New York Academy of General Practice. New York, NY, October 17, 1963.
9. Palmer CE. Studies of the center of gravity in the human body. *Child Develop* 1944;15(2/3):99–180.
10. "tensegrity." *Dictionary.com Unabridged.* Random House, Inc. Available at: http://dictionary.reference.com/browse/tensegrity (accessed: January 21, 2010).
11. Brownstein B, Bronner S, eds. *Functional Movement in Orthopaedic and Sports Therapy.* New York, NY: Churchhill Livingston, 1997:14–32.
12. Kappler RE. Postural balance and motion patterns. In: Peterson B, ed. *Postural Balance and Imbalance (1983 AAO Yearbook).* Newark, OH: American Academy of Osteopathy, 1983:612.
13. Kuchera ML, Kuchera WA. Postural decompensation. In: *Osteopathic Principles in Practice.* 2nd Ed. Rev. Columbus, OH: Greyden Press, 1994.
14. *Dorland's Medical Dictionary.* Philadelphia, PA: WB Saunders, 1989.
15. Kuchera ML. Gravitational stress, musculoskeletal strain, and postural alignment. *Spine State Art Rev* 1995;9(2):463–490.
16. Calliet R. *Low Back Syndrome.* 3rd Ed. Philadelphia, PA: FA Davis, 1981:24.
17. Beal MC. Biomechanics: A foundation for osteopathic theory and practice. In: Northup GW, ed. *Osteopathic Research: Growth and Development.* Chicago IL: American Osteopathic Association, 1987:37–58.
18. Fryette HH. Physiologic movements of the spine. *J Am Osteopath Assoc* 1917;18:1–2.
19. Cohen LA. Role of eye and neck proprioceptive mechanisms in body orientation and motor coordination. *J Neurophysiol* 1961;24:1–11.
20. Levin SM. A different approach to the mechanics of the human pelvis: tensegrity. In: Vleeming A, Mooney V, Dorman T, et al., eds. *Movement, Stability and Low Back Pain: The Essential Role of the Pelvis.* New York, NY: Churchill Livingstone, 1997:157–167.
21. Cummings CH. A tensegrity model for osteopathy in the cranial field. *Am Acad Osteopath J* 1994;4:(2 summer):9–13, 24–27.
22. Giles GF, Taylor JR. Lumbar spine structural changes associated with leg length inequality. *Spine* 1981;6:510–521.
23. Heilig D. *Patterns of Still Lesions and an Evaluation of Some Diagnostic Criteria in Altered Vertebral Postural Patterns* [master's thesis]. Philadelphia, PA: Philadelphia College of Osteopathy, 1957.
24. Dunnington WP. A musculoskeletal stress pattern: observations from over 50 years' clinical experience. *J Am Osteopath Assoc.* 1964;64:366–371.
25. Zink JG, Lawson WB. An osteopathic structural examination and functional interpretation of the soma. *Osteopath Ann* 1979;7:12–19.
26. Beal MC. The sacroiliac problem: review of anatomy, mechanics, and diagnosis. *J Am Osteopath Assoc* 1982;81(10):667–679
27. Jungmann M. *The Jungmann Concept and Technique of Antigravity Leverage.* Rangeley, ME: Institute for Gravitational Strain Pathology, Inc., 1982.
28. Willard FH. The muscular, ligamentous and neural structure of the low back and its relation to back pain. In: Vleeming A, Mooney V, Dorman T,

et al., eds. *Movement, Stability and Low Back Pain: The Essential Role of the Pelvis*. New York, NY: Churchill-Livingstone, 1997:3–35.

29. Kuchera ML, Irvin RE. Biomechanical considerations in postural realignment. *J Am Osteopath Assoc* 1987;87(11):781–782.

30. Denslow JS, Chase JA, Gardner DL, et al. Mechanical stresses in the human lumbar spine and pelvis. *J Am Osteopath Assoc* 1962;61:705–712.

31. Travell JG, Simons DG. *Myofascial Pain and Dysfunction: A Trigger Point Manual*. Vol II. Baltimore, MD: Williams & Wilkins, 1992.

32. Kuchera ML. Diagnosis and treatment of gravitational strain pathophysiology: research and clinical correlates (parts I & II). In: Vleeming A, ed. *Low Back Pain: The Integrated Function of the Lumbar Spine and Sacroiliac Joints*. Proceedings of the 2nd Interdisciplinary World Congress, University of California (San Diego), November 9–11, 1995:659–693.

33. Cathie AG. Some applied anatomy of postural changes. In: Peterson B, ed. *Postural Balance and Imbalance (1983 AAO Yearbook)*. Newark, OH: American Academy of Osteopathy, 1983:44–46.

34. Irvin RE. Suboptimal posture: the origin of the majority of idiopathic pain of the musculoskeletal system. In: Vleeming A, Mooney V, Dorman T, et al., eds. *Movement, Stability and Low Back Pain: The Essential Role of the Pelvis*. New York, NY: Churchill-Livingstone, 1997:133–155.

35. Kuchera ML, Bemben MG, Kuchera WA, et al. Athletic functional demand and posture (abstract). *J Am Osteopath Assoc* 90(9):843–844.

36. Denslow JS, Chase JA. Mechanical stresses in the human lumbar spine and pelvis. In: Peterson B, ed. *Postural Balance and Imbalance (1983 AAO Yearbook)*. Newark, OH: American Academy of Osteopathy, 1983:76–82.

37. Wolff J. Die innere Architekur der Knochen. *Arch Anat Phys* 1870;50.

38. Gofton JP, Trueman GE. Studies in osteoarthritis of the hip: part II. Osteoarthritis of the hip and leg-length disparity. *Can Med Assoc J* 1971;104:791–799.

39. Travell JG, Simons DG. *Myofascial Pain and Dysfunction: A Trigger Point Manual*. Vol II. Baltimore, MD: Williams & Wilkins, 1992:47.

40. Kuchera ML. Aging, postural decompensation and low back pain. *J Am Osteopath Assoc* 1986;86(10):74.

41. Zink JG. Respiratory and circulatory care: the conceptual model. *Osteopath Ann* 1977;5(3):108–112.

42. Gossman MR, Sahrmann SA, Rose SJ. Review of length-associated changes in muscle. *Phys Ther* 1982;62(12):1799–1807.

43. Travell JG, Simons DG. *Myofascial Pain and Dysfunction: A Trigger Point Manual*. Vol II. Baltimore, MD: Williams & Wilkins, 1992:547.

44. Hackett GS. *Ligament and Tendon Relaxation Treated by Prolotherapy*. 3rd Ed. Springfield, IL: Charles C Thomas, 1958.

45. Janda V. Muscle weakness and inhibition (pseudoparesis) in back pain syndromes. In: Grieve GP, ed. *Modern Medicine Therapy of the Vertebral Column*. Edinburgh, Scotland: Churchill Livingstone, 1986:197–200.

46. Kuchera ML. Treatment of gravitational strain patholophysiology. In Vleeming A, Mooney V, Dorman T, et al., eds. *Movement, Stability and Low Back Pain: The Essential Role of the Pelvis*. New York, NY: Churchill Livingstone, 1997:477–499.

47. Kuchera ML. Gravitational strain pathophysiology and "Unterkreuz" syndrome. *Manuelle Med* 1995;33(2):56.

48. Strong R, Thomas PE, Earl WD. Patterns of muscle activity in leg, hip, and torso during quiet standing. *J Am Osteopath Assoc* 1967;66:1035–1038.

49. Vleeming A, Snijders CJ, Stoeckart R, et al. The role of the sacroiliac joints in coupling between spine, pelvis, legs and arms. In: Vleeming A, Mooney V, Dorman T, et al., eds. *Movement, Stability and Low Back Pain: The Central Role of the Pelvis*. New York, NY: Churchill-Livingstone, 1997:53–71.

50. Thomas PE, Korr IM, Wright HM. A mobile instrument for reading electrical skin resistance patterns of the human trunk. *Acta Neuroveg* 1958;VVII (1–2):97–100.

51. Thomas PE, Korr IM. Relationship between sweat glands and electrical resistance of the skin. *J Appl Physiol* 1957;10:505–510.

52. Waxman SG. Aging, degeneration, regeneration, and plasticity. In: *Correlative Neuroanatomy*. 24th Ed. New York, NY: Lange/McGraw-Hill, 2000:282.

53. Osterman AL. The double crush syndrome. *Orthop Clin North Am* 1988;19(1):147–155.

54. Kuchera ML. Osteopathic considerations in neurology; In: Oken BS, (ed). *Complementary Therapies in Neurology: An Evidence-Base Approach*. London: Parthenon Publishing, 2004:49–90; chap 4.

55. Karachalios T, Sofianos J, Roidis N, et al. Ten-year follow-u[evaluation of a school screening program for scoliosis. Is the forward-bending an accurate diagnostic criterion for the screening of scoliosis? *Spine (Phila Pa 1976)* 1999;24(22):2318–2324.

56. Greenman PE. Lift therapy: use and abuse. *J Am Osteopath Assoc* 1979; 79:238–250.

57. Travell JG, Simon DG. *Myofascial Pain and Dysfunction: The Trigger Point Manual*. Vol II. Baltimore, MD: Williams & Wilkins, 1992: 22–88.

58. Willman MK. Radiographic technical aspects of the postural study. *J Am Osteopath Assoc* 1977;76:739–744.

59. Kuchera ML, Bemben MG, Kuchera WA, et al. Comparison of manual and computerized methods of assessing postural radiographs. *J Am Osteopath Assoc* 1990;90(8):714–715.

60. Peterson B, ed. *Postural Balance and Imbalance (1983 AAO Yearbook)*. Newark, OH: American Academy of Osteopathy, 1983.

61. Mense S, Simons DG. *Muscle Pain: Understanding Its Nature, Diagnosis, and Treatment*. Philadelphia, PA: Lippincott Williams & Wilkins, 2001.

62. Friberg O. The statics of postural pelvic tilt scoliosis: a radiographic study on 288 consecutive chronic LB patients. *Clin Biomech* 1987;2: 211–219.

63. Henrad J-Cl, Bismuth V, deMolmont C, et al. Unequal length of the lower limbs: measurement by a simple radiographic method: application to epidemiological studies. *Rev Rheum Mal Osteoartic* 1974;41: 773–779.

64. Morrissy RT, Goldsmith GS, Hall EC, et al. Measurement of the Cobb angle on radiographs of patients who have scoliosis. Evaluation of intrinsic error. *J Bone Joint Surg Am* 1990;72:320–327.

65. Lapadula G, Covelli M, Numo R, et al. Iliolumbar ligament ossification as a radiologic feature of reactive arthritis. *J Rheumatol* 1991;18: 1760–1762.

66. Tilley P. Radiographic identification of the sacral base. *J Am Osteopath Assoc* 1966;65:1177–1183.

67. Juhl JH, Ippolito Cremin TM, Russell G. Prevalence of frontal plane pelvic postural asymmetry—part 1. *J Am Osteopath Assoc* 2004;104(10): 411–421.

68. Kuchera ML, Miller K. Postural measurements in L4 degenerative spondylolisthesis. *J Am Osteopath Assoc* 1995;95(8):496.

69. Fernand R, Fox DE. Evaluation of lumbar lordosis: a prospective and retrospective study. *Spine* 1985;10(9):799–803.

70. Kuchera ML, Gitlin R, Frey-Gitlin K. Aging, lumbar lordosis and low back pain. *J Am Osteopath Assoc* 1992;92(9):1182.

71. Kuchera ML. *Conservative Management of Symptomatic Spondylolisthesis*. On file with the American Academy of Osteopathy (Newark, OH) in partial fulfillment of FAAO, 1987.

72. Kuchera ML. Diagnosis and treatment of gravitational strain pathophysiology: research and clinical correlates (parts I & II). In: Vleeming A, ed. *Low Back Pain: The Integrated Function of the Lumbar Spine and Sacroiliac Joints*. Proceedings of the 2nd Interdisciplinary World Congress; November 9–11, 1995:659–693; University of California (San Diego).

73. Levin S. Continuous tension, discontinuous compression; a model for biomechanical support of the body. *The Bulletin of Structural Integration*. 1982;8(1):31–33.

74. Steele KM, Essig-Beatty DR, Comeaux Z, et al., eds. *Pocket Manual of OMT: Osteopathic Manipulative Treatment for Physicians*. Philadelphia, PA: Lippincott Williams & Wilkins, 2008:4.

75. Semon RL, Spengler D. Significance of lumbar spondylolysis in college football players. *Spine* 1981;6(2):172–174.

76. Gallant R, ed. *The Jungmann Concept and Technique of Anti-Gravity Leverage: A Clinical Handbook*. 2nd Ed. Rev. Rangeley, ME: Institute for Gravitational Strain Pathology, Inc., 1992:46.

77. Travell JG, Simons DG. *Myofascial Pain and Dysfunction: The Trigger Point Manual*. Vol I. Baltimore, MD: Williams & Wilkins, 1983:680.

78. Negrini S, Zaina F, Romano M, et al. Specific exercises reduce brace prescription in adolescent idiopathic scoliosis: a prospective controlled cohort study with worst-case analysis. *J Rehabil Med* 2008;40: 451–455.

79. Negrini A, Verzini N, Parzini S, et al. Role of physical exercise in the treatment of mild idiopathic adolescent scoliosis. *Eur Med Phys* 2001:181–190.

80. Weiss HR. Rehabilitation of adolescent patients with scoliosis—what do we know? A review of the literature. *Pediatr Rehabil*, 2003; 6(3–4):183–194.

81. Rigo M, Quera-Salva G, Villagrasa M, et al. Scoliosis intensive outpatient rehabilitation based on Schroth method. *Stud Health Technol Inform* 2008;135:208–227.

82. Luibel GJ. Lordosis. *J Am Osteopath Assoc.* 1954;54(3):126–130.

83. Grieve GP. Lumbar instability. *Physiotherapy* 1982;68(1):29.

84. Dorman T. Pelvic mechanics and prolotherapy. In: Vleeming A, Mooney V, Dorman T, eds. *Movement, Stability and Low Back Pain: The Essential Role of the Pelvis.* New York, NY: Churchill Livingstone, 1997: 501–522.

85. Cruickshank JL, Koike M, Dickson RA. Curve patterns in idiopathic scoliosis: a clinical and radiographic study. *J Bone Joint Surg* 1989;71B(2): 259–263.

86. Morscher E. Etiology and pathophysiology of leg length discrepancies. *Prog Orthop Surg* 1977:9–19.

87. Kuchera ML, Kuchera WA. *Osteopathic Considerations in Systemic Dysfunction.* 2nd Ed. Rev. Columbus, OH: Greyden Press, 1994.

88. Hunt W. Inequality to length of the lower limbs, with a report of an important suit for malpractice; and also a claim for priority. *Am J Med Sci* 1879;77:102–107.

89. Cox WC. On the want of symmetry in the length of opposite sides of persons who have never been the subject of disease or injury to their lower extremities. *Am J Med Sci* 1875;69:438–439.

90. Garson JG. Inequality in length of lower limbs. *J Anat Physiol* 1879;13:502–507.

91. Hilton J. *Rest and Pain.* 6th Ed. Philadelphia, PA: JB Lippincott Co., 1950:404.

92. Dott GA, Hart CL, McKay C. Predictability of sacral base levelness based on iliac crest measurements. *J Am Osteopath Assoc* 1994;94(5): 383–390.

93. Nichols PJR, Bailey NTJ. The accuracy of measuring leg-length differences. *Br Med J* 1955;2:1247–1248.

94. Clarke GR. Unequal leg length: an accurate method of detection and some clinical results. *Rheum Phys Med* 1972;11:385–390.

95. Beal MC. A review of the short-leg problem. *J Am Osteopath Assoc* 1950;50:109–121.

96. Beal MC. The short-leg problem. *J Am Osteopath Assoc* 1950;50: 109–121.

97. Friberg O, Nurminen M, Korhonen K, et al. Accuracy and precision of clinical estimating of leg length inequality and lumbar scoliosis and comparison of clinical and radiological measurements. *Int Disabil Study* 1988;10:49–53.

98. Hoskins ER. The development of posture and its importance: III. Short leg. *J Am Osteopath Assoc* 1934;34:125–126.

99. Strong R, Thomas PE. Patterns of muscle activity in the leg, hip, and torso associated with anomalous fifth lumbar conditions. *J Am Osteopath Assoc* 1968;67:1039–1041.

100. Hackett GS. *Ligament and Tendon Relaxation Treated by Prolotherapy.* 3rd Ed. Springfield, IL: Charles C Thomas, 1958:27.

101. Sutton SE. Postural imbalance: examination and treatment utilizing flexion tests. In: Peterson B, ed. *Postural Balance and Imbalance (1983 AAO Yearbook).* Newark, OH: American Academy of Osteopathy, 1983: 102–112.

102. Denslow JS, Chace JA, Gutensohn OR, et al. Methods in taking and interpreting weight-bearing x-ray films. In: Beal MC, ed. *Selected Papers of John Stedmen Denslow (1993 AAO Yearbook).* Indianapolis, IN: American Academy of Osteopathy, 1993:109–120.

103. Travell JG, Simons DG. *Myofascial Pain and Dysfunction: A Trigger Point Manual.* Vol II. Baltimore, MD: Williams & Wilkins, 1992:47.

104. Irvin RE. Reduction of lumbar scoliosis by use of a heel lift to level the sacral base. *J Am Osteopath Assoc* 1991;91(1):34–44.

105. Beal MC. A review of the short-leg problem. In: Peterson B, ed. *Postural Balance and Imbalance (1983 AAO Yearbook).* Newark, OH: American Academy of Osteopathy, 1983:26–38.

106. Fryette HH. Some reasons why sacroiliac lesions recur. *J Am Osteopath Assoc* 1936;36:119–122.

107. Heilig D. Principles of lift therapy. In: Peterson B, ed. *Postural Balance and Imbalance (1983 AAO Yearbook).* Newark, OH: American Academy of Osteopathy, 1983:113–118.

108. Kuchera WA, Kuchera ML. Postural decompensation. In: *Osteopathic Principles in Practice.* 2nd Ed. Rev. Columbus, OH: Greyden Press, 1994:343–356.

109. Greenman PE. Lift therapy: use and abuse. In: Peterson B, ed. *Postural Balance and Imbalance (1983 AAO Yearbook).* Newark, OH: American Academy of Osteopathy, 1983:123–134.

110. Patriquin DA. Lift therapy: a study of results. In: Peterson B, ed. *Postural Balance and Imbalance (1983 AAO Yearbook).* Newark, OH: American Academy of Osteopathy, 1983:119–122.

111. Giles LGF, Taylor JR. Lumbar spine structural changes associated with leg length inequality. *Spine* 1982;7:159–162.

112. Lenssinck M-LB, Frijlink AC, Berger MY, et al. Effect of bracing and other conservative interventions in the treatment of idiopathic scoliosis in adolescents: a systematic review of clinical trials. *Phys Ther* 2005;85(12):1329–1339.

113. Zaina F, Negrini S, Atanasio S, et al. Specific exercises performed in the period of brace wearing can avoid loss of correction in Adolescent Idiopathic Scoliosis (AIS) patients: Winner of SOSORT's 2008 Award for Best Clinical Paper. *Scoliosis* 2009;4:8 doi:10.1186/1748-7161-4-8.

114. Carlson JA, Carlson JM, Earl DT. Three-dimensional counterstrain lifts (3-DCL)–theoretical concept and applications. *Am Acad Osteopath J* 1995;5(2):23–27.

115. Ferguson AB. The clinical and recent roentgenographic interpretation of lumbosacral anomalies. *Radiology* 1934;22:548–588.

116. Barbor R. Sclerosant therapy, the theory of treatment of ligamentous disturbance by a dextrose sclerosant. *Reunion Sobre Patologia tie la Columina Vertebral.* Murcia, Spain. March 30, 1977.

117. Wiltse LL, Newman PH, MacNab I. Classification of spondylolysis and spondylolisthesis. *Clin Orthop* 1976;117:23–29.

118. Friberg S. Studies on spondylolisthesis. *Acta Chir Scand* 1939;82(suppl 55):1440.

119. Wiltse LL, Widell EH, Jackson DW. Fatigue fracture: the basic lesion in isthmic spondylolisthesis. *J Bone Joint Surg* 1975;57A:1722.

120. Wiltse LL. Spondylolisthesis in children. *Clin Orthop* 1961;21: 156–163.

121. Rosenberg NJ. Degenerative spondylolisthesis–predisposing factors. *J Bone Joint Surg (Am)* 1975;57(4):467–474.

122. Kuchera ML. Postural decompensation in isthmic spondylolisthesis. *J Am Osteopath Assoc* 1987;87(1l):781.

123. Finneson BE. *Low Back Pain.* Philadelphia, PA: JB Lippincott Co., 1973:276–288.

124. Krauss H. Effect of lordosis on the stress in the lumbar spine. *Clin Orthop* 1976;117:56–58.

125. Newman PH. The etiology of spondylolisthesis. *J Bone Joint Surg* 1963;45B:39–59.

126. Wynne-Davies R, Scott JHS. Inheritance and spondylolisthesis: a radiographic family survey. *J Bone Joint Surg* 1979;61B:301–305.

127. Troup DG. Mechanical factors in spondylolisthesis and spondylolysis. *Clin Orthop* 1976;117:59–67.

128. Farfan HF, Osteria V, Lamy C. The mechanical etiology of spondylolysis and spondylolisthesis. *Clin Orthop* 1976;177:40–55.

129. Jackson DW, Wiltse LL, Cirincione RJ. Spondylolysis in the female gymnast. *Clin Orthop* 1976;117:68–73.

130. Magora A. Conservative treatment in spondylolisthesis. *Clin Orthop* 1976;117:74–79.

131. Boxall D, Bradford DS, Winter RB, et al. Management of severe spondylolisthesis in children and adolescents. *J Bone Joint Surg* 1979;61A: 479–495.

132. Lowe RW, Hayes TD, Kaye J, et al. Standing roentgenograms in spondylolisthesis. *Clin Orthop* 1976;117:80–91.

133. Hensinger RN, Lang JR, MacEwen GD. Surgical management of spondylolisthesis in children and adolescents. *Spine* 1976;1:207–216.

134. Meyerding HW. Spondylolisthesis. *Surg Gynecol Obstet* 1932;54: 371–377.

135. Taillard WF. Le spondylolisthesis chez l'enfant et l'adolescent. *Acta Orthop Scand* 1955;24:115–144.

136. Eisenstein S. Spondylolysis: a skeletal investigation of two population groups. *J Bone Joint Surg (Br)* 1978;60:488–494.

137. Kuchera ML, Barton J. Sagittal plane postural measurements. *J Am Osteopath Assoc* 1990;90(10):932.

138. Hoyt H, Bard D, Shaffer F. Experience with an antigravity leverage device for chronic low back pain: a clinical study. *J Am Osteopath Assoc* 1981;80(7):474–479.

139. Laurent LE, Oskman K. Operative treatment of spondylolisthesis in young patients. *Clin Orthop* 1976;117:85–91.

140. Phalen GS, Dickenson JA. Spondylolisthesis and tight hamstrings. *J Bone Joint Surg* 1961;43A:505–512.

141. Fisk JR, Noe JH, Winter RB. Scoliosis, spondylolysis, and spondylolisthesis. *Spine* 1978;3(3):234–245.

142. Phalen GS, Dickenson JA. Spondylolisthesis and tight hamstrings. *J Bone Joint Surg* 1961;43A:505–512.

143. Newman PH. A clinical syndrome associated with severe lumbosacral subluxation. *J Bone Joint Surg* 1965;47B(3):472–481.

144. Freeman JT. Posture in the aging and aged body. *JAMA* 1957;165(7):843–846.

145. Kimberly P. Visceroptosis: an osteopathic explanation of cause and symptoms. *J Am Osteopath Assoc* 1944;43(6):270–273.

146. Fisk JR, DiMonte P, Courington SM. Back schools—past, present and future. *Clin Orthop* 1983;179:18–21.

147. Gramse RR, Sinaki M, Ilstrup DM. Lumbar spondylolisthesis—a rational approach to conservative treatment. *Mayo Clin Prac* 1980;55:681–686.

148. Wiltse LL. The etiology of spondylolisthesis. *J Bone Joint Surg* 1962;44A:536–569.

149. Cochran A. Useful exercises for pelvis and spine. Derived from "Physiosynthesis." Handout distributed at Kirksville College of Osteopathic Medicine, Kirksville, MO: 1983.

150. Lay EM. Personal communication. Lectures delivered annually while teaching at Kirksville College of Osteopathic Medicine, Kirksville, MO: 1976–1982.

151. Pheasant HC. Practical posture building. *Clin Orthop* 1962;25:83–91.

152. Simons DG, Travell JG, Simons LS. *Travell and Simons' Myofascial Pain and Dysfunction: The Trigger Point Manual.* Vol I. Baltimore, MD: Williams & Wilkins, 1999.

153. Schwab WA. Principles of manipulative treatment—low back problem. In: Barnes MK, ed. *1965 AAO Yearbook.* Carmel, CA: Applied Academy of Osteopathy, 1965:90–94.

154. Cathie AG. Structural mechanics of the lumbar spine and pelvis. In: Barnes MW, ed. *1965 AAO Yearbook.* Carmel, CA: Applied Academy of Osteopathy, 1965:14–20.

155. Magoun HI Sr. Mechanics of chronic spinal lesion. *J Am Osteopath Assoc* 1943;42:489–500.

156. Luk KDK. The iliolumbar ligament. *J Bone Joint Surg* 1986;68B:197–200.

157. Kuchera ML, Jungmann M. Inclusion of levitor orthotic device in the management of refractive low back pain patients. *J Am Osteopath Assoc* 1986;86(10):673.

158. Dorman T, Ravin T. *Diagnosis and Injection Techniques in Orthopedic Medicine.* Baltimore, MD: Williams & Wilkins, 1991:34–35.

159. Kuchera ML. Alteration of intrapelvic spatial relationships utilizing an external pelvic orthosis in patients with low back pain. Originally published in *Proceedings of the International Society for Prosthetics and Orthotics.* June 1992:291. Also see *J Am Osteopath Assoc* 1992;92(9):1182.

37 Head and Suboccipital Region

KURT P. HEINKING, ROBERT E. KAPPLER, AND KENNETH A. RAMEY

KEY CONCEPTS

- Osteopathic manipulative treatment can improve functional outcomes in patients with sinus, eye, and ear disorders.
- Understanding the drainage patterns of the paranasal sinuses, the lymphatic channels, and the venous system assists the clinician to find possible points of connective tissue blockage.
- Knowing the parasympathetic and sympathetic innervation of head and neck as well as the consequences of autonomic nerve dysfunction can guide the clinician in treatment
- Evaluation of osteopathic cranial motion and the consideration of dural continuity are important when treating the head region.
- Somatic dysfunction plays a significant role in sinusitis, middle ear infections, and disorders of hearing and equilibrium.
- Somatic dysfunction may contribute to tension, migraine, and cluster headaches.
- Cranial dysfunction may contribute to facial nerve irritation and Bell palsy.
- Temporomandibular joint dysfunction is a common problem that responds well to manipulative treatment.

INTRODUCTION

Osteopathic manipulative treatment (OMT) in the head region is based on anatomy and physiologic function of the neurologic, vascular, muscular, articular, and lymphatic systems. Somatic dysfunction occurs in the head and face. Clinicians need to be as comfortable diagnosing and treating this region as they are in other regions of the body. Treatment of somatic dysfunction of the involved structures of the head is thought to diminish tissue congestion, improve sinus drainage, resolve motion restrictions, normalize autonomic tone, and decrease pain. Diagnosis for somatic dysfunction in this region is integrated with evaluation of the other HEENT structures. OMT may be used as a primary treatment, or as an adjunctive treatment with pharmacologic agents, hot or cold compresses, gargles, dental appliances, corrective lenses, hearing aids, creams or ointments, shampoos, eye or eardrops, massage, acupuncture, or other treatments. This chapter will demonstrate how the diagnosis of somatic dysfunction is critical to treating patients with HEENT disorders. Many studies have shown that diagnosis of somatic dysfunction and OMT improves patient outcome in a variety of conditions.

DESCRIPTIVE AND FUNCTIONAL ANATOMY

The Adult Skull

The adult skull is composed of 29 bones (Figs. 37.1–37.7). These are summarized in Table 37.1. From an osteopathic cranial perspective, they can be divided into midline and paired bones. During osteopathic cranial flexion, the midline bones (sphenoid, occiput, ethmoid, and vomer) move into flexion around their respective transverse axes. The paired bones externally rotate during osteopathic cranial flexion. During osteopathic cranial extension, the reverse occurs (1).

The Infant's Skull

The infant's skull is divisible into two parts: the neurocranium (vault and base) surrounds and protects the brain and consists of eight

bones; the facial skeleton or viscerocranium (face) consists of 13 bones. The neurocranium (vault and base) can be divided into two parts: the vault or calvaria, from a membranous origin; and the base, from a cartilaginous origin (23). The bones of the vault are separated by membranous spaces, the sutures. The fontanels are present at the angles of the parietal bones and at the junctions between several sutures of the calvarial bones. There are six fontanels: two are medial and unpaired (the anterior or bregmatic, posterior or lambdatic) and four are lateral and paired (the sphenoid and mastoid), two on either side (23). At birth, the skull is quite large in proportion to the other parts of the skeleton, and the neurocranium (vault and base) is, in turn, much larger than the viscerocranium (face).

There is a significant difference in the growth rate of the neurocranium as compared to that of the viscerocranium. The neurocranium grows quickly from birth to about the seventh year. At about 5 years of age, although brain growth is almost complete, the face has grown to only half its adult size (23). The bones of the orbital cavity—the frontal, lacrimal, palatine, zygomatic, ethmoid, maxilla, and sphenoid—develop in membrane and are very reactive to trauma and growth.

Most individual bones of the skull arise from multiple centers of ossification. The cartilaginous portion of the occipital bone is not fused at birth and is derived from five primary centers of ossification. The sphenoid bone is a more complex structure with multiple centers of ossification that unite to result in the three units. The occiput, sphenoid, and temporal bones demonstrate both *endochondral and intramembranous* types of ossification. When developed, the ossification centers form the bones of the calvaria. They are the frontal bones, the parietals, the squamous portions of the temporal bones, and the upper portion of the occipital (supraoccipital) squama (23).

The sutures separating these bones are the sagittal suture between the parietal bones, the metopic suture between the frontal bones, the paired coronal sutures between the two frontal and two parietal bones, the paired lambdoidal sutures between the supraoccipital and parietal bones, and the squamous sutures between the parietal, temporal, and sphenoid bones.

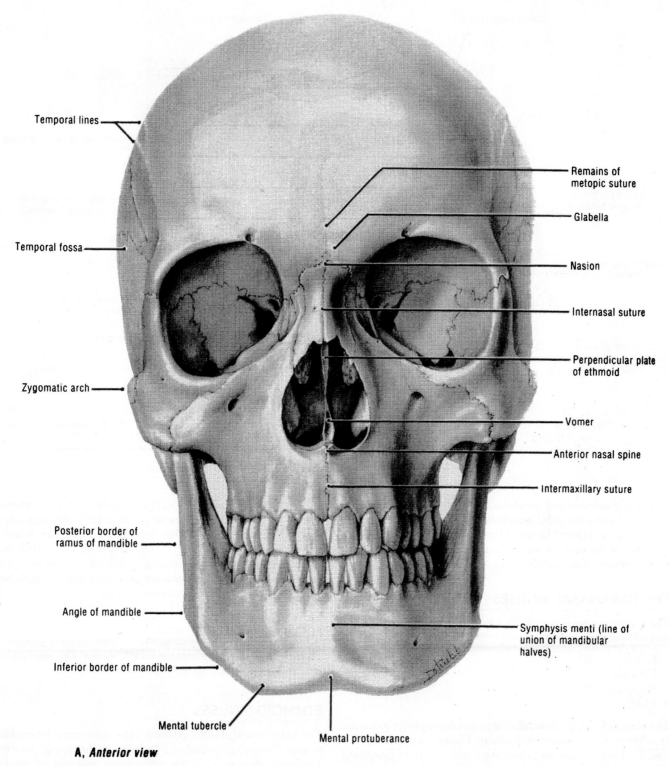

A, Anterior view

Figure 37-1 Frontal view of skull. (From Agur AMR. *Grant's Atlas of Anatomy*. 9th Ed. Baltimore, MD: Williams & Wilkins, 1991:452.)

At birth, ossification is not yet complete for most of the bones and they still consist of several component parts. For example, consider the occiput, sphenoid, and temporals. At birth, the occiput consists of four portions: the basiocciput, two "exocciputs," and the squama. The different articulations of the cranial base are named synchondroses. By definition, synchondroses are cartilaginous joints in which two bones are united by a fibrocartilage. At birth, the sphenoid presents essentially as three main parts: a central part that is the body and the lesser wings, and two lateral parts, each consisting of a greater wing and the associated pterygoid process. At birth, the temporal bones each consist of four parts: the squamous, petrous and tympanic portions, and the styloid process. The petrous portion is cartilaginous in origin; the squamous and tympanic portions are membranous in origin (23).

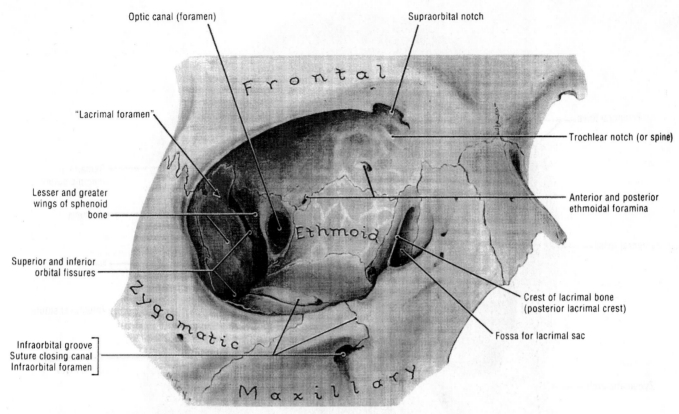

Figure 37-2 Orbital view of skull. (From Agur AMR. *Grant's Atlas of Anatomy.* 9th Ed. Baltimore, MD: Williams & Wilkins, 1991:482.)

During delivery and expulsion of the fetus, the occiput is positioned under the pubic symphysis around which extension of the craniocervical junction takes place. The superior and the inferior parts of the occipital squama may be stressed with resultant cranial somatic dysfunction.

THE PARANASAL SINUSES

The paranasal sinuses are air-filled extensions of the nasal cavity into the following cranial bones:

- Frontal
- Ethmoid
- Sphenoid
- Maxillae

The paranasal sinuses are small at birth and development proceeds at different rates, between individuals. The maxillary and sphenoidal sinuses develop first, about the fourth month of gestation. This is followed by frontal and ethmoidal sinus development, in the 6th month. The ethmoidal air cells reach mature size at 12 to 13 years of age. The maxillary sinuses assume their pyramidal shape between 5 and 8 years, reaching full size by age 15. The sphenoidal sinuses become pneumatized, at about 5 years of age (23).

The sinuses are lined with mucous membranes and connect via openings within the nasal cavities. All of the paranasal sinuses drain directly or indirectly into the nasal cavity. The balance of parasympathetic and sympathetic tone determines the nature of the mucosal secretions. Parasympathetic fibers from cranial nerve (CN) VII synapse in the sphenopalatine ganglion and promote thin, watery, saliva-like secretions. Sympathetic fibers from T1-T4

synapse in the cervical ganglia and promote thick, sticky secretions. Frontal and sphenoidal sinuses are absent at birth, although a few ethmoid cells and small maxillary sinuses are present. The ethmoid and maxillary sinuses enlarge during childhood. The frontal and sphenoidal sinuses develop during childhood and adolescence. Sinus headache referral patterns are predictable because branches of the trigeminal nerve innervate the sinuses.

FRONTAL SINUSES

The frontal sinuses drain into the middle meatus. The innervation is from the supraorbital nerves (4).

ETHMOID SINUSES

The anterior and middle ethmoid cells drain into the middle meatus. The posterior ethmoid cells drain into the superior meatus. The innervation is from the anterior and posterior ethmoidal nerves (sensory supply) and orbital branches of the pterygopalatine ganglion (parasympathetic secretomotor fibers) (4).

SPHENOID SINUSES

These drain into the sphenoethmoidal recess in close approximation to the cavernous sinuses. The innervation arises from the posterior ethmoidal nerves (sensory) and orbital branches of the pterygopalatine ganglion (secretomotor fibers) (4). Infections of the sphenoid sinus are especially dangerous because of close association with the pituitary, brainstem, cavernous sinus, and CNs.

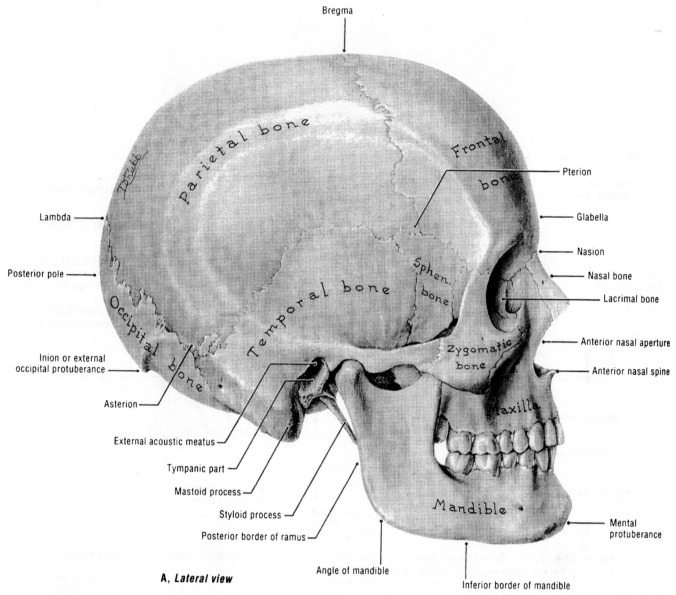

Figure 37-3 Lateral view of skull. (From Agur AMR. *Grant's Atlas of Anatomy.* 9th Ed. Baltimore, MD: Williams & Wilkins, 1991:454.)

Sphenoidal sinusitis is usually severely disabling and is associated with severe, deep head pain.

MAXILLARY SINUSES

The largest of the paranasal sinuses drain into the middle meatus. The innervation is derived from the infraorbital and the anterior, middle, and posterior superior alveolar nerves (4).

Sinus dysfunction (acute and chronic sinusitis and chronic postnasal drip) may result from dysfunction in the cranium. The physician should focus on improving the general health of the mucous membranes by correcting ventilation and circulation, restoring autonomic balance, and eliminating stagnant secretions by removing mechanical hindrances (1). Associated dysfunction in the upper thoracic spine, cervical spine, and sacrum should also be treated. (See *Osteopathy in the Cranial Field* by Magoun (1) and *Osteopathic Considerations in Systemic Dysfunction* by the Kucheras (2) for specific techniques.)

OCCIPUT (C0)—ATLAS (C1) ARTICULATION

The occiput-atlas joint is unique and has atypical motion. The condyles of the occiput are convex, while the articulating surfaces of the atlas are concave. This allows for a small gliding motion into flexion and extension. It also allows for an anterior/posterior translation as well as sidebending.

THE TEETH

When considering the effect of the dentition on somatic dysfunction of the head, face, and jaw, the clinician must understand basics of dental anatomy and malocclusion. There are two sets of teeth that develop in a lifetime. The primary teeth (also called the baby, milk, or deciduous teeth), and the permanent teeth (also called the adult or secondary teeth). Children have 20 primary teeth; they are replaced by the permanent teeth by about age 13. Adults have 32 permanent teeth. Most infants are born with no visible teeth—the

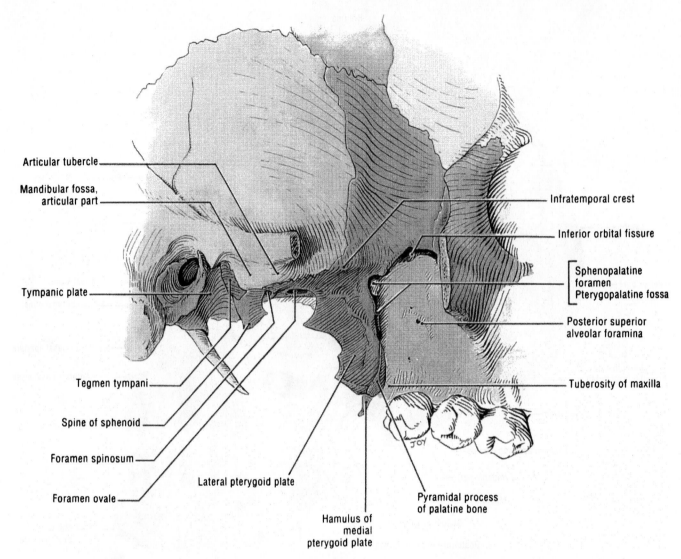

Figure 37-4 Lateral view of skull (close-up of sphenoid and temporal bones). (From Agur AMR. *Grant's Atlas of Anatomy.* 9th Ed. Baltimore, MD: Williams & Wilkins, 1991:502.)

teeth are forming inside the gums. The 20 primary teeth erupt over the time from when a baby is approximately 6 months to a year old. Primary teeth fall out and are replaced by 32 permanent teeth. This happens over the time from when a child is approximately 6 to 14 years old. Wisdom teeth (also called the third molars) are molars that usually erupt from the ages of 17 to 21. When examining teeth, the part of the tooth that is seen on the surface of the gum is the crown. It is made up of the enamel, dentine, and the pulp. The front incisor teeth have a straight edge and are used for cutting. The canine or "eye teeth" are the pointed long teeth between the incisor and the premolar teeth. Premolar teeth (bicuspids) have two cusps. Molar teeth each have four or more cusps. The enamel is the white hard covering over the crown of the tooth. It is the hardest material in the body and does not have a nerve or blood supply. Chipping or damage to enamel only will not be painful. Enamel cannot heal or repair itself as bone or dentine can. Dentine is an off white colored hard material that makes up the bulk of the tooth. Dentine can heal itself, and it can also register pain. The tooth becomes sensitive to temperature changes and feels painful, when the dentine is exposed. The nerves and the blood vessels of the tooth are called the pulp. When the pulp is exposed to infection, by decay or injury, it will die and cause severe pain.

An abscess will develop on the root. The roots are embedded in the tooth socket in the mandible. Roots are covered by cementum and held in place by the periodontal ligament. The periodontal ligament attaches the roots to the alveolar surface of the mandible. It has both a nerve and blood supply. The ligament provides an elastic cushion between the tooth and the bone. Slight movement of a tooth is made possible by the ligament. Teeth are not rigidly joined to bone. There is flexibility. Teeth change their position based on stresses and occlusion patterns.

Occlusion refers to the alignment of teeth and the way that the teeth fit together. Ideally, the points of the molars fit the grooves of the opposing molar. All teeth are aligned, straight, and spaced evenly. Malocclusion is the most common reason for referral to an orthodontist. Very few people have perfect occlusion. By treating moderate or severe malocclusion, the teeth are easier to clean and there is less risk of tooth decay and periodontal diseases. Malocclusion has a hereditary component, as well as an acquired due to habits, bruxism, and strains of the sphenobasilar synchondrosis (SBS). When hereditary, malocclusion may be from a disproportion between the size of the upper and the lower jaws or tooth size resulting in overcrowding of teeth. During infancy and childhood, personal habits like thumb sucking, tongue thrusting, pacifier use

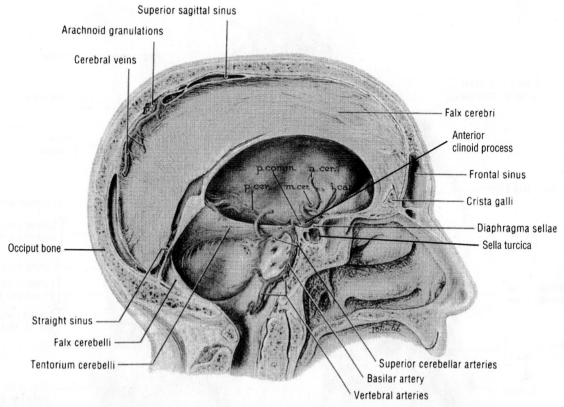

Figure 37-5 Lateral view of interior of skull. (From Agur AMR. *Grant's Atlas of Anatomy*. 9th Ed. Baltimore, MD: Williams & Wilkins, 1991:466.)

beyond the age of three, and prolonged use of a bottle can greatly affect the shape of the jaws as well. Even in the adult, improper fit of dental fillings, crowns, appliances, retainers, or braces may contribute to malocclusion. The position of the teeth and jaw will affect motion of the cranial mechanism. Receiving cranial treatment will change bite patterns and jaw position. Braces and retainers can decrease the palpable motion of the primary respiratory mechanism, causing headaches, jaw pain, and many other

complaints. Osteopathic physicians need to work closely with dentists to achieve the best functional outcome for their patients.

THE MANDIBLE

The mandible forms the lower jaw. The mandible is not part of the neurocranium, nor is it part of the viscerocranium. The mandible develops from membranous ossification (23). It has a horizontal

Figure 37-6 Interior view of nasal cavity. (From Agur AMR. *Grant's Atlas of Anatomy*. 9th Ed. Baltimore, MD: Williams & Wilkins, 1991:519.)

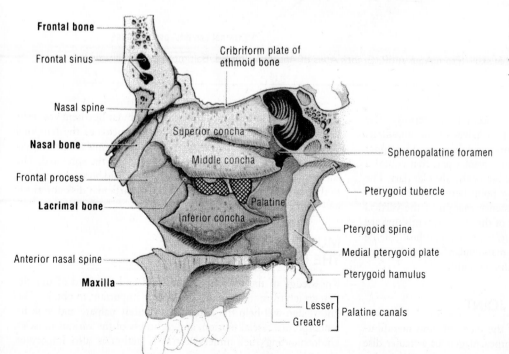

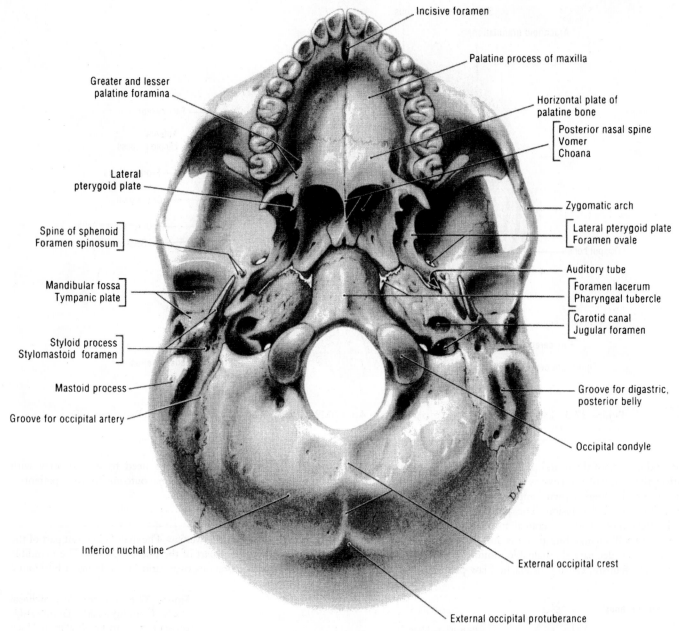

Figure 37-7 Inferior view of skull. (From Agur AMR. *Grant's Atlas of Anatomy*. 9th Ed. Baltimore, MD: Williams & Wilkins, 1991:582.)

body convex anteriorly and two rami ascending posteriorly. The *symphysis menti* is the union of the two halves of the mandible. It is prominent inferiorly as the mental protuberance. The upper part of the body of the mandible is the alveolar part that contains the teeth. A mental foramen is visible below the alveolar part. The angle of the mandible is the meeting point between the inferior margin of the mandible and the posterior margin of the vertical mandibular ramus. The superior part of the ramus extends upward to form a *coronoid process* and a *condylar process*. The head of the condylar process articulates with the mandibular fossa of the temporal bone to form the temporomandibular joint.

THE TEMPOMANDIBULAR JOINT

The TMJ is formed by the head of the mandible and mandibular fossa of the temporal bone. A fibrocartilagenous articular disc

separates these structures. The stylomandibular ligament connects the angle of the mandible to the styloid process of the temporal bone and the sphenomandibular ligament connects the lingula (medial aspect) of the mandible to the spine of the sphenoid. The lateral pterygoid muscle arises from the sphenoid bone and attaches to the articular disk. This muscle draws the articular disk anteriorly when the mouth is opened.

MUSCLES AND FASCIA OF THE HEAD AND FACE

Knowledge of the muscles of the head and face and of muscles that attach from the spine to the head is important to obtain. This knowledge will help the clinician accurately palpate and look for tenderpoints, fascial tension, and tightness of the various muscles. Understanding their innervation and action is also important,

TABLE 37.1		
Bones of the Adult Skull		
Cranial Group (8)	Facial Group (14)	Miscellaneous (7)
Occiput	Vomer	Six middle ear ossicles
Sphenoid	Mandible	Hyoid bone
Ethmoid	Paired maxillae	
Frontal	Paired palatine	
Paired temporals	Paired zygoma	
Paired parietals	Paired lacrimal	
	Paired nasal	
	Paired inferior conchae	

especially if the student physician is studying plastic surgery, neurosurgery, or otolaryngology.

MYOFASCIAL TRIGGERPOINTS

The myofascial system is often involved in head symptoms. Travell and Simons have described various myofascial trigger points (TPs) that may refer pain to and/or cause dysfunction of structures of the head (2) (Fig. 37.8 and Table 37.2). Somatic dysfunction and TPs are closely related and potentiate one another. Emotional stress may be associated with clenching of the teeth and may produce TPs in the masseter and pterygoid muscles. Frowning or squinting may set up TPs in the orbicularis oculi and occipitalis muscles. TPs in the sternocleidomastoid muscle may refer pain to the eye and may be associated with balance abnormalities. Motor vehicle accidents, especially from the rear, may produce TPs in the sternocleidomastoid, splenius cervicis, and trapezius muscles. TPs in the orbicularis oculi muscle may produce such ipsilateral visual disturbances as blurred vision, decreased light perception, tears, and conjunctival reddening. TPs in the occipitalis muscle may refer pain behind the eye and orbit. TPs in the trapezius muscle may refer pain to the orbit (2).

CONNECTIVE TISSUE

The dura mater lines the skull and produces folds, or intracranial membranes, that act as partitions between, and support for, the cerebral hemispheres and cerebellum (Figs. 37.9 and 37.10) (1). These structures form the reciprocal tension membrane and are integrally involved in osteopathic cranial motion. The dura lining the skull extends through the cranial sutures and becomes continuous with the periosteal covering of the skull. The falx cerebelli extends inferiorly from the straight sinus and firmly attaches to the foramen magnum. It attaches to the bodies of the second and the third cervical vertebrae and extends downward as a tube that ultimately attaches to the second sacral segment (Fig. 37.11). The dura becomes continuous with the extracranial fascia at various foramina in the base of the skull and continues outward as sheaths (perineurium) surrounding various cranial and spinal nerves. Extracranial and

intracranial dural continuity explain why dysfunction in the periphery can be referred to the head (1).

NEUROLOGIC STRUCTURES

Cranial Nerves

Knowledge of CN anatomy and function is important in treating patients with a variety of disorders referable to the head, eyes, ears, nose, and throat. CNs can become inflamed, infected, entrapped, and traumatized. Cranial strains/dysfunction of the sphenobasilar synchrondosis can affect their function as well. Table 37.3 highlights important aspects of the CNs.

Parasympathetics

Parasympathetic nerve fibers to the pupil are supplied by CN III (oculomotor nerve) (Fig. 37.12). They innervate the ciliary muscle and cause constriction of the pupil. Parasympathetic activity shortens the focal length of the lens and is associated with visual disturbance. Parasympathetic fibers to the lacrimal gland and nasopharyngeal mucosa originate in CN VII (facial nerve). They synapse in the sphenopalatine ganglion (Fig. 37.13). The postganglionic fibers then travel in the maxillary branch of CN V to the lacrimal gland. Parasympathetic hyperactivity resulting from sphenoid, maxilla, and palatine dysfunction results in excessive tear production and profuse, clear, thin secretions from the mucosa of the nasopharynx and sinuses. Parasympathetic nerves to the thyroid gland arise from the superior and inferior laryngeal nerves, a branch of the main vagus nerve (CN X) (2).

Sympathetics

The structures of the head and neck obtain their sympathetic innervation from cell bodies located at spinal cord levels T1-T4 (Fig. 37.14). Preganglionic and postganglionic fibers synapse in the upper thoracic region and/or cervical sympathetic ganglia. Sympathetic fibers to the head generally form sympathetic plexi that follow the course of the arterial supply (2). The superior, middle, and inferior cervical paraspinal ganglia lie in the fasciae of the cervical region at levels C2, C6, and C7, respectively. Upper thoracic, upper rib, and cervical somatic dysfunction can increase sympathetic tone to the structures of the head.

Visceral afferent nerves stimulated by organ dysfunction usually follow the same fascial pathways as the efferent sympathetic fibers of innervation. Excessive afferent input from head and neck structures is a factor in the production of facilitation in upper thoracic cord segments. Facilitation of cord segments is associated with excessive sympathetic outflow from the affected regions of the cord (T1-T4 to head and neck). Hypersympathetic stimulation to associated viscera, over time, produces physiologic changes in the viscera and in the somatic tissues innervated by the involved cord segments (2). Relevant palpatory changes mediated by viscerosomatic reflexes from HEENT structures can therefore be found in T1-T4 paraspinal tissues and in predictable anterior Chapman points on the anterior chest wall above rib 2.

Palpatory changes in the upper thoracic and cervical paraspinal tissues can therefore be a clue to structural or functional involvement of the head and neck structures innervated by sympathetic fibers. Conditions such as Horner syndrome (constricted pupil, ptosis, and facial anhidrosis on the affected side) indicate significant structural involvement or blockage of the sympathetic nervous system. Increased sympathetic tone also leads to functional photophobia,

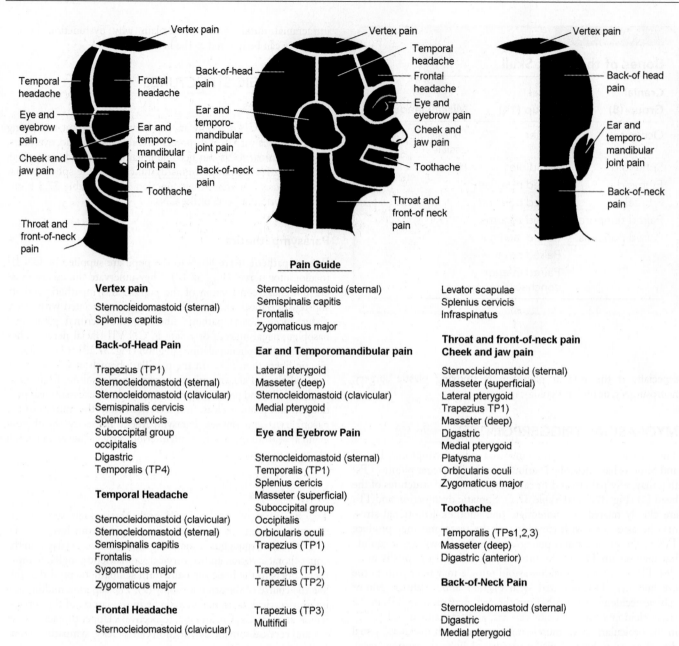

Pain Guide

Vertex pain

Sternocleidomastoid (sternal)
Splenius capitis

Back-of-Head Pain

Trapezius (TP1)
Sternocleidomastoid (sternal)
Sternocleidomastoid (clavicular)
Semispinalis cervicis
Splenius cervicis
Suboccipital group
occipitalis
Digastric
Temporalis (TP4)

Temporal Headache

Sternocleidomastoid (clavicular)
Sternocleidomastoid (sternal)
Semispinalis capitis
Frontalis
Sygomaticus major
Zygomaticus major

Frontal Headache

Sternocleidomastoid (clavicular)

Sternocleidomastoid (sternal)
Semispinalis capitis
Frontalis
Zygomaticus major

Ear and Temporomandibular pain

Lateral pterygoid
Masseter (deep)
Sternocleidomastoid (clavicular)
Medial pterygoid

Eye and Eyebrow Pain

Sternocleidomastoid (sternal)
Temporalis (TP1)
Splenius cericis
Masseter (superficial)
Suboccipital group
Occipitalis
Orbicularis oculi
Trapezius (TP1)

Trapezius (TP1)
Trapezius (TP2)

Trapezius (TP3)
Multifidi

Levator scapulae
Splenius cervicis
Infraspinatus

Throat and front-of-neck pain
Cheek and jaw pain

Sternocleidomastoid (sternal)
Masseter (superficial)
Lateral pterygoid
Trapezius TP1)
Masseter (deep)
Digastric
Medial pterygoid
Platysma
Orbicularis oculi
Zygomaticus major

Toothache

Temporalis (TPs1,2,3)
Masseter (deep)
Digastric (anterior)

Back-of-Neck Pain

Sternocleidomastoid (sternal)
Digastric
Medial pterygoid

Figure 37-8 Muscle trigger points pain guide **(left)** and areas of referred pain **(right)** in the head and neck. (From Travell JG, Simons DG. *Myofascial Pain and Dysfunction: The Trigger Point Manual. The Upper Extremities.* Vol 1. Baltimore, MD: Williams & Wilkins, 1983:166–167.)

unsteadiness, and tinnitus. Hyperesthesia of the pharyngeal tissues causes patients to cough and expectorate in an attempt to rid themselves of an imaginary foreign body in the throat (2).

Increased sympathetic activity alters the normal physiologic responses the tissues can provide. Vasoconstriction results in decreased nutrient supply to and reduced lymphatic and venous drainage from target organs and tissues. The body's ability to mount an immune response and obtain effective concentrations of medications is reduced in areas of vasoconstriction and tissue congestion (2).

Prolonged sympathetic stimulation changes the composition of the cells of the respiratory epithelium resulting in nasal and pharyngeal secretions that are thick and sticky, thereby reducing effective cleaning and clearing by the pseudostratified ciliated epithelium of the mucosa. Epithelial hyperplasia is present,

with a relative increase in the activity and number of goblet cells, constriction of arterioles, decreased vascular and lymphatic drainage of the tissues, and the mechanical difficulty in moving the mucus. Sympathetic stimulation also produces vasoconstriction and inhibits secretion, leading to dryness of the nasopharyngeal mucosa. Dryness and cracking of the mucosa break down the normal mucosal defenses, thereby permitting secondary bacterial infection (2).

Dilation of the pupil (mydriasis) also occurs with increased sympathetic activity to the eye. This elevates intraocular pressures in patients with narrow angle glaucoma. Prolonged upper thoracic and cervical dysfunctions have been associated with the development of cloudiness of the lens (2). The Barr-Lieou syndrome (vertigo, ataxia, vasodilation, and eye pain) results from hypersympathetic activity and proprioceptive dysfunction that often follows whiplash injuries.

TABLE 37.2

Myofascial TPs

Eye symptoms and/or pain
  Sternal division of the sternocleidomastoid muscle
  Splenius cervicis muscle
  Occipitalis muscle
  Orbicularis oculi muscle
  Trapezius muscle
Ear pain, tinnitus, and/or diminished hearing
  Deep portion of the masseter muscle
  Clavicular portion of the sternocleidomastoid muscle
  Medial pterygoid muscle
  Occipitalis muscle
Eustachian tube dysfunction
  Medial pterygoid muscle
Nose pain
  Orbicularis oculi muscle
Maxillary sinus pain and/or sinus symptoms
  Lateral pterygoid muscle
  Masseter muscle
  Sternal division of the sternocleidomastoid muscle
Throat pain and/or difficulty swallowing
  Medial pterygoid muscle
  Digastric muscle
CN entrapment
  V: (buccal nerve branch), lateral pterygoid muscle
  XI: sternocleidomastoid muscle

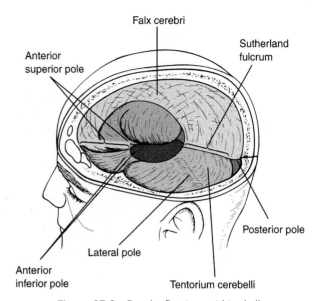

Figure 37-9 Dural reflections within skull.

The sympathetics innervate blood vessels that supply the thyroid and innervate the cells that produce thyroid secretions. Increased sympathetic stimulation may alter thyroid gland secretion (2).

Dorsal Rami of the Upper Cervical Nerves

Understanding the anatomy of the dorsal rami of the cervical nerves is important in understanding how somatic dysfunction at C2 and C3 may be related to tension headaches and "occipital neuritis." The greater and lesser occipital nerves have been implicated in the production of tension headaches, so this region is a common area of OMT. These branches of the dorsal rami of the upper cervical segments pierce through the fascia just below the superior nuchal line. Tension in this fascia has been implicated to cause compression and irritation of the greater occipital nerve.

The *greater occipital nerve* is the medial branch of the dorsal ramus of the second cervical nerve. It ascends between the muscles of the suboccipital triangle and the semispinalis capitis. The greater occipital nerve pierces the semispinalis capitis and the trapezius near their attachments to the occipital bone and ascends on the back of the scalp with the occipital artery. The greater occipital nerve supplies the skin of the occipital part of the scalp lateral to the median line and as far superiorly as the vertex of the skull. Its lateral branches communicate with those of the lesser occipital nerve. The greater occipital nerve gives off muscular branches

to semispinalis capitis joins with *occipitalis tertius*, the cutaneous branch of the third cervical nerve. The *occipitalis tertius* supplies the skin of the upper part of the back of the neck, near the median line, and the skin of the scalp over the external occipital protuberance.

The cutaneous branches of the cervical plexus are *the lesser occipital, the great auricular, the transverse cervical, and the supraclavicular nerves*. The lesser occipital nerve (C2, sometimes also C3) ascends in the neck along the posterior border of the sternocleidomastoid muscle. It pierces the superficial layer of cervical fascia near the insertion of the muscle and divides into branches, which supply the skin and subcutaneous tissue of the scalp behind and above the ear and of the upper portion of the cranial surface of the ear. The *great auricular nerve* (C2, C3) arises in the posterior triangle at the lateral border of the sternocleidomastoid muscle. It travels below the lesser occipital nerve and crosses obliquely in a course toward the ear and the angle of the mandible.

ARTERIAL SUPPLY

Internal Carotids

The face and the scalp are supplied by branches of the external carotid artery (primarily the facial artery) (3). The internal structures of the head are primarily supplied by the internal carotid and vertebral arteries (Fig. 37.15). The internal carotid artery passes through the carotid canal in the petrous portion of the temporal bone. It supplies the anterior portions of the cerebrum (3). Cranial dysfunction in the articulations between the temporal bones, occiput, and sphenoid can alter the normal function of these arteries (3). This can produce symptoms including weakness and altered sensation on the opposite side of the body.

External Carotids

The external carotid artery travels from the upper border of the thyroid cartilage to the neck of the mandible. Here, it divides into the superficial temporal and maxillary arteries. It is relatively superficial in the carotid triangle, where it is covered by the superficial layer of cervical fascia and is overlapped by the anterior border of

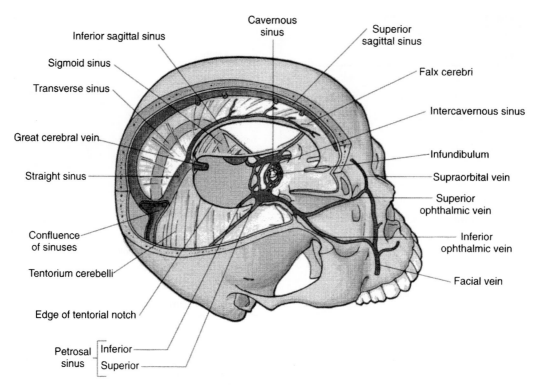

Figure 37-10   Median section of head and relationship of dural folds to intracranial structures. Superolateral view. (From Moore KL, Agur AMR. *Essential Clinical Anatomy*. Baltimore, MD: Williams & Wilkins, 1996:359.)

the sternocleidomastoid muscle. Leaving the carotid triangle, the artery is crossed by the posterior belly of the digastric and the stylohyoid muscles and separates these muscles from the stylopharyngeus muscle. The facial nerve crosses both vessels. The external carotid artery has eight branches. Of these, four arise in the carotid triangle: the superior thyroid, the lingual, and the facial arteries. Two posterior branches, the occipital and posterior auricular arteries, arise at the level of the posterior belly of the digastric muscle; and two terminal branches, the superficial temporal and maxillary arteries, take origin behind the neck of the mandible (24).

Vertebral Arteries

The vertebral arteries arise from the subclavian artery and ascend through the transverse foramen of C6-3. At C2, they make several right angle turns before piercing the dura to angle anteriorly and enter the skull through the foramen magnum (3). The vertebral arteries supply the visual area of the cerebrum (occipital lobe), brainstem, and cerebellum. Dysfunctions affecting this artery can be associated with visual abnormalities and dizziness (3).

Circle of Willis

The vascular interconnections of the brain, known as the cerebral arterial circle (Circle of Willis), serve to equalize the blood supply to the various parts of the brain under conditions of fluctuating pressure through the major vessels. This anatomic design is unique and vital whenever a major source vessel becomes thrombosed or has to be ligated. The vertebral arteries join to form the basilar artery. The basilar artery splits into the two posterior cerebral arteries. The anterior and posterior communicating arteries indirectly connect the internal carotid arteries of the two sides and the basilar system, so that an

arterial circle is formed at the base of the brain (24). The terminal vessels in and on the brain anastomose, but the larger arteries do not, except in this arterial circle. Effects from an occlusion of one vertebral artery may be dampened by these vascular interconnections.

Venous Drainage

Venous blood flows peripherally via superficial cerebral veins and centrally via the deep cerebral veins into the venous sinuses, which lie between the outer endosteal and the inner meningeal layer of the dura. The cerebral veins are thin walled and have no valves. There are numerous venous connections between cerebral veins and dural sinuses and venous systems of the meninges, skull, scalp, and nasal sinuses. This anatomic arrangement not only allows the spread of infection, but also allows cranial techniques to affect the venous drainage of the cerebral vessels. The venous drainage of the brain begins with the superior and inferior sagittal sinuses, as they drain into the transverse then sigmoid sinuses and finally into the internal jugular vein. The ophthalmic veins from the orbit drain backward to the cavernous sinus or forward to the facial vein. The cavernous sinus drains to the pterygoid plexus of veins, through the superior petrosal sinus to the transverse sinus and through the inferior petrosal sinus to the internal jugular vein. The veins of the scalp drain through veins that accompany the arteries, or through emissary veins, which connect the venous plexus of the scalp with the dural venous sinuses. The maxillary and superficial temporal veins form the retromandibular vein behind the angle of the mandible. The retromandibular vein communicates with the external jugular vein and the internal jugular vein. The facial vein drains into the internal jugular vein. The internal jugular vein lies in the carotid sheath and as it passes down the neck it receives the superior and middle thyroid veins. The external jugular vein lies subcutaneous

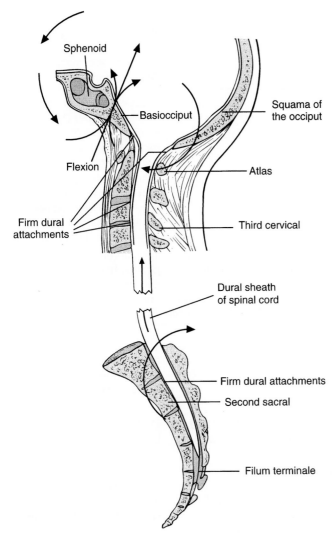

Figure 37-11 Dural continuity of skull, cervical vertebrae, and sacrum. (Adapted from Magoun H. *Osteopathy in the Cranial Field.* 3rd Ed. Kirksville, MO: The Journal Printing Co., 1976.)

on the sternocleidomastoid muscle. It joins the subclavian vein. The internal jugular vein and the subclavian vein form the brachiocephalic veins on the right and left.

Approximately 85% of the venous drainage from the head occurs via the internal jugular veins (Fig. 37.16). These veins pass through the jugular foramen, which is formed by both the occiput and the temporal bones and is located along the occipitomastoid suture. CNs IX to XI course along with the internal jugular vein and exit through jugular foramen as well, which is located between the occiput and the temporal bones. Suboccipital tension of this area is thought to cause fascial obstruction to flow and venous congestion. Specifically, an occipitomastoid compression can compromise venous flow through the jugular foramen, leading to congestion of the large valveless venous sinuses within the head. Sacral, upper thoracic, cervical, and associated regional connective tissue dysfunction can also contribute to congestion and impaired venous flow from the head (2).

Lymphatic Drainage

Understanding the lymphatic drainage patterns assists the physician in localizing pathologic conditions in the head (Fig. 37.17). There

are no lymphatic channels inside the skull. Lymphatic vessels in the forehead and anterior part of the face drain into the submandibular lymph nodes. Lymph vessels from the lateral face and eyelids drain inferiorly toward the parotid lymph nodes and ultimately drain into the deep cervical lymph nodes (3). The superficial lymph nodes of the head include the submandibular, occipital, retroauricular, and superficial parotid lymph nodes.

Lymph from the occipital region of the scalp drains into the occipital lymph nodes. The temporoparietal region drains into the retroauricular lymph nodes. The frontoparietal region drains into the superficial parotid lymph nodes. Lymph from the superficial lymph nodes eventually drains into the cervical lymph nodes. The deep cervical lymph nodes are located along the internal jugular vein. Lymph from the deep cervical structures passes through the jugular trunk into the left (thoracic duct) and right lymphatic trunks (Fig. 37.18) (3).

All drainage from the head passes through the neck, cervical fasciae, and thoracic inlet to return to the general circulation. Dysfunction in any of these structures can hinder the pathways and lead to lymphatic congestion. Increased sympathetic stimulation constricts the smooth muscle of the larger lymphatic vessels of the head and neck (associated with upper thoracic and cervical dysfunction), leading to decreased lymphatic drainage (2).

SENSORY ORGANS

Eye

Each orbit is composed of seven bones (see Fig. 37.2) (1):

- Frontal
- Sphenoid
- Maxilla
- Zygomatic
- Palatine
- Ethmoid
- Lacrimal

Four of the eye muscles (superior, inferior, medial, and lateral rectus) originate from a common tendinous ring surrounding the optic canal in the lesser wing of the sphenoid. The superior oblique muscle arises from the body of the sphenoid bone superomedial to the common tendinous ring and the inferior oblique muscle originates on the maxilla in the floor of the orbit. All are involved in eye movements (Fig. 37.19) (3).

Dysfunction of the frontal, sphenoid, and maxillae may produce muscle imbalance of the eye (1). Restrictions of the orbital bones, through fascial connections, contribute to venous stasis in head structures (1). A lateral stain pattern, maintained by unilateral condylar compression, is often associated with strabismus. A vertical strain pattern, maintained by bilateral condylar compression, is often associated with either myopia or hyperopia. Dysfunction of the occipital bone can obstruct the jugular foramen, leading to backward venous pressure in the orbit. These factors may contribute to such conditions as (1):

- Amblyopia
- Astigmatism
- Diplopia
- Hyperopia
- Myopia
- Strabismus

The patient receives clinical benefit from removal of cranial somatic dysfunction. Gentle eye mobilization using indirect techniques may also decrease ocular tension resulting from glaucoma.

TABLE 37.3

Cranial Nerves

CN	Anatomic Location	Innervation	Dysfunction
I. Olfactory	Foramina of the cribriform plate of the ethmoid bone		Crosses the lesser wing of the sphenoid (1). Altered sense of smell Impression of an odor that does not exist (2).
II. Optic	Optic canal (in the lesser wing of the sphenoid)		Lesions of the sphenoid or membranous tension may affect the optic nerve anywhere between the sphenoid and occiput (1).
III. Oculomotor	Midbrain, lateral wall of cavernous sinus, top of the petrosphenoidal ligament, superior orbital fissure	Levator palpebrae extraocular muscles of the eye (except the superior oblique and lateral rectus). Parasympathetic fibers supply the smooth muscle in the sphincter pupillae and ciliary muscles (3).	Tension on the petrosphenoid ligament causes potential compression
IV. Trochlear	Passes through the petrosphenoidal ligament, and enters the orbit via the superior orbital fissure		The most common symptom, diplopia, occurs when the patient looks downward.
V. Trigeminal			
V1 ophthalmic branch	Passes through the lateral wall of the cavernous sinus Enters the orbit through the superior orbital fissure	Upper eyelid, scalp, forehead, eyeball, ethmoid sinus, nasal cavity, lacrimal gland and conjunctiva.	Dysfunction of temporal bone may affect the function of this nerve.
V2 maxillary branch	Courses through: Inferior portion of cavernous sinus Middle cranial fossa Foramen rotundum Pterygopalatine fossa Infratemporal fossa Inferior orbital fissure	Supplies sensory fibers to the dura, maxillary sinus, maxillary premolar and molar teeth, nasal septum, lower eyelid, nose, and upper lip.	Tic douloureux may be associated with dysfunction of this nerve
V3 mandibular branch	Exits the middle cranial fossa via the foramen ovale	It contains both motor and sensory fibers. Supplies the teeth, gingiva, skin of the temporal region, the ear, lower face, muscles of mastication, floor of the oral cavity and tongue	Trigeminal neuralgia affecting this division. Sensory information from structures innervated by the trigeminal nerve (sinuses) may be perceived as headache
VI. Abducens	Courses underneath the petrosphenoid ligament, through the cavernous sinus, enters the orbit via the superior orbital fissure (3).	The abducens nerve supplies the lateral rectus muscle of the eye	Nerve most often affected and may result in medial strabismus
VII. Facial	Arises from the pons, enters the internal acoustic meatus of the temporal bone, joins the facial canal, and exits the skull via the stylomastoid foramen (3)	The sensory root anterior two thirds of tongue, soft palate, and a small area around the external auditory meatus. Secretory to the salivary glands and sensory to the lacrimal glands The motor root supplies the muscles of facial expression and muscles of the scalp, auricle, buccinator, platysma, staprdius, stylohyoid, diagastric	Dysfunction of the sphenoid,occiput (condylar or occiptomastoid compression) cervical and upper thoracic spine, and cervical fascia (1).

(continued)

TABLE 37.3 (*Continued*)

VIII. Auditory	Both divisions arise in a groove between the pons and medulla and course through the internal acoustic meatus with the facial nerve (3).		Lesions of the sphenoid, occiput, and temporals may affect the functioning of this nerve, producing vertigo or hearing dysfunctions (1).
IX. Glossopharyngeal	It arises from the medulla and leaves the skull through the jugular foramen (3)	Stylopharyngeus muscle Secretomotor to the parotid gland Sensory to the pharynx, tonsils, and posterior portion of the tongue.	Dysfunctions affecting the jugular foramen (temporal, occiput, occipitomastoid suture, or cervical fascia) may interfere with normal function of this nerve (1).
X. Vagus	Arises from the medulla and exits the skull via the jugular foramen (3).	Head, Neck, Thorax, abdomen, half of colon	Referred pain and parasympathetic reflexes headache, nausea, bradyarrythmia, cough
XI. Accessory	It arises from both the cervical spinal cord and the medulla, and exits the skull through the jugular foramen	Sternocleidomastoid and trapezius muscles; it also supplies muscles in the pharynx and palate.	Dysfunctions affecting the jugular foramen Sternocleidomastoid dysfunction
XII. Hypoglossal	It arises from the medulla and exits the skull via the foramen magnum. It courses through the hypoglossal canal in the occipital bone (3).	The hypoglossal nerve is the motor nerve of the tongue.	Dysfunction of the condylar parts of the occipital bone may affect functioning of this nerve (1), Suckling disorders in infants Dysphagia, dysarthria, and swallowing difficulties in adults

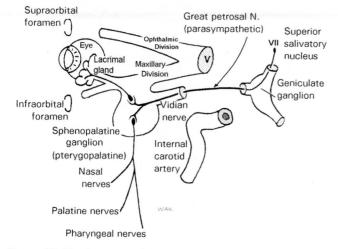

Figure 37-12 Parasympathetic nerves to orbital and nasal areas. (Modified from Kuchera ML, Kuchera WA. *Osteopathic Considerations in Systemic Dysfunction.* 2nd Ed. rev. Columbus, OH: Greyden Press, 1994.)

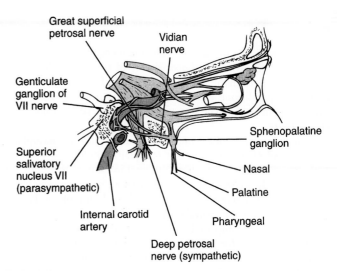

Figure 37-13 Sphenopalatine ganglion. (Modified from Kuchera ML, Kuchera WA. *Osteopathic Considerations in Systemic Dysfunction.* 2nd Ed. Rev. Columbus, OH: Greyden Press, 1994.)

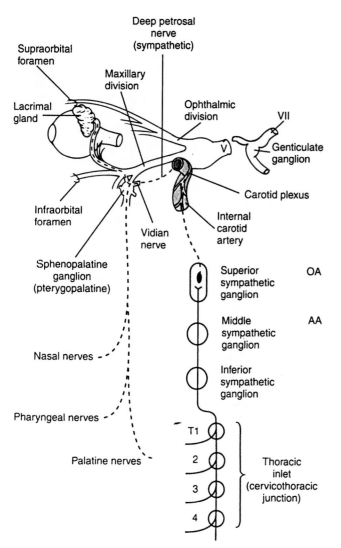

Figure 37-14 Sympathetic nerves to head. OA, occipitoatlantal; AA, atlantoaxial. (Modified from Kuchera ML, Kuchera WA. *Osteopathic Considerations in Systemic Dysfunction*. 2nd Ed. Rev. Columbus, OH: Greyden Press, 1994.)

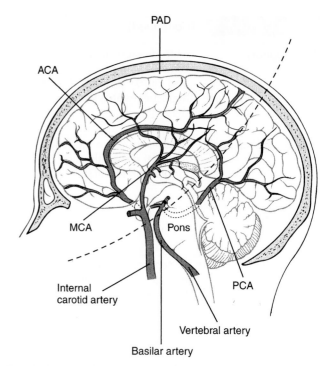

Figure 37-15 Major arterial supply to brain. Areas above *dotted line* are supplied by internal carotid arteries; areas below dotted line are supplied by vertebral arteries. ACA, anterior cerebral artery; MCA, middle cerebral artery; PCA, posterior cerebral artery; PAD, pia, arachnoid, and dura.

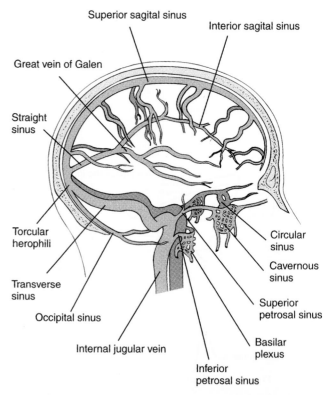

Figure 37-16 Venous drainage of skull. (Adapted from Magoun H. *Osteopathy in the Cranial Field*. 3rd Ed. Kirksville, MO: The Journal Printing Co., 1976.)

Ear

The ear serves two major functions: maintenance of equilibrium and hearing (3). Most of the structures of the ear reside within the petrous portion of the temporal bone. Hence, dysfunction of the temporal bone can be a factor in impaired hearing and asynchrony of temporal bone motion can be associated with vertigo (Fig. 37.20).

The Eustachian tube connects the middle ear to the nasopharynx (Fig. 37.21) (3). It functions to equalize middle ear pressure with atmospheric pressure. Fixed internal rotation of the temporal bone, typically secondary to occipitomastoid or sphenosquamous compression, maintains partial or complete closure of the Eustachian tube. This is associated with two effects: perception of high-pitched noises and impaired drainage from the middle ear, thereby producing a media for recurrent ear infections. Fixed external rotation maintains patency of the Eustachian tube and is associated with the perception of a roar or low-pitched noises (1). Eustachian tube dysfunction is the most common precursor of otitis media and is often responsive to treatment of somatic dysfunction affecting

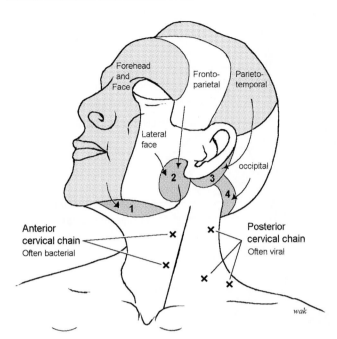

Figure 37-17 Lymph drainage from regions of the head and scapula. (Courtesy of William A. Kuchera, D.O., F.A.A.O.)

the cranium, cervical and thoracic spine, medial pterygoid muscle, cervical fasciae, and sacrum. Dysfunction affecting the ganglion impar is often associated with asthma, chronic otitis media, and chronic sinusitis. The ganglion impar is formed by the convergence of the pelvic sympathetic trunks and lies anterior to the coccyx. This ganglion ultimately communicates with thoracic sympathetic chain (4). Sacral and/or coccygeal restrictions may irritate this ganglion, contributing to increased tension in the upper thoracic and cervical spine. Treatment of sacral and/or coccyx somatic dysfunction will allow the ganglion impar to optimally function. Dysfunction of the ganglion impar is especially responsive to the vibratory percussion hammer techniques developed by Robert C. Fulford, D.O.

Throat

Impaired arterial supply to and venous and lymphatic drainage from the throat predisposes this region to infection. Dysfunction of the sacrum, upper thoracic and cervical spine, and/or hyoid bone is often seen in patients with pharyngitis and tonsillitis.

BIOMECHANICS AND MOTION

Suboccipital Region

A thorough knowledge of the suboccipital region is important, both in the infant and the adult. In the infant, asymmetric molding of the bones can cause functional disturbances such as strabismus, poor feeding, and recurrent otitis media (8). Cranial dysfunctions and asymmetries can cause membranous strain and lead to CN entrapments. Table 37.3 includes dysfunction of the CNs. In the infant, the occiput is formed in four parts. Each part is separated by a synchondrosis, a cartilage union that usually ossifies before adult life. In infants, somatic dysfunction can be classified as *interosseous* (occurring between different bones) or *intraosseous* (occurring between different parts of the same bone) (8). Therefore, diagnosis

of the suboccipital region in an infant or child is different than an adult.

In an adult, dysfunction occurs between the occiput (C0) and the atlas (C1). Knowledge of the anatomy of the region is important to understand the motions that occur.

Functional Anatomy

The occipitoatlantal articulation consists of the superior articular facets of the atlas and the two occipital condyles. The superior facets of the atlas face backward, upward, and medially, and are concave. The surfaces of the occipital condyles match the facets of the atlas, and the joint is best thought of as a sphere (the occiput) gliding in a shallow cup (the articular surfaces of the atlas).

Motion

Flexion-extension of the occiput is the primary motion, producing a small-amplitude nodding "yes" of the head. Approximately 50% of cervical flexion/extension occurs at the occipitoatlantal joint. However, the motion at the occipital condyles is more complex than a small flexion and extension movement. Because the occipital joint surface is convex and the articulating surfaces of the atlas are concave, there is a considerable amount of anterior-posterior glide as well. Flexion of the occiput on the atlas is accompanied by a posterior translatory glide of the occiput; extension is accompanied by an anterior translatory glide (7). During coupled sidebending and rotation, one condyle glides anterior and the other glides posterior.

Dysfunction

Somatic dysfunctions of the occipitoatlantal joint most often involve the minor motions of sidebending and rotation. The dysfunctional pattern between occiput and atlas demonstrates an atypical pattern of coupled sidebending and rotation in opposite directions. The sidebending and rotation of the occipitoatlantal joint in opposite directions occurs in part because of the position of the lateral atlanto-occipital ligament (7). When the occiput rotates left on the atlas, the lateral atlanto-occipital ligament causes the occiput to slide (translate) to the left and therefore sidebend to the right (7). Because sidebending-rotation mechanics between C0 and C1 occur in opposite directions, some authors mistakenly state that this is Fryette Type I mechanics. This is not correct, as C0 and C1 are not typical vertebral segments and, therefore, do not demonstrate Fryette Type I mechanics. In the Chicago model, clinicians refer to a posterior occiput and an anterior occiput. The muscle energy system refers to a flexed occiput (Chicago posterior occiput because the posterior occiput resists extension) or an extended occiput (an anterior occiput resists flexion) (Table 37.4).

Diagnosis

Clinically, the lateral translation test is commonly used (physiologic motion: rotation and sidebending to opposite sides). The clinician will translate the occiput (entire head) to the right and to the left. Freer translation right suggests the dysfunction to be sidebending left, rotation right; or probably a posterior occiput right (or anterior occiput left). The clinician then uses tissue texture abnormality and tenderness to reach a conclusion of which side is dysfunctional. An additional motion test is a posterior occiput resists extension on that side; an anterior occiput resists flexion on that side. Some clinicians use a "figure of 8" motion testing process to determine

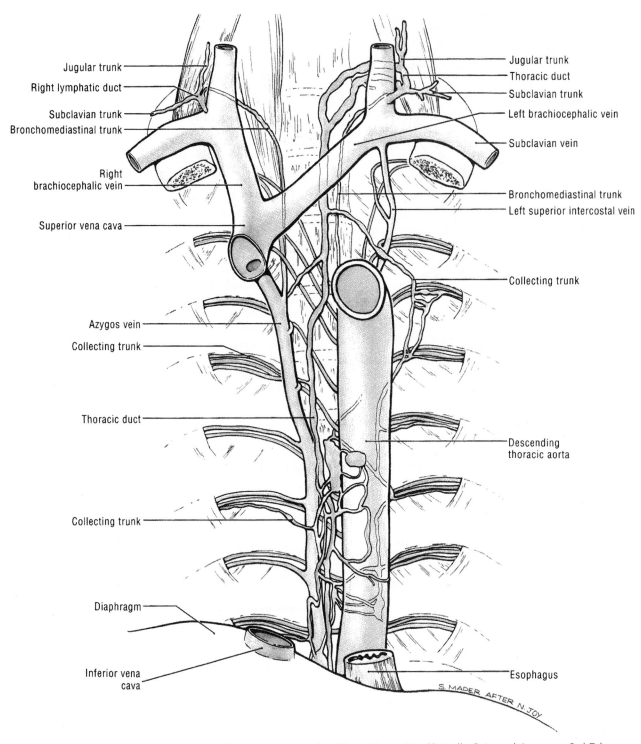

Figure 37-18 Lymphatic drainage through thoracic inlet. (From Moore KL. *Clinically Oriented Anatomy.* 3rd Ed. Baltimore, MD: Williams & Wilkins, 1985:78.)

the type of dysfunction. This process simultaneously evaluates the sidebending, rotation, and flexion/extension components.

EXAMPLE

Occiput rotated right, sidebent left. This pattern may be the result of a posterior/flexed occiput on the right or an anterior/extended occiput on the left.

Posterior/Flexed Occiput Right

- Pattern: O-A rotated right, sidebent left
- Right O-A translates posteriorly and will resist anterior translation. (This is the "open" side, and it will resist extension.)
- Left O-A translates freely both posteriorly and anteriorly
- Tissue texture change and tenderness to palpation is greater on the right

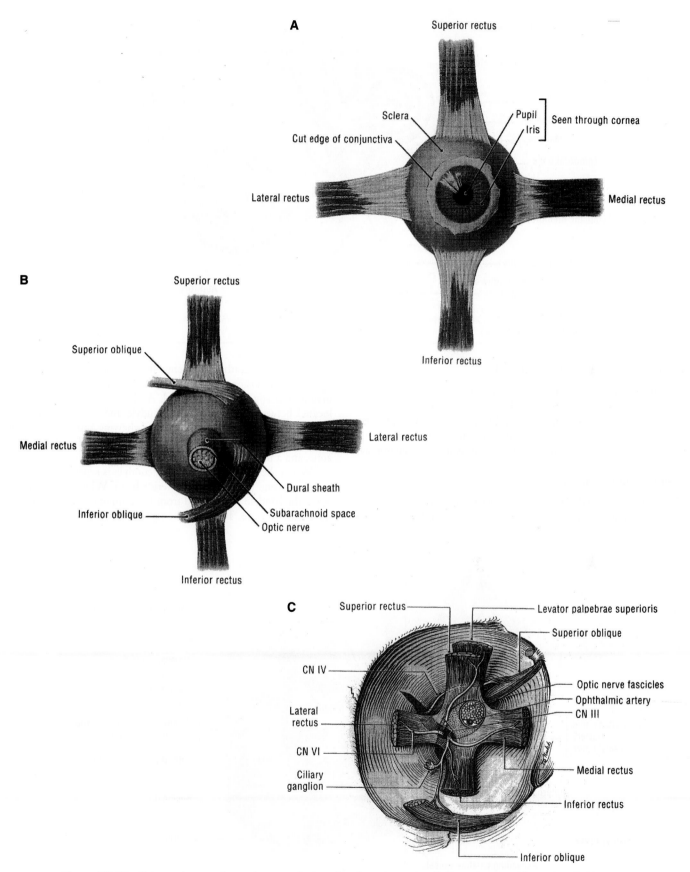

Figure 37-19 Extraocular muscles and nerves. **A.** Anterior view of muscles. **B.** Posterior view of muscles. **C.** Nerves of the orbit. *CN*, cranial nerve. (From Agur AMR. *Grant's Atlas of Anatomy.* 9th Ed. Baltimore, MD: Williams & Wilkins, 1991:486.)

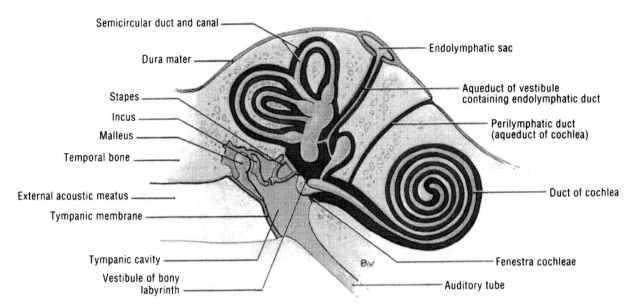

Figure 37-20 Internal structures of the ear. (From Agur AMR. *Grant's Atlas of Anatomy*. 9th Ed. Baltimore, MD: Williams & Wilkins, 1991:534.)

Anterior/Extended Occiput Left

- Pattern: O-A rotated right, sidebent left
- Right O-A translates freely both posteriorly and anteriorly
- Left O-A translates anteriorly and will resist posterior translation. This is the "closed" side, and it will resist flexion.
- Tissue texture change and tenderness to palpation is greater on left

Tempomandibular Joint

The TMJ has been described as the most complex joint in the body because it not only acts as a hinge joint but also permits a gliding movement (11). Both movements are necessary for adequate jaw opening and closing. The articular surface of the condyles of the mandible is smooth and spherical. A fibrocartilagenous meniscus located between the mandibular condyle and the temporal bone acts as a cushion to absorb the shock of chewing and speaking. The meniscus has three parts, a thick anterior band, a thin intermediate zone, and a thick posterior band (11).

When the mouth is closed, the condyle is separated from the temporal bone by the thick posterior band. When the mouth is open, the condyle is separated from the temporal bone by the thin intermediate zone. The articular surface of the temporal bone is

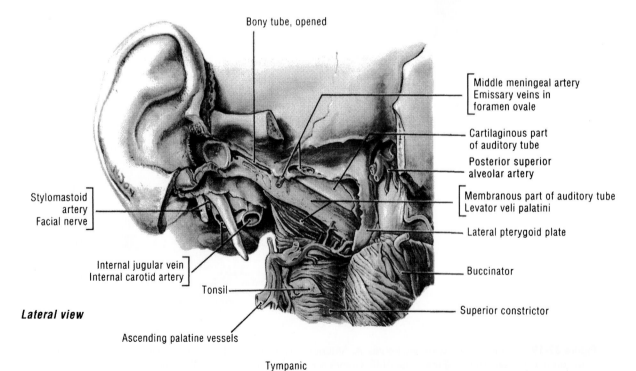

Figure 37-21 Connection of middle ear to nasopharynx. Lateral view. (From Agur AMR. *Grant's Atlas of Anatomy*. 9th Ed. Baltimore, MD: Williams & Wilkins, 1991:541.)

TABLE 37.4

Occiput Diagnosis

Chicago Terminology	Alternate Terminology
Posterior ("open") occiput	Flexed occiput
Anterior ("closed") occiput	Extended occiput

also complex, consisting of a convex articular eminence anteriorly and a concave articular fossa posteriorly.

When the jaw begins to open, there is a hinge movement like a drawbridge lowering. Then as further opening occurs, the condyle of the mandible glides along the squamous portion of the temporal bone until the mouth is wide open. Opening the mouth activates the suprahyoid muscles (mylohyoid, geniohyoid, and digastric muscles), which provide the hinge-like movement. Anterior condylar glide is provided by the inferior division of the lateral (external) pterygoid muscles (11). Then, as closing begins, a posterior glide of the condyles ensures proper placement of the condyles back into its fossa. Elevation of the mandible (closing the mouth) is accomplished by the temporalis, masseter, and medial (internal) pterygoid muscles (11). The meniscus should stay in contact with both bones during this hinge and glide motion. If it does not, it may slip forward or backward causing a click, or even the patient's jaw becoming locked in position. The jaw can become locked in an open or a closed position, depending on the position of the meniscus and the tension of various muscles. Strachan called "open lock" an anterior lesion. It was characterized by an uneven and painful forward glide (on the affected side); chin deviation toward the contralateral side, and inability to close the mouth. Strachan also termed the "closed lock" a posterior lesion (10,11).

SPHENOBASILAR SYNCHRONDOSIS

Assessment of motion of the SBS is important in any complaint referable to the head, eyes, ears, nose, and throat. In both the pediatric patient and adult, motion of the SBS is assessed through gentle palpation of the cranium. The quality, quantity, symmetry, and type of motion are evaluated. The trained clinician can evaluate gross patterns of articular, membranous, and fluid motion. The astute clinician can evaluate more specific individual bone motion, specific suture restrictions, and cranial related motion in other parts of the body. Individual motion of the temporals and their sutures is an important skill to obtain, especially in HEENT disorders.

Students of osteopathic medicine base the hypothetical biomechanics of the SBS on the observations and writings of William Garner Sutherland, as well as the clinical experience of many other osteopathic physicians. The exact physiology of the cranial rhythmic impulse is still under study; however, there is mounting evidence that this phenomenon is related to the Traube–Herring-Meyer wave. The biomechanical model of the primary respiratory mechanism has as its driving force, the inherent motion of the brain and spinal cord, the fluctuation of the cerebrospinal fluid, and the inherent motion of the intracranial and spinal membranes. In this hypothetical model, there is motion between the sphenoid and the occiput. As the SBS rises during cranial flexion, tension is placed on the dura and is transmitted to the sacrum. This upward pull on the sacrum causes cranial flexion (anatomic extension, or counternutation) of the sacral base. During the cranial extension phase, the SBS descends and tension is relieved to the dura sheath. During flexion, paired bones exter-

nally rotate, and during extension paired bones internally rotate. The primary respiratory mechanism is palpable throughout the body, due to the dural motion and fascial continuity.

PATIENT EVALUATION

Obtaining the history of the patient with a complaint referable to the head, eyes, ears, nose, throat, face, or jaw requires a knowledge of common clinical syndromes, anatomy of the region, and the physiologic function of the tissues involved. When a patient enters the office with the above type of complaint, the clinician must find out the primary problem, its duration, location, radiation, severity, associated symptoms, and what has been done so far. It is very important to find out if the patient had sustained any trauma to the head or face. Be sure to delineate if they had a closed head injury or witnessed loss of consciousness. If an injury was involved, the clinician should document all possible information regarding where and when the event occurred, how it happened, who was involved, and the patient's initial course of action (did they go to the emergency room?) The clinician must eliminate any urgent conditions that need to be expediously treated. They also need to use proper judgment in deciding when and how to utilize OMT and when not to. Evaluating the head, face, eyes, ear, nose, and throat in an infant or child is quite different than an adult or elderly patient. The most commonly encountered clinical conditions change as well. The diagnostic and treatment approach used with OMT is also variable based on the patient's age. The clinical application of knowledge and skills over a diverse and varied patient population takes a long time to learn and perfect.

HISTORY

Adult

In the adult patient with a chief complaint referable to the head, eyes, ears, nose, throat, face, or jaw requires the clinician to question the patient regarding:

- Pain
- Traumas
- Infections
- Allergies
- Surgeries
- Exposure to chemicals, irritants, alcohol, or drugs
- Tobacco
- Nutrition
- Emotional health
- Hormonal changes
- Last dental and eye exam

If the patient is found to have occupational risk of injury or reinjury, then appropriate preventative measures need to be in place. Some of these include Ear plugs/ear protection:

- Safety glasses/face shields
- Bite guards/dental protection
- Helmets
- Appropriate respirator masks
- Welding masks

When considering effects of the injury or illness on the cranial mechanism, the following needs to be obtained:

- A thorough birth history
- Dental history and dental surgeries

- Eye injuries and visual acuity
- Glasses, type of correction
- Face lift and/or Botox injections
- Head or neck (including sinus surgery)
- History of concussions

Many times, the history will point to the diagnosis prior to performing the physical exam. For example, with proper questioning of a pharyngitis patient, the patient may state that the sore throat is worse upon arising in the morning. When deriving a differential diagnosis from the history alone, this information could point to post nasal drip as a potential cause, as well as acid reflux disease (nocturnal acid secretion). At this point, the clinician would need to examine the posterior pharynx, the abdomen, and the thoracic and cervical spine for areas of related somatic dysfunction. With the additional information from the physical exam, clinicians can either confirm their suspicions, or go back and reprioritize their differential diagnosis.

Infant

Obtaining the history for an infant comes from the mother and or father, other family members, and caregivers. Sometimes, there is a discrepancy in information if multiple people are involved. A simple look at the child can tell the experienced clinician if the child is "sick" or "toxic" appearing. With infants, they can become ill very quickly, so time is of the essence if one suspects a serious condition, like an intracranial bleed. Any trauma case must be fully evaluated, and if there is any indication from the history or physical findings to suspect abuse (or negligence), the appropriate actions need to be taken. In the pediatric patient with a chief complaint referable to the head, eyes, ears, nose, throat, face, or jaw requires the clinician to question the family or medical staff regarding.

Prenatal history

- Maternal health
- Maternal infections
- Use of tobacco, alcohol, or illicit drugs
- Term, preterm, post dates
- Any intrauterine illnesses
- Epidural

Birth history

- Vaginal delivery or c-section
- Forceps
- Vacuum extraction
- Complications

Head Shape

- Craniosynostosis
- Caput secundum
- Cepahlohematoma
- Plagiocephaly

Head Control

- Age
- Favors one side

Acute Versus Chronic Illness

- Hospitalizations
- Antibiotic usage

- Immunizations
- Congenital anomalies
- Vision/gaze
- Hearing loss
- Suckling/difficulty latching on

Geriatric

Obtaining the history for a geriatric patient comes partly from the patient as well as other family members and caregivers. Sometimes, there is a discrepancy in information if multiple people are involved. The patient might have dementia and a poor recall of how they are doing or what had occurred in the short term. Similar to the child, a simple look at the elder can tell the experienced clinician if the elder is eating, drinking, or sleeping well. With geriatric patients, they may not seek medical care on their own. Many times, it is a family member who calls for them, concerned that they are not doing well. Any trauma case must be fully evaluated. It is common for elders to fall and strike their head. Many are on blood thinners, so that increases their risks for an intracranial bleed. If there is any indication from the history or physical findings to suspect elder abuse, the appropriate actions need to be taken. In the geriatric patient with a chief complaint referable to the head, eyes, ears, nose, throat, face, or jaw requires the clinician to question the family or medical staff regarding:

- Dizziness
- Fall risk "weakness"
- Visual acuity
- Tearing
- Nocturnal eye pain
- Hearing loss
- Dentures
- Closed head injuries
- Last dental and eye exam

PHYSICAL EXAMINATION

Adult

The physical exam always starts with an interpretation of vitals including height and weight. Comparison is made to past-recorded findings. Observation of the face, head, and neck is important. The clinician needs to look at head position, shape, and symmetry. The same holds true for the face. The clinician needs to look at facial position, shape, and symmetry. A unilateral facial droop may indicate a stroke or Bell palsy. An orbit that is larger or smaller and a protruding ear may indicate torsion of the SBS. The scalp and the hair need to be evaluated. Is the hair dry and brittle? If so they might have hypothyroidism. The skin needs o be evaluated for scars, rashes, and skin lesions. A red nose and cheeks may indicate rosacea or possibly lupus. A dark appearing mole on the top of the ear or near the hairline may be a melanoma. Patients who have had a craniotomy have a curvilinear scar on their scalp near the hairline. The temporal arteries need to be palpated, and sometimes ausculated. Tenderness in a 70-year-old patient with headaches, shoulder and hip stiffness, and elevated sedimentation rate may indicate polymyalgia rheumatica and/or temporal arteritis.

Eyes

Start with observation. An orbit that is larger with an ipsilateral protruding ear suggests torsion of the SBS. Unequal pupils (anisocoria) can be congenital or acquired. More than 3 mm is significant.

There are many causes, from sympathetic dysfunction, Horner syndrome, to brain tumors. Obtain a visual acuity test with and without correction. Check each part of the eye—the lids, pupils, iris, conjunctiva, sclera, lacrimal gland, tear duct, etc. Check the function of the extrocular muscles. Then perform an opthalmoscopic exam. Check the patient's cranial mechanism with their glasses on and off, focusing on both near and far objects (ceiling).

Ears

When examining the ears, look at their position during the standing structural exam. An ear that protrudes might be related to an externally rotated temporal bone. Look at the skin of the pinna, tragus, and antitragus. If you suspect otitis externa from your history, pull gently upward and posteriorly on the pinna. This will elicit pain if an otitis externa is present. Perform the otoscopic exam. The canal should be clear of wax, if not clean it out and get a good look at the drum. The drum should be pearly-white with a good reflection of light. The drum can be evaluated for motion by insufflation or a tympanogram. A hearing test is appropriate for specific complaints and for the occupational medicine visit.

Nose

The nose (and face) is a common place to get skin cancers, due to sun exposure. Look at the skin for erythema (rosacea, alcoholism, lupus), acne, scars, etc. Examine the nasal cavity. The nasal mucosa and turbinates should be pink, not red or bluish. The septum should be midline and not swollen. Sites of bleeding need to be found. Polyps appear as clear fleshy protrusions in the nasal cavity and may be related to asthma and aspirin sensitivity.

Sinuses

Palpation of the face over the frontal and maxillary sinuses reveals tenderness when they are full of fluid. The tissues may fell boggy or puffy as well also indicating this. If the frontal and maxillary sinuses are transilluminated, in a dark room, a defect in light transmission is seen in either the frontal bone (frontal sinuses) or in the palate (maxillary sinuses) when a sinus infection is present. This author has found that resistance to a light springing pressure over the maxillary or frontal sinuses can correlate with a sinus infection. Determining if there is involvement of the sphenoid or ethmoid sinuses is more difficult clinically. If the majority of mucus is running down the back of the patient's throat and they are not blowing it out through their nose, the deep sinuses may be involved. If they are tender between the eyes to palpation, this is an indicator as well. The patient usually has a severe deep headache. If the clinician questions involvement of the sphenoid and ethmoid sinuses, then a sinus computed tomography (CT) scan can be done.

Oral Cavity

Examine the lips first for signs of celosias (cracking near the corners), cyanosis, and herpes simplex lesions. Now look at the bubal mucosa, teeth, and gums. Receding gum lines, bleeding, and discoloration may indicate gingival/periodontal disease. Broken teeth, asymmetrically worn cusps, and crooked teeth may indicate bruxism. Palpate the tempomandibular joint as the patient opens and closes his or her mouth. Feel for clicking, grinding, and local tenderness. Watch the teeth hit when the mouth closes. If the jaw deviates to the right, palpate the cranial mechanism and look for an externally rotated temporal bone. Look at the tongue, posterior pharynx, tonsils, and uvula. Have the patient close his or her mouth and open it while palpating his or her CRI. Does it change? How so? If patients have a bite guard, check the motion of their SBS with the guard in and out. If you find that a specific position or motion locks up their mechanism, you know what to have them avoid or change.

Infant

The physical exam of the infant's head, face, eyes, ears, nose, and throat is much different than the adult. Many times, the infant will be sleeping or feeding, which allows a more thorough exam of the head, including the SBS. When the infant is crying, a view of the open mouth and posterior pharynx is possible. Examination should evaluate and document:

- Symmetry and shape of the head
- Head circumference
- Craniosynostosis
- Caput secundum
- Cepahlohematoma
- Plagiocephaly
- Fontanel's
- Dilated scalp veins
- Face, paralysis, asymmetry, color, texture
- Head control position and movement
- Eyes, red reflex, hypertelorism
- Visual acuity in children age 3: Snellen E game
- Shape, size, position of ears

Geriatric

The face of the elderly patient tells a lot about his or her health. Sunken eyes and cheeks may indicate dehydration or malnutrition. Geriatric patients tend to not drink much water and their mucus membranes may be dry and thin. Skin lesions are common especially actinic keratoses, seborrheic keratoses, basal cell cancers, and moles. Pupils may be hazy indicating cataracts. Many elderly patients have poor dentition, dentures, and bridges. Evaluate their cranial mechanism and occiput with their dentures in place, as this helps jaw position and facial appearance. When evaluating the cranial mechanism, the hearing aids may need to be removed so they do not whistle. When the patient lies supine, always keep enough pillows under his or head. This is due to their increased kyphosis as well as the patient with spinal stenosis.

COMMON CLINICAL SYNDROMES

Common Cold

Osteopathic treatment of the common cold should have an objective to accomplish. The objective can be based on the patients' symptoms, the pathophysiologic process, the structural findings, or a combination thereof. The primary etiologic factor in the common cold is the loss of physiologic and anatomic integrity resulting in vasomotor imbalance, dry mucus membranes, and a functionally impaired immune system (12). Predisposing factors include patients who are not well hydrated, have dry/irritated mucous membranes, have lowered resistance of the immune system, are exposed to others who are ill, have poor nutritional status, and are not sleeping well. Every patient has a normal amount of bacterial and viral flora of their mucous membranes; however, when this barrier becomes compromised, nosocomial flora can become "invaders." The viral etiology of the common cold, as well as a bacterial superinfection, needs to be considered as a "secondary infection," due to a *primary physiologic dysfunction*. OMT can address the primary physiologic dysfunction and allow the body's own immune system to fight the invading organism(s).

The process starts with compromised mucous membranes. The mucous membranes are under autonomic control. The vasodilator nerves come from the parasympathetic nervous system via CN seven, by way of the sphenopalatine ganglion. The vasoconstrictor nerves come from the sympathetics. The preganglionic fibers of the sympathetics to the head and neck arise in the upper thoracic spinal cord (T1-4). From here, they follow the great vessels into the neck to synapse at the superior cervical ganglion. From the superior cervical ganglion, postganglionic fibers supply the mucous membranes of the nose and throat as well as other structures of the face and neck. Osteopathic evaluation needs to start in the upper thoracics and ribs. Somatic dysfunction in this area can affect sympathetic tone to the head and neck. This with increasing fluid consumption will decrease the viscosity of the nasal secretions and bronchial mucus, allowing expectoration. It will also shrink the swelling and edema of the mucous membranes (making it easier to breathe) and normalize autonomic tone to the bronchi and lungs. According to Becker, articulatory treatment of the lower thoracic and lumbar spine will effect vasomotor tone to the abdominal viscera and provide better circulation to the skin of the entire body. He felt that there was a direct relationship between the vasomotor innervation of the nasal mucosa and that of the circulation in the skin (12). Following treatment of the thoracic spine and ribs, the thoracic inlet and cervical spine are treated. Eliminating fascial restrictions of the thoracic inlet can improve lymphatic drainage from the head and neck (2). Treatment of the sternoclavicular joints, first rib, and shoulders may be necessary to free the thoracic inlet. The suboccipital region is usually tender and reactive to palpation. If so, gentle indirect techniques are an appropriate choice. Treatment of the face, and neck, encourages drainage from the sinuses, ears, nose, and posterior pharynx. Tender reflex points are located over the branches of the trigeminal nerve (V1, V2, and V3) as well as in the masseters, temporalis, sternocleidomastoid, and anterior chest wall. Circular inhibitory pressure applied to these points causes vasoconstriction and improves nasal congestion draining of the sinuses. Facial effleurage and lymphatic pump procedures augment drainage. Treatment of cranial dysfunction assists in managing a patient with sinus congestion. If significant frontal sinus congestion is present, performing a frontal lift may be beneficial to facilitate drainage as well.

In summary, osteopathic treatment:

1. Improves the blood supply to the skin, head, and neck
2. Increases venous and lymphatic drainage from the affected area
3. Relieves muscle spasm, thereby improving breathing
4. Relieves pain
5. Reduces reflex disturbances
6. Improves circulation to and from the reticuloendothelial system and thereby improves immune function
7. Normalizes autonomic and somatic nerve function

Sinusitis

Acute sinusitis is a self-limiting problem. Chronic or recurrent sinusitis is more of a diagnostic and treatment dilemma. Always consider anatomic obstruction of drainage. This could be an abnormal osteomeatal complex, a polyp, swollen membranes, nasal septal deviation, or even a tumor. The paranasal sinuses are air-filled extensions of the nasal cavity into the frontal, ethmoid, sphenoid, and maxillary bones. All of the paranasal sinuses drain directly or indirectly into the nasal cavity. The frontal and sphenoidal sinuses are absent at birth and develop during childhood and adolescence. Sinus headache referral patterns are predictable because branches of the trigeminal nerve innervate the sinuses. Sinus dysfunction (acute and chronic sinusitis and chronic postnasal drip) may result from cranial dysfunction. Removing dysfunctional cranial motion patterns may allow the sinuses to drain more freely and provide symptomatic relief. In cases of bacterial sinusitis, improving blood flow to and lymphatic drainage from the sinuses may allow antibiotics to work more efficiently. Allergy may predispose to swelling, obstruction, mucus production, and superinfection.

The frontal sinuses drain into the middle meatus and are innervated by branches of the supraorbital nerves (CNV1 branch of the trigeminal nerve). Impaired drainage from the frontal sinuses may result from frontal bone restriction. Frontal sinusitis may be associated with palpable tissue texture changes over the supraorbital foramen. Frontal sinusitis may respond to frontal lift technique.

The ethmoid sinuses drain into the superior and middle meatus and are innervated by branches of the ophthalmic nerve (CNV1 branch of the trigeminal nerve). Impaired drainage may result from ethmoid bone restriction. This ethmoid bone restriction usually occurs secondary to frontal bone restriction, sphenoid dysfunction, or maxilla dysfunction. Ethmoid bone restriction may respond to frontal lift technique, vomer pump, and other facial articulatory techniques.

The sphenoid sinuses drain into the sphenoethmoidal recess, in close approximation to the cavernous sinuses, and are innervated by the posterior ethmoid nerve (CNV1 branch of the trigeminal nerve). Infections of the sphenoid sinuses are especially dangerous due to close approximation with the pituitary gland, brainstem, cavernous sinus, and CNs. Impaired drainage may result from motion restrictions affecting the sphenoid bone (torsion, sidebending/rotation, vertical strain, lateral strain, and SBS compression). Impaired drainage may respond to correction of the dysfunctional motion pattern.

The maxillary sinuses drain into the middle meatus and are innervated by branches of the maxillary nerve (CNV2 branch of the trigeminal nerve). Maxillary sinusitis may be associated with palpable tissue texture changes over the infraorbital foramen. The maxillary bone articulates with and is driven by the frontal bone and sphenoid. Maxillary sinusitis may improve with correction of dysfunctional maxillary, sphenoid, and/or frontal bone motion.

Increased sympathetic tone from the upper thoracic region can cause vasoconstriction and a reduction of medication distribution. It will also thicken mucus, decrease lymphatic response and lymphatic flow. Parasympathetic imbalance can cause increased tearing (watery eyes) and a runny nose. Dysfunction of the suboccipital region can irritate the vagus nerve producing a "vagal" headache and nausea. Sinus congestion may irritate the trigeminal nerve producing a headache. Lymphatic and venous stasis contributes to the pressure sensation and headache in these patients. T1-4 is the focus of sympathetic activity for the head and neck. Tissue texture changes at these thoracic levels and especially over the costotransverse area and the rib angles are significant. Parasympathetic innervation to the head and neck is via CNs III, VII, IX and X. Cranial somatic dysfunction can affect the function of these nerves. The occiput, atlas, and C2 should be considered a functional unit. Tissue texture abnormality is significant in this region in the sinusitis patient; this is partly due to the relationship of this area to the vagus nerve.

Tissue texture abnormality at the cranial base and occipitomastoid area can impair jugular drainage from the head. Thoracic inlet fascial restrictions can also impair lymphatic and venous drainage from the head. Cranial dysfunction, especially the temporal bone, can affect the autonomic nervous system, drainage from the eustachian tube and CN function.

Goals for Osteopathic Manipulative Management

1. Adequate treatment of sinus infections centers around three principles:

   - Drainage
   - Treat the offending organism or condition
   - Support the host

2. *Drainage* can be accomplished through a variety of techniques. Opening the thoracic inlet and decreasing sympathetic tone prior to sinus techniques works well. Inhibitory pressure over the branches of the trigeminal nerve may decrease nerve sensitivity to the underlying structures. Facial effleurage mobilizes lymph and increases circulation. Percussion over the sinuses loosens mucus. Articulation of the nasal bones opens the osteomeatal complex.

3. *Supporting the host* is directed at balancing sympathetic/parasympathetic tone, removing mechanical restrictions of lymphatic flow, relaxing soft tissue tensions, and improving motion restrictions.

OMT will help drain the sinuses and liquefy mucus. Without achieving adequate drainage and liquefaction of the mucus, antibiotics alone will not work. Suboccipital tissues contain significant (and very tender) tissue findings. Treat the upper thoracic and ribs first prior to addressing the suboccipital region. Dr. McCarty found numerous reflex tenderpoints associated with acute sinusitis (13). He felt that treating these reflex tenderpoints with inhibitory pressure breaks into the autonomic disturbance. Following treatment of these tender reflex points, the patient may feel warm and sweaty. This signifies adequate treatment (13). In addition, cranial dysfunction may result in sinus pain without the presence of infection. It is important to remember the associated neural innervations and treat the associated dysfunctional patterns. Additionally, trigeminal nerve stimulation will help with sinus drainage. Ethmoid articulation will facilitate sphenoid and ethmoid sinus drainage. Lymphatic decongestion of the pterygopalatine fossa area improves overall sinus drainage and eustachian tube function via the sphenopalatine ganglion. Addressing somatic dysfunction in the neck and upper thoracic regions improves lymphatic drainage from the sinuses including drainage through the thoracic outlet and diaphragmatic motion (T-L jct. and rib raising).

Tension Headache

Headache is one of the most common conditions seen in a primary care practice. Every year, 40 to 50 million Americans seek treatment for headaches (5). This condition can be caused by a number of intracranial and extracranial abnormalities. The underlying cause of many headaches is often described as "unknown" or "idiopathic."

Tension headaches are the result of the body's response to stress, anxiety, depression, fatigue, and emotional conflicts (work, school, family, and marriage). The body responds by contracting the skeletal muscles of the head, neck, and face. Tension-type headaches usually occur bilaterally and are described as a fullness, tightness, or pressure sensation in the forehead, temporal area, or back of the head or neck (especially in the suboccipital area). They may also be described as a band-like sensation around the head. Tension-type headaches are not usually associated with nausea or vomiting. They may be associated with sleep disturbances. Headaches in combination with anxiety may result in difficulties falling asleep. Headaches in combination with depression may be associated with early and frequent awakening.

A good history and physical exam is necessary to classify headaches. Quality and severity of pain, localization of pain, timing of headaches, associated symptoms (e.g., auras), dental history, and musculoskeletal pain and/or neurologic symptoms should all be investigated. Has he taken anything for the pain? Is he on any new medications? Has his social history changed (e.g., quit drinking coffee)? What are his current psychosocial issues? A detailed history is vital to the diagnosis and treatment of headache, especially if they are recurrent or chronic in nature. Information regarding the patient's birth history (length of mother's pregnancy, maternal complications, length of labor, method of delivery, use of forceps, pitocin or vacuum extraction, neonatal complications) and childhood growth and development may shed light on the precipitating factors for headache. A history of trauma is often important. Clinical experience has revealed that a forgotten fall or head injury that has resulted in a sacral shear has often been overlooked and is the key to providing effective treatment of a chronic headache. Family history should be obtained (5), including information about:

- Headache: onset, frequency, location, duration, and severity
- Associated symptoms
- Trigger factors
- Previous medical, surgical, and dental history
- Prior headache therapy

A thorough knowledge of anatomy and physiology and ability to diagnose structural abnormalities of the cranium, neck, upper thoraces, and sacrum often allows a physician to logically explain and treat previously unknown causes of headache. The implementation of a rational treatment plan significantly reduces suffering of the patient and improves overall functioning.

The head and scalp contain many pain-sensitive structures. These include:

- Skin and its blood supply
- Muscles of the head and neck
- Great venous sinuses and their tributaries
- Portions of the dura mater at the base of the brain
- Dural arteries
- Intracranial arteries
- Cervical nerves
- Trigeminal (V), abducens (VI), and facial (VII) nerves

The pathophysiology of tension-type headaches remains controversial but may involve the trigeminal neurovascular system and unstable serotonergic neurotransmission. Recent evidence supports the hypothesis that the basic pathophysiology of tension-type headache is qualitatively similar to but quantitatively different from migraine. The brain parenchyma itself is not sensitive to pain. Pain from structures above the tentorium cerebelli travel via the trigeminal nerve, so pain referred from structures above the tentorium cerebelli is perceived in the frontal, temporal, and parietal regions of the head. Pain fibers from structures below the tentorium cerebelli travel via the glossopharyngeal (IX) and vagus (X) nerves and the upper cervical spinal nerve roots. Therefore, pain referred from structures below the tentorium cerebelli is perceived in the occipital region (5).

A complete physical examination is performed, including a neurologic evaluation, in addition to the structural examination. The neurologic exam is mandatory, but likely to be normal. Carefully document your findings. Always rule out serious organic causes of headache, such as brain tumor, aneurysm, arteriovenous malformation, hemorrhage, and temporal arteritis. Neuroradiologic studies such as CT, magnetic resonance imaging (MRI), and/or magnetic resonance angiography are needed if any of the aforementioned is suspected (5).

From an osteopathic perspective, is there a postural component to this patient's problem? What are the specific mechanics of his upper body while he performs his job? Is there something noxious in the work place? Is he feeling anxious about his work performance? Structural abnormalities, usually acting via the fasciae, place tension on pain-sensitive structures and cause discomfort. For example, parietal bone dysfunction produces strain on the superior sagittal sinus, producing discomfort in the parietal region. Upper cervical dysfunction leads to discomfort in the occipital region. Gastrointestinal abnormalities result in headache in the occipital region via vagal transmission.

Upper thoracic and cervical muscle spasm may produce paresthesias in the upper extremity, but there are often limited objective findings for this on exam. Along with upper thoracic and cervical findings, suboccipital tissue texture changes and tenderness will be present as well. Somatic dysfunction in the upper thoracics, cervicothoracic junction, and cranium (internally rotated temporal bone) may result in increased sympathetic tone to the head. This will make the muscles in the upper back and neck tight. Poor posture can contribute to somatic dysfunction in the upper thoracic spine. Many people who work at a desk or computer develop a kyphotic posture where the scapulas are protracted and the shoulders are rolled forward. The upper neck backward bends and the suboccipital muscles tighten. The pectoralis minor muscle subsequently tightens. Workstation problems need to be addressed. Computer screens may need to be raised to eye level to promote good posture. Chair height may need to be altered to promote good posture. The patient may benefit from performing daily postural exercises, scapular stabilization exercises, pectoralis minor stretches, and scalene stretches. Patients with hypermobility affecting the neck may respond to cervical isometric exercises.

Is there an emotional component to the patient's condition? How does the patient look in general? Is his or her affect appropriate? Does the content and the manner of his speech give any clues to how he is feeling emotionally? Ask if he feels "stressed out." If so, acknowledge the patient's feelings; this may facilitate an important part of the patient's therapy.

Tension-type headache is the ideal situation in which to utilize osteopathic manipulation while addressing the underlying triggers (Table 37.5). Educating the patient regarding postural mechanics, appropriate footwear, and tension-relieving exercises will help reduce the frequency of his headaches. Stress management counseling should be offered to assist the patient in dealing with the emotional component of his condition. By identifying the patient's specific stressors and current coping mechanisms, you can individualize your recommendations to the patient's specific needs. This is also the opportunity to counsel the patient regarding the importance of smoking cessation. It has been clearly demonstrated that smokers experience more pain and heal more slowly. Is it possible that altered respiratory motion with utilization of accessory muscles of respiration is contributing to his headaches? Could hypoxia be playing a role as well?

MIGRAINE HEADACHE

Migraine headaches are a common cause of functional disability in the United States. The annual cost of lost productivity in the United States has been estimated to range from $1.2 billion to $17.2 billion. Migraine headaches are frequently described as a unilateral throbbing, pounding pain. They can radiate to the opposite side. They may be associated with nausea, vomiting,

---

TABLE 37.5

Treatment algorithm for Tension-Type Headache

Treatment Plan	Objective	Technique
Treat upper thoracic and rib dysfunction	Eliminate upper thoracic dysfunction involved in perpetuating the pain; balance autonomic tone	Soft tissue, MFR, ME, FPR, Counterstrain, HVLA, rib raising
Treat cervical dysfunction, particularly involving the occiput, C1, and C2	Eliminate cervical mechanics and soft tissue tension involved in exacerbating the pain	Soft tissue, Occipitoatlantal MFR, FPR, ME, HVLA
Treat cranial dysfunction including TMJ dysfunction	Eliminate cranial strain patterns affecting the trigeminal neurovascular system	Direct and indirect cranial osteopathy; MFR and ME technique for TMJ dysfunction
Treat lumbar, sacrum, and pelvis	Eliminate compensatory or contributing strain patterns from below	Soft tissue, MFR, ME, HVLA, Counterstrain
Address postural mechanics	Reduce exacerbating factors	Core strengthening, scapular retractions, cervical isometric exercises, proprioceptive training
Stress reduction counseling	Reduce exacerbating factors while enhancing overall well-being	One-on-one counseling to identify specific stressors and individualize stress management strategies
Health promotion and disease prevention	Reduce risk of future illness; enhance overall well-being	Smoking cessation, exercise and nutrition counseling; health screening (e.g., fasting lipids, immunizations)

diarrhea, vertigo, dizziness, tremors, photophobia (light sensitivity), phonophobia (sound sensitivity), sweating, and chills. Migraines may be preceded by scotomas (blind spots in the eyes); photopsia (flashing lights); vertigo; paresthesias (abnormal sensations); visual, olfactory, and auditory hallucinations; or syncope (passing out). Migraine headaches are recurrent and vary widely in intensity, frequency, and duration.

The initial episode most often occurs during puberty but can occur at any age between 5 and 40 years. Migraine headaches may be triggered by (5):

- Head injury or other trauma
- Stress
- Hormone fluctuations
- Fasting
- Oversleeping and under sleeping
- Vasoactive substances in foods (wine and cheese, cold foods)
- Changes in weather and temperature (bright light, poor ventilation)
- Physical stimuli (smoking), caffeine

Migraine headaches are thought to occur by the following mechanism. The production of migraine symptoms involves two major events: vasoconstriction and vasodilation. The cerebral blood vessels can be divided into two major systems: the innervated (adrenergic) system and the noninnervated arterial system. The large innervated vascular system consists of the arteries at the base of the brain and the pial arteries. These have a rich adrenergic nerve supply and respond to catecholamines. The noninnervated vascular system consists of the parenchymal arteries and the terminal high-resistance arteries. They respond to local metabolic factors.

Trigger factors (listed above) produce unilateral cerebral vasoconstriction via the adrenergic nervous system. Platelets systemically aggregate and release serotonin, which augments vasoconstriction of these adrenergically innervated blood vessels. The overall result is vasoconstriction with a reduction in cerebral blood flow. When blood flow is sufficiently reduced, an aura develops with symptoms occurring as a consequence of which brain region is affected by the constriction. The vasoconstriction phase causes local anoxia and acidosis and a systemic drop in serotonin. Serotonin sensitizes the pain receptors in the blood vessels. In response to local metabolic factors (anoxia and acidosis), the vessels of the noninnervated arterial system dilate, increasing cerebral blood flow and promoting local vasomotor changes resulting in a combined dilation of the innervated extracranial and intracranial arteries on the same side. This vasodilation, along with the sensitization of pain fibers, produces the pain of migraine (5).

A trigeminal vascular reflex may also explain some of the events seen in the production of migraines. Afferent pain fibers from the cortex, thalamus, hypothalamus, and cervical roots C1-3 communicate with the spinal nucleus of the trigeminal nerve. These impulses can then travel via the facial nerve (CN VII) to produce parasympathetic dilation of the internal and external carotid arteries. Pain perception is increased when the effects of this dilation feed back into the spinal nucleus of the trigeminal nerve. Stimulation of the trigeminal ganglion, through vasodilation, can also produce edema in the dura (5).

The biologically sensitive nervous system is confronted with trigger factors (listed above) that can provoke a migraine. The neurochemical balance of the nervous system changes and symptoms, recognized as *prodromal*, may occur. This change progresses until the migraine threshold is crossed and an area in the brainstem called the "migraine generator" is activated. This may initiate a wave of neuronal depression to move across the cortex and activate

trigeminal afferents and the vascular structures they innervate. As branches of the first division of the trigeminal nerve are activated, neuropeptides are released at the neurovascular junction. The neuropeptides produce a sterile inflammation of the meningeal arteries associated with platelet aggregation and release of serotonin, which may potentiate the migraine process. Bidirectional conduction conducts nerve impulses back into the CN V nucleus located in the brainstem. These impulses are then routed to various neurons in the thalamus and cerebral cortex. The upper cervical cord gets involved through this nucleus, too, and that explains the neck pain that is often involved. Brainstem reflexes are activated that produce the migraine-associated symptoms, including nausea, vomiting, photophobia, and phonophobia. Autonomic activation occurs via the facial nerve and results in nasal congestion, rhinorrhea, and lacrimation. Pain in the face over the sinus cavities is also common and may be due to CN V2 activation. Researchers have found evidence of breakdown products of serotonin in the urine of those who have just experienced a migraine headache. They have also found that injecting anyone with a *serotonin-depleting chemical* can produce a migraine headache, even if the person has never had a migraine in the past. Medications (Imitrex and Zomig—5HT1 receptor agonists) are effective in treating a migraine headache even during the attack. The pain from a migraine seems to be due to cerebral vasodilatation. In migraine patients, local vasodilatation of cerebral vessels seems to be produced when platelets line up in a portion of a cerebral artery and release humoral vasodilating substances. The vasodilatation is not autonomic—it is humoral.

Somatic dysfunction in the upper thoracic spine increases the level of sympathetic tone to the innervated blood vessels of the head. Increased sympathetic tone produces vasoconstriction and a resultant decrease in cerebral blood flow. This results in a relative anoxia and may lower the threshold for vasodilation, thereby contributing to the production of migraine symptoms. Cranial dysfunction affecting the cortex, thalamus and hypothalamus, and upper cervical dysfunction affecting cervical nerve roots C1-3 may result in the transfer of afferent pain stimuli to the spinal nucleus of the trigeminal nerve. The trigeminal nerve courses through various portions of the sphenoid bone. An elevated greater wing of the sphenoid (torsion) may apply dural pressure resulting in irritation of the trigeminal nerve, thereby feeding into the trigeminal vascular reflex. A sphenosquamous compression can compromise the function of the middle meningeal artery. The facial nerve courses through the temporal bone. Dysfunction of the temporal bone, such as internal rotation, can result in reflex vasodilation of the internal and external carotid arteries via the facial nerve. Occipitomastoid compression can result in reduced venous drainage through the jugular foramen, thereby producing congestion and dysfunction in the cortex, thalamus, and hypothalamus as well as CNs IX and X.

Migraine headaches are more than just a problem with the head. They are a total body problem. Myofascial strain patterns stored within the abdomen or elsewhere in the body can cause tension changes on the base of the skull contributing to the disorder. Excessive tension around the sacrum and coccyx can contribute to increased tension in the upper back and neck. Vasodilation of cranial vessels during a classic migraine is a local phenomenon. Patients with common migraine or mixed tension-type headaches often have upper thoracic somatic dysfunction associated with (autonomic) dysfunction to the head and neck. An extended upper thoracic somatic dysfunction is typically acutely painful; keep muscle tone of the head, suboccipital, and neck increased and motion restricted. It is common to find suboccipital dysfunction related to upper thoracic and rib somatic dysfunction. Treating the upper thoracics and ribs with Counterstrain or myofascial release techniques improves suboccipital tissue texture abnormality.

Somatic dysfunction of the sphenoid, temporal, and occiput may also be involved in trigeminal dysfunctions and headaches. The trigeminal ganglion provides sensory nerves from the forehead and upper and lower jaw. According to Magoun, normal movement of the temporals is critical, especially in migraine patients—they must move properly. It is difficult to treat a patient during an acute migraine. Treatment of a patient with a migraine can reduce the severity and frequency of acute migraine attacks, but the immediate treatment of an acute migraine in progress is medical.

OMT will enable many patients to either reduce the dosage or frequency of their medication. Several patients, when treated, may only occasionally require Motrin or Tylenol for rare minor headache. Does OMT work when the patient is actively having a migraine headache? Usually. It is always best to treat the patient between headaches. It is possible, however, to provide some relief while the patient is presently having a headache. It does take some time, however, for the inflammatory mediators and other chemicals involved in migraine headaches to be removed from the head by the lymphatics.

Most patients will be placed on a home exercise program that focuses on stretching exercises to reduce the amount of tension in the body (especially in the upper back and neck) and to help return balance to the body. OMT is used to improve motion in the body. The patient's responsibility is to maintain the improvements by performing the prescribed home exercise program. Stretches seem especially important.

TMJ SYNDROME

An estimated 10 million people in the United States (1 in 25) have TMJ disorder. The greatest incidence is in adults aged 20 to 40 years. The female-to-male ratio is 4:1 (11).

TMJ dysfunction is the most frequent source of facial pain after toothache. Patients with TMJ syndrome commonly complain of facial pain and jaw range of motion (ROM) restriction. Earache is fairly common. Facial pain is usually periauricular, worsened by chewing. The patient may also have clicking, popping, and snapping sounds, headaches, or neck pain.

The current diagnostic criteria divide TMJ dysfunction into three categories: myofascial pain dysfunction (MPD) syndrome, internal derangement (ID) injury, and degenerative joint disease (DJD) (11). MPD syndrome is best characterized as a psychophysiologic disease primarily involving the muscles of mastication, frequently provoked by tension as well as somatic dysfunctions elsewhere in the body (11). ID is defined as an abnormal relationship between the articular disc and the mandibular condyle (11). Dental procedures are a common source of trauma (particularly work on molar teeth) and can cause ID.

A common example includes acute and chronic disc displacement. Anterior disc displacement is the most common cause of ID. The disc dislocation reduces upon opening of the jaw, which causes an *opening click*. The disc dislocates again upon closing of the jaw, which causes a *closing click*. If the condyle cannot override the displaced disc, jaw locking occurs. DJD involves arthritic degeneration of the articular surfaces within the TMJ. This occur with long-standing dental malocclusion, bruxism, and ID of the TMJ. The other causes of DJD are osteoarthritis, rheumatoid arthritis, ankylosis, infections of the bone or joint, and neoplasia.

The TMJ has been described as the most complex joint in the body because it not only acts as a hinge joint but also permits a gliding movement, in which the condyle of the mandible slides along the squamous portion of the temporal bone (11). The articular surface of the temporal bone is similarly complex, consisting of a convex articular eminence anteriorly and a concave articular fossa posteriorly. The stylomandibular ligament connects the angle of the mandible to the styloid process of the temporal bone and the sphenomandibular ligament connects the lingula (medial aspect) of the mandible to the spine of the sphenoid. The condyle and the temporal bone are separated by an articular disc or meniscus that divides the joint cavity into two small spaces. The meniscus has three parts: a thick anterior band, a thin intermediate zone, and a thick posterior band (11). When the mouth is closed, the condyle is separated from the temporal bone by the thick posterior band. When the mouth is open, the condyle is separated from the temporal bone by the thin intermediate zone. The suprahyoid muscles (mylohyoid, geniohyoid, and digastric muscles) provide a hinge-like movement to open the mouth. Anterior condylar glide is provided by the inferior division of the lateral (external) pterygoid muscles. Closing the mouth is accomplished by the temporalis, masseter, and medial (internal) pterygoid muscles. Lateral displacement (grinding movement) activates the ipsilateral temporalis and the contralateral medial and lateral pterygoids and masseter muscles.

During the physical exam of the patient, observe for lateral tracking of the mandible away from midline as the mouth is slowly opened. A deflection of the jaw to one side may occur in a C- or S-shaped pattern. While testing jaw ROM, palpate for clicking or popping of the joint as well as crepitus. Sometimes, the jaw will become locked when opening or closing. Strachan called the open lock position an *anterior lesion*, characterized by an uneven and painful forward glide on the affected side, and chin deviation toward the contralateral side, with an inability to close the mouth (9). He called the closed lock a *posterior lesion*. He describes manipulative techniques for treating each condition.

When considering the work-up of patients with TMJ, laboratory and imaging studies generally are not indicated. MRI, although costly, is the study of choice if articular or meniscal pathology is suspected and an endoscopic or surgical procedure is contemplated and in a case of traumatic TMJ syndrome (11). If the patient has associated tinnitus, hearing loss, or other neurologic complaints, an MRI of the brain should be ordered.

Treatment needs to address the pathology present, the exacerbating factors, and the symptoms that the patient is suffering with. Pain is usually controlled with medications; however, reducing tension in the jaw muscles, decreasing swelling and inflammation, and improving tissue congestion can reduce pain. The key to relaxing jaw muscles is keeping the teeth slightly apart. Nonsteroidal anti-inflammatory drugs can reduce inflammation and control pain, especially after dental procedures. Gabapentin (Neurotin) and its new analog pregabalin (Lyrica) have been prescribed for chronic TMJ syndrome (11). Any chronic painful condition, such as chronic TMJ syndrome, will worsen any pre-existing anxiety or depression. Therefore, treatment should include stress management, relaxation techniques for the face and neck, as well as medications when necessary. According to Nelson, benzodiazepines and codeine have no place in chronic TMJ syndrome (11). Exercise sheets and other resources can be obtained online from the TMJ Association. With long-standing dysfunction, the joint capsule may stretch, making the joint unstable. In this instance, injection of a proliferating agent into the joint (sclerotherapy) may tighten the capsule and help normalize motion.

Improving somatic dysfunction of the cranium, upper cervical and upper thoracic region is of great benefit in TMJ patients.

These are common regions of dysfunction in these patients; however, somatic dysfunction of any region may contribute to the TMJ patient through the continuity of the fascia. Postural imbalance from short leg syndrome has also been associated with TMJ (2).

When considering cranial somatic dysfunction, evaluation of the occiput and temporals is critical. In a study of 130 TMJ patients, nearly all presented with at least one type of biomechanical cranial dysfunction. Since the mandible hangs from the temporals, asymmetric tension of the jaw muscles, bruxism, and malocclusion will affect the position and motion of the cranium. Cranial dysfunction can affect TMJ motion because as the temporal bone externally rotates, the ipsilateral mandibular fossa moves posteriorly and medially. Internal rotation allows the ipsilateral mandibular fossa to move anteriorly and laterally. The mandible will deviate toward the side of the externally rotated temporal bone or away from the side of the internally rotated temporal bone. Sphenoid dysfunction can affect the TMJ through its direct articulation with the temporal bone or by its articulation with the mandible through the sphenomandibular ligament. Occlusal splints (mouth orthotics) are controversial (8). Manipulative treatments should be given before and after fitting for occlusal splints and before and after restorative dentistry. Normalize function of the temporal bone, since the squamous portion of that bone directly affects articular function of the TMJ.

Dysfunction of the occiput and atlas is commonly associated with the temporal bone. Tender points located in the soft tissues between the ramus of the mandible and the mastoid process are commonly found. Sometimes referred to as atlas Counterstrain points, treatment of this area with Counterstrain, effleurage, or the William Galbreath technique is useful. Articular dysfunction of the occiput on atlas usually has an upper thoracic component maintaining it. The occiput dysfunction will return if adequate treatment of the upper thoracics is neglected. Treatment of the upper thoracic spine is important in TMJ patients.

Bell Palsy

Bell palsy is caused by an inflammation and compression of the facial nerve and results in unilateral paralysis or paresis of the face. The condition affects approximately 23 in 100,000 persons; with onset typically occurring between the ages of 10 and 40 years (15). Bell palsy affects men and women at a roughly equal rate of occurrence (15). Many patients recover within 1 to 3 weeks. The cornea must be protected and kept lubricated while the condition is resolving (6).

The physiologic mechanism responsible for Bell palsy appears to involve inflammation of the facial nerve within the osseous facial canal, causing compression and ischemia of the nerve (15). A viral cause of Bell palsy has been suspected since the mid-1990s. Herpes simplex virus–type 1 was isolated from the facial nerve in patients affected by Bell palsy (16).

Symptoms of Bell palsy may be mild or quite severe (15). Severe symptoms of facial paralysis and ineffective tear production sometimes progress to corneal ulcerations. Physical signs of Bells palsy include drooping of the corners of the mouth, indistinct skin folds and facial creases, and an unfurrowed forehead. The clinical presentation is worrisome, in the outpatient setting, as Bell palsy has signs similar to a stroke. When patients eat, food may collect between their teeth and lips, and they may drool from the corner of their mouth. Smiling may reveal a marked contrast between the two sides of the face, with the affected side drawn without wrinkles. Depending on where the lesion occurs in the osseous facial canal, a patient's taste reception in the anterior two thirds of the tongue

may be altered. A patient may also experience pain in or behind the ear and hyperacusis (15).

When considering treatment for Bell palsy, the conventional treatment involves the use of oral prednisone (60 to 80 mg daily) for 5 days, followed by a tapering in dosage for 5 additional days (15).

Understanding the anatomy of the facial nerve and facial canal is important prior to treating patients with OMT. When using OMT to treat a patient who has Bell palsy, knowledge of the anatomy of the facial nerve as it traverses the temporal bone is important in understanding the nature of symptoms. The facial nerve travels through the internal acoustic meatus, located in the petrous portion of the temporal bone. It travels through the temporal bone via the facial canal. Here lies the geniculate ganglion, which supplies taste to the anterior tongue and cutaneous sensation of the external acoustic meatus. Branches of the facial nerve include:

- the greater petrosal nerve
- the stapedius nerve
- the nerve of the chorda tympani

The petrosal nerve provides parasympathetic innervation of the lacrimal gland. The stapedius nerve innervates the stapedius muscle, allowing dampening of loud sounds, and the chorda tympani supplies taste to the anterior two thirds of the tongue and parasympathetic innervation of the submandibular and sublingual glands (15). The facial nerve exits the cranium through the stylomastoid foramen to give rise to six terminal motor branches leading to the muscles of facial expression (17).

The osteopathic treatment plan should include treatment of the whole person, not just the face and head. Dysfunction of the sacrum, upper thoracic and cervical spine, and osteopathic cranial mechanism can contribute to impaired lymphatic drainage from the facial canal, leading to inflammation of the facial nerve. Start by treating the patient's lymphatic system by freeing up restrictions found in four key diaphragms: the thoracic outlet, respiratory diaphragm, suboccipital diaphragm, and cerebellar tentorium. Treatment of the patient began in the area of the thoracic duct and thoracic outlet with myofascial release of the supraclavicular fascia and use of the thoracic pump technique. The respiratory diaphragm was treated to allow for deeper breathing, thus creating greater pressure gradients to aid in lymphatic flow (18). Primary respiratory mechanism and osteopathy in the cranial field were used to release restrictions in the cerebellar tentorium, which attaches to the temporal bone and allows for physiologic temporal motion. Osteopathic physicians commonly find restricted ipsilateral motion of the temporal bone and upper cervical restrictions in patients with Bell palsy (19). Another area commonly restricting temporal motion is at the occipitomastoid suture. Look for a compression of the occipitomastoid maintaining an internally rotated temporal bone on the side of facial paralysis. OMT can decrease the severity of symptoms and help speed recovery. In one case study, the application of OM procedures focusing on the enhancement of lymphatic circulation resulted in complete relief of the patient's unilateral facial nerve paralysis within 2 weeks—without the use of pharmaceuticals (16).

OTITIS MEDIA

Ear pain is a common patient complaint in the practice of the primary care physician. Acute otitis media is a significant worldwide problem commonly affecting children between 6 and 18 months. Otitis media is the most frequent reason for a childhood visit to a physician in the United States. By 3 years of age, 50% to 70% of children will have had one episode, while one third will have had more than three (20). Acute otitis media can affect a person of any age, although it is more often seen in children than in adults. The disease is usually caused by Streptococcus pneumoniae or Haemophilus influenzae. The standard of care for otitis media is based on following the 2004 AAP/AAFP Guidelines. The standard care for recurrent acute otitis media includes long-term antibiotic prophylaxis and surgery. The risks of standard care are recognized, and alternative means of treating acute disease and preventing recurrent otitis media are needed. For over a century, osteopathic physicians have reported favorable clinical outcomes in children treated with osteopathic manipulative medicine in addition to standard medical care. During the birth process, the forces of labor can affect the position and function of the cranial bones. These forces can alter the position and motion of the cranial bones. If left untreated, these cranial dysfunctions are thought to predispose the child to middle ear infections. Multiple studies have shown a beneficial effect of cranial osteopathy on children with otitis media (20–22). In regard to recurrent otitis media, OMT has shown a potential benefit when used as adjuvant therapy to the standard of care (20–22). Benefits included fewer tubes, improved tympanography, and less frequent use of antibiotics.

The manipulative techniques chosen are based upon the physician's skill and training, the type of dysfunction found, and the patient's presentation. The objectives to be accomplished are the following:

- Improve lymphatic drainage from the inner ear
- Decrease inner ear effusion
- Improve function of the Eustachian tube
- Improve cranial and temporal bone motion
- Decrease pain

OMT should be applied to only structures surrounding the ear. The upper thoracic spine and ribs, the thoracic inlet, the sacrum and pelvis, and the abdominal diaphragm may need to be treated as well. Locally, improving motion of the suboccipital region, releasing the occipitomastoid suture, and balancing the temporal bones are beneficial. One manipulative technique, called the *Galbreath technique*, is useful as well. First described in 1929 by William Galbreath, D.O., this technique involves mandibular manipulation, causing the eustachian tube to open and close in a "pumping action" that allows the ear to drain fluid more effectively.

REFERENCES

1. Magoun HI. *Osteopathy in the Cranial Field*. 3rd Ed. Kirksville, MO: The Journal Printing Co., 1976.
2. Kuchera ML, Kuchera WA. *Osteopathic Considerations in Systemic Dysfunction*. 2nd Ed. Columbus, OH: Greyden Press, 1994.
3. Moore KL. *Clinically Oriented Anatomy*. 3rd Ed. Baltimore, MD: Williams & Wilkins, 1992.
4. Williams PL. *Gray's Anatomy*. 38th Ed. Edinburgh, Scotland: Churchill-Livingstone, 1995.
5. Diamond S. *Clinical Symposia: Head Pain, Diagnosis and Management*. Summit, NJ: Ciba-Geigy Corp., 1994.
6. Taylor RB. *Family Medicine Principles and Practice*. 5th Ed. New York, NY: Springer-Verlag, 1998.
7. DiGiovanna EL, Schiowitz S, Dowling DJ. *An Osteopathic Approach to Diagnosis and Treatment*. 3rd Ed. Philadelphia, PA; Baltimore, MD: Lippincott, Williams & Wilkins, 125–126.
8. Nelson K, Glonek T. *Somatic Dysfunction in Osteopathic Family Practice*. Lippincott Williams & Wilkins, Copyright 2007:88–89.
9. Fryette HH. *Principles of Osteopathic Technique*. 2nd Ed. Kirksville, MO: Journal Printing Company, 1980:27–30.
10. Larson NJ. Osteopathic manipulative contribution to treatment of TMJ syndrome. *Osteopath Med* 1978;10(8):16–26.
11. Nelson KE, Glonek TG. *Somatic Dysfunction in Osteopathic Family Medicine*. Lippincott Williams, and Wilkins, Philadelphia, PA: Lippincott, Williams & Wilkins, Copyright 2007:208–216.
12. Becker AD. Osteopathic treatment of the common cold, in reprint. *JAOA* 2001;101(8):461–463.
13. Heinking KH, Hampton W. *Osteopathic Manipulative Treatment for the Head, Eye, Ear, Nose, and Throat Patient*. Philadelphia, PA; Baltimore, MD: Downers Grove, IL: H&H publishing.
14. Chaudhary A, Appelbaum J. Temporomandibular joint syndrome. Emedicine web page. Last updated June 30, 2004. Available at: http://www.emedicine.com/neuro/topic366.htm. Accessed April 10, 2005.
15. Lancaster DG, Crow WT. Osteopathic Manipulative Treatment of a 26-Year-Old Woman With Bell's Palsy From private practice in Dallas, Tex (Lancaster), and the Philadelphia College of Osteopathic Medicine in Pa (Crow).
16. Murakami S, Mizobuchi M, Nakashiro Y, et al. Bell palsy and herpes simplex virus: identification of viral DNA in endoneurial fluid and muscle. *Ann Intern Med* 1996;124(1 pt 1):27–30. Available at: http://www.annals.org/cgi/content/full/124/1_Part_1/27. Accessed March 28, 2006.
17. Moore KL, Dalley AF. *Clinically Oriented Anatomy*. 4th Ed. Philadelphia, PA: Lippincott Williams & Wilkins, 1999:1097–1102.
18. Ward RC, ed. *Foundations for Osteopathic Medicine*. Baltimore, MD: Williams & Wilkins, 1997:4, 720–721, 780–790, 843–849, 955–959.
19. Magoun HI. *Osteopathy in the Cranial Field*. 3rd Ed. Boise, ID: Northwest Printing, 1976:27–28, 269.
20. Degenhardt BF, Kuchera ML. Osteopathic Evaluation and Manipulative Treatment in Reducing the Morbidity of Otitis Media: A Pilot Study From the A.T. Still Research Institute and Kirksville College of Osteopathic Medicine of A.T. Still University of Health Sciences, Mo (Degenhardt); and the Department of Osteopathic Manipulative Medicine and the Human Performance & Biomechanics Laboratory at Philadelphia College of Osteopathic Medicine in Pa (Kuchera).
21. Pintal WJ, Kurtz ME. An integrated osteopathic treatment approach in acute otitis media. *J Am Osteopath Assoc*. Philadelphia, PA; Baltimore, MD: 89(9):1139–1139.
22. Mills MV, Henley CE, Barnes LLB, et al. The use of osteopathic manipulative treatment as adjuvant therapy in children with recurrent acute otitis media. *Arch Pediatr Adolesc Med* 2003;157:861–866.
23. Sergueef N. *Cranial Osteopathy for Infants, Children, and Adolescents*. New York, NY; Philadelphia, PA; St. Louis, MO: Churchill Livingstone, Elsevier, 2007:23–35, 45–47, 301.
24. Woodburne RT. *Essentials of Human Anatomy*. 7th Ed. Oxford University Press, 1983:147–148, 160–161, 283–284.

SUGGESTED READING

Headaches. In: DiGiovanna, Schiowitz, eds. *An Osteopathic Approach to Diagnosis and Treatment*, 2nd Ed. 1997; Lippincott; Philadelphia, PA; Baltimore, MD: 430–432.

Hoyt WH. Osteopathic manipulation in the treatment of muscle contraction headache. *JAOA* 1979;86:322–325.

Hruby RJ. The total body approach to the osteopathic management of temporomandibular joint dysfunction. *JAOA* 1985;85:502–510.

Lay EM. The osteopathic management of trigeminal neuralgia. *JAOA* 1975;75:373–389.

Mills MV, Steele et al. The use of osteopathic manipulative treatment as adjuvant therapy in children with recurrent acute otitis media. *Arch Pediatr Adolesc Med* 2003;157:861–866.

38 Cervical Region

KURT P. HEINKING AND ROBERT E. KAPPLER

KEY CONCEPTS

- Neck pain, second only to low back pain, is one of the most common complaints of patients seeing a primary care physician.
- Accurate diagnosis and treatment of the cervical spine is an important aspect of patient care.
- Dysfunction of the cervical spine is very common and may be related to numerous mechanical, systemic, and traumatic situations.
- Diagnosis of the cervical spine should consider basic imaging deemed necessary by any questionable clinical presentation or history.

INTRODUCTION

The cervical spine is of great significance to those who use manipulative treatment. The cervical region is a pathway between the head and the thorax with neural, vascular, and musculoskeletal communication. Injury, pathology, or dysfunction may interfere with these vital communications.

Accurate, gentle diagnosis and treatment of the cervical spine is an important aspect of patient care. Dysfunction of the cervical spine is very common and may be related to head and neck infections, trauma, stress, posture, sleeping, overuse, breathing, and orthopedic or rheumatologic conditions. The cervical spine is diagnosed based upon the patient's history and the circumstances present at the time of the evaluation. For example, the cervical spine evaluation of a young athlete in the emergency department following a head or neck injury is different than a 50-year-old patient with chronic neck stiffness upon arising in the morning. Some basic principles hold true, however. One caveat for the clinician is to have little reluctance to image the cervical spine in any patient in which the history, presentation, or situation deems it necessary or appropriate. An undiagnosed cervical spine fracture can have devastating consequences. This chapter will provide the reader with a basic understanding of cervical spine anatomy, physiology, dysfunction, and common conditions that would necessitate osteopathic diagnosis and/or manipulative treatment of cervical somatic dysfunction.

EPIDEMIOLOGY OF CERVICAL SPINE PAIN

Neck pain is one of the most common complaints of patients seeing a primary care physician. It is only second to low back pain for patient's seeking manual treatment (1). When discussing cervical spine pain, one must consider if it is acute or chronic and if it is related to a trauma. Acute neck pain by definition is pain on most days that has been present for at least 2 weeks. Chronic neck pain by definition needs to be present for 6 months. Posttraumatic neck pain needs to have ample history to support the mechanism of injury. Knowing these elements, the clinician has a better grasp of the epidemiologic statistics. The incidence of neck pain peaks between 20 and 40 years of age (2). Females present with neck and upper back pain more than males. The lifetime prevalence of neck pain is 71% (2–5). Patients with multiple medical problems, significant job stress, and occupational factors tend to have a

higher incidence of neck pain. Neck pain has been associated with psychological factors, such as high quantitative job demands. The combination of chronic illnesses adds to the severity of neck pain. Motor vehicle accidents are a common etiologic factor in patients with neck pain. Neck pain is the most frequently reported symptom in whiplash injury (6). It has been estimated that 66% to 82% of neck injuries seen clinically result from rear-end collisions (6). There is general agreement that acute neck injuries are more frequent among front seat passengers than among rear seat passengers. If head restraints are present, the use of seat belts alone results in fewer injuries. Without head restraints, the use of seat belts alone appears to cause a slight increase in injuries. A majority of studies show a higher incidence of whiplash injuries in women; some studies show the frequency of neck injury among women to be twice as high as among men (6). Lightweight people appear to be more susceptible to acute neck injury than heavier people. There is also a positive correlation between increased height and neck injuries. Neck somatic dysfunction was the most commonly reported somatic dysfunction found by a cohort of osteopathic physicians board certified in neuromusculoskeletal medicine, over a 6-month period (7).

HISTORY

Taking a thorough history is critical. This is especially true when it comes to neck trauma or closed head injuries, as many times these cases can have catastrophic outcomes and frequently become legal cases. Remember that assessment and treatment of the cervical spine is useful for a variety of presenting complaints, not necessarily just neck pain or headache. The type and specific location of the pain needs to be characterized, as well as the duration and severity. What has the patient tried to make it better? What has worked and what hasn't? Do certain activities make it worse? Have they ever had anything like this in the past? If so when and how did it resolve? Have they seen any other practitioners, or received any other treatments for their condition? Have they had any imaging of their cervical spine? If so, what is their understanding of their condition? Is their condition getting better, worse, or staying the same? How does their condition affect their day-to-day functioning?

An important aspect to the history of a cervical spine–related complaint is the involvement of trauma. Cervical spine trauma can be repetitive overuse, blunt trauma, or even emotional trauma. Multiple traumas may be layered upon one another. Delineating the mechanism of the trauma is important. This will explain the forces introduced into the tissues at specific direction, rate, and amount. The specifics of each trauma need to be quantified and subjective complaints separated from objective physical findings. Documentation of any neck pain or issue prior to a trauma is important, as well as resolution or persistence of symptoms.

Many times, there are elements in the history that point to a specific clinical condition. For example, consider the patient with "cervicogenic angina" (8). Pain may radiate to the left shoulder or arm and be accompanied by upper extremity numbness. The patient seeks out medical advice thinking that they might be having a "heart attack"; however, it is found that the causative condition is orthopedic in nature. In this condition, compression of cervical nerve roots or cervical spondylosis (9) causes pain to be referred to regions innervated by the C5-T1 nerve roots, most commonly the C7 nerve root (10,11). It is important to elicit a history of shoulder and arm pain that is related to position or movement of the arm as this may be more of an orthopedic etiology. Pain that radiates from the neck into the arm at night, which improves with placing the arm overhead ("Bakody's sign"), is more suggestive of a cervical nerve root irritation as well (26). Patients with cervical spondylosis commonly have palpable findings in the high thoracic region (12).

In contrast, consider "shoulder-hand syndrome" in which patients with acute coronary events or stroke develop pain, stiffness, and edema of the shoulder, arm, wrist, and hand. In this situation, the mechanism is different. Both local neurogenic inflammation and a hyperactivity of the sympathetic nervous system (upper thoracic spinal cord T1-4) are thought to cause the upper extremity symptoms. Interestingly, tissue texture changes in the soft tissues covering the upper thoracic spine and ribs may persist for years. Larson (13), Beal (14), and Nicholas et al. (15) have reported these tissue texture changes from T2-5 on the left in patients with cardiac disorders.

From the history, a differential diagnosis of the patient's current problem is made and then the physical examination, imaging, and other diagnostic studies are used to rule out conditions within the differential. Prior to the physical examination, a clinician needs to recall the anatomy of the region, pertinent physiologic principles, and relevant biomechanics. This section will highlight important concepts in each of these areas.

FUNCTIONAL ANATOMY OF THE CERVICAL SPINE

Skeletal Structures

The cervical spine consists of seven vertebral segments. The atlas (C1) and the axis (C2) are atypical. The atlas does not have a vertebral body; instead it rotates around the dens (16). The dens contacts the inner anterior surface of the ring-like atlas. The atlas consists of an anterior and posterior arch, joining to form the heavy lateral masses that bear the superior and inferior articular surfaces. The superior facets articulate with the occiput, and the inferior facets articulate with the axis. The axial articular masses are broader and deeper than other masses because they bear the weight of the skull without assistance from the odontoid process. The atlas has a facet for articulation with the dens on its internal surface, as well as an anterior tubercle for muscular attachments. The posterior arch is longer and bears a small posterior tubercle in place of a spinous process. The transverse processes of the atlas, called lateral masses, are modified and palpable. Each transverse process has a transverse foramen for the vertebral artery. The vertebral arteries traverse through the foramina of C6 through the atlas and pierce

the tectoral membrane to enter the foramen magnum. The second cervical vertebra, or axis, is identified by the projection of the odontoid process, or dens, which develops from the embryologic body of the first vertebra. The dens acts as a pivot point about which the atlas rotates. The posterior surface of the dens has a facet that accommodates the synovial bursa that separates it from the transverse band of the cruciate ligament. The axis does not form a neural foramen for spinal roots. Its transverse processes are the only ones in the cervical spine that are not grooved to allow exit of a nerve root (16). The spinous process of the axis (C2) is larger, palpable, and prominent on x-ray.

The cervical vertebrae from C2-7 are saddle shaped and contain a specialized set of synovial joints on the lateral surface of the vertebral bodies. These are known as uncovertebral joints (or uncinate) joints of Luschka and provide stability to the cervical spine. They may also decrease the likelihood of herniated nucleus pulposus in the cervical region. The joints of Luschka are not synovial; thus, inflammatory arthopathies spare these areas. However, the facet joints and atlantal-axial joint have synovial membranes that can be involved in inflammatory arthopathies. The articulations between C2, C3, and the remainder of the cervical joints are considered typical.

The cervical transverse processes are unique and different than the transverse processes in the thoracic and lumbar spine. The lateral portions of the cervical vertebra (C1-6) are modified to contain a foramen through which the vertebral artery passes. The anterior portion of the transverse process is developmentally a rib, whereas the posterior portion is a true transverse process (16). These portions fuse, but between them persists the transverse foramen, which allows for passage of the vertebral artery. Although this provides protection for the vertebral artery, it also creates the possibility of trauma to the artery from bony insult.

The transverse processes contain a gutter that runs obliquely from anterior to posterior through which the spinal nerves traverse. These nerves exit the spine through the neural foramina, which are largest at the C2-3 level and decrease in size progressively to the C6-7 level. Flexion of the cervical spine increases the vertical diameter of the neural foramen, whereas extension decreases it.

The bone between the facets, which can be palpated, is known as the articular pillar. The lateral portions of the atlas are known as lateral masses. The lateral portions of the cervical vertebra (C1-6) are modified to contain a foramen through which the vertebral artery passes. Although this provides protection for the vertebral artery, it also creates the possibility of trauma to the artery from bony insult. The cervical facets are in a plane that points on a 45-degree angle toward the eye. Rotation motion of the typical cervical segments follows the plane of the facets. Anterior or forward rotation is toward the eye rather than rotation in a horizontal plane. The facet joints are enclosed in a fibrous capsule that is lax to allow movement in multiple planes. Synovial tissue lines the joint capsules. They contain menisci that protect articular surfaces from damage during cervical motion. These menisci may become entrapped in the joint and cause cervical dysfunction. The C7 vertebra has anatomic characteristics that are similar to those of T1. The transverse process of the seventh vertebra does not contain a foramen for the vertebral artery and its accompanying veins and sympathetic nerves (16). The bone between the facets, which can be palpated, is known as the articular pillar.

Ligamentous Structures

The cervical vertebrae comprise a smooth lordosis, held in position by muscles and ligaments. The anterior and posterior longitudinal ligaments run along both sides of the spinal column and give support to the bony structure. They also help to contain the intervertebral discs. The anterior longitudinal ligament is a broad, strong ligament on the anterior aspect of the vertebral bodies from the atlas to the sacrum. Superiorly, the ligament attaches to the anterior arch of the atlas and the anterior atlanto-occipital membrane. The posterior longitudinal ligament lies on the posterior surface of the bodies of the vertebrae from the axis to the sacrum. The posterior longitudinal ligament is wider in the upper cervical spine and narrower in the lower cervical spine. Its lateral expansions over the discs are thin, weak, and represent a vulnerable area for disc herniation as compared to its strong central band. At the base of the skull, the tectoral membrane (occipital-axial ligament) is a continuation of the posterior longitudinal ligament and lies immediately behind the body of the axis. The alar ligaments are short, strong bundles of fibrous tissue directed obliquely superior and laterally from both sides of the superior portion of the odontoid process and attach to the medial aspect of the occipital condyles. They are often referred to as the "check" ligaments. The transverse ligament of the atlas is a broad, strong, triangular ligament arching across the ring of the atlas and anchored firmly on each side to a tubercle on the medial surface of both lateral masses of the atlas. The transverse ligament has two fascicles layered in a crosswise fashion, which gives it a cruciate configuration. The transverse ligament portion of the cruciate ligament complex supports the atlas in rotating about the dens. The anterior surface of the spinal cord lies immediately posterior to the transverse ligament. Rupture of this ligament (or laxity, which may occur with rheumatoid arthritis) creates the possibility of the dens contacting the spinal cord, causing catastrophic neurologic damage.

The remaining cervical vertebrae, C2-7, have a similar ligamentous configuration. The supraspinous and interspinous ligaments, found between adjacent spinous processes, attach each spinal vertebra to one another. The highly elastic ligamentum flavum (yellow ligament) lies posterior between adjacent lamina. There are two ligamentum flavum at each spinal level, separated by a small cleft posterior medially.

Intervertebral Discs

Each disc is situated between the cartilaginous endplates of two consecutive vertebrae. In the cervical spine, the discs are thicker anteriorly than posteriorly and are entirely responsible for the normal cervical lordosis. Positions of the cervical spine affect intradiscal pressure. Pressure is least in the supine position, and extension of the cervical spine results in the greatest intradiscal pressure (16). Each intervertebral disc is composed of a gelatinous nucleus pulposus surrounded by a laminated, fibrous annulus fibrosus. Successive layers of the annulus fibrosus slant in alternate directions so that they cross each other at different angles depending on the intradiscal pressure of the nucleus pulposus. At birth, the disc has a high water content (88%), which mechanically allows it to absorb a significant amount of stress; however, with age, the percentage of water decreases, and the ratio of proteoglycans changes. After 50 years of age, the nucleus pulposus becomes a fibrocartilaginous mass that has characteristics similar to those of the outer zone of the annulus fibrosis.

Muscular Structures

The majority of neck problems are muscular in nature. The majority of patients with neck complaints will have significant muscular tension in their neck. Palpation of the following muscles for tissue texture change, tension, Jones tender points, and myofascial trigger points is commonplace for practicing clinicians.

Posterior Neck Muscles

The posterior muscles of the neck are divided into superficial, intermediate, and deep groups. The posterior spinal muscles are continuous from the cervical spine to the sacrum. Superficial posterior muscles that attach to the cervical spine include the trapezius, erector spinae group (semispinalis cervicis, longissimus cervicis, longissimus capitus, and interspinalis), and the levator scapulae. The intermediate group contains splenius cervicis and splenius capitus. The deep group contains iliocostalis cervicis laterally; longissimus cervicis and longissimus capitis centrally; and spinalis cervicis, semispinalis capitis, and semispinalis cervicis medially.

Trapezius

The trapezius muscle is the most superficial muscle of the posterior group and is innervated by the spinal accessory nerve, cranial nerve 11. The trapezius posteriorly and sternocleidomastoid (SCM) anteriorly are jointly protected by a general investing fascia. Because the trapezius muscle attaches to the scapula, it is the primary connection between the head, neck, and the shoulder girdle. The trapezius stabilizes and elevates the scapula and extends the head. The process of lifting with the upper extremity distributes force to the cervical spine via the trapezius and corresponding fascial elements.

Levator Scapulae

The levator scapula muscle originates from the transverse processes of the atlas, axis, and the 3rd and 4th cervical vertebrae and inserts on the upper medial border of the scapula. The levator scapulae elevates the medial scapula and rotates it medially.

Intermediate Posterior Group

The intermediate muscles surrounding the spine function primarily as spinal extensors. This group includes the splenius capitis and splenius cervicis. The muscles originate from the spinous processes of the lower cervical and upper thoracic spine and insert on the transverse processes of the upper cervical spine and the mastoid process. Biomechanical studies have documented the importance of the splenius capitis and cervicis as prime muscle for extension of the head and neck.

Deep Posterior Group

In the deep layer, the erector spinae muscles from the thoracolumbar spine continue to the cervical region including the iliocostalis cervicis laterally; longissimus cervicis and longissimus capitis centrally; and spinalis cervicis, semispinalis capitis, and semispinalis cervicis medially.

The iliocostalis extends from the angles of the upper 6 ribs to the posterior tubercles of the transverse processes of the lower cervical vertebrae. The longissimus group extends from the transverse processes of the upper thoracic vertebrae to the posterior tubercles of the transverse processes of the lower cervical vertebrae. This anatomic relationship links thoracic spine mechanics with cervical dysfunction.

The semispinalis group arises on the posterior tubercles of the transverse processes of the upper thoracic and lower cervical vertebrae and inserts into the area between the superior and the inferior nuchal line of the occiput. Beneath the semispinalis muscles lies the multifidus from C4 to C7. The small rotatores muscles cross one segment of the spine and extend from the transverse process to the spinous process. In the upper cervical spine, suboccipital muscles (the rectus capitis posterior major and minor and the obliquus capitis superior and inferior) attach from the occiput to the C2 vertebra. These deep posterior cervical muscles are arranged in between each vertebra and form the suboccipital triangle at the base of the skull. Significant modification of these muscles occurs at C2, with a group of oblique muscles traversing from atlas and axis to the occiput. These muscular relationships make the occiput, atlas, and C2 a functional unit.

Anterior Neck Muscles

The anterior muscles of the neck are considered "strap muscles" and attach the sternum to the hyoid bone and the hyoid bone to the skull. There are also attachments from the upper ribs to the neck and skull. The anterior scalene muscles traverse from the lateral tubercles of the cervical spine (C3-5) and insert on the 1st rib. The middle and posterior scalene have a similar origin and insert on the 2nd rib. The scalenes as a group act as lateral stabilizers, as well as accessory muscles of respiration. Anteriorly, many muscles travel from the mandible to the hyoid, sternum, and clavicle. The anterolateral cervical muscles function to flex and rotate the head and neck. These muscles include the platysma, SCM, and hyoid muscles; strap muscles (of the larynx); scalenes, longus colli, and longus capitis. The platysma depresses the lower jaw and lip and tightens the skin of the anterior neck. The SCM is the dividing boundary for the anterior and posterior triangles of the neck. Similar to the trapezius, the sternocleidomastoid muscle is innervated by the spinal accessory nerve. The hyoid muscles do not contribute to the motion of the cervical spine, but they are important in controlling movement of the hyoid bone and larynx. The "strap muscles" attach to the hyoid, thyroid cartilage, and sternum and transverse medial to the SCM (except for the posterior aspect of the omohyoid muscle). The prevertebral muscles of the neck are the longus colli and longus capitis. The longus colli muscles extend from C1 to T3, spanning the lateral portions of the vertebral bodies and attaching at the anterior tubercles of the lateral masses of C3-6. The longus capitis muscles arise on the anterior tubercles of C3-6 and extend cephalad to the basiocciput.

Fascia

The three fascial layers of the cervical spine are superficial, intermediate, and deep. The superficial fascia exists as a single sheet over the anterior and posterior cervical triangles. The superficial fascia surrounds subcutaneous fat, the platysma muscle, the external jugular vein, and cutaneous sensory nerves.

The intermediate fascia layer contains the alar fascia. The alar fascia spreads behind the esophagus and surrounds the carotid sheath.

The deep layer of fascia has an outer, middle, and inner layer. The outer layer of the deep fascia extends from the trapezius muscle over the posterior triangle and then splits to enclose the sternocleidomastoid muscle. The middle layer of the deep cervical fascia encloses the strap muscles and extends laterally to the scapula. The inner layer of the deep fascia is the prevertebral fascia, which covers the scalenes muscles, the longus colli muscle, and the anterior longitudinal ligament. Fascia from the cervical spine follows a "tube within tube" structure and continues into the mediastinum to blend with the pericardium and great vessels.

Neural Structures

In the adult, the spinal cord extends from the medulla in the brain through the cervical and thoracic spine to the L2 level of the lumbar spine. The cervical spinal canal is widest at the atlantoaxial level and narrows maximally at the C6 level. The cervical cord itself is wider from C3 to T2, corresponding to the increase in nerves supplying the upper extremities. The spinal canal can be congenitally narrowed (spinal stenosis) due to orthopedic disease such as osteoarthritis, disc protrusions, and spondylolisthesis. Osteophyte formation contributes to stenosis, as does instability with excess front-to-back or side-to-side translation. A cervical disc may protrude posteriorly into the cord. If this occurs, the term myelopathy is used to indicate long tract signs are present. Patients who have congenitally small spinal canals, disc herniations, Arnold-Chiari malformation, syringomyelia, etc. are at increased risk for cervical cord injury, given the right circumstances. Additionally, damage to the cord may be ischemic as well as physical. Spinal cord injuries may occur from a number of different traumatic events, including:

- Automobile and motorcycle accidents
- Gunshots and stabbings
- Diving into an empty swimming pool
- Football and other violent contact sports

Cord injury due to any etiology can have catastrophic consequences.

Cervical Nerve Roots

The cervical spinal cord gives rise to the cervical plexus and the brachial plexus. Because the brachial plexus innervates the upper extremity, nerve root impingement at the cervical intervertebral foramen produces neck pain and upper extremity neurologic symptoms. Impingement of the nerve roots commonly occurs from disc protrusion or osteophyte encroachment. The mixed spinal nerve contains motor fibers, sensory axons of the dorsal root ganglia, and preganglionic fibers from the autonomic nervous system.

There are eight cervical nerve roots. In contrast with the nerves in the thoracic and lumbar spine, the nerves in the cervical spine take the name of the pedicle above which they exit. For example, the C5 nerve root exits between the fourth and the fifth cervical vertebra. The exception is the C8 nerve root, which exits between the seventh cervical and the first thoracic vertebrae. The C1 nerve root exits the vertebral canal from an orifice in the posterior occipital-atlanto membrane just above the posterior arch of the atlas and posterior medially to the lateral mass of the atlas. The C1 ventral primary ramus unites with the C2 ventral primary ramus to contribute fibers to the hypoglossal nerve. The dorsal primary ramus of C1 enters the suboccipital triangle supplying the muscles of this region. The C1 nerve root has no cutaneous branches. The C5 nerve root provides sympathetic innervation to the arteries of the head and neck. The C6 nerve root has fibers to the subclavian artery and brachial plexus. The C7 nerve root has components supplying the cardio aortic plexus, the subclavian and axillary arteries, and the phrenic nerves.

Cervical Sympathetic Nerves

The cervical sympathetic system consists of preganglionic and postganglionic autonomic fibers, as well as three cervical sympathetic ganglia. The preganglionic fibers originate in the intermediolateral gray column of the T1-5 spinal cord segments. In addition to efferent fibers, small, nociceptive afferents (C fibers) travel with the sympathetics and synapse in the upper thoracic cord as well. Nociceptive input (pain transmission) from the cervical spine produces palpable musculoskeletal changes in the upper thoracic spine and ribs, as well as increased sympathetic activity from this area (17,18). The three ganglia are the superior cervical ganglion, the middle cervical ganglion, and the inferior cervical ganglion. The first thoracic and inferior cervical ganglia are fused, and this structure is referred to as the stellate ganglion. The largest ganglion is the superior ganglion, located at the C2-3 level. The middle ganglion, the smallest, is located at C6. The inferior ganglion lies between the transverse process of C7 and the 1st rib.

Sinuvertebral Nerve

The sinuvertebral nerve emerges distal to the dorsal root ganglion, but prior to the division into dorsal and ventral rami. This small branch recurs into the intervertebral foramen to reach the vertebral canal. The terminal branches supply the posterior longitudinal ligament, the periosteum on the posterior aspect of the vertebral body, the outer layers of the intervertebral discs, and the anterior surface of the spinal dura. The cervical sinuvertebral nerves supply the level of entry and the disc above.

Irritation of the small caliber primary afferent fibers in the sinuvertebral nerve can refer pain several segments up or down the spinal cord, as well as to the contralateral side of the body.

The sinuvertebral nerve does not supply skeletal muscle or skin, so compression or damage to this nerve alone does not present with signs of denervation, weakness, or cutaneous analgesia. The sinuvertebral nerve contains only sensory and sympathetic fibers, and is very sensitive to stretch and possibly ischemia. This anatomic correlation may be why cervical spine dysfunction can refer pain to the periscapular region, chest wall, and shoulder.

Proprioceptive Reflexes

Cervical spine position has a dramatic influence on proprioception and balance. There are more joint proprioceptors in the cervical facet joint capsules than in the thoracic and lumbar spine. Proprioceptive reflexes from the cervical spine create a muscle response in the lower extremity. Rotation of the cervical spine in unconscious subjects causes involuntary, external rotation of the lower extremity in the direction of cervical rotation (20). Another phenomenon is cervical vertigo (21–23), in which proprioceptive input from suboccipital muscles and ligaments or the sternocleidomastoid muscle can produce vertigo.

Vascular Structures

The carotid, vertebral, and subclavian arteries supply the head and neck with arterial blood. The carotid arteries lie anterior to the cervical vertebra. The carotid pulse may be palpated for diagnostic purposes. Avoid pressure over the carotid arteries while palpating the cervical spine. The vertebral artery is the major source of blood supply for the cervical spine and the cervical portion of the spinal cord. The vertebral arteries typically originate off the subclavian artery (right vertebral) and aorta (left vertebral) and travel through the intervertebral foramen. They then enter the cranium through the foramen magnum. Just before joining, one or both of the vertebral arteries gives off a branch that joins with the branch from the other side and descends in the ventral medial fissure on the anterior aspect of the spinal cord as the anterior spinal artery. The vertebral arteries join together after passing through the foramen magnum to form the basilar artery. The vertebral artery can become occluded by thrombosis, which may be precipitated by injury to the artery as it passes through the intervertebral foramina and over the atlas. If patients complain in the history of symptoms referable to the vertebral artery, or there are related physical signs, vertebral artery tests should be done. Signs and symptoms that may indicate vertebral artery problems are listed in Box 38.1 (24). If there is

---

Signs and Symptoms That May Indicate Possible Vertebral-Basilar Artery Problems

Signs and Symptoms That May Indicate Possible Vertebral-Basilar Artery Problems (43,46)

- Malaise and nausea
- Vomiting
- Dizziness/vertigo
- Unsteadiness in walking, incoordination
- Visual disturbances
- Severe headaches
- Weakness in extremities
- Sensory changes in face or body
- Dysarthia (difficulty with speech)
- Unconsciousness, disorientation. Light headedness
- Dysphagia (difficulty swallowing)
- Hearing difficulties
- Facial paralysis

---

clinical suspicion of vertebral artery compromise by the history, and physical findings, high velocity low amplitude (HVLA) manipulation of the cervical spine should not be attempted.

The venous system includes a valveless complex of veins in the spine that forms a continuous connection between the pelvis and the cerebral sinuses, connecting with the caval and azygos systems. The absence of valves allows the reversal of blood from the pelvis to the cervical spine. The venous system of the cervical spine drains into the brachiocephalic veins. Disorders such as heart failure may cause jugular venous distension, which is visible and palpable.

Disturbance of the vascular supply produces neurologic symptoms. Occlusion of a vertebral artery by thrombosis, dissection, or mechanical insult can cause a posterior circulation stroke with permanent neurologic sequelae. Thoracic outlet syndrome is a condition arising from compression of the vascular and neural components of the brachial plexus in the thoracic outlet. It is a diagnosis of exclusion. The brachial plexus and the subclavian artery pass through this space. There are three anatomic regions of compression. These include between the anterior and middle scalene, between the clavicle and 1st rib, and between the pectoralis minor muscle and the costal cage. There are provocative tests used to differentiate the site of compression; however, they lack clinical specificity and reliability (25). The tests must reproduce the patient's symptoms as well as decrease his or her pulse. Symptoms such as paresthesia or hand weakness typically affect the ulnar side of the hand after an inciting activity or position is performed. Typically, shoulder abduction and external rotation worsen the symptoms. Symptoms resolve within minutes of cessation of the activity. Occasionally, distal pulses are absent or decreased and digital cyanosis can be present. Tenderness may be present in the supraclavicular fossa. Some forms of thoracic outlet syndrome are associated with sympathetic autonomic dysfunction, which produces upper extremity symptoms. In this case, somatic dysfunction of the upper thoracic spine and ribs is etiologic. Venous return from the upper extremity is not impaired by scalene tension, as the subclavian vein passes in front of the anterior scalene muscle.

Lymphatic Structures

The brain is devoid of lymphatic channels; vascular return from the cranium is venous. However, cervical lymphatic drainage is important. Infections and inflammation from the head, ear, nose, and throat require effective lymphatic drainage. Superficial nodes must penetrate the general investing fascia to connect with the deep channels that return lymph to the vascular compartment in the thorax. The thoracic inlet must be free of motion restrictions to allow lymph to return. The use of fascial soft tissue stretching/release facilitates lymphatic return, as lymph channels pass through the general investing fascia.

MOTION, POSTURE, AND BIOMECHANICS

The cervical spine is well suited for mobility and is less suited for bearing heavy loads. The saddle shape of each cervical vertebra provides its mobility and stability. The anterior column is composed of the vertebral body, longitudinal ligaments, and intervertebral disc and provides some weight-bearing capacity, shock absorption, as well as a flexible structure. The posterior elements, composed of the osseous canal, the zygapophyseal joints, and the erector spinae muscles, protect the neural elements, act as a fulcrum, and guide movement of the functional unit. Precise control of head position and unrestricted movement is essential for normal functioning of the special senses.

Alterations in the degree of curvature in one area of the spine result in reciprocal alterations in curvature in other areas of the spinal column to preserve the orientation of the body over the center of gravity. For example, an increase in lumbar lordosis results in increased cervical lordosis.

Gross Motion

The posterior longitudinal ligament limits flexion of the cervical spine. Extension of the cervical spine is limited by the direct contact of the vertebral lamina, the zygapophyseal joints, and the poster superior spinous process. In cervical flexion, the vertebral bodies separate, thereby opening the neural foramina. Compression of the nerve root is minimized because the flexion of the neck not only angulates the nerve but also allows greater space for the neural elements by widening the neural foramina.

In cervical extension, the foramina narrow. The spinal cord ascends and descends in the spinal canal as the neck is flexed and extended, respectively. In lateral bending or rotation, the foramina close on the side toward which the neck moves, while opening on the contra lateral side. The neural foramina is 20% to 30% larger in flexion than extension (26). Normal cervical flexion is 90 degrees, extension is 70 degrees, and rotation is 70 to 90 degrees (26).

Occipito-Atlantal Joint

The major motions at the occipito-atlantal (O-A) joint are flexion and extension. Side bending and rotation are considered minor movements. There is approximately 20 to 25 degrees of flexion/extension at the occipito-atlanto-axial complex. The occipital condyles converge anteriorly. The lateral portion of the atlas articulation is more cephalad than the medial portion. Due to this anatomy, the occiput rotates and side bends in opposite directions. This gliding motion is considered a minor movement of the joint and is the motion involved in occipital joint restriction.

Atlas-Axis Joint

The major motion of the atlas-axis joint is rotation. Half of the rotation of the cervical spine occurs at the atlas. Atlanto-axial (A-A) rotation averages 45 to 50 degrees, which represents about 50% of the axial rotation in the neck, with the lower cervical spine contributing the other 50% of rotation. Cineradiographic studies

show a significant amount of flexion and extension occurring at the atlas (27,28). This motion does not seem to be involved in somatic dysfunction of the atlas. Side bending is not a significant component of atlas movement. Cineradiographic studies have shown that during rotation, the atlas moves inferiorly on both sides, maintaining a horizontal orientation (29). Side-bending restriction is usually not diagnosed or treated. The atlas rotates about the dens, and motion restriction of the atlas involves rotation. Motion testing primarily involves rotation testing.

C2-7

Motion of the typical cervical segments (C2 through C7) is similar to type II mechanics. Cineradiography shows that the cervical spine rotates and side bends to the same side. Type I (neutral) mechanics have not been identified on cineradiography (30,31). The vertebral bodies of typical cervical segments are saddle shaped rather than flat on the superior and the inferior surfaces. Side bending of the cervical spine can produce lateral translation into the convexity. Some osteopathic physicians call this motion sideslip. The motion of the cervical spine as previously described is echoed by Bogduk and Mercer (32).

PHYSICAL EXAMINATION

There are important anatomical landmarks that help one to identify cervical structures. For instance, the angle of the mandible is at the level of the first cervical vertebra. The transverse process of the second cervical vertebra is located between the angle of the mandible and the mastoid process. The hyoid bone is anterior to the third cervical vertebra. The thyroid cartilage is anterior to the fourth cervical vertebra. The sixth vertebra is at the level of the cricoid cartilage (16).

Inspection

The first part of the physical examination of the neck involves observation/inspection. Surgical scars on the anterior portion of the neck most often indicate previous thyroid surgery or cervical fusion. Additionally, torticollis causes the head to be tilted toward the side with the contracted sternocleidomastoid muscle with rotation in the opposite direction. Observe the skin for color changes. Look for asymmetry of position, including:

- Flexion or extension
- Side bending to the right or left
- Rotation to the right or left
- Anterior/posterior curves
- Relationship of the head to the lateral weight-bearing line

The standing osteopathic structural exam does not exclude the neck. Therefore, it is important to perform a structural exam and look at the head and neck position in relation to body posture as well as gait. Following a structural examination, a neurologic examination should be performed. Following the neurological exam, active then passive range of motion is assessed.

ACTIVE MOTION TESTING

If the patient has neurological complaints or has sustained a significant neck trauma, first determine the amount the patient can move by active motion testing.

With the patient seated, ask him or her to:

- Rotate to the right and left
- Side-bend right and left (attempt to touch the ear to the shoulder)

- Flex or touch the chin to the chest
- Extend or backward bend

If any of these motions produce neurological symptoms, imaging should be reviewed or obtained prior to further testing or treatment. The motions obtained during active motion testing should be recorded in degrees. On follow-up visits, physicians may elect to bypass active motion testing and proceed directly to passive motion testing.

NEUROLOGICAL EXAM

The neurological exam delineates upper motor neuron versus nerve root and/or peripheral nerve lesions.

SENSORY

Sensory changes are a subjective clinical finding and are affected by the patient's emotional state, level of pain, and other factors. The sensory exam primarily involves testing the dermatomes from C5-T1, which are found on the upper extremity. The sensory distribution of the upper cervical segments involves the neck, scalp, and suboccipital region. During nerve compression, sensory changes occur first, followed by reflex changes, motor weakness, and ultimately, muscle atrophy.

DEEP TENDON REFLEXES

Deep tendon reflexes should be bilaterally symmetric and equal between the upper and the lower extremities. It is not uncommon for the patellar reflex to be brisk; however, brisk reflexes in the upper extremities points to cervical spinal stenosis, or an upper motor neuron lesion. With age, reflexes are more difficult to elicit. The biceps reflex has components from both C5 and C6. The brachioradialis reflex is primarily C6. The triceps reflex is C6-7. The C8 root has no reflex, so muscle strength is used to determine the integrity of the C8 nerve root.

Similarly, T1 has no deep tendon reflex, so it is evaluated for its motor and sensory components only. The scapulohumeral reflex tests the integrity of the cord segments from C4 to C6. The reflex is elicited by striking the lower end of the medial border of the scapula. The response is adduction and lateral rotation of the arm. This reflex tests the supply of the suprascapular (axillary) nerve to the infraspinatus and teres minor muscles.

MOTOR

True muscle weakness is one of the most reliable indicators of persistent nerve compression.

Motor strength quantification by physical examination is not precise; there are different grading regimes and considerations such as age of the patient and whether the muscle is weight bearing or not. A significant amount of motor strength must be absent before any consistent detection of weakness is made on the basis of a physical examination. Motor strength testing of the lower cervical spine (C5-T1) is routinely used during the clinical exam. Performing strength testing in sequence of each nerve root is time efficient. Start with the muscles supplied by the C5 root and progress to the T1 level. The upper cervical segments and their nerve roots are clinically tested less frequently. Table 38.1 summarizes each nerve root, the muscle it supplies, and the motion required to test it.

Upper Motor Neuron Tests

Upper motor neuron lesions present with hyper-reflexia, spasticity of the involved muscles, and a loss of fine motor control. Patients also develop a positive Babinski reflex or a Hoffmann reflex.

The Hoffmann sign can be elicited by placing the patient's middle phalanx of the third digit across the DIP joint of the examiners third digit on the dominant hand, with the palm facing down. Next, by placing the patient's 3rd digit in slight extension, the DIP joint is "flicked" downward by the examiner's thumb. An involuntary flexion of the DIP joints of the patient's thumb and little finger is a positive test (47). This sign is equivalent to the Babinski sign in the lower extremity.

TABLE 38.1

Neurology of the Cervical Nerve Roots

Disc	Root	Reflex	Muscle	Motion to Test	Sensation	Nerve
C4-5	C5	Biceps	Deltoid	Shoulder abduction	Lateral arm over	Axillary
				Shoulder flexion	Deltoid	
				Shoulder extension		
			Biceps	Elbow flexion		
C5-6	C6	Brachioradialis	Biceps	Elbow flexion	Lateral forearm	Musculocutaneous
			Wrist extensors			
C6-7	C7	Triceps	Triceps	Elbow extension	Middle finger	C7
			Wrist flexors	Wrist flexion		
			Finger extensors	Finger extension		
C7-T1	C8	None	Finger flexors	Finger flexion	Ring/little finger	C8
					Distal forearm	
T1-2	T1	None	Finger abductors	Finger abduction	Medial arm	Medial brachial cutaneous

Source: Hoppenfeld S. *Physical Examination of the Spine and Extremities.* Appleton, WI: Century, Crofts, 1976:120–124; chap 4.

Nerve Roots

Testing the muscles innervated by the brachial plexus begins with the deltoid and biceps muscles. The deltoid is innervated almost entirely by C5, while the biceps has a dual innervation from both C5 and C6 (34). The next muscle group that should be tested is the wrist extensors. This muscle group has primarily C6 innervation, with some innervation from the C7 nerve root (34). Elbow extension, a function of the triceps, as well as the wrist flexor group can be used to test the C7 nerve root. The next motor group to be tested is the finger flexors. The two muscles that flex the fingers are the flexor digitorum superficialis and the flexor digitorum profundus. These muscles are tested by having the patient curl the fingers around the examiner's index and 3rd digit while the examiner tries to pull out of the grip. Examining the intrinsic muscles of the hand tests the T1 neurologic level. The finger abductors, innervated by the ulnar nerve and largely the T1 root, consist of the dorsal interossei and abductor digiti quinti (34).

SPECIAL TESTS

Distraction Test

This test demonstrates the effect of neck traction in relieving a patient's neck pain. By widening the foramina, distraction relieves pain caused by a narrowed neural foramina and resulting nerve root compression. Distraction also relieves pain in the cervical spine by decreasing pressure on the joint capsules around the facet joints (34).

Compression Test

Compression can cause increased pain by narrowing the neural foramen, putting pressure on the facets, or initiating muscle spasm (34).

Valsalvas Test

This test increases the intrathecal pressure. If a space-occupying lesion, such as a herniated disc or tumor, is present in the cervical canal, the patient may develop pain in the cervical spine secondary to increased pressure (34).

Spurling Maneuver

This is a test of nerve root compression or irritation. This maneuver is designed to provoke the patient's symptoms. The test is done in three stages, each of which is more provocative. If symptoms are produced, one does not proceed to the next stage. The first stage involves compression with the head in neutral. The second stage places the head in extension then adds compression. The final stage places the head in Sidebending away from the effected side then toward the effected side and adds compression. A positive test is indicated by dermatomal pain down the arm in the distribution of the nerve root indicating nerve root compression. The Spurling test had a sensitivity of 30% and a specificity of 93%; thus, it is useful in confirming the absence of a cervical radiculopathy when negative (35).

Lhermitte Sign

The patient is in the long sitting position on the examiner's table. The patient's head and hip are flexed simultaneously. A sensation of lightning-like paresthesias or dysesthesias in the hands or legs upon cervical flexion is a positive test. This sensation is most often caused by multiple sclerosis or a large disc herniation impinging the anterior spinal cord, causing a cervical myelopathy (35).

Scapular and shoulder movements should also be tested.

PERIPHERAL NERVES

There are three common syndromes associated with compression of the median nerve. These include the pronator syndrome, carpal tunnel syndrome, and the anterior interosseous syndrome. These syndromes can mimic radiculopathy from the C6-8 and even T1 nerve roots. The ulnar nerve has two common areas of entrapment. The most common location of ulnar nerve entrapment is the elbow in the cubital tunnel. The ulnar nerve may also be compressed at the wrist in Guyon canal (36). These syndromes can mimic radiculopathy from the C6 and C7 nerve roots. The radial nerve is most commonly compressed at the elbow. Radial tunnel syndrome is a compression neuropathy of the radial nerve between the supinator muscle and the radial head just proximal to its entrance into the supinator muscle.

HEENT AND ANTERIOR NECK EXAM

It is possible for the temporomandibular joint, dental disease, upper respiratory infections, thyroid conditions, and problems of the shoulder to refer pain to the neck. Therefore, it is important to examine the eyes, ears, nose and throat, the thyroid, and the cervical lymph nodes in patients with neck pain.

SHOULDER EVALUATION

In cases in which it is difficult to differentiate intrinsic shoulder pathologic changes from referred cervical pain, it is possible to do an intra-articular injection of lidocaine (with or without steroid). Within 10 to 15 minutes of injection, it is generally possible to eliminate the component of pain that is due to intrinsic shoulder pathologic changes.

Palpation and Terminology

The cervical spine may be palpated in the seated position or in the supine position. Tissues on the anterior and lateral portions of the neck can be comfortably assessed with the patient seated and the physician standing behind the patient. Palpate muscle tension, tenderness, and tissue texture abnormality (scalenes, SCM, and trapezius). Passive motion testing to evaluate the ability of muscles to lengthen is sometimes performed (e.g., sidebend the cervical spine to evaluate scalene tension).

Palpation of the cervical spine with the patient supine allows for a detailed evaluation of tissue texture abnormality and tenderness surrounding the cervical spine. The suboccipital region contains muscles that are more lateral than the mid and lower cervical region, so paraspinal palpation must involve a more lateral placement of the fingers. Significant suboccipital tissue texture abnormality is usually associated with changes in the ipsilateral upper thoracic and rib angle area. Palpation over the posterior portion of the articular pillars reveals local muscle hypertonicity, tenderness, and tissue texture abnormality associated with segmental dysfunction. These changes are usually apparent with rotational restriction.

Palpate the lateral margins of the articular pillars (locate fingers laterally and direct the palpatory force medially) to reveal tenderness and tissue texture abnormality over the convex (anterior component) side of segmental dysfunction. For example, given C4 rotated and side-bent right (restriction rotation and side-bending left), the posterior portion of the articular pillar is tender on the right side; the lateral margin of the articular pillar is tender on the left side.

The terms open facet and closed facet are sometimes applied as positional descriptors of cervical spine somatic dysfunction. Flexion motion (in a normal spine without motion restriction) causes the facets to open, and extension motion closes the facets. Sidebending motion with coupled rotation to the same side produces a concave side and a convex side. The facets on the concave side are closed while the facets on the convex side are open. Given a condition of C5 extended, rotated, and side-bent right (restriction of flexion, rotation, and side-bending left), the right side is the concave side and the left side is the convex side. In motion testing, extension is free, so both facets close. During flexion motion testing, the facet on the right side is closed and resists opening. This produces palpable asymmetry in which the right transverse process (technically, the articular pillar) is more posterior, and the paraspinal muscle over C5 right is tight and palpable.

Segmental Diagnosis by Passive Motion Testing

Regional Motion

Test the range of regional cervical rotation, side bending, flexion, and extension with the patient in the supine position. Evaluate these motions by contacting the head bilaterally and introducing the motions through the head. The range of extension may be difficult to evaluate with the patient supine because the table gets in the way.

Segmental Motion

The experienced clinician tests those segments in which palpation and screening motion tests suggest a problem. The suboccipital area can be confusing. Neurologically, C1 and C2 are considered a common neurologic segment. Hyperactivity of the C1-2 segment potentially involves three joints: the O-A joint, the A-A joint, and C2/3. Therefore, positive palpatory findings in the suboccipital region demand testing of these three joints. Each joint is different in its motion, so they must be individually tested.

Occipital Motion Testing of C0–1

Lateral Translation Test

The physician stands or sits at the head of the supine patient. Grasp the head with both hands, with the fingertips of the index and middle fingers over the occipital articulation (Fig. 38.1).

Translate the head to the right and to the left, evaluating freedom or resistance. A more precise method is to perform the lateral translation test in flexion and in extension. Flex the occiput (O-A), and then translate to the right and to the left. Then extend the occiput and translate to the right and to the left. Restriction of right translation with freedom of left translation suggests an occiput rotated left and side-bent right (occiput posterior left). If translation is done in flexion and extension, restriction is encountered when the barrier is engaged. Restriction of right translation in the flexed position suggests an occiput that is extended, rotated left, and side-bent right with restriction of flexion, rotation right, and side bending left.

There are two O-A joints, one on each side. Given a condition of occiput rotated right and side-bent left, the dominant restriction, tenderness, and tissue texture abnormality may be on the right side or it may be on the left side. In treating this dysfunction with high-velocity technique, it may be appropriate to localize force precisely to one side or the other. The terminology that has been used by the osteopathic profession for years is positional terminology. This in no way implies that positional diagnosis is preferred; identification of motion restriction is imperative. In the above

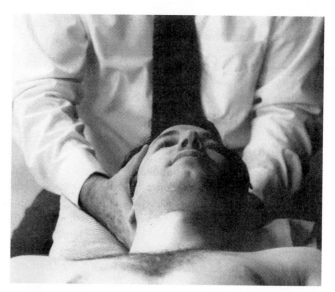

Figure 38-1 Lateral translation test for occipital motion.

example of the occiput rotated right and side-bent left, the right side is called posterior occiput and the left side is called anterior occiput. A posterior occiput right exhibits motion restriction, tissue texture abnormality, and tenderness on the right side. An anterior occiput left exhibits motion restriction, tissue texture abnormality, and tenderness left. Do confirmatory motion tests. Focusing on one side at a time, assess freedom of flexion and extension. The posterior occiput side exhibits restriction of extension. The anterior occiput side exhibits restriction of flexion.

Atlas Motion Test

The atlas rotates in relation to the axis and becomes restricted in rotation. The motion test of atlas function is a rotation test. It is convenient to isolate cervical rotation to the atlas by flexing the cervical spine prior to rotation. This produces physiologic locking of C2-7. This is an example of the third principle of physiologic motion of the spine. Flexion of C2-7 effectively eliminates rotation in this area.

Stand or sit at the head of your supine patient. Grasp the head with fingertips contacting the lateral mass of the atlas. Flex the cervical spine. Rotate to the right and to the left, assessing the range of motion and freedom or resistance (Fig. 38-2).

A right-rotated atlas exhibits restriction of left rotation. Osteopathic positional terminology for this dysfunction is posterior atlas right. Flexion, extension, and side-bending motions are not tested.

Some osteopathic physicians refer to an anterior atlas. The anterior side is opposite the posterior atlas. Given an example of atlas rotated right with restriction of left rotation, the right side would be the posterior atlas side. If the left side exhibited tenderness and tissue texture abnormality, it would be referred to as an anterior atlas left. These are not common, but when present, they are very symptomatic and tender. Retro-orbital pain is often associated with an anterior atlas.

C2-7 Motion Testing

Flexion and Extension Test

At a segmental level, C2-7 motion is difficult to assess by directly flexing and extending, although this has been the method used by

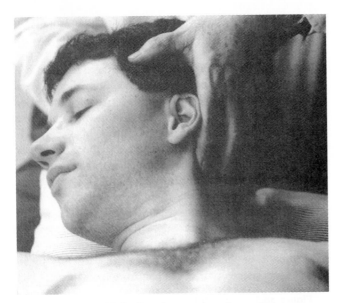

Figure 38-2   Rotation test for atlas motion.

many osteopathic physicians in the past. The lateral translation test, which was used extensively by the muscle energy tutorial committee (15), provides a more precise method of evaluating flexion and extension while evaluating side bending.

Lateral Translation Test

The lateral translation test is similar to the occiput lateral translation test, except that the hand placement is on the cervical region with the fingertips over the lateral portion of the articular pillars. Stand or sit at the head of the supine patient. Support the patient's head with your hands while palpating the lateral border of the articular pillars. Localizing the force to one segment, test lateral translation to the right and to the left with the segment flexed and with the segment extended. Restriction of right translation in the flexed position suggests extension. Right side bending suggests right rotation with restriction of flexion, left side bending, and left rotation (Fig. 38-3).

Rotation Test

Applying force to one segment at a time can do a rotation test. Rotation movement should follow the planes of the facets;

therefore, the force is directed up toward the eye, rather than in a horizontal plane. Stand or sit at the head of the supine patient. Support the patient's head, with your fingertips contacting the posterior surface of the articular pillars. Rotate (following the plane of the facets) to the right and to the left, assessing restriction or freedom. Remember, any normal segment should rotate both ways with equal range and freedom. Restriction of right rotation of C5 suggests a positional diagnosis of C5 left rotated, left side bent, with restriction of right rotation and right side bending. The posterior transverse process is on the left (Fig. 38-4).

DIAGNOSTIC MODALITIES

Indications for Imaging

Patients with acute neck pain who are older than 60 years of age (malignant tumor) or younger than 15 years of age (benign bone tumor) should be considered for plain roentgenograms of the cervical spine and determination of the erythrocyte sedimentation rate. Patients who sustain blunt trauma to the head or neck, those involved in high-speed motor vehicle accidents, or sports-related injuries should be imaged. There are imaging guidelines, such as the Nexus criteria, for use in the emergency department; however, these are only guidelines, and *an adequate history* is crucial to obtain when determining whether or not to image a patient. Although it is important to be cost effective, if there is any question about orthopedic injury in the patient's neck, image the patient.

Cervical Spine X-rays

Plain roentgenograms remain the initial step in diagnostic imaging of the cervical spine because of their availability, speed, relatively low exposure of tissue to radiation, and reasonable costs. A cervical spine x-ray series includes a lateral view, an A-P view, an open mouth view, and two oblique views. Plain cervical spine x-ray films are commonly used to evaluate the bony detail, alignment, disc space height, the neural foramina, and the facets. The lateral view of the cervical spine is the single most important view in evaluating degenerative conditions. The AP view of the cervical spine shows the cervical vertebrae from C3 through T1. The first two cervical vertebrae are generally hidden from view by the superimposed mandible and occiput and must be evaluated separately on an open-mouth (odontoid) view. The open-mouth (odontoid) view is useful for evaluating

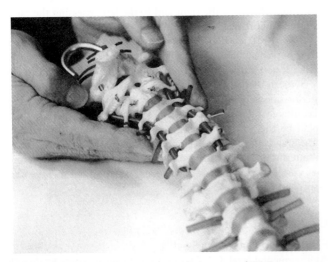

Figure 38-3   Lateral translation test of C2-7.

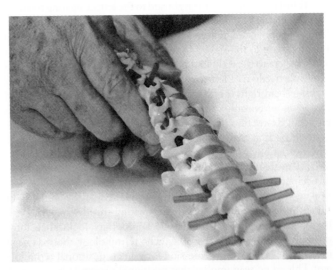

Figure 38-4   Rotation test of C2-7.

the relationship of the occiput, atlas, and axis. In addition, this view detects erosive changes found with inflammatory arthopathies. Oblique views are used to evaluate the intervertebral foramina, the pedicles, the lateral masses, and apophyseal joints.

In a neck-injured patient, the lateral x-ray is obtained first and cleared before the other views are taken. The anterior retropharyngeal space should also be evaluated (should not exceed 5 mm). The posterior margins of the vertebral bodies, the facet joints, and the contour of the spinolaminar line should be evaluated for congruity. As a general rule, on a standard lateral cervical spine film, the spinal canal as measured from the posterior aspect of the vertebral body to the narrowest point on the spinolaminar line should be about 17 mm. If this distance is narrowed by a posterior osteophyte to a diameter of 13 mm or less, it is likely that there is spinal cord compression. An intervertebral disc space separation increase with traction of more than 1.7 mm is also abnormal. A difference in angulation more than 11 degrees between two cervical segments on a lateral radiograph also suggests instability (37).

Determination if a radiographic finding is an acute injury, an older injury, or due to degenerative changes is often difficult (37). A common finding in an older patient with chronic neck pain includes decreased disc space height, marginal osteophytes, narrowing of the neural foramina, sclerosis of the vertebral endplates and facets, and poor alignment of the spinolaminar line. The combined findings indicate cervical spondylosis, a degenerative arthritic condition of the cervical spine. A common radiographic finding in acute neck spasm/pain includes a reversal of the cervical lordosis. This straightening of the cervical spine usually indicates muscle spasm; however, it may indicate an underlying disc injury, fracture or other problem.

CT Scan

CT scan provides more bony detail than plain films and provides a better understanding of spatial relationships. CT is helpful in evaluation of spinal stenosis, infections with paraspinal abscesses, postsurgical epidural scarring, facet and uncovertebral joint arthritis, primary metastatic tumors of the cervical spine, and trauma to the spinal column. CT can also visualize the medullary portion of the vertebral body and detect bone destruction before changes are visible on plain roentgenograms.

CT is particularly useful in the diagnosis and assessment of trauma because the patient is stationary during the procedure, limiting the hazards of moving the patient. Small fragments of bone that may not be detectable by plain roentgenogram are more easily seen on CT scan (38). A CT scan is better than an MR image for bone detail in identifying bone tumors. CT scans may be combined with myelography to outline the spinal cord and nerve roots. Evaluation of the craniocervical and cervicothoracic junctions can be difficult on a plain roentgenogram but is much easier with the CT examination.

MRI

The MR image of the cervical spine visualizes the vertebral column, intervertebral discs, spinal canal, spinal cord, and cerebrospinal fluid (CSF). Although more expensive, it is the preferred study in the evaluation of the discs and spinal cord. It is the preferred imaging modality for syringomyelia, cord atrophy, cord infarction, traumatic injury to the cord, and intramedullary tumors or multiple sclerosis affecting the spinal cord. When evaluating disc herniations, MRI can differentiate the annulous fibrosus from the nucleus pulposis. The MRI is also useful to evaluate postoperative scarring. Many asymptomatic patients have disc protrusions on MRI; therefore,

the history, physical findings, and scan should always be correlated together before embarking on a treatment plan (38).

Treatment of Neck Pain: General Treatment Guidelines

In the treatment of neck pain, the clinician must rule out urgent conditions that need expeditious treatment. He must determine if neurologic compromise is present, and if the patient needs to be seen in the emergency department, or if they can be treated as an outpatient.

The following are treatment guidelines for symptomatic, unstable cervical spine problems:

1. Avoid high-velocity manipulation of the cervical spine.
2. Decrease muscle tension. Treatment of the upper thoracic spine and ribs is essential to accomplish this goal.
3. Counterstrain, cranial, and indirect techniques are the least traumatic to the neck. Muscle energy technique, if done without pain, is appropriate.
4. Traction, with proper direction of force, is appropriate.

If the initial conservative treatment fails, symptomatic patients may be separated into two groups.

If no symptomatic improvement is achieved after 6 weeks of medical nonoperative therapy, plain roentgenograms should be taken and carefully examined. Patients who have no specific diagnosis and have pain that is resistant to a 12-week trial of medical nonoperative therapy are considered to have chronic neck pain. The primary goal for therapy with chronic neck pain is maximum function, not pain relief.

Common Treatments for Neck Pain
Injections

If there is no significant improvement in symptoms in 3 to 4 weeks in patients with local neck pain, local injections into palpable tender points or trigger points can be beneficial. Patients with chronic neck pain may undergo facet injections, or epidural steroid injections. A pain specialist usually performs these. Some patients with chronic neck pain may benefit from a stellate ganglion (sympathetic) block. A successful sympathetic block is manifested by the development of Horner's syndrome, including ptosis, miosis, and anhidrosis.

Collars

Collars are needed in a small proportion of patients. The collar initially should be worn continuously, day and night. The use of collars can cause the patient's neck muscles to become weak, so use the collar for as brief of a time as beneficial. For patients with acute intervertebral disc problems, the use of a collar is generally used for 2 to 3 weeks, slowly decreasing the time worn. Isometric strengthening exercises should be instituted as their pain permits to allow enough neck muscle strength for them to return to full activity. Some patients with acute cervical spine fractures may require immobilization of the neck with a hard plastic collar. These are generally worn from 1 to 3 months, or until bony fusion is seen on x-ray.

Medications

Another component of the initial treatment plan is drug therapy. Anti-inflammatory drugs, analgesics, and muscle relaxants usually improve patient comfort and are commonly used in conjunction with gentle OMT, stretches, ice or heat, and cervical spine support. The use of muscle relaxers is indicated for short-term painful muscular conditions. They can cause drowsiness and decrease a patient's reaction time, so caution should be exercised if the patient is driving or caring for young children. It is better to prescribe these for night time use to help the patient sleep. Analgesics help decrease the pain-spasm-pain cycle that can maintain a patient's symptoms. Anti-inflammatory drugs (NSAIDs) are useful, if the patient does not have a history of gastritis, reflux, or peptic ulcer disease.

Treatment of Specific Clinical Syndromes

Cervical Myelopathy

Cervical myelopathy occurs secondary to compression of the spinal cord (and nerve roots) in the cervical spinal canal. Historical questions should include a change in gait, balance, paresthesia, or loss of agility in their hands (39). Progressive and profound upper motor neuron signs, including weakness, spasticity, and gait abnormalities, are the clinical manifestations of myelopathy. The main lower motor neuron (radicular) signs are weakness with loss of tone and volume of the muscles in the upper extremity. Pressure on the spinal cord may produce pyramidal tract signs and spasticity in the lower extremities. The most frequent presentation of myelopathy is a combination of arm and leg signs and gait disorder (39). Patients who have the above signs, but do not have cervical myelopathy, should be evaluated for an underlying systemic medical illness as the cause of their neck pain. OMT in these patients may occur postoperatively, or if not a surgical candidate, with caution. Avoid positions that close down the cervical canal, such as cervical extension and rotation. Keep a few pillows under the patients' neck and have them place their feet on the treatment table to keep down dural tension. Indirect techniques and cranial techniques may help symptomatically.

Cervical Radiculopathy

Cervical root irritation from compression by osteophyte or disc protrusion produces nerve-related symptoms in the upper extremity, such as pain, numbness, or muscle weakness. The hallmark of this condition is that the pain and physical findings usually follow a specific nerve root (39). Careful neurologic testing reveals the nerve root dysfunction (see Table 38.1). Look for sensory loss, motor weakness, and decreased deep tendon reflexes. Palpable flaccidity of arm muscles may be present. Correlate the sensory dermatome, deep tendon reflex, palpatory findings and motor weakness with the specific disc level in the cervical spine. Remember that sometimes the nerve root irritation is intermittent and insufficient to produce any neurologic deficit. Occasionally, cervical radiculopathy may be confused with a brachial plexopathy. In the latter, irritation of the plexus in the axilla due to lymphadenopathy, radiation, traction, or trauma will also produce arm/hand symptoms. Remember that the upper portion of the brachial plexus innervates the thumb and the lower portion of the brachial plexus innervates the small finger.

In the acute situation, HVLA technique should be avoided at the level of herniation, as this vertebral level is considered to be unstable. HVLA may be used for articular dysfunctions distant from this spinal level, particularly the upper thoracic spine and ribs, as treating the upper thoracic spine and ribs is crucial in this scenario. Cervical root irritation usually produces a reflex change in the interscapular area, which then produces arm symptoms. A recalcitrant interscapular problem might be due to a reflex from the cervical spine. Many patients with cervical root problems experience shoulder pain when they lie supine on the table. Often, extension of the neck exacerbates the symptoms. In addition to spinal nerve root encroachment, diseases that directly affect the brachial plexus may result in a variety of upper extremity symptoms that must be distinguished from cervical root syndromes. The

patients with arm pain predominant (brachialgia) refractory to nonoperative management may have symptoms due to mechanical pressure from a herniated disc or hypertrophic bone and secondary inflammation of the involved nerve roots.

Systemic Concerns

Constitutional symptoms of fever or weight loss are suggestive of an infection or tumor. Infiltrative lesions of the spinal cord and tumors of the spinal column are associated with nocturnal increase in pain. Benign tumors tend to involve the posterior elements of vertebrae, whereas malignant tumors affect the vertebral bodies. Acute localized bone pain is usually associated with either fracture or expansion of bone. Localized cervical bone pain may be secondary to a systemic process that replaces bone (Paget disease) or a local tumor (osteoblastoma). Any condition that replaces bone with abnormal cells (tumor or sarcoidosis) or increases mineral loss from bone (hyperparathyroidism) weakens bone to the point at which fracture may occur spontaneously or with minimal trauma.

Morning stiffness of the neck lasting for hours is a common symptom of patients with spondyloarthropathies, or rheumatoid arthritis. Patients with this symptom should have cervical x-rays including a flexion-extension view of the cervical spine to detect subluxation. Patients with rheumatoid arthritis of the neck should not have HVLA of the cervical spine, as they are prone to AA instability and subluxations.

Patients with visceral pain have neck pain secondary to disorders in the cardiovascular, gastrointestinal, or neurologic systems. Patients with a visceral cause of their neck pain (angina, thoracic outlet syndrome, and esophageal disorders) have symptoms that affect structures distal to the cervical spine and recur in a regular pattern. Patients may complain of neck and arm pain that occurs with exertion.

Patients with neck pain and fever should be evaluated for any change in mental status or severe headaches. These individuals should have a lumbar puncture and their CSF examined for inflammatory cells, increased protein, or decreased glucose concentration compatible with meningitis.

Somatic Dysfunction

The osteopathic physician needs to determine if somatic dysfunction is present and significant. The clinician also need to determine if OMT is indicated or not, and potentially beneficial. Magee (38) discusses a précis of cervical spine assessment that includes joint play considerations in the evaluation of the patient with neck pain. It must be understood that OMT is used to treat somatic dysfunction, not just "neck pain." If no somatic dysfunction is present, no OMT is required. If a diagnosis of somatic dysfunction has been made and there is no contraindication, OMT may be performed. The type of OMT should be based on the patient's clinical condition and physician's experience and skill. The technique(s) should be safe, effective, and appropriate for the diagnosis made.

Concern has arisen over the years for the safety of cervical HVLA technique. HVLA in the cervical spine is a safe technique and indicated for articular somatic dysfunctions in the neck that have a distinct firm end-feel to their restrictive barriers. It needs to be performed precisely, gently, and in the appropriate patient. The American Osteopathic Association (AOA) has published a position paper on HVLA manipulation in the cervical spine. After considerable review of the literature, they have concluded that HVLA manipulation of the neck is a safe procedure with an incidence of severe injury to be 1/400,000 manipulations (40). It is the position of the AOA that all modalities of OMT for the cervical spine, including HVLA (thrust), should be taught at all levels of education, and that this method of treatment should be offered to patients. Other forms of osteopathic manipulation used for the cervical spine have not been shown to cause significant injury or harm to patients.

Suboccipital Pain

Suboccipital symptoms of tension and tissue change are almost always associated with upper thoracic and rib problems on the same side. It is important to treat the upper thoracic area first because of sympathetic influence and muscle connections. Testing the sub-occipital area before and after treatment of the upper thoracic reveals a significant decrease in suboccipital findings. Always diagnose and treat the atlas, as 50% of cervical rotation comes from its articulations. Cranial osteopathy is very useful in this situation as well. Cranial base dysfunction is related to the cervical spine, as the occiput, atlas, and C2 is a functional unit. O-A myofascial release is a simple, direct procedure that improves motion of these articulations and soft tissues.

Whiplash

Whiplash injuries occur primarily after rear-end motor vehicle collisions but may also occur during sports, falls, or on-the-job injuries. The mechanism is an acceleration-deacceleration event that leads to soft tissue injury and other "whiplash associated disorders" (WAD) (41). Acute extension trauma (whiplash) with injury to flexor muscles takes prolonged time to treat. Counterstrain, indirect fascial release, and cranial techniques are most appropriate for initial treatment. The sequence of treatment is as follows: the thoracic spine, the suboccipital area, and finally, the rest of the cervical spine. The upper thoracic acts as a functional base for the neck. The clinician should always look for an extended (flexion restriction) upper or midthoracic somatic dysfunction and initially treat it with indirect techniques. Gross cervical motion testing reveals restriction of rotation and side bending to the same side. The cervical prevertebral muscles (scalenes, longus group) are usually involved in acute neck problems and should be addressed only after the upper thoracic spine has been treated. For example, SCM shortening causes rotation and side bending to opposite sides. Counterstrain of the SCM and other anterior/posterior cervical tender points is a valuable initial treatment. In addition, releasing the abdominal diaphragm (redoming) by gentle ventral abdominal inhibition is a useful consideration. This resets the autonomics, removes traumatic myofascial strain, and lets the patient breathe more fully. Cranial treatment for any strains or simply to relax the autonomic nervous system can be used. When the patient can tolerate more direct treatment of the upper thoracic spine, treatment of the commonly found single segment extended dysfunction with HVLA technique is critical to his or her overall improvement.

Acute Spastic Torticollis

Acute Torticollis with massive neck muscle spasm causes motion to be painful and limited. The SCM is usually involved. The SCM is innervated by the spinal accessory nerve, a cranial nerve. Treat the cranial base with a direct myofascial release in hopes to alleviate any fascial compression to this nerve. Then use a muscle energy technique. Position the head at the midpoint of pain-free motion. Hold the head and ask the patient to turn the head toward the restriction and relax. Reposition the head a few degrees toward the restriction and repeat. Sometimes, a significant improvement in range of motion is achieved. This technique is not classified as direct or indirect, in that the barrier is not engaged nor is the neck positioned in the other direction. Instead, the neck is positioned in the middle, with the ultimate objective of reaching the barrier.

BEST EVIDENCE FOR NECK PAIN

The medical literature on neck pain from 1980 to 2006 has been critically reviewed by the Bone and Joint Decade 2000–2010 Task Force on Neck Pain and its associated disorders. Results of their comprehensive, systematic literature reviews have been published in *Spine*. They have evaluated the following topics related to neck pain (41–48):

- Effectiveness and safety of noninvasive interventions
- Course, risk factors, and prognosis of WAD
- Gaps in the current literature
- Epidemiology, assessment, and classification of neck pain
- Nonmodifiable and modifiable prognostic factors in neck pain
- Course and prognosis of neck pain in the general population

The following statements regarding neck pain are derived by review from a best-evidence synthesis of the current published literature (41–48):

- Neck pain is more common in middle-age women.
- Genetics, poor psychologic health, and exposure to tobacco are risk factors to neck pain in the general population.
- Manual therapies, patient education, and exercise are more effective than alternative strategies for patients with neck pain.
- Cervical spine manipulation and mobilization provided short-term benefits for patients with acute neck pain and headache (40).
- For subacute and chronic neck pain, spinal manipulation is more effective when compared with muscle relaxants or the usual medical care. Efficacy was enhanced when combined with other modalities, such as exercise (40).
- There are gaps in the literature when it comes to neck pain in children, neck pain related to culture and social policies, and the prevention of neck pain–related activity limitations.
- Patients who undertook general exercise had a better prognosis; those with little influence on their own work, those with psychological stress had a poorer prognosis.
- Fifty percent of patients with whiplash associated neck pain will report neck symptoms 1 year after the injury.
- Headrest, car seats (aimed at elimination head extension) in rear-end impacts were associated with less repeating of "whiplash-associated disorders," as was eliminating insurance payments.

The reader is recommended to review the best evidence on neck pain as this knowledge is important in directing the care of patients.

RISKS AND BENEFITS OF MANUAL MANIPULATIVE TECHNIQUES IN PATIENTS WITH NECK PAIN

Risks

The potential risk from manual manipulative techniques used in the cervical spine is from thrust-type (HVLA) procedures. The potential risk is from hyperextension and rotation forces causing a vertebral artery dissection and stroke. Although a few case reports have been published on this topic in the past 100 years, the natural occurrence of spontaneous dissection and stroke is higher than that reported with thrust-type procedures (40). Because of concern over this topic in the literature, the AAO (March 2003) and AOA (August 2004) developed position papers on osteopathic manipulation of the cervical spine. Their consensus after review of the literature was that they supported the appropriate use of cervical manipulation and the use of HVLA technique. (40) There have not been any complications from any of the manipulative treatment procedures, provided in clinical trials, over the past 25 years (over 100 publications) (40). There is still controversy in the medical literature on when or when not to use cervical thrust (HVLA) manipulation.

Benefits

There are many benefits to cervical manipulation. Some of the primary benefits include increased range of motion, decreased pain, improved activities of daily living, and shortened disability time (quicker return to work). Some secondary benefits include reduced reliance on medications (especially narcotics) and improved postural efficiency (40).

These benefits may decrease the need and cost for physical therapy and, in some cases, prevent unnecessary injections or surgery.

SUMMARY

Manipulative treatment of the cervical spine can greatly assist healing of injury, pathology, pain, or dysfunction of the cervical region. Appropriate treatment of the cervical spine requires a thorough understanding of the anatomy, somatic dysfunction, and orthopedic and systemic conditions. OMT should be integrated throughout the treatment plan of patients with neck pain. Improving motion and tissue restrictions of the neck has far-reaching effects to other regions of the body.

REFERENCES

1. Cote P, Cassidy JD, Carroll U, et al. The annual incidence and course of neck pain in the General population: a population-based cohort study. *Pain* 2004;112:267–273.
2. Hartvigsen J, Christensen K, Frederiksen H. Back and neck pain exhibit many common Features in old age; A population-based study of 4,486 Danish twins 70–102 years of age. *Spine* 2004;29: 576–580.
3. Walker-Bone K, Reading I, Coggon D, et al. The anatomical pattern and determinants of pain in the neck and upper limbs: an epidemiologic study. *Pain* 2004;109:45–51.
4. Chapline JF, Ferguson SA, Lillis RP, et al. Neck pain and head restraint position relative to the driver's head in rear-end collisions. *Accid Anal Prev* 2000;32:287–297.
5. Vogt MT, Simonsick EM, Harris TB, et al. Neck and shoulder pain in 70- to 79-year-old men and women: findings from the Health, Aging and Body composition Study. *Spine J* 2003;3:435–441.
6. Bilkey WJ. Manual medicine approach to the cervical spine and whiplash injury. Phys Med *Rehabil Clin North Am* 1996;7:749–759.
7. Sleszynski SL, Glonek T. Outpatient osteopathic SOAP note form: preliminary results in osteopathic outcomes-based research. *J Am Osteopath Assoc* 2005;105:181–205.
8. Grgic V. *Lijec Vjesn;* 2008;130(9–10):234–236.
9. Jacobs B, *N Y State J Med* 1990;90(1):8–11.
10. Ito Y, Tanaka N, Fujimoto Y, et al. *J Spinal Disord Tech* 2004;17(5): 462–465.
11. Wells P. *Am Fam Physician* 1997;55(6):2262–2264.
12. Heinking K. The geriatric athlete. In: Karageanes S, ed. *Principles of 9 Manual Sports Medicine.* Lippincott Williams & Wilkins, 2005:635–636; chap 42.
13. Larson NJ. Summary of site and occurrence of paraspinal soft tissue changes of patients in the intensive care unit. *JAOA* 976;75: 840–842.

14. Beal MC. Viscerosomatic reflexes: a review. *JAOA* 1985;85:786–801.
15. Nicholas AS, DeBias DA, Ehrenfeuchter W, et al. Kirschbaum: a somatic component to myocardial infarction. *Brit Med J* 1985;291: 13–15.
16. Warwick R, Williams PL, eds. *Gray's Anatomy*, British 35th Ed. Philadelphia, PA: WB Saunders, 1973:235.
17. Payan D. Peripheral neuropeptides, inflammation and nociception. In: Willard FW, Patterson MM, eds. *Nociception and the Neuroendocrine-Immune Connection, 1992 International Symposium.* Indianapolis, IN: American Academy of Osteopathy, 1992:3446.
18. deGroat W. Spinal cord processing of visceral and somatic nociceptive input. In: Willard FW, Patterson MM, eds. *Nociception and the NeuroendocrineImmune Connection, 1992 International Symposium.* Indianapolis, IN: American Academy of Osteopathy, 1992:4773.
19. Aston-Jones G, Valentino R. Brain noradrenergic neurons, nociception and stress: basic mechanisms and clinical implications. In: Willard FH, Patterson MM, eds. *Nociception and the Neuroendocrine-Immune Connection, 1992 International Symposium.* Indianapolis, IN: American Academy of Osteopathy, 1992:107–132.
20. Wing L, Hadephobes WW. Cervical vertigo. *Aust N Z J Surg.* 1974;44(3):275–277.
21. Jepson O. Dizziness origination in the columna cervicalis. *J Can Chiropractic Assoc.* 1967;11(1):78.
22. Hargrave WW. The cervical syndrome. *Aust J Physiother* 1972: 144–147.
23. Greenman P. *Principles of Manual Medicine.* Baltimore, MD: Williams & Wilkins, 1989:125.
24. Magee DJ. *Orthopedic Physical Assessment.* 4th Ed. Philadelphia, PA: Saunders, 2002:152–155.
25. Magee DJ. *Orthopedic Physical Assessment.* 4th Ed. Philadelphia, PA: Saunders, 2002:286–289.
26. Magee DJ. *Orthopedic Physical Assessment.* 4th Ed. Philadelphia, PA: Saunders, 2002: 133–135.
27. Hosono N, Yonenobu K. Cineradiographic motion analysis of atlantoaxial instability in os odontoideum. *Spine* 1991;16(suppl 10): S480–S482.
28. Van Mameren H, Sanches H. Cervical spine motion in the sagittal plane II. *Spine* 1992; 17(5):467–474.
29. Kirksville College of Osteopathic Medicine. *Cineradiographic Studies of the Atlas.* Kirksville, MO: Kirksville College of Osteopathic Medicine, 1970; Videocassette. [This tape was later erased and lost.]
30. Felding J. Cineroentgenography of the normal cervical spine. *J Bone Joint Surg* 1957;39A:1280–1288.
31. Ochs C, Romine J. Radiographic examination of the cervical spine in motion. *U S Naval Med Bull* 1974;64:2129.
32. Bogduk N, Mercer S. Biomechanics of the cervical spine. I. Normal kinematics. *Clin Biomech (Bristol, Avon)* 2000;15:633–648.
33. Magee DJ. *Orthopedic Physical Assessment,* 4th Ed. Philadelphia, PA: Saunders, 2002:47.
34. Hoppenfeld S. *Physical Examination of the Spine and Extremities* Appleton, WI: Century, Crofts, 1976:105–132;chapter 4.
35. Magee DJ. *Orthopedic Physical Assessment.* 4th Ed. Philadelphia, PA: Saunders, 2002:145–153.
36. Magee DJ. *Orthopedic Physical Assessment.* 4th Ed. Philadelphia, PA: Saunders, 2002:406.
37. Watkins RG. *The Spine in Sports.* St. Louis, MO: Mosby, 1996: 130–131.
38. Magee DJ. *Orthopedic Physical Assessment.* 4th Ed. Philadelphia, PA: Saunders, 2002:174–176.
39. Watkins RG. *The Spine in Sports.* St. Louis, MO: Mosby, 1996: 76–79.
40. Seffinger MA, Hruby R. *Evidence Based Manual Medicine: A problem Oriented Approach.* Philadelphia, PA: Saunders, 2007:184–187.
41. Hurwitz E, et al. Treatment of neck pain: noninvasive interventions. *Spine* 2008;33(45):S123–S152.
42. Carroll LJ, et al. Research priorities and methodological implications. *Spine* 2008;45(45):S214–S220.

43. Carroll LJ, et al. Methods for the best evidence synthesis on neck pain and its associated disorders. *Spine* 2008;33(45):S33–S38.

44. Carroll LJ, et al. Course and prognostic factors for neck pain in workers. *Spine* 2008;33(45):S93–S100.

45. Carroll LJ, et al. Course and prognostic factors for neck pain in the general population. *Spine* 2008;33(45):S75–S82.

46. Carroll LJ, et al. Course and prognostic factors for neck pain in whiplash-associated disorders (WAD). *Spine* 2008;33(45):S83–S92.

47. Holm LW, et al. The burden and determinants of neck pain in whiplash-associated disorders after traffic collisions. *Spine* 2008;33(45): S52–S59.

48. Hogg-Johnson S, et al. The burden and determinants of neck pain in the general population. *Spine* 33(45):S39–S51.

39

Thoracic Region and Rib Cage

RAYMOND J. HRUBY

INTRODUCTION

Because the heart and lungs are contained in the thorax, this region's unique significance in life has long been recognized. The inability to draw breath or the perception of pain in the thorax often constitutes real or imagined immediate and life-threatening problems. Movement of the thorax is necessary for normal function in both obvious and not-so-obvious ways. Because much of the regulatory outflow of the sympathetic nervous system originates in the thoracic spinal cord, disturbances in the muscles and joints of the thoracic region often mimic life-threatening problems. Injury to thoracic vertebrae can cause long-term sequelae for health and survival.

The most vital role of the thoracic region and rib cage is the contribution this region makes to the process of respiration. Respiration is a process involving the participation of several systems of the body, none the least of which is the musculoskeletal system. As Cathie (1) noted, "Respiratory activity requires motion in a greater number of articulations and with a greater frequency than any other musculoskeletal function." This not only includes the intervertebral joints of the thoracic spine but also the costovertebral and costotransverse joints at the posterior aspects of the ribs. In addition to the articular motion, optimal respiration also requires a degree of elasticity of the ribs and costal cartilages. The biomechanical architecture among the vertebrae and ribs may be thought of as a complex system of levers; anything that alters the normal movement of this system of levers may impair respiration.

The complexities of the thoracic region and the vital importance of its organ systems underscore the necessity for the osteopathic physician to understand its many functions, diagnoses, and potential treatment approaches. In diagnosis and treatment, it cannot be considered as separate from the other body regions, because dysfunction in it or other regions is always interdependent.

DEFINITION

The thoracic region (also commonly referred to as the *chest*) is that portion of the trunk between the neck and the abdomen that contains such structures as the heart, lungs, esophagus, the aorta and its branches, superior and inferior vena cavae, the trachea and primary bronchi, the thoracic duct, azygous and hemiazygous veins, and the sympathetic chain ganglia. The rib cage is the bony enclosing wall of the chest. It is a structure formed by the thoracic vertebrae, the ribs, the sternum, and the costal cartilages.

ANATOMY AND PHYSIOLOGY

Skeletal Anatomy

The thoracic cage includes 12 thoracic spinal vertebrae, 12 pairs of ribs, and the sternum (Fig. 39.1). Although the scapula overlies the posterior portion of the rib cage, is connected to the sternum through the clavicle, and is often involved in thoracic injuries and pain syndromes, this structure is more properly considered a part of the upper extremity.

White and Panjabi, the noted clinical anatomists and authors, divide the thoracic spine into three anatomical regions:

- Upper (T1-4)
- Middle (T4-8)
- Lower (T8-L1)

It is also helpful to divide the thoracic and upper lumbar spine into four functional divisions that roughly correspond to the thoracolumbar outflow of the sympathetic system:

- T1-4: Sympathetics to head and neck, with T1-6 to the heart and lungs
- T5-9: All upper abdominal viscera: stomach, duodenum, liver, gall bladder, pancreas, and spleen
- T10-11: Remainder of the small intestines, kidneys, ureters, gonads, and right colon
- T12-L2: Left colon and pelvic organs

This functional division is often very useful to the osteopathic physician, because visceral afferent (generally nociceptive) neurons usually follow the same pathway as the sympathetic outflow. Visceral disturbances often cause increased musculoskeletal tension in the somatic structures that are innervated from the corresponding spinal level through the viscerosomatic reflexes. Manipulative treatment at that spinal level is used to reduce somatic afferent input from the associated facilitated segments, which, in turn, reduces somatosympathetic activity to the affected viscus (3).

Generally, the thoracic spine has a mildly kyphotic, forward-bending curve that varies from person to person. In the osteoporotic or older patients, the angle of this curve can become more acute, causing biomechanical problems and necessitating compensatory adaptation in other regions of the spine and in general posture. Individual thoracic vertebrae are parts of a continuum with the cervical and lumbar vertebrae; size increases from cervical to lumbar to account for increased weight bearing. The spinous processes

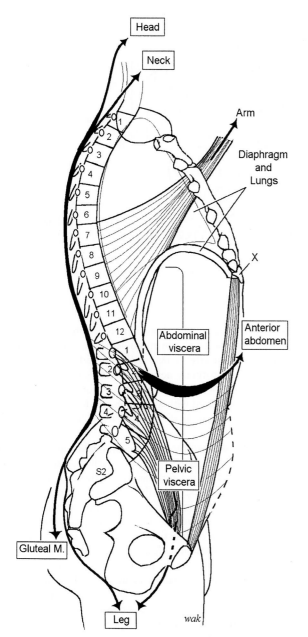

Figure 39-1 The thoracic region and its relationships.

BUM, BUL, BUM from cervical to thoracic to lumbar. In the lower portion of the thoracic spine, the superior facet surface begins to face more posteriorly than laterally, and at T12, it may even face medially, as part of a functional transition to the lumbar spine. The inferior facet of each thoracic vertebra faces in the opposite direction from the superior and has a slightly concave surface.

The thoracic vertebrae are separated by discs, as are the cervical and lumbar vertebrae. The discs act as shock absorbers and permit flexibility between the vertebrae. Each disc is composed of an outer anulus fibrosus and an inner nucleus pulposus, a gel at the center of the disc that acts like a semifluid hydrophilic ball bearing that, under sustained compression, becomes less hydrated and broader. The anulus fibrosus is composed of concentric lamellae of fibrocartilage, running at right angles to the fibers of adjacent layers. Its structural arrangement is more vulnerable to tears posteriorly, where the lamellae are thinner and less numerous. However, the restricted motion of the thoracic spine due to the attachments of the rib cage and the fairly broad posterior longitudinal ligament makes ruptured thoracic discs relatively uncommon. On the other hand, discopathy from trauma, aging, and degenerative disease is relatively common in the thoracic area.

The 12 sets of ribs correspond with the 12 thoracic vertebrae. All ribs are composed of a bony segment and a costal cartilage. Each rib has a cup-shaped depression in its bony segment where the costal cartilage fits into the costochondral joint and where the periosteum of the rib joins the perichondrium of the rib cartilage. The rib heads join with the thoracic vertebrae at the costovertebral articulations. The heads of ribs 2 through 9 articulate with a demifacet on the vertebra above and below. For example, rib 2 articulates by demifacets with T1 and T2. Unlike ribs 2 to 9, the heads of ribs 1 and 10 to 12 articulate with unifacets on their corresponding vertebrae. The transverse processes of vertebrae T1-10 all form synovial costotransverse joints with the tubercle of the corresponding rib.

Ribs 1, 2, 11, and 12 are called *atypical ribs*. Rib 1 is the flattest, shortest, broadest, strongest, and most curved. The subclavian artery and the cervical plexus are vulnerable to muscular compression where they pass over the 1st rib between the tubercles and attachments of the anterior and the middle scalene muscles (the so-called scalenus anticus syndrome). The latter is one of several conditions clinically labeled as *thoracic outlet syndrome*. The subclavian vein may also be compressed between the 1st rib and the clavicle. Rib 2 is considered anatomically atypical because of its tuberosity that attaches to the proximal portion of the serratus anterior muscle. Ribs 11 and 12 are anatomically atypical because they do not have tubercles, do not attach to the sternum or other costal cartilages, and have tapered ends. These 2 ribs are also called *floating* or *vertebral ribs*. Rib 10 is sometimes considered atypical because of its single articulation between the rib head and T10.

The anatomy of the rib cage is shown in Figure 39.2. Anatomically typical ribs (3 to 9, and in most respects 10) have heads, necks, tubercles, angles, and shafts that connect directly or via chondral masses to the sternum. Rib 1 and ribs 2 to 7 connect directly with the sternum by their own individual cartilaginous synovial joints (rib 1 with a stable synchondrosis); therefore, they are often called the *true ribs*. Ribs 8 to 10 merge into a single cartilaginous mass that attaches to the sternum; therefore, these are called *vertebral chondral ribs*. Ribs 11 and 12 do not connect with the sternum and are hence called *floating ribs*. Because ribs 8 to 12 do not connect directly to the sternum, they are often called the *false ribs*.

The costovertebral joints between the heads of the ribs and the vertebral bodies allow gliding or sliding costal motions. The costotransverse joints at the tubercle of the typical ribs, with the facets at

of the thoracic vertebrae are particularly large and easily palpated, pointing increasingly caudad from T1 through T9 and back to an almost anteroposterior orientation from T10-12.

Thoracic vertebral facet joints are plane-type synovial joints. The interarticular surfaces of these joints are smooth, shiny, compact bone that is covered with hyaline cartilage. The joints are surrounded by a thin, loose articular capsule that is lined with synovial membrane. The facet joints guide and limit gross, segmental, and coupled movements. The superior facets of each thoracic vertebra are slightly convex and face posteriorly ("backward"), somewhat superiorly ("up"), and laterally. Their angle of declination averages 60 degrees relative to the transverse plane and 20 degrees relative to the coronal plane. A tool to remember the facet facing is the mnemonic BUL (backward, upward, and lateral). This is in contrast to the cervical and lumbar regions, where the superior facets face backward, upward, and medial (BUM). Thus, the *superior facets* are

Figure 39-2   The bony anatomy of the rib cage and the naming of rib types.

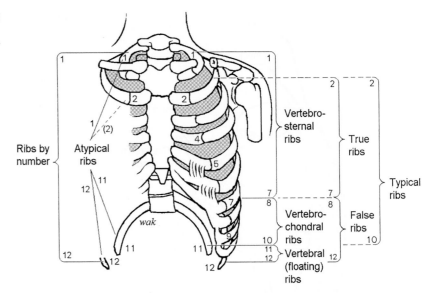

the tip of the transverse processes of their own vertebra, a synovial membrane, and a thin articular capsule, allow gliding and slight rotational motions. When these motions are restricted, respiratory movements are commonly impeded.

The sternum has three parts:

■ Head or manubrium
■ Body or gladiolus
■ Tail or xiphoid process

The superior portion of the manubrium cradles the clavicles at the sternoclavicular joints, forming the sternal notch or jugular notch, which is a landmark for several anterior thoracic strain/counterstrain tender points. The sternal notch lies almost directly anterior to the T2 vertebral body. The manubrium joins the sternal body via a fibrocartilaginous symphysis, or secondary cartilaginous joint, called the *sternal angle* or *angle of Louis*. This joint lies anterior to the fourth thoracic vertebra. Because the 2nd rib attaches to the manubrium and sternal body with a synovial joint, the sternal angle is an anterior landmark for counting the ribs. The xiphisternal joint is located anterior to the ninth thoracic vertebra. It is also a hyaline cartilage symphysis that fuses into a synostosis in the fifth decade.

Musculature

The muscles of the thoracic area are involved in:

■ Actions of the ribs and vertebrae
■ Posture
■ Head and neck control
■ Breathing
■ Locomotion
■ Stabilization of the extremities
■ Visceral function

Table 39.1 lists the major muscles of the thoracic area, with the action, proximal and medial attachments, distal and lateral attachments, and innervation of each (4). It is especially important to note the action of each muscle, because altered tone in these muscles can affect the function of not only the bones to which the muscles are attached but other body areas as well. In addition, increased or decreased tone has the capacity to alter both general and microcirculation in a myriad of ways, such as altered homeostatic regulation and cellular immunity.

As with all muscles, the thoracic muscles are fed not only by circulatory elements but also by physiologically active trophic substances delivered directly by nerves (5). In addition, there is evidence that the sympathetic nerve supply to striated and smooth muscles alters muscle tone and contractile forces. Therefore, the palpatory cues associated with altered muscle tone imply the presence of many differential diagnostic factors that are discussed throughout this text.

The larger muscles of the head, neck, shoulder girdle, and thorax control much of the activity of the thoracic cage and help stabilize the cervical and cranial areas, as well as the arms and shoulder girdle themselves. For example, the splenius capitus and cervicis muscles originate on the lower cranial and upper cervical areas and attach distally along the middle thoracic spine, as low as T6-T8 in some cases. Vertebral dysfunction in the upper thoracic areas can affect the action of these muscles, causing problems with motion outside the thoracic area in the head and neck. Lower down, the internal and external oblique muscles are generally viewed as trunk rotators, but they also attach to the lower ribs along with the diaphragm. Altered tone in these muscles can alter diaphragmatic and respiratory function and vice versa. Experienced palpation readily identifies these relationships.

Of special note are the erector spinae groups (Fig. 39.3), which extend and side-bend the vertebral column, and allow smooth flexion by gradually decreasing resistance to forward bending. These muscles are often involved in group or multiple movement dysfunction (i.e., altered coupling or non-neutral vertebral unit dysfunction), and are vulnerable to insult with unplanned movements or trauma. The deep back muscles, especially the rotatores and multifidus, are also implicated in this type of problem. These small muscles are richly innervated with muscle spindles, which provide proprioception. In fact, one of their primary tasks is to signal position and speed of motion of the vertebral column. (This task makes them important in the maintenance of posture and in directing movement.) They are also very vulnerable to sudden stretch and unplanned movement, which appears to alter the sensory input to the spinal cord and brain, with resultant development of altered motion and pain typical of vertebral somatic dysfunction (6–8).

The abdominal diaphragm is the primary muscle of respiration. It forms the floor of the thorax and attaches to the xiphoid process, the internal surface of the inferior 6 ribs, the upper two (left) or three (right) lumbar vertebrae, and their intervertebral

TABLE 39.1

Regional Thoracic Muscles

Muscle	Action	Proximal/Medial Attachments	Distal/Lateral Attachments	Innervation
Pectoralis major	1. Clavicular head: flexion, adduction, horizontal flexion, and medial rotation of the humerus at the shoulder. 2. Sternocostal head: flexion, adduction, medial rotation, and horizontal flexion of the humerus at the shoulder. Also extends flexed humerus. Through its action on the humerus, it depresses, protracts, and rotates downward.	1. Clavicular division: anterior surface of the medial 1/2 of the clavicle. 2. Sternocostal head: sternum to 7th rib, cartilages of true ribs and aponeurosis of external abdominal oblique muscle.	1. Clavicular division: lateral lip of the intertubercular groove of the humerus. 2. Sternal division: lateral lip of the intertubercular groove of the humerus.	1. Clavicular head: lateral pectoral, C5, C6. 2. Sternocostal head: pectoral, C7, C8, T1.
Pectoralis minor	Depresses scapula and rotates scapula inferiorly. Important anterior shoulder stabilizer.	Anterior surfaces of 3rd, 4th, and 5th ribs near the costal cartilages.	Coracoid process of the scapula.	Medial pectoral, C6, C7, C8.
Teres major	Adducts and medially rotates humerus at the shoulder. Extends the shoulder joint.	Dorsal surface of inferior angle of the scapula.	Medial lip of intertubercular groove of humerus. Medial to latissimus dorsi tendon.	Lower subscapular, C6, C7.
Teres minor	Lateral rotation of humerus at the shoulder. Stabilization of head or humerus.	Superior 2/3 of dorsal surface of lateral border of scapula.	Inferior aspect of greater tubercle of the humerus, capsule of the shoulder joint.	Axillary, C5, C6.
Trapezius	1. Lower fibers: depress the scapula. Retract the scapula. Rotate the scapula upward so the glenoid cavity faces superiorly. Give inferior stabilization of scapula. Help maintain spine in extension. 2. Middle fibers: retract and aid in elevation of scapula. 3. Upper fibers: elevate the scapula as in shrugging the shoulders. Rotate the scapula upward so the glenoid cavity faces superiorly. When acting with the other sections of the trapezius, it retracts the scapula.	1. Lower fibers: spinous processes of 6th–12th thoracic vertebrae. 2. Middle fibers: spinous processes of 1st–5th thoracic vertebrae. 3. Upper fiber: external occipital protuberance, medial 1/3 of superior nuchal line, ligamentum nuchae, and spinous process of the 7th cervical vertebra.	1. Lower fibers: medial 1/3 of spine of the scapula. 2. Middle fibers: superior border of spine of scapula. 3. Upper fibers: lateral 1/3 of clavicle and acromion process.	1. Lower division: spinal root of accessory and anterior primary rami C3, C4. 2. Middle division: spinal root of accessory and anterior primary rami C3, C4. 3. Upper division: spinal root accessory and anterior primary rami C3, C4.

(continued)

TABLE 39.1 (Continued)

Muscle	Action	Proximal/Medial Attachments	Distal/Lateral Attachments	Innervation
Latissimus dorsi	Extends, retracts, and medially rotates the humerus at the shoulder. Through its action on the humerus, it depresses, retracts, and rotates the scapula downward. Assists in forced expiration.	Flat tendon that twists on itself to insert into the intertubercular groove of the humerus, just anterior to and parallel with tendon of pectoralis major.	Broad aponeurosis that originates on the spinous processes of lower 6 thoracic and all lumbar vertebrae; posterior crest of ilium, posterior surface of sacrum, lower 3 or 4 ribs, and an attachment to the inferior angle of the scapula.	Thoracodorsal C6, C7, C8.
Levator scapulae	Elevates the scapula and rotates the scapula downward so the glenoid cavity faces inferiorly. Working with the upper fibers of the trapezius, it elevates and retracts the scapula. *Reversed action:* when the scapula is fixed, it laterally flexes and slightly rotates the cervical spine to the side.	Transverse processes of first four cervical vertebrae.	Vertebral border of scapula between superior angle and scapular spine.	Dorsal scapular C5 and anterior primary rami C3, C4.
Rhomboid	1. *Minor:* retracts and elevates the scapula. Assists in rotating the scapula downward. 2. *Major:* retracts and elevates the scapula. Inferior fibers aid in rotating the glenoid cavity inferiorly.	1. *Minor:* lower part of ligamentum nuchae, spinous processes of C7 and T1. 2. *Major:* spinous processes of T2-5.	1. *Minor:* medial border of scapula at the root of the spine of the scapula. 2. *Major:* medial border of scapula from spine to inferior angle.	1. *Minor:* dorsal scapular, C4, C5. 2. *Major:* dorsal scapular,C4, C5.
Quadratus lumborum	Lateral flexion of lumbar vertebral column; helps the diaphragm in inspiration.	Iliolumbar ligament, posterior part of the iliac crest.	Inferior border of the 12th rib and transverse processes of the upper four lumbar vertebrae.	Anterior primary rami T12, L3.
Serratus anterior	1. Accessory muscle of respiration. 2. Protraction of the scapula.	Superior lateral surfaces of upper 8 ribs at the side of the chest.	Costal surface of the medial border of scapula.	Long thoracic, C7.
Serratus posterior (superior/inferior)	Accessory muscles of inspiration. Superior elevates superior ribs; inferior depresses inferior ribs.	1. *Superior:* lower portion of ligamentum nuchae and spinous processes of the 7th cervical and 1st, 2nd, and 3rd thoracic vertebrae. 2. *Inferior:* spinous processes of 11th and 12th thoracic and 1st, 2nd, and 3rd lumbar vertebrae, and the thoracolumbar fascia.	1. *Superior:* superior borders of 2nd–5th ribs distal to the angles. 2. *Inferior:* inferior borders of lower 4 ribs just beyond their angles.	1. *Superior:* anterior primary rami T2-5. 2. *Inferior:* anterior primary rami T9-12.

Muscle	Action	Origin	Insertion	Nerve
Intercostals	1. Keep the intercostal spaces from bulging and retracting with respiration. 2. Elevate the ribs anteriorly with inspiration.			
External intercostals				
Internal intercostals				
Innermost intercostals				
Subcostals	Depress the ribs.			
Transversus thoracis	Depress the 2nd to 6th ribs.			
Levatores costarum	Elevate the ribs.	Transverse processes of the 7th cervical and upper 11 thoracic vertebrae.	The outer surface of the rib immediately below the vertebrae from which it takes origin, between the tubercle and the angle.	Anterior primary rami of the corresponding intercostal nerves.
Splenius	1. *Capitis*: acting bilaterally, extends the head and neck. Acting unilaterally, laterally flexes and rotates the head and neck to the same side. 2. *Cervicis*: laterally bends and rotates the neck.	1. *Capitis*: spinous processes of C7-T3, inferior half of ligamentum nuchae. 2. *Cervicis*: spinous processes of 3rd–6th thoracic vertebrae.	1. *Capitis*: mastoid process and lateral third of the superior nuchal line. 2. *Cervicis*: transverse processes of 1st, 2nd, 3rd, and 4th cervical vertebrae on the posterior aspect.	1. *Capitis*: posterior primary rami of the middle cervical spinal nerves. 2. *Cervicis*: posterior primary rami of the lower cervical spinal nerves.
Spinalis	1. *Cervicis*: laterally bends and rotates the neck. 2. *Thoracis*: acting unilaterally, lateral flexion of the spine. Acting bilaterally, extension of the spine.	1. *Cervicis*: lower portion of ligamentum nuchae, spinous processes of the 7th cervical and 1st and 2nd thoracic vertebrae. 2. *Thoracis*: spinous processes of the 1st and 2nd lumbar vertebrae, thoracic vertebrae 11 and 12.	1. *Cervicis*: spinous process of the axis and the 3rd and 4th cervical spinous processes. 2. *Thoracis*: spinous processes of upper thoracic, vertebrae T4-8.	1. *Cervicis*: posterior primary rami of the spinal nerves. 2. *Thoracis*: posterior primary rami of the spinal nerves.
Semispinalis	Extends the thoracic and cervical region and rotates it toward the opposite side.	1. *Capitis*: between superior and inferior nuchal lines of the occipital bone. 2. *Cervicis*: spinous processes of 2nd–5th cervical vertebrae. 3. *Thoracis*: spinous processes of the 1st–4th thoracic vertebrae and 6th and 7th cervical vertebrae.	1. *Capitis*: 7th cervical and 1st–6th thoracic transverse processes, and articular processes of 4th, 5th, and 6th cervical vertebrae. 2. *Cervicis*: transverse processes of the 1st–6th thoracic vertebrae. 3. *Thoracis*: transverse processes of 6th–10th thoracic vertebrae	1. *Capitis*: posterior primary rami of cervical spinal nerves. 2. *Cervicis*: posterior primary rami of cervical spinal nerves. 3. *Thoracis*: posterior primary rami of thoracic spinal nerves, T1-6.

(continued)

TABLE 39.1 (Continued)

Muscle	Action	Proximal/Medial Attachments	Distal/Lateral Attachments	Innervation
Longissimus	1. *Capitis:* acting bilaterally, extends the head; acting unilaterally, laterally flexes and rotates the head to the same side. 2. *Cervicis:* acting unilaterally, laterally flexes the neck. Acting bilaterally, laterally flexes the vertebral column. Acting bilaterally, extension of vertebral column; draws ribs down.	1. *Capitis:* transverse processes of the 1st–5th thoracic vertebrae and the articular processes of the 4th–7th cervical vertebrae. 2. *Cervicis:* transverse processes of the 1st–5th thoracic vertebrae. 3. *Thoracis:* the common broad thick tendon with the iliocostalis lumborum, fibers from the transverse and accessory processes of the lumbar vertebrae and thoracolumbar fascia.	1. *Capitis:* the posterior margin of the mastoid process. 2. *Cervicis:* transverse processes of the 2nd–6th cervical vertebrae and transverse process of the atlas. 3. *Thoracis:* the tips of transverse process of all thoracic vertebrae and the lower 9 or 10 ribs between the tubercles and angles.	1. *Capitis:* posterior primary rami of spinal nerves. 2. *Cervicis:* posterior primary rami of spinal nerves. 3. *Thoracis:* posterior primary rami of spinal nerves.
Iliocostalis	1. *Cervicis:* acting bilaterally, extension of the spine; acting unilaterally, laterally flexes the vertebral column. 2. *Thoracis:* acting bilaterally, extension of the spine; acting unilaterally, laterally flexes the spine. 3. *Lumborum:* acting bilaterally, extension of the spine; acting unilaterally, laterally flexes the spine.	1. *Cervicis:* the posterior tubercles of the transverse processes of the 4th, 5th, and 6th cervical vertebrae. 2. *Thoracis:* into the angles of the upper 6 or 7 ribs and into the transverse process of the 7th cervical vertebra. 3. *Lumborum:* inferior borders of the angles of the lower 6 or 7 ribs.	1. *Cervicis:* superior borders of the angles of the 3rd–6th ribs. 2. *Thoracis:* superior borders of the angles of lower 6 ribs medial to the tendons of insertion of the iliocostalis lumborum. 3. *Lumborum:* anterior surface of a broad and thick tendon, which originates from the sacrum, spinous processes of the lumbar and 11th and 12th thoracic vertebrae, and from the medial lip of the iliac crest.	1. *Cervicis:* posterior primary rami of spinal nerves, C8. 2. *Thoracis:* posterior primary rami of spinal nerves. 3. *Lumborum:* posterior primary rami of spinal nerves.
Rotatores	Rotate the vertebral column	1. *Brevis:* bases of the spinous processes (lamina) of the 1st vertebra above. 2. *Longus:* bases of the spinous processes (lamina) of the 2nd vertebra above.	1. *Brevis:* transverse processes of the vertebrae. 2. *Longus:* transverse processes of the vertebrae.	1. *Brevis:* posterior primary rami of spinal nerves. 2. *Longus:* posterior primary rami of spinal nerves.

Muscle	Proximal/medial attachment	Distal/lateral attachment	Action	Nerve supply
Multifidus	Spinous processes of all the vertebrae except the atlas.	Posterior surface of the sacrum, the dorsal end of the iliac crest, the mammary and transverse processes of lumbar and thoracic vertebrae, and the articular processes of the 4th–7th cervical vertebrae.	1. Rotate the vertebral column toward the opposite side. 2. Stabilize the vertebral column.	Posterior primary rami of spinal nerves.
Interspinales	Pairs of small muscles joining the spinous processes of adjacent vertebrae, one on each side of the interspinous ligament. Continuous in the cervical region extending from the axis to the 2nd thoracic vertebra and in the lumbar region from the 1st lumbar vertebra to the sacrum.	*See proximal/medial attachment.*	1. Unite the spinous processes. 2. Produce slight extension of the vertebral column.	Posterior primary rami of spinal nerves.
Intertransversarii	Unite transverse processes of consecutive vertebrae. Well developed in the cervical region.	*See proximal/medial attachment.*	1. Unite the transverse processes. 2. Produce lateral bending of the vertebral column.	Anterior and posterior primary rami of spinal nerves.
Diaphragm	The central tendon, which is an oblong sheet forming the summit of the dome.	An approximately circular line passing entirely around the inner surface of the body wall: 1. *Sternal portion:* two slips from the back of the xiphoid process. 2. *Costal portion:* the inner surfaces of the cartilages and adjacent portions of the lower 6 ribs on either side, interdigitating with the transversus abdominis. 3. *Lumbar portion:* medial and lateral arcuate ligaments and right and left crura from the anterolateral surfaces of the bodies and discs of the upper three lumbar vertebrae.	Contracts into the abdomen with inhalation and relaxes into the thorax with exhalation.	Phrenic nerve, C5.
Obliquus capitis inferior	Apex of the spinous process of the axis.	The inferior and dorsal part of the transverse process of the atlas.	Rotates the atlas, turning the face toward the same side.	Posterior primary rami of C1.
Subclavius	1st rib at junction with costal cartilage.	Groove on the inferior surface of the clavicle, between the costoclavicular and conoid ligaments.	Depresses clavicle, draws it medially.	Subclavius, C5, C6.

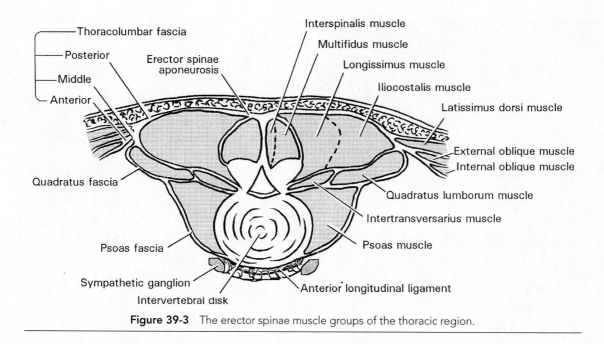

Figure 39-3 The erector spinae muscle groups of the thoracic region.

discs. Its fibers converge into a common central tendon that has no bony attachment. When the diaphragm contracts with inhalation, it descends into the abdomen; when it relaxes during exhalation, it moves superiorly into the thorax. This up-and-down movement produces pressure gradients between the thoracic and abdominal cavities, and is important for both efficient respiration and circulation. Because there are one-way valves in the larger lymphatic vessels, the pressure gradients also enhance the movement of lymph and venous blood toward the heart. When the dome of the diaphragm is flattened because of asymmetric load and/or tonus, respiration and lymphatic drainage from anywhere in the body become less efficient. Thus, for example, it would not be surprising to have a lymphatic component in the lower extremity edema of COPD as well as vascular.

Three apertures occur in the diaphragm: one for the vena cava at about the level of T8, another for the esophageal hiatus at T10, and the third for the aorta at the level of T12 (Fig. 39.4). Diaphragmatic muscle fibers are arranged so that when it contracts in inspiration, the vena caval opening dilates, permitting more venous blood to pass from the abdomen to the thorax; at the same time, the esophageal hiatus constricts to prevent gastric contents from rising in the esophagus. Its contraction has no influence on the aortic hiatus, which lies posterior to the diaphragm and does not truly pierce the diaphragm.

The diaphragm does most of the work of breathing under normal conditions and during moderately forced inspiration. With increased respiratory demands, accessory muscles of respiration become involved to move the ribs even more. The scalene muscles, attached to the upper 2 ribs, assist inhalation. Hypertonicity or hypotonicity of segmental intercostal muscles alters rib behavior, making breathing less efficient. Actual spasm in these muscles can result in pain at rest or especially with each deep breath or cough. Quiet exhalation creates passive recoil of the lung as the diaphragm relaxes. Forced exhalation also involves the inferior internal intercostal and abdominal muscles, including the trunk rotators and erector spinae.

Osteopathic manipulative treatments can often restore or partially rehabilitate altered diaphragmatic function. These treatments

are designed to increase motion of the lower costal cage by freeing the diaphragm for better excursion. This, in turn, helps improve breathing mechanics and assists in venous blood return and lymphatic flow. This approach can be especially helpful for individuals with asthma, respiratory infections, loss of general lung compliance, and associated disorders.

Lymphatics

As blood moves through the capillaries, fluid filters into the interstitial tissues. The return of interstitial fluid through the lymphatic system is necessary for health and proper function, and is even more important when the patient has disease. The lymphatic system is illustrated in Figure 39.5. Lymphatic drainage from the lower half of the body is supplied by the thoracic duct (or left lymphatic duct). Smaller lymphatic vessels drain into the cisterna chyli in the abdomen. Trunks from the left side of the head, the left arm, and the thoracic viscera also empty into the thoracic duct before it drains into the junction of the left internal jugular and left subclavian veins. In approximately 20% of the population, three trunks, the right jugular, the right subclavian, and the right transverse cervical, join to form the right lymphatic duct. The remainder of the population varies in the way the three trunks empty into the jugulosubclavian junction in the anterior neck. The right lymphatic duct enters the junction of the right internal jugular and right subclavian veins (9).

In general, the superficial lymph vessels of the thoracic wall ramify subcutaneously and converge on the axillary nodes (2,3). The lymph nodes from the deeper tissues of the thoracic wall drain into three groups of nodes:

1. The parasternal (internal thoracic) lymph nodes. These are four or five pairs of nodes located at the anterior ends of the intercostal spaces.
2. The intercostal lymph nodes, located in the posterior parts of the intercostal spaces in relation to the heads and necks of the ribs.
3. The diaphragmatic (phrenic) lymph nodes, located on the thoracic surface of the diaphragm.

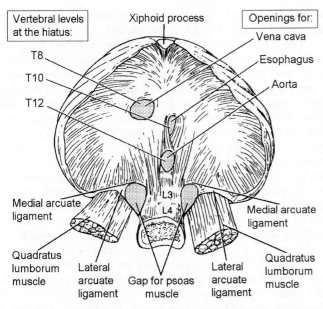

Vertebral levels at the hiatus:	Xiphoid process	Openings for:

- Vena cava
- Esophagus
- Aorta

T8

T10

T12

Medial arcuate ligament

Medial arcuate ligament

L3
L4

Quadratus lumborum muscle

Lateral arcuate ligament

Gap for psoas muscle

Lateral arcuate ligament

Quadratus lumborum muscle

Figure 39-4 Apertures of the abdominal diaphragm.

Connective Tissue and Fascia

Connective tissue unites and surrounds all other tissues. It is found between the cells of organs, as tendons of muscles, and as ligaments joining skeletal parts. Of special importance to the osteopathic physician are the fasciae of the body. These connective tissues surround virtually all organs, muscles, and vessels (10). Fascial elements called the *pericardium* and *pleura* even surround the heart and lungs, respectively. Fascia is a fibrous tissue that is effectively wound around the invested organs at various angles.

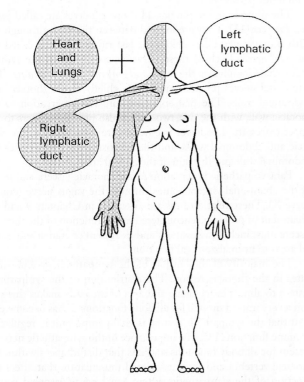

Heart and Lungs

Left lymphatic duct

Right lymphatic duct

Figure 39-5 The lymphatic system of the body.

The muscles of the thoracic cage are also invested with fascia. The internal thoracic wall is covered by a parietal layer of fascia called the *endothoracic fascia*. This deep fascia invests the internal intercostal, subcostal, and transversus thoracis muscles (10). This fascia blends with the periosteum of the ribs and sternum and with the perichondrial tissue of the costal cartilages. The endothoracic fascia also covers the superior surface of the diaphragm, thus becoming the superior diaphragmatic fascia. The endothoracic fascia is also continuous with the prevertebral layer of the cervical fascia and with the scalene fascia (also called *Sibson fascia*), where it attaches along the inner border of the 1st rib. Behind the sternum, it is also continuous with the fascia of the infrahyoid muscles. This parietal thoracic fascia proceeds through the openings of the diaphragm to become continuous with the transversalis fascia of the abdomen. In addition, there are specialized fascial elements that comprise the pericardium, pleura, and mediastinum.

Trauma, chemical alterations of the bathing fluids (immune changes), and other pathologic agents alter the angles of the fascial bands and change cross-linkages between the bands, causing altered tensions of the fasciae throughout the body. An increase in tension in the fascial sheets leads to altered interstitial fluid (lymph) flows, decreased blood flow, and decreased efficiency of organ function. Normalization of the fascial tensions returns the body to more efficient function, thereby using less energy. Osteopathic manipulative techniques, including direct and indirect myofascial release, have been developed to address these problems in ways not generally found to be effective with most other manipulative techniques. The thoracic fasciae are often involved in dysfunction due to thoracic trauma.

Vascular Structures

The arterial blood supply to the thoracic viscera comes largely from branches of the descending thoracic aorta. These include the pericardial, bronchial, mediastinal, phrenic, posterior intercostal, and subcostal arteries. The venous drainage of the thoracic visceral structures is accomplished by way of a corresponding system of veins that parallel the arteries. Several other structures that participate in the venous drainage of the thoracic regional viscera are the superior vena cava, a short section of the inferior vena cava, and the azygous and hemiazygous system of veins.

The thoracic portion of the spinal cord derives its arterial blood supply from three longitudinal structures: a single anterior and two posterior spinal arteries. In addition, the posterior intercostal arteries make contributions to the longitudinal arterial system (10).

The arterial blood supply to the walls of the thoracic cage comes from three main sources: the axillary and subclavian arteries, and the aorta. The axillary artery provides its contribution to the arterial blood supply of the thoracic cage walls by way of two of its branches: the superior thoracic and lateral thoracic arteries. The subclavian artery gives rise to the internal thoracic artery, which in turn provides arterial blood to the thoracic cage from the following branches: anterior intercostal, perforating, and musculophrenic arteries. It also gives rise to the superior intercostal artery. The aorta gives rise to the posterior intercostal arteries. The superior intercostal artery branches into the first and second intercostal arteries and then anastomoses with the third intercostal artery.

The venous drainage of the thoracic walls is accomplished by way of several venous structures. These include the internal thoracic veins, the anterior, posterior and superior intercostal veins, and the azygous and hemiazygous veins.

The arterial supply of the thoracic vertebrae and musculature is derived from branches of the posterior intercostal arteries. Each posterior intercostal artery gives rise to a spinal branch, which provides arterial blood to its corresponding spinal vertebra, along with the spinal cord and meninges at that vertebral level. The spinal branch then further divides into medial and lateral musculocutaneous branches. The medial branch provides arterial blood to the spinalis and longissimus thoracis muscles and a corresponding area of skin; the lateral branch provides arterial blood for the longissimus thoracis and iliocostalis muscles, the medial aspects of the latissimus dorsi and trapezius muscles, and a corresponding area of skin.

There is a corresponding network of veins to provide for venous drainage of the thoracic spinal region. These include the anterior and posterior internal plexus of vertebral veins, the anterior and posterior external plexus of vertebral veins, and the basivertebral and intervertebral veins (10).

Neural Structures

The neural connections of the thoracic area are of vital importance to all body functions. Not only do the usual connections to the musculoskeletal system exit the spinal cord in the thoracic region, but a large part of the sympathetic nervous system also originates in the thoracic region. The sympathetic innervation of the body is shown in Figure 39.6. An understanding of the relationships between the thoracic nerves, as well as their relationships to the bony landmarks is vital to understanding neurologic problems associated with the thoracic region.

The spinal cord, which runs from the brainstem to about the level of L3, is a continuous structure with no segmentation. During embryologic development, the spinal nerve bundles are gathered into spinal nerve roots that course between the encircling bones through the intervertebral foramina. This imposes what appears

to be a dermatomal segmentation effect. Inherently, however, the function of the spinal cord is not segmented.

The spinal nerves exit through the intervertebral foramina, which identify their vertebral level. Each spinal nerve is numbered at the level at which it exits, except in the cervical region, because there are eight cervical nerve roots and seven cervical vertebra. Spinal nerve C1 exits above the atlas, and the eighth root exits below C7. All other roots exit below their corresponding vertebrae. Because the intervertebral foramen is a bounded space and the nerve roots share that space with other tissues, the roots are especially vulnerable to pressure from herniated nucleus pulposus and even edema. Somatic dysfunction in a thoracic area may cause local edema and tissue tightening, which can exert pressure on the nerve root and, importantly, can alter blood and fluid flows to and from the nerve sheaths. Such pressure can alter neural conductivity in the affected roots, although the lack of proper blood and fluid flow to the sheaths can cause irritability in the nociceptors of the sheath, causing pain along the nerve distribution (11). Local disturbances can often be relieved with proper manipulative treatment that is designed to restore proper motion and fluid flow to the region. As stated previously, radiculopathy is somewhat rare in the thoracic region, although discopathy is less rare. These problems in the thoracic area are not easy to diagnose because of overlapping dermatomes and a lack of readily testable deep tendon reflexes.

The abdominal diaphragm receives its motor innervation through the phrenic nerves coming from C3-5. Perhaps more importantly, sensory nerves of the diaphragm innervate the mediastinal pleura, the fibrous pericardium, and the parietal layer of the serous pericardium (10). This relationship helps explain the very common palpatory findings of cervical tension and somatic dysfunction associated with pericardial or diaphragmatic irritation that are mediated via the viscerosomatic reflexes. Manipulative treatment of the involved cervical segments is designed to ameliorate thoracic and diaphragmatic dysfunction through somatovisceral reflex pathways.

The ventral rami of the first 11 thoracic nerves are called *intercostal nerves* (13). They are located between the ribs, although the 12th thoracic nerve lies below the last rib and is thus called the *subcostal nerve*. Each of these nerves is connected to the sympathetic chain ganglia via the *white and gray rami communicantes*. The intercostal nerves provide innervation chiefly to the thoracic and abdominal walls. The first six nerves provide innervation to the thoracic wall, with the first two nerves also providing fibers to the upper extremity. The lower five nerves are distributed to the thoracic and abdominal walls, and the subcostal nerve innervates the abdominal wall and the skin of the gluteal area.

Parasympathetic innervation to the thoracic viscera and many of the abdominal viscera comes through the vagus nerve (cranial nerve X). These relationships are discussed in Chapters 9 and 10. Treatment of problems encountered in the function of the thoracic viscera must include assessment and treatment of cranial and cervical areas to normalize vagal function.

The majority of the outflow of the sympathetic system originates in the thoracic region. The distribution of the sympathetic system to almost every tissue and area of the body makes this system a very important one for all body functions. It has become evident that the sympathetic system is vitally important in regulating immune function (13). The importance of the sympathetic nervous system for all body functions suggests that disturbances within the thoracic vertebra and their associated musculature that affect the function of the sympathetic system can have widespread consequences. Identification and treatment of somatic dysfunction in the

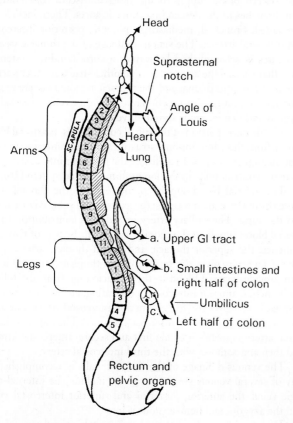

Figure 39-6 The sympathetic innervation of the body.

thoracic region is especially important in treating problems ranging from infectious processes to functional abnormalities.

Visceral Considerations

Visceral dysfunction that alters input to the spinal cord not only increases the sympathetic outflow back to the visceral areas through viscerovisceral reflex pathways but also alters somatic outflow in often unexpected patterns. Understanding this phenomenon provides insight on how to treat many painful and/or functional problems. Due to the overlap of visceral afferents onto spinal pathways that also receive somatic afferents, the sensory experience of visceral irritation is often one of referred pain to a somatic structure, with concomitant increased somatic muscle tone. One of the most common of these patterns is the shoulder pain and muscle tension associated with acute myocardial infarction. The nociceptive input from the compromised myocardium is experienced as shoulder or chest pain. Often, a vicious circle of increased somatic involvement results, as increased somatic activity also increases sympathetic outflow to the heart, further exacerbating the pathologic process. Although obviously not the only course of treatment, treating the somatic component of the process can be beneficial. Recognition of the visceral origin of referred pain patterns can save the osteopathic physician much time and missed diagnoses. Likewise, recognizing that osteopathic treatment of the involved somatic structures can also help the course of the problem. Understanding the somatic areas likely to show effects of underlying visceral pathologic conditions through viscerosomatic reflexes (3) provides the osteopathic physician with another important diagnostic and treatment tool.

BIOMECHANICAL CONSIDERATIONS

Physiologic Motion

In general, thoracic spinal motion occurs according to the mechanical principles formulated by Fryette. In other words, when the thoracic spine is in the neutral position, sidebending of spine in one direction results in rotation of the thoracic vertebrae in the direction opposite to the sidebending. When the thoracic spine is in a non-neutral position (i.e., flexed or extended), sidebending of spine in one direction results in rotation of the thoracic vertebrae in the same direction as the sidebending.

However, there are times when variations from Fryette principles occur in thoracic vertebral motion. Upper thoracic vertebrae may exhibit neutral (type I) motion, which may occur as low as T4, and movements are similar to normal cervical spine behavior. Some suggest that these motions are associated with the interdependent combination of asymmetrical vertebral and upper rib shapes and attachments and their interactions with cervical muscles (such as the splenius cervicis) that attach as low as T5 and T6. Middle thoracic vertebral motion is commonly a mix of neutral (type I) and non-neutral (type II) movements, which may produce rotation to either the formed convexity or to the formed concavity. Lower thoracic vertebral motion is more apt to be similar to lumbar neutral (type I) mechanics.

During inhalation, the thoracic cage widens its vertical, transverse, and anteroposterior dimensions as the diaphragm contracts (14). With deep inhalation, the anterior ends of the superior ribs move more anteriorly and superiorly along with the sternum (Fig. 39.7).

Typical ribs are attached to the sternum by the costal cartilage, and their movements displace the anterior component of the costosternal system superiorly and anteriorly. This motion is described as pump-handle motion. (See Glossary for more detailed defini-

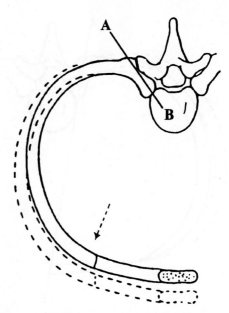

Figure 39-7 Functional transverse rib axis. (From *Gray's Anatomy.* 35th Ed. Edinburgh, Scotland: Churchill Livingstone, 1973:421, with permission.)

tion.); the rib shaft is the handle of the pump, and the vertebral column is the pivot point (Fig. 39.8).

The vertebrosternal ribs (1 and 2) and vertebrochondral ribs (8 to 10) move about functional pivots posteriorly and anteriorly. Functionally, their shafts move laterally and superiorly during inhalation, increasing the transverse diameter of the costal cage (Fig. 39.9). This motion is referred to as *bucket-handle motion* (Fig. 39.10). The anterior/posterior diameter of the chest is increased as the anterior ends of ribs 8 to 10 are elevated by the contraction of the diaphragm. Ribs 11 and 12 are called *vertebral ribs*, because they do not attach to the sternum or the chondral mass. These two atypical ribs have a pincer-type motion. The types of rib motion described clinically are depicted in Figure 39.11.

Nonphysiologic Motion

Both neutral (type I) and non-neutral (type II) vertebral unit dysfunction is common in the thoracic spine. Neutral (type I) asymmetries typically involve three or more segments that are neither flexed nor extended; they are mildly scoliotic. Non-neutral (type II)

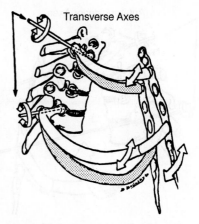

Figure 39-8 Pump-handle rib motion.

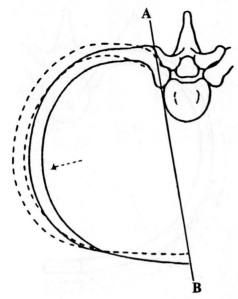

Figure 39-9 Functional anteroposterior rib axis. (From *Gray's Anatomy*. 35th Ed. Edinburgh, Scotland: Churchill Livingstone, 1973:421, with permission.)

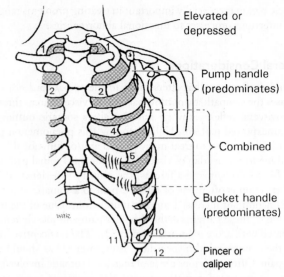

Figure 39-11 Clinical rib movement.

vertebral unit dysfunction generally involves a single vertebral unit and can have proximal and distal neutral (type I) responses.

Asymmetry of motion in any of the rib cage areas indicates the presence of respiratory rib dysfunction in that region. Respiratory rib dysfunction has either inhalation or exhalation restriction. There is usually one rib within a group of ribs that is responsible for maintaining the inhalation or exhalation restriction. This rib is referred to as the *key rib* and is the rib that must be identified and treated to remove a group restriction. Inhalation restrictions involve a rib or group of ribs that first stops moving during inhalation. The key rib is the most superior rib in the group. Exhalation restrictions involve a rib or group of ribs that first stops moving during exhalation. The key rib is the most inferior rib in the group.

Clinical Characteristics of Thoracic Region and Rib Cage Movement

Available thoracic spinal motion is generally less than in the cervical or lumbar areas. This is because all planes of motion are affected by costal cage mechanics and their complicated relationships with

Anteroposterior Axes

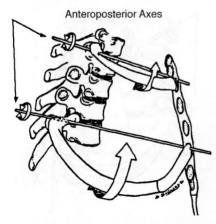

Figure 39-10 Bucket-handle rib motion.

head, neck, shoulder girdle, and lumbopelvic anatomy. Thoracic spinal motion is further complicated by a number of other factors that go beyond basic costovertebral configuration and mechanics. A few of the elements include configuration characteristics of the anteroposterior curves in the sagittal plane, such as:

■ Kyphosis
■ Costal cage asymmetries, such as pectus excavatum and pectus carinatum
■ Osteoporosis/osteoarthritis effects
■ Increased chest wall diameter associated with a variety of cardiopulmonary problems
■ Cervical, shoulder girdle, rotator cuff influences (i.e., anterior muscles are generally tighter than posterior groups); under these circumstances, anteroposterior curves tend to become more kyphotic
■ Effects of lifestyle and affective states, such as slumping with depression
■ Characteristics of primary and secondary lateral deviations include
    ■ Scoliosis with and without kyphosis
    ■ Effects of upper and lower motor neuron lesions
    ■ Effects of repetitive motion activities
    ■ General thoracic spinal motion characteristics

Because of configuration changes in size and shape, thoracic spinal motion characteristics vary markedly from the cervicothoracic to thoracolumbar junctions. The upper and middle portions demonstrate greater rotation than elsewhere in the spine, with the exception of the atlantoaxial joint. Generally, flexion capability is greater than extension. Side-bending capability is even less, because of rib cage constraints. In the lower portions, flexion and extension capacities are greatest, although side-bending abilities exceed those of rotation (i.e., they are more like lumbar spine mechanics).

Clinically, there is a constant tendency for spinal flexion because of the effects of gravity and the tendency for the back extensors to become inhibited while flexors tend toward contraction. Clinically, it seems that the rotatores, intertransversarii, and multifidi are often involved in postural stress, somatosomatic, and viscerosomatic reflexes. When these muscles are reflexively affected by facilitation, they are often responsible for maintaining non-neutral somatic dysfunction of the vertebral units that are innervated by the involved muscle, neural network, or viscera. Some refer to this phenomenon as the *somatic* component of impairment, illness, or disease.

Neurologic pathologic conditions, trauma, visceral disease, and intrinsic mechanical asymmetries are common sources of spinal dysfunction. Trauma, for example, often flexes, extends, and/or twists the spine simultaneously in such a way that the accumulated forces localize around a vertebral unit, thereby disturbing the mechanics of both the single vertebral segment and the vertebral units. Deforming injuries of this type often alter physical shapes; that is, they cause plastic deformations with permanent stretching of ligaments and distortions in facet joints and osseous-ligamentous relationships. Not surprisingly, recurring non-neutral/type II vertebral unit dysfunction is common under these circumstances. This type of vertebral unit change is sometimes associated with altered visceral functions; for example, somatic dysfunction is superimposed on vertebral segment and vertebral unit changes with resulting facilitated peripheral, autonomic, and centrally mediated reflex activities. Patients report many clinical symptoms when these processes occur.

The most important function of the rib cage is respiration. The ribs, along with the sternum, and the diaphragm move in a manner that increases and decreases the size of the thoracic cavity during inspiration and expiration. Because of the negative pressure produced with respiratory movements, the rib cage may also assist in returning venous blood back to the heart. The rib cage also protects the organs located within its cavity.

The motion of the ribs has been described earlier as either the pump-handle or bucket-handle type. More specifically, the upper rib cage, from approximately ribs 1 through 5, exhibits predominantly pump-handle motion, while ribs 6 through 10 provide increasing amounts of bucket-handle motion, until the lowest ribs of this group move predominantly in bucket-handle fashion. Ribs 11 and 12 move in a pincer-like fashion.

Rib cage mechanics can also be influenced because of its relationships with head, cervical, shoulder girdle, lumbar, and pelvic anatomical structures. Rib cage motion can be further complicated by a number of other factors beyond basic costal anatomy, configuration, and mechanics. Some of these factors include:

- Thoracic scoliosis or kyphosis
- Rib cage asymmetries, such as pectus excavatum or pectus carinatum
- Effects of bony diseases such as osteoporosis or osteoarthritis
- Increased chest wall diameter associated with illnesses such as chronic obstructive pulmonary disease
- Effects of abnormal tensions in cervical, rotator cuff, or shoulder girdle musculature
- Effects of trauma to the rib cage
- Effects of lifestyle and affective states, such as slumping with depression

Clinically, somatic dysfunction of the rib cage is often present secondary to somatic dysfunction of the thoracic vertebrae. Thus, the restricted motion in these combined structures may result in some of the same clinical characteristics as occur with problems associated with the thoracic spine.

SUMMARY

The thoracic and rib cage regions together form a complex region of the body, containing and protecting many vital organs. Osteopathic physicians must understand the proper function, diagnosis, and treatment of this area. Osteopathic manipulation is used to improve sympathetic and parasympathetic factors, diaphragm excursion, spinal and rib mechanics, and vascular and lymphatic flow (which improves breathing). The goal is to decrease sympathicotonia and energy wasted on inefficient breathing by decreasing abnormal mechanoreceptor and nociceptive input to the central nervous system (decreasing pain) and assisting the body in mobilizing the immune system.

Manipulative treatment of somatic dysfunction of this region can help the patient to heal from injury or pathology of this area. In addition, osteopathic palpatory diagnosis can be used to help differentiate the cause of sometimes difficult to interpret signs and symptoms with which patients may present.

REFERENCES

1. Cathie AG, Physiological motions of the spine as related to respiratory activity. *AAO Yearbook.* Colorado Springs: American Academy of Osteopathy, 1974:59.
2. White AA, Panjabi MM. *Clinical Biomechanics of the Spine.* Philadelphia, PA: JB Lippincott Co., 1990.
3. Patterson MM, Howell JN, eds. *The Central Connection: Somatovisceral/Viscerosomatic Interaction.* Indianapolis, IN: American Academy of Osteopathy, 1992.
4. Kendall FP, McCreary EK, Provance PG, et al. *Muscles Testing and Function with Posture and Pain.* 5th Ed. Philadelphia, PA: Lippincott Williams & Wilkins, 2005.
5. Korr IM. The spinal cord as organizer of disease processes. IV. Axonal transport and neurotrophic function in relation to somatic dysfunction. *J Am Osteopath Assoc* 1981;80(7):451–459.
6. Korr IM. Proprioceptors and somatic dysfunction. *J Am Osteopath Assoc* 1975;74(7);638–650.
7. Patterson MM, Steinmetz JE. Long-lasting alterations of spinal reflexes: a basis for somatic dysfunction. *Man Med* 1986;2:38–42.
8. Van Buskirk RL. Nociceptive reflexes and the somatic dysfunction: a model. *J Am Osteopath Assoc* 1990;90(9):792–804.
9. Chickly, B, *Silent Waves: Theory and Practice of Lymph Drainage Therapy.* Scottsdale, AZ: I.H.H. Publishing, 2002.
10. Sandring, S, ed. *Gray's Anatomy.* 39th Ed. Edinburgh, Scotland: Elsevier Churchill Livingstone, 2005.
11. Budgell B, Sato A. Somatoautonomic reflex regulation of sciatic nerve blood flow. *J Neuromusculoskeletal Sys* 1994;2:170–177.
12. Moore KL, Dalley AF. *Clinically Oriented Anatomy.* 5th Ed. Philadelphia, PA: Lippincott Williams & Wilkins, 2006.
13. Willard FH, Patterson MM, eds. *Nociception and the Neuroendocrine-Immune Connection.* Indianapolis, IN: American Academy of Osteopathy, 1994.
14. Guyton AC, Hall JE. *Textbook of Medical Physiology.* 11th Ed. Philadelphia, PA: Elsevier Saunders, 2006.

40

Lumbar Region

KURT P. HEINKING

KEY CONCEPTS

- Delineate a thorough and accurate history; this allows the development of a differential diagnosis.
- Consider serious and life-threatening conditions that require urgent evaluation, and or treatment of the lumbar spine.
- Knowledge of the functional anatomy, normal spinal motion, and somatic dysfunction of the lumbar region improves diagnosis and manipulative treatment.
- Develop an efficient integrated physical examination of the lumbar spine.
- Diagnose and evaluate viscerosomatic and somatovisceral reflexes, Chapman's points, Jones tenderpoints, and myofascial triggerpoints.
- Review the imaging studies of the lumbar spine and relate them to the known palpatory findings.
- Know when and how to utilize OMT in the treatment of somatic dysfunction of the lumbar spine.

INTRODUCTION

An efficient and accurate diagnosis and an effective treatment plan, are critical skills for an osteopathic physician to have. Because of the unique training and expertise in musculoskeletal medicine, many patients and clinicians seek out osteopathic physicians for a variety of concerns.

Common patient complaints that require evaluation of the lumbar spine include, but are not limited to: abdominal pain, lower back pain, and neuralgia of the lower extremities. In each of these situations, the lumbar spine needs to be examined and possibly treated with osteopathic manipulation. An evaluation for somatic dysfunction of the lumbar spine is integrated with the other physical exam procedures. If significant somatic dysfunction is found, and potentially related to the patient's condition, OMT may be utilized in the treatment plan along with analgesics, anti-inflammatories, muscle relaxers, and stretches or active exercises. This chapter will highlight how the diagnosis and treatment of somatic dysfunction is crucial in the overall treatment of the patient with lumbar spine pain.

EPIDEMIOLOGY OF LOW BACK PAIN

The lifetime prevalence of having lower back pain approaches 70%, so it is important for osteopathic physicians to be able to evaluate the lumbar spine. Lower back pain is the second leading cause of work absenteeism (after upper respiratory tract complaints) and results in more lost productivity than any other medical condition. Each year there are 13 million physician visits for lower back pain, with the highest prevalence in the 45 to 60-year-old Caucasian population. Back pain is the most frequent cause of activity limitation in people younger than 45 years of age, the second most frequent reason for physician visits, the fifth most frequent for hospitalization, and the third ranking reason for surgical procedures (1). Osteopathic physicians need to completely understand the anatomy and physiology of the lumbar spine in the healthy, diseased or injured, and postoperative patient. Patients with chronic back pain will search out osteopathic physicians for treatment after having lumbar spine surgery. About 1% of the U.S. population is chronically disabled because of back pain (1). Osteopathic physicians need to be able to diagnose the lumbar spine in people of all ages, body types, and sizes.

Anthropometric data are contradictory with no strong relationship between heights, weight, body build, and low back pain. Physical fitness is not a predictor of acute low back pain. The physically fit have a lesser risk of chronic low back pain and tend to recover faster than patients who are not physically fit (1). Many physicians consider obesity as a cause of low back pain, but epidemiologic studies have reported both positive and negative associations (1). In summary, most episodes of low back pain or sciatica resolve spontaneously within the first 2 weeks and a relative minority take 6 to 12 weeks. Only 1% to 2% of cases should require evaluation for operative management. Osteopathic physicians should be able to diagnose and treat the lumbar spine of patients of all ages and sizes, paying particular attention to the presentation based on a thorough understanding of the epidemiology.

HISTORY

An appropriate and thorough history of the patient's chief complaint is critical. It is always important to consider urgent, emergent, or other potentially serious conditions. Patients with worrisome historical findings need more comprehensive and expeditious treatment. Emergent disorders associated with acute paraplegia include spinal cord tumors, epidural hemorrhage, epidural abscess, embolus, spinal artery thrombosis, and central herniation of a nucleus pulposus (cauda equina syndrome) (2). The history of severe, tearing pain, and dizziness associated with an abdominal pulsatile mass alerts the physician to the problem of an expanding aneurysm. Patients with the cauda equina syndrome present with acute paraplegia, saddle anesthesia, and rectal or urinary incontinence (2). From the patient's history alone, the clinician should have a pretty good idea of what is going on and then develop a differential diagnosis. The astute clinician allows patients to tell their story in their own words and also steers them in directions that elicit the essential information needed for the diagnostic process. The clinician knows when the history must be abbreviated or prolonged, based on the patient's presentation. If not all the information is obtained during the initial evaluation, it is worthwhile to review the history on subsequent visits.

Pain needs to be evaluated by documenting a description of the pain, including its intensity, duration, location, radiation, alleviating or aggravating factors, and response to treatment. Not every chief complaint is pain. The chief complaint can be stiffness, a decrease in athletic performance, postural or muscular asymmetry, a localized mass, a skin lesion, etc. The important aspect to consider is: how does the chief complaint disturb the patient's day-to-day functioning?

Quality and Intensity

Initially patients should describe the quality of pain themselves without suggestions from the examining physician. Listed below are useful documents that assist with clinician documentation of pain, one of which is the McGill Pain Questionnaire. If the McGill Pain questionnaire is not used, the examining physician should include a line drawing of the body in the patient's history. The pictorial representation of the patient's pain helps delineate its extent. The "visual analogue scale" is a visual way to quantify pain based upon a 10-cm line drawing (2).

Another differentiation is between organic and psychogenic pain. A standardized way to differentiate psychogenic from organic pain is to use the Minnesota Multiphasic Personality Inventory (MMPI). The MMPI is a 566-question, self-administered true-false test formulated to identify psychological traits, for example, hypochondriasis, depression, hysteria, or psychopathic deviance, associated with elevated scale scores in patients with chronic pain (2).

A test that validates the presence of pain is the Mensana Clinic Back Pain Test (MPT). MPT is a 15-item questionnaire that takes about 10 minutes to complete. Patients are classified as objective-pain patients, exaggerating-pain patients, and affective-pain patients corresponding to increasing test scores (2). The MPT is more successful than MMPI in differentiating organic from function low back pain and is useful for patients with chronic low back pain. Roland and Morris developed a questionnaire consisting of 24 items (2). The test not only measures disability resulting from back pain but also measures response to therapy.

Consideration of the onset, duration, and progression of a complaint is essential. An inventory by systems is taken, especially those systems that could be related to the lumbar region. Although the history is discussed as an entity that precedes the physical examination, further questioning (history) may take place as positive clues are obtained during the physical exam. This approach to history taking will prompt the physician to ask questions about areas that the patient does not consider important.

The ability to visualize the underlying anatomy and apply that knowledge as the physician palpates is an important skill to develop. An understanding and recall of the physiologic spinal motion patterns is also necessary before performing the physical examination. Using this knowledge, the physical exam will help the clinician rule out specific conditions on the differential diagnosis list.

A prior knowledge of Chapman reflexes, viscerosomatic reflexes, and the autonomic innervation of the viscera is also useful during the physical exam. For example, if a patient complains of lumbar dysfunction, questions about bowel and bladder function, whether the urinary stream is full and forceful, and whether there is any pain or burning on urination are all functionally relevant questions to ask. During the physical examination, if the patient complains of acute tenderness when the iliotibial bands are palpated, questions about bowel habits and function are relevant, if the clinician understands Chapman reflexes. In women, these findings should also initiate questions about menses and pelvic discomfort; in men, questions about prostate or penile discomfort or deep, uncomfortable pressure in the perineal region are indicated. Asking if chilling or muscle-stressing activities increase the symptom might alert the physician to consider and examine for select *myofascial trigger points* related to the symptomatology.

Trauma History

When planning total management of patients with lumbar complaints, it is also important to ask the patient about past injuries or accidents that could have produced significant lumbar or sacroiliac (SI) dysfunctions, atypical spinal mechanics, or have affected the craniosacral mechanism. Most patients forget about these types of accidents.

Historical Points May Point to a Specific Etiology

Ask the patient about unexplained weight loss, night sweats, breast changes or masses, hematuria or hematochezia (blood in the stool). These questions explore the possibility of cancer of the organs that usually metastasize to bone and can produce pain in the back. The patient with nonspecific mechanical lower back pain usually has significant somatic dysfunction of the lumbar, sacral, and pelvic regions. If they do not, clinical suspicion for a visceral cause may be heightened. In evaluation of the patient with lumbar pain, understanding the "Red Flags" for more serious conditions is important (Fig. 40.1). These include:

- Age 50 years or older
- Previous history of cancer
- Unexplained weight loss
- Failure to improve with 1 month of therapy
- No relief with bed rest.

An algorithm to guide the initial assessment of acute low back pain symptoms is shown in Figure 40.1.

If the patient has leg pain or paresthesia, ask the patient to show exactly where it is located, and then decide if this could represent a dermatomal, myotomal, sclerotomal, or radicular pain pattern. Sclerotomes and myotomes have been documented and mapped (3). They are important and are often overlooked pain patterns. A radicular pattern would indicate that there may be nerve root pressure, perhaps related to a herniated intervertebral disc or a tumor in the cauda equina. In this particular case, traditional orthopedic and neurologic testing, which includes deep tendon reflex assessment, assessment of muscle strength/weakness, and testing key dermatomes for sensation and/or pain, is important.

When evaluating the lumbar region in a low back pain patient, it is imperative to consider the psychosocial stresses the patient is under. Emotional tension, stress, and job dissatisfaction are contributing and sometimes causative factors in lumbar spine pain. Psychological and psychosocial work factors including monotony at work, job dissatisfaction, and poor relations with coworkers have been found to increase complaints about low back pain (1). Prospective studies have concluded that these psychological risk factors were more predictive than any of the physical risk factors. In contrast to pain from nerve root irritation, psychogenic pain is not well localized. Large nondermatomal areas are affected. In this situation, radiation of pain follows no consistent pattern (1). Physical factors found to be associated with increased risk of low back pain include heavy work, lifting, static work postures, bending with twisting, and vibration.

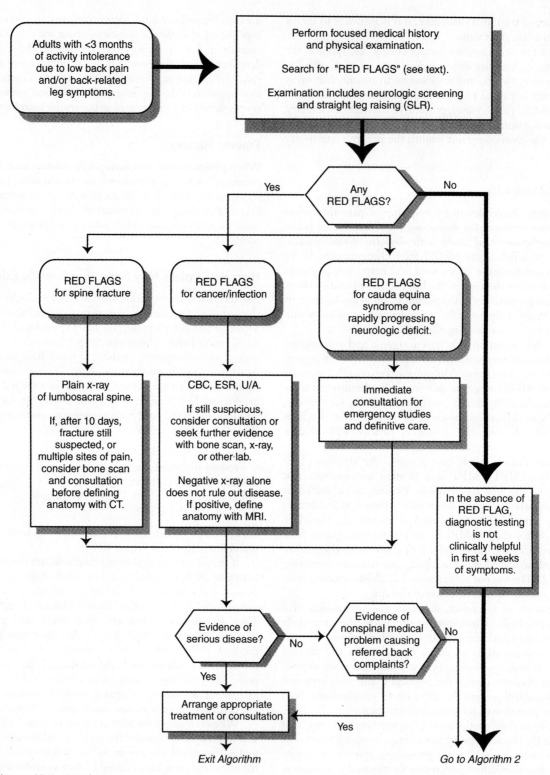

Figure 40-1 Initial assessment of acute low back pain symptoms. CT, computed tomography; CBC, complete blood count; ESR, erythrocyte sedimentation rate; U/A, urine analysis. (From Bigos S, Bowyer O, Braen G, et al. *Acute Low Back Pain Problems in Adults.* Clinical Practice Guideline, No. 14, Rockville, MD: U.S. Department of Health and Human Services; December 1994. Publica Health Service Agency for Health Care Policy and Research AHCPR publication 95-0642, with permission.)

Consider the Following:

- Job dissatisfaction
- Preexisting depression or anxiety
- Stressful, monotonous work

- Low control over work
- Unappreciated/unsupported at work
- Low level employment
- Low socioeconomic status

Stress plays a major role in the treatment of the low back pain patients well. When patients are stressed, their muscles tighten and become less flexible. Techniques that foster relaxation, improve soft tissue tension, and help the patient relax are useful. When patients are stressed, GI complaints are frequent, and these can produce viscerosomatic palpatory changes in the thoracic and lumbar spine.

An adequate social history is important to take in the patient with low back pain. There is a definite link between smoking and low back pain that increases with the duration and frequency of the low back pain. Several investigators have found an association between smoking, herniated discs, and low back pain (1).

The age of the patient can affect the clinician's ability to formulate a differential diagnosis. For example, spondyloarthropathies, including ankylosing spondylitis, reactive arthritis, and spondylitis associated with inflammatory bowel disease, and benign tumors of the spine occur between the third and the fourth decades (2). Diseases of middle age include diffuse idiopathic skeletal hyperostosis, gout, Paget disease, and osteomyelitis. A different set of diseases occurs more commonly during and following the sixth decade. These diseases include malignant disease (metastases), metabolic disease (chondrocalcinosis), and degenerative diseases (expanding aortic aneurysm) (2). Approximately 80% of patients with malignant disease affecting the lumbar spine are older than 50 years of age (2). The causes of back pain are outlined in Table 40.1.

TABLE 40.1

Causes of Back Pain

Mechanical	Tumor
Spinal arthritis	Primary
Degenerative disk disease	Myeloma
Facet arthritis	Sarcoma
Fracture	Neural tumor
Spondylolysis	Secondary (metastatic)
Spondylolisthesis	Prostate
Congenital	Lung
Genetic malformations	Breast
Achondroplasia	Kidney
Nonmechanical	Rheumatologic
Viscerogenic	Seronegative spondyloarthropathy
Renal colic	Ankylosing spondylitis
Inflammatory bowel disease	Psoriatic arthritis
Endometriosis	Reiter syndrome
Vasculogenic	Behçet syndrome
Aortic aneurysm	Fibromyalgia
Ischemic spinal claudication	Polymyalgia rheumatica
Epidural venous anomalies	Rheumatoid arthritis
Infection	Metabolic
Discitis	Osteoporosis
Herpes zoster	Paget disease
Osteomyelitis	

FAMILY HISTORY

In the presence of a particular histocompatibility locus antigen (27), members of a family are at risk of developing ankylosing spondylitis, reactive arthritis, psoriatic spondylitis, and spondylitis associated with inflammatory bowel disease. Each of the conditions can cause low back pain.

OCCUPATIONAL HISTORY

Workers doing heavy lifting at their job are at risk of developing mechanical low back pain, but this symptom also occurs in sedentary workers. Lifting a light object from a rotated position or stretching far overhead to reach an object on a shelf may be associated with the onset of low back pain.

It is incumbent on the physician not to assume that, because workers' compensation is involved or litigation is pending, the patient's symptoms are fictitious or exaggerated. Physicians should give the patient the benefit of the doubt. A self-employed individual may push the physician into cutting corners of evaluation and therapy to obtain the "quick fix" needed to allow a return to normal activities. On the other hand, the salaried employee may delay return because of the fear of reinjury.

Social History

Increased consumption of alcohol, coffee, or cigarettes is associated with osteoporosis, and illicit drug use results in immunosuppression and predisposition to infection. Marital discord causes severe stress and the propensity for muscles of the lower back and neck to tighten. Job stress and dissatisfaction has been linked to lower back pain.

Review of Systems

The presence of constitutional symptoms is a worrisome finding and requires a more thorough evaluation. Fever in the setting of new-onset neck or back pain may be associated with influenza, pyogenic discitis, or osteomyelitis to 83% for spinal epidural abscess (2).

Review of the integumentary system may reveal a history of scaling patches over the elbows (psoriasis), vesicular lesions following a dermatome (shingles), or a tick bite (Lyme disease). Each of these conditions can be related to lower back pain. Poor sleep habits, anxiety, or depressive symptoms can also clue the physician in toward an emotional etiology for the low back pain.

Aggravating and Alleviating Factors

Characteristically, mechanical lesions of the lumbosacral sine improve with rest and worsen with increased activity. Prolonged sitting with forward flexion causes back pain if the patient has a herniated disc, and prolonged standing in the extended position causes back pain if the patient has spinal stenosis.

Older patients with spinal stenosis will "lean on the shopping cart" because this forward bending of the spine opens the canal and foramina reducing nerve root pressure. Pain from tumors involving bone, muscle, or the spinal cord is often increased with recumbency. Patients with tumors seek relief by sleeping in a chair or pacing (2). However, other patients find relief of pain only with absolute immobility. This is a sign of acute infection, compression fracture related to metabolic bone disease, or pathologic fracture secondary to a tumor or infiltrative disease. Disc herniation causes radiating pain at rest, while with spinal stenosis radiating pain occurs in positions that extend the spine and decrease room in the spinal canal for the neural elements. Once the disc is extruded and the pressure on the annulus from disc protrusion is relieved, leg pain continues while back pain resolves (2).

In contrast to pain from nerve root irritation, psychogenic pain is not well localized. Large nondermatomal areas are affected. Radiation of pain follows no consistent pattern. Patients with psychogenic pain have difficulty describing factors that relieve or worsen their pain. The pain is present all the time. There is no position that is comfortable (2). Activities that involve little physical effort have an exaggerated effect on their pain. In general, patients with chronic spinal conditions experience some variability of symptoms that can be correlated with changes in barometric pressure and temperature.

Time of Day

Classically, inflammatory arthropathies cause morning stiffness. Patients have great difficulty getting out of bed in the morning because of stiffness and pain. Benign tumors, a prime example being an osteoid osteoma, cause severe nocturnal pain. The risk of disc herniation is greatest in the morning when the disc is extended to its greatest degree (2). At the end of the day, when the disc is less tense, symptoms related to joint compression are more likely.

SUMMARY

The history allows the clinician to select those parts of the physical examination that will help the clinician most efficiently make the

correct diagnosis from the possibilities included in the differential diagnosis list. Special tests, such as labs or MRI scans, can support or refute the differential diagnosis and help with the treatment plan. Prior to performing the physical exam and ordering tests, the physician needs to recall their descriptive and functional anatomy.

DESCRIPTIVE AND FUNCTIONAL ANATOMY

The lumbar spine normally consists of five vertebrae and forms a smooth lordotic curve just above the pelvis. The five lumbar vertebrae are the most massive individual segments of the vertebral column. This is perfectly logical, in that the lumbar spine carries the weight of the upper half of the body. The area is functionally compensatory for the relative immobility of adjacent spinal areas (thoracic cage and pelvis). This creates quite a dilemma. As mobility is gained, stability tends to be lost. Yet, the lumbar region accommodates for both stability and mobility. Understanding the functional relationship between the individual vertebral segments, and between the vertebrae and their associated soft tissues, is the first step in understanding somatic dysfunction of, as well as the impact of disease upon, the region. This understanding comes directly from a thorough knowledge of anatomy. Both the normal anatomy and the abnormal anatomy need to be appreciated as some patients require spinal surgery or have lumbosacral anomalies that disrupt anatomic relationships.

Lumbosacral anomalies are fairly common (Fig. 40.2). Sometimes during embryologic development, the lumbar spine may

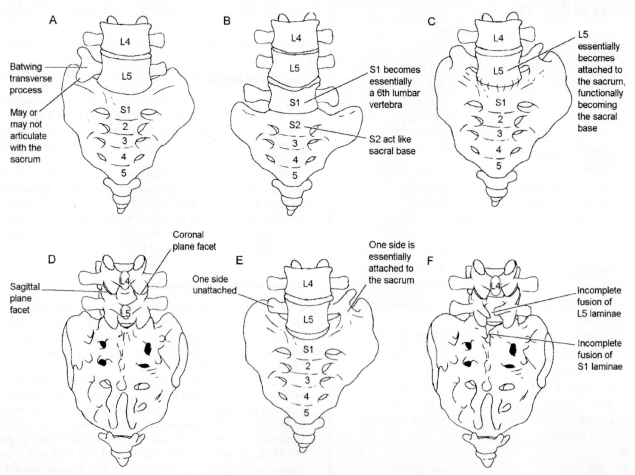

Figure 40-2 Common lumbosacral abnormalities: **A.** Batwing transverse processes of L5. **B.** Lumbarization of S1. **C.** Sacralization of L5. **D.** Facet asymmetry (zygopophyseal tropism) of L4. **E.** Partial sacralization of L5 (Bertolotti). **F.** Spina bifida occulta of both L$_s$ and of S.

form six vertebra. Even more rare is the patient with four lumbar vertebrae. Although this alters muscular attachments, it usually does not hinder stability during activity. The lumbar region normally has a lumbolumbar lordotic angle extending from L2-5 that averages 43 degrees. The normal lordotic curve of the lumbar spine functionally permits more extension than flexion.

The lumbar spine occupies half to two thirds of the posterior skeletal and myofascial wall of the true abdomen. It is directly linked to the thoracic and pelvic regions. Because of its functional anatomic connections, it can influence the head and neck, the upper extremities, the lower extremities, and even the viscera. This means that the location of symptoms does not necessarily indicate the region of their etiology. Problems in the pelvis, abdomen, leg, arm, head and thoracic regions, as well as the lumbar region, need to be considered.

Although the lumbar facets are relatively aligned in the sagittal plane, analysis reveals that the lumbar and thoracolumbar regions provide most of the motion of the trunk. The facets of the thoracic region, oriented in a coronal plane, would seem to allow more motion around all three axes. However, the rib cage hinders the ability of the thoracic region to rotate, side-bend, flex, or extend.

The Anterior Elements

Vertebral Body
A lumbar vertebra is larger than other spinal vertebrae. It is distinguished by the absence of costal facets (like the thoracic vertebrae) and transverse foramina (like the cervical vertebrae). The vertebral body is wider transversely and deeper anteroposteriorly than any other vertebrae (4). This large, cross-sectional area and its longitudinal and vertical trabecular arrangement increase its strength and stability. Lumbar vertebrae are capable of sustaining the heavy, functional, longitudinal loads that will surely be acting on them. The vertebral bodies also act as accessory organs for hematopoiesis.

Intervertebral Disc
An intervertebral disc is located between each lumbar vertebra. If all the intervertebral discs were stacked up one on another, they would normally account for one fourth of the length of the spine. Lumbar discs are large and built to tolerate and dissipate heavy loads. They are composed of glycosaminoglycans, mucopolysaccharides, proteoglycans, and collagen.

Intervertebral discs are named according to their region (lumbar in this case) and numbered according to the vertebral unit of which they are a part (i.e., the number corresponds to the first vertebra of the vertebral unit). Example: The intervertebral disc for the L2 vertebral unit would be the second lumbar disc. Each disc is joined to the inferior plate of the vertebra above it and the superior plate of the vertebra below it.

There is a compressible nucleus pulposus located at its center, and this is surrounded by layers of the anulus consisting of concentric lamellae of collagenous fibers. These anular fibers are oriented 65 degrees from vertical, and the layers alternate in a right/left direction as they encircle and contain the nucleus pulposus (5). Clinically, it is important to note that the anulus of a lumbar disc is fairly thick anteriorly but is noticeably thinner posteriorly. Historically, L4 and L5 intervertebral discs are at the greatest risk for rupture. Operation rates for herniated lumbar discs vary. It is estimated that the rate per 100,000 is 100 in Great Britain, 350 in Finland, 200 in Sweden, and more than 450 in the United States. More than 95% of operations are at the L4 and L5 levels. The mean age of surgery is 40 to 45 years, with men being operated on twice as often as women (1).

The nucleus pulposus is composed of 70% to 90% water, and is semifluid and hydrophilic. It is deformable, but not compressible. With postural weight bearing, the nucleus expands laterally against the anulus, and these two parts work together mechanically to act as a shock absorber between each vertebral body of the spine. When load is applied and the nucleus is compressed, it loses water. This results in a 1.5-mm creep in the first 2 to 10 minutes of compressive stress (5). Resting supine with the lower extremities flexed and raised is the optimal position for rehydrating the discs. With this rest, discs normally return to their full or optimal height. With aging, however, the hydrophilic properties of a disc are reduced, just as is its ability to reform after being stressed by prolonged pressure or a sudden and severe stress. The intervertebral discs are innervated by fibers from an elaborate plexus supplied by the sinu vertebral nerve on the posterior longitudinal ligament and the somatosympathetic nerve on the anterior longitudinal ligament. In initial stages of compression, the sinu vertebral nerve on the posterior longitudinal ligament irritated giving rise to lower back pain (3,5). In a normal healthy disc, branches from this plexus penetrate through the outer one third to reach the middle third of the annulus fibrosus. The annulus fibrosus receives nocioceptive innervation to its outer fibers (3). However, degenerative disc material obtained at the time of surgery shows that the small-caliber fibers have expanded their territory into the center of the disc. In patients with degenerative discs, discography is painful (generally a nonpainful procedure in normal individuals), as this might indicate some small-caliber fibers have expanded their territories in these patients.

The Posterior Elements

Pedicles
Pedicles connect the posterior elements to the vertebral body and mark the site where the posterior vertebral elements begin. In the lumbar region, pedicles are located on the superior third of the posterior surface of the vertebral body. This protects the nerve root of a vertebral unit from being injured by a significantly herniated intervertebral disc of that same unit. The nerve winds around the pedicle and exits its intervertebral foramen before it crosses the intervertebral disc.

Anatomically and radiographically, all of the posterior elements of a vertebra can be accurately identified if the pedicles of that vertebra are first identified. On an anteroposterior (AP) radiograph, the pedicles appear as two longitudinal rows of opaque ovals on the lateral, superior third of the vertebral bodies. These are used as landmarks for finding the other posterior elements (Table 40.2).

Transverse Processes
A transverse process projects laterally from the region of each pedicle. In the lumbar region, these processes are anatomically located directly lateral (in the same horizontal plane) to the spinous process of the vertebra of their origin. This fact helps in locating and palpating the pair of associated lumbar transverse processes after palpating and identifying a specific lumbar spinous process. This also permits accurate testing of the proper vertebra for rotational motion of a specific lumbar vertebral unit.

Superior and Inferior Articular Processes
An inferior articular process projects in a caudad direction from the region of the pedicle, and its articular facet faces laterally. A superior articular process projects cephalad from the same pedicle, and its facet faces medially (4). The joint space of an intervertebral synovial joint is formed by the facet of an inferior articular process of one vertebra and the facet of a superior articular process of the

TABLE 40.2

Osterior, Middle, and Anterior Spinal Elements Related to Back Pain

Elements	Possible Etiologies
Posterior elements—most common	
Spinous process, transverse processes, lamina, pedicles, ligaments, and joining capsule, intervertebral joints	Somatic dysfunction–TART[a]
	Especially the "half-dirty dozen"
	Age-related and activity-related strains–arthritis, overuse
	Severe or chronic twists
	Strains and sprains
	Spondylosis, overuse, or chronic trauma
	Spondylolisthesis
	Severe trauma and twists
	Fractures of pedicle, transverse process, or spinous process[b]
Middle elements	
Central spinal canal, meninges, spinal cord, and nerves	Compression of the spinal canal or nerve root
	Cauda equina syndrome[b]
	Intrinsic
	Intradural tumors
	Meningeal infections
	Extrinsic pressure through foramen and/or the thecal sac
	Metastatic tumors
	Ruptured disc with contents free in spinal canal
	Neurofibromas
	Spurs or other symptom, of aging or degenerative conditions (osteoarthritis)
	Benign tumors or fibromas
	Reflex etiologies—visceral dysfunctions and diseas
Anterior elements	
Posterior longitudinal ligament, vertebral body, anterior longitudinal ligament, and intervertebral disk	Compression fractures of the vertebral body
	Vascular causes—abdominal aneurysm[b]
	Traumatic disc disruption with pressure on nerve root or thecal sac
	Infection

[a]Glossary of osteopathic terminology. *AOA Yearbook and Directory.* Chicago, IL: American Osteopathic Association, 2000:869.
[b]Emergency.

next vertebra. Zygapophyseal joint tropism is the most common lumbar congenital abnormality and is found in 30% of patients. This term describes a composite arrangement where the articular pillars on one side of a vertebral unit are twisted so that the plane of the resulting synovial intervertebral joint on that side does not match the orientation of the synovial joint on the other side. However, asymmetric joints at the same level may be associated with asymmetric muscle tensions and altered spinal motions.

Lumbar Facet Joints

Lumbar facet joints have long been thought to represent a source of low back pain. Figure 40.3 shows sagittal plane standing postural radiographic measurements and their normal ranges. The facet joint is innervated by branches from the medial divisions of the dorsal rami above and below the joint. Inflammatory or degenerative diseases of any facet joint will activate multiple segments in the spinal cord. Pain from the facet joints may be referred to the lower extremity. The lumbar facet joints contain both nociceptive and proprioceptive innervation. Some studies have also found sympathetic axons detected in the joint capsule separate from the vasculature (6).

Lamina

A lamina projects medially and caudad from each pedicle, and normally meets its partner in the posterior midline to form a typical rectangular lumbar spinous process. In some instances, the laminae will not completely meet in the midline, and a spina bifida is

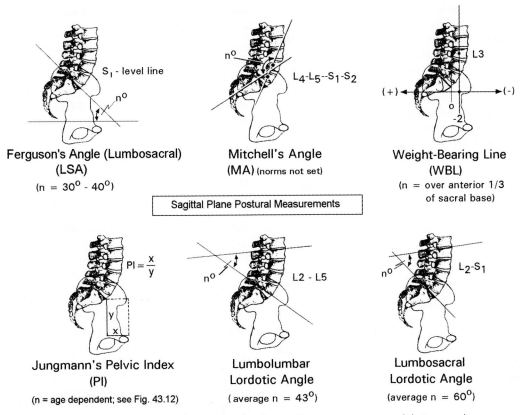

Figure 40-3 Sagittal plane standing postural radiographic measurements and their normal ranges.

produced. The most common congenital anomaly of this type is the "hidden" spina bifida, called spina bifida occulta. Spina bifida occulta is frequently found at the L5-S1 level of the spine. The only physical clue to its presence may be a midline patch of coarse hair on a patient's skin over its site (7). In this type of spina bifida, the skin is intact and there are no meningeal components. It may modify muscle attachments, however, and can be associated with a higher incidence of other posterior vertebral anomalies, including congenital or acquired spondylolisthesis. In the more serious forms of spina bifida, meningocele and meningomyelocele, the spinal membranes protrude, with or without cord tissue. These are disabling.

Spinous Processes

Clinically, the spinous process of a lumbar vertebra is located in the same horizontal plane as its associated transverse processes. Lumbar spinous processes are distinguished by their palpable, thick, quadrangular, "spade-like" distal ends. This is in contrast to the fingertip-shaped palpatory characteristic of the thoracic spinous processes. Their distinguishing shape provides palpatory evidence of where the lumbar region begins and where the thoracic spine ends. This also aids in counting lumbar or thoracic vertebrae. There is one exception; the spinous process of the fifth lumbar vertebra is smaller, lies in a hollow just above the sacral base, and its distal end is about one-third smaller than the rest of the lumbar spines (4). It feels more like a thoracic than a lumbar spinous process. This L5 spinous process characteristic helps to identify it as the last lumbar vertebra and not the first spinous process of the sacrum. Another, less accurate way of counting lumbar vertebrae is to find the most superior portion of the iliac crests and then follow a horizontal plane from there to the midline. This should cross the spinous process of L4, and counting can begin from there.

Spinal Canal

The spinal canal is actually an anatomic space between the posterior margin of a vertebral body and parts of its posterior elements (i.e., its two pedicles, and the laminae). It contains the dural tube, spinal cord, and origins of the spinal nerves down to approximately the L2-3 level, where the spinal cord ends. From that level on, the dural tube contains the cauda equina and the filum terminalis interna. The entire spinal canal is wider transversely than it is anteroposteriorly. In the lumbar spine, it is also triangular. The spinal cord usually terminates at the L2 level as the conus medullaris. Each of the remaining dorsal and ventral roots of the lumbar, sacral, and coccygeal nerves hangs in the dural tube and spinal canal, forming the cauda equina (horse's tail); they exit the conus medullaris or the dural tube as they approach their appropriate intervertebral foramen.

The Intervertebral Foramen

Intervertebral foramen (one on the right and one on the left) are formed by two adjacent vertebrae of a vertebral unit. They are defined by:

- Two adjacent vertebral bodies and the intervertebral disc between them
- Two adjacent pedicles
- The inferior articular process of one vertebra and the superior articular process of the next, including the synovial joint between them

A spinal nerve and a recurrent meningeal nerve, each carrying the same identification number as the vertebral unit, pass through a lumbar foramen (4). The recurrent meningeal nerve then reenters the foramina. These nerves only occupy 35% to 40% of the foramina area. A lumbar intervertebral foramen is normally two to three times larger than the area taken up by the lumbar nerves, so it seems that compression of the nerve would be difficult. With flexion, the facets and pedicles glide away from one another, and the size of the intervertebral foramen increases. With extension, the pedicles glide toward one another, and the foramen is reduced in size. Reduction of the foramen size also results from arthritis or spurs, hypertrophy of the posterior longitudinal ligament, extrusion of the nucleus pulposus, tissue congestion or edema, inflammation, and perineural edema. Removal or reduction of the effect produced by any of these factors may be enough to allow a symptomatic patient to become asymptomatic—pain free and able to work. This is important to remember when considering management of patients with back pain etiologies, paresthesias, or radiculopathies.

Ligaments

The ligamentous structures of the lumbosacral connection form a continuous, dense connective tissue stocking that houses the lumbar vertebrae and sacrum and provides attachment sites for the associated muscles. This complicated ligamentous structure plays a key role in the self-bracing mechanism of the pelvis, a mechanism that functions to maintain the integrity of the low back and pelvis during the transfer of energy from the spine to the lower extremities (6). The ligamentous support mechanism of the lumbosacral region is influenced by several major muscle groups in the low back and pelvis.

Ligamentum Flavum

The ligamentum flavum attaches the posterior elements of each vertebra together. It runs from each pedicle and lamina to the next, and makes up the posteriolateral boundary of the neural foramen. Thickening and calcification of this ligament can cause foraminal narrowing, spinal stenosis, and nerve root compression.

The ligamentum flavum is the main opposition to flexion loading of the lumbar spine. The ligamentum flavum can be injured with excessive spinal flexion. Unfortunately, there is little or no regenerative capacity in the elastic tissue of the ligamentum flavum; thus, a damaged ligament is replaced by a dense connective tissue cicatrix (6). The innervation of the ligamentum flavum and its potential role in the genesis of low back pain is of special note. Nerve fibers have been detected in the sections of the flaval ligament stained with protein ×100, a calcium-binding protein that is not entirely specific for neural tissue. Small-caliber sensory nerve fibers immunoreactive for protein gene product 9.5 (a pan-neuronal marker) were detected in a sample of flaval ligaments taken from patients with low back pain at surgery. Previous studies had failed to detect innervation of the ligamentum flavum. It is a hypothesis that the normal ligament has a paucity of sensory fibers that could increase in distribution in pathological conditions (6).

Interspinous Ligament

This ligament anchors the thoracolumbar fascia and multifidus sheath to the facet joint capsules, and becomes the central support system for the lumbar spine. Condrification of the interspinous ligament occurs after the third decade of life. These pathologic events occurring to the interspinous ligament should diminish the ability of the thoracolumbar fascia to influence the alignment of the lumbar vertebrae and thereby increase their risk of injury. Both proprioceptive and nociceptive axons have been described in the supraspinous and intraspinous ligaments (6).

Anterior Longitudinal Ligament

The anterior longitudinal ligament courses along the anterior vertebral bodies from the second cervical down to the sacral base, where it blends into the ligamentous encapsulation of the sacrum (4). The lateral borders of the anterior longitudinal ligament are attachment sites for the psoas muscle. In the lumbar spine, the anterior longitudinal ligament is thicker than the posterior longitudinal ligament. The anterior longitudinal ligament may generate pain, as Substance P has been detected in the small fibers of anterior longitudinal ligament samples from degenerate lumbar discs (6).

The Posterior Longitudinal Ligament

This ligament extends from the basiocciput to the sacrum caudally. The attachments are strongest to the outer layer of the annulus fibrosus of the intervertebral disc and the weakest to the vertebral body where the ligament arches over the opening of the foramen for the central vein. The posterior longitudinal ligament is broad in the cervical region and begins to narrow when it reaches the first lumbar vertebra (4). It takes on a scalloped appearance and is only one-half its original width when it reaches L5. The scallops produce a deficiency in the posterior longitudinal ligament that is located over the posterolateral portions of each lumbar intervertebral disc. The posterior portion of the intervertebral disc is also the thinnest portion of the anulus. Therefore, this is the region of a lumbar disc that is most likely to rupture; if it does, it is most likely to be associated with nerve root pressure. An extensive nerve plexus is present in the posterior and anterior longitudinal ligaments of the lumbar region. Very few large fibers with encapsulate endings have been found. Small primary afferent axons containing neuropeptides have been identified in the posterior longitudinal ligament and the peripheral portion of the annulus fibrosus.

The Iliolumbar Ligament

This ligament is located in the lumbosacral region. It is attached to the transverse processes of L4 and L5, and extends to the iliac crest and the anterior and posterior regions of the SI joint. It has been reported that this "ligament" may consist of muscle fibers in neonates and children and gradually becomes ligamentous over the next 30 years, but this has recently been disputed by some anatomists. The major function of the iliolumbar ligament is to restrict motion at the lumbosacral junction, particularly that of sidebending. Bilateral transection of the iliolumbar ligament, rotation is increased by 18%, extension by 20%, flexion by 23%, and sidebending by 29% (6).

Clinically, the iliolumbar ligament is typically the first ligament to become tender to palpation when there is lumbosacral postural stress and decomposition (6). A tender point on the iliac crest, located 1 inch superior and lateral from the inferior margin of the PSIS and in the iliolumbar ligament, becomes acutely tender to palpation. The tenderness palpated at the insertion of the iliolumbar ligament has been thought by some to be related to irritation of the cutaneous dorsal ramus of the L1/2 spinal nerve (7). Patients with early postural decompensation may not realize that the iliac attachment of this ligament is tender until it is palpated. Its tenderness is a physical clue that should prompt the physician to ask questions about posture and to carefully examine the spine, lower lumbar region, and SI joints for somatic dysfunction, scoliosis, and/or evidence of sacral base unleveling. An example would be an adult who has, for years, been successfully compensating for continuous low back strain secondary to a congenital sacral base unleveling or an acquired short leg. As a result of decompensation in the lumbosacral region, this patient finally becomes symptomatic with back pain. The first complaint of a patient with irritation of

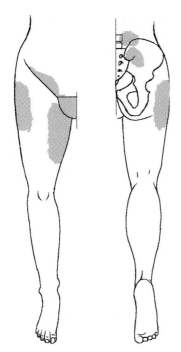

Figure 40-4 Referral pain pattern of a patient with an irritated right iliolumbar ligament syndrome.

the iliolumbar ligament may be groin pain, concerning the patient that they have a hernia (Fig. 40.4).

Muscles and Fascia

The first few lumbar vertebrae provide posterior attachments for the abdominal diaphragm. The left crura of the diaphragm attaches to the first two, and the right crura attaches to the first three lumbar vertebral bodies. The diaphragm then arches cephalad past these and the lower thoracic vertebrae, with its apex sometimes as high as the fifth intercostal space. It then curves caudad to attach to the xiphoid process. For this reason, somatic dysfunction of the first three lumbar vertebrae can be associated with a flattened, ineffective, dysfunctional, resting abdominal diaphragm. A flattened diaphragm is often associated with a lumbar lordosis and/or psoas and quadratus muscle spasms. In this flattened resting condition, the diaphragmatic dome is unable to develop efficient, appropriate pressure gradients between the thorax and abdomen during contraction and relaxation, and this results in decreased lymphatic flow and venous return from anywhere in the body. The physician should also remember that the innervation to the diaphragm is the phrenic nerve, which originates from nerve roots C3-5 of the spinal cord. Therefore, cervical somatic dysfunction can be involved in diaphragmatic dysfunction.

The lumbar spine also supplies partial origin for the erector spinae mass of muscles that extend from the pelvis all the way to the occiput. Unilateral contraction of extrinsic or intrinsic muscles of the back will side bend or rotate the spine. When working together, these muscles extend the spine. Through the lumbosacral aponeurosis and fascial divisions, the lumbar region is functionally attached to the gluteal muscles, the hamstrings, and via the iliotibial band, to the lower extremity. Through the lumbodorsal fasciae, with its continuity surrounding the external and internal oblique muscles and the rectus abdominus muscle, the posterior lumbar region is functionally related to the lateral and anterior abdominal wall.

Iliopsoas Muscle

A key muscle in lumbar spine complaints is the psoas major. The psoas muscle originates off the anterior portions of the upper lumbar vertebrae, near the insertion of the diaphragmatic crura, and joins with the iliacus inserting on the lesser trochanter of the femur as the iliopsoas. The psoas minor muscle (absent in 40% of patients) connects the lumbar spine to the pelvis. The iliopsoas muscle balances the lumbar spine and pelvis on the femur (8). The iliopsoas muscle is a primary hip flexor; however, it also has a role in postural balance. Iliopsoas tension is a common etiologic culprit in the patient with lower back pain. Bilateral iliopsoas spasm can increase pressure across the disc spaces as well as cause the patient to lean forward. Unilateral spasm will give the classic psoas posture, a listing to one side and forward bent. A tight psoas typically has a vertebral type II somatic dysfunction maintaining it both mechanically and through neurologic facilitation. The iliacus muscle may be considered separately, or in unison, with the psoas. Unilateral tension in an iliacus has been implicated in the production of a recurrent anterior ilium dysfunction.

"CORE Muscles"

In recent years, emphasis has been placed on training the "core" muscles of the abdomen, trunk, and pelvis in order to stabilize and support the lower back. However, there is still controversy as to what muscles make up the "core" and exactly how to train them. It is generally accepted that training certain muscles is critical in providing a stable lumbar spine. The transverse abdominus is one such muscle. The multifidus is another important muscle to train as well as the gluteus. The gluteus maximus tends to be a muscle that is weak and inhibited. This may be related to disuse, lumbar or sacral somatic dysfunction, or chronic nociception from the lumbar spine. These muscles are strengthened in many physical therapy programs for patients with back pain. Equally important is the gluteus medius muscle. The gluteus medius is typically inhibited and commonly has Jones tenderpoints in it. The Trendelenberg test is useful in assessing for unilateral weakness of the gluteus medius muscle.

Multifidus Muscle

The multifidus is divided into five bands each band arising from each lumbar vertebrae and associated tissues. Its distal attachments are the sacrum, interosseous SI ligaments, thoracolumbar fascia, and extreme medial edge of the iliac crest. Tendinous slips of the multifidus muscle pass under the long dorsal SI ligament to join with the sacrotuberous ligament. These connections integrate the multifidus into the ligamentous support system of the SI joint. The fibers of the multifidus are aligned in the vertical plane with only very slight horizontal deviations. This arrangement is specific for movement in the sagittal plane, making the multifidus a significant lumbar spine extensor muscle, along with the erector spinae muscles. The long fibers in the body of the muscle span multiple segments, thus giving the portion of the multifidus muscle an additional role as a stabilizer of the lumbar spine. Finally, by increasing tension of the thoracolumbar fascia, SI ligaments and sacrotuberous ligaments, activation of the multifidus also contributes to the self-bracing mechanism of the pelvis and to the transfer of energy from the upper body to the lower extremities (6). The multifidus muscle plays an important role in standing or seated posture, gait, trunk movement, and when lifting of carrying a load. Dysfunction of the multifidus muscle can lead to injury of the low back and to low back pain. Scoliosis and lumbar disc herniation have been associated with histochemical changes in the multifidus muscle.

Latissimus Dorsi

Although it is not a prime mover of the lumbar spine, the latissimus dorsi is clinically important to discuss. The latissimus dorsi muscle is one of the muscles which anchors the upper extremity to the trunk. The latissimus dorsi muscle has its axial attachment to the thoracolumbar fascia, iliac crest, and to the caudal three or four ribs. It attached to the humerus in the intertubercular groove between the pectoralis major anteriorly and the teres major posteriorly. The muscle can be divided into four parts: the thoracic portion attaches to the lower six thoracic spines, a transitional portion attaches to the upper two lumbar spines, a raphe portion attaches to the lateral raphe of the thoracolumbar fascia, and an iliac portion that attaches to the iliac crest (4). For osteopathic physicians, the latissimus dorsi muscle is the link between shoulder problems and low back problems.

Thoracolumbar Aponeurosis

There is continuity of the abdominal wall fascia and the thoracolumbar fascia posteriorly. The rectus sheath splits around the rectus abdominus and is continuous with the transversalis fascia as well as the deep fascia of the lumbar spine. The lumbar vertebrae act as anchors for the fascia. The thoracolumbar deep fascia surrounds, compartmentalizes, and protects all of the lumbar muscles and bones (Fig. 40.5). This fascia gives attachment to the latissimus dorsi muscle, which extends to the proximal end of the humerus. Next to the spine, it compartmentalizes the interspinalis, multifidi, and rotatores muscles. More laterally, but still near the midline, it encloses the longissimus muscle. Even more laterally, it encloses the iliocostalis muscle group that inserts on and provides a landmark for locating the angles of the ribs. The angle of the ribs marks the most lateral extent of the erector spinae mass. Deeper layers of the deep fascia form compartments for the intertransversarii. Anterior to the transverse processes, the deep fascia surrounds the psoas and quadratus lumborum muscles. The quadratus lumborum muscle can clinically and functionally be thought of as the posteroinferior extension of the abdominal diaphragm. Disturbances in vertebral motion or position place asymmetric tension on this three-dimensional fascial structure. The thoracolumbar fascia contains a small-caliber fiber system typical of nociceptive and sympathetic axons, and a large-caliber fiber system capable of proprioception (6).

Self-Bracing Mechanism

Activation of these muscles helps to tighten the connective tissue support structures, stabilizing the lumbosacral spine, and thereby contributing to a mechanism that has been referred to as self-bracing. The multifidus, gluteus maximus, and biceps femoris muscles play major roles, while the piriformis and latissimus dorsi play a lesser role. This arrangement of muscles and fascia facilitates the transfer of energy generated by movement of the upper extremities through the spine and into the lower extremities. The close coupling of these extremity and back muscles through the thoracolumbar fascia and its attachments to the ligamentous stocking of the spine, allow the motion of the upper limbs to assist in rotation of the trunk and movement of the lower extremities in gait, creating an integrated system (6). A summary of the "core" muscles affecting the lumbar spine is provided in Table 40.3.

Mesenteries

Approximately 30 ft of small intestines and portions of the ascending and descending colon are located anterior to the lumbar region. The abdominal mesenteries are formed by reflections of the parietal peritoneum from the posterior abdominal wall. These mesenteries carry arteries and efferent autonomic nerve fibers to the viscera. They also carry veins, lymphatic vessels, and visceral afferent nerves away from the viscera. In this way, somatic dysfunction of the myofascial tissues of the lumbar region can functionally influence the local environment of the abdominal viscera.

Myofascial trigger points in the gluteus medius, rotatores, multifidi, iliopsoas, quadratus lumborum, and the piriformis muscles

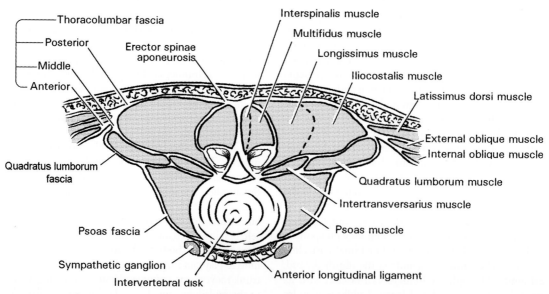

Figure 40-5 The deep fascia and thoracolumbar aponeurosis of the low back. It compartmentalizes, protexts, and gives attachments for the erector spinae mass and lumbar muscles.

Lumbar Spine Muscles Origin, Insertion, Action, and Innervation

Muscles	Origin	Insertion	Action	Innervation
Spinalis dorsi	Spinous processes of lumbar/thoracic vertebrae	Spinous process of four to eight vertebrae above	Extends vertebral column	Dorsal rami of spinal nerves
Semispinalis dorsi (most medial of erector spinae muscles)	Transverse processes of the 6th to the 10th thoracic vertebrae	Spinous processes of the upper four thoracic and lower two cervical vertebrae	Extends and rotates vertebral column	Dorsal rami of spinal nerves
Longissimus thoracis/lumborum (intermediate muscle of erector spinae muscles)	Transverse process of lumbar/thoracic vertebrae	Transverse processes of all the thoracic vertebrae into ribs 2–12 between their tubercles and angles	Extension, lateral flexion of vertebral column, rib rotation	Dorsal rami of spinal nerves
Iliocostalis thoracis/lumborum (most lateral of erector spinae muscles)	Upper borders of the angles of the lower six ribs	Upper borders of the angles of the upper six ribs and into the transverse process of the seventh cervical vertebra	Extension, lateral flexion of vertebral column, rib rotation	Dorsal rami of spinal nerves
Rotatores thoracis	Transverse processes of thoracic vertebrae	Spinous process of vertebrae above	Extends and rotates vertebral column	Dorsal rami of spinal nerves
Interspinales	Spinous processes of lumbar, thoracic and cervical vertebrae	Spinous process vertebrae of above	Extension, flexion and rotation of vertebral column	Dorsal rami of spinal nerves
Intertransversarii	Transverse processes of lumbar, thoracic and cervical vertebrae	Transverse process of vertebrae above	Lateral flexion of trunk	Dorsal rami of spinal nerves
Multifidus	Sacrum, Erector spinae Aponeurosis, PSIS, Iliac crest, and transverse processes of lumbar, thoracic and cervical vertebrae	Spinous processes of 1–4 vertebrae above	Stabilizes vertebrae in local movements of vertebral column	Dorsal rami of spinal nerves
Latissimus dorsi muscle	Spinous processes of thoracic T6–12, thoracolumbar fascia, iliac crest and inferior 3 or 4 ribs	Floor of intertubercular sulcus of humerus	Extends, Adducts, and medially rotates humerus (depresses, retracts, and inferiorly rotates scapula)	Thoracodorsal nerve

(continued)

TABLE 40.3 (Continued)

Muscles	Origin	Insertion	Action	Innervation
Quadratus lumborum	Iliac crest and iliolumbar ligament	Last rib and transverse processes of lumbar vertebrae	Unilateral: lateral flexion of vertebral column. Bilateral: depression of thoracic rib cage	The twelfth thoracic and first through fourth lumbar nerves
Psoas muscle	L1-5 transverse processes	Lesser trochanter of the femur	Lumbar plexus via anterior branches of L2-4 nerves	Flexes and rotates laterally thigh
Iliacus muscle	Iliac fossa	Lesser trochanter of the femur	Femoral nerve	Flexes and rotates laterally thigh
Rectus abdominus	Pubis	Costal cartilage of ribs 5–7, xiphoid process of sternum	Segmentally by thoracoab-dominal nerves (T7-12)	Flexion of trunk/lumbar vertebrae
Transverse abdominus	Ribs and the iliac crest	The pubic tubercle via the conjoint tendon, also known as the falx inguinalis	Compress the ribs and viscera, providing thoracic and pelvic stability	Lower intercostal nerves, as well as the iliohypogastric nerve and the ilioinguinal nerve
Internal oblique	Inguinal ligament, Iliac crest, and the Lumbodorsal fascia.	Linea alba, Xiphoid process, and the inferior ribs	Compresses abdomen and rotates vertebral column.	Lower intercostal nerves, as well as the iliohypogastric nerve and the ilioinguinal nerve
External oblique	Lower eight ribs	Iliac crest and ligamentum inguinale	Both flexion and rotation of the vertebral column.	Innervated by ventral branches of the lower six intercostal (thoracoabdominal) nerves and the subcostal nerve on each side.

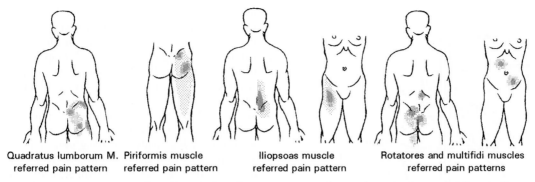

Quadratus lumborum M.   Piriformis muscle   Iliopsoas muscle   Rotatores and multifidi muscles
referred pain pattern   referred pain pattern   referred pain pattern   referred pain patterns

Figure 40-6   Pain patterns produced by myofascial trigger points in the quadratus lumborum, piriformis, iliopsoas, rotatores, and multifidi muscles of the back.

produce pain patterns in the lumbar region and sometimes into the sacral region and lower extremities (9,10) (Fig. 40.6).

Innervation of the Lumbar Region

Spinal Cord

In an adult, the spinal cord usually terminates at the L2 level as the conus medullaris (terminal range T12-L2, and some say to L3). The dural sac and a string of fibrous tissue and pia, known as the filum terminalis internus, continue on. The dural sac terminates by attaching to the spinal canal at the S2 level. Fibrous tissue and cells from the dura continue on as the filum terminalis externa, which attaches to the first coccygeal segment. Remember that the posterior longitudinal ligament is anterior to the spinal cord and has lateral deficiencies in the areas of the lumbar discs. The dural sac of the spinal canal, below the conus medullaris, contains the filum terminalis internus and lower lumbar, sacral, and coccygeal dorsal and ventral rootlets of the cauda equine (Fig. 40.7).

The lumbar spinal canal takes on a triangular configuration and normally decreases in its AP dimension as it progresses from L1 to L5 (4). As a person ages, the diameter of the lumbar spinal canal or intervertebral canal may be further compromised by factors that include hypertrophy of the posterior longitudinal ligament, thickening of the ligamentum flava on its anterior wall, osteoarthritis, exostoses, osteophytes, tumors, and ruptured lumbar intervertebral discs.

Tissue congestion, frank edema, and perineural edema can also compromise the nerves in the spinal canal or an intervertebral foramen, especially if the region already has somatic dysfunction and/or an anatomic/pathologic deformity. If there is enough pressure on the spinal cord or the nerves in the cauda equina, there will be loss of reflexes, weakness of muscles, and paralysis of the lower extremities and sphincters of the bladder and rectum. This symptom complex describes a severe form of spinal stenosis called cauda equina syndrome.

Spinal Nerve Roots and Spinal Nerves

The lumbosacral spinal cord gives rise to numerous nerve rootlets from the dorsolateral and ventrolateral sulci. In the subarachnoid space of the vertebral canal, between five and seven dorsal rootlets form each lumbar segment bundle together to form a dorsal spinal nerve root, which joins with a similarly derived ventral spinal nerve root. These nerve roots descend in the vertebral canal, exiting at each intervertebral foramen. At the level of the foramen, a complex relationship occurs. The nerve roots enter a funnel-shaped lateral recess of the spinal canal that narrows to form the lumbar nerve root canal. The distal end of the root canal is the intervertebral foramen. The walls of the nerve root canal are composed of the pedicle and

the pars interarticularis of the vertebra, the ligamentum flavum, and the lateral aspect of the intervertebral disc, the obliquity of the canals and their length increase. As the nerve root enters this canal, it is enveloped by a sheath of spinal dura termed the epineurium. In the canal, the nerve root is deflected laterally around the pedicle and over the surface of the intervertebral disc. The dorsal root ganglion is located at the point where the root passes around the pedicle and can leave an impression in the bony structure of the pedicle. The dorsal root ganglion contains the primary afferent cell bodies distal to this structure, the dorsal and ventral roots fuse to form the spinal nerve and the dural layer seals to the spinal nerve. In the lumbar region, as the spinal nerves leave their canals, they are attached to the foramen by several fibrous expansions of the canal wall. As the nerve root traverses the canal and foramen,

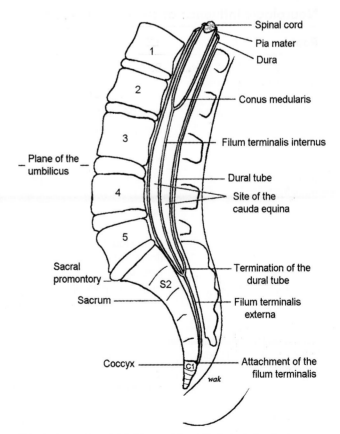

Figure 40-7   The relationships of the spinal cord, dural tube, conus medullaris, filium terminalis internus, cauda equine, and filum terminalis externa to the lumbar and sacral regions.

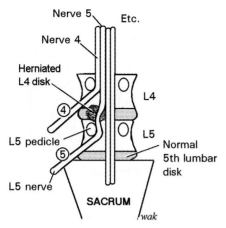

Figure 40-8 Pedicles located on the superior third of the posterior side of a lumbar vertebra protect the nerve from being injured by a herniated disc at its own level. It is more likely that a lumbar nerve would be affected by a herniated disc of the previous vertebral unit. That is why an S1 nerve root is usually affected by a herniated L5 intervertebral disc.

it is at risk from several structures: the pedicles and intervertebral discs, the ligamentum flavum, the capsule of the facet joint, and the foraminal ligaments (Fig. 40.8) (6).

In addition, the intervertebral canal transmits branches of the spinal artery into the spinal canal along with veins drain-

ing the epidural plexus and associated lymphatic vessels. Venous congestion, arteriovenous malformation, and epidural hematoma have all been demonstrated to mimic disc herniation or lumbar spinal stenosis. Whether by mechanical compression or fluid congestion, the traumatized lumbosacral nerve roots experience edema and ischemia, which lead to inflammatory and fibrotic alterations in the neural tissue with concomitant loss of motor function, paresthesia, and hypesthesia. Finally, an additional nonmechanical method for irritating neural tissue in the foraminal area appears to involve the release of nuclear fluids containing proinflammatory compounds as the proteoglycans and tumor necrosis factor-alpha from a leaky disc (6). Although we tend to think of disc herniation as the etiology of nerve root compression/irritation, there are certainly others. Table 40.4 reviews the lumbar roots, their dermatomes, innervated muscles, and physical findings.

Lumbosacral Dorsal Rami

The dorsal ramus leaves the spinal nerve as the nerve exits the lumbar intervertebral canals. As this ramus wraps around the facet joint directly below, it divides into several main branches: (I) Lateral branch that innervates the lateral fascial compartment containing the longissimus muscle; (II) Medial branches that innervate the medial fascial compartment containing the multifidus muscles. Specifically, the medial compartment contains the multifidus, interspinalis, and intertransversarii medialis muscles. It also contains skeletal elements such as the interspinous ligament, the facet joints,

TABLE 40.4

Neurologic Influence of the Lumbar Roots

Root	L1	L2	L3	L4	L5	S1
Sensory dermatome	Back to trochanter	Back	Back	Inner calf to medial portion of foot (first two toes)	Lateral lower leg	Sole
	Groin	Anterior thigh to the level of knee	Upper buttock to anterior thigh		Dorsum of foot	Heel
			Medial lower leg		First two toes	Lateral edge of foot
Innervated muscle(s)	Iliopsoas	Iliopsoas	Iliopsoas	Tibialis anterior	Extensor hallucis	Gastrocnemius
		Sartorius	Quadriceps femoris	Gluteus medius	Tibialis posterior	Gluteus maximus
		Hip adductors (longus, brevis, pectineus, magnus, gracilis)	Sartorius	Gluteus minimus	Hamstrings	Hamstrings
			Hip adductors	Tensor fasciae latae		Peroneus
				Quadratus femoris		
Functional limitation	Hip flexion	Hip flexion	Hip flexion	Knee extension	Toe extension	Ankle plantarflexion
		Hip adduction	Hip adduction		Ankle dorsiflexion	Knee flexion
			Knee extension			
Affected reflex	Cremasteric	Cremasteric	Patellar	Patellar	Tibialis posterior	Ankle
		Adductor		Gluteal	Gluteal?	Hamstring

and the ligament flavum (6). Inferiorly, the dorsal and possibly ventral rami of L5 and of the sacral roots provide innervation of the SI joint capsule. Irritation of the small-caliber primary afferent fibers of the dorsal ramus results in the perception of pain. This perception is usually a sharp, burning pain that is similar to spinal root pain and can refer to the area supplied by the corresponding ventral ramus, thus mimicking sciatica (6). As the dorsal ramus also innervates muscle groups in the back, compression or damage to this nerve can present with signs of denervation weakness, as well as with pain.

Lumbar Plexus

The lumbar plexus is composed of nerve roots L1-4 and a branch from T12. Lumbar nerve roots enter directly into the psoas muscle, where the lumbar plexus is formed. Lumbar nerves emerge from the borders and surfaces of the psoas muscle. (4) Psoas muscle spasm can compress these nerves producing pain referred into the anterior thigh.

Sympathetic Nervous System

The sympathetic nervous system has thoracolumbar outflow. Therefore, somatic dysfunction of the lumbar spine can affect the sympathetic nervous system. Somatic dysfunction in the thoracic spine can affect the lumbar spine via this neural pathway as well. Abdominal and pelvic viscera stimulate general visceral afferents that synapse near the sympathetics in the lumbar spinal cord. Therefore, visceral disease or dysfunction can cause palpatory findings in the lumbar spine. Sympathetic axons have been detected in the posterior longitudinal ligament, the ventral dura, the periosteum of the vertebral body, the intervertebral disc, and the vertebral body where they reach into the marrow cavity. The lumbar sympathetic trunk courses along the border of the psoas attachment.

Sinu Vertebral Nerves

The sinu vertebral nerve emerges distal to the dorsal root ganglion but prior to the division into dorsal and ventral rami. This small branch recurs into the intervertebral foramen to reach the vertebral canal. The terminal branches supply the posterior longitudinal ligament, the periosteum on the posterior aspect of the vertebral body, the outer layers of the intervertebral discs, and the anterior surface of the spinal dura. This nerve can travel up or down the vertebral canal at least two or three segments from the point of entry. Additionally, it can cross the midline to innervate tissue on the contralateral side. Some fibers cross the vertebral canal and subsequently pass outward through the contralateral intervertebral foramina. Dissection has demonstrated that the L1 and L2 roots have a complex array of multiple branches re-entering the intervertebral foramen, whereas the low lumbar vertebrae had only a few branches (6).

Small-caliber, primary afferent nociceptors—as well as sympathetic fibers—appear to be contained within the sinu vertebral nerve. Irritation of the small-caliber primary afferent fibers in the sinu vertebral nerve can refer to pain several segments up or down the spinal cord, as well as referring pain to the contralateral side of the body (6).

The sinu vertebral nerve does not supply skeletal muscle or skin, so compression or damage to this nerve alone does not present with signs of denervation weakness or cutaneous analgesia.

Somatosympathetic Nerves

No somatic nerves (direct branches of the dorsal or ventral rami or spinal nerves) reach the anterior aspect of the vertebral bodies. However, this area is richly supplied by sensory fibers traveling in branches of the sympathetic trunk. These small-caliber, primary afferent nociceptors, wrap around the anterior longitudinal ligament and the periosteum on the anterior aspect of the vertebral body and penetrate into the outer layers of the intervertebral discs. The pathway of return of these sensory fibers to the spinal cord follows the sympathetic trunk and appears to use the white rami in gaining access to the spinal nerve and dorsal root ganglia. Therefore, sensory fibers entering the trunk below L2 pass upward to reach the L1-2 white rami. Noxious stimuli in the lower lumbar and sacral levels will ascend in the sympathetic trunk and enter the spinal cord at the thoracolumbar junction. This results in the referral of pain, subsequent facilitation, and palpatory findings in the spinal segments at the thoracolumbar junction (6).

Somatosympathetic axons do not supply any skeletal muscle or skin, so damage to these nerves alone will not present with signs of denervation weakness or cutaneous analgesia.

While these nerves do not innervate muscle or skin, once facilitation has been established, the muscles are hypertonic and the skin is hypersensitive.

Dermatomes, Myotomes, and Sclerotomes

Lumbar dermatomes are located on the posterior lumbar paraspinal region and the anterior part of the thigh, leg, and foot. Pain or paresthesia in these areas of skin provides clues to the level of nerve root involvement and nerve dysfunction and/or irritation. One method is for the physician to mentally construct three oblique lines, from superolateral to inferomedial, on the anterior thigh, dividing it into three equal sections. The inferior of these three oblique lines must go through the patella. From superior to inferior, these lines delineate dermatomes L1, L2, and L3. A line visualized from the patella to the big toe delineates the medial L4 dermatome from the lateral L5 dermatome. A small section on the lateral side of the foot is the first sacral dermatome. Figure 40.9 approximates the location of lumbar dermatomes of any patient. Note that different books illustrate dermatomal patterns of various complexities. However, remembering that these divisions will vary slightly from person to person, this method provides an easy to recall, good general clinical pattern from which to work.

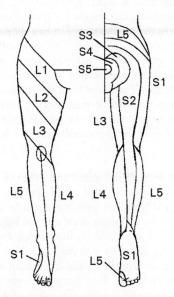

Figure 40-9 Dermatomal or radicular (nerve root) patterns. (Illustration by W. A. Kuchera.)

Myotomal pain is associated with cramps, weakness, and myofascial trigger points in the muscles that share innervation from the same irritated nerve roots.

Sclerotomal pain is described as vague, deep, toothache-like pain. It arises from ligaments, bones, or joints that share innervation from the same irritated nerve root. Knee pain, for example, can be the result of irritation of the L3 vertebra, ligaments in the L3 region, the pubic symphysis, the hip, or the knee. All of these sites have the same L3 sclerotomal origin.

Vasculature and Lymphatics

Blood Vessels

The lumbar spinal cord receives its arterial blood supply from segmental radicular arteries. In the lumbosacral region, one of these radicular arteries, the arteria radicularis magna, is larger than the rest and is the source of blood for the inferior two thirds of the spinal cord (4). The rest of the cord receives blood from associated segmental arteries. Arteries supplying a lumbar vertebra enter around the circumference of the vertebral body, especially near its transverse processes.

Evaluation of the patient with lower back pain should include an abdominal exam. Abdominal bruits over the renal arteries, iliac arteries, or the aorta indicate disease. A pulsatile mass to deep palpation always warrants investigation. Although more commonly seen in the elderly, an abdominal aortic aneurysm can be seen in young people with certain conditions (such as Marfan disease). The back pain in a dissecting aortic aneurysm is described as "ripping" in nature; however, it may be progressive and less intense as well.

Venous blood drains the spinal cord via a profuse plexus of thin-walled veins that communicate with the profuse, valveless venous plexus in the vertebrae and the anterior and posterior longitudinal veins of the dura. Venous blood from the profuse vertebral plexus of valveless veins drains into a large basivertebral vein (4), which exits from a foramen located in the posterior surface of each vertebral body. *All of these veins are valveless.* Venous blood from the spinal cord can drain into radicular veins or can drain cephalad into the large, valveless venous sinuses of the dura.

The profuse, valveless venous plexus of the spinal cord, vertebrae, communicating veins, and large, intracranial venous sinuses are of great clinical importance. An increase in intra-abdominal or intrathoracic pressures, as occurs with coughing, Valsalva maneuvers, or fascial tensions, can reverse the flow of venous blood and become a factor in the metastasis of primary abdominal and pelvic malignancies to the spine and brain. This mechanism also explains headaches and other central nervous system symptoms from increased venous pressure associated with visceral, spinal cord, or vertebral dysfunction. The blood from the muscles of the lumbar region drains into the inferior vena cava. It does not drain into mesenteric veins or pass through the portal system of the liver, as the venous blood from the abdominal and pelvic viscera does.

Lymphatics

Lymphatic fluid from all abdominal and pelvic viscera drains into the thoracic duct, which is also called the left lymphatic duct (LLD). All somatic lymphatic vessels at and inferior to a horizontal plane through the umbilicus drain into the inguinal nodes, the deep pelvic external and common iliac nodes, the preaortic and lateral aortic nodes, and then into the LLD. Note that lymphatic vessels from the gonads or the viscera *do not* drain into the inguinal region, but drain into the deep lymphatic vessels of the pelvis and then into the cisterna chyli. Therefore, gonadal and prostate inflammation or malignancy is not associated with enlarged,

palpable inguinal nodes. The LLD passes through the fasciae of the left side of the thoracic inlet twice before emptying into the left brachiocephalic vein. All lymphatic fluid (from anywhere in the body) must pass through the fasciae of the thoracic inlet on its way to the venous circulation and the heart.

Biomechanics Motion

The Vertebral Unit

From a functional anatomic or osteopathic perspective, a vertebral unit "is composed of two adjacent vertebrae with their associated disc, arthrodial, ligamentous, muscular, vascular, lymphatic, and neural elements" (11) (Fig. 40.10). In *Clinical Biomechanics of the Spine*, White and Panjabi label a vertebral unit as a functional spinal unit (FSU) (12). They define FSU as "two adjacent vertebrae and the connecting ligamentous tissues." Therefore, the vertebral unit is different and more comprehensive than the FSU of the orthopedic specialist; the two should not be confused when communicating or when reading the literature. With stress, a vertebral unit behaves according to its structure, strength, flexibility, and the functional ability of its ligaments, muscular, neural, vascular, and lymphatic connections. Both the vertebral unit and the FSU are given the same number as the cephalad vertebra of the unit. For example, the third lumbar unit is named L3. According to the vertebral unit definition, however, it not only indicates L3 moving on L4, but also includes their associated disc, arthrodial, and ligamentous, muscular, vascular, lymphatic, and neural elements.

Normal Motion

Moore (4) cites that the cervical and lumbar regions of the vertebral column are the most mobile and the most common sites of aches and pains. Lumbar motion is especially visible when the vertebrae of the lumbar spinal region move together as a group. The major motions are flexion, extension, side-bending, and rotation.

Note that side-bending and rotation are coupled motions. Their direction of motion may be opposite (type I motion) or in the same direction (type II motion), but side-bending and rotation occur together in the lumbar spine; one cannot occur without the other.

There are also minor translatory motions occurring in opposite directions on each of the three planes of motion. A vertebral unit normally has 12 possible movements available to it and, therefore, 12 movements that can be restricted in a somatic dysfunction of a joint. Somatic dysfunction usually involves these minor motions,

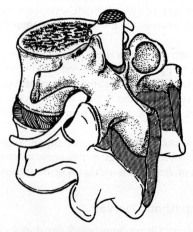

Figure 40-10   Vertebral unit.

and that dysfunction then affects the major motions that are possible for that joint. The pattern for multiple plane motion of a vertebral unit depends on the position of the sagittal plane of the spine when a vector of rotation or side-bending is introduced.

When the spine is in its neutral positional range, side-bending and rotation normally occur to opposite sides in multiple units, and this is called type I motion or type I mechanics. Type I motion occurs when it is predominately the vertebral bodies and discs that influence spinal action.

When the lumbar spine is flexed far enough or extended far enough that it is out of the neutral sagittal plane range and into the nonneutral sagittal plane range, rotation and side-bending normally occur to the same side, usually in the vertebral unit where the forces are localized. This is called type II motion or type II mechanics. Type II motion occurs when the facets exert the major influence on spinal motion.

There is another way of stating these two normal motion principles. In the neutral mechanical range for the sagittal plane (where multiple plane motion is predominately directed by the vertebral bodies and discs), side-bending and then rotation occur to opposite sides in a group of vertebrae, or rotation occurs toward the convexity of the curve. This is type I motion and is expected to occur in a group of vertebral units because of the joint facings, as well as the construction and ligamentous attachments of the lumbar vertebrae. In the lumbar region, this type of multiple plane motion occurs through a greater arc of extension than flexion.

If the lumbar sagittal plane is in a mechanical range where flexion or extension is sufficient to engage the facets as the prime movers of the spine, multiple plane motion will result in rotation and then side-bending occurring to the same side. This can also be stated as rotation into the concavity of the intended side-bending and is type II motion or type II mechanics. Positioning in the sagittal plane that is sufficient to induce type II mechanics with multiple plane motion is usually localized in a single vertebral unit. After type II motion occurs in that one vertebral unit, the other vertebral units involved in the group side-bending curve normally move according to type I mechanics.

Neutral, type I, and non-neutral, type II, motions are a usual and normal biomechanical occurrence during the performance of daily activities. When an activity is over, the spinal units that are free of somatic dysfunction will return to their neutral, resting positions. If motion is tested, they will exhibit ease of motion in all of their usual planes of motion.

Although the lumbar spine can normally flex about 40 degrees and extend about 30 degrees, non-neutral, type II motion is more likely to occur in the lumbar and thoracic spine when the spine is in a straightened configuration. Therefore, non-neutral mechanics with type II motion for the lumbar spinal region are more likely to occur when the lumbar spine is flexed. However, it is possible to produce type II motion with extreme lumbar hyperextension, as might occur when a high diver enters the water, when a gymnast does a back walkover, or when a painter stands on a ladder and reaches up to paint a high ceiling.

Atypical Motion

Atypical motion patterns found during motion testing of single spinal segments do exist. These are typically thought to be traumatically introduced, or due to disc disease, facet tropism, or asymmetric muscle tensions. Palpating motion of L5 reveals many different findings. L5 has normal Type II physiologic motion (as described by Fryette) where sidebending and rotation occur to the same side when significant flexion or extension is introduced. When testing L5 in a neutral position: sidebending and rotation may occur to

opposite sides. This may be due to a group curve, or to congenital facet tropism, or a sacral torsion. When L5 is part of a forward torsion dysfunction of the sacrum its diagnosed motion is found to be rotated in an opposite direction to the rotation of the sacrum and sidebent toward the involved oblique axis.

INTEGRATED PHYSICAL EXAMINATION

A complete physical examination is performed, with special emphasis on regions that are spotlighted by the history, or that have a functional association. Examining the part of the body that is painful is best left for the last portion of the evaluation. Do not forget to evaluate the vital signs in a patient with low back pain. Vital signs can document the presence of fever associated with an infection or neoplasm. Tachycardia may be the sympathetic nervous system's response to the patient's pain. Many times, objective physical examination findings do not correlate with lower back pain. However, reliable physical examination signs consist of measurements of lordosis, flexion range, determination of pain location on flexion and lateral bend, measurements associated with straight leg raising (SLR) test, determination of pain location in the thighs and legs, and sensory changes in the legs (7). Repeat re-examination is needed to correlate the validity and reproducibility of physical findings with other components of patient evaluation for low back pain. There also are ways to evaluate for functional deficits and disabilities in low back pain patients. The following physical examination functional assessment questionnaires evaluate for disabilities:

- Oswestry disability index
- Roland-Morris disability questionnaire
- Hendler 10-minute screening test

Prior to the examination, evaluate the patient's body type and anticipate positions you will need to have the patient in to obtain the physical findings. Obtain as much information in each position as possible. Be efficient. Portions of various exams will need to be integrated based on the patient position. Obtaining palpatory information is integrated with the other aspects of the physical exam. There is not an "add-on" osteopathic exam at the end of the patient encounter. In this chapter, only the more common points related to the lumbar spine and low back pain are described. The physical examination is extremely important in formulating a differential diagnosis.

Observation and Gait

What is the patient's appearance? Observation of posture and activity often provide the first clue to dysfunction. Posture mimics a patient's inner self more than his or her complaints or responses to direct questioning. An example would be the slumped posture of a depressed patient. During observation, it is important to expose the skin of the area in question in a professional manner. Be sure to evaluate the skin, especially in a back pain patient. A number of the spondyloarthropathies cause dermatologic abnormalities. Psoriasis causes erythematous raised plaques with overlying scales that occur on extensor surfaces (elbows and knees) and on the scalp. Painful vesicles distributed in a dermatomal pattern may indicate herpes zoster. Erythema migrans, a large, raised erythematous skin lesion, is the cutaneous hallmark of Lyme disease. Abnormalities of any superficial structures are noted. These abnormalities include a tuft of hair over the spine, which may indicate a congenital abnormality, such as spina bifida occulta. Café au lait spots are associated with neurofibromatosis.

Is there asymmetry of a region of the body when the whole body is observed? Clues to lumbar dysfunction may be indicated by observing the spacing difference between the arms and the hip/waist on each side of the body. This sign may indicate the presence of scoliosis, strain from sacral base unleveling, or a unilateral muscle spasm. If the protective spasm is unilateral owing to injury of the tissues on one side of the spine, scoliosis develops. The spine is tilted to one side because of one-sided muscle spasm. If the patient likes to stand in a forward-bent position, consider bilateral psoas muscle spasm, or a condition that is putting pressure on lumbar nerves in the intervertebral foramen. If the patient is leaning forward, to one side and has the ipsilateral foot everted when standing or walking, consider a unilateral psoas spasm. If this develops into a full psoas syndrome on one side, the patient may also complain of pain in the contralateral hip and leg, rarely past the knee. When a patient stands very erect and dislikes bending forward, he or she may be protecting a herniated disc or be suffering the effects of spinal stenosis, especially if there are other symptoms, such as muscular weakness, reflex changes, or muscle atrophy. Patients with legitimate back pain tend to resume the erect position with a fixed lordosis and without any spine movement (7). Arching the back and increasing the lordosis forces the facet joints together, narrows the foramen through which the nerves exit the spine, and compresses the disc posteriorly.

Patients with herniated discs have changes in their posture and gait. Disc herniation can also cause scoliosis by irritating nerves on one side of the spine. This usually occurs at the L4-5 level. Herniation of a nucleus pulposus *lateral* to the corresponding nerve root causes a sciatic list away from the side of the irritated nerve root. Herniation of a nucleus pulposus *medial* to the corresponding nerve root causes a sciatic list toward the side of the irritated nerve root (7). Patients do not like to bear weight on the leg that has sciatica or radicular pain.

Evaluating gait is important in evaluation of the lumbar spine and in the patient with back pain. In normal gait, the following events occur: Heel strike, Pronation, Midstance, Swing Phase, Loading medial foot, and the Push-off. Deficiencies in each of these phases may mean different things. Patients with an abnormal gait may limp, lurch, turn their foot outward, or hike their hip. Neurologic disorders such as Parkinson disease can cause a fenestrating or shuffling type of gait.

Standing Postural Examination

The standing postural examination gives useful information prior to evaluating the lumbar spine. There are specific findings to consider from the standing structural exam that will help you diagnose and treat the lumbar region. The presence of paravertebral muscle humping on one side or the other may be indicative of a group lateral curve (scoliosis). Unequal iliac crests, unequal greater trochanters, and asymmetric sacral sulcus depth may indicate a short leg syndrome and sacral base unleveling. During the lateral view, an increased or decreased lumbar lordosis is important to note. The presence of pelvic sideshift may correlate with an iliopsoas spasm on the side opposite the shift.

Active Motion Testing

Active motion is motion performed by the patient without assistance. It is always a good idea (especially after an injury) to have the patient actively move (prior to passive testing) to see his or her limits due to pain. The normal lumbar range of motion for forward flexion is 40 to 60 degrees, for extension 20 to 35 degrees,

for lateral bending 15 to 20 degrees, and for rotation 3 to 18 degrees (7). Passive motion testing is performed by the physician with the patient remaining relaxed. It is important that the physician observe not only the quantity of motion, but also the quality of motion.

Examination of Other Body Systems

In the low back pain patient, always evaluate heart, lungs, and abdomen on each patient visit. Auscultate the four quadrants of the abdomen to determine the presence, location, frequency, and pitch of peristaltic waves. An intermittent, low, occasional slow gurgle is normal. Conversely, high-pitched tinkling sounds may denote a developing bowel obstruction. Absence of bowel sounds may indicate a paralytic ileus. A bruit in the midline of the abdomen between the xiphoid process and the umbilicus could indicate renal stenosis or abdominal aortic aneurysm (especially when associated with a pulsating abdominal mass). A bruit at the junction between the middle and outer two thirds of the inguinal region could indicate a significant atherosclerosis of the common iliac or femoral artery. A bruit over the umbilical region could indicate a saddle thrombosis or severe atherosclerosis at the bifurcation of the abdominal aorta. The abdomen is also palpated for masses. Palpation is aided by mental visualization of the liver, kidneys, stomach, small intestines, bifurcation of the aorta at the level of the umbilicus, and the colon. The midline region between the xiphoid and umbilicus should be palpated for any pulsating tumor (abdominal aneurysm). Anteriorly occurring pulsations are normal, but lateral pulsations of the aorta suggest an aneurysm, especially if it is widened greater than 1 in (a normal adult abdominal aorta should not be wider than 1 in). Anterior Chapman points related to organs associated with symptoms in the lumbar region are located around the umbilicus, the pelvis, and in the iliotibial bands. Tender points in these locations may be associated with hypersympathetic activity resulting from viscerosomatic reflexes initiated in an irritated colon or pelvic organ, and the physician should question the patient regarding dysfunction of the organ most likely to be associated with that particular tender point. A positive response to specific questioning helps position a somatic clue according to its significance and rank when considering a differential diagnosis. Other physical examination tests for the abdomen of a patient are covered in other chapters.

If you suspect an arthritic process or other rheumatologic presentation, the eye examination may reveal the presence of conjunctivitis (reactive arthritis) or iritis (ankylosing spondylitis). Examination of the oropharynx may reveal painless (reactive arthritis) or painful (Behçet syndrome) oral ulcers. Lymphadenopathy may be associated with neoplastic processes (lymphoma) infectious processes (tuberculosis and subacute bacterial endocarditis) or idiopathic processes (sarcoidosis).

Neurologic Testing and Muscle Strength

It is important to perform a good thorough neurologic examination prior to evaluating the lumbar spinal segments. Attention is paid to the sensory, motor, and deep tendon reflex aspects of the neurologic examination. It is common practice to evaluate for muscle atrophy (lower motor neuron), dural tension signs and nerve root irritation (radiculopathy), and muscle spasticity with clonus (upper motor neuron). The differentiation of upper motor neuron, nerve root, and peripheral nerve lesions is an important one. Here are some clinical pearls that are helpful in evaluating sensation, strength, and deep tendon reflexes (DTRs).

Sensation

The clinician can evaluate gross sensory loss, or more specific sensory loss. A knowledge of the dermatomes is important as well as a knowledge of the distribution of the peripheral nerves. The best way to evaluate sensation is by two-point discrimination. Many clinicians use a bent paper clip for this test. Testing for hot/cold evaluates the spinothalamic tract. Evaluation for balance and proprioception evaluates the dorsal column/medial lemniscal system.

Muscle Strength

Of the possible neurologic abnormalities, true muscle weakness is the most reliable indication of persistent nerve compression with loss of nerve conduction (5). The patient should perform 10 toe raises on both feet and 10 more on each foot separately. Repeated testing causes fatigue, which accentuates differences in strength in the lower extremities. Patients may also be asked to walk on their heels to test for strength of the dorsiflexors of the foot (L5), or walk on their toes, which test the gastrocnemius/soleus complex (S1).

Deep Tendon Reflexes

DTRs are monosynaptic. Performing them correctly and symmetrically is important. You can reinforce the reflex by having patients attempt to pull apart their locked hands will distract them, allowing for relaxation of muscles. Unilateral loss of an ankle reflex is a significant neurologic sign, irrespective of age (5). Hyperactive reflexes may indicate an upper motor neuron lesion. Certain metabolic conditions can affect the deep tendon reflex (thyroid disease, calcium, and magnesium abnormalities).

Abdominal Reflexes

The superficial abdominal reflex is elicited by rubbing a sharp object in a rhomboid shape on the abdomen. A positive abdominal reflex, results in the retraction of the umbilicus in the direction of the quadrant stroked. Unilateral absence of the reflex suggests a lesion of an ipsilateral nerve root between T7 and L2, depending on the quadrant affected. If a positive Babinski reflex is present, the absence of abdominal reflexes takes on greater significance.

The clinician who evaluates the patient with low back pain needs to understand sensory, motor, and reflex changes that can occur at the L1 through S1 levels (see Table 40.4).

Autonomic Dysfunction

Nocioception from the low back, and especially the low lumbar spine, is transmitted to the cord by way of the C-fibers. These fibers travel with the sympathetic chain, enter the thoracolumbar area, synapse in the intermediolateral cell columns, and produce significant thoracolumbar irritability. To the palpating clinician, the muscles are hyperactive, hypertonic, and irritable. The sympathetic chain terminates in the ganglion impar, which is the lowest level of sympathetic ganglia in the spinal area.

Palpation and Motion Testing

The lumbar region is assessed during the physical examination in the same fashion as all other regions of the spine. Regional and segmental mechanics should be identified by evaluating the patient's overall body pattern; looking for tissue texture change, asymmetry of position, restriction of motion, and tenderness. As a rule, osteopathic physicians treat functional restrictions of motion, not only positional changes. Therefore, the lumbar spine's relationship to mechanics above and below must be evaluated.

Palpation of Tissue Texture Changes

Palpation for tissue texture changes and motion testing of the lumbar spinal segments is typically done seated or prone. Sometimes, palpation of the lumbar spine is done in the supine position, especially in the hospitalized patient. Tissue texture changes are palpable evidence of physiologic dysfunction. This may be due to positional change of a vertebral segment or perhaps from a viscerosomatic reflex from the kidneys, ureters, colon, or pelvic viscera. These patterns called viscerosomatic reflexes may or may not be related to the patient's chief complaint. Finding such reflexes may require the physician to perform a more detailed history or modify the patient's work-up.

Once an area of tissue texture change is found, segmental motion testing in that region is performed. This includes determining rotational, sidebending/translation, and flexion/extension motion restrictions. Determination is made if the findings support the diagnosis of a type II single segment dysfunction or a type I group curve dysfunction. For dysfunction to be present, the components of Tissue texture change, Asymmetry, motion Restriction, and Tenderness need to be present. The more of these that are present indicates the stronger association with somatic dysfunction. Besides palpation for restrictions in spinal joint motion, the astute clinician will also check for the presence and significance of Jones tenderpoints, Chapman's points, and myofascial restrictions. The presence of Chapman reflexes and puffy or boggy tissue texture changes may indicate that a viscerosomatic reflex is present. Motion of the lumbar spine when significant viscerosomatic reflexes are present is described as a "reluctance to motion," as contrasted to an absolute restriction. The barrier is "rubbery", as if more and more tight muscles are being engaged as the end point of permitted motion is reached. When motion testing, the clinician may find less segmental findings and more muscle/group findings.

Group Curve: Fryette Type 1 Mechanics

Group Curves are best identified with the patient standing or seated. The curve appears as prominent muscle mass over the convexity. The prominent muscle mass is a reflection of the rotational component of the curve. Curves can be tested for rotation and sidebending (seated position preferred). Standing behind the seated patient, control the patient's upper torso with one hand over the patient's shoulder girdle with your forearm in front of the other shoulder. (e.g., the physician's left hand would be over the patient's right shoulder, while the physician's left forearm would be in front of the patient's left shoulder) For gross motion testing, the physician's right hand would contact the patient's lumbar paraspinal area. The physician, using both the upper torso control and pushing directly over a lumbar transverse process, would introduce left rotation. To test right rotation, the physician has to change hands (right hand and forearm controlling the upper torso, left hand on left paraspinal area). Sidebending can be evaluated by providing a sidebending force through the upper torso and monitoring movement at the lumbar segments. Lateral curves are relatively free when attempting to increase the curve and somewhat resistant when attempting prone motion testing.

Sacral base unleveling from inequity of leg length, among other things, will result in lumbar type I mechanics. Typically, the resulting curve will be convex on the low side of the sacral unleveling. Pelvic sideshift to one side usually results in a lumbar curve convex on the opposite side. A type I lumbar curve may also develop as compensation for group curve mechanics above, as in idiopathic scoliosis. In idiopathic scoliosis, if the primary curve is thoracic, the convexity will commonly be on the right side. Typically, the

compensatory lumbar curve will be convex on the side opposite the thoracic primary scoliotic convexity. A thoracolumbar convexity may also be seen with idiopathic scoliosis. In this case, the curve may be convex left or right (Fig. 40.11). If a lumbar curve is the primary curve (greater as determined by Cobb method) (Fig. 40.12), the compensatory thoracic curve will be on the

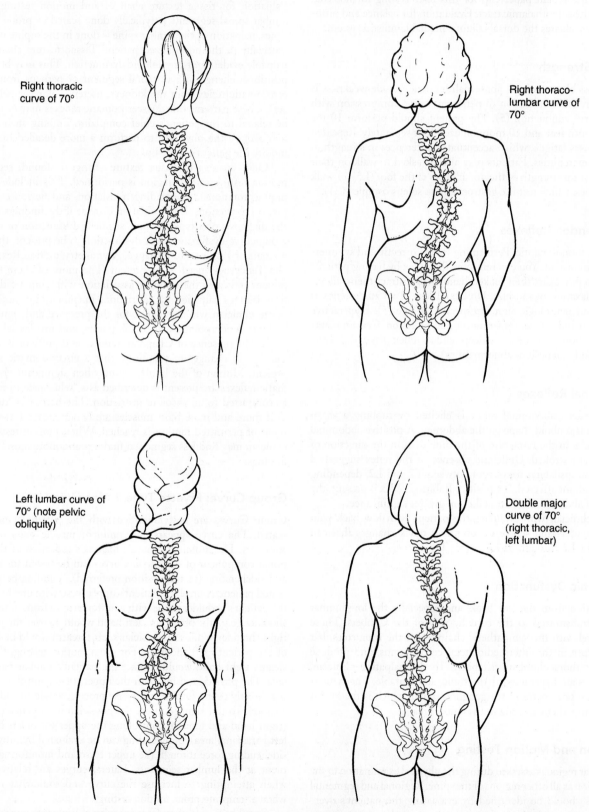

Right thoracic
curve of 70°

Right thoraco-
lumbar curve of
70°

Left lumbar curve of
70° (note pelvic
obliquity)

Double major
curve of 70°
(right thoracic,
left lumbar)

Figure 40-11 Curve patterns in idiopathic types of scoliosis classified by location.

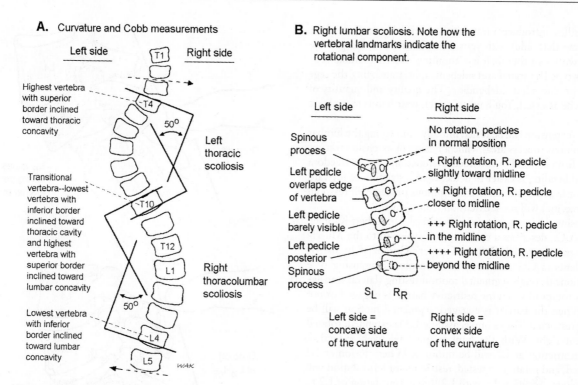

A. Curvature and Cobb measurements

Left side   T1   Right side

Highest vertebra
with superior
border inclined
toward thoracic
concavity

T4

50°

Left
thoracic
scoliosis

Transitional
vertebra--lowest
vertebra with
inferior border
inclined toward
thoracic cavity
and highest
vertebra with
superior border
inclined toward
lumbar concavity

T10

T12

L1

Right
thoracolumbar
scoliosis

Lowest vertebra
with inferior
border inclined
toward lumbar
concavity

50°

L4

L5   WAK

B. Right lumbar scoliosis. Note how the
vertebral landmarks indicate the
rotational component.

Left side   Right side

Spinous
process

No rotation, pedicles
in normal position

Left pedicle
overlaps edge
of vertebra

+ Right rotation, R. pedicle
slightly toward midline

++ Right rotation, R. pedicle
closer to midline

Left pedicle
barely visible

+++ Right rotation, R. pedicle
in the midline

Left pedicle
posterior
Spinous
process

++++ Right rotation, R. pedicle
beyond the midline

S_L   R_R

Left side =
concave side
of the curvature

Right side =
convex side
of the curvature

Figure 40-12 Measurement of curvature and rotation using the Cobb method. In the Cobb method, identification of the top and bottom of each curve is most important.

opposite side. In both these examples, the lumbar spine will demonstrate type I mechanics as described above.

Diagnosis of group curves involves a significant component of inspection. On forward bending, the rotational component of the curve produces a "humping" of the paravertebral muscle mass. In the thoracic spine, the scapula protrudes posteriorly. A group curve is group motion (two or more segments), with rotation and sidebending to opposite sides. Motion of a group curve can be evaluated by sidebending the curve. A lateral curve will increase with sidebending toward the concavity and will resist sidebending toward the convexity. A rotational test may yield confusing results depending on which part of the curve you are trying to rotate. If you push on the convex side from the apex down, you will experience resistance to rotation. However, if testing a segment above the apex, you will have to push on the concave side to encounter motion restriction. Relative to tissue texture change, there is muscle hypertonicity on the convex side, greatest at the apex. The muscles on the convex side of a lumbar group curve have been stretched. The muscles on the concave side of a group curve are shortened. Remember, palpate from side to side to pick up these tight superficial muscles. Relative to clinical problem solving, you need to ask the question: What is the cause of the curve? Some curves have existed for a long period of time so that anatomic adaptation has taken place. Given an anesthetic and curare (which paralyses muscles), the curve will persist. The cause is often from postural imbalance, scoliosis, or trauma. Some curves are not fixed, and are of short duration. The cause may be postural imbalance. However, sometimes a focal muscle contraction on the concave side is the cause of the curve. This focal contraction may be associated with a type II dysfunction with rotation into the concavity of the group curve. The curve represents a positional adaptation to the local muscle pull from a single segment dysfunction. If you treat the cause of the local muscle pull (or "kink"), the curve will disappear (13).

Segmental Dysfunction: Fryette's Type II Mechanics

Most students of the ostepathic medical profession prefer the *prone* position for determination of type II mechanics of the lumbar spine. The prone position is ideal for evaluating tenderness and tissue texture abnormality. To diagnose the lumbar spine in the prone position, place your thumbs over the transverse processes. "Grab some torso" with the rest of the hand. Instead of attempting to rotate a segment by pushing on a transverse process, rotate the torso with your hands in addition to applying pressure over the transverse process. Rotation is evaluated by grasping the patient's torso with the thumbs over the transverse process area. Rotation testing of each of the five lumbar vertebrae is the most accurate and time-efficient method of screening for lumbar somatic dysfunction, because the transverse processes are directly lateral to the spinous process of the lumbar vertebra being tested. Instead of simply pushing anteriorly over the transverse process, attempt to rotate the entire segment and the torso. Compare freedom versus resistance. Remember from a terminology issue, the direction of movement of the most anterior superior portion of the vertebral body is the direction of rotation. Additionally, you should be able to palpate tissue texture abnormality in an area of motion restriction. Sidebending with the patient in the prone position is tested using the same physician hand placement, but lateral translation is applied instead of rotation. Right translation is similar to left sidebending. Flexion and extension are tested with downward (anterior) pressure over the spinous process. Resistance to anterior pressure suggests a flexed dysfunction, while excess freedom with anterior pressure suggests extension. Most psoas dysfunctions are associated with a flexed upper lumbar dysfunction.

For *seated* segmental motion testing, force can be localized to a segment by placing your thumb on the side of a lumbar spinous process. Evaluating translation is particularly effective. In addition to introducing and controlling motion through the patient's shoulder girdles, introduce a translatory motion by contacting the patient's torso (left side) with your torso. While you can provide some force with your thumb, it is a "monitor." Given a lumbar segment that is type II, rotated and sidebent right, translating the segment right produces left sidebending. The quality and quantity of motion can be assessed. You have to switch your hands to evaluate the left side.

Flexion/extension can be tested initially monitoring the lumbar segment (spinous process area) while a flexion or extension force is introduced from above. For extended dysfunctions, excess freedom of backward bending is easier to detect than restriction of forward bending. For flexed dysfunctions, the spinous process will resist an anterior force, and will resist extension from above.

Diagnosing flexion vs. extension is critical. Dr. Robert Kappler, D.O., F.A.A.O., describes a corollary he developed to the Muscle Energy diagnostic model. Called "Kappler's Corollary" by osteopathic students in Chicago, the process involves diagnosing type II dysfunctions through segmental motion testing (lateral translation and/or rotation) when the restrictive barrier is engaged or not engaged. When the barrier is engaged, segmental motion will be excessively restricted. For example, assume L2 is extended, rotated and sidebent right. With the lumbar spine relatively extended, rotational restriction at L2 will be minimal. When flexion at L2 is introduced, and rotation is tested, restriction of left rotation will be very obvious. Additionally, with L2 flexed, translation of L2 to the right will be significantly restricted. Remember, treatment of type II (non-neutral) dysfunctions requires a proper diagnosis of the flexion/extension component as well as the rotation and sidebending component.

Atypical Findings

It is not uncommon to find single segment dysfunction that does not obey Fryette's principles of spinal motion. This is especially true at the L5 level. Variations in anatomy (facet tropism, transitional segments etc.) can cause atypical mechanics as well as traumatic injuries to the area. Figure 40.13 shows palpatory findings of spondylolisthesis. Disc protrusions with local muscle splinting/guarding can also make accurate diagnosis of the mechanical pattern inconsistent. When atypical segmental mechanics are present at L5, look for group curve mechanics and if a forward torsion is present. L5 may have single segment dysfunction, be part of a group curve, or be part of a forward or backward torsion.

Specific Tests

Straight Leg Raising Test (Lasègue Test)

The classic test of sciatic nerve (L1-5, S1) irritation is the SLR test (Fig. 40.14). Its purpose is to stretch the dura. The more useful SLR test is done by raising the leg with the knee extended. When the sciatic nerve is stretched and its nerve roots and corresponding dural attachments are inflamed, the patient experiences pain along its anatomic course to the lower leg, ankle, and foot. The test is performed with the patient in the supine position and the hip medially rotated and adducted, with the knee extended, the examiner flexes the hip until the patient complains of pain in the back of the symptomatic leg (18). Symptoms should not be produced in the lower leg until the leg is raised to 30 to 35 degrees. Initiation of the radicular pain at a lower angle of leg elevation (i.e., 30 degrees) is associated with a larger disc protrusion documented at the time of surgery (7). Until 30 degree elevation, there is no dural movement. Between 30 and 60 to 70 degrees, tension is applied to

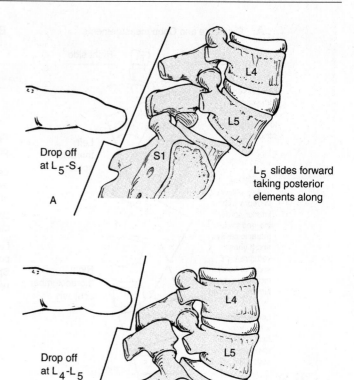

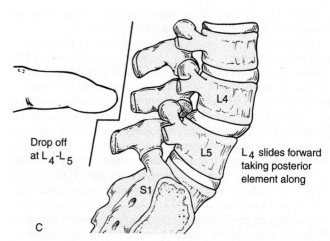

Figure 40-13 Location of anteriorly located spinous process (drop-off sign) depends on underlying mechanism of spondylolisthesis. **A.** In dysplastic spondylolisthesis, L5-S1 horizontal facets allow entire spine to glide forward creating drop-off between L5 and S1. **B.** In isthmic spondylolisthesis, pars defect between L5 and S1 allows anterior elements of L5 to slide forward along with the rest of the spine. Posterior elements of L5 remain behind with the sacrum, creating drop-off between L4 and L5. **C.** Degenerative spondylolisthesis at L4-5 does not affect anterior and posterior elements of the vertebral unit and therefore the drop-off sign is located between L4 and L5.

the dura and nerve roots. Symptoms produced at elevations above 70 degrees may represent nerve root irritation, but may also be related to mechanical low back pain secondary to muscle strain or to joint disease (7). The test is considered positive when the patient's radicular symptoms are reproduced. The diagnostic

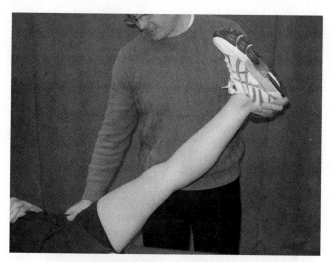

Figure 40-14   Straight leg raising.

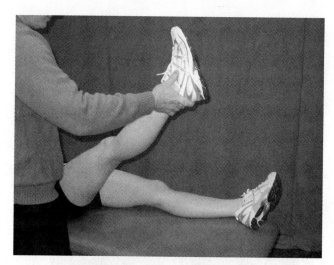

Figure 40-16   Contralateral SLR.

accuracy of the SLR test is limited by its low specificity. The diagnosis of a radiculopathy should not be based on an SLR test alone but on the totality of evidence from all the physical findings.

Bragard Test

A modification of the SLR test, called Bragard test, involves dorsiflexion of the patient's ankle (Fig. 40.15). As the leg is lowered back toward the table, until the patient experiences no pain, the examiner then dorsiflexes the ankle. If the dorsiflexion movement of the ankle reproduces the patient's symptoms, then the test is positive indicating a radiculopathy (18).

Contralateral—Straight Leg Raising Test

A positive contralateral SLR test is when the clinician lifts the uninvolved leg and the patient experiences radicular symptoms down the involved leg (Fig. 40.16). A positive contralateral SLR test is less sensitive but more specific than the SLR test for disc herniation (1). The test is usually indicative of a large disc herniation usually medial to the nerve root affecting both exiting roots (18).

Nachlas Test (Prone Knee Bending Test)

For "high" discs (L2-3 and L3-4), dural irritability is checked by the *Nachlas test*, which assesses irritation of the roots of the femoral

nerve—L2, L3 (Fig. 40.17) (1,18). With the patient prone, the L2-3 nerve roots are stretched by bending the knee until the heel reaches the ipsilateral buttocks. In patients who cannot achieve this, the examiner should flex the patient's knee as far as possible, then passively elevate the thigh up from the examining table. The flexed knee position should be maintained for 45 to 60 seconds. The test is positive if unilateral pain is reproduced in the lumbar area, buttocks, and or posterior thigh (18). If unilateral pain is produced in the front of the thigh (femoral stretch test), this indicates tight quadriceps muscles or a stretching of the femoral nerve (18).

Slump Test

The slump test adds more specificity to the SLR test by placing more dural tension on the affected nerve roots. The seated patient is asked to slump all the way forward and extend the neck (Fig. 40.18). If no symptoms are produced by this position, the examiner then holds the patient's head down (keeping the patients's shoulders slumped) to see if patient's pain is produced. If no pain is present, the clinician extends one of the patient's knees. If still no symptoms are produced, then the clinician should passively dorsiflex the patient's foot (18). Each of these provocative maneuvers applies more tension causing impingement of the dura and spinal cord or nerve roots.

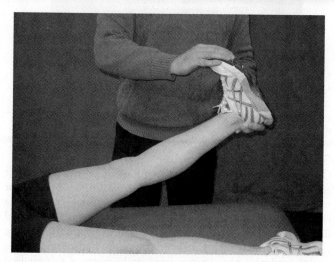

Figure 40-15   Bragard test.

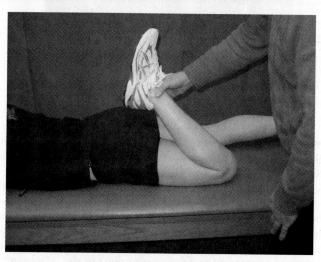

Figure 40-17   Nachlas test.

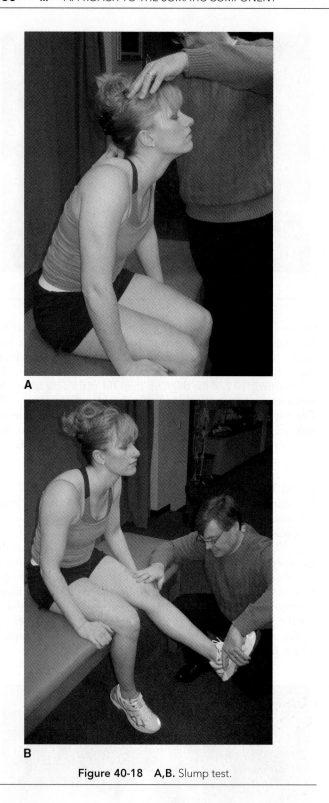

A

B

Figure 40-18   A,B. Slump test.

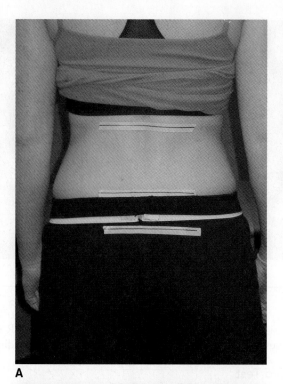

A

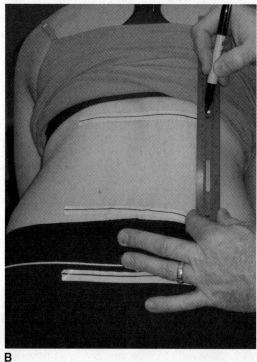

B

Figure 40-19   A,B. Schober test.

Schober Test

Schober test is typically used to measure the amount of lumbar flexion (Fig. 40.19). A point between the sacral dimples (level of S2) is marked with a horizontal line. The second point is marked 5 cm below this line. A third point 10 cm superior to the sacral dimples is also marked. The patient is asked to bend forward and the distance is measured. Patients with less than 4 cm of movement have decreased lumbar flexion. Lumbar extension can also be measured in this fashion. Patients with spondyloarthropathies have abnormal measurements and an abnormal Schober test (18).

Cauda Equina Syndrome

Cauda equina syndrome is a condition of spinal nerve root compression, usually by a massive disc protrusion, fracture or tumor that results in bowel and/or bladder dysfunction. Cauda equina syndrome requires emergent management and surgical decompression within 48 hours or permanent neurologic damage can ensue. Although there is not one single test to determine cauda equina syndrome, the clinician needs to be aware of this medical emergency. In suspected cases, sensory loss of the perineum (saddle anesthesia) and decreased anal sphincter tone are found. If these findings are present, additional tests and emergent management must be undertaken.

Tests for Malingering

To evaluate patients with these functional disorders, a list of physical signs was developed by Waddell and colleagues (7). Any of the individual signs count as one if positive. A finding of three or more of the five types is clinically significant. Isolated positive signs are ignored. The physical signs include Nonanatomic/nonorganic tenderness, thoracic, or low back pain with vertical pressure on the skull of a patient who is standing, neck or back pain reported when the shoulders and pelvis are passively rotated in the same plane, numbness in the forearm in the supinated and pronated positions, and over reaction to a normal stimulus.

Testing the Abdominal Diaphragm

This test is for the diagnosis of abdominal diaphragmatic dysfunction, or testing for evidence of flattening of the dome of the diaphragm. Diaphragm somatic dysfunction can occur in relationship to upper lumbar dysfunction. The physician grasps the lateral sides of the patient's lower rib cage and tests for right and left rotational preference of the deep fasciae. Freedom of rotation in both directions is a negative test. The patient is instructed to, "Take a deep breath in and out." At this point, if the patient has a flattened diaphragm, movement can be detected on only one side of the thoracoabdominal region.

Hip Drop Test

This test is a screening procedure to determine how well the lumbar spine compensates to sacral base declination. It is performed by having the patient stand on one leg and observing the position of the pelvis. *Negative test:* The iliac crest on the unsupported side drops 20 to 25 degrees, and there is a smooth lumbar curvature toward the weight-bearing side of the body. *Positive test:* The iliac crest *does not* drop 20 to 25 degrees on the non–weight-bearing side, and there is an angled, uneven, or poor lumbar spinal curve toward the weight-bearing side. A positive test indicates that the lumbar and/or thoracolumbar spine has difficulty side-bending toward the weight-bearing side of the body (i.e., the side *opposite* the positive test) (5).

Thomas Test

The Thomas test for psoas tension (hip flexion contracture) is the standard evaluation tool in physical therapy and orthopedics (Fig. 40.20). Patients are tested in the supine position. The patient

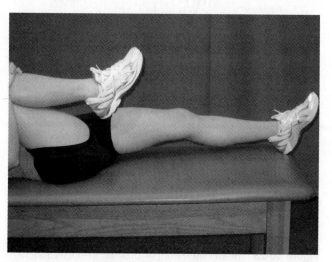

Figure 40-20   Thomas test.

lies supine on the examination table and holds the uninvolved knee to his or her chest, while allowing the involved extremity to lie flat. Holding the knee to the chest flattens out the lumbar lordosis and stabilizes the pelvis. If the iliopsoas muscle is shortened, or a contracture is present, the lower extremity on the involved side will be unable to fully extend at the hip (i.e., the thigh and popliteal region will not lay flat on the table). Degrees of hip flexion can be measured with a goniometer. The Thomas test is a "positional test," and unlike the prone evaluation of hip extension provides limited "end feel."

Evaluation of the Iliopsoas Muscle

Evaluation of the psoas muscle is a critical component to the evaluation of the lumbar spine. Iliopsoas hypertonicity is a common finding in acute and chronic lower back pain. Though a patient with chronic or subacute shortening of the psoas muscle can usually lie prone, the patient with acute psoas spasm or shortening cannot usually lay prone (flat) on the table. In this case, the physician can have the patient turn to the lateral recumbent position and attempt to extend the leg at the hip.

Iliopsoas hypertonicity has a neurologic component in the upper lumbar spine (L1, L2 FRS dysfunction). Treatment of psoas problems must not neglect this upper lumbar component (8). Clinicians need to diagnose this and treat the L1, L2 region, in addition to treating or stretching the tight psoas muscle. Psoas tightness may be reflex from disc herniations as well. Sometimes, psoas tension causes pelvic side shift so that the painful side bears less weight. For example, right lumbosacral pain will result in side shift right.

The basic biomechanical function is hip flexion. The psoas muscle is a long restrictor muscle. Long restrictors span two or more joints. Hypertonicity/shortening of the psoas compresses the hip joint, the SI joint, and the lumbar spine. When the psoas muscle is dysfunctional, it may also be weak. Attempting to exercise the psoas major simply compounds the problem. The hypertonicity and shortening (with resistance to lengthening) is the problem. Psoas problems can produce anterior thigh neurologic symptoms. The lumbar plexus passes through the psoas muscle, and anterior thigh discomfort results from nerve irritation.

Since the psoas is a muscle of postural balance, postural imbalance is a consequence of psoas problems. Pelvic side shift occurs with psoas tension; contraction of the left psoas produces pelvic side shift right. With pelvic sideshift right, a lumbar curve convex left is produced. Psoas hypertonicity causes restriction of SI motion, from compression and sometimes sideshift. If the seated flexion test is positive, you must evaluate the psoas as a possible cause. Diagnosis of psoas problems involves two separate components:

1. Restriction of hip extension, and
2. Ipsilateral upper lumbar (L1 or L2) which is flexed, rotated, and sidebent to the side of the shorter psoas.

Jones Tender Points, Chapman Reflexes

In a thorough physical examination of the lumbar spine, the clinician should evaluate for the presence of Jones tenderpoints. Remember that Jones tenderpoints correlate to lumbar segmental dysfunction. If a Jones L5 anterior tenderpoint is present, the clinician should evaluate the L5 segment for somatic dysfunction and vice versa. Treatment of the tenderpoint may improve or resolve the segmental dysfunction at L5. Treatment of the lumbar spine and/or sacrum may resolve the anterior L5 tenderpoint. So, Jones tenderpoints can give the clinician a clue of where articular dysfunction exists. Jones tenderpoints can also give the clinician a clue

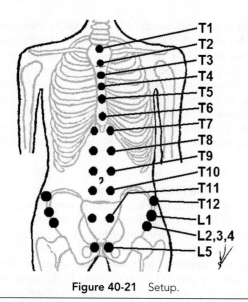

Figure 40-21 Setup.

of which muscle is dysfunctional and what muscles need exercises or stretches (Figs. 40.21 and 40.22).

Chapman reflex points are palpated to determine if there is a visceral relationship to the patient's lumbar spine complaint. Chapman reflex points are one of the early diagnostic clues to irritation and dysfunction of viscera. If Chapman reflex points for the lumbar region are to be evaluated, palpate for them at the beginning of the physical examination, because motion and repeated palpation or stretching of the myofascial tissues in their location will decrease their sensitivity and diagnostic value; their tenderness to palpation will disappear, at least for a period of time. Chapman points found around the umbilicus may be related to the bladder, kidney, or adrenal glands. Those over the pubic symphysis may be related to gonadal tissue. Posterior Chapman points to the large intestine lie in a triangular area on either side of the lower lumbar spine. If large bowel problems are suspected, do not give lumbar soft tissue treatment until you have palpated the anterior points related to the colon (found in the iliotibial bands) to secure data that would help confirm this suspicion. Chapman points should be carefully correlated with history, palpation, tenderness of the collateral

abdominal ganglia, and spinal somatic dysfunction, as well as with the palpation of the suspected organ system to determine their significance. (Figs. 40.23 and 40.24).

DIAGNOSTIC IMAGING

Diagnostic imaging of the lumbar spine is useful especially in young patients (<18 years old), patients >50 years old (malignancy might be a concern), trauma cases, or patients who have a neurologic deficit. For patients with uncomplicated lower back pain and no other medical issues, radiographs should be reserved until patients have documented that they are refractory to conservative management (14).

Asymptomatic patients commonly have some x-ray and MRI changes in the lumbar spine. It is important to remember that just because anatomic change is present and identifiable on radiographs, it is not necessarily the cause of any particular component of a patient's pain. A study that highlights this point is one performed by Friedenberg and Miller. They found that in asymptomatic patients between 30 and 70 years of age, 35% had radiographic evidence of spondylosis (14). Jensen and coworkers found only 35%

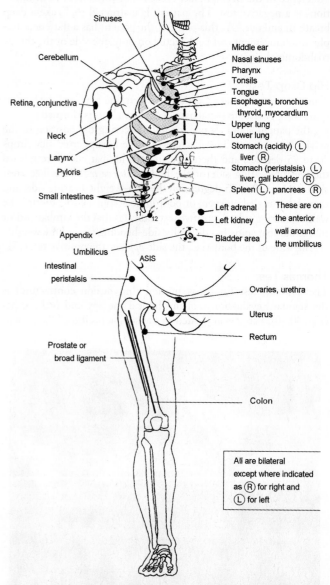

Figure 40-23 Treatment for upper thoracic type II dysfunction.

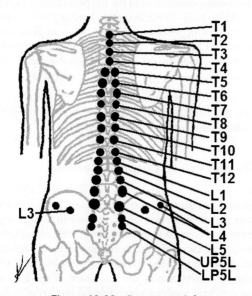

Figure 40-22 Rotation to left.

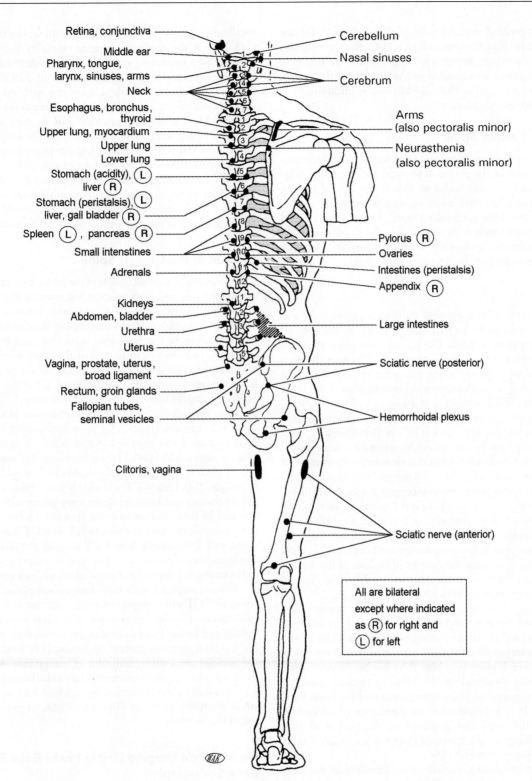

Retina, conjunctiva — Cerebellum

Middle ear — Nasal sinuses

Pharynx, tongue, larynx, sinuses, arms — Cerebrum

Neck

Esophagus, bronchus, thyroid — Arms (also pectoralis minor)

Upper lung, myocardium — Neurasthenia (also pectoralis minor)

Upper lung

Lower lung

Stomach (acidity) (L)

liver (R)

Stomach (peristalsis) (L)

liver, gall bladder (R)

Spleen (L), pancreas (R) — Pylorus (R)

Small intestines — Ovaries

Adrenals — Intestines (peristalsis)

— Appendix (R)

Kidneys

Abdomen, bladder

Urethra — Large intestines

Uterus

Vagina, prostate, uterus, broad ligament — Sciatic nerve (posterior)

Rectum, groin glands

Fallopian tubes, seminal vesicles — Hemorrhoidal plexus

Clitoris, vagina

— Sciatic nerve (anterior)

All are bilateral except where indicated as (R) for right and (L) for left

Figure 40-24   Treatment for lower thoracic, type I dysfunction. **A.** Anterior and **B.** Posterior view.

of 98 asymptomatic individuals (mean age, 42.3 years) had normal lumbar MR scans (14).

Most neurodiagnostic imaging studies have a high sensitivity (the ability to detect anatomic abnormalities) but a low specificity (the ability to remain negative in the absence of clinical disease). The CT scan and MRI of the lumbosacral spine detect anatomic changes that are not associated with symptoms in a significant proportion of patients. Strict adherence to the 1994 Acute Low Back Pain Guidelines to obtain plain roentgenograms for

individuals with fever, unexplained weight loss, cancer history, neurologic deficits, drug abuse history, an age older than 50 years, or trauma results in overutilization of roentgenograms compared to usual ordering patterns (14). As patients reach age 50, up to 95% of adults who come to autopsy show evidence of aging changes in the lumbosacral spine with disc space narrowing calcification, or marginal sclerosis. Therefore, not everyone with acute low back pain requires a set of plain roentgenograms. If the clinician is comfortable with diagnosis of an acute low back strain in a young patient, treatment may proceed without radiographic evaluation for the first 4 to 6 weeks after the onset of pain (14). Roentgenograms are indicated if there is no response to the treatment. On the other hand, roentgenograms are indicated on the first visit if the patient is older (>50 years of age) or there is additional medical information that requires investigation.

X-Ray of the Lumbar Spine

When interpreting roentgenograms, an organized and orderly process should be used by the physician to avoid missing subtle findings. It is generally recommended to look at the area of highest interest last. In general, three roentgenographic views are all that are required to assess the lumbosacral spine. An AP view, a lateral view, and spot lateral view to better visualize the lower two interspaces. When a lumbar spine series is ordered, two oblique views are also taken in order to help identify spondylolysis.

AP View

When looking at an AP radiograph of the lumbar region, the transverse processes will not be located directly lateral to the spinous process of their parent vertebra. The primary soft tissue structure seen in the AP projection is the psoas muscle. The psoas forms a triangular shape with the top at the transverse process of L1 and the base on the iliac crests. Asymmetrical visualization of the psoas muscle indicates clinical pathology in a minority of patients since positioning, muscle contraction, and rotation may affect the definition of the muscle border. The loss of a pedicle ("winking-owl" sign) is frequently seen in patients with metastatic disease to the spine. Scoliosis is commonly seen in this view and measurement of the degree of curvature using the Cobb method may be useful.

The lateral view is useful for evaluating for spondylolisthesis, an anterior slippage of one vertebra on the spinal segment below. When the vertebrae slips posterior, it is termed a retrolisthesis. Disc space narrowing, compression fractures, facet joints, vertebral endplate changes, and Schmorl nodes are evaluated in this view. It is also possible to measure the amount of lordosis of the lumbar spine using Cobb method as was done in the AP view. Normal lumbar lordosis ranges from 35 to 50 degrees.

The close-up view (spot view) of the L5-S1 area provides information about the status and alignment of the L5-S1 intervertebral disc space, and the upper portion of the sacrum. The L5-S1 disc space and intervertebral foramina are narrower than the spaces between the other lumbar vertebrae. The lumbar intervertebral foramina are best visualized in the lateral projection. Another radiographic interpretation is the determination of Ferguson lumbosacral angle. It is a measurement of the degree of lordosis or anterior tilt of the sacral base in relation to the horizontal. It is usually 35 to 45 degrees. An increased Ferguson lumbosacral angle relates to lumbosacral instability (5).

The oblique projection is obtained to demonstrate the facet joints and pars interarticularis. In this view, the posterior elements outline a shape that is reminiscent of a "Scotty dog." A collar on the "dog" suggests the presence of spondylolysis, or a stress fracture of the pars interarticularis, an area between the superior and inferior articular facets. The Scotty dog eye is the pedicle, its nose is the transverse process, its fore leg is the inferior articular facet, and its hind leg is the spinous process.

MRI (MR) of the Lumbar Spine

MR has been clinically available since the middle 1980s. Since then, MR has been used increasingly for evaluation of the musculoskeletal system, including low back and neck pain (14). MR is an excellent technique to view the spinal cord within the spinal canal (14). MR is the preferred imaging modality for syringomyelia, atrophy, cord infarction, traumatic injury, intramedullary tumors, or multiple sclerosis affecting the spinal cord. MR also shows early changes in discs and vertebral endplates with infectious discitis (14). The sensitivity of MR is equal to or greater than that of myelography. Most studies suggest that MR is more accurate in the detection of degenerative disc disease than discography or myelography (14). MR is better at imaging soft tissue structures, whereas CT is superior for imaging bony structures. MR is more sensitive than CT for the diagnosis of herniated discs (14). MR, especially when used with gadolinium, has clear advantages for demonstrating intraspinal tumors, detecting disc space infection, and distinguishing recurrent disc herniation from postoperative scar (14).

CT Scan of the Lumbar Spine

CT creates cross-sectional images of the internal structure of the spine at various levels, and, with reformatting, one can also obtain coronal and sagittal sections. The CT scan assesses not only the bony configuration and structure–space relationship but also the soft tissue in graded shadings so that ligaments, nerve roots, free fat, and intervertebral disc protrusions can be evaluated as they relate to their bony environment in a single scan. The CT scan has the great advantage of being noninvasive and safely administered. CT is the study of choice for delineating the bony detail of the lumbar spine. CT is useful in the diagnosis and assessment of trauma, and tumors of the lumbosacral spine. CT scan can visualize the medullary portion of the vertebral body and can detect bone destruction before changes are visible on plain roentgenograms (14). Fragments of bone that may not be detectable by plain roentgenograms are localized to the spinal canal by CT techniques (14). Helical CT scanning is the technique that allows for the continuous spiral motion of the x-ray gantry tube. Helical CT is not used for the evaluation of spinal disorders. However, for detection of viscerogenic causes of low back pain, helical CT is an effective diagnostic tool. For example, helical CT imaging surpasses conventional roentgenograms for detection of ureteral stones and is used commonly in the emergency department in patients with back pain.

When compared with two-dimensional planar imaging (CT scan), SPECT offers improved image contrast and more accurate localization of lesion. For example, in patients with a spinal tumor, activity can be localized to specific positions, such as the vertebral body, pedicle, spinous process, or lamina (14). Lesions that affect the pedicles are a strong indicator of malignancy, whereas lesions in the apophyseal joints are more likely to be benign (14). SPECT scan is useful in the evaluation of vertebral lesions, spondylolysis, stress fractures, facet arthritis, sacroiliitis, pseudoarthrosis, and spinal fusion status.

Radionuclide Imaging (Triple Phase Bone Scan or Bone Scintigraphy)

Radionuclide imaging is a sensitive yet not specific technique for the detection of bone abnormalities. Any process that disturbs the normal balance of bone production and resorption can produce an abnormality on bone scan. Increased osteoblastic activity (hot spot) is associated with greater concentration of radionuclide tracer on the bone scan. Interruption of the blood flow to the bone results in the absence of tracer on the scan (cold spot). The most useful study is a form of three-phase scan that involves an immediate blood pool image that is obtained by sequential images 3 to 5 seconds apart. Images are then obtained after several minutes, at 2 to 4 hours after injection, and occasionally at 24 hours to detect residual increase of bone activity (14). The most commonly used radiopharmaceutical for bone scanning is technetium 99m. A bone scan is particularly useful in circumstances of radiographic changes lagging behind increased bone activity. A bone scan will be positive in infection, inflammation, acute fracture, or malignancy. Because of this, the bone scan has been used most commonly for detecting metastatic disease. Approximately 80% of metastatic lesions are found in the axial skeleton (14). One notable exception to early detection of metastatic bone lesions by bone scan is multiple myeloma. Therefore, the lytic lesions of myeloma do not cause increased activity on bone scan until a fracture occurs (14).

In regard to infections of the bone (osteomyelitis) or discs (discitis), bone scans are useful because radiographs may not be positive for 10 to 14 days after the onset of the disease, whereas the bone scan may be abnormal within the first day (14).

In regard to fractures, trauma to bone, particularly stress fractures, may be difficult to detect by conventional radiography. Bone scintigraphy can detect lesions within 3 days of fracture. In children, the epiphyseal and metaphyseal growth plates are sites of active bone turnover in the areas of increased radionuclide concentration. Other diseases associated with abnormal bone scans include Paget disease, hemoglobinopathies, and aseptic necrosis of bone. Patients with sickle cell anemia have positive bone scans. In patients with acute infarcts of bone, the bone scan may demonstrate a cold spot.

LABORATORY TESTS

The vast majority of individuals with spinal pain do not require laboratory studies with their initial evaluation. Laboratory tests should be used in the situation in which a physician has developed a differential diagnosis by means of a history and physical examination for which laboratory data are needed to confirm or reject specific diagnoses. Laboratory test results should never replace a careful history and physical examination in the evaluation of the patient with spinal pain.

Obtaining baseline lab tests does have a role in separating mechanical from systemic diseases. They are also useful in distinguishing metabolic-endocrinologic disorders from those with more inflammatory characteristics. Patients who are candidates for laboratory evaluation include a patient who fails to respond to medical therapy; a patient who develops a significant change in the character of his or her pain; a patient with a known or suspected history of infectious or rheumatic condition; or an elderly patient with new onset spinal pain. The laboratory tests that are important in the study of disorders associated with spinal pain include acute-phase reactants, complete blood counts, blood chemistries, urinalysis, immunologic studies (cellular and humoral), body fluid analysis, cultures, and tissue biopsy.

Acute-Phase Reactants

Acute-phase reactants are a group of plasma proteins that increase or decrease by at least 25% during an inflammatory disorder (12). The degree of increase is greatest with cancer, severe infections, vasculitis, and burns. However, from a diagnostic or therapeutic orientation, the measurement of inflammatory cytokines does not help identify specific disorders. The most useful test in helping to differentiate medical from mechanical spinal pain is the erythrocyte sedimentation rate (ESR) (15). In general, an elevated ESR suggests the presence of inflammation in the body. The ESR is elevated with tissue injury, whatever the source. The ESR is used to screen for inflammatory disease and to follow the response to therapy. The ESR is normal in mechanical spinal pain. The ESR value must be interpreted according to the sex and age of the patient. The upper limit continues to rise as patients grow older. The change in ESR

may be more important than the absolute value when a patient is evaluated by a clinician.

Markedly elevated ESR (≥100 mm/hr) is most commonly associated with malignancies, particularly those that are metastatic (15). Other diseases associated with markedly increased ESR include connective tissue disease (polymyalgia rheumatica-temporal arteritis), acute bacterial infection (meningitis), and vertebral osteomyelitis with epidural abscess. The ESR also has utility as a means of following the progression or resolution of an inflammatory disorder. The ESR may be normal in patients with systemic diseases, including cancer. The ESR may remain elevated for up to 3 to 5 weeks after spinal surgery, in the absence of infection.

C-reactive protein (CRP) is an acute-phase protein synthesized by hepatocytes. CRP increases within hours of an inflammatory stimulus. CRP usually reaches a peak in 2 to 3 days and then recedes in 3 to 4 days. CRP is more accurate than ESR in detection of infections after spinal surgery because it returns to baseline more quickly than ESR (15). Serial determinations of CRP may also be helpful in following the course of acute and chronic inflammatory illnesses (15). Elevated CRP after disc surgery has been associated with retrodiscal infection that has been detected with magnetic resonance evaluation (15).

The Complete Blood Count

The hematocrit (Hct) level is normal in mechanical spinal pain, including herniated nucleus pulposus, spinal stenosis, and muscle strain. A decrease in Hct is a common finding associated with disorders mediated through chronic inflammation. A decreased Hct level should be evaluated with RBC indices, reticulocyte count, serum iron level, total iron-binding capacity, haptoglobin level, and examination of the stool for occult blood.

The white blood cell (WBC) count is normal in mechanical spinal pain. The WBC count is also normal in many forms of medical spinal pain. An elevated WBC (leukocytosis) count suggests the presence of an infection, particularly if early forms of polymorphonuclear leukocytes (band) are present. Increased numbers of WBCs are also seen in malignancies, particularly those of bone marrow or lymphatic origin. Patients on corticosteroids for their lower back pain have an increased WBC count in the 12,000 to 20,000 cells/mm³ range.

Platelets are normal in mechanical spinal pain and most medical causes as well. In malignancies, platelets are commonly abnormal and may be elevated (thrombocytosis). Platelet levels are frequently decreased in bone marrow and lymphatic tumors (15).

The Chemistry Panel

Calcium and phosphorus levels are also unaltered in osteoarthritis and mechanical causes of spinal pain. However, malignancies are associated with hypercalcemia. Malignancies with elevated serum calcium levels include those with parathormone activity (parathyroid adenoma and oat cell carcinoma of the lung), bone metastases, and multiple myeloma. In patients with lower back pain potentially related to inflammation, infection, or malignancy, (i.e., positive bone scan) indicating osteoblastic activity, one must consider evaluation of alkaline phosphatase (ALP). ALP is produced to the greatest extent by osteoblasts. Any condition that increases osteoblastic activity increases ALP (15). Disorders associated with ALP elevations include Paget disease, metastatic carcinoma, hyperparathyroidism, osteomalacia, fractures (during healing phase), and hypophosphatemia. Of the illnesses that cause spinal pain, metastatic tumors and Paget disease cause the greatest increases (2 to 30 times normal). Up to 86% of patients with metastatic prostate carcinoma and 77% with metastatic breast cancer to bone have ALP elevations (15). Not all elevations of ALP are associated with bone disease. Disease of the hepatobiliary system may be associated with marked increases of ALP activity.

In patients with lower back pain potentially related to chronic inflammation, infection or malignancy, the total protein may be increased. Patients with increased total protein should be evaluated with a serum protein electrophoresis. Marked increase in total protein associated with elevated globulin levels should raise the possibility of multiple myeloma.

The Urinalysis and Renal Function Tests

Abnormalities detected during a routine urinalysis are most helpful in identifying those individuals with viscerogenic-referred lumbar spine pain of genitourinary origin. The presence of proteinuria on a dipstick determination requires further evaluation. Twenty-four-hour urine collections may be helpful in patients with proteinuria to see if they have nephrotic syndrome. If multiple myeloma is suspected, a negative dipstick protein does not rule out the diagnosis because myeloma proteins are not detected by dipstick methods. Elevations in blood urea nitrogen (BUN) and serum creatinine are associated with decreased renal function. Patients with visceral back pain of genitourinary origin may have elevations of these parameters. The drug history is important in a patient with abnormalities of BUN and creatinine.

Rheumatologic Studies

The three tests most commonly ordered are the rheumatoid factor (RF), antinuclear antibody, and uric acid level. The predictive value of these tests is only 35% in a population of individuals with joint disease and an estimated combined prevalence of the three resulting illnesses of 10% (15).

RFs are a group of autoantibodies to human immunoglobulin G. The classic rheumatoid factor is an IgM antibody. Rheumatoid factors occur in a wide range of autoimmune and chronic infectious diseases. Approximately 80% of patients with rheumatoid arthritis are seropositive for RF. RF in low titer may also be identified in and increasing proportion of normal individuals as they grow older. More than 40% of healthy individuals who are 75 years of age have detectable RF (15).

ELECTRODIAGNOSTIC STUDIES

Electromyography with Nerve Conduction Velocity

Electromyography (EMG) with nerve conduction velocity is the study of how action potentials propagate to their corresponding muscle fibers. Electrodiagnostic studies are commonly used in the evaluation of diseases affecting the peripheral nervous system. These studies are extensions of the neurologic examination and provide an objective measure of nerve damage. They can confirm the clinical impression of nerve root compression, define the severity and distribution of involvement, and document or exclude other illnesses of nerves or muscles that could contribute to the patient's symptoms and signs. These studies are also useful in differentiating abnormalities associated with entrapment neuropathies, distal peripheral neuropathies, myopathies, and myelopathies (16). An abnormal EMG is corroborative evidence of organic disease and helps the surgeon select patients who are candidates for surgery. In many patients, electrical signs of nerve damage do not appear until 21 days after the initial insult. EMG

examination done too quickly in the course of events misses the lesion. The test is painful but usually does not require sedation or analgesics. Conduction is measured in the fastest-conducting fibers only. In addition, the extent of EMG abnormalities does not necessarily correlate with the extent of nerve damage. These studies may identify a specific nerve root lesion when clinical symptoms suggest abnormalities at two levels. Electrodiagnostic examination has a degree of accuracy in identifying patients with nerve root compression similar to that of myelography and clinical examination.

Osteopathic Manipulative Approach to Clinical Conditions

When a clinician treats a patient for acute or chronic lower back condition, the treatment approach chosen should follow the medical evidence supporting the most appropriate course of action. It should also take into consideration the clinician's experience, skill, time available, cost, and safety. The efficacy of spinal manipulation has not been clearly demonstrated in either acute or chronic nonspecific low back pain. Tables 40.5 and 40.6 outline nonsurgical treatment guidelines based on clinical evidence.

Acute Lumbar HNP

In patients with acute lumbar herniated discs, OMT can still be used and is quite helpful. Using HVLA technique at the level of herniation is a relative contraindication, especially if neurologic signs are present. Lumbar spinal segments that have an acute disc herniation are considered to be unstable, so mobilization by applying an impulse is counterintuitive. A more appropriate approach is to work on areas of dysfunction above and below the symptomatic area, to off-load pressure across the disc space. Relieving iliopsoas tension will reduce compressive load across the disc spaces. Counterstrain is a great way of reducing muscle irritability and decreasing pain in an acute setting. Working on the patient in a supine "constant rest" position with his or her hips and knees flexed can be beneficial. Most patients with acute lumbar pain syndromes have somatic dysfunction in the mid-to-upper thoracic spine and ribs. Treating this area, as well as the cranial region, helps reduce overall facilitation and the sympathetic nervous systems response to pain.

Acute Low Back Pain Due to "Psoas Syndrome"

A patient with psoas syndrome will walk into the office flexed forward and listing to one side. They will have significant central lower back pain. They may or may not have sciatic type pain down the opposite leg. In patients with psoas syndrome, the psoas muscle has become significantly tight as demonstrated by restricted hip extension. Acute, severe cases may have a hip flexion contracture and an inability of the patient to lie prone. The causes of an acute psoas spasm are varied; some considerations include prolonged sitting (long car ride), reflex mechanisms from nociceptors (disc protrusion), or a visceral etiology (endometriosis, ureteral stone). The key in this situation is to treat the flexed upper lumbar component of the problem (8). This can be done by direct or indirect methods. After treating the flexed lumbar component, the psoas muscle itself may be treated with any number of techniques, including muscle energy, Still technique, counterstrain, direct stretching, etc. Giving the patient home exercises to stretch the psoas may be helpful. If an underlying disc protrusion is causing the spasm, the constant rest position, ice, and medications are usually required as well to control

TABLE 40.5

Nonsurgical Treatment for Acute, Nonspecific Low Back Pain

Recommended	Efficacy Unclear	Not Recommended
Patient education	Back school	Bed rest
Continue usual activity	Narcotic analgesics	Trunk strengthening exercises
Moderate aerobic activity	Lumbar corsets/belts	Systemic steroids
Acetaminophen	Spinal manipulation	Antidepressants
NSAID or COX-2	Massage	TENS
Muscle relaxants	Multidisciplinary biopsychosocial rehabilitation	Traction
Local ice or heat		Trigger point injections
Cognitive-behavioral		
		Epidural steroids
		Facet joint injections
		Acupuncture

the symptoms and provided some relief to the patient. In cases where an underlying visceral issue is causing the psoas hypertonicity, then treatment of the visceral condition must be undertaken as well.

Iliolumbar Ligament "Syndrome"

The iliolumbar ligament is a small, yet clinically important, ligament that originates from the iliac crest and inserts on the transverse process of L4 and L5. The iliolumbar ligament is pain sensitive and refers pain to the groin, SI region, and lateral thigh. The ligament located on both sides of the lower lumbar spine acts as guide wires to stabilize the lower segments. In patients with L5 disc protrusions, instability, or spondylolisthesis, the iliolumbar ligament may become irritated and painful. There is tissue texture change at the ilial insertion of the ligament. Pelvic sideshift toward the iliolumbar ligament is common. The adductor muscle on the side of the tender ligament is commonly tight. Manipulative techniques for tenderness on or near this ligament primarily include an indirect/

counterstrain approach. Treating this ligament and its surrounding tissues with counterstrain has significant clinical value.

Lumbar Compression Fractures

Despite their apparent strength, the lumbar spine is the most common site for compression fracture. This is because there is a weak spot located in the anterior portion, where the trabecular arrangement and density is reduced. Sufficient flexion with anterior stress can result in a compression fracture of the vertebral body. This anterior area fractures at 75% of the force needed to fracture the posterior portion of the vertebral body. With or without lifting, compression fractures occur most frequently in persons who have reduced calcium and/or frank osteoporosis. Risk factors include Caucasian race, osteoporosis, cigarette smoking, poor diet, prolonged steroid use, prolonged inactivity, or hypoparathyroid disease. Compression fractures may also be a consequence of a malignancy. Even in the absence of risk factors, a compression fracture may be

TABLE 40.6

Nonsurgical Treatment for Chronic, Nonspecific Low Back Pain

Recommended	Efficacy Unclear	Not Recommended
Patient education	Trigger point injections	Bed rest
Continue usual activity	Epidural steroids	Systemic steroids
Moderate aerobic activity	Facet joint injections	TENS
Acetaminophen	Narcotic analgesics	Traction
NSAID or COX-2	Lumbar corsets/Belts	Acupuncture
Trunk strengthening exercises	Spinal manipulation	
Local ice or heat	Massage	
Cognitive-behavioral	Antidepressants	
Multidisciplinary biopsychosocial rehabilitation	Muscle relaxants	
Back school		

produced in anyone by forceful flexion, for example, in automobile accidents, and jumping off or falling from a considerable height. Early clues to a vertebral compression fracture are provided by the history and physical examination—not radiographs. The history will most likely reveal activities or risk factors like the ones described. If a compression fracture is suspected, do not ask the patient to perform flexion or side-bending. Instead, place the person in a lateral recumbent position for an examination. The physical examination will reveal discomfort, even with light palpation, percussion, or vibration over the spinous process of the involved vertebra. Palpatory discomfort and a history of discomfort with certain spinal motions will be out of proportion to the physical signs of injury. Pain is usually increased by leaning on the patient's shoulders, causing compression of the spinal column, and is eased by pulling cephalad from under the patient's arms, or by holding a gentle extension to the patient's spine. Although pain in the low back is usually immediate, it will be several days after the accident before a routine lateral lumbar radiograph will show a compression deformity of the vertebral body. The spine then angulates at the site of the compression fracture, and the spinous process at that vertebral unit becomes more prominent than normal. For treatment, the patient is given instructions and exercises that encourage gradual extension of the lumbar region, and/or a brace that is specifically ordered for the patient and is applied to prevent active flexion and maintain slight extension. Adequate pain relief medication is provided, taking care not to induce dependency or habituation. The use of codeine in lumbar fractures may be counterproductive, as both the pharmacologic properties of the medication and the nociceptive thoracolumbar reflex facilitation from the injury tend to constipate the patient. Most types of direct osteopathic manipulative treatment over the site of a compression are contraindicated, although classic direct and indirect myofascial treatment may be used to improve lymphatic flow, to reduce segmental facilitation, and to comfort the patient. Pain and Nociception are also reduced by myofascial treatment directed toward relief of sympathicotonia and general improvement of lymphatic drainage. Secondary sites of somatic dysfunction that develop as a result of the injury are treated to reduce their secondary facilitation of related cord segments. Only methods and activations that are comfortable for the patient and that do not stimulate the site of injury are used to reduce discomfort and promote normal healing (5).

REFERENCES

1. Borenstein DJ, Wiesel SW, Bowden SD. *Low Back and Neck Pain.* Philadelphia, PA: WB Saunders, 2004:41–45; chap 2, Epidemiology.
2. Borenstein DJ, Wiesel SW, Bowden SD. *Low Back and Neck Pain.* Philadelphia, PA: WB Saunders, 2004:89–101; chap 4, History.
3. Borenstein DJ, Wiesel SW, Bowden SD. *Low Back and Neck Pain.* Philadelphia, PA: WB Saunders, 2004:49–84; chap 3, Sources of Spinal Pain.
4. Moore KL. *Clinical Oriented Anatomy.* 2nd Ed. Baltimore, MD: Williams & Wilkins, 1985.
5. Ward R. *Foundations for Osteopathic Medicine.* 2nd Ed. Lippincott Williams & Wilkins; chap 50. Kuchera W., Lumbar Spine.
6. Vleeming A, Mooney, Stoeckart R. The muscular, liagamentour, and neural structure of the lumbosacrum and its relationship to low back pain. In: Willard FH, ed. *Movement, Stability and Lunbopelvic Pain.* 2nd Ed. Elsevier, 2007; chap 1.
7. Borenstein DJ, Wiesel SW, Bowden SD. Physical examination. In: *Low Back and Neck Pain.* Philadelphia, PA: WB Saunders, 2004:117–135; chap 5.
8. Kappler RE. The role of the psoas muscle in postural imbalance. *J Am Osteopath Assoc.* 1973:72:794–801.
9. Travell JG, Simon DG. *Myofascial Pain and Dysfunction: The Trigger Point Manual The Lower Extremities.* Vol II. Baltimore, MD: Williams & Wilkins, 1992.
10. Travell JG, Simon DG. *Myofascial Pain and Dysfunction: The Trigger Point Manual.* Vol 1. Baltimore, MD: Williams & Wilkins, 1999.
11. Glossary of osteopathic terminology. *AOA Yearbook and Directory.* 91st Ed. Chicago, IL: American Osteopathic Association, 2000:869.
12. White AA, Panjabi MM. *Clinical Biomechanics of the Spine.* 2nd Ed. Philadelphia, PA: JB Lippincott, 1990:45.
13. Ward R. *Foundations.* 1st Ed., 979; chap 70.
14. Borenstein DJ, Wiesel SW, Bowden SD. Radiographic evaluation. In: *Low Back and Neck Pain.* Philadelphia, PA: WB Saunders, 2004:146–175; chap 7.
15. Borenstein DJ, Wiesel SW, Bowden SD. Laboratory tests. In: *Low Back and Neck Pain.* Philadelphia, PA: WB Saunders, 2004:137–145; chap 6.
16. Borenstein DJ, Wiesel SW, Bowden SD. Miscellaneous evaluations. In: *Low Back and Neck Pain.* Philadelphia, PA: WB Saunders, 2004:177–187; chap 8.
17. Mainge JY, Mainge R. Painful iliolumbar ligament insertion or cutaneous dorsal ramus pain? An anatomic study. *Arch Phys Med Rehabil* 1991;72: 734–737.
18. Magee DJ. *Orthopedic Physical Assessment.* 4th Ed. St. Louis, MO: Saunders-Elsevier, 2006:452, 513–526, 631.

Pelvis and Sacrum

KURT P. HEINKING AND ROBERT E. KAPPLER

INTRODUCTION

Accurate and efficient diagnosis of the pelvic girdle is of great importance to practitioners of manual medicine. The pelvis holds a central role in coupling the mechanical forces of the lower extremities with the axial skeleton above, as it is the foundation for body support and locomotion. Alterations and restrictions of motions in the pelvic girdle may have a profound effect on vertebral function, the thoracoabdominal diaphragm, the urogenital diaphragm, the craniosacral mechanism, and the lower extremities. Somatic dysfunction of the pelvic girdle may be causative, contributory, or diagnostic for a wide range of patient complaints. Such complaints may be somatic, visceral, or emotional in nature. Common patient complaints that require evaluation of the sacrum and pelvis include, but are not limited to abdominal pain, pelvic pain, dysmenorhhea, lower back pain, urinary tract complaints, lower gastrointestinal issues and neuralgia of the lower extremities. In each of these situations, the sacrum and pelvis needs to be examined and possibly treated with osteopathic manipulation. An evaluation for somatic dysfunction of the lumbar spine is integrated with sacral-pelvic diagnosis and the other physical exam procedures. If significant somatic dysfunction is found, and potentially related to the patient's condition, osteopathic manipulative treatment (OMT) may be utilized in the treatment plan along with other appropriate therapies. The role of manual medicine in the management of the pelvic girdle is the restoration of functional symmetry between the arthrodial, neural, vascular, lymphatic, and connective tissue elements.

EPIDEMIOLOGY OF LOW BACK PAIN RELATED TO THE SACROILIAC JOINT

Although lower back pain is only one clinical condition related to dysfunction of the sacroiliac joint (SIJ), it is important to understand the correlation from an epidemiological standpoint. The lifetime prevalence of a patient having lower back pain approaches 70%, so it is important for osteopathic physicians to be able to evaluate the lumbar spine. Each year there are 13 million physician visits for lower back pain, with the highest prevalence in the 45- to 60-year-old Caucasian population (1). Back pain is the most frequent cause of activity limitation in people 45 years of age, the second most frequent reason for physician visits, the fifth most frequent for hospitalization, and the third ranking reason for surgical procedures (1). The incidence of sacroiliac (SI) dysfunction in persons with low back pain is highly variable depending upon the population being studied (2).

HISTORY

A history is not just the complaint, the symptoms, and the history of the disease, but it is the history of the patient who has the disease. In the diagnosis of pelvic girdle dysfunction, the importance of taking a complete history and performing an in-depth physical examination cannot be overemphasized. An appropriate and thorough history of the patient's chief complaint is critical. It is always important to consider urgent, emergent, or other potentially serious conditions. From the patient's history alone, the clinician should have a pretty good idea of what is going on, and then develop a differential diagnosis. If the physician listens carefully, the patient's history usually reveals the diagnosis (3).

Allow patients to tell their story in their own words and steer them in directions that elicits the essential information. The clinician knows when the history must be abbreviated or prolonged, based on the patient's presentation. Although the history is usually discussed as an entity that precedes the physical examination, further questioning (history) may take place as positive clues are obtained during the physical exam. This approach to history taking will prompt the physician to ask questions about areas that the patient does not consider important. If not all the information is obtained during the initial evaluation it is worthwhile to review and document the history on subsequent visits. In patients with pelvic girdle complaints, physicians should always be aware of their expressions, remarks, and gestures. A diseased organ does not walk into the physician's office, but an anxious and fearful patient does, who may misinterpret or be sensitive to the issues at hand.

THE CHIEF COMPLAINT

A physician should never assume that a patient's low back or pelvic pain has a solely muscular cause. The history should always clarify if a visceral or an emotional cause exists. Because the pelvic region includes the sexual organs, the patient's sexual history needs to be obtained when the patient presents with a complaint in the pelvic region. Considerations of the chief complaint should include several questions (4). Initially, patients should describe the quality of pain themselves without suggestions from the examining physician. Pain needs to be evaluated by documenting a description of the pain, including its intensity, duration, location, radiation, alleviating or aggravating factors, and response to treatment. Not every chief complaint is pain. The chief complaint can be stiffness, a decrease in athletic performance, a missed menstrual period, postural or muscular asymmetry, a localized mass, a skin lesion, etc. The important aspect to consider is how does the chief complaint disturb the patient's day-to-day functioning?

In addition, ask the following questions:

- Are there any associated symptoms?
- Have the symptoms stopped you from performing any activities?

- Have there been any changes in bowel or bladder habits?
- Have you had any diagnostics or received any medical care for this condition?
- What was the diagnosis and treatment outcome?
- Are you taking any medications, for the condition?
- Are your symptoms improving, staying the same or worsening?

Even when pain is the primary complaint and clinical suspicion centers on musculoskeletal causes, the physician remembers that pain is a "liar" and they should address the contributory topics listed in Table 41.1. Following obtaining the medical history, an inventory by systems is taken, especially those systems that could be related to the sacral and pelvic region.

HISTORY OF SACROILIAC DYSFUNCTION

There is no pathognomonic clinical picture, of SIJ dysfunction; however, pain referred to the groin is suggestive. Pain referred to the medial buttock, laterally to the sacrum, and below the iliac crest is a reasonable indication of SIJ dysfunction (26). The quality of pain that patients have with SIJ dysfunction is usually described as sharp, dull, or aching. The pain can refer to the groin, buttocks, posterior thigh, and occasionally below the knee. Symptoms are usually unilateral, are aggravated by sitting and are relieved by standing or walking (26). It is rare to have associated neurologic symptoms. Hamstring tightness is frequently present in SIJ dysfunction. Patients with short leg syndrome and sacral base unleveling complain of lower back or SIJ pain that is worse as the day goes on. Patients with a backward sacral torsion have significantly more pain than other sacral dysfunctions. Because of the location of the pain, patients will describe SI pain to the physician as "hip" pain. Since the hip joint affects position and motion of the ilium, it also

---

TABLE 41.1

Considerations for Complaints of Pelvic Pain

In Male and Female Patients	In the Female Patient	In the Male Patient
Employment risks	Menstrual history	Difficulty maintaining or achieving erection
Exercise risks/contact sports	Obstetric history	Difficulty with ejaculation
Hernia	Cleansing routines	Discharge or penile lesion
Past genitourinary surgeries	Douching history	Infertility
Cancer of the genitourinary tract	Abnormal vaginal bleeding	Urinary symptomatology
Chronic illness	Vaginal discharge	Urinary stream, good or poor
Family history	Date of last pelvic examination	Enlargement of the inguinal area
Psychiatric history	Date of last Pap smear and results	Testicular pain or mass
Medications, including contraceptive use	Past gynecologic procedures or surgery	Testicular self-examination practices
Sexual activity history		
Sexual orientation		
Sexually transmitted diseases		
Cancer of the reproductive organs		
Infertility		
Significant and related medical history (e.g., diabetes)		
Urinary tract symptoms		

Source: Seidel HM, Ball JW, Dains JE, et al. Mosby's Guide to Physical Examination. St. Louis, MO: CV Mosby Co., 1987.

affects the sacrum. When obtaining historical information for "hip pain," the clinician needs to include in the questioning any medical issues of the hip joint, the SIJ and the lower back. SIJ dysfunction has a relatively unknown incidence and variable clinical findings and takes skill and time to develop a consistent clinical diagnosis.

FUNCTIONAL ANATOMY

Skeletal/Ligamentous Anatomy

The pelvis consists of three bones and three joints forming an open ring shape. The false pelvis is a part of the lower abdomen and is walled laterally by ilia. The true pelvis is located inferior and posterior to the abdomen. It begins at the level of the sacral promontory, arcuate line, pectinate line, and pubic bones, ending with the inferior fascia of the pelvic diaphragm.

Growth and Development

In Vleeming's book, *Movement Stability and Low Back Pain*, the growth and development of the SIJs is described in detail (26). The following paragraphs based on this reference summarize this topic (26). The SIJ develops slowly; as cavitation is delayed until the 8th to 10th week of intrauterine life and is not well established until the second trimester. Since the ilium is the first bone to ossify in the pelvis, and the SIJ is late in developing. There are also very distinct microscopic differences between the sacral and iliac sides of the joint. On the iliac side of the joint, the cartilage is thinner. As a child grows, the SIJ undergoes unique age-related changes. Before puberty, the iliac side is rough in texture and looks bluish in color. The sacral surface appears smooth, glistening and creamy-white in color. The sacral surface has characteristics of hyaline cartilage, the iliac side, that of fibrocartilage. These differences in gross appearance are maintained throughout life. After puberty, there is considerable difference between the SIJ of men and women. In men, these ligaments remain well developed and strong. In women, the SIJ ligaments are not as well developed, thereby allowing the mobility required during childbirth. By the second decade of life, a crescent-shaped ridge develops along the iliac surface that interdigitates with a corresponding depression on the sacral side of the joint. By the third decade, this interdigitation is more pronounced, which further limits SIJ motion. In males, degenerative changes can occur on the iliac side of the SIJ as early as the third decade of life. However, similar changes do not affect the sacral side until the fourth or fifth decade of life. By the fourth and fifth decades, fibrous ankylosis can further limit joint motion. The SIJs can develop "accessory articulations" that may be acquired due to repetitive stress. These partial parallel accessory joints are estimated to be present in approximately 8% to 35% of the population. It is not known whether the presence of these joints changes palpable sacral motion.

The Ilia

Functionally, each innominate can be viewed as a lower extremity bone; and the sacrum, as a component part of the vertebral axis. In the past, the hip bones were referred to as the innominate bones because each was composed of three bones joined together at the acetabular notch. Initially there is a single cartilaginous model for the entire element, and the ischium, ilium, and pubis are the primary ossification centers before birth. Epiphyseal centers form in the cartilaginous iliac crest, anterior superior iliac spine (ASIS), and ischial tuberosities (at puberty) and eventually fuse in the late

teens or early 20s. The only remnants of the original cartilaginous model are the bilateral SIJs (26).

The acetabulum occupies the lateral aspect of the ilium and articulates with the head of the femur to create the hip joint. The two innominates are joined anteriorly by the symphysis pubis and cephalically with the sacrum via the bilateral SIJs. The female pelvis is less robust than the male pelvis, with smaller weight-bearing areas and less height.

Spinal Articulations

The three joints of the pelvis include the symphysis pubis and the two SIJs. The sacrum is attached to the lumbar vertebra by a lumbosacral disc, two lumbosacral synovial joints, and ligaments. The superior articular processes of the sacrum are concave and face posteromedially. They articulate with the inferior articular processes of the fifth lumbar vertebrae. Anomalous development commonly results in asymmetric lumbosacral facets (facet tropism) and, less commonly, incomplete separation and differentiation of the fifth lumbar vertebrae (sacralization). When the transverse processes of the fifth lumbar vertebra are atypically large, a pseudoarthrosis may occur with the sacrum or ilia (um). When this occurs bilaterally, it is termed a bat-wing deformity.

The Pubic Bones and Pubic Symphysis

The pubic symphysis is a fibrocartilagenous joint that has motion determined by its anatomic shape, ligaments, and muscular attachments. Muscular forces acting on each pubic ramus can cause rotation upon each other at the symphysis, about a transverse axis.

The Sacrum and Coccyx

The sacrum is shaped like an inverted triangle with the superior aspect being the base and the inferior aspect being the apex. The most anterior and superior portion of the first sacral vertebral body is called the sacral promontory. The anterior surface is concave, and the posterior surface is convex with palpable spinous tubercles. The medial row of tubercles is formed by fusion of the sacral articular processes. The lateral row is formed by the fusion of sacral transverse processes and inferiorly ends in a curve of the bone called the inferolateral angle. The sacrum contains the sacral canal and four bilateral sacral foramina for the passage of the ventral and dorsal rami of the first four sacral spinal nerves. The sacral hiatus is a defect near the apex, formed by a failure of laminal closure of the fifth sacral vertebra. It is at this location that sacral epidural nerve blocks are performed. The coccyx attaches to the sacral apex via the sacrococcygeal joint. The ganglion impar (where the right and left sympathetic chains join) rests on the anterior surface of the coccyx.

The Pelvic Articulations

The SIJs have been described as L- or C-shaped and are contoured with a shorter upper arm and longer lower arm, with the junction occurring approximately at S2. The articular surfaces are subject to a great deal of variation even in opposite sides of the same bone (5). The apex, or junction of the two arms of the SIJ, points anteriorly. The SI articulation is typically convex at the upper arm and concave at the lower arm. The longer arm of the joint surface is directed posteriorly and caudally, and the shorter arm faces posteriorly and cranially, therefore the SIJs converge inferiorly and posteriorly. It is a diarthrodial joint because it contains synovial fluid and matching articular surfaces. The articular surfaces, however, are different from those in any other joint in the body. It is in this joint alone that hyaline articular cartilage faces and moves against fibrocartilage. On the sacral side, this hyaline cartilage is usually 1 to 3 mm in depth. On the ilial side, there is fibrocartilage (26). The sacrum decreases in width from above downward; it is wedged between the two ilia. The predominant direction of fibers of the SI ligaments is such that they prevent excessive separation of the innominates and downward gliding of the sacrum (5).

The lumbosacral facets are predominantly coronal with the surface of the inferior lumbar facet slanting posteriorly. The sacral sulcus is a palpable groove just medial to the PSIS (Fig. 41.1). Much variation exists between anatomic description and an individual patient's anatomy. Weisl's work (6) demonstrates the varying contours of the articular surfaces of the sacrum and the ilia at their articulation with each other.

Frazier Strachan, D.O. (5), studied the anatomy of the sacrum extensively. He found that there was significant anatomic variation of the sacrum. Some sacrums are significantly curved, while others are relatively flat. After studying the anatomy of numerous sacrums, he came to the conclusion that there were three basic types, which he labeled type A, type B, and type C. The type A sacrum was wide dorsally and more narrow on the ventral surface. Type B was more wide ventrally than dorsally, and type C was a combination of both. The anatomic asymmetry will effect how the sacrum seats against the ilia and its stability (see concept of *form closure*). This will also affect the type of dysfunction and treatment required (5).

Ligaments

The sacrum is suspended between the innominate bones by three true and three accessory ligaments. The true pelvic ligaments include the anterior SI ligaments, interosseous SI ligaments, and posterior SI ligaments. The accessory pelvic ligaments include the sacrotuberous, sacrospinous, and iliolumbar ligaments. The iliolumbar ligaments attach from the anterior surface of the iliac crest and the anterior surface of the sacral base to the transverse processes of L4 and L5 (Fig. 41.2). The lower fibers blend in with the anterior SI ligament, thus integrating SI mechanics with the lumbar spine. There are anterior and posterior portions to the SI ligaments. The anterior ligaments are flat bands, while the posterior ligaments are thicker with multiple layers. The long dorsal SI ligament, which connects the PSIS to the lateral aspect of the third and fourth sacral segments, has a close anatomic relationship with the erector spinae muscles, posterior layer of the thoracolumbar

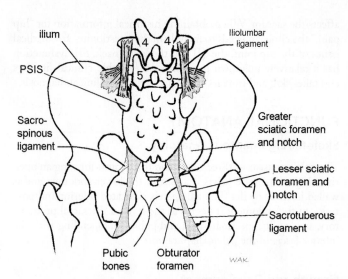

Figure 41-2 Pelvic ligaments and foramen. (Modified from Kuchera WA, Kuchera ML. *Osteopathic Principles in Practice.* 2nd Ed. Rev. Columbus, OH: Greyden Press, 1994.)

fascia, and a specific part of the sacrotuberous ligament (27). Another significant relationship of the long dorsal SI ligament is that this ligament becomes stretched when the sacrum is rotated in a posterior manner relative to the ilium (27). Thus, in situations where there is a decrease in lumbar lordosis, such as in the early stages of pregnancy or in aging, backward torsions, or unilateral/bilateral sacral extensions, this ligament may be stretched.

Accessory Ligaments

The bilateral sacrotuberous ligaments run from the inferior medial border of the sacrum and insert on the ischial tuberosities and the posterior margins of the sciatic notches. The bilateral sacrospinous ligaments lie anterior to the sacrotuberous ligaments and attach to the ischial spines, dividing this space into a greater and a lesser sciatic foramen. The sacrospinous and sacrotuberous ligaments restrain the anterior movement of the sacrum within the pelvic bones. The long head of the biceps femoris, piriformis, and gluteus maximus muscles often have direct attachments to the sacrotuberous ligament. It has been hypothesized that these muscles, interacting with the sacrotuberous ligament, have a role in SIJ mobility and stability. Detailed dissections of anatomic material by Vleeming et al. (1989) noted that, in all the sections, the gluteus maximus fascia was connected to the sacrotuberous ligament. In most dissections, a portion of the long head of the biceps femoris tendon is in continuity with the sacrotuberous ligament, traversing the ischium (27).

In the weight-bearing position, without strong pelvic ligaments, the sacral base tends to rock anteriorly. The downward effects of gravity, combined with environmental and genetic factors, can stress the tensile strength of these ligaments. These ligamentous stresses can create lumbosacral imbalance, chronic back pain, and joint degeneration. The iliolumbar ligament is prone to irritation by lumbosacral instability. When an iliolumbar ligament becomes irritated, its attachments to the crest and transverse processes of L4-5 become tender to palpation. Pain may be referred to the groin via the ilioinguinal nerve, mimicking the pain felt in an inguinal hernia. The iliolumbar ligament has also been implicated in a nerve entrapment syndrome under the iliolumbar ligament (Fig. 41.3). Palpatory diagnosis should therefore always include these ligamentous attachments.

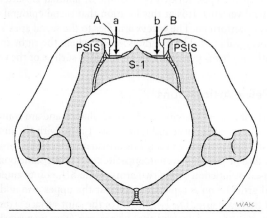

Figure 41-1 Cross-section of pelvis. Differential static landmarks for determining sacral sulcus depth (*A* and *B*) versus sacral base anterior or posterior (*a* and *b*). (Illustration by W.A. Kuchera.)

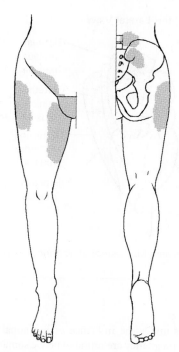

Figure 41-3   Pain referral pattern from iliolumbar ligament. (Modified from George S. Hackett, MD.)

Muscles and Connective Tissue

Muscles and connective tissue of the thoracoabdominal wall, aid in coordinating movements and pressures between the thoracic cage and the pelvic girdle. Muscles acting on or through the pelvis can be classified as primary (intrinsic muscles of the pelvic diaphragm) and secondary (muscles considered to have partial attachment to the true pelvis).

Primary Intrinsic Pelvic Muscles

Primary muscles and connective tissue intrinsic to the pelvic girdle include the pelvic and urogenital diaphragms. The pelvic diaphragm consists of the levator ani and coccygeus muscles, which form a basin, supporting the pelvic viscera and closing the pelvic outlet. The levator ani group includes the pubococcygeus, puborectalis, and iliococcygeus muscles. The urogenital diaphragm spans the area between the ischiopubic rami and is formed by the deep transverse perineal and sphincter urethrae muscles and their fasciae. The pelvic diaphragm slants downward from the lateral wall to the midline perineal structures while the urogenital diaphragm is rather level. This creates a small potential fingerlike space (ischiorectal fossa) on either side superior to the urogenital diaphragm and inferior to the pelvic diaphragm, which may provide an anterior avenue for the spread of perineal infections. The pelvic floor muscles work in a synergistic way with the abdominal diaphragm to increase intra-abdominal pressure. They also provide support during defecation, inhibit bladder activity, and assist in providing lumbosacral pelvic support (25).

SECONDARY MUSCLES (PARTIAL PELVIC ATTACHMENT)

Secondary muscles include:

- Rectus abdominis
- Transverse abdominis
- Internal and external oblique
- Quadratus lumborum

The external abdominal oblique muscle forms the inguinal ligament as it courses between the ASIS and the pubic tubercle.

The lower extremity may influence the pelvic girdle through its musculature and connective tissue.

Each compartment of the lower extremity has unique actions on the sacrum and pelvis. The anterior and medial compartments of the thigh may affect iliac and pubic motion and contain the following muscles:

- Quadriceps femoris
- Sartorius
- Gracilis
- Adductor group
- Iliopsoas (functionally)

The muscles of the "lateral compartment" of the leg include only the tensor fascia lata muscle and the iliotibial band. The deep fascia of the thigh (fascia lata) is continuous with the superficial thoracolumbar fascia of the thorax and splits to form the compartments of the lower extremity.

The muscles of the posterior compartment of the leg and gluteal region include:

- Glutei maximus, medius, and minimus
- Piriformis
- Obturator externus
- Superior and inferior gemelli
- Biceps femoris
- Semimembranosus
- Semitendinosus

Dysfunction of muscles or fascia of the posterior compartment or gluteal region may affect function of the pelvic girdle. The fascia covering the posterior aspect of the piriformis muscle and the biceps femoris have been found to be continuous with the posterior SI ligament. The implication of these findings is that physical activity and diagnostic tests, such as the straight leg raising tests, could stress the SIJ due to this arrangement. Inflammation of the SIJ could affect the piriformis muscle and biceps femoris through resultant reactive muscle spasm.

Collectively, the muscles of the gluteal region, the quadratus femoris, and the iliopsoas comprise the rotator cuff of the hip (Fig. 41.4).

According to anatomic dissections by Vleeming et al. (27), in all specimens, traction on the posterior layer of the thoracolumbar lumbar fascia transmitted force to the contralateral side, specifically into the fascia of the gluteus maximus. He related that the contralateral latisimus dorsi to the involved gluteus maximus could affect the stability of the SIJ owing to the connecting fascia. Stability of the SI region is achieved by a combination of ligamentous and dynamic muscular function crossing the SIJs (27). Through anatomic study, the gluteus maximus tendon has fibers that blend with the posterior iliosacral ligaments and it overlies the lower half of the SIJ. The tendons of the erector spinae run inferiorly from the paraspinal areas to attach to the posterior surface of the sacrum directly through the perimysial membranes of the multifidus muscles. The multifidus muscle takes its origin from the median sacral crest and runs laterally to attach to the medial PSIS (7).

Integrated Function

There is an integrated function between the muscles of the gluteal region, the abdominal diaphragm, and the muscles of the pelvic and urogenital diaphragms. The pelvic diaphragm consists of the

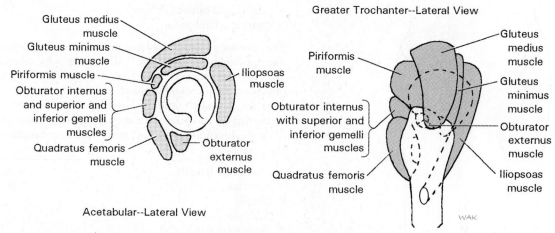

Figure 41-4   Rotator cuff muscles of right hip. (Modified from Kuchera WA, Kuchera ML. *Osteopathic Principles in Practice*. 2nd Ed. Rev. Columbus, OH: Greyden Press, 1994.)

levator ani and coccygeus muscles, which form a basin, does not rhythmically contract, but when relaxed, it works synchronously with the abdominal diaphragm. This synchronous movement with the abdominal diaphragm preserves interstitial fluid homeostasis in the true pelvic region. A relaxed pelvic diaphragm is absolutely necessary for the efficient movement of lymphatic fluids away from the pelvis and perineal tissues. Somatic dysfunction of the symphysis pubis or disturbed ilioilial mechanics (asymmetry of the relationship between the two innominates) can place asymmetric tensions on the pelvic and urogenital diaphragms. These tensions may result in tension myalgia or pain of the pelvic floor, low back pain, dyspareunia, and painful defecation with associated constipation (8). The muscles of the gluteal region become tense and tender to the touch. Tension on the pubovesicular and puboprostatic fascia from innominate dysfunction (especially pubic shears and compressions) may produce urinary tract symptoms such as burning, frequency, fullness, and a weak stream. Such tensions on the inguinal ligament from disturbed ilioilial mechanics can affect the lateral femoral cutaneous nerve, resulting in anterior thigh pain.

Dysfunction of any of the abdominal muscles or their fasciae may disturb respiratory excursion, compromising the intra-abdominal pressure changes that promote lymphatic and venous return. The thoracolumbar and lumbosacral fasciae contribute to the origin of the internal abdominal oblique and the transverse abdominis muscles. Fascial restrictions in these areas can restrict both thoracolumbar and sacral motion. The inner-membranous layer of the superficial thoracolumbar fascia (Scarpa) attaches to the iliac crest and pubic symphysis. It is continuous with the fascia of the thigh inferior to the inguinal ligament (fascia lata), the posterior perineal membrane, and the tunica dartos scrota. Fascial restrictions along its course may affect the thigh, perineum, or abdomen, as fluid collections can traverse along these planes.

Dysfunction of the rectus femoris, the iliacus, or the ipsilateral adductor group may cause an anterior rotation of the innominate and inferior shear at the pubes. Adductor dysfunction may be related to reflex changes at the ipsilateral iliolumbar ligament, while a pubic shear may affect the pelvic and urogenital diaphragms. Gait may be affected by lumbosacral somatic dysfunction, affecting the superior gluteal nerve (L4-5, S1) and the gluteus medius and minimus. Piriformis hypertonicity related to sacral somatic dysfunction may produce benign sciatica. Hamstring tension may cause a posterior rotation of the innominate and affect pelvic mechanics.

Female patients under the influence of hormonal and structural changes during pregnancy are prone to pelvic somatic dysfunction. There are many biomechanical causes such as changes in their center of gravity, an increased lumbar lordosis, and anterior rotation of the pelvis.

Vascular/Lymphatic Anatomy

Following the bifurcation of the abdominal aorta at the approximate level of the umbilicus, the right and left common iliac arteries diverge and descend to the lumbosacral junction. Here they divide into the internal and external iliac arteries. The internal iliac arteries have two trunks that supply the pelvic viscera, perineum, and gluteal region. The proximal anterior trunk supplies the urinary bladder, uterus, vagina, and rectum. Distally, the artery branches into the internal pudendal artery, supplying the genitalia and perineum, and the inferior gluteal artery, supplying the gluteal region. The posterior trunk contains the iliolumbar, lateral sacral, and superior gluteal arteries collectively supplying the intrinsic muscles of the pelvis, the sacrum, and the superior gluteal region.

Veins of the pelvic girdle form venous plexi encircling the pelvic organs and the sacrum and generally following the arterial distribution. The rectal venous plexus communicates with the portal system via the superior rectal vein, which is valveless (Fig. 41.5).

Lymphatic drainage from the pelvic girdle generally follows the corresponding arteries. Lymphatic flow from the lower extremities and pelvic viscera (apart from the gut) passes through the pelvic girdle, terminating ultimately in the lateral aortic groups. Organs and tissues drained by these groups include:

- Testes
- Ovaries
- Fallopian tubes
- Uterus
- Kidneys
- Ureters
- Posterior abdominal, pelvic, and perineal walls

Lymph from the remaining viscera (bladder) and gluteal region passes initially to regional nodes along the internal iliac arteries. The external genitalia drain to the inguinal nodes and then deeper into the external iliac and the intermediary lumbar groups.

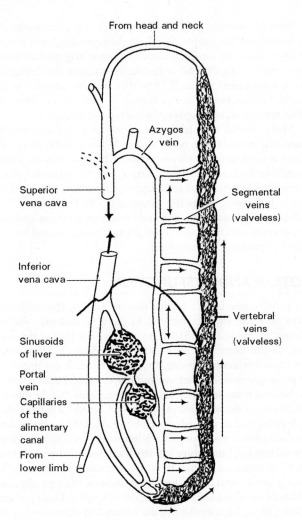

From head and neck

Azygos vein

Superior vena cava

Segmental veins (valveless)

Inferior vena cava

Vertebral veins (valveless)

Sinusoids of liver

Portal vein

Capillaries of the alimentary canal

From lower limb

Figure 41-5 Valveless vertebral venous plexus. (Illustration by W.A. Kuchera; adapted from G. Zink.)

Lymphatic drainage of the rectum and anal canal is unique in that, above the pectinate line, lymph follows a deep course to the internal iliac nodes and preaortic nodes. Below the pectinate line, the lymph drains superficially to the inguinal nodes. As lymph flows through a number of intermediary groups in the lumbar region, on up to the cisterna chyli and thoracic duct, the diameter of the thoracic duct and lymphatic channels is under sympathetic control similar to blood vessels. Hypersympathetic activity can reduce lymphatic flow capacity. Accumulation of pelvic lymph may occur in the preaortic, lateral aortic, or retroaortic lymph node groups. Peripherally compromised lymphatic drainage has been linked to the pathogenesis of atherosclerosis and to the development of hypertension (9). Correction of pelvic girdle dysfunction, as well as piriformis tension, may allow improved lymphatic venous return, blood flow, and gait for a patient whose activities of daily living are already compromised by a cardiovascular condition.

Nerves

The nervous system may influence the pelvic girdle through one of four areas. These are the:

- Lumbar plexus
- Sacral plexus
- Coccygeal plexus
- Autonomic nerves of the pelvis

The lumbar plexus lies between the anterior and posterior masses of the psoas major, anterior to the transverse processes of the lumbar vertebrae. The plexus is formed by the contributions of the ventral rami from T12 to L4 with only partial contributions from T12. The lumbar plexus gives motor supply to muscles in the abdomen and thigh, which act on the pelvic girdle. These muscles include the:

- Psoas major and minor
- Iliacus
- Pectineus
- Internal abdominal oblique
- Transverse abdominis
- Quadriceps group
- Adductor group
- Sartorius
- Gracilis

The lumbar plexus also supplies sensation to the thigh, buttocks, lower abdomen, and pubic area. The sacrum contains sacral foramen for passage of the sacral nerve roots, which exit anteriorly and posteriorly. The innervation of the SIJ and its ligaments is derived exclusively from the dorsal branches of the sacral spinal nerves. The joint capsule contains complex encapsulated and unencapsulated nerve endings capable of providing position sense and pressure information. The numerous thick myelinated axons in the nerve branches to the SIJ ligaments indicate the presence of special encapsulated mechanoreceptors and nociceptors (26,27). The posterior innervation to the SIJ is from the posterior primary rami of L4 through S3 (26). The anterior innervation arises from branches of the anterior primary rami from L2 to S2. The posterior and anterior rami are variable and this may account for the inconsistent pain referral pattern seen with SIJ syndrome (2). Since the SIJs have a wide distribution of innervation, it is possible that pain referred from the SIJ will not be associated with any motor, reflex, or sensory deficit on physical examination.

The lumbosacral trunk (ventral rami of L4 and L5), the first three sacral ventral rami, and a portion of the fourth form the sacral plexus. The ventral rami divide into anterior and posterior branches. The anterior branch forms anterior nerves that innervate the flexors and adductors; the posterior branch forms posterior nerves that innervate the extensors and abductors.

The sacral plexus has motor and sensory innervations in the pelvis and lower extremities and contains parasympathetic fibers (S2, S3, and S4) for innervation of the left colon and pelvic organs. The sciatic nerve is a muscular branch of the lumbar and sacral plexi composed of fibers from the ventral rami of L4-S3. Pathology at the L4-5 or L5-S1 level is the usual cause of nerve root compression, as it is uncommon within the sacrum. The sciatic nerve is closely associated with the piriformis muscle. Eighty-five percent of the time the sciatic nerve passes through the greater sciatic notch just inferior to the piriformis; it passes through the muscle in <1% of the population. Since injections are sometimes given in myofascial triggerpoints when the muscle is spastic, it is important to realize that more than 10% of the time the peroneal portion of the sciatic nerve passes through the muscle, and in 2% to 3% of instances it exits above the piriformis and passes posterior to the piriformis muscle (10) (Fig. 41.6). Piriformis hypertonicity can cause sciatica. Evidence indicates that this may not be due to pressure, but to a chemical reaction that irritates peroneal fibers of the sciatic nerve. For this reason, there is referred pain down the posterior thigh.

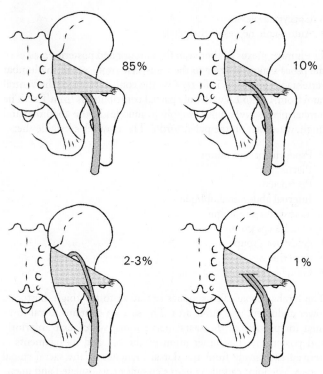

Figure 41-6 Position of sciatic nerve in relationship to the piriformis muscle. (Adapted from Beaton LE, Anson BJ. The sciatic nerve and the piriformis muscles: their interrelation as a possible cause of coccygodynia. *J Bone Joint Surg (Br)*. 1938;20:686–688.)

The coccygeal plexus is located on the pelvic surface of the coccygeus muscle and formed by the coccygeal nerve with contributions from S4 and S5. This plexus gives rise to the anococcygeal nerve that pierces the sacrotuberous ligament to supply the skin over the coccyx.

The autonomic nerves of the pelvis include the sacral sympathetic trunks, the parasympathetic nerves of the pelvic splanchnics, and the inferior hypogastric plexus. The right and left sacral sympathetic trunks are extensions of the lumbar sympathetic chain ganglia and are located on the ventral surface of the sacrum medial to the sacral foramina. They contain four or five ganglia and eventually fuse over the coccyx to form the single ganglion impar. The sacral sympathetic trunks have gray rami communicantes that follow the sacral and coccygeal nerves for innervation of blood vessels and sweat glands in the body wall and extremities. Because the sacral and coccygeal nerves do not have white rami, visceral afferent impulses returning from sites of sympathetic innervation by the sacrum and coccyx refer viscerosomatic symptoms to the thoracolumbar region of the body. Examples include anterior lower thoracic or sacral exostoses and anterior disc protrusions or ruptures. Contractions of the uterus refer pain to the thoracolumbar region, as the visceral afferent nerves travel to this level from the uterine body. The sacral splanchnics come off the chain and contribute to the formation of the inferior hypogastric plexus. The pelvic splanchnics arise directly off the ventral rami of S2-4 and supply parasympathetic innervation to the left colon and inferior hypogastric plexus for pelvic viscera. Visceral afferent nerves following parasympathetic nerve pathways produce viscerosomatic symptoms over the sacrum. An example is sacral pain and pressure from uterine contractions. The inferior hypogastric plexus contains both sympathetic and parasympathetic fibers; it gives rise to smaller plexi to the rectum, bladder, prostate, uterus, and vagina.

Somatic dysfunction of the lumbar spine may affect the lumbar plexus and produce symptoms in both the pelvis and lower extremity. Dysfunction of the Quadratus lumborum may produce symptoms similar to a groin pull or hernia, by irritating the ilioinguinal and iliohypogastric nerves (L1) as they pass just anterior to this muscle. Dysfunction of the piriformis, or sacrum, can affect the sciatic nerve and cause signs and symptoms of sciatica.

Many visceral complaints are related to an imbalance in the autonomic control of the pelvic viscera. When irritable bowel syndrome is dominated by parasympathetic hyperactivity (headache, nausea, diarrhea, and cramps), relaxation of the pelvic diaphragm through ischiorectal fossa techniques relieves the congestion and pain by influencing the pelvic parasympathetic (S2, S3, S4). Normalizing parasympathetic tone and encouraging venous and lymphatic return with firm continuous pressure over the sacral base can help treat primary dysmenorhhea.

MOTION AND DYSFUNCTION

The pelvic girdle holds a central role in coupling the mechanical forces from the lower extremities to the axial skeleton. The two primary functions of the SIJ are to dissipate the load of the upper trunk to the lower extremities and to facilitate childbearing by ligamentous relaxation during pregnancy. Somatic dysfunction of the pelvis occurs when there are motion preferences during activity that become restricted when activity is completed and the joint has returned to an abnormal resting position. Consider a patient bending forward and to one side, to pick tomatoes. The sacrum flexes initially, and then moves posteriorly into extension. With prolonged forward bending (at the hips and low back) the sacrum can become "stuck" in extension. When the patient stands up and walks they develop lumbosacral pain. Clinical examination will typically reveal a bilateral sacral extension or a backward torsion. During normal walking, physiologic motions of the sacrum and ilium occur around various theoretical axes of motion. Somatic dysfunction affecting any of these axes hinders gait, requires compensatory changes, and increases energy expenditure.

Individual axes of the pelvic bones are described in the following paragraphs, as well as the motion about or around those axes. This is followed by a discussion of the biomechanical stability of the SIJs, and an integration of the coupled movements during the motion cycle of walking.

Innominates

The innominates can be functionally considered as part of the lower extremity. The innominates rotate anteriorly and posteriorly about the inferior transverse axis of the sacrum. The innominates may also be considered to rotate posturally around an axis passing through the greater trochanters of the femur. Reynolds (11) demonstrated that there were multiple varying instantaneous axes of rotation of the ilium about the sacrum when the thigh was used to introduce motion at the SIJ.

If the clinician considers the ilium functionally, each lower extremity, including the attached innominate, is likely to shear superiorly or inferiorly as well as have rotation around a horizontal/transverse axis. Innominate motion can be induced by hip motion as during gait, or by muscular forces from below or above. When the innominate rotates anteriorly, it glides in the direction of the short arm of the "L" and posteriorly along the longer length of the "L." When the innominate rotates posteriorly, it glides in the direction of the longer length of the "L" and superiorly up the short length of the "L" (25). According to Fryette (12), it is thought that the sacrum follows the motion of the ilia, however to a lesser degree.

Pubes

Pubic bone motion is complex. The pubic bones are thought to correspond to ilial motion by rotating anteriorly and posteriorly about a transverse axis. With anterior rotation of the ilium the ipsilateral pubic bone is commonly found to be inferior. With posterior rotation of the ilium the ipsilateral pubic bone is commonly found to be superior. However, the pubic bones may also be sheared (subluxed) superiorly or inferiorly along with the rest of the respective innominate. Pubic somatic dysfunctions usually occur when iliac movement is maximal. Strachan came to these conclusions in the SI research in the 1930s (5,14). Anterior and posterior pubic shears can also occur, as well as a "gapped" pubic symphysis. These are rare and usually result from a significant traumatic event.

Sacrum

Ordinarily, SI motion is a result of mechanical forces acting on the sacrum. These forces can come from above, associated with changes of position or center of gravity within the torso, or from below, as in walking. While muscles are attached to the sacrum, sacral motion is not caused by sacral flexors, extensors, lateral flexors, or rotators (13). Describing motion of the sacrum about certain theoretical axes is a model by which the osteopathic physician explains how the sacrum seems to work as a result of the forces acting upon it. The osteopathic physician is also able to gather palpatory information, use this model, and describe the motion present and motion restricted. The palpatory findings become objective evidence of SI motion disturbances. It is then possible to design methods of manipulative treatment to remove the dysfunctions. By palpating landmarks and passive motion testing after manipulation the effectiveness of treatment can be evaluated.

Theoretical Axes of Motion

Mitchell (13) describes three transverse axes. The *superior transverse axis* is at the level of the second sacral segment, posterior to the SIJ, in the spinous process area. This is the respiratory axis where flexion and extension associated with respiration occur, as well as nutation and counternutation when using this terminology. The *middle transverse axis* is located at the anterior convexity of the upper and lower limbs of the SIJ. Sacral postural flexion and extension occur about this axis. The *inferior transverse axis* is located at the posterior-inferior part of the inferior limb of the SIJ and is the axis about which innominate (ilial) rotation occurs. Conceptually, one can consider each axis to roughly correspond to the anatomical remnants of the embryological transverse processes of the S1, S2, and S3 vertebrae, found on the sacral side of the SIJ (7).

There are two oblique axes of the sacrum, named according to the side of the body toward which the superior end of the oblique axis is located. Motion about an oblique axis may actually result through motions occurring about a vertical, anterior-posterior (AP) and transverse sacral axis (combination of rotation and side bending). Sacral movement can occur around an individual axis or simultaneously around multiple axes. Sacral shears do not rotate around an axis. Many studies of sacral/pelvic motion document movement of the SIJ and movement of the ilia in relation to the sacrum (14). However, many of the studies do not assess SI motion that is evaluated passively during clinical motion testing, or other osteopathic diagnostic procedures.

Sacroiliac Motion Research

There has been considerable debate over the years as to the mobility of the SIJs. Both in vivo and in vitro kinematic studies have demonstrated various types of motion in the SIJ, including rotation, gliding, tilting, nutation, and translation (27). In the late 1930s, Fraser Strachan, D.O., (CCO anatomy professor) et al. (14) conducted a cadaveric SI motion study. One innominate was encased in concrete. The sacrum and other innominate were free to move. Steel pins were fixed in all the bones. Forces were applied to the lumbar spine. C.R. Nelson, D.O., an engineer, made all the measurements and calculations. There are two excellent reports of this study (14). Strachan's research looked at how the sacrum moved in relation to the ilium when forces were applied to the cadaveric spine. The following summarize his findings:

- All of the movements of the sacrum on the ilium are gliding movements. Theses include flexion, extension, rotation, lateral flexion, and a gliding upward and downward.
- When force is transmitted vertically downward from the lumbar region, the sacrum glides downward and flexes. When traction is applied, the sacrum glides upward and extends.
- When rotation to one side is applied from above through the lumbar spine, the sacrum rotates to the same side and laterally flexes to the opposite side.
- When lateral flexion to one side is applied from above through the lumbar spine, the sacrum laterally flexes to the same side and rotates slightly, but the direction of rotation is inconsistent.
- When rotation to one side is applied from above through the lumbar spine, the sacrum rotates to the same side and laterally flexes to the opposite side.
- When lateral flexion to one side is applied from above through the lumbar spine, the sacrum laterally flexes to the same side and rotates slightly, but the direction of rotation is inconsistent.
- Freedom of movement is greater in flexion-extension and in gliding upward and downward than in rotation or lateral flexion.
- The ilium always moves in the same direction as the sacrum, but to a lesser degree.

Studies on SI motion in living subjects were performed by Weisl with lateral x-rays in the 1950s (6). Weisl noted a 6 mm displacement between end points of motion, but the error of measurement was calculated to be 3 mm (6). Colachis et al. (1963) performed a study with rods in the iliac bones and reported 5 mm of translation but no other results (28). Selvik, in 1974, described a technique called roentgen stereophotogrammetric analysis (RSA), by which it was possible to measure sacral movement in all three planes (28). The RSA technique could measure very small SIJ movements with a high degree of accuracy and specificity. According to Vleeming, the RSA technique could not identify SI dysfunction. While treatment was effective in relieving symptoms, the bony relationships were not altered. The research could not find significant differences of motion between movements of symptomatic and asymptomatic joints (28). However, these studies did not assess passive motion induced to the patient's SIJ by the physician, as is done in the clinical arena.

According to Vleeming, in 1983, Grieve used a RSA method to analyze movements of skin markers placed on the PSISs and sacrum. She measured iliac and sacral movement between standing and standing with one leg in flexion. She found the average movement at approximately 10 mm between the two positions. The sacrum was shown to rotate anterior relative to the ilia when standing up from lying supine. There was also an inward movement of the iliac crests, noted as positive values around the Z-axis for the left side and negative values for the right (28).

An *in vivo* SI motion study was carried out by Sturesson et al. (28). It used the RSA technique. In this technique, small metal balls were implanted in skeletal structures under local anesthetic. The motion between the metallic reference points of the ilium and the sacrum were measured in various positions by dual radiographic techniques. He found that in healthy young people, moving from a normal posture to hyperextension produced the greatest degree of motion. This was slightly more than 2 degrees on average, with a maximum of 4 degrees (15).

In 1990, Vleeming performed a similar study showing range in motion from zero to about 4 degrees, on individuals who had been found to have SI dysfunction based on a consensus from two physiotherapists, an orthopedic surgeon, and a chiropractor.

Sacroiliac Joint Stability

Much attention and research has been placed on stability of the SIJs. This is primarily due to the clinical finding of SIJ dysfunction in the patient with lower back pain, as well as the general medical consensus that the majority of back pain suffers have poor lumbar-pelvic motion and stability. Therapeutic exercise and osteopathic treatment for the core lumbar and pelvic musculature helps patients with low back pain and SI syndrome. The SIJ is one in which a small amount of motion is desirable, as excessive motion is much more difficult to treat clinically.

Click-clack Phenomenon

This postural transition from lumbar lordosis to lumbar kyphosis is called the lumbopelvic "click-clack" phenomenon. The click-clack phenomenon implies unfavorable loading of the lumbosacral and SI region. This motion occurs when a patient goes from a seated position to a standing position. It is thought that the intermediate position between kyphosis and lordosis is unfavorable, because of a lack of stability. This positional change, as well as counternutation (anatomic sacral extension), is unfavorable because of loading of the long dorsal SI ligaments. This ligament has been reported to be painful in 42% of patients with peripartum pelvic pain, and 46% with nonspecific low back pain. Control of the click-clack phenomenon depends on the rate of muscle action: the muscle forces must be generated at precisely the right time. This process may be viewed as a joint protecting or an arthrokinetic reflex. Weakness or tightness of involved muscles of the kinetic chain may delay muscle reaction and impair the functional stability of the SIJs.

Self-Bracing Mechanism

When considering the biomechanics of the sacrum, the forces applied to the joint and the shape of the joint surfaces must be taken into account. Gravitational force is applied to the SIJs in the standing position. Unlike other joints, this force is almost parallel to the surfaces of the SIJs. Because of this, there is considerable shear loading in the SIJ and a risk of damaging the ligaments. In general, the strong ligamentous structures surrounding the SIJ are assumed to be sufficient to prevent shear force and stabilize the joints. However, Vleeming et al. states that the ligaments alone are not capable of transferring lumbosacral load effectively to the iliac bones during standing and sitting. Research has shown that muscles and fascia contribute to the self-bracing or self-locking mechanism of the SIJ. The muscles involved apply a tension cross-brace to the SIJs, similar to the effect of wearing a SI belt. The muscles includethe latisimus dorsi, the thoracolumbar fascia, gluteus maximus, and the iliotibial tract. Ventrally the muscles involved include the external

abdominal obliques, the linea alba, the internal abdominal obliques, and the transverse abdominals. In both standing and sitting, the activity of the oblique abdominal muscles, especially the internal obliques, was found to be significant. Interestingly, research showed that leg crossing correlates with a significant decrease in activity of the internal obliques, causing an unstable situation. The psoas muscles are continuously active in erect postures acting as muscles of postural balance (16,23). This muscle, however, produces shear loading of the SIJs as well, because its orientation is almost parallel to the SIJ surfaces. Clinically, the authors find this muscle to be the most common culprit in restrictions of SI motion.

Form and Force Closure

According to the self-locking mechanism, *resistance against shear* results from the specific properties of the articular surfaces of the SIJ (form closure) and from the compression produced by body weight, muscle action, and ligament force (force closure). Different aspects of this mechanism operate depending on if the patient is standing, sitting, walking, or lifting. According to this model, the SIJ becomes especially prone to shear forces if loaded in anatomic sacral extension. This position with flattening of the lumbar spine, is thought to lead to abnormal loading of the lumbar discs and, in the end, herniation. The SIJs remain in place by friction forces between, and tangential to, the contact surfaces. These forces are generated by compression. The SIJs have symmetric ridges and grooves in the joint surfaces that apply friction. Form closure refers to a stable situation with closely fitted joint surfaces, in which no extra force is needed to maintain the state of the system, given the actual load situation. Form closure requires the proper size, shape, and attitude of the articulating surfaces, on which the load is dependent.

Additional compressive forces are needed to resist high load situations when shearing of the SIJ surface occurs. Force closure by this musculotendinous cross-bracing system is essential when form closure is absent, or insufficient. Vleeming described three muscle slings (one longitudinal and two oblique) that can be activated differently, based on the load applied. Compression by these slings can be produced by muscle forces, in combination with forces in ligaments and fascia that cross the SIJ surfaces. For example, consider postural scoliosis with unlevelness of the sacral base. To counter the torque that results from sacral unlevelness, muscular force is necessary to stabilize the situation by formation of scoliosis.

SACRAL MOTION

Considering these principles, four general categories of sacral motion can be described. These include:

- Postural
- Respiratory
- Inherent
- Dynamic

Postural Motion

In the standing or seated patient, postural motion of sacral flexion or extension occurs about a middle transverse axis. Flexion and extension of the sacrum correspond to anatomic nomenclature, with a reference point at the anterior portion of the sacral base. Flexion (forward bending, nutation) occurs when the sacral base is moving forward or anteriorly. Extension (backward bending, counternutation) of the sacral base occurs when the sacral base moves posteriorly. Terminology for sacral motion uses the same reference point as terminology for spinal motion, the most anterior superior part of the body (in the case of the sacrum, the sacral base). Postural flexion/extension of the sacrum is sometimes referred to as sacral base anterior (for flexion) or posterior (for extension). This prevents confusion of understanding sacral motion that occurs during flexion and extension of the Sphenobasilar synchrondosis during craniosacral motion (see "Inherent Motion"). When a person is seated and the torso is forward bent, the sacral base moves anteriorly. When a person is standing and begins forward bending, the sacral base begins to move anteriorly, tightening the sacrotuberous ligaments. As forward bending continues, the pelvis moves posteriorly in relation to the feet. This shift in the base of support causes the sacral base to move posteriorly.

Respiratory Motion

Respiratory motion also affects the sacrum, partially because the diaphragm is attached to the top three lumbar vertebrae (L1-2 on the left and L1-3 on the right). Mitchell and Pruzzo (17) showed that the sacrum moves in response to respiration along the superior transverse axis at the second sacral segment. As inhalation occurs, the lumbar lordotic curve decreases, and therefore the sacral base moves posteriorly. As we exhale, the lumbar lordosis increases and the base of the sacrum moves slightly forward.

Inherent Motion

Cranial terminology defines cranial sacral flexion/extension as the position of the sacrum when the sphenobasilar synchondrosis (SBS) is in flexion or extension. In flexion, the sacral base moves backwards (posteriorly). Therefore, cranial flexion is anatomic extension. Students were taught that relative to the sacrum, cranial flexion or extension was the opposite of anatomic flexion or extension. If anyone was referring to sacral motion from a cranial perspective, it was imperative to state cranial flexion or cranial extension. Because of this confusion, the Educational Council on Osteopathic Principles (ECOP) has encouraged the use of the terms *nutation* and *counter-nutation* to describe sacral movement in the cranial cycle of flexion/extension. Nutation means nodding forward, referring to anterior motion at the sacral base. During the flexion phase (of craniosacral inherent motion), the sacrum counternutates. During the extension phase (of craniosacral inherent motion), the sacrum nutates.

ECOP added the term to the Glossary to satisfy those ECOP members who felt that use of this term would clarify the difference between anatomic flexion and cranial flexion. The Glossary of Osteopathic Terminology (created by ECOP and published in Foundations) defines **nutation** as "nodding forward; anterior movement of the sacral base around a transverse axis in relation to the ilia, occurring during sphenobasilar extension of the craniosacral mechanism." This definition clearly implies that nutation, and counter-nutation, are terms to be used in describing sacral motion/position in relation to the cranial concept. With the expanded use of these terms, our profession has created a new set of confusions. Nutation is also being used to describe and name biomechanical flexion (sacral base moving forward) of the sacrum. Another term approved by ECOP concerns tissue texture abnormality, asymmetry, restriction of motion, and tenderness (TART Criteria), as outlined in Table 41.2.

Dynamic Motion

Dynamic motion of the sacrum and pelvis occurs during walking. As weight bearing shifts to one leg, unilateral lumbar sidebending engages the ipsilateral oblique axis by shifting weight to that SIJ. The sacrum now rotates forward on the opposite side, creating a deep sacral sulcus. With the next step, this process reverses as weight bearing changes to the other leg. The sacral base is constantly moving forward on one side, then the other, about the oblique axes. As this occurs, the two innominates are rotating in opposite directions to each other about the inferior transverse sacral axis. One side rotates anteriorly as the other side rotates posteriorly. With the next step, this process reverses as the anteriorly rotated ilium moves into posterior rotation. Interacting with the bony and ligamentous structure during this motion are the viscera, the weight of the upper body, the muscles of locomotion and balance, and the pelvic diaphragm, all revolving around the constantly changing instantaneous axes at the pelvis.

NORMAL MOTION OF WALK CYCLE

In the following passage from his paper, "Structural Pelvic Function," Mitchell (13) described the interplay of locomotion and balance as being the walking cycle:

> The cycle of movement of the pelvis in walking will be described in sequence as though the patient were starting to walk forward by moving the right foot out first.

TABLE 41.2

Tart Criteria for Identifying Somatic Dysfunction

Tissue Texture Abnormalities	How the Tissue Feels to the Palpating Hand	Classify as Acute or Chronic
Asymmetry	Apparent relationship of landmarks and tissues	Made by observation, not palpation; is generally static positional asymmetry
Restriction of motion	How the tissue moves	Arthrodial, muscular, or fascial elements
Tenderness	Pain elicited by palpation	Generalized as in traumatic tissue damage, such as contusion, or specific for individual muscles or sclerotomal levels, as in tender point diagnosis

To permit the body to move forward on the right, trunk rotation in the thoracic area occurs to the left accompanied by lateral flexion to the left in the lumbar with movement of the lumbar vertebrae into the forming convexity to the right. There is a torsional locking at the lumbosacral junction as the body of the sacrum is moving to the left, thus shifting the weight to the left foot to allow lifting of the right foot. The shifting vertical center of gravity moves to the superior pole of the left SI, locking the mechanism into mechanical position to establish movement of the sacrum on the left oblique axis. This sets the pattern so the sacrum can torsionally turn to the left, thereby the sacral base moves down on the right to conform to the lumbar C curve that is formed to the right.

When the right foot moves forward there is a tensing of the quadriceps group of muscles and accumulating tension at the inferior pole of the right SI at the junction of the left oblique axis and the inferior transverse axis, which eventually locks as the weight swings forward allowing slight anterior movement of the innominate on the inferior transverse axis. The movement is increased by the backward thrust of the restraining ground, tension on the hamstrings begins; as the weight swings upward to the crest of the femoral support, there is a slight posterior movement of the right innominate on the inferior transverse axis. The movement is also increased by the forward thrust of the propelling leg action. This iliac movement is also being influenced, directed and stabilized by the torsional movement on the transverse axis at the symphysis. From the standpoint of total pelvic movement one might consider the symphyseal axis as the postural axis of rotation for the entire pelvis.

As the right heel strikes the ground and trunk torsion and accommodation begin to reverse themselves, and as the left foot passes the right foot and weight passes over the crest of the femoral support, and the accumulating force from above moves to the right, the sacrum changes its axis to the right oblique axis and the sacral base moves forward on the left and torsionally turns to the right.

The cycle on the left is repeated identically to the right half movements. The shifting vertical center of gravity moves to the superior pole of the left SI locking the mechanism into mechanical position to establish movement of the sacrum on the left oblique axis.

Somatic dysfunctions may accentuate and retain portions of the motion described above. These are called physiologic somatic dysfunctions, because the muscles, connective tissue, and joints remain in positions that are normally a part of physiologic motion but are dysfunctional when the body should have returned to a neutral position but did not do so. Nonphysiologic somatic dysfunction is generally induced by trauma. It is evidenced by the joint, muscle, and connective tissue elements being in positions and/or relationships that are not part of the physiologic range of motion and do not involve the physiologic axes of motion. Examples include sacral, innominate, and pubic shears.

Integrated Physical Examination

The osteopathic examination is not a traditional history and physical with a palpatory examination added to it. An osteopathic examination strives to provide a time- and cost-effective diagnosis while encompassing the interrelationship between structure and function. Integration of the physical findings with the emotional, environmental, and genetic factors allows the osteopathic physician to understand their impact on body unity. An understanding and recall of the physiologic spinal motion patterns is also necessary before performing the physical examination. Using this knowledge, the physical exam will help the clinician rule out specific conditions on the differential diagnosis list. A prior knowledge

of Chapman reflexes, viscerosomatic reflexes, and the autonomic innervation of the viscera are also useful during the physical exam. While performing the physical exam, osteopathic physicians may discover paraspinal tissue texture changes that have characteristic palpatory qualities and conclude that these changes are due to visceral disturbances. These tissue texture changes are palpated in the subcutaneous tissue, and superficial and deep fascia, rather than in the muscle. Palpation leads to motion testing of tissues. Passive motion testing is performed as part of the integrated physical exam. In this fashion, through palpation and motion testing, an osteopathic physician examines the homeostatic reserve of each patient, an area crucial in determining prognosis, treatment design, and prevention. *To find health is the object of the physician, anyone can find disease* (18).

Begin with observation of the patient's gait. Do they turn one foot outward or inward? Do they hike a hip, lean to one side, or limp? Any of these findings can relate to dysfunction of the sacrum and pelvis. Perform a structural examination including a standing flexion test, a pelvic sideshift test, and a seated flexion test. Look for un-level iliac crests as well as greater trochanters. If they have a low greater trochanter, low iliac crest, and deep sacral sulcus on the same side, and have pelvic sideshift away from this side, they probably have a leg length inequality. This situation will un-level the sacral base, and affect pelvic stability. Do they have a group curve in the thoracic or lumbar region? This finding correlates with sacral base unleveling and is commonly seen with forward sacral torsions. Look for a reversal of their A-P curves. A flattened upper lumbar spine and an increased lumbar lordosis of the lower segments correlate with bilateral iliopsoas tension. If the entire lumbar spine is flattened, look for a sacral base that is held in extension (counternutation). If they have a significant increase in their lumbar lordosis, their sacrum will be bilaterally flexed, almost parallel to the ground. In this situation L5 frequently is unstable and may develop disc protrusions or other orthopedic changes. A Trendelenberg test can be done to evaluate for gluteus medius weakness (Table 41.3). As an addition to this examination, some physicians (and physical therapists) include a scanning examination for myofascial triggerpoints or tenderpoints. The assessment and treatment of myofascial trigger points is important when dealing with pelvic pain and dysfunction. If performed properly, a standing structural exam and evaluation of gait can provide useful clinical information to aid in the diagnosis and treatment of sacral and pelvic dysfunction.

Have the patient sit on the table and perform a cardiopulmonary examination. The palpatory examination should include an assessment of the patient's cardiovascular status. Pulses should be palpated and ascultated for bruits bilaterally. An abdominal pulse should be palpated, identified, classified, and ascultated. Peripheral edema, sacral edema, and trophic changes in the skin should be evaluated. In addition to the auscultation over arteries in the periphery, auscultation of the heart, lungs, and abdomen should accompany any patient evaluation. If atheromatous disease is suspected, auscultation over the carotid and femoral arteries is imperative, if an abdominal aneurysm is suspected, the diameter of the abdominal aorta is evaluated carefully.

While the patient sits on the table, perform a neurologic examination. Muscle testing and sensation are the primary focus of the neurologic examination of the pelvis and hip (21).

Muscle Testing

Muscles of the lower extremity and buttocks require assessment when evaluating the pelvis and hip. Descriptions of the innervation, functional anatomy, and dysfunction are discussed in the chapters

TABLE 41.3

Special Orthopedic and Physical Therapy Tests Performed on the Pelvis

Orthopedic Tests of the SIJs	Characteristics
Ipsilateral prone kinetic test	Prone
Gapping test	Supine, compress/IR both ilia Positive test = SI pain
Approximation test	Supine, or prone, ER both ilia Positive test = SI pain
SI rocking test	Supine, passively flex, and extend sacrum Positive test = SI pain
Squish test	
Femoral shear test	Supine, Flex hip and knee, compress Positive test = SI pain
Prone springing test	Prone, anterior pressure, springing motion Positive test = pain

Special Tests of the Pelvis (30)	Characteristics
Straight leg raising test	Supine, flex hip, knee extended Positive = radicular pain 30–70 degrees
Prone knee bending test (Nachlas)	Prone, Flex knee, extend hip Positive = pain anteriorly
Gillet test	Standing, flex hip and knee maximally Positive = asymmetry of PSIS, sacral spines
Ipsilateral anterior rotation test	Standing, side-lying, Passively rotate ilium Positive = pain
Flamingo test	Standing, hip flexed, abducted, ER, knee flexed Positive = pain
Leg length tests	Supine, Measure ASIS to medial malleolus Positive = discrepancy
Sign of the buttock	Supine, Flex hip with knee extended, then flex knee Positive = knee flexion does not allow further hip flexion
Gaenslen test	Side-lying, Flex lower hip, hold. Examiner extends top hip. Positive = pain in SIJ
Leaguer sign	Supine, flex, abduct, laterally rotate symptomatic hip with overpressure Positive = positive = pain in SIJ
Supine-to-sit (long sitting) test	Supine, legs straight, patient sits up. Positive = one leg moves proximal farther than the other = pelvic dysfunction
Yeoman test	Prone, flexes knee to 90 degrees, extend hip Positive = pain anterior SI ligaments
Thomas test	Supine, flex hip, hold knee to chest, allow other leg to extend Positive = un-held hip remains semiflexed
Trendelenberg test	Standing, one leg stance, evaluate pelvic position, evaluates stance leg: gluteus medius strength Positive = hip drops on nonstance side

on lumbar spine and lower extremity. Primary intrinsic muscles of the pelvis, although not tested for strength, may be palpated for tension, tissue texture changes, and tender points. Lumbar and pelvic muscles that may have triggerpoints referring pain to the pelvis should also be investigated (19,20).

Sensation Testing

The dermatomal distribution of sensory nerves to the pelvic girdle ranges from T10 to S5, involving nerve roots from the thoracic, lumbar, and sacral regions (Fig. 41.7). Dermatomes of the anterior abdominal wall run in transverse and oblique bands. These dermatomes begin at the umbilicus with the T10 strip followed inferiorly by the T11 strip. The T12 strip lies just superior to the inguinal ligament, while L1 lies just inferior to it. Inferior to the L1 dermatome lie the L2 and L3 strips covering the anterior thigh and ending at the patella. The buttocks, PSISs, and iliac crest are supplied by the cluneal nerves (21) (posterior primary divisions of L1, L2, and L3). The posterior femoral cutaneous nerve (S2) supplies sensation to a longitudinal band traversing the posterior thigh.

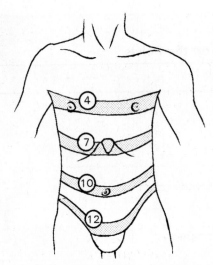

Figure 41-7 Anterior thoracic dermatomes. (Reprinted from Kuchera WA, Kuchera ML. *Osteopathic Principles in Practice.* 2nd Ed. Rev. Columbus, OH: Greyden Press, 1994, with permission.)

The lateral femoral cutaneous nerve (S3) supplies sensation to the lateral thigh. The cutaneous innervation of the perineum is arranged in concentric rings around the anus: the outermost (S2), middle (S3, S4), and innermost (S5).

Orthopedic Sacroiliac Joint Testing

In addition to observation of landmarks for asymmetry, palpation for tissue texture changes, and passive motion testing of joints and tissues; the orthopedic and physical therapy literature also stresses the performance of pain provocative tests, kinetic tests, and special tests. Pain provocative tests include traditional orthopedic tests, motion demand tests and ligament tension tests (25). Kinetic tests can be assessed either weight bearing or non–weight bearing. These tests assess SI motion during patient-generated movements.

DIAGNOSIS OF ILIOSACRAL AND PUBIC SOMATIC DYSFUNCTION

Iliosacral Somatic Dysfunctions

Iliosacral somatic dysfunctions include:

- Innominate rotations, anterior and posterior
- Innominate subluxations (shears), superior and inferior
- Innominate flares (inflares and outflares)
- Pubic shears (subluxations), superior and inferior
- Unequal hamstring length
- Unequal iliopsoas length

Anterior Innominate Rotation

This exists when the dysfunctional side has the following positional characteristics:

- Entire innominate appears to be rotated in a direction anterior to the other hip bone.
- ASIS is more inferior (caudad).
- PSIS is more superior (cephalad).

Subjective complaints may include ipsilateral hamstring tightness and spasm and sciatica (secondary to piriformis dysfunction). Palpatory findings may include the following:

- Tissue texture changes at the ipsilateral ILA of the sacrum.
- Iliolumbar ligament tenderness
- Positive ASIS compression test on the involved side (Fig. 41.8)
- Positive standing flexion test on the involved side
- Motion characteristics should indicate freedom of anterior rotation, about an inferior transverse axis, on supine motion testing, and resistance to posterior rotation.

Posterior Innominate Rotation

This exists when the dysfunctional side has the following positional characteristics:

- Entire innominate appears to be rotated in a direction posterior to the other hip bone.
- ASIS is more superior (cephalad).
- PSIS is more inferior (caudad).

Subjective complaints may include inguinal/groin pain (secondary to rectus femoris dysfunction) and/or medial knee pain (secondary to sartorius dysfunction).

Palpatory findings may include:

- Inguinal tenderness
- Tissue texture change (TTC) at the ipsilateral sacral sulcus
- Positive ASIS compression test on the involved side (see Fig. 41.8)
- Positive standing flexion test on the involved side
- Motion characteristics include freedom of posterior rotation about an inferior transverse axis on supine motion testing and resistance to anterior rotation.

Superior Innominate Shear (Subluxation)

This exists when the dysfunctional side has the following characteristics:

- ASIS is more superior (cephalad).
- PSIS is more superior (cephalad).
- Pubic ramus may be more superior (cephalad).
- Positive ASIS compression test on the involved side
- Positive standing flexion test on the involved side

Note: The reciprocal positioning of the ASIS and PSIS exists only if there is a pure superior shear without any rotation of the innominate.

The two innominates appear to be sheared so that the one hip bone is subluxed superiorly to the other.

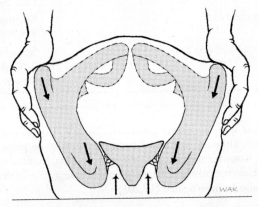

Figure 41-8 ASIS compression test. (Modified from Kuchera WA, Kuchera ML. *Osteopathic Principles in Practice.* 2nd Ed. Rev. Columbus, OH: Greyden Press, 1994.)

Subjective complaints may include pelvic pain. Palpatory findings may include tissue texture changes at the ipsilateral SIJ and ipsilateral pubes. Motion characteristics include freedom of superior translation.

Inferior Innominate Shear (Subluxation)

This condition exists when the dysfunctional side has the following characteristics:

- ASIS is more inferior (caudad).
- PSIS is more inferior (caudad).
- Pubic ramus may be more inferior.
- Positive ASIS compression test on the involved side
- Positive standing flexion test on the involved side

The two innominates appear to be sheared so that the one ilium is subluxed inferiorly to the other. This condition is rare, and walking tends to reduce it. Subjective complaints may include pelvic pain. Palpatory findings may include tissue texture changes at the ipsilateral SIJ and ipsilateral pubes. Motion characteristics include freedom of inferior translation.

Innominate Flares

This condition is a positional change of an innominate in which the ASIS is medial or lateral to its usual position. This may be thought of as rotation of an innominate in relation to a vertical axis. If the ASIS is more lateral on the dysfunctional side, the patient has an innominate outflare. If the ASIS is more medial on the dysfunctional side, the patient has an innominate inflare. Inflares and outflares tend to occur simultaneously with innominate rotation. It would be common to see an anterior rotation of the ilium with a component of an inflare. It would also be common to see a posterior innominate with a component of anoutflare. Subjective complaints may include pelvic or SI pain. Palpatory findings may indicate greater laxity in the muscles on the side that is more lateral and more tautness on the side that is more medial.

Pubic Somatic Dysfunction

Vertical Pubic Shears

Isolated vertical pubic shears (subluxations) may or may not actually exist. There may be evidence of a rotation or subluxation that is difficult to diagnose. However, there are times when the ASISs appear to be equal, the PSISs appear to be equal, and yet the pubes are definitely displaced so that one is detectably superior and the other inferior. Since the ASISs and PSISs are equal, it does not appear that the ilium is rotated or sheared. When the dysfunctional side is superior, it is said to be a superior pubic shear; if the dysfunctional side is inferior, it is an inferior pubic shear. More commonly, the clinician will find a superior pubic shear with an associated posterior ilium or an upslip. The same hold true for an inferior pubic shear and an anterior ilium or a down slip. Anterior pubic shears are uncommon, and are usually associated with trauma. In these cases, one side of the symphysis is anterior to the other.

Pubic Symphysis Compressions/Gapping

Pubic symphysis compressions occur, evidenced by bilateral tenderness of each pubic rami as well as tenderness centrally over the symphysis. Using the adductor muscles of the thigh in a muscle energy technique can reduce these compressions.

The L5 anterior counterstrain point is also located on the pubes. Treatment of this tender point with counterstrain technique may be appropriate and necessary in treating pubic symphysis symptoms because what appears to be a pubic dysfunction may actually be reflexive evidence of L5 dysfunction.

Gapping or subluxation of the pubic symphysis can occur after childbirth, after pelvic fractures, or other traumas. Pelvic x-rays clearly document the degree of gapping. These are usually quite painful, and not easily treated. Treatment of the SIJs, core muscles, and applying lateral and anterior compression to the lateral aspects of the ilia with a SI belt may help. To review iliosacral and pubic diagnoses (Tables 41.4 and 41.5).

Other Considerations of the Pelvis

Unequal Hamstring Length

Unequal hamstring length can be considered either a pelvic or a lower extremity somatic dysfunction because the hamstrings are attached to both the pelvis and the lower extremity. If the hamstrings are of unequal length, standing flexion test results may be either falsely positive or negative. Therefore, it is imperative to treat the hamstrings and retest. If the standing flexion test and pelvic landmark positions normalize, the dysfunctional hamstrings were the problem. Otherwise, treat as indicated by the second diagnosis. If an innominate is anterior, it will separate the origin and insertion of the hamstrings, making the muscle tight and irritable.

Unequal Iliopsoas Length

Unequal psoas length may be suspected when pelvic side shift is present, when the upper lumbar lordotic curve is flattened, or when seated or prone evaluation suggests upper lumbar flexed somatic dysfunction. To test the ability of the psoas muscle to lengthen, place the patient in a prone position. Stand at the side of the table. Stabilize the ipsilateral pelvis with your free hand. Grasp the thigh just above the knee and extend the hip until the ASISs begin to rise off the table. Note the ease and degrees (quality and quantity) of hip extension on both sides. Also, on the tighter side, the leg appears heavier. Compare the two sides.

TABLE 41.4

Pubic Symphysis Dysfunctions

Diagnosis	Characteristics
Superior right	Positive right standing flexion test Superior right pubic tubercle Tense, tender right inguinal ligament
Superior left	Positive left standing flexion test Superior left pubic tubercle Tense, tender left inguinal ligament
Inferior right	Positive right standing flexion test Inferior right pubic tubercle Tense, tender right inguinal ligament
Inferior left	Positive left standing flexion test Inferior left pubic tubercle Tense, tender left inguinal ligament

TABLE 41.5

Iliosacral Somatic Dysfunction

Diagnosis	Characteristics
Anterior rotation right	Positive right standing flexion test Inferior right ASIS Superior right PSIS
Anterior rotation left	Positive left standing flexion test Inferior left ASIS Superior left PSIS
Posterior rotation right	Positive right standing flexion test Superior right ASIS Inferior right PSIS
Posterior rotation left	Positive left standing flexion test Superior left ASIS Inferior left PSIS
Outflare right	Positive right standing flexion test Lateral right ASIS Medial right PSIS
Outflare left	Positive left standing flexion test Lateral left ASIS Medial left PSIS
Inflare right	Positive right standing flexion test Medial right ASIS Lateral right PSIS
Inflare left	Positive left standing flexion test Medial left ASIS Lateral left PSIS
Superior shear (upslip) right	Positive right standing flexion test Superior right ASIS Superior right PSIS
Superior shear (upslip) left	Positive left standing flexion test Superior left ASIS Superior left PSIS
Inferior shear (down slip) right	Positive right standing flexion test Inferior right ASIS Inferior right PSIS
Inferior shear (down slip) left	Positive left standing flexion test Inferior left ASIS Inferior left PSIS

DIAGNOSIS OF SACROILIAC JOINT SOMATIC DYSFUNCTION

The most common and standard diagnoses of SI somatic dysfunction include (but are not limited to):

- Sacrum anterior
- Sacrum posterior
- Forward torsions (rotation of the sacrum on the same oblique axis):
  - Left rotation on left oblique axis
  - Right rotation on right oblique axis
- Backward torsions (rotation of the sacrum on the opposite oblique axis):
  - Right rotation on left oblique axis
  - Left rotation on right oblique axis

- Bilateral sacral flexion
- Bilateral sacral extension
- Unilateral sacral flexion (sacral shear)
- Unilateral sacral extension (sacral shear)

In the osteopathic profession, several models of SI dysfunction have been described. Three systems of nomenclature currently used to define sacropelvic mechanics are those described by Strachan (HVLA), Mitchell (muscle energy), and Van Buskirk (Still technique). The HVLA system is described in Walton's text, *Osteopathic Diagnosis and Technique, Sacroiliac Diagnosis* (22). Both the Chicago and Mitchell models describe similar events, but from differing points of reference. Both systems are based on physiologic motion of the sacrum, pelvis, and lumbar spine. However, the Strachan model does not describe or identify what the Mitchell system refers to as backward sacral torsions; just as the Mitchell system has no equivalent for Strachan's posterior sacrum.

The Still (Van Buskirk) model looks at the sacrum in a unique way (7). It looks at sacral dysfunction as more of a myofascial restriction that is present after the lumbar spine and pelvis has been already treated. The student of osteopathic medical profession needs to understand these three approaches in dealing with SI and pelvic somatic dysfunction.

Table 41.6 outlines the examination for somatic dysfunction of SI articulation.

The Mitchell Model

The model of SI motion and dysfunction most commonly taught in Colleges of Osteopathic Medicine is that developed by Fred Mitchell, Sr., D.O. and amplified by his son Fred Mitchell, Jr., D.O., and others. Mitchell introduced a new vocabulary, new concepts regarding SI motion, and new diagnostic tests. The first publication was an article in the 1958 *AAO Yearbook* entitled "Structural Pelvic Function" and republished in 1965. The following paragraph summarizes the new vocabulary, concepts and diagnostic tests contributed by Mitchell.

In the paper, the nomenclature never defined a relationship between the sacrum and the ilium, although he recognized that during the motion cycle of walking the ilia move back and forth in opposing directions. The focus was more centered of what was occurring between the sacrum and L5. The paper explained how the motion cycle of walking was utilized to analyze sacral, lumbar, and ilial motion. Three transverse axes of sacral motion were identified (superior, middle, inferior) and an oblique axis (upper pole on one side and lower pole on the opposite side). The Seated flexion test indicated the side of the SI dysfunction while the Standing flexion test indicated the side of the iliosacral dysfunction.

Mitchell described sacral torsions as oblique axis dysfunctions. They are named for the rotation of the sacrum in relation to L5. The terminology of sacral torsions does not name ilial motion/position in relation to the sacrum, although this is described in the diagnostic findings of sacral torsions. In torsions, lumbar side-bending engages the oblique axis, and the sacrum rotates about an oblique axis. *Forward torsions* were named right on right; or left on left with L5 following neutral mechanics. *Backward torsions* were named right on left, or left on right with L5 following nonneutral mechanics.

In relation to unilateral flexions, he described that they have a shallow sulcus and a posterior/inferior inferior lateral angle (ILA) on the same side.

TABLE 41.6

Examination for Somatic Dysfunction of SI Articulation

Position	Examination	Results
Step 1. Patient standing	Evaluate anatomic landmarks, standing flexion test	A positive standing flexion test means dysfunction in the leg and/or pelvis on that side.
Step 2. Patient seated	Perform seated flexion test	Will specifically determine whether there is a SI dysfunction, and if so, which side (but not which arm) of the SIJ is dysfunctional.
Step 3. Patient supine	Positional assessment of ASISs, pubic tubercles, and medial malleoli	Helps determine the etiology of the problem and whether it is purely sacral or a "mixed" problem, incorporating iliac and pubic dysfunction.
Step 4. Patient prone	Palpate for tissue texture changes, motion testing of the sacrum, motion testing of L5, ligamentous tension testing	Helps the physician discover which axis is involved, find what portion of the SIJ is restricted, determine L5 motion and position, and evaluate pelvic ligamentous tensions.

In the Mitchell muscle energy model of diagnosis, two assumptions are made when determining an iliosacral diagnosis. The first is that the dysfunction is due to neuromuscular imbalance, with the muscle(s) on one side being hypertonic and their opposites being hypotonic. The second is that the side of dysfunction is the side of the positive standing flexion test.

With regards to the innominates Mitchell's paper described the inferior transverse axis for innominate rotation. The anterior and posterior innominate rotation was basically unchanged from the older models. He also discussed the innominate upslip (superior translation or shear) as first described by Fryette. He also commented on pubic shears.

The Mitchell model, being based on the motion cycle of walking, teaches that a pubic shear prevents normal motion of the pelvis, lumbar spine, and sacrum during walking.

The following are the diagnostic tests he described:

- Standing and Seated flexion test
- Lumbosacral spring test
- Backward bending test
- Positional assessment was utilized
- All motion testing is limited to sagittal plane motion
- Palpation for tissue texture abnormality was not described in 1958.

The Mitchell model uses positional asymmetry and the backward bending and spring tests to obtain a diagnosis of sacral dysfunction. Palpation for TTC and passive motion testing of sacral motion about the oblique axes was not part of their diagnostic process.

Following introduction of his concepts to the osteopathic profession, a Muscle Energy Tutorial Committee was created. The Muscle Energy Tutorial Committee met for a number of sessions, and developed a curriculum for teaching the "Mitchell Model" and muscle energy technique. With the development of new schools of osteopathic medicine (in addition to the five existing schools), the faculty of the new schools received tutorial training in the Mitchell muscle energy model. By sheer numbers, the Mitchell model became the language of the osteopathic profession.

The Chicago Model

The Chicago model dates back to the late 1930s, when Strachan, D.O. (CCO anatomy professor) et al. conducted a cadaveric SI motion study. Strachan's findings are discussed in the section on Biomechanics and motion. The Chicago/HVLA system is described in Walton's text, *Osteopathic Diagnosis and Technique, Sacroiliac Diagnosis* (22). Strachan's model describes sacral dysfunction in relation to the ilium rather than to L5. Historically, prior to Mitchell's paper in 1958 on structural pelvic function (13), SI problems were described as the sacrum in relation to the ilium, or the ilium in relation to the sacrum. Dysfunctions include anterior sacrum and posterior sacrum. Sacral movement is around an oblique axis: motion may be restricted at either the upper or lower arm of the L- (C-) shaped SIJ. Note that the ILA is not the lower arm of the joint, but a portion of the sacrum used for palpation and positional reference. The sacrum is diagnosed as either anterior or posterior to the ipsilateral ilium (Table 41.7).

Any discussion of the Chicago model must begin with an understanding that the sacrum is described in relation to the ilium. This seems a very logical approach when discussing the SIJ. There are two SIJs, one on either side. It is entirely logical when evaluating the relationship of the sacrum to the ilium that both sides can and should be explored for diagnostic findings. It always has depended on palpation for tissue texture changes as well as looked at anatomic asymmetry. In the early days, Philadelphia preferred to name the ilial position in relation to the sacrum. The Chicago model recognized a right and a left SIJ. SI dysfunctions were further classified as upper pole dysfunctions and lower pole dysfunctions. The model uses asymmetry of position, tissue texture change, and motion testing about each oblique axis to arrive at the diagnosis. In the Chicago model, the relationship between the sacrum and L5 (the lumbosacral joint) is not defined. Assessment of L5 requires a separate assessment. L5 position is not a part of the terminology of a Chicago SI lesion. Ordinarily, L5 rotates in the opposite direction of the sacrum. The term "compensated L5" has been applied to this relationship. (See Nelson, the Sacrum, a bone of contention.) The Chicago model delineates two primary sacral dysfunctions; the anterior sacrum and the posterior sacrum. Both dysfunctions involve the oblique axis. Described below are the clinical findings of each.

An anterior sacrum left would be described as an upper pole dysfunction on the left. The left sacral sulcus would be deep in relation to the ilium. The sacrum dysfunction would be described as sacral rotation right, sidebending left, with a deep sulcus left,

TABLE 41.7

Chicago Model Sacral Dysfunctions

Diagnosis	Characteristics
Anterior right	Positive seated flexion test right Deep and tender right sacral sulcus Left ILA immobile to downward/anterior compression
Anterior left	Positive seated flexion test left Deep and tender left sacral sulcus Right ILA immobile to downward/anterior compression
Posterior right	Positive right or left seated flexion test Deep left sacral sulcus Posterior and inferior right ILA TTC over lower pole of SI joint Right ILA immobile to downward/anterior compression
Posterior left	Positive right or left seated flexion test Deep right sacral sulcus Posterior and inferior left ILA TTC over lower pole of left SI joint Left ILA immobile to downward/anterior compression

tenderness and tissue texture abnormality were found in the deep sulcus. In the early days, the term oblique axis was not used. However, sacral rotation right and sidebending left would be motion about a right oblique axis.

A posterior sacrum is a lower pole dysfunction. A posterior sacrum right involves sacral rotation right and sidebending left. However, the right ILA is posterior, with tissue texture abnormality and tenderness over the lower pole of the SIJ on the right. A posterior sacrum is a form of oblique axis dysfunction in which the deep sulcus and posterior ILA are on opposite sides.

Both the anterior sacrum left and a posterior sacrum right could be described as "right on right" dysfunctions. Yet they are quite different. From the perspective of someone who understands the difference, treatment can be very specific. The muscle energy technique for torsions is a form of lumbar sidebending technique.

What about unilateral flexions and extensions? Strachan reported in 1938 "When a force is transmitted vertically downward from the lumbar region, the sacrum glides downward and flexes. When traction is applied from above, the sacrum glides upward and extends." Strachan has defined the motion of unilateral flexions and extensions. If a downward force causes the sacrum to glide and flex, and for some reason the sacrum gets "stuck" on that side, a unilateral flexion exists. Positionally, the sulcus will be deep, and the ILA is posterior/inferior on the same side. Since gravity is always producing a downward force, unilateral flexions are reasonably common.

Unilateral extensions are rare, because a traction-type force from above is necessary to glide the sacrum upward. Strachan also stated that the major motions of the sacrum are flexion-extension and gliding up and down. He considered restrictions of the minor motions (rotation and sidebending) to be treated first.

Pelvic Sideshift

The Chicago model also describes the concept of pelvic sideshift. The model looks at pelvic side shift as an etiology and a maintaining factor of SI dysfunction.

Pelvic side shift is not a part of the Mitchell model. Pelvic side shift is a significant cause of SI dysfunction. If the pelvis is side shifted to the right, the body compensates by shifting lumbar mass to the left. A curve, convex left, is created. The sacrum must sidebend to accommodate the curve. The sacrum side bends left. Since the sacrum normally rotates to the opposite side of sidebending, the sacrum rotates right. This will produce an anterior sacrum left or a posterior sacrum right (or a right on right torsion). What causes pelvic sideshift? There are two general causes: (a) muscle-pull mechanics, dominantly psoas, and (b) postural imbalance from short leg, curves, trauma, etc. Since sideshift is not a part of the Mitchell model, many students are not taught to test for pelvic side shift. Side shift is a condition where the base of support (sacrum) is lateral to the midline. Significant side shift can be determined by simple inspection. Given the reality that positional change and freedom of motion are in the same direction, sliding the pelvis to one side or another will reveal freedom in one direction and restriction in the other direction. Dysfunctions are named for the freedom (which is also the position).

Side shift can also be evaluated with the patient prone. Simply grasp the pelvis and translate it to either side.

Chicago Philosophic Approach

The Chicago model is more than just two sacral dysfunctions and the pelvic sideshift test. The philosophic approach taught for generation's stems from the teachings of Robert Kappler, D.O., F.A.A.O. His pragmatic clinical approach cuts through the didactic biomechanical models and focuses on the patient. The approach starts with the clinician looking for an answer to the question, "Why is the sacrum in trouble?" It also stresses palpation for TTC as they signify altered physiology. Lastly, the philosophy stresses the concept of repeating the seated flexion test at the end of treatment to objectify the treatment response. In conclusion, anterior sacrum's and posterior sacrum's are definite clinical entities. Understanding these conditions, and knowing how to diagnose them, will provide a more specific and comprehensive understanding of the SI problem, and its causes.

Approach by Edward G. Stiles, DO, FAAO

Dr. Edward G. Stiles has put forth the idea that in the normal physiological relationship between the ilia and the sacrum each of these three axes performs a different function (personal communication). According to his research the superior pole corresponds to the axis of rotation for craniosacral motion and the cranial rhythmic impulse. Dr. Stiles proposes that the middle poles have to do with sacral flexion and extension (e.g., lumbosacral flexion and extension). The middle pole is therefore the natural axis for iliosacral interaction. The inferior poles are proposed to be the axes for diagonal rotation of the sacrum in relation to the innominates and the lumbar spine.

Contributions of Richard L. VanBuskirk, D.O., F.A.A.O.: The Still Technique Model

Another important concept that is the emerging nature of SI disturbances which remain after treatment of the lumbar spine and pelvis is ligamentous and fascial and contrasted to a bony positional change of the sacrum and the ilium. A. T. Still commented (Research and Practice) that after a technique is done, and the restriction comes back, the problem is the ligaments and fascia. (Still) The Still model demonstrates that after treatment of lumbar and innominate somatic dysfunctions, only two types of sacral dysfunctions seem to remain. Both of these sacral dysfunctions behave as if the sacrum was fixated at two of four restriction points, one superior, and one inferior on each side. The two superior restrictive axis points are on the sacral base just medial to the PSISs of the ilia and inferior to L5. The two inferior restrictive axis points are in the area of the origins of the sacrotuberous ligaments on the lower part of the sacrum, the ILA. (7) A restriction in one of the two superior axis points is identified during a seated flexion test in which the sensing fingers are firmly placed on the sacral sulcus. If there is a restriction the sacral sulcus will ride superior during the patient's flexion at the waist. A restriction in one of the inferior axis points can be identified by tightness of the tissues to any form of direct motion testing, tightness in the sacrotuberous ligament, and by inferior and/or posterior position of the ILA.

The seated flexion test as done by Van Buskirk differs from the Mitchell model seated flexion test. The tips of the sensing fingers are placed over the SI joint just medial to the PSIS at the level of the sacral base or sulcus. A positive test is indicated when the patient bends forward and the sensing finger travels superior in relation to the other side.

The second test is the position of the ILA, with the patient seated. This is checked at the sacrotuberous ligament. This is said to be positive if one ILA is posterior and doesn't move anteriorly, if the sacrotuberous ligament is tight on that side, or if the ILA is more inferior on that side. The positive side is that of restriction.

A positive seated flexion test on one side and a positive ILA test on the other side are diagnostic of a *diagonal sacrum*. Van Buskirk describes that whenever a diagonal SI dysfunction is found, there will be a corresponding single segment lumbar neutral dysfunction. This neutral lumbar dysfunction commonly will be found at L5.

If the positive seated flexion test and the positive lateral angle test are on the same side, the diagnosis is a *unilateral sacrum* (Table 41.8. The sacral diagnosis will be named for the pattern of free axis points (i.e., whether they are diagonal to each other or on the same side) and the free direction of rotation of the sacral base. These dysfunctions are effectively treated with a Still technique.

Despite the differences of the various models of SI dysfunction, from a clinical perspective, there is a generalized agreement among practicing physicians that the pubes, pelvis, and lumbar spine must be effectively treated before treating the SIJ.

Ilia

Innominate function and dysfunction involve shifts in iliosacral motion among the three described axes. Van Buskirk finds that most of the motion is across the superior and inferior axes with little or no motion in the middle axis (7). The Still Model uses the following five tests to evaluate the ilia:

- PSIS position
- ASIS
- Pelvic translation or ASIS compression test

TABLE 41.8

Still Model Sacral Dysfunctions

Diagnosis	Characteristics
Diagonal right	Positive right seated flexion test Positive left ILA test
Diagonal left	Positive left seated flexion test Positive right ILA test
Unilateral right	Positive right seated flexion test Positive right ILA test
Unilateral left	Positive left seated flexion test Positive left ILA test

- ASIS tenderpoint
- Standing flexion test

There is no single test or even pair of tests that predict the nature of the iliosacral somatic dysfunction. Van Buskirk finds that innominate somatic dysfunctions act as if the normal axis of motion at the middle pole of the SIJ has been transferred to the other axes. The anterior innominate dysfunction, characterized by PSIS superior and ASIS inferior on the affected side, acts as if there were a restriction at the inferior pole of the SIJ. That is, attempts to move the innominates seem to isolate to the inferior SI pole rather than the normal middle pole. The posterior innominate dysfunction, characterized by PSIS inferior and ASIS superior on the affected side, acts as if there were a restriction at the superior pole of the SIJ.

The Still model also recognizes up slipped and down slipped innominates. Down slipped innominates are rare in clinical practice, and are usually created by a traumatic pull to the leg. Listed below, Van Buskirk relates how up slipped innominates can occur:

- Asymmetrical weight bearing on one leg for a prolonged time
- Upward shear on the side of the shoe lift
- Longer leg may develop an upward pelvic shear.
- Trendelenberg gait (see gluteus medius below) or a limb can cause an up slipped innominate.

No single treatment using the Still Technique has been found which resolves the up slipped innominate completely. According to Van Buskirk, the only complete success requires treating each of the three restriction poles. When treatments focused on each of the three poles are performed during the same session, the dysfunction seems fully released, and does not reoccur as readily.

Pubes

Regarding the pubes, Van Buskirk feels that pubic ramus evaluation is a poor test for iliosacral dysfunction. With the Still technique model, treatment of innominate dysfunctions often reduces pubic ramus dysfunctions. For that reason, Van Buskirk typically evaluates and treats the innominate dysfunctions first. Clinically, Van Buskirk will evaluate and treat the external abdominal oblique and the ilioinguinal ligament when there is a pubic dysfunction. When diagnosing these muscles and the pubes, evaluation includes palpating for tenderpoints on the ASIS and lateral pubes. If a tenderpoint is present at both sites the dysfunction will involve the external abdominal oblique. If the tenderpoint includes only the insertion on the lateral pubes, the ilioinguinal ligament is involved.

The pubic dysfunction is treated before the external abdominal oblique and/or the ilioinguinal ligament.

Psoas

With psoas dysfunction, leg extension will be markedly restricted and the foot will tend to be everted. Leg extension is evaluated with the ilium stabilized. Another finding related to psoas dysfunction is a referred tenderpoint found on the anterior-lateral aspect of the thigh, just inferior and about 1 cm medial to the inferior ASIS (7). Van Buskirk finds this tenderpoint routinely when there is a psoas restriction.

Clinical Application of the Models

SI dysfunction is described in this chapter using the most consistent criteria of all three systems. No matter which model is used, to integrate the following information into the clinical arena, the physician must consider three questions:

1. Is the sacrum in trouble?
2. Why is the sacrum restricted?
3. What are we going to do for the patient?

Somatic Dysfunction of the Sacrum

Sacral Torsions

The Mitchell system, based on the cycle of walking (as previously detailed), describes sacral motion relative to L5. The sacrum can move forward or backward about left and right oblique axes depending on the individual's center of gravity and gait, can flex or extend around a transverse axis, or can shift in the L- (C-) shaped articulation, causing a shear. Mitchell's dysfunctions include sacral torsions Sacral torsions refer to motion at the lumbosacral junction where the sacrum and L5 are rotating in opposite directions. Rotation of the sacrum is movement about an oblique axis or diagonal axis. Sacral torsion does not describe a relationship between the sacrum and the ilium.

Forward Torsions

Forward torsions occur when the lumbar spine is in neutral. In this example, side bending of the lumbar spine to the left (during the motion cycle of walking) engages the left oblique axis. The lumbar spine, in neutral, rotates right with left side bending. Since the left oblique axis is engaged, the sacrum rotates left about the left oblique axis, producing a deep sacral sulcus on the right. Torsion implies that the sacrum has rotated left, while the lumbar spine has rotated right. (Note that, with neutral lumbar mechanics, left side bending produces rotation right.) The term forward torsion is derived from the observation that, in the erect posture, the sacrum is in a flexed forward position (45 to 55 degrees from the vertical, or 35 to 45 degrees from the horizontal). The Ferguson lumbosacral angle is measured from the horizontal. There are two forward torsions: left rotation on a left oblique axis (left on left), and right rotation about the right oblique axis (right on right). Positional findings with each of the two forward torsions include those shown in Table 41.9.

In the normal motion cycle of walking, the sacrum rotates from side to side. Dysfunction in the form of a forward torsion occurs when the sacral base rotates forward, becomes restricted, and does not rotate back as far as it should. The forward sacral torsion and anterior sacrum have several findings in common. Subjective complaints include SI, inguinal, or groin discomfort and low back pain. Objective findings include freedom of rotation anteriorly about

TABLE 41.9	
Mitchell Model SI Somatic Dysfunction	
Diagnosis	**Characteristics**
Unilateral flexion right	Positive right seated flexion test Deep right sacral sulcus Inferior/posterior right ILA
Unilateral flexion left	Positive left seated flexion test Deep left sacral sulcus Inferior/posterior left ILA
Unilateral extension right	Positive right seated flexion test Shallow right sacral sulcus Superior/anterior right ILA
Unilateral extension left	Positive left seated flexion test Shallow left sacral sulcus Superior/anterior left ILA
Left on left torsion	Positive right seated flexion test Deep right sacral sulcus Posterior left ILA L5 rotated right, sidebent left Left base restriction
Right on right torsion	Positive left seated flexion test Deep left sacral sulcus Posterior right ILA L5 rotated left, sidebent right Right base restriction
Right on left torsion	Positive right seated flexion test Shallow right sacral sulcus TTC right sulcus Posterior/inferior right ILA L5 rotated left, sidebent left, nonneutral Left base restriction
Left on right torsion	Positive left seated flexion test Shallow left sacral sulcus Posterior/inferior left ILA L5 rotated right, sidebent right, nonneutral Right base restriction
Bilateral flexion	Bilateral positive seated flexion test Bilaterally deep sacral sulcus Bilaterally posterior/ILA Middle pole restriction
Bilateral extension	Bilateral positive seated flexion test Bilaterally shallow sacral sulcus Bilaterally anterior ILA Inferior pole restriction

an oblique axis, with sacral side bending and rotation in opposite directions. There is an increased lordotic curve. Spinal asymmetry and postural imbalance are noted: The sacrum has rotated in a direction opposite to the supported lumbars. There is an ipsilateral positive seated flexion test, deep sacral sulcus with tissue texture abnormality, possible psoas tension, and short leg. Neutral mechanics apply to L5, with side bending and rotation to the opposite side. However, rotation of L5 is also in a direction opposite to that of the sacrum.

Backward Torsions

Backward torsions (nonneutral) occur when the lumbar spine is in nonneutral (flexion or, where the curve exceeds normal lordosis, extension) and the sacral base rotates posteriorly about the opposite oblique axis. While they do not occur within the cycle of walking, they are associated with physiologic motion when a person forward bends and then side bends. Consider a patient in the standing position who bends forward. The sacrum actually extends or backward bends at this time. The lumbar spine is flexed to a point where any multiple plane motion results in nonneutral multiple plane motion. The patient reaches sideways to pick up an object. The lumbar spine side bends to the right from the nonneutral sagittal plane position. The right oblique axis is engaged as a result of the right side bending. L5 rotates right according to nonneutral lumbar mechanics. The sacral base moves posteriorly at the left base as the sacrum rotates to the left according to sacral nonneutral mechanics. This example is called left on right (left rotation about the right oblique axis). There are two types of backward sacral torsions: right rotation on a left oblique axis (right on left), and left rotation on a right oblique axis (left on right). Positional findings with each of the two backward torsions include those shown in Table 41.9.

A backward torsion is not the same as a posterior sacrum. A posterior sacrum is a type of forward torsion in which the inferior portion of the sacrum is posterior. In a backward torsion, the posterior portion is at the sacral base (the shallow sulcus).

Subjective complaints include low back pain or SI discomfort that gets worse when bending forward or walking. Objective findings include those listed above, plus a decreased lordotic curve. Palpatory findings include tissue texture abnormality and a shallow sacral sulcus on the side of the dysfunction, with tissue texture abnormality at L5. Nonneutral mechanics apply to L5, with rotation and side bending occurring to the same side and opposite the side of the sacrum's rotation. According to Kappler, his experience treating backward torsions involves the following findings (R.E. Kappler, *personal communication*):

- Significant tissue texture abnormality and tenderness is located over the shallow sulcus.
- Sacrum resists applied flexion, and it is painful.
- There is usually a mid-lumbar flexed type II dysfunction on side opposite the shallow sulcus.
- Psoas tension is usually not a factor.
- Treatment of backward torsions:
  - Treat the innominates
  - Treat the mid-lumbar flexed dysfunction

Bilateral Sacral Flexion

If the sacrum is flexed forward, with the sacral base anterior, the lumbar lordosis appears to be increased, the seated flexion test is negative, the sacral sulci are bilaterally deep, and the ILA's are posterior. It is postulated that this motion occurs about a middle transverse axis of the sacrum. This is called a bilateral sacral flexion. When the lumbosacral spring test is performed, there is good spring (a negative test) because the sacral base, already anterior, moves forward easily. If the backward bending test is done, the sacral sulci is still deep (if not deeper), and the ILAs are still posterior (or more posterior) because the base of the sacrum normally moves forward and the apex moves posteriorly during backward bending of the lumbar region.

This is an extremely common dysfunction in the postpartum female because of birth mechanics. Subjectively, the patient complains of low back pain that becomes worse when bending backward. Objective findings include:

- Increased lumbar curve
- Deep bilateral sacral sulci with tissue texture changes
- Bilateral ILAs posterior
- Negative lumbar spring test
- No change with the hyperextension test

Motion characteristics include resistance to posterior rotation of the base of the sacrum if pressure is placed on the apex.

Bilateral Sacral Extension

In some cases, the patient does not have a positive seated flexion test, yet complains of low back pain, and the sacrum seems to be at the center of the problem. At that time, the sacral sulci should be examined, the ILA's checked, the spring test and backward bending test performed, and a careful analysis made of the relationship of the sacrum to the lumbar spine. The lordotic curve may be increased or decreased. With postural flexion at the lumbar spine (forward bending), the sacrum extends (the base moves posterior), and there is a decrease in the lumbar lordotic curve. If the lordotic curve seems to be decreased, it may be that there is a posterior sacral base. In a bilateral extension, the sacrum is held in a backward bent position and does not easily bend forward. The lumbosacral spring test is therefore positive, which means there is either poor spring or no spring. Sacral sulci and ILAs should appear symmetric in either prone or backward bending positions, and, if there is any difference on the backward bending test, the sulci look more shallow, and the ILAs more anterior.

Subjectively, the patient complains of low back pain or fatigue that becomes worse with forward bending. Objective findings include:

- Decreased lumbar curve
- ILAs equal and perhaps anterior
- Positive lumbar spring test
- ILAs stay equal during hyperextension test (superior/inferior)
- Sacral sulci are bilaterally shallow, with tissue texture changes
- Sacrum resists posteroanterior pressure at base, but yields to posteroanterior pressure on apex

Sacral Shears

The sacrum can appear as if it has slipped anteriorly or posteriorly around a transverse axis that allows it to shift within the L- (C-) shaped SIJ. If it slips forward, it produces a finding called a sacral shear or unilateral sacral flexions and extensions. ECOP has concluded that "shears" and unilateral sacral flexions and extensions are the same thing.

Unilateral Sacral Flexion

If there is a positive seated flexion test, with the base of the sacrum anterior on the dysfunctional side (sacral sulcus deep on that side) and the ipsilateral ILA is posterior, the patient has a unilateral sacral flexion. The ipsilateral medial malleolus is more inferior, and the transverse process of L5 is more posterior on the dysfunctional side. Both sides of the sacral base move anteriorly with exhalation but do not move easily in a posterior direction with inhalation. The spring test should be negative, since the base of the sacrum moves anteriorly easily when it is flexed. The backward bending test should show improvement because, while the one side is flexed forward, making the sacral sulcus deep, when the patient bends backward the other side of the sacral base should be pulled forward, increasing symmetry.

Unilateral Sacral Extension

If there is a positive seated flexion test, with the base of the sacrum posterior on the dysfunctional side (sacral sulcus shallow), and the ipsilateral ILA is anterior, the patient has a unilateral sacral extension. To confirm this, test the patient with the spring test and the backward bending test. The spring test should be positive, since the base of the sacrum does not move anteriorly easily when the sacrum is held in an extension position. On the backward bending test, the sulci and ILAs should look even less symmetric because, while the one side is held backward, making the sacral sulcus shallow, when the patient bends backward; the other side of the sacral base should be pulled forward, making the results look worse.

Anterior Sacrum

An anterior sacrum is a positional term describing a somatic dysfunction in which the sacral base has rotated forward and side bent to the side opposite the rotation. The upper limb of the SIJ has restricted motion, and the dysfunction is named for the side on which forward rotation occurs. An anterior sacrum is probably one type of Mitchell's forward torsion. For example, anterior sacrum left describes a condition in which the sacrum is rotated right and side bent to the left, the directions of ease of motion. (This could also be considered right rotation about a right oblique axis.) There is restriction of left rotation and right side bending. The sacral sulcus is deep on the left, with tenderness and tissue texture abnormality in the left sulcus. When downward pressure is applied over the right ILA, attempting to rotate the sacrum about the right oblique axis, the left superior portion of the sacrum resists moving posteriorly, toward the ilium.

The anterior sacrum is clearly an "oblique axis dysfunction". Therefore, it is one form of a forward torsion with motion restriction, tissue texture abnormality, and tenderness associated with the deep sulcus side. An anterior sacrum (e.g., anterior sacrum left) has the following characteristics:

- Deep sulcus left, (right ILA posterior)
- Tissue texture abnormality and tenderness in the deep sulcus
- Right rotated, left sidebent
- Positive seated flexion test left
- Left sacral base will not move posteriorly when pressure is applied to right ILA.
    - (This motion test would involve the right oblique axis.)
- The conceptual model is that anterior sacrum's are an upper pole dysfunction (upper part of the "L" shaped articulation.).
- Because the sacrum is sidebend left, the left SI is the "compressed side". In the standing position, the left sacral base will be lower (inferior).
- Gluteus medius hypertonicity and tenderness were commonly found on the side of the anterior sacrum.

Posterior Sacrum

A posterior sacrum is diagnosed when the sacrum has rotated backward and is side bent to the side opposite of rotation. It is named for the side of the backward or posterior rotation. This rotation side bending to the opposite side could be considered rotation about an oblique axis. The posterior sacrum is on the side opposite the deep sulcus at the inferior pole of the joint. The patient

experiences discomfort at the inferior arm of the SIJ and possibly sciatic pain. There is a pelvic side shift to the side of dysfunction, spinal asymmetry, and postural imbalance. The seated flexion test may be positive on either side of a posterior sacrum dysfunction. There is ipsilateral piriformis tension, and the ipsilateral ILA is posterior and inferior. There may be contralateral psoas tension, and there is generally a contralateral short leg. For example, a posterior sacrum right has rotated right and side-bent left, the directions of ease of motion; rotation left and side-bending right are restricted. A posterior sacrum involves restriction of motion at the lower limb of the SI articulation. Tissue texture abnormality and tenderness are located over the inferior portion of the dysfunctional SIJ; in this example, the tenderness is on the right. The rotation, in this case, is in relation to the right oblique axis. A posterior sacrum is probably a form of forward torsion in which the major joint motion restriction is on the side opposite the deep sulcus. A motion test for lower pole (lower limb of the L) restriction (e.g., posterior sacrum right) is to contact the inferior borders of the sacrum with both thumbs and apply a cephalad/anterior force, attempting to glide the sacrum in the direction of the lower limb of the joint. Restriction is felt on the posterior sacral side. Although there are similarities between the posterior sacrum and the forward torsion, there is no true Mitchell equivalent to Strachan's posterior sacrum. A posterior sacrum should not be confused with a backward torsion, a posterior sacral base, or an extension of the sacrum.

The posterior sacrum is an oblique axis dysfunction. Therefore, it is a form of forward torsion with tissue texture abnormality, tenderness, and motion restriction on the side of the lower pole. A posterior sacrum (e.g., posterior sacrum right) has the following characteristics:

- Right ILA posterior (deep sulcus left)
- Tissue texture abnormality and tenderness at the right inferior pole (lowest part of the SI joint)
- Right rotated, left sidebent.
- Positive seated flexion test on right (usually)
- Confirmatory motion test, patient prone. Pressure on the inferior surface of the sacrum applied in a superior-anterior direction, trying to glide the sacrum superiorly along the lower limb of the "C"-shaped articulation, is met with resistance. The ILA is inferior, and resists moving superiorly. The conceptual model is that of a lower pole SI restriction.
- From a sidebending perspective, the posterior sacrum is on the "stretch side" of the SI problem
- A posterior sacrum is not included in the Mitchell model.
- Piriformis muscle hypertonicity and tenderness is commonly found on the side of the posterior sacrum.

Unilateral Sacrum

A positive seated flexion test on one side and a positive ILA test on the other side are diagnostic of a *diagonal sacrum*.

Diagonal Sacrum

If the positive seated flexion test and the positive lateral angle test are on the same side, the diagnosis is a *unilateral sacrum*. To review sacral diagnoses, refer to Table 41.8.

Integrated Diagnosis of the Lumbar Spine, Sacrum, Pelvis

Understanding all the above-mentioned portions of the physical examination, and the characteristics of the specific dysfunctions, the clinician now needs to evaluate the sacrum and lumbar spine. Start with interpreting the standing flexion test, pelvic sideshift and the seated flexion test. Before diagnosing the sacrum, diagnose the lumbar spine in the prone position. To review the specifics of this see the chapter on lumbar spine. It is a good time to evaluate for segmental dysfunction and Jones tenderpoints. In addition to generalized changes in the pelvic girdle tissues, the physician may detect small myofascial tender points. Such areas may be characterized by a small, palpable, circumscribed thickening of tissue that is tender with moderate to deep palpation. These tender points may be associated with autonomic dysfunction or refer pain to a neurologic distribution. Muscles containing tender points reveal pain with active or passive range of motion. There may be areas of patchy weakness in the range of motion of muscles containing painful tender points. Joints controlled by muscles with tender points may have a diminished range of motion. The pelvic girdle contains many of these myofascial tender points because myofascial structures are constantly working to maintain postural balance. Numerous authors (18–20) have indicated continuous postural strain as the cause of precipitating and/or perpetuating myofascial tender points. Tenderpoints also correspond to segmental dysfunction.

Segmental dysfunction in the upper lumbars (L1-2) that is flexed is typically involved with a tight psoas muscle (23). A tight psoas muscle is characterized by a decrease in hip extension on physical examination. A tight psoas will cause pelvic sideshift and apply a compressive load across the SIJ, contributing to the dysfunction (23). Another relationship commonly found by Kappler (R.E. Kappler, *personal communication*) is a flexed lumbar segment at L2 or L3 is seen in conjunction with a backward torsion. The segment will be rotated in the opposite direction of the torsion. Treatment of this segment, many times will improve the backward torsion. When there is a forward sacral torsion, there is usually a group curve convex opposite to the side of sacral rotation. For unilateral sacral flexions, L4 or L5 may be extended rotated and sidebent to the same side. For unilateral sacral extensions, L5 may be flexed or significantly restricted. Sometimes in these dysfunctions, there is unilateral muscle hypertonicity over and along the whole SIJ. In this situation, there is usually significant ipsilateral thoracolumbar tension/findings as well as findings in the upper thoracic spine and cranium. Many times in patients with significant SI restrictions, there are alternating single segment lumbar dysfunctions (e.g., L1 left, L2 right, L3 right, L5 left). In the patient with significant SI dysfunction that has little or no findings in the lumbar spine, carefully check L5. It is not uncommon for disc herniations to have minimal lumbar somatic dysfunction, yet maximal leg symptomology. Another evaluation method is to apply the lumbosacral spring test to the L5 spinous process. Decreased spring indicates a backward torsion. If sharp or severe pain occurs with the spring test, they may have a disc protrusion or a spondylolisthesis. In either situation, they will commonly have bilateral muscle tension from T10-L1 as well as an anterior L5 Jones tenderpoint. With significant pain the sympathetics become involved and travel up to the low thoracic cord, cause facilitation and this produces palpable muscular tension. Patients with L5 discs, spondylolisthesis, backward torsions, or any significantly painful L5 condition, will have the anterior Jones tenderpoint nearly 100% of the time. If no pain occurs with springing L5, look more closely at the ilia and pubes, as well as the cranium. Palpable strains in the cranial mechanism correlate to sacral motion restrictions due to the continuity of the dural membrane. Skilled osteopathic physicians are able to palpate inherent motion of the human body. Physicians trained in craniosacral diagnosis can palpate this motion in the sacrum as the craniosacral mechanism moves the sacrum between the two ilia.

Following assessment of the lumbar spine, check for restriction of hip extension, indicating a tight psoas muscle. From here, evaluate the sacrum for position and motion. Check the sacral sulci for depth, tenderness and tissue texture change TTC. A deep sulcus may indicate an anterior sacrum or forward torsion. A shallow sulcus with diffuse TTC and significant tenderness usually correlates with a backward torsion. A positive backward bending test confirms this. Then motion test the sacrum on each theoretical oblique axis. Look for the restriction of motion, but name it for the freedom of motion. Palpate for TTC over the upper and lower poles of the SIJs, as well as for tenderness/tension of the piriformis muscle. From here, the clinician will attempt to glide the lower aspect of the sacrum cephalad along the joint by applying a firm pressure alternating between the thumbs. Resistance to motion is seen with a posterior sacrum dysfunction, or any dysfunction in which the lower pole of the sacrum is involved. If a posterior sacrum is present, check the piriformis for tenderness, and the pelvic floor on that side. Checking for tension in the ischiorectal region is important, especially in patients with pelvic pain, and postoperative cases. When the patient coughs muscular tension, or pressure, is bilaterally palpated. If no movement occurs, the SI dysfunction is affecting the movement of the pelvic floor musculature. If there are findings associated with a backward torsion such as a shallow sulcus with diffuse TTC and significant tenderness, confirmation can be done with the backward bending and spring tests.

Have the patient lie supine and perform an abdominal examination. For evaluation of the pelvic girdle, a complete examination of the abdomen is required. Following inspection, auscultation, and palpation, the physician can percuss the liver, spleen, and stomach, and palpate for any pelvic masses. A rectal examination, a pelvic examination in the female, and a prostate examination in the male should be a part of a complete examination of the pelvic/sacral region.

At this point, evaluate the ilia in the supine position. Start with the position of the ASISs by evaluating their position at the inferior portion of each ASIS. Perform the ilium compression test, pushing downward, cephalad, and lateral to the ASIS. An assessment of rotational restriction of the pelvis can be performed as well. At this point, palpate for tension of the musculature of the inguinal region. The more localized areas of tension usually have more tenderpoints. Assess for Jones anterior tenderpoints, and correlate them to what was found segmentally in the lumbar spine. Assess the pubic ramus for asymmetry and motion. Evaluate to see if one pubic ramus is superior or inferior, as well as anterior or posterior (rare). A direct motion test on the pubes can be performed if necessary. If the pubes is anterior the pelvis will rotate away from the dysfunctional side. Screen the hip joints for restrictions in internal rotation, flexion, and abduction/external rotation. Special orthopedic tests of the hips SIJs, and ilia can be performed at this time. See Table 41.10 for these tests. Check the attitude of the feet, the levelness of the medial malleoli, and fascial drag in each extremity by a brief light internal rotation motion.

Evaluation of the sacrum and or pelvis can be done in the seated position for those patients who cannot lie down. The seated flexion test should be done before treatment and at the end of treatment. Although a positive seated flexion test is not a very sensitive or specific test, its greatest utility is that it returns to negative after manipulative treatment is completed. Kappler, D.O., F.A.A.O. (R.E. Kappler, *personal communication*) has devised a translation test performed in the seated position that assess motion at the sacral sulci by translating the lumbar spine back and forth. The authors find this a very useful test in older, obese, and pregnant patients. In the seated position, the motion of the abdominal diaphragm

TABLE 41.10

Commonly Used Osteopathic SI Tests

Osteopathic SI Tests	Characteristics
Standing flexion test	PSIS moves cephalad Indicates SIJ dysfunction
Seated Flexion test	PSIS moves cephalad Indicates SIJ dysfunction
Pelvic sideshift	Pelvis shifts off to one side Indicates contralateral psoas or lumbar dysfunction
Hip drop	One leg standing produces lumbar curve Indicates lumbar dysfunction
Backward bending test	Prone, prop-up alters sulcus depth Asymmetry of sulcus depth increases
Spring test	Prone, anterior springing of L5 Poor spring = positive test
Iliac compression test	Supine, posterior/lateral compression Poor motion = positive test
Posterior sacrum confirmatory test	Prone, superior glide of sacral lower pole Restricted superior glide = positive test
Kappler Seated Translation Test	Seated, palpate sacral sulci for motion as the lumbar spine is translated toward the sulci. Restricted motion = positive test

(as well as its excursion) can be evaluated, which many clinicians assess when evaluating the pelvic region.

TOP 10 CAUSES OF SACROILIAC DYSFUNCTION

Cause No. 1: Psoas

Treatment of psoas dysfunction is the first step in treating SI dysfunction (R.E. Kappler, *personal communication* (23). Psoas muscle tension compresses the lumbosacral area and the SIJs. Psoas tension will also cause pelvic sideshift, another cause of SIJ dysfunction. The sacrum cannot function properly with excessive psoas tension. There are two components to a tight psoas: (a) tight psoas and (b) a flexed Type II dysfunction at L1 or L2, with rotation to the side of the tight psoas (23). To check psoas tension, in the prone patient, grasp the thigh just above the knee, and extend the hip. Compare both sides. This method of testing provides excellent "end feel". If the psoas is tight, examination of the upper lumbar spine is essential. Treatment of the upper lumbar dysfunction by itself will many times resolve the psoas tension and improve hip extension. Some clinicians utilize the Thomas test for psoas assessment. This test is mostly a test of inspection, and does not provide the clinician with proper end feel. Additionally, it fails to evaluate

the flexed upper lumbar dysfunction. Management of SI problems always involves checking the psoas. Clinicians who fail to remove the psoas component and pelvic sideshift will find that the SI dysfunction will recur very quickly (23).

Cause No. 2: Lumbar Somatic Dysfunction

Lumbar somatic dysfunction, particularly type II flexed dysfunctions, may contribute to SI dysfunction. Effective treatment of the lumbar somatic dysfunction will often release the SI restriction. Lumbar group curves can be due to sacral base declination, or they can be there prior to the SI dysfunction, such as in idiopathic scoliosis. In either situation, improving the group's function as a whole can help with dysfunction of the SIJs or pelvis.

Cause No. 3: Short Leg Syndrome/Postural Imbalance

The first symptoms of short leg syndrome are usually SI discomfort or pain. Symptoms are worse with excessive walking or running. Examination of the sacrum usually reveals a deep sacral sulcus on the short leg side with significant tissue texture abnormality and tenderness. Short leg and postural imbalance are a cause of SI dysfunction. The typical pattern for an anatomic short leg is a chronic, recurrent anterior sacrum (or forward torsion) on the short leg side, pelvic side shift to the long leg side, and lumbar curve convex on the short leg side (31). A chronic anterior sacrum on the side of the short leg is a classic finding of short leg syndrome. The status of the sacrum, the depth of the sacral sulci, and pelvic sideshift can be used clinically to evaluate progress of lift therapy. Psoas tension may exist in a patient with a symptomatic anatomic short leg. Depending on which psoas tightens, psoas tension can help compensate for a short leg, or it can exacerbate a short leg problem. Given an anatomic short leg left with a chronic left anterior sacrum and pelvic side shift right, tightness of the right psoas will correct the pelvic side shift tendency and improve the patient's condition. However, tightness of the left psoas will exaggerate the side shift right and make the problem worse.

Cause No. 4: Pelvic Side Shift

Pelvic sideshift is usually assessed with the patient standing. It can be assessed with the patient lying prone as well, although gravity is not a factor. When the patient is standing observation may show that the pelvis is shifted from midline. When a slight lateral force is applied to the pelvis in either direction, the pelvis will sideshift away from the tight psoas or if a group curve is already present, away from the convexity of a lumbar group curve. For example, with pelvic side-shift right, the compensatory change is for body mass to be moved to the opposite side producing a lumbar curve convex left. In this example, the sacrum has to side bend left to accommodate the lumbar curve. When the sacrum side bends left, it rotates right, producing SI dysfunction. This is one mechanism of SI dysfunction associated with the tight psoas, a lumbar group curve, or a short leg problem.

Cause No. 5: Simple Traumatic Sacral Somatic Dysfunction

It is not uncommon to see patients following simple traumatic somatic dysfunction. Two common mechanisms are patients who slip and fall on their buttocks, or are involved in a motor vehicle accident where the force of the impact travels through their brake leg into their pelvis. The trauma causes the SIJ to become wedged or "stuck" in an abnormal position. Depending on the severity and duration of their injuries, these patients usually "limp into the office and leap out," and are forever grateful for the one-treatment cure.

Cause No. 6: Pubic and Pelvic Floor Dysfunction

It is very important to assess and treat the pubic symphysis in sacral and pelvic dysfunction. When treated, improved pubic motion will allow each ilium to move as it is supposed to during gait and daily activities. Pubic dysfunction is also related to pelvic floor tension/dysfunction. With pubic dysfunction, fascial tension on the urogenital diaphragm can affect genitourinary function. Pelvic floor dysfunction is thought to cause congestion to the pelvic viscera, such as the prostate or uterus.

Cause No. 7: Reflex Causes

Reflex causes such as viscerosomatic reflexes from pelvis or unilateral sympathetic nervous system dysfunction are causes of SI pain. Viscerosomatic reflexes are associated with tissue texture abnormality along the SIJ, which is puffy and warm. This is similar to acute tissue texture abnormality found in the thoracic area from abdominal or thoracic visceral problems.

Cause No. 8: Cranial Dysfunction

Sacral motion restriction and somatic dysfunction can be related to strains or compression of the SBS. An evaluation of the sacrum should include an evaluation of the cranial mechanism. An evaluation of tension in the anterior abdominal wall, and the respiratory diaphragm is important to assess with the cranial mechanism. Poor abdominal diaphragm motion, compression of the SBS, and SIJ restriction are commonly found co-existing in the same patient. In this clinical situation, the clinician must treat each of these regions to affect change of the whole mechanism.

Cause No. 9: Lumbosacral Instability

SI pain may be caused by orthopedic problems of the L5-S1 segment (spondylolysis, spondylolisthesis); congenital anomalies can predispose the patient to SI dysfunction. In these cases, mobilization of the SIJ does not relieve the pain. Many times with the above-mentioned conditions, there is lumbosacral instability. However, lumbosacral instability may also occur with poor force and form closure of the joint (26,28). In cases of lumbar L5-S1, the iliolumbar ligament insertion on the ilium may become very tender. Other causes of iliolumbar ligament tenderness include ipsilateral lumbothoracic irritability, anterior rotation of L5, and pelvic side shift to that side. In orthopedic disease of L5, such as a spondylolisthesis, bilateral tenderness of these ligaments is commonly found. This may be the first ligament to be strained with postural decompensation. L5 is a frequent site of disc disease and may be unstable, as well as painful. In an unstable L5 situation, manipulative treatment needs to address the adjacent segments that are restricted. Avoid excessive HVLA to L5, especially if it is thought to be an unstable segment.

Cause No. 10: Disc Protrusions

Lumbar disc protrusions at L4 or L5, in the early stages, radiate pain into the buttock region that is interpreted as SI pain. Often the sacrum is restricted from secondary muscle hypertonicity. In these cases, treating the SI restriction is not associated with the relief of pain.

Treatment

Treatment of the sacrum and the pelvic region needs to be individualized, based on the location, duration, and severity of the somatic dysfunction present. Taken into consideration is the age of the patient, and concurrent medical or orthopedic conditions. The techniques chosen need to be matched to the type of somatic dysfunction present, and the skills of the physician. The techniques should be safe, effective, and well executed. Dysfunction of the sacrum, ilium, pubes and lumbar spine commonly co-exist and affect one another. Dysfunction distant from the sacrum and pelvis may be critical to resolving the sacral or pelvic dysfunction.

Sequencing Lumbar-Sacrum-Pelvis Treatment

The sequence of treatment is important; however, this is not the always the same from patient to patient. It is generally accepted (and taught) to treat the lumbar spine, psoas, ilium and pubes prior to treating the sacrum. There is some controversy as to which region listed above to start with. Starting with the greatest area of restriction is appropriate, as long as it was not acutely injured. Since the sacrum and SIJs respond to forces directed from above (gravity) and also from those coming from below (ground reactive force), leaving it to last in the treatment scheme seems logical.

The muscle energy model (24) bases SI dysfunction on the motion cycle of walking. Dysfunction of the pubes significantly affects this motion cycle, thus sacral-pelvic motion. Because of this the muscle energy model stresses the importance of treating the pubes is first. The muscle energy approach does not consider pelvic side shift. The muscle energy diagnostic approach also does not include tissue texture abnormality. The remainder of the muscle energy model is to treat the pelvis, then the lumbar spine, before the sacrum.

The Chicago Model as proposed by Kappler insists that the pelvis and lumbar spine must be treated first (23). The psoas muscle is included with the lumbars. The psoas must be effectively treated first. There are a number of different techniques which can be used for dysfunction of the psoas. Sometimes the thoracolumbar area must be treated, or included in the process.

The Still technique approach is very specific that the pelvis and lumbar area must be treated first. If they are treated appropriately, then the Still model of oblique sacrum dysfunction (R, L) and unilateral sacrum dysfunction (R, L) is all that remains. (The Still Technique model treats innominate up-slip as a unique entity.)

Specific technique procedures are beyond the scope of this chapter; however, listed below are goals to accomplish when treating the sacrum and pelvis.

Goals of treatment include:

- Treat segmental upper lumbar dysfunctions
- Improve hip extension (iliopsoas tension)
- Improve asymmetry/alignment of the innominates
- Treat any pubic dysfunction
- Level the sacral base
- Improve cranial motion
- Improve abdominal and pelvic diaphragm motion
- Resolve anterior or posterior lumbar tenderpoints
- Obtain a negative seated flexion test

OMT is not just the application of a technique. During treatment, the experienced physician will constantly reassess the "change" that is being made in the tissues and adjust the treatment accordingly. One of the more difficult things to master for students of osteopathy is being able to tell if they made "change" or not. Another difficulty is when to say: "enough treatment for today." The amount of dosage given to an anatomic area must be monitored.

OMT is a critical element in returning a patient to health and wellness; however it is only one aspect to the overall care of the patient. It treating sacral and pelvic problems, corrective exercises for weak inhibited muscles and stretches for tight muscles can be beneficial.

Assessing Muscle Function and Stability of the Pelvic Girdle

Addressing these muscular issues with appropriate stretches and exercises will contribute to the improvement of the patient. Assessing the neuromuscular firing patterns that occur when the patient extends their hip is also useful. The common pattern for patients is the following sequence of muscle activation as the patient extends their hip from a prone position (24):

1. Hamstring
2. Gluteus maximus
3. Contralateral erector spinae
4. Ipsilateral erector spinae

The most common sequence seen in patients with sacral, pelvic, and lumbar somatic dysfunction is:

1. Hamstrings
2. Upper lumbar and low thoracic erectors
3. Inhibited gluteus maximus

Treatment of somatic dysfunction and addressing muscle weakness and tightness helps to normalize these patterns and resolve sacral and pelvic somatic dysfunction. According to Janda, specific muscles become tight and others become weak and inhibited. Listed below are the "phasic" muscles of the pelvic girdle that commonly become weak or inhibited.

Weak phasic muscles of the trunk and pelvic girdle:

- Gluteus maximus, medius, minimus
- Transverse abdominis
- Multifidus
- Vastus medialis, lateralis

Janda also described muscles that become tight. It is not only important to address the strength of the muscles, but also their length.

Tight "postural" muscles of the trunk and pelvic girdle:

- Iliopsoas
- Hamstrings
- Lumbar erector spinae
- Quadratus lumborum
- Rectus femoris
- Tensor fascia lata/iliotibial band
- Thigh adductors
- Piriformis

In addition to evaluating muscle groups that are inhibited or tight, co-contraction of groups of muscles acting together will affect the stability of the SIJs. Muscles of the pelvic floor act together with the transverse abdominus to stabilize the pelvis during lifting (25). Groups of muscles contribute to the force closure mechanism proposed by Vleeming. An "inner muscle unit and an outer muscle unit" have been described as providing stabilizing forces for the pelvis. It is important that these groups work synchronously with sufficient recruitment and balanced muscle function (25). They are comprised of the following groups of muscles:

Inner Muscle Units

- Pelvic floor
- Transverse abdominus
- Multifidus
- Abdominal diaphragm

Outer Muscle Units

- Posterior oblique system (Latissimus dorsi, gluteus maximus, thoracolumbar fascia)
- Deep longitudinal system (Erector spinae, deep laminae of thoracolumbar fascia, sacrotuberous ligament, biceps femoris)
- Anterior oblique system (External and internal oblique, contralateral thigh adductors, anterior abdominal fascia)
- Lateral system (gluteus medius and minimus, contralateral adductors)

There are many other ways to help treat your patient besides OMT and exercises. These can include foot orthotics, heel lift therapy, acupuncture, injections, massage, physical therapy, etc. Find the best combination for your patient. Consider cost, time required, access to care, and availability.

SUMMARY

OMT is a critical component of the overall treatment of patients with conditions found attributable to sacral and pelvic somatic dysfunction. Manipulative treatment should be applied with an objective to accomplish, and for a given diagnosis. Manual techniques can restore functional symmetry between the arthrodial, vascular, lymphatic, and connective tissue elements of the pelvic girdle. When coupled with corrective exercises and other treatment modalities, it is a powerful, safe and efficacious tool for the clinician to use when treating a wide variety of patients.

REFERENCES

1. Borenstein DJ, Wiesel SW, Bowden SD. *Low Back and Neck Pain.* Philadelphia, PA: WB Saunders, 2004:41–44.
2. Mooney V. Sacroiliac joint dysfunction. In: Vleeming A, ed. *Movement, Stability and Lumbopelvic Pain.* Churchill Livingstone, 1997: 37–43:chap 2.
3. Kuchera WA, Kuchera ML. *Osteopathic Principles in Practice.* 2nd Ed. Rev. Columbus, OH: Greyden Press, 1994.
4. Seidel HM, Ball JW, Dains JE, et al. *Mosby's Guide to Physical Examination.* St. Louis, MO: CV Mosby Co., 1987.
5. Strachan WF. Applied anatomy of the pelvis and perineum. *J Am Osteopath Assoc* 38(8):57–58.
6. Weisl H. The articular surfaces of the sacroiliac joint and their relationship to the movements of the sacrum. *Acta Anat* 1954;22:1–14.
7. VanBuzkirk RL. *The Still Technique Manual.* 2nd Ed. Indianapolis, IN: American Academy of Osteopathy, 2006.
8. Thiele GH. Coccygodynia: cause and treatment. *Dis Colon Rectum* 1963;6:422–436.
9. Korr IM. Sustained sympathicotonia as a factor in disease. In: *The Collected Papers of Irvin M. Korr.* Newark, OH: American Academy of Osteopathy, 1979:77–89.
10. Beaton LE, Anson BJ. The sciatic nerve and the piriformis muscle: their interrelationship as a possible cause of coccygodynia. *J Bone Joint Surg (Br)* 1938;20:686–688.
11. Reynolds HM. Three dimensional kinematics in the pelvic girdle. *J Am Osteopath Assoc.* 1980;80:277–280.
12. Fryette HH. *Principles of Osteopathic Technique.* Carmel, CA: Academy of Applied Osteopathy, 1954.
13. Mitchell FL. Structural pelvic function. In: *American Academy of Osteopathy Yearbook.* Indianapolis, IN: American Academy of Osteopathy, 1958: 71–90.

14. Strachan WF, Beckwith CG, Larson NJ, et al. A study of the mechanics of the sacroiliac joint. *J Am Osteopath Assoc* 37(12):575–578.

15. Sturesson B, Selvik G, U'den A. Movements of the sacroiliac joints: a roentgen stereophotogrammetric analysis. *Spine* 1989;14:162–165.

16. Bachrach RM. The relationship of low back pain to psoas insufficiency. *J Orthop Med* 1991;13:34–40.

17. Mitchell FL, Pruzzo NA. Investigation of voluntary and primary respiratory mechanism. *J Am Osteopath Assoc* 1971;70:1109–1112.

18. Truhlar RE. *Doctor A.T. Still in the Living.* Privately published, Cleveland, OH: 1950. Distributed, Indianapolis, IN: American Academy of Osteopathy, 62.

19. Travell JG, Simons DG. *Myofascial Pain and Dysfunction: The Trigger Point Manual.* Vol 1. Baltimore, MD: Williams & Wilkins, 1983.

20. Travell JG, Simon DG. *Myofascial Pain and Dysfunction: The Trigger Point Manual The Lower Extremities.* Vol II. Baltimore, MD: Williams & Wilkins, 1992.

21. Hoppenfeld S. *Physical Examination of the Spine and Extremities.* Norwalk, CT: Appleton & Lange, 1976:151–152, 164.

22. Walton WJ. *Osteopathic Diagnosis and Technique, Sacroiliac Diagnosis.* 1st Ed. St. Louis, MO: Matthews Book Co., 1966:187–197. Distributed, Colorado Springs, CO: American Academy of Osteopathy; reprinted, 1970.

23. Kappler RE. The role of the psoas muscle in low back complaints. *J Am Osteopath Assoc* 1973;72:794–801.

24. Greenman PE. *Principles of Manual Medicine.* Baltimore, MD: Williams & Wilkins, 1989:226–227.

25. Dutton M. The sacroiliac joint. In: *Orthopedic Examination, Evaluation, Intervention.* McGraw-Hill, 2004: chap 27.

26. Bernard TN. The role of the sacroiliac joints in low back pain: basic aspects of pathophysiology and management. In: Vleeming A, ed. *Movement, Stability and Lumbopelvic Pain.* Churchill Livingstone, 1997:73–86.

27. Vleeming A, Snijders CJ, Stoeckart R, et al. The role of the sacroiliac joints in coupling between spine, pelvis, legs and arms. In: Vleeming A, ed. *Movement, Stability and Lumbopelvic Pain.* Churchill Livingstone, 1997:53–71.

28. Sturesson B. Movement of the sacroiliac joint: a fresh look. In Vleeming A, ed. *Movement, Stability and Lumbopelvic Pain.* Churchhill Livingstone, 1997:53–71.

29. Snijders CJ, Vleeming A, Stoeckart R, et al. Biomechanics of the interface between spine and pelvis in different postures. In: Vleeming A, ed. *Movement, Stability and Lumbopelvic Pain.* Churchill Livingstone, 1997:103–113:chap 6.

30. Magee DJ. *Orthopedic Physical Assessment.* 3d Ed. Philadelphia, PA: Saunders, 1997:567–605;chap 10.

31. AAO Yearbook. "Postural balance and imbalance". Newark, OH: 1983:7.

Lower Extremities

MICHAEL L. KUCHERA

INTRODUCTION

The lower extremities provide for support and facilitate locomotion through the use of strong bones and powerful muscles. In each foot alone, there are 126 muscles and ligaments, 33 joints, and 26 bones (plus 2 sesamoid bones under the first metatarsophalangeal joint).

The structure and function of the lower extremities also allow them to play several other significant roles. They contribute to balance and the body's postural strategies as well as housing the muscular "pumps" involved in locomotion. The latter function means that the lower extremities are a major contributor in the returning of venous and lymphatic fluids back to the central vascular system. Furthermore, their condition is a key factor in designing a number of exercise protocols that are important for a person's general health. Because of their many roles, structural pathologies and somatic dysfunction in the lower extremities have local, postural, *and* systemic implications.

Basic clinical screening evaluation of the lower extremities (as a discrete region) typically includes an initial observation of the region during normal walking as well as walking on toes or on heels; standing with both eyes open or eyes closed; squatting; bending, integrated with a standing flexion test evaluation of PSIS motion; one-legged stork (or modified Trendelenburg) test; and joint range of motion including straight-leg raising test. These musculoskeletal screening tests are integrated with standard screening functional tests for neural, lymphatic, and vascular disorders. A positive finding in any of these screening examinations, or an indication in the history of a need for closer examination of the region, indicates the need for palpation; assessment of the end-feel during range-of-motion testing of each joint; and assessment of muscle strength, stability, and flexibility. Often in recognition of the biomechanical-postural model, a standing flexion test will be repeated *after* correction of somatic dysfunction above the pelvis in order to screen for possible biomechanical influence of the lower extremities on the structures above.

System ic Relevance

The regional structure and the function of the lower extremities are inexorably linked to systemic clinical issues. Possessing motor, sensory, and autonomic innervations that extend from the lower thoracic region to the sacrum, the lower extremities are often targets of referred pain from the somatic structures in the lumbar and pelvic regions or from certain abdominopelvic viscera. (Although these relationships are mentioned in this chapter, readers are

encouraged to also consult those chapters in this text associated with the primary region or disorder.)

Furthermore, while many clinicians consider the pelvis to be the foundation on which the spine balances, the lower extremities actually form the final common platform for postural alignment (1). In order to keep upright, the body slightly sways over its base of support using the ankles and hips especially to counter imbalance. Sway is caused by actions of the ankle musculature that attempt to keep the center of mass over the base of support. This *ankle strategy* focuses on minor disturbances in balance; while the body's *hip strategy* manages major balance disturbances. Hip strategy uses the trunk musculature to bring postural center of mass over the base of support; it is quicker than the ankle strategy and can overcome larger variances in balance. In the most extreme circumstances, the body will step in the opposite direction of the disturbance to prevent a fall, which moves the base of support in order to maintain balance (2). For these reasons, osteopathic manipulative treatment (OMT) and lower extremity rehabilitation (including foot orthotics, ankle exercises, and other lower extremity adjunctive strategies) are used to address local, regional issues—such as a pronated foot or an anatomically shortened femur—to affect the more systemic postural issues. (Refer to Chapter 36: for lower extremity diagnostic and management issues associated with this biomechanical model.)

In clinical practice, the osteopathic practitioner seeks to ensure and enhance those structure–function relationships that are important to the biomechanical, bioenergic, neuromusculoskeletal, and circulatory functions of the lower extremities. Clinical goals include:

- Promotion of energy-efficient, painless locomotion
- Maintenance of optimal stability-flexibility balance in and around the joints
- Reduction of mechanical stress on somatic (skeletal, arthrodial, myofascial) structures
- Motor, sensory, proprioceptive, and autonomic neural balance
- Elimination of nociceptive drive
- Elimination of afferent referral from the colon or pelvic organs
- Elimination of entrapment phenomena and compartmental syndromes
- Safe, effective venous, and lymphatic return

Regional Relevance

Functionally, the lower extremities extend to the iliosacral joint; anatomically, most texts begin at the hip. Regardless of the systemic implications, this chapter will limit its review to the functional anatomy and basic examination of the lower extremities while emphasizing the following regional relationships:

1. Skeletal, arthrodial, and ligamentous structure and function
2. Neuromuscular structure and function
3. Vascular and lymphatic structure and function

Throughout this chapter, these relationships will be linked to a number of regional clinical considerations ranging from ankle sprains (with techniques detailed in a case study at the end of this chapter) to the impact of piriformis syndrome.

SOMA: SKELETAL, ARTHRODIAL, LIGAMENTOUS STRUCTURE AND FUNCTION

Embryologically, limb development begins with the activation of a group of mesenchymal cells in the lateral mesoderm that in turn gives rise to bone, cartilage, and ligamentous structures. Limb buds adjacent to the lumbar and sacral sclerotomes will first be seen at about 4 weeks' gestation. As the limbs elongate, mesenchymal models of the bones are formed. Chondrification centers appear in the fifth week and by the end of the sixth week, the entire limb skeleton is cartilaginous.

Osteogenesis of long bones begins in the seventh week from primary ossification centers located in the middle of the cartilaginous models of the long bones. Ossification centers are present in all long bones by the 12th week, although ossification of the foot bones and of the tibial tuberosites is not complete until approximately 20 years of age.

Tibial tuberosity ossification begins at 7 to 9 years. Clinically, this is worthy of notice because the patellar tendon attachment at the chondro-osseous junction of the tibial tuberosity is the site of one of the most common apophysitides, Osgood-Schlatter disease (3). This exercise-induced growth disorder affects boys aged 10 to 15 and girls aged 8 to 13 years causing pain, especially in the physically active individual, but is also occasionally severe at night thereby warranting consideration of a malignancy in the differential diagnosis.

The bony skeleton and joints of each lower limb are depicted and named in Figure 42.1. The bones making up these joints are covered in articular cartilage. The majority are synovial joints consisting of a capsule and synovial membrane; however, the distal tibiofibular joint is a fibrous syndesmosis with an interosseous membrane. Each of these joints is stabilized by ligaments, which limit joint motions and are a part of the normal end-feel sensed when palpating joint motion.

Differential Diagnosis of Lower Extremity Joints

Several systemic or nonregional disorders might manifest with signs and symptoms in the lower extremities and must be differentiated

Figure 42-1 Bones and joints of the lower extremity.

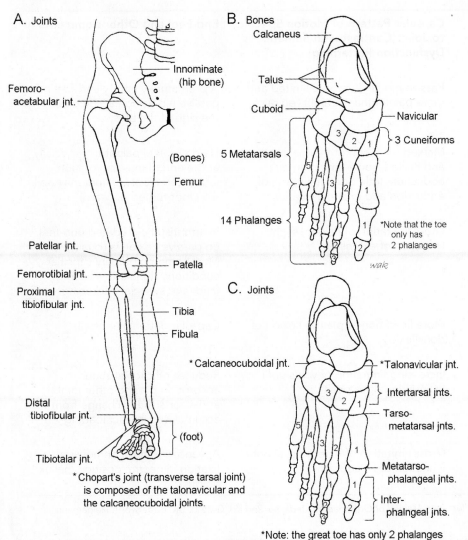

from alternative local diagnoses. Differential diagnosis of a given lower extremity symptom begins with a clinical interpretation of the patient's history and a physical examination that integrates the osteopathic palpatory structural examination. Each of the major structure-function models that are available to osteopathic physicians for interpreting their findings is capable of adding relevant information with respect to this region; the neurological and biomechanical models are particularly useful.

Application of the neurological model, for example, requires a thorough understanding of the lower extremity pain patterns that are associated with pain referral from skeletal, arthrodial, ligamentous, and myofascial structures as well as from a variety of neural, vascular, and visceral structures. In applying the respiratory-circulatory model to this region, the more pertinent knowledge comes from understanding lymphaticovenous drainage patterns and the compartmentalization of the lower extremity.

In order to apply the biomechanical model, lower extremity joint function should be examined and treated while recognizing that each joint has both major and minor motions that are distinct to the structure and function of that joint, each being adapted for an optimal balance between flexibility and stability. Major motions of the lower extremity joints are best recognized by the patient; minor joint motions are glides that are often not able to be produced voluntarily in isolation and that are typically assessed with end-feel palpation. It is often the minor motion of the joint that is responsible for somatic dysfunction and often the failure to address the minor motion of a joint with OMT leads to failure in fully restoring normal joint motion. The pattern of major and minor joint motions helps in the differential diagnosis of each joint. That is, is the pattern one of orthopedic origin (e.g., absent end-feel), rheumatologic origin (e.g., a capsular pattern), or biomechanical origin (e.g., a somatic dysfunction "STAR" pattern)? (Sensitivity, Tenderness, Asymmetry, and Restricted motion are "STAR" objective findings commonly used in making the diagnosis of somatic dysfunction, with the restricted motion pattern of barriers and freedoms providing the greatest differential diagnostic component in this discussion.)

Pain Quality and Referral

Joint capsules are subject to pathological and inflammatory processes. Such processes result in *capsular patterns* of restricted motion in which all or most passive movements of the joint prove painful and limited (Table 42.1). A capsular pattern due to inflammation or

---

TABLE 42.1

The Capsular Patterns

Region Involving Capsular Pattern (Common Diagnoses)	Capsular Pattern of Motion Specific to Joint (Contrast with Somatic Dysfunction Patterning)	End-Feel and Other Comments
"Sign of the Buttock"		
Indicates major lesion such as osteomyelitis, ischiorectal abscess, iliac neoplasm, etc.	Passive hip flexion more limited and more painful than straight-leg raise	A prematurely empty end-feel on passive hip flexion accompanies the sign of the buttock
Hip		
Rheumatoid, traumatic, or spondylitic arthritis; osteoarthrosis	Marked limitation of internal rotation and flexion, some limitation of abduction, little or no limitation of adduction and external rotation	Hard end-feel palpated especially at the end of internal rotation (advanced cases: patient may walk with foot turned outward)
Knee		
Traumatic arthritis, rheumatoid arthritis, osteoarthritis, Baker cyst	Gross limitation of flexion, slight limitation of extension	In arthritis, the palpated end-feel on passive flexion is usually hard. Most common primary capsular conditions signaled by warmth, fluid, and synocial thickening
Ankle		
Osteoarthrosis, reactive arthritis	More limitation of plantar flexion of dorisflexion	Capsular patterns unusual
Talocalcaneal Joint		
Osteoarthrosis, rheumatoid or subacute rheumatoid arthritis	Increasing limitation of varus until fixation in valgus position	Reduces efficacy of shock absorption placing other joints at risk for arthritic change from accumulated impact loading
Big Toe		
Rheumatoid arthritis, osteoarthrosis, gout	Gross limitation of extension, slight limitation of flexion	Advanced pattern demonstrates fixation in neutral position (hallux rigidus)

Source: From Cyriax JH, Cyriax PJ. *Cyriax's Illustrated Manual of Orthopaedic Medicine.* 2nd Ed. Oxford, UK: Butterworth-Heinemann Ltd., 1993:6–8.

pathology is palpably different from the patterns of tenderness and restricted motion assessed in somatic dysfunction (4). Palpation of the capsular pattern is also dramatically different from the laxity assessed in ligamentous sprains. Thus, palpation of the end-feel provides significant information about the differential diagnosis of a painful or improperly functioning joint. Many rheumatological diagnoses present with deep-seated, toothache-like, sclerotomal pain and a capsular palpatory pattern.

Pain is also used in making a presumptive diagnosis of the temporal-pathophysiological condition of a joint. Pain occurring prior to resistance to movement might indicate an acutely inflamed joint, that pain that is synchronous with resistance might indicate a less acutely inflamed joint, and that pain occurring after resistance might indicate a noninflamed joint. Pain upon active motion that disappears when the joint is passively moved might reflect that the pain generator lies in muscles around the joint rather than within the joint itself.

Ligamentous Sprain Classification
In the diagnosis of ligamentous sprains, the joint line and stabilizing ligaments should be palpated directly for tenderness followed by end-feel assessment for arthrodial motion or laxity. The greater the structural damage due to ligamentous spraining, the greater the laxity that results in a loss of normal end-feel and stability. Palpation of joint play end-feel is, therefore, useful in classification of traumatic and orthopedic conditions such as sprains and in differentiating these from somatic dysfunction.

Ligamentous sprains are generally classified by degree. A first-degree sprain assumes that the integrity of the ligament is undisturbed, which results in generally intact tensile strength. Some label this degree of injury a *strain*, while others reserve the term, *strains*, for muscle injuries. A first-degree sprain, while tender to specific palpation and painful when stressed, is generally stable to most orthopedic ligamentous tests. Patients with first-degree sprain respond well to conservative osteopathic care focusing on functional strategies and might even return to activity within days of the injury (5,6). With proper care, such sprains typically recover with normal function and no ligamentous laxity.

A third-degree sprain (also known as a *grade III sprain*) indicates complete disruption of the ligament with no remaining tensile strength. Orthopedic testing indicates the "sloppy" end-feel of complete instability. Good splinting and early surgery may offer the best prognosis when dealing with third-degree ligamentous sprains around the structurally unstable knee. With ligaments of the inherently more stable ankle joint, surgery may be delayed or unnecessary to reestablish stability; recovery can be as long as 4 months (7).

Second-degree sprains make up the ligamentous injuries in between these two diagnoses. Second-degree sprains may be further divided into grade I (partial tearing with slight laxity) and grade II (more complete tearing and moderate laxity) sprains. Second-degree sprains, even when grade II, do not usually require surgical repair if they are immobilized for a duration that is appropriate to stabilize the amount of structural damage. Prolotherapy (8) or certain rehabilitative procedures may be employed to restore a component of the laxity and lost joint stability.

HIP: Femoroacetabular Joint

Structure
The hip, or *coxa*, is a term used loosely to indicate the articulation of the femoral head with the acetabular socket of the innominate bone. (Recognize that the term, *hip*, may also be used by patients

to refer to any part of the region between the waist and the thigh.) Throughout this chapter the term, *hip*, will be interchangeable with the structural and functional elements associated with the femoroacetabular joint itself.

The hip is a ball-and-socket synovial joint with a socket deeper than the glenoid fossa of the shoulder that reflects the characteristic stability of the joint. In a newborn with a congenitally shallow acetabulum, this lack of stability can be evaluated using the *Ortolani test* for dislocation (Fig. 42.2) and the *Barlow test* for reduction (Fig. 42.3). Early discovery permits satisfactory results with triple diapering or conservative brace management. Failure to perform a satisfactory examination risks a late diagnosis and the necessity for surgical correction.

Femur
The femur is the longest and heaviest bone in the body, attaining a length about one-fourth the height of an adult (9). This fact allows the forensic pathologist or archaeologist to estimate an individual's height from the femur alone. The angle formed by the intersection of the anatomic axis of the shaft of the femur and the longitudinal

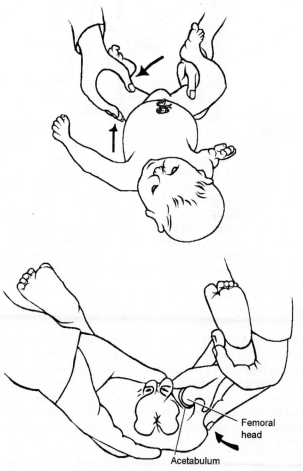

Figure 42-2 Ortolani test for hip dislocation. Used in the first few weeks of life, in neonates with a subluxated hip, this maneuver creates resistance felt at 45 to 60 degrees. A positive sign is a palpable click (not heard) when resistance is overcome and the femoral head reduces. (**Top:** From Kuchera ML, Kuchera WA. *Osteopathic Principles in Practice.* 2nd Ed. Rev. Columbus, OH: Greyden Press, 1994:636, illustration by W.A. Kuchera. **Bottom:** Modified from Burnside JW. *Physical Diagnosis: An Introduction to Clinical Medicine.* 16th Ed. Baltimore, MD: Williams & Wilkins, 1981:246.)

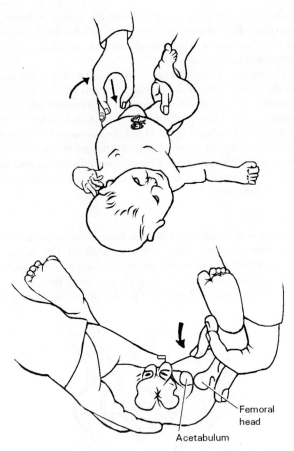

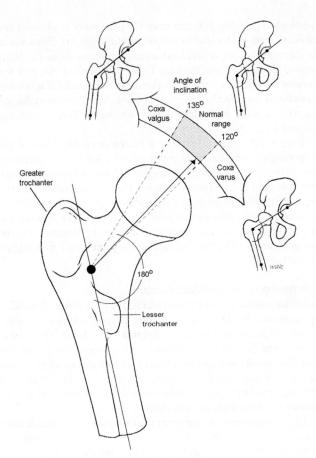

Figure 42-3 Barlow test for hip reduction. Test for hip reduction is a modification of the Ortolani test; it is used to identify an unstable hip in infants up to 6 months of age. The Ortolani test is first performed followed by a posterolateral pressure over the inner thigh. If the femoral head slips out over the posterior lip of the acetabulum and reduces spontaneously when the pressure is released, then the joint is not dislocated but is unstable. (**Top:** From Kuchera ML, Kuchera WA. *Osteopathic Principles in Practice.* 2nd Ed. Rev. Columbus, OH: Greyden Press, 1994:636, illustration by W.A. Kuchera. **Bottom:** Modified from Burnside JW. *Physical Diagnosis: An Introduction to Clinical Medicine.* 16th Ed. Baltimore, MD: Williams & Wilkins, 1981:246.)

Figure 42-4 Angle of inclination. Measures less than 120 degrees in coxa varus; greater than 135 degrees in coxa valgus. (Illustration by W.A. Kuchera.)

axis of the neck of the femur is called the *angle of inclination*. This angle normally measures 120 to 135 degrees. If the angle of inclination is larger than 135 degrees, the condition is referred to as *coxa valgus*. If it measures less than 120 degrees, the condition is called *coxa varus* (Fig. 42.4). The femoral shaft is twisted so that the condyles of the distal femur are in a transverse plane even though the femoral neck angles forward 12 to 15 degrees; this is called the *angle of anteversion*.

Ligaments

The *iliofemoral ligament* on the anterior aspect of the hip joint is the strongest ligament in the body. Because it is shaped like the letter Y, it is also called the Y-ligament of Bigelow. This ligament tenses with full hip extension and helps to maintain posture in the military at-ease position with minimal muscle activity. On the posterior side, the *ischiofemoral ligament* attaches to the ischial portion of the acetabular rim and wraps over the posterior and superior part of the hip joint where it attaches just medially to the base of the greater trochanter of the femur. This important anatomic

configuration tends to screw the femoral head into the acetabulum with extension, which prevents hyperextension. Normal extension is typically limited to less than 35 degrees. Functional hip ligaments are illustrated in Figure 42.5.

Structure–Function Relationships

Motion

The major motions of the hip (femoroacetabular) joint that the patient can voluntarily create and are grossly tested are shown below along with ranges and approximate means for a 30 to 40 year old population (10):

- Flexion 120 degrees (range: 90 to 150 degrees)–extension 10 degrees (range 0 to 35 degrees)
- Abduction 40 degrees (range: 15 to 55 degrees)–adduction 30 degrees (15 to 45 degrees)
- External rotation 35 degrees (range: 10 to 55 degrees)–internal rotation 30 degrees (range: 20 to 50 degrees)

Minor joint motions of the hip assessed with end-feel palpation include:

- Anterior glide occurring with external rotation
- Posterior glide occurring with internal rotation

Gross hip ranges of motion and passive assessments of end-feel are usually tested with the patient supine and the pelvis stabilized. Ranges of motion vary from individual to individual and differ in different populations tested. For example, expect different averages

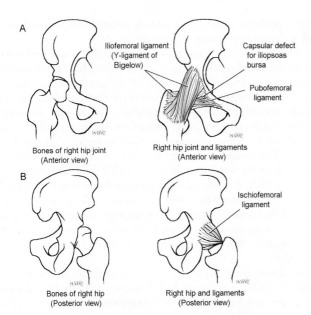

Figure 42-5 Functional hip ligaments. **A.** Bones and ligaments of the right hip joint (anterior views). Iliofemoral ligament (Y-ligament of Bigelow) and pubofemoral ligament. The iliofemoral ligament on the anterior aspect of the joint is the strongest ligament in the body and is used in military posture. **B.** Bones and ligaments of the right hip joint (posterior views). The ischiofemoral ligament on the posterior side of the joint limits extension to less than 35 degrees. (Illustration by W.A. Kuchera.)

when testing male collegiate football players compared to teenage female gymnasts. Therefore, a side-to-side comparison of both symmetry and the quality of the barrier at the end of motion is much more important than measuring the absolute number of degrees in the range of motion. Moreover, such side-to-side comparisons can be reliably counted upon (11). This holds true as well for the assessment of all of the lower extremity joints. In the presence of asymmetric motion, the quality and pattern of the barriers helps to differentiate hypomobility on one side from hypermobility on the other hand to distinguish somatic dysfunction from pathology.

The character and pattern of the end-feel of each hip motion may be springy (physiologic) or it might suggest a capsular, traumatic, or dysfunctional pattern. Subtle differences in somatic dysfunction of myofascial rather than articular origin may also be appreciated by evaluating the quality of the end-feel of the hip joint.

The muscles and soft tissues of the hip typically limit flexion more than the ligaments. Straight-leg raising at the hip around a transverse axis is limited by the hamstring muscles to approximately 85 to 90 degrees. If the knee is bent in order to remove the hamstring influence, the thigh can normally be flexed up to 150 degrees at the hip. If significant improvement in range of motion is not seen after flexing the hip, the situation is not consistent with a biomechanical cause. Thus, when more pain and limitation of motion coupled with an empty end-feel coincides with bent-knee hip flexion rather than with straight-leg raising, serious conditions including septic bursitis, ischiorectal fossa abscess, osteomyelitis or neoplasm of the upper femur, or other significant pathology of the ilium must be ruled out (12) (see Table 42.1).

Extension while the subject is prone and their legs are extended might measure as much as 35 degrees; bending the hip and knee of the opposite lower extremity relaxes some of the muscular restriction to hip extension and should increase this measurement.

Around an anteroposterior (AP) axis through the femoral head, the hip might abduct and adduct by as much as 55 and 45 degrees, respectively. To test adduction in a supine patient with the knee locked, the leg must be lifted to cross over the opposite leg.

Around a functional longitudinal axis, hip external rotation might measure up to 55 degrees and internal rotation up to 50 degrees.

In summary, the major motions of the hip and the minor motion glides of anterior glide (with external rotation) and posterior glide (with internal rotation) should be assessed and their pattern evaluated. A physiological end-feel to one motion compared to a barrier in the opposite direction is consistent with a dysfunctional pattern. A capsular pattern of marked limitation to internal rotation and limitation to flexion and abduction as well should raise suspicions of an underlying inflammatory process. If the initial findings from the examination of the hip do not follow functional biomechanical principles, they warrant further evaluation.

Longitudinal Axis

The anatomical longitudinal axis that runs down the shaft of the femur is not its functional axis. The *functional longitudinal axis* of the femur runs distally from the femoral head to a point midway between the condyles. With internal rotation at the hip on this functional axis, the femoral head glides posteriorly; with external rotation, the femoral head glides anteriorly. Internal rotation with posterior glide and external rotation with anterior glide represent the linked minor motions of the femoroacetabular joint.

Because arthritic change modifies gliding motions and occurs early in the minor motions of the joint (13), screening for hip problems should combine the standard Patrick screening test (Fig. 42.6) with evaluation for a hip capsular pattern. The acronym FABERE is often used to describe the order in which the *Patrick FABERE* test is performed:

- *F*lexion
- *Ab*duction
- External *R*otation
- *E*xtension

As a screening test, the Patrick FABERE test is more reliable for hip pathology than sacroiliac dysfunction (14). Hip joint pathology, such as osteoarthritis, will usually create pain in the inguinal region. A positive Patrick test that lacks a hip capsular palpatory pattern or has pain limited to the posterior pelvis is more likely to reflect sacroilitis or pain arising from the sacroiliac joint or anterior sacroiliac ligament than hip pathology.

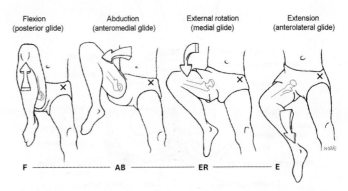

Figure 42-6 Patrick FABERE test of the hip. X, opposite hand should stabilize the left ASIS. Test may reproduce back or buttock pain from sacroilitis or severe SI joint dysfunction; groin pain is often indicative of hip joint pathology. (Illustration by W.A. Kuchera, D.O., F.A.A.O.)

Arthritic change progresses from functional demand accentuated by biomechanical stress to pathophysiological response and structural change. For example, the biomechanical stress placed on the hip joint by a short lower extremity results in a higher incidence of greater trochanteric bursitis and of osteoarthritis (15,16), both occurring on the long leg side. Somatic dysfunction and arthritic pathology often coexist within this structure-function spectrum; each should be addressed with appropriate therapeutic tools that are integrated into a regimen for total patient treatment (17).

KNEE: FEMOROTIBIAL AND PATELLOFEMORAL JOINTS

Structure

The true knee, *genu*, or femorotibial joint is a double condylar, complex synovial articulation formed by the femoral condyles and the tibial plateau (Fig. 42.7). This joint contains medial and

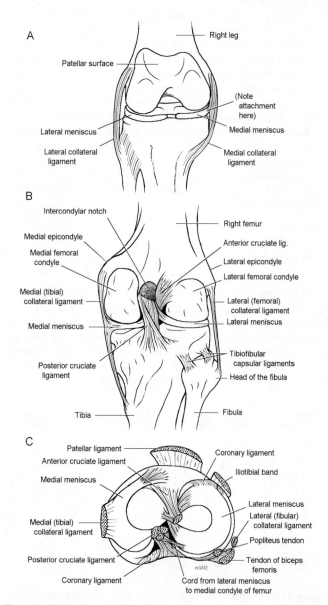

Figure 42-7 Knee joint. **A.** Anterior view. **B.** Posterior view. **C.** Relationship of collateral ligaments to knee cartilage (anterior view). (Illustration by W.A. Kuchera.)

lateral semilunar cartilages to provide some stability, smoothness, and resilience to pressure.

The medial condyle of the knee is longer than the articular surface of the lateral condyle (Fig. 42.8). This structural configuration affects joint function and the end result is dependent upon whether the tibia is moving on the femur (seated) or the femur is moving on a stationary tibia (standing). With extension of the knee, the lateral condyle reaches its physiologic limit of motion, whereas the medial condyle of the femur continues to track posteriorly on the tibial plateau. This results in a posterolateral glide of the tibia with full extension of the knee. Full extension locking requires this minor rotational glide. The opposite (anteromedial glide) occurs with full flexion of the knee. These minor motions of the joint should be checked for somatic dysfunction by adding an anteromedial glide while inducing external rotation of the tibial plateau and a posterolateral glide while inducing internal rotation of the tibial plateau (Fig. 42.9).

In testing the gross range of motion of the knee, the median motions will be approximately 145 degrees (115 to 160 degrees) for flexion and for extension or hyperextension, –2 degrees (0 to –10 degrees) (18).

This section also covers the patellofemoral joint in the area of the true knee joint.

Ligaments and Cartilage

Lateral and medial collateral ligaments, adapted to limit lateral glide of the tibia with adduction and medial glide of the tibia with abduction, stabilize the true knee joint. The lateral (fibular) collateral ligament does not attach to the lateral semilunar cartilage (*lateral meniscus*), while the medial (tibial) collateral ligament does attach to the medial semilunar cartilage (*medial meniscus*) (see Fig. 42.7). This anatomic arrangement makes the medial meniscus more susceptible to tears. It also predisposes the structure to displacement, especially from a blow to the knee that comes through the knee from the lateral to the medial side or to twisting injuries of the knee.

Valgus stress testing of the knee at 30 degrees (Fig. 42.10A) induces abduction of the tibia with medial glide and provides information on stability of the medial collateral ligament. Varus stress testing at 30 degrees (Fig. 42.10B) induces adduction of the tibia with lateral glide and provides information on stability of the lateral collateral ligament. In addition to ligamentous evaluation, these positions permit assessment for medial and lateral glide somatic dysfunction.

A palpable click accompanied by pain while performing *McMurray meniscal tests* (Fig. 42.11) strongly suggests displacement or a meniscal tear, but the test may only be positive in 35% of cases. Although the most sensitive (but least specific) single assessment is actually palpation of a tender meniscus at the joint line (19), usually a combination of maneuvers based upon pain provocation with compression, traction, or shear forces is required to confirm the diagnosis (20).

It is important to understand that one function of the menisci is to limit extreme knee flexion and extension. In extreme knee extension during the screw-home motion, the menisci are forced anteriorly and the anterior horns of the menisci block further extension. In full flexion, the posterior horns of the meniscus are driven posteriorly and block knee flexion (21). Therefore, during meniscus testing, if the pain or snapping occurs near maximum knee flexion, the posterior horns are probably involved, and if the pain or clunk occurs toward knee extension, the middle to anterior portion of the meniscus is probably involved. Again, sensitivity for meniscal damage is less impressive than specificity with each

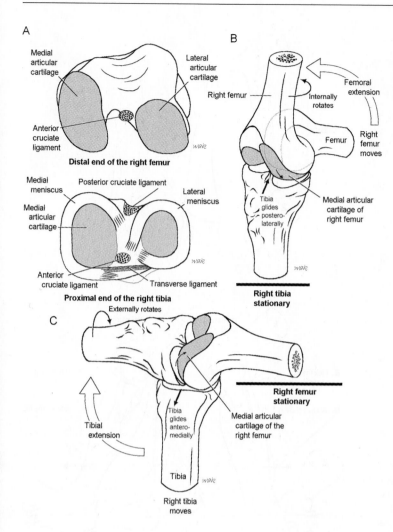

Figure 42-8 Longer medial condyle influences knee joint function. Structure–function relationship of the medial condyle. In knee extension, the medial, but not the lateral, femoral condyle will continue to track posteriorly, resulting in internal rotation of the femur (if the tibia is stationary) or external rotation of the tibia (if the femur is held stationary). The condylar glide occurring with external rotation of the tibia is called the *anteromedial glide*. (Illustration by W.A. Kuchera.)

given test (22,23)—Fouche variation (see Fig. 42.11), for instance, is almost pathognomic for a posterior meniscal tear (24), but such tears are only detected with physical examination in about % of cases.

In addition to pain, patients with a meniscal tear experience swelling, popping, or clicking, limited knee motion, and occasional joint locking during walking. Meniscal tears decrease the shock-absorption properties of the knee joint and can predispose to arthritic change in the joint itself over time.

Interestingly, treatment of locking due to displacement or medial meniscal tear might be accomplished by modifying the McMurray test, starting from the flexed neutral knee position. First, gently externally rotate, abduct, and gap the medial side of the knee joint until a slight bulge is felt at the joint line; follow with pressure over the medial meniscus (and the medial collateral ligament to which all or a fragment of the meniscus may be attached) to reduce the bulge. Complete the procedure by holding firm digital pressure over the medial meniscus during knee extension and internal rotation.

The cruciate ligaments run between the tibia and the femur and are named according to their tibial attachments. The posterior cruciate ligament attaches to the posterior part of the tibia and prevents excessive posterior glide. The anterior cruciate ligament attaches to the anterior part of the tibia and prevents excessive anterior glide of the tibia at the knee joint. Stability of the anterior cruciate ligament (Fig. 42.12A) is checked with an anterior drawer test (knee flexed toward 90 degrees) or, with greater specificity, a *Lachman test* (knee flexed up to 30 degrees). Stability of the posterior cruciate ligament is checked with a *posterior drawer test* (Fig. 42.12B). These maneuvers also permit assessment of anterior and posterior glide end-feel for dysfunction.

The combination of torn anterior cruciate and medial collateral ligaments along with a torn medial meniscus occurs predictably from certain traumas featuring valgus stress forces such as a tackle

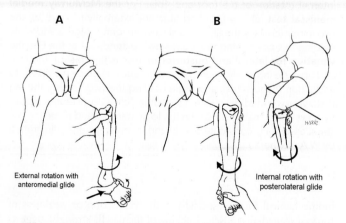

Figure 42-9 Physical examination of minor tibial glides. Physical examination of anteromedial glide with external rotation **(A)** and posterolateral glide with internal rotation **(B)** of the knee. (Illustration by W.A. Kuchera.)

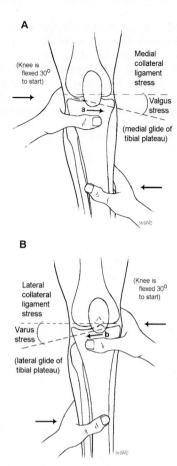

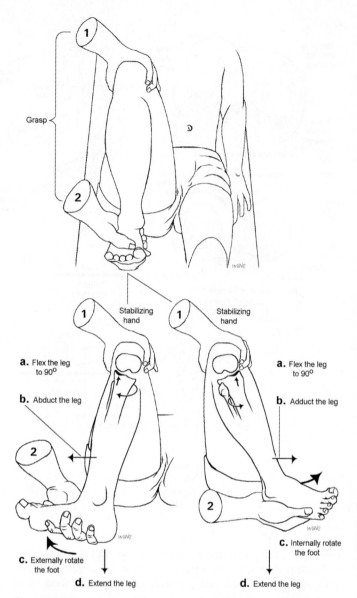

Figure 42-10 Valgus and varus testing. Tests for collateral ligament injury at the knee. **A.** Tibial abduction with medial glide or genu valgus stress also tests for medial collateral ligament stability. **B.** Tibial adduction with lateral glide or genu varus stress also tests for lateral collateral ligament stability. (Illustration by W.A. Kuchera.)

Figure 42-11 Meniscal diagnostic tests. Tests for medial, lateral, or posterior meniscus injuries: In these tests, start with the knee fully flexed. One hand (1) palpates the knee at the medial and lateral joint line. The other hand (2) holds the foot to control external and internal rotation of the foot and tibia. For the **McMurray medial meniscal test** (a), the foot and tibia are externally rotated (b), the two hands (c) place the tibia into abduction (genu valgus), and while holding this positioning the leg is slowly extended. For the **Fouche variation for lateral and posterior meniscus injuries** (b), the foot and tibia are internally rotated, the two hands (c) place the tibia into adduction (genu varus), and while holding this positioning, the leg is slowly extended. Pain with a palpable "click" constitutes a positive test. Note that starting with the leg extended and reversing the steps essentially constitute Steinmann I meniscal signs. (Illustration by W.A. Kuchera.)

to the outside of the knee with the knee extended fully and the foot fixed. Because this injury causes significant knee instability, historically many clinicians referred to this constellation as *O'Donaghue's triad* or more commonly as the *unhappy (or terrible) triad* (25).

Q-Angle and the Patella

The angle formed by the intersection of the functional longitudinal axis of the femur and the tibial longitudinal axis is referred to as the *Q- (or Quadriceps-) angle*. Normally, the Q-angle measures 10 to 12 degrees (Fig. 42.13). An angle of 20 degrees or more is definitely abnormal with some practitioners suggesting an increased biomechanical risk for individuals with Q-angles greater than 15 degrees (26). As the Q-angle increases, the patient appears more "knock-kneed," a condition referred to as *genu valgus*. A "bowlegged" appearance is known as *genu varus*. Biomechanically, coxa varus increases the Q-angle, as does a pronated foot, and both enhance the possibility of genu valgus.

The Q-angle has a major effect on the tracking of the patella, a sesamoid bone in the tendon of the quadriceps femoris muscle group. Patellofemoral joint dysfunction and structural change may each arise from abnormal tracking of or pressure on the patella.

Accentuated Q-angles might be associated with symptoms of patellar pain due to ligamentous stress at the knee or through secondary development of muscle imbalance and trigger points (TrPs). The patella might even sublux laterally with these

biomechanical forces, especially with dysfunction or weakness of the vastus medialis muscle. Locking of the patella strongly suggests myofascial trigger points (MTrPs) in the vastus lateralis muscle. Complete locking of the patella immobilizes the knee joint in slight flexion, while partial locking causes difficulty in straightening the knee after sitting in a chair.

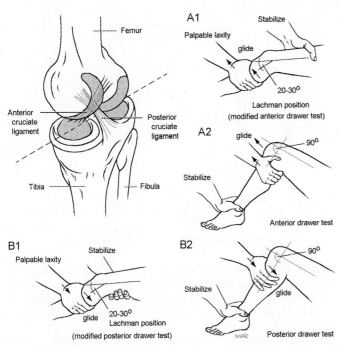

Figure 42-12 Testing cruciate ligaments and A-P glide dysfunction. Structure-function tests of the anterior **(A)** and posterior **(B)** cruciate ligaments using the Lachman (1) and drawer (2) tests.

Prolonged patellofemoral dysfunction, due to these biomechanical factors, predisposes an individual to structural changes including irregular or accelerated wearing or roughening of the articular surface on the posterior surface of the patella (*chondromalacia patellae*) (27). This coexistence of structural and functional disorders must be considered, appropriately diagnosed,

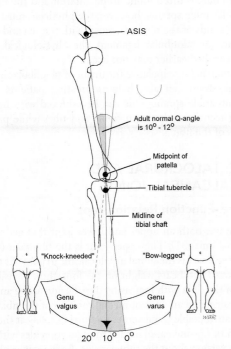

Figure 42-13 Q-angle. Q-angle (quadriceps angle) normally measures 10 to 12 degrees. Key landmarks for establishing the Q-angle are the ASIS, the patella, and the tibial tuberosity. Note the change in the Q-angle in genu valgus and varus.

and treated to encourage optimum healing. When the tracking disorder is secondary to muscular imbalance, it is very important to consider neural agonist–antagonist relationships and, therefore, to sufficiently stretch any tight hamstrings prior to trying to strengthening weak quadriceps (28).

Patellar structural problems also arise from:

- Patellar dislocation
- Chronic or direct patellar trauma
- Fracture of the lower extremity

Structural problems of the patella are evaluated, in part, by palpating over and around the patella. Look for subpatellar tenderness, crepitus, grinding or clicking with compression against the underlying femur (patellar grind test) when gliding the patella medially, laterally, superiorly or inferiorly. Effusion within the knee joint also strongly suggests structural change.

As a consequence of secondary bony alignment and muscular imbalance, functional patellar tracking difficulties may also be the presenting symptom of postural disorders.

Motion

The major motions of the knee joint are flexion and extension. Because of the irregular shape of the joint surfaces, these two motions are combined with some minor involuntary glides, rolling, and rotational motions. Minor motions of the tibial plateau at the knee include:

- Anterior and posterior glides
- Medial and lateral glides
- Internal rotation with posterolateral glide
- External rotation with anteromedial glide

Complete extension of the knee creates a bony lock. Testing of minor motions of the joint and ligament assessment should therefore be performed with the knee in variable degrees of flexion. Abduction and adduction of the tibia are passive motions of the knee that cannot be voluntarily created by the patient. A varus stress motion applied in an attempt to create adduction of the tibia produces a lateral glide (with slight internal rotation). A valgus stress motion–inducing abduction of the tibia produces a medial glide (with slight external rotation) of the tibia. Restriction of glide in one direction suggests somatic dysfunction; laxity in one direction suggests ligamentous sprain or tear.

The knee should move into full extension and lock, freely and without restriction. This is tested by grasping the foot of the supine patient with one hand and raising that lower extremity just off the table. The knee is flexed slightly with the other hand and then released, allowing it to extend. A normal knee drops freely into extension and bounces off the ligaments. Structural injuries, especially medial meniscal tears, might result in inability to extend fully or in guarding on extension.

The hyperextended knee is referred to as *genu recurvatum*.

Diagnostic Testing

The osteopathic palpatory examination of the knee incorporates standard knee testing positions and maneuvers while noting the presence and pattern of these findings:

- Gross range of motion
- Restricted gliding minor motions (end-feel)
- Hypermobility and loss of stability (end-feel)

As with other lower extremity joints, all findings are compared from side to side for asymmetry and the quality of the end-feel motions.

The same testing maneuvers needed to diagnose somatic dysfunction offer orthopedic and rheumatologic information about knee structure. In general during testing, if the asymmetrical end-feel of the test is too loose, there is an orthopedic diagnosis. If generally restricted in both directions of a given paired motion (e.g., flexion–extension), there is often a rheumatologic diagnosis. If a pattern of paired motions are assessed to be physiologically free in one direction but ends too abruptly in the other, the diagnosis is joint somatic dysfunction. Thus, interpreting each test for the available dual structure-function information provides twice the diagnostic power in the same amount of time that is usually spent on examining the knee structure alone.

A knee with gross limitation of flexion and slight limitation of extension is consistent with a capsular pattern of that joint. This palpatory finding, correlated with history and other physical findings, leads to an appropriate differential diagnosis of varying types of arthritis and synovitis affecting the knee. The capsular pattern of the knee (29) differs significantly from a somatic dysfunction, in which minor motions of the joint are restricted in one aspect of each paired motion and free in the opposite direction.

Fibular Motion

The proximal tibiofibular joint is a separate synovial joint at the knee (Figs. 42.14 and 42.15). Although the angulation of the articulation actually permits the minor motions of anterolateral and posteromedial glide of the fibular head, clinicians simply report fibular head glide as *anterior* or *posterior*. The fibular head lies in the same horizontal plane as the tibial plateau.

The distal tibiofibular articulation is a syndesmosis. This joint allows the fibula to move laterally from the tibia to accommodate the increased width of the talus presented during dorsiflexion. Restricted dorsiflexion of the ankle warrants examination and treatment of this syndesmosis.

When the fibular head glides anteriorly, reciprocal motion is initiated at the distal fibula (lateral malleolus), which glides posteriorly. Posterior fibular head motion is accompanied by anterior motion at the distal fibula. External rotation of the tibia and ankle carries the distal fibula posteriorly and elevates and glides the proximal fibular head anteriorly. The opposite occurs with internal rotation of the tibia and ankle (see Fig. 42.15).

With pronation of the foot, ligamentous attachments glide the distal talofibular joint posteriorly with reciprocal glide of the head of the fibula anteriorly. The opposite occurs with supination.

Fibular Head Dysfunction

Fibular head dysfunction is checked by gliding the fibular head posteriorly (and slightly medial) and anteriorly (and slightly lateral). In grasping the fibular head, the physician must take care not to cause undue pressure on the peroneal (fibular) nerve, which lies directly posterior to this structure. Posterior fibular head somatic

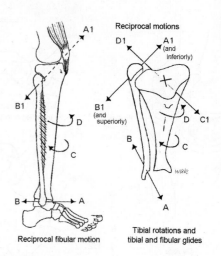

FIGURE 42-15 Reciprocal motions. External rotation of the tibia (C) moves the distal fibula posteriorly (B) and reciprocally is associated with the fibular head moving anteriorly (B1). The opposite is true (A, A1) with internal rotation (D) of the lower leg. (Illustration by W.A. Kuchera.)

dysfunction can itself cause symptoms related to entrapment neuropathy or compression of the common peroneal (common fibular) nerve. (Habitual crossing of one leg over the opposite knee—"crossed leg peroneal palsy"—can also lead to this condition due to prolonged pressure on the nerve against the fibular head. It is especially prevalent in patients with cachexia who have lost significant soft tissue "padding" in this region.)

Fibular head dysfunction often occurs in recurrent ankle sprains and responds well to manipulative procedures (30). In the more common ankle sprain in which the foot tends to supinate, the distal fibula is often found to be anterior and the fibular head posterior. In ankle sprains, however, the physician must be sure to check both ends of the fibula, because, with trauma and disruption of the anterior talofibular ligament, the physiological, reciprocal motion described earlier may not occur.

Palpation and manipulative treatment of tibiofibular interosseous membrane strain can also help in treating patients who have incurred an ankle sprain. This can be achieved with ligamentous balancing techniques between fibula and tibia while palpating at both ends of the fibula.

ANKLE: TALOCRURAL AND TALOCALCANEAL JOINTS

Structure–Function Relationships

The ankle has both an upper and lower joint that act together as a functional unit (31). The upper joint is the tibiotalar (talocrural) joint and the lower is the subtalar (talocalcaneal) joint. As the patient walks forward and bears weight on the foot, there is visible medial rotation of the tibia with increasing dorsiflexion at the ankle. However, the calculated amount of medial rotation of the tibia is greater than that attributable to movement occurring solely at the tibiotalar joint (32,33). The increased medial rotation coincides with a relative calcaneal eversion about the subtalar axis. As the stance phase of the walking cycle continues to the toe-off interval, the tibia externally rotates with simultaneous calcaneal inversion about the subtalar axis. Without movement at the subtalar joint, it would be difficult for a person to balance their body over one lower limb (34).

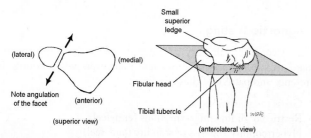

Figure 42-14 Proximal tibiofibular joint. Note that the fibular head and the tibial tuberosity are on the same horizontal plane.

Tibiotalar/Talocrural Joint

The tibiotalar (or talocrural joint) involves the talus moving in the ankle mortise. Until the publication of Inman's studies (35,36), the axis of the tibiotalar joint was thought and described in anatomy textbooks to be a horizontal axis that corresponded with the articular surfaces of the joint. Inman demonstrated that the single empirical (functional) axis in 80% of his specimens was not horizontal. He described an oblique axis directed laterally and downward (average 8 degrees) on a coronal plane and laterally and posteriorly (average 6 degrees) on a transverse plane. Despite this knowledge, the major motions of the tibiotalar joint are simply described as dorsiflexion and plantar flexion. Minor motions occur with each; posterior glide with dorsiflexion and anterior glide with plantar flexion. These minor motions are important when setting up manipulative techniques of the talus or of the fibula.

The gross ranges of motion for the ankle average 15 degrees (range: 5 to 40 degrees) for dorsiflexion and 40 degrees (range: 10 to 55 degrees) for plantar flexion (37). Interesting for patient care, studies suggest that people with inflexible ankles have nearly five times the risk of ankle sprain of people with an average flexibility (38). As in all other lower extremity joints, a side-to-side comparison for symmetry and quality of the end-feel of motion is recommended.

Recurrent somatic dysfunction of the ankle at the tibiotalar joint is more commonly found to prefer plantar flexion with anterior glide with a resistant barrier to posterior glide at the end of dorsiflexion. The tibiotalar capsular pattern is, however, restricted in both directions and especially resistant to plantar flexion. Ankle sprains, more likely to occur when the tibiotalar joint is plantar flexed, are discussed with foot position (supination and pronation) later in this chapter and were classified by severity earlier in the chapter.

Adduction, toeing-in, and some supination of the foot accompany plantar flexion. This motion carries the lateral malleolus anteriorly. Through reciprocal action of the fibula, the proximal fibular head also glides posteriorly and inferiorly. The talus glides anteriorly, placing the narrow portion of the talus in the ankle mortise, a less stable position.

Since the tibiotalar axis passes distally to the tip of each malleolus, its position may be estimated by placing the fingertips at the most distal ends of the malleoli. At this position, the fingers are over the transverse axis of the tibiotalar joint.

Abduction, toeing-out, and some pronation of the foot accompany dorsiflexion. This type of motion carries the lateral malleolus posteriorly and, through reciprocal action, glides the fibular head anteriorly and superiorly. With dorsiflexion, the talus glides posteriorly. Because the talus is structurally wider anteriorly, it fits more securely with the posterior glide component in the ankle mortise. Dorsiflexion is, because of its structure, a more functionally stable position. This stability is the reason taping techniques to treat or prevent ankle sprains usually emphasize a dorsiflexed position. Major and minor ankle motions are shown in Figure 42.16.

Subtalar/Talocalcaneal Joint

The subtalar or talocalcaneal joint (Fig. 42.17) has been called the main *shock-absorber* joint (39,40) of the lower extremity. It earned this designation because, in coordination with the intertarsal joints, it determines the distribution of forces upon the skeleton and soft tissues of the foot. This synovial joint has a single oblique axis that declines backward and laterally; it is stabilized by the strong talocalcaneal ligament.

The shock-absorbing function of this joint is particularly important in absorbing *accumulated impact loading* (calculated by multiplying the number of steps times the person's body weight times an activity "magnifier" ranging from a factor just above 1 for walking activities to up to 10 to 12 times the person's weight for jumping; the magnifying factor for running varies from 1.5 to 5 times body weight) (41). Such calculations become important in predicting outcomes such as aggravation of the lower extremity arthritis pain from prescriptive treadmill activity to risk of tissue injury in athletes with heavy running or jumping activities. Running is one of the most widespread activities during which overuse injuries of the lower extremity occur and the majority of biomechanical risk factors for such injury stem from this rear portion of the foot (42). Examples of overuse injuries that commonly occur during running include stress fractures, medial tibial stress

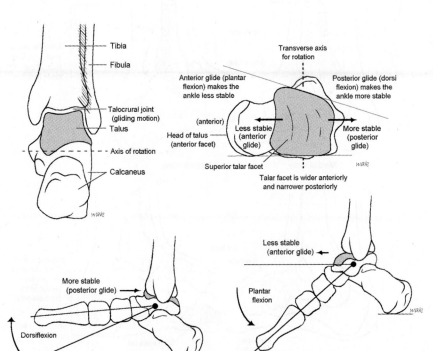

Figure 42-16 Major and minor ankle motions. Dorsiflexion with posterior glide is the more stable joint position because the wedge-shaped talus is engaged. (Illustration by W.A. Kuchera.)

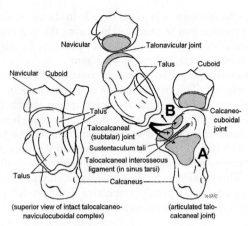

Figure 42-17   Subtalar joint. Persons with flat feet have a more horizontal axis and greater foot motion. Those with a more vertical axis have a more rigid, pes cavus foot. **A.** Posterolateral glide. **B.** Anteromedial glide. (Illustration by W.A. Kuchera.)

(shin splints), chondromalacia patellae, plantar fasciitis, and Achilles tendinitis.

Normal subtalar joint function is, therefore, critical to normal foot and lower-extremity functions (43); it should be a major focus of sports medicine physicians. In addition to its shock-absorbing function, the subtalar joint acts like a mitered hinge by allowing triplanar translation of motion between the foot and the lower extremity. Movement of the calcaneus produces leg rotation—inversion of the calcaneus produces external rotation of the tibia, and causes the talus to glide posterolaterally over the calcaneus; eversion of the calcaneus produces medial rotation of the tibia and anteromedial glide of the talus on the calcaneus. Clinically, these mechanics seem to explain the palpable talocalcaneal motions:

posterolateral glide of the talus when the ankle is supinated and the anteromedial glide at the talocalcaneal joint when the ankle is pronated.

Inman (44) found the average inclination of the subtalar axis from the horizontal plane on the sagittal plane to be 42 degrees (ranging from 20 to 68 degrees). If the inclination of the axis is 45 degrees, rotation of the tibia and calcaneus has a one-to-one relationship. The more horizontal the axis, the more the calcaneus rotates and the less the leg rotates. Because the metatarsals of the forefoot appear to remain stationary, this calcaneal rotation is not very obvious during walking. Inman's studies concluded that approximately half of the population has some linear displacement of the talus along the axis with movement in the subtalar joint.

Ankle Sprains
Lateral Stabilizing Ligaments and Ankle Sprains
Ankle sprains are very common in a general practice. When a patient presents with ankle trauma, the Ottawa ankle rules (45) help determine when a radiograph is needed to rule out a fracture (Fig. 42.18). This test has a sensitivity of nearly 100% and a modest specificity; its use calculated to reduce unnecessary radiographs by 30% to 40% (46).

Approximately 80% of all sprains are of the supination type (47). The supination position, which includes the less stable tibiotalar plantar flexion position, simply predisposes the ankle to ligamentous sprain injuries (especially the lateral stabilizing ligaments of the ankle). Additionally, somatic dysfunction occurs during the mechanism of injury, which extends well beyond the local ligamentous stress (Fig. 42.19).

In a supination sprain, eversion of the calcaneus and posterolateral glide at the talocalcaneal joint occurs. Abrupt stretching of the lateral and anterior compartments often initiates peroneus (fibularis) or other MTrPs (Fig. 42.20) (48). The distal fibula may be drawn anteriorly with reciprocal posterior glide of the fibular

Figure 42-18   Ottawa ankle rules for suspected fracture.

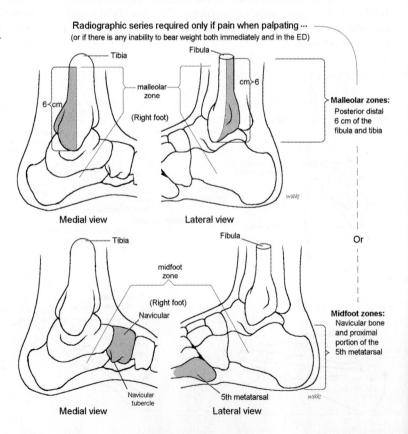

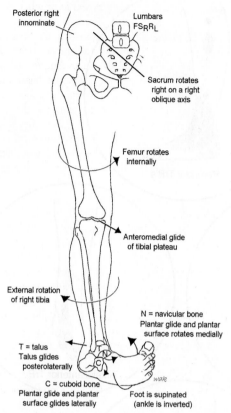

Movements activated by a right ankle strain

Posterior right innominate

Lumbars
F S R R L

Sacrum rotates right on a right oblique axis

Femur rotates internally

Anteromedial glide of tibial plateau

External rotation of right tibia

N = navicular bone
Plantar glide and plantar surface rotates medially

T = talus
Talus glides posterolaterally

C = cuboid bone
Plantar glide and plantar surface glides laterally

Foot is supinated (ankle is inverted)

Figure 42-19 Supination sprain dysfunctions. Somatic dysfunctions and structural stress occurring in the more common supination ankle sprain.

head. If the anterior talofibular ligament is torn, the distal fibula can move posteriorly with anterior glide of the fibular head. Because sprains are traumatically induced, somatic dysfunction might not follow simple biomechanical predictions.

Somatic dysfunction does not stop here. The tibia often externally rotates with an anteromedial glide of the tibial plateau. The femur internally rotates. Myofascial forces (postural forces) then continue upward into the pelvis and spine. Failure to diagnose and treat or rehabilitate beyond the ankle itself increases recurrence rates and prolongs the healing and rehabilitation processes. It also increases complaints in distant sites due to the patient's involuntary attempts to compensate for continued dysfunction.

Three separate ligaments stabilize the lateral side of the ankle (Fig. 42.21). From anterior to posterior, these are the:

- Anterior talofibular ligament
- Calcaneofibular ligament
- Posterior talofibular ligament

Because the biomechanical stresses associated with a supination strain progress from anterior to posterior, ankle sprains are often named by type according to the extent of ligamentous involvement: Type 1 involves anterior talofibular ligament only; Type 2 involves the anterior talofibular and calcaneofibular ligaments; and Type 3 involves all three lateral supporting ligaments.

Classification of sprains by severity was discussed earlier in this chapter; a clinical treatment scenario with useful techniques for treating a supination sprain appears near the end of this chapter.

A pure inversion sprain can result in sprain of the calcaneofibular ligament alone. This occurs in basketball players during rebounding when they land—without any plantar flexion—directly on the lateral aspect of the foot. An understanding of the biomechanics of the foot and ankle explains why this is an uncommon ankle sprain.

MEDIAL STABILIZING LIGAMENTS

The deltoid ligament (Fig. 42.22) stabilizing the medial side of the ankle is so strong that trauma stressing this structure is more likely to fracture a piece of medial malleolus than tear the ligament. The Ottawa Ankle Rules for palpatory pain that prompts strong consideration of an ankle radiograph for fracture recognize this (see Fig. 42.18). Fortunately, pronation sprains are uncommon. This is due both to the strength of the deltoid ligament and the stability imparted by gliding the wide portion of the talus into the tibiotalar joint during dorsiflexion.

Foot Bones, Joints, and Arches

Structure–Function relationships

The movement of the foot (or *pes*) is a composite movement of the talocalcaneal joint of the hind foot and movement of the forefoot about the talonavicular and calcaneocuboid joints. Inversion is that movement in which the heel (calcaneus) faces medially as the inside edge of the foot is lifted. Eversion occurs when the heel faces laterally as the outside edge of the foot is lifted. In the nonweightbearing foot, inversion and eversion can be applied to the forefoot as it moves more medially or more laterally, respectively (Fig. 42.23.).

Gray's Anatomy has described pronation and supination in the foot as movements of the forefoot that do not include movement of the calcaneus. This is not true with weightbearing and active motion. In the upper extremity, pronation and supination are movements of the forearm and muscles of the forearm produced by supinator and pronator muscles. In the foot, however, there are no muscles anatomically labeled as *pronators* or *supinators*. An active attempt to supinate the foot results in a combination of adduction, plantar flexion, and inversion. Likewise, an attempt to pronate the foot results in abduction, dorsiflexion, and eversion.

With weightbearing, supination of the foot is accompanied by eversion of the calcaneus and posterolateral glide of the talus with respect to the navicular at the talocalcaneal joint.

The foot plays a major role in gait; typically by reciprocally reflecting stability and flexibility characteristics with the ankle. For example, while providing less stability at the ankle, supination locks the foot. This allows stabilization at heel strike and propulsion at toe-off. Pronation during weightbearing stabilizes the ankle and creates eversion of the calcaneus with anterolateral glide of the talocalcaneal joint. Pronation unlocks the foot for surface adaptation and shock absorption during running. The various stages being described with respect to the structure–function relationships during gait include (Fig. 42.24):

- **Contact stage**—The contact stage begins with heel strike on the lateral border of the calcaneus. The tibia internal rotation occurs to the tibia as the foot pronates at the subtalar joint through the contact phase. Contact is made by the fifth metatarsal with the ground as the foot continues rolling medially until the metatarsals become fully loaded at the conclusion of the contact phase. The contact phase is designed to convert the foot into a mobile adaptor and shock absorbing mechanism

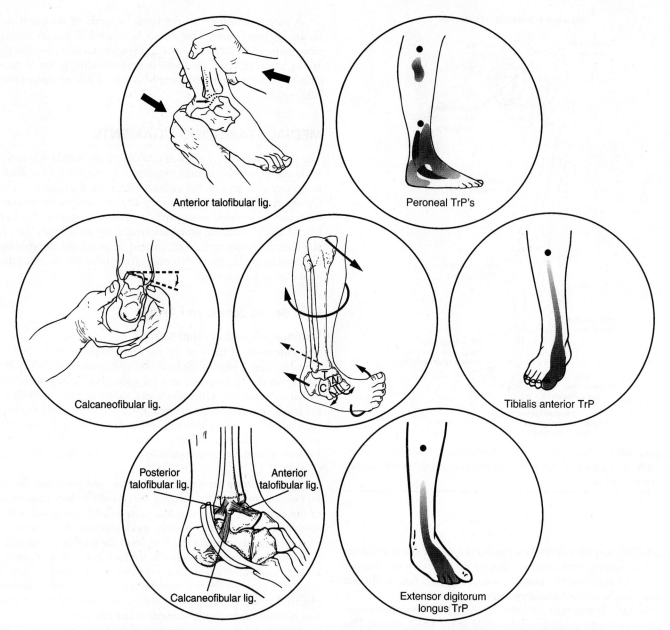

Figure 42-20 Supination somatic sources of pain in common supination injury. Muscles are stressed (in order)—peroneus, tibialis anterior, and extensor digitorum longus—leading to strain or TrPs. Ligaments (*lig.*) stressed are (in order): anterior talofibular, calcaneofibular, and anterior tibiotalar. *T*, talus; *N*, navicular; *C*, cuboid leading to sprain.

■ **Midstance stage**—The midstance phase converts the foot from a mobile adaptor into a rigid lever. The tibia externally rotates during this phase and the foot supinates at the subtalar joint preparing the foot for the propulsive phase

■ **Propulsive phase**—Heel lift commences the propulsive phase. The subtalar joint should approach the neutral position just prior to heel lift. It is at this point that the forefoot and the rearfoot lock together to enable effective toe-off. Supination continues during toe-off with the resultant external tibial rotation

TRANSVERSE TARSAL JOINT

The transverse tarsal joint contains the talonavicular and calcaneo-cuboid articulations, which are separate joints that act together as a functional unit. Because it responds to eversion or inversion of the

heel, the functional unit has its greatest influence during the stance phase of the walking cycle. The talonavicular and calcaneocuboid joints plus the two small talocalcaneal joints are collectively called *Chopart joint*. When amputating a foot, the surgeon follows the articulations of the Chopart joint.

Between the intertarsal joints and the subtalar joint is a groove called the *sinus tarsi*. Attached along this groove is the very strong interosseous talocalcaneal ligament that provides stability for the subtalar and intertarsal joints. Following injury or overuse, an inflammatory sinus tarsi syndrome may occur leading to medial or lateral heel pain on weightbearing; a conservative biomechanical approach is typically successful (49).

With internal rotation of the leg and inversion of the heel, the lines of the talonavicular and calcaneocuboid axes coincide. This produces enough freedom in the transverse tarsal joint so that

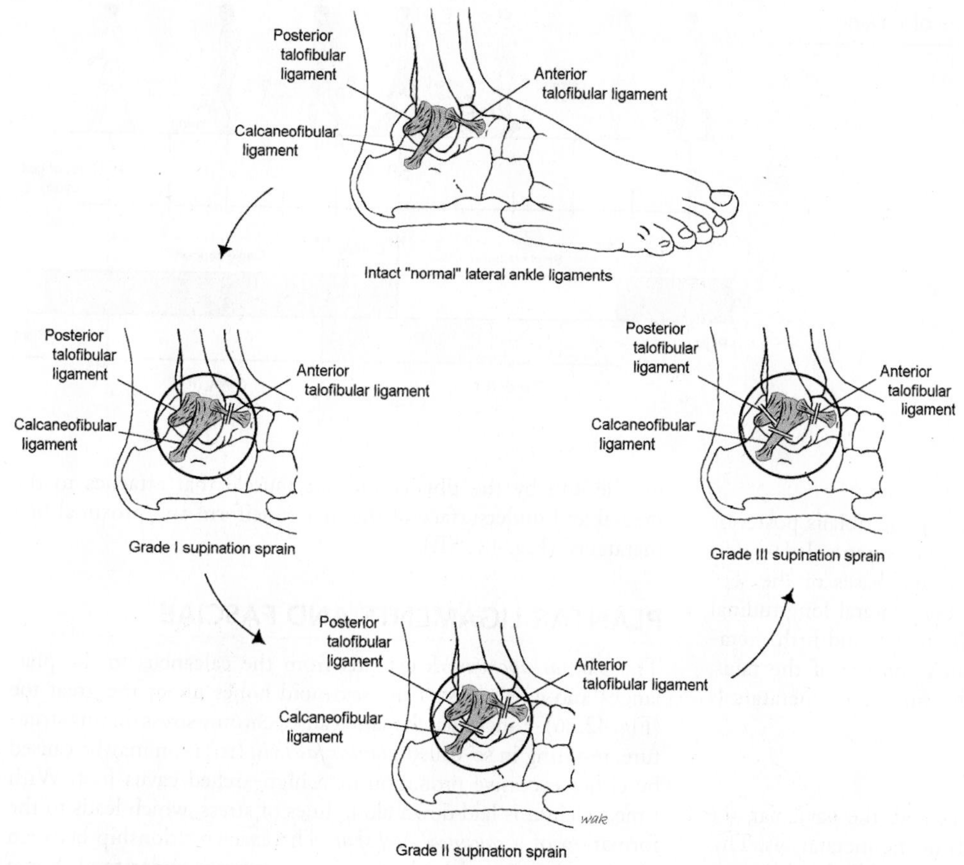

Figure 42-21 Ligamentous stability of the lateral ankle. *Consider discussing types in legend*

Posterior talofibular ligament

Anterior talofibular ligament

Calcaneofibular ligament

Intact "normal" lateral ankle ligaments

Posterior talofibular ligament

Anterior talofibular ligament

Calcaneofibular ligament

Grade I supination sprain

Posterior talofibular ligament

Anterior talofibular ligament

Calcaneofibular ligament

Grade III supination sprain

Posterior talofibular ligament

Anterior talofibular ligament

Calcaneofibular ligament

Grade II supination sprain

the forefoot can evert or invert to accommodate for an uneven terrain.

When the leg rotates externally and everts the heel on a weightbearing forefoot, the transverse tarsal joint appears to become more rigid. This is because the two axes do not coincide. In this position, the forefoot no longer accommodates for an uneven terrain.

As the heel rises in plantar flexion, the transverse tarsal joint must follow the movement about the subtalar axis and invert with the heel to assist the toe-off interval.

FUNCTIONAL ARCHES OF THE FOOT

The two main functional arches of the foot are the longitudinal arch (with medial and lateral components) and the transverse arch. They are maintained by:

- Interlocking articular facets of the bones
- Interosseous ligaments
- Special fascial sheaths
- Plantar ligaments
- Muscles and muscle tendons

A so-called metatarsal arch is not a functional arch; it refers to the heads of the five metatarsals. Restrictions or altered relationships here are usually secondary to dysfunction of the other foot arches (50).

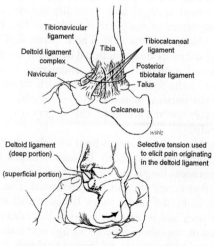

Tibionavicular ligament

Deltoid ligament complex

Tibia

Tibiocalcaneal ligament

Navicular

Posterior tibiotalar ligament

Talus

Calcaneus

Deltoid ligament (deep portion)

(superficial portion)

Selective tension used to elicit pain originating in the deltoid ligament

Figure 42-22 Deltoid ligament.

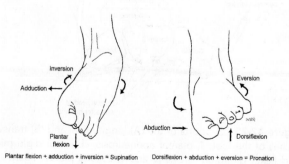

Inversion

Adduction

Plantar flexion

Eversion

Abduction

Dorsiflexion

Plantar flexion + adduction + inversion = Supination   Dorsiflexion + abduction + eversion = Pronation

Figure 42-23 Combined motions (left foot): Inversion versus eversion, supination versus pronation.

Figure 42-24   Feet in the motion cycle of walking.

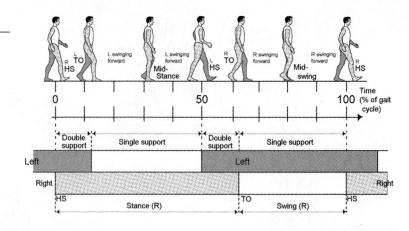

Longitudinal Arch

The *longitudinal arch*, which is supported by the tibialis posterior muscle, is divided into medial and lateral components. Its tendon attaches to the navicular, first cuneiform and bases of the second, third, and fourth metatarsals. The bony lateral longitudinal arch is the calcaneus, the cuboid, and the fourth and fifth metatarsals. The bony medial longitudinal arch consists of the talus, navicular, the three cuneiforms, and the first three metatarsals (Fig. 42.25A).

Transverse Arch

The *transverse arch* is composed of the cuboid, the navicular, the three cuneiforms, and the proximal ends of the metatarsals. This arch is supported inferiorly by the peroneus (fibularis) longus

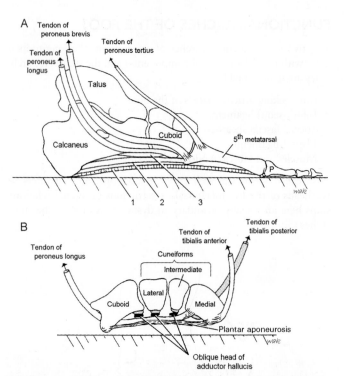

Figure 42-25   Supports of the **(A)** longitudinal and **(B)** transverse arches of the foot. *1*, plantar aponeurosis, abductor digiti minimi, and flexor digitorum brevis IV and V; *2*, long plantar ligament; *3*, short plantar ligament; *P*, phalanges. (From Hamilton JJ, Ziemer LK. Functional anatomy of the human ankle and foot. In: *AAOS Symposium on Foot and Ankle.* St. Louis, MO: CV Mosby, 1983:13.)

muscle and by the tibialis anterior muscle that attaches to the medial and undersurface of the first cuneiform and proximal first metatarsal (Fig. 42.25B).

PLANTAR LIGAMENTS AND FASCIAE

The *plantar aponeurosis* extends from the calcaneus to the phalanges and encompasses the sesamoid bones under the great toe (Fig. 42.26). Functional demand causes chronic stress on this structure, resulting in so-called *plantar fasciitis*. Irritation may be caused by either excessive pronation or a high-arched cavus foot. With time, calcium is laid down along lines of stress, which leads to the formation of a *calcaneal heel spur*. The exact relationship between plantar fasciitis and heel spurs is not entirely understood. Some argue that the regional condition is a "degenerative fasciosis without inflammation" (51), rather than a true fasciitis that would also bring the use of steroid injections as a treatment for either condition into question. Consider as well that 60% to 70% of patients with plantar fasciitis have a heel spur that can be seen on an x-ray; however, many patients without symptoms of pain can have a heel spur.

Plantar fasciitis affects approximately 10% of runners and a similar proportion of the general population at some point in life (52). It is typically worse in the morning and after sitting for a long period. Approximately one third of patients have the condition bilaterally and only about 20% have flat feet (53). MTrPs in the soleus muscle will also refer to pain to the heel and must be considered in the differential diagnosis of heel spurs and plantar fasciitis (54). Even in absence of soleus TrPs, studies document strength and flexibility deficits in the supporting musculature of the posterior calf and foot on the side affected by plantar fasciitis (55). These anatomical and physiological alterations create a functional deficit in the normal foot biomechanics. Correction of such underlying biomechanical dysfunctions in the foot and calf along with weight reduction for overweight patients is the treatment of choice; surgery is rarely necessary and the scar from the surgery may even aggravate the condition.

The *long plantar ligament* runs from the calcaneus to the lateral three metatarsals (see Fig. 42.26). It forms a tunnel for the passage of the peroneus longus muscle as that tendon passes under the foot to the first cuneiform and first metatarsal. The short plantar ligament is, by definition, short. It lies medial to the lateral longitudinal arch and is attached between the calcaneus and the proximal end of the cuboid. The *spring ligament* (calcaneonavicular), which strengthens the medial longitudinal arch, runs from the sustentaculum tali of the calcaneus to the navicular.

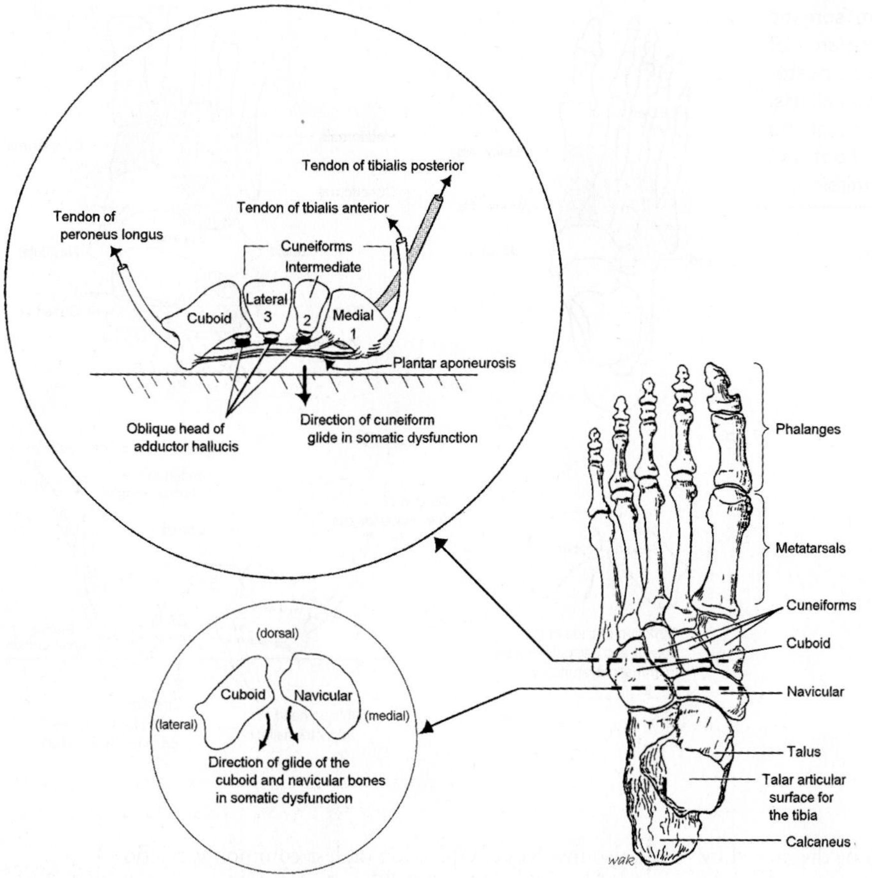

Figure 42-26 Plantar ligaments supporting the arches of the foot.

Pes Planus and Pes Cavus

By observation alone, most experienced clinicians are able to agree if a foot is pronated (flat), supinated (cavus), or rectus (normal) (56); unfortunately, observation of the static foot is much less relevant than its dynamic properties (57).

Persons with *pes planus* (flat foot) have a defect of the foot that eliminates their arch; they have a more horizontal subtalar axis and greater motion in their feet. This explains why they break down their shoes quickly and prefer to go barefoot. The condition is most often inherited; however, arches can also fall in adulthood, in which case the condition is sometimes referred to as *posterior tibial tendon dysfunction*. This occurs most often in women over 50, but it can occur in anyone. Risk factors for developing pes planus include obesity, diabetes, surgery, injury, rheumatoid arthritis, or use of corticosteroids; some studies suggest that the earlier in life that children start wearing shoes, the more likely the risk of a flat foot later on. Unilateral flat foot can sometimes account for a genu valgus and knee pain or a functional short leg on the same side with secondary postural changes above. It can also be problematic if the foot is unable to supinate during the propulsive phase of gait.

Persons with *pes cavus* (high arch) have a more vertical subtalar axis angle; biomechanically, they have a more rigid foot and a less stable ankle. Therefore, athletes with pes cavus have a greater risk of lateral foot injuries such as stress fractures of the fifth metatarsal and ankle sprain (58).

METATARSAL AND PHALAGEAL FINDINGS

Hallux valgus and bunions have a significant hereditary component; hammer toes are acquired. Each of these manifests structural changes with associated biomechanical effects and related somatic dysfunction.

Hallux Valgus, Bunions, and Hammer Toes

Hallux valgus is a structural deformity resulting from the contracture of various periarticular structures of the first metatarsophalangeal joint—it is progressive.

Bunion protrusion is accentuated by varus deviation of the first metatarsal. Muscle imbalance aggravates symptoms, but surgical intervention of the structure may be required for symptomatic relief. Applying counterstrain OMT to a tender point on the medial aspect of the great toe often provides symptomatic relief.

Hammer toes are often functional and can be associated with MTrPs in the dorsal interossei. Deformation might disappear after treatment of this particular somatic dysfunction (59).

Somatic Dysfunction–Related Elements

Tarsal Somatic Dysfunction

Somatic dysfunction of the tarsal bones (cuboid, navicular, or cuneiforms) is relatively common. In middle- and long-distance runners, these bones might even sublux.

Somatic dysfunction of the cuboid involves the edge nearest the middle of the foot. This edge glides toward the plantar surface of the foot and rotates laterally around its AP axis; somatic dysfunction of the navicular involves the edge nearest the middle of the foot gliding toward the plantar surface and rotating medially around its AP axis (Fig. 42.27). Cuneiform somatic dysfunction usually manifests as a consequence of the second cuneiform gliding directly plantarward.

Figure 42-27 Navicular, cuboid, and cuneiform somatic dysfunction; relation to supports of the transverse arch of the foot. Stippled tube represents tendon of tibialis posterior; black areas represent oblique head of adductor hallucis. (From Hamilton JJ, Ziemer LK. Functional anatomy of the human ankle and foot. In: *AAOS Symposium on Foot and Ankle*. St. Louis, MO: CV Mosby, 1983:13, with permission.)

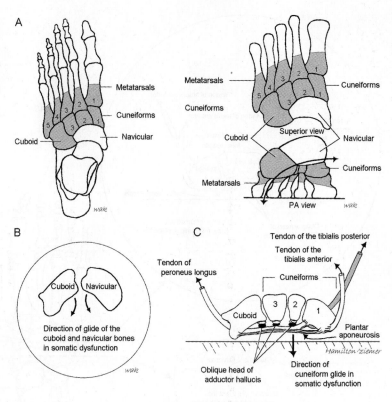

Somatic dysfunction of these tarsal bones can be diagnosed by the combination of tenderness and increased tissue tension over the plantar surface of each of these bones. Osteopathic manipulative treatment (OMT) is effective, although some patients find orthotics to modify predisposing biomechanical factors useful as well.

There are five metatarsophalangeal joints. As the forefoot inverts with plantar flexion, the body weight is transferred to these articulations for push-off. Foot structure provides two functional axes for push-off: an oblique axis that passes through the heads of the second through fifth metatarsals, and a transverse axis that passes through the heads of the first and second metatarsals.

Structurally, a *Dudley J. Morton foot* is characterized by a short first metatarsal that is not designed to accept the normal weight-bearing function involved in the push-off portion of gait. Callus forms under the second and third metatarsal heads as they assume the weightbearing function. Increased functional demand remodels bone. This results in thickening of the second metatarsal; the thickening is evident on x-ray films. Painful walking in 76% of soldiers suffering as a consequence of this condition was relieved by treatment of an in-shoe orthotic (60) to add support under the short first metatarsal to modify the structure–function relationships and OMT to permit realignment. This foot configuration has been identified as one of the perpetuating and precipitating factors of Travell MTrPs and muscle imbalance as distant as the temporomandibular joint (61). Figure 42.28 shows an orthotic used to modify structure–function relationships in Morton foot.

Somatic Dysfunction

Somatic dysfunction of the tarsometatarsal, metatarsophalangeal, and interphalangeal joints involves their minor motions:

- Plantar or dorsal glide
- Internal or external rotation
- Lateral or medial glide

It also involves compression or, less commonly, traction.

Indirect stacking OMT techniques are especially helpful in jammed toes. A stacking technique is one where the physician moves a joint in the direction of preference in all of its planes, stacking one motion upon the other. Compression or traction is then applied to that combined position. The technique may require holding the position of ease for 90 seconds or until the joint tensions relax. The joint is then slowly returned to a neutral position and rechecked for motion.

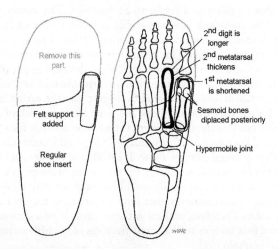

Figure 42-28 Orthotic used to modify structure–function relationships in Dudley J Morton foot. Toe portion of the sole insert is removed so support is under only the first metatarsal head. Lateral side of the support must not extend under second metatarsal head. Insert should reach to the distal end of the first metatarsal.

SOMA: NEUROMUSCULAR STRUCTURE AND FUNCTION

With respect to the lower extremities, the osteopathic *neurological model* considers the motor and sensory innervations of somatic structures in the region as well as the influence of spinal facilitation, proprioceptive function, the autonomic nervous system, and the various processes leading to the phenomenon of pain referral. Therapeutic application of OMT within this model focuses on the reduction of mechanical stresses, balance of neural inputs, reduction of pain with elimination of nociceptive drive, and coordination of processes in the motion cycle of walking.

Differential Diagnosis of Neuromuscular Conditions

A traditional neurological examination used to rule out associated neurological diseases or structural problems affecting the nervous system is a part of the lower extremity work-up. At a minimum, this should include Achilles and patellar deep tendon reflexes, assessment for ankle clonus, straight-leg raising assessment, and evaluation of lower extremity muscle tone, strength, flexibility, and coordination. Palpation of potential entrapment structures or sites is important. Evaluation of sensation can be indicated as well.

Upper motor neuron disorders are characterized by hyperreflexia and associated pathological reflexes such as ankle clonus or Babinski upgoing toe reflex. Lower extremity muscles may demonstrate spasticity or rigidity.

Lower motor neuron disorders are generally characterized by hyporeflexia accompanying muscle weakness or flaccidity. Dermatomal patterns of pain and/or dysesthesia associated with radicular (nerve root) problems in the lower extremities follow general patterns as depicted in Figure 42.29. Depending on the location of the lower motor neuron problem, the pattern might be that of a plexopathy, a neuropathy, or a peripheral neuropathy instead of a radiculopathy. In any case, reviewing the lumbar and pelvic regions is necessary to thoroughly understand the neuromuscular problems affecting the lower extremities.

Radicular Patterns

Radiculopathy might have as its cause, for example, a herniated nucleus pulposus, osteoarthritic spur, advanced spondylolisthesis,

or mass lesion. Regardless of the cause, there are relatively predictable structural and functional effects that need to be evaluated in the lower extremities. History and physical findings will uncover patterns of lower extremity sensory changes, pain, and reflex changes as well as muscle weakness, atrophy, predisposition to TrPs, and imbalance. The diagnosis of lumbar or upper sacral radiculopathies by electromyography focuses on the discovery of fibrillation potentials in patterns of lower extremity muscles sharing a common involved nerve root.

L4 radiculopathy is suspected when there is a reduction of the patellar deep tendon reflex, dysesthesia in the L4 distribution and patterns of weakness, cramping, or TrPs in those muscles innervated by the L4 nerve root, such as the quadriceps and tibialis anterior. Often, a patient exhibiting these symptoms will complain that a knee gives way or that climbing stairs is difficult.

L5 radiculopathy has no abnormal deep tendon reflex; it is suspected when there is dysesthesia in the L5 distribution and patterns of weakness, cramping or TrPs in the gluteus medius and ankle dorsiflexors, such as tibialis anterior, extensor hallucis, and extensor digitorum brevis. This patient may often complain of tripping over carpets or "small cracks in the sidewalk" because of a foot drop.

S1 radiculopathy is suspected with reduction of the Achilles deep tendon reflex, dysesthesia in the S1 distribution, and patterns of weakness, cramping, or TrPs of intrinsic foot muscles, the gastrocnemius-soleus complex and the buttock/gluteal muscles. This is the most common radiculopathy, often resulting from a herniated disc between L5 and S1.

Acute lumbosacral radiculopathies are capable of disturbing efficient gait and have a significant impact on the bioenergic and biomechanical structure-function models of osteopathic care. Even after their resolution, chronic changes such as atrophy and residual lower extremity muscle weakness can continue to disturb efficient gait. Muscles in the particular radicular pattern are also at high risk to develop MTrPs.

Other Neural Patterns

Pain descriptions and pattern distributions extend beyond dysesthesia or anesthesia associated with a nerve root or dermatomal pattern. Other lower extremity patterns of pain occur in sclerotomal and myotomal distributions. Often, the pain quality and patterns are mixed. For example, pain patterns referred from the facet joints of the lumbar spine (sclerotomal structures) overlap MTrP pain (Fig. 42.30) that arises from the following muscles (myotomal structures) (62):

- Multifidi
- Quadratus lumborum
- Glutei
- Piriformis
- Obturator internus

Myotomal pain referral often results in a sensation described as a *charley horse* or a crampy sensation that *reaches out and grabs* with a particular movement. A myotomal distribution is associated with the location of muscles that share the same neural innervation and the trophic substances conveyed by neural axoplasmic flow. Muscle innervations are reviewed in Tables 42.2 to 42.4. Pathological or biomechanical entrapment of a nerve root, plexus, or peripheral nerve can leave weakness or TrPs in the muscles distal to that site in the particular neural pattern associated with the involved structure, even after the pain resolves. Reinnervation associated with processes leading to axonotmesis (or higher degree injury) typically occurs at a rate of one inch per month; muscles not supported by

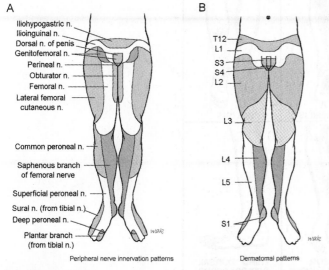

A.
- Iliohypogastric n.
- Ilioinguinal n.
- Dorsal n. of penis
- Genitofemoral n.
- Perineal n.
- Obturator n.
- Femoral n.
- Lateral femoral cutaneous n.
- Common peroneal n.
- Saphenous branch of femoral nerve
- Superficial peroneal n.
- Sural n. (from tibial n.)
- Deep peroneal n.
- Plantar branch (from tibial n.)

Peripheral nerve innervation patterns

B.
T12 — L1 — S3 — S4 — L2 — L3 — L4 — L5 — S1

Dermatomal patterns

Figure 42-29 A. Peripheral nerve patterns. **B.** Dermatomal or radicular (nerve root) patterns. (Illustration by W.A. Kuchera.)

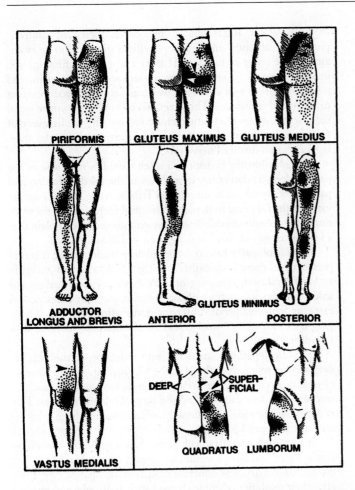

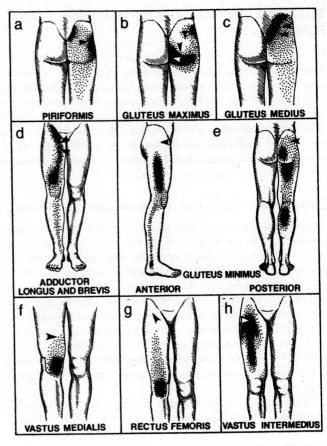

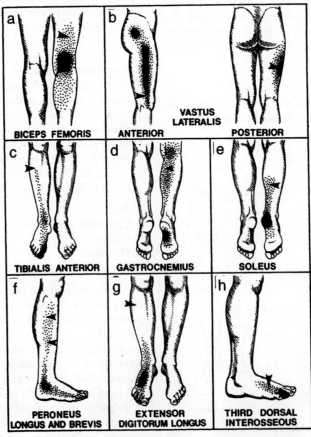

Figure 42-30 Travell MTrP patterns.

TABLE 42.2

HIP Joint Myofascial Dysfunction: Structure and Clinical Impact

Structure → Functional Anatomical Features	Clinical Implications of Somatic Dysfunction
Hip Flexors	
Iliopsoas (*L1-4; innervation from ventral rami*)—attachments L12-5 to femoral lesser trochanter • Activation: strongest flexor of thigh; flexes spine to bend • Activation with feet planted: bends spine forward • Standing normally extends lumbar lordosis	Postural muscle (hypertonic when stressed) • History/Symptoms: Activated by sit-ups or bending over a low table; Aggravated by weight-bearing; relief recumbent with knees bent • Referral: To back and anterior groin • Exam: Positive Thomas test; psoas posturing or psoas syndrome; tender over iliacus or psoas counterstrain points; may have L1 or L2 Fryette II dysfunction; chronic psoas contracture might demonstrate lumbar hyperlordosis and a loud audible pop (psoas tendon) during the Thomas test
Pectineus (*L2-3; femoral ± obturator n*) • Activation: flexion and adduction of thigh at hip • Designed for power not speed	Postural muscle (hypertonic when stressed) • Referral: As deep-seated groin ache
Other contributors to hip flexion: **sartorius; thigh adductors; tensor fascia latae;** and **rectus femoris** (only when knee extended)	Sartorius is the "tailor muscle" flexes, abducts, and externally rotates the hip; TFL tightens the iliotibial band to increase power of hip flexors and it steadies the trunk on the thigh
HIP Extensors	
Gluteus maximus (*L5-S2; inferior gluteal n*) • Activation: Most powerful extensor of thigh • Location/size unique; provides anatomic basis for upright posture; Type I (slow twitch) ms fibers suited for continuous postural use	Phasic muscle (inhibited when stressed) • History/Symptoms: Restlessness; sit or walk uphill = pain • Referral: To buttock • Exam: Antalgic gait
Hamstrings (*L5-S2; sciatic nerve*) • Activation: Extension during walking • Activation: Restrains hip flexion produced by body weight during stance phase of walking	Postural muscle (hypertonic when stressed) • History/Symptoms: Perpetuated by chair pressure under thighs; pain sitting and walking; disturbs sleep • Referral: To posterior thigh • Exam: Decreased hip flexion with straight-leg raising test
Adductor magnus—ischiocondylar portion (*L4-S1; sciatic innervation*) • Only portion of adductor magnus assisting flexion and then only when the femur is flexed more than 70°	Postural muscle (hypertonic when stressed) • Referral: To inner thigh
HIP Abductors	
Gluteus medius (*L4-S1; superior gluteal innervation*) and **Gluteus minimus** (*L4-S1; superior gluteal n*) • Activation: Stabilizes pelvis during single limb stance = Prevents nonstance innominate from falling inferior (negative Trendelenburg) • Activation: internal rotators of the hip	Phasic muscles (inhibited when stressed) • History/Symptoms: TrPs aggravated by walking, slouching in chair, or lying on back • Referral: G. medius to posterior iliac crest, sacroiliac joint, sacrum, and minor to buttock • Referral: G. minimus to buttock, lateral and posterior thigh; mistaken for L5 or S1 radiculopathy (but may coexist) • Exam: Positive Trendelenburg test = weakness in hip abductors; antalgic Trendelenburg gait = "abductor lurch"
Piriformis (*S1-2; piriformis nerve innervation*) • Activation: Acts as abductor when thigh flexed (only externally rotates with knee extended) • Location: Might entrap entire or peroneal portion of sciatic nerve	Postural muscle (hypertonic when stressed) • History/Symptoms: Perpetuated by sacroiliac somatic dysfunction (especially sacral shear) or irritation (sitting on billfold); might have fallen/missed step; may see foot drop

(continued)

TABLE 42.2   (*Continued*)

	• Referral: to pelvic floor; sciatica to knee if entrap sciatic n.
	• Associated with pelvic floor dysfunction, dyspareunia, prostatodynia
Hip abductors to lesser extent: **Sartorius, gluteus maximus, iliopsoas,** and **obturator internus** (when thigh is flexed only)	
HIP Adductors	
Adductor longus, brevis, and magnus (*L2-4; obturator innervation*)	Postural muscle (adductor magnus hypertonic when stressed)
• Activation: Early in swing phase, muscles pull limb toward midline	• Referral: To inguinal ligament, inner thigh, and upper medial knee
HIP External Rotators	
Obturator internus (*L5-S2; n to obt. Internus*)	Phasic muscles (inhibited when stressed)
• Activation: When the thigh is extended, causes external rotation at hip (when flexed, causes abduction)	• History/Symptoms: Responsible for pelvic floor symptoms (fullness in rectum)
	• Referral: to anococcygeal region (some to posterior thigh)
Piriformis (*S1-2; innervation from branches of S1-2 ventral rami*)	Postural muscle (hypertonic when stressed)
• Activation: External rotator *only when femur is extended* (acts as abductor when thigh flexed)	• History/Symptoms: Perpetuated by sacroiliac somatic dysfunction (especially sacral shear) or irritation (sitting on billfold); might have fallen or missed step; may see foot drop
• Location: Might entrap entire or peroneal portion of sciatic nerve	• Referral: To pelvic floor; sciatica to knee if entrap sciatic n.
	• Associated with pelvic floor dysfunction, dyspareunia, prostatodynia
HIP Internal Rotators	
Gluteus medius and **gluteus minimus** (*L4-S1*)	See hip abductors above
Hip internal rotation also from: **gemelli** and **quadratus femoris** (*L4-S1*); less from **piriformis** (*S1-2*)	

TABLE 42.3

Knee Joint Myofascial Dysfunction: Structure and Clinical Impact

Structure → Functional Anatomical Features	Clinical Implications of Somatic Dysfunction
Knee Flexors	
Biceps femoris (*L5-S2; sciatic n. long head = tibial portion; short head = peroneal portion*); Attachment—both heads plus semimembranosus establish a tripartite anchor on the fibular head	Postural muscle (hypertonic when stressed)
• Long head crosses both hip and knee	• History/Symptoms: Often wakes patient at night
• Short head crosses only knee	• Referral: Distalward from TrPs in the posterior thigh to the back of the knee or to the region of the fibular head
• Short head active in knee flexion for toe clearance during walking	
• Active contraction also induces some external rotation of the knee	

(continued)

TABLE 42.3 *(Continued)*

Semimembranosus and **semitendinosus** (*L5-S2; sciatic n. tibial portion*) • Also hip extensors • Hamstrings are not consistently active for knee flexion during walking (passive knee motion when the hip is flexed is more common) • Active contraction also induces some internal rotation of the knee	Postural muscle (hypertonic when stressed) • History/Symptoms: aggravated by walking often causing limp; TrPs often misdiagnosed as "sciatica" or "osteoarthritis of the knee" or "growing pains"[a]; TrPs remaining post-op often cause of "postlaminectomy syndrome" • Referral: proximally to lower buttock • Exam: Tightness in the hamstrings is associated with secondary inhibition and laxity of the gluteal muscles
Also **popliteus** and **gastrocnemius** • Popliteus initiates flexion from fully extended knee before hamstrings act	
Knee extensors	
Quadriceps (*L2-4; femoral n.*); Attachments—All four tendons unite into patellar tendon with patella; anchored to tibial tuberosity by patellar ligament • **Rectus femoris** crosses both hip and knee joints (proximal attachment to anterior posterior iliac spine [ASIS]); also a hip flexor • Three **vasti** cross only knee joint • *Q-angle* is the quadriceps angle measured from ASIS to midpatella to tibial tuberosity	Rectus femoris is a postural muscle (hypertonic when stressed); the other quadriceps are phasic muscles (inhibited when stressed) • History/Symptoms: Thigh and knee pain and weakness of knee extension especially going up stairs; may interrupt sleep. TrPs in v. medialis cause "buckling knee" and may cause patient to fall; TrPs in v. lateralis may restrict motion of the patella; pain with walking; TrPs in v. intermedius create difficulty straightening knee after prolonged sitting • Referral: Anterior knee pain is referred from v. medialis and rectus femoris; Posterior knee pain and pain anywhere along the lateral thigh to the iliac crest referred from v. lateralis • Exam: Include Q-angle and patellar grind tests; Imbalance in quadriceps with one another or with the hamstrings predispose to chondromalacia patellae (as does an increased Q-angle); Direct trauma to the quadriceps should be observed for myositis ossificans
Knee external rotator	
Biceps femoris (*L5-S2; sciatic n.*) • Also a knee flexor	See description with Knee Flexors above
Knee internal rotators	
Popliteus (*L4-S1; tibial n.*) • Unlocks knee at the start of weight bearing by "externally rotating the thigh on the fixed tibia"; internally rotates tibia when thigh is fixed • Prevents posterior glide of tibia relative to femur while crouching	• History/Symptoms: Aggravated by braking forward motions during twists (e.g., skiing), high heels by excessive foot pronation and by training on uneven ground • Referral: Pain behind the knee when crouching, walking down stairs, or running downhill • Exam: Mimics symptoms of Baker cyst but no associated swelling in the region
Semimembranosus and **semitendinosus** • Also knee flexors (primary)	See description under Knee Flexors above
Also **sartorius** (*L2-3; femoral nerve*) and **gracilis** (*L2-3; obturator n.*) • Sartorius is the longest muscle in the body crossing both hip and knee; it is a hip flexor and knee internal rotator • Gracilis is the second longest muscle in the body crossing hip and knee	• Pain from the sartorius in the anterior thigh is superficial and described as tingling or sharp; may exhibit symptoms of meralgia paresthetica (entrapment of lateral femoral cutaneous nerve)[e] • Pain from gracilis is a hot stinging, superficial pain in the medial thigh; it may be relieved by walking

TABLE 42.4

Ankle-Foot Joints Myofascial Dysfunction: Structure and Clinical Impact

Structure → Functional Anatomical Features	Clinical Implications of Somatic Dysfunction
Ankle dorsiflexors	
Tibialis anterior (*L4-S1; deep peroneal n.*) • An anterior compartment muscle • A dorsiflexor at the talotibial joint • Also supinates foot at the talocalcaneal and transverse tarsal joints	Phasic muscle (inhibited when stressed) • History/Symptoms: Might complain of tripping over carpets, dragging foot, or "foot slap". Weakness in muscle may be caused by L5 radiculopathy, peroneal mononeuropathy, the habit of crossing the legs at the knee, or posterior fibular head somatic dysfunction • Referral: Pain and tenderness referred into great toe and anteromedial ankle • Exam: Weakness leads to varying degrees of foot drop (rule out other causes)
Extensor digitorum longus (*L4-S1; deep peroneal n.*) • Also everts the foot balancing inversion of tibialis anterior • Helps prevent posterior postural sway	• History/Symptoms: Dysfunction often results in foot slap after heel strike • Referral: Dorsum of foot and ankle • Exam: TrPs might entrap deep peroneal n fibers; Ms imbalance → formation of hammer toes
Peroneus tertius (*L5-S1; deep peroneal n.*); Attachment—Tendon passes in front of lateral malleolus to insert on proximal 5th metatarsal • An anterior compartment muscle • A dorsiflexor at the talotibial joint • Also everts foot	Phasic muscle (inhibited when stressed) • History/Symptoms: Weakness in ankle dorsiflexion predisposing to ankle instability and repeat sprains; Might be mistaken for ankle arthritis. Weakness in muscle might be caused by L5 radiculopathy, peroneal mononeuropathy, the habit of crossing the legs at the knee, posterior fibular head somatic dysfunction or prolonged immobilization (as in an ankle cast) • Referral: Anterolateral ankle and sometimes to lateral heel • Exam: Failure to identify and treat TrPs post-ankle sprain can prolong rehabilitation process
Ankle plantar flexors	
Gastrocnemius (*L5-S2; posterior tibial n.*); Attachment—shares Achilles tendon attachment to calcaneus • Gastrocnemius-soleus complex referred to as triceps surae; constitutes close functional unit	Postural muscle (hypertonic when stressed) • History/Symptoms: Often nocturnal leg cramps; "tennis leg" (partial tearing of gastrocnemius) with a sudden intense calf pain, as if kicked, followed by swelling and local tenderness • Referral: Upper posterior calf and/or to instep • Exam: Failure to recognize "tennis leg" might lead to a posterior compartment syndrome
Soleus (*S1-2; tibial n.*); Shares Achilles attachment to calcaneus • Gastrocnemius-soleus complex constitutes close functional unit • Soleus function during gait is to add to knee and ankle stability • Acts as "second heart"[g] in moving venous and lymphatic fluid from lower extremity (e.g., fainting with military "attention" position) • Also aids in inversion of foot and extension of knee	Postural muscle (hypertonic when stressed) • History/Symptoms: pain severe walking up hill or stairs; May cause growing pains in children • Referral: Heel pain with TrPs in this muscle and/or may refer proximally to sacroiliac joint or even temporomandibular joint • Exam: May restrict dorsiflexion at ankle; Soleus TrPs easily mistaken for Baker cyst, thrombophlebitis, and/or Achilles tendinitis

(continued)

TABLE 42.4 (Continued)

Peroneus (Fibularis) longus and brevis (*L4-S1; superficial peroneal n.*) Attachments—**p. longus** attaches to fibular head and to upper 2/3 of lateral fibula, crosses behind the lateral malleolus over the cuboid, and divides to attach to the 1st cuneiform and the base of the 1st metatarsal; **p. brevis** travels with **p. longus** but inserts on the lateral aspect of the 5th metatarsal • Lateral compartment muscles • Plantar flex and pronate foot	Phasic muscles (inhibited when stressed) • History/Symptoms: TrPs initiated by inversion twisting of ankle or prolonged immobilization in ankle cast; Predispose to weak ankles and recurrent sprains; Pain easily mistaken for arthritis in ankle; numbness often noted in web of great toe • Referral: Lateral malleolus and some of lateral leg • Exam: May have deep peroneal nerve entrapment with some foot drop; p. longus and brevis aggravated by Morton foot structure; TrPs in p. longus can entrap the common peroneal nerve and weaken both anterior and lateral compartment muscles
Foot supinators	
Tibialis anterior (*L5-S1; deep peroneal n.*) • An anterior compartment muscle • Supinates foot at talocalcaneal and transverse tarsal joints • Also dorsiflexes at the talotibial joint	Phasic muscle (inhibited when stressed) • History/Symptoms: patients may complain of tripping over carpets, dragging foot, or "foot slap." Weakness in muscle may be caused by L5 radiculopathy, peroneal mononeuropathy, the habit of crossing the legs at the knee, or posterior fibular head somatic dysfunction • Referral: Great toe and anteromedial ankle • Exam: Weakness leads to varying degrees of foot drop
Foot pronators	
Peroneal (Fibularis) muscles (*L5-51; deep peroneal n.*); Attachment—Tendon passes in front of lateral malleolus to insert on proximal 5th metatarsal (p. longus and brevis are lateral compartment ms's; p. tertius is an anterior compartment muscle) • All pronate the foot (eversion and abduction) • p. tertius also dorsiflexes at the talotibial joint • p. brevis and longus also plantar flex	Phasic muscles (inhibited when stressed) • History/Symptoms: May be mistaken for ankle arthritis. Weakness in muscle may be caused by L5 radiculopathy, peroneal mononeuropathy, the habit of crossing the legs at the knee, posterior fibular head somatic dysfunction, or prolonged immobilization (as in an ankle cast) • Referral: Lateral ankle and foot; sometimes to lateral heel • Exam: Failure to identify and treat TrPs post-ankle sprain can prolong rehabilitation process Weakness in ankle dorsiflexion predisposing to ankle instability and repeat sprains
Foot and/or toe flexors	
Flexor digitorum longus (*L5-S1; tibial n.*)	• History/Symptoms: TrP perpetuation by Morton foot, running on uneven ground, or barefoot in the sand; Pain worse with walking • Referral: Sole of foot
Flexor hallucis longus (*L5-S2; tibial n.*)	• History/Symptoms: TrP perpetuation by Morton foot, running on uneven ground or barefoot in the sand • Referral: Plantar surface of great toe and first metatarsal head
Also intrinsic foot muscles	• History/Symptoms: Intolerably sore feet, limited walking range, limp
Foot and/or toe extensors	
Extensor digitorum longus (*L4-S1; deep peroneal n.*)	See above under Ankle Dorsiflexors
Extensor hallucis longus (*L4-S1; deep peroneal n.*)	• Dysfunction makes foot less adaptable to the ground while walking • History/Symptoms: TrPs may be perpetuated by L4-5 radiculopathy; often created following anterior compartment syndrome, prolonged jogging, or dorsiflexed ankle position during sleep • Referral: Dorsum of foot at the base of the great toe
Also intrinsic foot muscles	• History/Symptoms: Intolerably sore feet, limited walking range, limp

this reinnervation growth or by local collateral sprouting within an 18-month time frame typically become connective tissue incapable of reinnervation (63).

Sclerotomal referral is a deep, achy sensation that is toothache-like in quality. Sclerotomal (bony/ligamentous) distribution has also been mapped out (Fig. 42.31), but it is often overlooked and patients might dismiss it as lower extremity arthritic pain. (Notice that different aspects of the knee and the hip joints share the L3 and L4 sclerotomes.)

In general, referred pain is reproducible; as a consequence, diagnosis can be enhanced by stimulating the postulated pain generator to cause the pain symptom and by anesthetizing (or deactivating) that structure to see if the pain is eliminated. An understanding of the patterns associated with each referral improves patient diagnosis and treatment design. Failure to appreciate nondermatomal patterns may lead a practitioner to ineffectively treat symptoms rather than causes or to incorrectly consider a patient with legitimate symptoms a malingerer.

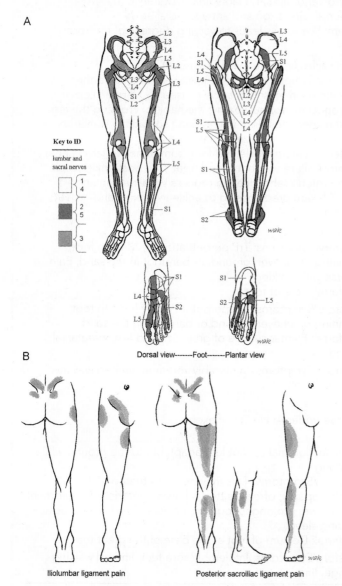

Figure 42-31 Sclerotomal pain patterns. **A.** Bone; **B.** Ligaments: 1. Iliolumbar (ILL); 2. PSI.

Referral from Lumbopelvic Structures

In addition to lumbar nerve roots and sclerotomes discussed earlier, a number of other lumbopelvic region myofascial, arthrodial, ligamentous, and visceral structures commonly refer pain to the inguinal area or hip. Somatic examples include iliolumbar and posterior sacroiliac (PSI) ligaments (64), quadratus lumborum muscle (65), and lumbar zygapophysial joints (66). Referral from visceral structures in this region are also often seen—as in a urinary tract stone passing down the ureter—radiating pain into the ipsilateral flank and the inner thigh region (67). Tissue texture changes in the form of Chapman reflexes may also occur as seen along the iliotibial band in patients with colon, prostate, or broad ligament viscerosomatic conditions (68).

Referral Originating in the Lower Extremities

Structures in the pubic or hip region often refer pain to the knee. For example, an adolescent male with knee pain and no sign of knee dysfunction or structural abnormality should have a hip x-ray to rule out a slipped capital epiphysis or other hip joint pathologies. Lower extremity MTrPs create predictable patterns of pain and dysfunction. In addition, nociceptive input from structures in the lower extremity may facilitate areas in the spine at the levels of T11-L2 that subsequently initiate symptoms from other structures sharing that same innervation (69).

Myofascial Trigger Point Patterns

Myofascial somatic dysfunction in this region leads to a number of patient symptoms that range from pain to weakness and that often limit range of motion and alter joint function. MTrPs as described by Travell and Simons also have predictable referral patterns not associated with dermatomes (see Fig. 42.30 for a synopsis of representative TrPs associated with the lower extremities). By definition, these points are a form of somatic dysfunction. They represent impaired or altered function of myofascial tissues with effects also in related neural, vascular, and lymphatic elements. TrPs respond to a wide range of treatment techniques: counterstrain, muscle energy, vapocoolant spray and stretch, dry needling, and procaine injection to name but a few. It is important however to identify any precipitating or perpetuating factors including coexistent lumbosacral radiculopathy, muscle imbalance, or poor ergonomics used in a repetitive manner.

Integrated Firing Patterns

Asymmetric postural stress creates recurrent and predictable patterns of lower extremity muscle somatic dysfunction that are characterized by neuromuscular imbalance or MTrPs. In neuromuscular imbalance, stressed postural (antigravity) muscles exhibit an increased irritability (short and tight), whereas their antagonists demonstrate inhibition (weak and atrophic) (Fig. 42.32) (70). When stressed, the iliopsoas, piriformis, hamstrings, gastrocnemius-soleus complex, adductor magnus, rectus femoris, and tensor fasciae latae all tend to tighten, while the vasti (especially the vastus medialis), glutei, peroneus, and tibialis anterior all tend to be inhibited and weak (71). Application of the biomechanical—postural model coupled with an understanding of the myotatic unit, muscle agonists and antagonists, and patterns of use is necessary for efficient diagnostic and therapeutic approaches to the treatment of lower extremity dysfunction that arise from this pattern of neuromuscular dysfunction.

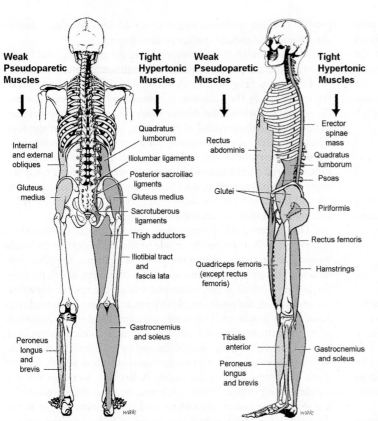

Figure 42-32 Muscle imbalance caused by biomechanical stressors.

Hip-Thigh Neuromuscular Considerations

Structure–Function Relationships

The muscles of the hip and thigh are generally large and powerful. They can be grouped according to their functional role (see Table 42.2).

The nerves innervating this region include the largest nerve in the body, the sciatic nerve, as well as the gluteal and femoral nerves. Based upon their location, some of these nerves are particularly vulnerable to trauma.

The sciatic nerve exits the pelvis through the greater sciatic notch and divides into a posterior tibial and a common peroneal nerve somewhere variably high in the thigh. In most individuals, it passes under the piriformis muscle; however, in approximately 10% of the U.S. population, the peroneal portion of the sciatic nerve actually passes through the piriformis muscle (72). (This anatomic variation occurs in one third of patients of Asian descent.) In the buttock or thigh, the sciatic nerve might be affected functionally by the piriformis muscle. Primary causes for such piriformis dysfunction can arise from direct trauma such as a fall onto one buttock or sitting for a prolonged period of time on a hard surface such as a toilet seat. Secondary dysfunction of the piriformis might be postural in origin or due to articular somatic dysfunctions involving the sacrum (sacral shears in particular) or the hip. Because of the close anatomical relationship between the two, biochemical irritation of the sciatic nerve is possible with irritation of the piriformis. Piriformis structure–function relationships are depicted in Figure 42.33.

Another source of iatrogenic trauma to the sciatic nerve comes from accidental injection into the nerve. Because the peroneal fibers are the more superficial, they are the most commonly involved in injection injuries; the resultant side effects include foot drop. Injections into the buttocks should be in the upper outer quadrant to avoid this problem in general injections; injections for piriformis TrPs should avoid steroids to decrease the risk of permanent damage from accidental introduction of the injected contents into the nerve. A more complete synopsis of the causes of foot drop may be found at the end of this chapter in the clinical section.

Numerous other lower extremity neural conditions can be found from the iliac region (*meralgia paresthetica*) to the toes (*Morton neuroma*). These and other conditions can arise from either trauma or somatic dysfunction and can be complicated by either. Meralgia paresthetica is a consequence of jeans that are too tight or pelvic somatic dysfunctions affecting the lateral femoral cutaneous nerve as it passes under the inguinal ligament near its attachment at the

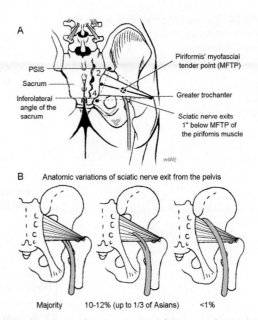

Figure 42-33 Piriformis structure–function relationships.

anterior superior iliac spine (ASIS); it manifests as superficial pain and numbness in the anterolateral thigh. Morton neuroma is an enlarged nerve that usually occurs in the interspace between the third and fourth metatarsals where the local pain is worsened by wearing shoes and by walking. Morton neuroma can be diagnosed by palpating this interspace and squeezing the forefoot from side to side to recreate the patient's pain or to palpate an audible click (*Mulder sign*).

Knee-Leg-Foot Neuromuscular Considerations

Structure–Function Relationships

Muscles of the thigh and leg that affect knee, ankle, and foot function (see Tables 42.3 and 42.4). Several thigh muscles have already been described in relation to their effect at the hip. These include the:

- Hamstrings
- Rectus femoris
- Tensor fasciae latae

The hamstrings and the short head of the biceps femoris are the chief flexors of the knee. The hamstrings, by definition the muscles that attach to the ischial tuberosity, attach to the leg below the knee and are supplied by the tibial division of the sciatic nerve (73). The head of the biceps femoris crosses the knee and is innervated by the peroneal portion of the sciatic nerve. Both heads of the biceps femoris also cause external rotation of the knee, while the remaining hamstrings cause internal rotation.

The quadriceps femoris group (three vasti and the rectus femoris) muscles are the chief extensors of the thigh; they are innervated by the femoral nerve. While the rectus femoris is a postural muscle and can become hypertonic on one side in relationship to tight hamstrings on the other side when there is pelvic rotation, the three vastus muscles are phasic and become pseudoparetic when stressed. Muscle imbalance that leads to MTrPs in the vastus muscles (especially vastus medialis) are often responsible for the so-called buckling knee syndrome (74). In this syndrome, no other reason except the trigger point for failure of the knee—which simply gives way without warning—can be identified; however, secondary

patellar tracking problems might be noted. (See the discussion of chondromalacia patellae earlier in this chapter.)

The remainder of the nerve supply in the thigh, leg, and foot is derived from the posterior tibial and common peroneal (common fibular) nerves (Fig. 42.34). A vulnerable site for entrapment or trauma exists as the common peroneal nerve (common fibularis nerve) passes behind the fibular head. The tibial nerve supplies the posterior compartment of the leg and the muscles of the foot. The deep peroneal nerve supplies the anterior compartment of the leg with sensation to the webbing between the first and second toes. The superficial peroneal nerve supplies the lateral compartment of the leg as well as the skin on the anterolateral side of the leg and the dorsum of the foot. OMT to the fibular head is often effective in treating this entrapment.

The posterior tibial nerve runs through the tarsal tunnel—a narrow space that lies on the inside of the ankle next to the ankle bones. The tunnel is covered with a thick ligament, the *flexor retinaculum*, that protects and maintains the structures, which includes the posterior tibial nerve, contained within the tunnel; therefore, compression of the posterior tibial nerve at this site is referred to as *tarsal tunnel syndrome*. This syndrome, that causes pain anywhere along the bottom of the foot, is often associated with diabetes, back pain, or arthritis. It can also be caused by an injury to the ankle, such as a sprain, or by a growth, abnormal blood vessels, or scar tissue that press against the nerve. A flat foot increases the risk for developing tarsal tunnel syndrome, because the outward tilting of the heel can produce strain and compression on the nerve. Treatment for tarsal tunnel syndrome includes in-shoe orthotics designed to help redistribute weight and take pressure off the nerve or corticosteroid injections. Tarsal tunnel syndrome caused by known conditions, such as tumors or cysts, might respond better to surgery than when the cause is not known.

Example of Differential Diagnosis Considerations: Foot Drop

There are numerous sites where structural or functional conditions could create weakness in the muscles that help to dorsiflex the foot.

Figure 42-34 Sciatic branches. Nerve supply of the lower extremity arising from the sciatic nerve and its branches.

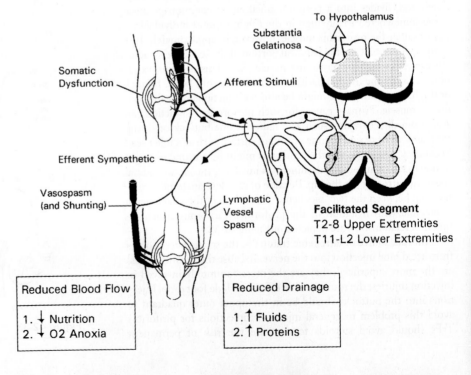

The differential diagnosis of foot drop is therefore quite extensive and encompasses systemic conditions such as multiple sclerosis to focal conditions such an L5 radiculopathy.

The most common regional neuromusculoskeletal conditions in the differential diagnosis include (75) from proximal to distal anatomical sites:

- L5 radiculopathy (e.g., secondary to herniated L4 disc)
- Cauda equina lesion (e.g., secondary to spinal adhesions)
- Lumbosacral plexopathy (e.g., secondary to colorectal carcinoma)
- Sciatic nerve injury (e.g., secondary to injection injury)
- Peroneal entrapment neuropathy
  - At piriformis (e.g., due to piriformis syndrome)
  - At fibular head (e.g., due to posterior fibular head somatic dysfunction or to Baker cyst)
- Peroneal or tibialis anterior MTrPs (e.g., due to prior severe supination ankle sprain)

The dorsiflexors of the foot are primarily phasic muscles (antagonists to postural muscles); dysfunction or trigger points in these muscles, especially the tibialis anterior, might also lead to weakness and a tendency for mild foot drop symptoms especially after using the muscle(s) for a period of time (76).

Techniques that remove joint or myofascial somatic dysfunction in the areas discussed above are considered helpful in reducing foot drop symptoms (77,78). Recommended techniques (depending on the site of entrapment) include:

- Counterstrain for the piriformis muscle after correction of the joints associated with this muscle's bony attachments (sacroiliac and femorohumeral joints)
- Balanced ligamentous and membranous tension for the fibular head and lower leg interosseous membrane

OTHER RELATED VASCULAR AND LYMPHATIC ELEMENTS

Enhancing homeostasis associated with vascular and lymphatic elements is a significant portion of an integrated osteopathic treatment regimen in the lower extremities. By definition, removal of somatic dysfunction is linked to its influence on related neural, vascular, and lymphatic elements (Fig. 42.35). As with other regions, the respiratory-circulatory model plays a central role in this aspect of care. In the respiratory-circulatory model, both diagnosis and treatment of the lower extremity begin proximally and move distally. Terminal lymphatic drainage sites are located just inferior to the inguinal ligament in the femoral triangle and as severity increases the congestion extends to fullness in the popliteal region and eventually to the tissues around the Achilles tendon. In addition to fullness or bogginess, dysfunctional drainage results in tissues that are tight, tender, or ticklish. Should one of these peripheral sites be congested without the more proximal site(s), this would indicate a localized trauma rather than a problem involving the entire lower extremity.

In the lower extremities, a number of potential spaces are subject to trauma and swelling. Therefore, this section will also focus on clinical understanding of compartment syndromes and a number of bursitis complaints in the lower extremity.

Arterial Supply

The inferior margin of the acetabulum is incomplete, forming an acetabular notch through which the hip joint receives its blood vessels (Fig. 42.36). These vessels could easily be disrupted by a femoral neck fracture, which creates the possibility of delayed healing or

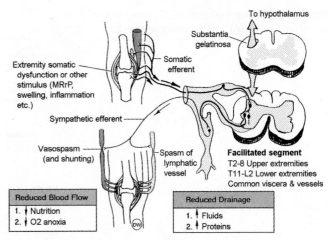

Figure 42-35 Segmental facilitation. Influence of somatic dysfunction on normal vascular and lymphatic elements of the lower extremity. (From Kuchera ML, Kuchera WA. *Osteopathic Considerations in Systemic Dysfunction.* 2nd Ed. Rev. Columbus, OH: Greyden Press, 1994, with permission.)

nonunion; somatic dysfunction rarely causes problems with these large vessels.

The femoral artery is the major vessel supplying the lower extremities. Easily located in the femoral triangle, this artery is bounded by the sartorius and adductor muscles and the inguinal ligament. The mnemonic NAVEL provides a reminder of the order, from lateral to medial, of the structures in the femoral triangle:

Nerve
Artery
Vein
Empty space
Lymphatics

The arterial pulse in the femoral triangle helps to establish all of the other palpatory landmarks in this region. Acute loss of pulses in the lower extremity is usually a contraindication to the use of OMT.

The vascular supply is very poor to the menisci in the knees (especially the central section) and to synovial joint tissues in general. In large part, nutrition to the joints depends on good blood flow to the region and subsequent diffusion into the synovial fluids. Metabolic waste products moving out of the arthrodial tissues likewise diffuse into the synovial fluid. This vascular supply limitation also affects decisions concerning surgery (79) in meniscal tears:

- If a tear is within 3 mm of the periphery, it is considered vascular and often heals with conservative care.
- The area 3 to 5 mm from the periphery is considered a gray zone and may benefit from OMT or heat to improve blood flow, but surgery may need to be considered.
- More than 5 to 7 mm from the periphery is considered to be avascular.
- Unstable tears or tears within the vascular zone are repairable.

Treatment of somatic dysfunction is postulated to improve blood delivery by reducing hypersympathetic activity. This is important for the nutritional status of the tissues in the lower extremities. It would also benefit the delivery of medications such as non-steroidal anti-inflammatory drugs to target tissues in the lower extremities where pharmacological effectiveness is proportionate

Figure 42-36 Hip vasculature. Anatomy of the acetabular notch (**A**) and femoral triangle (**B**).

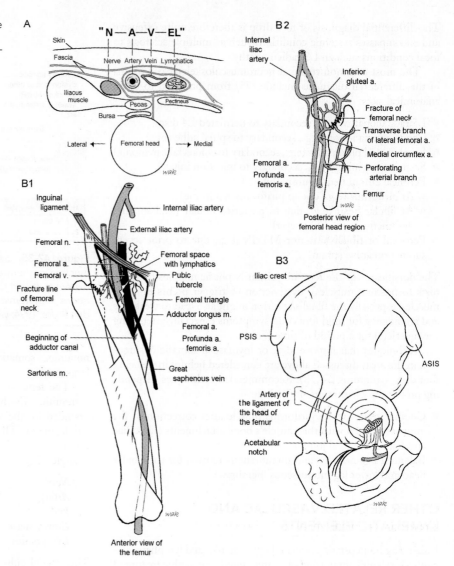

to tissue or synovial concentration of the drug. Cell bodies for the sympathetic nerve supply to the lower extremities' vasculature are found at the level of T11-L2.

Venous and Lymphatic Drainage

The very act of locomotion plays an important role in lymphatico-venous return. Use of the lower extremity muscles in walking and running moves these fluids through one-way valves back toward the central vascular system. OMT to open fascial pathways and eliminate MTrPs can improve venous and lymphatic drainage of the extremities. Drainage can also be enhanced using a variety of lymphatic pump techniques such as those performed on the chest cage to maximize pressure gradients between the thorax and abdomen or directly through the lower extremities as with the pedal pump (Dalrymple) technique (each is described more fully in Chapter 51). Lymphatic pumps performed in this manner have been shown to be as effective as treadmill or bicycling exercise and to release nitric oxide at levels consistent with those produced through the upregulation of endothelial nitric oxide synthase (80). The Dalrymple pump is contraindicated in patients with positive Homans or Moses tests or other findings that suggest deep vein thrombosis (81).

Drainage using the respiratory-circulatory model is the most likely added osteopathic component to be used in the treatment of swelling in the various compartments and bursae of the lower extremities.

Bursae and Bursitis

Bursae are small, synovial tissue-lined structures that help different tissues glide over one another, such as a tendon sliding over another tendon or bone. A number of bursae are located around the hip, knee, and ankle (Fig. 42.37). They may swell and become painful when infected or when irritated as a response to direct trauma or stresses placed on the joints of the lower extremities.

Bursitis is inflammation of a bursa. There is palpable swelling that can be defined and that is sensitive to deep pressure. Pain alone in the region of the bursa often leads to misdiagnosis.

Trochanteric Bursitis

In the hip region (see Fig. 42.37), *trochanteric bursitis* is a common clinical diagnosis or, in many cases, a misdiagnosis. The subgluteus maximus (trochanteric) bursa lies at the root of the iliotibial tract. Here, it separates the greater trochanter of the femur from the converging fibers of the gluteus maximus and the tensor fasciae latae.

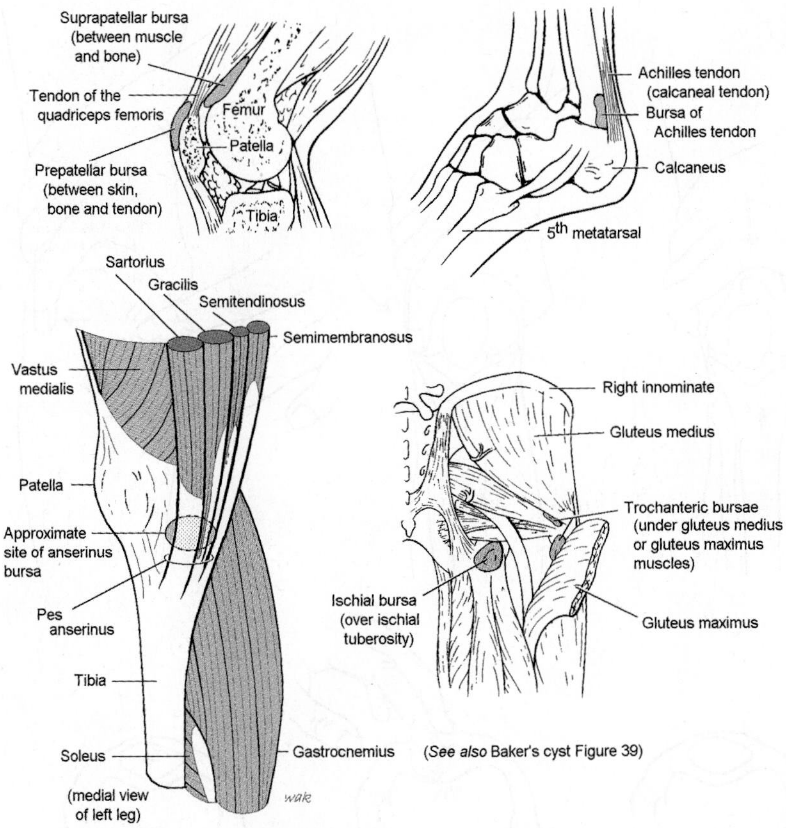

Figure 42-37 Bursae of the lower extremity.

The bursa also separates these fibers from the origin of the vastus lateralis muscle. TrPs in any of these muscles can refer pain to this site and are commonly misdiagnosed as a trochanteric bursitis; this is also the case in quadratus lumborum TrPs (82) and in the ligamentous pain referral from iliolumbar ligament (83).

True inflammation and swelling of the trochanteric bursa (trochanteric bursitis) causes an intense pain over the bursal location that radiates into the lateral thigh. Palpation of the bursa just below the greater trochanter reveals the swelling and heat. Pressure applied to this site increases the pain that can be further aggravated by walking, hip abduction, or internally rotating the hip. Injection of the bursa with a local anesthetic with or without accompanied steroids quickly and significantly reduces pain. A higher incidence of trochanteric bursitis is found on the long leg side of individuals with unequal leg length (84).

Patellar Bursitis

The knee is a common site for trauma to the bursa designed to protect the relatively exposed superficial structures from injury against those underlying them. A large prepatellar bursa separates the patella from the skin anterior to it. Inflammation of this bursa from long-term kneeling or from other trauma results in a condition known as *housemaid's knee*.

The suprapatellar bursa connects to the synovial cavity of the knee joint and can be used in physical diagnosis to determine if knee trauma has caused significant swelling. The physician first milks any fluid in this bursa from the medial to the lateral side. Then, by palpating anteromedially for a fluid wave initiated by a gentle squeeze from the anterolateral side of the suprapatellar tendon, it is possible to detect 10 to 15 mL of effusion in the knee. This *bulge test* is used for small effusions (Fig. 42.38A). If the effusion is so large that the tissues become turgid, a fluid pulse might not be able to create a bulge and the test can provide a false-negative result. Large effusions are more accurately diagnosed with a ballottement test (Fig. 42.38B) in which the kneecap is tapped gently (ballotted). A palpable transmission of bony contact is palpated if the effusion is large enough to have distanced the patella from the bone behind it.

The superficial and deep infrapatellar bursae are less often involved in clinical problems.

A *Baker cyst* arises from enlargement of either the semimembranosus bursa or the bursa behind the medial head of the gastrocnemius (Fig. 42.39). The swollen cyst is often painful, especially with flexion of the knee, and the swelling is more prominent in the standing position. Both of these bursae commonly communicate with the synovial cavity of the knee. For this reason, knee trauma such as a meniscal tear, or diseases such as rheumatoid arthritis, can initiate the cyst. Rupture of a Baker cyst may be misdiagnosed as thrombophlebitis; extension of a Baker cyst may compress the common peroneal nerve near the fibular head and lead to a foot drop.

Pes Anserine Bursitis

Pes anserine bursitis is a common finding in patients or athletes who present with complaints of anterior knee pain. The pes anserine bursa, along with its associated medial hamstring tendons, is located along the proximomedial aspect of the tibia (see Fig. 42.37). This condition is usually found in patients who have tight hamstrings, although it also can be caused by trauma (as in a direct blow). In most patients, pes anserine bursitis is a self-limiting condition that responds to a program of hamstring stretching and quadriceps strengthening.

Figure 42-38   Tests for effusion in the knee. The bulge test (**A**) is useful for finding a minimal amount of effusion in the knee. The ballottement test (**B**) is positive if there is a large amount of effusion present. (Illustration by W.A. Kuchera.)

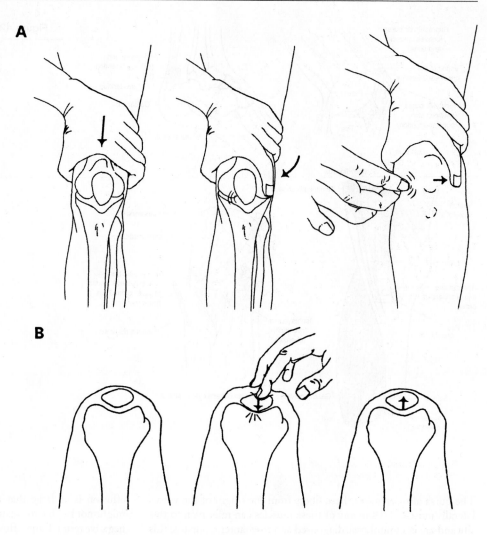

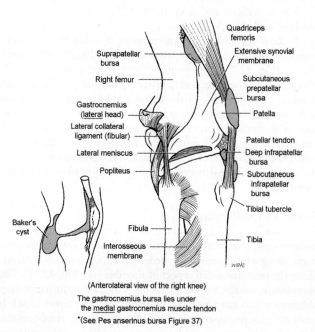

Figure 42-39   Bursae of the knee and Baker cyst.

Bursa of the Achilles Tendon

In the ankle region, the superficial bursa of the Achilles tendon can be irritated by poorly fitting shoes and can swell (see Fig. 42.37). This results in a tender *pump bump*.

Compartments in the Lower Extremity

The lower leg is divided into three compartments (Fig. 42.40):

- Anterior osseofibrous compartment
- Lateral osseofibrous compartment
- Two posterior osseofibrous compartments—deep and superficial

Clinically, a compartment syndrome can arise from trauma or vigorous overuse, leading to a rise in intracompartmental pressure. This in turn compromises the circulation, including venous return, within that compartment.

Recurrent mild compartment symptoms are managed with ice and OMT. Ice decreases pain and metabolic demand after activity. OMT also decreases pain and improves venous and lymphatic return. Management of coexisting TrPs is also helpful but not with injections; they would increase pressure in an already tight compartment. Modification of the running surface or the running shoe may also be required in order to prevent recurrent compartment syndromes.

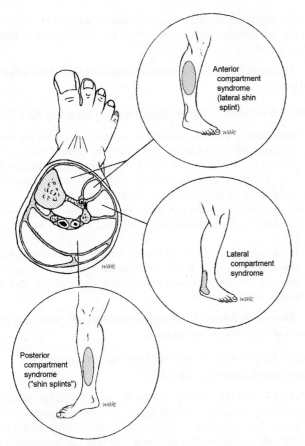

Figure 42-40 Fascial compartments of the lower extremity.

Anterior Compartment

The anterior compartment is covered anteriorly by a relatively nonexpansile fascia. Structurally, this creates the potential for development of an anterior compartment syndrome. Bleeding into this compartment from a fracture or other trauma creates increased pressure in this enclosed space. For runners, sometimes muscle swelling impairs venous outflow, which results in a rise in intracompartmental pressure. If intracompartmental pressure becomes great enough, arterial circulation is reduced, and ischemia with potential necrosis of muscle in the compartment can occur. An *acute compartment compression* is a surgical emergency requiring fasciotomy. Such a situation is more likely to occur in the anterior compartment than in other divisions of the leg. The acute compartment compression may occur in runners where symptoms of intense pain develop during the run but do not subside afterward.

Palpation reveals the entire tibialis anterior muscle to be hard and tender. Anterior compartment muscles may also exhibit weakness upon testing and peripheral pulses are usually present. Decreased sensation is often present between the first and second toes as a result of entrapment of the deep peroneal nerve. While primarily a clinical diagnosis, intracompartmental pressure can be measured with a wick catheter (85). Because of the location of the pain on the anterolateral side of the leg, recurrent anterior compartment syndrome is also sometimes called *anterior shin splints*.

Lateral Compartment

In the lateral compartment syndrome, pain is located diffusely along the lateral aspect of the lower leg. It recurs in runners with excessive pronation of the foot or might result from rupture of the peroneus longus muscle.

Posterior Compartment

The posterior compartment syndromes typically refer pain anteromedially. While some reserve the term *shin splints* only for periostitis along the line of attachment of a repeatedly overloaded muscle (86), others include posterior compartment syndrome in the differential diagnosis along with stress fractures of the tibia and chronic periostitis (the soleus syndrome). Posterior compartment syndromes are often bilateral and difficult to manage conservatively.

CLINICAL PATTERNS AND OSTEOPATHIC MANAGEMENT

To this point in the chapter, the lower extremity has been discussed as a series of component parts; in reality, each of these parts interact. Somatic dysfunction or pathology in any one skeletal, arthrodial, or myofascial component affects the rest of the somatic structures as shown in both the common compensatory malalignment syndrome (87) and a traumatically induced problem such as an ankle sprain (88).

Case Management 1: Supination Ankle Sprain

A 22-year-old amateur rugby player presents with acute swelling and lateral ankle pain after twisting his ankle by stepping in a small pothole in the playing field 24 hours earlier. The description of his injury matches that of a classic supination sprain. He has his right ankle wrapped with an over-the-counter elastic bandage using a figure-of-eight pattern extending from metatarsals to mid-calf. He is able to bear weight gingerly, but prefers to use a set of crutches from a prior ankle injury 1 year ago on the same side. He has been icing and elevating the ankle, which had been his only care in the prior injury.

Examination incorporating the Ottawa ankle rules (see Fig. 42.18) suggests no ankle or forefoot fracture. In addition to the tenderness, swelling, and ecchymosis over the anterior talofibular ligament, he has the typical somatic dysfunction pattern depicted/summarized in Figure 42.19.

One fourth of all individuals who have experienced a significant ankle sprain will continue to have pain, instability, and sprain recurrence (89). Two theories, each with valid support, explain why. One theory blames mechanical instability due to damaged support structures while the other blames functional instability owing to dysfunctional neural-proprioceptive pathways that inaccurately report ankle position. Regardless, somatic dysfunction is thought to play a role in both.

The somatic dysfunction associated with a supination sprain was previously described (see Fig. 42.19) (90). OMT as part of the biomechanical-postural model is prescribed to improve ankle dorsiflexion—reduced ankle dorsiflexion increasing the risk of recurrent ankle sprains by 500% (91)—and to remove somatic dysfunction in joints and muscles known to impair proprioceptive balance mechanisms (92). Furthermore, osteopathic treatment for this condition involves opening and implementing the respiratory-circulatory model to provide reduction of the swelling, loss of function, and residual dysfunction seen in acute ankle trauma (93). Outcomes associated with the use of manual treatment suggest more rapid resolution of pain, swelling, and dysfunction and might reduce the risk of reinjury (94–99). Consideration of the biopsychosocial model is also part of the osteopathic approach in this (and other cases)—what, if any, health impact might be associated with the inability of an athlete to miss a key game; to ignore advice and play on an injured ankle; or to fail to regain function with subsequent loss of scholarships and self-image?

What follows is a safe and effective method for the local hands-on treatment of an acute supination ankle sprain on the right side; it is also an effective combination for use in chronic conditions where OMT was perhaps not part of the rehabilitation process. All use balanced ligamentous and balanced membranous techniques (BLT/BMT) appropriate even immediately after a sprain. In chronic conditions or when the swelling recedes in a recent ankle sprain, gentle direct muscle energy technique to the talocrural joint may be added if needed.

With practice, transitioning from the subtalar joint into the talocalcaneal joint (Figs. 41A,B) and from that balanced anatomy carrying the indirect fascial unwinding technique up through the anterior talofibular ligament into the interosseous membrane can be done seamlessly without changing hand positions around the talocalcaneal joint. Fascial unwinding from the foot-ankle up and from the hip down (Fig. 41D) is also a time-effective approach to this injury.

Diagnosis: Supination with posterolateral glide of the talocalcaneal joint.

OMT: Balanced Ligamentous Tension of Forefoot to Hind Foot and Talus to Calcaneous (see Fig. 42.41A)

1. Doctor takes the right foot in the right hand with the thumb and first digit pinching the talus; the remainder of the fingers holding the arch of the foot. The left hand stabilizes the calcaneous between fingers and thenar eminence. (Patient is supine)
2. Using a motion between the two hands like "wringing out a wet cloth," glide the talus posterolateral on the calcaneous to the point of BLT. The right hand will move slightly counterclockwise while the left hand moves clockwise; the right hand will also slightly increase the foot's arch

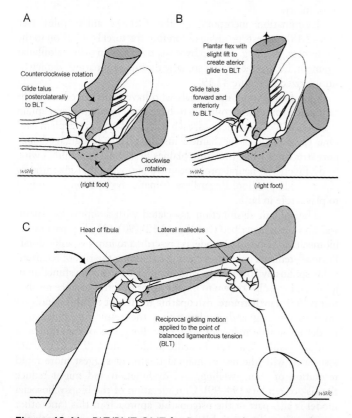

Figure 42-41 BLT/BMT OMT for Patients with Supination Sprain **(A)** Posterolateral talocalcaneal SD; **(B)** Plantar flexion with anterior glide SD; **(C)** Fibular SD with interosseous strain.

3. Concentrating on the persistent yielding between the talus and the calcaneous, continuously adjust the BLT until a release is palpated

Diagnosis: Plantar flexion with anterior glide of the talocrural joint.

OMT: Balanced Ligamentous Tension (see Fig 42.41B):

1. Maintaining the same hand hold as above, gently lift the lower extremity off the table to create a gentle anterior glide of the talus in the ankle mortise and add just enough plantar flexion (and additional anterior glide) to feel BLT between the talus and the rest of the lower leg at the ankle
2. Concentrating on the persistent yielding between the talus in the mortise, continuously adjust the BLT until a release is palpated
3. If the doctor wishes a slight shift of focus can be made at this point to gently pull in an anteromedial direction through the anterior talofibular ligament into the distal fibula and the interosseous membrane

Diagnosis: Fibular head dysfunction (usually posterior) with strain of interosseous membrane.

OMT: BLT of Fibula and BMT of the Interosseous Membrane (see Fig. 42.41C):

1. Doctor's left thumb pad contacts the right fibula just posterior to the fibular head; the right thumb pad is placed just posterior to the lateral malleolus. The supine patient's hip and knee on that side are bent so that the lower extremity sits comfortably on the doctor's thumbs. The weight is adjusted to avoid compression over these thumbs. (The doctor may use fingers or even a forehead to help take weight off of the thumbs.)
2. The lower extremity is adjusted by modifying the hip and knee bend (and perhaps a bit of external rotation at the hip) so that the fibula at both ends feels as if the same slight weight is resting on each thumb. (The doctor will typically have their elbows both resting on the table.)
3. The fibula is then balanced (to BLT) with either a slight amount of inferior-superior glide from the lateral malleolus thumb to move the fibular head posterior to balance -OR- with a slight amount of superior-anterior pressure from the fibular head thumb to glide the fibular head anterior to balance
4. Final fine tuning usually consists of an inferior longitudinal balancing force through both thumbs along the long axis of the fibula that often also needs slight medial glide of the distal fibula (in the direction of the sprained anterior talofibular ligament) to the point of BMT
5. Concentrating on the persistent yielding of the fibular head in the direction it first preferred, and along the interosseous membrane between the tibia and fibula adjust the BLT/BMT until a release is palpated

Diagnosis: Edema, inflammation, and fascial torsion in lower extremity.

OMT: Popliteal Spread, Fascial Unwinding, and Lateral Fluctuation of the Lower Extremity to Enhance Homeostasis to Handle Inflammation and Edema:

1. Patient is supine with leg slightly flexed and abducted to allow the doctor (standing at the end of the table) to place the patient's ankle/foot between his or her lower thighs to help control the patient's leg

2. Using the fingers of both hands, the doctor contacts the medial and lateral edges of the hamstring muscle tendons and gently spreads these away from the midline of the popliteal region. ("Popliteal spread technique.")

3. Abduct/adduct, flex/extend, and internally/externally rotate at the hip to the point of balanced ligamentous tension

4. Maintain hip but stack major and minor motions at the knee (flex/extend, abduct/adduct, and externally/internally rotate with anteromedial or posterolateral glides, respectively)

5. Maintain hip and knee balanced tensions and now add an approximation of pronation/supination of the foot

6. Add a little traction or compression along the longitudinal axis of the lower extremity again to BLT

7. As "fascial unwinding" is performed, ask where the patient feels warmth. It should progress from thigh to knee to calf to foot to toes over a period of a minute or less. (If the progression stops, it indicates a site of significant somatic dysfunction that may require specific OMT.)

8. Place the patient's feet flat on the table with knee flexed to 90 degrees and hip flexed to 45 degrees

9. The doctor's caudad hand holds the dorsum of the patient's foot and ankle and the cephalad hand rests on top of the patient's knee

10. The patient's knee is moved medial and lateral at the knee to find the position of greatest ligamentous balance

11. From that point of balance, the doctor institutes a small rhythmic medial to lateral excursion that is maintained until treatment is finished

After appropriate diagnosis of the patient (including his ankle), osteopathic treatment of the patient focuses first to limit pathophysiology and promote inherent motions during the "PRICE" (Protection, Relative rest, Ice, Compression/support, Elevation) approach in the acute state; indirect OMT plays a role at this point. Subsequently, strategies shift to effective rehabilitation including early mobilization, correction of somatic dysfunctions that could limit shock absorption, ankle range of motion (especially dorsiflexion), or muscle-proprioceptive imbalance. Patient education and exercise (strengthening, range of motion, and proprioceptive) (100,101) often play a role in this stage for full return of function and prevention of recurrence.

SUMMARY

A thorough understanding of the functional anatomy of the lower extremities, coupled with grounding in osteopathic practice principles, establishes a foundation for the osteopathic approach to the lower extremities and their effect on the whole person. Palpation assists in differential diagnoses of a wide range of structural and functional disorders in this region. The osteopathic physician then seeks to balance and improve biomechanical and homeostatic functions to influence a wide range of patient conditions.

From a sports medicine practice to the care of patients with deep vein thrombosis in an internal medicine practice, the osteopathic approach to the lower extremities offers an effective approach to diagnosis, prevention, and treatment.

REFERENCES

1. Irvin RE. Suboptimal posture: the origin of the majority of idiopathic pain of the musculoskeletal system. In: Vleeming A, Mooney V, Dorman T, et al., eds. *Movement, Stability, and Low Back Pain: The Essential Role of the Pelvis.* New York, NY: Churchill-Livingstone, 1997:133–155.

2. Horak F, Nashner L, Diener H. Postural strategies associated with somatosensory and vestibular loss. *Exp Brain Res* 1990;82:167–177.

3. Peirce N. Patellofemoral disorders, chondromalacia dysfunction, maltracking and plica syndrome. In: Hutson M, Ellis R, eds. *Textbook of Musculoskeletal Medicine.* Oxford, UK: Oxford University Press, 2006;297–308.

4. Cyriax JH, Cyriax PJ. *Cyriax's Illustrated Manual of Orthopaedic Medicine.* 2nd Ed. Oxford, UK: Butterworth-Heinemann Ltd., 1993:6–8.

5. Seffinger MA, Hruby RJ, Kuchera WA. *Evidence-Based Manual Medicine: A Problem-Oriented Approach.* Philadelphia, PA: Saunders, 2007:291–311.

6. Kerkhoffs GMMJ, Rowe BH, Assendelft WJJ, et al. Immobilisation and functional treatment for acute lateral ankle ligament injuries in adults. *Cochrane Database Syst Rev* 2002;(3):CD003762.

7. Wexter RK. The injured ankle. *Am Fam Physician* 1998;57:474–480.

8. Dorman TA. Refurbishing ligaments with prolotherapy. *Spine*: State of the Art Reviews. 1995;9(2):509–516.

9. Moore KL. *Clinically Oriented Anatomy.* 2nd Ed. Baltimore, MD: Williams & Wilkins, 1985:403.

10. Roaas A, Anderrson GBJ. Normal range of motion of the hip, knee and ankle joints in male subjects, 30–40 years of age. *Acta orthop. scand.* 1982; 53, 205–208.

11. Roaas A, Anderrson GBJ. Normal range of motion of the hip, knee and ankle joints in male subjects, 30–40 years of age. *Acta orthop. scand.* 1982; 53, 205–208.

12. Cyriax JH, Cyriax PJ. *Cyriax's Illustrated Manual of Orthopaedic Medicine,* 2nd Ed. Oxford, England: Butterworth-Heinemann Ltd; 1993:81.

13. Christmann OD. Biomechanical aspects of degenerative joint disease. *Clin Orthop.* 1969;64:77–85.

14. Slipman CW, Sterenfeld EB, Chou LH, et al. The predictive value of provocative sacroiliac joint stress maneuvers in the diagnosis of sacroiliac joint syndrome. *Arch Phys Med Rehabil.* 1998;79(3):288–92.

15. Gofton JP, Trueman GE. Studies in osteoarthritis of the hip, Part II: osteoarthritis of the hip and leg-length disparity. *Can Med Assoc J.* 1971;104:791–799.

16. Brody DM. Running injuries. *CIBA Clin Symp* 1980;32(4):25.

17. Kuchera WA, Kuchera ML. *Osteopathic Principles in Practice.* 2nd Ed. Rev. Columbus, OH: Greyden Press, 1994.

18. Roaas A, Anderrson GBJ. Normal range of motion of the hip, knee and ankle joints in male subjects, 30–40 years of age. *Acta Orthop Scand* 1982;53:205–208.

19. Strobel M, Stedtfeld HW. *Diagnostic Evaluation of the Knee.* New York, NY: Springer-Verlag, 1990:166–182.

20. Solomon DH, Simel, Bates, et al. The rational clinical examination. Does this patient have a torn meniscus or ligament of the knee? Value of the physical examination. *JAMA* 2001;286(13):1610–1620.

21. Renstrom P, Johnson J. Anatomy and biomechanics of the menisci. *Clinics Sports Med* 1990;9:523–538.

22. Jackson JL, O'Malley PG, Kroenke K. Evaluation of acute knee pain in primary care. *Ann Intern Med* 2003;139:575–588.

23. Corea JR, Moussa M, al Othman A. McMurray's test tested. *Knee Surg Sports Traumatol Arthrosc* 1994;2(2):70–72.

24. Strobel M, Stedtfeld HW: *Diagnostic Evaluation of the Knee.* New York, NY: Springer-Verlag, 1990:166–182.

25. O'Donoghue D. The unhappy triad: Etiology, diagnosis and treatment. *Am J Orthop* 1964;6:242–247.

26. Cowan DN, Jones BH, Frykman PN, et al. Lower limb morphology and risk of overuse injury among male infantry trainees. *Med Sci Sports Exerc* 1996;28:945–952.

27. Hoerner EF. Injuries of the lower extremities. In: Vinger PF, Hoerner EF, eds. *Sports Injuries: The Unthwarted Epidemic.* Littleton, MA: PSG Publishing Company, Inc., 1986:235–249.

28. Kuchera ML. Treatment of gravitational strain pathophysiology. In: Vleeming A, Mooney V, Dorman T, eds. *Movement, Stability and Low Back Pain: The Essential Role of the Pelvis.* Edinburgh, UK: Churchill Livingstone, 1997;477–499; chap. 39.

29. Ombregt L, ter Veer HJ. Disorders of the inert structures: capsular and non-capsular patterns. In: Ombregt L, Bisschop P, ter Veer HJ, et al., eds. *A System of Orthopaedic Medicine.* London, UK: WB Saunders, 1995:783–800.

30. Blood SD. Treatment of the sprained ankle. *J Am Osteopath Assoc* 1980;79:680–692.

31. Inman VT. *Joints of the Ankle.* Baltimore, MD: Williams & Wilkins, 1976:42.

32. Inman VT, Mann RA. Biomechanics of the foot and ankle. In: *DuVries' Surgery of the Foot*. 3rd Ed. St. Louis, MO: 1973:17.

33. Levens SA, et al. Transverse rotation of the segments of the lower extremity in locomotion. *J Bone Joint Surg* 1948;30A:859–872.

34. Hicks JH. The mechanics of the foot, I: the joints. *J Anat* 1953;87:345–357.

35. Inman VT. *Joints of the Ankle*. Baltimore, MD: Williams & Wilkins, 1976:42.

36. Inman VT, Mann RA. Biomechanics of the foot and ankle. In: *DuVries' Surgery of the Foot*. 3rd Ed. St. Louis, MO, 1973:17.

37. Roaas A, Anderrson GBJ. Normal range of motion of the hip, knee and ankle joints in male subjects, 30–40 years of age. *Acta Orthop Scand* 1982;53,205–208.

38. de Noronha M. Refshauge KM. Herbert RD. et al. Do voluntary strength, proprioception, range of motion, or postural sway predict occurrence of lateral ankle sprain? [Review]. *Br J Sports Med* 2006;40(10):824–828; discussion 828.

39. Kuchera WA, Kuchera ML. *Osteopathic Principles in Practice*. 2nd Ed. Rev. Columbus, OH: Greyden Press, 1994.

40. Nack JD, Phillips RD. Shock absorption. *Clin Podiatr Med Surg* 1990;7(2):391–397.

41. Nigg BM, Denoth J, Neukomm PA. Quantifying the load on the human body: problems and some possible solutions. In: Morecki A, Fidelus K, Kedzior K, et al. eds. *Biomechanics VII-B*. Baltimore, MD: University Park, 1981:88–99.

42. Hreljac A. Impact and overuse injuries in runners. *Med Sci Sports Exerc* 2004;36(5):845–849.

43. Kirby KA. Biomechanics of the normal and abnormal foot. *J Am Podiatr Med Assoc* 2000;90(1):30–34.

44. Inman VT, Mann RA. Biomechanics of the foot and ankle. In: *DuVries' Surgery of the Foot*. 3rd Ed. St. Louis, MO, 1973:17.

45. Stiell IG, McKnight RD, Greenberg GH, et al. Implementation of the Ottawa ankle rules. *JAMA* 1994;271:827–832.

46. Bachmann LM, Kolb E, Koller MT, et al. Accuracy of Ottawa ankle rules to exclude fractures of the ankle and mid-foot: systematic review. *BMJ* 2003;326:417; doi:10.1136/bmj.326.7386.417.

47. Roy S, Irvin R. *Sports Medicine: Prevention, Evaluation, Management, and Rehabilitation*. Englewood Cliffs, NJ: Prentice-Hall, 1983:380.

48. Kuchera WA, Kuchera ML. *Osteopathic Principles in Practice*. 2nd Ed. Rev. Columbus, OH: Greyden Press, 1994.

49. Shear MS, Baitch SP, Shear DB. Sinus tarsi syndrome: the importance of biomechanically based evaluation and treatment. *Arch Phys Med Rehabil* 1993;74:777–781.

50. Greenman PE. *Principles of Manual Medicine*. 2nd Ed. Baltimore, MD: Williams & Wilkins, 1996:411–446.

51. Lemont H, Ammirati KM, Usen N. Plantar fasciitis: a degenerative process (fasciosis) without inflammation. *J Am Podiatr Med Assoc* 2003;93:234–237.

52. D'Maio M, Paine R, Mangine RE, et al. Plantar fasciitis. *Sports Med Rehabil Ser* 1993;16(10):137–142.

53. Furey JG. Plantar fasciitis. The painful heel syndrome. *J Bone Joint Surg Am* 1975;57:672–673.

54. Travell JG, Simons DG. *Myofascial Pain and Dysfunction: The Trigger Point Manual. The Lower Extremities*. Vol II. Baltimore, MD: Williams & Wilkins, 1992:429–459.

55. Kibler WB, Goldberg C, Chandler TJ. Functional biomechanical deficits in running athletes with plantar fasciitis. *Am J Sports Med* 1991;19:66–71.

56. Dahle LK, Mueller MJ, Delitto A, et al. Visual assessment of foot type and relationship of foot type to lower extremity injury. *J Orthop Sports Phys Ther* 1991;14(2):70–74.

57. Razeghi M, Batt E. Foot type classification: a critical review of current methods. *Gait Posture* 2002;15:282–291.

58. Kennedy JG, Knowles B, Dolan M, et al. Foot and ankle injuries in the adolescent runner. *Curr Opin Pediatr* 2005;17:34–42.

59. Travell JG, Simons DG. *Myofascial Pain and Dysfunction: The Trigger Point Manual. The Lower Extremities*. Vol II. Baltimore, MD: Williams & Wilkins, 1992.

60. Harris RJ, Beath T. The short first metatarsal, its incidence and clinical significance. *J Bone Joint Surg* 1949;31A:553–565.

61. Simons DG, Travell JG, Simons LS. *Travell and Simons Myofascial Pain and Dysfunction: The Trigger Point Manual. Volume 1, Upper Half of Body*. Baltimore, MD: Williams & Wilkins, 1999:178–235.

62. Travell JG, Simons DG. *Myofascial Pain and Dysfunction: The Trigger Point Manual. The Lower Extremities*. Vol II. Baltimore, MD: Williams & Wilkins, 1992.

63. Donoff RB. Nerve regeneration: basic and applied aspects. *Crit Rev Oral Biol Med* 1995;6(1):18–24.

64. Hackett GS. *Ligament and Tendon Relaxation Treated by Prolotherapy*. 3rd Ed. Springfield, IL: Charles C Thomas, 1958.

65. Travell JG, Simons DG. *Myofascial Pain and Dysfunction: The Trigger Point Manual. The Lower Extremities*. Vol II. Baltimore, MD: Williams & Wilkins, 1992:28–88.

66. Travell JG, Simons DG. *Myofascial Pain and Dysfunction: The Trigger Point Manual. The Lower Extremities*. Vol II. Baltimore, MD: Williams & Wilkins, 1992:23–27.

67. Walsh PC, ed. *Campbell's Urology*. 7th Ed. Philadelphia, PA: WB Saunders, 1998:2698.

68. Kuchera ML, Kuchera WA. *Osteopathic Considerations in Systemic Dysfunction*. 2nd Ed. Rev. Columbus, OH: Greyden Press. 1994.

69. Kuchera ML, Kuchera WA. *Osteopathic Considerations in Systemic Dysfunction*. 2nd Ed. Rev. Columbus, OH: Greyden Press, 1994:159–167.

70. Janda V. Muscle weakness and inhibition (pseudoparesis) in back pain syndromes. In: Grieve GP, ed. *Modern Medicine Therapy of the Vertebral Column*. Edinburgh, Scotland: Churchill-Livingstone, 1986:197–200.

71. Kuchera ML. Treatment of gravitational strain pathology. In: Vleeming A, Mooney V, Dorman T, et al, eds. *Movement, Stability, and Low Back Pain: The Essential Role of the Pelvis*. New York, NY: Churchill-Livingstone, 1997:477–499.

72. Travell JG, Simons DG. *Myofascial Pain and Dysfunction: The Trigger Point Manual. The Lower Extremities*. Vol II. Baltimore, MD: Williams & Wilkins, 1992:186–214.

73. Basmajian JV. *Grant's Method of Anatomy*. 9th Ed. Baltimore, MD: Williams & Wilkins, 1975:327–328.

74. Travell JG, Simons DG. *Myofascial Pain and Dysfunction: The Trigger Point Manual. The Lower Extremities*. Vol II. Baltimore, MD: Williams & Wilkins, 1992:248–288.

75. Steiner C, Staubs C, Ganon M, et al. Piriformis syndrome pathogenesis, diagnosis, and treatment. *J Am Osteopath Assoc* 1987;87(4):318–323.

76. Travell JG, Simons DG. *Myofascial Pain and Dysfunction: The Trigger Point Manual. The Lower Extremities*. Vol II. Baltimore, MD: Williams & Wilkins, 1992:355–369.

77. Travell JG, Simons DG. *Myofascial Pain and Dysfunction: The Trigger Point Manual. The Lower Extremities*. Vol II. Baltimore, MD: Williams & Wilkins, 1992.

78. Kuchera ML: Chapter 4. Osteopathic considerations in neurology; In: Oken BS, ed. *Complementary Therapies in Neurology: An Evidence-Base Approach*. London: Parthenon Publishing, 2004:49–90.

79. Wheeless CR, ed. *Wheeless' Textbook of Orthopaedics*. Available at: http://www.wheelessonline.com/ortho/medial_meniscus. Retrieved December 2009.

80. AJ Hoyt Masters Ref or most recent ref when published.

81. Kuchera ML, Kuchera WA. *Osteopathic Considerations in Systemic Dysfunction*. 2nd Ed. Rev. Columbus, OH: Greyden Press, 1994; for contraindication to Dalrymple.

82. Travell JG, Simons DG. *Myofascial Pain and Dysfunction: The Trigger Point Manual. The Lower Extremities*. Vol II. Baltimore, MD: Williams & Wilkins, 1992:28–88.

83. Hackett GS. *Ligament and Tendon Relaxation Treated by Prolotherapy*. 3rd Ed. Springfield, IL: Charles C Thomas, 1958.

84. Brody DM. Running injuries. *CIBA Clin Symp* 1980;32(4):25.

85. Travell JG, Simons DG. *Myofascial Pain and Dysfunction: The Trigger Point Manual. The Lower Extremities*. Vol II. Baltimore, MD: Williams & Wilkins; 1992.

86. Travell JG, Simons DG. *Myofascial Pain and Dysfunction: The Trigger Point Manual. The Lower Extremities*. Vol II. Baltimore, MD: Williams & Wilkins, 1992.

87. Schamberger W. *The Malalignment Syndrome: Implications for Medicine and Sport*. China: Churchill Livingstone, 2002.

88. Kuchera WA, Kuchera ML. *Osteopathic Principles in Practice*. 2nd Ed. Rev. Columbus, OH: Greyden Press, 1994.

89. Kiblcr WB. Coiegio norteamericano de medieina deportiva: manual A.C.S.M. dc medieina depotiiva. Isi ed. Barcelona: Editorial l'aidotribo, 1998.

90. Kuchera WA, Kuchera ML. *Osteopathic Principles in Practice*. 2nd Ed. Rev. Columbus, OH: Greyden Press, 1994.

91. de Noronha M. Refshauge KM. Herbert RD. et al. Do voluntary strength, proprioception, range of motion, or postural sway predict occurrence of lateral ankle sprain? [Review]. *Br J Sports Med* 2006;40(10):824–828; discussion 828.

92. Travell JG, Simons DG. *Myofascial Pain and Dysfunction: The Trigger Point Manual. The Lower Extremities*. Vol II. Baltimore, MD: Williams & Wilkins, 1992; and ankle strategy ref.

93. Eisenhardt AW, Gaeta TJ, Yens DP. Osteopathic manipulative treatment in the emergency department for patients with acute ankle injuries. *J Am Osteopath Assoc* 2004;103:417–421.

94. Blood SD. Treatment of the sprained ankle. *J Am Osteopath Assoc* 1980;79:680–692.

95. Eisenhardt AW, Gaeta TJ, Yens DP. Osteopathic manipulative treatment in the emergency department for patients with acute ankle injuries. *J Am Osteopath Assoc* 2004;103:417–421.

96. Pellow JE, Brantingham JW. The efficacy of adjusting the ankle in the treatment of subacute and chronic grade I and grade II ankle inversion sprains. *J Manipulative Physiol Ther* 2001;24:17–24.

97. Lopez-Rodriguez S. Fernandez de-Las-Penas C. Alburquerque-Sendin F. Rodriguez-Blanco C. Palomeque-del-Cerro L. Immediate effects of manipulation of the talocrural joint on stabilometry and baropodometry in patients with ankle sprain [Clinical Trial. Journal Article]. *J Manipulative Physiol Ther* 2007;30(3):186–92.

98. Bleakley CM, McDonough SM, MacAuley DC. Some conservative strategies are effective when added to controlled mobilisation with external support after acute ankle sprain: a systematic review [Review] [75 refs] [Journal Article. Review]. *Aust J Physiother* 2008;54(1):7–20.

99. Seffinger MA, Hruby RJ, Kuchera WA. *Evidence-Based Manual Medicine: A Problem-Oriented Approach*. Philadelphia, PA: Saunders, 2007: 291–311.

100. Higgins R. The ankle joint. In: Hutson M, Ellis R, eds. *Textbook of Musculoskeletal Medicine*. Oxford, UK: Oxford University Press, 2006: 331–337.

101. Seffinger MA, Hruby RJ, Kuchera WA. *Evidence-Based Manual Medicine: A Problem-Oriented Approach*. Philadelphia, PA: Saunders, 2007: 291–311.

Upper Extremities

KURT P. HEINKING

INTRODUCTION

The upper extremities are vital to performing the activities of daily living. Even minor injuries may produce disabilities that significantly affect overall function. Effective diagnosis and treatment necessitates a thorough understanding of the structure and function of this important region.

FUNCTIONAL ANATOMY

Skeletal and Arthrodial Structures

Functionally, the upper extremity can be divided into the (2):

- Acromioclavicular joint (A-C joint)
- Sternoclavicular joint
- Scapulothoracic joint
- Glenohumeral joint
- Elbow (ulnohumeral joint)
- Wrist (radiocarpal joint)
- Intercarpal, carpometacarpal, metacarpophalangeal (MP), and interphalangeal (IP) joints

Motion restrictions in one joint will require compensatory movement in the other joints. Painful joints can be restricted in their motion or have excessive motion beyond their usual functional requirement. Excessive motion or inflammation of a joint will cause the surrounding muscles to contract in an attempt to stabilize or protect the joint.

Scapulothoracic Joint

The scapulothoracic joint is formed by the articulation of the anterior surface of the scapula with the posterior thorax. It is a pseudoarticulation. The position of the scapula is controlled by muscular forces. The scapula is attached to the spine and ribs by the rhomboids, trapezius, serratus anterior, pectoralis minor, and levator scapulae. Tension in these muscles controls the position of the scapula. The levator scapulae and trapezius provide postural support, while the middle trapezius and rhomboids retract the scapulae. The serratus anterior protracts the scapulae, and when contacting with the upper trapezius, these muscles will cause upward rotation and elevation (27). The position and motion of the scapula controls the glenohumeral joint. Abnormal position of the ribs, such as that seen in scoliosis, will affect the positional alignment of the scapula, bringing it more into a protracted and elevated position on the side of the convexity of the scioliotic curve. Motion of the shoulder on the convex side of the scoliotic curve will be different than on the concave side. Somatic dysfunction of a single rib, or a group of ribs, will affect the smooth gliding motion of the scapula over the posterior rib age. The rotator cuff muscles attach the humeral head to the scapula. If the position of the scapula is abnormal, these muscles are required to function differently, based on their length/tension relationships. The various motions of the scapula are:

- Elevation (upper trapezius and levator scapula)
- Depression (lower trapezius, lower rhomboids)
- Protraction (serratus anterior)
- Retraction (rhomboids and middle trapezius)
- Rotation about a transverse axis

A-C Joint

The A-C joint is formed by the articulation of the lateral end of the clavicle with the acromion process of the scapula. The A-C joint is a planar joint with a crescent-shaped rudimentary incomplete meniscus (22). The acromion has a variable shape and slope, and forms the roof of the coracoacromial arch (26). The coracoacromial ligament attaches from the outer portion of the coracoid process to the undersurface of the acromion and makes up the anterior portion of the coracoacromial arch (26). Under the coracoacromial arch is the subacromial bursa and rotator cuff tendons. This is the region in which extrinsic or outlet impingement of the rotator cuff occurs. The A-C joint depends on its ligamentous attachments for stability; these are the A-C and coracoclavicular ligaments. The strongest ligament between the clavicle and scapula is the coracoclavicular ligament. It has two portions. The coronoid portion of this ligament prevents anterior rotation of the distal clavicle; the trapezoid portion resists posterior rotation of the distal clavicle. Although a planar joint, functionally, this joint acts similar to a ball and socket, providing anteroposterior, superoinferior, and rotational motion. A small, yet important, amount of clavicular motion occurs with shoulder movement; there is controversy over the amount of motion occurring at this joint. Large amounts of axial motion have been described, as well as rotation axially less than 10 degrees over the arc of shoulder abduction (27).

Sternoclavicular Joint

The sternoclavicular joint is formed by the articulation of the medial end of the clavicle with the manubrium of the sternum. The sternoclavicular joint has a saddle-shaped articular surface. The clavicular notch on the sternum is shallow and small compared to the articular surface of the medial end of the clavicle. Fortunately, this is a complex synovial joint that contains a cartilaginous meniscus. This provides needed stability. The interclavicular ligament resists superior displacement of the sternal end of the clavicle. The costoclavicular ligament attaching to the first costal cartilage acts as a fulcrum and limits upward movement of the lateral end of the clavicle (22). As the clavicle abducts, this ligament helps produce a downward glide to the sternal end of the clavicle. The subclavius muscle depresses and pulls the medial end of the first rib forward when the lateral end of the clavicle is elevated.

Glenohumeral Joint

The glenohumeral joint is formed by the articulation of the head of the humerus with the glenoid fossa of the scapula. The humeral head is large, smooth, slightly elliptical, and covered in articular cartilage. The glenoid is small, concave, and has a cartilaginous lip (labrum) that helps locate the humeral head into the glenoid. The proximal humerus is separated anatomically into four parts: the articular surface, the lesser tuberosity, the greater tuberosity, and the diaphyseal humeral shaft (27). The humeral head is angulated medially 45 degrees to the long axis and retroverted 30 degrees. The joint has significant mobility, but lacks stability due to its design. The joint undergoes spinning, sliding, and rolling. The joint is synovial and enclosed by a strong ligamentous capsule. The joint capsule has a superior, middle, and inferior glenohumeral ligament complex. The capsule is weak anteriorly and inferiorly (inferior glenohumeral ligament complex), allowing for instability or dislocation to commonly occur in that direction. The posterior capsule is commonly tight, which causes anterior translation and elevation of the humeral head. This situation can cause secondary impingement of the rotator cuff (26). The fibrocartilagenous labrum surrounds the periphery of the glenoid. The labrum acts as an attachment site for the capsuloligamentous structures, and as a "cup" to increase the surface area of the glenoid, as well as providing a negative intracapsular pressure that helps to center (or capture) the humeral head.

Ulnohumeral Joint

The ulnohumeral joint is the true elbow joint (6). The hinge-like elbow joint allows for motion around a transverse axis. It has a ligamentous capsule that is thickened on the medial and lateral sides, yet is weak anteriorly and posteriorly. For anterior and posterior stability, muscles such as the biceps brachii and triceps serve the function as ligaments.

The trochlear notch of the ulna is closely fitted to the trochlea of the humerus. The surfaces are lined with articular cartilage and fit together in a spiraled fashion. This is so that as the elbow is extended, the hand is held away from the body (carrying angle) and when the elbow is flexed the hand is close to the mouth. The motion occurs without requiring any rotation of the humerus at the shoulder. The minor motions (such as abduction/adduction) are allowed by the relative looseness of the fit of the trochlea in the trochlear notch, and the presence of articular cartilage (22).

Proximal Radioulnar Joint

The head of the radius at the proximal end of the radial bone near the elbow is not a part of the elbow joint. The pivotal motion for pronation and supination of the forearm is provided by the proximal radioulnar joint. The radial head rotates on the capitellum during pronation and supination. During elbow extension, the radial head glides posteriorly on the capitellum. During elbow flexion, the radial head glides anteriorly on the capitellum (22).

The Wrist (Radiocarpal) Joint

The wrist is formed by the junction of the ulna, radius, and the carpal bones. The joint is considered an ellipsoidal synovial articulation. The true wrist joint is the radiocarpal joint, formed by the distal end of the radius and the three proximal carpal bones: the scaphoid, lunate, and the triquetral. The convexity of the scaphoid, lunate, and the triquetral fit into the concavity of the radius and the articular disc. The disc separates the distal radioulnar joint from the wrist joint cavity and attaches the ulna to the radius. The capsular ligaments are sufficiently loose to allow some minor movements of the carpal bones (22). Possible motions include flexion, extension, abduction, and adduction, as well as supination and pronation of the hand and forearm. Flexion and adduction of the wrist are typically freer.

Table 43.1 outlines the major motions of the shoulder, elbow, wrist, and MP joints.

THE HAND

Intercarpal Joints

The scaphoid, lunate, and the triquetral articulate with the greater and lesser multiangular bones, the capitate and hamate. Motion between these rows of bones is more free in flexion. If bony point tenderness is present in the face of hand trauma, always x-ray the hand to make sure a scaphoid fracture is not present.

Carpometacarpal Joints

The first carpometacarpal articulation is cavoconvex, and classified as a saddle-shaped joint. It is freely movable in two planes and rarely subject to dysfunction. The second to fifth carpometacarpal joints are gliding joints. The fifth is the most mobile, then the fourth. The second and third are fairly restricted in motion.

TABLE 43.1

Major Motions of the Shoulder, Elbow, Wrist, and MP Joints

Glenohumeral Joint	Elbow	Wrist	Metacarpophalangeal
Abduction 180 degrees	Flexion 135 degrees	Supination 90 degrees	Flexion 90 degrees
Adduction 45 degrees	Extension 0–5 degrees	Pronation 90 degrees	Extension 30–45 degrees
Flexion 90 degrees		Flexion 80 degrees	
Extension 45 degrees		Extension 70 degrees	
Internal rotation 55 degrees		Ulnar deviation 30 degrees	
External rotation 40–45 degrees		Radial deviation 20 degrees	

Source: From Hoppenfeld S. *Physical Examination of the Spine and Extremities.* New York, NY: Appleton-Century-Crofts, 1976, with permission.

TABLE 43.2

Major Motions of the Proximal and Distal IP Joints

Proximal IP Joint	Distal IP Joint
Flexion 100 degrees	Flexion 90 degrees
Extension 0 degrees	Extension 20 degrees

Source: From Hoppenfeld S. *Physical Examination of the Spine and Extremities.* New York, NY: Appleton-Century-Crofts, 1976, with permission.

TABLE 43.3

Major Motions of the Joints of the Thumb

Thumb	Thumb MP Joint	Thumb IP Joint
Palmar abduction 70 degrees	Flexion 50 degrees	Flexion 90 degrees
Palmar adduction 0 degrees	Extension 0 degrees	Extension 90 degrees

MP Joints

These joints allow for more mobility than the carpometacarpal joints. These joints are commonly affected by rheumatoid and osteoarthritis, and can become enlarged and stiff. Flexion, extension, abduction, and adduction occur, as well as a slight amount of rotation. There is a joint capsule surrounding each joint as well as a synovial membrane.

IP Joints

The proximal IP joints are called the "PIP joints," the distal IP joints are called the "DIP joints." The DIP joints can become enlarged with firm nodules (Herberden nodes) on either side of the dorsal midline. These are usually painless and indicate osteoarthritis. The PIP joints and metacarpal phalangeal joints are usually involved in rheumatoid arthritis and demonstrate Haygarth nodes. The joint may be thickened, inflamed, and tender, with a fusiform appearance. In males, the ring finger is typically longer than the index finger, in females, the opposite holds true.

Table 43.2 outlines the major motions of the proximal and distal IP joints, and Table 43.3 includes the major motions of the joints of the thumb.

Muscles

Muscles generally act in groups to produce specific motions. Detailed assessment of the upper extremity necessitates an understanding of these groups and their innervations (2). Tables 43.4 through 43.7 present the muscles and nerves of the following joints (2):

> Glenohumeral joint (Table 43.4)
> Scapulothoracic joint (Table 43.5)
> Elbow (Table 43.6)
> Wrist (Table 43.7)

The rotator cuff muscles are critical to maintaining stability of the glenohumeral joint, as well as providing precision movements and propulsion in throwing or swinging motions. The cuff is formed by the confluent tendon of the supraspinatus, infraspinatus, teres minor, and subscapularis. The supraspinatus, infraspinatus, and teres minor insert on the greater tuberosity. The subscapularis inserts on the lesser tuberosity of the humerus. The supraspinatus has been thought to initiate abduction; however, it is currently felt that it is more of a glenohumeral joint stabilizer. Because of its angle of insertion (70 degrees from the glenoid), the supraspinatus acts as a fulcrum, applying a compressive force to hold the humeral head in the glenoid, as the synergistic action with the deltoid causes abduction. The supraspinatus is active during the entire arc of abduction; paralysis of the suprascapular nerve causes a 50% reduction in abduction torque (27). Without a properly functioning supraspinatus, impingement of the cuff between the humeral head and undersurface of the acromion occurs.

The teres minor and infraspinatus depress, extend, and externally rotate the humerus. The infraspinatus is more active with the arm at the side, the teres minor is more active with the shoulder in 90 degrees of elevation. The subscapularis internally rotates, flexes, and depresses the humeral head. The tendinous insertion is

TABLE 43.4

Muscles and Nerves of the Glenohumeral Joint and Shoulder

Primary Flexors	Deltoid (Anterior Portion) Muscle	Axillary Nerve	C5
	Coracobrachialis muscle	Musculocutaneous nerve	C5-6
Secondary flexors	Pectoralis major muscle (clavicular head)		
	Biceps		
Primary abductors	Deltoid (midportion) muscle	Axillary nerve	C5-6
	Supraspinatus muscle	Suprascapular nerve	C5-6
Secondary abductors	Deltoid muscle (anterior, posterior)		
	Serratus anterior muscle via scapula		
Primary adductors	Pectoralis major muscle	Anterior thoracic nerve (medial, lateral)	C5-T1
	Latissimus dorsi muscle		
Secondary adductors	Teres minor muscle		
	Anterior deltoid muscle		
Primary extensors	Latissimus dorsi muscle	Thoracodorsal nerve	C6-8
	Teres major muscle	Lower subscapular nerve	C5-6
	Deltoid (posterior portion)	Axillary nerve	C5-6
Secondary extensors	Teres minor muscle		
	Triceps (long head) muscle		
Primary external rotators	Infraspinatus	Suprascapular nerve	C5-6
	Teres minor	Axillary branch	C5
Secondary external rotators	Deltoid muscle (posterior portion)		
Primary internal rotators	Subscapularis muscle	Subscapular nerves (upper and lower portion)	C5-6
	Pectoralis major muscle	Anterior thoracic nerves (medial and lateral)	C5-T1
	Latissimus dorsi muscle		
	Teres minor muscle		
Secondary internal rotators	Deltoid muscle (anterior portion)		

TABLE 43.5

Muscles and Nerves of the Scapulothoracic Joint

Primary Elevators	Trapezius Muscle	Accessory Nerve	CN XI
	Levator scapulae muscle	Dorsal scapular nerve C5 (plus)	C3-4, C5
Secondary elevators	Rhomboid major muscle		
	Rhomboid minor muscle		
Primary protraction	Serratus anterior muscle	Long thoracic nerve	C5-7
Primary retraction	Rhomboid major muscle	Dorsal scapular nerve	C5
	Rhomboid minor muscle	Dorsal scapular nerve	C5
Secondary retraction	Trapezius muscle		

continuous with the anterior capsule, helping to limit anterior instability. During throwing and eccentric activity, the subscapularis and infraspinatus are the two most important stabilizing forces of the shoulder (26,27).

The long head of the biceps is intimately associated with the rotator cuff and has been considered the "fifth tendon" of the rotator cuff (26). The biceps tendon is intra-articular, yet extrasynovial, and passes deep to the "rotator interval" a space between the supraspinatus and subscapularis tendon insertions. The coracohumeral ligament and the superior glenohumeral ligament complex surround the biceps tendon and act as a pulley as it enters the intertubercular groove. The long head of the biceps

TABLE 43.6

Muscles and Nerves of the Elbow Joint

Primary flexors	Brachialis muscle nerve	Musculocutaneous	C5-6
	Biceps muscle nerve	Musculocutaneous	C5-6
Secondary flexors	Brachioradialis muscle		C6
	Supinator muscle		
Primary extensor	Triceps muscle	Radial nerve	C7
Secondary extensor	Anconeus muscle		

TABLE 43.7

Muscles and Nerves of the Wrist

Primary flexors	Flexor carpi radialis m.	Median n.	
	Flexor carpi ulnaris m.	Ulnar n.	
Primary extensors	Extensor carpi radialis longus m.	Radial n.	C6(7)
	Extensor carpi radialis brevis m.	Radial n.	
	Extensor carpi ulnaris m.	Radial n.	
Primary supinators	Biceps m.		
	Supinator m.	Radial n.	
Secondary supinator	Brachioradialis m.		
Primary pronators	Pronator teres m.	Median n.	C6
	Pronator quadratus m.	Median n. (ant. interosseous branch)	
Secondary pronator	Flexor carpi radialis m.		

tendon then travels in the intertubercular sulcus, which has a variable shape and slope. Because of differences in the shape and slope of this groove, the tendon can translate back and forth causing degenerative changes in the tendon. The biceps function is controversial as some believe it is a humeral head depressor; others feel it is a passive player in most shoulder motions (26).

The teres major muscle is not considered a rotator cuff muscle. It is sometimes used as a donor muscle in shoulder surgeries. The teres major acts in synergy with the latissimus dorsi muscle, to cause humeral extension, internal rotation, and adduction (27).

Arterial Supply

The left subclavian artery arises from the posterior part of the aortic arch. It passes posterior to the left sternoclavicular joint. The right subclavian artery arises from the brachiocephalic trunk (3). The subclavian arteries pass over the top of the first rib between the anterior and middle scalene muscles. This is an area of compression in thoracic outlet syndrome. The subclavian artery becomes the axillary artery at the lateral border of the first rib. The axillary artery passes posterior to the pectoralis minor muscle and becomes the brachial artery at the inferior border of the teres major muscle. Branches from the axillary and brachial arteries supply the structures of the shoulder, arm, forearm, and hand. Somatic dysfunction of the following structures may affect arterial supply:

- Anterior and middle scalenes
- Upper thoracic vertebrae
- Upper ribs
- Clavicles
- Fascia of the upper extremity

The vascular supply of the rotator cuff has been extensively studied. There is a "critical zone" of anastamotic blood supply to the rotator cuff muscles; in this critical zone, it is hypothesized that rotator cuff tears begin. One such area is in the supraspinatus tendon immediately proximal to its insertion of the greater tuberosity of the humerus (26).

Venous Supply

The axillary vein lies on the medial side of the axillary artery. The axillary vein receives tributaries that correspond to the branches of the axillary artery and receives venae comitantes of the brachial artery. It ends at the lateral border of the first rib, where it becomes the subclavian vein (3). The subclavian vein passes over the first rib anterior to the anterior scalene muscle (3). The subclavian vein unites with the internal jugular vein to become the brachiocephalic vein (3). The left brachiocephalic vein passes posterior to the left sternoclavicular joint and crosses the midline. The right brachiocephalic vein passes posterior to the right sternoclavicular joint. The right brachiocephalic vein joins the left brachiocephalic vein to form the superior vena cava (3). Dysfunction in the upper thoracic vertebrae (causing increased sympathetic tone to the upper extremities), upper ribs, clavicles, and fascia of the upper extremities may impair venous return. Because the vein passes anterior to the scalene muscles, scalene tension does not create venous distention of the upper extremity. A thrombosis in the subclavian vein can cause swelling in the breast and upper extremity due to venous obstruction.

Lymphatic Drainage

The major lymph nodes of the upper extremities are found in the fibrofatty connective tissue of the axilla. They are arranged in five groups, four of which lie inferior to the pectoralis minor tendon and one which lies superior to it (Fig. 43.1). These groups are:

- Pectoral
- Lateral
- Subscapular
- Central
- Apical

The pectoral group of axillary lymph nodes lies along the medial wall of the axilla. This group receives lymph mainly from the anterior thoracic wall and breast. The efferent vessels from these nodes pass to the central and apical groups of axillary lymph nodes (3).

The lateral group of lymph nodes lies along the lateral wall of the axilla. This group receives lymph from most of the upper limb.

The subscapular group of axillary lymph nodes is located along the posterior aspect of the thoracic wall and scapular region. Efferent vessels pass from here to the central group of axillary lymph nodes.

The central group of axillary lymph nodes is situated deep to the pectoralis minor near the base of the axilla. This group receives lymph from the other axillary lymph nodes. Efferent vessels pass lymph to the apical lymph nodes.

The apical group of axillary lymph nodes is situated in the apex of the axilla. This group receives lymph from the central lymph nodes. The efferent vessels from this group unite to form the subclavian lymphatic trunk. The right subclavian lymphatic trunk drains into the right lymphatic duct. The left subclavian lymphatic trunk drains into the thoracic duct. Somatic dysfunction affecting the venous system may also affect lymphatic drainage, thereby producing congestion in the upper extremity. Fascial restriction of the thoracic inlet and pectoral fascia can also cause lymphatic stasis of the upper extremity.

Sympathetics

The sympathetic innervation to the upper extremities arises from the upper thoracic spinal cord. The sympathetic ganglia lie anterior to the rib head, in the fascia common to both structures. Dysfunction in the upper thoracic spine and ribs may increase sympathetic tone to the upper extremity and produce altered motion, nerve dysfunction, and lymphatic and venous congestion (28). Increased sympathetic tone is accompanied by palpatory findings in the upper thoracic/rib area and increased sensitivity to painful stimulus. It also prevents arterial blood from getting to the structures of the arm and reduces the amount of lymphatic fluid returning from the arm via the lymphatic vessels. The cause of these musculoskeletal findings may be viscerosomatic; they may be primary somatic in the area, or they may be reflex from the cervical spine. Nociceptive afferents from the cervical spine travel in the sympathetic chain and synapse in the intermediolateral cell columns of the upper thoracic cord. This produces an irritable focus in the cord, with resulting somatic and sympathetic hyperactivity (28).

Brachial Plexus

Nerve roots C5-8 and T1 form the brachial plexus. These nerve roots pass through the intervertebral foramen of the cervical vertebrae and pass between the anterior and the middle scalene muscles (3). The roots unite to form successive trunks, divisions, cords, and branches. The nerve trunks extend from the scalene triangle (formed by the anterior and middle scalenes and the clavicle) to the clavicle. Nerve divisions extend from a position posterior to the clavicle to the axilla. Nerve cords are found in the axilla. Nerve cords divide into branches that innervate various structures in the upper extremity. The neurovascular bundle of the arm contains the subclavian artery, subclavian vein, brachial plexus, and the sympathetic nerve plexus.

Peripheral Nerves and Nerve Entrapment

The three main peripheral nerves of the upper extremity include the median nerve, the ulnar nerve, and the radial nerve. Understanding the innervation of each and site of potential compression is important.

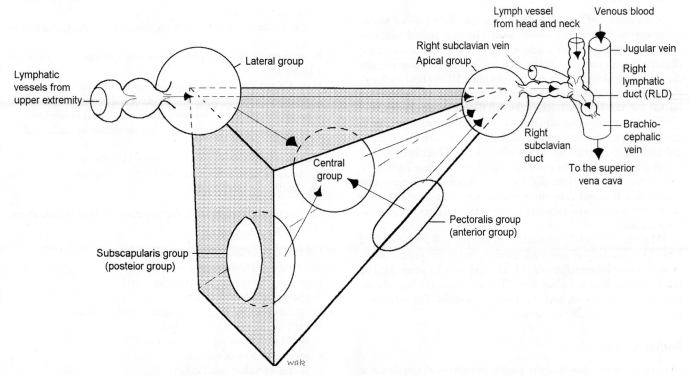

Figure 43-1 Lymphatic drainage of upper extremity. (Illustration by W.A. Kuchera.)

Median Nerve

The most proximal level of compression of the median nerve may produce the pronator syndrome, which is a compression of the median nerve as it passes through the pronator teres muscle, or under the ligament of Struthers (29). It is associated with pain in the proximal volar forearm and sensory signs and symptoms in the radial 3½ digits of the hand. Symptoms are generally aggravated by flexion of the elbow against resistance. Sensory symptoms and signs of the pronator syndrome typically mimic C6 and C7 radiculopathy. The pronator syndrome may affect the function of the median nerve innervated muscles in the C6 and C7 distribution (29).

The median nerve has a motor branch called the anterior interosseous nerve. In anterior interosseous syndrome, there are no sensory abnormalities. Pain in the proximal forearm is typically aggravated by exercise and abates with rest. Motor abnormalities are manifested as weakness and are referred to those muscles innervated by this nerve (flexor pollicis longus, pronator quadratus, and flexor digitorum profundus of the index finger). This syndrome may mimic a C8 radiculopathy because this is the root through which they are all innervated (29).

The next region of compression for the median nerve is at the carpal tunnel at the wrist. Compression of the median nerve in the carpal tunnel (carpal tunnel syndrome) typically causes sensory symptoms such as night pain, paresthesias, and numbness in the hand in the radial 3½ digits. Symptoms may be referred proximally from the hand toward the forearm and even the elbow and may be reproduced or elicited by Phalen maneuver or Tinel sign. Thenar muscle weakness and atrophy represent advanced disease. Sensory symptoms may mimic C6 and C7 radiculopathy, but no C6 or C7 muscle demonstrates abnormalities because they are all innervated proximal to the carpal canal. Thenar motor weakness may mimic T1 radiculopathy because of abnormalities of the opponens pollicis and the abductor pollicis brevis; however, other T1-innervated muscles are normal (29).

Ulnar Nerve

The ulna nerve can become entrapped at the elbow (cubital tunnel syndrome) or at the wrist (Guyon canal). The most typical symptom of cubital tunnel syndrome is aching pain on the medial aspect of the elbow, although radiation of the pain and paresthesia may migrate distally on the ulnar forearm and into the ulnar 1½ digits of the hand. Symptoms may be elicited by percussion of the nerve behind the medial epicondyle or by acute, prolonged flexion of the elbow (29).

The ulnar nerve may also be compressed at the wrist in Guyon canal. Compression at this level usually affects both the superficial and the deep branches of the ulnar nerve. Therefore, sensory symptoms are referred to the volar aspect of the ulnar 1½ fingers. The dorsal aspect of these digits remains unaffected because that area of skin is supplied by the dorsal sensory branch of the ulnar nerve, which originates proximal to the wrist and does not traverse Guyon canal.

The deep branch is essentially all motor, and the superficial branch is essentially all sensory. Therefore, motor symptoms, weakness, and atrophy are referrable only to those muscles innervated by the deep branch of the ulnar nerve. These include the hypothenar muscles, the interossei, and the abductor pollicis. The syndrome may mimic T1 and C8 radiculopathy (29).

Radial Nerve

The radial nerve has a deep motor branch that can become compressed in the radial tunnel (posterior interosseous syndrome).

The all-motor deep branch, the posterior interosseous nerve, supplies the brachioradialis, extensor carpi radialis longus and brevis, and supinator muscles, and then splits into a superficial sensory branch that does not enter the radial tunnel. Because only the motor branch is compressed, sensory symptoms are rare, although aching over the site of compression is felt and may be elicited by full extension of the elbow with the which may be caused by an extra cervical rib or by tightened scalene muscles. Compression may occur at the thoracic outlet where the artery passes between the chest and the upper extremity (29).

Osteopathic diagnosis largely involves the assessment of both quality and quantity of motion. General ranges of motion permit effective screening of the skeletal and arthrodial components of this region. Somatic dysfunction typically involves restriction and the end of a range of motion. It is most likely to be found in the minor motion(s) of each joint. Orthopedic problems associated with disruption of joint stabilizers commonly involve laxity and instability at the end of a range of motion. The most time-effective, yet thorough examination involves screening ranges of motion with careful attention to end-motion palpatory finding.

DIAGNOSIS

History

The clinician must determine the exact nature of the chief complaint, its duration, location, severity, and associated symptoms. The presenting complaint may be pain; however, it may also be weakness, swelling, or stiffness. Obtain as much information as possible in a time-efficient manner. Experienced clinicians continue to pursue historical questions while simultaneously examining the patient.

The following questions will assist the clinician in obtaining a thorough history:

- What is the complaint? For example: (numbness, pain, stiffness, weakness, swelling, coolness/color change) Is there more than one in different areas?
- If pain is the complaint: location, duration, severity, and radiation
- If stiffness is the complaint: morning stiffness greater than 1 hour?
- If swelling is the complaint: unilateral or bilateral?
- If weakness is the complaint: diffuse or a specific muscle?
- If restricted motion is the complaint: articular or muscular?
- If neuralgia is the complaint: what dermatome? unilateral or bilateral?
- If a rash is the complaint: characterize/describe it.
- If coolness or a color change is the complaint: history of Raynaud?

No matter what the complaint, the clinician needs to inquire about the following:

- Location, duration, severity, radiation
- Mechanism of intermittent or constant?
- Improving, worsening, staying the same?
- Aggravating/alleviating factors?
- What has been done so far (diagnosis and treatment)?
- What was the mechanism of injury?
  - Blunt trauma or repetitive overuse?
  - revious history of trauma?
  - Is this a work-related injury?
  - What are the functional limitations (what they can or can't do)?

When is arm pain something more? Upper extremity discomfort cannot always be attributed to an orthopedic condition or somatic dysfunction in this area. A good clinician must determine whether the discomfort is primarily caused by dysfunction in the extremity or referred from another area.

If the cause lies in the upper extremity itself, there is generally restricted motion. Pain is usually localized to specific dermatomes and may be described as acute, sharp, and severe. Discomfort is usually improved by rest, is frequently reproduced by motion, and may lead to the perception of strength loss.

If the discomfort is referred from another area (e.g., the lungs, diaphragm, stomach, intestines, heart, or cervical spine), passive motion does not appear to be restricted. Pain is diffuse, poorly localized, and may be described as nagging, achy, or dull. Discomfort is usually worse at night. Discomfort is frequently related to symptoms in other areas (difficulty breathing, chest pain, cough, gastrointestinal upset) and may not be reproduced by motion. Motion is generally good, but decreased strength or muscle atrophy is possible (e.g., disc herniation).

Pain is not the only presenting complaint. The patient may relate stiffness, swelling, and weakness as well. Specific points in the history may indicate the diagnosis. For example, pain radiating into the deltoid insertion at night, and an inability to lie on the involved shoulder correlates with a rotator cuff tear. Pain or numbness radiating into the hand when lying down, relieved with pulling the arm overhead may indicate cervical radiculopathy.

Physical Examination

The physical examination of the upper extremities also includes an examination of the cervical spine, the thoracic spine and rib cage, the heart, the lungs, the nervous system, the skin, and the abdomen. A rheumatologic and orthopedic examination is also an important part of the exam of the upper extremities. The examination for somatic dysfunction is integrated with all other parts of the physical exam.

Observation

Observation begins the moment the patient walks into the room. Observe overall posture and motion. Is there any abnormality? Observe the patient in the standing position. Look at the height of the shoulders. A low shoulder may be the result of a short leg or a lateral curve. Look at the spine from the side. Is the thoracic kyphotic curve normal, increased, or decreased? A local area of thoracic spine flattening ("pothole") may indicate the presence of an extended somatic dysfunction. Begin at the shoulder and examine the skin of the upper extremity. Are there any scars from prior injuries? A transverse scar on the anterior neck may indicate a cervical fusion. Is there any asymmetry? Areas that appear reddened or have pigment changes may have somatic dysfunction. Observe the various muscle groups bilaterally. Is there evidence of hypertrophy or atrophy? Look for the presence of fasciculation (small tremors) in the muscle. Look to see if the clavicles are symmetric. Did the patient ever fracture his or her clavicle or have a acomioclavicular separation? A visual and palpable deformity is usually present. Look at the hands. Is there deformity of the patient's knuckles or fingers?

Structural Exam

A structural examination is an important part of the evaluation of the patient with an extremity complaint. Postural strain, muscle imbalance, scoliosis, and forward head position can all contribute to or be the etiologic factor in upper extremity complaints. To review the components of the structural exam, review Chapter 34.

Palpation

Palpation for tissue texture change or tenderness should be focused to a few specific areas.

Begin in the upper thoracics. The upper thoracics usually have significant palpatory findings.

Palpate laterally to the scapula near the posterior axillary fold. In this location, muscles such as infraspinatus and teres minor are usually tender. Anteriorly, tissue texture change and tenderness is found over the pectoralis minor, anterior ribs, and biceps tendon. Palpate the neck for scalene hypertonicity and tissue texture change over the lower cervicals. Now, palpate into the deeper tissues. Look for signs of acute or chronic tissue texture change. Remember to compare the right side with the left side and areas located superiorly with areas located inferiorly. Compare muscle groups bilaterally for size and tone. Palpation needs to include not only the cervical and thoracic spine but also the ribs, clavicles, and scapula. All muscles affecting the upper extremity need to be palpated, especially those which the history indicates. Fascia of the thoracic inlet, pectorals, and latissimus dorsi needs to be assessed. The interosseous membrane of the forearm is important to evaluate in situations where repetitive overuse is a consideration.

Pulses

Thorough examination of the upper extremities necessitates an examination of the brachial and radial pulses. The brachial pulse is found on the medial surface of the arm just medial to the biceps tendon. The radial pulse is best palpated over the lateral and ventral side of the wrist. Examine the arterial pulses with the distal pads of the second, third, and fourth fingers. Palpate firmly but not so hard that the artery is occluded. Arterial pulses can be examined for:

- Heart rate and rhythm
- Pulse contour (wave form)
- Amplitude (strength)
- Symmetry

Lack of symmetry between the left and the right extremities suggests impaired circulation. In thoracic outlet syndrome, the clinician may find that the radial pulse diminishes with specific positioning of the arm and neck.

Table 43.8 outlines the standard method for recording amplitude of the pulse.

Reflexes

The three basic reflexes that evaluate the integrity of the nerve supply to the upper extremity are the biceps reflex, the brachioradialis reflex, and the triceps reflex (Table 43.9). Each of these is a deep tendon reflex (lower motor neuron reflex) transmitted to the cord as far as the anterior horn cells and returning to the muscle via the peripheral nerves. Reflexes may be increased in the presence of an upper motor neuron lesion or may be decreased in the presence of a lower motor neuron lesion (bulging disc with radiculopathy).

Biceps Reflex

This reflex primarily tests the integrity of neurologic level C5. Place the patient's arm over your opposite arm so that it rests on your

TABLE 43.8

Deep Tendon Reflexes of the Upper Extremity

Reflex	Biceps	Brachioradialis	Triceps
Stimulus site	Biceps tendon	Brachioradialis tendon or just distal to the musculotendinous junction	Distal triceps tendon above the olecranon process
Typical response	Biceps contraction	Flexion of elbow and/or pronation of forearm	Elbow extension/muscle contraction
Central nervous system correlate	C5-6	C5-6	C7-8

TABLE 43.9

Standard Method for Recording Amplitude of the Pulse

4/4	Bounding
3/4	Full, increased
2/4	Expected
1/4	Diminished, barely palpable
0	Absent, not palpable

TABLE 43.10

Standard Method for Recording Amplitude of a Reflex

0	Absent
1/4	Decreased but present
2/4	Normal
3/4	Brisk with unsustained clonus
4/4	Brisk with sustained clonus

forearm. With your elbow supporting the patient's arm under the elbow's medial side, place your thumb on the tendon of the biceps in the cubital fossa. Instruct the patient to rest the arm on your forearm and relax. Tap your thumbnail with a neurologic hammer. The biceps should jerk slightly. You should be able to see or feel its movement.

Brachioradialis Reflex

This tests neurologic level C6. Support the patient's arm in the same manner used to test the biceps reflex. Tap the brachioradialis tendon at the distal end of the radius with the neurologic hammer.

Triceps Reflex

This reflex tests neurologic level C7. Use the same position as above. Tap the triceps tendon where it crosses the olecranon fossa (2). Remember to use bilateral comparison.

Reflexes may be graded as shown in Table 43.10.

Motor Strength

The strength of various muscle groups can be evaluated by applying force in a manner that loads the muscle as the patient resists. Remember to test the uninjured side first. Table 43.11 shows a standard method of recording motor strength.

Differences in muscle strength may be subtle. Compare the strength of various groups in different positions to get the full clinical picture. There are some simple screening procedures that are useful. For cervical root or brachial plexus problems, perform a grip strength test by asking the patient to squeeze two of your fingers. Another simple test is to ask the patient to squeeze the thumb and

index finger together while you try to pull them apart. If normal strength is present, it is difficult to pull them apart. Although not a test of strength, palpation for flaccidity may reveal muscles that should be tested. Observation, palpation, and measurement (with a tape measure) for muscle atrophy are important in the right clinical situation.

Sensation

This can be tested by light touch, pinprick, or two-point discrimination. Compare both sides and areas located superiorly with areas located inferiorly. Look for areas of either decreased or increased sensation. Sensation around the upper extremity is provided by five different nerve supplies:

1. C5 supplies the lateral arm
2. C6 supplies the lateral forearm
3. C7 supplies the index finger
4. C8 supplies the medial forearm
5. T1 supplies the medial arm

Articular Configuration and Physiologic Motion

The Glenohumeral Joint

The glenohumeral joint has been compared to a beach ball on a seal's nose. It has significant mobility, but little stability. The depth of the glenoid is increased by a cartilaginous cup or labrum. The joint capsule is normally quite lax and loose, particularly anteriorly and inferiorly, providing for excess movement. Joint stability is maintained by the attachment of the rotator cuff muscles (supraspinatus, infraspinatus, teres minor, and subscapularis) to the articular capsule. Movement then occurs in flexion, extension, internal rotation, and external rotation. In the horizontal plane, with the

TABLE 43.11

Standard Method for Recording Motor Strength

5/5	Normal	Complete range of motion against gravity with full resistance
4/5	Good	Complete range of motion against gravity with some resistance
3/5	Fair	Complete range of motion against gravity
2/5	Poor	Complete range of motion with gravity eliminated
1/5	Trace	Evidence of slight contractility; no joint motion
0	Zero	No evidence of contractility

humerus at 90 degrees to the trunk, it is also possible to have flexion, extension, internal rotation, and external rotation (23).

Gross Motion Assessment of the shoulder can involve general screening tests or specific motion tests. Perform active *gross motion testing* first, especially if an injury is present. Having the patient raise the arms overhead and touch the back of the hands together is an excellent screening test. Ability to comb the hair tests for external rotation and abduction. Reaching over the shoulder, as if to touch the opposite scapula (Apley scratch test), tests horizontal abduction. Having the patient reach behind his or her back, as if reaching for the patient's pocketbook, tests internal rotation. Shoulder motions can also be screened by the seven motions of Spencer (5).

A gross passive test of stability of the glenohumeral joint is to stabilize the scapula and translate the head of the humerus anteriorly and posteriorly. Compare both sides. An unstable joint moves too freely; with adhesive capsulitis, there is no motion. Orthopedic testing for laxity of the glenohumeral joint will determine if there is unidirectional or multidirectional laxity. Motion of the entire pectoral girdle can be evaluated without stabilizing the scapula to isolate glenohumeral motion. Additional motions can be tested, such as how freely does the arm move overhead? How freely does the arm reach across the torso? It is important to always compare both glenohumeral joints for asymmetry of position and motion. A summary of screening motions is found in Table 43.12.

Specific Motion Tests

Individual motions can be tested with the patient seated. Testing of the shoulder can be localized to the glenohumeral joint by stabilizing the scapula with one hand as the arm is moved with the other. It is important to hold (stabilize) the acromion so glenohumeral motion is assessed, as contrasted to scapulothoracic motion. Flexion and extension motions are simple to test. For abduction, pay attention to the quality and end feel of motion as well as the actual quantity. Lateral (external) rotation can be tested with the humerus parallel to the torso, moving the patient's hand/wrist laterally. From this position, medial (internal) rotation cannot be effectively tested because the forearm contacts the torso. Abduct the arm to 90 degrees. Lateral rotation involves raising the hand superiorly.

Medial rotation involves lowering the hand (with the humerus remaining in the abducted position).

The Scapulothoracic Joint

In evaluating total shoulder girdle motion, observe the amount of scapulothoracic motion as the shoulder girdle moves. For the initial 30 degrees of abduction, glenohumeral motion is greater than scapulothoracic motion. Thereafter, both joints tend to move about the same amount. The ratio of motion in that first 30 degrees has been reported to range from 4:1 to 7:1, the glenohumeral joint moving more (27). Therefore, smooth uninhibited function of both joints is important for shoulder abduction. Malposition of the scapula alters the working length of the shoulder girdle muscles. The scapula glides medially and laterally, superiorly and inferiorly, and rotates over the posterolateral chest cage. The position of the scapula can be evaluated in a seated or standing examination. Asymmetry of position of the scapula usually indicates asymmetry of motion. Scapular motion can be tested with the patient sidelying. Grasp the scapula with both hands and take it through the various motions. The scapula can (5):

1. Glide forward and separate each vertebral border 15 cm and glide backward to bring the vertebral borders closer
2. Glide 10 to 12 cm superiorly and inferiorly
3. Rotate to elevate or depress the glenoid fossa 30 degrees each way

Costovertebral Joints of the First Rib

The costovertebral and costotransverse joints of the first rib are synovial. The first rib is an atypical rib and only articulates with the body of T1. The common somatic dysfunction of the first rib is elevation: the rib moves freely in elevation and has a restriction of motion to depression. Motion is tested by placing your thumbs over the posterior aspect of the rib and instructing the patient to take a deep breath. Assess the quality of motion in both inhalation (elevation) and exhalation (depression). Frequently, T1 is rotated and side-bent to the side opposite the side of the elevated first rib.

Costosternal Joint of the First Rib

This is a synchondrosis, not a synovial joint. It is therefore very stable. Its functional purpose is more for support than for motion. Because of this stability, somatic dysfunction is not often found in this area; however, local tenderpoints do occur.

Sternoclavicular Joint

The sternoclavicular joint is the only true joint that attaches the upper extremity to the thoracic cage. In general, motion at this joint is minimal, yet palpable, and often correlates to visual asymmetry as well. Because of anatomic proximity and ligamentous attachments, somatic dysfunction of the first rib and the sternoclavicular joint is related. The sternoclavicular joint has a saddle-shaped articular surface. The clavicular notch on the sternum is shallow and small compared to the articular surface of the medial end of the clavicle (22). Fortunately, this is a complex synovial joint that contains a cartilaginous meniscus. This provides some needed stability. The interclavicular ligament resists superior displacement of the sternal end of the clavicle. The costoclavicular ligament, attached to the first costal cartilage, acts as a fulcrum and limits upward movement of the lateral end of the clavicle (22). As the clavicle abducts, this ligament helps produce a downward glide to

TABLE 43.12

Active and Passive Range of Motion of the Upper Extremity Components

Area	Active	Passive
Finger	Flexion (MCP: 85–90 degrees; PIP: 100–115 degrees; DIP 80–90 degrees) Extension (MCP: 30–45 degrees; PIP: 0 degrees; DIP 20 degrees) Abduction (20–30 degrees) Adduction (0 degrees)	Flexion Extension Abduction
Thumb	Flexion (CMC: 45–50 degrees; MCP: 50–55 degrees; IP: 85–90 degrees) Extension (MCP: 0 degrees; IP: 0–5 degrees) Abduction (60–70 degrees) Adduction (30 degrees)	Flexion Extension Abduction Adduction
Wrist	Abduction or radial deviation (15 degrees) Adduction or ulnar deviation (30–45 degrees) Flexion (80–90 degrees) Extension (70–90 degrees)	Abduction or radial deviation Adduction or ulnar deviation Flexion Extension
Forearm	Pronation (85–90 degrees) Supination (85–90 degrees)	Pronation Supination
Elbow	Flexion (140–150 degrees) Extension (0–10 degrees)	Flexion Extension
Shoulder	Elevation/abduction (170–180 degrees) Elevation/forward flexion (160–180 degrees) Elevation/plane of scapula (170–180 degrees) Lateral (external) rotation (80–90 degrees) Medial (internal) rotation (60–100 degrees) Extension (50–60 degrees) Adduction (50–75 degrees) Horizontal adduction/abduction (cross-flexion/cross-extension; 130 degrees) Circumduction (200 degrees) Scapular protraction Scapular retraction	Elevation/forward flexion of arm Extension/abduction of arm Elevation/abduction of only Glenohumeral joint Lateral rotation of arm Medial rotation of arm Extension of arm Adduction of arm Horizontal adduction/ abduction of arm Quadrant test

the sternal end of the clavicle. The subclavius muscle depresses and pulls the medial end of the first rib forward when the lateral end of the clavicle is elevated.

There are three types of motion in the sternoclavicular joint. Greenman states these are abduction, horizontal flexion, and rotation (23). During abduction, the proximal clavicle moves inferior in the frontal plane. Abduction and external rotation are linked, as is adduction and internal rotation. The fulcrum for superior–inferior movement is the costoclavicular ligament, located approximately 1 inch lateral to the sternoclavicular joint (21). In the horizontal plane, the proximal clavicle translates anterior or posterior. Axial rotation also occurs down a theoretical long axis through the bone, as motion is transmitted through the humerus and scapula. It is important to note that the clavicle is not supplied with any rotator muscles, so it will rotate only as much as determined by motion introduced through the scapula.

A-C Joint

A-C function is important in overall shoulder motion. The A-C joint is a planar joint with a crescent-shaped rudimentary incomplete

meniscus. It depends on its ligamentous attachments for stability. The strongest ligament between the clavicle and scapula is the coracoclavicular ligament (22). The conoid portion of this ligament prevents anterior rotation of the distal clavicle; the trapezoid portion resists posterior rotation of the distal clavicle (22). The A-C joint has motion about three axes, each of which is subtle and takes skill to palpate. The motions that occur include abduction (a superior-inferior movement) and rotation about a long axis down the clavicle. When testing motion, it is important to realize that the small flat downward surface of the clavicle faces downward and laterally. According to Greenman, the joint is approximately angled 30 degrees; therefore, treatment needs to be performed in 30 degrees of horizontal flexion (23). When the clavicle is dysfunctional, there will be local tenderness at the A-C joint, but negative orthopedic shoulder separation tests.

Although Strachan (22) describes a mild elevation of the distal end of the clavicle as a somatic dysfunction, a true A-C separation goes beyond somatic dysfunction and is a traumatic injury, often occurring when patients fall on their shoulder. In this situation, the A-C joint can be tested for separation by palpating. With the patient seated, palpate the A-C joint so that the fingers contact acromion as well as clavicle. With the arm at the patient's side, pull inferiorly. This will gap the joint. A normal joint will resist gapping; a separated joint will gap easily. In an orthopedic injury to the joint, there is typically visual asymmetry, depending on the grade of ligamentous sprain.

Thoracic Inlet

The thoracic inlet can be considered anatomically and functionally. The anatomic boundaries include the manubrium of the sternum anteriorly, the first thoracic posteriorly, and the first rib laterally. When considering the definition functionally, the thoracic inlet comprises the manubrium of the sternum anteriorly, the first four thoracic segments, and the first and second ribs.

Thoracic Outlet

The thoracic outlet is the space between the anterior scalenes, where the subclavian artery and brachial plexus pass.

ELBOW AND FOREARM

Configuration and Physiologic Motion

The ulnohumeral joint is the true elbow joint (6). The head of the radius at the proximal end of the radial bone near the elbow is not a part of the elbow joint. Primary motion of the normal elbow is 160 degrees of flexion and 0 degrees of extension about a transverse axis (10 degrees of hyperextension is found in some individuals). The elbow joint is stable medially and laterally but weak anteriorly and posteriorly. Its anteroposterior stability and strength depends on the muscles that pass anteriorly and posteriorly to the elbow joint and on how firmly the trochlea of the humerus fits into the trochlear notch of the ulna. The medial side of the ulnar notch is anatomically elongated and there is a slight ridge in its joint surface. There is also a grooved spiral in the humeral joint surfaces. The groove/spiral anatomic characteristic causes the hand to normally move toward the mouth when the elbow is flexed and to the lateral side of the hip when it is extended. This structural configuration also produces the normal carrying angle of the arm, greater in the female than in the male. This carrying angle is not very noticeable if the arm is hanging at the side of a person because in this position, the forearm has a natural partial pronation. The elbow also "wobbles" into ulnar adduction during its normal motion.

WRIST AND HAND

Configuration and Physiologic Motion

The hand joins the forearm by way of the true wrist joint. This is a stable joint composed of the radius, three carpal bones, and the attached cartilage. The basic configuration of the true wrist (the radiocarpal joint) is illustrated in Figure 43.2. This joint has two major axes of motion: the transverse axis, around which there is flexion and extension, and an anteroposterior axis, about which there is abduction and adduction. All motions are named according to the anatomic position of the joint and not according to the position in which the physician is holding the hand in relation to the body of the patient. Movement of the wrist toward the thumb side is abduction and toward the little finger is adduction.

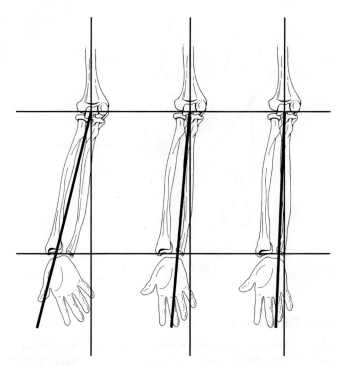

Figure 43-2 Right radiocarpal joint (true wrist joint) and distal radioulnar joint. R, radius; U, ulna; S, scaphoid; L, lunate; T, triquetral. (Illustration by W. A. Kuchera.)

Each motion of the wrist has a normal range of motion. The wrist can flex 90 degrees and extend 70 degrees about its transverse axis and can abduct 20 degrees and adduct 50 degrees about its anteroposterior axis. Combined motion about both of these axes permits a motion called circumduction. Figures 43.3 and 43.4 illustrate normal motion of flexion and extension.

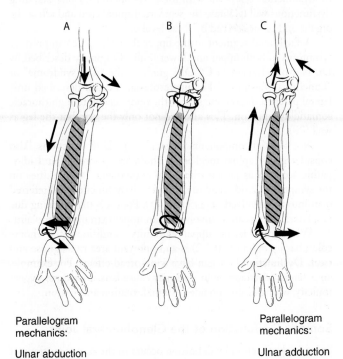

Parallelogram mechanics:

Ulnar abduction

Parallelogram mechanics:

Ulnar adduction

Figure 43-3 Wrist flexion: dorsal glide of proximal carpal bones. (Illustration by W. A. Kuchera.)

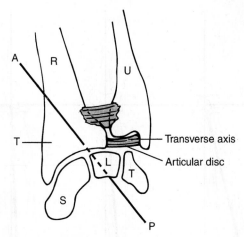

Figure 43-4 Wrist extension: anterior (ventral) glide of proximal carpal bones. (Illustration by W. A. Kuchera.)

Axial Component

The axial component to the patient's upper extremity complaint needs to be the first step in the evaluation of an extremity complaint. Key areas to evaluate include the upper thoracic spine (T1-6) and the ribs, the thoracolumbar junction (T10-L2), and the midlower cervical spine (C4-7). Segmental motion restrictions in any or all of these areas need to be evaluated.

Vertebral and rib somatic dysfunction can cause increased sympathetic tone to the upper extremity. Increased sympathetic tone to the upper extremity causes nondermatomal paresthesias, pain, muscular tension/irritability, vascular reactivity, and sweat gland dysfunction. Increased sympathetic tone can occur with any facilitated segment; however, extended single segment dysfunctions tend to be more symptomatic than flexed ones (30). Bilateral rib dysfunction can occur with these dysfunctions. Long-standing dysfunctions will facilitate the segmental spinal cord and affect the organs and tissues served by these levels.

A facilitated segment in the upper thoracic spine can produce symptoms in both upper and lower limbs. Originally described by Dr. Norman Larson (a CCOM grad) as the "T_{2-3} syndrome" or "Functional Vasomotor Hemiparesthesia," Larson described unilateral paresthesias on one side of the body related to high thoracic somatic dysfunction. This affected not only the arm but the leg as well (28).

Not all axial components are single type II dysfunctions. Also consider group spinal mechanics, short leg syndrome, and idiopathic scoliosis as part of the "axial component." Convexities on the symptomatic side tend to maintain rib dysfunction and referred pain into the involved upper extremity. Poor scapular tracking due to a lateral curve can be involved in an upper extremity complaint.

When considering upper extremity conditions, the thoracolumbar junction (T10-L2) is an important area to diagnose and treat. Dysfunction here can have widespread effects. For example, an extended dysfunction at T12 may cause latissimus dorsi hypertonicity, which limits shoulder external rotation and flexion.

Somatic Dysfunction of the Glenohumeral Joint

Somatic dysfunction by definition occurs in the minor motions of the joint. Due to the ball-and-socket nature of the glenohumeral joint, this would include restrictions of translatory motions, which can occur in many directions. Some authors call this "joint play," "translation," or "glide." For the glenohumeral joint, the osteopathic profession does not name specific somatic dysfunctions based on this concept. Dysfunctions of the shoulder joint are active or passive exaggerations of its cardinal movements (22). Many osteopathic physicians will evaluate each single plane motion (i.e., extension) and treat restrictions of motion in that single plane. In addition to articular restrictions, there are fascial restrictions that traverse the shoulder joint that can limit shoulder motion. Jones strain-counterstrain points and Simons and travel myofascial tenderpoints occur in the muscles controlling the glenohumeral joint. Dysfunctions elsewhere in the body can produce symptoms referable to the shoulder joint. For example, an A-C joint dysfunction can cause deltoid muscle tension, just as a sacroiliac dysfunction can cause latissimus dorsi tightening. Both situations will produce shoulder pain. Greenman feels that the primary motion loss involves abduction and external rotation. The humeral head moves cephalad and caudad on the glenoid during abduction. Loss of this ability is significant in shoulder function (23).

Somatic Dysfunction of the Clavicle

Although motion is understood, standard terminology of clavicle motion is not well described in the osteopathic literature. It is thought that there is reciprocal motion between the distal end and the proximal end of the clavicle. Anterior motion at the distal end of the bone results in posterior motion at the proximal end. Superior motion that occurs at the distal end of the clavicle results in inferior motion at the proximal end. Rotation of the entire clavicle (anterior or posterior) occurs about a theoretical long axis. Motion at the sternoclavicular joint and the A-C joint is not to the same degree, due to their anatomic configuration. More motion is available at the distal end of the clavicle, due to the type of joint present and the S-like shape of the bone. Motion of the clavicle is important during respiration where it must remain mobile during each phase of respiration, as it is related to the mechanics of the first rib. When there is dysfunction of the first or second rib, assessment of the clavicle is important. The physician needs to determine if an orthopedic injury exists (sprain) versus a subtle motion restriction as seen with somatic dysfunction.

Somatic Dysfunction of the A-C Joint

The primary somatic dysfunction diagnosed at the A-C joint occurs when rotation of the clavicle (about a long axis) becomes restricted. When the humerus is fully flexed, the clavicle will rotate posteriorly. When the humerus is fully extended, the clavicle rotates anteriorly. This subtle motion can be palpated with one finger on the acromion and a second on the clavicle. Restriction of humeral flexion is related to an anterior clavicle dysfunction. In this situation, the supraclavicular space feels wider and the associated fascia is tense. Restriction of humeral extension is related to a posterior clavicle dysfunction. In this situation, the supraclavicular space feels narrower and the associated fascia is less tense.

Greenman determines rotation restriction of the A-C joint differently. According to the orthopedic literature, the A-C joint is inclined in the coronal plane, approximately 20 to 50 degrees (27). Greenman assesses the A-C by placing the glenohumeral joint in 30 degrees of horizontal flexion and abduction to the first barrier. He then applies introduces internal and external rotation of the glenohumeral joint until motion or a restrictive barrier is found at the A-C joint. Greenman describes another dysfunction of the A-C joint, in which he describes restricted abduction. The A-C joint is evaluated with the glenohumeral joint placed in 30 degrees of horizontal flexion and abduction is introduced until a restrictive barrier is found (23).

Despite the different methodologies of determining dysfunction, the easiest treatment approach for these A-C restrictions is to use the humerus as a lever. Flexing/extending or internally/externally rotating the arm transmits force to the acromion and then through the A-C joint. If the arm exhibits restriction of motion, engage the barrier, hold, and have the patient contract against your holding force (using principles of muscle energy technique).

Somatic Dysfunction of the Sternoclavicular Joint

The proximal clavicle can move/glide anteriorly or posteriorly, superiorly or inferiorly, as well as rotate anteriorly/posteriorly. Motions at the sternoclavicular joint can be palpated as the patient's arm is horizontally flexed, shrugged, or internally/externally rotated. Small gliding motions can also be directly introduced with your fingertips, looking for restriction (or freedom) of motion. Both Strachan and Greenman describe two primary dysfunctions of the sternoclavicular joint (22,23): One in which there was upward displacement of the proximal clavicle and one in which there is anterior displacement of the clavicle. Although terminology is not consistent, the dysfunction is the same. Abduction dysfunction (upward displacement of the proximal clavicle) is tested by having the patient "shrug their shoulders." The normal finding is for the medial end of both clavicles to move caudad. If an abduction restriction is present, the medial end of one will stay superior, in the original position. To test for a restriction of horizontal flexion (anterior displacement), the medial ends of the clavicles are palpated while the supine patient is instructed to reach toward the ceiling. The normal finding is for the medial end of the clavicles to move posteriorly. If a horizontal flexion is present, the medial end of one (or both) will stay anterior in the original position (23). Although not a primary dysfunction, to test for rotation, the patient's arm is placed in 90 degrees abduction, with the elbow flexed. While palpating the sternoclavicular joint, internal/external rotation of the humerus is introduced, transmitting motion to the sternoclavicular joint. At the end range of internal rotation, the proximal clavicle should rotate anteriorly. At the end range of external rotation, the proximal clavicle should rotate posteriorly. Strachan also discusses an element of impaction that occurs with clavicular dysfunction and hypermobility with chronic dysfunctions (22).

Somatic Dysfunction of the Elbow Joint

Somatic dysfunction of the elbow joint is named according to the minor motion that is present of the ulnohumeral joint, that is, ulnar abduction, or ulnar adduction (Fig. 43.5). An abduction somatic dysfunction appears as though the arm is more angulated, as there would be an increased carrying angle. In an adduction somatic dysfunction, the arm appears straighter, decreasing the carrying angle (producing a "gunstock deformity") (Fig. 43.6). Patients may complain of forearm tightness or wrist pain with either dysfunction. Patients occasionally have point tenderness of the lateral or medial epicondyle, confusing this condition with epicondylitis. There is reciprocal motion between the elbow and the wrist. If the elbow prefers abduction, the wrist will prefer adduction and vice versa. Somatic dysfunction of the elbow will affect full flexion and extension of the elbow. An elbow that does not go completely into extension typically has somatic dysfunction, an orthopedic condition, or both. The "smoothness" or quality of flexion and extension of the elbow may also be affected.

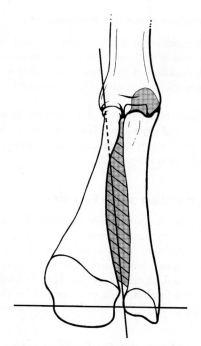

Figure 43-5 **(A)** Ulnar abduction, **(B)** ulnar neutral, and **(C)** ulnar adduction. (Illustration by W. A. Kuchera.)

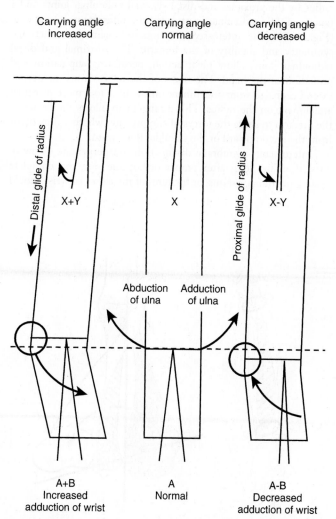

Figure 43-6 Carrying angle and parallelogram effect. (Illustration by W.A. Kuchera.)

Several principles govern the elbow joint area:

1. Somatic dysfunction of the extremity is found in the minor gliding motions of the joint, not the major motions
2. Somatic dysfunction of the ulnohumeral joint is usually primary and somatic dysfunction of the radioulnar joints is usually secondary
3. Impaired function of any joint of the arm produces compensatory changes in all other joints. If total functional demand overtaxes any one of the other joints, secondary somatic dysfunction is also produced in those joints

Somatic Dysfunction of the Forearm

Patients who repetitively use their forearms (D.O.s, carpenters, mechanics, etc.) may have increased tension and tenderness in the whole forearm muscular "system." This type of finding may be related to increased sympathetic tone from upper thoracic/rib somatic dysfunction, as well as overuse. However, repetitive overuse may strain the forearm, wrist, or elbow and can also very easily strain the forearm muscles and interosseous membrane.

Interosseous Membrane Dysfunction

The true elbow and wrist joints are functionally linked with the radius by the proximal and distal synovial radioulnar joints and a fibrous middle radioulnar joint called the interosseous membrane (Fig. 43.7). The interosseous membrane maintains functional symmetry and stability of the forearm. The proximal and distal radioulnar joints allow pivot action, permitting supination and pronation of the hand. The fibers of the interosseous membrane extend cephalad from attachment on the ulna to a more proximal attachment on the radius. This arrangement allows the bones of the forearm to share the forces of compression whether they occur from the hand upward or the shoulder downward.

Interosseous membrane dysfunction can perpetuate elbow or wrist disability long after proper orthopedic care and complete healing of strains, sprains, or fractures of the elbow or wrist should

have taken place. In some unknown way, the collagen tissues often retain stress patterns of past injury. This means that clinically, it is important to treat forearm dysfunction right away before these patterns have a chance to develop. In such cases, palpation of the interosseous membrane reveals increased tension and elicits areas of subjective tenderness. Interosseous strains may be treated with direct or indirect fascial treatments.

Ulnohumeral and Radiocarpal Dysfunction

The radius and ulna are held in a parallelogram arrangement by the radiocarpal joints (Fig. 43.8). The ulna is part of the elbow joint, and the radius is part of the wrist joint. The radius is able to move more freely than the ulna. With the ulna relatively fixed at the ulnohumeral joint and the radius fairly fixed at the radiocarpal joint (especially with the scaphoid), abduction or adduction of the ulna results in a reciprocal positioning of the hand. During abduction of the ulna, the radius glides distally and the wrist is literally pushed into increased adduction. During adduction of the ulna, the radius glides proximally and the wrist is pulled into a more abducted position, compared with the position of the opposite wrist. If this reciprocal positioning principle of the elbow and the wrist is incorporated in the direct and indirect treatment of ulnar abduction or adduction somatic dysfunctions, these techniques will become more effective and efficient. The parallelogram arrangement of the forearm bones with the action of the proximal and distal radioulnar joints permits forearm/wrist motions. As these motions occur, the interosseous membrane (a radioulnar fibrous joint) provides stability to the forearm and prevents stress of the ligaments and/or bony compression in the forearm or the wrist.

Strachan described an internal and external rotation dysfunction of the ulna in relation to the humerus (22). This dysfunction was assessed by moving the forearm into complete supination and pronation and attempting to spring it further. When considering somatic dysfunction of the forearm, inspection by itself is usually not very helpful, although it may be helpful when the carrying angle has been affected by somatic dysfunctions of the

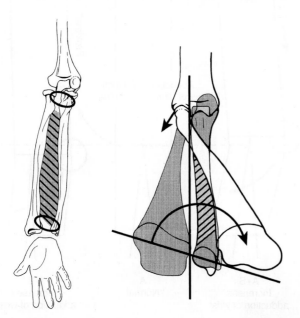

Figure 43-7   Forearm: interosseous membrane. (Illustration by W.A. Kuchera.)

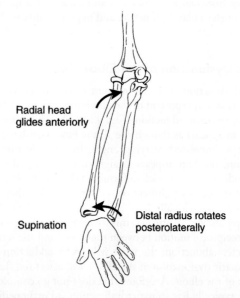

Figure 43-8   Right forearm: parallelogram effect. (Illustration by W.A. Kuchera.)

ulnohumeral joint. Increased abduction of the ulna would increase the carrying angle and encourage adduction of the hand at the wrist. Increased adduction of the ulna at the elbow encourages some abduction of the hand at the wrist. This is noticed as less adduction of the hand at the wrist.

If all ulnohumeral joint somatic dysfunction has been treated, there is no inflammation in the elbow joint, and the elbow still cannot be flexed completely, the problem is most likely one of the radioulnar joints, usually the proximal one. The interosseous membrane may also be involved.

Radial Head Somatic Dysfunction

There is reciprocal motion of the radius. When the hand is pronated, the distal end of the radius crosses over the ulna as it moves anteriorly and medially (Fig. 43.9). Near the end of full pronation, the head of the radius glides posteriorly, that is, there is reciprocal motion of the radial head relative to the distal radius. Motion in an arc opposite from the position of the pronated hand is called supination (Fig. 43.10). When the forearm is supinated, the distal end of the radius moves posteriorly and the radial head glides anteriorly.

Posterior radial head somatic dysfunction is usually produced by a fall forward onto the palm of an outstretched hand because the anterior motion of the distal radius, started by the pronation, is accentuated. Though a fall forward is on the hand, the hand is in a pronated position, and the forward vector of the hand and body pushes the distal radius into a more anterior rotation, causing the radial head to move posteriorly (Fig. 43.11).

An anterior radial head somatic dysfunction is likely to result from a fall backward, where the patient extends the arm posteriorly to break the impact of the fall, lands on the palm, and forces the distal end of the radius posteriorly. In this type of injury, the forearm is in the supinated anatomic position (Fig. 43.12).

These motions are best palpated near the end of full supination or pronation of the hand. They are palpable if the operator's fingers

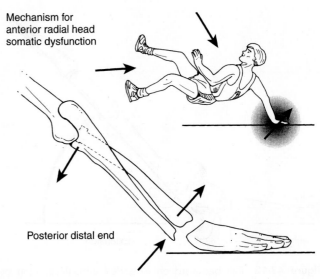

Mechanism for anterior radial head somatic dysfunction

Posterior distal end

Figure 43-10   Forearm: supination. (Illustration by W.A. Kuchera.)

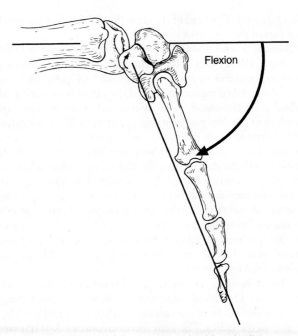

Flexion

Figure 43-11   Forward fall on outstretched hand. (Illustration by W.A. Kuchera.)

are under the patient's elbow and the thumb of that hand is palpating the radial head while the other hand supinates or pronates the patient's hand. Motion in the symptomatic forearm is compared with motion in the opposite or normal forearm.

Somatic Dysfunction of the Wrist

If the wrist hurts, look at the elbow. The only sign of somatic dysfunction of the elbow may be a complaint of wrist pain. The true wrist is the ellipsoid synovial radiocarpal joint formed by a concavity in the distal end of the radius, three proximal carpal bones of the wrist (the navicular or scaphoid bone in the snuffbox of the wrist, the lunate, and the triquetral bones), and an articular disc. The articular disc separates the true wrist joint from the distal

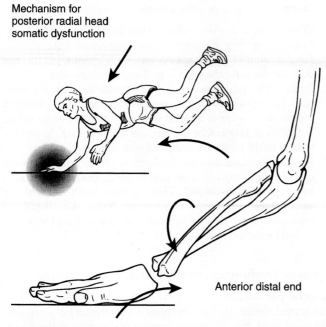

Mechanism for posterior radial head somatic dysfunction

Anterior distal end

Figure 43-9   Forearm: pronation. (Illustration by W.A. Kuchera.)

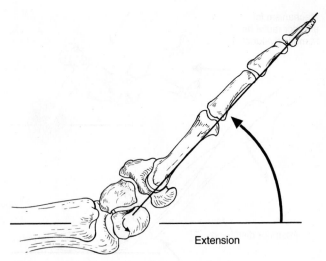

Figure 43-12 Fall backward on extended arm. (Illustration by W.A. Kuchera.)

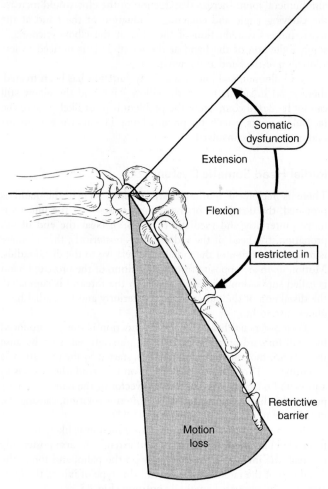

Figure 43-13 Wrist extension: somatic dysfunction. (Illustration by W.A. Kuchera.)

radioulnar joint. The head of the ulna (the distal end of the ulna) is not a part of the true wrist joint.

Somatic dysfunction is not related to the gross motions of the wrist but to dysfunction of the slight gliding motions of the carpal bones on the radius as the wrist is moved. In Figures 46-11 and 46-12, notice the direction of glide of the carpal bone during each of these wrist motions. Somatic dysfunction of the wrist is named according to the direction of motion preference. If a wrist extends and is restricted in its full flexion, it is an extension somatic dysfunction (Fig. 43.13), with the wrist restricted in flexion. In this extension somatic dysfunction, the three carpal bones glide ventrally and are restricted in gliding dorsally. The opposite is true for a flexion somatic dysfunction of the wrist; similar relationships occur for the other wrist motions. Restriction of wrist extension is more common than restriction of wrist flexion. This is probably due to a more developed and dominant flexor muscle mass. A restriction of wrist extension is typically seen with increased tension of the forearm flexors.

The scaphoid, lunate, and triquetral bones fit into the concavity of the radius. The articular disc between these bones also separates these articulations from the radioulnar articulation and binding of the ulna to the radius. The joint moves around an A/P transverse axis and allows for the movements of flexion/extension and abduction/adduction. Flexion is more prominent as is adduction. The carpals can move slightly forward, backward, medially, or laterally. Carpal bones can be displaced toward the palm or dorsally. When this occurs, there is usually some visual and also palpatory evidence. There may be associated motion restriction of the wrist. Dorsally displaced carpal may impede wrist extension. Carpals displaced toward the palm can narrow the carpal tunnel. The scaphoid, lunate, and triquetral articulate with the distal row of carpals or the trapezium, trapezoid, capitate, and hamate. Movement is freer in flexion than in extension. There is a slight amount of side-to-side rocking allowed by the gliding between the two rows of bones. Additionally, there may be dysfunction of the intercarpal joints. Actually, this is more of a partial dislocation of a carpal bone.

Dysfunction at the wrist follows the motion restrictions seen at the elbow. There is reciprocal motion. If the elbow moves freely into abduction, the wrist will move freely into adduction and vice versa. Restriction of wrist extension is more common than restriction of wrist flexion. This is probably due to a more developed and

dominant flexor muscle mass. Other factors such as osteoarthritis, cartilage tears, or occult fractures can limit wrist extension as well.

Several principles describe somatic dysfunction of the wrist:

1. Observation is not very helpful when looking for somatic dysfunction; swelling of the wrist is an inconsistent sign
2. Painful compression means dysfunction is present, but this test does not diagnose the specific problem that is present
3. Radial glide and limited parallelogram motions are not obvious until the opposite motion is attempted. If there is an adduction somatic dysfunction at the wrist with a proximal shift of the radius, the problem may not be evident until abduction of the wrist is tested and the results are compared with the opposite side
4. Flexion/extension somatic dysfunction of the wrist is usually caused by a trauma that overcomes the ligamentous restraints and opposing muscle pull. This can often result if a strain or sprain exceeds the extent of a somatic dysfunction. Restricted extension of the wrist is its most common major motion loss caused by dysfunction

Somatic Dysfunction of the Hand

Intercarpal Joints

Intercarpal somatic dysfunction often occurs from a fall on an outstretched hand. For this reason, somatic dysfunction in these areas is very likely to have a compression component. If the wrist joint is swollen, the physician must rule out fracture of the navicular bone (scaphoid). This is also true if there is pain on pressure over the snuffbox, or if there is persistent pain and dysfunction after proper conservative care, even if the initial posttrauma radiographs showed no evidence of fracture. Sometimes, the scaphoid does not reveal evidence of fracture until the disruption in its blood supply slowly produces degeneration of the bone.

Carpometacarpal Joints

All of these joints, except the thumb, are classified as plane synovial joints, which share a common joint cavity with the intercarpal joints. Their main type of somatic dysfunction is a dorsal glide with restriction in ventral glide. Palpation at the base of the suspected metacarpal may reveal an abnormal anterior or posterior position in relation to the carpals. Mobility is assessed by moving the metacarpal heads back and forth. A restriction of both motions indicates an impaction or compression type of dysfunction.

The carpometacarpal joint of the thumb is different; it is a separate saddle-type joint, having both a concave and a convex articular surface. This configuration permits angular movements in almost any plane with the exception of limited axial rotation. Only a ball-and-socket joint has more motion than the carpometacarpal joint of the thumb. Because it has very good motion, it is more likely to have compression strain or sprain of the ligaments than to have somatic dysfunction.

MP and IP Joints

The MP joints and all the IP joints of the hand are gliding joints. The fifth MP joint has the most motion; there is less motion in the fourth MP joint, and the third and second MP joints have the least motion. The MP and IP joints may develop somatic dysfunction in any one of a combination of six gliding motions:

- Anteroposterior glide
- Mediolateral glide
- Internal-external rotational glide
- All of these motions are minor and cannot be initiated directly by muscle action

Compression is always part of MP and IP somatic dysfunctions, as when a ring on a finger gets caught as a person jumps over a wire fence. Intermetacarpal cramps and pain may be a sign of MP or IP somatic dysfunction. Pain in the metacarpal joints may be referred from an ulnohumeral joint somatic dysfunction. Dysfunction of the fingers typically involves the fascial components. There are usually restrictions of fascial rotation, abduction/adduction, or compression/distraction. These types of problems manifest as impediments in finger flexion, swelling of the digits, or pain. Jones tenderpoints occur in the upper extremity as well. A common tenderpoint called CM1 (thenar point) is found in the thenar muscle mass. It is commonly found in patients who use their hands repetitively.

Special Tests for the Upper Extremity

There are many special tests of the upper extremity that are useful to determine if orthopedic, neurologic, or vascular compromise is present.

OSTEOPATHIC TREATMENT: COMMON CLINICAL CONDITIONS

Carpal Tunnel Syndrome

This condition is most commonly described as an entrapment neuropathy of the median nerve at the wrist producing paresthesia and weakness of the hands (9). Carpal tunnel syndrome is frequently associated with repeated or sustained activity of the fingers and hands. Incidence rates are reported as high as 25.6 cases per 200,000 work hours (10) and involving 10% of workers. Medical cost estimates vary from $3,500 to $60,000 per case (11).

Patients experience numbness or paresthesia on the palmar surface of the thumb, index, and middle fingers, and radial half of the ring finger. Numbness and paresthesia of the whole hand may also occur. Pain may be referred to the forearm and, less commonly, to the neck and forearm regions. Pain or tingling of the fingers often occurs at night and is relieved by shaking or exercising the hand. Weakness and atrophy of the thenar muscles usually appear late and can occur without significant sensory symptoms. On examination, symptoms may be reproduced by percussion over the volar surface of the wrist (Tinel sign) or by full flexion of the wrist for one minute (Phalen maneuver). Decreased touch may be demonstrated over the fingers supplied by the median nerve. Nerve conduction studies are considered to be the gold standard for the diagnosis of this condition (9).

The syndrome is traditionally described as resulting from pressure on the median nerve where it passes with the flexor tendons of the fingers through the tunnel formed by the carpal bones and the transverse carpal ligament (9). Additional explanations exist. Single compressions of dog sciatic nerves have failed to produce significant conduction loss. Both proximal and distal compressions have produced conduction blocks in 50% of test animals (12).

In 1973, Upton and McComas (13) proposed the existence of the "double crush syndrome." This syndrome hypothesizes that neural function is impaired when single axons that are compressed on one region become especially susceptible to damage in another area. The authors report that a slight compression may cause a reduction in axoplasmic flow that is too small to result in denervation changes, but when coupled with the onset of a slowed lesion, might further reduce axoplasmic flow below the safety margin for prevention of denervation at a distal lesion, and clinical symptoms ensue (13). Abramson et al. demonstrated that decreased blood supply to a nerve alters conduction (14). Larson suggested that upper thoracic dysfunction alters upper extremity vasomotion (15). Hurst et al. demonstrated a relationship between cervical arthritis and bilateral carpal tunnel syndrome (16). Sunderland has suggested that lymphatic and venous congestion contributes to this disorder (17).

The treatment of carpal tunnel syndrome has traditionally involved the use of wrist splints, anti-inflammatory drugs, and local injection of steroids. Surgical decompression of the carpal tunnel with release of the transverse carpal tunnel ligament is used if symptoms persist or if motor abnormalities are present (9,18). Evidence in the preceding paragraph suggests that the hand symptoms may be related to dysfunctions in the upper extremity, and the cervical and thoracic spine. Osteopathic treatment incorporates the modalities described above and should also include:

1. Reducing sympathetic tone to the upper extremity by correcting upper thoracic and upper rib dysfunctions. This directly affects nerve function by improving blood flow and reducing congestion through improved lymphatic and venous drainage. An internally rotated temporal bone may be associated with increased sympathetic tone in the upper thoracic spine and, if it is diagnosed, should also be treated.
2. Removing cervical somatic dysfunction to improve brachial plexus function
3. Removing myofascial restrictions in the upper extremity, thereby removing potential sites of additional compression
4. Increasing space within the carpal tunnel using direct release techniques

Tennis Elbow

Tennis elbow is also known as lateral epicondylitis. This condition is thought to be an inflammatory response to overuse of the extensor muscle group attached to the lateral epicondyle of the humerus. There is also the thought that this condition may be related to a degenerative tendonosis and/or ischemic phenomenon. It is usually caused by repeated overload of the musculotendinous units. This condition produces pain that may be localized to the lateral epicondyle or may radiate down the forearm extensor group or up into the brachioradialis muscle. The pain is intensified by resistive extension of the wrist and fingers, or by shaking hands. Pressure over the lateral epicondyle is painful (7,8).

Common areas of somatic dysfunction include the ipsilateral upper thoracic spine and ribs, the radial head and ulnohumeral joint, the lower cervical spine, and the pronator teres muscle. OMT directed to the upper thoracic spine and counterstrain for the affected ribs will decrease muscle tension of the forearm as well as tenderness of the lateral epicondyle. Counterstrain for the extensor tendons is useful as well. Treatment of a radial head dysfunction or an abducted ulna may completely resolve symptoms in patients with lateral epicondyle pain, but not true epicondylitis.

Rotator Cuff Tendonitis

Rotator cuff disease and impingement syndromes are commonly seen disorders in occupational, athletic, and traumatically injured patients. They are also common in the aging athletic or active patient, who becomes more sedentary. Rotator cuff disease can be caused by repetitive overuse (micro trauma), a single traumatic event (macro trauma), instability of the glenohumeral joint, or musculotendinous fiber failure. Most rotator cuff problems are muscular and result from a degenerative tendonopathy due to intrinsic muscular fatigue. The muscles that comprise the rotator cuff include the supraspinatus, infraspinatus, teres minor, and subscapularis. Supraspinatus is the most commonly involved muscle in rotator cuff injury. Each cuff muscle plays a unique and important role in stabilizing the shoulder. Impingement syndromes are biomechanical causes of, or the effects of, rotator cuff disease. The classic concept of impingement involves "outlet impingement" between the greater tuberosity and the acromion. Narrowing of this subacromial space produces soft tissue encroachment, edema, and tendonitis. Neer classified impingement and rotator cuff disease into three stages: inflammation and edema (I), fibrosis and tendonitis (II), and partial or complete tearing (III) (26). In younger athletes, this type of impingement can occur due to ligamentous laxity and muscle imbalance. Another form of impingement exists, primarily in throwing athletes. Called internal impingement, it involves impingement of the surface of the rotator cuff under the posterior-superior glenoid rim (26).

Posture, core muscle strength, and anatomic position of the scapula are critical factors in rotator cuff impingement. It is a total body problem, not an isolated joint inflammation. Somatic dysfunction of the upper thoracic spine and ribs contributes to abnormal rotator cuff firing patterns and fatigue. Cervical somatic dysfunction can impair nerve function to the muscles of the rotator cuff, also impairing muscle strength. Sacroiliac and lumbar dysfunction can affect the shoulder through tension in the latissimus dorsi muscle. In patients with poor posture, weak core muscles and somatic dysfunction, muscles of the cuff (and surrounding the shoulder) tend to develop Jones tender points or Simon-Travell myofascial trigger points. Left untreated, these points perpetuate the problem by maintaining muscle inhibition, tightness, and pain. OMT needs to address the axial spinal component, improve scapular mobility, decrease fascial tensions, improve local blood flow, and reduce pain. The addition of physical therapy is critical, but at the right time, and in the correct fashion. Exercises work better when areas of somatic dysfunction have been improved and inflammation has diminished. Proper strengthening and stretching will decrease the chances of somatic dysfunction reoccurring as well.

Adhesive Capsulitis

Also known as "frozen shoulder," this condition is characterized by pain and restricted movement of the shoulder, usually in the absence of intrinsic shoulder disease. Adhesive capsulitis may follow bursitis or tendonitis of the shoulder or may be associated with systemic disorders, such as chronic pulmonary disease, myocardial infarction, and diabetes mellitus. Prolonged arm immobility contributes to the development of this condition. Reflex sympathetic dystrophy is thought to be a pathogenic factor. The capsule of the shoulder is thickened, and a mild, chronic, inflammatory infiltrate and fibrosis may be present.

Pain and stiffness usually develop gradually over several months to a year, but may progress rapidly in some patients. Pain may interfere with sleep. The shoulder is tender to palpation, and active and passive motions are restricted (9).

Early mobilization after an injury to the arm or shoulder may help prevent the development of this condition. Local injection of corticosteroids and administration of nonsteroidal anti-inflammatory drugs and physical therapy may help (9). Osteopathic manipulation should be directed to the upper thoracics, upper ribs, and entire shoulder complex. The objective is to improve motion. Avoid taking the patient into the "crampy" pain zone. This only slows progress. Only progress as fast as the patient can respond. Indirect techniques may be especially effective in the initial treatment phases.

Thoracic Outlet Syndrome

This condition results from compression of the neurovascular bundle (subclavian artery, subclavian vein, and brachial plexus) as it courses through the neck and shoulder. Several dysfunctions may compress the neurovascular bundle as it passes from the thorax to the arm, including:

- Cervical ribs
- Excessive tension in the anterior and middle scalene muscles
- Dysfunction of the clavicle, upper ribs, or upper thoracics
- Abnormal insertion of the pectoralis minor muscle
- Patients may develop
- Shoulder and arm pain
- Weakness
- Paresthesia
- Claudication
- Raynaud phenomenon
- Ischemic tissue loss
- Gangrene

Examination is often normal unless provocative maneuvers are performed. Occasionally, distal pulses are decreased or absent and digital cyanosis and ischemia may be evident. Tenderness may be present in the supraclavicular fossa (9). Some forms of thoracic outlet syndrome are associated with sympathetic autonomic dysfunction, which produces upper extremity symptoms. Sympathetic dysfunction has accompanying palpatory findings in the upper thoracic or rib area. Most patients can be conservatively managed. Patients should avoid positions that aggravate symptoms. Osteopathic treatment should be directed toward improving mechanics in the:

- Cervical region
- Upper thoracics
- Upper ribs
- Clavicles
- Scalene muscles
- Muscles of the shoulder and pectoral girdle
- Surgical intervention is a last resort.

SUMMARY

Osteopathic clinical examination of the upper extremity includes the diagnosis of somatic dysfunction integrated into the examination procedure. The relationship between anatomic structure and physiologic function is considered prior to deciding a treatment plan. Osteopathic treatment needs to address the specific diagnosis, incorporating the innate ability of the patient to heal given the appropriate environment of improved tissue function. OMT directed at the somatic component of the patient's condition will improve the tissue's function and thus the patient's own ability to heal himself or herself.

REFERENCES

1. Truhlar RE. *Doctor A. T. Still in the Living.* Published by the author, 1950.
2. Hoppenfeld S. *Physical Examination of the Spine and Extremities.* Norwalk, CT: Appleton & Lange, 1976:25.
3. Moore KL. *Clinically Oriented Anatomy.* 3rd Ed. Baltimore, MD: Williams & Wilkins, 1992:528.
4. Seidel HM, Ball JW, Dains JE, et al. *Mosby's Guide to Physical Examination.* St. Louis, MO: Mosby, 1987:309–311.
5. Kuchera WA, Kuchera ML. *Osteopathic Principles in Practice.* 2nd Ed. Rev. Columbus, OH: Greyden Press, 1994:539.
6. Kuchera WA, Kuchera ML. *Osteopathic Principles in Practice.* 2nd Ed. Rev. Columbus, OH: Greyden Press, 1994:615–629.
7. Roy S, Irvin R. Throwing and tennis injuries to the shoulder and elbow. In: *Sports Medicine: Prevention, Evaluation, Management, and Rehabilitation.* Salt Lake City: Prentice Hall, 1983:221–222.
8. Gunter-Griffin, Letha Y. *Athletic Training and Sports Medicine.* 2nd Ed. Rosemont, IL: The American Academy of Orthopedic Surgeons, 1991:274.
9. Wilson JD, et al. *Harrison's Principles of Internal Medicine.* 12th Ed. New York, NY: McGraw-Hill, 1991:1487.
10. Armstrong TJ. *An Ergonomics Guide to Carpal Tunnel Syndrome.* Ergonomics Guide Series. Akron, OH: American Industrial Hygiene Association, 1983.
11. Hiltz R. Fighting work-related injuries. *Natl Underwriter* 1985;89:15.
12. Nemoto K. Experimental study on the vulnerability of the peripheral nerve. *Nippon Sea Gakkai Zasshi* 1983;57:1773–1786.
13. Upton A, McComas AJ. The double crush in nerve entrapment syndromes. *Lancet* 1973;2:359.
14. Abramson DI, Rickert BL, Alexis JT, et al. Effects of repeated periods of ischemia on motor nerve conduction. *J Appl Physiol* 1971;30: 636–642.
15. Larson NJ. Osteopathic manipulation for syndromes of the brachial plexus. *J Am Osteopath Assoc* 1972;72:94–100.
16. Hurst LC, et al. The relationship of double crush syndrome to carpal tunnel syndrome (an analysis of 1000 cases of carpal tunnel syndrome). *J Hand Surg* 1985;10:202.
17. Sunderland S. The nerve lesion in the carpal tunnel syndrome. *J Neurol Neurosurg Psychiatry* 1976;39:615.
18. Anonymous. Carpal tunnel syndrome: getting a handle on hand trauma. *Occup Hazards* 1987;42:45–47.
19. Ward RC. Upper extremities. In: *Foundations for Osteopathic Medicine.* 2nd Ed. Philadelphia, PA: Lippincott, Williams & Wilkins, 690–704; Chap 47.
20. Ward RC. Muscle energy techniques. In: *Foundations for Osteopathic Medicine.* 2nd Ed. Philadelphia, PA: Lippincott Williams & Wilkins, 906–907; Chap 57.
21. Ward RC. Balanced ligamentous tension techniques. In: *Foundations for Osteopathic Medicine.* 2nd Ed. Philadelphia, PA: Lippincott Williams & Wilkins, 926–927; Chap 59.
22. Fryette HH. *Principles of Osteopathic Technique.* 2nd Ed. Kirksville, MO: Journal Printing Company, 1980:154–232.
23. Greenman PE. *Principles of Manual Medicine.* 2nd Ed. Baltimore, MD: Williams & Wilkins, 1996:271–285.
24. Walton WJ. *Osteopathic Diagnosis and Technique Procedures.* Colorado Springs, CO: American Academy of Osteopathy, 1970:201–203, 463–473.
25. DiGiovanna EL, Schiowitz S, Dowling DJ. *An Osteopathic Approach to Diagnosis and Treatment.* 3rd Ed. Philadelphia, PA: Lippincott Williams & Wilkins, 364–373, 409–464.
26. DeLee JC, Drez D. *Orthopaedic Sports Medicine Principles and Practice.* Vol 2, 2nd Ed. Philadelphia, PA: Saunders, Copyright 2003:1065–1095.
27. DeLee JC, Drez D. *Orthopaedic Sports Medicine Principles and Practice.* Vol 2, 2nd Ed. Philadelphia, PA: Saunders, Copyright 2003:840–850.
28. Nelson K, Glonek T. *Somatic Dysfunction in Osteopathic Family Practice.* Philadelphia, PA: Lippincott Williams & Wilkins, Copyright 2007: 349–350.
29. Borenstein DJ, Wiesel SW, Bowden SD. *Low Back and Neck Pain.* Philadelphia, PA: WB Saunders, 2004.
30. Karagenas S. *Principles of Manual Sports Medicine.* Philadelphia, PA: Lippincott Williams & Wilkins. Copyright 2005:628–640.

Abdominal Region

RAYMOND J. HRUBY

HISTORICAL PERSPECTIVE AND SUPPORTIVE EVIDENCE

Osteopathic manipulative techniques can be used as part of a complete treatment approach to abdominal visceral problems. Such techniques have been part of osteopathic practice since the time of Andrew Taylor Still, the founder of osteopathic medicine. One early description of abdominal visceral treatment by Still is that of his first case of "flux," or dysentery, in a 4-year-old boy. He describes his examination of the child, noting that the child's back was hot while the abdomen was cold to the touch. In writing about his treatment, he states

> I began at the base of the brain, and thought by pressures and rubbings I could push some of the hot to the cold places, and in so doing I found rigid and loose places on the muscles and ligaments of the whole spine, while the lumbar was in a very congested condition. I worked for a few minutes on that philosophy, and told the mother to report next day, and if I could do anything more for her boy I would cheerfully do so. She came early next morning with the news that her child was well (1).

Still described having treated many other similar cases with a high degree of success. His knowledge of the structure–function relationships involved with abdominal conditions was extensive enough to warrant an entire chapter of one of his books being devoted to this topic (2).

Other osteopathic physicians since the time of Still have promoted the use of osteopathic manipulative techniques directed toward the abdominal viscera. Hazzard described how to examine the abdomen and discussed treatment approaches for various abdominal visceral diseases (3). Conrad (4) devoted a section of his book to diseases of the abdomen, specifically diseases of the stomach, intestines, liver, kidneys, and spleen. He described and illustrated specific osteopathic manual techniques for these organs. In a rather extensive treatise on the abdomen, McConnell (5) talked about the osteopathic approach from the ventral plane of the body, and described "ventral technique." Tender points, described as "gangliform contractions," were noted by Frank Chapman, D.O., and came to be known as "Chapman's reflexes." The only known reference text on this topic was published by Owens (6).

In later years, other osteopathic researchers published studies illustrating the use of osteopathic manipulative techniques for abdominal conditions. For example, Hermann (7) demonstrated that osteopathic manipulative treatment (OMT) prior to abdominal surgery greatly reduced the incidence of postoperative ileus. He also demonstrated that OMT could be successfully used to treat postoperative ileus when it did occur. In a recent study, Radjieski et al. (8) demonstrated the use of OMT could significantly reduce the length of hospital stay in patients with acute pancreatitis.

Researchers in other health care professions have also noted the clinical relationship between the soma and the viscera. As an example, Pikalov and Kharin (9) found using spinal manipulative techniques as part of the treatment plan for duodenal ulcer disease resulted in pain relief and clinical remission much sooner than conventional medical treatment alone. Travell and Simons (10) have noted that abdominal myofascial trigger points may produce visceral symptoms such as diarrhea, vomiting, belching, food intolerance, and infantile colic. Barral has published extensively on the use of manual techniques for treatment of the abdominal viscera (11,12). Other authors in this area include Finet (13) and Lossing.

Thus, it becomes apparent that optimum treatment of abdominal visceral conditions requires an understanding of the underlying structure–function relationships and of the segmental viscerosomatic reflex phenomena that are involved. An understanding of osteopathic philosophy and principles, and the ability to use OMT as part of a complete treatment approach to abdominal disease, is one of the most unique characteristics of the osteopathic physician.

Definition

The abdomen may be defined simply as the region of the trunk below the thoracic diaphragm. This area consists of two parts: an upper part, the *abdomen proper*; and a lower part, the *lesser pelvis* (14) (Fig. 44.1). These two areas are continuous at the plane of the inlet of the lesser pelvis. This inlet is bounded by the sacral promontory, the arcuate lines of the innominate bones, the pubic crests, and the upper border of the symphysis pubis.

Functional Anatomy

The *abdomen proper* is bounded *superiorly* by the thoracolumbar diaphragm; *inferiorly* it becomes continuous with the pelvis or, as some anatomists describe it, the abdominopelvic portion of the abdominal cavity (15), by way of the superior aperture of the lesser

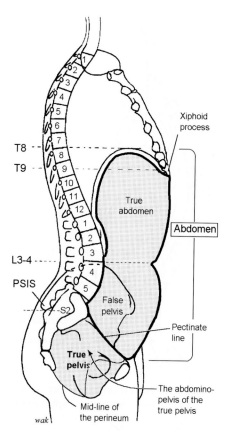

Figure 44-1   Boundaries and skeletal elements of the abdomen.

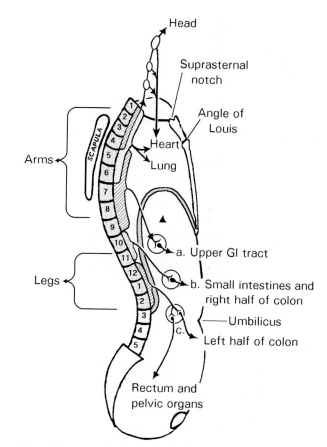

Figure 44-2   Primary sympathetic (efferent) nerves of the body.

or true pelvis. *Anteriorly* the abdomen is bounded by the abdominal muscles, which include the rectus abdominis, the pyramidales, the external obliques, the internal obliques, and the transversus abdominis. *Posteriorly* the abdomen is bounded by the lower thoracic and the lumbar vertebrae, the crura of the diaphragm, the psoas and quadratus lumborum muscles, and the posterior parts of the iliac bones.

The *lesser pelvis* or abdominopelvic portion of the abdomen is shaped somewhat like an inverted cone. Its *anterolateral* boundary consists of those parts of the hip bones below the arcuate lines and the pubic crests, and the obturator internus muscles; its superior and dorsal boundary includes the sacrum, coccyx, and the piriformis and coccygeus muscles; and its *inferior* boundary includes the levator ani muscles and fascial coverings (which together form the pelvic diaphragm).

The abdominal structures of interest in this chapter are the stomach, small intestine, large intestine, liver, gallbladder, spleen, pancreas, kidney, parts of the ureters, suprarenal glands, and numerous blood and lymph vessels, lymph nodes, and nerves. The lower ureters, the urinary bladder, and internal genitalia are not covered in this chapter.

Skeletal Structures

The skeletal elements of the abdomen are the lumbar vertebrae, the sacrum, coccyx, and the innominate bones (see Fig. 44.1).

Muscular Structures

The muscles of the abdominal region may be divided into anterolateral and posterior groups. The anterolateral group includes the rectus abdominis, the pyramidalis, the external oblique, the internal oblique, and the transversus abdominis; the posterior group consists of the quadratus lumborum, psoas major, psoas minor erector spinae and iliacus (14). The reader should note that somatic dysfunctions of these posterior muscles may mimic the pain of certain abdominal disorders or may be painful because of viscerosomatic reflex activity associated with abdominal problems. The thoracoabdominal diaphragm, while not usually considered part of the abdominal wall, should nevertheless be considered when evaluating the abdomen for somatic dysfunction.

Neurological Structures

Primary sympathetic fibers for innervation of all organs below the diaphragm, except the descending colon and pelvic organs, pass from the intermediolateral cells in the thoracic spinal cord through the thoracoabdominal diaphragm. In the abdomen, these primary fibers enter the celiac, superior mesenteric, and the inferior mesenteric collateral ganglia where they synapse (Fig. 44.2). Secondary or postganglionic fibers continue on to innervate specific groups of organs in the abdomen and pelvis. Parasympathetic innervation is supplied from the craniosacral outflow. All abdominal organs down to the midtransverse colon are supplied by the vagus nerve (cranial nerve X); the rest of the abdominal organs and all of the pelvic viscera receive their parasympathetic innervation from the pelvic splanchnic nerves (S2-4).

Visceral afferent impulses travel back to the cord using the same course used by the sympathetic efferent nerves to that organ (Fig. 44.3). This pain tends to be vague and gnawing, deep, poorly localized, and midabdominal. Visceral afferent fibers from the root of the mesentery report to the somatic cord segment of that organ's sympathetic innervations (14). This type of sensory input produces the paraspinal tissue changes that help the physician to locate

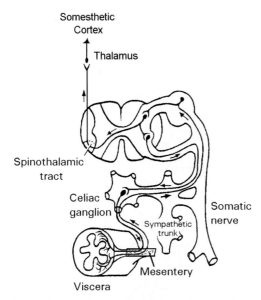

Figure 44-3   Neurologic pathway of visceral pain (afferent fibers).

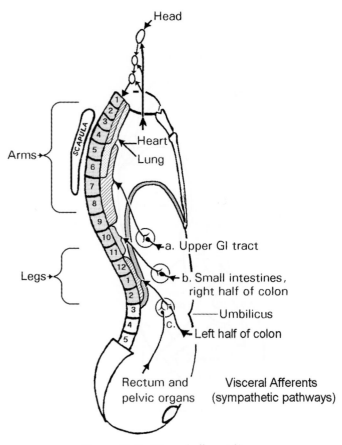

Figure 44-5   Visceral afferent fibers.

the viscus that is most likely dysfunctional. The tissue changes are *t*enderness, *a*symmetry, *r*ange-of-motion differences, and *t*issue texture changes (TART). The pain and tissue texture changes are primarily localized at the paraspinal level consistent with the organ's sympathetic innervation (Figs. 44.4 and 44.5).

Somatic pain may also be caused by what is known as the percutaneous reflex of Morley. This type of somatic pain is usually located directly over the inflamed organ and is produced by direct contiguous irritation of the parietal peritoneum and the abdominal wall (Fig. 44.6). It is responsible for rebound tenderness and abdominal guarding associated with more severe abdominal pain.

Vascular Structures
Arteries
The thoracic aorta lies along the anterior and left anterolateral side of the thoracic vertebrae. It enters the abdominal cavity through the aortic hiatus in the abdominal diaphragm at the level anterior to the 12th thoracic vertebra. Here, it becomes the abdominal aorta. Its main abdominal branches are the celiac, superior mesenteric, renal, and inferior mesenteric arteries (14).

Veins
Various small veins and plexuses in the pelvis eventually flow into the external and internal iliac veins. The two pairs of external and internal iliac veins unite to form the left and right common iliac veins, and these in turn unite to form the inferior vena cava, which conveys blood to the right atrium of the heart (Fig. 44.7). The veins that collect blood from the digestive tract, spleen, pancreas, and gallbladder join to form the portal vein. The portal vein carries blood to the liver, where this vein branches out into a series of very

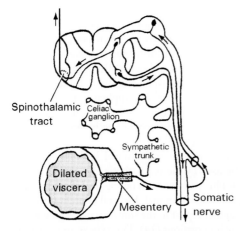

Figure 44-4   Neurologic pathway of viscerosomatic pain.

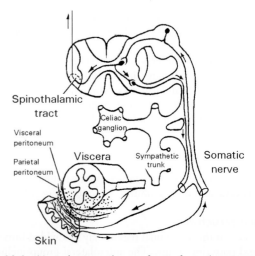

Figure 44-6   Neurologic pathway of pain from the percutaneous reflex of Morley.

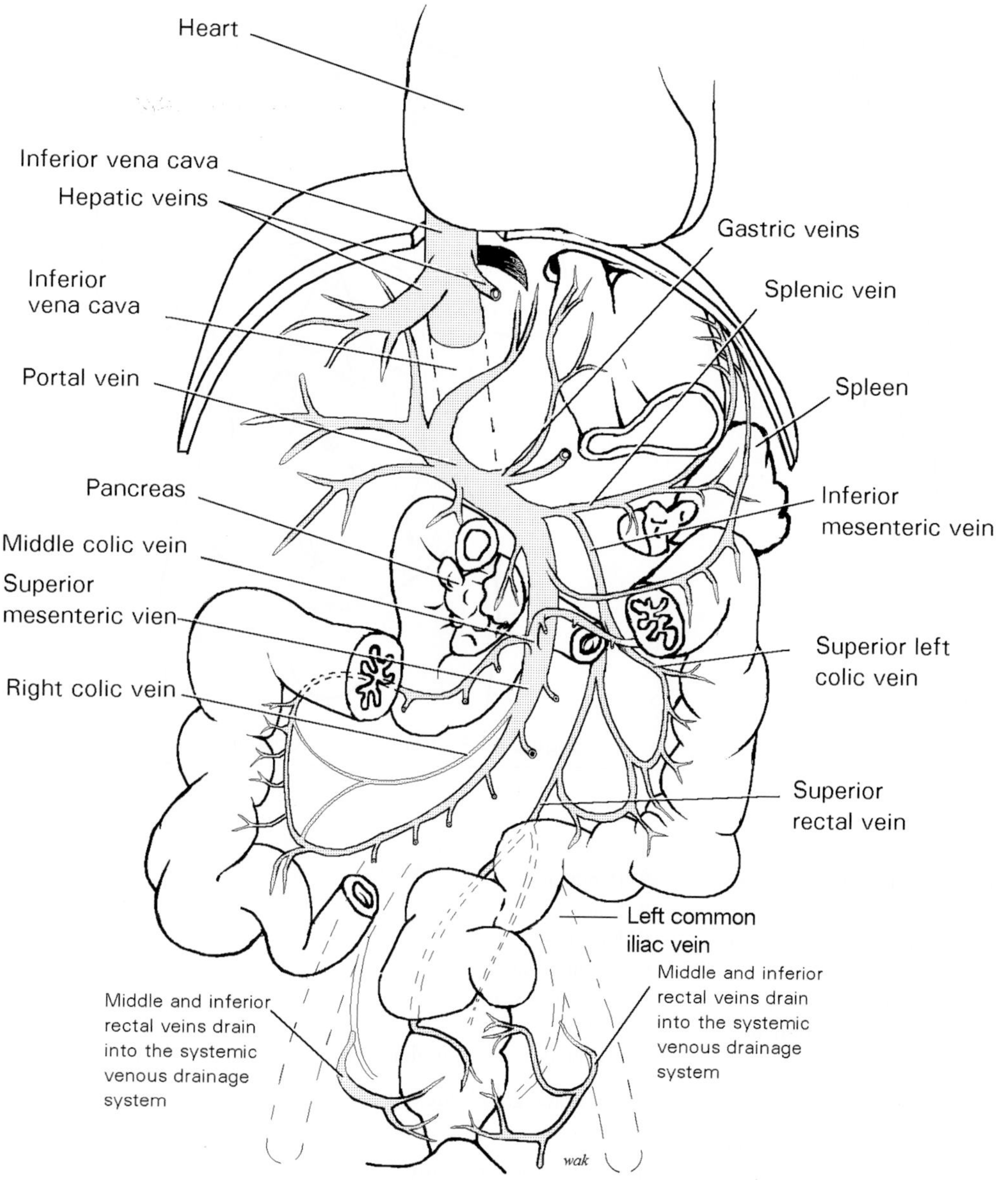
Heart
Inferior vena cava
Hepatic veins
Inferior
vena cava
Portal vein
Pancreas
Middle colic vein
Superior
mesenteric vien
Right colic vein
Gastric veins
Splenic vein
Spleen
Inferior
mesenteric vein
Superior left
colic vein
Superior
rectal vein
Left common
iliac vein
Middle and inferior
rectal veins drain
into the systemic
venous drainage
system
Middle and inferior
rectal veins drain
into the systemic
venous drainage
system
wak

Figure 44-7 Venous drainage: portal venous system for the viscera.

small vessels called sinusoids. From here, hepatic veins convey the blood to the inferior vena cava (14).

Lymphatic Structures

The left lymphatic duct (the thoracic duct) drains interstitial fluids from the lower extremities, the pelvic and abdominal viscera, the left arm, and the left side of the head (Fig. 44.8). It begins as the *cisterna chyli*, a 2-inch, yellowish, cylindrical structure that lies just to the left of the thoracolumbar junction at about the level of the first lumbar vertebra. It receives lymphatic vessels that drain interstitial fluids from all the abdominal organs, the pelvic organs, the lower extremities, and all of the superficial lymphatic vessels located below a horizontal plane of the body running through the umbilicus. The superficial lymphatic vessels drain lymph into superficial inguinal nodes. Lymph then travels into the deep nodes, the deep trunks along the common iliac arteries and the aorta, and finally into the cisterna chyli. It should be noted that lymph from the ovary, testicles, and prostate does not drain into the inguinal nodes but drains into the deep pelvic nodes (16).

Connective Tissue and Fascial Elements

The muscles of the abdominal region have associated fascial sheaths. The deep fascial layers have names associated with the various abdominal regions. Table 44.1 shows these fascial layers and their associated abdominal regions.

The *peritoneum* is a large serous membrane that consists of two layers: the *parietal* layer, which lines the abdominal wall; and a *visceral* layer, which is reflected over the abdominal viscera. The parietal peritoneum angles from the posterior wall of the abdomen to form very defined mesenteric connections to the abdominal viscera. These mesenteries carry the sympathetic and parasympathetic fibers and arteries to the viscera. They also carry visceral afferent fibers, veins, and lymphatic vessels away from the viscera. The visceral peritoneum is sensitive to stretch. It produces visceral pain only when the distention of the viscus exceeds the length of the visceral peritoneum on the outside of the mesentery.

The root of the mesentery for approximately 30 ft of small intestines is only 6 inches long and is located on the posterior wall of the abdominal cavity, posterior to a point about 1 inch to the

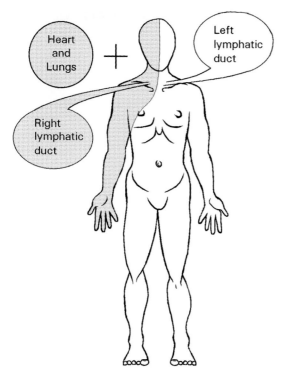

Figure 44-8   Main lymphatic ducts of the body.

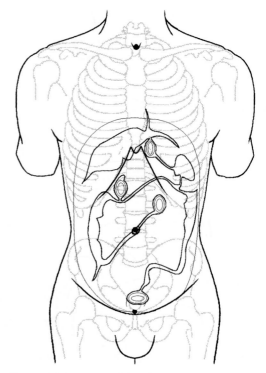

Figure 44-9   Roots of the abdominal mesenteries.

left of and 1 inch above the umbilicus (Fig. 44.9). The root of the mesentery runs inferolaterally to a second point just anterior to the right sacroiliac joint (14). Mental visualization of these mesenteries allows a physician to determine more accurately the origin of palpable masses and the origin of auscultated abnormal sounds. It is also important when performing visceral manipulation to free fascial pathways and improve visceral function.

Visceral Structures
The visceral structures with which we are concerned in the abdomen are the following (Fig. 44.10):

- Stomach
- Liver
- Gallbladder
- Pancreas
- Spleen
- Kidneys
- Urinary bladder
- Small intestine
- Colon
- Aorta and common iliac arteries

The adrenal glands are not palpable.

Topographic Anatomy
There are certain surface landmarks of the abdomen that are palpable (17). These landmarks are shown in Figure 44.11 and include:

- Costal margins
- Xiphoid process
- Iliac crests
- Anterior superior iliac spines
- Pubic crests and tubercles
- Inguinal ligaments
- Umbilicus
- Linea alba

For purposes of locating abdominal structures and describing abnormalities, the abdomen is conventionally divided into four quadrants (Fig. 44.12). Another method divides the regions of the abdomen into nine sections (see Fig. 44.10B). Either method may be used, although division into quadrants is most commonly seen.

OSTEOPATHIC ABDOMINAL DIAGNOSIS

History

While beyond the scope of this chapter, it must be emphasized that a thorough history is a critical element in making a correct

---

TABLE 44.1

Abdominal Regions and Their Associated Deep Fascial Layers

Region	Fascial Layer
Internal surface of the transversus abdominis	Transversalis fascia
Inferior surface of thoracolumbar diaphragm	Diaphragmatic fascia
Psoas and iliac areas	Iliac fascia
Anterior surface of the quadratus lumborum muscles	Anterior layer of the thoracolumbar fascia
Muscles of the pelvis	Pelvis fascia

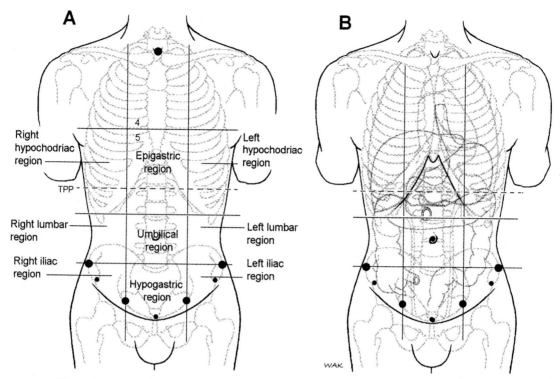

Figure 44-10   A. Approximate location of visceral organs. **B.** The nine-quadrant abdomen.

diagnosis of a patient's abdominal problem. The history should include at least the following information:

1. Chief complaint
2. History of the chief complaint
3. Past medical history
4. Past surgical history
5. Current medications
6. Nutritional history
7. Allergies
8. Family and social history
9. Review of systems

The reader is referred to standard textbooks on patient interviewing for more information on this topic.

Physical Examination

A complete physical examination is performed with special emphasis on regions that are spotlighted by the history or that might have functional association with the symptoms expressed by the patient. In this chapter, only the more important points as related to a patient with abdominal symptoms are considered.

General

Before beginning the abdominal examination, care must be taken to ensure that the patient is as relaxed as possible and in a comfortable position. The examination of the abdomen is commonly done with the patient in the supine position, resting comfortably on an examination table or bed. A pillow supports the patient's head; a patient with increased thoracic kyphosis may require more than one pillow for support of the head and shoulders. A pillow may be placed under the patient's knees for additional comfort. If orthopnea is present, raise and support the trunk with a back rest to relax the abdominal muscles (18). The patient should be draped in a manner that allows the abdomen to be exposed from the xiphoid region to the

pubes. The examining room temperature should be adjusted for the patient's comfort, and the room should be adequately illuminated for the performance of the examination. The physician may stand on either side of the patient for the examination. The only instruments required for performing the abdominal examination are the physician's warm hands and warm stethoscope head. The examination should employ the methods of physical examination in the following sequence: observation, auscultation, palpation, and percussion. The osteopathic physician includes examination for the elements of somatic dysfunction commonly noted by the TART acronym.

Observation

For this part of the examination, the examiner should be seated in a chair at the side of the patient so that the examiner's head is only slightly higher than the abdomen. Ideally, there should be a single source of light that shines across the patient's abdomen toward the examiner, or lengthwise over the patient (18). The abdomen is observed for the following:

- Symmetry
- Contour
- Scars
- Pulsations
- Visible masses
- Engorged veins
- Visible peristalsis
- Unusual pigmentation
- Hair distribution
- Distention

Auscultation

Auscultate the four quadrants of the abdomen to determine the presence, location, frequency, and pitch of peristaltic waves. This could reveal the intermittent, low-pitched, occasional slow gurgle

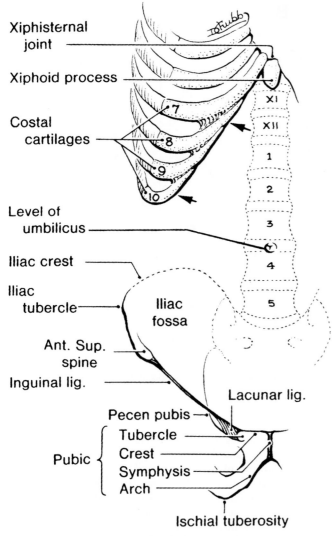

Figure 44-11 The abdominal landmarks.

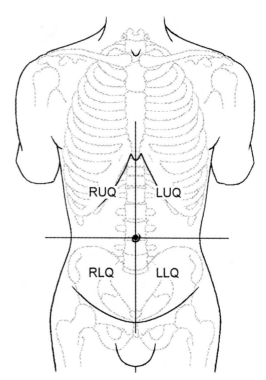

Figure 44-12 The four-quadrant abdomen.

that is normal, or the high-pitched, tinkling sounds of developing obstruction. Bowel sounds may be absent, indicating possible paralytic ileus. The midline of the abdomen between the xiphoid process and the umbilicus is auscultated for bruits. These could indicate an aneurysm and/or renal artery stenosis. The periumbilical region and the junction between the middle and outer two thirds of the inguinal region are auscultated for a bruit that could be associated with a significant atherosclerosis of the common iliac or femoral artery.

Percussion

Percussion of the abdomen is more commonly performed in the asymptomatic patient, since, in the interest of patient comfort, painful conditions of the abdomen may preclude the use of percussion. Ordinarily percussion is used to outline the borders and help to determine the approximate size and position of solid organs, such as the liver, and hollow fluid-filled organs such as the urinary bladder. In general, the hollow viscera that occupy most of the abdomen contain gas and are usually resonant to percussion.

Palpation

Palpation of the abdomen begins with a touch that is light yet firm, using the palmar surfaces of the approximated fingers to contact the abdominal wall. The physician lightly palpates each quadrant,

checking for tenderness, any cutaneous or subcutaneous masses, and any unusual sensitivity. If the patient is apprehensive or is unable to relax during palpation of the abdomen, it is useful to ask the patient to flex his or her hips and knees in order to facilitate relaxation of the abdominal muscles.

During light palpation, the physician can assess the abdominal wall for somatic dysfunction. Each quadrant of the abdomen can be palpated for abnormal myofascial tension, and the presence of tender points such as counterstrain points and Chapman reflex points (Fig. 44-13). One should note that Chapman reflex points related to abdominal visceral pathology are located next to the sternum in the intercostal spaces of ribs 5 through 11 and at the tip of rib 12, along the lateral thigh areas, and posteriorly along the thoracic and lumbar vertebral columns.

After performing light palpation, the osteopathic physician proceeds to deep palpation of the abdomen. Each quadrant is examined for tenderness, masses, or enlarged organs. At this time, the physician also assesses the deep fasciae and soft tissues of the abdomen, looking for abnormal tissue tensions that might indicate disturbance related to the collateral ganglia or mesenteries. The mobility and motility of the various abdominal organs may be assessed according to the theory and techniques described by Sutherland (19), Barral (11), and others.

Osteopathic Manipulative Treatment for Abdominal Disorders

Treatment Goals

As with OMT to any other body region, OMT should be applied to the abdominal region with specific goals in mind. The goals of treatment will vary with each individual patient. Some of these goals include:

■ Addressing asymmetries, motion restrictions, and tissue texture abnormalities that are viscerosomatic reflections of homeostatic disturbances

Palpatory findings:

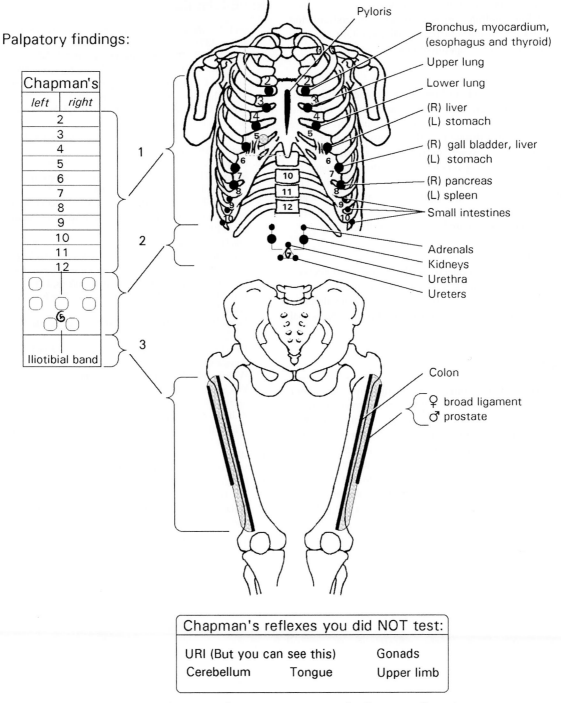

Figure 44-13 Thirty-second screening examination for Chapman reflex points.

- Decreasing or eliminating pain
- Removing segmental motion restrictions
- Improving altered skeletal vertebral unit and myofascial motion arising from aberrant visceral and autonomic activity
- Decreasing or eliminating segmental facilitation
- Decreasing or eliminating trigger point and tender point activity
- Decreasing pathophysiologic musculoskeletal and neuroreflexive factors influencing circulation
- Enhancing musculoskeletal and neuroreflexive-mediated circulatory functions

- Improving organ function
- Altering any or all of the previously mentioned situations as either contributing to, or predictive of, future health problems

Approaches to Using Osteopathic Manipulative Techniques on the Abdomen

Spinal Approach

Any spinal somatic dysfunctions that may relate to an abdominal problem should be treated in order to improve spinal motion and therefore restore normal nerve function in segmentally related areas. This approach includes typical manipulative methods such as high velocity/low amplitude, muscle energy, counterstrain, and others. Paraspinal rib raising and paraspinal inhibition are used effectively for treatment of sympathicotonia.

Peripheral Approach

This approach includes such techniques as thoracic and pedal lymphatic pumps, diaphragmatic redoming, and thoracic inlet and pelvic diaphragm releases. These techniques are used to improve the ability to move fluids throughout the abdominal region, thus improving the delivery of oxygen, nutrients, and arterial blood to affected areas, and facilitating venous and lymphatic drainage for the removal of the waste products of cellular metabolism. This approach also includes the use of diagnostic Chapman reflexes and their soft tissue treatment, such as treatment of Chapman points for the large bowel that are located on the lateral thigh areas.

Direct Approach

These techniques are applied directly to the abdomen to alleviate TART changes in the abdominal wall structures. Some techniques are applied more deeply to affect structures such as the abdominal mesenteries, the collateral ganglia, or specific abdominal organs.

SUMMARY

One should not forget that somatic dysfunction may be present with abdominal visceral conditions. Optimum treatment of these conditions should be based on osteopathic philosophy and principles, and should include appropriate OMT. Using osteopathic manipulation as part of a complete treatment approach to the patient with an abdominal visceral disorder serves several purposes. It provides a more holistic, total body approach to the treatment of a patient's medical problems, it addresses important structure–function relationships, and it helps to optimize the patient's self-healing and self-regulatory mechanisms.

REFERENCES

1. Still AT. *Autobiography of A.T. Still*. Kirksville, MO: Published by the author, 1897.
2. Still AT. *The Philosophy and Mechanical Principles of Osteopathy*. Kansas City, MO: Hudson-Kimberly Publishing Company, 1902.
3. Hazzard C. *The Practice and Applied Therapeutics of Osteopathy*. Kirksville, MO: The Journal Printing Company, 1901.
4. Conrad CF. *A Manual of Osteopathy*. 4th Ed. New York, NY: The University Book Company, 1919.
5. McConnell CP. *Ventral Technique*. Indianapolis, IN: The American Academy of Osteopathy, Yearbook, 1951.
6. Owens C. *An Endocrine Interpretation of Chapman's Reflexes*. Carmel, CA: Reprinted by the American Academy of Osteopathy, 1932.
7. Hermann E. *The DO*. 1965;163–164.
8. Radjieski JM, Lumley MA, Canteri MS. Effect of osteopathic manipulative treatment on length of stay for pancreatitis: a randomized pilot study. *JAOA* 1998;98:15.
9. Pikalov AA, Kharin VV. Use of spinal manipulative therapy in the treatment of duodenal ulcer: a pilot study. *J Manipulative Physiol Ther* 1994;17:5.
10. Travell JG, Simons DG. *Myofascial Pain and Dysfunction: The Trigger Point Manual*. Baltimore, MD: Williams & Wilkins, 1999.
11. Barral JP, Mercier P. *Visceral Manipulation*. Rev. Ed. Seattle, WA: Eastland Press, 2006.
12. Barral JP. *Visceral Manipulation II*. Rev. Ed. Seattle, WA: Eastland Press, 2007.
13. Finet G, Wiallame C. *Treating Visceral Dysfunction*. Portland, OR: Stillness Press, 2000.
14. Williams PL, Warwick R, eds. *Gray's Anatomy*. 39th Ed. Philadelphia, PA: WB Saunders, 2004.
15. Spraycar M, ed. *Stedman's Medical Dictionary*. 26th Ed. Baltimore, MD: Williams & Wilkins, 1999.
16. Chikly B. *Silent Waves: Theory and Practice of Lymph Drainage Therapy*. Scottsdale, AZ: International Health & Healing Inc. Publishing, 2002.
17. Willms JL, Schneiderman H, Algranati PS. *Physical Diagnosis*. Baltimore, MD: Williams & Wilkins, 1994.
18. LeBlonde RF, DeGowin RL, Brown DD. *DeGowin's Diagnostic Examination*. 8th Ed. New York, NY: McGraw-Hill, 2004.
19. Sutherland WG. In: Wales AL, ed. *Teachings in the Science of Osteopathy*. Fort Worth, TX: The Sutherland Cranial Teaching Foundation, 1990.

45

Thrust (High Velocity/Low Amplitude) Approach; "The Pop"

JOHN G. HOHNER AND TYLER C. CYMET

KEY CONCEPTS

- The high-velocity/low-amplitude (HVLA) (thrust) approach is characterized by positioning to engage the restrictive barrier, followed by a corrective maneuver to move through the barrier.
- Accurate diagnosis is the key to performance of HVLA (thrust) techniques.
- Positioning against the restrictive barrier in all planes is followed by a rapid and brief corrective thrust.
- HVLA (thrust) techniques can be taught and learned easily. The necessary motor coordination for effective use requires extensive practice and experience.

CASE STUDY

D.J. is a 27-year-old female who presented with right-hand numbness of 1 month duration. She started a new job, as a cashier, about 2 months ago. She stated that at first, her entire right hand started to "fall asleep" occasionally while working at her cash register. At the time of her visit, the numbness occurred within five minutes of working and was relieved with rest. She had also noted right-sided upper back pain over the past month. There was no history of injury or previous numbness. There was no past medical or surgical history. She tried ibuprofen and a wrist splint without improvement.

Physical examination revealed normal vital signs, normal cardiac and pulmonary exams. Neuromusculoskeletal exam revealed normal motor, reflexes, and sensation of the right upper extremity. Tinel and Phalen tests were negative. Acute tissue texture changes and tenderness were noted over the transverse process area of T3 right. Motion changes were noted at T3 consistent with somatic dysfunction at T3 E SR right with a *distinct barrier* found at attempts to flex, side bend, and rotate T3 to the left.

The presence of distinct barrier mechanics means that this type of somatic dysfunction would be amenable to HVLA treatment.

DEFINITION OF TECHNIQUE

The Glossary of Osteopathic Terminology defines high-velocity/low-amplitude (HVLA) technique as, "An osteopathic technique employing a rapid, therapeutic force of brief duration that travels a short distance within the anatomic range of motion of a joint, and that engages the restrictive barrier in one or more planes of motion to elicit release of restriction. Also known as thrust technique."

VARIABILITY OF THRUST TECHNIQUES

"Thrust techniques" are a collection of direct method manipulative treatments that move a restricted joint through its dysfunctional barrier (1). These techniques vary widely in the amount, speed, localization, and application vectors of the treatment forces that are applied. The common treatment goal is that, after the thrust, appropriate physiologic motion is restored to the dysfunctional joint. The term *direct* refers specifically to positioning the restricted

joint(s) to engage the restrictive barrier and then applying a corrective force to move through that dysfunctional barrier. Simply stated, one moves the restricted joint in the direction it won't move. When speaking of osteopathic HVLA thrust manipulation, after precise positioning against the restrictive barriers in all planes, the final force is a quick (high-velocity), short (low-amplitude) thrust. The velocity of the actual thrust is rapid and brief. The amplitude is sufficient to move through the restrictive barrier but precise enough to stop short of or at the anatomic barrier. Greenman (2) describes this force as an "impulse." Often, a click or pop is heard at the time the force is applied. Upon reassessment of the treated joint, there should be an immediate increase in both the range of motion and the freedom of motion. *Indirect* treatments, involving positioning into the direction of ease, are described elsewhere (3).

HISTORIC PERSPECTIVE

Thrust styles of manipulation have been documented worldwide throughout recorded history (4). The European immigrants brought the techniques of the "bone setters" to America with them (5). The ensuing American schools of osteopathic medicine and chiropractic medicine developed since (Chapter 3).

Robert Kappler, D.O., has theorized on the development of HVLA as a distinctly osteopathic modality as follows:

> Thrust technique has been the major type of technique taught in colleges of osteopathic medicine and has been practiced by osteopathic physicians for years. In the 1970s, the osteopathic medical school curricula began to include other types of techniques. Until recently, however, osteopathic manipulation and high-velocity technique were essentially synonymous. Graduates are now exposed to a complete spectrum of direct and indirect techniques; therefore, osteopathic manipulation is no longer synonymous with thrust technique.

It is interesting to speculate why osteopathic manipulative techniques taught in the colleges evolved into the exclusive domain of thrust techniques and remained that way for so many years. Faculty may have been responsible for the change. Students, in the early days, assisted in the teaching of techniques. These students may have played a major role in moving the curriculum to thrust techniques. Thrust techniques can be taught by precisely describing the nature of the restriction and providing techniques for treating the dysfunction. These techniques can then be memorized and practiced. In contrast, fascial release and indirect techniques require skill in assessing motion patterns in the tissues. The technique is difficult to describe because the physician is responding to tactile and proprioceptive input from his or her hands. Faculty find release techniques difficult to teach and students may perceive them as abstractions. Thrust techniques are easier to teach and to learn. However, although thrust techniques can be described in a precise manner, the motor coordination necessary to use these techniques effectively requires extensive practice and experience.

DIAGNOSIS AND SOMATIC DYSFUNCTION

It cannot be stated strongly enough that the key to properly performing thrust manipulation with the greatest efficacy and the least side effects is the ability to diagnose accurately and to only use HVLA technique when the diagnosis warrants it. The practitioner first must learn to perform a palpatory diagnosis (see Chapter 33) and understand what these findings mean. Only then can the treating physician use those findings to determine the best treatment methodology. Somatic dysfunction is the term used to describe the areas of impaired or altered function of related components of the somatic system which are identified by the palpatory diagnosis. By necessity, this term encompasses a wide variety of musculoskeletal disorders.

"Somatic dysfunction" can include disordered changes among some or all of the bones, muscles, fascia, arthrodial structures and their associated neural vascular and lymphatic components. This variety of etiologic elements is reflected both in the wide variance between the possible palpatory somatic dysfunction diagnoses and in the possible treatment choices. This plethora of disparate diagnostic possibilities gives rise to the need for a methodology to differentiate them and thus to be able to choose the optimal treatment modality. Manipulation is much more efficacious when the modality chosen is correctly matched to the type of somatic dysfunction that is found. When examining an area for somatic dysfunction, identify changes from the norm by using the mnemonic TARt:

- Are there palpable tissue texture changes (T)?
- Is there visually observable asymmetry (A)?
- Is there a restriction of motion (R)?
- Does the palpatory exam elicit tenderness (t)?

BARRIER MECHANICS

To understand the type of somatic dysfunction that is amenable to HVLA manipulation, one has to understand the Barrier Concept (Fig. 45.1). The Barrier Concept refers to the movement capabilities of a joint during normal and restricted motion. These movement capabilities are evaluated, during the palpatory exam, by both their quantity and quality of motion. The quantity is the amount of movement from the joint's midline or neutral point of motion to a motion barrier. The neutral point of motion is that position of a nondysfunctional joint at rest, with equal myofascial forces pulling it in all directions. Quantity of motion is determined by the amount of movement from the neutral point (Fig. 45.1).

When a healthy joint is actively moved during normal activity, the end of motion is at the physiologic barrier. When the range of motion of a joint is tested passively during a physical examination, the end of the furthest motion is the anatomic barrier. Motion beyond the anatomic barrier implies disruption of osseous or ligamentous structures of that joint. Both the anatomic and

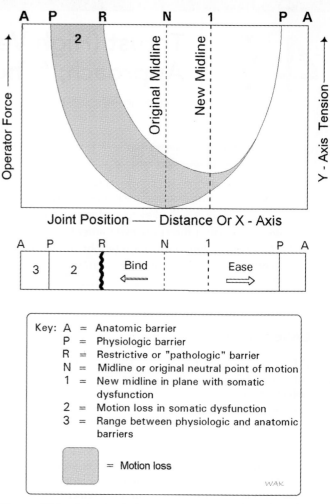

Figure 45-1 Somatic dysfunction: quantity and quality of joint motion. (*Foundations for Osteopathic Medicine*. 2nd Ed., p. 853)

the physiologic barriers are present in healthy joints without any dysfunction. A third barrier, the restrictive or pathologic barrier, is found when a joint experiences the motion loss of somatic dysfunction. The quantity of motion to arrive at the restrictive barrier is less than the amount traveled to reach the physiologic barrier. This shifts the midline of joint motion away from the restrictive barrier. The palpatory experience, when the examiner feels the restricted motion, is that the joint will move better in one direction than in the other. One of the goals of manipulative treatment is to aid a return to normal, unrestricted motion.

The quality of motion refers to the palpatory sense of how smoothly a joint can be moved through its range of motion. A resistance or hesitance through motion implies some type of dysfunction of the joint. End feel is a term describing the quality of motion that is felt by palpation of a joint when it is brought passively to its final barrier of motion. End feel can be a function of both the focal tissue turgor at the region of the somatic dysfunction and the tethering actions of the muscle and fascia which is being stretched. The end feel is nebulous or rubbery with reflex somatic dysfunctions. The end feel is firm and distinctive with mechanical-type arthrodial dysfunctions.

The quantity and quality of motion, along with the end feel, allow the examiner to determine the Restriction of motion in the diagnostic TARt mnemonic mentioned earlier. It is TARt that defines somatic dysfunction. The components of TARt that predominate for any given dysfunction then can dictate how to treat that dysfunction with manipulation. In this author's opinion, HVLA or thrust manipulation would be the modality of choice in a dysfunction that has distinctive barrier mechanics with a palpable loss of motion at a restrictive barrier and with a firm end feel. HVLA is designed to remove motion loss, regain normal motion, and restore normal barriers in somatic dysfunction. If one were to weight the importance of the TARt components in the diagnosis of a somatic dysfunction to be treated with HVLA, it would look like this TARt. Similarly weighted, the TARt for Counterstrain diagnosis might look like TARt. All TARt is not created equal.

MECHANISM OF TREATMENT

To understand why HVLA works on an area of somatic dysfunction, one must first understand *why* the dysfunctional segment won't move. A somatic dysfunction exhibiting barrier mechanics is *not* "subluxed," "out of place," "out of joint," or "dislocated." Like a door that will not fully close, it is inhibited from completing its full normal motion. What *is* going on is that some external or internal force or factor has caused local segmental irritation sufficient to create focal edema and swelling in a small discrete area (6). This in turn causes a tightening of the fascial structures, myofascial component, and capsular components of a specific arthrodial joint. The articular distortion results in reflex hypertonicity of the musculature crossing the given joint. There is thus a resultant decrease to the range of motion around that area. This is discussed in the osteopathic and scientific literature on proprioceptors and somatic dysfunction (7–12). The palpatory experience is described earlier. In more simplistic terms, on motion testing, "it *will* go this way, it *won't* go that way." Restoration of motion of the articulation results in restoration of normal proprioceptive input from the joint and reflex relaxation of muscles surrounding the joint.

There are special considerations when treatment is applied to a vertebral joint as opposed to an appendicular joint. The "typical" vertebral joints (C2-L5) are assessed in the three cardinal planes of motion. Restrictions are classically found in sidebending, rotation, and flexion/extension. The thrust treatment however is along a summed vector of all these findings. The unique motion patterns found in the sacroiliac (SI), atlantoaxial, and occipitoatlantal joints are addressed in the cervical and sacral chapters. The HVLA treatments for SI and occipitoatlantal joint dysfunctions also tend to be along a summed vector. Atlantoaxial dysfunctions are diagnosed and treated in a rotational manner along a vertical axis. The entire gamut of appendicular motion patterns does not lend itself to treatment generalizations, but a few trends do predominate. Many appendicular joints have a predominant major joint motion and lesser minor joint motions. The patient presents with loss of, and pain with, the major joint motion. This is frequently the result of a restricted minor joint motion and treatment is focused along a single vector of the minor joint motion loss.

The mechanism of the audible pop or snap, which is frequently heard at the moment of the thrust, is a subject of great debate (13). It is frequently, but not always, the harbinger of a successful treatment. The production of noise may merely be the incidental result of treatment forces spilling over to a joint above or below the targeted dysfunction. Similarly, a lack of an audible articulation does *not* mean that the restrictive barrier was not successfully treated. In any case, the treatment should always be followed with thorough reassessment. Box 45.1 addresses the issue of joint noise.

Joint Noise The Manipulative Crack/Pop/Click/ Snap/Grind or Thud

Tyler Cymet, D.O.

Joints make noise. Joint noise may occur with regular use of the joint by an individual, and it may occur with motion of the joint induced by a health care provider moving or treating a specific area.[i]

The noises that emanate from joints have intrigued and confounded physicians. Laennec was unclear as to the reason for these sounds and noted the presence of joint noise in his treatise on lung sounds.[ii]

It is the noises that are evident to the patient and provider that attract the most attention, but there are noises that emanate from the joint that are not apparent to the unaided ear. Auscultation of joints can be performed with a myodermato-osteophone, which was developed by Heuter in 1885 to help physicians locate areas where joint activity was not fluid.[iii]

Studies on joint sounds have focused on objective analysis of the sound or vibration signals, also known as vibroarthrographic signals that are measureable.[iv]

There is also a theory that joints that make noise are more likely to develop medical issues. This theory arose from a study by Walters linking joint noise and early development of arthritis that was published in 1929.[v]

Some people argue that a noise or sound is a necessary part of a manipulation, and the occurrence of noise along with a manipulative medicine procedure is what differentiates a manipulation from mobilization of a joint.[vi] Others contend that the presence or absence of a noise is irrelevant to the effect of a mobilization or manipulation.[vii]

The reason for joint noise is unclear. A hypothesis explaining the reason for joint noise suggests eventration of gas into the synovial fluid with the breaking of the surface tension of the fluid causing the pop sound.[viii] It may also be that the noise comes from the snapping or releasing of ligamentous adhesions in the joint,[ix] or that the bone itself is being pulled out of place and snapping back into a neutral position.[x] It may also be a ballooning of the joint capsule that causes the noise to occur (Ehrenfeutchter W, Nicholas AS, *personal communication*).

While we do not know what the relationship is between joint noise and effective manipulative treatments, acknowledging what is seen and experienced by the patient and provider is a necessary part of a good treatment. We may need to reassure our patients that a joint noise isn't necessary for a successful treatment, and presence of a noise isn't considered to be an issue.

[i]Protoppapas M, Cymet TC. Joint cracking and popping: understanding noises that accompany articular release. *JAOA* 2002;102(5):283–287.

[ii]Laennec RTH. *A Treatise on the Diseases of the Chest and on Mediate Auscultation*. London: Underwood, 1848.

[iii]Mollan RAB, McCullagh GC, Wilson RI. A critical appraisal of auscultation of human joints. *Clin Orthop Relat Res* 1982;170:231–237.

[iv]McCoy GF, McCrea JD, Beverland DE, et al. Vibration arthrography as a diagnostic aid in disease of the knee. *J Bone Joint Surg* 1987;69-B(2):288–2931.

[v]Walters CF. The value of joint auscultation. *Lancet* 1929;1:920–921.

[vi]Mierau D, Cassidy JD, Bowen V, et al. Manipulation and mobilization of the third metacarpophalangeal joint-a quantitative radiographic and range of motion study. *Man Med* 1988;3:135–140.

[vii]Reggars JW. Multiple channel recording of the articular crack associated with manipulation of the metacarpophalangeal joint: an observational study *Aust Chiropr Osteopath* 1999;8(1):16–20.

[viii]Unsworth A, Dowson D, Wright V. Cracking joints: a bioengineering study of cavitation in the metacarpophalangeal joint. *Ann Rheum Dis* 1972;30:348–358.

[ix]Hood W. Symposium. Manipulative treatment. *Med J Aust* 1967;1(25):1274–1280. Cited by Heilig D. The thrust technique. *J Am Osteopath Assoc* 1981;81:247.

[x]Hood W. Symposium. Manipulative treatment. *Med J Aust* 1967;1(25):1274–1280. Cited by Heilig D. The thrust technique. *J Am Osteopath Assoc* 1981;81:247.

TECHNIQUE METHODOLOGY

The HVLA approach involves:

- Initial positioning
- Engagement and stacking of barriers
- Accumulation of forces
- Final corrective thrust

Initial Positioning

Initial positioning refers to both the physician's own position and that of the patient. Once the physician is in a relaxed and balanced position, his or her cortex will be freed up to pay attention to the diagnostic input from the fingers and hands as he or she continually fine-tunes the technique during its application. If the physician's own proprioceptors are firing due to imbalance from an awkward stance during the treatment, or straining to hold up more weight than one's own strength allows, it is difficult to focus on the treatment at hand.

Position the patient comfortably at the start of the treatment. This allows the patient to relax. In turn, this decreases the tonicity of the longer muscles overlying the dysfunction and the pull from muscles above and below the dysfunction. A patient will feel imbalance on the part of a treating physician and tense his or her own muscles in anticipation of a fall or drop. When performing a treatment using HVLA, one wants to focus the vector forces as precisely as possible and use only the minimum force that is necessary. The more variables that can be eliminated from the manipulative equation, the more likely one will obtain a successful solution.

Engagement and Stacking of Barriers

Engage barriers in sidebending, rotation, and flexion/extension. The physician "stacks" these individual components to address each component of the somatic dysfunction just as one would with muscle energy or myofascial release techniques. Maintain each previously engaged barrier as the next barrier is engaged and the forces accumulate. As a clinician becomes experienced, this summation of vector forces, along with the arrival at a single summed vector, becomes very fast and efficient. Experienced physicians sense how the tissues are responding to the force being applied and make subtle alterations in the direction of force to effectively engage the barrier in all planes. If this set up is painful to the patient or the physician, then something is wrong! Move the patient back to his or her neutral position and reassess. The technique set up may be incorrect or the patient may have a somatic dysfunction of a type that is not amenable to HVLA. In that case, use some other modality! One may simply need to treat some overlying soft tissue dysfunction first and then retry the HVLA.

Accumulation of Forces

The basis of most HVLA treatment is that one is treating the dysfunctional relationship between two bones. To treat them, the physician holds one bone still and moves the other the way it would really rather not go at the moment. The discomfort, if any, that a patient experiences during an HVLA treatment, is at the moment when all of the forces are stacked against the restrictive barrier. This is a natural conclusion to correct stacking as mentioned above. A novice frequently runs into trouble at this stage,

by losing concentration and relaxing the forces on the segment. If this happens, do not continue with the thrust. Forces that do not accumulate at the dysfunctional segment dissipate into adjacent structures and could result in an iatrogenic side effect. Instead, reassess and set up the stacking again. The accumulation of forces is not a separate phase. It should be viewed, instead, as an instantaneous transit point between the final summation of forces and the thrust.

Final Corrective Thrust

HVLA thrust techniques use a short, rapid thrust, hence the words high velocity. Once the barrier is engaged, the final force is applied quickly from that position. The proper application has been described as a tack hammer blow, sudden but not forceful. The term *impulse* applied to HVLA technique recognizes that the force is a sudden acceleration and deceleration. Do not back off before delivering the corrective thrust. The exhalation phase of respiration is the relaxation phase, and the final force is often applied during exhalation. If intuition tells one not to thrust, then don't. The physician's "intuition" is probably based on proprioceptive feedback that some part of the treatment is not balanced properly.

Some thrust techniques are not executed at high velocity and some have a larger or variable amplitude of motion during the articulation. Consider an experience where the patient is set up to treat a joint restriction, the joint goes click, and the restriction is released as the physician is positioning the patient and localizing forces. Sometimes, one may instead tease a joint with carefully and slowly applied forces. Again, experience is very beneficial in applying the proper force. Although HVLA is described as thrust technique, the actual speed and force may be modified to fit the patient's needs.

DOSAGE

Give the patient time to respond to the treatment; the sicker the patient, the less the dose. Older patients respond more slowly; young patients respond more quickly. In most circumstances, treating the same segment more than once a week using thrust technique is discouraged (14). When treating hospital patients on a daily basis, Larson (N.J. Larson, *personal communication*, 1967, 1978) would vary the technique, so he did not repeat the same technique on a given area. If the same somatic dysfunction keeps recurring, then the physician needs to assess why this is happening and address that factor first. In this author's opinion, continual thrust treatment on the same segment, without improvement, is a good recipe for hypermobility but not much else.

BENEFITS OF HVLA

HVLA is well tolerated and extremely time efficient in the hands of a skilled practitioner. It is a modality of choice when addressing somatic dysfunction with distinct, firm barrier mechanics. The patient usually experiences immediate relief, with decreased pain and increased freedom of motion.

PRECAUTIONS AND CONTRAINDICATIONS

Some joints are unstable and hypermobile. Within the numerous joints of the spine, a pattern of alternating hypomobility and hypermobility may exist. The loose, hypermobile joints are overworked while the stiff, hypomobile joints escape excess motion. A normal physiologic reaction to a painful hypermobile joint is for muscles surrounding the joint to splint the joint and protect it from excess motion. Physical examination reveals restriction of motion. Underneath that protective muscle splinting is an unstable joint. A high-velocity thrust technique may work, as evidenced by a decrease in pain and improvement in motion. Unfortunately, the treatment contributes to the joint instability. The more HVLA technique is used, the looser the joint becomes.

Most of the concerns with HVLA center on treatment of the cervical spine (15). Both advanced rheumatoid arthritis and Down syndrome diagnoses should cause the practitioner to consider alar ligament instability. Dislocation of the dens associated with rupture or laxity of the transverse ligament of the atlas can cause death or quadriplegia. Cervical manipulation has been associated with vertebral basilar thrombosis (15). Advanced carotid disease should cause one to be careful with any form of cervical manipulation. With all this having been said, the Position Paper on Cervical Manipulation by the American Osteopathic Association speaks on the overwhelming safety of cervical manipulation in general (16).

General contradictions to HVLA include local metastases and osseous or ligamentous disruption. Apprehension on the part of the patient is a relative contraindication. In other circumstances, consider the risk/benefit ratio. If the risk of harming the patient exceeds the potential therapeutic benefit, the technique is not indicated. Risk also relates to the skill of the physician. There is more risk with an unskilled physician. If forceful, direct techniques may harm the patient, gentle indirect release techniques might be considered.

DIAGNOSES AND TECHNIQUES

739.0 Head-Suboccipital Somatic Dysfunction

OA E RR SL (Anterior/Extended Occiput)

Dysfunction: Anterior left occiput (The occiput is rotated to the right and sidebent to the left, with tissue texture change on the left.).

Objective: To improve left rotation and right sidebending of the occiput.

Discussion: When the occiput is rotated right and sidebent left, the left OA joint is held in a facet "locked closed" position. The OA joint on the right side is held in a "facet locked open" position. This technique addresses the "facet locked closed" position by opening the joint with the applied corrective force. An anterior occiput is a "pull" technique (translate the head toward the "locked close" side, to accumulate force at the anterior occiput).

Patient Position: Supine.

Physician Position: Standing at the head of the table.

Procedure (Fig. 45.2):

1. Place your right 2nd metacarpal-phalangeal joint against the right posterior lateral aspect of the patient's occiput with your fingers projecting around the posterior skull and your thumb angled up toward the patient's eye
2. The head and neck are raised from the table and a small amount of extension is introduced (over your right fulcrum hand) to allow localization of forces between the occiput and atlas
3. Grip the most inferior/lateral aspect of the patient's left occiput with your left fingertips, allowing the patient's head to lie in your left hand. Using a coordinated movement of your two hands, gently rotate the head to the left until the barrier is engaged

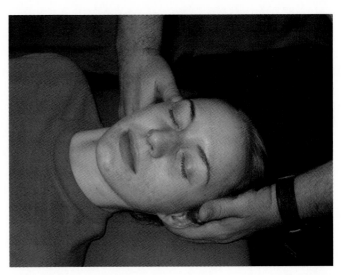

Figure 45-2 Occiput on atlas—anterior/extended dysfunction.

4. To localize to the dysfunction, simultaneously exert a cephalad pulling force with your left fingertips and a mild translation force to the left with your right 2nd metacarpophalangeal joint. At this point, you should feel all the forces accumulate at the left OA joint
5. A small amount of additional posterior translation from your left fingers is necessary to localize forces to the OA joint
6. The final corrective movement is a quick rotatory thrust to the left, with more of a "pull" through your left hand and a slight "push" with the right
7. Reassess

OA F RR SL (Posterior/Flexed Occiput)

Dysfunction: Posterior right occiput (The occiput is rotated to the right and sidebent to the left, with tissue texture change on the right).

Objective: To improve left rotation and right sidebending of the occiput.

Discussion: When the occiput is rotated right and sidebent left, the left OA joint is held in a facet "locked closed" position. The OA joint on the right side is held in a "facet locked open" position. This technique addresses the "facet locked open" position by closing the joint with the applied corrective force. The posterior occiput is a "push" technique (translate in the direction of the nose to engage localization at the posterior occiput).

Patient Position: Supine.

Physician Position: Standing at the head of the table.

Procedure (Fig. 45.3):

1. Place your right second metacarpal-phalangeal joint (index finger) over the posterior lateral aspect of the patient's occiput with your fingers projecting around the posterior skull and your thumb angled up toward the patient's eye
2. The head and neck are raised (one inch or less) from the table and a small amount of extension is introduced (over your right fulcrum hand) to allow localization of forces between the occiput and atlas
3. Cradle the left side of the patient's face on the anterior aspect of your left forearm and palm. Contact the soft tissues under the patient's left mandible with the fingertips of your left hand. Gently rotate the head to the left until the barrier is engaged

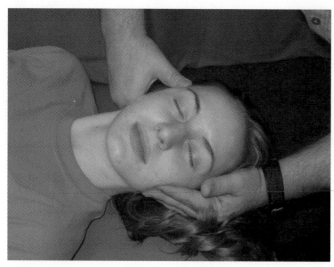

Figure 45-3   Occiput on atlas—posterior/flexed dysfunction.

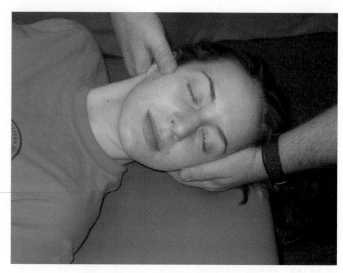

Figure 45-4   Atlas on axis dysfunction.

4. Using your left forearm as a lever, slightly lift the head, while simultaneously applying a mild translation force downward with your right index finger. At this point, you (and the patient) should feel all the forces accumulate at the right OA joint

5. A small anteriorly directed translatory force helps to localize forces to the OA joint

6. The final corrective movement is a quick rotatory thrust to the left through your right MCP joint. This is actually more of a "push technique" with left rotation achieved by translation toward the nose, pushing the posterior occiput anteriorly

7. Reassess motion

739.1 Cervical Somatic Dysfunction

AA N RR (Posterior Atlas)

Dysfunction: Atlas (C1) on axis (C2) rotated right (posterior atlas right).

Objective: Improve atlas (C1) rotation to the left.

Discussion: Unlike other cervical vertebrae, somatic dysfunction of the atlas occurs in its major motion—rotation. A posterior atlas has tissue texture change and tenderness on the freer side of rotation. An anterior atlas has tissue texture change on the restricted side of rotation.

Patient Position: Lying supine.

Physician Position: Standing at the head of the table.

Procedure (Fig. 45.4):

1. Place the lateral aspect of your right index finger over the right posterior aspect of the atlas. The fingers of your right hand are allowed to encircle the posterior aspect of the patient's neck, just below the occiput. Your right thumb should be pointing across the patient's cheek, contacting the lateral aspect of the right zygomatic process

2. Your left hand is placed over the patient's left temporo-occipital area, with your fingers spread to provide comfortable control of the head. Your left index and middle finger should contact the left atlantoaxial joint to maintain localization of forces

3. With hands positioned as above, the head and neck are raised from the table, to a neutral position, and a *small* amount of

extension (backward bending) is introduced between the atlas (C1) and the axis (C2), to facilitate localization of forces

4. Employing a combined motion with your right and left hands, rotate the head and atlas vertebra to the left until the barrier is engaged. Check to be sure that the right index finger is applying force over the atlas (C1) and has not "slipped" down onto the axis (C2)

5. With the barrier engaged, apply a short, quick, final corrective thrust of left rotation

6. Return the patient's head and neck to the neutral position

7. Reassess motion

C2-7 Dysfunction (Posterior Cervical)

Dysfunction: (C5 F RR SR) C5 on C6 flexed (forward bent), rotated right, sidebent right (tissue texture change, motion restriction, and tenderness on the right)—also called a "posterior C5 right."

Objective: Improve left rotation, sidebending, and extension at C5-6.

Discussion: The most common error in this technique is to lose localization as the head and neck are rotated. It is important to sense your way into the barrier prior to applying corrective forces. If well localized, only minimal corrective force is necessary. The physician must control the head at all times.

Patient Position: Lying supine.

Physician Position: Standing at the head of the table.

Procedure (Fig. 45.5):

1. Palpate for tissue texture abnormality over the posterior component (C5 right). Place the lateral aspect of your right index finger over the posterior component. Your right thumb should point towards the patient's eye

2. Your left hand (passive) cradles the left side of the patient's head maintaining comfortable control of the head and neck throughout the procedure

3. With your right hand, introduce segmental anterior translation (an "extension break" of the neck) at the C5 on C6 level

4. Maintain this extension break over the index finger of your right hand

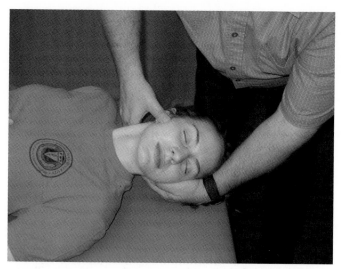

Figure 45-5   Cervical dysfunction—vertebral segments C2-7.

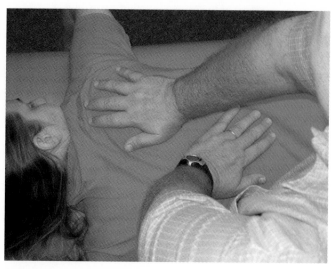

Figure 45-6   Patient prone, thoracic thrust—for a flexed thoracic dysfunction.

5. While maintaining this extension break, rotate the head and neck to the left (down to and including C5) until the restrictive barrier is reached. Sidebending left is achieved by keeping the patient's left temple close to the table. Caution—lifting the head away from the table will introduce sidebending in the wrong direction

6. It may be necessary to move your body slightly to the right side of the able to keep yourself "behind your work", which provides more comfort and control

7. The final corrective force is a quick, gentle, short rotational force through your right hand directed anteriorly and superiorly toward the eye. Do not apply excessive force to the cervical spine. Be very gentle and specific

8. Reassess

Considerations: Do not pivot the head on the table. Do not attempt to control cervical motion by placing your passive hand on the top of the head.

739.2 Thoracic Somatic Dysfunction

Patient Prone, Flexed Thoracic Thrust (Texas Twist/Cross Hand Pisiform Thrust)

Dysfunction: T5 flexed, rotated right, sidebent right; (T5 F RR SR)—posterior component right.

Objective: Improve extension, left sidebending, and left rotation.

Discussion: REMEMBER: Diagnose a dysfunction before attempting a thrust! This technique is useful for flexed dysfunctions but is not appropriate for an extended dysfunction. There are a number of variations in this technique. The placement of hands varies. Some physicians prefer to stand on one side of the table and treat dysfunction on either side of the spine. A modification of this technique may be used to thrust on the rib angle. PRECAUTION: Excessive force may crack ribs, particularly if osteoporosis is present. **This technique is contraindicated for osteoporotic patients or for an extended dysfunction.**

Patient Position: Prone.

Physician Position: Standing at the side of the table, opposite to the posterior component.

Procedure (Fig. 45.6):

1. Place your right thenar eminence over the right posterior transverse process of T5. Place your left hypothenar eminence on the opposite side of the spine contacting the left transverse process of T6

2. With firm contact over the transverse processes (refer to diagram on the previous page), push down (anterior) and superiorly on T5 right while simultaneously pushing down (anterior) and inferiorly on the left

3. Downward pressure introduces extension

4. Now translate the lesion right that effectively localizes the side-bending barrier and applies a "twist" to the soft tissues

5. Final corrective force: With your elbows locked, apply a quick, light, HVLA thrust anteriorly, predominately on the posterior transverse process of T5

6. Reassess motion

Flexed Upper Thoracic Dysfunction (Spinous Process Thrust)

Dysfunction: T2 on T3, flexed, rotated right and side bent right (T2 F RR SR)

Objective: To restore motion in extension, rotation, and side bending left.

Discussion: The upper thoracic spine is difficult to treat. This technique is useful on thoracic vertebrae 1-4, flexed and extended dysfunctions. It offers great therapeutic specificity for this problem area. This technique is most effective when the restriction is predominately sidebending. Both the hand on the spinous process and the hand on the patient's head and neck are working in synchrony to rotate and sidebend the dysfunctional segment in the same direction.

Patient Position: Seated.

Physician Position: Standing behind the patient.

Procedure (Fig. 45.7):

1. Place your right foot on the table several inches to the right of the patient's right hip

2. Drape the patient's right axilla over your right knee. You may place a pillow between your knee and the patient's axilla

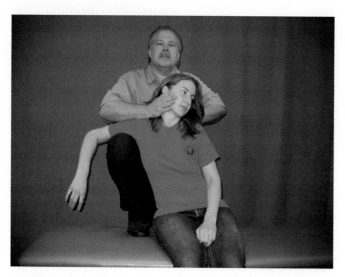

Figure 45-7 Spinous process thrust—for a flexed upper thoracic dysfunction.

3. With the fingers of your left hand loosely over the patient's left shoulder, place your left thumb in contact with the tissues on the left side of the spinous process of T2

4. Apply a downward pressure with your left hand directed toward your right knee to aid in localizing forces between T2 and T3

5. While maintaining the patient's shoulders parallel to the table-top, use your knee to translate the patient's upper torso to the right. This introduces left side bending between T2 and T3 from below

6. Place your right elbow over the patient's right shoulder with your forearm stabilizing the patient's neck/head. Your hand drapes over the top of the patient's head. This allows greater control and localization. Physicians with large hands may place their right hand, widespread, over the right side of the patient's face

7. With your right hand, translate the patient's head and neck posteriorly, moving the cervical spine as a unit, introducing extension between T2 and T3

8. With your right hand/arm, sidebend the head and neck to the left until you feel left side bending between T2 and T3

9. Rotate the head and neck to the left until you feel left rotation between T2 and T3

10. Your final corrective force is a short, transverse thrust with the thumb of your left hand producing left rotation and sidebending of T2. Raising your left elbow above the patient's shoulder will enhance the corrective force

11. Reassess

739.3 Lumbar Somatic Dysfunction

Lumbar Flexed Dysfunction (Patient on Side/Lumbar Roll)

Dysfunction: Lumbar type II somatic dysfunction. L2 rotated left, sidebent left, and flexed (L2 F RL SL).

Objective: To improve the ability of L2 to rotate and sidebend right and extend.

Discussion: Many variations of this technique exist. Some schools use patient on side technique for Fryette type I, or II dysfunctions. The mechanics of this technique may be difficult to understand,

because the corrective force is applied to the bottom segment of the vertebral unit. Dr. Kappler uses the analogy of a "two-wrench system" to loosen a bolt/nut in comparison to this technique.

The Chicago side lumbar technique for type II dysfunctions emphasizes sidebending. The applied sidebending opens the "closed facet" or "single segment concavity." The posterior component ("facet closed") is placed down. Placing the posterior component down on the table relatively fixes L2 so that "the bottom is brought around to meet the top." *The bottom of the spine is stretched out; the upper side is compressed.*

Note: Many side lumbar techniques "scissor" the patient with the upper shoulder maximally rotated. The scissor approach stretches the upper side producing inappropriate sidebending. This approach might be ok if treating a group curve.

The sequence of events in this technique is to set up the bottom (pelvis), obtain an extension break from above down, then to thrust.

Patient Position: Lying on left side facing the physician (dysfunctional side, the left side in this case, must be down) with pillow(s) supporting head. *It is crucial (especially in women with a wider pelvis) that in the side lying position, the left side of the lumbar spine is stretched, so it is in contact with the table.*

Physician Position: Standing at the side of the table, facing the patient. The table height is commonly placed at (or below) the level of the physician's hips/pelvis.

Procedure (Fig. 45.8):

1. With the patient lying on his or her left side, palpate over the posterior component and interspinous space of L2 on L3 with your right hand

2. With the patient's hips and knees flexed, grasp both of his or her lower legs and flex the patient's hips until motion is isolated at the L2-L3 interspace. Flex the patient's top leg forward over the edge of the table. The patient's top foot may hook behind his or her other knee. Lock or pin this leg to the table using your left thigh. This will maintain your localization from below

3. Switch hands so that you palpate the L2-3 vertebral unit with your left hand. Grasp the patient's lower arm (above the elbow) with your right hand

4. Extension from above down to the somatic dysfunction is obtained by pushing the patient's lower arm posteriorly and

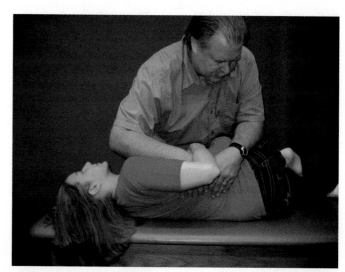

Figure 45-8 Patient on side, "Lumbar Roll"—for a flexed lumbar dysfunction.

cephalad, while monitoring the accumulation of forces at L2. Rotation from above down to L3 can be obtained by pulling the patient's arm anteriorly and superiorly. Monitor accumulation of force at L2

5. Additional rotation to "take out the slack" is only appropriate if the patient is excessively mobile

6. Slip your right hand underneath the patient's right arm, contacting the anterior shoulder region with your forearm, or the palm of your right hand, while monitoring the dysfunction with your left fingertips

7. Contact the patient's lateral right ilium with your left forearm, while palpating for localization of your force. If you have done a good job setting up the bottom, you don't need much more motion on the pelvis. The terminal objective of this positioning is simply to "stretch out the bottom and compress the top," achieving right lumbar sidebending

8. Prior to the thrust, ask the patient to turn his or her head toward the ceiling. Maintain the holding force with your right forearm or hand to keep the patient's right shoulder from rolling forward during your final localization and thrust. To further localize from below, rolling the patient's hips toward the table is often useful. The final corrective force, through your left forearm, is a combined vector force in an anterior and cephalad direction, dropping your weight downward onto your contact. This directed force is on the patient's pelvis with your left forearm, emphasizing right sidebending of the lumbar spine

9. Reassess motion

Lumbar Flexed Dysfunction (Seated/Walk Around)

Dysfunction: L1 on L2, rotated right and sidebent right, flexed (L1 F RR SR). This technique is useful for lower thoracic and all lumbar somatic dysfunctions.

Objective: Improve rotation and sidebending left and extension of L1 on L2.

Discussion: This technique is especially useful for flexed dysfunctions in the thoracolumbar junction. Much of the rotational force is from above, and extension is maintained throughout the movement. Localize the barrier through lateral translation. When performing this technique, it is important to keep *both* of the patient's ischial tuberosities in contact with the table. Instructing the patient to turn his or her head to the side opposite to the dysfunction may enhance results by adding more rotation from above.

Physician Position: Standing behind the seated patient.

Patient Position: Patient sitting astride the end of the table with his or her back toward the physician. Keep the patient's pelvis close to the edge. An electric table is useful for proper technique execution.

Procedure (Fig. 45.9):

1. Instruct the patient to clasp his or her hands behind his or her neck

2. With your left arm, reach beneath the patient's left axilla (just below the shoulder), crossing the chest anteriorly. Place your left hand over the patient's right arm, grasping the area just below the right humeral head

3. Place the heel of your right hand over the right transverse process of L1. Instruct the patient to slump forward slightly until gaping (flexion) is palpated with your right hand. Now ask the patient to "sit up as straight as possible." Take up the extension with your right hand. Ask the patient to "relax" while you maintain the extension at L1

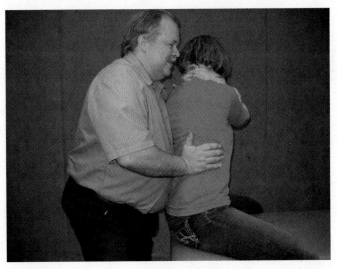

Figure 45-9 Patient seated, "Walk Around"—for a flexed lumbar dysfunction.

4. Using the heel of your right hand, translate the entire lumbar and low thoracic area across the midline to the right, by applying pressure with your body against the patient's left axilla. This right translation engages the barrier and localizes the left sidebending force to L1 on L2

5. Keep the patient's shoulders level and ischial tuberosities on the table

6. While maintaining your lateral translation, rotate L1 to the left. This is accomplished by pushing with your right hand, and by taking a step or two, or "walking around," the end of the table to the right. Maintain the localization by pressure through your right hand until the barrier is engaged. Your right arm should be functionally fixed to your torso, or you may fix your right elbow to your right side

7. Your right arm keeps the patient's torso extended. Do not allow the L1 somatic dysfunction to flex during the corrective force, as this will probably render the technique ineffective

8. The final corrective force is a quick increase in left rotation of L1 with an anterolaterally directed force through the heel of your right hand by shifting your body around to the restrictive barrier. At this point, your feet don't move. Use your entire body as a unit and maintain good body mechanics. Be sure to engage the barrier prior to your thrust. Do not "wind up and thrust"

9. Reassess motion

739.4/739.5 Sacroiliac Somatic Dysfunction

Trunk Rotation Ilium Thrust—Patient Supine

Dysfunction: Right posterior sacrum (sacrum rotated right on the right oblique axis, restriction of the right SI joint, inferior pole).

Objective: Improve motion of the SI joint.

Discussion: A posterior sacrum is an inferior pole restriction of the SI joint, wherein the ILA on the side of restriction is more posterior/inferior. A posterior right sacrum will be rotated right on a right oblique axis. The sacrum will be sidebent left.

Patient Position: Supine.

Physician Position: Standing at the level of the patient's waist, opposite the side of the posterior sacrum.

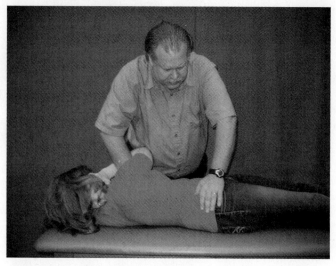

Figure 45-10 Ilium thrust, trunk rotation, patient supine—for a posterior sacrum.

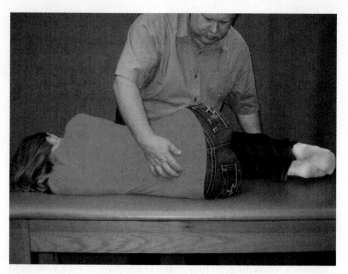

Figure 45-11 Ilium thrust, patient on side—for an anterior sacrum.

Procedure (Fig. 45.10):

1. Slide the patient's upper torso away from you to introduce the proper sidebending. The patient's left shoulder should now be lying in the midline of the table. Leave the patient's legs in the middle of the table
2. Have the patient place the hands behind the neck and interlace the fingers
3. Take your cephalad hand and insert it through the triangle formed by the patient's right arm. The dorsum of your cephalad hand should rest on the sternum
4. Place your caudad hand over the patient's right iliac crest stabilizing the pelvis
5. Rotate the patient's torso to the left with your cephalad arm by pivoting the patient on the patient's left shoulder. Make sure to keep the patient's left shoulder in the middle of the table throughout this arc of motion. Do not flex the patient's torso
6. As the patient's torso is rolled toward you, take up all the slack in the tissues until localization is felt down at the sacrum. The final corrective force is a quick thrust posteriorly on the ilium, moving the ilium to approximate with the posterior right sacrum
7. Reassess motion

Note: If the technique is unsuccessful, do not apply more force. The technique "will go or won't go."

Ilium Thrust—Patient on Side (Anterior Sacrum)

Dysfunction: Right anterior sacrum (sacrum rotated left on the left oblique axis, restriction of the right SI joint, superior pole).

Objective: To improve motion of the right SI joint.

Discussion: This technique moves the ilium to "meet up with" the anterior sacrum.

Repeat the seated flexion test following treatment to evaluate the techniques efficacy.

Patient Position: Lying on his or her left side.

Physician Position: Standing in front of the patient at waist level.

Procedure (Fig. 45.11):

1. Place the fingertips of your right hand in the right sacral sulcus to monitor localization of forces at the right SI joint

2. With your left hand, grasp under the patient's ankles, flexing his or her knees and hips together until motion is appreciated (and localized to) the right SI joint with your right index finger
3. Drop the patient's right leg off the front of the table. This results in proper sidebending of the SI joint
4. Place your left forearm posterior to the patient's right iliac crest
5. While monitoring the SI joint with your left hand, place your right forearm in the patient's right axilla and rotate his or her torso posteriorly until you appreciate motion at the SI joint. Your right arm is now a holding force
6. With your left forearm roll the patient's lower torso toward you so that your body weight is above the patient's pelvis. The table must be low enough to do this
7. The final corrective force is a thrust through your left forearm directed anteriorly down the patient's leg (toward the floor), moving the innominate anteriorly and inferiorly to approximate with the anterior sacrum
8. Reassess motion

739.6 Lower Extremity Somatic Dysfunction

Posterior Fibular Head Thrust

Dysfunction: Example: left posterior fibular head. That is, the head of the left fibula is in a position of posterior displacement in relation to the tibia.

Objective: Improve anterior translation of fibular head.

Discussion: The fibular head and lateral malleolus often have reciprocal motions. In this example, it would be common to find an associated anterior lateral malleolus.

Patient Position: Supine.

Physician Position: Standing at the patient's left side at the level of his or her knee.

Procedure (Fig. 45.12):

1. Place the lateral portion (of the proximal end) of your right index finger directly behind the head of the left fibula
2. Your right thumb should project over the anterior surface of the fibula
3. Grasp the patient's left ankle with your left hand positioned anterior to the malleoli (thumb projects downward just above

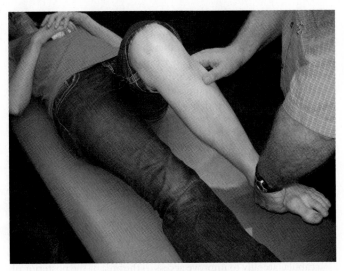

Figure 45-12 Posterior fibular head thrust.

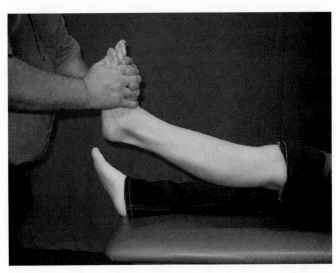

Figure 45-13 Tibio-talar tug technique.

the lateral malleolus and the fingers project downward above the medial malleolus)

4. Position the patient's left knee in extreme flexion. This will engage the barrier as your right index finger acts as a fulcrum
5. Corrective movement is then applied by anterior pressure against the posterior fibular head using the right hand as a fulcrum, while simultaneously externally rotating the ankle
6. Reassess fibular motion

Tibio-Talar Tug

Dysfunction: Anterior tibia dysfunction—tibia is translated anteriorly on the talus.

Objective: To restore normal motion of the ankle.

Discussion: This technique is useful in the treatment of the common anterior tibia dysfunction. When the tibia is anterior, the talus is relatively posterior and prefers dorsiflexion. This technique involves engaging the restrictive barrier into plantar flexion and "tugging" the talus anterior to correct the dysfunction.

Patient Position: Supine.

Physician Position: Standing at the foot of the table.

Procedure (Fig. 45.13):

1. The physician grasps the patient's foot by interlacing his or her fingers of both hands over the dorsum of the foot allowing the thumbs to project under the plantar surface of the foot
2. The foot and leg are lifted from the table with the foot held at right angles and the foot is supinated and inverted
3. The physician then applies a slight traction force through the foot to disengage the tibial-talar joint
4. The patient is asked to relax and the physician applies a corrective force of a quick tug increasing the supination, inversion, and traction

739.7 Upper Extremity Somatic Dysfunction

Anterior Radial Head Thrust (Radioulnar)

Dysfunction: The right radial head is restricted in posterior motion and external rotation of the forearm is restricted (supination).

Objective: Restore free posterior motion of the radial head and improve supination.

Discussion: The anterior radial head is relatively rare.

Patient Position: Seated.

Physician Position: Standing facing patient.

Procedure (Fig. 45.14):

1. Grasp patient's right hand with your right hand, as if shaking hands
2. Grasp patient's right elbow in such a way that the fingers of your left hand contact the olecranon process. Place your left thumb (alternatively you may use the fingers of your left hand) in the antecubital space applying a firm posterior directed pressure over the radial head. Your thumb will act as a wedge to thrust the radial head posteriorly
3. Use your right hand to induce pronation and flexion of the patient's forearm and wrist while introducing rapid flexion of the elbow. This flexion results in the simultaneous posterior thrust of the radial head through the wedging action of

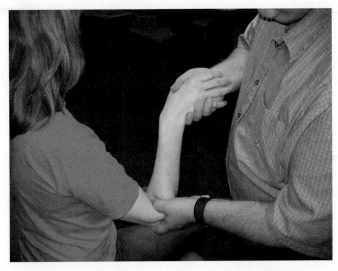

Figure 45-14 Anterior radial head thrust (radioulnar).

your left hand or thumb between the radius and the biceps muscle

4. Reassess motion of the radial head

Posterior Radial Head Thrust (Radioulnar)

Dysfunction: Right radial head is restricted in anterior motion relative to the ulna and is free in posterior motion. A restriction of internal rotation (pronation) may also be found.

Objective: Restore free anterior motion of the radial head and restore pronation.

Discussion: The posterior radial head is relatively common.

Patient Position: Seated.

Physician Position: Standing facing patient.

Procedure (Fig. 45.15):

1. Grasp patient's right hand with your right hand, while stabilizing the wrist
2. Hold patient's proximal forearm in your left hand, with your thumb applying an anteriorly directed pressure to the posterior aspect of the radial head
3. Now, while maintaining the anterior pressure on the radial head, with the arm in a pronated position and the elbow flexed, the corrective technique should be a fluid movement supinating the forearm and wrist and extending the elbow
4. Just before reaching complete extension, apply a HVLA thrust through your left thumb on the proximal radial head moving it anteriorly
5. Reassess motion

739.8 Rib Somatic Dysfunction

Elevated Upper Rib Thrust (Reverse Rib)

Dysfunction: Left 3rd rib is prominent with tissue texture abnormality and restricted motion to an anterior and inferior applied force. Associated limitation of right rotation and sidebending of T2 on T3 is present.

Objective: To restore normal motion to the rib and associated thoracic segment.

Discussion: This is a Chicago technique introduced by Norman J. Larson, D.O., F.A.A.O. This technique may be used for 2nd, 3rd, and 4th "structural" rib dysfunctions. This rib dysfunction is associated with a primary thoracic dysfunction. This technique is most effective with a flexed upper thoracic dysfunction and less effective with extended dysfunctions. As such, the primary thoracic dysfunction should be treated first before you employ this technique. In the situation in which the left 3rd rib is dysfunctional, T2 is rotated and sidebent left with the body of T2 pushing against the head of rib 3, straining the costotransverse articulation.

Patient Position: Seated.

Physician Position: Standing behind the seated patient.

Procedure (Fig. 45.16):

1. Place your right foot on the table several inches to the right of the patient's right hip. Place your right knee under the patient's right axilla and drape the patient's arm over your knee. Place a pillow between your knee and the patient's axilla. The patient's left arm may be drawn across his or her lap. This moves the scapula laterally to improve access to the area of the posterior rib angle. Stabilize the patient against your leg and torso. Maintain the patient's shoulders parallel to the table
2. Drape your left hand over the patient's left shoulder with your thumb contacting the angle of the dysfunctional 3rd rib. Apply a firm fixing force inferiorly and medially over the rib
3. Place your right hand (and forearm if necessary), with widespread fingers, over the right side of the patient's neck, cheek and zygoma. Your third digit should contact the face just inferior to the zygoma. Avoid placing your fingers in the patient's eyes and nose
4. With your right hand, translate the cervical spine as a unit, posteriorly until motion is noted at the T2-3 spinal level. Gently extend the cervical spine until motion is appreciated at the T2-3 spinal level. Rotate the patient's head to the right until forces accumulate at the level of T2. You may make minor adjustments to further enhance localization. These can include small amounts of sidebending or rotation to help localize the barrier
5. The final corrective force is a quick increase in right rotation of the patient's head and neck while maintaining firm fixation with your left hand on the rib. A counter thrust is not executed on the rib. The corrective force has moved T2 in relation to T3 and to the head of rib 3. The rib is usually felt to become suddenly freer following the execution on the technique. Instructing

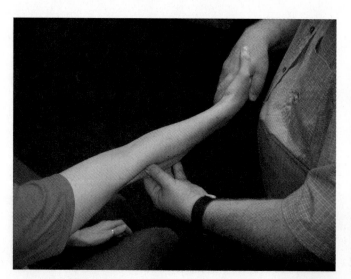

Figure 45-15 Posterior radial head thrust (radioulnar).

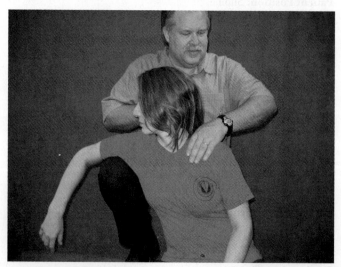

Figure 45-16 Elevated upper rib thrust, "reverse rib."

the patient to shake his or her head "no" before applying the final correcting thrust may enhance results
6. Reassess motion

REFERENCES

1. The Glossary Review Committee of the Educational Council on Osteopathic Principles. Glossary of osteopathic terminology. In: Allen TW, ed. *AOA Yearbook and Directory of Osteopathic Physicians.* Chicago, IL: American Osteopathic Association, 1994.
2. Greenman PE. *Principles of Manual Medicine.* Baltimore, MD: Williams & Wilkins, 1989:94.
3. Bowles CH. Functional technique: a modern perspective. In: Beal MC, ed. *The Principles of Palpatory Diagnosis and Manipulative Technique.* Newark, OH: American Academy of Osteopathy, 1992:174–178.
4. Schiotz EH, Cyriax J. *Manipulation. Past and Present.* London, England: William Heinemann Medical Books, Ltd., 1975.
5. Harris JD, McPartland JM. Historical perspectives of manual medicine. In: Stanton DF, Mein EA, eds. *Physical Med Rehabil Clin North Am* 1996;7(4):679–692.
6. Denslow JS. Pathophysiologic evidence for the osteopathic lesion: the known, unknown, and controversial. *J Am Osteopath Assoc* 1975;74:415–421.
7. Hargrove-Wilson. Symposium: manipulative treatment. *Med J Aust* 1967;24:274–280.
8. Kappler R. Role of psoas mechanism in low back pain. *J Am Osteopath Assoc* 1973;72:784–801.
9. Korr IM. *The Collected Papers of Irwin Korr.* Colorado Springs, CO: American Academy of Osteopathy, 1979.
10. Korr IM. Proprioceptors and somatic dysfunction. *J Am Osteopath Assoc* 1975;74:638–650.
11. Patterson M. A theoretical neurophysiologic mechanism for facilitated segment. *J Am Osteopath Assoc* 1978;77(5):399.
12. Patterson M. A model mechanism for spinal segmental facilitation. *J Am Osteopath Assoc* 1976;(1):62–72.
13. Van Buskirk R. Nociceptive reflexes and the somatic dysfunction: a model. *J Am Osteopath Assoc* 1990;(9):792–809.
14. Kimberly PE. Formulating a prescription of osteopathic manipulative treatment. In: Beal MC, ed. *The Principles of Palpatory Diagnosis and Manipulative Technique.* Newark, OH: American Academy of Osteopathy, 1992:146–152.
15. Hamann G, Haass A, Kujat D, et al. Cervicocephalic artery dissection and chiropractic manipulation. *Lancet* 1993;20:34(8847):764–765.
16. Hamann G, Haass A, Kujat D, et al. Position Paper on Osteopathic Manipulation Treatment of the Cervical Spine, Adopted by American Osteopathic Association's House of Delegates July 14, 2005.

46

Muscle Energy Approach

WALTER C. EHRENFEUCHTER

KEY CONCEPTS

- Muscle energy is a plan of diagnosis and treatment which relies on active patient effort through muscular contraction.
- This approach requires active use of the patient's muscles, on request, from a precisely controlled position, in a specific direction, and against a distinctly executed counterforce.
- Postisometric relaxation is a mobilization technique that applies gentle force to improve "articulation" and thereby restore previously restricted motion.
- The versatility of this approach allows combination with any of the other osteopathic manipulative techniques in total patient management.

CASE STUDY

A.J., a 54-year-old male, presents with recent onset lower back pain. The pain began while he was attempting to push a heavy automobile. The worst pain is located in the region of the lumbosacral junction and spreads across the top of the right iliac crest and into the right groin. The pain is worse with truncal flexion and improves with truncal extension. The pain is a constant dull ache with sharp exacerbations. He denies radicular pain, sensory loss, paresthesias, or lower extremity weakness.

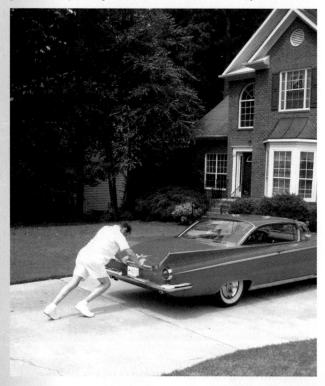

Physical examination reveals normal vital signs, normal cardiac and pulmonary exams. Neuromusculoskeletal exam reveals normal motor, reflexes, and sensation. Gross motion testing notes mildly restricted lumbar range of motion. The standing flexion

test is positive on the right suggesting a possible innominate dysfunction. This is confirmed by palpating passively induced iliosacral motion and discovering loss of right iliosacral motion. The posterior superior iliac spine on the right is more cephalad than on the left. The sacral sulcus on the right is shallow. The diagnosis is a right anteriorly rotated innominate somatic dysfunction.

Mechanism of Injury:

Excessive contraction of the rectus femoris muscle on the right against an unyielding resistance has resulted in the innominate bone being rotated anteriorly relative to the sacrum.

Treatment:

The appropriate muscle energy technique is utilized to treat the right anterior innominate somatic dysfunction. Reassessment reveals restoration of symmetric passively induced iliosacral motion and a normal standing flexion test. Additionally, the patient reports immediate substantial pain relief.

DEFINITION

Muscle energy technique has been defined as a form of osteopathic manipulative treatment in which the patient's muscles are actively used on request, from a precisely controlled position, in a specific direction, and against a distinctly executed counterforce.

Muscle energy techniques involve the patient's active cooperation to contract a muscle or muscles, inhale or exhale, or move one bone of a joint in a specific direction relative to the adjacent bone. For these reasons, muscle energy cannot be used if the patient is in a coma, uncooperative, too young to cooperate, or unresponsive (8).

HISTORY

Muscle energy is a system of osteopathic diagnosis and treatment with roots extending back to Andrew Taylor Still. Dr. Still did not record the way that he treated, preferring to insist that his students conduct an exhaustive study of anatomy while absorbing the osteopathic philosophy. He told students that if they knew anatomy and understood osteopathic philosophy, they would know what to do. As the osteopathic profession sought to increase the efficiency of teaching students how to treat patients, certain key individuals made contributions by developing a particular type of technique into a plan. Fred Mitchell, Sr. contributed by developing a plan of diagnosis and treatment that he called muscle energy because of its reliance on active patient effort through muscular contraction

Mitchell (1) credited Kettler as the first to focus (his) attention on the importance of the vast amount of tissue involved between joints, muscle, and fascia, and the changes it undergoes in the lesioning process. Kettler also emphasized that without establishing bilateral myofascial harmony, the lesion pattern is not obliterated and returns again and again. Mitchell also quoted Still, showing that he knew about this: "The attempt to restore joint integrity before soothingly restoring muscle and ligamentous normality was putting the cart before the horse" (1).

Some sources allege that muscle energy techniques are an outgrowth of a method developed by T. J. Ruddy (2) called resistive duction. In Ruddy's method, the physician offers resistance to the patient's active movement, but the patient is required to move quickly, often at a rate of 60 excursions per minute, or equal to the patient's pulse rate. Ruddy's purpose in asking the patient to contract muscle quickly and repetitively was twofold:

1. To increase blood (and other tissue fluid) movements to remove metabolic waste products from the cells and circulate oxygen
2. To tone inactive muscles that might be weak

Mitchell and Kettler must have been unaware of the proprioceptive neuromuscular facilitation (PNF) techniques developed by Kabat, Knott, and Voss at the Kabat-Kaiser Institute during the late 1940s. These techniques were not widely known. PNF uses skills to reeducate muscle for several reasons (3):

> *"To gain inhibition in muscles which may be in a protective spasm."*
> *"To improve range (of motion) at an intervertebral level."*

Mitchell first published his work in the *Yearbook of the American Academy of Osteopathy* in 1958 after receiving requests for a written description of the work he had developed in the 1940s and 1950s. He described one method of correction that used the effort of an extrinsic guiding operator as the activating force plus the intrinsic respiratory and muscular cooperation of the patient. He wrote about the direct method treatments of soft tissues (with attention to fasciae) and treatment using Neidner's fascial release prior to articular correction. Muscular energy technique, he wrote, with its many ramifications, is a most useful tool in preparation of the soft tissues. Ligamentous stretching may also be of use before articular correction is attempted (1).

Lewit and Simons (4) wrote that the use of postisometric relaxation was pioneered by Mitchell Sr. and clearly described by F. L. Mitchell Jr. as a mobilization technique that applies gentle force to improve "articulation" and thereby restore previously restricted movement. Later authors believed that Mitchell's muscle energy approach did this more quickly than PNF techniques. Probably because Mitchell's work was not recorded in indexed allopathic literature, Travell and Simons (5) credited Lewit in their text by stating that the concept of applying postisometric relaxation in the treatment of myofascial pain was presented for the first time in a North American journal in 1984.

Mitchell taught his techniques in tutorials to numerous physicians. The first 5-day Mitchell tutorial was held in Fort Dodge, IA, in 1970 and was attended by John Goodridge, Philip Greenman, Rolland Miller, Devota Nowland, Edward Stiles, and Sara Sutton—all osteopathic physicians. Several tutorials followed across the country. In 1972, Mitchell's examination and treatment procedures were videotaped at Michigan State University's College of Osteopathic Medicine. After Mitchell's death in 1974, the American Academy of Osteopathy organized a committee of physicians who had taken a tutorial with Mitchell and developed a manual for the presentation of 5-day courses to familiarize others with Mitchell's work. Additional tutorials were conducted for new faculty at the newly established colleges of osteopathic medicine from 1977 to 1981. The five earlier established osteopathic colleges began to integrate muscle energy procedures into their curriculum. In 1979, Mitchell et al. (6) published the manual that was and is still used as a reference in most osteopathic medical colleges. In 1999, Mitchell, Jr. completed publication of an exhaustive text on the muscle energy approach (7). Muscle energy diagnostic and treatment procedures developed by Mitchell, Sr. are currently a standard part of the osteopathic manipulative medicine curriculum and are also used by many physical therapists.

INDICATIONS AND CONTRAINDICATIONS

The muscle energy approach is indicated in the presence of somatic dysfunction in the absence of contraindications. Postisometric relaxation and joint mobilization using muscle force type techniques should not be applied to acutely injured or painful muscles. These would be better treated using a reciprocal inhibition technique.

Postisometric relaxation and joint mobilization using muscle force muscle energy techniques should not be requested of a patient with low vitality that could further be compromised (e.g., by provoking internal bleeding) by adding active muscle exertion. Examples would include a postsurgical patient or a patient in an intensive care unit immediately following a myocardial infarction. These patients could still be candidates for the use of those techniques requiring the use of respiratory assistance, oculocephalogyric reflex, reciprocal inhibition, or the crossed extensor reflex as these are exceptionally gentle techniques. Oculocephalogyric reflex techniques are contraindicated in anyone who has undergone recent eye surgery or has recently sustained trauma to the eye.

Muscle energy techniques are contraindicated for any individual who is unable or unwilling to follow the verbal directions of the physician. Examples here would include the very young child or infant; those not able to understand the physician due to a language barrier, or hearing loss; as well as the mentally ill who are unable to cooperate.

Complications: When both the patient and the type of muscle energy technique are chosen properly, no serious complications occur. Minor complications such as posttreatment muscle or joint soreness tend to be self-limiting and resolve within 24 to 36 hours without additional treatment.

Use of inappropriately excessive force has been reported to result in the complications of tendon avulsion from bone (in an 85-year-old man) and rib fracture (in a patient with osteoporosis). Inappropriate application of oculocephalogyric reflex cervical range of motion muscle energy techniques has resulted in anterior chamber intraocular hemorrhage in a single patient postcataract removal and lens implant surgery (C. Walter Ehrenfeuchter, D.O., F.A.A.O.—*personal communication*).

FACTORS INFLUENCING THE SUCCESSFUL APPLICATION OF MUSCLE ENERGY TECHNIQUES

Good results depend on accurate diagnosis, appropriate levels of force, and sufficient localization. Poor results are most often caused by inaccurate diagnosis, improperly localized forces, or forces that are too strong.

Diagnosis

An inaccurate diagnosis may lead to inappropriate treatment and does not achieve the desired improvement in the patient's condition. Even if a segmental diagnosis is accurate, complicating factors and the entire clinical picture of the patient need to be considered. For example, a careful diagnosis may indicate that side-bending is restricted at a segment superior to the one identified for treatment; this then interferes with the localization required, and the superior segment may need to be treated before the inferior segment.

Localization

The localization of force is more important than the intensity of force. Localization depends on the physician's palpatory perception of movement (or resistance to movement) at or about a specific articulation. Such perception enables the physician to make subtle assessments about a dysfunction and create variations of suggested treatment procedures.

Monitoring the localization of forces and confining the direction of force by the diagnosed muscle group to the level of somatic dysfunction are important to achieve desired results. When the physician introduces motion into an articulation that is a segment or two below the dysfunctional one, the probability of success greatly decreases because the forces have been directed to the wrong muscles.

Amount of Force

Using excessive force is the most common mistake made in applying muscle energy technique. This is not a wrestling match between patient and physician. Excessive force recruits other muscles to assist in stabilization of the body part being treated and may completely negate the intent of the technique. Excessive forces used on older patients may result in tendon avulsion from bone.

Asymmetrical Muscle Strength

Where asymmetry of range of motion occurs, consider and test the possibility of asymmetrical strength. Some ranges of motion may be asymmetrical because of weakness of a group of muscles rather than the shortness of the antagonist group. If asymmetry of muscle strength is present, employ a method to increase the strength of the weak muscle group. Progressive resistance exercises are used to strengthen weakened muscle groups. If weakness and shortness occur in different muscle groups but on the same side, attend to the shortness first. Jull and Janda (10) feel the agonists spontaneously increase their strength if the shortened or hypertonic fibers are lengthened.

TYPICAL SEQUENCE OF STEPS IN TECHNIQUE

Diagnosis

The physician should make an accurate diagnosis prior to initiating any treatment sequence. Although a diagnosis of somatic dysfunction from the muscle energy perspective has some unique elements, they are well described in the chapters on regional examination of the body. The reader is referred to those chapters to learn the appropriate diagnostic techniques.

Sequence

Based on an accurate diagnosis, a muscle energy procedure follows these principles:

1. The physician positions the body part to be treated at the position of initial resistance. It is important that only the "feather edge" of the restrictive barrier is engaged for maximal efficacy of these techniques. The "feather edge" of the restrictive barrier is the point where the restrictive barrier is just beginning to be engaged or where the tissue tension is just palpable.
2. The physician instructs the patient about his or her participation and helps the patient to obtain an effective direction of movement for the limb, trunk, or head. The patient is instructed in the intensity and duration of the muscle contraction.
3. The physician directs the patient to contract the appropriate muscle(s) or muscle group.
4. The physician uses counterforce in opposition to and equal to the patient's muscle contraction.
5. The physician maintains forces until an appropriate patient contraction is perceived at the critical articulation or area. This generally takes 3 to 5 seconds, but the duration varies with the size of the muscle being treated.
6. The patient is directed to relax by gently ceasing the contraction while the physician simultaneously matches the decrease in patient force.
7. The physician allows the patient to relax and senses the tissue relaxation with his or her own proprioceptors.
8. The physician takes up the slack permitted by the procedure. The slack is allowed by the decreased tension in the tight muscle, allowing it to be passively lengthened. The physician notes increased range of motion.
9. Steps 1 to 8 are repeated three to five times until the best possible increase in motion is obtained. The quality of response often peaks at the third excursion, with diminishing return thereafter.
10. The physician reevaluates the original dysfunction.

PHYSIOLOGIC PRINCIPLES

There are nine different physiologic principles of muscle energy technique:

1. Joint mobilization using muscle force
2. Respiratory assistance
3. Oculocephalogyric reflex
4. Reciprocal inhibition
5. Crossed extensor reflex
6. Isokinetic strengthening
7. Isolytic lengthening
8. Using muscle force to move one region of the body achieve movement of another bone or region
9. Postisometric relaxation

The following section describes the goals, physiologic basis, and contraction force for each of these principles. Examples of treatment of somatic dysfunction using each of these principles will be found under the treatment section. (Note: Example numbers correspond to the examples in the techniques section.)

Postisometric Relaxation

Goal
To accomplish muscle relaxation.

Physiologic Basis

Mitchell Jr. (9) postulated that immediately after an isometric contraction, the neuromuscular apparatus is in a refractory state during which passive stretching may be performed without encountering strong myotatic reflex opposition. All the operator needs to do is resist the contraction and then take up the slack in the muscles during the relaxed refractory period. With muscle contraction, there may also be increased tension on the Golgi organ proprioceptors in the tendons; this inhibits the active muscle's contraction.

Force of Contraction

Sustained gentle pressure (10 to 20 lb of pressure)

Example

See 739.5 pelvic somatic dysfunction

Example 5—Hip girdle dysfunction—hamstring muscles

Joint Mobilization Using Muscle Force

Goal

To accomplish restoration of joint motion in an articular dysfunction.

Physiologic Basis

Distortion of articular relationships and motion loss results in a reflex hypertonicity of the musculature crossing the dysfunctional joint, similar to thrust (HVLA) technique. This increase in muscle tone tends to compress the joint surfaces, and results in thinning of the intervening layer of synovial fluid and adherence of the joint surfaces. Restoration of motion to the articulation results in a gapping, or reseating of the distorted joint relations with reflex relaxation of the previously hypertonic musculature.

Force of Contraction

Maximal muscle contraction that can be comfortably resisted by the physician (30 to 50 lb of pressure)

Example

See 739.5 pelvic somatic dysfunction

Example 6—Innominate dysfunction—anterior rotation

Respiratory Assistance

Goal

To produce improved body physiology using the patient's voluntary respiratory motion.

Physiologic Basis

The muscular forces involved in these techniques are generated by the simple act of breathing. This may involve the direct use of the respiratory muscles themselves, or motion transmitted to the spine, pelvis, and extremities in response to ventilation motions. The physician usually applies a fulcrum against which the respiratory forces can work.

Force of Contraction

Exaggerated respiratory motion

Example

See 739.4 sacral somatic dysfunction

Example 4—Sacral dysfunction—unilateral extended sacrum

Oculocephalogyric Reflex

Goal

To affect reflex muscle contractions using eye motion.

Physiologic Basis

Functional muscle groups are contracted in response to voluntary eye motion on the part of the patient. These eye movements reflexively affect the cervical and truncal musculature as the body attempts to follow the lead provided by eye motion. It can be used to produce very gentle postisometric relaxation or reciprocal inhibition.

Force of Contraction

Exceptionally gentle

Contraindications

Fracture, dislocation, or moderate to severe segmental instability in the cervical spine. Evocation of neurologic symptoms or signs on rotation of the neck.

Example

See 739.1 cervical somatic dysfunction

Example 2—Restriction of regional cervical rotation

Reciprocal Inhibition

Goal

To lengthen a muscle shortened by cramp or acute spasm.

Physiologic Basis

When a gentle contraction is initiated in the agonist muscle, there is a reflex relaxation of that muscle's antagonistic group.

Force of Contraction

Very gentle (think ounces, not pounds of pressure)

Example

See 739.1 cervical somatic dysfunction

Torticollis due to acute sternocleidomastoid muscle spasm

Crossed Extensor Reflex

Goal

Used in the extremities where the muscle that requires treatment is in an area so severely injured (e.g., fractures or burns) that it is directly unmanipulable or inaccessible.

Physiologic Basis

This form of muscle energy technique uses the learned cross pattern locomotion reflexes engrammed into the central nervous system. When the flexor muscle in one extremity is contracted voluntarily, the flexor muscle in the contralateral extremity relaxes and the extensor contracts.

Force of Contraction

Very gentle (think ounces, not pounds of pressure)

Example

See 739.5 pelvic somatic dysfunction

Example 2—Severe acute hamstring strain

Special types of muscle contractions may be used in addition to the classic isometric contraction for special situations. Two specific examples are given below.

Isokinetic Strengthening

Goal

To reestablish normal tone and strength in a muscle weakened by reflex hypertonicity of the opposing muscle group.

Physiologic Basis

Where asymmetry of range of motion exists, there is also the potential for asymmetry in muscle strength. If there is shortening of an antagonist muscle, attend to that first. Jull and Janda (10) feel the agonists spontaneously increase their strength if the shortened or hypertonic fibers are lengthened first.

Once this is accomplished, further restoration of strength can be accomplished through the use of an Isokinetic contraction. In Isokinetic contractions, the length change occurs at a constant velocity. Typically concentric contractions are used, where the muscle is permitted to shorten, but at a controlled slow rate.

Force of Contraction

Sustained gentle pressure (10 to 20 lb of pressure)

Example

See 739.5 pelvic somatic dysfunction

Example 3—Hamstring shortening resulting in reflex quadriceps weakness

Isolytic Lengthening

Goal

To lengthen a muscle shortened by contracture and fibrosis.

Physiologic Basis

It is postulated that the vibration used here has some effect on the myotatic units in addition to mechanical and circulatory effects (11).

Force of Contraction

Maximal Contraction that can be comfortably resisted by the physician (30 to 50 lb of pressure)

Example

See 739.5 Pelvic Somatic Dysfunction

Example 4—Hamstring contracture

Using Muscle Force to move one region of the body achieve movement of another bone or region

Goal

To treat somatic dysfunction.

Physiologic Basis

For some dysfunctions, especially those involving the pelvis, it is often more effective to move one body structure by moving another body structure adjacent to it. Muscular force is used to move the first structure and that body part's response to the muscle force is transmitted to yet another part of the body.

Force of Contraction

Sustained gentle pressure (10 to 20 lb of pressure)

Example

See 739.4 sacral somatic dysfunction

Example 3—Bilaterally extended sacrum

DIAGNOSES AND TECHNIQUES

739.0 Craniocervical Somatic Dysfunction

Example 1—Acute cervical sprain and strain (Whiplash)

Diagnosis

Position: Occiput is flexed on C1
   Restriction: Occiput is restricted in extension on C1

Type of Muscle Energy

Reciprocal inhibition

Treatment Position

Patient: Supine
   Physician: Seated at the head of the table

Procedure

1. The physician's one hand is placed beneath the patient's occiput with the fingers in contact with the suboccipital musculature
2. The index and middle fingers of the physician's other hand are placed on top of the patient's chin (Figs. 46.1 and 46.2)
3. The patient is instructed to very gently tilt the head backward so that their chin comes up against the physician's fingers. The physician should be able to palpate the contraction of the suboccipital muscles with the hand beneath the occiput
4. This contraction is maintained for a full 3 to 5 seconds
5. The patient is instructed to relax, simultaneously ceasing your counterforce. Wait 2 seconds for the tissues to relax

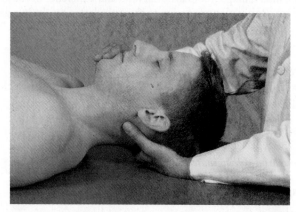

Figure 46-1 Occipitoatlantal (C0-1) dysfunction example C0 ESLRR—Post-isometric relaxation. (Reprinted from Atlas of Osteopathic Technique by Nicholas & Nicholas Published by LWW, 2008 with permission.)

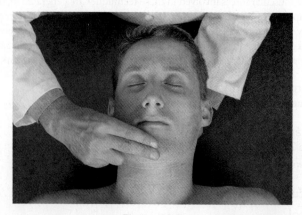

Figure 46-2

6. The physician shifts his fingers from the front of the chin to just below the chin
7. The physician lifts the chin cephalad, simultaneously pressing caudad with the hand beneath the occiput until the new restrictive barrier is engaged
8. The physician then shifts his fingers once again to the anterior surface of the chin
9. Steps 3 to 8 are repeated three to five times
10. Success of the technique is determined by retesting occipitoatlantal segmental motion

739.1 Cervical Somatic Dysfunction

Example 1—Cervical segmental somatic dysfunction: C5NRS_L

Diagnosis

Position: C5NRS_L; C5 is neutral, rotated left, and sidebent left
  Restriction: C5 Restricted in right rotation and right sidebending

Type of Muscle Energy

Oculocephalogyric Reflex

Treatment Position

Patient: Supine
  Physician: Seated at the corner of the head of the table

Procedure (Fig. 46-3)

1. Cradle the head and neck in both hands and with the middle or index fingers palpate the C5-6 facet joints
2. Lift the head forward until you straighten the cervical spine
3. Let the head extend backward from above downward until C5 is positioned in neutral relative to C6
4. Rotate C5 to the right until initial resistance to segmental motion is palpated. Sidebending will occur automatically because sidebending and rotation of coupled motions in the cervical spine. (The left hand is mostly supporting the head and neck while the right hand monitors movement at the C5-6 facet joint.)
5. Instruct the patient "look far to your left."
6. Maintain this contraction for a full 3 to 5 seconds
7. Direct the patient to "look straight ahead and relax."
8. Wait 2 seconds for the tissues to relax, then rotate C5 to the right until the new restrictive barrier is engaged

9. Steps 5 to 8 are repeated three to five times
10. Success of the technique is determined by retesting segmental motion at the C5-6 level

Example 2—Restriction of regional cervical rotation

Diagnosis

Position: Cervical region rotated left
  Restriction: Cervical region restricted in right rotation

Type of Muscle Energy

Oculocephalogyric reflex.

Contraindications

Fracture, dislocation, or moderate-to-severe segmental instability in the cervical spine. Evocation of neurologic symptoms or signs on rotation of the neck.

Treatment Position

Patient: Supine
  Physician: Seated at the head of the table

Procedure (Fig. 46.4)

1. The patient's head and neck are rotated to the right to the feather edge of the regional motion barrier
2. The patient is instructed "look as far as you can to your left"
3. This position is held for a full 3 to 5 seconds
4. Direct the patient to "look straight ahead again and relax"
5. Wait 2 seconds for the tissues to relax and then rotate the head and neck further to the right, engaging the new regional restrictive barrier
6. Steps 2 to 5 are repeated three to five times
7. Success of the technique is determined by reassessing cervical regional rotation

Example 3—Torticollis due to Acute Sternocleidomastoid Muscle Spasm

Diagnosis

Acute left sternocleidomastoid spasm

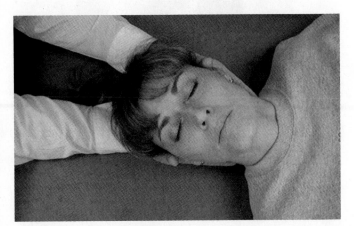

Figure 46-3 Treatment for cervical segmental dysfunction, C2-6.

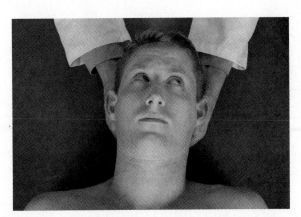

Figure 46-4 Cervical range of motion: oculocervical reflex. (Reprinted from Atlas of Osteopathic Technique by Nicholas & Nicholas. Published by LWW 2008 with permission.)

Type of Muscle Energy

Reciprocal inhibition

Contraindications

Fracture, dislocation, or moderate-to-severe segmental instability in the cervical spine. Evocation of neurologic symptoms or signs on rotation of the neck.

Treatment Position

Patient: Supine with the head positioned off the end of the table

 Physician: Seated at the head of the table supporting the patient's head

Procedure (Fig. 46.5)

1. The patient's head is flexed approximately 45 degrees, then rotated so that the hypertonic sternocleidomastoid muscle is positioned superiorly
2. The patient's head is now lowered straight toward the floor until the restrictive barrier produced by this hypertonic muscle is engaged
3. Instruct the patient "push your head very gently directly toward the floor"
4. During this contraction, the physician is palpating the involved muscle with one hand to ensure that adequate relaxation is occurring. The contraction is held for 3 to 5 seconds
5. The patient is instructed to relax. After 2 seconds of relaxation, the head is again lowered toward the floor until the new restrictive barrier is engaged
6. Steps 3 to 5 are repeated three to five times
7. Success of the technique is determined by palpating the involved Sternocleidomastoid muscle for reduction in tone and by observing the patient's head position in the erect posture for improved body carriage

739.2 Thoracic Somatic Dysfunction

Example 1—Thoracic segmental somatic dysfunction

Diagnosis

Position: T8ERS$_R$; T8 is extended, rotated, and sidebent right

 Restriction: T8 is restricted in flexion, rotation, and sidebending left

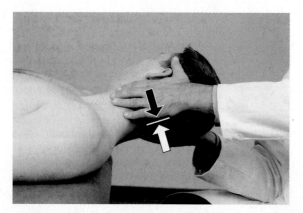

Figure 46-5 • Left sternocleidomastoid spasm (acute torticollis): reciprocal inhibition. (Reprinted from Atlas of Osteopathic Technique by Nicholas & Nicholas, LWW, 2008 with permission.)

Type of Muscle Energy

Postisometric relaxation

Treatment Position

Patient: Seated on the side of the treatment table, arms crossed grasping their own shoulders

 Physician: Standing behind the patient on the side opposite the direction of rotation

Procedure (Fig. 46.6)

1. Place the pads of your right fingers between the spinous processes of T8 and T9. Have the patient slowly bend forward until you feel a slight separation of these spinous processes
2. Maintaining this forward bent posture, place your left axilla over the top of the patients left shoulder. Your left hand reaches across the front of the patient to grasp the right shoulder
3. Lean down onto the patient's left shoulder until you feel this sidebending force reach the T8 level
4. You do not have to position the patient in rotation as sidebending and rotation are coupled motions in the thoracic spine
5. Instruct the patient "pull your right shoulder down toward the floor"
6. This contraction is held for a full 3 to 5 seconds
7. Direct the patient to relax, simultaneously ceasing your counterforce
8. Further flex and left sidebend the patient until you reach the new segmental restrictive barrier for T8
9. Steps 5 to 8 are repeated three to five times
10. Success of the technique is determined by retesting segmental motion at the T8 level

739.2 Lumbar Somatic Dysfunction

Example 1—Lumbar segmental somatic dysfunction

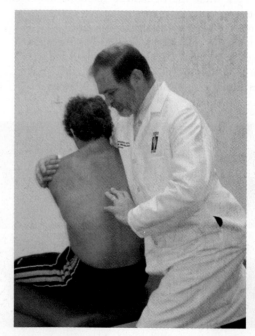

Figure 46-6 Treatment of thoracic segmental somatic dysfunction.

Diagnosis

Position: L5FRRSR; L5 (a type II dysfunction) is flexed, rotated right, and side bent right.

Restriction: L5 is restricted in extension, right rotation, and right side-bending.

Type of Muscle Energy

Postisometric relaxation

Treatment Position

Patient: Lateral recumbent and lying with the rotational component closest to the table (in this case on the right side). The hips are flexed 45 degrees and the knees are flexed 90 degrees.

Physician: Standing facing the patient

Procedure (Fig. 46.7)

1. The physician palpates the interspinous space between L5 and S1 with the cephalad hand
2. The patient's lumbar spine is passively flexed and extended by flexing and extending the hips until the dysfunctional segment is positioned in neutral relative to flexion and extension
3. The patient's upper leg is flexed slightly further at the hip and dropped off the side of the table cephalad to the lower leg
4. The patient's pelvis is rotated anteriorly until the initial resistance reaches the segment to be treated
5. The L5-S1 interspinous space is now palpated with the physician's caudad hand while the patient's upper shoulder is carried posteriorly again until the initial resistance reaches the segment to be treated
6. The patient is instructed to "pull gently forward with your shoulder." This contraction is held for a full 3 to 5 seconds. After 2 seconds of relaxation, the shoulder is carried posteriorly until a new restrictive barrier is met
7. The patient is then instructed to "pull your hip gently backward." This contraction is held for a full 3 to 5 seconds. After 2 seconds of relaxation, the hip is carried forward until a new restrictive barrier is met
8. Each sequence of contraction/relaxation/repositioning is repeated three to five times or as long as further segmental

motion is being gained. If coordinated enough, the patient may contract muscles at both the hip and shoulder simultaneously.
9. Success of the technique is determined by reevaluating segmental motion at the dysfunctional lumbar segment

739.4 Sacral Somatic Dysfunction

The diagnosis of sacral dysfunction generally requires just two types of information:

1. *The relative position of the two sacral sulci and the two inferior lateral angles (ILAs)* (Fig. 46.8). The two sacral sulci are designated as feeling either deep or shallow compared with each other. The ILAs are designated as being posterior/inferior or anterior/superior relative to each other. For unilateral sacral dysfunction, when the deep sulcus and the posterior/inferior ILA are on opposite sides of the sacrum, you have torsion. When the deep sulcus and the posterior/inferior ILA are on the same side of the sacrum, you have a unilateral sacral flexion (shear) or extension
2. *A motion test.* Several different motion tests have been devised over the years to assess unilateral sacroiliac dysfunction
   - *Lumbar spring test.* In this test, the patient is prone, and a springing force is directed anteriorly into the lumbar spine

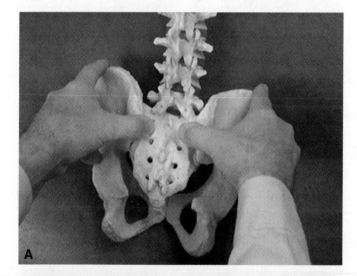

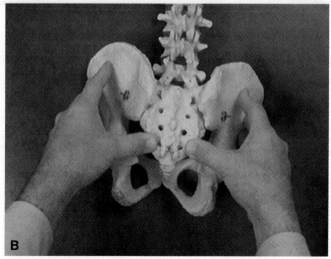

Figure 46-8 Sacral landmarks. **A**. the sacral sulci. **B**. the ILAs.

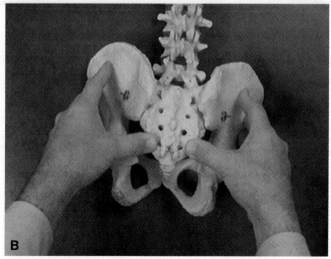

Figure 46-7 Treatment for lumbar, type II segmental dysfunction, lateral recumbent position.

(Fig. 46.9). Normal spring (negative spring test) indicates the presence of an anterior torsion or a unilateral flexion. Increased resistance to pressure (positive spring test) indicates the presence of either a posterior torsion or a unilateral extension

- *Sphinx test,* also called lumbopelvic hyperextension, employs observation in changes in asymmetry at the sacral sulci (Fig. 46.10). When going from the prone position to the sphinx position, if the sacral sulci become more symmetric, you have an anterior torsion or a unilateral flexion. If the sacral sulci become more asymmetric, you have a posterior torsion or a unilateral extension
- Seated flexion test (see Chapter 41)
- *Seated assessment of ILA asymmetry* (Figs. 46.11 and 46.12). This test is performed in a manner similar to a seated flexion test (special tests of the pelvis), but the ILAs are monitored. As in the sphinx test, if the asymmetry increases, you have a posterior torsion or unilateral extension. If the asymmetry decreases or stays the same, you have an anterior torsion or unilateral flexion
- *Four-digit contact* (Fig. 46.13). Contact the four corners of the sacrum as depicted. Assess motion of the sacrum by direct

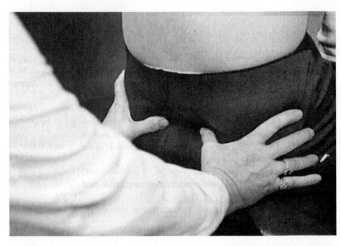

Figure 46-11 Test for inferior lateral angle asymmetry, starting position.

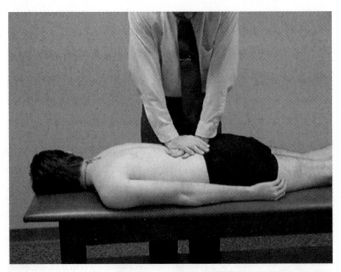

Figure 46-9 Lumbar spring test.

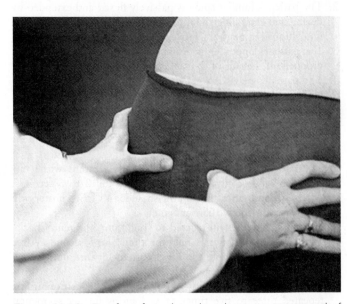

Figure 46-12 Test for inferior lateral angle asymmetry, at end of flexion.

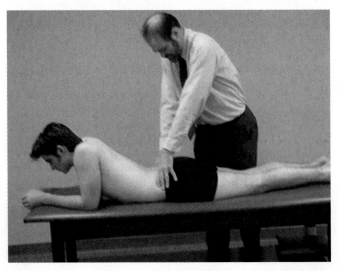

Figure 46-10 Sphinx test.

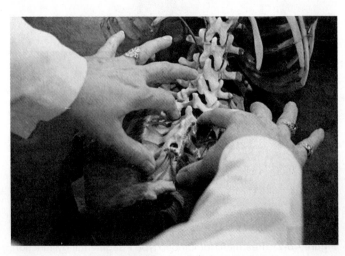

Figure 46-13 Four-digit contact.

pressure on the sacrum, moving it about its various axes, or quietly palpate sacral motion while the patient respires.

Example 1—Sacral dysfunction—anterior torsion

Diagnosis

Example: A left on left sacral torsion.

Position: Anterior torsion about a left oblique axis; an L on L sacral torsion (the first L designates the direction of sacral rotation, the second L designates the oblique axis on which this rotation is occurring).

Restriction: Posterior rotation about the left oblique axis is restricted. The oblique axes are not free to alternate during the gait cycle.

Type of Muscle Energy

Complex: the experts are still debating exactly what happens during this technique, but it is likely a combination of multiple muscles simultaneously going through postisometric relaxation.

Treatment Position

Patient: Left lateral modified Sims' position (lying on the side of the axis)

Physician: Stands at the side of the table facing the patient

Procedure (Fig. 46.14)

1. The patient's right shoulder is pressed as close to the table as it will go. Postisometric relaxation technique may be used to obtain optimal positioning
2. The physician's cephalad hand palpates over the right sacral sulcus
3. The patient's hips and knees are flexed to 90 degrees. Both legs are then dropped off the side of the table. A pillow may be necessary to cushion the distal thigh against the table edge
4. The physician's caudad hand is placed just proximal to the lateral malleolus of the upper leg
5. The patient is instructed to "lift your legs straight up toward the ceiling"
6. This contraction is held for a full 3 to 5 seconds

7. Direct the patient to relax, simultaneously ceasing your counterforce
8. Wait 2 seconds for the tissues to relax, and then press both legs toward the floor until a new restrictive barrier is reached
9. Steps 5 to 8 are repeated three to five times
10. Success of the technique is determined by rechecking the symmetry of the sacral sulci and ILAs, and by retesting sacral motion

Example 2—Sacral dysfunction—posterior torsion (Fig. 46.15—treatment of posterior sacral torsion)

Diagnosis

Example: A left on right sacral torsion.

Position: Posterior torsion about a right oblique axis; an L on R sacral torsion (the L designates the direction of sacral rotation, the R designates the oblique axis on which this rotation is occurring).

Restriction: Anterior rotation about the right oblique axis is restricted. The oblique axes are not free to alternate during the gait cycle.

Type of Muscle Energy

Complex: the experts are still debating exactly what happens during this technique, but it is likely a combination of joint mobilization using muscle force and postisometric relaxation.

Treatment Position

Patient: Right lateral recumbent position (lying on the side of the axis)

Physician: Stands at the side of the table facing the patient

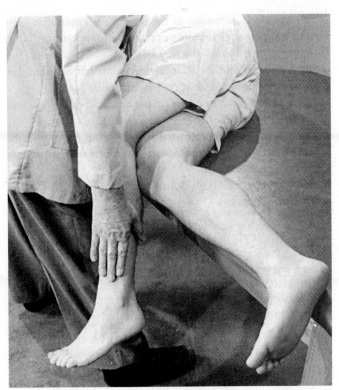

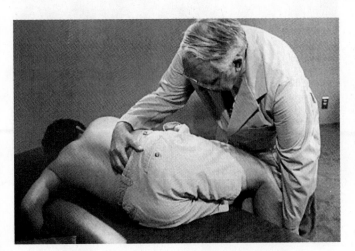

Figure 46-14   Treatment of anterior sacral torsion.

Figure 46-15   Treatment of posterior sacral torsion.

Procedure (Fig. 46.15)

1. The patient's left shoulder is carried posteriorly until the initial restriction is sensed
2. The physician's cephalad hand palpates over the left sacral sulcus
3. The patient's hips are flexed to 45 degrees and the knees to 90 degrees
4. The patient's upper leg is flexed further at the hip and dropped off the table cephalad to the lower leg
5. The physician grasps this leg just above the lateral malleolus.
6. The patient is instructed to "lift your ankle up toward the ceiling as hard as you can"
7. This contraction is maintained for a full 3 to 5 seconds
8. Direct the patient to relax, simultaneously ceasing your counterforce
9. Wait 2 seconds for the tissues to relax, and then press the leg further toward the floor until a new restrictive barrier is reached
10. Steps 6 to 9 are repeated three to five times
11. Success of the technique is determined by rechecking the symmetry of the sacral sulci and ILAs and by retesting sacroiliac motion

Example 3—Bilaterally extended sacrum

Diagnosis

Position: Bilaterally extended sacrum
    Restriction: Sacrum restricted in flexion on both sacroiliac joints

Type of Muscle Energy

Using muscle force to move one region of the body achieves movement of another bone or region. (In this case, muscles will move the lumbar spine that will in turn move the sacrum.)

Treatment Position

Patient: Seated on a low stool at the end of the treatment table, with the feet together and the knees separated.
    Physician: Seated at the end of the treatment table behind the patient.

Procedure

1. A pillow or pad is placed on the patient's sacral base and the physician's one knee is placed against this, exerting a continuous anterior pressure against the sacral base
2. The patient is instructed to reach back and grasp the edges of the table
3. The physician gently restrains the patient by both shoulders
4. The patient is instructed to "lift the lower end of your sternum up toward the ceiling." (This has the effect of increasing the lumbar lordosis, arching the back in the manner of "an old sway backed horse." Increasing the lumbar lordosis normally makes the sacrum move into flexion, the desired effect here.)
5. This contraction is held for 3 to 5 seconds
6. The patient is instructed to relax while the physician maintains anterior pressure on the base of the sacrum
7. Steps 4 to 6 are repeated three to five times
8. Success of the technique is determined by reassessing sacral motion (sacral rock test) as well as the depth of the sacral sulci and position of the ILAs

Example 4—Sacral dysfunction—unilateral extended sacrum

Diagnosis

Example: Unilateral extended sacrum—right
    Position: Unilateral extended sacrum—right
    Restriction: Right sacroiliac joint restricted in flexion

Type of Muscle Energy

Respiratory assistance

Treatment Position

Patient: Sphinx position (prone with the elbows supporting the upper body)
    Physician: Standing at the side of the patient opposite the side of dysfunction

Procedure (Fig. 46.16)

1. The hypothenar side of the heel of the physician's right hand is placed in the region of the right sacral sulcus exerting a steady pressure directed toward the table. It is reinforced by the physician's left hand
2. The patient is instructed to "inhale and then exhale quickly"
3. During exhalation, the physician follows forward nutation of the sacrum
4. During inhalation, the physician resists posterior nutation of the sacrum
5. Steps 2 to 4 are repeated three to seven times
6. Success of the technique is determined by rechecking symmetry of the sacral sulci and the ILAs, and by retesting sacroiliac motion

739.5 Pelvic Somatic Dysfunction

Example 1—Superior pubic bone somatic dysfunction

Diagnosis

Position: Pubic bone on side of dysfunction is displaced superiorly

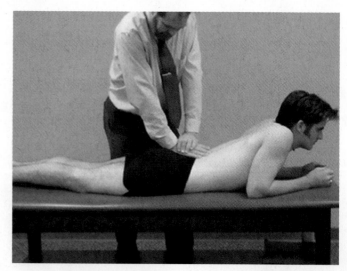

Figure 46-16   Treatment of unilateral extended sacrum.

Restriction: Pubic bone on side of dysfunction resists inferior movement

Type of Muscle Energy

Joint mobilization using muscle force.

Treatment Position

Patient: Supine, lying near the edge of the table
  Physician: Standing at the side of the table on the side of dysfunction

Procedure (Fig. 46.17)

1. The physician abducts the patient's ipsilateral thigh so that the leg and thigh can hang off the side of the table
2. The physician's cephalad hand is placed on the patient's contralateral anterior superior iliac spine to prevent the patient from rolling off the table during the technique
3. The physician's caudad hand is placed just proximal to the patient's ipsilateral knee
4. The physician presses downward on the thigh until the restrictive barrier is engaged
5. The patient is instructed to "lift your knee up toward the ceiling and slightly toward the table"
6. This isometric contraction is maintained for a full 3 to 5 seconds
7. The patient is instructed to relax
8. Wait 2 seconds for the tissues to relax, then reposition the patient's thigh further down toward the floor until the new restrictive barrier is engaged
9. Steps 5 to 8 are repeated three to five times
10. Effectiveness of the technique is determined by reexamining the position of the pubic tubercles and by repalpating passively induced iliosacral motion

Example 2—Severe acute hamstring strain

Diagnosis

Severe acute right hamstring strain with spasm

Type of Muscle Energy

Crossed extensor reflex

Treatment Position

Patient: Supine
  Physician: Standing at the side of the table on the side of acute spasm

Procedure (Fig. 46.18)

1. The patient's *right* hip is flexed to the initial resistance while keeping the knee in extension
2. If the range of motion permits, the leg may be placed atop the physician's shoulder
3. The physician's hands are placed on top of the patient's thigh to maintain the knee in extension throughout the technique
4. The patient is instructed to "very gently push your *left* knee down against the table"
5. This contraction is held for a full 3 to 5 seconds
6. Direct the patient to relax
7. Wait 2 seconds for the tissues to relax, then further flex the *right* hip until the new restrictive barrier is engaged
8. Steps 4 to 7 are repeated three to five times or until no additional motion can be gained
9. Effectiveness of the technique is assessed by retesting *right* hip range of motion in flexion with the knee extended

Example 3—Hamstring shortening resulting in reflex quadriceps weakness

Diagnosis

Reflex weakness of the right quadriceps

Type of Muscle Energy

Isokinetic strengthening

Treatment Position

Patient: Prone
  Physician: Standing at the side of the table on the side of the weakened quadriceps

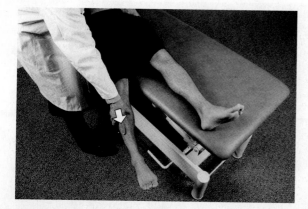

Figure 46-17 Right Superior Pubic Shear Dysfunction: Muscle Contraction Mobilizes Articulation. (Reprinted from Nicholas & Nicholoas with permission.)

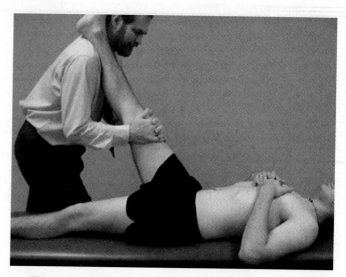

Figure 46-18 Treatment of hypertonic hamstring muscle.

Procedure

1. The right knee is flexed until the motion barrier for the quadriceps is reached. The physician restrains the leg just proximal to the ankle
2. The patient is instructed to "gently push your leg against my hand"
3. While the patient is pushing, slowly, allow the knee to extend through the middle of its normal range of motion. This typically takes 3 to 5 seconds
4. Instruct the patient to stop pushing
5. Steps 1 to 4 are repeated three to five times
6. Success of the technique is determined by retesting quadriceps strength

Example 4—Hamstring contracture

Diagnosis

Hamstring contracture

Type of Muscle Energy

Isolytic lengthening
   Treatment position
   Patient: Supine
   Physician: Standing at the side of the table on the side of the contractured hamstring

Procedure

1. The patient's hip is flexed to the initial resistance while keeping the knee in extension
2. The patient's leg is then placed atop the physician's shoulder
3. One hand is placed on the thigh, just proximal to the knee; the other is placed just proximal to the ankle posterior to the Achilles tendon
4. The patient is instructed to "push your knee down toward the table as hard as you can"
5. While the patient is pushing, the physician creates an oscillatory motion with both hands. This repeatedly stretches the muscle at a rate of about four times per second (4 Hz)
6. This combined forceful contraction and vibratory stretching is continued for 3 to 5 seconds
7. The patient is instructed to relax and the oscillatory motion is stopped
8. Wait 2 seconds for the tissues to relax and then further flex the hip to the new restrictive barrier
9. Steps 4 to 8 are repeated three to five times
10. Success of the technique is determined by retesting hip range of motion in flexion with the knee extended

Example 5—Innominate dysfunction—anterior rotation

Diagnosis

Position: Innominate rotated anteriorly
   Restriction: Innominate restricted in posterior rotation

Type of Muscle Energy

Joint mobilization using muscle force

Treatment Position

Patient: Supine
   Physician: Seated on the table on the side of dysfunction

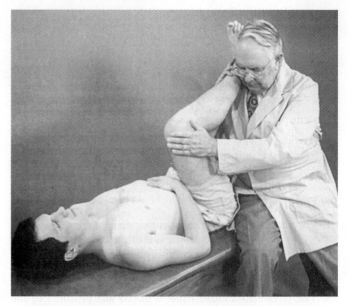

Figure 46-19   Treatment for anteriorly rotated innominate.

Procedure (Fig. 46.19)

1. The patient's leg on the side of dysfunction is flexed at the hip and the knee, and the foot is placed on the physician's shoulder
2. The physician's hands are placed against the hamstring muscles just proximal to the popliteal region
3. The patient is instructed to "push your thigh against my hands"
4. This contraction is held for a full 3 to 5 seconds
5. Direct the patient to relax, simultaneously ceasing your counterforce
6. Wait 2 seconds for the tissues to relax, and then reposition the innominate into further posterior rotation by further flexing the hip until the new restrictive barrier is engaged
7. Steps 3 to 6 are repeated three to five times or until a sudden release of the innominate dysfunction is palpated
8. Effectiveness of the technique is assessed by rechecking iliosacral motion

739.6 Lower Extremity Somatic Dysfunction

Knee—Proximal Fibula Posterior (Fig. 46.20)

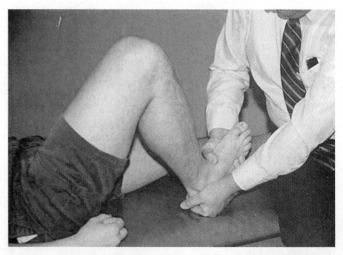

Figure 46-20   Treatment of proximal fibula posterior.

Diagnosis

Position: The proximal fibula is posterior.

Restriction: The proximal fibula is restricted in anterior glide.

Type of Muscle Energy

Joint mobilization using muscle force

Treatment Position

Patient: Supine with hip flexed 45 degrees and knee flexed 90 degrees

Physician: Standing at the foot of the table facing the patient

Procedure (Fig. 46.20)

1. The physician's medial hand is placed on the dorsum of the foot with his or her thumb on the lateral aspect and the fingers on the medial aspect
2. The physician's lateral hand anchors the calcaneus
3. The ankle is inverted to the initial resistance
4. The patient is instructed to "push your foot sideways into my thumbs and up into my hand." This eversion/dorsiflexion of the ankle is thought to contract the extensor digitorum longus and the tibialis anterior muscles, drawing the fibula forward
5. This contraction is held for a full 3 to 5 seconds
6. Direct the patient to relax, simultaneously ceasing your counterforce
7. Wait 2 seconds for the tissues to relax, and then further invert the foot until a new restrictive barrier is met
8. Steps 4 to 7 are repeated three to five times or until no additional motion can be gained
9. Effectiveness of the technique is determined by retesting motion at the proximal tibiofibular articulation

739.7 Upper Extremity Somatic Dysfunction
Diagnosis

Hypertonicity of the rhomboid causing medial scapular displacement

Position: Scapula medially displaced

Restriction: Scapula resists lateral displacement

Type of Muscle Energy

Postisometric relaxation

Treatment Position

Patient: Seated on the side of the table

Physician: Standing behind the patient and to the left

Procedure (Fig. 46.21)

1. The physician reaches in front of the patient with the left hand and grasps the patient's right forearm
2. The patient's right arm is drawn across the front of the body from right to left, and downward in a direction paralleling the direction of the fibers of the rhomboid major and minor
3. The physician's right hand is placed to the left of the spine to provide a counterforce to truncal rotation
4. The patient is instructed to "pull your right elbow toward the right," while the physician provides an unyielding counterforce
5. This contraction is maintained for 3 to 5 seconds
6. The patient is instructed to relax

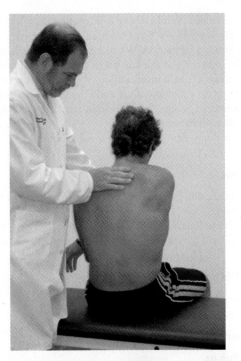

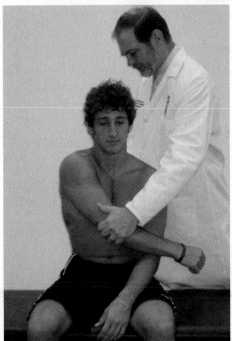

Figure 46-21 Treatment of hypertonic rhomboid, from behind and from the front.

7. After a second or two of relaxation, the physician puts increased tension on the rhomboid musculature by drawing the right arm further across the front of the body until the new restrictive barrier is engaged
8. Steps 4 to 6 are repeated three to five times
9. Success of the technique is determined by repalpating the rhomboid musculature and retesting scapular motion

739.8 Costal Somatic Dysfunction

In general, costal somatic dysfunction is divided into two groups: ribs held in inhalation (inhalation ribs) and ribs held in exhalation

(exhalation ribs). While many rib dysfunctions occur singly, occasionally you will see three or more ribs in a group, all having the same motion restriction. When a group of ribs is held in inhalation, the lowest rib is the key rib to treat. For example, let's say ribs 6, 7, and 8 are held in inhalation. When you treat rib 8, it will in turn draw rib 7 down with it and 7 will draw 6 along as well. Similarly, when a group of ribs is held in exhalation, the upper most rib is the key rib to treat.

Rib dysfunction—ribs 7 to 10 held in inhalation

Diagnosis

Position: Inhalation rib; a rib moves fully in inhalation; a rib is held in inhalation.

Restriction: Restriction of exhalation; rib stops early in exhalation; extent and duration of exhalation movement are decreased.

Type of Muscle Energy

Respiratory assistance

Treatment Position

Patient: Supine.
Physician: Standing at the side of the table

Procedure (Fig. 46.22)

1. The patient's upper body is side-bent to the side of dysfunction until tension is taken off the dysfunctional rib
2. The web formed by the physician's thumb and index finger is placed in the lateral aspect of the intercostal space above the dysfunctional rib on its superior surface
3. The patient is instructed to inhale and exhale deeply
4. On exhalation, the physician exaggerates the bucket handle motion of the rib being treated
5. On inhalation, the physician resists motion of the rib
6. Steps 4 and 5 are repeated three to seven times until maximal motion of the rib has been achieved
7. Success of the technique is determined by retesting motion of the dysfunctional rib

Rib dysfunction—ribs 1 and 2 held in exhalation

Diagnosis

Position: Exhalation rib; the rib moves fully in exhalation; the rib is held in exhalation.

Restriction: Restriction of inhalation; rib stops early in inhalation; extent and duration of inhalation motion are decreased.

Type of Muscle Energy

Joint mobilization using muscle force and reciprocal inhibition

Treatment Position

Patient: Supine
Physician: Standing at the side of the patient opposite the side of the dysfunctional rib

Procedure (Fig. 46.23)

1. The patient's head is turned about 30 degrees away from the side of the dysfunctional rib
2. The patient's arm on the side of the dysfunction is placed with the dorsum of the wrist against the forehead
3. The physician's caudad hand reaches under the patient and grasps the angle of the dysfunctional rib exerting continuous traction in a caudad and lateral direction
4. The patient is instructed to "lift your head straight up toward the ceiling." This is done without altering the 30 degree rotation of the head
5. This contraction is held for a full 3 to 5 seconds
6. Direct the patient to relax, simultaneously ceasing your counterforce
7. Wait 2 seconds for the tissues to relax, and then exert increasing caudad and lateral traction with your caudad hand beneath the rib
8. Steps 4 to 7 are repeated three to five times
9. Success of the technique is determined by retesting motion of the dysfunctional rib

739.9 Other Somatic Dysfunction

Redoming the diaphragm

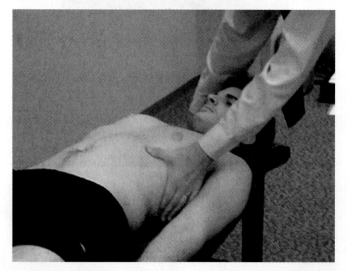

Figure 46-22 Treatment for ribs 7 to 10, held in inhalation.

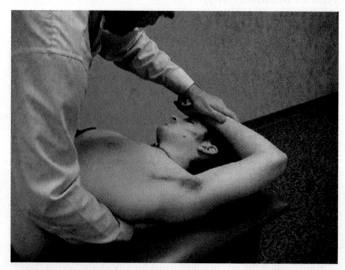

Figure 46-23 Treatment for ribs 1 and 2, held in exhalation.

Diagnosis

Position: Diaphragm held in Inhalation
   Restriction: Diaphragm restricted in Exhalation

Type of Muscle Energy

Respiratory assistance.

Contraindications

Recent ingestion of a large meal
Hiatus hernia, gastroesophageal reflux disease (relative)
Friability of the liver or spleen (cirrhosis, mononucleosis, leukemia, lymphoma)

Treatment Position

Patient: Supine with hips and knees flexed, feet flat on the table
   Physician: Standing at the side of the table facing the head of the table

Procedure (Fig. 46.24)

1. The physician places the thumbs and thenar eminences 2 to 3 in below the costal margin with thumbs pointing toward the Xiphoid process
2. The patient is instructed to "take a deep breath and then breathe all the way out"
3. The physician's thenar eminences follow the diaphragm in its exhalation motion, exaggerating it by placing a cephalad pressure on the upper abdominal viscera
4. The patient is again instructed to inhale as the physician maintains this pressure on the diaphragm

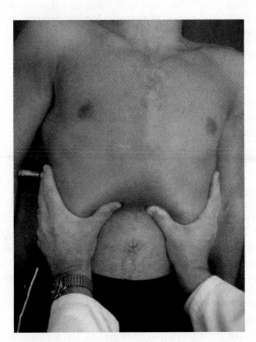

Figure 46-24   Redoming the diaphragm.

5. As the patient again exhales, further cephalad excursion of the diaphragm is encouraged
6. This procedure is repeated for three to five respiratory cycles
7. Success of the technique is determined by retesting excursion of the diaphragm

SUMMARY

Although muscle energy techniques may be used as standalone techniques for the treatment of somatic dysfunction, they are often combined with other techniques. They can be useful in creating the soft tissue relaxation necessary to accomplish HVLA Thrust techniques. Many muscle energy and HVLA techniques are done in the same position, so no repositioning of the patient is required when moving from one technique to the other.

Used another way, muscle energy techniques are used to lengthen muscles shortened by both hypertonicity and contracture. Once the hypertonicity has been eliminated using the muscle energy technique, the patient is in perfect position to begin applying direct myofascial release techniques to the passive connective tissue elements of that same muscle.

Muscle energy techniques are used to balance muscle tone, strengthen reflexly weakened musculature, improve symmetry of articular motion, and enhance the circulation of body fluids (blood, lymph, and interstitial fluid).

Although these are some of the more common uses, the versatility of muscle energy techniques allows them to be combined with any of the other osteopathic manipulative techniques in total patient management.

REFERENCES

1. Mitchell FL Sr. Structural pelvic function. In: Barnes MW, ed. *Yearbook of the Academy of Applied Osteopathy.* Indianapolis, IN: American Academy of Osteopathy, 1958:79.
2. Ruddy TJ. Osteopathic rhythmic resistive duction therapy. In: Barnes MW, ed. *Yearbook of the Academy of Applied Osteopathy.* Indianapolis, IN: American Academy of Osteopathy, 1961:58.
3. Guyer AF. Proprioceptive neuromuscular facilitation for vertebral joint conditions. In: Grieve GP, ed. *Modern Manual Therapy of the Vertebral Column.* New York, NY: Churchill Livingstone, 1986:626.
4. Lewit K, Simons DG. Myofascial pain: relief by post-isometric relaxation. *Arch Phys Med Rehabil* 1984;65:453–456.
5. Travell JG, Simons DG. *Myofascial Pain and Dysfunction: The Trigger Point Manual.* Vol 2. Baltimore, MD: Williams & Wilkins, 1992:10.
6. Mitchell Jr FL, Moran PS, Pruzzo NA. *An Evaluation and Treatment Manual of Osteopathic Muscle Energy Procedures.* Valley Park, MO: Mitchell, Moran, and Pruzzo, 1979.
7. Mitchell Jr FL. *The Muscle Energy Manual.* East Lansing, MI: MET Press, 1999.
8. Goodridge, JP. Muscle energy technique: definition, explanation, methods of procedures. *J Am Osteopath Assoc* 1981;81:249–254.
9. Mitchell Jr FL, Moran PS, Pruzzo NA. *An Evaluation and Treatment Manual of Osteopathic Manipulative Procedure.* 2nd Ed. Kansas City, MO: Institute for Continuing Education in Osteopathic Principles, Inc., 1973:325.
10. Jull GA, Janda V. Muscles and motor control in low back pain; assessment and management. In: Twomaey LT, Taylor JR, eds. *Physical Therapy for the Low Back.* New York, NY: Churchill Livingstone, 1987:272.
11. Mitchell FL Jr. *The Muscle Energy Manual.* Vol 1. East Lansing, MI: MET Press, 1999:14.

KEY CONCEPTS

- This approach emphasizes appreciation and recruitment of the innate and inherent motion of the myofascial structures.
- Patterns of motion and ease are identified across proximal and distal structures, diaphragms, compartments, viscera, and organ systems.
- Techniques of this type are myofascial release (MFR), integrated neuromusculoskeletal release, fascial-ligamentous release, and bioelectric fascial activation and release.
- Respiratory assistance, fulcrums, body position, neuroreflexive activities, oscillation, passive progressive motion, and muscular contractions may aid in the progression of MFR.

CASE STUDY

JM is a 49-year-old Caucasian male who has been suffering with right sciatica for 3 months after beginning a cardiac fitness program. He describes the pain as an ache from his right buttock to posterior thigh, but not below the knee. He notices it with walking and standing and it decreases with rest or sitting. He denies any numbness or tingling in his legs, or any weakness with activities. He has noticed that he is wearing out the sole on his left shoe and has had to replace them more frequently. He denies any recent trauma. Ibuprofen helps the pain temporarily.

The rest of his review of systems is noncontributory. Past medical history is negative for neuromusculoskeletal issues other than the present chief complaint and is positive for elevated blood pressure. Family history is positive for hypertension both maternal and paternal. Medications are occasional ibuprofen for sciatica.

Physical Exam

BP: 130/72; Pulse: 70 regular; Resp: 12 and regular and in moderate distress.

Gait:

Antalgic with limp right and pain in right sacroiliac (SI) joint with full weight bearing on right leg and reproduction of sciatica right

Postural exam:

Posterior view: right iliac crest low, right PSIS low with lateral curve changes convex right lumbar and left thoracic with downward tilt of right shoulder. Greater trochanter is low right with externally rotated right hip. Pain in right SI joint with change in position seated to standing.

Palpatory exam:

Pain on palpation of the right piriformis with reproduction of chief complaint of sciatica. Tenderness and tightness of left quadratus lumborum and right thoracolumbar fascia with torsion to the left of the torso on the pelvis and contralateral pattern through the rectus abdominus fascia.

Inhibited right hamstrings with tight right quadriceps femoris and right piriformis.

Neurologic exam:

No signs of peripheral or central compromise and is otherwise normal.

Vascular exam:

Normal

Diagnosis:

- Postural imbalance with short right leg
- Sciatica
- Somatic dysfunction of thoracic, lumbar, sacrum, pelvis, and lower extremity

Treatment:

- Myofascial release (MFR) to the thoracic, lumbar, sacrum, pelvis, and lower extremity
- Postural x-rays
- Consider heel lift after review of x-rays
- Home exercise program

DESCRIPTION OF TECHNIQUES

MFR is a system of diagnosis and treatment first described by Andrew Taylor Still and his early students, which engages continual palpatory feedback to achieve release of myofascial tissues (1). It can be applied as a *direct or indirect technique*. In a direct technique, a restrictive barrier is identified in the myofascial tissues and is engaged with a loaded, constant, directional force until the tissue releases and motion is restored. In an indirect technique, the tissues position of ease is identified and is engaged with directed pressure guiding the tissues along this line of least resistance until free movement of all tissues is achieved. A *combined procedure* (2), whereby the practitioner's hands engage both a barrier and point of ease simultaneously, allows the MFR to occur through the application of both direct and indirect methods interactively.

Activating forces used in MFR techniques are as follows (3–5):

1. *Inherent (intrinsic) force*: using the body's natural tendency to seek homeostasis, inherent force is the rhythmic activity in all tissues that works to improve the hydrodynamics and bioenergetic factors around restricted tissues and articulations

2. *Respiratory force (cooperation/assist)* may be used in four ways:
   (a) While using a direct or indirect position, *full cycle respiratory effort* is used as a fascial and/or articulatory activating force
   (b) Once positioned, a *particular phase of respiration* enhances the position of the area being treated
   (c) *Breath holding* for the maximum time that a patient can tolerate causes air hunger and triggers a generalized relaxation of soft tissues
   (d) *Coughing or sniffing on command* produces a respiratory impulse to assist in the release of restrictions

3. *Patient cooperation*: the patient is requested to move in specific directions in various planes of an articulation to aid in mobilizing an area of restriction

4. *Physician-guided force*: after engaging a barrier or point of ease, the physician sequentially guides the tissue or joint through various positions following a shifting pattern of easy motion until the path of dysfunction is retraced and released

5. *Springing/vibration*: placing the hands or percussion hammer on a dysfunction and applying variable degrees of pressure and/or frequency of force causing springing or vibration in the structure activating releases of the tissues

TYPES OF MFR

Fascia is ubiquitous connective tissue, enrobing the body in a *big bandage* (6) contributing to form and function that is accessed by manipulative techniques to alleviate somatic dysfunction. Muscular relationships to the fascia contribute to the shifting tightness and looseness identified through range of motion changes and palpation as direct and indirect barriers. Appreciation and recruitment of the *innate and inherent motion* of the myofascial structures allow for the identification and treatment of patterns of motion and ease across proximal and distal structures, diaphragms, compartments, viscera, and organ systems. The *bioresponsive electrical potentials of the fascia* (7) produce palpable changes in fascial motion and ease related to the status of the internal environment of homeostasis and the biomechanical response to the external environment aiding in the diagnosis and treatment of visceral as well as musculoskeletal disorders and diseases. Respiratory assistance, fulcrums, body position, neuroreflexive activities, oscillation, passive progressive motion, and muscular contractions may aid in the progression of MFR (8–10). Techniques of this type are *MFR, integrated neuromusculoskeletal release (INR), fascial-ligamentous release, and bioelectric fascial activation and release*. Related techniques (facilitated positional release, functional release, counterstrain, balanced ligamentous tension, progressive inhibition of neuromuscular structures, soft tissue, articulatory, Still method, osteopathy in the cranial field and visceral) are discussed in other chapters in this text. Other related techniques in present use are facilitated oscillatory release, Fulford percussion vibrator, and balanced membranous tension.

Soft tissue techniques are related techniques that are *not* in the family of MFR techniques discussed in this chapter. They treat the soft tissues of the body with inhibitory pressure, stretching and kneading, petrissage and skin rolling, deep friction, tapotement, and effleurage.

HISTORY

> *As this philosophy (osteopathy) has chosen the fascia as a foundation of which to stand, we hope the reader will chain his patience for a few minutes on the subject of the fascia, and it's relation to vitality. It stands before the philosopher as one of, if not the deepest living problem ever brought before the mind of man (11).*

Dr. Still spent a great deal of time writing and pondering on the importance of fascia in health and disease as he developed the science of osteopathy. Dr. Still did not write detailed instructions on how to perform a treatment; instead in *Research and Practice*, he provided a rationale for applying osteopathic principles and integrating osteopathic manipulative treatments into the medical management of diseases. Even though Dr. Still did not leave a technique manual and we only have a short video of him performing a treatment, his emphasis on the fascia affected the development of early osteopathic methods, which are the foundation for this class of technique today. He directed his students and colleagues to hunt in the fascia as *"The ground in which all causes of death do the destruction of Life"* (12), and many did.

Pioneers in early osteopathic thought and education (13,14) continued to develop methods of diagnosing and treating the fascia by applying the principles of osteopathy: the body is a unit with the innate ability to heal where structure and function are reciprocally interrelated. Such osteopathic luminaries as Sutherland, Kaufman, Snyder, Cathie, Cole, Smoot, Zink, Becker (Alan and Rollin), and Fulford all expanded our understanding of fascia and laid the foundation for a renaissance of technique development beyond a joint centric model of manipulation.

In the 1980s, Peckham, Chila, and Ward began to discuss how to describe in a more significant way what was developing as MFR (15). Two models emerged from these discussions, the *biomechanical model* of Ward and the *big bandage of fascial continuum model* of Chila. The *biomechanical model* emphasizes the muscular–fascial relationship and developed the techniques known as MFR and integrated INR that emphasizes mechanics, anatomic relationships, tight and loose relationships, tethering and interdependent neural influences as the base for diagnosis and treatment. The *fascial continuum model of the big bandage* emphasizes the fascia and developed into fascial release and fascial-ligamentous release techniques that use the integrity of the fascial continuum to treat proximal to distal, a fulcrum with leverage, torsion and traction, respiratory assistance, and reflexive neurologic reset. Both Ward and Chila began teaching their respective models influencing the next generation of osteopathic techniques.

Within this resurgence of interest in the myofascia, Sutherland's teachings on the treatment of the membranes and ligaments and Fulford's percussion vibrator techniques were being taught and incorporated into osteopathic education. Harakal and Becker taught the importance of enlisting the aid of the *physician within* a patient in all osteopathic treatments (16). Fulford challenged the osteopathic physician to treat a patient's life force with proper intention and attention to achieve positive results (17). An increased interest in innate motions of connective tissues, vibratory changes across tissues, the bioenergy discussions of Sutherland, Becker and Fulford, and the fluid properties of palpation and treatment emerged. A renaissance of osteopathic thought and technique was fueled by this focus shift from joint-based models to the evolving connective tissue models.

In the 1990s, influenced by osteopathic teachings of Still, Kappler, Larson, Chila, Ward, Harakal, Alan and Rollin Becker, Sutherland and Fulford, O'Connell explored bioenergetic research

TABLE 47.1

Models of MFR Techniques

Models of MFR	Techniques	Tissue Focus	Emphasizes
Biomechanical model	MFR, integrated INR	Muscular–fascial relationships	Mechanics, anatomic relationships, tight/loose concepts, tethering and interdependent neural relationships
Fascial continuum of the big bandage model	Fascial-ligamentous release, fascial release	Fascia	Fascial continuum, treat proximal to distal, fulcrum with leverage, torsion and traction, respiratory assistance and reflexive neurologic reset
Bioenergetic model	Bioelectric fascial activation and release, fascial release, MFR	Fascia, holographic interface in homeostasis	Bioresponsive electrical potentials, diaphragms, longitudinal cables and tubes, fascial interface in homeostasis, holographic diagnosing and treating

as it applies to diagnosing and treating in the fascia. What emerged was the *bioenergetic model* that emphasizes the bioresponsive electric potentials of the fascia, primary and compensatory patterns of dysfunction, the fascial continuity of diaphragms with longitudinal cables and tubes, the fascial interface of internal (ECF) and external (biomechanical) environmental factors on homeostasis, a treatment process of intention, attention, and activation of the bioenergetic fascia with holographic palpation, diagnosis and treatment. This approach allows the totality of the human being to be accessed through a single hand placement, or portal of entry (18). These models are summarized in Table 47.1.

MECHANISM OF ACTION

Embryologic development of the mesodermal germ layer gives rise to connective tissues and muscles. The largest mesodermal derivative is connective tissue encompassing blood, cartilage, bone, and connective tissue proper. Histologically, these tissues are distinguished by the proportions of fiber, cells, and extracellular matrix into six types: areolar, white fibrous, yellow elastic, mucous, retiform, and basement membrane. The principal cell types are fibroblasts, fat cells, fixed macrophages, mast cells, plasma cells, and leukocytes. The extracellular matrix contains collagenous, elastic and reticular fibers, mucopolysaccharides, proteoglycans, and molecules of

collagen, elastin, mucin, reticulin, chondroitin sulfate, keratin sulfate, heparin, chondroitin acid, and hyaluronic acid (19). Collagen is a major component of connective tissue proper and more specifically white fibrous tissue. Fascia, the largest component of white fibrous tissue, contains linear sheets of collagen found in superficial, deep, and subserous layers (Fig. 47.1).

A special property of connective tissue cells is *embryologic plasticity* (20). This property allows differentiated connective tissue cells, when properly stimulated, to dedifferentiate to a polypotential root cell and redifferentiate into another type of connective tissue cell. Histologically, some traumatized tendon or muscle tissues demonstrate islands of cartilage or bone exemplifying this process. Experiments by Becker et al. (21) document that disruption in the collagen of the periosteum creates a bioelectric current that affects the *charge* of the cell membrane of fibroblasts, which triggers their *embryologic plasticity* as part of the healing process in fractures. This cell membrane charge signals changes in the DNA and RNA resulting in cell dedifferentiation into a primitive polypotential root cell. These cells then redifferentiate into the cells needed during the healing process. These expressions of the connective tissues embryologic plasticity illustrate that in the face of traumatic biomechanical stress, connective tissue responds by changing its cell type to meet the demand on the tissue mediated by bioelectric changes at the tissue, cell, and nuclear levels.

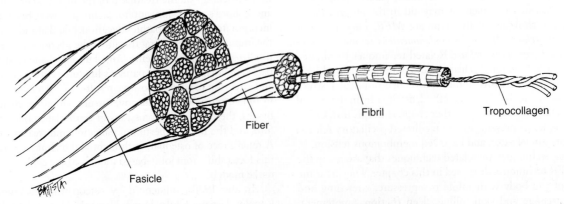

Figure 47-1 Mobility of collagen is demonstrated in its structure.

The extracellular matrix of connective tissue contributes to homeostasis through diffusion, absorption, secretion, diffusion gradients, modification of absorbed substances, metabolism and catabolism, and the excretion of metabolic end products and waste (22). All cells contribute to this extracellular fluid (ECF) interfacing with nerve endings, hormones, vascular and lymphatic structures. This organization allows for coordination of the internal (metabolic, cellular, and organ systems) components of homeostasis within the structure of connective tissues.

The muscles are divided into smooth, cardiac, and skeletal types. They are related embryologically to connective tissue, the vascular system, cranial nerves (CN), and the autonomic and peripheral nervous systems through *migratory segmental differentiation* (Fig. 47.2). Skeletal muscle fibers develop from the mesodermal myotomes and regional mesenchyme and migrate in a sea of connective tissue in response to lines of stress in the developing embryo. Skeletal muscle myofibrils extend along these lines of stress in a linear fashion and become bundled as fascicles by the perimysium. Between the fascicles, the endomysium contains the nerves, blood and lymph vessels, and acts as lubricant and cushion. Fascicles are bundled by the epimysium and the tendons develop connecting the muscles to the developing skeleton. This creates a compact integration of multiple systems residing within a connective tissue container (Fig. 47.3).

Earlier authors like Cathie (23) and Becker (24) suggested that fasciae move independently. A 1987 soft tissue dissection done by Frank George, D.O., in the anatomy laboratories of Michigan State University demonstrates that fascia and muscle are anatomically inseparable and suggests that complex muscle activities act on bones, ligaments, tendons, associated with joints as well as the fasciae.

Fascia is associated with all organs, tissues, cells, and structures. The superficial and deep layers are found everywhere in the body as complete ensheathments. The subserous layer lies innermost on the deep layer anywhere there is a body cavity. The deep layer of fascia is the most complicated of the three, being two layered with intervening septa.

Clinically, it is possible to conceptualize such wrapping as being a *big bandage* of the body. Such an analogy is implied in osteopathic literature. One can find reference to the idea that the body retains form even if everything except the connective tissue framework is removed. If this is so, then it is also reasonable that form permits the consideration of motion. The continuity of this arrangement and considerations of structural–functional interrelationships make it possible to discuss biomechanical attributes of fascia in relation to manipulative treatment. Fascia supports and stabilizes, helping to maintain balance. It assists in the production and control of motion and the interrelation of motion of related parts in concert with muscles. Many of the body's fascial specializations have postural functions in which stress bands can be demonstrated. Finally, the dura mater is a special connective tissue surrounding the central nervous system. Bony anchors for this tissue exist in the skull and at the sacrum. Stiles began teaching an application of Buckminster Fullers tensegrity systems to human anatomy, which has further contributed to the growing understanding of the connective tissue continuum.

Collagen, fibrin, and reticulin of connective tissue act as the body's reactor to motion and stress and coupled with the skeletal muscle interact to produce *irritability, contractility, relaxation, distensibility, and elasticity* (Table 47.2) (25). *Irritability* is the ability of the muscle fiber to react to stimulation. *Contractility* is the ability to actively create tension between its origin and insertion, and the opposing passive state is *relaxation*. *Distensibility* is the ability of

the associated connective tissue to be stretched or deformed by an outside force, and if the force does not exceed the tensile strength of the connective tissue, the muscle will not be injured. *Elasticity* is the ability of the connective tissue to return to its original resting shape when forces are removed (26).

Other force effects in connective tissue of importance are *plastic deformation, elastic deformation, viscosity, stress, strain, and creep* (Table 47.3). In plastic deformation, a stressed, formed, or molded tissue *preserves* its new shape; and in elastic deformation, a stressed, formed, or molded tissue *recovers* its original shape. Viscosity is the capability of a solid to continually yield under stress with a measurable rate of deformation. *Stress* is the effect of a force normalized over an area. *Strain* is a change in shape as a result of stress. *Creep* is the continued deformation of a viscoelastic material under constant load over time (Fig. 47.4). *Hysteresis*, or *stress-strain*, is defined as a connective tissue response to loading and unloading in which the restoration of the final length of the tissue occurs at a rate and to an extent less than during deformation (loading) representing energy loss in the connective tissue (Fig. 47.5) (27). Generally speaking, the body's connective tissues are under some degree of load and extension (expansion). The increase and subsequent reversal of extension produces a degree of tissue response less than the relatively unloaded state. This phenomenon is referred to as *hysteresis*. It implies the occurrence of some flow and dissipation of energy throughout the loaded tissue. Hysteresis occurs less with successive cycles of extension, indicating stabilization of response (28).

It is now clear that the physical properties of fascia and muscles explain how physical laws of adaptability apply to MFR techniques. *Hooke law* (29) states that stress applied to stretch or compress a body is proportional to the strain, or change in length thus produced, so long as the limit of elasticity of the body is not exceeded. Palpatory diagnosing and treating is the systematic application of directed mechanical pressures and motions while monitoring the tissue response. Perceived alterations in motions, symmetry, tissue texture, and tenderness define somatic dysfunction (30). The response in intact fascia to mechanical stress is predictable, detectable, and when dysfunctional, it is treatable with MFR techniques. These physical properties coupled with Hooke law are the foundation for the characteristic palpatory findings of barriers and ease, tight and loose, and strain patterns.

Wolff law of bone transformation (31) states: every change in the function of a bone is followed by certain definite changes in internal architecture and external conformation in accordance with mathematical laws. Function dictates structure. Every change in the form and the function of a bone is followed by certain changes in its internal architecture and secondary alterations in its external conformation. Structure dictates function. Multiple studies examined the application of this law. In the 1950s, Yasuda and Fukada and Bassett and Becker demonstrated that bone is *piezoelectric*. Piezoelectricity is a current produced by a substance that transforms mechanical stress to electrical energy. Piezoelectric substances act as transducers and are able to discharge electrical current when physically stressed, and when placed in an electric current, they vibrate at a frequency dependent upon their crystal lattice structure. Further studies identified *collagen* as the piezoelectric substance in bone (32). *Fascia is a collagen-rich connective tissue*. The piezoelectric properties of collagen are outlined in Table 47.4.

Piezoelectricity is important in the maintenance of bone as well as responses to stress. Studies investigating Wolff law noted that a bioelectric gradient is formed in bone in response to stress. The electronegative charge in the compressed bone stimulates

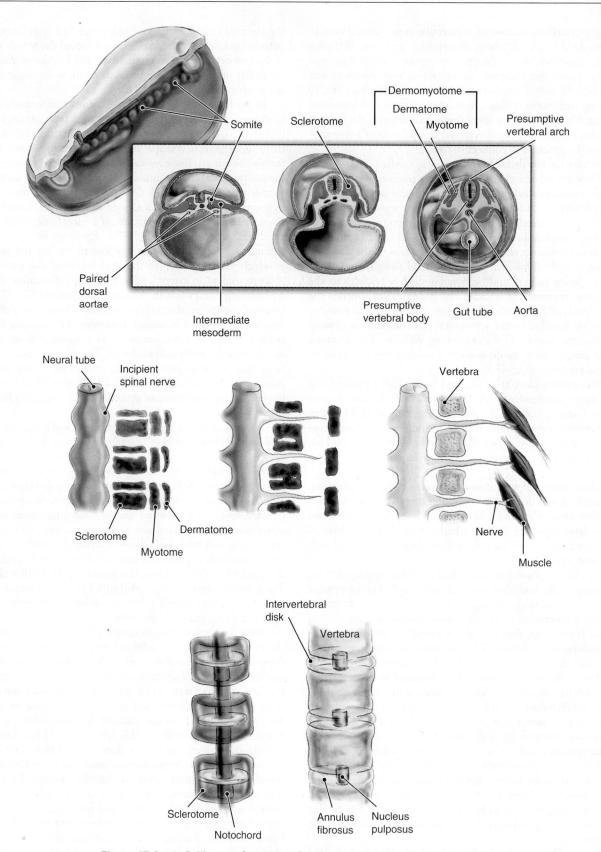

Figure 47-2 A–C. The transformation of paraxial mesoderm into its derivatives.

osteoblasts, and the electropositive bone stimulates osteoclasts directing the remodeling of the bone. This was further clarified when Becker and Bachman (33) discovered that when mechanically stressed, collagen in bone produces a biphasic signal, negative with stress (load), and positive with release (unload). This stress-release signal is rectified to a direct current at the junction between the apatite and collagen in the bone. *The strength of this signal indicates the amount of stress and the polarity changes identify the*

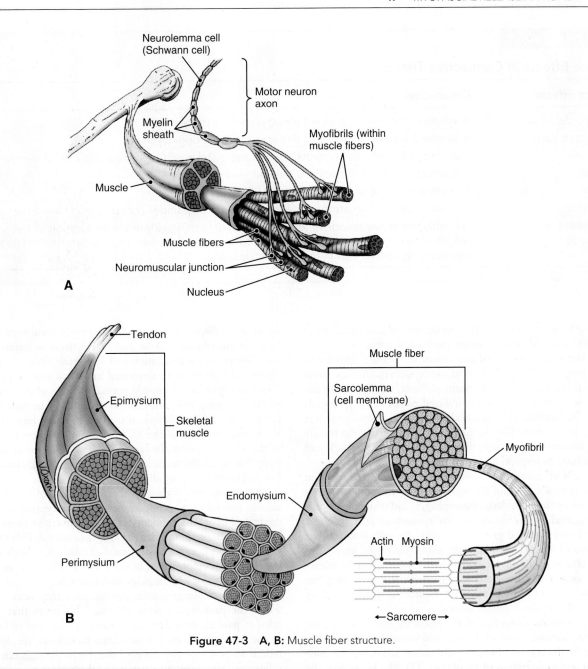

Figure 47-3   A, B: Muscle fiber structure.

TABLE 47.2

Physical Properties of Muscle

Properties	Description
Irritability	Ability of the muscle fiber to react to stimulation
Contractility	Ability to actively create tension between its origin and insertion
Relaxation	Ability to reduce tension between its origin and insertion
Distensibility	Ability of the associated connective tissue to be stretched or deformed by an outside force, and if the force does not exceed the tensile strength of the connective tissue, the muscle will not be injured.
Elasticity	Ability of the connective tissue to return to its original resting shape when forces are removed

TABLE 47.3

Force Effects in Connective Tissue

Force Effects	Description
Plastic deformation	A stressed, formed, or molded tissue *preserves* its new shape
Elastic deformation	A stressed, formed, or molded tissue *recovers* its original shape
Viscosity	Capability of a solid to continually yield under stress with a measurable rate of deformation
Stress	The effect of a force normalized over an area
Strain	A change in shape as a result of stress
Creep	The continued deformation of a viscoelastic material under constant load over time
Hysteresis or stress-strain	A connective tissue response to loading and unloading where the restoration of the final length of the tissue occurs at a rate and to an extent less than during deformation (loading) representing energy loss in the connective tissue

direction of the stress. This signal triggers osteocyte activity, allowing the bone to remodel to adapt to the mechanical stress.

The electronegative signal also caused the linear alignment of collagen perpendicular to the lines of compressive mechanical stress (Figs. 47.6 and 47.7). This alignment of the collagen becomes the base for ossification. Also, stress-induced piezoelectric potentials are short in duration while the healing current of bone growth is sustained in duration. This healing current stimulates electrically sensitive connective tissue cells that are embryologically plastic and allow the bone to respond to growth or stress appropriately.

The cells of connective tissue are mobile, allowing migration of cells to meet the needs of the organism. This ameboid motion is exemplified by the fibroblasts, macrophages, and white blood cells and is triggered by positive or negative chemotaxis or in response to a bioelectric potential gradient directing the cells into and out of the area of need. This movement allows tissues to respond to changes in their environment, both internal and external, by releasing chemotactic factors, creating a gradient and activating the movement of connective tissue cells facilitating the clearing of debris and the repair of injured tissues.

Disruption and distortion of the fascia triggers a repair process directed at correction of damage and strengthening of tissue mediated by the release of chemotaxic factors activating the congregation and proliferation of fibroblasts. The fibroblasts coat the injured area and collagen is then deposited in a linear fashion along lines of mechanical tension in the tissue (34). Mechanical tension creates bioelectric current changes that guide the orientation of the

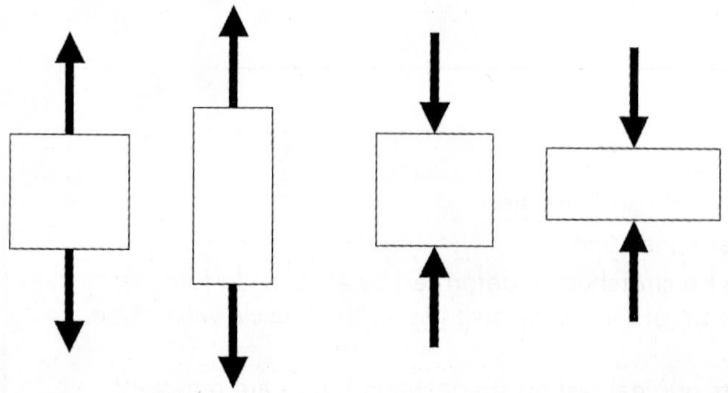

fibrin and collagen. If neurologic integrity is compromised or the tissue is immobilized, dense connective tissue is formed. Edema and disruptions in circulation and lymphatic drainage also cause fibrin and collagen to be deposited in a thick and haphazard scar. These thickened areas impede normal function of the linear sheets of fascia causing stiffness, changes in range of motion, pain, and further edema (35). Chronic alterations in fascial integrity impede the normal function of the ECF with consequences to the health of the whole organism. In Dr. Still's words: "I know no part of the body that equals the fascia as a hunting ground ... By its actions we live and by its failure we die" (36).

Other research highlights the importance of fascia in maintaining general proprioception. Since proprioception is ultimately controlled by interdependent neural and muscular elements, after joint and muscle spindle activity is accounted for, 75% of remaining proprioception occurs in fascial sheaths (37). Such responses were actually demonstrated in the 1960s by Earl (38) and Wilson (39) in their work with muscles under stretch.

Patients challenged with chronic pain may seek a position where the pain lessens or is relieved. This infers that positional relief of pain allows a decrease in some critical level of facilitation in the nervous system. Fascial release techniques are designed to reduce afferent input to the cord directly or through central brain influences. Muscle proprioceptors and the gamma motor system are affected with reduction of excitation of the muscle spindle, and the resumption of normal length and motion (40). Further rationales for the mechanism of releases of dysfunction with OMT are found in the works of Korr (41), Becker (42), and Patterson (43).

Collagen is the source of stress-related electrical potentials through its piezoelectric nature as a transducer. Collagen communicates the presence, location, direction, and strength of mechanical stress by producing a biphasic electric current. This bioelectric current affects the charge-sensitive cells that move and change in response. Studies demonstrate how collagen is the ultimate communicator between biomechanical events, bioelectric changes, cellular function, and the ECF. MFR techniques harness the power of collagen through diagnosing and treating in the fascia, the largest collagen pool in the body.

FASCIA AND HOMEOSTASIS

Homeostasis is both a state of equilibrium and the process by which this balance is maintained. It is a dynamic, ever-adapting,

Figure 47-4   Deformation under load.

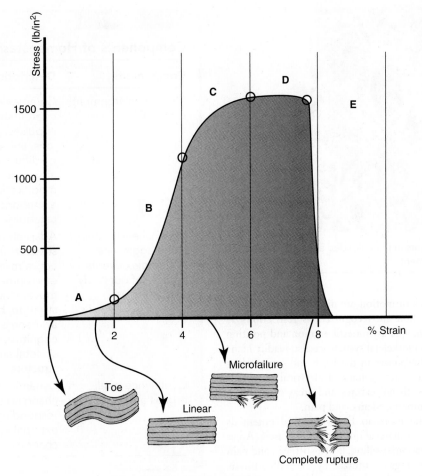

Figure 47-5   The stress-strain response.

and changing series of events responding to internal and external environmental changes (Table 47.5). *The challenge of homeostasis is to recognize all events, external and internal, communicate needs for adaptation throughout the organism, and direct responses both internal and external.* Nothing is isolated (44).

As previously discussed, fascia responds to biomechanical stress, through its collagen fibers, by producing microelectrical potential changes. These changes communicate the biomechanical events through electrical changes in the ECF to cellular, neural, vascular, and lymphatic components. These stress-generated potentials are predictable and precise whether traumatic or intentional.

Palpation introduces compressive and distraction forces into fascial tissue, which responds in predictable patterns of motion produced by adaptations to the mechanical stress. Alterations in

TABLE 47.4

Piezoelectric Properties of Collagen

Properties	Description
Transducer	Able to discharge electrical current when physically stressed and when placed in an electric current, vibrate at a frequency dependent upon its crystal lattice structure
Biphasic signal	Negative with stress (load) and positive with release (unload)
Stress related signal	Strength of this signal indicates the amount of stress and the polarity changes identify the direction of the stress
Stimulates osteocytes	Electronegative charge in the compressed bone stimulates osteoblasts, and the electropositive bone stimulates osteoclasts directing the remodeling of the bone
Stimulates and directs the migration of electrically sensitive cells	By releasing chemotactic factors, creating a gradient and activating the movement of necessary connective tissue cells facilitating the clearing of debris and the repair of injured tissues
Activates cells	Stimulates electrically sensitive connective tissue cells which are embryologically plastic

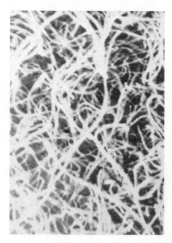

Figure 47-6 Collagen fibers in the unloaded state demonstrating a multidirectional arrangement.

normal patterns and ranges of motion are diagnostic parameters. Abnormal patterns of motion are recognized as restrictions to motion and ease of motion. The asymmetric motion and position of components of the musculoskeletal system are also readily identified through palpation. Responses in the ECF and surrounding structures to adaptations to stress-generated electrical potentials produce acute and chronic tissue textures and areas of stiffness, looseness, tenderness, asymmetry, edema, and pain.

In systemic disease alterations in ECF, electrical potentials result in changes in the biomechanical integrity of the fascia. Areas of acute and chronic congestion, swelling, laxity, stiffness, and pain are produced. Palpatory findings are utilized by the skilled physician to identify the disease produced somatic dysfunction. Integrating an understanding of the patterns of viscerosomatic and somatovisceral relationships adds a deeper diagnostic and therapeutic dimension to the palpatory exam (45).

Homeostasis involves a complex series of events and interfaces between all systems and the internal and external environment. Neuroreflexive coordination is essential in this endeavor. Autonomic, especially sympathetic tone, affects not only pain perceptions but also the balance of neurovascular exchange affecting edema and effusions. This in turn affects motion and tissue function. Proprioception integrated with the special senses of

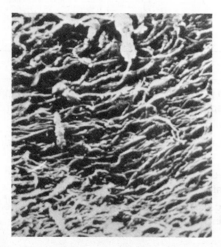

Figure 47-7 • Collagen fibers in the loaded state demonstrating a linear rearrangement.

TABLE 47.5

Components of Homeostasis

Components	Description
Internal environment is the ECF	Complex activities coordinating hormones, nerve impulses, gases, nutrients, ions, and electrical potentials by diffusion, gradients, absorption, secretion, modification of substances, excretion, metabolism and catabolism
External environment is the aggregate of complex events outside of our body that affect us	Adaptation to external stressors and accommodates active manipulation of the environment with posture, movement, coordination, strength, balance, and awareness coordinating cognitive, neural, muscular, skeletal and vascular structures.
Confluence of all organs and systems	Dynamic, ever-adapting, and changing series of events responding to internal and external environmental changes

sight, hearing, and touch is essential to balance, posture, and gait. Evaluating the patient in multiple positions (standing, seated, prone, supine) and activities (walking, standing, squatting, changing positions, bending, work positions) adds another dimension to fascial diagnosis and treatment. Dysfunctions in these areas are important contributors to chronic recurring somatic and visceral dysfunctions. Identification of such patterns and their neuromyofascial components allows the clinician the opportunity to affect and extinguish self-perpetuating cycles. Once this is accomplished, repatterning the neuromyofascia into a more physiologic response is appropriate.

McEwen at the Rockefeller Institute has postulated that the shift from homeostasis to the disease state is related to the systems response to stress, whether traumatic, psychological, emotional, physiologic, or environmental. The body under stress of any source enters a state of allostasis, where epinephrine and cortisol are released. If this state becomes long term, an allostatic load ensues with physiologic consequences such as elevated blood pressure and heart rate with increase risk of cardiovascular disease. Cortisol levels can suppress the immune system, affect organ function, alter metabolism, and contribute to depression. The allostatic load may become somaticized and be expressed as somatic dysfunction with *body language significance* (46), which may help in identifying the nonsomatic cause of chronic, recurrent dysfunction in light of appropriate treatment. Examples of this are when the body seems to act out its underlying stress condition. A patient with chronic emotional stress may have low back pain; mental and emotional feelings of "shouldering" a heavy burden may cause shoulder pain; refusing to change behaviors leads to a stiff neck. Understanding homeostasis now is expanded to include the interface and interaction between the physical, emotional, mental, and spiritual bodies. Insights into these connections can be found in many sources outside the medical literature. One very helpful little book in understanding and interpreting connections between thought patterns and disease is *Heal Yourself* by Louise Hay who has been working with patients with cancer, AIDS, and other life-altering diseases.

Disease occurs when one or more system(s) fail to maintain their part in homeostasis. It begins as a clinically undetectable change in ECF and progresses until clinically detectable signs and symptoms appear making the diagnosis apparent (47). The goal of the clinician is to detect the disease and institute appropriate treatment as early as possible. This will limit the amount of damage to the systems and organs as well as enhancing the bodies healing capabilities. Learning to diagnose and treat with MFR techniques is a clinical advantage for **in the fascia, no disease escapes notice and no cure occurs without its assistance**.

INDICATIONS, CONTRAINDICATIONS, AND COMPLICATIONS

Indications

Diagnosing in the Fascia

The skilled physician is able to identify altered fascial patterns from any source, internal or external, as somatic dysfunction. Once identified, the pattern, location, and type of somatic dysfunction assist in the diagnosis of visceral and somatic disease, which is then treated with the appropriate application of MFR technique and/or combination of osteopathic techniques with standard medical/surgical care. Monitoring changes, immediate and distant (over time), in the form and function of fascial structures indicate the status of diseases and their response to all treatment endeavors.

Treating in the Fascia

MFR techniques are used to alleviate the visceral and somatic components of somatic dysfunction in the connective tissues of the body, with a focus on fascia, muscles, and related structures (neuroreflexive, circulatory, lymphatic, respiratory, bioenergetic, systemic, holographic, and homeostatic). In systemic disease, MFR techniques address structural imbalances and somatic dysfunction indicative of and pursuant to changes in homeostasis and aid in the normalization of function in all systems. MFR techniques address somatic dysfunction by normalizing motion, relieving edema, reestablishing symmetry, relieving pain, aiding circulatory and lymphatic function, normalizing neuroreflexive activity, supporting visceral function, restoring bioenergetic balance, and supporting homeostatic function.

The key to clinical success is the systematic development and application of the MAN acronym—*M*echanics, *A*natomic relationships, and interdependent *N*eural influences with tethering, tight-loose relationships, three-dimensional patterns (Ward), harnessing a fulcrum, balanced points of tension, expanding releases of dysfunction over time within the connective tissue continuum (Chila), utilizing the holographic fascial structure of tubes, diaphragms, and longitudinal cables, identifying primary somatic and visceral dysfunctions with their related patterns, and activating releases in the bioenergetic fascial continuum supporting homeostasis. (O'Connell) Treatment is enhanced when the clinician addresses the patient with proper *intention* (humility and respect of the patients process), *attention* (mindfulness of the individuals needs), and with appropriate application of technique, *activation* of releases (supporting the healing process) (Chila, Ward, and O'Connell).

Contraindications

Absolute contraindications include absence of somatic dysfunction, lack of patient consent, and/or cooperation. Relative contraindications may be regional or local.

The safe introduction of motion depends upon multiple factors: integrity of the tissues (open wounds, fractures, recent surgery), the amount of traumatized tissues (thermal injury, contusions, crushing), concomitant diseases (deep vein thrombosis, disseminated or local neoplasms, aortic aneurysm, uncontrolled diabetes), or internal injuries (ruptured viscera or vascular structures), surgical interventions, infections, cooperation of the patient, and the skill of the physician (48).

Complications

A word of caution: overly aggressive interventions are counterproductive. Care should be taken to ensure that any treatment respects the limits of dysfunctional and injured tissues. Exceeding these limits creates a traumatic event. Somatic dysfunction resulting from iatrogenic trauma layered on already dysfunctional or traumatized tissue is the most difficult dysfunction to treat (49).

Patients commonly experience a temporary worsening of discomfort following the first treatment or two. This possibility should be communicated to the patient. The phenomenon is similar to postexercise muscle soreness. Older age groups and general deconditioning are common contributors to the problem. Those with autoimmune, inflammatory, and rheumatologic disorders such as lupus erythematosus and fibromyalgia can experience repeated flare-ups.

SPECIAL CONSIDERATIONS IN DIAGNOSTICS

Subtle Palpatory Skills

Dr. Still: For many years, immersed in extensive study of normal and abnormal positions of the human anatomy, Still had formed in his mind a perpetual image of every articulation in the framework of the human body. Before William Roentgen's discovery of the X-ray machine, visualization, good observation skills, a delicate sense of touch—and that perpetual image—were the only tools Still had to assist him in detecting the abnormal from the normal. He also claimed to see an aura around all of his patients—vibrations emanating from the body—giving him additional clues about his patient's conditions. The Old Doctor, skeptical of the new instrument (x-ray machine), stated to some students, "The x-ray by tremendously increasing the vibrations enables us to see under the surface what our eyes will not discover. Why can't we train our minds to do that?" (50) (Andrew Taylor Still, p. 176).

Ward: Inherent tissue motions are palpably evident, asymmetrically patterned, neuroreflexive activities in the soft tissues. They constantly move, often at variable rates. Palpation that focuses on these motions should readily identify patterns of shifting asymmetric tightness and looseness. Asymmetrically perceived end-feels are commonly referred to as *direct* and *indirect barriers*. As a rule, inherent movements are easier in some directions, less so in others. Myofascially, shifting tightness and looseness identifies unevenly distributed direct and indirect barriers. Many are independent of joint mechanics. Others are tightly linked to joint mechanisms (51).

During treatments with MFR techniques, there is a link between the intrinsic body movements of both the patient and the operator at some level. How this occurs is unknown, but it is likely that both conscious and subconscious brain-mediated factors are at play. In 1989, Grinberg-Zylerbaum and Ramos reported on their studies of nontouching, silent communication between two or more individuals. Electroencephalography (EEG) was used as a means for studying silent communication patterns between two individuals. Partners who reported feelings of being blended with one another altered their EEG patterns to the point of being virtually identical. Similar blending effects are reported during MFR encounters. Whether these experiences are in any way similar to the Grinberg-Zylerbaum and Ramos work has not been investigated. Skilled palpation in the fascia enables the clinician to "see" anatomic and mechanical detail, much like a blind person senses the environment. As improvements appear, appreciation for seemingly obscure, but important, subtleties emerge (52).

Chila: MFR techniques require refinement of palpatory skills to appreciate subtleties of stress patterns and motion characteristics. Technique application allows the patient to manifest their own potency rather than using blind external force and overpower its assistance. The clinician uses palpation to listen to the effects of the biokinetic energies and forces while allowing the biodynamic intrinsic force to manifest (53). The corrective forces engage the identified resistance to motion and direct it to a point of simultaneous balance and decreased tension, allowing the intrinsic force of the tissues to correct the imbalance. The focus is on the quality of movement, particularly on initiation of motion. The correct gauging of force and velocity provides infinite variation in the delivery of technique. Control minimizes force. The effective physician should be able to vary the applications of force over time during a single manipulative treatment. Appropriate use of a fulcrum and leverage can refine the physician's diagnostic touch and treatment effectiveness.

Visualization and synthesis of messages received through the fingers are the basis for clinical behavior. Conceptualization of anatomic-physiologic dysfunction peculiar to a given patient is the key to maximizing manipulative responses. The sustained effective response following treatment is contingent on selective and controlled variation of force from an appropriate fulcrum. When these conditions are met, inherent neuroregulatory mechanisms acting in accordance with the capacity of the patient will facilitate the resolution of dysfunction (54).

O'Connell: Fascia can be viewed as an "Intelligent Tissue" functioning as the interface between internal and external events and playing a key role in homeostasis. As discussed previously, embryologic plasticity gives connective tissue the unique ability to respond by cellular adaptation to meet the changing needs of the organism (18). Through the use of "thinking fingers" Sutherland), intelligent palpation interfaces with the fascia in a clinical dialogue giving access to peripheral and central structures, viscera and soma, and the biological and bioenergetic bodies. The body, mind, and spirit are all available to the skilled clinician as the whole of the human condition is recorded and assessable in the holographic fascia. As clinicians improve their palpatory skills, there is an awareness that from any portal of entry into the fascia the whole of the patient's condition, body, mind, and spirit is available for diagnosis and treatment. Once this skill level is achieved, the practitioner is able to identify the primary dysfunction rapidly from contact at any site within the anatomy. *Within the holographic fascia, the primary dysfunction is not limited to connective tissue structures and may be anywhere in the body, mind, and spirit continuum.* Focused clinician *intention* to assist in healing and *attention* to the homeostatic fascial holographic interface allows for the *activation* of far reaching releases and healing dynamics. This level of skill has been described by many master osteopaths and healers as a "knowing" sensation or viewing an image or movie like projection that flashes into a stilled mind. The power and potency of techniques at this level

demand of the clinician an attitude of humility, respect, suspended expectations, and compassion (55). It is within the patient that the capacity to heal resides.

> **Dr. Still:** "*Don't believe for one second that this was the limit of his vision. According to many who studied with him and others who have spent years studying his works it was his hope that the experience of living, dynamic anatomy would awaken dormant centers of perception in the student. Gradually, over a period of years of focused attention, conscious intention of purpose and deep non-judgmental concentration on the experience of life as manifested in the patient, the physician would evolve to a higher level of interaction with the dynamic mechanism of the patient. He would evolve into an osteopath.*" (Osteopathy Research and Practice, p. xix)

THE TECHNIQUES

Fascial Ligamentous Release-Chila

Fascial ligamentous release is a dynamic and expansile form of MFR emphasizing the cybernetic loop between the physician and patient. Selective, controlled reciprocal variation of force and appropriate leverage coupled with inherent neuroregulatory mechanics impact the resolution of dysfunction within the capacity of the patient. Key elements of this dynamic process are as follows:

- Application of force is variable
- Utilization of time is variable
- Visualization and synthesis are mandatory
- Conceptualization is paramount
- Tolerance and response are individual
- Inherent capacity is the standard for health or disease
- Dynamic interchange where the patient allows the physician to enter bodily territorial space
- Physician is a facilitator and observer
- Implication is that the patient's life story is available through examination and evaluation of body tissues
- Energy flows from thought (56)

In conjunction with these elements, the patient provides breath assistance and/or muscular assistance in the corrective procedure. The establishment of a fulcrum is sought within the physician's body to match or balance the fulcrum within the patient's body; this facilitates a continuum of reflex release from within the patient's body. Once local and regional dysfunctions have been addressed by the establishment of an appropriate fulcrum, expanding leverage is achieved through torsion and traction applied to the extremities. It is the ongoing analysis of dysfunction within this connective tissue continuum that makes possible the integration of multiple manipulative approaches through variable applications of force.

The establishment of an appropriate fulcrum facilitates *diagnostic touch*. The placing of the hands and fingers on the tissues under examination is done with the idea that the fingers can mold themselves to the patient's body. The initiation of the pattern within the area of complaint is realized by a slight compression at the fulcrum points. The application of the principle of the fulcrum varies with the complaints of the patient. *The use of this method is not a time-consuming process.* Harnessing internal patient mechanisms are used, and it is necessary only to contact them to sense them speaking for themselves. The point(s) of contact is(are) listening posts. Let the tissues tell the story; be quiet and listen. Biokinetic (dysfunctional) energies or forces are always at work in all physiologic and pathologic processes. With the appropriate use of diagnostic touch, the biodynamic (healing) intrinsic force within is allowed to manifest itself.

Special consideration of respiration-circulation function is essential in diagnosing and treating. Compromised respiratory-circulatory effectiveness is the result of generalized fascial-ligamentous tension throughout the body. For that reason, the character of respiration provides information about such tension. Observe four factors about respiration:

1. *Type of respiration:* diaphragmatic, costal, or mixed
2. *Abdominal wall motion:* visible to the level of the umbilicus; visible to the level of the symphysis pubes
3. *Rate:* slow, rapid; documented before and after treatment
4. *Duration of cycle:* inspiration and expiration equal, inspiration shorter in duration than expiration, inspiration longer in duration than expiration, dilation of the nares during respiration

Generally speaking, the body's connective tissues are under some degree of load and extension (expansion). As previously discussed, connective tissues under sustained load will extend (expand) in response to the load. In biomechanical terms, this continued extension is referred to as *creep.* An imposed constant load will result in relaxation, as the extension remains constant. In either situation, the tissue displays less subsequent resistance to extension than in the original state. Patterns of previous mechanical events affect the tissue's response to load and extension. Physician-applied extension effects tend to revert to their pre-extension responses, whether functional or dysfunctional, if the neuroreflexive processes are not altered. This observation is useful in appreciating recurrence of dysfunctional complaints and patterns. The timed release of tissues associated with the fascial-ligamentous release model considers these factors as the sequential and expanding progression of releases allows the patient to tolerate central nervous system modulation by the lowering of afferent inputs. Significant reduction or elimination of sensitization is proportional to the patient's capacity to appropriately respond. This view is attuned to the idea that central nervous system conditioning over time may be the vehicle for the retention as well as the reduction of dysfunctional states. The physician's role is that of a facilitator. By appropriate facilitation, the physician is able to observe the capacity for change while the patient is enabled to expand the power of the change. The standard for the successful outcome of this interchange is the motivation of the patient.

Integrated INR-Ward

The ability to identify tethering effects that persistently create and maintain pathologic asymmetries is essential. *Tightness suggests tethering, while looseness suggests joint and/or soft tissue laxity with or without neural inhibition.* Sometimes, tethering relates directly to changes in coupled vertebral motions and altered joint play causing the motion segment to be altered. Knowing the difference between neutral and nonneutral vertebral mechanics is essential. Both local soft tissue, neuroreflexive and neurocirculatory changes, such as viscerosomatic reflex changes, are common contributors to tethering. Tethering arises from many sources, as shown in Box 47.1.

Painful sensations are common at loose sites, particularly in chronic cases. Typically, there is little muscle spasm or tightening. Under these conditions, associated muscles are commonly weak and inhibited. Some practitioners refer to these sites as *hypermobile,* implying that ligamentous laxity and joint instability are the fundamental problems. An alternative idea concludes that loose, painful muscles are weak and inhibited over large, often ill-defined areas, including vertebral mechanics.

Common Causes of Tethering

The spine, with altered coupled vertebral motions from any source

Altered soft tissue mechanics (remembering that all tissues and their inherent motions are intrinsically asymmetric)

The synovial joints and their influences on joint play

Asymmetric neural inputs arising from:

Multiple levels of the central nervous system, including CN, brainstem, midbrain, thalamus, and cortex; limbic system and reticular activating system; primary spinal cord; peripheral nervous system at any level

Viscerosomatic reflexes, somato-visceral reflexes, and somato-somatic reflexes

Neurohumoral activities of all kinds

Lowered reflex thresholds from sites of disease, injury, and degeneration

Biobehavioral and sociocultural factors, environmental stressors

From a clinical perspective, whole-body effects are the rule rather than an exception. Loosened sites are often vulnerable to injury under relatively trivial circumstances. Repeated ankle and lumbosacral sprains, as well as neck and shoulder problems arising from altered lumbopelvic and lower limb mechanics, are common examples. The tight-loose concept can be quickly appreciated by the exercise given in Box 47.2.

Tightness of any kind suggests tethering and direct barriers. It also implies the presence of direct barriers and "bind." Some are of bony origin, but many are not. Whether these tethers and areas of bind should be removed requires careful assessment.

One form of tethering is acute muscle spasm, which is almost always self-limited. Another relates to generally tight muscles, which are not always sources of pain and altered function. Stressful lifestyles and personality issues are common in this group. True spasticity, centrally mediated neural tethering, arises from upper motor neuron pathologies. Cerebral palsy, central spinal stenosis, strokes, and effects of head injuries are common examples.

Tight-Loose Concept Exercise

A simple laboratory exercise readily demonstrates the tight-loose concept. With the patient lying supine, the operator grasps the patient's wrists. By slowly raising the upper limb toward full overhead extension, one gets a sense of shifting three-dimensional tightness or looseness that begins at the wrists and eventually involves the whole of the patient's body. By carefully attending to both the quality and the amplitude of these passively induced operator forces, clearly defined mechanically asymmetric sites of tightness and looseness become apparent.

As each limb is moved separately and together, tight-loose relationships vary considerably and their end-feels are different. Some are abrupt, almost like hitting a wall. Others are soft, like either falling into or fluffing a pillow. Importantly, these asymmetric shifts rarely follow classic anatomic patterns. With practice, variable tensions and loads are readily sensed from the hands and wrists distally into the lumbodorsal fascia and pelvis.

Scar tissue implies the presence of passive mechanical tethering that may actually stabilize an otherwise unstable site. Scar tissue changes the ability of a tissue to respond and move in normal planes and produces a new focus of motion patterning. Acute localized muscle tension and tethering generally imply peripheral neural involvement. A history of direct trauma is common for this group.

Looseness generally occurs in association with indirect barriers, neural inhibition, and painful sites. Since inhibition often accompanies neural injury and Wallerian degeneration, pain reports and muscle weaknesses are a common theme with this group.

Three-dimensional vertical, horizontal, and wraparound patterns are the rule and can be identified with some practice. Looking for three-dimensionally related areas of tightness and looseness is the key.

Tightness and looseness should be evaluated from a patterned three-dimensional context that includes:

- Skeletal and soft tissue configurations
- Upper and lower motor neuron influences
- Effects of mechanical modeling and remodeling of bones, joints, and soft tissues
- Effects of general skeletal factors
- Injury history
- Effects of repetitive daily activities
- Psychoemotional states
- Limiting psychosocial and socioeconomic factors

Locating direct and indirect barriers is a useful method for understanding tightness, looseness, and tethering effects. The general goal is to release tightness and restore three-dimensionally patterned functional symmetry to the extent possible without aggravating hypermobility. As forces against direct and indirect barriers are sequentially applied, an experienced operator can efficiently *treat the whole body in a reasonably short time.*

Integrated neuromuscular and MFR approaches and treatment processes are used to diagnose and modify altered reflex and mechanical patterns anywhere in the body. Applying this form of treatment depends on one's ability to palpate and interactively respond to shifting reflex and mechanical changes as they occur. Recognition of active and passive elements influencing both local and general myofascial and skeletal patterns is an important element in the process. The key to clinical success is the systematic development and application of the MAN acronym—*M*echanics, *A*natomic relationships, and interdependent *N*eural influences.

Bioelectric Fascial Activation and Release-O'Connell

MFR techniques apply compression and distraction forces into the affected fascia directed toward or away from a barrier of motion. Once the barrier or point of ease is engaged, the fascia responds with a decrease in resistance and motion resumes. *The fascia responds rapidly to the light forces applied by all MFR techniques.* As previously discussed, this rapid response is the result of the multiple properties of myofascial tissue: irritability, distensibility, contractility, relaxation, plasticity, elasticity, viscosity, stress, strain, creep, hysteresis, piezoelectric responses, and neuroreflexive activity within the fascial continuum.

During the technique, the fascia releases its restrictions in stages and leads the physician through a pattern of motion. Depending on the skill of the clinician, releases occur in two dimensions, three dimensions, or holographically. This pattern component of motion is often complex and traverses any direction or plane, structure or region, organ or system, within the body-mind-spirit continuum.

Viewing this from the bioenergetic model, the response of the fascia is directed and mediated by microelectrical potential changes. Internal or external trauma and dysfunction leaves a pattern of bioelectric potential changes in the fascia that record the direction, strength, and location as somatic dysfunction (see mechanisms mentioned earlier). The application of the diagnostic and corrective forces also produces bioelectric potentials. This activation of bioenergetic tissues opens a diagnostic dialogue within the fascial continuum. Clinician-induced patterns interact with the dysfunctional pattern differently than the normal tissue. This discernable difference unmasks the dysfunctional pattern as it leads the physician along its path to the primary dysfunction. With practice, the dysfunctional pattern becomes rapidly obvious, the primary dysfunction is evident, and releases begin almost immediately.

The MFR technique of activating a bioenergetic response and following, both diagnostically and therapeutically, as the pattern releases is *bioelectric fascial activation and release*. BFAR builds on the principles of integrated INR/MFR and fascial-ligamentous release within the family of MFR techniques.

The fascia is a holographic system with a physical structure of a continuum of tubes, diaphragms, and longitudinal cables that contain the record of all events, internal and external, biologic and bioenergetic, in any patient. This design is similar to a transportation system with many connections, lines, and stations allowing the rider to enter at any point and travel throughout the whole system. Understanding the fascia as a readily accessible portal of entry, the clinician has the opportunity to engage in a meaningful and far-reaching diagnostic dialogue with the patient. As dysfunction from any cause occurs, its effects are transported throughout the whole organism via this continuum interfacing with homeostatic mechanisms from the bioenergetic to the systemic to the intracellular. To optimize this dialogue, the clinician needs to have the appropriate *intention* to assist the innate healing properties of the patient to alleviate or eliminate the effects of disease processes and the restoration of the patient's ability to resume command of the clinical situation (Chila), *attention* to the type, structure and pattern of dysfunction diagnostically and therapeutically (Ward) and to *activate* the holographic homeostatic response throughout the patient facilitating the release of dysfunction. (O'Connell) The physician is a partner in this process and the patient's mechanisms are in control. Healing, therefore, is an internal dynamic of the patient and is not imposed by the well-meaning endeavors of clinicians.

Tensegrity systems are another way of looking at the responsiveness of the fascia. As discussed by Edward Stiles, D.O., a tensegrity structure consists of multiple nontouching rods (compression struts) and a continuous connecting system (tension system) embedded or islanding the compression struts. He references Donald Ingber, M.D., Ph.D.'s research suggesting that the bones of the body are compression struts and the continuous tension system is the myofascial and ligamentous tissues of the body representing a tensegrity structure. These totally integrated systems exhibit balanced tension and system wide adaptation when a force is introduced anywhere in the structure. This is accomplished by integrated multilevel hierarchical systems in which an introduced force can influence any part of the total system, from the macro to the micro and vice versa. In this way, the force can be distributed throughout the system in a nonlinear manner. Ingber's research further demonstrates that distortions altering cellular shape and function affect cell differentiation and specialization, biochemical activity, and genetic expression of the affected cells. Stiles stresses the importance of these concepts in the application of OMT in the removal of somatic dysfunction and enabling patients to realize their optimal health potential by restoring their tensegrity potential (57).

Considering the concepts of holographic fascia and tensegrity, diaphragms are especially good portals of entry to the fascia because they occur at important anatomical crossroads where curves change, cavities change, and passage points for major circulatory and lymphatic vessels and organs occur. The central diaphragms are the tentorium, thoracic inlet/outlet, respiratory diaphragm, and pelvic diaphragm. Secondary diaphragms occur in the extremities at the palmer and plantar fascia. Diaphragms are muscular and fascial structures giving shape and form to the tubular structure of the body and counter the physical effects of gravity, entropy, and enthalpy while preserving the body's ability to function and perform in space. Myofascial structures act as longitudinal cables connecting all diaphragms allowing a coordination of motion throughout the system.

Choosing a portal of entry to the fascia is based on the patient's history, test and imaging results, consults, exams, and the provisional diagnosis coupled with knowledge of anatomy and mechanics. This may lead to a very specific structure such as an organ, tendon, or muscle, or need further delineation through active diagnostic palpation. In the case of the latter, choose a diaphragm that you feel the most comfortable palpating or the closest diaphragm to the region of suspected dysfunction to begin diagnostic palpation. In all cases, test tightness, looseness, local tissue quality, and range of motion.

Using compression, distraction, or the *full deep respiration cycle*, induce motion and note the different patterns of interaction between the normal (predictable) and the dysfunctional (unpredictable) tissue response. This discernable difference makes the dysfunctional pattern obvious, and following it leads to the primary dysfunction that may be proximal or distal, in any organ or system, biological and/or bioenergetic, and be a barrier or point of ease. With practice, the dysfunctional pattern, whether a barrier or point of ease, becomes rapidly obvious, making the primary dysfunction evident and releases begin almost immediately. In using BFAR, no more than *three deep respiratory cycles* are needed to activate the release in a progressive fashion. With each respiratory cycle, motion in the tissue begins as a release occurs and a new end point of motion manifests. Each successive deep respiratory cycle continues this process until the release is complete. Return to the original portal of entry and reassess for symmetry and resolution of that pattern of dysfunction.

"Peeling an Onion" of Layered Dysfunctional Patterns

Often, upon reassessing after releasing a primary dysfunction pattern, a new primary pattern of dysfunction is evident. Throughout life, the body is exposed to many traumatic and stressful events that produce a distinct primary dysfunction pattern. Just as the most dysfunctional segment within a pattern of dysfunction is primary, so too the most dysfunctional of the layered patterns is the *primary pattern of dysfunction*. As this pattern resolves, the next most dysfunctional pattern becomes primary. This process is much like *peeling an onion* (58). This onion layer effect continues until all dysfunctional patterns are resolved. A word of caution, after the release of a primary dysfunction pattern, the body needs time to respond and adjust. If the clinician immediately begins the release of other emerging patterns of dysfunction, the system tends to decompensate. To avoid this, address the next emerging primary dysfunction pattern in another treatment session.

Another important consideration is when a pattern of dysfunction is associated with an acute condition, such as, but not limited to, pneumonia, a cardiac event, or uncontrolled diabetes.

These acute patterns are always considered primary and should be addressed first.

There are occasions when a new traumatic event exacerbates an old pattern and makes it primary, such as heading a soccer ball and exacerbating the birth primary dysfunction pattern. In adults, these very early chronic patterns are closest to the core of the onion and all other patterns and dysfunctions are layered on top of it. In releasing these activated primordial patterns, the clinician must be very careful because the changes in the body will be monumental, with both wondrous and devastating effects possible. Another possibility of interaction between multiple traumas is an accumulated trauma vector. This vector is created by a reaction between existing vectors and does not follow the physical pattern of trauma. When releasing these accumulation vectors, changes will occur in the reactive old trauma patterns as well, so be careful to take this into consideration. Gradual releases and close follow-up are necessary to safely harness the body's innate ability to heal.

Be patient: The effects of disorderly and aggressive treatment disrupt the hierarchal balance of dysfunction patterns and systemic chaos results. These patients present significant challenges to first relieve the iatrogenic effects and then to reconstruct and treat the layered dysfunctional patterns in the body. The intelligence of the tissue knows the needs of the system, and it is the prudent physician who honors this and applies the process of releases in peeling the onion of dysfunctional patterns accordingly (Box 47.3).

Trauma Patterns

The effects of trauma and the ensuing trauma patterns are special dysfunctional patterns and warrant further discussion. Trauma and alterations in the ECF precipitate a cascade of events mediated by bioelectric potential changes in the collagen-laden fascia. These events have local and distant effects, ultimately affecting homeostasis. All musculoskeletal treatment medical, surgical, rehabilitative or manipulative engages these properties, whether passively or actively.

Disruption and distortion of the fascia triggers a repair and strengthening process mediated by the release of chemotaxic factors activating the congregation and proliferation of fibroblasts. The fibroblasts coat the injured area with a fibrin matrix and collagen is then deposited in a linear fashion along lines of mechanical tension in the tissue (59). These lines of stress produce bioelectric potential changes that direct the repair of the damaged tissue

---

Concepts for Peeling an Onion of Dysfunctional Patterns

Always treat the *primary pattern of dysfunction*

　　Space out treatments to allow the system to rebalance

　　Acute patterns are always considered primary

　　Identify and treat the next primary pattern of dysfunction and continue this process as the layered patterns of dysfunction emerge allowing recuperation time between treatments

　　Release activated primordial patterns very careful as the changes in the body will be monumental, with both wondrous and devastating effects possible

　　Treat the effects of disrupted hierarchal balance of patterns of dysfunction by first relieving the iatrogenic effects and then to reconstruct and treat the layered dysfunctional patterns in the body with respect for the mechanical lines of force affecting the tissue. *Healing therefore takes into account the function of the injured tissue as it repairs its structure.*

If neurologic integrity is compromised or the tissue is immobilized, dense connective tissue is formed. Without the lines of tension and motion, edema and disruptions in circulation and lymphatic drainage also cause fibrin and collagen to be deposited in a thick and haphazard scar. These thickened areas impede normal function of the linear sheets of fascia causing stiffness, changes in range of motion, pain, and further edema (60). This process increases the tissue scarring in a vicious self-perpetuating cycle. Chronic alterations in fascial integrity impede the normal function of the ECF with consequences to the health of the whole organism. *Movement is essential to the appropriate, functional repair of fascia.*

The following healing concepts apply to all connective tissue when injured:

- Linear fibrin and collagen is deposited in response to tension in the tissue and directed by bioelectric potential changes
- Immobilization causes collagen and fibrin to be condensed and haphazard
- Motion improves circulation, exchange of lymphatic fluids and metabolites, and encourages the normal distribution of fibrin and collagen

- It is essential that motion, whether passive or active, be introduced into traumatized tissue as soon as possible
- Appropriate application of OMT will help to restore normal function in traumatized tissue

Tensegrity concepts help to explain relationships between trauma and chronic pain (61). As previously discussed, the body can be viewed as a tensegrity system where trauma affects the whole system and adaptations occur as the body rebalances. As the trauma is distributed, the area of the most intense adaptation is not always at the site of trauma. This site is often the location of the pain complaint, which is secondary by adaptation to the original site of trauma and its related dysfunction pattern. Therefore, evaluation of the whole patient is necessary to identify the site and pattern of the traumatic event, not just the site of pain. Treating the cause of the pain is more efficient and will yield better results than treating the adaptive effect which is pain.

Trauma History

To understand the patient's complaints and condition, a good trauma history is essential (62). Table 47.6 outlines the components of a trauma history; this information will help to identify areas and patterns of related dysfunctions and the state of health of the patient.

TABLE 47.6

Components of a Trauma History

Components	Description
Chronology of trauma	When, where, and what happened during the trauma
Events surrounding the time of the trauma	Circumstances, state of health, state of mind, age, life changes, etc.
Progression of the trauma-related symptoms	Radiation or migration of pain or symptoms, development of other symptoms, etc.
Mechanism of trauma	Motor vehicle accident, birth trauma, fall, surgery, etc.
Direction and motion of trauma	As detailed as possible, e.g., pivoting left on right foot when tackled on the outside of the right knee
Type of trauma	Blunt, sharp or cutting force, compression, traction, active motion against resistance, repetitive, etc.
Original signs and symptoms	Bruising, pain, swelling, asymmetry, fractures, motion changes, organ symptoms, etc.
Changes in signs and symptoms	Progressing, developing or continuing pain, functional changes, neurologic, mental or emotional symptoms, improving symptoms, etc.
Types and responses to treatments	Surgery, medication list, physical therapy, supplements, alternative care, etc.
Pretrauma diseases and changes since the trauma	Any changes in types of disease and response to treatment
Posttrauma diseases	New conditions and response to treatment
Previous trauma	List and any residuals still present at time of present trauma
Subsequent trauma	Relationship to the presenting trauma, e.g., repetitive work injuries, falls due to unstable joints, etc.
Disabilities related to the presenting trauma	Achieved or applied for, e.g., social security, personal injury, worker's compensation, private disability
Disabilities *not* related to the trauma	Achieved or applied for, e.g., social security, personal injury, worker's compensation, private disability

The creation of a treatment plan for the dysfunctional and/or traumatized patient incorporates these concepts. Osteopathic management of these patients addresses the trauma and its effects with OMT integrated with medical, surgical, rehabilitative, and alternative interventions. Treating somatic dysfunction enhances and supports healing and homeostasis in all levels, body, mind, and spirit. "*To find health should be the object of the doctor. Anyone can find disease*" (63) (*Philosophy of Osteopathy*, A.T. Still, p. 28).

CLINICAL CASES

CASE 1: BIOMECHANICAL MODEL OF WARD

Refer to the chapter-opening case.

CASE 2: "THE BIG BANDAGE" MODEL OF CHILA

P.R. is a 46-year-old African American female who presents with pain in the right shoulder, neck, and upper back after gardening this weekend. She spent a day weeding and planting in her gardens and went to bed stiff and woke up this morning in pain with poor motion of her neck and right shoulder without radiation of pain or numbness. She denies any other recent traumas. She did have a similar problem last spring when she began to garden again and was helped by osteopathic manipulative treatments.

Review of systems is positive for ovarian cysts and is otherwise noncontributory.

Past medical and family histories are unchanged from last year.

Tests: x-rays of the cervical spine a year ago demonstrated mild degenerative changes at the facets and discs at C5-6.

Medications: ibuprofen 200 mg 2 po every 6 hours since yesterday with relief of stiffness but not the pain. Aleve 1 to 2 q12 prn prior to her periods and at midcycle for ovarian pain.

Physical exam: BP: 120/80; Pulse: 76 in acute moderate distress.

Neurologic: normal reflexes and sensation of upper extremities; strength intact with pain with end points of exertion.

Peripheral vascular: pulses normal with good capillary refill and no edema of all extremities.

Musculoskeletal: range of motion of right shoulder limited in abduction with pain, and otherwise both shoulders normal; cervical spine spasms with rotation of head and neck greater than 20 degrees left, otherwise motion intact; thoracic spine limited by pain in all planes of motion with spasms.

Diagnosis

Sprain/strain right shoulder
Sprain/strain cervical spine
Sprain/strain thoracic spine
Somatic dysfunction of the cervical, thoracic spine, and right upper extremity

Treatment

MFR
Stretches
Continue ibuprofen

CASE 3: BIOENERGETIC MODEL OF O'CONNELL

E.G. is a 3-week old female infant brought in by her parents for problems with sucking, torticollis, and inability to move her right arm. She is the product of an uncomplicated term pregnancy that was augmented with pitocin for failure to progress due to being in an occiput posterior position. Labor lasted 22 hours and she was delivered without further assistance. She weighed 8 lb 2 oz and had APGARS of 7 and 9. Mom states that E.G. had problems latching on from the start and cried a lot keeping her from nursing at the breast or with bottles with expressed milk. They noticed that she did not move her right arm like her left and that her head was always turned left and tilted onto her right shoulder. The pediatrician reassured them that this would resolve on its own. Since it did not, they have brought her to seek osteopathic manipulative treatments at the advice of their lactation consultant.

The rest of the review of systems shows steady weight gain in the 25th percentile, no reflux, and is otherwise noncontributory.

Family history is negative for similar conditions and both parents are healthy and 22 years old.

Physical exam: Pulse 140 regular, respirations nonlabored, distressed with certain positions, nursing and changing clothes.

Neurologic: Inability to actively, grossly move right shoulder; movement of elbow and wrist and grip are maintained but weak on the right with the left being normal. Torticollis with head turned left with upward gaze and inability to actively rotate right. Suck is disorganized with posterior tongue position and inability to maintain suction on digit, nipple, or breast with aerophagia and discomfort. The rest of her neurologic exam is appropriate for age.

Musculoskeletal: Torticollis rotated left with spasm of right sternocleidomastoid (SCM) muscle with pain with passive motion of head and neck right past midline. Group curve cervical spine has the most significant loss of motion at C5 and C1-occiput. Ribs 1 to 2 elevated right with depression of the acromioclavicular joint with a click with motion. Position of ease is head rotated left with upward tilt with right shoulder internally rotated. Cranial motion demonstrates a compression of the mastoidal suture and occipital condyle on the right. T1-3 are extended and any attempt at flexion in this region is painful.

The rest of the physical exam is normal and appropriate for age.

Diagnoses

Erbs palsy
Torticollis, spasmodic
CN trauma of birth (9–12)
Feeding problems of the newborn
Somatic dysfunction head, cervical, thoracic, ribs, upper extremity right

Treatment

MFR
Set up for physical therapy
Discussed positional support when feeding
Continue with lactation consultant to support breast feeding

DIAGNOSES AND TECHNIQUES

Techniques are divided according to somatic dysfunction body regions. Ward's, Chila's, and O'Connell's techniques will be described separately.

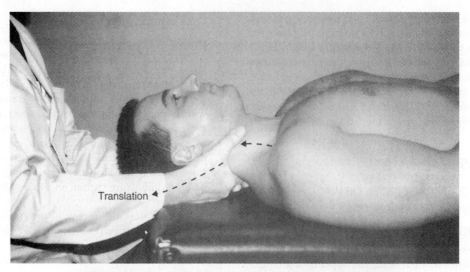

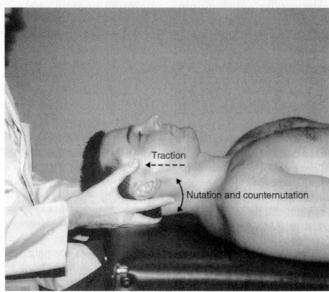

Figure 47-8   A, B. Craniocervical technique.

TECHNIQUES BY WARD

739.0 and 739.1: Head and Cervical Region

Craniocervical Spine

Patient Supine

This process is shown in Figure 47.8. The goal is to establish three-dimensional movement symmetry in the cervical spine from basiocciput to upper thoracic influences. Particular emphasis is placed on restoration of adequate side bending and rotation, both generally and in relation to single segment mobility. This technique is usually more effective after lower cervical, cervicothoracic junction, and upper thoracic, upper limb factors have been released beforehand.

Note: To protect the vertebral arteries, take particular caution to avoid simultaneous side-bending and extension maneuvers. *While important for all age groups, most injuries have occurred under age 35.*

Procedure

1. The patient lies supine with heels on the table, arms comfortably at the sides. This basically ensures that unusual mechanical stresses transmitted through the Achilles tendons and ankles will be neutralized. For those patients with significant kyphosis, it is helpful to use a large pillow to minimize cervical and thoracolumbar problems

2. Sit at the patient's head

3. Two hand positions, among many possibilities, are particularly useful:
   (a) One hand overlapping the other—this permits carefully controlled and focused, twist, traction, and side-bending maneuvers. The maneuvers are used both separately and with patient cooperation
   (b) By grasping the basiocciput with the palms of each hand, the fingers are left free to sort out both superficial and deep mechanisms

4. From either hand position, traction, turning, and side-bending maneuvers assess myofascial and joint-related tightness and looseness
   (a) Pay particular attention to tightness, remembering that loose joints with surrounding inhibited muscle groups are common sources of pain and disability. In more acute situations, on the other hand, loose joints are usually associated with tight muscles as they work to protect and stabilize the system. The opposite findings are also common, such as tight joints with accompanying inhibition of overlying muscles

(b) Facet joints are often tight on one side, loose on the other. Side-to-side motion testing with only a little rotation will determine which facets are failing to effectively open or close

(c) The procedure's focus is to carefully, but persistently, apply well-focused stress against tight sites with and without patient assistance

(d) INR CN and upper limb activities such as finger tapping and hand rolling are commonly helpful. They also save the practitioner time

5. Linking subtle translatory maneuvers (e.g., combinations of distraction and extension with flexion, extension, side-bending, and rotation) is usually helpful. In particular:

(a) Release deep upper cervical muscles by combining CN activities with occipitoatlantal nutation and counternutation. Remember that SCM, trapezius (CN XI), and scalene mechanics are easily accessible primary neck stabilizers that are often asymmetric in relation to each other. For example, the left SCM mechanism is typically tighter than the right from origin to insertion. Commonly, the underlying scalene system is looser (i.e., tightness and looseness occur among ipsilateral layers as well as from side to side, front to back, and circumferentially)

6. In the process:

7. Atlantoaxial joints and surrounding attachments are carefully rotated against tightness

8. Middle and lower cervical attachments and coupled joint movements are stressed using translatory movements with combinations of side bending, flexion, and extension that avoids a lot of rotation (Remember the vertebral arteries!)

9. Treatment is complete when symmetric movements are restored to facet joints and surrounding soft tissues within the ability of the patient to adapt

739.2 and 739.8: Thoracic Region and Ribs

Thoracic Cage, Spine, Diaphragm, and Lower Costal Cage: Supine

This process is shown in Figure 47.9.

Objective

The goal is to three dimensionally balance scapulothoracic, thoracic spine, and costodiaphragmatic relationships.

Procedure

Supine

1. The patient lies supine with heels on the table, arms comfortably at the sides. This basically ensures that unusual mechanical stresses transmitted through the Achilles tendons and ankles will be neutralized. For those patients with significant kyphosis, it is helpful to use a large pillow to minimize cervical and thoracolumbar problems

2. Sit at the head of the table

3. Resting your elbows on the table, reach under the patient and place the hands firmly against inferior costothoracic attachments on either side of the thoracic spine. Be sure to maintain whole-hand contact across and along the erector spinae as well as around the costal cage

4. Both positional and movement-related tight-loose asymmetries will become apparent

5. Focus on the following:

(a) Diaphragmatic asymmetries that become apparent as the patient slowly but deeply inhales and exhales

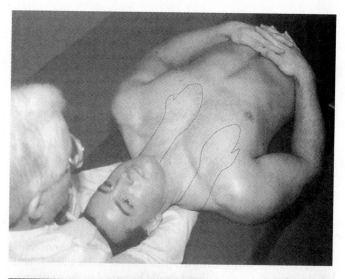

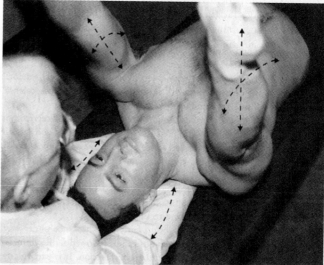

Figure 47-9 A, B. Thoracic and rib technique.

(b) Upper limb asymmetries that occur as the patient actively moves the upper limbs in a variety of directions

(c) Repeat the procedure by passively moving each arm and shoulder with one hand remaining behind the patient

(d) Thoracolumbar junction asymmetries are assessed by having the patient move the lower limbs in a variety of directions; focus on the proximal iliopsoas as well more distal, lumbopelvic relationships as they respond to active patient movements

6. As inherent tissue movements become apparent, gently, but firmly, lift the thoracolumbar attachments anteriorly and laterally. Shifting sites of tightness and looseness are balanced against each other until inherent movements become quietly symmetric. Sometimes, considerable traction and twist are needed to release asymmetrically tight areas

7. As tightness releases, varieties of release-enhancing activities are helpful. Examples are:

(a) Three-dimensional upper and lower limb movements

(b) Breath holding at neutral, during moderate and deep inhalation, and then during moderate and deep exhalation, which can be combined with three-dimensional upper and lower limb movements

8. Treatment is complete when thoracocostal movements are as functionally symmetric as can be expected

739.3: Lumbar Region

Thoracolumbar Release

Figure 47.10 illustrates this process.

Objective

To balance the thoracolumbar junction three dimensionally in relation to lumbopelvic, thoracocostal, and diaphragmatic mechanics.

Review

Review cervical, trapezius, shoulder girdle, and costal cage anatomy for their three-dimensional perspectives and functional relationships to the area.

Procedure

Prone

1. The patient's feet should be off the end of the table to minimize lower limb stresses in relation to the pelvis and low back
2. Initially, the patient's head should be turned to the most comfortable side. Holding it exclusively in the midline, as many wish to do, often obscures tight-loose effects at the thoracolumbar junction

3. The hands and arms are comfortably placed either over the sides of the table, or on the table beside the hips and thighs
4. Stand beside the patient's hip, facing cephalad
5. Place your hands at the thoracolumbar junction, covering posteroinferior rib, trunk rotator, and diaphragmatic sites
6. Place hands widely open with the thumbs pointed cephalad along either side of the spinous processes, while the remainder of each hand spreads over the posteroinferior costodiaphragmatic and upper lumbar areas
7. Identify superficial and deep tightness and looseness patterns three dimensionally
8. Firmly separate the thumbs across the midline as the left hand creates clockwise and the right hand creates counterclockwise traction. The hands should not slide on the skin
9. As the skin is stretched between the thumbs, it will initially blanch. As compression, traction, and twist are maintained, tissues begin to relax both reflexively and mechanically in accordance with principles discussed earlier in this chapter. After initial blanching, the site of major soft tissue tension commonly becomes reddened and warmer, the so-called blush phenomenon
10. Typical releases occur three dimensionally with sustained traction and twist, and they can occur singly or in multiples. The latter often creates a wormlike sensation under the palpating hands. As multiple releases continue, so-called unwinding phenomena often occur, as shifting patterns of tightness and looseness alter three-dimensional relationships. With practice, one learns to feel deeply into the areas surrounding facet joints. Symmetric segmental movements to passive three-dimensional stressing suggest that the procedure is complete. Treatment is complete when repetitive stressing of selected sites no longer creates release activity

739.4: Sacrum

Focused Prone Sacral Base Release: Two-Handed Technique

This process is shown in Figure 47.11.

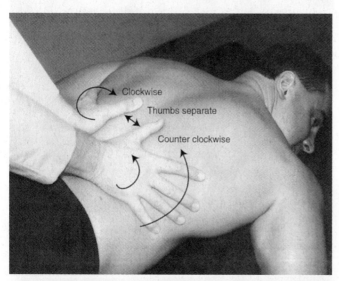

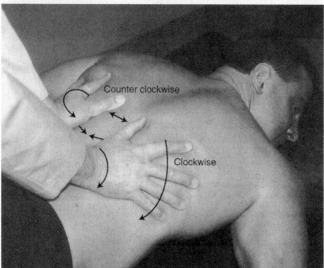

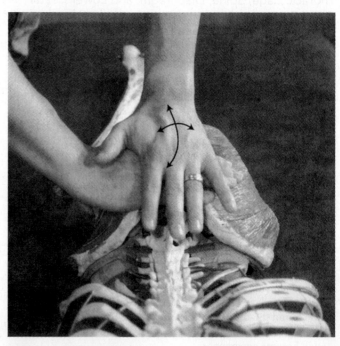

Figure 47-10 Lumbar technique. **A.** Operator stands beside patient's hip, with head to side. **B.** Head right.

Figure 47-11 Sacral technique. Using a rocking motion, induce lumbosacral joint distraction.

Objective

The goal is to three dimensionally balance the sacral base in relation to L4-5 mechanics, the iliolumbar ligament, and positional innominate asymmetries.

Review

Review lumbopelvic anatomy, L4-5 mechanics in relation to the sacrum and pelvis, iliolumbar ligament, and innominate, hip rotator, and pelvic diaphragm relationships, including distal iliopsoas and piriformis muscle influences.

Procedure

Prone

1. The feet should be off the end of the table to minimize lower limb stresses in relation to the pelvis and low back
2. The head should be turned to the most comfortable side
3. The hands and arms are comfortably placed either over the sides of the table or on the table beside the hips and thighs
4. If right handed, stand at the patient's left shoulder, facing caudad
5. Place one hand either horizontally, or transverse to the sacrum, contacting the posterior superior iliac spines and medial gluteus maximus attachments bilaterally
6. Place the other hand over the bottom hand along the long axis of the sacrum between the two innominates, with the index finger overlying one SI joint and inferior lateral angle as the ring finger covers the other. By using this hand placement, the long finger falls naturally over the sacral spines and sacral hiatus
7. Evaluate patterns of tightness and looseness by rocking the sacrum in multiple planes:
   (a) Proximally and distally, by distracting the sacrum and lumbar spine at the sacral base along the long axis of the spine
   (b) Circumferentially, by transversely translating each hand across the pelvis in opposite directions
8. Using a rocking nutation-counternutation gapping motion, induce lumbosacral joint distraction. Be sure to create the motion by moving the distal hand caudally as well as up and over the natural curve of the sacrum. Some sacrums are in a more or less straight-line relationship with the spine. Others are sometimes acutely angled with the plane of the sacral base virtually perpendicular to the flow of the operator-imposed forces
9. Both light- and heavy-handed force can be used, depending on your skill. A key to success is the ability to monitor, induce, and enhance both inherent tissue and craniosacral activities
10. As both static and dynamic loading is applied, inherent tissue movement-related tightness and looseness usually becomes apparent. Static forces load the system against direct and indirect barriers without superimposing oscillating movements. Dynamic forces load the system with subtle operator-induced forces that:
    (a) Follow along behind inherent tissue and craniosacral movements
    (b) Systematically seek out three-dimensional shifts of direct and indirect barriers as releases occur
11. Success is more apt to occur when special attention is given to the sacral base in relation to L4-5 mechanics, iliolumbar ligament anomalies, degenerative changes, and nonneutral vertebral mechanics.)
12. Treatment is complete when L5 and sacral base mechanics and associated inherent motions are as symmetric as can reasonably be expected

739.5: Pelvis

Pubic Symphysis Release

Treatment procedures for the pelvis are shown in Figure 47.12.

Objective

The goal is to restore symmetry to the pubic symphysis.

Review

Review the functional three-dimensional relationships among the proximal thigh adductors, anterior and posterior innominates and their asymmetries, as well as changes involving the rectus sheath and transverses abdominis muscles, where they attach to the pubic symphysis.

Procedure

Supine

1. The patient lies supine with heels on the table and the arms comfortably at the sides or on the abdomen. Short-armed individuals should keep the arms on the table to avoid stressing shoulder and thoracolumbar systems. This more or less ensures that unusual mechanical stresses transmitted through the Achilles tendons and ankles will be neutralized. For those with significant kyphosis, it is helpful to use a large pillow to minimize cervical and thoracolumbar problems

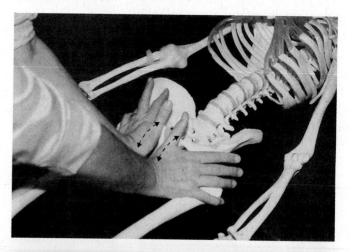

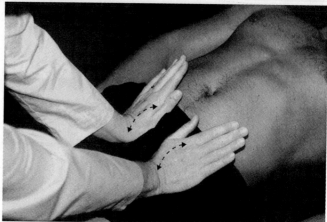

Figure 47-12 Pelvic technique. **A.** Symphysis release. **B.** Thenar eminences are placed on either side of symphysis pubis, thumbs pointed superiorly and anteriorly.

2. Facing cephalad, the practitioner sits or stands beside the patient's right thigh, near the knee

3. First, assess for symphyseal shear and positional asymmetry. Some prefer visual analysis, while others prefer a combination of palpation and vision. Tightness and looseness in the rectus sheath often identify the most problematic site. Sometimes tightness will be on the inferior side, sometimes the superior. Usually, there are strong correlations with innominate positioning, but there are enough exceptions that one must be alert

4. Place the thenar eminences on either side of the symphysis pubis, thumbs pointed superiorly and anteriorly. Proximal adductor and iliacus tendon attachments should be palpably evident under the thenar muscles

5. Induce firm, slow forces that either exaggerate (indirect barriers) or decrease (direct barriers) symphysis asymmetry. Direct rocking back and forth, similar to an articular maneuver, is often effective. Hold against the barriers until releases occur. Mild oscillations usually become evident as the rectus fasciae, bony pelvis, pelvic diaphragm, trunk rotators, and thigh adductors become more symmetric

739.6: Lower Extremity

Treatment procedures for the lower limb are shown in Figure 47.13.

Goal

The goal is to release each lower limb from lumbopelvic and hip rotator attachments to the foot and ankle.

Review

Review the following:

1. Functional neurology of the lower limb, including pelvic girdle, low back, trunk rotators, and lumbodorsal fascia, latissimus dorsi, scapulocostal stabilizers in relation to the low back, brachial plexus influences through shoulder girdle structures, as well as diaphragmatic-phrenic influence. Remember that the limbs are precisely represented in cerebellopontine functions as well as in multiple areas of the homunculus and precentral gyrus, among many

2. Functional neuromuscular anatomy of the foot, ankle, knee, and their myofascial elements

3. Functional neuromuscular anatomy of the hips and upper leg

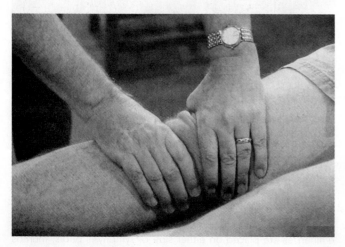

Figure 47-13   Lower extremity technique.

4. Circulatory anatomy of both the lumbopelvic system and the lower limbs

5. The effects of common medical problems, such as arthritis, diabetes, and effects of trauma and surgery

Note 1: Smoking-related circulatory problems, arthritis, and diabetes are among the most common sources of lower limb dysfunctions.

Note 2: Proprioceptive instability on one leg is a common signal of unilateral muscle weakness and neural inhibition anywhere from the low back to the plantar surface of the ipsilateral foot. Pain is a common presenting complaint.

Procedure

Supine

1. To begin, the heels should be on the table with knees extended to minimize lower limb stresses. The head and neck should be comfortable with minimal stress on the spine and pelvis

Note: Remember to check for leg-length inequalities and altered hip mechanics both prone and supine. It is common to find differences supine, prone, and seated. Pelvic obliquities are common when these inconsistencies occur.

2. The hands and arms are comfortably placed either on the abdomen or at the sides

3. Sit or stand beside the patient

4. Grasp distal femur and distal patellar/proximal tibial attachments

5. Using firm, passive, circumferential movements, assess each fully extended knee for three-dimensional tightness and looseness. Particular care is taken in assessing medial hamstring as well as lateral hamstring/iliotibial band/proximal fibular head tight-loose relationships

Note: Myofascially, this is a fairly ambiguous area to assess and treat, so one must subjectively rely on tight-loose end-feels. Remember that both lumbopelvic and foot-ankle mechanics significantly influence the system.

6. Assess hip function in the same way, with the leg in full extension and then with varieties of flexion, internal and external rotation, abduction, and adduction

7. Passively twist the knee in opposite directions (axial twist), being sure that the hand and fingers are firmly in contact with areas of maximum tightness. Usually, maximum tightness is in two places:
   (a) Laterally around distal iliotibial band attachments and proximal fibular head
   (b) Medially and posteriorly near and around distal hamstring attachments

8. Asymptomatic lateral knee/fibular head problems (tightness) in response to medial complaints where the knee is generally more mobile are common. Distal tensor fasciae latae problems are also common in this group in conjunction with ipsilateral gluteus medius weakness. A positive standing Trendelenburg test is the most common signal of gluteus medius weakening
   (a) Remember that proximal SI joint and sacrotuberous-sacrospinous ligamentous factors are also common sources of distal difficulties, and vice versa

739.7: Upper Extremity

Treatment procedures for the upper limb are shown in Figure 47.14.

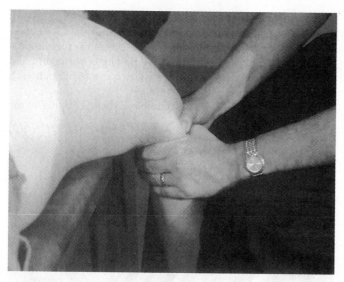

Figure 47-14 Upper extremity.

Upper Limb and Shoulder
Rotator Cuff and Partially Frozen Shoulder Dysfunctions
Goal

The goal of this treatment is to three dimensionally balance cervical, shoulder, scapulocostal, anterior chest wall, rotator cuff-glenohumeral, upper arm, elbow, wrist, and hand influences.

Review

Review the following:

1. Functional neurology of the neck in relation to the upper limb, including brachial plexus and cervical autonomic elements, as well as CN sensory and motor functions
2. Rotator cuff, glenohumeral, elbow, wrist influences
3. Craniocervical spine relationships with particular reference to large and small muscle influences from basiocciput to upper thoracic and related scapulothoracic, scapulocostal influences

Procedure

The procedure is carried out with the patient prone, with their arm and shoulder off table. Most of the time, this position is used to deal directly with compromised shoulder and scapulocostal mechanics (see also "Spencer Techniques"). Direct myofascial stressing occurs across and around the rotator cuff, acromioclavicular joint, distal glenohumeral attachments, and inferior subscapularis, latissimus dorsi, infraspinatus, teres major and minor attachments:

1. The patient's feet should be off the end of the table to minimize lower limb stresses in relation to the pelvis and lower limb
2. The patient's head should be turned to the most comfortable side. Note the effect of head turning on tightness and looseness across the shoulder in question. Proximal and superior cervical attachments are often compromised and need to be released along with the shoulder

Note: Keeping the head in the midline readily neutralizes craniocervical asymmetries, but also reduces the chance that significant tight-loose asymmetries will be missed.

3. The patient's hands and arms are comfortably placed either over the sides of the table or on the table beside the hips and thighs. If the hands are over the sides of the table, be sure to note any asymmetric scapulocostal effects
4. The operator sits on a rolling stool that allows movement in response to shifting sites of tightness and looseness
5. Holding the affected arm between the knees allows the operator use of the rolling stool to guide movements as specific stressing against tight barriers occurs
6. Initially, place both hands firmly around the glenohumeral attachments immediately lateral to the acromioclavicular joint. The fingers of one hand firmly contact pectoralis major attachments anteriorly, while the other hand contacts teres/infraspinatus attachments posteriorly
7. Assess tightness and looseness by three dimensionally stressing the system using distraction, compression, twist, and shear
8. Direct and firm stressing against tightness gets the process under way. For example, approximately 5 to 15 lb of load are common before initial releases begin
9. Pay particular attention to posterior and inferior glenohumeral restrictions close to the scapula
10. Long-term problems usually require firmly held movements that assertively stretch the area without interfering with neuro-circulatory functions
11. A well-organized home exercise and/or physical therapy program is usually needed to maintain improvement
12. Side-lying techniques using a similar approach are also helpful

TECHNIQUES BY CHILA

739.0: Head and Suboccipital Region

Cranium
Treatment procedures for the cranium are shown in Figure 47.15.

Occipitoatlantal Articulation
1. One hand contacts the posterior tubercle of the atlas
2. The opposite hand contacts the vertex of the patient's head. The fulcrum is established by the placement of the elbow on the tabletop

Basilar Axes of the Skull
The patient's head rests on the interlaced or overlapped fingers of the physician. The physician's thumbs extend above the ears toward the forepart of the head. The fulcrum is established by the placement of the elbows on the tabletop.

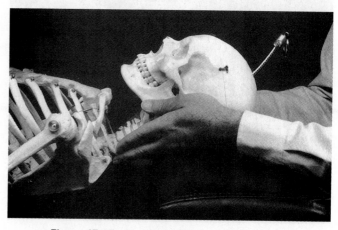

Figure 47-15 Head and suboccipital technique.

739.1, 739.2, and 739.8: Cervical Region, Thoracic Region, and Ribs

Rib Cage

1. Place one hand beneath the rib cage, with the fingertips just beyond the spinous processes of the associated thoracic vertebrae (Fig. 47.16)
2. Place the other hand on the anterior ends of the ribs. The fulcrum is established by the elbow on the knee

Lower Thorax

Place both hands beneath the patient at the level of the 12th thoracic segment (T12) (Fig. 47.17). This area corresponds to the level of the insertion of the trapezium muscles bilaterally. The fulcrum is established bilaterally by the elbows resting on the tabletop.

Upper Thorax

The patient's head rests on a pillow. One hand and arm contact the upper thoracic spinous processes, with the fingers spread slightly to contact the ribs on each side (Fig. 47.18). Place the opposite hand on the sternum. The fulcrum is established by the elbow on the tabletop, beneath the patient's head.

Cervical Area

Both hands bridge the entire cervical area from the base of the skull to the upper thorax (Fig. 47.19). The fulcrum is established bilaterally by the elbows and forearms resting on the tabletop.

739.3: Lumbar Region

The patient's knees are flexed, and the feet placed flat on the table. Lateralization of the feet, with inversion of the toes, helps to stabilize the pelvis.

Upper Lumbar, Psoas Muscle

Place one hand under the upper lumbar area (Fig. 47.20). The opposite arm and hand bridge the flexed knees. The fulcrum is established by the elbow on the knee (upper lumbar area).

739.4 and 739.5: Sacrum and Pelvis

The patient's knees are flexed, and the feet placed flat on the table. Lateralization of the feet, with inversion of the toes, helps to stabilize the pelvis.

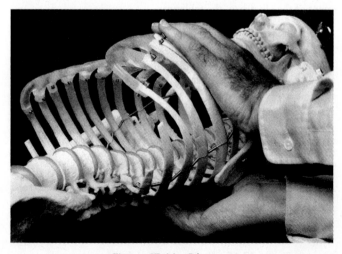

Figure 47-16   Rib cage.

Sacrum and Pelvis

1. Mold with the patient's sacrum with one hand
2. Place the fingertips of this hand at the level of the spinous process of the fifth lumbar segment (L5). The opposite arm and hand bridge the anterior superior iliac spine (ASIS) on each side of the pelvis (Fig. 47.21)
3. The fulcrum is established by the elbow, which is leaning on the treatment table

Sacrum, Iliosacrum, Lower Lumbar

1. Mold with the patient's sacrum with one hand (Fig. 47.22)

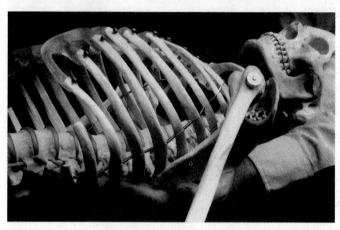

Figure 47-17   Lower thorax.

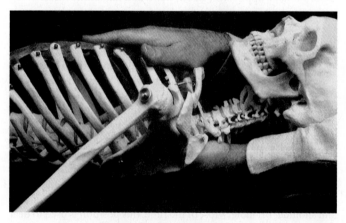

Figure 47-18   Upper thorax.

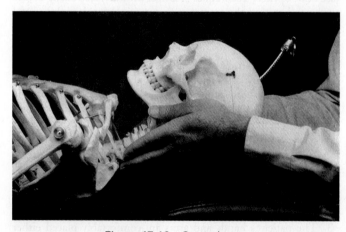

Figure 47-19   Cervical area.

2. Place the opposite hand under the iliosacral articulation. The fingertips of this hand contact the spinous process of the lower lumbar segments (L3, L4, L5). Both elbows establish the fulcrum: one leaning on the treatment table (sacrum), the other leaning on the physician's knee (iliosacrum; lower lumbar)

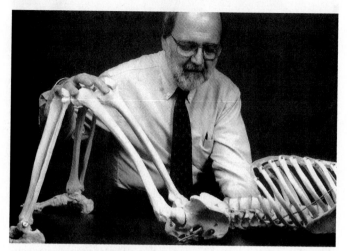

Figure 47-20   Upper lumbar, psoas muscle.

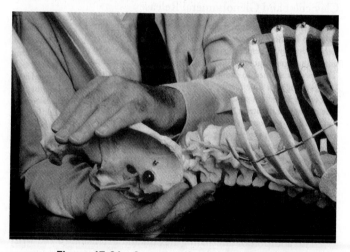

Figure 47-21   Sacrum and pelvis. Bridge ASIS.

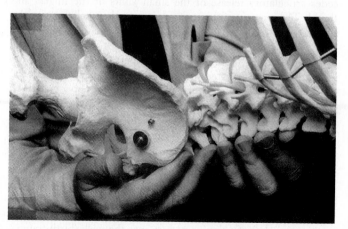

Figure 47-22   Sacrum, iliosacrum, lower lumbar.

739.6: Lower Extremity

Lower Extremity
Selectively employ torsion (rotation) and traction in two phases to release muscular, fascial, ligamentous, and articular dysfunction. The fulcrum is established by the elbows of the physician's arms in supporting the motions of the patient's foot, lower leg, and knee.

Abduction Phase (Lower Leg)
Invert the plantar surface of the foot (Fig. 47.23). Introduce torsion between the ankle and the knee. Advance the effect of torsion by slowly moving the knee across the lower abdomen, resulting in progressive abduction of the lower leg. The torsion will be felt in the lateral malleolar area, the medial compartmental area of the knee, the tensor fascia lata area, and the trochanter area. Upon completion of this phase, gradually extend the lower extremity and slowly return it to the tabletop.

Adduction Phase (Lower Leg)
Evert the plantar surface of the foot (Fig. 47.24). Introduce torsion between the ankle and the knee. Steadily advance the effect of torsion by slowly moving the knee away from the lower abdomen, resulting in progressive adduction of the lower leg. The torsion will be felt in the medial malleolar area, the lateral compartmental area of the knee, the medial thigh area, and the inguinal area. Upon

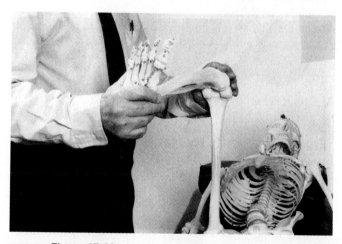

Figure 47-23   Lower extremity, abduction phase.

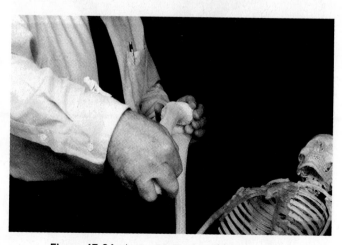

Figure 47-24   Lower extremity, adduction phase.

completion of this phase, gradually extend the lower extremity and slowly return it to the tabletop.

Foot

Note tenderness to palpation in the plantar myofascial tissues. Give particular attention to such findings along the medial longitudinal arch. The contour of the foot can be analogized to the spinal complex:

The calcaneus represents the sacrum
The tarsal bones represent the lumbar region
The tarsometatarsal area represents the thoracolumbar junction
The metatarsal area represents the thoracic region
The metatarsophalangeal area represents the cervicothoracic junction
The phalangeal area represents the cervical region

Tender points can be analogized to the ipsilateral spinal level, including paraspinal tissues.

Treatment is by increased plantar flexion of the foot about the point of greatest tenderness (Fig. 47.25). Perform articulatory release of the small joints of the toes in sequence, from the great toe to the small toe.

739.7: Upper Extremity

Upper Extremity
Scapulofascial Release
Accomplish this by exploring ease and resistance to motion in several planes: cephalad, caudad, medially, laterally, clockwise, and counterclockwise (Fig. 47.26). Both hands are used to grasp the scapula completely, both medially and laterally.

Axillary Release
Accomplish this by manual decongestion of the posterior axillary tissues and the pectoral tissues.

Expansion of the Inferior Thoracic Aperture
Accomplish this by supporting the elbow region with one hand and the wrist region with the other hand. For this and all subsequent procedures, the fulcrum is established by the elbows of the physician's body in support of the motions of the patient's upper extremity. Bring the extended upper extremity of the patient closer

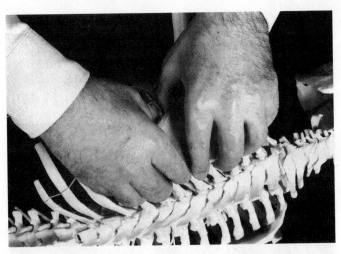

Figure 47-26 Upper extremity, scapulofascial release.

to the side of the body. Sustained supination as the upper extremity is carried toward the posterior thorax facilitates release of the thoracolumbar junction. Sustained pronation as the upper extremity is carried toward the xiphoid process facilitates musculofascial release along the costal margin. The cumulative effect of these forces contributes to ligamentous articular release of the elbow region.

Clavicular and Glenohumeral Release
Accomplish this by placing the extended upper extremity in a neutral position, with respect to the side of the body, and abducting to the point where a continuum exists between the upper extremity and the position of the clavicle. Sustained pronation as the upper extremity is carried toward the manubrial region facilitates release of the manubrial area and the sternoclavicular articulation. Sustained supination as the upper extremity is carried toward the posterior thorax facilitates release of the acromioclavicular articulation and the glenohumeral area.

Radioulnar, Wrist, Hand, and Fingers Release
Accomplish this by sustained alternating supination and pronation. This facilitates the release of fascial ligamentous tension along the course of the interosseous membrane to the flexor retinaculum (Fig. 47.22).

The addition of alternating flexion and extension of the wrist facilitates the release of articular dysfunctions of the carpal bones (Fig. 47.23). Fascial ligamentous release of the palmar area precedes articulatory release of the small joints of the fingers and thumb. The progress of the sequence is from the small finger to the thumb (Fig. 47.24).

Expansion of the Superior Thoracic Aperture
Accomplish this by grasping the deep webbing between the index finger and thumb of the patient's extended upper extremity. Sustained alternating supination and pronation facilitates the release of congestion in this area and contributes to release of the cervicothoracic junction (Figs. 47.27–47.29).

TECHNIQUES BY O'CONNELL

739.0 and 739.1:   Head and Cervical Region

Head/cervical: Release across diaphragms (tentorium cerebelli to thoracic inlet) of a trauma pattern into the neck (birth trauma, personal injury, or MVA) (Fig. 47.30).

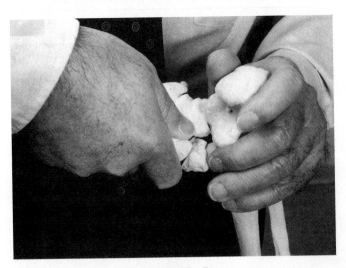

Figure 47-25 Foot

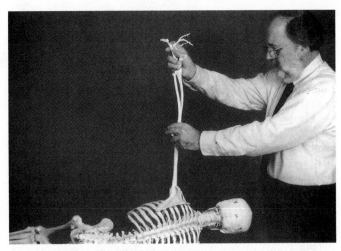

Figure 47-27   Upper extremity, radioulnar.

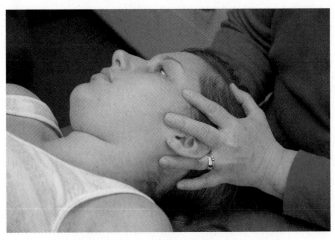

Figure 47-30   Head and neck technique.

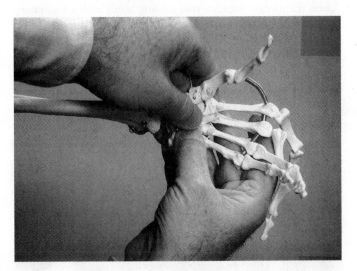

Figure 47-28   Upper extremity, wrist.

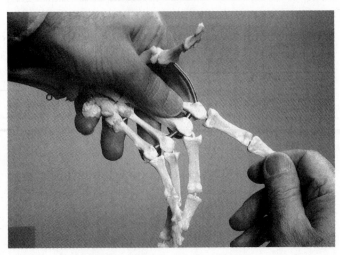

Figure 47-29   Upper extremity, hand and fingers.

Place the patient in the supine position and sit at the head of the treatment table.

Place your hands on the head with the index fingers above the zygomatic process, the middle finger below the process, and the ring fingers behind and contacting the pinnae, taking care not to overlay the mastoidal suture, while placing the little finger on the occipital squama. Then lay the palms of your hands lightly on the head with your thumbs on the parietals. This captures the tentorium between your hands while allowing contact with the suboccipital fascia.

Sense the motion of the tentorium and note the asymmetries in motion between temporalis and occiput. Now focus on the motion of the posterior external fascial planes of the head into the neck as you continue to monitor the tentorium.

Introduce a compressive or distractive force into the tissues and a pattern of motion will become evident that travels between the tentorium and the thoracic inlet. Following this pattern along its ease or oppose the pattern and engage the motion barrier of this pattern. Since the fascia is a continuum, the trauma pattern will follow a distinct path and move across multiple structures, organs, and regions as the fascia responds intelligently to the forces. This pattern of motion reflects the traumatic pattern of strain in the tissues and reproduces the positions of trauma.

Choose a direct or an indirect approach and follow the pattern along its responsive moving barrier or point of ease as the pattern releases. Three deep respiratory cycles facilitate the release with repositioning continuously as the pattern releases.

Return the patient to neutral and retest as above taking note as to whether the pattern is extinguished.

Trauma patterns are not limited to normal physiologic motion patterns and may be confusing to the clinician, but with practice, can aid the clinician in diagnosis as well as treatment.

739.2, 739.7, and 739.8: Thoracic Region, Upper Extremity, and Ribs

Thoracic/Ribs/Sternum/Clavicle/Upper Extremity

This approach allows for anatomical access to all structures that converge at this diaphragm, the longitudinal connections between diaphragms and an excellent technique to experience a holographic release (Figs. 47.31 and 47.32).

The complexity of the motions that interface and are accessed here usually cause more complex and grosser levels of motion sensed by the clinician and the patient and is referred to as "the dance."

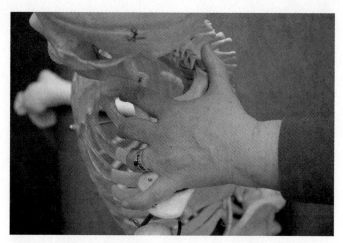

Figure 47-31 Thoracic inlet approach to thoracic, ribs, and upper extremities technique.

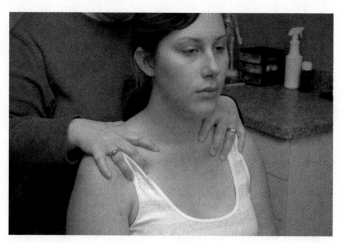

Figure 47-32

It is important to note that this approach allows the clinician to travel the fascial continuum both diagnostically and therapeutically.

Position the patient seated on the table. The clinician stands directly behind the patient making sure the patient is slightly lower so that the clinician is able to place their hands on the thoracic inlet in a comfortable position.

The handhold is designed to capture the whole thoracic inlet with contacts on the bony anchors to the inlet. Place your hands on top of the patient's shoulders with your thumbs posteriorly with the tips pointing toward the spinous processes of C7 and T1. Anteriorly, your third and fourth fingers overly the clavicle with the tip of the fingers contacting the first rib and second rib anteriorly. Place the second finger along the shaft of the clavicle pointing toward the sternoclavicular joint. Place the fifth finger laterally toward the acromioclavicular joint. In this position, relax the hands so that the palms overly and contact the tops of the shoulders.

Assess the motion patterns in both hands simultaneously, remembering that it is usual that motion may occur in different planes and directions. With a respiratory cycle, identify the patterns of motion and choose a direct or indirect approach. With three deep respiratory cycles, follow the shifting release pattern with both hands and stabilizing the patient's torso with your own epigastrium remembering not to limit the motion, but to

dance with the patient's release. Return the patient to neutral and reevaluate the resolution of the pattern.

739.3: Lumbar Region

Lumbar: Iliopsoas release (lifting injury, short leg accommodation) (Figs. 47.33 and 47.34).

Place the patient prone on the table and stand at the side of the patient. Place your hand that is closest to the patient's head perpendicular to the long line of the spine with the spinous processes of T11-L1 in the midline of the palm of your hand. Lay your hand down with your fingers on the contralateral side of the spine and your thenar and hypothenar eminences on the ipsilateral side of the spine. This allows for the capture of the posterior fascial attachments of the respiratory diaphragm and the posterior longitudinal fascial planes of the lumbar spine/torso.

Place your other hand parallel to the long line of the spine with the palm of your hand at the sacral base and your fingers extending cephalad and spread capturing the lumbopelvic spine and fascia.

The motion is this region is more tubular in character, and as the release occurs, both hands will be moving in different directions. Assess the motion between your sensing hands with a respiratory cycle, or with palpatory listening to the innate fascial motion. Identify areas of restriction and ease between these listening posts and choose a direct or indirect approach.

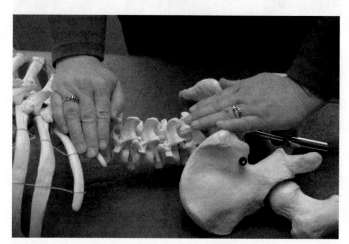

Figure 47-33 Lumbar technique.

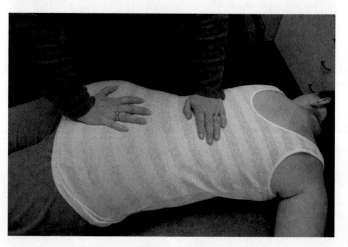

Figure 47-34

Augment the motion with three respiratory cycles and follow the shifting pattern as it releases.

Return to neutral and reevaluate the motion.

739.4 and 739.5: Sacrum and Pelvis

Sacrum/pelvis: Sacral sling release in three dimensions (fall, pregnancy pain, postdelivery pain) (Figs. 47.26 and 47.35).

Place the patient in the supine position and stand or sit next to the patient facing the pelvis.

Place one hand under the pelvis, perpendicular to the long line of the spine, with the spinous processes in midpalm with your finger tips across to the contralateral SI joint and your thenar/hypothenar eminences on the ipsilateral SI joint and relax your hand.

With your other hand, reach across the ilia grasping the contralateral anterior ilia with your finger tips and contact the ipsilateral ilia with your forearm or elbow.

With your upper arm and hand, compress the ilia toward midline, disengaging the sacrum posteriorly, which now floats in the lumbosacral fascia.

With a deep breath set the fascia in motion, identifying positions of ease and barriers to motion of the sacrum within the fascia. Become aware of the relationship between the posterior fascia and the anterior fascia, the motion into the pelvic floor and the fascial loop up into the rectus, transversalis, internal and external obliques fascia. Now become aware of the bony pelvis within this fascial container and with a deep breath, with your entry into this system, using the sacrum as a guide, go through three respiratory cycles following the three-dimensional release of the structures as direct, indirect, or combined.

Return to neutral and reassess the motion in the structures for resolve of the dysfunctions (Fig. 47.36).

739.6: Lower Extremity

Lower extremity: Tubular release of knee using heel-to-hip approach (twist of knee trauma with a stable knee) (Fig. 47.37).

Place the patient in the supine position and stand at the foot of the table.

Grasp the heel placing it in the palm of your outside hand and grip the calcaneous between your hypothenar eminence and fingers keeping the leg on the table. Place your other hand on the dorsum of the foot with your thumb wrapped under the arch.

Place the ankle in neutral position and maintain this throughout the release. Begin the release in segments from the distal to proximal extremity allowing a gradual accumulative release below and above the injured joint.

With the above handhold, lean back placing a traction force into the ankle to calf and follow the stress pattern in the tissue by positioning of the leg, taking care to make small arc motion adjustments. Continue the release with increased traction to the tibial plateau allowing for the positional pattern adjustments. Repeat this process of gradually increasing traction and following the pattern to the lower femur, mid femur and end at the hip.

Hold this position and have the patient take three deep breaths and follow the shifting pattern throughout. Return the limb to neutral and reevaluate motion, pain, and edema of the knee.

739.9: Abdomen/Other

Abdomen/other: Prostate release through the pelvic floor. Pelvic floor fascial motion is important to the proper placement and

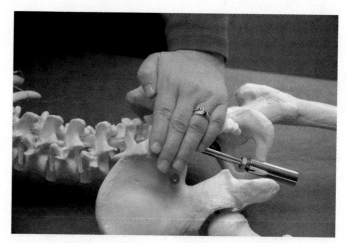

Figure 47-35 Sacrum and pelvis technique.

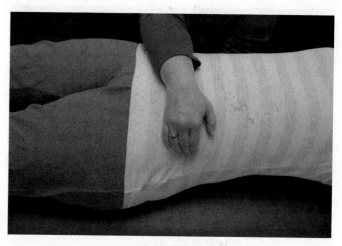

Figure 47-36

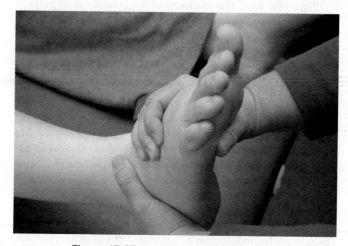

Figure 47-37 Lower extremity technique.

function of the prostate that sits on top of the diaphragm. Congestion is encouraged by a lack of tone and motion in this diaphragm (Figs. 47.38 and 47.39).

Place the patient supine on the table and sit next the side of the pelvis.

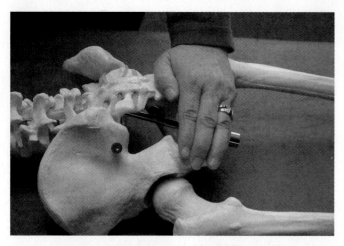

Figure 47-38 Abdomen and viscera technique.

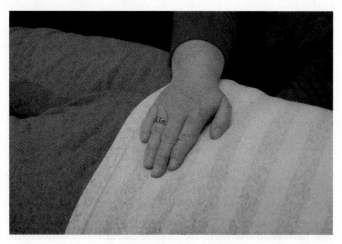

Figure 47-39

Place your hand that is closest to the patient's head perpendicular to the long line of the spine with the coccyx in the palm of your hand and contact the ischial tuberosities, contralaterally with your fingers and ipsilaterally with your hypothenar eminence capturing the posterior pelvic diaphragm.

Place your other hand parallel to and in contact with the edge of your fifth digit with the pubic symphysis. Lay your hand down flat now contacting the lower abdominal wall fascia.

Bring your awareness to the fascial motion loop between the anterior and posterior fascial planes as they converge in the pelvic diaphragm. Traveling that loop, become aware of the motion and tension in tissues, allowing a three-dimensional motion to occur between your sensing hands.

Sense the placement of the prostate (or bladder, vagina, uterus, or rectum) and the tension or ease in the fascia surrounding them.

Identify the pattern of motion ease and restriction. Choose a direct or an indirect approach, and with three respiratory cycles, follow the shifting pattern as it releases. Maintain your awareness of the viscera while you allow both of your hands to move in response to the tissue tension changes as the release progresses with the three deep respiratory cycles. Remember that these motions may take different directions and traverse multiple viscera and are diagnostic as well as therapeutic.

At the end of the release, return to neutral and reassess the motion pattern.

REFERENCES

1. Glossary of Osteopathic Terminology.
2. Ward R, et al. *Foundations for Osteopathic Medicine.* 2nd Ed. Philadelphia, PA: Lippincott Williams & Wilkins, 2003:931–932.
3. Kimberly PE. *Outline of Osteopathic Manipulative Procedures, The Kimberly Manual.* Marceline, MO: Walsworth Publishing Company, 2006:30–31.
4. Ward R, et al. *Foundations for Osteopathic Medicine.* 2nd Ed. Philadelphia, PA: Lippincott Williams & Wilkins, 2003.
5. O'Connell J. *Bioelectric Fascial Activation and Release, The Physician's Guide to Hunting with Dr. Still.* Indianapolis, IN: American Academy of Osteopathy, 2000.
6. O'Connell J. *Bioelectric Fascial Activation and Release, The Physician's Guide to Hunting with Dr. Still.* Indianapolis, IN: American Academy of Osteopathy, 2000:909.
7. O'Connell J. *Bioelectric Fascial Activation and Release, The Physician's Guide to Hunting with Dr. Still.* Indianapolis, IN: American Academy of Osteopathy, 2000:59.
8. Ward R, et al. *Foundations for Osteopathic Medicine.* 2nd Ed. Philadelphia, PA: Lippincott Williams & Wilkins, 2003;909, 936.
9. O'Connell J. *Bioelectric Fascial Activation and Release, The Physician's Guide to Hunting with Dr. Still.* Indianapolis, IN: American Academy of Osteopathy, 2000:65.
10. ECOP Myofascial Release Outline, revised 4/07.
11. Still AT. *Philosophy of Osteopathy.* Indianapolis, IN: American Academy of Osteopathy, 162.
12. Still AT. *Philosophy of Osteopathy.* Indianapolis, IN: American Academy of Osteopathy, 23.
13. Page LE. The role of the fasciae in the maintenance of structural integrity. In *The American Academy of Osteopathy Yearbook.* Indianapolis, IN: American Academy of Osteopathy, 1952:70.
14. Snyder GE. Fasciae—applied anatomy and physiology. In: *The American Academy of Osteopathy Yearbook.* Indianapolis, IN: American Academy of Osteopathy, 1956:65.
15. Personal communication with Anthony Chila, DO, FAAO 2/07.
16. Personal Attendance. *Sutherland Cranial Teaching Foundation.* Introductory Course 1981.
17. Fulford RC. *Touch of Life.* New York, NY: Pocket, 1997.
18. O'Connell J. *Bioelectric Fascial Activation and Release, The Physician's Guide to Hunting with Dr. Still.* Indianapolis, IN: American Academy of Osteopathy, 2000:61.
19. Gray H. *Anatomy, Descriptive and Surgical.* 1901 Ed. Philadelphia, PA: Running Press, 1974:1086–1092.
20. Patten BM. *Human Embryology.* 3rd Ed. New York: McGraw-Hill Inc., 1968:59.
21. Patten BM. *Human Embryology.* 3rd Ed. New York: McGraw-Hill Inc., 1968:156.
22. Patten BM. *Human Embryology.* 3rd Ed. New York: McGraw-Hill Inc., 1968:1090–1091.
23. Cathie AG. The fascia of the body in relation to function and manipulative therapy. In: *The American Academy of Osteopathy Yearbook.* Indianapolis, IN: American Academy of Osteopathy, 1974:81–87.
24. Becker RF. The meaning of fascia and fascial continuity. *Osteopath Ann* 1975:3:8–32.
25. Gowitzke BA, Milner M. *Scientific Basis of Human Movement.* 3rd Ed. Baltimore, MD: William & Wilkins, 1998:143–145.
26. Gowitzke BA, Milner M. *Scientific Basis of Human Movement.* 3rd Ed. Baltimore, MD: William & Wilkins, 1998:145.
27. Ward R, et al. *Foundations for Osteopathic Medicine.* 2nd Ed. Philadelphia, PA: Lippincott Williams & Wilkins, 2003:1158.
28. Ward R, et al., eds. *Foundations for Osteopathic Medicine.* 2nd Ed. Philadelphia, PA: Lippincott Williams & Wilkins, 2003:909.
29. *Stedman's Medical Dictionary.* 23rd Ed. Baltimore, MD: William & Wilkins Company.
30. Kottke FJ, Stillwell GK, Lehman JF. *Krusen's Handbook of Physical Medicine and Rehabilitation.* 3rd Ed. Philadelphia, PA: W.B. Saunders Company, 1971:391.
31. *Stedman's Medical Dictionary.* 23rd Ed. Baltimore, MD: William & Wilkins Company.

32. Becker RO, Seldon G. *The Body Electric*. New York: Quill, 1985: 152–155.
33. Becker RO, Seldon G. *The Body Electric*. New York: Quill, 1985:156.
34. Kottke FJ, Stillwell GK, Lehman JF. *Krusen's Handbook of Physical Medicine and Rehabilitation*. 3rd Ed. Philadelphia, PA: W.B. Saunders Company, 1971:390.
35. Kottke FJ, Stillwell GK, Lehman JF. *Krusen's Handbook of Physical Medicine and Rehabilitation*. 3rd Ed. Philadelphia, PA: W.B. Saunders Company, 1971:391.
36. Still AT. *Philosophy of Osteopathy*. Indianapolis, IN: American Academy of Osteopathy.
37. Bonica JJ. *The Management of Pain*. 2nd Ed. Philadelphia, PA: Lea and Febiger; 1990:66.
38. Earl E. The dual sensory role of muscles spindles. *Phys Ther J* 1965;45:4.
39. Wilson VJ. Inhibition in the central nervous system. *Sci Am* 1966;5: 102–108.
40. Chila AG. *Connective Tissue Continuity: Membranous and Ligamentous Articular Dysfunction*. Athens, OH: Ohio University College of Osteopathic Medicine, 2006:48.
41. Korr IM. The spinal cord as organizer of disease processes—some preliminary perspectives. *JAOA* 1976;76:35–45.
42. Becker RF. The gamma system and its relation to the development and maintenance of muscle tone. *JAOA* 1975;75:170–187.
43. Patterson MM. A model mechanism for spinal segmental facilitation. *JAOA* 1976;76:62–72.
44. O'Connell J. Bioelectric responsiveness of fascia: a model for understanding the effects of manipulation. In: *Techniques in Orthopaedics*. Vol 18(1). Philadelphia, PA: Lippincott Williams & Wilkins, Inc., 2003: 67–73.
45. O'Connell J. Bioelectric responsiveness of fascia: a model for understanding the effects of manipulation. In: *Techniques in Orthopaedics*. Vol 18(1). Philadelphia, PA: Lippincott Williams & Wilkins, Inc., 2003:17–18.
46. Stiles E. Stylized osteopathic seminars. Stiles DO on Web.
47. O'Connell J. *Bioelectric Fascial Activation and Release, The Physician's Guide to Hunting with Dr. Still*. Indianapolis, IN: American Academy of Osteopathy, 2000:15.
48. ECOP Myofascial Release Outline Revised 4/07.
49. O'Connell J. Bioelectric responsiveness of fascia: a model for understanding the effects of manipulation. In: *Techniques in Orthopaedics*. Vol 18 #1. Philadelphia, PA: Lippincott Williams & Wilkins, Inc., 2003:12.
50. Trowbridge C. *Andrew Taylor Still, 1828–1917*. Kirksville, MO, The Thomas Jefferson University Press, 1991:176.
51. Ward R. et al., eds. *Foundations for Osteopathic Medicine*. 2nd Ed. Philadelphia, PA: Lippincott Williams & Wilkins, 2003:934.
52. Ward R. et al., eds. *Foundations for Osteopathic Medicine*. 2nd Ed. Philadelphia, PA: Lippincott Williams & Wilkins, 2003;933.
53. Chila AG. *Connective Tissue Continuity: Membranous and Ligamentous Articular Dysfunction*. Athens, OH: Ohio University College of Osteopathic Medicine, 2006:48.
54. Chila AG. *Connective Tissue Continuity: Membranous and Ligamentous Articular Dysfunction*. Athens, OH: Ohio University College of Osteopathic Medicine, 2006:25.
55. O'Connell J. *Bioelectric Fascial Activation and Release, The Physician's Guide to Hunting with Dr. Still*. Indianapolis, IN: American Academy of Osteopathy, 2000:59–61.
56. Chila AG. *Connective Tissue Continuity: Membranous and Ligamentous Articular Dysfunction*. Athens, OH: Ohio University College of Osteopathic Medicine, 2006:69.
57. Stiles E. Stylized Osteopathic Seminars. Stiles DO on Web.
58. O'Connell J. *Bioelectric Fascial Activation and Release, The Physician's Guide to Hunting with Dr. Still*. Indianapolis, IN: American Academy of Osteopathy, 2000:66.
59. Kottke FJ, Stillwell GK, Lehman JF. *Krusen's Handbook of Physical Medicine and Rehabilitation*. 3rd Ed. Philadelphia, PA: W.B. Saunders Company, 1971:390.
60. Kottke FJ, Stillwell GK, Lehman JF. *Krusen's Handbook of Physical Medicine and Rehabilitation*. 3rd Ed. Philadelphia, PA: W.B. Saunders Company, 1971:391.
61. Stiles E. Stylized Osteopathic Seminars. Stiles DO on Web.
62. O'Connell J. *Bioelectric Fascial Activation and Release, The Physician's Guide to Hunting with Dr. Still*. Indianapolis, IN: American Academy of Osteopathy, 2000:68–69.
63. Still AT. *Philosophy of Osteopathy*. Indianapolis, IN: American Academy of Osteopathy, 28.

48 Osteopathy in the Cranial Field

HOLLIS H. KING

KEY CONCEPTS

- Osteopathy in the cranial field (OCF) delineates an anatomically based understanding of range and vector of motion and physiologic dynamics of cranial bones and intracranial structures.
- The primary respiratory mechanism (PRM) is a functional unit based on the accommodative actions of cranial articular surfaces.
- The traditional model of OCF includes five phenomena: the inherent rhythmic motion of the brain and spinal cord, fluctuation of cerebrospinal fluid, mobility of intracranial and intraspinal membranes, articular mobility of cranial bones, and involuntary mobility of sacrum between ilia.
- Evidence-based research appears to support the vast majority of the PRM phenomena and the palpatory experience of osteopathic practitioners who utilize OCF in medical practice. Ongoing research recognizes the need to provide answers to more questions.

CASE STUDY

R.R. is a 26-year-old female who presents with right-sided facial weakness, which she said she had for 1 week, accompanied by a dulled sense of taste and some trouble hearing. She reported that the day before the onset of symptoms she had been up all night studying. Her medical history was notable for an incident of facial weakness that lasted for one month when she was 7 years old. The physical exam revealed weakness of her right eyelid with delayed blinking, along with right-sided facial droop and lips that remained flat on the right side when she attempted to smile. The patient's appearance was most notable for facial asymmetry with decreased tone on the right side. The structural exam also revealed a side-bending/rotation dysfunction on the right side of the cranium. Cervical vertebrae C2 and C5 were side-bent and rotated right. The diagnosis of Bell palsy was made and osteopathic manipulative treatment (OMT) applied.

The OMT applied integrated muscle energy, myofascial release, soft tissue, and cranial manipulation. The patient's right anterior innominate was treated with muscle energy until symmetry of innominates was achieved. Thoracic outlet and respiratory diaphragms were treated with myofascial release, followed by thoracic lymphatic pump. Cervical rotation dysfunctions were treated with muscle energy. The suboccipital area was treated with soft tissue, occipitoatlanta, and condylar decompression techniques that lead to application of the Galbreath treatment (1) for mandibular drainage, which supports lymphatic drainage and temporal bone-related structure alignment. Finally, osteopathy in the cranial field (OCF) was used to balance the cranial intradural tension membranes and promote symmetry in temporal bone and sacral motion. The cerebellar tentorium served as the focus of this treatment because of its attachments—specifically its lateral attachments to the temporal bones along the petrous ridge enclosing the superior petrosal sinuses, its posterior attachments to the occipital bone forming the transverse sinuses, and its apical attachment to the cerebral falx forming the straight sinus.

The day after the treatment, the patient reported that most of her muscle tone had returned and her sense of taste was normal again. She received a second treatment, and one week after the second treatment, the patient was asymptomatic.

Central to the success of this case is the knowledge of the anatomy of the facial nerve as it traverses the temporal bone. The facial nerve exits the cranium through the stylomastoid foramen to give rise to six terminal branches leading to the muscles of facial expression. This anatomic knowledge allowed the deduction to be made that the patient's lesion was most likely at the chorda tympani. This deduction was also supported by the patient's altered sense of taste and auditory disturbances.

For further information on this interesting case, refer to the article upon which it is based (2).

INTRODUCTION

OCF has its roots in the origins of osteopathic principles, practices, and philosophy going back as far as 1899 when William G. Sutherland observed a disarticulated skull and conceived the notion of the potential for cranial bone motion (3). It has been stated that Sutherland did for the head that which Still did for the rest of the body, which was to delineate an anatomically based understanding of range and vector of motion and physiologic dynamics of cranial bones and intracranial structures. Sutherland's cranial anatomic observations and applications of the osteopathic structure-function tenet regarding cranial neuroanatomy have had reported benefit in clinical practice and have the potential to revolutionize the treatment of many neurological disorders. This chapter surveys the key concepts of OCF, its clinical applications, and the research underlying its theory and clinical applications.

HISTORY

William G. Sutherland, D.O., D.Sc. (Hon) (1873 to 1954), was an early student of Dr. A.T. Still. Sutherland graduated from the

American School of Osteopathy in Kirksville, Missouri, in 1899. While a student, he observed a mounted disarticulated skull. The sphenoid and the squamous portions of the temporal bones caught his attention, and he states, "As I stood looking and thinking in the channel of Dr. Still's philosophy, my attention was called to the beveled articular surfaces of the sphenoid bone. Suddenly there came a thought; I call it a guiding thought—beveled like the gills of a fish, indicating articular mobility for a respiratory mechanism."[3] He dismissed the thought but it kept returning, as if goading him to study the details of the various articulations of the skull.

Sutherland was an original thinker, and his application of Still's philosophy is recognized as "one of the most innovative ideas to be advanced by a member of the osteopathic profession" (4). Anatomy books at that time stated that the sutures of the cranium were immovable. This, however, did not deter Sutherland. He was determined to understand why the articular surfaces have such a unique design, and he persevered until he understood that the design was accommodative to the function of the central nervous system (CNS), cerebrospinal fluid (CSF), and dural membranes, all of which function as a unit. He named this functional unit the *primary respiratory mechanism* (PRM).

Sutherland established his practice in Minnesota and devoted 30 years to study, original research on himself, and observation of his patients before he began to share his discovery with his colleagues. The remarkable results he obtained with patients aroused the interest of other physicians. They prevailed upon him to teach them his method of treatment. He agreed to do so, and classes began at his home. The classes and the interest grew, slowly but steadily, because those who were able to learn the concept and apply this method of osteopathic diagnosis and treatment had similar results of relieving patients of pain and distressful conditions when other forms of treatment failed to help.

Development of the Concept

As more physicians studied and practiced Sutherland's method of osteopathic treatment, they formed an organization, the Osteopathic Cranial Association, for the purpose of joining together to promote further study, support research, and publish literature to help educate physicians and laypersons. This membership organization later changed its name to the Cranial Academy and became a component society of the American Academy of Osteopathic Medicine.

Another, little known, pioneer of the cranial concept was Charlotte Winger Weaver, D.O. (1884–1964), a 1912 graduate of the American School of Osteopathy. Dr. Weaver was reintroduced to the profession by Margaret A. Sorrel, D.O., in the 1998 Sutherland Memorial Lecture. Dr. Weaver considered the cranial bones as modified vertebrae possessing articular surfaces and she taught her concepts through the Doctor Weaver Foundation established in 1927. Dr. Weaver did many dissections of skulls and dural membranous structures, and she had a special interest in the relationship between lesions of the basicranium and neuropsychiatric disorders. She taught that the basicranium could be distorted by birth trauma. Apparently, Dr. Sutherland knew Dr. Weaver, but their researches into the cranium were from two different perspectives and done independently (5).

In 1953 Dr. Sutherland, with Drs. Chester Handy and Harold I. Magoun, Sr, established the Sutherland Cranial Teaching Foundation, Inc., for the purpose of continuing the teaching of the cranial concept. Dr. Sutherland had established that an accurate diagnosis and successful treatment required sensitive and proficient palpation that could not be learned from a book; expert instructors using hands-on teaching and repeated verification were needed.

Dr. Sutherland's discovery and teachings have supplied knowledge and methods that clarify and expand on the science of osteopathy. Prior to Dr. Sutherland's work, the body was treated as if the head was incapable of having somatic dysfunction.

OCF is osteopathy of the entire person because the inherent force that manifests from within the head region functions throughout the body. Therefore, this form of diagnosis and treatment affects the whole person rather than being limited to the cranium. Furthermore, the position of the head atop the vertebral column affects the postural balance of the entire neuromusculoskeletal system. For example, if the cranial bone structures have been brought into a state of imbalance through trauma, the cranium will cause compensatory changes throughout the neuromusculoskeletal system in order to keep the equilibrium apparatus efficient in its function.

Progression and Integration of OCF in Medical Education and Clinic Practice

The teaching and practice of OCF was continued after Sutherland's death by the Sutherland Cranial Teaching Foundation (SCTF) and The Cranial Academy. In the past 55 years of teaching and practice of OCF, there emerged a number of leaders who have preserved and advanced Sutherland's cranial concept through their teachings sponsored by these organizations. Magoun, D.O., wrote *Osteopathy in the Cranial Field* (6), a text that for many years has been a primary reference for those studying OCF. Howard Lippincott, D.O., and his wife Rebecca Lippincott, D.O., taught with Sutherland for many years and published the first work on ligamentous articular strain based on Sutherland's teaching (7,8). Rollin E. Becker, D.O., succeeded Lippincott, D.O., as President of the SCTF and was considered the leading teacher of OCF for many years. His writings are also a primary reference for those studying OCF (9,10). Robert C. Fulford, D.O., was a contemporary of Becker and also studied with Sutherland; his writings elaborate many cranial principles and elucidate many of the subtle aspects of OCF (11–13). Anne L. Wales, D.O., along with her husband Chester Handy, D.O., taught OCF with Dr. Sutherland and she brought into print many of Sutherland's recorded lectures (14). Beryl E. Arbuckle, D.O., was a pediatrician and researcher who, as part of her research on OCF, attended hundreds of autopsies at the hospital of Philadelphia College of Osteopathic Medicine. These autopsies involved gross or microscopic study of the skull. Dr. Arbuckle was noted for her application of OCF on special needs children, particularly those with cerebral palsy (15). Viola M. Frymann, D.O., F.A.A.O., was also a student of Sutherland and has championed OCF with children (16). She has been instrumental in teaching and research on OCF internationally as well as in the USA (17,18). Edna M. Lay, D.O., F.A.A.O., has also been a leader in teaching OCF and working with children, and her writings have shaped the form of this very chapter in previous editions (19).

The insights and techniques derived by Dr. Sutherland's expansion of basic osteopathic principles are increasingly integrated into osteopathic teaching and clinical care (20–22). *The International Classification of Disease, Ninth Revision (ICD-9-CM)*, delineates coding for somatic dysfunction of the cranium, and *Current Procedural Terminology* provides coding for OMT of the head. In recent years, the American Osteopathic Association (AOA) has received numerous research grant proposals from both clinicians and basic scientists to study the mechanisms and/or efficacy of this approach; the AOA has funded several of these projects (23–26).

Instruction in OCF, also commonly referred to as cranial osteopathy (CO), has been a part of standard training in departments of osteopathic principles, practice, and manipulative medicine in all osteopathic medical schools. Concepts and terminology pertaining to OCF/CO have been developed and defined by the Educational Council on Osteopathic Principles of the American Association of Colleges of Osteopathic Medicine. They have been published in the *Glossary of Osteopathic Medical Terminology*, which is updated annually and is easily accessed online (27).

As the federally recognized accrediting body for residency training programs within the osteopathic medical profession, the AOA has approved the *Basic Standards for Residency Training in Neuromusculoskeletal Medicine and Osteopathic Manipulative Treatment*. OCF/CO is one of the OMT models within these basic standards. The AOA also is the federally recognized body charged with approval of certifying boards within the osteopathic medical profession. The AOA has chartered the American Osteopathic Board of Neuromusculoskeletal Medicine. This certifying board administers written, oral, and practical examinations that include items relating to OCF/CO. Questions pertaining to principles of OCF/CO appear on the written portions of the Comprehensive Osteopathic Medical License Examination (COMLEX-USA) administered by the National Board of Osteopathic Medical Examiners, and COMLEX-USA results are accepted for medical licensure in all 50 of the United States.

PRIMARY RESPIRATORY MECHANISM

Central to Sutherland's cranial concept is his integration of anatomic structure and physiologic processes into the PRM model. Many components of this model have garnered scientific verification over the last 3 decades while the rest, though plausible, await empirical demonstration.

Primary refers to first in importance and precedes thoracic respiration in importance. Dr. Sutherland posited that physiologic centers, located in the floor of the fourth ventricle, which regulate pulmonary respiration, circulation, digestion, and elimination, and depend on the function of the CNS, were primary in the maintenance of life (6) Respiratory refers to the exchange of gases and other metabolites at the cellular level. Mechanism implies an integrated machine, each part in working relationship to every other part. The PRM is described as having five anatomic-physiologic components, also often referred to as the five phenomena of OCF. These five components or phenomena are described in the following sections and include:

1. The Inherent Rhythmic Motion of the Brain and Spinal Cord
2. Fluctuation of Cerebrospinal Fluid
3. Mobility of Intracranial and Intraspinal Membranes
4. Articular Mobility of Cranial Bones
5. Involuntary Mobility of Sacrum Between Ilia

The Inherent Rhythmic Motion of the Brain and Spinal Cord

The inherent motion of the CNS is a subtle, slow, pulse-wavelike movement. It is described as having a biphasic cycle, which may have a rhythmic nature. The entire CNS shortens and thickens during one phase and lengthens and thins during the other (6). In words still relevant today, Lassek described the brain as being "vibrantly alive … incessantly active … dynamic … highly mobile, able to move forward, backward, sideward, circumduct and to rotate." He further stated, "The normal, human brain is a wondrous, enormously complex, master organ which can be only made by nature. There are probably approximately twenty billion neurons

in the CNS of man and it runs on a mere 25 W of electrical power" (6, p. 23). As the cerebral hemispheres develop in fetal life, they grow, lengthen, and curl or coil within the developing cranium in the shape of a pair of ram's horns. Specific motion characteristics of cranial palpation are attributed to this configuration of brain structures.

Since the publication of Magoun's text, the delineation of embryological development principles by Jealous (28), based in large measure on the work of Blechschmidt(29,30), has increased the understanding of Sutherland's formulation of the PRM and enhanced the detailed application of OCF in clinical practice through the appreciation of the anatomic positional changes of human structures as they develop from embryonic to adult human configuration and location.

Fluctuation of Cerebrospinal Fluid

The CSF is formed by the choroid plexuses and circulates through the ventricles, over and around the surface of the brain and spinal cord through the subarachnoid spaces and cisternae and is reabsorbed in the choroid plexus. Thus, the CSF is inside and outside of the CNS, bathing, protecting, and nourishing it. Fluctuation is defined as a wavelike motion of fluid in a natural or artificial cavity of the body observed by palpation or percussion (31). From the perspective of Sutherland's concept of the PRM, as the CNS shortens and lengthens in a biphasic rhythmic motion, the ventricles of the brain change shape slightly and the fluid moves concurrently. Furthermore, the combined motility of the CNS and the fluctuation of CSF manifests as a hydrodynamic activity as well as a bioelectric interchange throughout the body. Stated simply, this combined activity of the CNS and CSF functions both as a pump and as a bioelectric generator. Recording of the bioelectric flow in fascia and connective tissue is in the piezoelectric range (32).

Mobility of Intracranial and Intraspinal Membranes

The meninges surround, support, and protect the CNS. The dura mater, the outermost of the three meningeal coverings, is composed of two layers of tough fibrous tissue. The outer layer of dura mater lines the cranial cavity, forming a periosteal covering for the inner aspect of the bones, and extends through the sutures of the skull to become continuous with the periosteum on the outer surface of the skull.

The inner layer of dura mater covers the brain and spinal cord and has reduplications named the falx cerebri and the tentorium cerebelli. These sickle-shaped structures arise from a common origin along the straight sinus and invest the various bones of the cranium. The two layers of dura mater are blended or fused in certain areas and are separated in other areas, forming the intradural venous sinuses.

The dura mater extends down the spinal canal with firm attachment around the foramen magnum and in the spinal canal of the sacrum at the level of the second sacral segment. There are also occasional attachments at C2 and C3 and the lower lumbar. The falx cerebri arises from the straight sinus, attaching to the occiput, parietals, frontals, and the crista galli of the ethmoid. The two halves of the tentorium cerebelli arise or originate at the straight sinus and attach to the occiput, temporals, and sphenoid bone.

The spinal and cranial dura with its reduplications respond to the inherent motion of the CNS and fluctuation of CSF and move through the biphasic cycle, influencing the bones of the cranium and the sacrum. Sutherland named this functional anatomic unit, consisting of the dura mater within the cranium and spinal canal, the reciprocal tension membrane (RTM) (6). It has also been referred to as the "core link" (6) because of the potential to transmit biomechanical forces by linking the cranium to the sacrum. Influences such as trauma and postural strains that affect one part of the mechanism have been clinically observed to affect other parts of the body via this "core link."

Articular Mobility of Cranial Bones

The most dramatic and debated phenomenon of the PRM has been the articular mobility of the cranial bones. Careful study of the design of the various articulations of the cranium and face and the RTM and its influence on the motion of the bones led Sutherland to an appreciation of the mechanical design of this anatomy and their relationship of the inherent motility of the CNS and CSF. At birth, the cranial bones are smooth-edged osseous plates with membrane and/or cartilage between them. With normal growth and motion of intracranial structures, the edges of the cranial bone plates develop and come together with sutures (joints) between them. These sutures allow for a minimal amount of motion while still providing protection for the brain. The remaining debate on the PRM model and research in support of the model are reported below.

Involuntary Mobility of Sacrum Between Ilia

The cranial dura is continuous with the spinal dura; the spinal dura extends through the vertebral canal into the sacral canal, attaching at the level of some cervical and lumbar segments and the second sacral segment. Careful study of the design of the articular surfaces reveals that the sacrum may move on one or several postural axes in relation to the ilia (pelvic bones). In addition to these voluntary or postural movements, the sacrum also responds to the inherent mobility of the CNS, to the fluctuation of the CSF, and to the pull of the intracranial and intraspinal membranes with an involuntary movement that can be observed by palpation in the living body. This slight rocking motion occurs around a transverse axis (called the respiratory axis). Normally, the involuntary motion of the sacrum is synchronous with the involuntary motion of the occiput, each bone being influenced by the rhythmic pull of the spinal and cranial dura mater.

Appreciation of the five phenomena of the PRM in theoretical and practical terms requires an integration of the anatomic and physiologic factors substantiated by empirical research, and experience-derived applications are discussed subsequently. It may help to visualize this physiologic unit of function with all five components moving slightly but steadily in the living body from before birth until death. Becker (33, p. 57) summarizes its influence on the total body economy as follows, "Health requires that the PRM have the capacity to be an involuntary, rhythmic, automatic, shifting suspension mechanism for the intricate, integrated, dynamic interrelationships of its five elements. It is intimately related to the rest of the body through its fascial connections from the base of the skull through the cervical, thoracic, abdominal, pelvic, and appendicular areas of the body physiology. Since all of the involuntary and voluntary systems of the body, including the musculoskeletal system, are found in fascial envelopes, they, too, are subjected to the 10 to 14 cycle-per-minute rhythm of the craniosacral mechanism in addition to their own rhythms of involuntary and voluntary activity. The involuntary mobility of the craniosacral mechanism moves all the tissues of the body minutely into rhythmic flexion of the midline structures with external rotation of the bilateral structures and, in the opposite cycle, extension of the midline structures

with internal rotation of the bilateral structures 10 to 14 times/min throughout life."

RESEARCH INDICATIVE OF THE PRIMARY RESPIRATORY MECHANISM

The Inherent Rhythmic Motion of the Brain and Spinal Cord

Much of the support for this phenomenon of the PRM derives from research done in basic science and medical laboratories outside the osteopathic profession. That the CNS anatomy moves has been proven and is not a matter of controversy. Representative studies demonstrating brain and spinal cord motion characteristics are presented next.

Greitz et al. (34), utilizing magnetic resonance imaging (MRI) technology, demonstrated brain tissue movement characterized by a caudal, medial, and posteriorly directed movement of the basal ganglia, and a caudad and anterior movement of the pons during cardiac systole. The resultant movement vectors created a "funnel shaped" appearance to the brain resulting in a "piston-like" remolding of the brain. The authors felt that this "piston-like" action of the brain during cardiac systole was the driving force responsible for compression of the ventricular system and thus the driving force for the intraventricular flow of cerebral spinal fluid.

Enzmann and Pelc (35) demonstrated brain motion during the cardiac cycle utilizing a similar MRI technology. Peak displacement of the brain ranged from 0.1 to 0.5 mm, except the cerebellar tonsils that demonstrated a displacement of 0.4 mm.

Poncelet et al. (36), using echo-planar MRI, were able to demonstrate pulsatile motion of brain parenchyma. Brain motion in Poncelet's study appeared to consist of a single displacement during systole and a slow return to baseline configuration during diastole. This displacement includes a descent of midbrain and brainstem toward foramen magnum with velocities ≤2 mm/s and medial compression of thalami onto the third ventricle with a velocity of ≤1.5 mm/s.

Feinberg and Mark (37) postulated that the pulsatile nature of CSF flow and brain motion was driven by the force of expansion of the choroid plexus. In their study, which involved observations of pulsatile brain motion via MRI, ejection of CSF into the ventricles occurred simultaneously with reversal of CSF flow in the basal cisterns. These observations suggest that the pumping force for CSF circulation may be a vascularly driven mechanism. They reported the velocity of anterior cortex and corpus callosum movement is 0.4 ± 0.25 mm/s and motion velocity of the basal ganglia and foramen of Monro is 0.63 ± 0.5 mm/s.

Maier et al. (38) demonstrated periodic brain and CSF motion associated with periodic squeezing of the ventricles due to the compression of the intracranial vasculature. They reported peak velocities up to 1 mm/s followed by a slower recoil. Having the subject do a Valsalva maneuver (exert pressure as if trying to defecate), the brain stem showed initial caudal and subsequent cranial displacement of 2 to 3 mm. Coughing produced a short swing of CSF in the cephalic direction.

Mikulis et al. (39) demonstrated movement of the cervical spinal cord in an oscillatory manner, conducted in a craniocaudal direction during cardiac systole. They also reported maximum rate of oscillation as 7.0 mm/s ± 1.4.

These dimensions of motion of cranial and spinal CNS structures suggest that the intracranial structures may not move as far or as fast as spinal cord structures, but these structures do all manifest motion of a precise measurable nature. This motion appears to be related to the vascular dynamics of the circulatory system and the cardiac cycle. This element of the PRM is not controversial as such motion has been well studied and established.

The PRM also postulates a deep cellular level, life-sustaining respiratory function that contributes to the rhythmicity of the PRM. Rhythmic motion suggestive of such a phenomenon has been identified in animals and possibly humans. As long ago as 1951, oligodendrocyte tissue from rat corpus callosum was placed in tissue culture medium and photographed by ciné-photomicrography (40). The authors state, "These cells show a characteristic rhythmic pulsatility apparently identical with that described in 1935 by Canti et al. (41) in the case of oligodendrocytes obtained from in culture from oligodendroglioma of the human brain. We believe also that we have seen similar cells in a few tissue culture preparations from the cortex of the normal human brain." (41, p. 114) In 1957, Wolley and Shaw (42) reported rhythmic contractions of the oligodendroglial cells of brain and spinal cord. In the early 1960s, Hyden (43) reported that glial cells, grown in a culture, pulsate continuously.

Using more modern technology, Vern et al. (44) were able to measure rhythmic oscillatory patterns related to intracellular oxidative metabolism in the cat and rabbit. They demonstrated a synchronous rhythm at about 7 cycles/min for the creation and then utilization of cytochrome oxidase within the cells of the cortex of the test animal subjects. Dani et al. (45) showed active waves of astrocytic Ca^{2+} in the rat hippocampus in response to neural activity. Propagation of the calcium wave was usually within 5 to 6 seconds from the beginning of neural stimulation, and under constant stimulation produced waves at the rate of 2/min. The findings of these studies are indicative of a regular periodicity propagated by biochemical activity of astroglia.

Whether or not there is any biomechanical impetus to the palpable characteristics of the PRM by cellular and intracellular activity, motility as well as mobility possibly associated with a primary respiration process has been identified.

Fluctuation of Cerebrospinal Fluid

That the CSF moves in a fluctuant flow pattern through the ventricles of the brain and within the subarachnoid space around the brain and spinal cord is also a noncontroversial and well-established phenomenon. In fact, much of research cited above, which demonstrated the motion of the brain and spinal cord, also identified features of the CSF fluctuant flow.

Summarizing over a century of research DuBolay et al. (46, p. 497) stated, "The majority of workers throughout these seven decades have become convinced that the 'cardiac' CSF pressure rise measured in the ventricles, at the cisterna magna and in the lumbar theca, is caused by the rhythmic arterial input of blood to the cranial cavity." DuBolay further states, "Most authors, e.g., Becher (47), had envisaged the arterial inflow to the head as causing an expansion of the brain and of the vessels within the basal cisterns. O'Connell (48) suggested that the brain's expansion, by compressing the third ventricle, might constitute a CSF pump."

Of particular interest to the OCF practitioner is the effect of spinal dural membranes (the third listed phenomenon of the PRM discussed below) on the flow of CSF. Levy et al. (49) reported that in healthy people the spinal CSF flow rate was 12.4 ± 2.92 mm/s. In patients with spinal dysraphism (conditions like spina bifida), the rate is much slower at 2.12 ± 1.69 mm/s. In patients with spinal cord compression (such as from traumatic injury or tumors), the rate was also slowed at 1.87 ± 1.4 mm/s. They concluded further that, "The origin of cord pulsations is compatible with a direct transfer of motion from brain pulsations."

Anatomic connection between CSF flow and the lymphatic system, a long-held hypothesis in OCF practice, appears to have been established. Research by Walter et al. (50) in which india ink particles injected into rat subarachnoid space were found distributed around the olfactory nerves and within the lymphatic vessels. The authors state, "This anatomical communication, thus, allows the CNS to connect with the lymphatic system. The presence of the route may play an important role in the movement of antigens from the subarachnoid space to the extracranial lymphatic vessels, resulting in inducement of an immune response of the CNS" (50, p. 388).

Based on the widely accepted nature of the fluctuant flow of CSF as demonstrated by decades of research and clinical application, this phenomenon of the PRM appears to be supported by the evidence and is not controversial.

Mobility of Intracranial and Intraspinal Membranes

The existence of the dura mater membrane around the brain and spinal cord is well documented and utilized in anatomic research and medical practice. Every medical student and anatomist who has dissected the central nervous has seen this membrane. Every physician who has done a lumbar puncture (or spinal tap) has felt the "pop" as the needle penetrates the dura in the procedure to obtain a sample of CSF. Those who practice OCF utilize this anatomy to treat cranial and cervical malalignment from the sacrum, or sacral malalignment from the base of the skull. These types of treatment are believed to be possible because of the hypothesized direct connection between the cranium and sacrum in the form of the dural membranes.

As a phenomenon of the PRM, the RTM anatomy has been proven useful by many clinicians in practice, but has received critical review even by cranial practitioners (51,52). Norton reported insignificant correlation between PRM rates palpated simultaneously at the cranium and sacrum (51). Chaitow (52) reported different length measurements for the spinal canal when a person was forward bent versus backward bent. While these reservations raise questions yet to be answered, other experimental and anatomic findings tend to lend support to the concept that dural membrane linkage between the sacrum and cranial base may be correct and have clinical value.

Kostopoulos and Keramidas (53) utilized a novel approach to anatomic research on a male cadaver that had been embalmed for 6 months. The brain tissue was removed through two cut windows, leaving intact the intracranial dural membranes. The measurement used was a piezoelectric element attached to the falx cerebri with the motion recorded by oscilloscope. Application of the frontal lift cranial treatment maneuver then produced a 1.44-mm elongation of the falx cerebri and a parietal lift maneuver produced a 1.08-mm elongation. Even on embalmed tissue, application of the sphenobasilar compression maneuver produced a –0.33 mm movement, and the sphenobasilar decompression maneuver a +0.28 mm movement of the falx cerebri. The Kostopoulos and Keramidas data suggest that for cranial structures there is an identifiable association between cranial maneuvers applied to the cranium and the movement of cranial dural membranes.

Based on MRI imagery of *in vivo* kinematic analysis of head and neck position in extension and flexion positions, Zhu et al. (54) reported relative displacements of brain with respect to skull as the head position changes. The displacements were on the order of 1 to 2 mm when the head changed positions voluntarily. The authors state, "These displacements over the normal range of head/neck flexion suggest free interfacial conditions between brain and skull" (54, p. 2).

A possible connection between the cranial structure motion and sacral motion was identified by Zanakis et al. (55). Utilizing infrared surface skin markers positioned over the subject's parietal and frontal bones, cranial bone motion was observed utilizing a three-dimensional kinematic motion sensitive system. During the study, there was simultaneous palpation of the sacrum by an experienced examiner. The findings reported a 92% correlation between the examiner who signaled perception of the flexion phase of sacral movement via a foot-activated switch and the movement of the cranial bone markers.

Given the relatively small numbers of subjects in both of the empirical studies (51,55) and the difficulties inherent in ascertaining reliable palpatory data (56), it appears that indeed further study is needed before the RTM concept can be established empirically. The implications of anatomy-based, spinal canal length differences in forward versus backward bending are also in need of further study.

Therefore, while there is no doubt as to the existence of the continuity of dural membranes around the CNS, the clinical applications of this anatomy, as postulated by the concept of the PRM, are in need of further validation. However, from the perspective of OCF practitioners who report treatment success using this particular formulation of OCF, there is little doubt of the clinical applicability of the cranial to sacral connection of the dural membranes.

Articular Mobility of Cranial Bones

The most controversial phenomenon of the PRM from a scientific perspective is the concept of palpable cranial bone motion. Misgivings have been expressed based primarily on the assumed anatomic impossibility of such motion (57,58). However, cranial sutures are constructed in such a way that motion is possible beyond simple bony compliance (Fig. 48.1). The basis of the traditional anatomic concept of cranial bone immobility is derived primarily from forensic anthropology research done to estimate the age of skeletal remains. However, there is a growing body of literature that brings into question this long-held anatomically based perspective. The challenge to the position that cranial bones are incapable of motion is based on examination of the basis for this conclusion in the first place and empirical evidence of cranial bone motion in the second place.

To appreciate the conceptual challenge implied by the concept of cranial bone motion, it is important to know that in the last century respected scientists, anatomists, and anthropologists posited

the fusion and inherent immobility of cranial bones. Most often cited are the works of Bolk (59), Melsen (60), Perizonius (61), Cohen (62), and Sahni et al. (63) all of whom state or are reported to have held the view that cranial sutures were fused and immobile. Based on thorough examination of this debate, it may turn out that this view has been an anatomic version of "the world is flat" debate of the last millennium.

With the exception of Bolk (59), all of the aforementioned anthropologists and anatomists cite as precedent for their work, that of Todd and Lyon (64,65) as central to the idea that cranial bones fuse and therefore are immobile. There is reason to question Todd and Lyon's conclusions based on a close reading of their lengthy manuscripts. Paul Dart, M.D. (66) states, "In interpreting this data, it must be noted that Todd and Lyon were attempting to establish 'modal' norms for sutural closure, and they discounted data that was clearly out of the modal pattern before creating their summary. 11.7% of their 307 white male specimens and 25.8% of their 120 negro male specimens were excluded from the data due to prolonged sutural patency."

Further reason to question the concept of universal sutural fusion was given by Singer (67). He found a high percentage of specimens with much less closure than Todd and Lyon's norms, including a 64-year-old specimen with no closure at sagittal, lambdoid, or left coronal sutures and three specimens aged early 40s with virtually no sutural closure in the coronal, lambdoid, or sagittal sutures. Also in the 1950s, Pritchard et al. commented to the effect that "Obliteration of sutures and synostosis of adjoining bones, *if it happens at all* (italics added), occurs usually after all growth has ceased. In great apes synostosis of all sutures occurs immediately after growth has ceased, but in man and most laboratory animals sutures may never completely close. These differences have been attributed to the differences in the degree of development of the masticatory apparatus" (68, p. 81).

A recent article by Sabini and Elkowitz (69) gives pictorial and systematic review of 36 human cadaver skulls ranging in age from 56 to 101 years, all well above the age when bone growth is complete. Twenty-six of the skulls showed more than 100% obliteration of the coronal suture, 31 of the skulls had unobliterated lambdoidal sutures, and 24 of the skulls had unobliterated sagittal sutures. The lambdoidal suture was the least fused on a majority of the skulls and the attachment of musculature on the occipital bone was cited as the probable cause of maintaining sutural patency. Similar to Pritchard et al. (68) Sabini and Elkowitz speculated that the chewing motion contributes to muscular tension on the bones, maintaining some degree of sutural patency. The endocranial (inner) surface of the skull was not evaluated so that no estimate of through and through fusion of each suture could be made. However, the finding of a significant amount of sutural patency (nonfusion) certainly brings into question the idea that all cranial sutures are fused and therefore cannot move.

Prior to the Sabini and Elkowitz publication, the work of Retzlaff and associates dealt directly with the nature of cranial suture morphology and cranial bone motion. Retzlaff et al. (70, p. 663) state, "Gross and microscopic examination of the parieto-parietal and parieto-temporal cranial sutures obtained by autopsy from 17 human cadavers with age range of 7 to 78 years shows that these sutures remain as clearly identifiable structures even in the oldest samples." Retzlaff et al. (71) identified sutural elements contradicting ossification and demonstrated the presence of vascular and neural structures in the sutures. These studies also showed the presence of nerve and vascular tissue substantial enough to supply the needs of connective tissue activated beyond mere bony sutural adhesions and ossification. Additionally, Retzlaff et al. (72) traced nerve endings

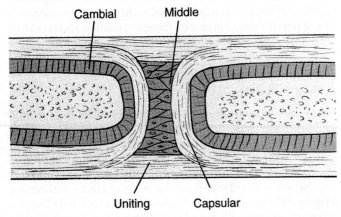

Figure 48-1 Histology of cranial sutures. (From Magoun HI. *Osteopathy in the Cranial Field*. 2nd Ed. Kirksville, MO: Journal Printing Company, 1966, with permission.)

Cambial   Middle

Uniting   Capsular

from the sagittal sinus through the falx cerebri and third ventricle to the superior cervical ganglion in primates and mammals. That such structures were found in cranial sutures brings further doubt to the idea that these sutures fuse and are immobile.

Empirically demonstrated cranial bone motion in animals is well documented. Michael and Retzlaff (73) demonstrated cranial bone (parietal) mobility in the squirrel monkey. In cats, parietal bone motion in the range of 200 to 300 μm was induced by laboratory-controlled changes in the CSF volume (74–76). Jaslow (77) demonstrated in goat skulls (*Capra hircus*) that patent cranial sutures in adult animals may play a role in shock absorption and redistribution of forces directed against the skull (e.g., ballistic forces directed against the goat's skull) and during chewing movements. Thus, a compliant skull is a stronger, more resilient skull in that it is capable of absorbing and redistributing forces directed against it.

Research involving assessment of human cranial bone motion has been done by neurologists, space physiologists, osteopathic medical profession physicians, and basic scientists. In work later cited by NASA scientists, Frymann (78) developed a noninvasive apparatus for mechanically measuring the changes in cranial diameter. Cranial motion was recorded simultaneously with thoracic respiration. On the basis of her extensive recordings on one human subject, she concluded that a rhythmic pattern of cranial bone mobility exists and moves at a rate that is different than that of thoracic respiration.

In a 1981 study on two comatose patients, Heifetz and Weiss (79) used a strain gauge device that demonstrated cranial vault expansion associated with an artificially induced rise in intracranial pressure (ICP). Utilizing a head-holding device similar to Gardner-Wells tongs, accompanied by a strain gauge meter, the skull device was inserted into the calvaria above the external auditory canal. The strain gauge device employed a "Wheatstone Bridge," which was designed to detect any expansion of the skull of about 0.0003 mm or greater, which when it occurred, would produce a voltage change of 1 μV. They performed 19 trials and each time ICP was artificially elevated, there was a voltage change. This voltage change indicated that the skull tong pins were being spread apart. This could only occur with expansion of the cranial vault.

A promising approach to assessing cranial bone motion before and after cranial manipulation was carried out utilizing x-rays (Dental Orthogonal Radiographic Analysis) on 12 subjects (80). The before to after changes in cranial bone position measured in degrees ranged from 0 to 8 degrees for atlas, mastoid, malar, sphenoid, and temporal bone position. The percentage of subjects with identifiable changes ranged 66.6% with the mastoid to 91.6 % for the atlas, sphenoid, and temporal bones. There are plans to expand this research utilizing a larger number of subjects.

Russian and United States Space Research

One of the strongest areas of research, which involved assessment of cranial bone motion, has been that carried out by the Russian and U.S. astronaut programs. The concerns that led to this research had to do with the nature of human response to prolonged weightlessness in space. Without gravity, would the human circulatory and CNSs function normally? In the process of assessing intracranial fluid dynamics, various types of radiographic and ultrasound equipment have been used to measure intracranial volume as well as cranial bone dimensions, and changes in these dimensions have been observed.

Yuri Moskalenko, Ph.D. (81,82), first published research on cats in space that described "third order waves" similar to that described above in glial cells. After being introduced to OCF by Frymann, D.O., Moskalenko and associates carried out several studies that showed cranial bone motion. One utilizing NMR tomograms, showed cranial bone motion between 380 μm to 1 mm, and cranial cavity volume increases by 12 to 15 mL, with a rhythmicity of 6 to 14 cycles/min (83). This work was followed by a study utilizing bioimpedence measures and transcranial ultrasound Doppler echography to demonstrate slow oscillations of the cranial bones at 0.08 to 0.2 Hz (84). Moskalenko demonstrated that these oscillations, "…were of intracranial origin and were related to the mechanisms of regulation of the blood supply to and oxygen consumption by cerebral tissue, as well as with the dynamics of CSF circulation" (84, p. 171). Moskalenko and Frymann have carried this work into a formulation of a theory that explains the physiology of the PRM (85).

In the mid-1990s, NASA was also concerned about intracranial fluid volume changes in astronauts in space. NASA carried out research and developed an ultrasound device, pulse-phase locked loop (PPLL), with sensitivity to 0.1 μm, to more precisely assess intracranial anatomy and physiology (86). This NASA team at the Ames Research Center carried out a series of studies (87–90).

On two fresh cadavera (<24 hours post mortem), female 83 and male 93, ICP pulsations were generated manually by infusing saline into the intracranial ventricular system at a rate of 1 cycle/s (1 Hz) (87). In this study, an increase in ICP of 15 mL Hg caused a skull expansion of 0.029 mm, and this was interpreted by the authors as similar to that found by Heisey and Adams (74), Frymann (78), and Heifetz and Weiss (79).

In another study, seven healthy volunteers fitted with the PPLL device were placed in 60 degree, 30 degree head-up tilt, supine, and 10 degree head-down tilt positions. The average path length from forehead to occipital bone increased 1.038 ± 0.207 mm at 10 degree head down tilt relative to 90 degree upright. "In other words, when intracranial pressure increases, arterial pulsation produces a higher amplitude ICP pulsation. Increased amplitude of ICP pulsations will be manifested by larger fluctuations in distance across the skull" (88, p. 3).

Summarizing their work to a certain point, the NASA research team stated, "Although the skull is often assumed to be a rigid container with a constant volume, many researchers have demonstrated that the skull moves on the order of a few micrometers in association with changes in intracranial pressure" (89, p. 66). In their last publication in this series, they state, "…analysis of covariance reveled that there was a significant effect of tilt angle on amplitude of cranial diameter pulsation ($p < 0.001$). . . . As a result, amplitudes of cranial distance pulsation increased as the angle of tilt decreased. The observed changes in cranial diameter pulsation are considered to be statistically significant" (90, p. 883).

Contemporary Osteopathic Research on Cranial Bone Motion

Research comparing palpatory assessment of cranial bone motion with simultaneous assessment by laser Doppler flowmetry technology has been done. Striking correlations have been found between cranial palpation reports and the technologically measured physiologic motion phenomena identified by the laser Doppler flowmetry. Nelson et al. (91–94) posit that it is the Traube-Hering and Meyer oscillations that they have identified. Based on laser Doppler flowmetry electronically recorded on humans, they described oscillations that occur about 4 to 6 cycles/min. In their studies, these oscillations have been shown to correlate with reports of phases of cranial bone motion as reported by osteopathic cranial practitioners.

These investigators proposed that Traube-Hering and Meyer oscillations comprise all or account for most of the cranial bone motion palpated by cranial practitioners. To have instrumented recordings of physiologic activity correlated to the palpatory experience of OCF practitioners constitutes support for the PRM and the concept of cranial bone motion.

Another approach to examining cranial bone motion was carried out by Crow et al. (95,96) This group utilized MRI imagery of eight slices each through the same calvarial plane on the heads of 20 healthy subjects. ImageJ (97) analysis from the National Institutes of Health showed that there were significant differences ($p < 0.003$) between the means for largest and smallest cranial bone dimensions for area. The mean difference was 122.69 mm^2 for the area analyzed on the outer table of the cranial bones. The significant differences in this intracranial dimension would not be possible if cranial bones were not capable of motion. The authors suggested the intracranial area change may be related to intracranial fluid volume changes.

The evidence for cranial bone motion is increasing in number and quality, but the nature of the motion has more questions to be answered. Commentary that holds to the "cranial bones are fused" perspective is particularly critical of the sphenobasilar junction mobility model (98). In answer, Cook (99), an OCF practitioner with a background in engineering and computational fluid mechanics, presents a plausible model based on cranial bone compliance and flexibility that would explain the palpatory experience of OCF practitioners.

Involuntary Mobility of Sacrum Between Ilia

That the sacrum moves in its position between the ilia is an anatomical fact. It would not be possible for humans to walk or run if the iliosacral joints did not allow motion. It is hard to imagine, but for centuries it was believed by scientists of the day that the pelvis was a solid array of bone and that there was no independent motion of the sacrum.

The biomechanical dimensions of iliosacral joint motion were delineated by Weisl in the mid-1950s (100). Elaboration on iliosacral motion characteristics was done by Kissling (101) who has subjects perform flexion and extension movements of the spine as well as one-legged stance to induce sacroiliac motion. The range of motion was 0.2 to 1.6 mm, with an average of 0.7 mm for males and 0.9 mm for females. Other research describes a number of different axes of sacral motion, a concept already well integrated into OMT training programs, with motion noted to be in the range of 1 to 3 mm (102).

As seen in the now-settled debate over sacroiliac joint motion, history may be repeating itself in the debate over cranial bone motion. It is unfortunate that today there is doubt about cranial bone motion despite the growing evidence for the reality of this phenomenon.

The controversy of sacral motion from the perspective of the PRM has to do with the nature of the impetus for the sacral motion. There is some evidence to support the contention of *involuntary active motion* of the sacrum between the ilia. Mitchell and Pruzzo (103–105) demonstrated a horizontal axis for sacral motion located anterior to the second sacral segment. Movement around this axis was measured at 0.9 to 4.7 mm at the sacral apex, and the impetus for this motion was simply breathing, which associated sacral motion with the normal respiratory excursion (103). While this research establishes normal respiratory motion as one impetus for sacral motion, other research describes the sacral motion induced by the PRM as separate and distinct from motion caused by respiratory excursion (78).

Furthermore, the correlation of sacral motion with cranial bone motion has not been established empirically (51), and may be related to the apparent differences in spinal canal length previously mentioned by Chaitow (52) who cites the work of Butler (106).

OCF Research Status

Evidence-based research appears to support the vast majority of the PRM phenomena and the palpatory experience of osteopathic practitioners who utilize OCF in medical practice. However, more questions need to be answered and these questions are subjects of ongoing research. Based on the preponderance of evidence supportive of OCF, the succeeding sections will elucidate the classic OCF concepts taught in osteopathic medical schools and osteopathic training programs worldwide.

MECHANICS OF PHYSIOLOGIC MOTION

The overall shape of the skull is that of a relative sphere with its inferior surface indented. The sphenoid and occiput meet to create this indentation, which is slightly convex on its superior surface. These two midline bones form the key articulation of cranial bone motion at the sphenobasilar symphysis (or synchondrosis) in the base of the skull. This is a cartilaginous union up to the age of 25 years and thereafter has the resiliency of cancellous bone (107).

The overall motion of the cranium is similar to the motion of the chest during respiration, but the two do not occur simultaneously. Thoracic respiration occurs 12 to 16 cycles/min in adults and up to 44 cycles/min in newborns (108); the most frequently encountered motion of the PRM normally occurs 10 to 14 cycles/min (6).

The terminology used to describe the directions of motion of the various bones is similar to that for the motions of the spine and extremities. Midline bones (the sphenoid, occiput, ethmoid, vomer, and sacrum) move through a flexion phase and an extension phase around a transverse axis, while paired bones move through external and internal rotation. They are moved through this biphasic cycle in response to the pull or influence of the dural membranes, which are influenced by the coiling and uncoiling of the CNS and the fluctuation of the CSF. This motion, initiated from within the living body, is referred to as inherent motion or involuntary motion.

With flexion of the sphenobasilar symphysis, there is slight increase in the convexity of the superior surface of the joint. At the same time, the area where the coronal and sagittal sutures join, called bregma, descends. Palpation in the flexion portion of the biphasic cycle senses that the head widens slightly in its transverse diameter and shortens slightly in its anteroposterior (AP) diameter as the paired bones move toward external rotation. With extension of the midline bones, the head narrows and lengthens slightly as the bregma ascends, and all paired bones move toward internal rotation.

During the biphasic cycle, the osseous cranium changes shape slightly but allows some intracranial fluid volume change. The research of Heisey and Adams (74) and Moskalenko (83) suggests there is enough cranial bone compliance and "sutural stretch" to allow as much as a 15-mL intracranial fluid volume change.

During flexion, the sacrum is influenced by the spinal dura and core link and moves posterosuperiorly at its base while the apex moves anteriorly toward the pubes. During extension, the base moves anteriorly and the apex moves posteriorly. This motion occurs around a transverse axis in the area of the second sacral segment posterior to the sacral canal and is called the respiratory axis of the sacrum. The other axes of sacral motion are postural axes (Fig. 48.2).

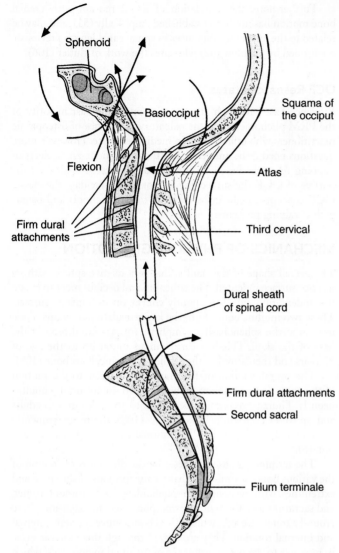

Figure 48-2 Craniosacral mechanism with *arrows* indicating direction of motion during flexion phase of physiologic motion. (From Magoun HI. *Osteopathy in the Cranial Field.* 2nd Ed. Kirksville, MO: Journal Printing Company, 1966, with permission.)

PALPATION OF THE PRIMARY RESPIRATORY MECHANISM

The inherent motion of the cranium is not visible but it is palpable. This motion is perceived as a subtle, soft, slight movement of fluid (CSF) and semifluid (CNS) inside an osseous case. The first attempts at this palpatory exercise may not reveal anything, or you may feel the subject's thoracic respiration transmitted through the neck to the head. If the breathing is a distraction, ask the patient to hold their breath for a moment. If you can still sense the rhythmic motion in the head, the inherent motion is coming from within the cranium. With palpatory experience, one learns to distinguish between these different motions.

Follow these steps to palpate this rhythmic motion:

1. Position the patient supine, with the head 8 to 10 in from the head of the table
2. Sit comfortably at the head of the table with your forearms resting on the table and your hands placed on the sides of the patient's head. Have the patient move up or down on the table to comfortably accommodate to your relaxed posture
3. Contact the patient's head lightly, allowing the fingers and part of the palms to gently conform to the curvature of the head. (It is essential that the palmar surface of all the fingers, but not the thumbs, contact the head because the nerve endings that sense the subtle cranial motion are proprioceptors located in tendons and around joints. The numerous tactile sensors in the fingerpads are not as receptive to this motion. Even though a gentle and light contact is essential, it is not a fingertip contact.)
4. Allow your mind to become quiet and direct your attention to the space between your hands, allowing what is sensed by your proprioceptors to be perceived by your brain. Continue to stay relaxed; do not try to feel something. If the patient's head has fairly normal motion, you may feel a slow, rhythmic swelling or widening followed by a receding or narrowing. This constitutes one cycle of inherent motion. This cycle is usually steadily repeated. The motion is so mild and subtle that it may actually feel as if the head is breathing

Subtle motion is easier for some physicians to palpate than for others. Some find this difficult to sense because they try too hard. Their intensity is so set, their effort so strong, that they block their own sensorium. It is essential to be relaxed, physically, mentally, and emotionally. Your attitude should be similar to one who is trying to hear a minor sound—complete attention is given to listening.

Keep the hand contact light. Pressure by the hands will suppress the inherent motion and/or distract the sensors (proprioceptors) in the hands. If excessive hand pressure is continued, the patient may get a headache.

If you have difficulty perceiving the motion in one patient, try other patients. The cyclic characteristics of the motion and its amplitude (strength or power) usually vary from one individual to another. The biphasic cycle of motion of the PRM most often encountered occurs 10 to 14 times/min, although it can occur at somewhat faster or slower rates. When observing the rate, allow one full minute and count the number of cycles (one flexion phase plus one extension phase equals one complete cycle).

Evaluating the amplitude, or quality rather than rate, of the PRM in patients who have clinical problems requires experience but has been found to be statistically possible (109) and may reveal the most useful clinical data about the patient. After palpating five or ten individuals, one can determine that the strength or vitality of the rhythm is stronger in one or two individuals, fair or medium in some, and weak or poor in others. Experience with palpation has shown that the rate and amplitude of the PRM, when considered in addition to clinical knowledge of the patient's history and symptoms, becomes an additional diagnostic indication of their state of health and is helpful in determining a prognosis.

There are many scenarios in which the rate and quality of the PRM may be increased slightly:

- Following vigorous physical exercise
- With systemic fevers
- Following effective OMT of the craniosacral mechanism

The rate and quality of the PRM may be decreased in the following situations:

- Stress (mental, emotional, physical)
- Chronic fatigue
- Chronic infections
- Mental depression and other psychiatric conditions (110)
- Chronic poisoning
- Other debilitating conditions

The cyclic, biphasic motion originating within the PRM, is most evident to palpation in the head region but is palpable in every part of the body. The impulse moves longitudinally through the body and extremities, with midline structures moving through flexion/extension and paired structures moving through external/internal rotation. Its presence or absence and its deviation from normal direction are useful diagnostic signs.

The body is subject to stresses and strains from before birth until death. Pressures and forces affect the developing fetus, the neonate during birth, and the individual through childhood, adolescence, and adulthood. These forces cause minor to major distortions of the cranium that result in strains of the sphenobasilar synchondrosis (SBS). With induced strain, the efficiency of the PRM is compromised. The compromise may be minor to major in its effect on the health of the individual.

STRAINS

Several types of strains of the SBS are known and frequently encountered in the practice. In order to understand a discussion of strain patterns, it is necessary to know some terminology and to recall some basic principles of anatomy. The portion of the occiput that is at the base of the skull and is part of the SBS is called the basiocciput. Likewise, the part of the sphenoid that lies at the base of the skull and is part of the SBS is the basisphenoid. When we discuss motion of these bones, we name the motion for what is occurring at the most anterior and superior portion of the structure. However, the major articulation that concerns us in the following discussion of strain patterns is composed of the anterior portion of one bone (the occiput) and the posterior portion of another bone (the sphenoid). So, when motion occurs in the same direction in the two bones, the two bones appear to move in opposite directions at the SBS. Keeping these principles in mind will help you understand the following discussion of strain patterns.

Torsion occurs around an AP axis of the skull that extends from nasion through the symphysis to opisthion (Fig. 48.3A). The sphenoid and related structures of the anterior cranium rotate in one direction about this axis; the occiput and related structures of the posterior cranium rotate in the opposite direction, producing a twist or torsion at the SBS. This strain is named for the side of the high wing of the sphenoid, right torsion (RT), or left torsion (LT).

Side bending/rotation (SBR) at the SBS occurs around an AP axis and around two parallel vertical axes. The AP axis is the same as the axis around which torsions occur. The vertical axes are through the body of the sphenoid and through the foramen magnum, perpendicular to the physiologic transverse axes and the AP axis (Fig. 48.3B). This is a compound movement similar to physiologic motion in the spine when rotation and side bending are concomitant movements. Because the sphenobasilar symphysis is slightly convex upward, as the two bones side bend away from each other (around the two parallel vertical axes), both bones rotate inferiorly on the convex side (around the AP axis) and superiorly on the concave side. This strain pattern is named for the side of the convexity, SBR right (SBR_R) or SBR left (SBR_L). These four strain patterns (RT, LT, SBR_R, SBR_L) are common and are considered physiologic if their presence does not interfere with the flexion-extension motion of the mechanism.

Extreme or exaggerated flexion with decreased extension of the SBS is considered a strain pattern. Conversely, marked or exaggerated extension with decreased flexion is considered a strain pattern. Normally, the PRM moves through the flexion and extension phases equally and fully.

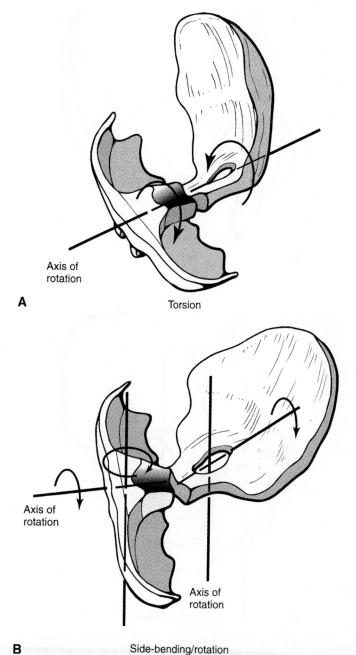

A Torsion

B Side-bending/rotation

Figure 48-3 Schematic patterns of sphenobasilar junction. In torsion and SBR, sphenoid and occiput rotate in opposite directions about axes indicated. **A.** Torsion with great wing high on the right. Occiput is lower on the side of high great wing. **B.** SBR with convexity to the left. Both great wings of sphenoid and occiput are lower on the side of convexity. (From Sutherland WG, Wales AL. *Teachings in the Science of Osteopathy.* Portland, OR: Rudra Press, 1990, with permission.)

Vertical and lateral strains or displacement occur at the SBS and can be superimposed on the above strains. Vertical strain at the SBS is present when the sphenoid and the occiput rotate in the same direction around their own transverse axes (Fig. 48.4A). This creates a superior or inferior strain at the SBS and disrupts normal flexion-extension. Vertical strain is named for the position of the basisphenoid relative to the occiput, superior, or inferior.

Lateral strain at SBS occurs when both bones rotate in the same direction, clockwise, or counterclockwise, around two parallel

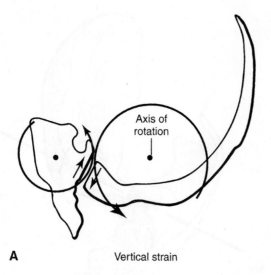

A Vertical strain

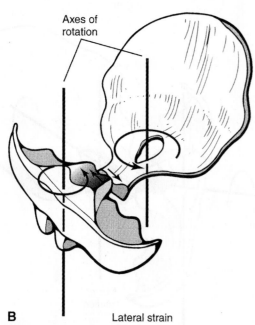

B Lateral strain

Figure 48-4 Schematic patterns of sphenobasilar junction. In vertical and lateral strain patterns, sphenoid and occiput rotate in the same direction around parallel axes. **A.** Superior vertical strain. As a result of rotation of the bones, the base of the sphenoid is relatively elevated with the base of the occiput relatively depressed. **B.** Right lateral strain. As a result of rotation of the bones, the base of the sphenoid is relatively displaced to the right with the base of the occiput relatively displaced to the left. (From Sutherland WG, Wales AL. *Teachings in the Science of Osteopathy.* Portland, OR: Rudra Press: 1990, with permission.)

vertical axes (Fig. 48.4B). Basisphenoid and basiocciput veer in opposite directions, producing a shearing type of motion. When this strain occurs *in utero* or during the birth process, it results in a parallelogram-shaped head in the infant. Lateral strain is named for the direction the basisphenoid shifts, right or left.

SBS compression is a strain in which the sphenoid and occiput have been forced together to such a degree that physiologic flexion-extension is impaired. Compression varies from mild to moderate to severe and occurs from a force to the back of the head, to the

front of the head, or from a circumferential compression (as during birth) that exceeds the resiliency of the tissues.

Strains of the SBS involve the entire cranial and facial structure and influence the position and motion of the sacrum by way of the RTM. The midline bones and paired bones accommodate to the strain(s) in the base of the skull. Trauma to the head, face, spine, sacrum, pelvis, or lower extremities is a common strain-producing factor. Pelvic function is affected by a strain in the base of the skull. Likewise, the function of the cranial bones is affected by strain in the pelvis. The body, including the head, truly functions as a unit.

PRINCIPLES OF DIAGNOSIS

The diagnosis of a pathologic condition or malfunction of the PRM is based on the history, observation, and palpation. Palpation by a well-trained and sensitive operator is the most reliable source of information.

Patient History

Taking the patient's history includes asking leading and pertinent questions to encourage the patient to recall relevant past events and to describe the complaint in some detail. In addition to the usual questions pertaining to heredity, childhood diseases, adult diseases, and surgeries, two other areas for questioning are pertinent to dysfunction of the craniosacral mechanism: trauma history and information about the delivery and newborn recovery period.

Trauma

Obtain the following information about trauma:

1. Age at which the trauma occurred; this includes birth trauma.
2. Type of force as well as amount, velocity, direction, and the area of impact; vehicular accidents, blows to the face or head, and falls on the tailbone or buttocks are common
3. Dental history including extractions, orthodontia, malocclusion, bruxism, and temporomandibular joint problems
4. Fractures, concussions, inertial injuries, coma
5. Habitual head pressures, such as sleeping positions, thumb sucking, ear phones, orthodontic head gear, new dentures, etc
6. Extremes of temperature: chilling of the face or head may precede Bell palsy; heatstroke or sunstroke may be related to headache
7. Surgical procedures involving the head such as the mouth gag, the bite block, the bronchoscope or gastroscope, or the anesthetic mask held over the nose-mouth for prolonged periods with a tight headband to keep it in place
8. Changes in appearance or personality following severe trauma

Adult patients tend to recall only injuries of the recent past. They believe that injuries from infancy, childhood, or adolescence are of no importance and tend to forget past trauma. They may need leading questions to elicit this information. Some patients have amnesia related to trauma to the head and cannot relate accurate information. A family member may be able to give additional history.

History of Delivery and Newborn Period

If the patient is an infant or child, a more detailed history from the parent(s) is essential. Questions concerning the health of the mother during pregnancy, the number and character of pregnancies, the details of the delivery, the appearance and action of the newborn, and the development of the infant should be asked. Signs and symptoms compatible with severe forces of labor and delivery are an indication for considering OMT in the care of these patients. Following is a list of signs and symptoms that might indicate that a newborn has experienced severe forces during labor and delivery:

- Distortion of the cranium
- Excessive molding
- Ridging or overriding along any suture
- Difficulty in suckling or swallowing
- Vomiting
- Respiratory distress
- Bradycardia
- Tachycardia
- Abnormal crying
- Strabismus
- Nystagmus
- Spasticity or flaccidity of the limbs
- Opisthotonos
- Drowsiness
- Cyanosis
- Convulsions
- Fever
- Tremors

Abnormal habits such as lying with the head turned to one side only, head banging, or constant rubbing of the back of the head against the sheet are indicative of strains of the cranium.

Diagnosis by Observation

Look for symmetry or distortion of the osseous structure beneath the soft tissues. Observe the face and head: the shape and contours of the head and face show hereditary influences as well as the combined effect of the forces of labor on the bones. At birth, the sphenoid, temporals, and occiput are made up of several osseous parts with cartilage between parts and between bones to allow for compression and molding of the head during birth. Strains within a bone may occur and are called intraosseous strains.

The flexion type of skull is round in shape with a wide transverse and a shortened AP diameter, with the temporals in relative external rotation (flared laterally). In this type of skull, the frontals are wide and sloping upward, the cheek bones are wide, and an open mouth view of the maxillary region of the hard palate reveals it to be wide and with a low arch to the vault. All paired structures are in a position of relative external rotation.

The extension type of skull is long and narrow with temporals in relative internal rotation, frontals narrow with the brow appearing more vertical, orbits and face narrow, and maxillae (hard palate) narrow with a high arched vault. All paired structures are in a position of relative internal rotation.

Note the positioning of the bones. The position of the sphenoid bone influences the position of the peripheral bones of the anterior cranium, which includes the frontals and all bones of the face except the mandible. The position of the occiput influences the position of the bones of the posterior cranium (the parietals and temporals) and in turn influences the position of the mandible.

With torsion and SBR of the SBS, the facial structures tend to appear asymmetric as they assume a position of relative external rotation on the side of the high wing and a position of relative internal rotation on the side of the low wing. If the sphenoid is rotated on an AP axis, the eyes and orbits will appear unleveled, as will the cheekbones and the maxillae.

Note the relative positioning of landmarks. It is sometimes difficult to determine if the occiput has rotated on the AP axis because it is hidden by hair. As the occiput tilts on this axis, it carries the temporals with it. The temporal on the low side of the occiput is positioned toward relative external rotation, and the temporal on the high side of the occiput is positioned toward relative internal rotation. Therefore, the relative position of the ears gives an indication of the tilt of the occiput. Compare right and left ear lobes to see if they are level; note flaring of the ears. A temporal positioned toward external rotation tends to be more flared; a temporal positioned toward internal rotation tends to be more flat. By combining the findings of the anterior and posterior cranium, the observer is able to arrive at a tentative or working diagnosis of torsion or SBR of the SBS.

Viewing the midline of the face, noting the nose, mouth, and center of the chin, provides additional information. Nasal deviation may indicate the relative position of the maxillae and sphenoid or may indicate past trauma or fracture. The chin (mandible) tends to deviate to the side of the externally rotated temporal bone. Heredity also influences facial characteristics and is a significant consideration for establishing a prognosis.

Strains of the cranial base occur during birth or from trauma. If trauma is induced into a prior strain pattern, the findings of observation are not reliable for diagnosis.

Diagnosis by Palpation

To become an expert at the art of palpation for diagnosis and treatment requires repeated experience, patience, and perseverance. These guidelines help improve palpatory skill:

1. Use a light hand contact. If your contact is stronger than the force of the inherent motion, you interfere with the mechanism you are attempting to diagnose or treat. Do not interject yourself into the patient's PRM

2. Have a clear visualization of the structure(s) beneath your hands. This requires a detailed study of the anatomy and physiologic motion of each of the bones of the body, including the cranium and face. The design of the articulations between bones and their mechanical and physiologic relationship is a complex study, but it is essential to providing accurate diagnosis and successful treatment

3. Understand that the job of the physician is to assist the patient to obtain or maintain optimal health. The physician does not do the healing; healing comes from within the patient. With knowledge and experience, one learns to tune into and be guided by the PRM of the patient to facilitate this healing process, assisting the patient's own inherent healing capacity to release biomechanical impediments. The automatic processes that promote healing are much more intelligent and efficient in the management of the health of the individual than any external force or person can be

CLINICAL CONSIDERATIONS

Neonatal

OMT of infants and children can be a rewarding experience for the patient and the doctor, because children respond to treatment faster than adults and because treatment in this stage of life can prevent dysfunction later in life.

Compromised function of the PRM is a cumulative process beginning *in utero* or during birth, combined with the various traumatic incidents of growing up, as well as one or more traumatic events sustained as an adult. The physician must keep this in mind when taking the history.

Consideration of the trauma of the birth process deserves further explanation. The base of the skull is formed in cartilage and

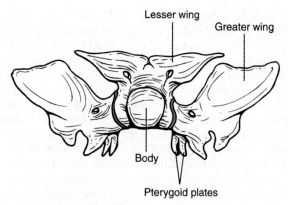

Figure 48-5 Sphenoid at birth in three parts. Cartilage intervenes between body-lesser wing unit and greater wing-pterygoid units. (From Sutherland WG, Wales AL. *Teachings in the Science of Osteopathy*. Portland, OR: Rudra Press, 1990, with permission.)

the vault is formed in membrane. At birth, the sphenoid is in three parts, the temporal is in three parts, and the occiput is in four parts, with cartilage intervening between the osseous elements (14). The frontal and mandible are in two parts and each maxilla is in two parts. This is nature's way of protecting the CNS and providing for compressibility of the head as it passes through the birth canal. The bones of the vault are osseous plates that overlap at the edges. The cartilaginous base tends to compress, bend, twist, or buckle depending on the amount and direction of compression and rotational forces of labor and birth. These various parts are vulnerable to misalignment; the brain, cranial nerves, and intracranial membranes are subject to possible injury or malfunction. One or more of the strain patterns of the SBS generally has its beginning during the birth process (Figs. 48.5 and 48.6).

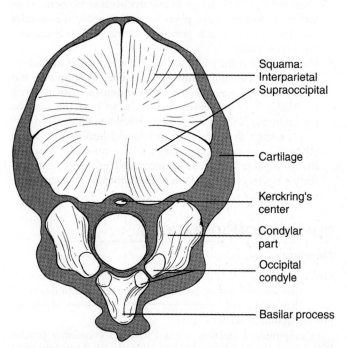

Figure 48-6 Occiput at birth in four parts within a cartilaginous matrix. Articular condyles receive contributions from both condylar and basilar parts of the occiput. (From Sutherland WG, Wales AL. *Teachings in the Science of Osteopathy*. Portland, OR: Rudra Press, 1990, with permission.)

The infant's first breath and subsequent crying with deep breathing, kicking, squirming, and suckling assist with decompression of the cranium, face, and pelvis (14). Decades of clinical experience have shown that if the activities of the neonate are not strong enough to open up the entire PRM to its optimal function, these neonates benefit from the assistance of an osteopathic physician trained in the cranial concept and in treatment procedures. Examination and treatment are best given during the first few days of life, at which time a great deal is accomplished by releasing the compressive forces of birth. If no treatment is provided, as time passes and growth progresses, the strains become more established. In time, the formative parts of the various bones of the base change from cartilage to osseous tissue. If overlapping of the osseous plates of the vault is allowed to remain, the plates grow together, forming a synostosis. Osteopathic physicians utilizing OCF have found that when synostosis pervades the vault, the osseous case cannot grow and expand at the same rate as the brain inside, and the brain function of that individual appears to be compromised. Expert treatment given early in the life of an individual can be one of the most important therapeutic measures in preventive medicine. Treatment given later is beneficial, but more can be accomplished in less time and with less effort and expense if treatment is given soon after the stresses and strains occur.

An example of disturbance of function directly related to the compressive forces of birth concerns the posterior part of the cranial base. There are four parts to the developing occiput:

- The basilar process
- Two condylar parts along the lateral sides of foramen magnum
- Squama extending from the posterior border of the foramen magnum to the lambdoid suture

The medulla oblongata rests on the basilar part, and the spinal cord extends through the space within the four parts. Cranial nerves IX, X, and XI and the jugular veins pass through the jugular foramina at the anterolateral border of each condylar part. Cranial nerve XII passes through the anterior condylar canals located within the condylar parts near the junction between the condylar parts and the basilar part. Compression with rotation of the posterior cranium during birth with distortion, displacement, and jamming of these four osseous plates and intervening cartilage is easily visualized (see Fig. 48.6). Knowing the function of these cranial nerves and their intimate relationships with the bones of the cranial base makes it easy to see how distortion of the cranial base could lead to symptoms such as vomiting, torticollis, or respiratory distress.

This abnormal mechanical stress on the brainstem, cranial nerves, and venous drainage is treated by gentle application of mild, sustained spreading of the formative parts of the base of the skull by a physician trained to apply OMT in this manner.

The relative position and motion of the temporal bones affect drainage from the middle ear through the pharyngotympanic tube; their somatic dysfunction is clinically capable of resulting in tinnitus, dizziness, and decreased auditory acuity. Treatment is aimed at releasing membranous strains of the cranial base, temporal bones, and upper cervical spine to help reestablish equal and synchronous motion to the temporals as well as the entire PRM. Consider these factors:

1. Without normal motion present, stasis of fluids and lack of oxygen provide an ideal medium for proliferation of microorganisms
2. When the inherent motion throughout the cranium and face is optimal, the movement of fluids and mucus is enhanced (a provision of nature for emptying the ethmoid, sphenoid, and maxillary sinuses)

3. The autonomic nerve supply to the nasal mucosa by way of the sphenopalatine ganglion is vulnerable to impingement by malaligned adjacent boney structures
4. Middle ear infections, sinusitis, pharyngitis, and other acute inflammatory processes are often associated with altered cranial functions (111)

Trauma

Trauma is by far the major cause of disruption and malfunction of the PRM. The force of trauma is extreme in vehicular accidents. The force from a fall is transmitted from the feet or ischial tuberosities upward through the body into the base of the skull. The vector of force established through the body or head is palpable (112,113) and is an important diagnostic sign. The direction of motion of the CSF and CNS is disrupted, and the function of the PRM is mildly to severely impaired, depending on the severity of the trauma and the response of the patient.

Trauma to the PRM can occur from mild, sustained force such as wearing a spring type of headset or from orthodontic appliances on the teeth (114). Also, wearing a tight hat or swim cap will augment or create or alter existing patterns. Trauma occurs in various degrees and in innumerable forms.

The PRM functions as a unit; trauma to one area affects the entire RTM. The PRM does its best to continue to function, but the quality of that function decreases with the passage of time and additional trauma. The rate and amplitude of the PRM is a most valuable diagnostic and prognostic indicator of the severity of the compromise and response to treatment (9). A slow rate and a low amplitude are dependable indicators of a longstanding and/or overwhelming problem during which the patient's vitality has been depleted, indicating more treatment over a longer period of time will be required (9). The reciprocal is also true. In the course of treatment, improvement is associated with a rate and amplitude increase toward a more normal pattern.

CLINICAL RESEARCH

The foregoing discussion of the types of conditions that benefit from application of OCF and the principles of treatment is based on the consensus of teachers of OCF with many years of successful clinical practice.

The development of clinical research on OCF has grown as resources for such research have become more available, but there has always been a scientific, systematic observational discipline applied by those who used OCF in the medical practice. Over the years, there have been a number of reports of the clinical applications of OCF. Some of the earliest appeared in the OCF text by Magoun (6, p. 112) with charts done by G. A. Laughlin, D.O., which showed an apparently reduced sweat production before and after application of the technique known as the compression of the fourth ventricle (CV_4). This appeared to reflect a decrease in sympathetic nervous system activity, which has also been demonstrated in more recent research (115). Also in the Magoun text are illustrations documenting, in a group of five patients, substantial lowering of blood sugar and white blood cell counts before and after application of the CV_4 (6, p. 113).

The Magoun text devotes a chapter to the "Practical Application of the Cranial Concept," and reports on a number of conditions in which application of OCF techniques has proven beneficial for the individuals involved. A number of these applications of OCF are amplified in other publications (116–118).

It is significant to note that OCF treatment is like any other modality of OMT in the hands of a capable osteopathic physician.

It is the specific attention to the anatomy of the particular part of the body being manipulated that facilitates the OMT and enhances the probability of benefit. Furthermore, it is the knowledge of anatomy and especially neuroanatomy in the cranial area that provides the basis for a strong rationale for how OCF might be beneficial. This point is exceedingly well illustrated in a series of articles by Magoun on the theme of entrapment neuropathy in the cranium (111,119,120). That is, if cranial bone motion exists and OCF maneuvers can affect cranial bone and intracranial structures such as cranial nerves, then there may be great utility in applying such technique in clinical practice.

From a philosophy of science perspective, appropriate application of OCF based on systematic observation of anatomic relationships palpated by the osteopathic physician and correlated with changes in the patient's symptoms is indeed scientific procedure. It remains for the osteopathic medical profession to develop documentation procedures that will facilitate collection of this type of data from many physicians utilizing OCF and thereby obtain large-scale population data appropriate for analysis. In the meantime, those who utilize OCF in clinical practice are following a tried and true scientific methodology in the application of OCF: practice based on proof of benefit to patients as reported by many clinicians on many patients. This is the principle of appeal to authority and precedence of success by practice. Gradually, empirical clinical practice studies are being carried out and published. Many of the clinical observations made at the time of Sutherland and the early cranial osteopaths have begun to receive scientific support.

Otitis Media

The location of the eustachian tube within the temporal bone and the possible derangement of the temporal bone during a difficult labor and delivery comprise the anatomy and life circumstance that have been described as the basis for the application of OCF to the treatment of otitis media. The clinical success reported by OCF clinicians has been validated by positive results in several studies and has resulted in plans for a multisite clinical trial (121–123). These studies showed improvement in health as measured by fewer ear tubes, improved tympanography assessment, and generally reduced need for antibiotics in children suffering from recurrent ear infections (otitis media).

Pregnancy, Labor, and Delivery

The prenatal application of OMT has been a staple of the osteopathic medical profession since its inception (124). Clinical research on the application of OMT in prenatal care has a long history too. As early as 1911, studies on 100 of women who received prenatal OMT were published, and benefits such as shorter durations of labor and fewer complications were reported (125). In a study where the application of OCF was not the only OMT modality applied in prenatal care, but was included in OMT delivered to virtually every patient, the results were statistically significant ($N = 321$ patients) for fewer preterm deliveries and fewer cases of meconium-stained amniotic fluid (126).

A promising pilot study that awaits a larger follow-up was done by Gitlin and Wolf (127) on women who were overdue to deliver and had not yet perceived uterine contractions. Eight women were treated using only the CV_4. Two were eliminated due to disruption during the posttreatment monitoring, while the other six all began uterine contractions within 34 minutes with an average of 17.5 minutes. The theory underlying the use of the CV_4 is that this maneuver "helps nature take its course." It is probably incorrect to be concerned about the use of the CV_4 in pregnant women out of fear of inducing contraction, as the women in this study were "over due" and the OCF only facilitated a normal gestational phase.

Pediatric Applications

Besides the previously mentioned research on otitis media, the general concern for the effects of a difficult labor and delivery involves many unfortunate outcome possibilities. Frymann (128) evaluated the cranial bone mechanics of 1,250 newborns and found that 88% had identifiable malalignment in the form of cranial bone strain patterns. Frymann (129) has gone on to present data indicating benefit of OCF in the treatment of children with learning problems, children with neurological deficits (130), and seizure disorders (131).

Inspired by Frymann's work, research was done in Russia by Lassovetskaia (132) on children with language and learning problems. In this study, 96 children undergoing neuropsychological tutoring in a large school program due to delayed academic performance were selected and compared to the performance of the rest of the children before and after receiving OCF for 6 to 12 weeks. The children who received the OCF were significantly higher in virtually all categories of academic performance compared to the comparable population of children who did not receive OCF.

As with all OMT, OCF is described as an effective means to correct anatomic malalignment and restore optimal physiologic function by improving the anatomic structures associated with those functions. For example, in the treatment of colic, the commonly found impingement of the tenth cranial nerve (which coordinates the peristaltic wave action of the gastrointestinal tract) as it passes through the jugular foramen, caused by compression of the nerve during the birth process, between the occipital and temporal (mastoid area) bones, can be relieved by gentle OCF to decompress and relieve the obstructed flow of coordinated nerve supply to its intended destination. In fact, a recent pilot study found that the OCF applied to infants with colic did significantly reduce the symptoms of colic (134). Obstructive sleep apnea in infants may also be reduced by osteopathic treatment employing OCF (135). Mobility in children with cerebral palsy has been improved with OMT including OCF (136).

Dental Applications

Because the teeth are cranial bones that move within their sockets, which are in turn housed in cranial bones, application of OCF for treatment of dental conditions can and has been used successfully in practice. In a series of articles, Magoun (137–139) gives case studies and specific technique for OCF treatment of individuals whose cranial malalignment involves dentition. Lay carried on this work on dental applications and described more case studies utilizing OCF with an emphasis on temporomandibular joint dysfunction (114). With the publication of these articles, many dentists have been attracted to study and even apply OCF in their practices. There is even a special membership section within The Cranial Academy for dentists.

Empirical research was done by Baker (140) who demonstrated measurable changes in the dental arch of a patient receiving OCF. Serially measured models of maxillary teeth over six months showed overall lateral dimensional changes between permanent second molars of 0.0276 of an inch. It is common in the practice of orthodontics today to move the maxillary arch this much and more, up to 2 mm by dental appliances, but in the case reported by Baker, the changes were brought about by OCF alone.

It is worthy of note that musculoskeletal deformities, specifically scoliosis and pronounced kyphosis dorsalis (Scheuermann disease), have now been associated with malocclusion (141). This finding substantiates emphasis on early childhood treatment and prevention championed by practitioners of OCF.

Effects of OCF on Vascular and Autonomic Nervous System Functions

A commonly applied OCF technique called the "venous sinus technique" has been reported by many who practice OCF to be successful in the relief of headache and sinus congestion symptoms. A study by Huard (142) suggests that the efficacy of this technique may be in the restoration of optimal intracranial vascular flow. Huard applied the venous sinus technique to 39 subjects, with 39 others receiving light touch only, and another group of 39 subjects received no touch at all. The outcome measure was a radiology procedure called the encephalogram, which utilizes ultrasound technology to record blood flow. Huard's results showed that the subjects receiving the OCF venous sinus technique had demonstrably improved blood flow in the area of the cranial base.

A study by Cutler et al. (115) showed statistically significant effects of application of the CV_4 on sleep latency and the reduction of sympathetic nerve activity. In a controlled environment, healthy subjects who received the CV_4 treatment went to sleep faster than subjects who received only a light touch control protocol or no touch at all. Sympathetic nerve activity, measured at the peroneal nerve in the popliteal fossa using standard microneurographic technique, was also significantly reduced in the CV_4 group compared to control or no treat groups.

Further evidence of the impact of OCF on physiological function is the work on healthy humans that showed a statistically significant improvement in heart rate variability. In this study, Giles et al. (143,144) used soft tissue manipulation to the cervical spine with emphasis on the occipitoatlantal decompression maneuver, a commonly OCF technique. With an $N = 24$ in a crossover design, heart rate variability was best when the OCF was applied compared with sham and time control conditions. Using a similar design, Henley et al. (145) also found alterations in heart rate variability as a result of OMT that utilized several OCF maneuvers. A study done in Israel evaluated the impact of cranial manipulation on urinary tract function and quality of life in outpatients with multiple sclerosis (146). Results showed statistically significant reductions in postvoiding residual volume, urinary frequency, urinary urgency, and improvement in quality of life. The nature of OCF suggests impact on parasympathetic centers in the lower brain stem and in the sacral spinal cord may be the likely mechanism of action in this study.

Clinical Research—Summary

OCF clinical research compares favorably with the amount of clinical research done on the other commonly used OMT modalities. From a technical perspective, the application of OCF takes longer than other OMT modalities and is often not applied due to time restraints. Critics of OCF cite lack of clinical evidence for benefits thereof and raise the question of risk-benefit ratio. However, there has been only one report of an adverse events from the application of OCF, and the teaching and practice of OCF have been modified to take into account factors that may cause adverse events (147). On the other hand, improvement reported in the reviewed clinical articles on OCF is certainly suggestive, if not compelling, evidence of benefit for OCF.

PRINCIPLES OF TREATMENT

The aim of treatment with OCF, as with any osteopathic procedure, is to normalize structure and function. The optimal function of the PRM affects not only the CNS but also every cell and tissue in the body. Regardless of which method or procedure a physician elects to use, this constant cyclic motion is at work behind the scenes every minute of every hour of every day of every year of an individual's life.

Goals of Treatment

The goals of treatment include:

- Normalizing nerve function, including all cranial and spinal nerves as well as the autonomic nervous system
- Counteracting stress-producing factors by normalizing function of the cerebrum, thalamus, hypothalamus, and pituitary body
- Eliminating circulatory stasis by normalizing arterial, venous, and lymphatic channels
- Normalizing CSF fluctuation
- Releasing membranous tension
- Correcting or resolving cranial articular strains
- Modifying gross structural patterns

Some hindrances to treatment are myofascial strains from below the cranium or from the sacrum, local or general infections, nutritional deficiencies, and organic poisons (6). For optimal management of the patient's health problems, the physician must address nonstructural hindrances to health, in addition to applying OMT. To use the power or potency of the inherent activity of the PRM within the patient to assist with the release of strains (somatic dysfunctions), it is necessary to understand balanced ligamentous tension and balanced membranous tension. Balanced ligamentous tension is used in treating any articulation supported and protected by ligaments. Balanced membranous tension refers to the dura mater (RTM) and is used to treat the articulations of the cranium, face, and sacrum.

The point of balanced membranous tension is defined as that point in the range of motion of an articulation where the membranes are poised between the normal tension present throughout the free range of motion and the increased tension preceding the strain or fixation that occurs as a joint is carried beyond its normal physiologic range (6). Thus, it is the most neutral position possible under the influence of all the factors responsible for the existing pattern. That is, all attendant tensions having been reduced to the absolute minimum.

This point is unique for each strain that occurs. It is the point at which the inherent force can move through the involved tissues at its maximum efficiency. The operator seeks to position the bones making up the articulation at the point of balanced membranous tension by keen, sensitive, knowledgeable palpation. Dr. Sutherland expressed this as palpating with seeing, feeling, thinking, knowing fingers.

Figure 48.7 illustrates arriving at the point of balanced membranous tension by positioning the components. The squares indicate two bones making up an articulation, and the arrows represent the directions the operator employs for positioning (6).

Figure 48.7A illustrates indirect action or exaggeration. This procedure is commonly employed from the age of 5 through adulthood. It is not used in acute trauma to the head when exaggeration of misalignment may produce or increase intracranial hemorrhage. To employ this method, increase the abnormal relationship at the joint by moving the articulation slightly further in the direction of malalignment.

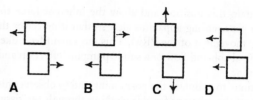

Figure 48-7 Methods for arriving at the point of balanced membranous tension. **A.** Indirect action (exaggeration). **B.** Direct action. **C.** Disengagement. **D.** Opposite physiologic motion. (From Magoun HI. *Osteopathy in the Cranial Field*, 2nd Ed. Kirksville, MO: Journal Printing Company, 1966, with permission.)

Figure 48.7B illustrates direct action. This treatment method is employed when exaggeration is not desirable, as in acute trauma and in young children in whom the sutural pattern has not yet developed. This treatment is also used when there are overriding sutures. The components are gently guided back toward their normal position.

Figure 48.7C illustrates disengagement. This treatment method is used when force or excessive membranous tension impacts the osseous components. Disengagement technique merely separates the opposing surfaces within the anatomic and physiologic limits of permitted motion.

Figure 48.7D illustrates opposite physiologic motion. This method is seldom used, but when needed it is employed to release a strain when a traumatic force has severely violated the physiologic pattern. One component is influenced by direct action; the other is influenced by indirect action.

The physician selects the method of choice according to the patient's age and history, as well as by palpatory diagnosis.

Respiratory cooperation may be used to enhance the effort of inherent motion. The patient is asked to hold their breath in full inhalation or exhalation after the physician has positioned the articulation at balanced ligamentous or membranous tension. Holding the breath at full inhalation is more commonly used, but if the articulation is held toward extension or internal rotation, holding the breath at full exhalation is more effective.

Example 1

An example would be a case in which the patient reports a history of a fall on their rear end, possibly from a slip on a banana peel.

Diagnosis

Somatic dysfunction of the lumbosacral junction (L5-S1 compression).

Treatment

Treatment is indirect method, using balanced ligamentous tension, exaggeration, and inherent force.

Procedure

1. Position the patient supine
2. Sit at the side of the table so that the operator's dominant hand (assume right hand) can be placed under the patient's sacrum
3. Place the right hand under the sacrum so that the patient's coccyx rests between the operator's thenar and hypothenar eminences. The finger tips should be placed at the sacral base with the 3rd and 4th digits just below L5
4. Place the left hand perpendicular to the right hand with the hypothenar eminence barely touching right hand fingers and in firm comfortable palpatory contact with L5

5. Maintain this position and allow the inherent force to work. Keep your sensing apparatus alert so that it perceives the slow cyclic movement of the PRM. This movement feels like a longitudinal ebb and flow or a subtle pumping effect up and down the spine

6. Continue to maintain the positioning and to observe this cyclic motion; the inherent force is working through the tissues that are maintaining the somatic dysfunction. As they accomplish their task for this articulation at this time, the amplitude of the inherent rhythm lessens and the pumping decreases, and the tissues beneath your palpating fingers seem to soften or melt. Once the tissues have softened, the flexion and extension motion of the sacrum begins to increase. As flexion and extension motion of the sacrum increases toward normal, it may be necessary to gently pull caudad on the sacrum before full motion is restored

7. At this time, cease to hold the articulation in the treatment position. Gently recheck the motion of the articulation to ascertain the therapeutic response. Physiologic motion is restored to varying degrees

A strain of the sacral base can be treated using the inherent forces and positioning for balanced membranous tension of the RTMs. This technique is applicable for an uncomplicated strain of the sacral base. If a strain of the sacral base is complicated by additional traumatic strains such as a compression in either sacroiliac (SI) joint, the technique as described will probably not be successful.

If SI joint compression is present, treatment position will vary slightly. If, for example, the patient's left SI joint is compressed, the doctor's left hand will be under the sacrum. This hand maintains the same position as for treatment of sacral base compression. However, the operator' other hand (in this case the right hand) would be placed under the ilium, perpendicular to the fingers of the left hand. The fingertips of the right hand would be at the medial border of the left ilium and would barely touch the 5th digit and hypothenar eminence of the left hand. As in step 6, maintain this position while observing the cyclic motion of the PRM. In this case, rather than providing caudad traction, it may be necessary to provide gentle lateral traction until normal balance between the motion of the sacrum and the motion of the ilium is restored.

Example 2
Another case is a patient who has been struck on the side of the head, possibly by a baseball bat or fist.

Diagnosis
Somatic dysfunction of the sphenobasilar symphysis is SBR right (SBS is SBR_R).

The sphenoid and occiput have rotated on an AP axis so that the right side of the cranium is relatively inferior (caudad) and the left side is relatively superior (cephalad). Concomitant with that position, the greater sphenoid wing and the lateral angle of the occiput on the right side are slightly spread and the greater sphenoid wing and the lateral angle of the left occiput are slightly approximated.

Treatment
Treatment is indirect method, balanced membranous tension, with exaggeration and inherent forces to balance the RTM.

Procedure
1. Position the patient supine
2. Sit at the head of the table

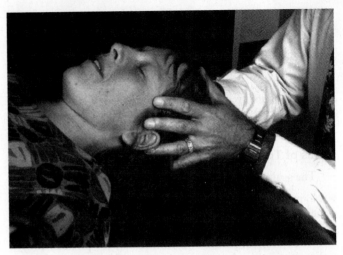

Figure 48-8 "Vault hold" for contact of the cranium. (From Hruby R. *Craniosacral Osteopathic Technique: A Manual.* 2nd Ed. Okemos, MI: The Institute for Osteopathic Studies, 1996:33l, with permission.)

3. Place your hands on the lateral sides of the patient's head with the index fingers contacting the greater wings of the sphenoid and the little fingers contacting the lateral angles of the occiput (vault contact) (Fig. 48.8)

4. Gently palpate the rhythmic activity of the patient's PRM and RTM

5. The right hand slowly moves slightly caudad with index and fifth fingers spreading slightly, while the left hand moves slightly cephalad as the fingers approximate slightly. This positioning is slight and must be accurate, being guided by the ease of tension in the membranes within the cranium. With the ease of membranous tension, the inherent forces begin to manifest with increased vigor. The amplitude of the PRM automatically increases

6. Maintain the positioning and carefully and continuously observe the increased activity of the inherent forces at work within the patient's mechanism. As the inherent forces work through the membranous strain, they gradually cease the increased activity and become quiet. This cessation of the inherent rhythm is called a still point (14)

7. After the still point occurs, cease to maintain the positioning of the bones and membranes and continue to observe the fluctuant activity by light palpation. The quiet period passes, the rhythmic fluctuation resumes, increasing slowly and steadily in amplitude until it has returned to a more normal flexion-extension of the SBS

8. Gently remove your hands

There is no substitute for thorough training and practice in the development of skill in OMT based on the principles of OCF/CO. Well-known and typically utilized treatment procedures based on the principles of OCF/CO are the compression of the fourth ventricle (CV_4) and the V-spread procedures.

The CV_4 (Fig. 48.9 A,B) is typically used to stimulate the body's inherent therapeutic capacity to deal with whatever dysfunction is present. By inducing extension (or internal rotation) of the PRM, the inherent capacity for self-regulation and healing is facilitated by a stimulation of CSF flow.

The technique is as follows:

1. Operator at head of table
2. Patient supine

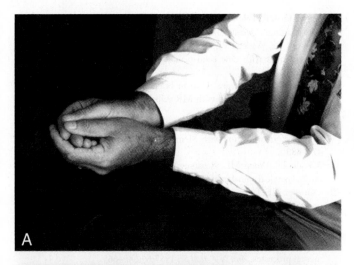

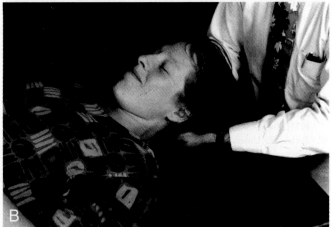

Figure 48-9 Compression of fourth ventricle (CV₄). **A.** Hand position for CV₄ technique. **B.** CV₄ technique. (From Hruby R. *Craniosacral Osteopathic Technique: A Manual,* 2nd Ed. Okemos, MI: The Institute for Osteopathic Studies, 1996, with permission.)

3. With both hands palm up, place one hand in the palm of the other so that the thenar eminences lie parallel to one another. Then slip the hands under the head, permitting the lateral angles of the occiput medial to the occipitomastoid suture to rest on the thenar eminences. The thenar eminences provide a cushion for the occiput that should be comfortable for the patient and operator. The fingers are free and not pressing on the neck. The weight of the head rests on the thenar eminences and thereby gently compresses the lateral angles

4. Become aware of the cyclic motion of the occiput. Follow it toward extension (i.e., as the hands rock gently toward the operator). Discourage flexion (hands moving away). The amplitude of the motion will get progressively smaller until the still point is reached. The still point may be difficult to detect because it passes so swiftly. However, it is followed by a sense of softening and warmth in the occiput and the gentle rocking motion of flexion and extension that should be more easily detectable. At the same time, thoracic respiration should become primarily diaphragmatic and approximate the same cycle as the PRM

5. Observe the cranial activity to be sure that it remains quiet and then very gently remove your hands and put the patient's head on the table. Figure 48.9 demonstrates the CV₄ via the occiput, but it is also possible to accomplish a CV₄ via the temporals, parietals, and sacrum

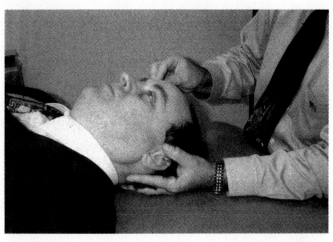

Figure 48-10 V-spread of occipitomastoid suture. (From Hruby R. *Craniosacral Technique: A Manual.* 2nd Ed. Okemos, MI: The Institute for Osteopathic Studies, 1996, with permission.)

The V-spread (Fig. 48.10) is a very simple, safe technique for releasing any peripheral suture such as frontonasal, nasomaxillary, or occipitomastoid. The technique is as follows:

1. Place the index and middle fingers of the ipsilateral hand on either side of the suture. For a linear suture like the occipitomastoid, use the palmar surface of the length of two fingers. For a small suture like the frontonasal, use the fingertips

2. Place the palm of the other hand on the patient's head at the other end of the longest diameter of the head from the suture (e.g., for the left occipitomastoid), place the hand on the right frontal only. You will soon perceive a gentle impulse coming into the palm of this hand. Now cluster the fingers at the site of that impulse. You have thereby localized the optimum place from which to direct a palpatory sensation of a "fluid wave" to the restricted suture. As long as the suture is restricted, the fluid sensation will "bounce" back, but as soon as it releases, you will feel a gentle, easy motion between your hands

Treatment procedures of the cranium should be used only by physicians experienced with palpation of the subtle activity of the PRM. Guidance by a physician experienced with the function of the PRM and the inherent forces is essential to learning this technique.

SUMMARY

Much research remains to be done in order to demonstrate the exact mechanisms involved in craniosacral dysfunction and recovery. However, more than 55 years of clinical experience has indicated that the use of OCF/CO has given relief to many patients in whom no other treatment was effective.

REFERENCES

1. Ward RC, ed. *Foundations for Osteopathic Medicine.* 2 Ed. Baltimore, MD: Lippincott Williams & Wilkins, 2003:378–380.
2. Lancaster DG, Crow WT. Osteopathic manipulative treatment of a 26-year-old woman with Bell's palsy. *J Am Osteopath Assoc* 2006;106:285–289.
3. Sutherland AS. *With Thinking Fingers.* Indianapolis, IN: Cranial Academy. Originally published by Journal Printing Company, Kirksville, MO: 1962:12–13.
4. Northup GW, ed. *Osteopathic Research: Growth and Development.* Chicago, IL: American Osteopathic Association, 1987:40.

5. DiGiovanna EL. *An Encyclopedia of Osteopathy.* Indianapolis, IN: American Academy of Osteopathy, 2001:100.

6. Magoun HI. *Osteopathy in the Cranial Field.* 2 Ed. Kirksville, MO: Journal Publishing Company, 1966.

7. Lippincott RC. Cranial osteopathy. *Amer Acad Osteopath Yearb* 1947:103–109.

8. Lippincott HA. The osteopathic technique of Wm. G. Sutherland, D.O. *Amer Acad Osteopath Yearb* 1949:1–41.

9. Becker RE. In: Brooks RE, ed. *Life in Motion.* Portland, OR: Stillness Press, 1997.

10. Becker RE. In: Brooks RE, ed. *The Stillness of Life.* Portland, OR: Stillness Press, 2000.

11. Fulford RC. *Touch of Life.* New York, NY: Pocket Books, 1996.

12. Fulford RC. In: Cisler TA, ed. *Are We On the Path? The Collected Works of Robert C. Fulford, DO, FCA.* Indianapolis, IN: The Cranial Academy, 2004.

13. Comeaux Z. *Robert Fulford, DO and the Philosopher Physician.* Seattle, WA: Eastland Press, 2002.

14. Sutherland WG. In: Wales AE, ed. *Teachings in the Science of Osteopathy.* Cambridge, MA: Rudra Press, 1990.

15. Arbuckle BE. *The Selected Writings of Beryl E. Arbuckle, D.O., FACOP.* Indianapolis, IN: American Academy of Osteopathy, 1994.

16. http://www.osteopathiccenter.org/ Accessed January 21, 2008.

17. King HH, ed. *The collected papers of Viola M Frymann, DO: Legacy of Osteopathy to Children.* Indianapolis, IN: American Academy of Osteopathy, 1998.

18. King HH, ed. *Proceedings of international research conference: Osteopathy in Pediatrics at the Osteopathic Center for Children in San Diego, CA 2002.* Indianapolis, IN: American Academy of Osteopathy, 2005.

19. Lay EM. Osteopathy in the cranial field. In: Ward RC, ed. *Foundations for Osteopathic Medicine.* Baltimore, MD: Lippincott Williams & Wilkins, 1997.

20. DiGiovanna EI, Schiowitz S, Dowling DJ. *An Osteopathic Approach to Diagnosis and Treatment.* 3 Ed. Baltimore, MD: Lippincott Williams & Wilkins, 2005.

21. Greenman PE. *Principles of Manual Medicine.* 3 Ed. Baltimore, MD: Lippincott Williams & Wilkins, 2003.

22. Kuchera ML, Kuchera WA. *Osteopathic Considerations in Systemic Dysfunction.* 2 Ed. Rev. Columbus, OH: Greyden Press, 1994.

23. Heisey SR, Adams T. Effects of cranial bone mobility on cranial compliance. In: *Thirty-sixth Annual AOA Research Conference Abstracts, 1992,* part 2; 1992. Also in: *J Am Osteopath Assoc* 1992;92(9):1284.

24. Heisey SR, Adams T, Smith MC, et al. The role of cranial suture compliance in defining intracranial pressure. In: *Thirty-seventh Annual AOA Research Conference Abstracts, 1993,* part 2; 1993. Also in: *J Am Osteopath Assoc.* 1993;93(9):951.

25. Norton JM, Sibley G, Broder-Oldack RE. Quantification of the cranial rhythmic impulse in human subjects. In: *Thirty-sixth Annual AOA Research Conference Abstracts, 1992,* part 2; 1992. Also in: *J Am Osteopath Assoc.* 1992;92(9):1285.

26. Sibley G, Broder-Oldach RE, Norton JM. Inter-examiner agreement in the characterization of the cranial rhythmic impulse. In: *Thirty-sixth Annual AOA Research Conference Abstracts, 1992,* part 2, 1992. Also in: *J Am Osteopath Assoc.* 1992;92(9):1285.

27. http://www.aacom.org/people/councils/Documents/OsteopathicTerminologyGlossary.pdf accessed February 10, 2008.

28. Jealous J. *Emergence of Originality.* 2 Ed. Farmington, ME: Biodynamic/Sargent Publishing, 2001.

29. Blechschmidt E. *Beginnings of Human Life.* Berlin, Germany: Springer-Verlag, 1977.

30. Blechschmidt E, Gasser RF. *Biokinetics and Biodynamics of Human Differentiation.* Springfield, IL: Charles Thomas Publishing, 1978.

31. *Dorland's Illustrated Medical Dictionary.* 26 Ed. Philadelphia, PA: WB Saunders, 1981.

32. Karki J. *Signaling Conditioning Piezoelectric Sensors.* Dallas, TX: Texas Instruments Application Report SLOA033A, September 2000.

33. Becker RE. Craniosacral trauma in the adult. *Osteopath Ann* 1976;4:43–59.

34. Grietz D, Wirestam R, Franck A, et al. Pulsatile brain movement and associated hydrodynamics studied by magnetic resonance phase imaging: the Monro-Kellie doctrine revisited. *Neuroradiology* 1992;34:370–380.

35. Enzmann DR, Pelc NJ. Brain motion: measurement with phase-contrast MR imaging. *Radiology* 1992;185:653–660.

36. Poncelet BP, Wedeen VJ, Weiskoff RM, et al. Brain parenchyma motion: measurement with cine echo-planar MR imaging. *Radiology* 1992;185:645–651.

37. Feinberg DA, Mark AS. Human brain motion and cerebrospinal fluid circulation demonstrated with MR velocity imaging. *Radiology* 1987;163:793–799.

38. Maier SE, Hardy CJ, Jolesz FA. Brain and cerebrospinal fluid motion: real-time quantification with M-mode MR imaging. *Radiology* 1994;193:477–483.

39. Mikulis DJ, Wood ML, Zerdoner OAM, et al. Oscillatory motion of the normal cervical spinal cord. *Radiology* 1994;192:117–121.

40. Lumsden CE, Pomerat CM. Normal oligodendrocytes in cell tissue: a preliminary report on the pulsatile glial cells in tissue cultures from the corpus callosum of the normal rat brain. *Exp Cell Res* 1951;2:103–114.

41. Canti RG, Bland JO, Russell DS. *Assoc Res Nerv Men Dis* 1935;16:1–5.

42. Wolley DW, Shaw EN. Evidence for the participation of serotonin in mental processes. *Ann N Y Acad Sci* 1957;66:649–665.

43. Hyden H. Satellite cells in the central nervous system. *Sci Am* 1961;205:62.

44. Vern BA, Leheta BJ, Juel VC, et al. Slow oscillations of cytochrome oxidase redox state and blood volume in unanesthetized cat and rabbit cortex: interhemisheric synchrony. *Adv Exp Med Bio* 1998;454:561–570.

45. Dani JW, Chernjavsky A, Smith SJ. Neuronal activity triggers calcium waves in hippocampus astrocyte networks. *Neuron* 1992;8:429–440.

46. DuBolay GH, O'Connell J, Currie J, et al. Further investigations on pulsatile movements in the cerebrospinal fluid pathways. *Acta Radiol Diagn* 1971;13:496–523.

47. Becher E. Untersuchen über die Dynamic der "Cerebospinalis." *Mitt Grenzgeb Med Chir.* 1922;35:329.

48. O'Connell JAE. Vascular factor in intracranial pressure and maintenance of cerebro-spinal fluid circulation. *Brain* 1943;66:204–228.

49. Levy LM, DiChiro GD, McCollough DC, et al. Fixed spinal cord: Diagnosis with MR imaging. *Radiology* 1988;169:773–778.

50. Walter BA, Valera VA, Takahashi S, et al. The olfactory route for cerebrospinal fluid drainage into the peripheral lymphatic system. *Neuropathol Appl Neurobiol* 2006;32:388–396.

51. Norton JA. Challenge to the concept of craniosacral interaction. *Amer Acad Osteopath J* 1996;6(4):15–21.

52. Chaitow L. *Cranial Manipulation Theory and Practice: Osseous and Soft Tissue Approaches.* 2 Ed. London: Elsevier Churchill Livingston, 2005.

53. Kostopoulos DC, Keramidas G. Changes in elongation of falx cerebri during craniosacral therapy techniques applied on the skull of an embalmed cadaver. *J Craniomand Pract* 1992;10:9–12.

54. Zhu Q, Dougherty L, Margulies SS. In vivo measurement of human brain displacement. Paper presented at June 2003 Summer Bioengineering Conference, Key Biscayne, FL.

55. Zanakis MF, Dimeo J, Madoma S, et al. Objective measurement of the CRI with manipulation and palpation of the sacrum [abstract]. *J Am Osteopath Assoc* 1996;96(9):55.

56. Nelson KE, Sergueef N, Glonek T. Recording the rate of the cranial rhythmic impulse. *J Amer Osteopath Assoc* 2006;106(6):337–341.

57. Ferre JC, Barbin JY. The osteopathic cranial concept: Fact or fiction. *Surg Radiol Anat* 1991;13:165–170.

58. Hartman SE, Norton JM. Interexaminer reliability and cranial osteopathy. *Sci Rev Altern Med* 2002;6:23–34.

59. Bolk L. On the premature obliteration of sutures in the human skull. *Am J Anat* 1915;17:495–523.

60. Melsen B. Time and mode of closure of the spheno-occipital synchondrosis determined on human autopsy material. *Acta Anat* 1972;83:112–118.

61. Perizonius WRK. Closing and non-closing sutures in 256 crania of known age and sex from Amsterdam (A.D. 1883–1909). *J Hum Evol* 1984;13:201–216.

62. Cohen MM Jr. Sutural biology and the correlates of craniosynostosis. *Am J Med Genet* 1993;47:581–616.

63. Sahni D, Jit I, Neelam, et al. Time of fusion of the basisphenoid with the basilar part of the occipital bone in northwest Indian subjects. *Forensic Sci Int* 1998;98:41–45.

64. Todd TW, Lyon DW. Endocranial suture closure, its progress and age relationship. I. Adult males of white stock. *Am J Phys Anthrop* 1924;7:325–384. II. *Am J Phys Anthrop* 1925;8:23–45.

65. Todd TW, Lyon DW. Endocranial suture closure, its progress and age relationship. III Endocranial closure in adult males of negro stock. *Am J Phys Anthrop* 1925;8:47–71. IV *Am J Phys Anthrop* 1925;8:149–68.

66. Dart P. An overview of research supporting the fundamental concepts of osteopathy in the cranial field. Unpublished manuscript, data and commentary given at the Cranial Academy Conference in Palm Springs, CA, June 20, 2000.

67. Singer R. Estimation of age from cranial suture closure: Report on its unreliability. *J Forensic Med* 1953;1:52–59.

68. Pritchard JJ, Scott JH, Girgis FG. The structure and development of cranial and facial sutures. *J Anat* 1956;90:73–86.

69. Sabini RC, Elkowitz DE. Significant differences in patency among cranial sutures. *J Am Osteopath Assoc* 2006;106:600–604.

70. Retzlaff EW, Upledger JE, Mitchell FL Jr, et al. Aging of cranial sutures in humans [abstract]. *Anat Rec* 1979;193:663.

71. Retzlaff EW, Mitchell FL Jr, Upledger JE, et al. Neurovascular mechanisms in cranial sutures [abstract]. *J Am Osteopath Assoc* 1980;80:218–219.

72. Retzlaff EW, Jones L, Mitchell FL Jr, et al. Possible autonomic innervation of cranial sutures of primates and other animals [abstract]. *Brain Res* 1973;58:470–477.

73. Michael DK, Retzlaff EW. A preliminary study of cranial bone movement in the squirrel monkey. *J Am Osteopath Assoc.* 1975;74:866–869.

74. Heisey SR, Adams T. Role of cranial bone mobility in cranial compliance. *Neurosurgery* 1993;33(5):869–876.

75. Heisey SR, Adams T. A two compartment model for cranial compliance. *J Am Osteopath Assoc* 1995;95:547.

76. Adams T, Heisey RS, Smith MC, et al. Parietal bone mobility in the anesthetized cat. *J Am Osteopath Assoc* 1992;92(5):599–622.

77. Jaslow CR. Mechanical properties of cranial sutures. *J Biomechanics* 1990;23(4):313–321.

78. Frymann VM. A study of the rhythmic motions of the living cranium. *J Am Osteopath Assoc* 1971;70:1–18.

79. Heifitz MD, Weiss M. Detection of skull expansion with increased intracranial pressure. *J Neurosurg* 1981;55:811–812.

80. Oleski SL, Smith GH, Crow WT. Radiographic evidence of cranial bone mobility. *J Craniomandib Pract* 2002;20(1):34–38.

81. Moskalenko YE, Cooper H, Crow H, et al. Variation in blood volume and oxygen availability in the human brain. *Nature* 1964;202(4926):59–161.

82. Moskalenko YE, Weinstein GB, Demchenko IT, et al. *Biophysical aspects of cerebral circulation.* Oxford: Pergamon Press; 1980.

83. Moskalenko YE, Kravchenko TI, Gaidar BV, et al. Periodic mobility of cranial bones in humans. *Human Physiology* 1999;25(1):51–58.

84. Moskalenko YE, Frymann VM, Weinstein GB, et al. Slow rhythmic oscillations within the human cranium: phenomenology, origin, and informational significance. *Human Physiology* 2001;27(2):171–178.

85. Moskalenko YE, Frymann VM, Kravchenko T. A modern conceptualization of the functioning of the primary respiratory mechanism. In King HH, ed. *Proceedings of international research conference: Osteopathy in Pediatrics at the Osteopathic Center for Children in San Diego, CA 2002.* Indianapolis, IN: American Academy of Osteopathy, 2005;12–31.

86. Hargens AR. Noninvasive intracranial pressure (ICP) measurement. 1999 *Space Physiology Laboratory.* Available at: http://spacephysiology.arc.nasa.gov/projects/icp.html

87. Ballard RE, Wilson M, Hargens AR, et al. Noninvasive measurement of intracranial volume and pressure using ultrasound. *American Institute of Aeronautics and Astronautics Life Sciences and Space Medicine Conference.* Book of Abstracts, pp. 76–77, Houston, TX, March 3–6, 1996.

88. Ueno T, Ballard RE, Cantrell JH, et al. Noninvasive estimation of pulsatile intracranial pressure using ultrasound. *NASA Technical Memorandum 112195.* 1996.

89. Ueno T, Ballard RE, Shuer LM, et al. Noninvasive measurement of pulsatile intracranial pressure using ultrasound. *Acta Neurochir* 1998;71(suppl):66–69.

90. Ueno T, Ballard RE, Macias BR, et al. Cranial diameter pulsation measured by non-invasive ultrasound decrease with tilt. *Aviat Space Environ Med* 2003;74(8):882–885.

91. Nelson KE, Sergueff N, Lipinski CL, et al. The cranial rhythmic impulse related to the Traube-Hering-Meyer oscillation: comparing laser-Doppler flowmetry and palpation. *J Am Osteopath Assoc* 2001;101(3):163–173.

92. Sergueef N, Nelson KE, Glonek T. Changes in the Traube-Hering-Meyer wave following cranial manipulation. *Amer Acad Osteop J* 2001;11:17.

93. Nelson KE, Sergueff N, Glonek T. The effect of an alternative medical procedure upon low-frequency oscillation in cutaneous blood flow velocity. *J Manipulative Physiol Ther* 2006;29:626–636.

94. Nelson KE, Sergueff N, Glonek T. Recording the rate of the cranial rhythmic impulse. *J Am Osteopath Assoc* 2006;106(6):337–341.

95. Crow WT, King HH, Patterson, RM, et al. Measuring inherent cranial bone motion in humans using MRI. Poster and Abstract presented at International Conference on Advancements in Osteopathic Research (ICAOR), September 2008.

96. Crow WT, King HH, Patterson RM, et al. Assessment of calvarial structure motion by MRI. *Osteopath Med Prim Care* 2009;3:8. Available at: http://www.om-pc.com/content/3/1/8

97. ImageJ 1.33u National Institutes of Health, USA (open access-rsbweb.nih.gov/ij/).

98. Hartman SE, Norton JM. Interexaminer reliability and cranial osteopathy. *Sci Rev Altern Med* 2002;6:23–34.

99. Cook A. The mechanics of cranial motion—the sphenobasilar synchondrosis (SBS) revisited. *J Bodywork Mov Therap* 2005;9:177–188.

100. Weisl H. The movement of the sacro-iliac joint. *Acta Anat* 1955;23:80–91.

101. Kissling RO, Jacob HA. The mobility of the sacroiliac joint in healthy subjects. *Bull Hosp Joint Dis* 1996;54(3):158–164.

102. Walker JM. The sacroiliac joint: a critical review. *Phys Ther* 1992;72:903–916.

103. Mitchell FL Jr, Pruzzo NL. Investigation of voluntary and primary respiratory mechanisms. *J Am Osteopath Assoc* 1971;70:149–153.

104. Mitchell FL Jr. Voluntary and involuntary respiration and the craniosacral mechanism. *Osteopath Ann* 1977;5:52–59.

105. Pruzzo NA. Lateral lumbar spine double-exposure technique and associated principles. *J Am Osteopath Assoc.* 1970;69:84–86.

106. Butler D. *Mobilisation of the Nervous System.* Edinburgh, UK: Churchill Livingston, 1991.

107. Williams PL, Warwick R, Dyson M. *Gray's Anatomy.* 37 Ed. Edinburgh, Scotland: Churchill-Livingston, 1988.

108. Bates B. *A Guide to Physical Examination,* 3 Ed. Philadelphia, PA: JB Lippincott Co., 1983:149.

109. Drengler KE, King HH. Inter-examiner reliability of palpatory diagnosis of the cranium [abstract]. *J Am Osteopath Assoc* 1998;98(7):387.

110. Woods JM, Woods RH. A physical finding related to psychiatric disorders. *J Amer Osteopath Assoc* 1961;60:988–993.

111. Magoun HI. Entrapment neuropathy in the cranium. *J Am Osteopath Assoc* 1968;67:643–652.

112. Magoun HI. Whiplash injury: a greater lesion complex. *J Amer Osteopath Assoc* 1964;63:524–535.

113. Harakal JH. An osteopathically integrated approach to the whiplash complex. *J Amer Osteopath Assoc* 1975;74:941–955.

114. Lay EM. The osteopathic management of temporomandibular joint dysfunction. In: Gelb H, ed. *Clinical Management of Head, Neck and TMJ Pain and Dysfunction; a Multidisciplinary Approach to Diagnosis and Treatment.* Philadelphia, PA: W.B. Saunders Co., 1985.

115. Cutler MJ, Holland BS, Stupinski BA, et al. Cranial manipulation can alter sleep latency and sympathetic nerve activity in humans: a pilot study. *J Altern Complement Med* 2005;11(1):103–108.

116. Feely RA, ed. *Clinical Cranial Osteopathy: Selected Readings.* Indianapolis, IN: The Cranial Academy, 1988.

117. King HH, ed. *The Collected Papers of Viola M Frymann, DO: Legacy of Osteopathy to Children.* Indianapolis, IN: American Academy of Osteopathy, 1998.

118. King HH, ed. *Proceedings of international research conference: Osteopathy in Pediatrics at the Osteopathic Center for Children in San Diego, CA 2002.* Indianapolis, IN: American Academy of Osteopathy, 2005.

119. Magoun HI. Entrapment neuropathy of the central nervous system: part II. Cranial nerves I-IV, VI-VIII, XII. *J Am osteopath Assoc* 1968;67:779–787.

120. Magoun HI. Entrapment neuropathy of the central nervous system: part III. Cranial nerves V, IX, X, XI. *J Am Osteopath Assoc* 1968;67:889–899.

121. Mills MV, Henley CE, Barnes LLB, et al. The use of osteopathic manipulative treatment as adjuvant therapy in children with recurrent acute otitis media. *Arch Pediatr Adolesc Med* 2003;157:861–866.

122. Steele KM, Kukulka G, Ilker CL. Effect of osteopathic manipulative treatment on childhood otitis media outcomes. Poster presented at the *American Osteopathic Association 102 Annual Meeting and Scientific Seminar* 1997 (Oct) grant # 94-12-400.

123. Degenhardt BF, Kuchera ML. Osteopathic evaluation and manipulative treatment in reducing the morbidity of otitis media: a pilot study. *J Amer Osteopath Assoc* 2006;106:327–34.

124. Still AT. *The philosophy and mechanical principles of osteopathy.* Kansas City, MO: Hudson-Kimberly Publishing Co., 1902.

125. Whiting LM. Can the length of labor be shortened by osteopathic treatment? *J Am Osteopath Assoc* 1911;11:917–921.

126. King HH, Tettambel MA, Lockwood MD, et al. Osteopathic manipulative treatment in prenatal care: a retrospective case control design study. *J Am Osteopath Assoc* 2003;103(12):577–82.

127. Gitlin RS, Wolf DL. Uterine contractions following osteopathic cranial manipulation [abstract]. *J Am Osteopath Assoc.* 1992;92(9):1183.

128. Frymann VM. Relation of disturbances of craniosacral mechanisms to symptomatology of the newborn: study of 1,250 infants. *J Am Osteopath Assoc* 1966;65:1059–1075.

129. Frymann VM. Learning difficulties of children viewed in the light of the osteopathic concept. *J Am Osteopath Assoc* 1976;76:46–61.

130. Frymann VM, Carney RE, Springall P. Effect of osteopathic medical management on neurologic development in children. *J Am Osteopath Assoc* 1992;92:729–744.

131. Frymann VM. The osteopathic approach to the child with a seizure disorder. In: King HH, ed. *Proceedings of international research conference: Osteopathy in Pediatrics at the Osteopathic Center for Children in San Diego, CA 2002.* Indianapolis, IN: American Academy of Osteopathy, 2005:89–96.

132. Lassovetskaia L. Applications of the osteopathic approach to school children with delayed psychic development of cerebro-organic origin. In: King HH, ed. *Proceedings of international research conference: Osteopathy in Pediatrics at the Osteopathic Center for Children in San Diego, CA 2002.* Indianapolis, IN: American Academy of Osteopathy, 2005:52–59.

133. Centers S, Morelli MA, Vallad-Hix C, et al. General Pediatrics. In Ward RC, ed. *Foundations for Osteopathic Medicine.* 2 Ed. Philadelphia, PA: Lippincott Williams & Wilkins, 2002:305–326.

134. Hayden C, Mullinger B. A preliminary assessment of the impact of cranial osteopathy for the relief of infantile colic. *Complement Therap Clin Pract* 2006;12:83–90.

135. Vandenplas Y, Denayer E, Vandenbossche T, et al. Osteopathy may decrease obstructive apnea in infants: a pilot study. *Osteopath Med Prim Care* 2008;2:8.

136. Duncan B, McDonough-Means S, Worden K, et al. Effectiveness of osteopathy in the cranial field and myofascial release versus acupuncture as complementary treatment for children with spastic cerebral palsy: a pilot study. *J Am Osteopath Assoc* 2008;108:559–570.

137. Magoun HI. Osteopathic approach to dental enigmas. *J Am Osteopath Assoc* 1962;62:34–42.

138. Magoun HI. Dental equilibration and osteopathy. *J Am Osteopath Assoc* 1975;74:115–125.

139. Magoun HI. The dental search for a common denominator in craniocervical pain and dysfunction. *J Am Osteopath Assoc* 1979;78:83–88.

140. Baker EG. Alteration in width of maxillary arch and its relation to sutural movement of cranial bones. *J Am Osteopath Assoc.* 1971;70:559–564.

141. Segatto E, Lippold C, Andras V. Craniofacial features of children with spinal deformities. *BMC Musculoskelet Disord* 2008;9:169. Available at: http://www.biomedcentral.com/1471/2474/9/169.

142. Huard Y. Influence of the venous sinus technique on cranial hemodynamics. In: King HH, ed. *Proceedings of international research conference: Osteopathy in Pediatrics at the Osteopathic Center for Children in San Diego, CA 2002.* American Academy of Osteopathy: Indianapolis, IN, 2005: 32–36.

143. Giles PD. Effects of cervical manipulation on autonomic control. Unpublished Master's Thesis University of North Texas Health Science Center, Fort Worth, TX, 2006.

144. Giles PD, Smith M, Hensel K. Effects of cervical manipulation on autonomic control. *J Compl Altern Med.* (In preparation).

145. Henley CE, Ivins D, Mills M, et al. Osteopathic manipulative treatment and its relationship to autonomic nervous system activity as demonstrated by heart rate variability: a repeated measures study. *Osteopathic Medicine and Primary Care* 2008;2:7.

146. Raviv G, Shefi S, Nizani D, et al. Effects of craniosacral therapy on lower urinary tract signs and symptoms in multiple sclerosis. *Complement Ther Clin Pract* 2009;15(2):72–75.

147. Greenman PE, McPartland JM. Cranial findings and iatrogenesis from craniosacral manipulation in patients with traumatic brain syndrome. *J Am Osteopath Assoc* 1995;95(3):182–192.

49

Strain and Counterstrain Approach

JOHN C. GLOVER AND PAUL R. RENNIE

KEY CONCEPTS

- Astute clinical observation (Jones) followed by progressive exploration of a line of thought represents the development of this approach.
- Treatment of somatic dysfunction can be enhanced by placing the patient's body in a position of maximum comfort. Effective use of this approach requires exploration of anterior and posterior body areas for appropriate diagnosis(es).
- Correlations between symptoms, history and physical examination, structural findings and associated tender points are necessary preparation for utilization of this approach.
- Tender points described and utilized in this approach are most commonly found in muscle tissue. Explorations of muscle involvement through research activity continue to elaborate the involvement of various body systems.

CASE STUDY

A 45-year-old male presents to the office with a complaint of non-radiating low back pain of 2 weeks' duration. The pain is described an intense deep pain at times and achy at other times. It is worse when he tries to stand upright. The problem began 2 weeks ago when he spent a day cleaning out his garage. After working most of the day bending and lifting to go through boxes and move them into a storage cabinet, he lifted a very heavy box of books. He was bent over at the waist and had barely lifted the box off the ground when he felt a sharp pain in his low back. He dropped the box and, as a reflex reaction, stood up quickly. He went inside to sit down to rest, and when he tried to stand up from the chair, he had a low back spasm and could not stand upright. Over the course of the last 2 weeks, he has tried hot showers, a heating pad, a topical analgesic cream, and Extra Strength Tylenol, all without much benefit. The patient denies any change in bladder or bowel function.

Physical examination:

Vital signs within normal limits (P: 72, R: 14, BP: 118/74, T: 98°F), HEENT, cardiovascular, pulmonary and abdominal exams are within normal limits. Neurological exam: normal lower extremity DTRs (2+/4+ bilaterally) and normal sensation in the lower extremities. Straight leg raising test is negative. Structural exam reveals a discrete area of intense tenderness to palpation and tissue texture abnormalities at the level of the anterior superior iliac spine (ASIS), one-third the distance to midline and deep in the abdomen bilaterally over the iliopsoas muscles with the left more tender than the right.

Diagnosis:

1. Lumbar strain, left greater than right
2. Somatic dysfunction—lumbar spine and abdomen

Plan:

Osteopathic manipulative treatment using counterstrain with good results and well tolerated by the patient.

Discussion:

The initial injury occurred when the patient used the erector spinae muscles from a stretched position as the agonist to lift a heavy load. Due to muscle fatigue from lifting and bending all day and the heavy load, he strained the erector spinae muscles that produced the pain. When he stood up rapidly to protect the strained erector spinae muscles from further damage, the rapid lengthening of the shortened antagonist iliopsoas muscles reported a strain to the central nervous system before an actual strain occurred. This resulted is hypershortened iliopsoas muscles containing Jones tender points. The lumbar strain (erector spinae) will heal, but the Jones tender points will remain in the muscles until the somatic dysfunction is treated.

INTRODUCTION

Initially, Lawrence H. Jones, D.O., F.A.A.O., referred to his new treatment approach as *spontaneous release by positioning* (5) but found this term to be cumbersome. Dr. Jones decided to use a shorter term, *strain-counterstrain*, describing what he believed was more descriptive of the underlying physiologic mechanism he used to treat somatic dysfunction. Jones, once he formalized its teaching, always referred to the manipulative treatment model he developed as strain-counterstrain. In this chapter, we refer to this method as *counterstrain*, the terminology used in the Glossary of Osteopathic Terminology (Educational Council on Osteopathic Principles, 2009) and by most practitioners.

Manipulative treatment models are divided into two primary divisions: direct and indirect, based on the initial positioning of the patient relative to the restrictive barrier. Counterstrain is an indirect model with the initial positioning away from the restrictive barrier. It has a unique advantage over other manipulative treatment models in that the patient can provide feedback to the physician to indicate when they are in the correct position for treatment. The model is also highly accessible to the student who has limited palpatory skills and treatment experience. In fact, counterstrain is often taught early in an osteopathic curriculum because it is a treatment model that novice students can use and experience success. Additionally, if the student pays attention to the tissue changes under their monitoring hand, they will learn to palpate the more subtle tissue changes needed to be effective in applying other manipulative treatment models. While counterstrain can be learned early in manual skills development, it can continue to be used effectively as the sole manipulative treatment model by experienced physicians and is also used in combination with other models.

HISTORY

Counterstrain began as an unexpected discovery in 1955. A young, athletic-looking man visited Lawrence H. Jones, D.O., F.A.A.O. (Jones, 1981), because he had developed a psoasitis 2½ months before seeking treatment that left him in pain and unable to stand erect. The injury was not caused by trauma, but it gradually worsened over the 2½ months. Since the onset, the man had received treatment by two chiropractors with no substantial improvement. Jones treated the man several times with thrust-type treatment over the course of 6 weeks with no better results.

At one visit, the man reported difficulty sleeping due to pain. Jones worked with the patient for 20 minutes to find a comfortable sleeping position. After finding the position, Jones left the young man in the position and went to treat another patient. When Jones returned, he assisted the young man to a standing position and to their mutual surprise, the patient stood erect and pain free for the first time in 4 months. Jones was impressed by the results and decided to investigate these findings.

Jones experimented by treating patients with whole-body positions of comfort. He had frequent success and wanted to shorten the time in the treatment position. He observed that there were discrete tender paravertebral areas prior to treatment that became pain free after time in the position of comfort. Dr. Jones then began positioning only the affected region of the body, and this reduced the time in the treatment position. He experimented with reducing the amount of time needed for treatment. Ninety seconds in the position of comfort proved to be the optimal time required to benefit the patient. Shorter periods of time did not always produce lasting relief, and longer periods did not necessarily yield greater benefit. He also began mapping the discrete areas of tenderness and correlating them to specific somatic dysfunctions identified by the traditional methods he learned in osteopathic medical school.

Jones found that he could only find the discrete paravertebral areas of tenderness in half of his patients. More answers came when Jones saw another patient he was treating for psoitis who thought he developed a hernia from an accident in his garden. Although the physical examination revealed no inguinal hernia, there was a discrete area of tenderness. Jones placed the man in a position of comfort to treat the psoitis and then palpated the tender area from the groin injury. To their mutual surprise, the tissue was no longer tender. Jones slowly returned the patient to a neutral position and palpated the area again. He found no evidence of tenderness.

Jones had discovered that there were anterior as well as posterior tender points. He began to search for tender points on the front of the body (Jones, 1966). This observation is consistent with the osteopathic principle of the body is a unit. The emphasis on spinal function and posterior diagnostic evaluation had eclipsed this connection.

Other treatment approaches to the musculoskeletal system have identified discrete areas of tense tender tissue. Travell (Travell and Simons, 1999) developed an approach and used the term *trigger point* to describe tense areas. Jones et al. (1995) initially used the same term, but later referred to these areas as *tender points*. Jones described over 300 specific tender points, and new tender points continue to be found. Through correspondence, Travell and Jones identified similarities and differences between their points. Table 49.1 provides a comparison of trigger and tender points.

Jones' theory for the mechanism of action in counterstrain is that the initial injury produces a sudden "panic" lengthening of the antagonist muscle to the originally strained and painful agonist muscle. Jones treated the tender point associated with the asymptomatic antagonist muscle by shortening this muscle, which also places the originally strained and painful muscle back into a stretched position, the position of the original strain, thus producing a counter to the strain.

Dr. Jones made two important discoveries:

1. Placing the body into a position of maximum comfort can treat somatic dysfunction
2. The anterior aspect of the patient must be evaluated, as well as the posterior, to effectively diagnose and treat somatic dysfunction

THEORETICAL PHYSIOLOGIC BASIS OF COUNTERSTRAIN

Physicians have demonstrated the clinical benefits of counterstrain for over 50 years (Anonymous, 1989; Bailey and Dick, 1992; Brandt and Jones, 1976; Cislo et al., 1991; Jacobson, 1989; Jones, 1973; Radjieski et al., 1998; Ramirez et al., 1989; Schwartz, 1986). Counterstrain basic research has been limited to only a few studies. (Howell et al., 2006; Luckenbill-Edds and Bechill, 1995; Wynne

---

TABLE 49.1

Comparison of Trigger Points and Tender Points

Trigger Point	Tender Point
Patient presents with characteristic pain pattern	Typically no characteristic pain pattern
Located in muscle tissue	Located in muscle, tendons, ligaments, and fascia
Locally tender	Locally tender
Elicits jump sign when pressed	Elicits jump sign when pressed
Elicits a radiating pain pattern when pressed	No radiating pattern when pressed
Present within a taut band of tissue	Taut band not present
Elicits twitch response with snapping palpation	Twitch response not present
Dermographia of skin over point	Dermographia not present

et al. 2006). One study showed a change in the muscle spindle following counterstrain treatment, supporting Dr. Jones hypothesis (Howell et al., 2006). More studies need to be done, especially electromyography studies of tissues containing the tender points, to demonstrate the specific muscles, ligaments, etc. associated with the somatic dysfunction.

Understanding muscle physiology provides some answers because tender points are most commonly found in muscle tissue. The neural system is another key component in the development and maintenance of somatic dysfunction. A third element important to understanding counterstrain is the role of the circulatory system.

At the time Jones was formulating his ideas about counterstrain, Korr (1974) published an article on proprioceptors and somatic dysfunction, which helped to explain the role of the proprioceptors in muscle tone and the response to injury. Another important part of the model is the gamma system and its role in muscle tone. Van Buskirk (1990) described the important role of nociception in somatic dysfunction. The role of the circulatory system has been described (Rennie et al., 2004) and needs further exploration and has not yet been adequately explained.

One of the most important characteristics of the counterstrain model is the relationship between tender points and somatic dysfunction. The location of a specific tender point is constant from one patient to another. This suggests a strong anatomic basis for their location. Different myofascial structures including tendons, ligaments, fascia, and muscle bellies have all been found to contain tender points. Myotomal, dermatomal, and sclerotomal relationships have been proposed to explain the relationship between a specific anatomic segment and the related tender points (Beal, 1985; Yates and Glover, 1994; Rennie et al., 2004). Another interesting anatomic correlation is the close location of tender points in areas where *motor points* are found (Rennie et al., 2004). A motor point is the site where the motor nerve pierces the investing fascia and enters the muscle it innervates.

Mapping the pathways of afferent nerves and the central system is important to understanding the role of the afferent nervous system. The bulk of afferent input comes from the soma (as opposed to the viscera). This difference is so great that nociceptive messages from the viscera are typically interpreted as being of somal origin. This unequal distribution can also be seen with the illustration of the homunculus in the cerebral cortex. The homunculus illustrates the proportional area in the cortex devoted to sensing and interpreting afferent input from different locations in the periphery. The neuronal "crosstalk" in the central nervous system between sensory and motor nerves is the source of the various reflexes between the viscera and the soma. It also provides an explanation for the effect counterstrain treatments have on visceral function and circulatory flow.

Normal function of the gamma efferent system is partly responsible for the change in muscle tone with changing demand. Jones proposed that the gamma system is responsible for the development of an inappropriate proprioceptive reflex associated with somatic dysfunction. A rapid lengthening of the myofascial tissue sets up the inappropriate reflex. An event occurs that produces rapid lengthening of a muscle. Afferent feedback indicates possible myofascial damage from a strain. The body tries to prevent the myofascial damage by rapidly contracting the myofascial tissue that may be strained. This produces a rapid lengthening in the antagonist muscle. It is proposed that the rapid lengthening of the antagonist produces the inappropriate reflex, which is manifest as a tender point. The theory is that the nociceptive feedback from the antagonist is interpreted as a muscle strain (although a strain

has not occurred). The end result is hypertonic myofascial tissue and restricted motion. A guarding reflex by the patient, without actual mechanical trauma, can also produce the inappropriate reflex. Although this model does explain the development of tender points in muscle tissue, it does not explain tender points in other types of tissue.

Trauma produces change in myofascial tissues at microscopic and biochemical levels (Mense, 1997). The force of the trauma causes damage to myofibrils and their microcirculation. Myofibril damage interferes with the actin-myosin bridges and changes the chemistry around them. Nociceptive information is carried to the central nervous system to alert the body to the tissue damage. The tissue disruption and subsequent chemical changes cause the tissue to become more sensitive to touch and may be part of the reason for the formation of a tender point. The damage to the microcirculation changes intramuscular pressure and muscle function. A small increase in intramuscular pressure can produce muscle fatigue due to decreased cellular metabolism (Mense, 1997). This change in metabolism changes the chemical matrix around the myofibrils and can produce nociceptive activity resulting in tenderness (Mense, 1997).

A tender point is sensitive to palpation and therefore must be related to nociceptive activity. The position of comfort used to treat a somatic dysfunction with counterstrain is a very specific three-dimensional position in space. When the optimal position of comfort is established, the tenderness of the tender point disappears or becomes insignificant. This seems to indicate a neural relationship between the tender point and the somatic dysfunction. Neural messages are rapidly transmitted and used by the body when quick responses are needed. Palpation of changes at the tender point and in the surrounding tissue suggests that in addition to the neural component, the position of comfort also produces changes in the myofascial tissue and small circulatory vessels.

A clue for the treatment time comes from the palpation of a pulsation, the *therapeutic pulse*, at a tender point location. The frequency of the pulsation is the same as the cardiac rate and would therefore suggest a circulatory relationship. Another important element is that the pulsation is not present before positioning; it develops only when the patient is moved close to the position of comfort and disappears after myofascial tissue relaxation. This process takes approximately 90 seconds to occur. The pulsation phenomenon does not occur with every tender point; however, when it is palpated, it does correlate with markedly improved treatment response.

Indications

Identification of the presence of a tender point is an indication for counterstrain. Tender points can be found in acute and chronic musculoskeletal conditions. They may also be found in association with a viscerosomatic reflex. The tender points may be the primary indication of somatic dysfunction or develop secondary to another primary cause for somatic dysfunction such as a joint restriction. Counterstrain is indicated for any patient who is hesitant about the forces used in other forms of manipulative treatment, a frail patient or a trial of manipulative treatment to access a patient's tolerance. Tender points have been identified in every region of body.

Contraindications

Absolute contraindications are rare when considering the use of counterstrain. The presence of a fracture in the area used to treat the somatic dysfunction would be a contraindication. Another would be the treatment of a patient with a torn ligament in the area to be treated where positioning for treatment would risk further tearing. All other contraindications for not using counterstrain are relative. Patients who cannot voluntarily relax are not good candidates for counterstrain. Children who cannot remain passive are poor candidates. Some of the elderly who confuse not moving with relaxation and cannot be taught the difference do not respond well to counterstrain. Severe osteoporosis where positioning the patient for treatment may risk a fracture is contraindicated, although this is typically not a problem because the position for treatment is within a patient's range of motion and therefore should not cause a problem. Treatment of the cervical spine in patient with vertebral artery disease may be contraindicated with severe disease. This applies especially to positions with marked rotation and/or hyperextension. In addition, severely ill patients who may not tolerate a treatment reaction are not good candidates although counterstrain has been used very effectively in the hospital setting, including intensive care units. An example of this situation is in the case of a patient who is having a myocardial infarction. A classic presentation with all the signs and symptoms would cause the physician to get the patient to a hospital for treatment, but if the signs and symptoms are not classic, a viscerosomatic reflex associated with the myocardial infarction may be treated, reducing the discomfort and delay getting prompt treatment for the myocardial infarction.

PHASES OF PALPATORY DEVELOPMENT

There are two basic phases in the development of palpatory and treatment skills used to treat patients with counterstrain. The first is to identify the various locations where tender points may be found by following the descriptions given in a counterstrain text, pressing the location, and asking the patient if it is tender. Initially, many students are unable to identify the tissue texture abnormalities associated with the presence of a tender point and rely on the patient's response to their pressing the tender point location. This same method is used to position the patient. The novice practitioner moves the patient in a direction that should shorten the dysfunctional myofascial tissue (or that reproduces the treatment position given in a text) and relies on the patient response of the level of tenderness to indicate if the treatment position is being approached. This method is effective, but time consuming.

A patient who does not perceive tenderness of a tender point despite the presence of a tender point is referred to as a *stoic* patient. Counterstrain is not effective on these patients if the student relies totally on the patient's response because the patient is incapable of providing an accurate response. The second phase of learning begins when the student can perceive the tissue texture abnormalities characteristic of a tender point. These tissue texture abnormalities will alert a student to the presence of a tender point before the patient experiences tenderness as the student presses the tender point.

Another important step for the student is the ability to palpate changes in the tissue texture abnormality of the tender point during treatment. A change of position of the patient toward the position of maximal comfort will cause decreased tension or softening of the tissue of the tender point. This allows the student to know immediately if they are moving the patient in the correct direction for treatment. Experience will also allow the student to correlate the degree of tissue change with the amount of positional change needed. The changes in tissue texture can also be used to determine when the time needed in the treatment position is sufficient.

DIAGNOSIS

Several different approaches can be used. History and observation can be an indicator of tender point location. If the patient can recount accurately the mechanism of the injury, it can lead the physician to the tender point. For example, a patient whose injury occurred in a flexed position typically has a tender point on the anterior aspect of the body and the treatment position is to approximate the position of injury. Observation of the patient's habitus provides valuable clues to the location of significant tender points. A patient who has difficulty standing upright and is more comfortable in a forward bent position typically has tender points on the anterior aspect of the body. The more forward or backward bend without sidebending and rotation the more likely the tender point will be located close to the midline. If the patient is most comfortable with a sidebent and/or rotated position, then the tender points are more likely to be located lateral to the midline. The report of pain patterns by the patient can be used to identify specific muscle groups that may contain tender points (Myers, 2006).

Another method is to do a neuromusculoskeletal exam and after segmental diagnosis is made to look for the tender points associated with the segment. If the segment is flexed, rotated, and sidebent to the right, there is commonly a tender point on the anterior aspect of the body on the left side, but there also may be tender points on the right anterior or either the right or left side on the posterior aspect of the body.

Still another method is to scan the tender points in the region of the complaint and one region above and below the area of the complaint. A thoracic complaint may yield significant tender points in the thoracic, cervical, lumbar, or costal regions as well as the upper extremities. It is always important not to narrow the evaluation of a patient just to the area of the complaint.

TREATMENT

Counterstrain is a very gentle technique that is well tolerated by most patients. The patient is not subjected to any external force other than gentle positioning. In addition, patients do not generate force from their own muscle contraction to produce effective treatment. It is an indirect technique, with positioning away from restrictive barriers; therefore, it is tolerated in both acute and chronic problems.

Counterstrain is based on identifying tender points associated with somatic dysfunction and positioning the patient to eliminate the tenderness of the point. Counterstrain is easy to understand and apply; however, mastery requires time to learn the location of tender points; skill in fine-tuning the treatment position for maximum results; and the clinical experience to understand the correlations between symptoms, structural findings, and associated tender points. The basic steps for treating somatic dysfunction with counterstrain after a relevant osteopathic neuromusculoskeletal exam are as follows:

1. Find the most significant/relevant tender point
2. Establish a tenderness scale
3. Continuously monitor tender point tenderness and tissue texture
4. Place the patient passively in a position that results in the greatest reduction of tenderness and tissue texture abnormality at the tender point (position of comfort/ease)
   (a) Slowly position the patient towards a position of comfort/ease, with large movement initially, while the patient remains passive
   (b) Then, fine-tune the position through small arcs of movement in multiple planes of motion to find the greatest position of comfort/ease

5. Maintain this position for 90 seconds while the patient remains passive
   (a) Continuously monitor the tender point for tissue texture changes
   (b) Periodically retest for tenderness
6. Slowly return the patient passively to the pretreatment position while maintaining contact with the tender point
7. Reevaluate for resolution of tenderness and tissue abnormality at the tender point

Step 1: Find the Most Significant/Relevant Tender Point

Tender points are typically located in tendinous attachments or in the belly of a muscle. Additional tender points are found in other myofascial tissues (tendons, ligaments, and myofascial sheets) associated with the joint dysfunction. Tender points are typically discrete, small, tense, and edematous. The areas are typically smaller than a fingertip, and they are exquisitely tender. A significant tender point is about four times more tender than the adjacent tissue. Tender point tissue changes may range from several inches to almost nothing. The tissue of the tender point is found to be more tense than the surrounding tissue.

It is essential to identify the most significant tender point associated with the somatic dysfunction rather than just finding a point that is tender. Due to the exquisite tenderness of significant tender points, a patient will typically jump, wince, guard, or push your hand away when you press the tender point. Patients are often surprised with the amount of tenderness, especially when they were unaware of the existence of the tender point. In rare cases, a patient does not perceive tenderness when a tender point is pressed, but they still can be treated with counterstrain by monitoring tissue changes, rather than the patient's reactions, that occur during treatment.

Palpate for a tender point with the pad of your finger or thumb. The pads of the fingers are profoundly more sensitive to tactile input and are better at identifying the location of tender points. Avoid using the fingertips, especially if you have long fingernails. Fingertips are less sensitive and can elicit iatrogenic tenderness.

Palpation should be slow and firm but gentle. The pressure used to elicit a tender point is typically a few ounces and not strong enough to elicit tenderness in normal tissue. Jones recommended using the amount of force needed to blanch under the fingernail of the palpating finger. The vector of pressure is also important. Typically, the tissue of the tender point is pressed onto more rigid tissue like bone or cartilage. Do not forget to check for other pathology that might produce tenderness that is not related to neuromusculoskeletal tender points, such as infection, inflammation, or pathology of visceral origin.

Before the physician begins palpating for tender points, ask the patient to report any tenderness as you palpate. The physician is palpating for tissue texture abnormalities, especially edema and tension before the patient experiences tenderness. Verify the presence of a tender point by asking the patient if the area is tender while the potential tender point is pressed briefly. The tenderness of a tender point is an objective sign elicited by physically palpating the dysfunctional area. In contrast, pain is a subjective symptom that the patient may experience without palpation. Jones found that tender points are often found in nonpainful areas.

One method to determine where tender points may be found is to perform an osteopathic structural examination noting any alteration of movement, asymmetry of paired landmarks, or tissue texture abnormalities. Palpating these areas for tender points is how Jones originally found many of the tender points he described. Evaluate the patient for variations from ideal posture and palpate those areas for tender points. For example, a patient presenting with flattening of the normal thoracic kyphotic curve is likely to have one or more posterior thoracic tender points associated with the extension in this region. Tender point locations can also be suggested based on clinical history and presenting complaints. By knowing the position in which the original injury occurred, the most likely places for significant tender points can be deduced. Many myofascial pain patterns have been described by Travell and may provide additional correlation.

The presence of a significant tender point will result in the patient attempting to obtain a comfortable posture to alleviate the functional distress. This is an unconscious attempt by the patient to shorten and relieve tense myofascial tissues. Patients tend to bend around a tender point. That is, tender points tend to be at the focal point of the concavity of the postural adaptation. If the patient is forward bent, tender points tend to be anterior. If a patient is backward bent, tender points tend to be posterior. Jones found that a patient who presents sidebent to one side usually has a tender point on the opposite side of the spine (L.H. Jones, *personal communication*, 1993).

Tender points are frequently found in areas other than the area of pain or discomfort. The primary or key strain may induce a secondary or compensatory strain elsewhere, which may be more symptomatic. For example, when the psoas muscle chronically stays in spasm, patients seldom complain of abdominal or anterolateral hip pain. Instead, they complain of pain in the lumbosacral or sacroiliac regions, due to the strain and compensation of those regions by the psoas spasm. Tender points may be 180 degrees around the body from the site of the presenting pain. For example, in a patient with pain between the shoulder blades, the tender point is often on the sternum. It is also possible to have both anterior and posterior or right and left tender points associated with the same anatomic segmental level. This is because tender points are mediated through the nervous system and can result in multiple points for a single somatic dysfunction. If there are multiple tender points in a given area, ask the patient which is the most tender. Then, treat the most severe tender point first. Associated but less significant tender points often disappear after successful treatment of the tender point.

If the tender point results from a viscerosomatic reflex, tenderness returns within minutes or hours, not days. When this is found, a thorough review of the patient's medical history and more careful physical examination are needed. Be sure all of the possible causes of the original tenderness have been considered. (For more information about viscerosomatic reflexes, refer to the discussion of viscerosomatic reflexes in the basic science section of this book, or read Beal's article (1985)). This information is also important when treating patients in the hospital. (Refer to the article by Schwartz (1986) on the treatment of hospital patients with counterstrain.)

Initially, the physician will palpate the anatomical location of a tender point as described by Dr. Jones and others and then test for the presence of a tender point. As the physician's skill grows, tissue texture abnormalities, typically increased tension, will become evident well before the patient reports any tenderness. The skilled palpating hand will zero in on the area of greatest tissue change and then confirm the identification of a significant tender point by pressing on the tissue to elicit tenderness from the patient. This ability to palpate the tissue changes associated with the tender point will also be used for more accurate positioning and will allow the physician to treat a stoic patient.

Step 2: Establish a Tenderness Scale

To facilitate the communication between physician and patient, it is important to establish a means of monitoring the level of tenderness of the tender point. Physicians typically use a tenderness scale to enhance verbal feedback with the patient. Several scales have been used effectively. The one most commonly used is a 0-to-10 scale, with 10 being equal to the level of tenderness prior to positioning for treatment and 0 representing the absence of tenderness. The scale represents a continuous range from the pretreatment tenderness (a 10) to the elimination of tenderness (a 0). The number does not represent a fixed quantity of tenderness. The 10 of one tender point is different to the 10 of another tender point. The scale allows the patient to communicate changes in tenderness and is correlated with palpatory changes. The same amount of pressure should be used each time the physician attempts to elicit tenderness of a specific point although different pressures are needed for different tender points due to different amounts of tissue over the tender points. It should be emphasized to the patient that this is not acupressure or a form of massage. Firm pressure is applied only when trying to determine the level tenderness. At other times, only light contact is maintained. This feedback provides a means for monitoring the effectiveness of positioning and treatment for both patient and physician.

Step 3: Monitor Tender Point Tenderness and Tissue Texture

It is important to maintain contact with the tender point throughout treatment. This allows the physician to palpate the tissue changes that occur at the tender point when establishing the optimal treatment position as well as the end point of treatment. The pressure used to monitor the tender point is less than what is used to test for tenderness. Monitoring pressure allows enough force to maintain contact with the myofascial tissues of the tender point without causing tenderness in the patient. A patient in pain does not relax well and therefore is more difficult to treat.

After a significant tender point is selected for treatment, it is monitored as the physician begins to move the patient toward the position of comfort described by Dr. Jones and others. The myofascial tissues of the tender point will begin to relax as the patient is moved toward the correct treatment position. About half way to the described treatment position, the physician stops and tests the level of tenderness. The pressure used to test for the level of tenderness is increased to the firm pressure used initially to test for the presence of a tender point. Jones found it requires about four times the pressure on normal tissue to produce tenderness as it does to elicit tenderness of a tender point (Jones et al., 1995). The pressure should be applied as a short quick push, not a long slow sustained amount of pressure. If the physician is moving the patient in the correct direction, the tenderness will decrease. The closer to the optimal position, the less tenderness is present. Once the physician is able to palpate changes in tissue texture, the changes can be used to determine if the patient is being positioned correctly. For example, if the physician is moving the patient toward the optimal position, the tissues typically relax. If the patient is moving away from the optimal position, the tissue tension typically increases. Experience will teach the physician the correlation between tissue changes and the level of tenderness. This is then used to find the optimal position of comfort more efficiently by taking less time to find the optimal position. Each new position is accompanied by retesting the tenderness of the tender point.

Step 4: Place Patient Passively in Position of Comfort

One of the advantages of counterstrain is that treatment is always in a position of comfort or ease. By placing the patient in a position of comfort, discomfort is avoided and further injury is unlikely to occur. Counterstrain can be used for patients with a wide variety of medical conditions, unless gently moving the patient into the specific treatment position is contraindicated. A word of caution: medical judgment must always be used to determine the appropriateness of any treatment. Every patient needs to be evaluated thoroughly on an individual basis. The only absolute requirement is that the patient must be relaxed while the physician places the dysfunctional area of the body into the position of comfort and maintains it during treatment.

The optimal position of comfort is a very specific position in space. The position is similar for the same tender point in different patients, but the exact position is unique for each patient. To find the optimal position, the physician uses a combination of palpation and feedback from the patient. Maintaining continuous light contact with the tender point during treatment is important for maximum effectiveness and efficiency.

The first step in positioning is to approximate the position expected. The expectation may be from previous clinical experience, patient history, or from looking at an illustration of the positioning in a counterstrain book. The purpose of the positioning is to reduce the tension on the dysfunctional myofascial structures. As a rule, the closer tender points are to the midline, the more flexed or extended is the patient's presenting posture, and more flexion or extension is required for the treatment position. With tender points more lateral to the midline, more sidebending and rotation are usually required for treatment. Sidebending and/or rotation of the body away from the tender point are the most common positions needed for effective treatment.

Slowly move the patient toward the described or expected position of comfort while monitoring the tender point for relaxation of the tissue. When marked relaxation of the tender point is palpated, stop moving the patient. Press the tender point and ask for the level of tenderness. If the level of tenderness is greater than 3 on the 10-point scale, continue to move the patient in the same direction. Then, as significant relaxation is palpated, stop movement and test again. Repeat this process until the tenderness level is three or less. If the number increases, return in the direction just traveled and retest. It may be necessary to change direction or add other directions to find the correct position. Figure 49.1 shows the changes in tenderness as the patient is moved from a neutral starting position to the position of comfort and beyond.

From the beginning of positioning to about half way to the position of comfort, large movements are typically used because the reduction in tenderness is small for the distance traveled. As you get close to the optimal position, fine-tuning the position with small motions is required. A small change in position at this point in the treatment markedly reduces tenderness. For example, several inches of movement close to the neutral position may reduce the tenderness by one on the scale, whereas it may take only one quarter inch of movement close to the optimal position to reduce the tenderness the same amount. Slow, small movements, constant light contact of the tender point for monitoring, and retesting the tender point for reduction of tenderness with each new position all allow the practitioner to find the precise position of optimal comfort. If the optimal position is overshot, the level of tenderness will increase. Fine-tune the position until the tenderness has been reduced by at least 70% (3 on the scale), preferably 100%. The

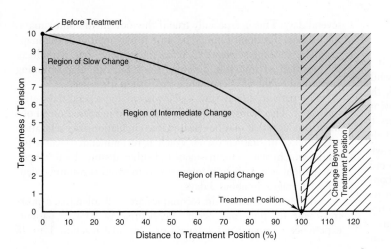

Figure 49-1 Tenderness scale-distance graph. (Courtesy of Johannes Liedtke)

position of comfort must be at least 70% improved over the initial tenderness, or the technique is ineffective. Jones recommended a reduction of two thirds, and other practitioners have suggested three fourths. An effort should be made to maximally reduce the tenderness. The extra time spent trying to eliminate the tenderness will significantly increase the effectiveness of the treatment.

A common mistake is to use constant firm pressure on the tender point throughout the treatment sequence. Instead, constant light contact should be maintained. Once the optimal treatment position has been determined, be sure to maintain only light contact with the myofascial tissue of the tender point. There are three important reasons for maintaining contact:

1. Tissue changes that occur in the tender point can be monitored more easily and aid in determining the end point of treatment
2. The tender point can continue to be fine-tuned while maintaining the optimal position of comfort, because the position may change slightly during treatment
3. Both the patient and the practitioner can be confident of the location of the tender point

The third reason may seem unimportant, but when contact with the tender point is lost, the patient may question whether the same point is being pressed. Also, the practitioner may have difficulty reestablishing contact with the point with enough confidence to allow an accurate recheck.

At times, a pulsation in the tender point may be palpated. This is referred to as the therapeutic pulse. Although its intensity may vary, it is often close to the intensity of the radial pulse. In fact, palpating the patient's radial artery with the other hand typically shows it to be synchronous with the therapeutic pulse. For this reason, it is postulated that the position of release results in a sympathetic vasodilation of the small arterioles in the myofascial tissue. At times, the therapeutic pulse can be palpated while attempting to find the optimal position of comfort, enabling the practitioner to establish the position more accurately. At other times, the therapeutic pulse will not be palpated until the treatment position has been maintained for a period of time. In either case, the appearance of the therapeutic pulse can be used to enhance the treatment.

Step 5: Maintain Position for 90 Seconds While Patient Remains Passive

Once the position of comfort has been established, hold it for 90 seconds. It is important to remember that the patient must remain

relaxed without contracting the dysfunctional myofascial tissue. The 90 seconds does not begin until the patient is completely relaxed. It may be necessary to remind the patient to stay relaxed several times during the 90 seconds, because often the patient contracts muscles unconsciously. An apparent decrease in the patient's weight as you support them in the treatment position is an indication that the patient is contracting muscles. Patients who are not comfortable will not be able to relax for the entire 90 seconds. Also, if the practitioner is not comfortable, it is difficult to hold the patient in the treatment position for 90 seconds. You may need to experiment to find the best way to remain comfortable during treatment. Each patient and clinical setting offers different challenges. It may be necessary to invent a new treatment position to enable both the patient and yourself to remain comfortable. This is especially true with pregnant patients, patients with some degree of paralysis, hospitalized patients, and with physician-patient size mismatches.

Dr. Jones used 120 seconds to treat rib dysfunctions. When asked if these tender points were different in some way to all the other tender points, Dr. Jones said they were not different. His stated reason for increasing the time to 120 seconds was purely behavioral. He felt that most patients were a little uncomfortable leaning up against the physician, so he gave them an additional 30 seconds to relax. Once the patient is in the position of maximal comfort for the rib tender point, the same 90 seconds is all that is needed to treat the dysfunction. The tender points are not different, but the physician must be aware of the patient's state of relaxation and comfort being close to the physician. This is critical in all areas of the body and a common reason for failure of a physician to get a good response using counterstrain.

Feel for tissue changes in the tender point and surrounding tissue. As time in the treatment position increases, the tissue relaxes and you should feel a softening. The myofascial tissue around the tender point may begin to move in a seemingly random pattern. This sensation is due to the relaxation of myofascial tissue in different planes. Although treatment time may not always be exactly 90 seconds, it is important to maintain the treatment position for 90 seconds when beginning to learn counterstrain. The ability to palpate myofascial release patterns enhances counterstrain treatment and can also be used to improve palpatory skills needed for myofascial release techniques. As discussed earlier, you may also feel the therapeutic pulse. Once the random motion becomes symmetrical or the therapeutic pulse disappears, it is time to move the patient back to the starting position. Once the tissue changes that signal the end of treatment can be palpated with confidence; watching a clock is no longer necessary.

Step 6: Passive Slow Return While Maintaining Tender Point Contact

After maintaining the position of comfort for 90 seconds, it is time to slowly return the patient to the starting position while monitoring the tender point. Before starting to move, ask the patient to remain passive and not assist you by actively moving. Patients may unconsciously try to help. If the patient starts to help or move, stop the return and remind the patient not to help. When the patient has relaxed, start moving again, more slowly. An apparent decrease in the patient's weight as you move them is another indication that the patient is contracting muscles. A common error when learning counterstrain is to move the patient too quickly. A slow return is critical. The first few degrees of motion during return are the most critical. Watch the patient for signs of flinching or other guarding gestures. Palpating for muscle contraction could also provide a sign that the patient is being moved too quickly.

Step 7: Reevaluate Tenderness and Tissue Texture

Once the patient has been returned to a relaxed position, reevaluate the tenderness and tissue texture of the tender point. To consider the treatment successful, no more than 30% (3 on the 10-point scale) of the original tenderness should remain. Ideally, all of the tenderness will have resolved. If more than 30% of the tenderness remains, several possible reasons may exist. The patient may not have been optimally positioned, the physician may have let the position change during treatment, the patient may have contracted the muscle being treated, or the physician may have lost contact with the tender point. Repeat the positioning, with particular attention to obtaining and maintaining the optimal position with the patient completely relaxed.

Another cause for failure may be that another tender point is the primary problem and, therefore, the most significant point was not treated. Evaluate the tender points in the area near the tender point just treated and the corresponding area on the opposite side of the body to see if another, more significant tender point is present. This is especially true if the point treated was part of a sequential line of tender points. Consider the possibility that the primary tender point is distant from the area evaluated or on the opposite side of the body from the reported problem. More than one treatment session may be necessary to completely resolve a tender point. Also, failure to completely resolve the tenderness does not necessarily indicate an ineffective treatment. Some of the most challenging tender points to treat are when both anterior and posterior tender points are present at the same level (e.g., AT4 and PT4).

Reevaluate the original structural findings to evaluate the effectiveness of the treatment. You are treating a somatic dysfunction, not just a tender point, so reevaluating cannot be overstated. Motion restrictions, asymmetry, and tissue texture abnormalities should improve or disappear after effective treatment. With chronic somatic dysfunction, the tissue changes may be slower to return to normal.

Clinical tips for providing strain and counterstrain techniques are found in Box 49.1.

PATIENT EDUCATION

It is important to start instructions before the patient gets off the treatment table. Patients are curious to see if the treatment eliminated the presenting complaint. Warn the patient not to test previously restricted motions and to avoid extremes of motion for several days. This is especially true if the movement approximates the original position of injury, because it may reproduce the inappropriate reflex just treated. Active movement that reproduces the position of injury is different from the careful positioning performed by the physician while the patient is passive.

The patient should stay well hydrated for several days after treatment. This helps with the elimination of increased metabolic waste products that may be released into circulation after relaxation of the tense myofascial tissue. Water is recommended over other fluids, which may contain sugar and other dissolved substances. The patient is especially recommended to avoid consuming alcoholic beverages for about 3 days.

Although counterstrain techniques are well tolerated, a posttreatment reaction may occur. Approximately 30% of patients experience a generalized soreness or a flu-like reaction 1 to 48

Clinical Tips

- A single somatic dysfunction may have more than one associated tender point
- Test for tenderness of a specific tender point with the same amount of pressure each time
- Use less pressure to monitor a tender point than to test it
- Physician's palpatory abilities are more reliable than a patient's report of tenderness
- Anterior points typically require flexion and posterior points typically require extension
- Midline points typically require pure flexion (if anterior) or pure extension (if posterior), whereas the more lateral a point is from midline, the more rotation and/or sidebending is required
- If there are multiple tender points in an area, usually the most tender one is the most significant and should be treated first
- If several tender points of equal tenderness occur in a row, treat the middle one first
- Spend a little extra time to fine-tune and completely eliminate the tenderness of a tender point
- The optimal position of comfort is obtained when the tender point is no longer tender and the tissue tension is maximally reduced
- Monitor changes in myofascial tension and adjust the treatment position to decrease the tension for maximum results
- Monitor the myofascial tissue of the tender point throughout the treatment
- For maximum results, the patient must be completely relaxed (passive) during treatment
- Recheck the tenderness of a point several times while in the treatment position
- Causative factors and mechanism of injury are unique to each patient. Therefore, the exact position of ease will vary depending on the response of the tissue during positioning
- Scan for both anterior and posterior tender points within a region/functional unit to determine the most significant
- Aim for a reduction of tenderness of less than or equal to 70% with a goal of 100%
- Use both tenderness and tissue texture abnormalities to find the best treatment position
- The presence of a therapeutic pulse indicates good myofascial relaxation
- If difficulty reducing the tenderness to zero is experienced, there usually is another more significant tender point that needs to be treated first or the patient is contracting muscles near the tender point

hours after treatment. This usually is experienced by the patient on the morning after treatment and may last 1 to 5 days, although 1 day is most typical. The reaction usually occurs only after the first treatment, but may be experienced after other treatments. The cause of the reaction is unclear, but may be related to the washout of metabolic waste products from the dysfunctional myofascial tissue. There also is a correlation with treating dysfunctions where the therapeutic pulse is palpated during treatment. In any case, the patient should be alerted to the possibility of a posttreatment reaction. Prescribing an analgesic for 1 or 2 days may help reduce the discomfort. This possibility of a posttreatment reaction also provides a reason for caution in using counterstrain to treat some gravely ill patients.

Patients want to know how often they need to be treated and how long it will take to resolve the complaint. As with all forms of manipulative treatment, there is no single, definitive answer. One treatment may eliminate the somatic dysfunction, although other dysfunctions require treatment over a more extended period of time. Jones had patients return in 3 to 7 days after the initial treatment, although 1 to 2 weeks may be more practical for many physicians. As the somatic dysfunction resolves, the time between treatments is increased. The end point of treatment depends on the cause of the problem, the underlying tissue damage, preexisting medical problems, the response of the patient, cooperation by the patient to avoid painful positions, and the skill of the physician.

EVOLUTION OF THE COUNTERSTRAIN MODEL

It is not the nature of an osteopathic physician to learn a manipulative model by memorizing a group of techniques and repeating them over and over. Andrew Still did not write a technique manual. Instead, he emphasized learning anatomy and concepts that can be applied to meet the unique needs of each patient. Therefore, it is no surprise that osteopathic physicians have modified Larry Jones' model. Classical counterstrain involves maintaining the position of release for 90 seconds, but this is not always necessary or the best option. Just as each patient is an individual, the time needed for treatment is not a constant. The physician's ability to accurately position the patient and the patient's ability to remain completely passive are two critical factors that affect the time needed. The best indicator that the treatment is complete is the palpatory response gained by monitoring the tender point. The tissues relax and rhythmic motion of the surrounding myofascial tissues returns, indicating the treatment is finished. If the myofascial tissues in the region being treated begin to unwind, the physician may choose to change from counterstrain to myofascial release to treat the somatic dysfunction. Counterstrain is classically a positional release model, but it is the physician's experience and choice whether remaining in one position or moving the dysfunctional area offers the best option for treatment.

Instead of treating a single tender point with a position of ease, Ross Pope, D.O., F.A.A.O., found stacking several regional tender points at once allows him to use a single position for treatment. This allows treatment of a region with a single position and greatly increases his efficiency. Paul Rennie, D.O., F.A.A.O., has found combining counterstrain with exercise is another approach that increases the efficiency of treatment and improves patient recovery. Specific exercises are combined with the treatment of specific tender points (Rennie et al., 2001).

Other alternatives may be used to speed up the time for the release to occur. With the patient in the counterstrain treatment position, the patient may contract the antagonist to the muscle being treated and attempt to move out of the treatment position. The contraction used is an isometric contraction commonly utilized with muscle energy technique and has been shown to be effective. Another option to decrease the time needed is to use a facilitating force applied by the physician. Compression is most commonly used, but distraction or a torque force can also be used. This approach blends well with Dr. Schiowitz' Facilitated Positional Release model. Dr. Van Buskirk used Jones' tender points as he worked on redeveloping the Still technique. He would identify a somatic dysfunction, find an associated tender point, position to eliminate the tenderness, add a compressive force, and then bring the joint from its indirect position in a continuous arc past neutral and through the restrictive barrier. He also uses distractive and torque forces as in Facilitated Positional Release. A number of osteopathic physicians, including Larry Jones, studied Janet Travell's myofascial pain syndromes and the associated trigger points described. A number of the trigger point locations described were identical to the tender point locations, so it was natural for physicians to try to treat trigger points with a counterstrain positional release approach and it was found to be quite effective (Myers, 2007; Ravin et al., 2008).

One component of the counterstrain model that has been a source of confusion for students is the nomenclature used for the tender points. Dr. Jones identified and named the points he found in several ways over a number of years. Some were named for the dysfunctional segment, others for a nearby landmark, some for an associated diagnostic finding, and a number for a muscle in which the point was located. Jones changed the names of a number of points between the publication of his two books (Jones, 1981; Jones et al., 1995), and in most cases, the change was to identify the muscle he felt was associated with the somatic dysfunction. It is time for an overall review of Jones tender points nomenclature to produce a more uniform standard for the tender point names. The basis of the system should be based on anatomy, predominately muscles. This will help students learn both the names and treatment positions more effectively.

DIAGNOSES AND TREATMENTS BY BODY REGION

The treatment illustrations that follow are intended as an introduction to the counterstrain technique model. An example from each of the 10 codable regions of the body has been chosen to illustrate a variety of treatment options. More in-depth counterstrain reference texts are available for more complete coverage of the body regions (Jones, 1981; Jones et al., 1995; Myers, 2007; Ravin et al., 2008; Rennie et al., 2004).

The treatment positions presented may be modified for the needs of the physician and the patient. Therefore, knowledge of the three-dimensional position that is typically used to treat a tender point is helpful to change the position from that described in a text. For example, a change to seated, supine, or sidelying may be preferred by either the physician or the patient. Certain conditions may necessitate changing a preferred position of treatment. For example, a pregnant patient in the third trimester may need to be treated in a side-lying position. As long as the treatment can be successfully performed, modifications may be helpful adaptations to these techniques. If you can position the patient and reduce the tenderness to zero it should be an effective treatment position.

Head (739.0): Head Region, Occipitocervical Region

Dr. Jones described a number of tender points on the head, many associated with cranial dysfunctions and the reader should refer to a counterstrain text for a description of these tender points. In addition, several of the cervical tender points are located on the skull. Two very common tender points found on the head are the anterior first cervical and posterior second cervical tender points.

Anterior First Cervical (AC1)

Tender Point Location

Found on the posterior surface of the ascending ramus of the mandible approximately 1 cm from the angle of the jaw pressing anteriorly (Fig. 49.2).

Treatment Position (Patient Supine)

Slight *flexion* of the head and upper neck, *rotation* away from the side of the tender point close to the end range of motion, and slight *sidebending* away from the side of the tender point.

Cervical Spine (739.1): Cervical Region, Cervicothoracic Region

The cervical spine has several maverick tender points (points where the position of comfort is different from what might be expected). Anterior tender points are typically located on the most anterolateral aspect of the anterior tubercles of the cervical vertebra. Posterior tender points are found on the occiput or associated with the tip of the spinous processes or lateral to the spinous processes.

Anterior Fourth Cervical (AC4)

Tender Point Locations

Found at the anterior-lateral surface of the anterior tubercle of the fourth cervical vertebrae pressing anterolateral to posteromedial (Fig. 49.3).

Treatment Position (Patient Supine)

Flexion of the head and upper neck to the fourth cervical vertebra (approximately 45 degrees). *Sidebend* and *rotate* the head and upper neck away from the side of the tender point.

Thoracic Spine (739.2): Thoracic Region, Thoracolumbar Region

Anterior thoracic spine tender points are located in two major areas. The first group of tender points, AT1-6, are located midline

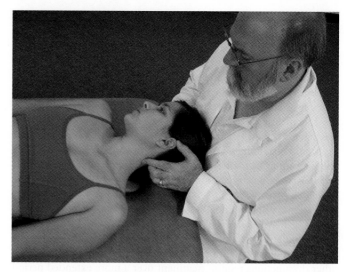

Figure 49-3   Anterior fourth cervical (AC4).

on the sternum. They can be located by palpating for tense, tender tissue overlying the sternum. The second group is located in the abdominal wall. Most are located in the rectus abdominis muscle and can be found an inch or two lateral to midline on the right or left. Posterior thoracic tender points are found on two parts of each vertebra. One location is associated with the spinous process, and is more tender on either the left or right side. The second location is on either transverse process.

The treatment described here is given for different spinal levels but are not hard and fast requirements. Extension, sidebending, and rotation to any level can be introduced either from above or below the segment. The physician's choice is based on the flexibility of the patient, patient comfort, and the relative size of the patient and physician.

Posterior Fifth Thoracic (PT5)

Tender Point Location

On the inferolateral side of the spinous process of the fifth thoracic vertebra pressing anteriorly (Fig. 49.4). Even though the spinous process is a midline structure, there will be more tenderness on one

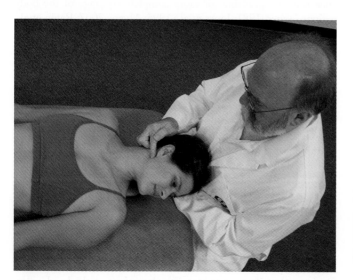

Figure 49-2   Anterior first cervical (AC1).

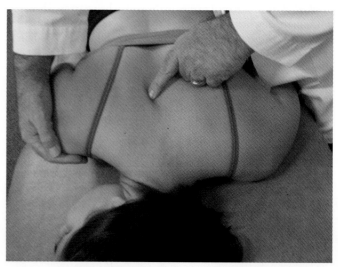

Figure 49-4   Posterior fifth thoracic (PT5).

side more than the other and also look for deviation of the spinous process.

Treatment Position (Patient Prone)
Sidebend the trunk away from the deviated side of the spinous process by pulling the opposite shoulder in a caudal and posterior direction. This creates extension with rotation and sidebending away from the deviated side.

Ribs (739.3): Rib Cage, Costochondral, Costovertebral, Sternochondral Regions

Jones used the terms "depressed" and "elevated" to refer to the tender points associated with rib somatic dysfunction. This was done to emphasize what was done with the patient to find a position of maximum comfort. The convention in current use is to name the tender points for their location on the body. In the example used here, both conventions have been combined.

Anterior tender points correspond to Jones depressed ribs and posterior tender points correspond to Jones elevated ribs. The anterior rib tender points start just below the medial end of the clavicle where the first rib attaches to the sternum and move laterally in an arc to the anterior axillary line. Most of the anterior rib tender points are on the ribs along the anterior axillary line. It is not common to find tender points below the sixth rib, but they do occur. The posterior tender points, with the exception of the first rib, are located on the angle of the ribs.

Anterior (Depressed) Third Rib (AR3)
Tender Point Location
On the third rib in the anterior axillary line, pressing from anterolateral to posteromedial (Fig. 49-5).

Treatment Position (Patient Seated)
Depression of the ipsilateral costal cage by *sidebending* that side, *flexion* of the thoracic cage, head, and neck with elevation of the contralateral shoulder and translation away from (sidebend toward) the tender point. Fine-tune with *rotation* of the body, usually toward the tender point. Sidebending can be increased with patients legs placed on the table opposite the elevated shoulder. The elevated shoulder is usually supported on the physician's thigh.

Lumbar Spine (739.4): Lumbar Region, Lumbosacral Region

Anterior lumbar spine tender points are mostly located around the rim of the pelvis anteriorly. They can be found in association with the ASIS, anterior inferior iliac spine, and anterior surface of the pubic rami. Posterior lumbar tender points are found mostly in the same places as in the thoracic spine, although the tender points found on the tips of the transverse processes need to be approached by pressing anteromedially at about a 45-degree angle.

The naming convention used for describing spinal dysfunction in the osteopathic profession is to describe the dysfunctional segment relative to the segment below it. If motion is introduced from below the dysfunctional segment, the vertebral segment below it moves first, producing a position relative to the dysfunctional segment that can seem confusing. As an example, if the vertebra below the dysfunctional segment is rotated to the right, then the relative position of the dysfunctional segment to the vertebra below is described as rotated left. This is important to understand when reading the treatment descriptions for this section.

Posterior Fifth Lumbar (PL5)
Tender Point Location
On the tip of the spinous process, testing right and left sides of the spinous process to identify the most tender side pressing anteriorly (Fig. 49.6).

Treatment Position (Patient Prone)
Extend the trunk on the ipsilateral side of the spinous process by lifting the pelvis in a posterior direction. This creates extension with the needed rotation of the lower vertebrae toward the tender point side.

Pelvis (739.5): Pelvic Region, Hip Region, Pubic Region

There are several anterior tender points and several posterior tender points that are important for diagnosis and treatment of pelvic somatic dysfunction. The anterior points typically require flexion. Rotation of varying amounts is also needed and, to a lesser degree, sidebending. Posteriorly, tender points are associated with sacral problems and muscles of the pelvis. Extension is the predominant motion associated with the posterior tender points, although several points require some degree of flexion.

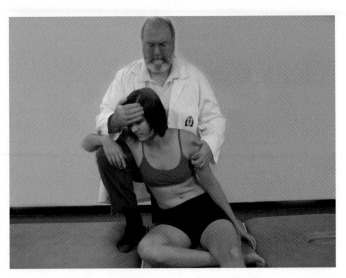

Figure 49-5   Anterior third rib (AR3).

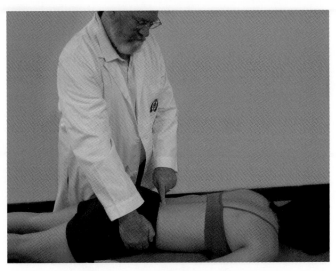

Figure 49-6   Posterior fifth lumbar (PL5).

Piriformis (PIR)
Tender Point Location
In the middle of the piriformis muscle, half way between the greater trochanter and where it attaches to the lateral side of the sacrum pressing posterolateral to anteromedial (Fig. 49.7).

Treatment Position (Patient Prone)
Marked flexion of the ipsilateral hip to about 135 degrees and marked *abduction*. *Lateral rotation* of the hip may also be required, particularly if tenderness is found more lateral on the piriformis muscle.

Pelvis (739.6): Sacral Region, Sacrococcygeal Region

A number of tender points are located on the sacrum and associated with the musculature of the posterior pelvis. The tender point locations and treatment demonstrate the counterstrain approach to the sacrococcygeal region. Because there are many tender points in the sacrococcygeal region, it is recommended that a text devoted to counterstrain is consulted for more extensive discussion of the tender points associated with this body region.

High Ilium Sacroiliac (HISI)
Tender Point Location
Found just lateral to the PSIS of the ilium, pressing lateral to medial (Fig. 49.8).

Treatment Position (Patient Prone)
Extension of the ipsilateral hip. Slight *external rotation* and *abduction* of the hip is also added.

Upper Extremity (739.7): Upper Extremities, Acromioclavicular, Sternoclavicular Regions

The tender point location and treatment demonstrates the counterstrain approach to the upper extremity. Because there are many tender points in the upper extremity, it is recommended that a text devoted to counterstrain is consulted for more extensive discussion of the tender points associated with this body region. Tender points may be found at attachment points for muscles or ligaments as well as in the belly of a dysfunctional muscle.

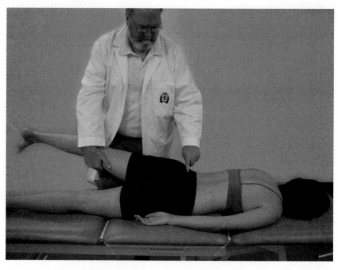

Figure 49-8 High ilium sacroiliac (HISI).

Supraspinatus (SPI)
Tender Point Location
In the middle of the supraspinatus muscle, superior to the spine of the scapula pressing cephalad to caudad (Fig. 49.9).

Treatment Position (Patient Supine)
Flexion and *abduction* to about 45 degrees and *external rotation* of the humerus.

Lower Extremity (739.8): Lower Extremities

The tender point location and treatment demonstrates the counterstrain approach to the lower extremity. Because there are many tender points in the lower extremity, it is recommended that a text devoted to counterstrain is consulted for more extensive discussion of the tender points associated with this body region. Tender points may be found at attachment points for muscles or ligaments as well as in the belly of a dysfunctional muscle.

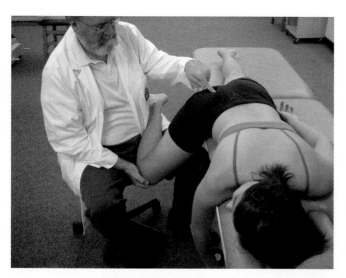

Figure 49-7 Piriformis (PIR).

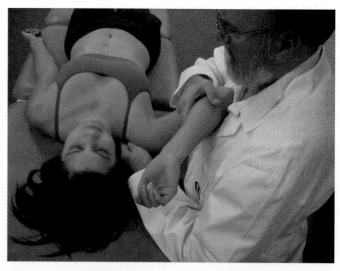

Figure 49-9 Supraspinatus (SPI).

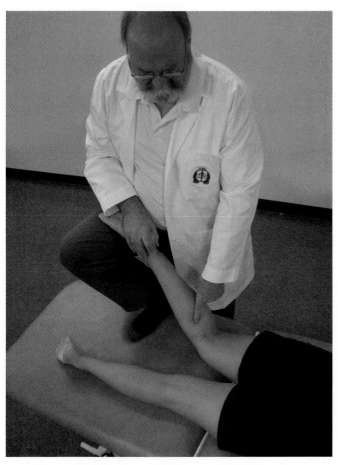

Figure 49-10   Extension ankle (EXA).

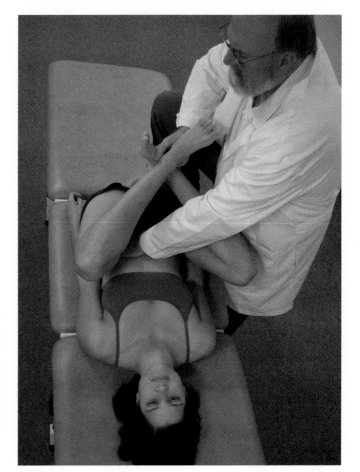

Figure 49-11   Iliacus (ILA).

Extension Ankle (EXA)

Tender Point Location
Within the two bellies of the gastrocnemius just below the lower popliteal margin, pressing posterior to anterior (Fig. 49.10).

Treatment Position (Patient Prone)
Marked *plantar flexion* of the ankle. This is usually accomplished with the patient prone and the dorsum of the involved foot supported on the physician's thigh. Pressure is put on the calcaneous to produce plantar flexion.

Abdomen (739. 9): Abdomen Region and Other

A number of tender points are found in the abdomen. These include anterior thoracic 7 to 11, iliacus and anterior lumbar 1 through 4. These tender points may also be related to viscerosomatic reflexes.

Iliacus (ILA)

Tender Point Location
At the level of the ASIS, one third of the way toward midline from the ASIS deep in the abdomen over the iliacus pressing anterior to posterior (Fig. 49.11).

Treatment Position (Patient Supine)
Marked *flexion* of the hips bilaterally to shorten the iliacus muscles. Both hips are *laterally rotated* with the knees *abducted* from the center of the body.

REFERENCES

Anonymous. Reader's thoughts on treating low back pain with counterstrain technique [Letter to the editor]. *J Am Osteopath Assoc* 1989;89:1379, 1384, 1387.

Bailey M, Dick L. Nociceptive considerations in treating with counterstrain. *J Am Osteopath Assoc* 1992;92(3):334, 337–341.

Beal MC. Viscerosomatic reflexes: a review. *J Am Osteopath Assoc* 1985; 85(12):786–801.

Brandt B Jr, Jones LH. Some methods of applying counterstrain. *J Am Osteopath Assoc* 1976;75(9):786–789.

Cislo S, Ramirez MA, Schwartz HR. Low back pain: treatment of forward and backward sacral torsions using counterstrain technique. *J Am Osteopath Assoc* 1991;91(3):255–256, 259.

Educational Council on Osteopathic Principles. *Glossary of Osteopathic Terminology* (Revised ed., p. 29). Chevy Chase, MD: American Association of Colleges of Osteopathic Medicine, 2009.

Dodd JG, Good MM, Nguyen TL. In vitro biophysical strain model for understanding mechanisms of osteopathic manipulative treatment. *J Am Osteopath Assoc* 2006;106:157–166.

Howell JN. Cabell KS, Chila AG. Stretch reflex and Hoffmann reflex responses to osteopathic manipulative treatment in subjects with achilles tendinitis. *J Am Osteopath Assoc* 2006;106: 537–545.

Jacobson EC, Lockwood MD, Hoefner VC Jr, et al. Shoulder pain and repetition strain injury to the supraspinatus muscle: etiology and manipulative treatment. *J Am Osteopath Assoc* 1989;89(8):1037–1040, 1043–1045.

Jones LH. Foot trauma without hand trauma. *J Am Osteopath Assoc* 1973;72(1):87–95.

Jones LH. Missed anterior spinal lesions: a preliminary report. *DO* 1966;6:75–79.

Jones LH. Spontaneous release by positioning. *DO* 1964;4:109–116.

Jones LH. *Strain and Counterstrain*. Newark, OH: American Academy of Osteopathy, 1981.

Jones LH, Kusunose R, Goering E. *Jones Strain-Counterstrain*. Boise, ID: Jones Strain-Counterstrain, 1995.

Korr IM. Proprioceptors and somatic dysfunction. *J Am Osteopath Assoc* 1974;74:638–650.

Luckenbill-Edds L, Bechill GB. Nerve compression syndromes as models for research on osteopathic manipulative treatment. *J Am Osteopath Assoc* 1995;95(5), 319–326.

Meltzer KR, Standley PR. Modeled repetitive motion strain and indirect osteopathic manipulative techniques in regulation of human fibroblast proliferation and interleukin secretion. *J Am Osteopath Assoc* 2007;107:527–536.

Mense S. Pathophysiologic basis of muscle pain syndromes: an update. *Phys Med Rehabil Clin N Am* 1997;8(1):23–53.

Myers H, Devine W, Glover J. *Clinical Application of Counterstrain*. Tucson, AZ: Arizona Osteopathic Association, 2006.

Radjieski JM, Lumley MA, Cantieri MS. Effect of osteopathic manipulative treatment of length of stay for pancreatitis: a randomized pilot study. *J Am Osteopath Assoc* 1998;98(5):264–272.

Ramirez MA, Haman J, Worth L. Low back pain: diagnosis by six newly discovered sacral tender points and treatment with counterstrain. *J Am Osteopath Assoc* 1989;89(7):905–906, 911–913.

Ravin T, Cantieri M, Pasquarello G. *Principles of Prolotherapy*. Denver, CO: American Academy of Manual Medicine, 2008.

Rennie PR, Glover JC, Carvalho C, et al. *Counterstrain and Exercise: An Integrated Approach*. Williamston, MI: RennieMatrix, 2001.

Rennie PR. Counterstrain tender points as indicators of sustained abnormal metabolism: advancing the counterstrain mechanism of action theory. *AAO J* 2007:17–23.

Schwartz HR. The use of counterstrain in an acutely ill in-hospital population. *J Am Osteopath Assoc* 1986;86(7):433–442.

Travell JG, Simons DG. *Myofascial Pain and Dysfunction: The Trigger Point Manual*. Vol 1. Baltimore, MD: Williams & Wilkins, 1999.

Van Buskirk RL. Nociceptive reflexes and the somatic dysfunction: a model. *J Am Osteopath Assoc* 1990;90(9):792–794, 797–809.

Woolbright JL. An alternative method of teaching strain/counterstrain. *J Am Osteopath Assoc* 1991;91(4):370, 373–376.

Wynne MM, Burns JM, Eland DC, et al. Effect of counterstrain on stretch reflexes, Hoffmann reflexes, and clinical outcomes in subjects with plantar fasciitis. *JAOA* 2006;106(9):547–556.

Yates HA, Glover JC. *Counterstrain: A Handbook of Osteopathic Technique*. Tulsa, OK: Y Knot Publishers, 1994.

Recommended References

1. Jones LH, Kusunose R, Goering E. *Jones Strain-Counterstrain*. Boise, ID: Jones Strain-Counterstrain, 1995.

2. Myers H, Devine W, Glover J, et al. *Clinical Application of Counterstrain*. Tucson, AZ: Arizona Osteopathic Association, 2007.

3. Nicholas A, Nicholas E. *Atlas of Osteopathic Techniques*. Philadelphia, PA: Lippincott Williams & Wilkins, 2008.

4. Ravin T, Cantieri M, Pasquarello G. *Principles of Prolotherapy*. American Academy of Manual Medicine, 2008.

5. Rennie PR, Glover JC, Carvalho C, et al. *Counterstrain and Exercise: An Integrated Approach*. 2nd Ed. Williamston, MI: RennieMatrix, 2004.

Soft Tissue/Articulatory Approach

WALTER C. EHRENFEUCHTER

CASE STUDY

A 54-year-old man presents to the office with a sore throat and dry cough. He complains of an ulcer on the buccal surface of his left cheek. He admits to having similar ulcers around his mouth in the past. He denies other complaints.

Physical examination:

Vital signs are normal. Exam of the buccal mucosa reveals a shallow ulcer with a red border approximately 2 mm in diameter; tongue is in the midline; there is no tonsillar hypertrophy or erythema; teeth in good repair. Small left submental node is palpable. CV, pulmonary, abdominal, and neurologic exams are noncontributory. Structural exam reveals rigid, tender, hypertonic paravertebral musculature from the C5 to T2 spinal levels bilaterally. Rib 4 on the left is held in exhalation.

Diagnosis

1. Acute herpetic stomatitis
2. Somatic dysfunction—cervical, thoracic, rib

Plan

1. Treatment with antiviral medication
2. Soft tissue technique on the hypertonic cervicothoracic musculature
3. Articulatory technique on the rib dysfunction

SOFT TISSUE TECHNIQUE (INHIBITION-VIDA INFRA)

Treatment Position

Patient: Supine
  Physician: Seated at the head of the table

Procedure

1. You place the pads of the fingers of both hands beneath the cervicothoracic junction, just lateral to the spinous processes (Fig. 50.1)
2. You extend the cervicothoracic junction until you feel the musculature relax under your fingers
3. You then maintain a deep sustained pressure over these muscles until they are further felt to soften (release). This may take anywhere from 30 seconds to several minutes
4. Success of the technique is determined through palpation to reassess the characteristics of the soft tissues that prompted

the selection of the technique to begin with. Success may also be determined in part by reassessing the patient's symptomatology (sore throat and cough)

ARTICULATORY TECHNIQUE

Dysfunction

Position: Rib 4 held in exhalation
  Restriction: Rib 4 is restricted in inhalation

Treatment Position

Patient: Lateral recumbent—lying on the right side
  Physician: Standing behind the patient at the side of the treatment table

Procedure

1. Place your caudad hand posterior to the left iliac crest to stabilize the body (Fig. 50.2)
2. Place your caudad knee against the angle of rib 4 on the left and maintain a firm steady pressure (a folded towel or small pillow may be needed between your knee and the rib to minimize patient discomfort) (Fig. 50.3)
3. With your cephalad hand, grasp the patient's left arm just proximal to the wrist
4. Smoothly carry the left shoulder into a combination of flexion and abduction in order to place the pectoralis minor muscle on passive stretch (Fig. 50.4). It is the tension on this muscle combined with the gapping force provided by the knee that allows the rib to easily articulate (Fig. 50.5)
5. Success of the technique is determined by reassessing respiratory motion of rib 4. Success may also be determined in part by reassessing the patient's symptomatology (sore throat and cough) (1)

INTRODUCTION

Soft Tissue Technique

Definition

Soft tissue techniques are defined as direct techniques that address the muscular and fascial structures of the body and associated neural and vascular elements.

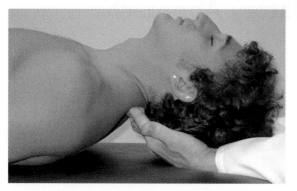

Figure 50-1   Cervicothoracic inhibition technique.

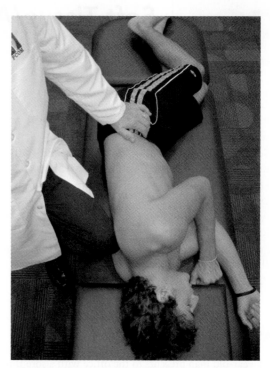

Figure 50-3   Articulatory technique. Upper rib: exhalation dysfunction, step 2.

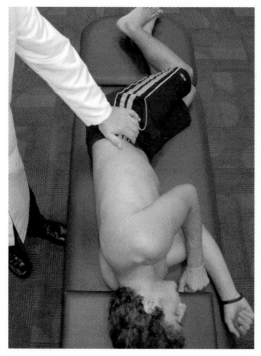

Figure 50-2   Articulatory technique. Upper rib: exhalation dysfunction, step 1.

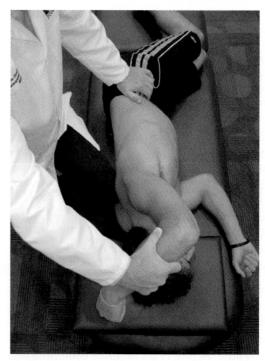

Figure 50-4   Articulatory technique. Upper rib: exhalation dysfunction, step 4.

History

Preparation of the soft tissues in order to achieve improved articular motion has been one of the basic tenets of the manipulative approach since the early days of A.T. Still. Based on descriptions provided by his students, it is believed that Dr. Still made extensive use of the soft tissue style—direct inhibitory pressure.

Indications

Soft tissue techniques may be applied in a number of different ways to:

- Relax hypertonic muscles and reduce spasm
- Stretch and increase the elasticity of shortened fascial structures
- Enhance circulation to local myofascial structures
- Improve local tissue nutrition, oxygenation, and removal of metabolic wastes
- Improve abnormal somato-somatic and somato-visceral reflex activities, thus improving circulation in areas of the body remote from the area being treated
- Diagnostically to identify areas of restricted motion, tissue texture changes, and sensitivity

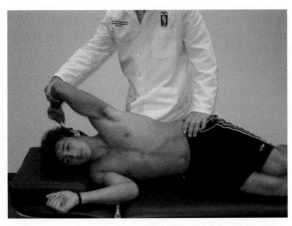

Figure 50-5 Articulatory technique. Upper rib: exhalation dysfunction, step 4.

- Observe tissue response to the application of manipulative technique
- Improve local and systemic immune response
- Provide a general state of relaxation
- Provide a general state of tonic stimulation by stimulating the stretch reflex in hypotonic muscles

Other techniques used on more superficial soft tissue structures include variations on techniques developed in the European massage movement. These include:

- Effleurage—a light stroking movement
- Petrissage—kneading of the muscles
- Tapotement—striking with the side of the hand
- Skin rolling—lifting the skin away from the deeper structures and "rolling" the skin fold along the body

Contraindications

Relative Contraindications
Individual techniques may be contraindicated in specific situations such as; in a patient with severe osteoporosis, prone pressure techniques may be contraindicated in the thoracocostal region, but lateral recumbent techniques could be easily applied.

Direct techniques that stretch acutely injured muscles, tendons, ligaments, or joint capsules may do additional damage to these structures, or increase the amount of pain the patient experiences and are therefore contraindicated.

Articulatory Technique

Definition
Articulatory techniques have also been called springing techniques and are defined as direct techniques. In these techniques, the physician gently and repetitively carries the body part being treated through the restrictive barrier. This form of technique could also be called low-velocity/high-amplitude technique. Many of these techniques use long lever forces to achieve their effects.

History
Articulatory techniques are at least as old as the osteopathic profession itself. In fact, the only film clip that exists of A.T. Still performing a technique is 9 seconds long and appears to be a shoulder or clavicular articulatory technique.

Indications
Articulatory technique is indicated when the restrictive barriers to motion appear to be in a joint itself or in the periarticular tissues. It can be used to affect a single joint (e.g., the Glenohumeral joint) or for an entire region (e.g., the thoracic cage). It is well tolerated by arthritic patients, elderly or frail individuals, as well as critically ill or postoperative patients. Also infants and very young patients, as well as others who are unable to cooperate with instructions for other techniques often derive great benefit from articulatory techniques.

Contraindications

Relative Contraindications
In the upper cervical region, due to the possibility of vertebral artery compromise, it is wise to avoid the combination of repetitive rotation and extension.

Absolute Contraindications to Both Soft Tissue and Articulatory Techniques
Many techniques including soft tissue and articulatory techniques are contraindicated for use in the local region of any of the following conditions:

- Fracture or dislocation
- Neurologic entrapment syndromes
- Serious vascular compromise
- Local malignancy
- Local infection (e.g., cellulitis, abscess, septic arthritis, osteomyelitis)
- Bleeding disorders

BASIC TECHNIQUE PRINCIPLES

Soft Tissue Technique
1. The patient should be comfortable and able to relax
2. The physician should also be in a position of comfort to minimize energy expenditure and make use of body weight and leverage rather than having to exert muscular force
3. Initially, the applied forces are very gentle and of low amplitude. The force is applied rhythmically, typically 1 or 2 seconds of stretch followed by a similar time frame releasing that stretch
4. As the soft tissues are palpated responding to the technique, the applied forces can be increased to increase the amplitude of the technique. The rate of application typically remains the same
5. The applied forces should be comfortable for the patient. Some patients experience some discomfort, but it is recognized by the patient as a good discomfort
6. Do not allow your hands to create friction by sliding across the skin or rubbing it. The physician's hand should carry the skin with it as the activating force is applied. Do not compress the musculature directly against a bone
7. The technique is continued until the desired effect is achieved. This typically means that the amplitude of excursion of the soft tissues has reached a maximum and has plateaued at that level

Articulatory Technique
1. The patient should be comfortable and able to relax
2. The physician should also be in a position of comfort to minimize energy expenditure and make use of body weight and leverage rather than having to exert muscular force

3. The physician moves the affected joint or body part through its range of motion until the restrictive barrier is engaged

4. A gentle but firm force is applied carrying the body part a short distance through the restrictive barrier. The distance is limited by the tissues being treated and the patient's tolerance to pain or fatigue

5. This force is applied rhythmically, typically 1 or 2 seconds of stretch followed by a similar time frame releasing that stretch. The joint is permitted to return to a point just short of its restrictive barrier

6. As the patient responds to the technique, the restrictive barrier will shift position within the physiologic range of motion. For each cycle of the applied technique, reengage the restrictive barrier and carry the affected body part a short distance further through that new barrier to normal motion

7. The applied forces should be comfortable for the patient. Some patients experience some discomfort, but it is recognized by the patient as a good discomfort

8. The technique is continued until the location of the restrictive barrier reaches a plateau; that is, no further increase in range of motion can be achieved by continuing the technique, or until full physiologic range of motion has been restored to the joint(s) being treated

9. At no time is the anatomic barrier to joint motion exceeded

TYPES OF TECHNIQUES

Soft Tissue Technique

Parallel Traction

In this type of soft tissue technique, the forces being applied are parallel to the myofascial structures needing treatment. This may be done by separating the proximal and distal attachments of the muscle (both hands moving in opposite directions like a taffy pull) or by anchoring one end of the muscle and pulling on the other (one hand or structure serving as a stationary anchor, the other one mobile) (Fig. 50.6).
Example: Intermittent cervical traction

Diagnosis
1. Hypertonicity of the cervical musculature
2. Bulging cervical disc
3. Cervical degenerative disc disease

Treatment Position
Patient: Supine on the treatment table
   Physician: Seated at the head of the table

Procedure
1. The physician's one hand cradles the occiput with the thumb and index finger spanning the region just caudad to the superior nuchal line

2. The physician's other hand cradles the chin. (In some patients, this will aggravate a preexisting temporomandibular joint or dental problem—for those cases, an alternative is to place this hand across the patient's forehead.) (Fig. 50.7)

3. The physician applies axial cephalad traction with both hands simultaneously, maintaining the head and neck in a neutral to slightly flexed position. The occipital hand must not squeeze the occiput or there is the risk of compressing the occipitomastoid suture

4. This technique is applied slowly and rhythmically with gradually increasing amplitude (Fig. 50.8)

5. The technique is continued until the desired soft tissue or disc response is obtained. This may take anywhere from 2 to 5 minutes

6. Success of the technique is determined through palpation to reassess the characteristics of the soft tissues that prompted the selection of the technique to begin with. Success may also be determined in part by reassessing the patient's symptomatology

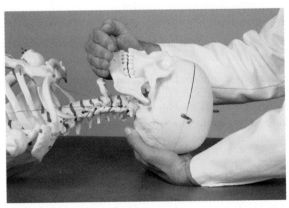

Figure 50-7 Intermittent cervical traction. (Used from Nicholas & Nicholas. *Atlas of Osteopathic Technique.* Philadelphia, PA: Lippincott, Williams & Wilkins, with permission.)

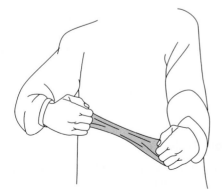

Figure 50-6 The taffy pull.

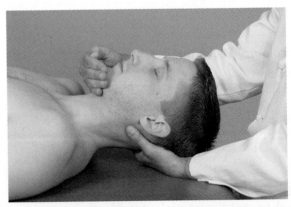

Figure 50-8 Intermittent cervical traction. (Used from Nicholas & Nicholas. *Atlas of Osteopathic Technique.* Philadelphia, PA: Lippincott, Williams & Wilkins, with permission.)

Perpendicular Traction

In this type of soft tissue technique, the myofascial structure being treated is contacted near its midpoint between the proximal and distal attachments, and a stretching force is applied at right angles to the muscle's longitudinal axis (e.g., similar to an archer stretching a bowstring) (Fig. 50.9).

Example: Contralateral traction

Diagnosis: Hypertonicity of the cervical paraspinal musculature

Treatment Position

Patient: Supine on the treatment table

 Physician: Standing at the side of the head of the treatment table

Procedure

1. The physician's cephalad hand bridges the forehead to stabilize and control head motion (Fig. 50.10)
2. The physician's caudad hand reaches around the side of the neck to contact the cervical paraspinal musculature just lateral to the spinous processes
3. While keeping the caudad elbow locked in extension, the physician rotates his/her upper trunk to draw that arm upward, drawing the paraspinal musculature ventrally. Force must be exerted with the cephalad hand to control the head and ensure that minimal cervical extension occurs
4. Care must be taken not to apply too much pressure to the lateral aspect of the cervical region as this may provoke bradycardia and hypotension due to a reflex carotid body response
5. This technique is applied slowly and rhythmically with gradually increasing amplitude
6. The technique is continued until the desired soft tissue response is obtained. This may take anywhere from 2 to 5 minutes

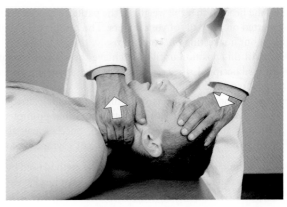

Figure 50-10 Contralateral traction. (Used from Nicholas & Nicholas. *Atlas of Osteopathic Technique*, Philadelphia, PA: Lippincott, Williams & Wilkins, with permission.)

7. Success of the technique is determined through palpation to reassess the characteristics of the soft tissues that prompted the selection of the technique to begin with. Success may also be determined in part by reassessing the patient's symptomatology

Note: By increasing the rotational force, this technique may be converted to an articulatory technique. By adding more of an axial milking motion, it may be used to enhance lymphatic drainage in the cervical lymph node chains.

Inhibition

In this type of soft tissue technique, the myofascial structure being treated is contacted over the musculotendinous portion of the hypertonic muscle and a force is directed straight into the muscle. Pressing into a hypertonic muscle belly can be painful and may bruise the muscle; therefore, pressure should be directed to the musculotendinous junction.

Example: Suboccipital inhibition

Diagnosis: Hypertonic suboccipital musculature

Treatment Position

Patient: Supine

 Physician: Seated at the head of the treatment table

Procedure

1. Places the pads of your fingers just inferior to the superior nuchal line in the suboccipital soft tissues (Fig. 50.11)

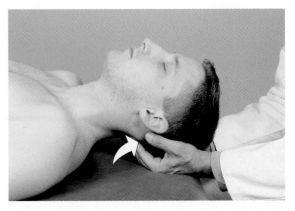

Figure 50-11 Suboccipital inhibition. (Used from Nicholas & Nicholas. *Atlas of Osteopathic Technique*. Philadelphia, PA: Lippincott, Williams & Wilkins with permission.)

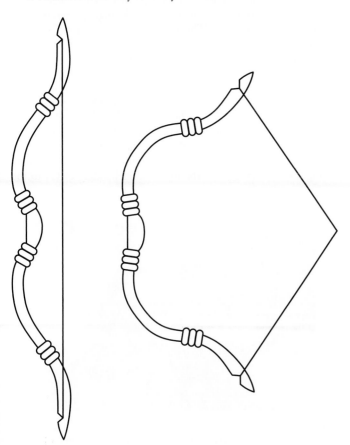

Figure 50-9 The bowstring.

2. Lifts the head so that the weight of the patient's head is entirely supported on the pads of your fingers. The head is held slightly above, but not resting on, your palms
3. Maintain this position until you achieve the desired relaxation of the suboccipital tissues. This may take anywhere from 30 seconds to several minutes
4. Success of the technique is determined through palpation to reassess the characteristics of the soft tissues that prompted the selection of the technique to begin with. Success may also be determined in part by reassessing the patient's symptomatology

Note: This technique is similar in position to the method used by A.T. Still when he created a rope sling to relieve his own headaches.

Articulatory Technique

Regional

Articulatory techniques may be applied to entire regions of the spine to improve regional range of motion when the restriction to motion is perceived by the physician to have an articular component to it.
Example: Cervical sidebending

Diagnosis

Position: Cervical spine is sidebent left.
 Restriction: Cervical region is restricted in right sidebending.

Treatment Position

Patient: Lateral recumbent, lying of the side of the positional diagnosis
 Physician: Sitting on the side of the table in front of the patient, facing the patient's head

Procedure

1. Take your left arm and place the patient's right shoulder in your left axilla (Fig. 50.12)
2. Your left hand will grasp the spinous process of T1 to serve as an anchor and a reference for motion during this technique
3. With your right hand, grasp the patient's head in the left occipitoparietal region and support it in a position neutral to the rest of the spine
4. Lift the patient's head up toward the ceiling until you palpate motion occurring at the T1 level. This is your initial restrictive barrier

5. Stretch the cervical spine through this motion barrier, using your left hand to anchor T1
 (a) Hold this position briefly (<1 second), then return the neck to a position just away from the restrictive barrier
6. Rhythmically repeat step 5 as many times as is necessary to achieve full physiologic range of motion for the cervical spine in regional sidebending
7. If you are unable to reach full range of motion, continue the technique until there is no further advancement of the restrictive barrier toward the physiologic barrier
8. Success of the technique is determined by retesting cervical regional sidebending range of motion

Segmental

Segmental articulatory techniques are applied to segmental motion restrictions that are perceived to be articular in nature in the vertebral column.
Example: Segmental somatic dysfunction—C4

Diagnosis

Position: C4 is rotated right and sidebent right.
 Restriction: C4 is restricted in left rotation and left sidebending.

Treatment Position

Patient: Supine
 Physician: Standing at the head of the treatment table

Procedure

1. Cradle the patient's head between your two hands (Fig. 50.13)
2. Place the pad of your right index or middle finger posterior to the articular process of C4. This is the articulating finger
3. Place the pad of your left index or middle finger posterior to the articular process of C5. This finger will serve as an anchor and a reference to palpate segmental motion at this level
4. Position the cervical spine so that the C4/5 motion segment is in neutral in the sagittal plane
5. Use your hands to turn the head to the left until you palpate the motion reach the C5 palpating finger. This is your initial restrictive barrier. (Remember that sidebending and rotation are always coupled motions to the same side in the C2-6 region. You cannot produce one without producing the other.)
6. Holding the head and neck stable, use your right articulating finger to exaggerate the rotation/sidebending of C4 to the

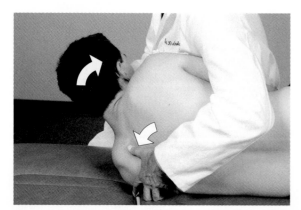

Figure 50-12 Cervical sidebending. (Used from Nicholas & Nicholas. *Atlas of Osteopathic Technique*. Philadelphia, PA: Lippincott, Williams & Wilkins, with permission.)

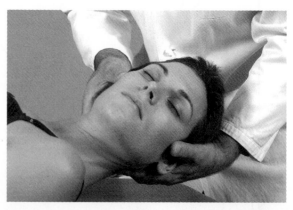

Figure 50-13 Segmental somatic dysfunction: C4. (Used from Nicholas & Nicholas. *Atlas of Osteopathic Technique*. Philadelphia, PA: Lippincott, Williams & Wilkins, with permission.)

left. Hold this position briefly (<1 second) and then allow the return of the C4 segment to its position just before engaging the restrictive barrier

7. Rhythmically repeat step 6 as many times as is necessary to achieve full physiologic range of motion for C4

8. If you are unable to reach full range of motion, continue the technique until there is no further advancement of the restrictive barrier toward the physiologic barrier

9. Success of the technique is determined by retesting segmental motion at the C4 level

Peripheral

Articulatory techniques are especially useful in treating restriction of motion of the peripheral limb joints.
Example: Radiocarpal joint restriction

Diagnosis

Position: Radiocarpal joint extended
 Restriction: Radiocarpal joint restricted in flexion

Treatment Position

Patient: Supine with dysfunctional arm extended toward the ceiling.
 Physician: Standing at the side of the treatment table on the side of dysfunction.

Procedure

1. The physician clasps the hand from both sides with his/her hands. The first hand clasps the patient's hand in a fashion similar to a grip taken in arm wrestling (Fig. 50.14)

2. Steady traction is exerted upward toward the ceiling by the physician. The hand is held pointing vertically toward the ceiling throughout the technique (Fig. 50.15)

3. The patient's wrist is flexed to the restrictive barrier by carrying the patient's shoulder toward flexion (Fig. 50.16)

4. The radiocarpal joint is carried further into flexion through the restrictive barrier and held there for a brief period of time (less than a second). The radiocarpal joint is then allowed to return to a position just before the restrictive barrier by slightly extending the shoulder (Fig. 50.17)

5. Rhythmically repeat step 4 as many times as is necessary to achieve full physiologic range of motion for the radiocarpal joint

6. If you are unable to reach full range of motion, continue the technique until there is no further advancement of the restrictive barrier toward the physiologic barrier

7. The same techniques can be carried out in radial or ulnar deviation and circumduction (Fig. 50.18A and B)

8. Success of the technique is determined by retesting radiocarpal range of motion

TECHNIQUE EXAMPLES

739.0: Head and Suboccipital Somatic Dysfunction

Soft Tissue Technique
Temporalis Muscle
Diagnosis
Hypertonicity of the temporalis muscle

Type of Soft Tissue Technique
Parallel traction

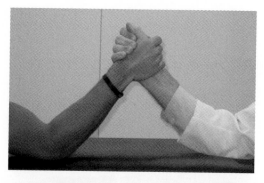

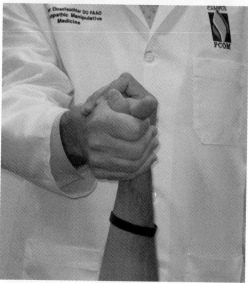

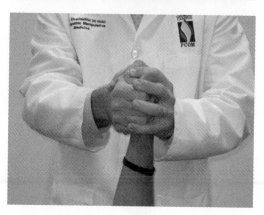

Figure 50-14   A–C. Radiocarpal restriction.

Treatment Position
Patient: Supine with head turned to place dysfunctional temporalis muscle superiorly
 Physician: Seated at the side of the table facing the patient.

Procedure
1. Place your cephalad hand beneath the patient's head to prevent excessive head movement (Fig. 50.19)
2. Take the thumb of your caudad hand and place it approximately 2 cm caudad to the temporal lines in the region of the temporalis muscle previously determined to be hypertonic. Your other fingers extend over the top of the skull

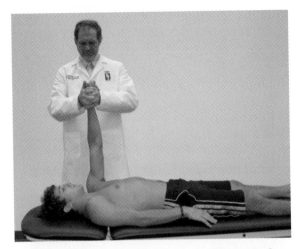

Figure 50-15   Radiocarpal joint restriction, step 2.

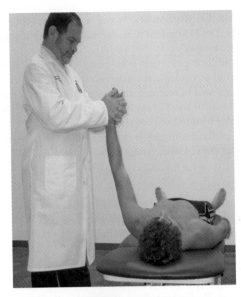

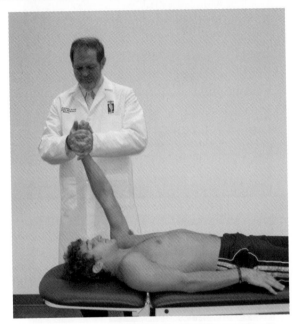

Figure 50-16   Radiocarpal joint restriction, step 3.

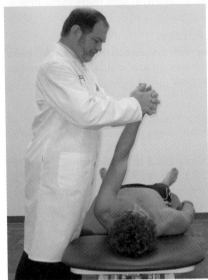

Figure 50-18   A-B. Radiocarpal joint restriction, step 9.

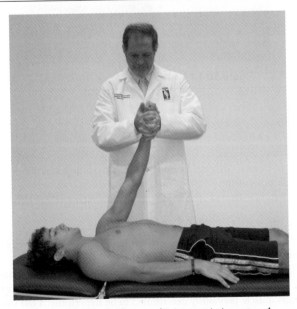

Figure 50-17   Radiocarpal joint restriction, step 4.

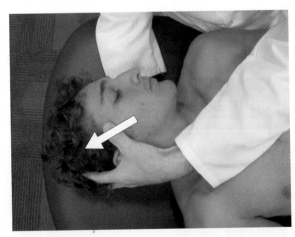

Figure 50-19   Temporalis muscle soft tissue.

3. The one end of the temporalis muscle is anchored by its attachment to the coronoid process. Your thumb then exerts a force directly toward the skull until sufficient pressure to engage the musculature is achieved
4. Exert a tractional force parallel to the muscle fiber direction toward the top of the skull
5. Apply this force gently and rhythmically every 1 to 2 seconds. Note the softening of the soft tissue structures as you continue this technique for 1 to 2 minutes. (The time frame is shortened here because of the smaller size of the muscle being treated.)
6. Success of the technique is determined by repalpating the previously hypertonic temporalis muscle

Articulatory Technique
Temporomandibular Joint
Diagnosis
Position: Mandible laterally translated to the right
   Restriction: Mandible restricted in left lateral translation

Type of Articulatory Technique
Peripheral

Treatment Position
Patient: Supine with the head turned with the side to be treated superior.
   Physician: Seated at the side of the head of the table facing the patient.

Procedure
1. The physician's cephalad hand is placed under the patient's head, elevating it slightly (Fig. 50.20)
2. The physician's caudad hand is positioned with the third, fourth, and fifth fingers along the posterior border of the ramus of the mandible and the hypothenar eminence along the body of the jaw
3. The patient is instructed to open the mouth slightly
4. The physician exerts pressure with the hand on the jaw so as to draw the jaw forward at the temporomandibular joint and deviate the jaw laterally to the left
5. This traction on the jaw is applied and released in a slow rhythmic pattern, continuing the technique for 30 seconds to 2 minutes
6. Success of the technique is determined by reassessing mandibular range of motion in lateral translation.

739.1 Cervical Somatic Dysfunction
Soft Tissue Technique
Cradling with Traction
Diagnosis
Hypertonicity of the cervical paraspinal musculature

Type of Soft Tissue Technique
Parallel traction

Treatment Position
Patient: Supine
   Physician: Seated at the head of the table

Procedure
1. The physician's fingers are placed under the patient's neck bilaterally, with the finger pads contacting the cervical paraspinal musculature overlying the articular pillars and just lateral to the spinous processes (Fig. 50.21)
2. The physician exerts pressure ventrally of sufficient force to engage the soft tissues without extending the cervical spine
3. The physician pulls the hands cephalad producing a longitudinal traction
4. This traction is slowly released
5. The physician's hands are repositioned along the cervical pillars and steps 2 to 4 are repeated in a gentle rhythmic manner
6. This technique is continued for 2 to 5 minutes
7. Success of the technique is determined by repalpating the previously hypertonic cervical musculature

Articulatory Technique
Segmental Cervical Extension
Diagnosis
Position: C4 flexed (flexed dysfunctions are commonly found following whiplash injuries)
   Restriction: C4 restricted in extension

Type of Articulatory Technique
Segmental
Treatment Position
Patient: Supine
   Physician: Seated at the head of the treatment table

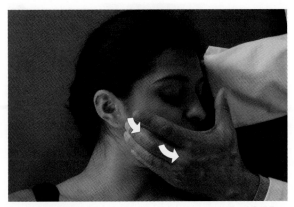

Figure 50-20 • Temporomandibular joint articulatory technique. (Used from Nicholas & Nicholas. *Atlas of Osteopathic Technique.* Philadelphia, PA: Lippincott, Williams & Wilkins, with permission.)

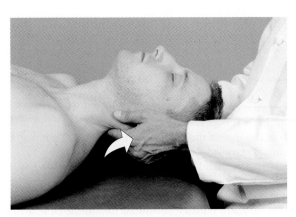

Figure 50-21 • Cradling with traction soft tissue technique. (Used from Nicholas & Nicholas. *Atlas of Osteopathic Technique.* Philadelphia, PA: Lippincott, Williams & Wilkins, with permission.)

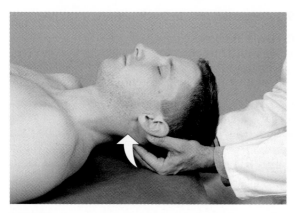

Figure 50-22 Segmental cervical extension articulatory technique. (Used from Nicholas & Nicholas. *Atlas of Osteopathic Technique.* Philadelphia, PA: Lippincott, Williams & Wilkins, with permission.)

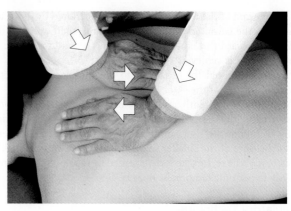

Figure 50-23 Prone pressure with counterpressure soft tissue technique. (Used from Nicholas & Nicholas. *Atlas of Osteopathic Technique.* Philadelphia, PA: Lippincott, Williams & Wilkins, with permission.)

Procedure

1. The physician's fingers are placed under the patient's neck bilaterally, with the finger pads contacting the C4 articular processes and lateral to the spinous processes (Fig. 50.22)
2. The physician exerts pressure ventrally of sufficient force to extend C4 on C5 to the initial restrictive barrier
3. C4 is carried through its restrictive barrier into further extension and held there for a brief period of time (less than a second). C4 is then allowed to return to a position just before the restrictive barrier by releasing the extension force
4. Rhythmically repeat step 3 as many times as is necessary to achieve full physiologic range of motion for C4
5. If you are unable to reach full range of motion, continue the technique until there is no further advancement of the restrictive barrier toward the physiologic barrier
6. Success of the technique is determined by retesting C4 segmental extension

739.2 Thoracic Somatic Dysfunction

Soft Tissue Technique
Prone Pressure with Counterpressure

Diagnosis
Thoracic paravertebral muscle hypertonicity

Type of Soft Tissue Technique
Parallel traction

Treatment Position
Patient: Prone with the head turned toward the physician
   Physician: Standing at the side of the table facing the patient's thorax.

Procedure

1. Place your caudad hand on the far side of the spine; the heel of your hand is over the transverse process of the thoracic vertebra at the level of the hypertonic musculature. Your fingers are pointing cephalad (Fig. 50.23)
2. Place your cephalad hand on the near side of the spine, with the heel of your hand over the opposite transverse process of that same vertebral segment. Your fingers are pointing caudad
3. Exert sufficient pressure downward toward the table to engage the myofascial structures of the spine
4. Once this has been accomplished, exert a longitudinal force simultaneously with both hands

5. This pressure is slowly released
6. The hands are both repositioned together either a segment cephalad or caudad depending upon the needs of the patient
7. Steps 3 to 6 are repeated in a rhythmic fashion for 2 to 5 minutes
8. Success of the technique is determined by palpating the previously hypertonic thoracic paravertebral musculature

Articulatory Technique
Thoracic Sidebending

Diagnosis
Position: T8 sidebent left
   Restriction: T8 restricted in right sidebending

Type of Articulatory Technique
Segmental

Treatment Position
Patient: Prone with the head turned toward the physician
   Physician: Standing at the side of the table facing the patient's thorax

Procedure

1. Place your caudad hand on the far side of the spine, the heel of your hand is over the transverse process of T8. Your fingers are pointing cephalad (Fig. 50.24)

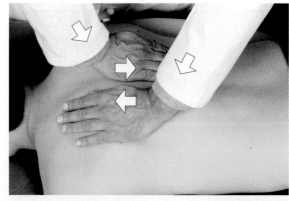

Figure 50-24 Thoracic sidebending articulatory technique. (Used from Nicholas & Nicholas. *Atlas of Osteopathic Technique.* Philadelphia, PA: Lippincott, Williams & Wilkins, with permission.)

2. Place your cephalad hand on the near side of the spine, with the heel of your hand over the opposite transverse process of T8. Your fingers are pointing caudad

3. Exert sufficient pressure downward toward the table to produce articular motion of the spine

4. Once this has been accomplished, exert a longitudinal force simultaneously with both hands to carry T8 through its restrictive barrier and hold it there briefly (<1 second). This pressure is slowly released allowing T8 to return to a position just before engaging the restrictive barrier

5. Steps 3 and 4 are repeated in a rhythmic fashion until full physiologic motion has been restored to T8

6. If you are unable to reach full range of motion, continue the technique until there is no further advancement of the restrictive barrier toward the physiologic barrier

7. Success of the technique is determined by reassessing segmental sidebending at T8

739.3 Lumbar Somatic Dysfunction

Soft Tissue Technique
Lumbar Seated Technique for Paraspinal Tissues
Diagnosis
Hypertonicity of the left lumbar paraspinal musculature.

Type of Soft Tissue Technique
Perpendicular traction

Treatment Position
Patient: Seated, straddling the treatment table with his/her back to the end of the table.
   Physician: Standing behind the patient toward the side opposite the side to be treated. Table height should be adjusted so that the physician stands roughly one head taller than the patient.

Procedure
1. Instruct the patient to place their left hand behind their neck. They are then instructed to grasp the left elbow with the right hand (Fig. 50.25)
2. Place the heel of your left hand on the patient's left paraspinal muscle mass, just lateral to the spinous processes
3. Take your right arm, pass it in front of the patient (under the right upper arm), and grasp the patient's left upper arm
4. Instruct the patient to lean forward and relax so that their weight will be carried by your right arm. The patient will have a natural tendency to rotate their trunk to the right

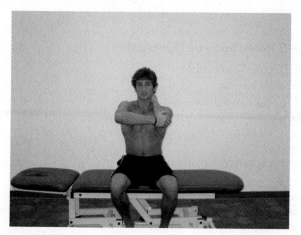

Figure 50-25   Lumbar seated technique for paraspinal tissues.

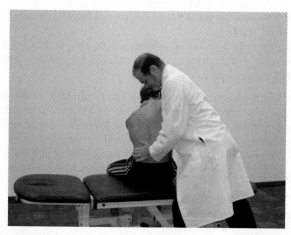

Figure 50-26   Lumbar seated technique for paraspinal tissues, step 6.

5. Carry the hypertonic paraspinal musculature laterally away from the spine with your left hand. Simultaneously turn your body to the right so that the rotation of the patient's trunk to the right is exaggerated

6. This traction and rotation is held for as short time and then it is released. The natural tension of the soft tissues will return the lumbar column to a position just inside the restrictive barrier (Fig. 50.26)

7. Reposition your left hand to engage a different portion of the lumbar paraspinal musculature

8. Repeat steps 5 to 7 in a rhythmic fashion for 2 to 5 minutes

9. Success of the technique is determined by palpating the previously hypertonic lumbar musculature

Articulatory Technique
Lumbar Regional Rotation: Seated Position
Diagnosis
Position: Lumbar region rotated left
   Restriction: Lumbar region restricted in right rotation

Treatment Position
Patient: Seated, straddling the treatment table with his/her back to the end of the table.
   Physician: Standing behind the patient toward the side opposite the side to be treated. Table height should be adjusted so that the physician stands roughly one head taller than the patient.

Procedure
1. Instruct the patient to place their left hand behind their neck. They are then instructed to grasp the left elbow with the right hand
2. Place the heel of your left hand to the left of the patient's spine, overlying the lumbar transverse processes
3. Take your right arm, pass it in front of the patient (under the right upper arm), and grasp the patient's left upper arm
4. Instruct the patient to lean forward and relax so that their weight will be carried by your right arm. The patient will have a natural tendency to rotate their trunk to the right
5. Turn your body to the right so that the rotation of the patient's trunk to the right is exaggerated. Simultaneously exert an anterior pressure with your left hand over the left lumbar transverse processes
6. This rotational force is held for as short time and then released. The natural tension of the soft tissues will return the lumbar column to a position just inside the restrictive barrier

7. Reposition your left hand to engage a different portion of the lumbar spine
8. Repeat steps 5 to 7 in a rhythmic fashion for 2 to 5 minutes
9. Success of the technique is determined by retesting lumbar regional range of motion in rotation

Note: This technique may be converted to a segmental lumbar rotation technique by isolating the forces of the left hand over a single transverse process and by limiting truncal rotation to that amount which specifically articulates that segment.

739.4 Sacral Somatic Dysfunction

Soft Tissue Technique
Bilateral Thumb Pressure: Sacral Region
Type of Soft Tissue Technique
Parallel traction

Diagnosis
Hypertonicity of the multifidus and erector spinae musculature overlying the sacrum

Treatment Position
Patient: Prone
    Physician: Standing at the side of the treatment table at the level of the patient's thighs

Procedure
1. Place your thumbs on either side of the spinous process of S1 (Fig. 50.27)

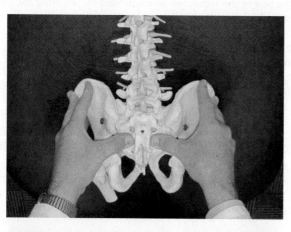

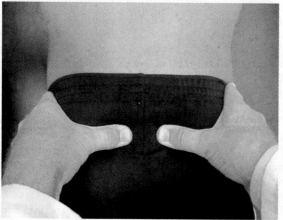

Figure 50-27   A-B. Bilateral thumb pressure—sacral region.

2. Gently press down toward the table until sufficient pressure is in place to engage the sacral paravertebral musculature. *Note:* Care must be taken not to exert excessive pressure as this will compress the muscle against the bone. This causes the patient unnecessary pain and may bruise the soft tissues
3. To the extent permitted by the soft tissues, slide your thumbs cephalad carrying the skin and musculature with them. At the end of longitudinal glide, separate your thumbs slightly exerting a lateral traction. *Note:* Do not slide over the surface of the skin
4. Hold this position for a short period of time and then gradually release the tension
5. Reposition your thumbs half to one segment lower on the sacrum
6. Repeat steps 2 to 4 for 2 or 3 minutes
7. Success of the technique is determined by palpating the degree of tissue tension in the previously hypertonic postsacral musculature

Articulatory Technique
Sacral Rock
Diagnosis
Restriction: Sacral motion with respiration is restricted.

Treatment Position
Patient: Prone
    Physician: Standing at the side of the patient at the level of the patient's pelvis

Procedure
1. Place your cephalad hand on the sacrum, heel of the hand at S1, fingers pointing toward the coccyx (Fig. 50.28)
2. Place your caudad hand on top of the other hand, heel of the hand at the S4/5 level, fingers pointing toward the lumbar spine (Fig. 50.29)
3. Instruct the patient to inhale deeply, and follow the sacrum into extension
4. At the end of inhalation, carry the sacrum slightly further into extension and hold it there for a second (Fig. 50.30)
5. Instruct the patient to exhale, and follow the sacrum into flexion
6. At the end of exhalation, carry the sacrum slightly further into flexion and hold it there for a second (Fig. 50.31)
7. Steps 3 to 6 are repeated for 2 or 3 minutes
8. Success of the technique is determined by reassessing sacral motion

739.5 Pelvic Somatic Dysfunction

Soft Tissue Technique
Piriformis Muscle
Type of Soft Tissue Technique
Inhibitory pressure

Diagnosis
Hypertonicity of the piriformis muscle

Treatment Position
Patient: Lateral recumbent with the hypertonic piriformis muscle away from the table.
    Physician: Standing at the side of the treatment table, facing the patient at the level of the patient's pelvis.

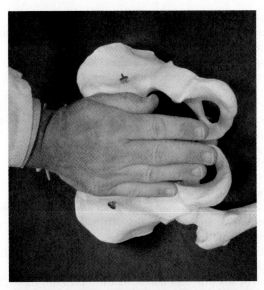

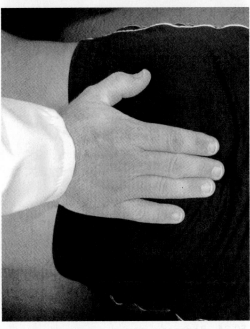

Figure 50-28   A-B. Sacral rock, step 1.

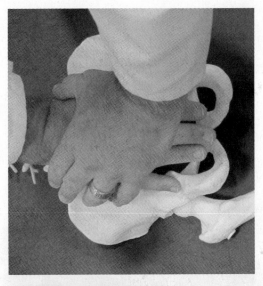

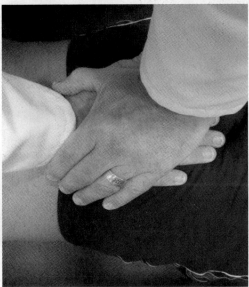

Figure 50-29   A-B. Sacral rock, step 2.

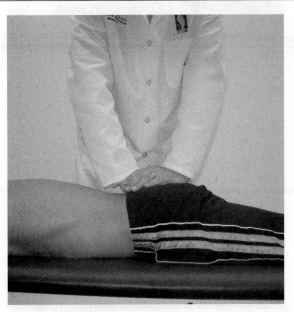

Figure 50-30   Sacral rock, step 4.

Procedure
1. Flex the patient's hips to 45 degrees and knees to 90 degrees
2. The hypertonic muscle can be located at the superior posterior corner of the greater trochanter (Fig. 50.32)
3. Place the olecranon process of your cephalad elbow on top of this hypertonic fascicle of muscle (Fig. 50.33)
4. Press gently down ward toward the table for 2 to 5 minutes or until a softening (release) of the muscle is felt. *Note:* Care should be taken with this technique as the olecranon is less sensitive to pressure than the hands and neophytes often exert too much force
5. Success of the technique is determined by repalpating the previously hypertonic piriformis muscle and/or by testing hip range of motion in internal rotation with the hip held in a neutral position

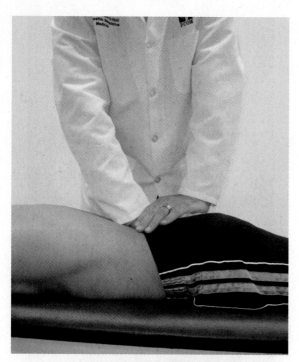

Figure 50-31 Sacral rock, step 6.

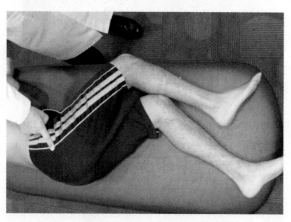

Figure 50-32 Piriformis muscle, step 2.

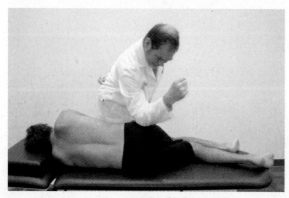

Figure 50-33 Piriformis muscle, step 3.

Articulatory Technique
Posteriorly Rotated Innominate: Modified Sims Position

Diagnosis
Position: Posteriorly rotated innominate
   Restriction: Innominate is restricted in anterior rotation

Treatment Position
Patient: Modified Sims position with the innominate to be treated away from the table (Fig. 50.34)
   Physician: Standing behind the patient at the level of the patient's pelvis

Procedure
1. Place the heel of your cephalad hand posterior to the posterior superior iliac spine on the side of the dysfunction and exert a continuous firm force
2. With your caudad hand, grasp the patient's shin just distal to the knee (Fig. 50.35)
3. With a smooth continuous motion, perform the following motions:
   Flexion of the hip to 100 to 120 degrees (Fig. 50.36)
   Abduction of the hip to 25 to 30 degrees (Fig. 50.37)
   Extension of the hip to 35 to 40 degrees (Fig. 50.38)
   Adduction of the hip to 0 degrees (Fig. 50.39)

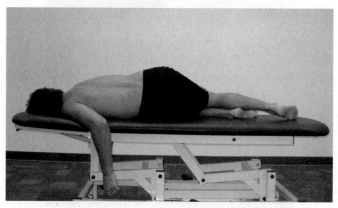

Figure 50-34 Posteriorly rotated innominate—modified Sims position.

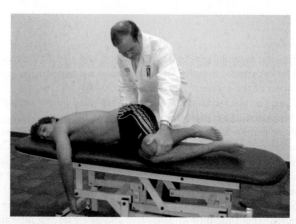

Figure 50-35 Posteriorly rotated innominate—modified Sims position, step 2.

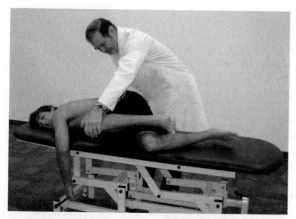

Figure 50-36 Posteriorly rotated innominate—modified Sims position, step 3.

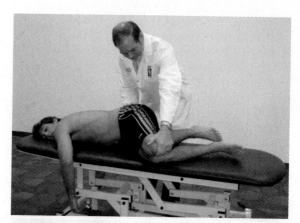

Figure 50-39 Posteriorly rotated innominate—modified Sims position, step 3, adduction.

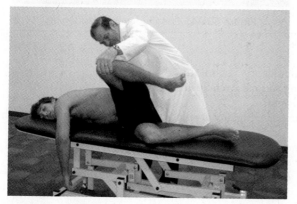

Figure 50-37 Posteriorly Rotated innominate—modified Sims position, step 3, abduction.

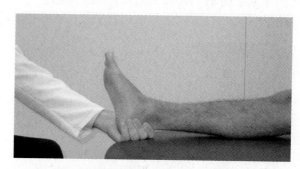

Figure 50-40 Plantar fascia soft tissue.

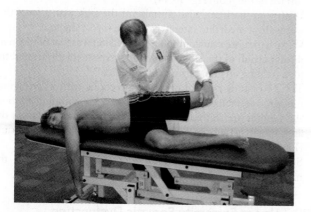

Figure 50-38 Posteriorly rotated innominate—modified Sims position, step 3, extension.

4. Repeat this series of movements three to five times
5. Success of the technique is determined by retesting iliosacral motion

739.6 Lower Extremity Somatic Dysfunction

Soft Tissue Technique
Plantar Fascia
Diagnosis
   Plantar fasciitis
   Rigid pes planus
   Need for general relaxation and sedation

Treatment Position
Patient: Supine
   Physician: Seated at the foot of the treatment table

Procedure
1. Place your other hand beneath the patient's heel to stabilize the foot (Fig. 50.40)
2. Make a loose fist with your dominant hand, and position your fingers so that a smooth spiraling arc of a surface is created by the proximal phalanges of your fingers (Fig. 50.41)
3. Contact the sole of the foot just proximal to the heads of the metatarsals with the proximal phalanx of your little finger (Fig. 50.42)
4. Maintaining a firm pressure against the arch, slide your fingers down the sole of the foot toward the medial calcaneal tubercle. Your proximal phalanges of your fingers should make sequential contact (little finger, ring finger, middle finger, index finger) with the sole of the foot proximal to the heads of the metatarsals (Fig. 50.43)
5. Upon reaching the heel, remove your hand and repeat steps 3 and 4
6. This technique is continued for 3 to 5 minutes
7. Success of this technique is determined by palpating for reduced tension in the plantar fascia, or reassessing the mobility of the longitudinal arch, or by auscultating a snoring sound from your patient

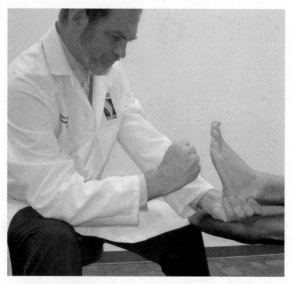

Figure 50-41   Plantar fascia soft tissue, step 2.

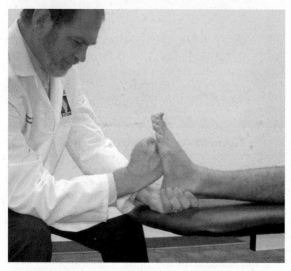

Figure 50-42   Plantar fascia soft tissue, step 3.

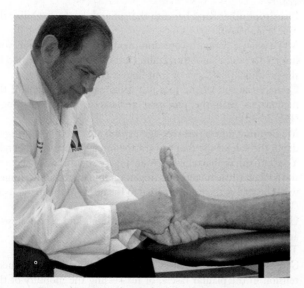

Figure 50-43   Plantar fascia soft tissue, step 4.

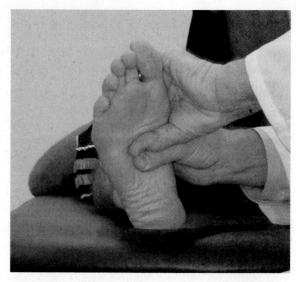

Figure 50-44   Longitudinal arch springing.

Articulatory Technique
Longitudinal Arch Springing
Diagnosis
Restriction: Rigidity or reduced motion of the longitudinal arch

Treatment Position
Patient: Patient lies supine
   Physician: Seated at the foot of table

Procedure
1. Place both thumbs under the arch of the foot from the medial aspect with the fingers of each hand fanning out on the dorsal surface of the foot (Fig. 50.44)
2. With your more cephalad thumb, lift the arch with a force that wraps from medial to lateral across the top of the foot
3. With your more caudad thumb, lift the lateral aspect of the more distal portion of the arch; your hand wraps medially around the foot creating an arch raising counterforce
4. The two hands twist in opposite directions with a "wringing" motion, reestablishing the arch. After each wringing motion, the thumbs are shifted slightly more proximal or distal on the arch, not twisting the foot in exactly the same way each time (Fig. 50.45)
5. Success of the technique is determined by reevaluating the mobility of the longitudinal arch

739.7 Upper Extremity Somatic Dysfunction

Soft Tissue Technique
Rhomboid Muscles
Type of Soft Tissue Technique
Parallel traction

Diagnosis
Hypertonicity of the rhomboid musculature

Treatment Position
Patient: Lateral recumbent technique with the rhomboid to be treated away from the table
   Physician: Standing facing the patient at the level of the patient's shoulder

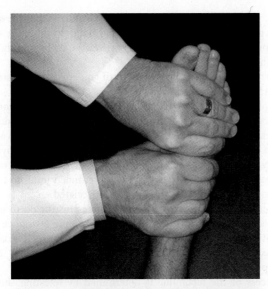

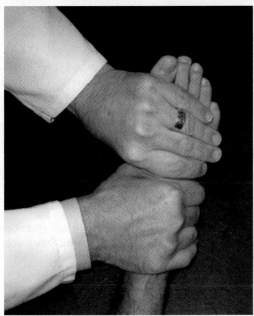

Figure 50-45   A-B. Longitudinal arch springing, step 4.

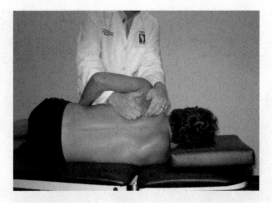

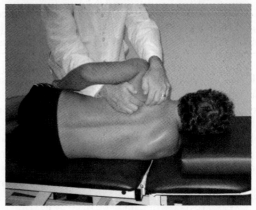

Figure 50-46   A-B. Rhomboid muscles.

Procedure
1. Extend the patient's shoulder to 45 degrees and have the patient's hand rest on the lateral abdomen (Fig. 50.46)
2. Pass your caudad hand under the patient's arm, and with the pads of your fingers, grasp the medial border of the scapula
3. With your cephalad hand, contact the anterior portion of the shoulder to provide an effective counterforce
4. With your caudad hand, draw the medial border of the scapula laterally and caudad, parallel to the fibers of the rhomboid musculature, hold for a second, and slowly release the tension
5. This technique is applied slowly and rhythmically gradually progressing along the medial border of the scapula
6. Continue this technique for 3 to 5 minutes
7. Success of the technique is determined through palpation of the previously hypertonic rhomboid musculature. Success may also be determined in part by reassessing the patient's symptomatology

Articulatory Technique
Seven Stages of Spencer
Historical note: These techniques were developed by Charles H. Spencer, DO of Los Angeles, CA. They were first presented before the Section on Technic at the Portland Session of the American Osteopathic Association Convention, August 1915, and published in the *Journal of the American Osteopathic Association.* The original version of these techniques was largely forgotten; as were the photos and many personal modifications were developed by osteopathic physicians over the ensuing years. One of the common modifications of stage 5 was taught by Angus Cathie, DO, in Philadelphia, hence the division of stage 5 into parts 5-A and 5-B. Stage 5-A is the technique as Spencer performed it (2–5). Another commonly taught modification is the addition of a postisometric relaxation muscle energy technique performed in the same position for those stages that permit this sort of modification.

Indications
> Bursitis of the shoulder
> Tendinitis and tenosynovitis of the shoulder
> Fibrous adhesive capsulitis

Treatment Position
Patient: Lateral recumbent with the shoulder to be treated away from the table
> *Physician:* Standing at the side of the table facing the patient at the level of the patient's chest

Procedure
Stage 1: Extension
1. Use your cephalad hand to stabilize the shoulder girdle by spanning with scapular and clavicle from the superior aspect with your thumb and fingers (Fig. 50.47).

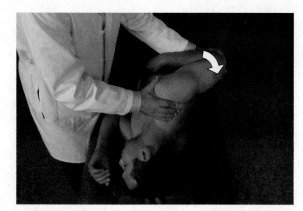

Figure 50-47 Seven stages of Spencer—stage 1—extension. (Used from Nicholas & Nicholas. *Atlas of Osteopathic Technique.* Philadelphia, PA: Lippincott, Williams & Wilkins, with permission.)

2. With your caudad hand, grasp the patient's forearm just distal to the elbow
3. Carry the shoulder into extension until you engage the restrictive barrier
4. Apply a gentle but firm force carrying the shoulder a short distance through its restrictive barrier. Hold for 1 or 2 seconds and release. Passive tissue tension will return the shoulder to a position just inside the restrictive barrier. Apply this force rhythmically, stretching 1 to 2 seconds, followed by a release of that stretch. This rhythmic stretching is continued until no further progress in shoulder extension can be appreciated
5. *Muscle energy modification:* The patient is instructed to flex the shoulder against the physician's unyielding resistance. This contraction is held for 3 to 5 seconds followed by a second of relaxation before the restrictive barrier is again engaged
6. Step 5 is repeated three to five times
7. Success of the technique is determined by retesting shoulder range of motion in extension. Success is determined in part by reassessing the patient's symptoms

Stage 2: Flexion
1. Draw the patient's arm across in front of their body toward flexion. At the same time, turn your body to face the head of the table, arm in front of you (Fig. 50.48)
2. Switch hands so that your hand farthest from the body grasps the patient's hand

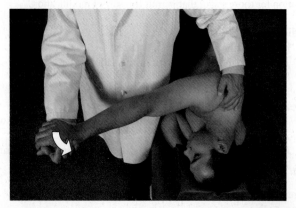

Figure 50-48 Seven stages of Spencer—stage 2—flexion. (Used from Nicholas & Nicholas. *Atlas of Osteopathic Technique.* Philadelphia, PA: Lippincott, Williams & Wilkins, with permission.)

3. Use your hand that is closest to the patient to anchor the shoulder girdle by placing the heel of your hand on the spine of the scapula and extending your fingers over the top of the shoulder to the clavicle
4. Carry the shoulder into flexion until you engage the restrictive barrier
5. Apply a gentle but firm force carrying the shoulder a short distance through its restrictive barrier. Hold for 1 or 2 seconds and release. Passive tissue tension will return the shoulder to a position just inside the restrictive barrier. Apply this force rhythmically, stretching 1 to 2 seconds, followed by a release of that stretch. This rhythmic stretching is continued until no further progress in shoulder flexion can be appreciated
6. *Muscle energy modification:* The patient is instructed to extend the shoulder against the physician's unyielding resistance. This contraction is held for 3 to 5 seconds followed by a second of relaxation before the restrictive barrier is again engaged
7. Step 5 is repeated three to five times
8. Success of the technique is determined by retesting shoulder range of motion in flexion. Success is determined in part by reassessing the patient's symptoms

Stage 3: Compression Circumduction
1. Return to your starting position for stage 1 (Fig. 50.49)
2. Abduct the patient's shoulder to approximately 90 degrees
3. Very gently compress the patient's elbow toward the glenoid fossa
4. Start making small clockwise circles, a circumduction motion. Gradually enlarge these circles creating larger and larger concentric circles as the patient's condition permits. This movement is continued for 15 to 30 seconds
5. Then reverse direction performing the same maneuver in a counterclockwise direction. There are occasions where a restriction may not be felt in one direction but may become quite evident in the reverse direction
6. It is not necessary to perform the entire circle every time. If an arc of motion is identified that is particularly restricted, movement can be limited to that restricted arc
7. *Muscle energy modification:* None for stage 3

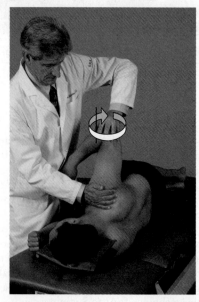

Figure 50-49 Seven stages of Spencer—stage 3—compression circumduction. (Used from Nicholas & Nicholas. *Atlas of Osteopathic Technique.* Philadelphia, PA: Lippincott, Williams & Wilkins, with permission.)

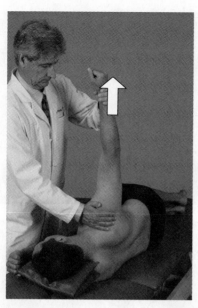

Figure 50-50 Seven stages of Spencer—stage 4—traction circumduction. (Used from Nicholas & Nicholas. *Atlas of Osteopathic Technique*. Philadelphia, PA: Lippincott, Williams & Wilkins, with permission.)

8. Success of the technique is determined by reassessing circumduction of the shoulder. Success is determined in part by reassessing the patient's symptoms

Stage 4: Traction Circumduction
1. Upon completion of stage 3, extend the patient's elbow and grasp the patient's arm at the wrist by encircling it with your hand (take care not to compress any of the neural or vascular structures crossing the wrist joints) (Fig. 50.50)
2. Place a gentle traction upward toward the ceiling on the wrist
3. Start making small clockwise circles, a circumduction motion. Gradually enlarge these circles creating larger and larger concentric circles as the patient's condition permits. This movement is continued for 15 to 30 seconds
4. Then reverse direction performing the same maneuver in a counterclockwise direction. There are occasions where a restriction may not be felt in one direction but may become quite evident in the reverse direction
5. It is not necessary to perform the entire circle every time. If an arc of motion is identified that is particularly restricted, movement can be limited to that restricted arc
6. *Muscle energy modification:* None for stage 3
7. Success of the technique is determined by reassessing circumduction of the shoulder. Success is determined in part by reassessing the patient's symptoms

Stage 5A: Adduction and External Rotation
1. Return to the starting position for stage 1 (Fig. 50.51)
2. Move your cephalad arm so that your forearm is at right angles to the long axis of the patient's body and parallel to the surface plane of the table
3. Slightly flex the shoulder so that the arm may pass just in front of the body
4. With your caudad hand, adduct the shoulder until the restrictive barrier is engaged

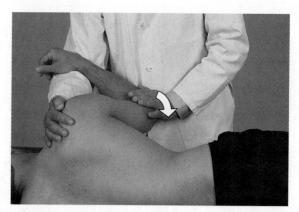

Figure 50-51 Seven stages of Spencer—stage 5A—adduction external rotation. (Used from Nicholas & Nicholas. *Atlas of Osteopathic Technique*. Philadelphia, PA: Lippincott, Williams & Wilkins, with permission.)

5. Apply a gentle but firm force carrying the shoulder a short distance through its restrictive barrier. Hold for 1 or 2 seconds and release. Passive tissue tension will return the shoulder to a position just inside the restrictive barrier. Apply this force rhythmically, stretching 1 to 2 seconds, followed by a release of that stretch. This rhythmic stretching is continued until no further progress in shoulder adduction can be appreciated
6. *Muscle energy modification:* The patient is instructed to abduct the shoulder against the physician's unyielding resistance. This contraction is held for 3 to 5 seconds followed by a second of relaxation before the restrictive barrier is again engaged
7. Step 5 is repeated three to five times
8. Success of the technique is determined by retesting shoulder range of motion in adduction. Success is determined in part by reassessing the patient's symptoms

Stage 5B: Abduction
1. Return to your starting position for stage 5 (Fig. 50.52)
2. With your caudad hand, abduct the shoulder until the restrictive barrier is engaged
3. Apply a gentle but firm force carrying the shoulder a short distance through its restrictive barrier. Hold for 1 or 2 seconds and release. Passive tissue tension will return the shoulder to a position just inside the restrictive barrier. Apply this force rhythmically, stretching 1 to 2 seconds, followed by a release of that

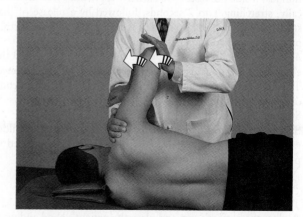

Figure 50-52 Seven stages of Spencer—stage 5B—abduction. (Used from Nicholas & Nicholas. *Atlas of Osteopathic Technique*. Philadelphia, PA: Lippincott, Williams & Wilkins, with permission.)

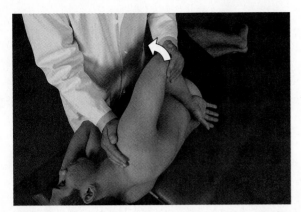

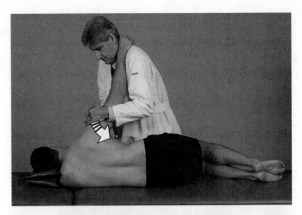

Figure 50-53 Seven stages of Spencer—stage 6—internal rotation. (Used from Nicholas & Nicholas. *Atlas of Osteopathic Technique*. Philadelphia, PA: Lippincott, Williams & Wilkins, with permission.)

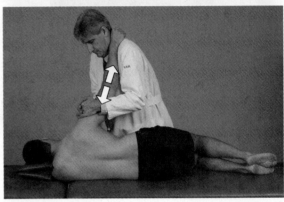

Figure 50-54 A & B. Seven stages of Spencer—stage 7—traction with inferior glide. (Used from Nicholas & Nicholas. *Atlas of Osteopathic Technique*. Philadelphia, PA: Lippincott, Williams & Wilkins, with permission.)

stretch. This rhythmic stretching is continued until no further progress in shoulder abduction can be appreciated

4. *Muscle energy modification:* The patient is instructed to adduct the shoulder against the physician's unyielding resistance. This contraction is held for 3 to 5 seconds followed by a second of relaxation before the restrictive barrier is again engaged
5. Step 5 is repeated three to five times
6. Success of the technique is determined by retesting shoulder range of motion in abduction. Success is determined in part by reassessing the patient's symptoms

Stage 6: Internal Rotation
Note: Patients with severely advanced fibrous adhesive capsulitis may not be able to be placed in position for this technique without significant modification (Fig. 50.53).

1. Abduct the patient's shoulder 45 degrees. Internally rotate the patient's shoulder 90 degrees (if possible). Place the dorsum of the patient's hand in the small of the back
2. Reinforce the anterior portion of the shoulder with your cephalad hand
3. Gently pull the patient's elbow forward until the restrictive barrier is engaged
4. Apply a gentle but firm force carrying the shoulder a short distance through its restrictive barrier. Hold for 1 or 2 seconds and release. Passive tissue tension will return the shoulder to a position just inside the restrictive barrier. Apply this force rhythmically, stretching 1 to 2 seconds, followed by a release of that stretch. This rhythmic stretching is continued until no further progress in shoulder abduction can be appreciated
5. *Muscle energy modification:* The patient is instructed to pull the elbow backward against the physician's unyielding resistance. This contraction is held for 3 to 5 seconds followed by a second of relaxation before the restrictive barrier is again engaged
6. Step 6 is repeated three to five times
7. Success of the technique is determined by retesting shoulder range of motion in internal rotation. Success is determined in part by reassessing the patient's symptoms

Stage 7: Traction with Inferior Glide
1. Turn and face the head of the table (Fig. 50.54)
2. Abduct the patient's arm and place the patient's hand and wrist on your shoulder closest to the patient
3. With fingers interlaced, place your hands just distal to the glenohumeral joint

4. Scoop the patient's humeral head in a caudad direction parallel to the table, creating a translatory motion toward the inferior edge of the glenoid fossa
5. Apply a gentle but firm force carrying the shoulder a short distance through its restrictive barrier. Hold for 1 or 2 seconds and release. Passive tissue tension will return the shoulder to a position just inside the restrictive barrier. Apply this force rhythmically, stretching 1 to 2 seconds, followed by a release of that stretch. This rhythmic stretching is continued until no further progress in shoulder abduction can be appreciated
6. *Muscle energy modification:* While maintaining the caudad traction on the patient's arm, instruct the patient to press their hand down against your shoulder. This contraction is held for 3 to 5 seconds followed by a second of relaxation before the restrictive barrier is again engaged
7. Step 6 is repeated three to five times
8. Success of the technique is determined by retesting shoulder range of motion. Success is determined in part by reassessing the patient's symptoms

739.8 Rib Somatic Dysfunction

Soft Tissue Technique
Scalene Stretching
Diagnosis
Hypertonicity of the scalene musculature maintaining ribs 1 and 2 in a position of inhalation on the left side of the neck

Type of Soft Tissue Technique
Parallel traction

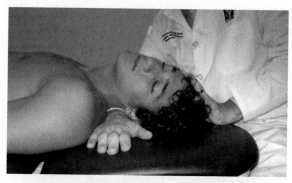

Figure 50-55 Scalene stretching.

Treatment Position
Patient: Supine
    Physician: Seated to the right side of the head of the treatment table

Procedure
1. Pass your caudad arm beneath the patient's neck with your hand adjacent to the opposite shoulder (Fig. 50.55)
2. Gently, using your more cephalad hand, roll the patient's head along your arm from your fingers toward your elbow, until it is rotated 45 to 60 degrees from the midline
3. Allow the patient's head to drop over your forearm, placing the anterolateral cervical musculature on stretch. (You may have to raise your elbow slightly off the table.)
4. Slowly, roll the head slightly further through the soft tissue restrictive barrier, simultaneously pressing the head gently down toward the table. Hold this position for a second and release, allowing the head to rise and roll back to just inside the restrictive barrier
5. This technique is applied slowly and rhythmically gradually increasing the amount of stretch
6. Continue this technique for 3 to 5 minutes
7. Success of the technique is determined by reassessing freedom of motion of the first and second ribs, and by repalpating the previously hypertonic scalene musculature. Success is in part determined by reassessing the patient's symptoms

Articulatory Technique
Rib Raising: Seated Position
Diagnosis
Restriction of motion of ribs 2 to 6. Motion will be created through traction on the pectoralis major muscle. (Motion may be imparted indirectly to rib 1 via its clavicular relations and ribs 7 to 10 through the attachments of the serratus anterior muscle.)

Treatment Position
Patient: Seated on the side or end of the treatment table.
    Physician: Standing facing the patient with one foot behind the other.

Procedure
1. Instruct the patient to cross his or her arms, hooking their thumbs into the antecubital fossae (Fig. 50.56)
2. Reach under the patients arms with both your hands, then pass them over the patient's shoulders
3. Make contact with the pads of your fingers at the level of the second costotransverse articulation, just lateral to that same joint

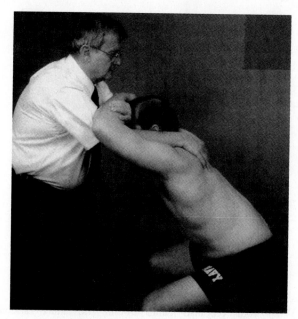

Figure 50-56 Rib raising—seated position.

Note: At each rib level, you will want to position the pads of your fingers between the costotransverse articulation and the angle of the rib.

4. Lean your weight onto your back foot, drawing the patient toward you. The patient's forearms should translate forward, parallel to the floor. At the same time, this should permit the shoulders to drop, increasing the tension on the pectoral musculature and drawing the anterior aspect of the ribs cephalad
5. Simultaneously press forward with the pads of your fingers to create a gapping pressure at the costotransverse articulations
6. Hold this position for 1 second, then release, allowing your weight to transfer to the more anterior foot, and the patient to spring back to a more upright position
7. Move the pads of your fingers down one rib level and repeat. Continue this stepwise down the rib cage until you can no longer comfortably reach the rib levels (usually in the range of ribs 6 to 8)
8. Reverse the procedure, working your way back up the rib cage until you again reach the second rib
9. Success of the technique is determined by retesting motion of the previously restricted costal levels

739.9 Abdominal: Other Somatic Dysfunction

Soft Tissue Technique
Lateral Abdominal Wall
Diagnosis
Hypertonicity of the lateral abdominal wall musculature

Type of Soft Tissue Technique
Perpendicular traction/parallel traction
(This depends upon which muscle layer you wish to talk about.)

Treatment Position
Patient: Prone
    Physician: Standing at the side of the table on the side opposite the hypertonic musculature

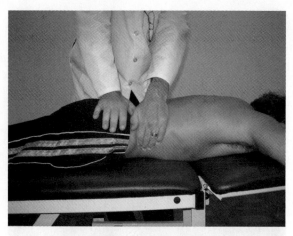

Figure 50-57   Lateral abdominal wall.

Procedure
1. Wrap your cephalad hand around the lateral abdominal wall. Make your palmar contact as complete as possible (Fig. 50.57)
2. Place your caudad hand on the iliac crest with the heel of your hand near the posterior superior iliac spine
3. Draw the abdominal wall toward you, simultaneously increasing the pressure on the iliac crest to maintain the pelvis in place
4. Hold this position for a second, then release, allowing the abdominal musculature to draw back to its position just inside the restrictive barrier
5. Reposition your hand slightly on the abdominal wall and repeat
6. Continue steps 3 to 5 rhythmically for 3 to 5 minutes
7. Success of the technique is determined by repalpating the previously hypertonic abdominal muscles

Articulatory Technique
Liver Articulation
Note: In this technique, the liver is considered to articulate with the diaphragm. Inflammatory conditions involving the liver may result in adherence of the liver to the diaphragm with subsequent restriction of diaphragmatic and lower right costal motion

Diagnosis
Restriction of hepatic motion relative to the diaphragm

Treatment Position
Patient: Seated on the side of the treatment table
    Physician: Standing behind the seated patient

Procedure
1. Reach under the patient's arms and bring your finger pads into contact with the abdominal wall 1.5 to 2 in. below the right costal margin (Fig. 50.58)
2. Have the patient slump back against you, relaxing the abdominal wall
3. Exert a posterior pressure with the pads of all of your fingers and then curl them upward against the inferior surface of the anterior edge of the liver
4. Instruct the patient to take a deep breath
5. Follow the liver edge as it glides slightly down and forward with downward motion of the diaphragm

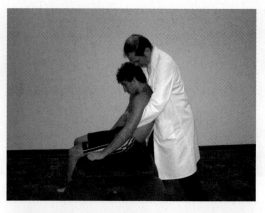

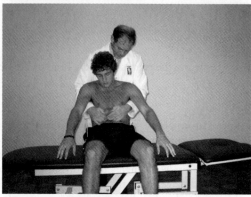

Figure 50-58   A, B. Liver articulation.

6. Instruct your patient to exhale. Again follow the liver edge as it glides superiorly and posteriorly with upward motion of the diaphragm
7. Increase your pressure against the liver margin and instruct the patient to breathe deeply again. Try not to allow the liver to move
8. Instruct the patient to exhale and follow the liver as it moves with exhalation
9. Repeat steps 7 and 8 until no further increase in liver motion is palpable
10. Success of the technique is determined by reassessing diaphragmatic and right lower costal motion

SUMMARY

Both soft tissue and articulatory techniques span a wide range of force levels and are therefore adaptable to a wide variety of patient types and problems, making them two of the most versatile treatment forms available. These techniques are often used to decrease muscle tension and increase joint mobility prior to use of high-velocity low-amplitude thrust techniques. They can be used alone, or in combination with any other manipulative technique.

REFERENCES

1. Hildreth AG. *The Lengthening Shadow of Dr. Andrew Taylor Still*. Kirksville, Missouri: Simpson Printing Company, 1942:186–189.
2. Spencer H. Shoulder technique. *J Am Osteopath Assoc* 1916;15:218–220.
3. Spencer H. Treatment of bursitis and tendosynovitis. *J Am Osteopath Assoc* 1926;25:528–529.

4. Patriquin DA. The evolution of osteopathic manipulative technique: the Spencer technique. *J Am Osteopath Assoc* 1992;92:1134–1146.

5. Nicholas AS, Evan N. *Atlas of Osteopathic Techniques*. Philadelphia, PA: Lippincott Williams & Wilkins, 2008.

6. Nicholas A. *Atlas of Osteopathic Techniques*. Philadelphia, PA: Philadelphia College of Osteopathic Medicine, 1981.

7. Rubenstein S, Eimerbrink JH, Heilig D, et al. *Osteopathic Techniques*. Philadelphia, PA: Osteopathic Publications, 1949.

8. Zink JG, Holistic approaches to homeostasis. In: Barnes MW, ed. *American Academy of Osteopathy Yearbook*. Indianapolis, IN: American Academy of Osteopathy, 1973.

9. Ehrenfeuchter W, Heilig D, Nicholas A. Soft tissue techniques. In: Ward RC, ed. *Foundations for Osteopathic Medicine*. 2nd Ed; Chap 54.

10. Patriquin D, Jones J. Articulatory techniques. In: Ward RC, ed. *Foundations for Osteopathic Medicine*. 2nd Ed; Chap 55.

51

Lymphatics Approach

MICHAEL L. KUCHERA

KEY CONCEPTS

- The lymphatic system plays a major role in numerous homeostatic mechanisms of the body.
- The lymphatic system is particularly vulnerable to fascial dysfunction in the region of the superior thoracic inlet.
- Initial draining of the lymphatic system must always be done through terminal areas.
- The risk-to-benefit ratio for lymphatic techniques is quite good. No known significant complications have resulted from osteopathic lymphatic treatment to date. Clinical judgment, however, should always be used when prescribing treatment for a patient in any disease state.

CASE STUDY

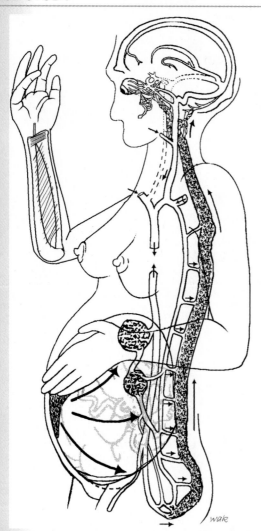

Pregnant Medical Transcriptionist With Finger Swelling and Tingling:

This chapter documents numerous benefits that could be derived from thoughtful osteopathic care centered about the respiratory-circulatory model and the systematic, sequential application of local, regional and systemic "lymphatic" osteopathic manipulative treatment (OMT) to facilitate fluid homeostasis.

Initial Case Presentation:

After 14 years at the same job without complaint, a 32-year-old transcriptionist now presents with 6-week progressive numbness and tingling in her right (dominant) hand. Awakening her nearly every night, the distribution of her dysesthesiae includes her thumb and the next 2½ digits. For the last month, she has had difficulty opening jars and has nearly dropped objects. Gravida I, para 0-0-0-1 and early in her second trimester, she takes no medications or nutritional supplements other than a prenatal vitamin.

Findings:

Her right thenar eminence appears smaller than the left and manifests reduced grip strength; all fingers on the right hand are puffy. On the right, positive neurological tests include Phalen's (at 20 seconds) and Tinel's (just distal to the wrist's flexor crease). There are no other historical or physical findings to indicate thyroid disorder, cervical radiculopathy, diabetes, vascular disease, or other significant health issue.

The common compensatory pattern (CCP) of Zink is violated by her superior thoracic inlet that prefers rotation and sidebending to the left. She has tender fullness in the right supraclavicular region and posterior axillary fold; in the supine position, her shallow, rapid breaths are seen to extend only halfway down to the umbilicus. Spinal palpatory reveals only grade I severity, Fryette type-I somatic dysfunctions; no Chapman points or collateral ganglion findings were identified. She has a right posterior radial head. Active myofascial trigger points (MTrPs) are palpated in the right pronator teres and in several forearm and finger flexor muscles.

Electromyography (EMG) consisting of nerve conduction studies (NCS) with needle examination confirmed moderate severity median entrapment neuropathy at the wrist with positive sensory and motor NCS but no fibrillation potentials in the thenar eminence; it also ruled out a concomitant cervical radiculopathy.

This case and its discussion at the end of the chapter were chosen to illustrate the rationale and manual components associated with applying the respiratory-circulatory model. The ultimate result of the OMT portion of her care in this regard included reduction of upper extremity edema, resolution of the signs and symptoms of her carpal tunnel syndrome (CTS), and increased function in both her arm and several other systems.

INTRODUCTION

The lymphatic system plays a major role in numerous homeostatic mechanisms of the body; it transports fats to the blood from digestive processes, facilitates immune function, is a vital component of the overall circulatory system of the body, and assists the body in removing interstitial tissue fluid and plasma proteins that accumulate as a result of tissue metabolism, inflammation, infection, trauma, or system dysfunction. For these reasons, a coordinated, systematic approach known as the "Respiratory-Circulatory model" and a number of lymphatic treatment techniques have been used clinically by osteopathic professionals to treat patients with a various conditions such as edema and infection. This model is indicative of one of the "structure-function framework" approaches commonly employed by osteopathic practitioners in their objective and subjective interpretation of the physical findings that lead to rational diagnoses and treatment. It also codifies a systemic osteopathic approach to deliver treatment that specifically and effectively accomplishes lymphaticovenous homeostatic goals; it may even provide useful respiratory-circulatory strategies aimed toward enhancing intrinsic, host-maintained health levels.

In order to systematically set and initiate clinical goals applying the "Respiratory-Circulatory model," osteopathic physicians incorporate a number of important principles that influence both the choice of OMT techniques and the order of their application.

History—Systematic

> The cells, which make up our body, have an internal environment also. The fluid matrix of it must be free of 'pollution.' Waste products of tissue metabolism must be constantly carried away by the veins and lymphatics. The health and life of cells and therefore the whole body depend on it—J. Gordon, Zink, DO, F.A.A.O. (1).

The lymphatic system, which is integral to the understanding of health and disease, was accurately first described as a system by Olaf Rudbeck (Sweden) in 1653 (2). The osteopathic profession, from its onset, embraced the importance of the lymphatic system and attempted to document its role in health. A. T. Still emphasized that diagnosis of the fascia and treatment of the lymphatic system was vital for maintaining health and treating disease (3); therefore, in 1898, his faculty in Kirksville used skiagraphy (an early form of x-ray) to research the distribution of the vascular and lymphatic systems (4).

Later, one of Still's students, Frederic Millard, D.O., researched the structure and functions of the lymphatic system and published *Applied Anatomy of the Lymphatics* in 1922 (5). The first DO to specifically describe physical examination of fluid and lymphatic status (6,7), Millard based aspects of his surgical versus nonsurgical recommendations on the state in which he found the lymph nodes. He noted that the lymph vessels were "pliable and readily compressed"; that "for every congested tissue there is a corresponding lymph disturbance"; and that "attempts to clear the lymph stream before clearing the edema in the clavicular regions is to over-tax the general lymph stream and cause profound reactions" (8). In addition, Millard also described a series of "lymphatic drainage" techniques (9–11) while admonishing the osteopathic practitioner to "never work over an enlarged or indurated lymph node," advocating instead to "free the efferents and the lymph will drain" (12).

J. Gordon Zink, D.O., F.A.A.O., acknowledging the work of Millard as his major inspiration, expanded the approach by popularizing the concept that "respiration and circulation are unifiable functions" (13), and that, for homeostasis, eternal respiration determines internal respiration. Zink's influence and teaching led to the profession's general adoption of the "Respiratory-Circulatory" model and

acceptance of technique sequences designed to enhance cellular level health (internal respiration) by maximizing external respiration. In his extensive teaching of the respiratory-circulatory model, Zink placed special emphasis on the fascial restrictions that limited venous and lymphatic return, the value of creating pressure differentials in the body cavities for effective venous-lymphatic flow, and the central importance of the thoracoabdominopelvic pump in the maintenance of lymphatic homeostasis (14–16). While the idea that respiration affected venous return was known at this time, it was only quantified and confirmed with Doppler studies in the 1980s (17).

Specific lymphatic treatments outside the osteopathic profession were first defined and described by Emil Vodder, a French Ph.D. in the 1930 and consisted largely of manual lymph drainage (18). Based upon manual therapies for draining lymphedema, Vodder method was developed further in Europe during the 1960s and applied to the treatment of lymphedema patients, as a part of Complex Decongestive Therapy (Complex Decongestive Therapy). Schools teaching therapists and physicians to perform the Vodder technique opened in the 1970s about the same time that Zink was popularizing a codified approach for osteopathic physicians to enhance the lymphatics.

Zink, and subsequently Bruno Chikly, M.D., described diagnostic sites for identification of regional lymphatic dysfunction (sites of "terminal lymphatic drainage") (19–21) and integrated concepts from osteopathy in the cranial field. In addition, Zink specifically linked "primary and secondary respiration" by talking about the "craniosternosacral mechanism"; as a consequence of his attempts to raise awareness of this approach, osteopathic students fondly referred to Zink as the "lymphomaniac."

History—Osteopathic Lymphatic Technique

> If we think ... and say that disease is only too much dirt in the wheels of life, then we see that 'Nature takes this method to wash out the dirt.'...Let the lymphatics always receive and discharge naturally, if so we have no substance detained long enough to produce fermentation, fever, sickness, and death. We strike at the source of life and death when we go to the lymphatics. ...Thus it behooves us to handle them (the lymphatics) with wisdom and tenderness, for by and from them, a withered limb, organ, or any division of the body receives what we call reconstruction, or is builded anew ....—A. T. Still (22).

Still preferred that his students create techniques to accomplish clinical goals, that is, techniques based upon their knowledge of anatomy rather than a memorized maneuver. ("*I am not here to teach a bunch of parrots*," he wrote) (23). Probably for this reason, the lymphatic techniques used by Still as early as the 1870s were not described by his students until later (24). Nonetheless, some specific osteopathic lymphatic techniques, using a few minutes of local manual pumping to reduce swelling in and around organs (such as the pressure-sensitive liver), were described in the profession's literature as early as 1898 (25).

Like that over the liver, rhythmic manual pumping over the spleen (a secondary lymphoid organ) was described and researched very early in the osteopathic profession; as it is even today. Clement A. Whiting, D.O., studied the effects of using splenic pump on immune function in 1910 (22) as did M.A. Lane, D.O. in 1920 (26), and Yale Castlio, D.O., and Louise Ferris-Smith, D.O., in the 1930s (27,28). Research, using modern methods to investigate lymphatic pump techniques to enhance immune function began again in earnest with the work of Measel (29,30) in the 1980s and continues today with funding from both NIH and the osteopathic profession. (Modern research outcomes are discussed later in this chapter.)

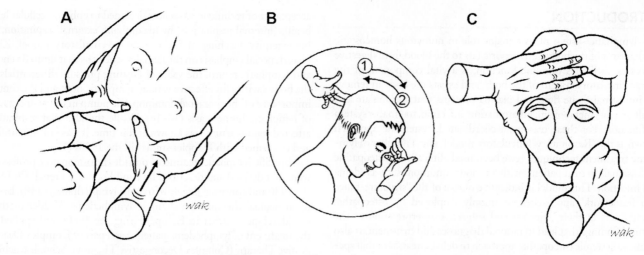

Figure 51-1 Examples of OMT techniques designed to move venous and/or lymphatic fluids.

Osteopathic techniques expanded to the use of muscle pumps and respiratory pumps; each enhancing normal homeostatic mechanisms to move fluids in the vascular-lymphatic system. C. Earl Miller in 1926 first described and then researched the effects of the classic thoracic lymphatic pump along with other lymphatic approaches (Fig. 51.1A) (31,32). T.J. Ruddy, M.D., D.O., developed a muscle pump system called "Rapid Rhythmic Resistive Duction" for treating lymphatic congestion in multiple areas (especially the head and neck) (33) that was the precursor to later development of muscle energy techniques (Fig. 51.1B). William Galbreath, DO, described the Galbreath technique, a method for mobilizing lymphatic fluid in the mandibular region and for draining accumulated fluid from the middle ear in 1929 (Fig. 51.1C) (34,35).

Another student of A. T. Still, D.O., and a contemporary of Millard, D.O., William Garner Sutherland, D.O., also focused on fluid diagnosis and treatment. Best known for his contributions to osteopathy in the cranial field, Sutherland emphasized the definition of Webster's definition of "fluctuation" as "the movement of a fluid within a natural or artificial cavity and observed by palpation or percussion" (36). The techniques he described and taught within the profession were simple and effective. He noted, "With the method I described of facilitating the movement of lymph and controlling the Tide by bringing the fluctuation to the short rhythmic period, you have the interchange of all the fluids of the body" (37).

The lymphatics were postulated by osteopathic practitioners to play a diagnostic and therapeutic role in visceral function. For example, Frank Chapman, D.O., another student of Still, elucidated a series of so-called neurolymphatic reflexes believed to correspond to visceral structures in the 1930s. These so-called Chapman's Reflexes (see "Chapman's Approach" in Chapter 52) are now more typically described as secondary tissue texture changes associated with viscerosomatic reflexes in a distribution associated with the sympathetic nervous system.

When all is said and done, Sutherland offered the most cogent insight, as true now as it was then:

> *The science of Osteopathy is simple. You realize you are a mechanic of the fluids of the body as well as of the skeletal system* (38).

STRUCTURE AND FUNCTION

Lymph and the structures making up the lymphatic system comprise approximately 3% of the body's total weight. Lymphatic structures may be divided into the lymphatic collecting system and the organized lymph tissue. In this chapter, organized lymph tissue includes the following structures (Fig. 51.2):

- Spleen
- Liver
- Thymus
- Tonsil
- Vermiform appendix
- Lymphoid tissues in the gastrointestinal and pulmonary tracts
- Lymph nodes

Lymph and the lymphatic system cleanse, purify, and defend the body; they also play a role in absorbing and transporting nutrients and maintaining fluid balance (Table 51.1).

Structural Components of Lymphatic System

Embryology

The lymphatics, along with other components of the immune system, begin to develop by the end of the fifth week and make significant and observable progress around the 20th week of gestation.

Lymphatic vessels, lymph nodes, the spleen, and myeloid tissue (the tissue in bone marrow responsible for production of various classes of blood cells, including lymph cells) all develop from lateral plate mesoderm. In contrast, both the thymus and the epithelial components of the tonsils differentiate from foregut endoderm.

Lymphatic vessels may arise from two different developmental trajectories; they can either form contingently as an outgrowth of the venous system or independently but still in close association with veins to create numerous lymphaticovenous connections throughout the body. Like blood vessels, large lymphatic vessels develop an endothelial lining and are capable of releasing nanomolar levels of nitric oxide (NO) by upregulating transcription of endothelial NO synthase (eNOS). They have a distinctive vasculature structure including a discontinuous basement membrane, open endothelial junctions, anchoring filaments, valves, and intrinsic contractility; features that both share similarities to and contrast with the blood vasculature.

Masses of lymphocytes accumulate about lymphatic vessels and organize as lymph nodes. The spleen is composed of somewhat similar tissue, but its channels are supplied with blood rather than lymph.

Continued lymphangiogenesis occurs after tissue damage and in pathological states such as myocardial infarction. The "driving force" for new lymphatic vessel development is the need for organized interstitial fluid flow homeostasis (39).

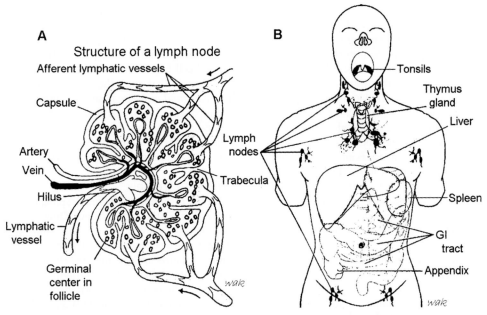

Figure 51-2   Organized lymphoid tissues and lymph nodes.

TABLE 51.1

Functions of the Lymphatic System in Regard to Homeostasis

Purification/cleansing of tissues

- Lymph bathes all body organs and cleanses extracellular space.
- Lymph is delivered to lymph nodes which act as purifying filters to remove waste (particulate matter, exudates, bacteria, etc.)
- Along with the fluid in lymph, waste products, proteins, postinjury biochemical by-products, etc. are removed.

Maintaining fluid balance

Daily about 30 L fluid moves from capillaries to the interstitial spaces.
- ~ 90% back into blood capillaries
- ~ 10% (3L) drains into lymphatic channels
- Fluid overload: Lymphatic system protects against damage

Lymphatics also return ~50% of plasma proteins diffusing out of vascular system (high molecular weight).

Defense/immunology

With so much contact with the body, the lymphatics provide a first-line defense against infection. The lymphatics carry antigen to the lymph nodes where the immune response is initiated.

Aging, lymphatics, and the immune system

- Immune system begins development at ~20 wk of gestation
- At birth, the immune system is still immature but lymphoid tissue is plentiful during infancy and increases in amount until 6–9 y of age.
- At puberty, the immune system matures; lymphoid tissues slowly regress until 15–16 years of age.
- Barring autoimmune dysfunction or disorders such as AIDS, lymphoid tissue and immune function levels are stable through most of the adult lifespan.
- In the geriatric patient, the system may decline to the point where they cannot mount a fever (silent infections).

Nutrition

Villi of small intestines absorb large amounts of long chain fats, chylomicrons, and cholesterol

After fatty meals, the thoracic duct may contain 2% fat; lymph-fat "chyle" changes color from clear yellow to milky white

Organized Lymph Tissues

The **spleen** is the largest single mass of lymphoid tissue in the body. This pressure-sensitive organ abuts the diaphragm, which provides movement from its inherent respiratory-circulatory activity that is important for the employment of its homeostatic function. The spleen can be detected deep to the left 9th to 11th ribs and can be located by percussion of the area for splenic dullness. In the absence of splenomegaly, the spleen should not be palpable or percussible below the costal margin. Functionally, the spleen destroys deformed or damaged red blood cells, clears particulate antigens and microorganisms (particularly poorly organized bacteria), and synthesizes immunoglobulin.

Half of the body's lymph is formed in the **liver**, which also has a functional role in the purging bacteria from the body. The liver, similar to the spleen, is also a pressure-sensitive organ abutting the diaphragm. Unless there is hepatomegaly, the liver's edge is palpable at approximately the right costal margin. The liver's venous-lymphatic drainage is shared between the gallbladder and the pancreas with the former serving as this region's "gatekeeper" to venous and lymphatic drainage.

In infancy, the **thymus** is a relatively large organ that peaks in size at age 2 years. It serves to provide immunologically potent cells needed to develop mature immune cells. It is also a preprocessing site for T-lymphocyte immune cells. After puberty, in adulthood, it involutes and is replaced by fatty tissue.

The palatine, lingual, and pharyngeal **tonsils** are organized lymph tissues that are considered to be important to the child, but nonessential in adult immunologic function. In early life, they provide cells that are essential to building immunity. The **vermiform appendix** is also additional organized lymph tissue that is viewed as nonessential to adult immune function.

There are two types of **visceral lymphoid tissues,** pulmonary and small intestinal. Pulmonary lymphoid tissues aid in the filtration of particulate matter and toxins from the lungs. The small intestinal mucosal lymphoid tissues (Peyer patches and lacteals) have an autonomic innervation stemming from the enteric nervous system (including the Auerbach and Meissner plexi).

Finally, there are 400 to 450 superficial and deep **lymph nodes** that differ from other organized lymphatic tissues because they are dispersed along the lymphatic vessels where they filter lymph and to synthesize lymphocytes. The lymph nodes might be the most highly organized of all lymphoid tissues (Fig. 51.2B)—with nodal reticuloendothelial cells to phagocytize bacteria, particulate matter, and cell fragments and with germinal centers to manufacture lymphocytes that enter the lymph as it passes through the node. The *superficial nodes* are located in subcutaneous connective tissues accompanying superficial veins and drain into three main groups: cervical, axillary, and inguinal. They receive lymph from skin and deeper tissues of the head, neck, and extremities. The *deep nodes* (Fig. 51.2A) drain into a system of collecting channels/trunks.

Lymphatic Vessels

With the exception of the brain, spinal cord, epidermis (including hair and nails), the endomysium of muscle and cartilage, bone marrow, and selected portions of the peripheral nerves—all of which are perfused by minute interstitial conduits or by direct diffusion—lymph channels are disseminated throughout the entire body. The lymph channels begin as blind endothelial tubes or capillaries composed of a single layer of leaky squamous epithelium that is supported by anchoring filaments (Fig. 51.3A); this site is associated with the formation phase of lymph.

The lymphatic collectors are approximately 100 to 600 μm in diameter and consist primarily of chains of muscular units called "lymphangions" (Fig. 51.3B), which possess two-leaflet bicuspid valves. Described as little "lymphatic hearts" (40), lymphangions work much like the body's heart pacemakers, contracting regularly throughout the lymphatic system (lymphangiomotoricity) and moving lymph in peristaltic waves. From the tunica media to the tunica externa, these muscular units have extensive autonomic (sympathetic and parasympathetic) innervation, which is somewhat similar to the alpha and beta receptor system found in blood vessels.

Peripheral lymph capillaries join to form capillary plexes that, in turn, form larger paired trunks that will eventually feed into either the right or left thoracic ducts (Fig. 51.4). On their way to the thoracic ducts, superficial lymph vessels follow the course of the superficial veins and lymph nodes and drain into deep lymphatic channels; deep lymphatic vessels follow the deep veins and deep

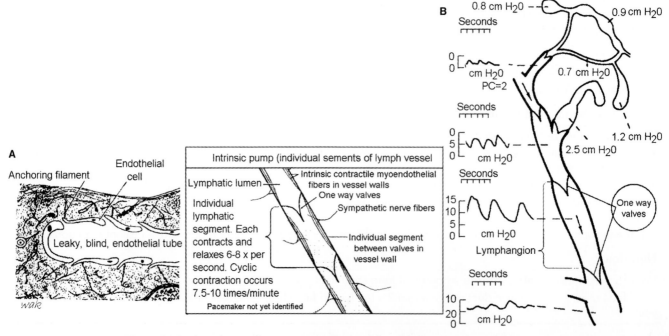

Figure 51-3 Lymphatic collection system: Terminal, lymphagion, vessels, and ducts.

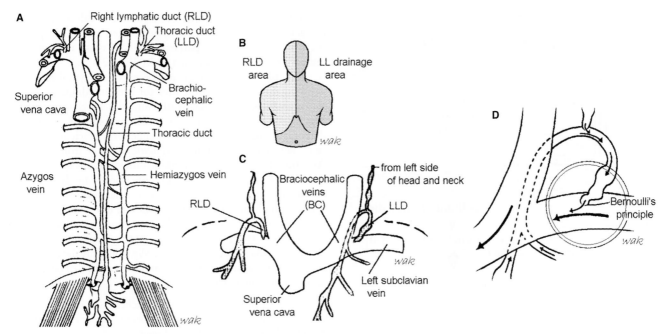

Figure 51-4 Terminal drainage phase: Lymphatic ducts, drainage regions, and Bernoulli principle.

lymph nodes that subsequently drain the deep structures of the neck, the perineum and pelvis, the abdomen and the thorax. These deep channels lie around all major organs of the body.

A distinct, centimeter-long right lymphatic duct (RLD) can be found in 20% of patients and will cross the anterior scalene muscle to empty into the region of the jugulosubclavian vein junction. In 80% of patients, the three major right-sided drainage trunks (right jugular, right subclavian, and right bronchopulmonary trunks) will empty here through two to three openings. There are semilunar valves at the lymphaticovenous juncture to prevent venous blood from refluxing into the RLD. The right side receives drainage from right side of the head and neck, right upper extremity, right chest, heart, and lungs with the possible exception of the left upper lobe. (Fig. 51.4B).

The left-sided thoracic duct (LLD) is the largest lymphatic channel in the body; it extends 38 to 45 cm in length from the first lumbar vertebra to the root of the neck. This thoracic duct drains lymph from the left arm and left side of the neck and head, thorax, upper abdomen (to umbilicus) as well as both sides of the abdomen below the umbilicus and both of the lower limbs. The LLD arises either from the confluence of several lymph trunks on the posterior abdominal wall or, in 20% of patients, from these lymph trunks draining into the cisterna chyli. The cisterna chyli, when present, is anterior to L1-2. The LLD then passes through the aortic opening in the diaphragm at the T12 level. It ascends in the posterior mediastinum to the right of the midline between the descending aorta (to its left) and the azygos vein (to its right). When the thoracic duct reaches the horizontal plane at the level of the sternal angle (T4), it inclines to the left. It then passes out of the thoracic cage into the neck through Sibson fascia, which covers this "superior thoracic inlet" and merges with scalene fascia, and then turns to pass a second time through the same fascia back into the chest cage where it terminates in either the junction of the left internal jugular or subclavian (brachiocephalic) veins. Before it terminates, the duct receives the left jugular trunk (draining lymph from left head and neck) and left subclavian trunk draining the left upper extremity).

The one-way valve that prevents venous blood from entering the LLD is under sympathetic control as is the smooth muscle in the wall of the LLD. It should be generally noted that large lymphatic vessels are affected by both autonomic control, which facilitates peristalsis, and upregulation of eNOS activity from the endothelial shearing forces caused by lymphatic movement (41).

Lymph Fluid

Lymphatic fluid (lymph) contains the cells produced in the lymph nodes as well as the fluid, electrolytes, small proteins, and cells that leak out of arterial capillaries into the blind-ended lymphatic capillaries. The primary cells in lymph are lymphocytes (2,000 to 20,000/mm in the thoracic duct). There are also macrophages and foreign antigens; bacteria and viruses found in peripheral lymph prior to being filtered are brought in close contact with the lymphatic immune cells. Lymph also carries clotting factors and after meals lymph coming from the left thoracic duct will carry chyle that is richly laden with emulsified water-soluble fats.

Increased capillary permeability as occurs in various inflammatory and infectious conditions allows fluid and proteins to escape into the interstitial tissues. These, along with the debris and by-products secondarily produced, must be removed by the lymphatic system. The inflammatory process will progress through a proliferative phase.

Lymphatic Physiology and Homeostatic Mechanisms

A plan for management of lymphatic stasis is based on the understanding of the mechanics of lymph formation and its propulsion. There are three lymph phases: (1) formation, (2) vascular, and (3) terminal.

The **formation phase** (Fig. 51.5) consists of the movement of extracellular fluid into blind endothelial tubes. This is not as automatic as it might sound. Circulatory forces (the hydrostatic and osmotic gradients, which produce capillary exchange) dissipate almost immediately beyond the edge of the vessel. Furthermore, Starling forces do not account for the movement of fluid through the interstitial matrix (gel) where **cellular respiration** takes place.

By the time fluid reaches these blind end pouches, a small uphill gradient must be overcome before lymph can form. This means that *motion* (including inherent tissue movements and fluctuation of extracellular fluid) is a vital interstitial mechanism that promotes interstitial interchange and thereby facilitates cellular respiration.

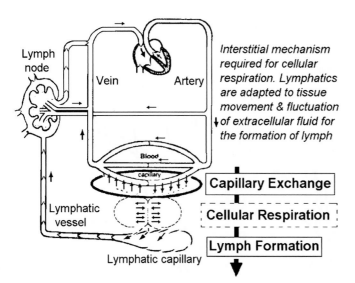

Figure 51-5 Formation phase involved in cellular respiration and lymph formation.

Lymphatics are adapted to utilize motion for the formation phase of lymph. Anchoring filaments attached to each of the endothelial cells (see Fig. 51.3A) produce a change in volume with alternating movements in the local interstitial tissue. With this structure, overlapping endothelial cells allow the ebb and flow of fluid fluctuation from the interstitium into the lymphatic system. Motion opens access to lymphatics; swelling increases the opening, and up to a certain point the anchoring filaments prevent collapse of the thin-walled capillaries. Unfortunately, too much swelling closes the initial lymphatic entry sites. So, a major limiting factor for overall lymphatic homeostasis is the movement of lymphatic fluid into the blind endothelial sacs and the initial lymphatic tubules during the formation phase.

The **vascular phase** consists of the movement of lymph through the lymphatic vessels (see Fig. 51.4). In this phase, the lymphangion is the functional unit with its smooth muscle, valves, and intrinsic peristalsis being under autonomic control.

The **lymphangion** can generate enough pressure to account for intravascular lymph movement (see Fig. 51.3B). Additionally, lymphatic propulsion from the vessels themselves is homeostatically accomplished with the help of muscle pumps, respiratory motion, and intrinsic movement of the viscera (such as the intestines). One-way valves encourage propulsion toward the heart. The walls of the lymphangion segments between the valves contain smooth muscle fibers; distention of the walls in these segments produces stimulation of stretch receptors resulting in rhythmic peristaltic waves that effectively move lymph toward the heart.

Unfortunately, the vascular phase can become dysfunctional with increased tissue tension and somatic dysfunction. Here, the thinnest-walled vessels, the lymphatics, are the first vascular structures affected by fascial dysfunction or torsion.

The lymphatic system is particularly vulnerable to fascial dysfunction in the region of the superior thoracic inlet. The vulnerability of the vascular phase of lymphatic function is most likely at this site because the thoracic duct must pass through this fascial diaphragm (Sibson fascia) twice before discharging lymph back in to the central cardiovascular system. Recalling the contiguous nature of the scalene and Sibson fascia in this region, congestion is especially prominent when coexisting with scalene muscular hypertonicity.

In the vascular phase, the large lymph vessels may also become dysfunctional with sympathicotonia, which impairs both their

peristalsis and the sympathetically controlled valves between the thoracic ducts and the venous system. Here too, trigger points in the scalene muscles are purported to also cause dysfunction by reflexly impeding thoracic duct peristalsis (42).

The **terminal drainage phase** refers to lymphatic drainage into regional collection sites for eventual drainage into the thoracic ducts and subsequently into the subclavian vein (see Fig. 51.4). These junctures are under sympathetic control. The diaphragm, Sibson fascia, and the superior thoracic inlet are once again key areas for terminal lymphatic drainage from all regions. As Millard noted, "The lymph stream must always be drained first through terminal areas. Attempts to clear the lymph stream before clearing the edema in the clavicular regions over-tax the general lymph stream and cause profound reactions."

Zink, who popularized the respiratory-circulatory model, referred to certain palpable sites of "terminal lymphatic drainage" dysfunction that could be used clinically to identify the first regional signs of compromised lymphatic homeostasis in this phase. These terminal sites include (Fig. 51.6):

- Supraclavicular for the region of the head and neck
- Posterior axillary fold for each respective upper extremity
- Subxiphoid for the abdominal region
- Inguinal for each respective lower extremity

In the respiratory-circulatory model, 35% to 60% of the drainage through the thoracic duct is said to be accounted for by various pumping activities associated with the act of respiration; external respiration determining internal respiration. The two main respiratory elements in this regard include the mechanical pump created by the diaphragmatic crura on the cysterna chyli and the Venturi Effect (Bernoulli Principle), which acts both as a "suction pump" and factor to reduce the outflow pressure against which lymph must drain (see Fig. 51.4D).

Quoting the Venturi effect, Zink linked venous with lymphatic return in the respiratory-circulatory model. He described a "**Warmth Provocative Test**" used to identify areas of spinal somatic dysfunction that he postulated were significant enough to impede effective segmental venous return (Fig. 51.7). Segmental or systemic, the model predicts that the greater the venous return, the greater the lymphatic return.

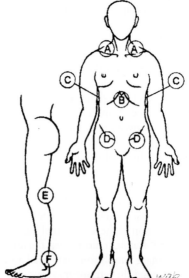

A. Supraclavicular space "head and neck"

B. Epigastric region "abdomen and chest"

C. Posterior axillary fold "arm"

D. Inguinal region "lower extremity"

E. Popliteal space "leg"

F. Achilles region "ankle and foot"

Figure 51-6 Palpation sites for terminal lymphatic drainage dysfunction from body regions.

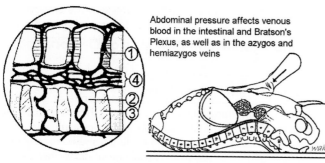

Figure 51-7 Zink "Warmth Provocative" test for a significant somatic dysfunction using the respiratory-circulatory model.

IMPLEMENTING THE RESPIRATORY-CIRCULATORY MODEL

The respiratory-circulatory model concerns itself with the maintenance and enhancement of extra- and intracellular environments through the unimpeded delivery of oxygen and nutrients and the removal of cellular waste products. In this model, the clinical goal is to identify and remove key tissue stresses interfering with the flow or circulation of body fluids in order to positively affect tissue health (43). Therapeutic application of OMT, as determined by this model, addresses somatic dysfunction affecting respiratory mechanics, circulation, and the flow of body fluids. Many of the techniques used in this model are designed to enhance the homeostatic mechanisms associated with the lymphatic system, and these are therefore sometimes broadly referred to as "lymphatic techniques" even though they may have other roles and other mechanisms.

Lymphatic techniques are those which are designed to remove impediments to lymphatic circulation and promote and augment the flow of lymph. The purpose of so-called lymphatic treatments is to improve the functional capacity of the lymphatic system, which includes maintenance of fluid balance in the body, purification and cleansing of tissues, and enhancement of immune response. As the lymphatic system is also involved in tissue nutrition and the absorption of macronutrients from the gastrointestinal tract and interstitial fluids, treatments enhancing lymphatic function can theoretically improve tissue nutrition.

Indications and Contraindications

With the foregoing aspects in mind, general indications for use of lymphatic treatment techniques within the framework of the respiratory-circulatory model include:

- Acute somatic dysfunction
- Sprains, strains
- Edema, tissue congestion, or lymphatic/venous stasis
- Pregnancy (Fig. 51.8)
- Infection
- Inflammation
- Pathologies with significant venous and/or lymphatic congestion.

The respiratory-circulatory approach is one of three arms used in the treatment of systemic dysfunction wherein coordinated, directed osteopathic manipulative treatment provides homeostatic enhancement (44). (The other two are strategies and techniques to modify sympathetic and parasympathetic activity—see ANS-Related Chapters 10 and 11). Examples of systemic implication can be found in Table 51.2 (45).

There are few absolute systemic contraindications to the approach other than conditions such as anuria (if the patient is not on dialysis) or in an area of necrotizing fasciitis. That said, clinical judgment must be used in employing lymphatic techniques with particular attention directed toward the patient's diagnosis, clinical condition, and medical therapy. It is obvious that local issues (such as a fracture at the sites where a given technique might transmit force) must be considered when deciding on any treatment approach. These and other pragmatic factors influence choice of the appropriate technique, site, dose, duration, and frequency of treatment.

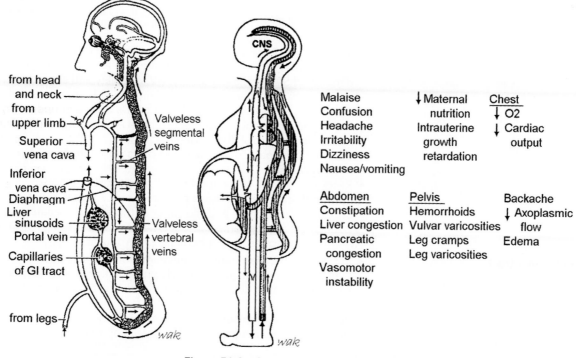

Figure 51-8 Congestive phase of pregnancy.

TABLE 51.2

Lymphatic Homeostatic Concerns in Systemic Disease and Dysfunction (Synopsis of *Osteopathic Considerations in Systemic Dysfunction*)

Systemic Region or Patient Population	Examples of Pathologies or Homeostatic Concerns
Eyes-ears-nose-throat (right side of head and neck drain to right thoracic duct; left side to the left thoracic duct)	• Glaucoma linkage to fluid drainage of eye • Endolymphatic hydrops ("glaucoma of the ear") • Meniere's: Fibrosis of edematous fluids in the endolymphatic duct • Foreign body (or wax) against the eardrum (vagal stimulation) may cause rapid shallow breathing (thereby compromising effectiveness of the respiratory-circulatory model) • Lymph node pattern helpful in noting site of inflammation/infection
Upper respiratory tract	• Tissue congestion increases "misery index" in URTI and decreases medication tissue distribution • Lymph node pattern helpful in noting site of inflammation/infection; also type of infection (viral vs bacterial infection: posterior cervical chain > anterior cervical chain)
Lower respiratory tract (Pleural sac and lung tissues drain to pretracheal nodes and then to the RLD)	• Minor diaphragm flattening decreases efficacy of respiratory-circulatory pump affecting all body systems • Flattened diaphragm in COPD changes contraction of the diaphragm from inhalation into exhalation • Increased fluids or infection in alveoli stimulate vagal afferents that reflexly decrease the depth of respiration • Coughing often leads to exhalation rib dysfunction → chest cage respiratory efficacy • COPD often leads to barrel chest, rigid chest cage mechanics with flattened diaphragm and hypertonicity in secondary muscles of respiration (especially sternocleidomastoid)
Cardiovascular conditions (heart and mediastinum drain to the right thoracic duct)	CHF → pulmonary edema with secondary rapid, shallow breathing (due to stimulation of vagal afferents in alveoli) as well as hepatomegaly (nonfriable type); electrolyte imbalance from peripherally sequestered fluid plays role in CHF morbidity; increases lymphatic functional demand up to 40× resting capacity • Thoracic duct dilation (up to 16× normal) may occur with additional backflow of lymphatic fluid; dilated thoracic duct may leak leading to ascites • Vagal stimulation from posterior-inferior wall myocardial infarctions may decrease depth of respirations • Impaired lymphatic drainage from myocardium causes EKG abnormalities similar to sick sinus syndrome as well as arrhythmias, diminished SA node automaticity, AV irritability and slowed AV conduction; increased mortality and morbidity from myocardial infarctions; increased colonization of bacteria in heart and valves • Prolonged lymphatic impairment to heart → endomyocardial fibrosis and endomyocardial fibroelastosis • Lymphatic drainage of vascular wall plays postulated role in atherosclerosis • Recognize for use of pectoral muscles that 60% of coronary artery/cardiac disease patients have pectoralis major trigger points • Superior mediastinum and the superior thoracic inlet anatomic boundaries are the same Hypertension increases peripheral lymph production
Gastrointestinal tract	• Irritation of the diaphragm by inflammation or perforation of 0upper GI structures may cause diaphragmatic hypertonicity (and C3-5 referral) that decreases efficacy of the respiratory-circulatory model • Irritation of the stomach's vagal receptors may cause decreased depth of respiration (rapid shallow breathing results)

(continued)

TABLE 51.2 *(Continued)*

	• Gall bladder and pancreas share same lymphatic drainage pathways; compromise of drainage increases risk of pancreatitis resulting from gall bladder disorder • Poor lymphatic function decreases absorption and distribution of nutrients from the gut (especially those that are fat soluble) • Increased tissue congestion in and around the bowel leads to bloating, more symptomatic pain in irritable bowel syndrome, increased fibrosis in colitis and Crohn disorders; fatigue, constipation and/or diarrhea, pain, and cramps • Decreased medication distribution, accumulation of active drugs and drug by-products in congested tissues, and reduced supply available to other needy tissues; accumulation of toxic by-products normally managed by the liver • Some upper gastrointestinal surgical procedures irritate the diaphragm (retractors or free air introduced in endoscopic procedures) → decreased diaphragmatic respiratory efficacy
Genitourinary tract	• Renal lymphatics drain capsule and parenchyma of kidney acting as a "safety valve" aiding in clearance of waste products as well as fluid, electrolytes, infectious, and drug byproducts • Lymphatic drainage maintains needed oncotic gradient for countercurrent salt/water exchange in kidneys; impaired lymphatics increase oncotic pressure and decreases ability of kidney to concentrate urine • In acute ureteral obstruction, renal hilar lymph flow increases 300% • Capsular lymphatics dilate to prevent renal damage in hydronephrosis • Pelvic congestion (in conjunction with hormonal basis) → dysmenorrheal, premenstrual syndrome, ovarian cysts, backache-headache-bloating of PMS, emotional instability and depression • Prostatic congestion decreases distribution of prostatic medications (if used) and may play a role in chronic nonbacterial prostatitis
OB patients	• Congestive phase is 28–36 weeks of gestation—partly mechanical, partly hormonal, partly biological • Breast engorgement (day 3 primipara or day 2 multipara) responds well to treatment of lymphaticovenous drainage of breasts
Pediatric patients	Heightened immune responsiveness suggests need to inform caregivers that lymphatic techniques intended to increase immune function may generate significant pyrogens and increase fever transiently (hours)
Geriatric patients	• Diminished immune function may not be as responsive to lymphatic techniques to improve immune response • Increased venous and lymphatic stasis of dependency and more common in the aged patient may cause misinterpretation of congestive findings as secondary to an acute or other local pathological process
Rheumatological patients	• Lymphatics remove waste products and immune complexes out of the region of inflamed joints; congested joints are more painful and have less synovial distribution of anti-inflammatory or disease-modifying medications • Swelling with poor lymphatic drainage leads to fibrosis around joints and further decreases range of motion • Tendons are very rich in lymphatics; tenosynovitis responds well to lymphatic techniques

Source: Kuchera M, Kuchera W. *Osteopathic Considerations in Systemic Function.* Columbus, OH: Greyden Press, 1994.

Relative contraindications to certain techniques exist; however, they are specific to the respiratory-circulatory model and certain lymphatic treatment techniques. These include the following examples:

- *Cancer:* There is some concern about enhancing lymphatic flow based upon potential lymphatic spread of cancerous cells rather than activating the immune system. Advocates point out the value of exercise in a number of cancerous conditions that is known to increase lymphatic flow. Because, to date, no risks of lymphatic treatment on patients with cancer have been demonstrated, judicious use in select cancer patients is supported by most authorities

- *Certain infections:* Splenic pump and hepatic pump techniques are probably contraindicated in Infectious mononucleosis patients or any patient who may have a fragile hepatosplenomegaly. The approach (especially applied directly over infected tissues or nodes) must be used with caution if at all in patients with overwhelming bacterial infections and an associated risk of dissemination or chronic infections that have a risk of reactivation (abscess, chronic osteomyelitis)

- *Certain circulatory disorders* (venous obstructions, embolism, hemorrhage) or *coagulopathies* (including patients on anticoagulants): For example, a technique like the Dalrymple pedal pump should be avoided if a patient has positive Homan or Moses signs or any other indication of deep vein thrombosis in one of his or her lower extremities

Safety and Efficacy

The risk-to-benefit ratio for lymphatic techniques is quite good. No known significant complications have resulted from osteopathic lymphatic treatment to date and multiple published studies have documented the efficacy of various lymphatic treatments. Nonetheless, clinical judgment should always be used when prescribing treatment for a patient in any disease state.

For example, in recognition of the highly effective immune function in the majority of the pediatric population, be sure to warn caregivers that a lymphatic treatment approach may transiently increase their child's fever; this being a normal response to the pyrogens produced in fighting infection. Treatment of the fever may or may not be necessary depending upon its level and duration.

Finally, a special comment will be made here regarding the safety of returning fluids back into an already fluid-overloaded condition such as that found in a patient with congestive heart failure (CHF). In such a state, the thoracic duct may be dilated sixteen times its normal size; subsequent leakage can cause ascites and congestive backflow can compromise other organs (e.g., pulmonary edema or hepatomegaly). In a study of severe CHF

patients where death was imminent, a surgical shunt was created between the thoracic duct and venous system; the clinical outcome was stabilization (fluid-electrolyte improvement) within 24 hours (46). This has been offered to suggest that homeostatic lymphatic fluid return will not overload the system even in severe CHF (47).

Principles of Diagnosis

Use of the respiratory-circulatory model or of lymphatic techniques in a coordinated systematic manner is based upon determining how much the patient would benefit relative to their risk of their application:

1. *Indications/risk-to-benefit ratio:* Obtain a history and physical examination relating to swelling, organ dysfunction and disease, shortness of breath, areas of swelling or puffiness, tissue trauma, and infection. Knowing whether a given pathological condition has a significant lymphatic component is helpful in deciding the degree of emphasis on the respiratory-circulatory model and the use of lymphatic techniques. Palpable tension, tenderness or ticklishness, or full, boggy tissue texture changes in the regional terminal lymphatic drainage sites are particularly useful in determining if regional tissue congestion exists (see Fig. 51.6). The initial history and examination should also cover possible absolute and relative contraindications for the use of lymphatic techniques

2. *Central myofascial pathways:* Palpate anatomical transition zones and consider the fascial compensated or noncompensated patterns described by Zink (Fig. 51.9) to describe common fascial restrictions such as torsion or rotational patterns, which may cause restriction of lymphatic flow. Restriction in any direction or pattern indicates dysfunction; however, a pattern of fascial motion restrictions that does not alternate in direction for adjacent regions is considered to be "uncompensated" or "traumatic" and is often a cause of congestive symptoms and an indication for treatment under this model. Even compensated patterns of fascial somatic dysfunction may cause symptoms; however, this is especially true in patients who are restricted to bed rest where the peripheral muscular pumps normally activated by walking fail to simultaneously alter the relationships between adjacent regions to permit free fluid flow. Other key myofascial somatic dysfunctions that can be associated with general reduction in lymphatic flow include trigger points in the scalene muscles

3. *Fluid pumps:* Observe and palpate muscular and fascial diaphragmatic function including thoracic inlet restrictions, for conditions that may limit lymphatic flow. In the supine position, the motion of respiration should be seen to extend all the way to the pubic symphysis in a patient who is breathing passively and in a nonselfconscious manner; failure to do so could

Figure 51-9 Regional diagnosis and transition zone relationship to the four major transverse diaphragms.

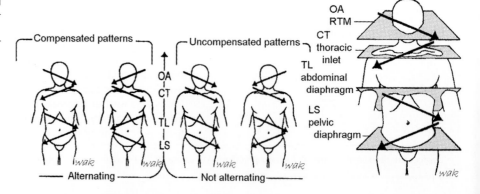

be interpreted as a need to address improvement of thoracic diaphragm function. Likewise, the pelvic diaphragm should be palpated. It should normally move passively and synchronously with the thoracic diaphragm and exhibit equal tension to the medial wall of both ischiorectal fossae. A poorly functioning thoracic diaphragm that does not respond to redoming OMT or treatment of the inferior thoracic outlet may warrant diagnosis and treatment of any C3-5 (phrenic) somatic dysfunction. Attempts to "redome" the pelvic floor with OMT should follow treatment of any bony-articular pelvic somatic dysfunctions

4. *Spinal Involvement:* After treatment of the central pathways and diaphragms, compression of the abdominal region by the physician's hand should create a uniform sensation of warmth down to the sacrum—Zink "Warmth Provocative test" (48) (see Fig. 51.7). A spinal area perceived to be warmer than others may be interpreted as a site of somatic dysfunction requiring treatment to maximize fluid return. Other key somatic dysfunctions interfering with the respiratory-circulatory model would include those thoracic, rib, and sternal dysfunctions that restrict motion of the chest cage (secondary respiration) and cranial base, C2 somatic dysfunction, and sacral somatic dysfunctions that restrict the depth of respiration (primary respiratory mechanism)

5. *Peripheral/Regional pathways:* Evaluate sites of terminal lymphatic drainage associated with early regional lymphatic congestion (see Fig. 51.6). Congestion in the terminal lymphatic drainage sites may constitute an indication for comprehensive treatment using the respiratory-circulatory model. Palpate other regional and local tissues to evaluate the presence of congestion and excess fluid in the interstitial tissues. This helps identify the region that might benefit from local fluid techniques as a last step in this model's protocol

Principles of Treatment

Treatment protocols using this model are typically designed to (1) remove impediments to lymphatic flow, (2) enhance mechanisms involved in respiratory-circulatory homeostasis, (3) extrinsically augment the flow of lymph and other immune system elements, and (4) further mobilize lymphatic fluids from local or regional tissues that would benefit from decongestion. These are summarized in Table 51.2.

Theoretically, all manipulative treatments can influence the lymphatic system through change in muscle tone, myofascial pathways, neural reflexes, autonomic tone, and effects of respiration. Certain osteopathic techniques however have been long identified as "lymphatic techniques" because of their efficiency and efficacy. Some of these techniques are postulated to remove somatic dysfunctions that interfere with various motions needed for lymph formation or lymph flow, others to remove key somatic dysfunctions that impede flow between or through somatic structures, and yet others do not remove somatic dysfunction but rather are considered to augment homeostatic mechanisms important in respiration and circulation.

Proposed Mechanisms of Treatment

To improve treatment outcomes, different strategies might be selected to enhance homeostatic mechanisms specifically linked to the different phases of lymphatic function (see Figs. 51.3 to 51.5). For example:

■ Any OMT technique that improves *local tissue motion* should enhance the *lymph formation phase*, consequently reducing edema and improving cellular level nutrition. While tensegrity principles suggest that this can be indirectly accomplished with almost any technique that removes somatic dysfunction throughout the body, the most effective choice should be specific local manual techniques that include oscillatory movement, various manual techniques focused upon the soft (myofascial) tissues, or any addition of a host of energy-transmitting physical therapy modalities (such as pulsed ultrasound or Fulford percussion hammer) that could increase local tissue motion

■ Application of other types of ancillary modalities such as rest, ice, compression, and elevation during acute edematous states should be properly timed to limit local swelling (to prevent it from overwhelming the local homeostatic mechanisms allowing entry into the blind-end lymphatic capillaries) and otherwise remove impediments to the lymph *formation phase*

■ Several OMT treatments affect lymphatic channels as they travel between fascial layers or body regions. Any treatment that reduces myofascial restriction can theoretically improve lymphatic flow by optimizing the *vascular phase* and thereby increasing the efficacy of intrinsic lymphatic pumps. Myofascial release (MFR), balanced ligamentous tension, and ligamentous articular strain techniques would seem to be especially suited to removing such local and regional fascial obstructions

■ Also numerous OMT treatment forms employ direct external forces that serve to act as extrinsic pumps that mobilize lymphatic fluid in the *vascular phase*. Some of these treatments improve the lymph flow by applying external pressure (soft tissue effleurage, massage, petrissage, etc.), whereas others remove somatic dysfunction that generally restricts fluid or employs directed muscle energy OMT to speed propulsion using muscle pumps. This latter mechanism is especially effective in the periphery when combined with Ruddy Rapid Resistive Duction OMT where contraction-relaxation rates may be two to three times the normal heart pulsation. (See as an example Ruddy technique using the sternocleidomastoid muscle.) Significant increases in lymphatic flow rates in the thoracic duct have been measured as well using both the muscle pumps involved in exercise and the passive pressure changes of various lymphatic pump OMT techniques (Fig. 51.10A)

■ Osteopathic treatment that seeks to enhance the efficacy of respiratory mechanisms (primary and secondary) in order to maximize venous and lymphatic return during either the *vascular* or the *terminal phase* typically focuses upon improving diaphragm or chest cage functions. (See as an example: thoracic diaphragm release technique, Fig. 51.10B.) Such respiratory approaches to circulation function largely through amplifying rhythmic pressure changes between compartments as well as the previously mentioned Bernoulli principle

■ Lymphatic pump manipulative techniques are also used over the spleen, liver, chest cage, or from the feet. The direct motion against the tissues could affect the *formation phase*; the systemic and rhythmic pumping could affect the *vascular phase*; and the additional pressure changes in intra-abdominal and intrathoracic cavities could affect the *terminal phase*. (See as examples: splenic pump and Dalrymple pedal pump, respectively.)

Other mechanisms of action for OMT have been postulated and are worthy of exploration. For example, the role of eNOS is of particular interest because of the mechanics of the lymphatic pumps. The intermittent movement associated with the previously mentioned Dalrymple pedal lymphatic pump has the potential to increase shear stress on the vascular endothelium (Fig. 51.10C). Such shear stresses applied at twice the typical heart rate were

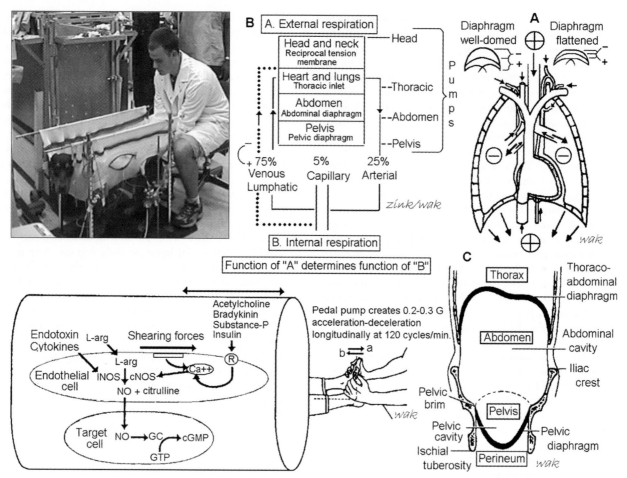

Figure 51-10 **A.** Mobilization of immune cells as a postulated mechanism for lymphatic pump OMT. **B.** Pressure changes, Bernoulli principle, and relationship between internal and external respiration as a postulated mechanisms for diaphragmatic lymphatic pump techniques. **C.** Upregulation of endothelial NO as a postulated mechanism for some of the action of OMT.

postulated to release an increased amount of NO (through upregulation of eNOS) from the blood vessels (49,50); a mechanism of action that has been postulated to account for many of the benefits of OMT (51). Release of NO through the same mechanism of action has similarly been postulated as an underlying mechanism for many of the benefits attributed to exercise (52). Interestingly, NO is not only produced in the walls of blood vessels but produced in the luminal wall of lymphatic vessels as well (53). This suggests that physiologic levels of NO produced by lymphatic endothelium may play a role in regulating lymphatic vascular tone.

As more is learned about the mechanisms of action for various OMT techniques, additional strategies may be found for the existing techniques as well as being able to finetune the frequency and duration of their application in order to accomplish the desired goals.

Evidence-Based Physiological Outcomes of Treatment

A wide range of lymphatic drainage techniques have been shown to be effective in reducing pain, edema, and tissue turgor secondary to numerous traumatically induced inflammatory processes. Furthermore, evidence is growing for the use of manual techniques and exercise to enhance immune function. Regardless of the professional degree of the healthcare practitioner, a growing number of techniques ranging from massage (including effleurage and petrissage) (54) to indirect OMT (such as counterstrain) (55,56) to mechanical tissue movement (such a vibration) (57) to exercise strategies have each been documented to accomplish particular physiological responses.

For many decades, it has been known that scarring or thickening of tissues might occur after trauma if only water is resorbed and interstitial proteins remain; poorly rehabilitated ankle sprains with thickening of the Achilles tendon is one example of this. Efficient lymphatic drainage facilitates removal of the proteins in edematous states and might effectively prevent this problem. Furthermore, removal of inflammatory cytokines and the subsequent resolution of the pain and sequelae associated with an inflammatory process depend on efficient lymphatic drainage. The evidence base for movement, early ambulation, use of compressive wraps to limit initial swelling, elevation to allow the effect of gravity to improve lymphatic drainage and various lymphatic drainage manual methods from those of Vodder to those of the massage therapists is extensive (58,59).

The osteopathic respiratory-circulatory model also depends upon the role of OMT to improve the compliance of the chest wall, diaphragmatic excursion, and efficacy of the respiratory process generally. Here, the logic is convincing but less extensive evidence has been published concerning the application. Nonetheless, examples of the evidence-base here include demonstration that restriction of chest wall excursion limits forced expiratory vital capacity and forced expiratory volume in 1 second (60) while treatment of chest wall somatic dysfunction with OMT has been shown to increase chest expansion, O_2 saturation, increase total lung capacity, and improve vital capacity as much as incentive spirometry or more (61–63). In patients with chronic obstructive pulmonary disease (COPD), manual treatment of the chest wall to increase respiratory efficacy has been shown "chest wall gymnastics" (64,65), and by osteopathic physicians using OMT (61).

With respect to immune function and the lymphatic model, a significant amount of documentation has been made in the last few decades and, based upon the emphasis of currently funded research in the osteopathic profession, tremendous advances are immediately ahead. It has been noted that the production of lymphocytes is increased greatly as lymph passes through the nodes. Research indicates that T-lymphocytes remain approximately 30 minutes in the blood circulation, about 5 to 6 hours in the spleen, and 20 hours in the lymphatic vascular system (66).

In the early 1980s, Measel (67) conducted experiments testing immune response in healthy individuals using the classic thoracic (Miller) pump technique. He found a greater immune response to several subserotypes of pneumococcal polysaccharide in the treatment group relative the control group. Since that study, several other groups have looked at immune function in response to different lymphatic pumps in isolation.

For example, in 39 healthy subjects provided with hepatitis B vaccine, one study (68) found a faster rise in antibody titers in those who also had lymphatic and splenic pump techniques three times weekly for 2 weeks compared to the control group. By 13 weeks, 50% of treated subjects versus only 16% of controls achieved protective antibody titers and at all points in time after 6 weeks, the antihepatitis titers in the treatment group were higher than in the control. However, by the end of the study period, both groups had similar numbers of individuals with protective antibody titers. In a different study using splenic pump alone in nursing home residents, the researchers failed to show improved influenza vaccine antibody titers after the use of splenic pump, but did document a reduction in antibiotic use during the influenza season (69).

Recent research studies conducted at the Osteopathic Research Center (ORC) located at the University of North Texas Health Sciences Center—Texas College of Osteopathic Medicine (UNTHSC-TCOM) clearly support the claim that lymphatic pump OMT techniques (thoracic or abdominal) are capable of enhancing both lymphatic flow and leukocyte flux. Innovative protocols employing dogs with surgically cannulated thoracic ducts were designed to answer the question of "How much lymph could a lymph pump pump if a lymph pump could pump lymph?" (70) The model (see Fig. 51.10A) permitted the researchers to directly measure approximately a three-fold increase in thoracic duct lymph flow as well as a five to seven-fold increase in the number of active immune cells per milliliter of lymph in response to the lymphatic pumps; similar to the increases seen in exercise. Researchers at the ORC are now studying the impact of lymphatic pump in reducing morbidity and mortality in rats infected with highly pathogenic pneumonia-causing bacteria as well as others with carcinomas in the lungs.

Using a human model at the Philadelphia College of Osteopathic Medicine (PCOM), researchers at the Human Performance and Biomechanics Laboratory of the Center for Chronic Disorders of Aging demonstrated that using the Dalyrimple pump created significant increases in NO at levels consistent with those expected from eNOS release (71) (see Fig. 51.10B). Furthermore, NO levels from this passive intervention were consistent with those levels produced by moderately intense exercise. Researchers at this site

are investigating the impact of pedal lymphatic pump OMT on NO levels and other parameters in subjects with conditions ranging from fibromyalgia syndrome to Parkinson disease. Preliminary studies performed collaboratively by these PCOM and UNTHSC-TCOM researchers using real-time NO probes in dogs have shown this biomarker to rise and fall in venous blood and thoracic duct lymph with each respiration and to be increased with application of a lymphatic pump maneuver.

At this point in time, there are also calls for osteopathic research based upon around the respiratory-circulatory model ranging from studies to reduce postmastectomy lymphedema (72,73) to those to reduce mortality risk in any future influenza pandemic (74).

Treatment Technique Order (Integrated into the Respiratory-Circulatory Model)

Following a common-sense order for most fluid systems, the order of the techniques used in the respiratory-circulatory model might be summarized by the following series of statements:

> *First open the pathways for fluid to flow; then turn on their thoracoabdominopelvic pump to its normal operating level. If you have congestion, turn the pumps up to "high" to clear any backflow in the system. When the backflow is cleared, then new fluid from targeted areas can be moved into the drainage system.*

With this simple mechanical process in mind, the order of integrating choices from the varying broad categories of "lymphatic treatment" techniques proceeds roughly in the order of the following goals:

(Goal 1) open myofascial pathways at transition areas of the body
(Goal 2) maximize normal diaphragmatic motions
(Goal 3) increase pressure differentials or transmit motion in order to pump or otherwise augment fluid flow beyond normal levels, and
(Goal 4) mobilize targeted tissue fluids into the lymphaticovenous system

Examples of these techniques appear in Tables 51.3 to 51.6 and are subdivided with relationship to each stepwise goal. Following each portion of the table, a few descriptive step-by-step techniques are offered to supplement the figures or provide alternative methods.

(Step/Goal 1) Techniques for Freeing Lymphatic Pathways

> *The lymph stream must always be drained first through terminal areas. Attempts to clear the lymph stream before clearing the edema in the clavicular regions (thoracic inlet) is to over-tax the general lymph stream and cause profound reactions.*—F. P. Millard, D.O. (75).

In the respiratory-circulatory model popularized by Zink, D.O., the first step of care should be to open the major fascial pathways (see Fig. 51.9). The four key sites used in diagnosis and treatment of this clinical goal are the:

1. Craniocervical junction
2. Cervicothoracic junction
3. Thoracolumbar junction
4. Lumbopelvic junction

These are transitional areas where anatomic structure changes (several related to transverse diaphragms between the regions). Therefore, these are the areas where function first changes.

TABLE 51.3

Integration into a Sequenced Respiratory-Circulatory Model Approach: Lymphatic Techniques to Open Pathways and Remove Restriction to Flow

Manipulative Approaches	Comments
Regional OMT of Zink's transitional areas • Craniocervical junction release • Cervicothoracic junction (superior thoracic inlet: T1-4, R1-2, manubrium) • Thoracolumbar junction (inferior thoracic outlet) • Lumbopelvic junction	Direct or indirect method OMT as appropriate to either the regions involved or to the separate structures contributing to the structure-function of the region (see Fig. 51.11 for Regional handholds adaptable to MFR, BLT, or muscle energy OMT techniques)
Sibson fascial release (helps to add OMT to scalenes and ribs 1 and 2)	Indirect or direct
Soft tissue techniques • Kneading—stretching • Direct MFR • Indirect MFR • Tapotement • Petrissage • Fascial unwinding • Fulford percussion hammer release • Directed self-stretching techniques/exercises	Specific technique less important than the goals of limiting entrapment and providing freedom for free lymphaticovenous flow; petrissage excellent at scar sites; fascial unwinding or Fulford percussion OMT excellent post trauma as in an MVA *Note: In the extremities, these techniques may follow "out-of-order" ... often just prior to the last step*
Anterior and posterior axillary fold techniques	Important in upper extremity lymphatic drainage; anterior fold—pectoral traction combination also increases lymph flow (see later)
Extremity popliteal fossa release (spread) Direct MFR (extension ME may be added)	Improves pathway from foot, ankle, and lower leg
Other considerations include: • Treatment of the first rib and clavicle and scalenes Including the targeted regionalized soft tissue pathways described in the fourth section earlier rather than later	Depending upon the amount of congestion and other clinical factors, treatment sequence may vary here

Manipulative Approaches	
Other **preparatory OMT** may include: • For thoracoabdominal diaphragm: OMT to C3-5 or phrenic; OMT lower rib attachments (esp R12) and quadratus lumborum; psoas or even hip also may affect • For pelvic diaphragm: OMT to innominate, sacral, pubic somatic dysfunctions may be needed first • Reducing exaggerated sagittal plane posture also affects both diaphragms—through quadratus lumborum and psoas as well as the posterior L1-2-(3) attachments for the thoracoabdominal diaphragm, but also for the pelvic diaphragm tension placed on the pelvic floor by gravity and the counter-rotation within the pelvis (see Chapter 36)	
Thoracic diaphragm "redoming"/indirect release	
Thoracic diaphragm "redoming"/direct release	
Ischiorectal fossa technique for the pelvic diaphragm	

If perfection is not possible (no somatic dysfunction), Zink noted that the natural homeostatic inclination of the patient was to develop an alternating pattern at the four transitional areas. The most common pattern involved the pelvis rotating to the right, thoracolumbar junction to the left, upper thoracic inlet area rotating to the right, and the occipitoatlantal region rotating to the left.

He described this pattern, seen in 80% of normal individuals, as the "CCP." The uncommon pattern (seen in 20%) has the opposite alternating fascial pattern.

Traumatically induced and/or highly dysfunctional fascial patterns were felt to significantly compromise the ability of the body to move venous or lymphatic fluids. Uncompensated patterns are

TABLE 51.4

Integration Into a Sequenced Respiratory-Circulatory Model Approach: Lymphatic Techniques to Maximize Diaphragmatic Functions

Manipulative Approaches	Comments
Thoracic diaphragm "redoming": direct or indirect release	For the thoracoabdominal diaphragm to respond, consider also: OMT to C3-5 or phrenic; OMT lower rib attachments (esp R12) and quadratus lumborum; psoas or even hip also may affect function
Ischiorectal fossa technique for the pelvic diaphragm	For pelvic diaphragm: OMT to innominate, sacral, pubic somatic dysfunctions may be needed first
Other preparatory OMT may include:	Reducing exaggerated sagittal plane posture also affects both diaphragms—through quadratus lumborum and psoas as well as the posterior L1-2-(3) attachments for the thoracoabdominal diaphragm, but also for the pelvic diaphragm tension placed on the pelvic floor by gravity and the counter-rotation within the pelvis (see Chapter 36: Postural Model)

TABLE 51.5

Integration into a Sequenced Respiratory-Circulatory Model Approach: Lymphatic Techniques to Accentuate Lymphatic Return and Augment Lymphatic Pumps

Manipulative Approaches	Comments
Thoracic pump—with and without modifications • Classic thoracic (Miller) pump: Takes advantage of rhythmic added passive recoil from chest wall for greater pressure differentials with each pumping motion • Atelectasis modification: Takes advantage of periodic sudden "explosive" recoil to refill collapsed alveoli • Pulmonary toilet variation: Takes advantage of continuous superimposed vibratory motion to mobilize secretions	Usual large amplitude component uses inherent respiratory rate for about 2 min; superimposed vibratory rate typically about 120/min. • Atelectasis variation contraindicated in emphysema patients (with hyperinflated blebs) • Avoid aspiration of secretions as well as gum or other intraoral objects
Splenic pumps • Immune function: Adult and pediatric versions • Also good for left lower lobe pneumonia • Abdominal pump version below costal margin	(See text for relative contraindications such as splenomegaly; Usual rate = 120/min for 2 min)
Liver pump: In reducing toxicity (a variation called the "liver flip" involves a quick release after taking up the passive range of the chest wall and may be useful in right lower lobe pneumonia with adhesion)	(See text for relative contraindications such as hepatomegaly)
Pedal (Dalrymple) pump	Usually 120/min for 2 min; (see relative contraindications in conditions such as deep vein thrombosis)
Ruddy rapid resistive duction (muscle pump) techniques • Specific or grouped isometric muscle pump against resistance moves fluid through one-way valves • Holding angle of the rib while patient intermittently activates/relaxes specific muscles attached to the rib(s) in question may be used to treat specific ribs and to improve rib cage dysfunction generally	Principle the same for all regions; rate typically twice the heart rate; muscle effort energy is minimal
Rib raising—seated and supine	

(continued)

TABLE 51.5 *(Continued)*

Pectoral traction	
Proximal lymphatic duct siphon technique and/or fluctuation at the distal cisterna chyli	
CV4 ("Compression of fourth Ventricle")	Links primary respiratory mechanism to secondary respiration; CV4 often results in slower, deeper respirations and empirically enhances fluid movement out of the body
Nasal sinus drainage and pump	Sometimes this is performed at the end of a sinus treatment
Exercise-Induced muscle pumps • Generally moves fluids with total body exercise (postulated mechanisms include muscle pump effect on one-way valves, enhanced depth of respiration, and/or release of eNOS) • Specific group muscle exercises my target tissues for drainage • Certain impact exercises (e.g., mini-trampoline) may be better for interregional pressure changes and eNOS release than nonimpact types	OMT to prepare the body for certain exercise types is recommended; placing exercise in the context of the Respiratory-Circulatory model is a very effective physician-patient decision for maintaining gains started in the office or hospital

TABLE 51.6

Integration into a Sequenced Respiratory-Circulatory Model Approach: Lymphatic Techniques to Mobilize Local Lymphatic Congestion

Manipulative Approaches	Comments
Mobilization (general and focused) from the head and neck region • Soft tissue OMT: Anterior cervical arches and hyoid • Soft tissues OMT: Lateral and posterior cervical tissues • Soft tissue, Ruddy OMT or counterstrain of the sternocleidomastoid ms • Submandibular and jugulodigastric drainage OMT • Mandibular and Eustachian drainage (Galbreath) OMT • Auricular drainage OMT	While some of these techniques could arguably be included in the first stage of opening pathways, they are usually performed either after that first step or at the end prior to effleurage depending on the degree of congestion
Mobilization (general and focused) from the upper extremity • Posterior axillary fold technique • Shoulder girdle OMT with goals of free clavicular and scapulocostal motions • Ulnoradial interosseous membrane release (LAS or BMT) • Removal of scalene and upper extremity MTrPs (etc.) causing entrapments	
Mobilization (general and focused) from the lower extremity • Fascial unwinding of the lower extremity • Tibiofibular interosseous membrane release • Removal of lower extremity MTrPs (etc.) causing entrapments	
Mobilization (focused) from the gastrointestinal tract	
Mobilization (focused) exercise from the uterus/pelvis • Uterine (Marion Clark) drainage exercise	Usually taught to do at home as self-exercise
Soft tissue OMT for fluid movement • Effleurage • Tapotement • Lateral fluid fluctuation (transmitted vibration)	After finding a BLT or BMT position, a lateral fluid fluctuation in any area may be introduced with greatly enhanced tissue reaction (e.g., adding oscillatory supination-pronation while performing the radioulnar interosseous membrane technique)

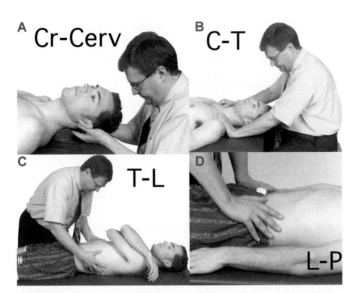

Figure 51-11 Hand placement for MFR or BLT to correct regional somatic dysfunctions compromising fluid drainage at the transition zones/major transverse diaphragms.

defined by the palpatory finding of even one nonalternating fascial preference between adjacent regions.

Many alternatives for opening fascial pathways exist to the indirect methods offered in Figure 51.11. Direct release method techniques for these transitional regions (and their transverse diaphragms) can also be supplied using the same hand placement and simply varying the level and type of the tissues contacted as well as the direction, tension, and type of release. An example for direct release of the very important superior thoracic inlet is offered as follows.

Direct Method Treatment of the Superior Thoracic Inlet (Cervicothoracic Diaphragm)

Example: Assume that the fascia at the patient's thoracic inlet has been diagnosed as being regionally $S_L R_L$.

Position: Patient is supine with arms across the chest (or comfortably along side) and the physician is seated at the head of the table.

Activating Force(s): Direct MFR, direct balanced regional ligamentous articular strain (or an adaptation for direct muscle energy) OMT:

1. Physician's hands are placed on the shoulders with fingers on the anterior chest wall below the clavicle and thumbs posterior behind the 1st to 2nd ribs
2. Physician applies caudad pressure to take the patient's right shoulder to its restrictive barrier (Inlet S_R)
3. While maintaining the right shoulder caudad pressure, the physician's left hand moves the patient's shoulder anteriorly and to the right to its restrictive barrier as the left hand contact simultaneously moves the patient's right shoulder posterior and medially (R_R). (The hands move simultaneously like turning a car's steering wheel.)
4. The patient is asked to take a deep breath in and out as the physician resists motion except for the direction described earlier

Continue until there is a myofascial or ligamentous release—depending upon the desired depth of the targeted tissues—resulting in equal right and left sidebending as well as equal right and left rotation. (If no release is sensed, it is possible to have the patient attempt to turn away from the barrier against resistance using standard

postisometric muscle energy steps.) Opening drainage pathways for the extremities may follow the opening of the transitional core regions in Step/Goal 1 (listed in Table 51.3 earlier); however, often when there is a lot of systemic congestion (as is the case for this chapter's pregnant transcriptionist), then this component is placed later in the series. Thus, opening local pathways for the extremities or a particular visceral structure may take place *after* core diaphragms are working (Step/Goal 2) and even *after* central congestion has been cleared (Step/Goal 3).

In mild cases, opening these more distal pathways can be done in conjunction with opening the core pathways.

(Step/Goal 2) Techniques for "Redoming" or Otherwise Maximizing Function of the Diaphragms

When the thoracoabdominal diaphragm contracts, it does so around its central tendon. It descends because of the stabilization offered largely by the quadratus lumborum muscle that stabilizes the 12th rib, a lower attachment of the diaphragm. A "flattened diaphragm" does not displace as much volume and is therefore a less effective pump (see Fig. 51.10B). In fact, in some conditions, the diaphragm is so flattened that it becomes a muscle of *exhalation* as it pulls the 11th and 12th calipered ribs medially.

In approaching the thoracoabdominal diaphragm with OMT, it is also helpful to recognize the posterior attachments of the crus of the diaphragm to L1-2-3 and lower ribs, the myofascial relationships of the diaphragm with the quadratus lumborum and psoas muscles, and the fascial continuity of the deep fascia of the abdomen and that underlying the diaphragm. Likewise in approaching the pelvic diaphragm, bony attachment and myofascial triggerpoints should be considered.

Table 51.4 presents lymphatic techniques for maximizing diaphragmatic function.

Two techniques are offered as examples for the thoracolumbar diaphragm; these are extensions of the previously mentioned inferior thoracic outlet techniques. Direct or indirect techniques that begin by using the handhold (themselves very effective for releasing the inferior thoracic outlet or thoracolumbar region) shown in Figure 51.11C can be transitioned into a thoracoabdominal diaphragm technique by simply concentrating on function and release of the diaphragmatic elements noted in steps 4 and 6 of the direct MFR technique.

Direct MFR to Open the Inferior Thoracic Outlet and Redome the Thoracoabdominal Diaphragm (see Fig. 51.11C)

Example: Assume that the region prefers sidebending and rotation left and that the diaphragm does not move as well on the left. Patient is supine with the patient standing on either side.

1. Position the lower ribs and thoracic cage to the "feather-edge" of the direct rotation barrier by moving both hands together to rotate to the patient's right
2. Add left translation with both hands simultaneously to create a right sidebending
3. Fine tune until the direct myofascial and ligamentous articular strain creep phenomenon begins (direct MFR/LAS)
4. At this point as the creep continues, shift attention to the diaphragm as the patient breathes. Add additional compression to the hemidiaphragm that moves most (in this example, the right moves best)
5. As the patient exhales, continue to follow the MFR/LAS release process (SB and rotate right more fully)
6. As the patient inhales, resist the most functional hemidiaphragm

7. Repeat steps 5 and 6 until diaphragmatic excursion begins on the poorly functioning side and the MFR/LAS release sensation is complete. Recheck with deep inhalation and exhalation for symmetry and functional excursion

Also, consider using the alternative anteroposterior hold to apply an indirect diaphragmatic redoming technique that has the advantage of being able to address the quadratus lumborum, psoas, and thoracolumbar lordotic curve as well. This technique is described as follows:

Indirect MMF to Redome the Thoracoabdominal Diaphragm

Example same as earlier and the same positions for physician and patient. For this technique:

1. Place one hand posteriorly to cup the L1-3 vertebral column (posterior diaphragmatic attachments) with fingers contacting paraspinal muscles on one side and the heel of the hand contacting the opposite muscles
2. Place fingers of the anterior hand to broadly contact the subxiphoid region compressing to sense the deep anterior abdominal fascia that is continuous with the fascia lining the undersurface of the diaphragm
3. Rotate one hand clockwise and opposite hand counterclockwise (whichever is indicated by testing fascial drag) to the point of indirect balanced tension
4. Fine tune balance by adding any superior-inferior and left-right translation between hands (moving in opposite directions) to establish full balance between the hands
5. Follow the release with normal respiration continuously maintaining the balance point until a release occurs in both hands

Multiple options for this vital area guarantee success when either the patient's status or presence of a surgical site might prevent a different technique.

(Step/Goal 3) Techniques to Accentuate Lymphatic Return and/or to Augment Lymphatic Pumps

This therapeutic step is all about changing pressures to move fluids through vessels with one-way valves, to enhance the siphon pump, or to transmit pressure changes into pressure-sensitive organs such as the liver or spleen. Typically, most pumps are performed at a rate of 120 beats/min and for the duration of 2 minutes.

Table 51.5 presents lymphatic techniques for accentuation of lymphatic return and augmentation of lymphatic pumps.

An interesting and effective fluid augmentation technique associated with this step is directed at the thoracic duct itself. A one-way valve is located at the proximal end of the thoracic duct. The thoracic duct can be stimulated at its proximal or its distal ends by directed, transmitted vibrations. Dr. Sutherland likened the thoracic duct to a siphon, indicating a functional turn at its superior end, allowing it to drain downward into the venous junction of the brachial and subclavian veins. The thoracic duct may be stimulated with a transmitted vibration at its proximal and distal ends.

Vibratory Methods for Treatment of the Thoracic Duct

Position: The patient is supine with knees flexed and feet on the table. The physician stands at the right side of the patient.

From the Distal End

1. Physician contacts the patient's upper right abdominal quadrant with one hand just below the costal margin and may reinforce this hand with the other hand.

2. A gentle, rhythmic vibration is instituted and directed toward the cisternal chyle. (This would be toward a midpoint of a line extending from the xiphoid process to the umbilicus.)

Toward the Proximal End

1. The physician's palm contacts the patient's left thorax over the second or third intercostal space at the midclavicular line and that hand is reinforced with the other hand.
2. A gentle, rhythmic vibration is instituted and directed posteriorly, laterally, and superiorly toward the junction of the thoracic duct to the left brachiocephalic vein.)

End point: A palpable sense of decongestion of tissues.

(Step/Goal 4): Mobilizing Targeted Lymphaticovenous Congestion

In the final goal, after the pathways are open and the body's homeostatic mechanisms are moving fluids, the osteopathic physician may select OMT techniques that decongest specifically targeted tissues. This step may incorporate manual lymphatic drainage techniques from other systems (such as the direct, light superficial effleurage strokes to move fluids through one-way valves toward the heart), the use of muscle pumping techniques (such as were packaged by Ruddy), gentle lateral fluctuation of fluids (as suggested by Sutherland), local MFR applied to the local somatic tissues, various visceral and mesenteric lifts applied to the viscera (76,77), or activation of reflex mechanisms to promote fluid movement.

Table 51.6 presents lymphatic techniques for mobilizing local lymphatic congestion.

The posterior axillary fold technique offers what Dr. Zink refers to as the "gateway to the upper extremity" (78). The mechanism of action for this technique has been postulated (79) to be reflex, autonomic, lymphatic, or a combination of parts of each. Palpation of the posterior and anterior axillary folds for evidence of myofascial dysfunction is clinically important in assessing the degree of lymphatic dysfunction affecting the upper extremities and/or breasts. The posterior axillary fold is the location of palpable myofascial points in the subscapularis, teres major, and latissimus dorsi muscles. It is also the site of terminal lymphatic drainage dysfunction for the upper extremities. Zink discusses diagnosis and treatment of this region to relieve lymphatic congestion in the upper extremity. Those findings closely parallel the palpatory and clinical findings described independently by Travell and Simons (80), using myofascial points located in the posterior axillary fold. Points higher in the posterior axillary fold correlate predominantly with shoulder referral, although lower points refer distally. Both Zink and Travell report that treatment of myofascial dysfunction in this area results in reduction of swelling, joint dysfunction, and dysesthesia. Likewise, appropriate treatment of anterior axillary fold dysfunction results in reduction of breast tenderness and congestive changes attributed to entrapment of breast lymphatics traveling around and through the pectoralis muscle toward the subclavicular lymph nodes (81).

Posterior Axillary Fold Technique

This technique is useful in patients who have increased lymphatic congestion of the upper extremity, as may occur in patients with shoulder discomfort, hand and/or arm paresthesias, patients with cool clammy hands, or patients who have had a radical mastectomy. It should probably be preceded by rib raising techniques or paraspinal inhibition to the patient's T1-8 thoracic region to calm segmental facilitation and insure that the large lymphatics are optimally functioning. This technique may also be used to treat tender myofascial points in the posterior axillary fold muscles. The more congested the tissues, the more tenderness there will be during the initial treatment with this treatment technique. **Note**: *This technique will be difficult to initiate in patients who are excessively ticklish, although thereafter it is "uncomfortable" enough generally to overwhelm the tickle.*

Position: The patient is supine and the physician stands or sits by the patient's shoulder and faces the patient's head on the side that is to be treated:

1. Physician caudad hand grasps the patient's posterior axillary fold with the thumb anteriorly and the fingers posteriorly. The total lateral length of the thumb and the index finger is snug against the patient's rib cage
2. The physician reinforces this grip of the caudad hand with the fingers and thumb of the cephalad hand
3. A steady, gentle, firm, squeezing pressure is applied through the entire length of the physician's thumb and held for about 10 to 15 seconds
4. The fingers are moved from the cephalad end toward the caudal end of the axillary fold and step 3 is repeated. This is repeated until the entire posterior axillary fold has been treated

Successful treatment: The patient, when asked, will feel warmth, not only in the arm but also to the finger tips, as good vascular flow is re-established. This warmth can be increased by having the patient clench and unclench the fist because this activates the peripheral muscular lymphatic pumps.

Lateral Fluctuation at the Forearm

This technique capitalizes on the use of motion in moving fluid out of the interstitial tissues into the blind lymphatics. As with all such local fluid mobilization techniques, pathways will have already have been cleared prior to using this technique. Note that for upper extremity OMT, the ulna is treated prior to the radius that is, in turn, treated prior to the wrist. If considered, LAS or BLT techniques for the interosseous membrane between the radius and the ulna could then be added. Lateral fluctuation of the forearm or effleurage is usually the last technique applied in applying the respiratory-circulatory model to this region.

Position: The patient is seated and the operator is seated and facing the patient:

1. Physician grasps the patient's hand as if to shake hands
2. The patient's elbow is supported by the other hand and the patient's elbow is flexed 90 degrees
3. Physician supinates and pronates the forearm until the position of greatest ligamentous balance is palpated
4. From this position of balance, the physician institutes a small rhythmic supination/pronation excursion that is continued during the entire treatment

Follow-Up and Self-Treatment Prescriptions

Neither the physician nor the patient should be surprised if a compensatory fascial somatic dysfunction pattern returns between clinic visits—few individuals are perfectly symmetrical. They can be informed that with normal walking activities, such alternating patterns are periodically aligned to permit fluid drainage. On the other hand, in hospitalized patients or individuals who are extremely sedentary, even compensatory fascial patterns may lead to symptomatic congestion and these individuals benefit from periodic treatment using the protocols discussed in Tables 51.3 to 51.6. Additionally, after a traumatic injury, core pathways may assume nonalternating, noncompensatory patterns compromising the respiratory-circulatory mechanism systemically or local pathways may be compromised leading to local congestive phenomena. Such symptomatic processes often benefit from osteopathic care using this model.

Patients may be educated to maximize their own respiratory-circulatory homeostatic mechanisms or to help prevent its dysfunction. These are important osteopathic goals designed to help patients raise their own health level or to be empowered to participate in their own ongoing care in a chronic condition. This may also be preventative in the previously mentioned sedentary individuals to keep them from needing to be "patients."

Depending upon the clinical situation, specific self-stretching exercises can be provided. The physician may choose to focus the patient on exercises that maintain open drainage pathways or exercises that are more general (systemic).

CASE STUDY (CONTINUED)

PREGNANT PATIENT WITH CARPAL TUNNEL SYNDROME

Initial Case Presentation:

After 14 years at the same job without complaint, a 32- year-old transcriptionist now presents with 6-week progressive numbness and tingling in her right (dominant) hand. Awakening her nearly every night, the distribution of her dysesthesiae includes her thumb and the next 2½ digits. For the last month she has had difficulty opening jars and has nearly dropped objects. Gravida I, para 0-0-0-1 and early in her second trimester, she takes no medications or nutritional supplements other than a prenatal vitamin. *The distribution of the numbness and weakness coupled with an almost pathognomonic night-wakening symptom is classic for CTS, a median entrapment neuropathy at the wrist.*

CTS occurs more commonly in individuals with (a) biomechanical risk factors (e.g., overuse on the computer, square wrists, forearm somatic dysfunction including triggerpoints, etc.); (b) neurological risk factors (e.g., double crush conditions including cervical radiculopathy or dysfunction, scalene entrapment, etc.); (c) hormonal risk factors (e.g., hypothyroidism, diabetes, etc.); and (d) fluid overload/edema (e.g., pregnancy) to name just a few causes bearing on the choice of osteopathic model that might be selected.

Findings:

Her right thenar eminence appears smaller than the left and manifests reduced grip strength; all fingers on the right hand are puffy. On the right, positive neurological tests include Phalen's (at 20 seconds) and Tinel's (just distal to the wrist's flexor crease). There are no other historical or physical findings to indicate thyroid disorder, cervical radiculopathy, diabetes, vascular disease, or other significant health issue.

The common compensatory pattern of Zink is violated by her superior thoracic inlet that prefers rotation and sidebending to the left. She has tender fullness in the right supraclavicular region and posterior axillary fold; in the supine position, her shallow, rapid breaths are seen to extend only half-way down to the umbilicus. Spinal palpatory reveals only grade I severity, Fryette type-I somatic dysfunctions; no Chapman points or collateral ganglion findings were identified. She has a right posterior radial head. Active MTrPs are palpated in the right pronator teres and in several forearm and finger flexor muscles.

EMG consisting of NCS with needle examination confirmed moderate severity median entrapment neuropathy at the wrist with positive sensory and motor NCS but no fibrillation potentials in the thenar eminence; it also ruled out a concomitant cervical radiculopathy. *The presence of both sensory and motor problems suggests that this problem is probably at least moderate in severity and that treatment is warranted. The EMG confirms this but without fibrillation potentials indicates that conservative management is possible in this case. The EMG also ruled out a cervical radiculopathy as might coexist in a low, but significant percentage of cases and could itself predispose that extremity to MTrPs.*

Coupled with several ruled-out risk factors, her pregnancy (including edema, signs of terminal lymphatic drainage dysfunction, poorly effective respiration, and multiple somatic dysfunctions impeding both optimal fluid return and optimal biomechanical efficiency) suggests that the optimal first conservative step might be a combination of applying the respiratory-circulatory model in conjunction with a biomechanical/ergonomical approach.

OVERVIEW OF APPROACH WITH OMT

Thus, while the findings in this particular case confirmed a neurological manifestational pathology, they also suggested that majority of the dysfunctional components (and perhaps the structural changes themselves) were related to overwhelming the patient's underlying myofascial and fluid homeostatic mechanisms. It was therefore determined that this particular case would best be "primarily" addressed conservatively by applying the **Respiratory-Circulatory model** instead of the **Neurological model** and emphasizing education and exercises derived from the **Biomechanical model.**

The primary goals selected for this particular pregnant transcriptionist included correcting somatic dysfunction (1) to remove pathway impediments to fluid return and (2) to maximize the use of respiratory and muscle pumps to augment that return. Additional goals to empower her through education to reduce ergonomic stress while self-exercising to keep fluid pathways open were also felt to be needed. The resultant homeostatic improvement in her ability to manage systemic fluid changes (seen in pregnancy) simultaneously with local edema (that may have resulted from overuse and trigger points associated with her job) eliminated her CTS symptoms and, in this case, modified several of the pathogenic causes of median entrapment so that self-healing mechanisms could take over.

Care in this case consisted of OMT at each of her remaining prenatal visits (employing from those techniques listed later only as needed to accomplish the clinical goals of the respiratory-circulatory model) and asking her to take a short rest with forearm-wrist stretches every few hours. This simple regimen successfully resolved her symptoms after the second visit even as she continued to work. After vaginal delivery and 1 month of maternity leave, she returned to work. Her thenar eminence on the right returned to normal and she had no further hand symptoms. With clinical improvement, she refused to repeat the EMG and she remained empowered with her prior education concerning wise ergonomics, self-stretch exercises for the neck and forearm, and breathing exercises (which also helped calm her "biopsychosocial" stressors that were related to being a working mom with a new child). She now seeks OMT occasionally "when she feels overly stressed at work" but is ultimately responsible for her own health.

RESPIRATORY-CIRCULATORY MODEL COMPONENTS USED IN THIS CASE

Opening the Pathways With Diaphragm Redoming

> *Direct MFR Thoracic Inlet OMT*
> *Direct MFR Thoracic Outlet Combined with Diaphragm Redoming Seated Muscle Energy of the Lumbopelvic Junction (no diagram)*
> *Soft Tissue Inhibition, Posterior Axillary Fold Technique*
> *Integrated Myofascial Spray and Stretch of Common* MTrPs (82)

AUGMENTING THE FLOW AND MOBILIZING REGIONAL CONGESTION

Pectoral Traction
BLT/BMT with Lateral Fluctuation of Arm

EXERCISE PRESCRIPTION FOR PATIENT

Self-Stretch (83,85)

EVIDENCE-BASED OUTCOMES OF OTM IN CTS CASES

Numerous osteopathic trials have been conducted in the care of patients with CTS (86–90). Sucher has even demonstrated the efficacy of the exercises recommended earlier in "opening" the carpal tunnel in cadaveric specimens (91). Currently, a large-scale study funded with NIH funding is underway at the ORC in Texas. (See Chapter 43 in this text for more information concerning CTS.)

COMMENT ON OTHER OSTEOPATHIC MODELS THAT COULD HAVE BEEN INVOLVED IN THIS CASE

Neurological Model:

Screening diagnosis identified the primary pathology to be related to probable median entrapment neuropathy at the wrist consistent with a unilateral CTS. However, there was no additional evidence of C5-C8 neural involvement as might exist from cervical disk disease, cervical ribs, scalene triggerpoints or entrapment, or significant cervical somatic dysfunction that might lead to a "double crush syndrome" augmenting CTS symptoms or to confusion with the sensory and motor supply of the hand. Furthermore, no segmental facilitation from viscera sharing the upper extremity's sympathetic segments (T2-8) was seen. In other cases of CTS, OMT to augment sensory, motor, and autonomic homeostasis might be the primary management strategy. Increased sympathetic tone decreases blood flow to the upper extremity, reduces the ability of large lymphatics to move fluid, and can play a role in the development of what was formerly called "reflex sympathetic dystrophy" but is now referred to as "complex regional pain syndrome." There is definitely an overlap between the respiratory-circulatory model and the neurological model

Biomechanical Model:

In pregnancy, many postural and biomechanical changes take place. Increasing sagittal plane curves have their effects on the transverse diaphragms and create additional myofascial forces all of which can overlap with the respiratory-circulatory model. From an ergonomic perspective, pregnant women often will modify how they perform tasks based upon growing uterine impediments to bending or positioning themselves to perform certain work tasks or activities of daily living,

Metabolic-Energy Model:

Hypothyroidism is more common in pregnancy and causes thickening of connective tissue that can predispose to CTS (up to 10% of bilateral CTS patients may have myxedema). The relaxin circulating in the pregnant patient may also interact with the postural and biomechanical model through changes in tensegrity. While the former was not a problem in this case, myxedema would need to be addressed prior to effectively applying the respiratory-circulatory model and the relaxin component in a pregnant patient influences choices of OMT techniques to use regardless of the model.

Behavioral Model:

This model mentioned the impact that respiratory instruction had in enhancing calmness and focus post-partum. (It did not mention the use of focused breathing this patient performed during her labor as a distraction from the pain of delivery). Optimal respiratory-circulatory homeostasis has a number of benefits important in the behavioral model including reduction of pain and anxiety by decreasing venous congestion around the central nervous system and enhancing the quality of sleep. Conversely, patients with heavy biopsychosocial stressors often have muscle tension and shallow breathing that compromise optimal respiratory-circulatory function.

In summary, an osteopathic approach to an individual case may not follow a single model, but identifying which model might have a primary impact permits the osteopathic practitioner to better focus his or her treatment plan in a time-efficient and effective manner. The outcome of applying the osteopathic respiratory-circulatory model to the chief complaint in this case accomplished much more than reduction of edema and thereby reduction of the signs and symptoms of "carpal tunnel syndrome."

REFERENCES

1. Zink JG, Applications of the osteopathic holistic approach to homeostasis. *Am Aca of Osteo Yearb* 1973;37–47.
2. Chikly B. Who discovered the lymphatic system? *Lymphology* 1997;30: 186–193.
3. Still AT. The lymphatics. In: *Philosophy of Osteopathy.* Kirksville, MO: A.T. Still, 1899:105–106.
4. Smith W. Skiagraphy and the circulation. *J Osteopath* 1899;3:356–378.
5. Millard FP. *Applied Anatomy of the Lymphatics.* Kirksville, MO: International Lymphatic Research Society, 1922.
6. Millard FP. New method of diagnosing various diseases by palpating lymphatic glands. *J Am Osteopath Assoc* 1920;19:405–408.
7. Millard FP. A lymphatic examination. *J Osteopath* 1922;29:78–81.
8. Millard FP. *Applied Anatomy of the Lymphatics.* Kirksville, MO: International Lymphatic Research Society, 1922:26–27.
9. Millard FP. *Applied Anatomy of the Lymphatics.* Kirksville, MO: International Lymphatic Research Society, 1922.
10. Goode GW, Millard FP. Manipulative lymphatic therapy [see comments]. In: *Selected Papers from the Section of Manipulative Therapeutics.* Indianapolis, IN: American Academy of Osteopathy, 1940;2:11–14.
11. Millard FP. Lymphatics: prevention of complications of diseases sought through clearance of stasis. *Osteopath Prof* 1945;13(3):20–23, 56.
12. Millard FP. *Applied Anatomy of the Lymphatics.* Kirksville, MO: International Lymphatic Research Society, 1922:43.
13. Zink JG. Respiratory and circulatory care: the conceptual model. *Osteopath Ann* 1977;5(3):108–112.
14. Zink JG. Respiratory and circulatory care: the conceptual model. *Osteopath Ann* 1977;5(3):108–112.
15. Zink JG, Lawson WB. The role of pectoral traction in the treatment of lymphatic flow disturbances. *Osteopath Ann* 1978;6(11):493–496.
16. Zink JG, Fetchik WD. The posterior axillary folds: a gateway for osteopathic treatment of the upper extremities. *Osteopath Ann* 1981;9(3):114–117.
17. Smith HJ. Ultrasonic assessment of abdominal venous return. I. Effect of cardiac action and respiration on mean velocity pattern, cross-sectional area and flow in the inferior vena cava and portal vein. *Acta Radiol Diagn* 1985;26(5):581–588.
18. Vodder E. *Le Drainage Lymphatique, Une Nouvelle Méthode Thérapeutique.* Paris, France: Santé Pour Tous, 1936.
19. Zink JG. Respiratory and circulatory care: the conceptual model. *Osteopath Ann* 1977;5(3):108–112.
20. Chikly B. *Silent Waves: Theory and Practice of Lymph Drainage Therapy-With Applications for Lymphedema, Chronic Pain and Inflammation.* I.H.H. Publishing, 2001.
21. Chikly B. Can practitioners be trained to manually identify lymphatic flow? Evidence from a case control study assessing skills in *Manual Lymphatic Mapping* (MLM).
22. Still AT. The lymphatics. Philosophy of Osteopathy. Kirksville, Mo: A.T. Still; 1899. Available at: http://www.meridianinstitute.com/eamt/files/still2/st2cont.html. Accessed July 13, 2007:105, 108–109.
23. Still AT. H.H. Gravett Papers. In: Trowbridge C, ed. *Andrew Taylor Still, 1828–1917.* Kirksville, MO: Thomas Jefferson University Press (NMSU), 1991:156.
24. Chikly BJ. Manual techniques addressing the lymphatic system: origins and development. *J Am Osteopath Assoc* 2005;105:457–464.
25. Barber ED. Diseases of the lymphatic system. In: *Osteopathy Complete.* Kansas City, MO: Hudson-Kimberly Publishing Co., 1898:131–146.
26. Lane MA. On increasing the antibody content of the serum by manipulation of the spleen. *J Osteopath* 1920;27:361–364.
27. Castilio Y, Ferris-Swift L. Effects of splenic stimulation in normal individuals on the actual and differential blood cell count, and the opsonic index [reprint]. 1932. *1955 Yearbook of the Academy of Applied Osteopathy.* Carmel, CA: Academy of Applied Osteopathy, 1955:111–120.
28. Castilio Y, Ferris-Swift L. The effect of direct splenic stimulation on the cells and the antibody content of the blood stream in acute infections diseases [reprint]. 1934. *1955 Yearbook of the Academy of Applied Osteopathy.* Carmel, CA: Academy of Applied Osteopathy, 1955:121–138.
29. Measel JW. The effect of the lymphatic pump on the immune response: I. Preliminary studies on the antibody response to pneumococcal polysaccharide assayed by bacterial agglutination and passive hemagglutination. *J Am Osteopath Assoc* 1982;82(1):28–31.
30. Measel JW, Kafity AA. The effect of the lymphatic pump on the B and T cells in peripheral blood [abstract]. *J Am Osteopath Assoc* 1986;86(9):608.
31. Miller CE. The lymphatic pump, its application to acute infections. *J Am Osteopath Assoc* 1926;25:443–445.
32. Miller CE. Osteopathic principles and thoracic pump therapeutics proved by scientific research. *J Am Osteopath Assoc* 1927;26:910–914.
33. Ruddy TJ. Osteopathic manipulation in eye, ear, nose, and throat disease. *Acad Appl Osteopath Yearb* 1962;133–140
34. Galbreath WO. Acute otitis media, including its postural and manipulative treatment. *J Am Osteopath Assoc* 1929;28:377–379.
35. Pratt-Harrington D. Galbreath technique: a manipulative treatment for otitis media revisited [review]. *J Am Osteopath Assoc.* 2000;100:635–639.
36. Sutherland WG. *Teachings in the Science of Osteopathy.* Fort Worth, TX: Sutherland Cranial Teaching Foundation Inc., 1990:13.
37. Sutherland WG. *Teachings in the Science of Osteopathy.* Fort Worth, TX: Sutherland Cranial Teaching Foundation Inc., 1990: 138.
38. Sutherland WG. *Teachings in the Science of Osteopathy.* Fort Worth, TX: Sutherland Cranial Teaching Foundation Inc., 1990: 127.
39. Swartz MA, Boardman KC Jr. The role of interstitial stress in lymphatic function and lymphangiogenesis [review]. *Ann N Y Acad Sci.* 2002;979:197–210; discussion 229–234.
40. Mislin H. Zur Funktionsanalyse der Lymphgefässmotorik. *Rev. Suisse Zool* 1961;68:228–238.
41. Leak L, Cadet J, Griffin C, et al. Nitric oxide production by lymphatic endothelial cells in vitro. *Biochem Biophys Res Commun* 1995;217: 96–105.
42. Simons DG, Travell JG, Simons LS. *Travell and Simons' Myofascial Pain and Dysfunction: The Trigger Point Manual—Volume 1. Upper Half of Body.* Baltimore, MD: Williams & Wilkins, 1999:504–537.
43. Degenhardt BF, Kuchera ML. Update on osteopathic medical concepts and the lymphatic system. *J Am Osteopath Assoc* 1996;96:97–100.
44. Kuchera M, Kuchera W. *Osteopathic Considerations in Systemic Function.* Columbus, OH: Greyden Press, 1994:189–235.

45. Kuchera M, Kuchera W. *Osteopathic Considerations in Systemic Function.* Columbus, OH: Greyden Press, 1994:18, 31, 50, 67, 68, 94, 107, 133, 134, 141, 227–231.

46. Dumont AE, Clauss RH, Reed GE, et al. Lymph drainage in patients with congestive heart failure. Comparison with findings in hepatic cirrhosis. *N Engl J Med* 1963;269:949–52.

47. Kuchera M, Kuchera W. *Osteopathic Considerations in Systemic Function.* Columbus, OH: Greyden Press, 1994:53–78.

48. Zink JG. Applications of the osteopathic holistic approach to homeostasis. *Am Acad Osteopath Yearb* 1973;37–47:42.

49. Sackner MA, Gummels E, Adams JA. Effect of moderate-intensity exercise, whole-body periodic acceleration, and passive cycling on nitric oxide release into circulation. *Chest* 2005;128:2794–2803.

50. Overberger R, Hoyt JA, Daghigh F, et al. Comparing changes in serum nitric oxide levels and heart rate after Osteopathic Manipulative Treatment (OMT) using the Dalrymple pedal pump to changes measured after active exercise. *J Am Osteopath Assoc* 2009;109(1):41–42.

51. Salamon E, Zhu W, Stefano GB. Nitric oxide as a possible mechanism for understanding the therapeutic effects of osteopathic manipulative medicine. *Int J Mol Med* 2004;14:443–449.

52. Green D, Maiorana A, O'Driscoll G, et al. Effect of exercise training on endothelium-derived nitric oxide function in humans. *J Physiol* 2004;561:1–25.

53. Leak L, Cadet J, Griffin C, et al. Nitric oxide production by lymphatic endothelial cells in vitro. *Biochem Biophys Res Commun* 1995;217:96–105.

54. Zainuddin Z, Newton M, Sacco P, et al. Effects of massage on delayed-onset muscle soreness, swelling, and recovery of muscle function. *J Athl Train* 2005;40(3):174–180.

55. Dodd JG, Good MM, Nguyen TL, et al. In vitro biophysical strain model for understanding mechanisms of Osteopathic Manipulative Treatment. *J Am Osteopath Assoc* 2006;106(3):157–166.

56. Meltzer KR, Standley PR. Modeled repetitive motion strain and indirect osteopathic manipulative techniques in regulation of human fibroblast proliferation and interleukin secretion. *J Am Osteopath Assoc* 2007;107(12):527–536.

57. Leduc A, Lievens P, Dewald J. The influence of multidirectional vibrations on wound healing and on the regeneration of blood- and lymph vessels. *Lymphology* 1981;14(4):179–185.

58. Didem K, Ufuk YS, Serdar S, et al. The comparison of two different physiotherapy methods in treatment of lymphedema after breast surgery. *Breast Cancer Res Treat* 2005;93:49–54.

59. Foldi E, Foldi M, Clodius L. The lymphedema chaos: a lancet. *Ann Plast Surg* 1989;22:505–515.

60. Cline CC, Coast JR, Arnall DA. A chest wall restrictor to study effects on pulmonary function and exercise. *Respiration* 1999;66:182–187

61. Howell RK, Allen TW, Kappler RE: The influence of OMT in the management of patients with COPD. *J Am Osteopath Assoc* 1975;75:757–760.

62. Sleszynski SL, Kelso AF. Comparison of thoracic manipulation with incentive spirometry in preventing postoperative atelectasis. *J Am Osteopath Assoc.* 1993;93:834–838, 843–845.

63. Pratt-Harrington D, Neptune-Ceran R. The effect of OMT in the post-abdominal surgery patient. *Acad Appl Osteopath J* 1995;9:9–13.

64. Kakizaki F, Shibuya M, Yamazaki T, et al. Preliminary report on the effects of respiratory muscle stretch gymnastics on chest wall mobility in patients with COPD. *Respir Care* 1999;44(4):409–414.

65. Minoguchi H. Shibuya M. Miyagawa T. et al. Cross-over comparison between respiratory muscle stretch gymnastics and inspiratory muscle training. *Int Med* 2002;41(10):805–812.

66. Chikly B. *Silent Waves: Theory and Practice of Lymph Drainage Therapy-With Applications for Lymphedema, Chronic Pain and Inflammation.* I.H.H. Publishing, 2001.

67. Measel JW Jr. The effect of the lymphatic pump on the immune response: I. Preliminary studies on the antibody response to pneumococcal polysaccharide assayed by bacterial agglutination and passive hemagglutination. *J Am Osteopath Assoc* 1982;82:28–31.

68. Jackson KM, Steele TF, Dugan EP, et al. Effect of lymphatic and splenic pump techniques on the antibody response to hepatitis B vaccine: a pilot study. *J Am Osteopath Assoc* 1998;98:155–160.

69. Noll DR, Degenhardt BF, Stuart MK, et al. The effect of osteopathic manipulative treatment on immune response to influenza vaccine in nursing home residents: a pilot study. *Altern Ther Health Med* 2004;10:74–76.

70. Gevitz N. Center or periphery? The future of osteopathic principles and practices. *J Am Osteopath Assoc* 2006;106(3):121–129.

71. Overberger R, Hoyt JA, Daghigh F, et al. Comparing changes in serum nitric oxide levels and heart rate after osteopathic manipulative treatment (OMT) using the Dalrymple pedal pump to changes measured after active exercise. *J Am Osteopath Assoc* 2009;109(1):41–42.

72. Ota KS. Postmastectomy lymphedema: a call for osteopathic medical research [Letter]. *J Am Osteopath Assoc* 2006;106(3):110–111.

73. Opipari MI, Perrotta AL, Essig-Beatty DR. Oncology. In: Ward RC, ed. *Foundations of Osteopathic Medicine.* 2nd Ed. Philadelphia, PA: Lippincott Williams & Wilkins, 2003:473–474.

74. Patterson MM. The coming influenza pandemic: Lessons from the past. *J Am Osteopath Assoc* 2005;105(11):498–500.

75. Millard FP. *Applied Anatomy of the Lymphatics.* Kirksville, MO: International Lymphatic Research Society, 1922:27.

76. Barral J-P, Mercier P. *Visceral Manipulation.* Eastland Press, 1988.

77. Stone CA. *Visceral and Obstetric Osteopathy.* Edinburgh, UK: Churchill Livingston Elsevier, 2007.

78. Zink JG, Fetchik WD, Lawson WB. The posterior axillary folds: a gateway for osteopathic treatment of the upper extremities. *Osteopath Ann* 1981;9(3):81–88.

79. Kuchera ML, McPartland JM. Myofascial trigger points as somatic dysfunction. In: Ward RC, ed. *Foundations for Osteopathic Medicine.* 2nd Ed. Baltimore, MD: Lippincott Williams & Wilkins, 2003:1034–1050.

80. Simons DG, Travell JG, Simons LS. *Travell and Simons' Myofascial Pain and Dysfunction: The Trigger Point Manual. Volume I: Upper Half of Body.* 2nd Ed. Baltimore MD: Williams & Wilkins, 1999.

81. Travell JG, Simons DG. *Myofascial Pain and Dysfunction: The Trigger Point Manual. Volume I. The Upper Extremities.* Baltimore, MD: Williams & Wilkins, 1983.

82. Foley WM, Kuchera ML, Lyons JB, et al. Effect of OMT on myofascial somatic dysfunction and objective parameters of severity in patients with carpal tunnel syndrome. *J Am Osteopath Assoc* 2006;106(8):477.

83. Sucher BM. Myofascial release of carpal tunnel syndrome. *J Am Osteopath Assoc* 1993;93(1):92–101

84. Sucher BM. Myofascial manipulative release of carpal tunnel syndrome: documentation with magnetic resonance imaging. *J Am Osteopath Assoc* 1993;93(12):1273–1278.

85. Nicholas AS, Nicholas EA. *Atlas of Osteopathic Techniques.* Philadelphia, PA: Wolters Kluwer Health/Lippincott Williams & Wilkins, 2008.

86. Sucher BM. Palpatory diagnosis and manipulative management of carpal tunnel syndrome. *J Am Osteopath Assoc* 1994;94:647–663.

87. Sucher BM. Myofascial manipulative release of carpal tunnel syndrome: documentation with MRI. *J Am Osteopath Assoc* 1993;93:1273–1278.

88. Strait BW, Kuchera ML. Osteopathic manipulation for patients with confirmed mild, modest and moderate carpal tunnel syndrome. *J Am Osteopath Assoc* 1994;94(8):673.

89. Ramey KA, Kappler RE, Chimata M, et al. MRI assessment of changes in swelling of wrist structures following OMT in patients with carpal tunnel syndrome. *J Acad Appl Osteopath* 1999;9(2):25–31.

90. Foley WM, Kuchera ML, Lyons JB, et al. Effect of OMT on myofascial somatic dysfunction and objective parameters of severity in patients with carpal tunnel syndrome. *J Am Osteopath Assoc* 2006;106:77.

91. Sucher BM. Hinrichs RN. Manipulative treatment of carpal tunnel syndrome: biomechanical and osteopathic intervention to increase the length of the transverse carpal ligament. *J Am Osteopath Assoc* 1998;98 (12):679–86.

91. Sucher BM, Hinrichs RN, Welcher RL, et al. Manipulative treatment of carpal tunnel syndrome: biomechanical and osteopathic intervention to increase the length of the transverse carpal ligament: part 2. Effect of sex differences and manipulative "priming". *J Am Osteopath Assoc* 2005;105:135–143.

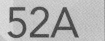

Representative Models

DENNIS J. DOWLING

This chapter contains a number of manipulative interventions currently practiced and taught by osteopathic physicians. Unlike the manipulative models presented in Chapters 45 to 51 inclusive, the models described in this chapter are not uniformly taught at all colleges of osteopathic medicine. The premises of the models are rationally based on accepted scientific principles. Their inclusion in this chapter demonstrates varying expressions of manipulative intervention within the somatic dysfunction diagnostic terminology developed by the osteopathic medical profession.

The contemporary approaches covered in this chapter include the following:
A. Balanced Ligamentous Tension and Ligamentous Articular Strain
B. Facilitated Positional Release
C. Progressive Inhibition of Neuromuscular Structures
D. Functional Technique
E. Visceral Manipulation
F. Still Technique
G. Chapman's Approach
H. Fulford Percussion

52A — Balanced Ligamentous Tension and Ligamentous Articular Strain

WM. THOMAS CROW

KEY CONCEPT

In this section, emphasis is placed on the role of ligaments in maintaining articular dysfunction. The cardinal principles of this approach are three: disengagement of the dysfunctional area (compression/decompression), exaggeration of the dysfunctional pattern (returning to the original position of injury), and balanced tension of ligaments (maintained until release). Retracing the path of injury via ligamentous tension and strain is done anatomically and facilitated by respiratory cooperation of the patient.

CASE STUDY

A 50-year-old male complains of pain in the left hip. It started several weeks ago after climbing six flights of stairs at work. The pain is worse in flexion and going up stairs. He tolerates going down stairs easier. The pain radiates from the groin mainly into the left thigh region. However, he is more functional and can bear weight on his left leg. Rest makes it better. It is worse at the end of the day than in the morning. Advil relieves most of his pain but it is now causing him some "stomach burn."

OBJECTIVE

Physical exam is normal except as follows. Neurological—no focal sensory or motor deficits, reflexes symmetrical. Less hypersensitivity to touch noted in the S1 S2 distribution. M/S muscle spasm noted in the L adductors. His gait is antalgic.

ASSESSMENT

719.45 JOINT PAIN-PELVIS
728.85 SPASM OF MUSCLE

Plan:
OMT to region

OSTEOPATHIC STRUCTURAL EXAM AND TREATMENT NOTE

Patient was found to have tenderness, asymmetry, restriction of range of motion, and tissue texture changes in the following areas:

Lumbar Spine:
Lumbar paraspinal muscles tight bilateral, L4–5 RLSRL

Sacrum and Innominates:
Posterior sacrum—left. **Inferior** pubic symphysis shear—right, Tight piriformis—left

Pelvis:
Adductors restricted in extension
739.4 SOMAT DYSFUNC SACRAL REG
739.5 SOMAT DYSFUNC PELVIC REG
739.3 SOMAT DYSFUNC LUMBAR REG

Plan:
Osteopathic manip, 3 to 4 body regn
PT treated with ligamentous articular strain (LAS) and balanced ligamentous tension (BLT) techniques. PT tolerated procedure well. No complications. Rest and ice to areas, if needed. He may continue to use **Tylenol** 1 PRN pain. Increase in PO fluids × 24–48 hours

INTRODUCTION

Balanced ligamentous and balanced membranous tension to treat LASs were concepts of Dr. Andrew Taylor Still. William G. Sutherland, D.O., a student of Still, reinforced these concepts in his teaching. Rebecca and Howard Lippincott wrote the principles and techniques down and subsequently published them as the "Osteopathic

Technique of Wm. G. Sutherland" in the 1949 *Year Book of the Academy of Applied Osteopathy* (1). Dr Anne Wales in the Northeast called what she was doing BLT techniques and Rollin Becker in Dallas called it LAS techniques. The terms come from the above-mentioned article where it states "Osteopathic lesions are strains of the tissues of the body. When they involve joints it is the ligaments that are primarily affected so the term 'ligamentous articular strain' is the one preferred by Dr. Sutherland. The ligaments of a joint are normally on a balanced, reciprocal tension and seldom if ever are they completely relaxed throughout the normal range of movement... Since it is the ligaments that are primarily involved in the maintenance of the lesion it is they, not muscular leverage, that are used as the main agency for reduction....This is the point of balanced tension" (1).

HISTORY

At the time that Dr. Sutherland received his osteopathic training at Kirksville, Dr. Still was still supervising the instruction given at the college. The principles that were taught had to conform exactly to his concept. Dr. Sutherland made good use of every opportunity to learn and understand them and has adhered closely in his thinking and practice to Dr. Still's principles throughout his professional career. "In consequence, the technique which he presented to us is a reflection of the clear vision of our founder" (2). During this course, Sutherland related the following: "Dr. Still gave me a lesson one day along with the rest of our class. A member of our class had stepped on a rusty nail. All the appropriate surgical management and cleansing had been used, but it would not heal. It began to look an angry red, so we called in the Old Doctor. He said, 'You damn fools!' and we were. We had not stopped to consider that when the patient stepped on that nail he drew his leg up away from it. The lasting problem was not the nail or the original wound; it was what occurred in the sudden jerk of the patient that caused a membranous strain between the fibula and the tibia (3). Sutherland's student H. A. Lippincott, D.O., elaborated on this: "Since it is the ligaments that are primarily involved in the maintenance of the lesion it is they, not muscular leverage that are used as the main agency for reduction. The articulation is carried in the direction of the lesion position as far as is necessary to cause tension of the weakened elements of the ligamentous structure to be equal to or slight in excess of the tension of those that are not strained. This is the point of balanced tension. Forcing the articulation back and away from the direction of lesion strains the ligaments that are normal and unopposed, and if it is done with thrust or jerks there is a definite possibility of separating fibers of ligaments from their bony attachments. When the tension is properly balanced the respiratory or muscular cooperation of the patient is employed to overcome the resistance of the defense mechanism of the body to the release of the lesion" (1). Sutherland is best remembered for his application of osteopathic techniques for the cranium and sacrum. However, it is clear that he had learned from Dr. Still techniques for treating the whole body, and was only expounding more on an area that was receiving insufficient attention at that time, that is, the motion of the individual bones in the cranium. This is why Sutherland, later in his life, held that he had just pulled back a veil so that others could see more clearly.

While LAS techniques may not be the only techniques used by Drs. Still and Sutherland, they are the ones that both of them described. For example, Dr. Still wrote: "Without going into detail further, I will say that all dislocations, partial or complete, can be adjusted by this rule: First loosen the dislocated end from other tissues, then gently bring it back to its original place" (4).

Carl Phillip McConnell, D.O., M.D., who had been treated by Still and was on the faculty at the American School of Osteopathy, described Still's treatment technique in his book, *The Practice of Osteopathy*, by writing "Disengage the articular points that have become locked. Reduce the dislocation by retracing the path along which the parts were dislocated. One can readily see that a dislocated ball and socket joint could be reduced only by the dislocated bone retracing the path through which it left its socket as the capsular ligament would at once prevent its returning to the socket by any path other than that taken when dislocated. This applies to all dislocations to a greater or lesser extent" (5).

In 1917, Edythe Ashmore wrote that there were two methods commonly employed by osteopaths in the correction of lesions, the older of which is the traction method, the latter the direct method or thrust (6). In a footnote, she wrote: "The term 'direct' is preferred for the reason that the imitators of osteopathy have given to the word 'thrust' an objectionable meaning of harshness" (6). As noted previously, the older method is now known as LAS techniques, while the newer methods refer to high velocity–low amplitude techniques. Of the former, she wrote: "Those who employ the traction method secure the relaxation of the tissues about the articulation by what has been termed exaggeration of the lesion, a motion in the direction of the forcible movement which produced the lesion, as if its purpose were to increase the deformity. C.P. McConnell states that this disengages the tissues that are holding the parts in the abnormal position. The exaggeration is held, traction made upon the joint, replacement initiated and then completed by reversal of the forces" (6).

RECIPROCAL TENSION

Sutherland coined the terms "reciprocal tension ligaments" and "reciprocal tension mechanism" to describe the role of ligaments in joints (3). An example of this is the wrist as it moves into flexion displacing the distal row of carpal bones toward the dorsal surface of the arm. During extension the reverse occurs. Each bone then rotates as the group is moved. The tension of the carpal ligaments remains constant and constantly shifts its balance. This is a key concept in Dr. Sutherland's approach.

The type of motion which may occur at any given articulation is determined by the shape of the joint surfaces, the position of the ligaments, and the forces of the muscles acting upon the joint. Ligaments do not stretch and contract as muscles do; consequently, the tension in a ligament has very little variation. The tension distributed throughout the ligaments of any given joint is balanced. In normal movements, as the joint changes position, the relationships between the joint's ligaments also change, but the total tension within the ligamentous articular mechanism does not. The distribution of tension between the ligaments is altered, however, when the joint is affected by injury, inflammation, and/or mechanical forces. This is what happens in somatic dysfunction. The distribution and vector of tension within any given ligament will change according to the position of strain in the joint. However, the shared tension within the ligamentous articular mechanism of any given joint remains constant as long as the ligament is not damaged. This has been called a reciprocal tension mechanism. Of course, the balance within the ligamentous articular mechanism can be strained if the joint is inappropriately moved beyond its physiologic range of motion. In the former case, it is the balance of tension, which is distorted. In the latter case, the fibers of the ligament are subjected to microscopic tears and stretch. While this (the latter case) will most assuredly result in a strain to the balance of the articular ligaments, the ligaments do not need to be disrupted for the balance to be distorted. The distortion in balance is a mechanical strain, which may or may not involve an anatomical one. In any somatic dysfunction, there is always a strain.

H.A. Lippincott, D.O., describes LAS as "Osteopathic lesions are strains of the tissues of the body. When they involve joints, it is the ligaments that are primarily affected so the term 'ligamentous articular strain' is the one preferred by Dr. Sutherland. The ligaments of a joint are normally on a balanced, reciprocal tension and seldom if ever are they completely relaxed throughout the normal range of movement. When the motion is carried beyond that range, the tension is unbalanced and the elements of the ligamentous structure that limit motion in that direction are strained and weakened. The lesion is maintained by the overbalance of the reciprocal tension by the elements that have not been strained. This locks the articular mechanism or prevents its free and normal movement. The unbalanced tension causes the bones to assume a position that is nearer that in which the strain was produced than would be the case if the tension were normal, and the weakened part of the ligaments permits motion in the direction of the lesion in excess of normal. The range of movement in the opposite direction is limited by the more firm and unopposed tension of the elements which had not been strained" (1).

FASCIA

Still looked to the fascia for the source of disease (4). Strains in the fascia not only pull bones out of position and impinge on nerves, vessels, and lymphatics but also impede the flow of the interstitial fluid. At the 1998 Cranial Academy Conference, the osteopathic anatomist Frank Willard, Ph.D., stated that the fascia should be defined and studied as a system unto itself and not simply as an obscuring material hiding more important tissues (7). From an embryological standpoint, fascia, bone, and all the connective tissues arise from the mesenchyme.

CONNECTIVE TISSUE

Connective tissue makes up about 16 percent of the body's weight and stores approximately 25% of the body's total water. It forms the biological building blocks of the skin, muscles, nerve sheaths, tendons, ligaments, fascia, blood vessels, joint capsules, periosteum, aponeuroses, bones, adipose tissue, and cartilage and the framework for the internal organs (8). Connective tissue, with a special emphasis on fascia for our purposes here, has unique deformative characteristics. The fascia derives its unique characteristics from its viscosity and elasticity, both of which are changed by manipulation to reinstate homeostasis in the body. Being viscoelastic in nature, the fascia has both permanent (viscous) and temporary (elastic) deformation characteristics (9,10). In addition, fascia has a plastic component that allows for permanent elongation and a mechanical component that allows it to contract; thus, the fascia and bones deform in the same four ways. Wolff law states: "Every change in form and function of a bone, or in its function alone, is followed by certain definite changes in its internal architecture and secondary alterations in its external conformations, for example, bone is laid down along lines of stress" (11).

This process apparently also applies to the fascia and all connective tissue.

CRIMPING

If there are abnormal stresses found in the collagen that makes up the tendons and ligaments, then the tendons and ligaments will be deformed and their basic functions will be affected. Tendons attach muscle fibers to bones and transmit muscle forces, and the ligaments check excess motion of the joints and guide joint motion (12). Ligaments have a less consistent parallel arrangement of collagen than tendons (13). The orientation of the ligament takes on an undulating configuration known as the crimp, which allows the

ligament to work like a spring and which is an essential function of normal ligaments. Upon injury to the ligament, the spring will be straightened, causing the ligament to function improperly.

IMMOBILIZATION

Scientific studies have shown that fascia and connective tissue have certain biochemical and physiologic responses to immobilization. Most of the currently available research is on animals, which may limit its application to the human population. Nevertheless, in the studies on animal connective tissues, laboratory animals were immobilized for various periods of time and then examined at different time intervals (14).

BIOCHEMICAL CHANGES SECONDARY TO IMMOBILIZATION

Fibrofatty infiltrates were found in the capsular folds and recesses, and the longer the joint was immobilized, the greater the amount of infiltration (15–17). There was a loss of water and of glycosaminoglycans in the ground substance, a lubricant found between the collagen fibers, which are the primary connective tissue fibers that compose the fascia. Collagen fiber lubrication is associated with the maintenance of a critical interfiber distance, which has to be maintained between the fibers in order for them to move smoothly. When this distance is not maintained, microadhesions form and new collagen is then laid down in a haphazard manner (15). Immobilization for >12 weeks resulted in an overall loss of collagen since its rate of degradation exceeded its rate of synthesis under these circumstances (16). Joint contracture occurs as the result of remodeling and shortening of connective tissues when connective tissue is immobilized in the presence of inflammatory exudates. When a limb is immobilized in the absence of inflammatory exudates, no contracture occurs. In addition, biochemical changes are noted (17,18).

PHYSIOLOGICAL CHANGES SECONDARY TO IMMOBILIZATION

The force needed to move an immobilized joint is ten times that of a normal joint. After several repetitions, the amount of force required to move the immobilized joint is reduced to three times that of a normal joint. Over time, the joint will usually regain normal joint mobility (19). Manipulation of experimentally immobilized rat knees by either high velocity techniques or range of motion resulted in the rupture of macroadhesions and the restoration of partial joint mobility. Movement restores the normal histological makeup of the connective tissue, but the chances of obtaining optimum results decrease as the immobilization period increases (19). All periarticular connective tissues responded in the same manner. Ligament and capsule surrounding the fascia all have the same basic response to immobilization. Manual manipulation of the tissues causes a reversal of effects, provided manipulation was done within three months of immobilization (17).

Every cell in the body is surrounded by fascia that fuse together to make bigger sheets of fascia. Eventually, these fuse together to form tendons and ligaments. When you look at the smallest fibers of a muscle, it is still surrounded by fascia. It is like plastic bags within plastic bags within plastic bags. It is through pressure on these "plastic bags" that we are causing a change in the body. Pascal law states that "Pressure applied to a liquid at rest from any point is transmitted equally in all directions" (20). The human body consists of many closed fluid systems like the plastic bags that respond exactly as predicted by Pascal principle, that is, an increase in the pressure of fluid in one of the plastic bags will distribute its pressure to other portions of the body.

The effects of the hydrodynamic fluctuation of body fluids restore motion and life to "dead spots," or somatic dysfunctions, changing the structure of the tissues. Research has shown that changes in the structure of the tissues of the body alter the structure of the cytoskeleton, which in turn can actually alter gene expression and cellular metabolism (21). Therefore, we believe that we can bring about significant change on all levels by manipulating the tissues of the body. This concept is echoed in the osteopathic literature.

Every organ in the body exhibits the phenomenon of pulsations or rhythmic action which is incessantly active, dynamic, and highly mobile, resulting in forward, backward, sideways, and rotational fluid movement (19). These pulsations appear to be ubiquitous. They propel the extra cellular fluids into and across the semipermeable membranes of cells everywhere and deliver nutrients and remove metabolic waste products even from synovial spaces, bursae, and other nonvascular compartments. Every cell membrane of the body is continuously and rhythmically bathed with these essential fluids in a fashion similar to the ebb and flow of the ocean upon the beach.

Fluid dynamics, joint physiology, fascia, and vectors of injury may look on the surface to be unrelated, but, on a deeper level, are found to be closely connected. As osteopaths, we are interested in continuously advancing our skills and studying the interrelatedness of biomechanics. As you expand your knowledge of osteopathy, you will move from a view of the human body as a skeleton, with other tissues hanging on as it were, to a view of the body as a moving, living organism with a skeleton found within it. As a result, your attention will move from bones and joints to the fascia and fluid dynamics. It is important to understand the scientific principles upon which these techniques are based in order to apply them most successfully. If you understand the principles, you can then create your own techniques.

PRINCIPLES OF CORRECTIVE TECHNIQUE

Look at a somatic dysfunction as an impediment to the flow of the interstitial fluid. The fluid moves around areas of dysfunction like a stream flows around a stone. The goal of your treatment is to remove the stone and let the stream flow through unimpeded. Take that which you palpate as hard and make it soft. When you feel the flow come through the dysfunctional area, your treatment of that area is complete.

Once an area of dysfunction has been located, compress or decompress the joint or fascial plane to disengage the injury so that the displaced bone can be moved. (This is similar to pushing in the clutch on a car to shift gears.) Then carry the injured part in the direction of least resistance, returning it to the original position to which it was forced during the injury. Carrying the injury the way it wants to go is an indirect method of treatment and is also one that follows the direction of the somatic dysfunction. Remember that just after the initial injury, the injured part sprang back toward a normal position but was caught in limbo—part way between the position of the injury and the normal functional position. So, when correcting the injury, you must carry the injured part back to the exact position of injury and maintain that position until the body rebalances all the connective tissue surrounding the dysfunction, and draws the part back to its normal functional physiologic position. This can be done using a direct technique, an indirect technique, or a combination of indirect and direct methods.

It is the act of disengagement, exaggeration, and balance that makes the techniques work. These are the three basic components to remember when utilizing LAS techniques: disengage, exaggerate, and balance:

1. Disengage: Compress or decompress the joint or fascial plane, increasing the pressure or traction until you are able to move the injured part
2. Exaggerate: Carry the injured part back to the original position of injury by, for example, rotating, flexing, "side bending," or "side shifting" until the balance point or still point is found. For example, if the right ankle is slightly inverted, you exaggerate the position of the ankle by taking it into a more inverted position, which is how the injury occurred originally
3. Balance: Maintain the area of dysfunction in the position of injury, that is, the balance point or still point, until a release occurs. The bone will move slightly farther in the direction of exaggeration. It then will move back to its normal functional position as the cranial rhythmic impulse or tide returns through the tissues that were injured. Once the correction has occurred, the injured ligaments will start their 3-month healing process

LAS Hip Technique

Symptoms/diagnosis: Hip pain, often due to a force transferred up from the lower extremity or a fall directly on the hip
Procedure (Fig. 52A.1):

Roll the knee medially to raise the symptomatic hip slightly off the table. Place the thenar eminence of your hand farthest from table between the greater trochanter and the table. Place the patient's knee in the fossa just below your coracoid process on the side nearest the patient to control the distal femur. Grasp the medial proximal aspect of the femur close to the femoral head with the index, middle finger, and thumb of your other hand. Use your shoulder to increase or decrease the flexion at the hip and to slightly internally or externally rotate the femur. The patient's foot is dangling just off the table. Compress the hip slightly anteriorly and medially with your thenar eminence on the greater trochanter. With your medial hand grasping the femur close to the femoral head, generate pressure posteriorly and laterally with your middle finger, index finger,

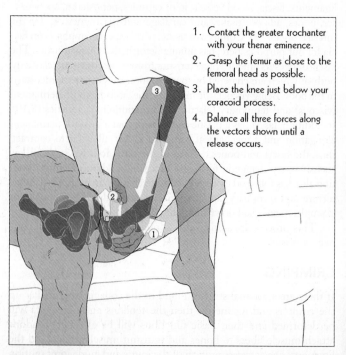

1. Contact the greater trochanter with your thenar eminence.
2. Grasp the femur as close to the femoral head as possible.
3. Place the knee just below your coracoid process.
4. Balance all three forces along the vectors shown until a release occurs.

Figure 52A-1 Las technique for the hip. (From LAS by William Thomas Crow and Conrad Speece. Used with permission of Eastland Press.)

and thumb. Using your shoulder, locate the direction of balanced tension in the hip by slightly increasing or decreasing the flexion of the femur and slightly internally or externally rotating the femur. Balance the forces at the hip joint from all three contact points. When the release occurs, the connective tissue surrounding the head of the femur will readjust itself, all three vectors of force will "melt," and the femur will move back to it functional physiologic position.

Active range of motion is assessed with the patient standing facing the physician, and the physician slowly moving the patient's foot into internal and external rotation. Restriction of active motion is noted by assessing movement at the pelvis. The treatment is performed with the patient sitting facing the physician. The leg to be treated is crossed so that the ankle rests over the contralateral knee.

Treatment for Externally Rotated Legs

The physician places one hand upon the medial aspect of the femur near the femoral neck to externally rotate the femur. The other hand grasps the patient's knee. The physician establishes a point of balance between the femoral head and the acetabulum. The patient also places his or her hands upon his or her knee. The patient holds the knee down and laterally while rotating the body away from the leg and backward.

Treatment for Internally Rotated Legs

In this instance, the physician's handhold is more proximal so that there is less torque at the acetabulum. The physician establishes a point of balance between the femoral head and the acetabulum. The patient draws the knee medially and upward while rotating forward and toward the affected side.

REFERENCES

1. Lippincott H. *The Osteopathic Technique of Wm. G. Sutherland, D.O.* Yearbook of the Academy of Applied Osteopathy, 1949.
2. Fox JPC, Crow WT, eds. San Antonio, TX, 1995.
3. Sutherland W. *Teachings in the Science of Osteopathy*. Rudra Press, 1990.
4. Still A. *Osteopathy: Research and Practice*. Kirksville, MO: The Journal Printing Company, 1910.
5. McConnell C. *Practice of Osteopathy*. Kirksville, MO: The Journal Printing Company, 1906.
6. Ashmore E. *Osteopathic Mechanics*. Kirksville, MO: The Journal Printing Company, 1915.
7. Willard F. Fascia as an organ system. In: *Cranial Academy*. San Diego, CA, 1995.
8. Ham A. *Histology*. Philadelphia, PA: JB Lippincott, 1979.
9. Stromberg DW, DA, Viscoelastic description of a collagenous tissue in simple elongation. *J Appl Physiol* 1969;26:857–862.
10. Hooley CM, NG, Cohen RE. The viscoelastic deformation of tendon. *J Biomech* 1980;13:521–528.
11. *Foundations for Osteopathic Medicine*. Ward R, ed. Baltimore, MD: Williams & Wilkins, 1997.
12. Frankel VN, M, *Basic Biomechanics of the Skeletal System*. Philadelphia, PA: Lea and Febiger, 1980.
13. Kennedy JH, RJ, Willis RB et al. Tension studies of human knee ligaments, yield point, ultimate failure and disruption of the cruciate and tibial collateral ligaments. *J Bone Joint Surg* 1976;58A:350–355.
14. Woo SM, JV, Akeson WH, et al. Connective tissue response to immobility. Arthritis Rheum 1975;18:257–264.
15. Akeson WAD, LaViolette D, Secrist D. The connective tissue response to immobility: an accelerated aging response. *Exp Gerontol* 1968;3(4):289–301.
16. Akeson WA, D. Immobility effects of synovial joints: the pathomechanics of joint contracture. *Biorheology* 1980;17;95–110.
17. Akeson WA, D, LaViolette D. The connective tissue response to immobility: a study of the chondroitin-4 and 6-sulfate dermatan sulfate changes in periarticular connective tissue of control and immobilized knees of dogs. *Clin Orthop Relat Res* 1967;51:183–189.
18. Amiel D, Akeson WH, Harwood FL, et al. Stress deprivation effect on metabolic turnover of medial collateral ligament collagen. *Clin Orthop Relat Res*. 1983;172:265–270.
19. Evans EE, G, Butler J, et al. Experimental immobilization and mobilization of rat knee joints. *J Bone Joint Surg (American Edition)*, 1960;42A(5): 737–758.
20. *Stedman's Medical Dictionary*. 26th Ed. Baltimore, MD: Williams & Wilkins, 1995.
21. Chen CI, DE. Tensegrity and mechanoregulation: from skeleton to cytoskeleton. *Osteoarthritis Cartilage* 1999;7(1):81–94.

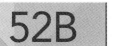

Facilitated Positional Release

DENNIS J. DOWLING

KEY CONCEPT

In this section, emphasis is placed on decreasing muscle hypertonicity involved in the maintenance of articular dysfunction. The dysfunctional region is initially placed in a relatively neutral position. Activating force of compression, traction, or torsion is applied to effect immediate release of tissue tension, articular restriction, or both. Subsequent positioning into resistance seeks to affect larger (regional) muscle groups or smaller (intrinsic) deep muscles involved in joint mobility.

CASE STUDY

The patient is a 48-year-old female who presented to the osteopathic physician's office with several complaints of chronic lower back pain, neck pain, left shoulder pain, and frequent headaches. She described these as originating in her early twenties with no noted precipitating event, but all of the symptoms have been gradually increasing over the years. The most recent symptom to appear has been intermittent radiating of pain and tingling from the left lower back to the left buttock and sometimes the left lower leg. The level of pain is a 3 to 4/10 pain and is worse in the morning after awakening. She has been married for 25 years, has three children, and works full time as a librarian. She describes that she is happy and satisfied in her private and professional life. In her free time, she exercises and does volunteer work at her church both of which she states helps often, but always, with her symptoms. She has been seen by several physicians and health practitioners, including orthopedists, a neurologist, a rheumatologist, physical therapists, massage therapist, an acupuncturist, and a nutritionist. The massage therapy has helped but was only of short benefit. Radiological findings included some mild degenerative changes in the cervical and lumbar spinal regions with a paracentral herniated disc on the left at L4-5. Neurophysiological (EMG/NCS) only demonstrated some involvement of the L5 paraspinal muscles. Blood serology has been negative. She has been prescribed a tricyclic antidepressant, a specific serotonin reuptake inhibitor, gabapentin, various nonsteroidal anti-inflammatories, muscle relaxants, and narcotic analogue medications. She discontinued all of the medications either because of side effects or ineffectiveness. She does occasionally take acetaminophen for her headaches, which she describes as tightness at the back of her head radiating to her temple area. She denies any aura or other symptoms associated with the headaches. She denies any other constitutional symptoms, is up to date with her gynecological, breast, and physical examinations, is not menopausal, is monogamous, and utilizes barrier methods for birth control. Her bone density studies have revealed minimal osteopenia. She has no known allergies, has never smoked or used recreational drugs, has only one to two glasses of wine per week, and has never had surgery. Her only hospitalizations were for her pregnancies, which were all full term and resulted in spontaneous vaginal deliveries. Family history is essentially negative with only a positive with her father's controlled hypertension.

On physical examination, the patient is a well-nourished, well-developed woman who appears to be younger than her stated age and is in no apparent distress. Gait and posture are normal. Regional demonstrates full range of motion and equal with the exception of reduced left shoulder flexion/abduction/internal rotation, lumbar side bending and rotation to the right, and cervical side bending and rotation to the right. Standing and seated flexion tests, straight leg-raising, and Spurling compression tests are negative. Motor strength is 5/5, reflexes are 2/4, and sensory is intact for touch/sharp/dull and is symmetrical throughout. The rest of the physical examination is benign and noncontributory. Specific structural findings include: left trapezius spasm, C3 $ES_L R_L$, C7 $FS_L R_L$, elevated first rib on the left, T6 $FS_L R_L$ lumbar paravertebral muscle spasm on the right, latissimus dorsi muscle spasm on the left, L3 $ES_L R_L$, and L4 $FS_L R_L$. A mild flexion pattern with a CRI of 8 was noted and the sacrum and pelvis were symmetrical and mobile. Diagnoses of cervical, rib, thoracic and lumbar somatic dysfunctions; lumbar herniated disc; lumbar radiculopathy; and lumbar and cervical strain and sprain were made. The shoulder pain and restriction of motion were determined to not be directly related to shoulder restriction or pathology but were secondary to the spasms of the trapezius and latissimus muscles and the cervical and rib segmental dysfunctions. The patient was treated primarily with soft tissue and facilitated positional release (FPR) techniques. After the first treatment, she described that the pain was a 1 to 2/10, less frequent, and she was having less frequent headaches. The course of treatment resulted in weekly treatments for three weeks, and then biweekly, followed by monthly intervals.

HISTORY

In the 1980s, Stanley Schiowitz, D.O., F.A.A.O., was an associate dean and chairman of the Department of Osteopathic Principles and Practices (OPP) at the New York College of Osteopathic Medicine. His clinic practice on campus gave the undergraduate OPP fellows a great opportunity to practice osteopathic manipulation under the supervision of an experienced practitioner. Time after time, they would describe the same experience: Dr. Schiowitz would enter the treatment room after each had treated a patient, they would describe some finding or restriction that was recalcitrant to treatment, Dr. Schiowitz would perform some quick maneuver that was unfamiliar to them, the patient would be improved, and Dr. Schiowitz would quickly exit to go see other patients. As they exchanged notes on what they observed and mimicked some of his treatments, the group found that they were able to successfully perform them. Whenever possible, Dr. Schiowitz taught them one on one or in small groups. It appeared that he had a cohesive approach for treatment that was, as of that time, nameless and without explanation. In order to record the description in the "Progress" section of the SOAP note, the OPP fellows would use the letters "IO" ("Instant Osteopathy") as an abbreviation. Because of his busy practice and time limitations, Dr. Schiowitz sought out and adapted methods of treatment that were rapid and effective and based on anatomical and physiological principles. Some of his students have remarked that he had to develop a quick approach to treatment since he couldn't stay in one place for 90 seconds. He has admitted that he may have seen some practitioners using some elements or on very specific diagnoses but not in a globally designed system. By 1990, Dr. Schiowitz had formulated the treatment to the extent that it was published in the JAOA (1) and taught at national meetings. The OPP fellows and some faculty members became his earliest table trainers at some of these sessions.

FPR is primarily an indirect method of treatment as has been published. Actually, as practiced by Dr. Schiowitz and those whom he has directly taught, FPR is a mixed indirect followed by direct treatment. The physician initially places the region or somatic dysfunction into a position between flexion and extension to approach the neutral position as defined by Fryette (2). An activating force, compression, traction, or torsion, is then applied to facilitate an immediate release of tissue tension, joint motion restriction, or both. This is followed by placing the region into its directions of dysfunction for a few seconds and then repositioned, if desired, in the barrier directions followed by rediagnosis. This latter aspect, the positioning into the barriers, brings FPR into greater resemblance with the Still technique (3). The goals of treatment are to decrease muscle hypertonicity that maintains somatic dysfunction whether by affecting larger regional groups or by modifying smaller more intrinsic deep muscles, which are involved in joint mobility.

FPR as a technique is easily applied, effective, and time efficient. Often, patients report immediate relief of tension and/or tenderness and restoration of function. Because treatment of specific dysfunctions is accomplished in seconds, repeat application can be attempted or other methods of treatment can be subsequently applied.

THEORY

Korr (4) wrote that the immobility of a lesioned segment was initiated or maintained by increased gain in gamma motor neuron activity of the muscles of that segment. The gamma motor neurons specifically innervate the intrinsic muscles, the muscle spindle apparatus that act as sensors for overall muscle tonicity. When a gamma motor neuron stimulates a muscle spindle, such as a nuclear bag fiber, the fiber shortens in length and the stretch receptor, either annulospiral or flower spray, becomes more sensitive to stretch than it was previously. Even if the overall extrinsic muscle is in a rest position, the length-sensing nerve fibers of the muscle spindles may be sending signals back to the spinal cord, which in turn stimulate alpha motor neuron fibers innervating the same muscles. In effect, the muscle may remain in tension even in a so-called neutral position and may worsen with further stretching. Bailey (5) proposed that this high gain-set of the muscle spindle results in changes of the soft tissues that are characteristic of somatic dysfunction. Because of these aspects, FPR is an indirect form of osteopathic manipulation in which the patient remains passive throughout treatment.

Carew's (6) discussion of the feedback mechanism of the muscle spindle stretch reflex indicated that compressing muscles into more than the neutral position results in an inverse spindle output. The afferent excitatory input to the spinal cord through the Group Ia and II fibers is eliminated. This results in a "quieting" of the gamma motor gain to the spindle, reduction of the stretch stimuli, and resultant elimination of the reflex activation of the alpha motorneuron. The tension and hypertonicity of the extrafusal muscle fibers is reset.

Specific diagnosis in three planes is required for accurate treatment with FPR. The primary step in the application of FPR is the placement of the region of somatic dysfunction into its neutral position. This unloads the joints and may also affect both proprioceptive and nocioceptive elements. The dysfunction can then respond more easily and rapidly to the applied therapeutic position, motion, and force. For the spine, the articular facets are placed into an idling position between the flexed and the extended extremes. A facilitating force, typically compression and/or torsion, is applied and maintained throughout the treatment. Generally, initial soft tissue relaxation is noted at this time. Using the triplanar diagnosis, further positioning of the somatic dysfunction is applied into all of the directions of relative freedom. Further easing of the dysfunction occurs at this point. This position is held for approximately 5 seconds after which the region is restored to neutral. In practice, Dr. Schiowitz often followed neutral by bringing the dysfunction into the barrier directions and then returned the region again to neutral. The dysfunction is then reassessed. The tension that was noted in the area is most typically is gone or at least reduced. Joint motion symmetry increases after treatment with the FPR modality if the etiology or maintenance of the dysfunction is due to muscular hypertonicity. If the asymmetry of joint motion is caused by other factors, such as arthritic or other degenerative changes, congenital malformation, meniscoid or synovial entrapment or ligamentous damage, the joint may remain restricted. Other modalities of osteopathic manipulation or repeated treatment with FPR may be necessary to complete treatment of the dysfunction.

DIAGNOSIS

The diagnostic methods used to determine somatic dysfunction can vary. The use of FPR treatment procedures does not require special diagnostic tests unique to FPR. However, diagnosis is a prerequisite to treatment. Mennell (7) has described a method of skin rolling. Mitchell et al. (8) have used the coupled motion of vertebrae as described by Fryette to conduct rotoscoliosis testing, while

Johnston (9) incorporates a method of scanning and screening to progressively narrow the findings to specific diagnoses.

Schiowitz utilizes a very rapid method of diagnosis that incorporates the introduction of small motions to test all cardinal planes of motion. The appreciated palpatory response indicating relative freedom and resistance results in a specific diagnosis. For superficial muscular diagnosis, the physician places the pads of his fingers on the area of dysfunction and determines elements of Sensitivity, Tissue Texture Changes, Asymmetry, and Restriction of Motion (S-T-A-R) (10). This can be accomplished in seconds and the FPR treatment applied. For specific segmental dysfunction, the physician introduces motion in all three planes by alternating forces in opposite directions. In the spine, the pads of the fingers apply anterior force to create rotation both to the left and to the right. When pressure is placed on the right transverse process, it creates a slight left rotation. Segmental dysfunctions will have directions of relative ease and restriction with the direction of restriction demonstrating greater resistance to the applied pressure and the freedom allowing less. Lateral motion, or side bending in the spine, is tested by applying pressure to deviate one transverse process into a more cephalad direction and the opposite side simultaneously into the caudad direction. Relative ease and restriction to the forces are noted and the opposite directions are tested. Sagittal planar motions of flexion and extension require observation of the resistance to anterior deviation of one vertebra with the next lower one. The pads of the fingers are pressed anteriorly on the superior surfaces of the upper vertebra's transverse processes for flexion and on the inferior surfaces for extension. The combination of all findings results in a triplanar diagnosis of segmental dysfunction. For the extremities, similar methods are utilized to determine flexion-extension, abduction-adduction, and rotation. The directions of ease will be the ones that will be introduced immediately after placing the joint into neutral and adding the facilitating force.

Using a combination of methods can further increase the accuracy of the diagnosis and therefore the treatment.

TREATMENT

FPR treatment can be used to address at abnormal superficial tissue texture as well as influence the deep intrinsic muscles involved in segmental joint mobility. When it is a clear diagnostic differentiation as to which is primarily involved in the somatic dysfunction, the superficial soft tissue changes should be initially treated. If the dysfunction persists after this treatment, FPR should then be directed toward treatment of the deeper muscular component involved in the specific joint motion restriction. FPR is primarily an indirect technique that requires the patient to remain passive. However, sometimes the patient can assist initially into attaining a neutral position, the physician braces the patient, and then the patient relaxes. The technique can be adapted to treat the patient in a supine, prone, side-lying, or upright position.

Tissue Texture Change Treatment

1. The physician monitors the region to be treated
2. The anteroposterior spinal curve of the treatment area is flattened. This position places that region of the spine into an idling position, which shortens and softens associated muscle. A palpatory softening is customarily noted immediately. The lordoses of the lumbar and cervical regions are slightly flexed while the thoracic spine is extended. When treating the patient

in the supine or prone positions, pillows can be used to attain approximation of neutral

3. A facilitating force is applied. This may be compression, torsion, or a combination of the two. At times, traction may be used with or without torsion
4. The physician places the patient (patient's musculature) into a relaxed position. This usually requires approximating the origins and insertions by further compression and/or torsion. Additional softening is often noted
5. The position is held for 3 to 5 seconds and then all facilitating forces are released
6. The patient's condition is reevaluated. In some cases, passive stretch can be introduced

Intervertebral Motion Restriction Treatment

The same basic procedures are used to address intervertebral motion restrictions, with the additional requirement that the physician place the vertebra into a position that allows freedom of motion in all planes. For the cervical spine, the patient can be treated in the seated position but more frequently in the supine position. The thoracic and lumbar regions are typically treated in the seated or prone positions, but the techniques can be adapted for side-lying positions:

1. The dysfunction is monitored continuously
2. The lordosis or kyphosis is flattened
3. A facilitating force, either compression, torsion, or a combination is applied specifically to the monitored dysfunction. Often, regional tension decreases immediately
4. The directions of the somatic dysfunction are added just to the level of the dysfunction. Further relaxation is noted. The sequencing can be varied depending on the skill and experience of the physician. In fact, motion into all directions can be applied simultaneously rather than in a stepwise fashion. Some clinicians have even found the treatment effective by placing the dysfunction into neutral, applying the directions of relative freedom, and then adding the facilitating force
5. The position is held for 3 to 5 seconds, the facilitating forces are released, and the region is returned to neutral
6. The dysfunction is reevaluated. When appropriate, movement can be introduced into the barrier directions

SIDE EFFECTS AND CONTRAINDICATIONS

There are few contraindications and most are relative in nature in the clinical application of FPR. If the patient is not able to tolerate the positioning or experiences discomfort, either alternative positioning of the region or alternative techniques should be used. FPR to the cervical region approximates a Spurling maneuver and if the patient experiences radicular pain, then repositioning or traction may be used. Lumbar techniques may put torsion into knees or hips that have degenerative changes or prosthetics. Performing lumbar discogenic treatment would be contraindicated with a patient who has had a hip replacement as the external rotation and torque forces may possibly disarticulate the joint. The same can be said for the use of the first rib technique with patients with shoulder pathology. The compression and twisting involved with the treatment may exacerbate conditions where there are new or chronic shoulder dislocations or separations. Any recent history trauma of any region should raise suspicion of fracture or dislocation. Compression, even the relatively small forces used in FPR, may make a stable fracture unstable. Accurate diagnosis and integration of clinical knowledge

should direct the use of any intervention with osteopathic manipulation. Caution but not contradiction should be used in case of osteoporosis, malignancy, rheumatological disorders, congenital malformations, stenosis, or other clinical diseases.

Generally, patients experience relief and few side effects when treated with FPR. As with any other treatment, there may be transient fatigue, soreness, or stiffness due primarily to restoration of circulation to previously dysfunctional tissue and release of muscular waste products. In rare cases, the patient experiences these discomforts on subsequent treatments.

SUMMARY

FPR is an easily administered, nontraumatic, and efficient technique. When it is properly performed, the patient often reports immediate relief of point tenderness and restoration of function. If complete normalization is not achieved, it can be repeated, or other methods of treatment can be applied immediately. This can mean treatments lasting a few minutes that can be easily incorporated into a busy clinical, non-manipulative specialist practice. Although primarily axial procedures have been described in this chapter, it is possible to use FPR for other regions of articular and soft tissue dysfunction.

DIAGNOSES AND TECHNIQUES

739.1-Cervical

Soft tissue treatment.

Findings

Posterior cervical muscle hypertonicity (soft-tissue texture abnormalities).

Patient Position

Supine on the table; the patient's head is beyond the end of the table, resting on a pillow on the physician's lap.

Procedure

1. The patient is supine and the physician sits at the head of the table (Fig. 52B.1)
2. The physician cradles the patient's neck in the palm of his hand utilizing the hand that is on the opposite side of the dysfunctional region. When treating the left side, the right hand is used.

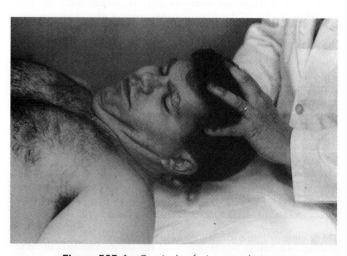

Figure 52B-1 Cervical soft tissue technique.

The pad of the index or other finger acts as both monitoring finger and fulcrum, on the contralateral muscular spasm

3. The physician's other hand is placed on the top of the patient's head. This hand then straightens the patient's cervical lordosis by slightly forward bending the neck
4. Using the hand that is on the top of the patient's head, the physician applies a compressive facilitating force to the neck, through the patient's head and sufficient enough to be appreciated and to create a relaxation of the tissue noted at the monitored location
5. Maintaining the compressive force, extension is introduced to the neck to the level of the monitoring finger. This should cause a further relaxation of the tissue being treated
6. Side bending and rotation, usually toward the side of the tense tissues, are added to the point that the tissues continue to soften
7. The position is maintained for 3 to 5 seconds before returning the neck slowly to a neutral position
8. The tissue being treated is reevaluated. A mild stretch can be applied into the barrier directions can be added while monitoring the tissue tension

Note: If tissue changes are found anteriorly, flexion instead is usually required. Some muscles, such as the sternocleidomastoid, have side-bending and rotation components in opposite directions. Knowledge of anatomy determines the direction that muscles must be placed into their individual shortened positions as determined by palpation and tissue response. Careful localization of the component motions of forward/backward bending, side bending/rotation, and compression to the area of tissue texture change will result in faster and more efficient results.

Cervical Segmental Somatic Dysfunction

Findings
C3 ES_LR_L and C7 FS_LR_L.

Patient Position
Supine, with the patient's head beyond the end of the table, resting on a pillow on the physician's lap.

Procedure
1. The physician sits at the head of the table (Fig. 52B.2)
2. The physician cradles the patient's neck in the palm of his hand. When treating the left side, the right hand is used. The pad of a finger monitors posterior to the left articular pillar of C3

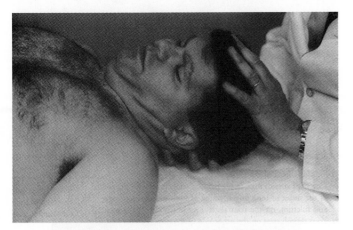

Figure 52B-2 Typical cervical C3 ES_LR_L left technique.

3. The physician's other hand is placed on the top of the patient's head. This hand then introduces straightening the patient's cervical lordosis by slightly flexing the neck down to the level of the monitoring finger on C3. This is the neutral component
4. The physician's hand on the top of the patient's head adds a compressive force directed through the head to the neck until noted at the monitored level
5. The physician adds slight extension to the neck through the level of the monitored C3 while maintaining the compression
6. The relative freedom of motion of the somatic dysfunction is added by side bending C3 to the left by introducing a translatory force to the right through your monitoring finger
7. Rotation of the head and neck only through the level of C3 is added. This places C3 into all three planes of freedom of motion
8. This position is held for 3 to 5 seconds and then the physician slowly returns the neck to neutral
9. The C3 motion freedoms and restrictions are reevaluated. Improved range of motion into the barrier directions can be applied

Note: If the diagnosis is flexion rather than extension (C7 FS_LR_L), step 5 is replaced by adding flexion through the level of C7 rather than adding extension. Similarly, if the diagnosis is one of right side bending and right rotation, the appropriate adjustments should be made to engage these relative freedoms.

This procedure to dysfunctions of the suboccipital area can be specifically applied to the occipitoatlantoid articulation. The flexion or extension component can be localized by introducing a nodding motion to the skull. Any further flexion or extension of the cervical spine is nonspecific. The typical and restrictive motions of the occipitoatlantoid joint involves side bending and rotation in opposite in opposite directions. The appropriate directions of relative freedom should be used.

739.2-Thoracic

Thoracic segmental somatic dysfunction.

Findings
T6 FS_LR_L.

Patient Position
The patient is seated on the end of the table.

Procedure
1. The physician stands behind and to the side of the dysfunction to be treated (in the T6 FS_LR_L somatic dysfunction as in the current case, this is to the left of the patient) (Fig. 52B.3)
2. The physician monitors at the left T6 transverse process with his right hand. The palm of the hand can be used to support the region during the next step
3. Although FPR is a passive technique, attaining a neutral position in the seated position requires patient cooperation. The patient is asked to sit up as straight as possible and push his or her chest forward. This will straighten the thoracic kyphosis and add to the initial neutral component
4. The physician places his left axilla over the patient's left shoulder. This should be as close to the cervicothoracic junction as is possible. The physician's forearm is placed across the patient's chest and his left hand should grasp the patient's right shoulder
5. The physician adds a downward compressive force through his left axilla onto the patient's left shoulder. This both adds the facilitating force and introduces a localized left side bending down through to the level of the monitoring finger at T6

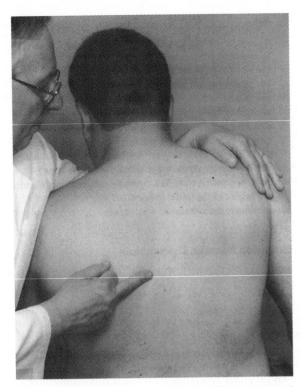

Figure 52B-3   Thoracic spine T6 FS$_L$R$_L$ technique, seated.

6. Flexion to the level of T6 is added by pulling forward on both of the patient's shoulders while maintaining the side bending
7. The physician rotates the patient's thoracic spine to the left down through the level of T6 by pulling the right shoulder forward
8. The position is held for 3 to 5 seconds, and then the patient is slowly returned to a neutral position
9. The somatic dysfunction is reassessed. Improved range of motion into the barrier directions can be applied

Note: If the diagnosis is extension rather than flexion (T6 ES$_L$R$_L$), the flexion in step 6 is replaced adding extension instead through the level of T6. This is accomplished by the physician pulling the shoulders backward. Similarly, if the diagnosis is side bending and rotation is to the right, the appropriate adjustments into the relative freedoms of the somatic dysfunction are made. If the somatic dysfunction is a neutral group curve, neither flexion nor extension is used. The physician stands on the side of the curve concavity, the side-bending side, and monitors at the apex of the curve. Adjustments are applied in order that the side bending and rotation are achieved in the opposite directions.

Alternative Thoracic Segmental Somatic Dysfunction (Extension Dysfunctions), Prone

Findings
T6 ES$_L$R$_L$.

Patient Position
The patient is prone, with pillows beneath the abdomen and head. This creates a flattening of the thoracic kyphosis. The patient's arms are placed at his sides.

Procedure
1. The physician stands at the side of the table opposite to the somatic dysfunction. For T6 ES$_L$R$_L$, the physician stands at the right side of the patient (Fig. 52B.4)

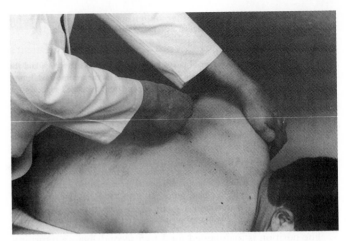

Figure 52B-4   Thoracic spine T8 ESRRR technique, prone.

2. The physician palpates and monitors the T6 posterior left transverse process with the fingers of his right hand
3. The physician's left hand grasps the patient's left shoulder. The patient's entire shoulder should be held with your fingers placed on the superior and lateral portion of the shoulder
4. The patient's left shoulder is compressed medially toward the spine (this flattens the spine in the anteroposterior plane) and then toward the patient's feet (this compressive force creates left side bending). The combination of forces creates a force vector that is parallel to the patient's thoracic spine
5. Some extension of the spine is created through the level of T6 by maintaining traction on the shoulder as the patient's shoulder is lifted from the table, until motion can be palpated at the level of the monitoring fingers
6. To create greater extension, the physician stands up straighter, pulling the patient's shoulder further posteriorly. This also creates some additional left rotation down through the level of T6

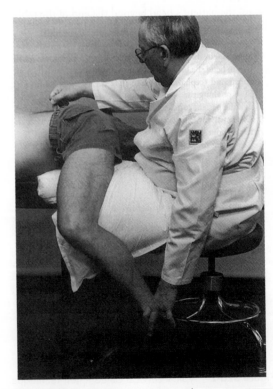

Figure 52B-5   Discogenic pain syndrome treatment.

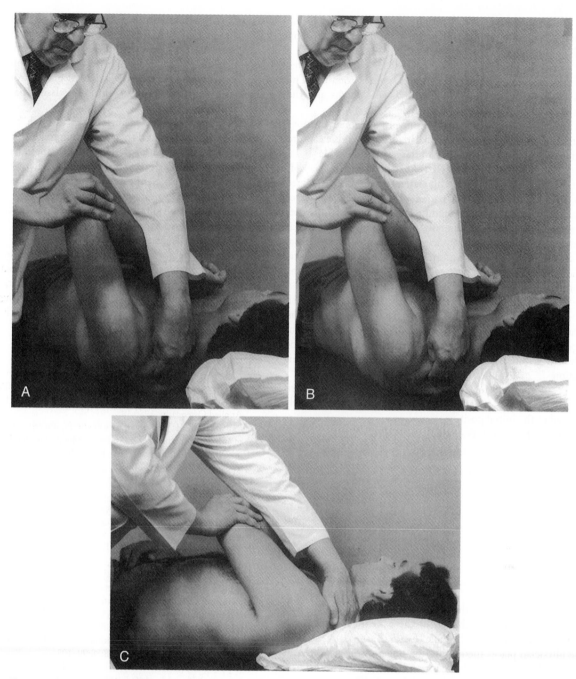

Figure 52B-6 Treatment for first rib. **A.** First rib elevated on left. **B.** Internal rotation and flexion introduced. **C.** Adduction and circumduction added.

7. This position is held for 3 to 5 seconds, and then the patient's shoulder and thoracic region are slowly returned to the neutral position
8. The T6 somatic dysfunction is then reevaluated

Note: If the diagnosis is a flexion somatic dysfunction, FPR is more easily accomplished with the patient in the seated position as described previously.

739.3-Lumbar

Discogenic pain syndrome treatment.

Findings
Left lumbar disk herniation or bulge with left radiculitis.

Position
The patient is prone, close to the left edge of the table, with a sufficient number of pillows beneath the abdomen to cause flattening of the lumbar lordosis.

Procedure
1. The physician sits on a rolling stool at the (left) side of table of the dysfunction, with the physician's thighs parallel to the table, at the level of the patient's pelvis, facing the patient's head (Fig. 52B.5)
2. The physician monitors the posterior transverse process (left) of the level to be treated (L4-5) with a finger of the (right) hand that is closer to the patient

3. The physician uses his nonmonitoring (left) hand to grasp the patient's (left) knee and flex the patient's (left) hip and knee on the involved side

4. The physician places the patient's upper leg across his anterior thighs. This creates abduction and external rotation. The patient's lower leg is lateral to the physician's thighs and the physician grasps the patient's (left) ankle

5. The physician localizes motion to the involved segment by moving the patient's upper leg in a cephalad direction. It is easiest to do this by rolling the stool closer to the head of the table

6. The physician raises his outer (left) knee by lifting his heel off the floor. The physician pushes the lateral part of his (left) knee into the popliteal fossa of the patient's (left) knee. This creates a traction force that can be modified, as the physician further raises and moves his knee laterally, until motion is palpated at his monitoring finger. The physician's knee is now at the medial surface of the popliteal fossa of the patient's knee and the medial surface of the knee and acts as a fulcrum for the rest of the technique

7. The physician uses his nonmonitoring (left) hand to push the patient's (left) lower leg toward the floor until motion is palpated at his monitoring finger. There may be a slight amount of tension noted at the monitored location. Often, the patient will state that the symptoms are reduced while in this position

8. The position is held for 3 to 5 seconds until there is a sudden release of the somatic dysfunction and then the patient is slowly returned to the initial position

9. The lumbar region is reevaluated

739.8-Rib

First Rib
Findings
First rib elevated on left.

Patient Position
The patient is supine.

Procedure

1. The physician stands on the side of the elevated rib. In the current example, this is to the left of the patient. The physician faces toward the head of the table (Fig. 52B.6)

2. The physician places the monitoring finger of the hand that is closer to the patient (left hand for an elevated left first rib) over the posterior portion of the elevated first rib. The finger serves

primarily as a monitoring component. The physician's forearm serves as a fulcrum for some of the subsequent steps

3. The physician's other (right) hand grasps the patient's left elbow. The shoulder is flexed to approximately 90 degrees and abducted slightly (10 to 20 degrees) from the vertical. This should be adjusted until the tissues soften maximally (Fig. 52B.6A)

4. A compressive force is introduced through the patient's left elbow directed toward the monitoring finger (Fig. 52B.6B)

5. Slight further flexion of the patient's shoulder is introduced by the physician deviating the patient's elbow more cephalad. This causes the patient's forearm to abut the physician's forearm and introduces some internal rotation into the shoulder. The absolute position should be determined by the relaxation of the monitored rib soft tissue

6. The position is held for 3 to 5 seconds

7. While maintaining the compressive force and the internal rotation, the physician adducts and further internally rotates the patient's upper arm. To complete the treatment, the physician circumducts the patient's arm through a curving motion and back into a neutral position alongside his torso (Fig. 52B.6C)

8. The first is reevaluated

REFERENCES

1. Schiowitz S. Facilitated positional release. *JAOA*. 1990;901:145–155.
2. Fryette HH. *Principles of Osteopathic Technic*. Carmel, CA: Academy of Applied Osteopathy, 1980:19.
3. Van Buskirk RL. Treatment of somatic Dysfunction with an osteopathic manipulative method of Dr. Andrew Taylor Still in Ward (ed.). *Foundations for Osteopathic Medicine*. 2nd Ed. Philadelphia, PA: Lippincott Williams & Wilkins, 2003:1094–1114.
4. Korr IM. Proprioceptors and somatic dysfunction. *JAOA*. 1975;75:638–650.
5. Bailey HW. Some problems in making osteopathic spinal manipulative therapy appropriate and specific. *JAOA*. 1976;75:486–499.
6. Carew TJ. The control of reflex action. In: Kandel ER, Schwartz JH, eds. *Principles of Neural Science*. 2nd Ed. New York, NY: Elsevier Science Publishing Co Inc., 1985:464.
7. Mennell JM. *Back Pain: Diagnosis and Treatment Using Manipulative Techniques*. Boston, MA: Little, Brown & Co, 1960:75.
8. Mitchell FL Jr, Moran PS, Pruzzo NA. *An Evaluation and Treatment Manual of Osteopathic Muscle Energy Procedures*. Valley Park, MO: Mitchell, Moran & Pruzzo Assoc, 1979:229–253.
9. Johnston WL. Segmental definition, Part 1: a focal point for diagnosis of somatic dysfunction. *JAOA*. 1988;88:99–105.
10. Dowling DJ. S.T.A.R.: a more viable alternative descriptor system of somatic dysfunction. *AAO J*. 1998; 8(2):34–37.

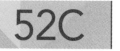

52C Progressive Inhibition of Neuromuscular Structures

DENNIS J. DOWLING

KEY CONCEPT

In this section, emphasis is placed on decreasing tissue tonicity. Clinical symptoms are assumed to be directly related to increased dysfunctional tone. A steady pressure (constant mild/moderate force) is applied to regions of dysfunction. The relationship between musculoskeletal structures and underlying visceral organs is also considered. In order to achieve efficacy and accuracy, a thorough knowledge of the typical and variant courses of nerves, fascial bands, and muscles is required. This knowledge must be augmented by clinical decision-making skills.

CASE STUDY

The author had headaches as a teenager and was brought by his parents for treatment to the family physician. Most of the treatments that were offered had a limited impact or had very undesirable side effects. Accompanying the cephalgia were other apparently related symptoms: a boring pain of the right eye; increased lacrimation; right-sided facial pain; nasal congestion; and scalp sensitivity. There was also frequent suboccipital pain that appeared to be related in onset to the periorbital pain, although no direct connection was apparent. Eventually, common precipitating events leading to the symptoms were discerned: prolonged reading; eyestrain due to exposure to bright sunlight; and dehydration. There were no sensory deficits. Some symptoms could occur independently and were usually worsened by stress. Having little knowledge of anatomy at the time, the author attempted self-treatment involving the application of manual pressure to various locations of the head. Pressing painful sites appeared to bring about only temporary relief when any were pressed singly. The pain could recur almost immediately after release of the pressure. Adjacent regions of the scalp also developed sensitivity during or after release of pressure. Eventually, some patterns appeared to develop as these secondary and even subsequent points became unmasked. The most successful approach appeared to be the sequential treatment of a series of points.

Much later, as an osteopathic student and physician, the author began to integrate osteopathic manipulative medicine theory along with personal clinical observations in the utilization of treatment of these apparently linear patterns. The method of self-treatment was converted into a treatment modality and taught to other students of osteopathy. Gradually, the rationale as well as further expansion of use of this specialized inhibitory technique beyond treatment of headaches became clearer (1). Some similarities and differences were noted in relationship to other manipulative methods of point or applied pressure techniques.

INHIBITION

Progressive Inhibition of Neuromuscular Structures (PINS) is most closely related to the osteopathic modality of inhibition. The *Glossary of Osteopathic Terminology* states that inhibition is "...a term that describes steady pressure to soft tissues to effect relaxation and normalize reflex activity" (2). The "steady pressure to soft tissues" is perhaps one of the oldest methods of manual treatment, regardless of the name applied. Classically, inhibition is a constant mild-to-moderate amount of force exerted by the fingers, elbow, knee, or even foot on regions of hypertonic muscle. Even though the patient's presenting complaint may be of pain or decreased function, the objective of the treatment is to decrease the tonicity of the tissues. Any symptoms that the patient has are assumed to be directly related to this increased dysfunctional tone (3). Larger, more superficial muscles are the most easily identified whether they are in the normal-relaxed or hypertonic states. Regional muscles can be selected and treated individually or in pairs. Typically, the patient is treated in either the supine or the prone positions. This may facilitate the process by reducing the use of some muscles for positional support of the trunk and neck. As an example, the trapezius, can be easily located in the cervical, shoulder, and upper thoracic regions. Some portion of the muscle can be grasped, pressed,

or pinched. A hypertonic muscle is commonly found to be firmer than the same muscle on the opposite side of the body and perhaps more than its antagonist. This finding, and perhaps greater sensitivity or tenderness, are noted as the pressure is introduced. As long as the applied pressure remains constant, the structures should reflexively relax. Attempts should be made to avoid altering the position or amount of pressure, as these will more likely be stimulatory.

In regard to inhibition, the relationship between musculoskeletal structures and the underlying visceral organs should also be considered. These organs receive innervations from the same spinal cord segment levels that service the skin, bones, joints, ligaments, and muscles. The sympathetic chain lies just anterior to the rib heads and dysfunction of the vertebral or rib joints may result in increased stimulation to related structures, visceral, and musculoskeletal (4). Acute responses to increased sympathetic activity are the same as to any new injury: redness (rubor), pain (dolor), swelling (tumor), heat (calor), and decreased function (funcio laesa) (5). More superficial structures such as the skin and subcutaneous tissue may have a "doughy" consistency and the pain noted by the patient would be typically sharp and throbbing. Chronic sympathetic hyperactivity in the absence of adequate treatment and/or recovery demonstrates altered signs and symptoms: the muscles may feel fibrotic ("ropy"); the skin is thinner, paler, and cooler; and pain responses can range from relative insensitivity ("anesthetic") to altered sensitivity ("paresthesia") to hypersensitivity. The pressure provided by the application of a modality, such as inhibition, may result in a transitory increase in the palpatory findings or symptoms followed by reduction of some or all of these components can be readily appreciated. When the visceral organs are the primary dysfunction, the persistence or recurrence of a musculoskeletal somatic dysfunction may indicate the viscerosomatic reflex. When a musculoskeletal injury is the etiology, manipulative treatment may result in a more persistent reduction or elimination of all pathological components.

Inhibitory techniques have a different visceral focus in the suboccipital and sacral regions. Rather than a sympathetic effect, the parasympathetic system predominates. Somatic dysfunction of the upper cervical, occipital, and sacral regions may reflect or result in prolonged inappropriate parasympathetic activity. Inhibitory treatment results in reduction of increased regional musculoskeletal tone and congestion, and theoretically downregulates the more internal mechanisms.

A thorough understanding of the structure and function of all of the factors related to somatic dysfunction is necessary in guiding accurate treatment with Inhibitory and **PINS** treatments. When correlated with somatic dysfunction findings, treatment patterns may be moved about several locations with the intent upon reducing all of the relevant dysfunctions.

When Andrew Taylor Still was a young man suffering from chronic headaches, he treated himself with a rope-swing by lowering the rope to a few inches above the ground. A blanket was slung across it and he positioned his neck with the base of the skull on this support and subsequently fell asleep. He awakened refreshed and pain-free. Whether intentionally or inadvertently, his self-treatment appears to represent an inhibitory treatment as much as a positional intervention (6). Despite an aversion to defining specific types of treatment in his writings, Dr. Still included some descriptions of both inhibition and stimulation methods (7).

Some of Dr. Still's early students likewise described inhibitory techniques as well as a rationale for their use. In his book, *A Manual of Osteopathy*, Eduard Goetz, D.O., described and illustrated Readership will be largely nonosteopathic, so we must not assume familiarity with Still so a brief background as to who he was would be helpful if you wish to keep this reference in inhibition for various conditions, both somatic and visceral (8). The accompanying photographs in this small handbook clearly demonstrate and detail inhibitory treatment of several regions. Of special note are the orbital and suboccipital regions of the head. A few minutes of pressure applied individually to each of these points was recommended.

A more extensive description appears in *The Principles of Osteopathy* by Dain L. Tasker, D.O. (9). Dr. Tasker described the rationale as to the effectiveness of inhibitory techniques, especially since inhibition appeared to be a natural phenomenon. Bodily functions such as defecation and urination could not come under conscious and unconscious control without the adapted or learned ability to perform inhibition. In discussing the effectiveness of externally applied inhibitory pressure directed toward decreasing hyperactivity, as is applied by an osteopathic physician, he stated that it is not the surface pressure that is effective but the initiation or alteration of the reflex arc that subsequently occurs. The initial response to the placing a pressure is, in effect, a form of stimulation since it is impacting on the soft tissue. However, steadily applied pressure results in a diminution of the stimulation and a resultant inhibition of the region sets in motion a lessening of the dysfunction. These may bring about some alterations both deep to and distant from the location of the applied pressure. In citing Hilton law "that the skin, muscles and synovial membrane of a joint, or the skin, muscles of the abdomen and contents covered by peritoneum, are innervated from the same segment of the cord," Tasker states that the "overstimulation" caused by inhibition results in diminution or elimination of the overreactivity.

An Expansion of His Rationale Here Would Be Good

Osteopathic Point and/or Pressure Techniques

Many types of passive direct and indirect systems of osteopathic treatment of somatic dysfunction exist. Some standard points and diagnoses are used as fulcrums and/or monitoring locations in practically all of these modalities. Constant palpation at these points is one of the best means for an osteopathic physician to experience feedback and monitor the success of the treatment when performing Jones' strain-counterstrain treatment (10–12). Often, the patient can likewise appreciate the alteration. The muscle spindle sensory organ is embedded into the larger extrafusal muscle. The sensory ends of nerve fibers to these small muscles are stimulated by stretch of any kind, whether it is static or dynamic. The result is a single spinal segment increase in alpha motorneuron activity, which results in contraction of the whole extrafusal muscle. As a means of preventing overstretching of the soft tissue, it is quite successful and should decrease as soon as the danger retreats. However, if the region is underprepared or overwhelmed, the reflex can persist longer than is appropriate. The signals from the spindle continue to fire as if the tissue were being too rapidly stretched or overstretched even though the overall length of the muscle may be normal or relatively short. The sensitivity of a "tender point" reflects increased underlying activity. The external pressure at the tender point often elicits the complaint while the positioning during strain-counterstrain technique shortens the whole muscle. This allows the spindle reflex mechanism to be reset and the sensitivity disappears.

Facilitated positional release (FPR) (13) is similar in many respects to strain-counterstrain. It differs in its use of an activating force, usually compression or torsion, after initially positioning

the region in neutral. Strain-counterstrain is a form of positional release while FPR utilizes an additional facilitating force. Both strain-counterstrain and FPR theoretically utilize the same neurophysiological mechanism, the muscle spindle. Richard Van Buskirk, Ph.D., D.O., F.A.A.O., also attributes the muscle spindle as the core activator that is treated by the Still technique (14). It shares many similar applications to strain-counterstrain and FPR. Based on his recovery of components of the technique on the writings of Charles Hazzard, D.O., (15) as well as Dr. Still himself, Dr. Van Buskirk describes the technique as initially utilizing the palpatory diagnosis of dysfunctions to place the region into the freedoms. Finally, the osteopathic physician introduces movement past the neutral point into the barrier directions. This low-velocity, relatively low-amplitude articulatory movement toward the barriers follows the positional treatment into the freedoms.

In the spinal regions, functional technique (16) utilizes diagnostic points to define the somatic dysfunction that exists at that level relative to its two adjoining vertebrae, the one above and the one below. Detection of somatic dysfunction is typically made by percussion and more specific testing to scan and screen the regions. Elaine Wallace, D.O., developed Torque unwinding, (17) she utilizes constructs whereby the body is imagined as a collection of adjacent or overlapping cubes. Theoretically, injuries direct forces into a whole "cube" that is typically in a state of torsion during the process. When the patient is twisted, the initial vector force may be straight, but the resultant pathway becomes arched or more twisted as the person and region straightens. In this manner, the fascia acts more colloid-like with disruption and a tissue memory of the force in the form of adaptation. Torque unwinding treatment involves the introduction of oscillating rhythmic balancing pressures directed centrally from two diametrically opposed theoretical cube faces. The intent is for the therapeutic forces to counteract the residual traumatic ones. Other variations of myofascial or fascial release techniques (18,19) that utilize point contacts as references, contact points, and/or diagnostic reflections occur in the osteopathic literature. Trigger band technique, as described by Steven Typaldos, D.O., (20) is a method of treating the pathological crosslinkages of fascial bands by exerting deep pressure along certain connective tissue pathways. Chaitow (21,22) describes neuromuscular technique that consists mostly of point localization and pressure followed by deep stroking and/or rolling of the tissue.

Chapman's point treatment (23) reflects a neurological/endocrine/lymphatic alteration reflected to specific points on the surface that should raise suspicion of a possibly latent visceral correlate. Some of the specific mapped points are similar in location and correlation to those of acupuncture.

Nonosteopathic Point and/or Pressure Systems

Cyriax method (24), Trigger point therapy (25,26), acupressure (27,28), reflexology, Rolfing, and Shiatsu (29,30) bear some similarities to typical inhibition and stimulatory techniques. The practitioner provides the treatment in each by pressing the patient's soft tissue.

The British medical orthopedist James Cyriax, M.D., practiced joint mobilization and massage and utilized a pinching technique on several locations. Trigger point therapy, developed by Janet Travell, M.D., maps out the relationship between a remote referral region and a damaged myofascial nexus. The methods of treatment can include manual pressure, dry needling, or a combination of anesthetic and/or steroid agents injected into the trigger point. A vapocoolant spray can be directed from the trigger point toward the referral zone in another form of the treatment. An apparent variant of the trigger point concept, Bonnie Prudden Myotherapy, consists of primary points, as well as satellite points. Both types of points are treated for short intervals several times per day over several sessions (31,32). Stretching may also be incorporated in either Bonnie Prudden myotherapy or trigger point therapy.

Acupressure utilizes surface points that represent reflections of energy or chi forces within the body aligned along meridians by specific point locations. The technique generally involves the application of pressure as well as circular motions. When treated with acupuncture needles, the practitioner may also burn incense or apply electricity to the outer tip of the acupuncture needles.

Ida Rolf, Ph.D., developed the eponymous system, Rolfing (33). Sometimes known as "Dr. Elbow," because of her use of that region to apply pressure, she proposed utilizing deeply applied forces on regions of the body. The actual amount of force applied in this modality exceeds that which is commonly employed in osteopathic inhibition. There is a great deal of emphasis placed on approximating ideal symmetry and alignment. Followers of Dr. Rolf made some alterations to the technique and integrated them into other modalities involving movement patterns (Hellerwork, Aston-Patterning).

One of the oldest forms of manual therapy, Shiatsu, attempts to reduce the amount of the tissue tension present. Although typically brief in duration, the amount of force can be quite intense. Specific treatment patterns are utilized for certain conditions. Reflexology also relates energetic or visceral components to resonant areas located on the hands, feet, and ear. As with acupuncture, the name of the organ is related more to a theoretical functional contribution to the integrity or energy component of the organ than the actual physical structure of the viscera.

PINS Method

PINS requires an osteopathic physician's capability to utilize anatomical and clinical knowledge to determine involved structures and sequence of treatment in the localization of points and the application of pressure in a logical fashion to treat persistent or resistant dysfunction. The osteopathic physician must have a thorough knowledge of the typical and variant courses of nerves, fascial bands, and muscles and augmented by clinical decision-making skills for efficacy and accuracy. This may involve the treatment of contiguous muscles, addressing the overlapping zones where more than one involved nerve, muscle, or fascial tissue may be contributing to the persistence of somatic dysfunction, and the development of a sequencing of **PINS** treatment. It is not as simple as locating a single sensitive point. Any patient can point to a location that hurts or that is sensitive to pressure. Shoulder pain can originate in the glenohumeral joint and specific treatment can be successful in increasing mobility and decreasing discomfort. However, when that is unsuccessful, more of the same treatment may not be the answer and this may prove frustrating to both the patient and the doctor. If the restrictions of motion of the shoulder involve the combination of flexion, abduction, and external rotation as well as reduction of scapulothoracic motion with freedoms in the opposite directions, the latissimus dorsi may be in spasm. It attaches in the bicipital groove of the humerus, pulls the arm into extension, internal rotation, and adduction, the motions directly opposite the restrictions. Treatment may have to go beyond this focus by including the upper ribs, pectoralis muscles, lower cervical spine, clavicle, thoracic spine, lumbar spine, pelvis, and lower extremity in the process. Fascial planes, and therefore fascial stresses, must also be considered.

In **PINS**, patients can offer feedback. They participate in the treatment by describing the amount of pain or other sensitivity at the palpated areas. As the treatment proceeds, the osteopathic physician takes note of the tissue changes that occur, as well as the integration of the patient's subjective experience. **PINS** can be used before or after other methods of treatment, manipulative or otherwise, as part of a comprehensive treatment regimen.

Procedure

The development of an appropriate and specific diagnostic and treatment protocol using **PINS** requires the following:

1. In most cases, the patient should be lying supine or prone. This is to allow postural muscles to be in a fairly relaxed state. However, treatment can be done with the patient seated or standing in some regions of the body

2. The osteopathic physician stands or sits near the region to be treated. The fingers of both hands should be able to contact the patient comfortably and accurately

3. Examine the patient. Determine any relationship between the patient's symptoms, somatic dysfunctions, and the soft tissue findings

4. Determine the components of the somatic dysfunction. The mnemonic "S-T-A-R" (34) can be used to track the different aspects:

   (a) Inquire about **[S] Sensitivity changes.** These are the patient's subjective responses to palpation. These can include tenderness, numbness, radiation, warmth, irritation, throbbing, etc

   (b) Locate **[T] Tissue texture changes.** They can be chronic (prolonged blanching of the skin, ropy or fibrous texture of the muscles and fascia, coolness, dryness, vascular changes) or acute (increased redness, swelling and edema, moist, and/or increased temperature). Palpation may initially worsen this component

   (c) **[A] Asymmetry** can be noted by visual inspection or by palpatory examination. The so-called nondysfunctional side is used as the standard of expected form. Theoretically, an imaginary line down the middle of the body should reveal symmetry of one side to the other in a nondysfunctional condition

   (d) Perhaps the most important determinant of somatic dysfunction is **[R] Restriction of Motion.** Restriction can be by quantity (number of degrees of motion), quality (i.e., stiffness, tremors, cogwheel rigidity, extraneous movement, etc.)

5. The site of subjective complaints of pain can be deceptive and may not help in the actual localization of the etiology. As an indicator that there is a problem, pain is fairly reliable. Tight muscles on one side may be relatively pain free while the contralateral stretched muscles may be more "attention-seeking." Symptoms may distract treatment from the more needy locations. Pain, or any other symptom, tells that there is a problem but may or may not correlate with the dysfunction

6. Locate a "primary sensitive" point by examination of the tissue in the region of the patient's complaint. If a significant one is not found, then knowledge of anatomical relationships is used to widen the search to adjacent areas

7. Using knowledge of anatomical structures, another point is located. This may be designated as the "end point" for **PINS** treatment purposes. It is located either distally or proximally to the primary point in a structure that links the two points. Having a thorough working knowledge and understanding of muscle origins/insertions, nerve and vascular pathways, and ligamentous attachments is a good beginning in determining

this pair of points. If the primary point is at a muscular origin, the end point may be at the insertion, or vice versa. Sometimes, one or the other point is located in the belly of the muscle. In that case, exploration of both ends of the attachments to bone may reveal the location of an end point. Ligaments, which are generally shorter and more fibrous, have points that are probably also fairly close to one another. Keep in mind that fascia encompasses all structures and the path between one point and another may seem to cross other structures. The more specialized the fascia, the more palpable and tendinous it is. Tracing superficial and deep pathways of nerves is useful when determining paths that apparently do not correlate with the other structures. Primary and end points may be found where a nerve passes out of a foramen, between or through muscles, or around bony protrusions. Sometimes, if more than one nerve innervates a region, the primary point can be found at the beginning of one nerve and the end point at the beginning of the other. In the case of nerve distribution of an extremity, one point will typically be found closer to the body, while the other will be closer to the end of the extremity. There are no exhaustive maps of points and sensitive point locations. There is no substitution for an excellent working knowledge of anatomy. The designated primary point will most likely be nearer to the patient's symptoms. The end point may also elicit the patient's presenting symptoms but usually to a lesser extent. Since the entire structure is in dysfunction, all intervening points between the primary and the end points must be addressed. In any case, the first steps are to make a determination of the two ends of the pattern. A patient's complaints of apparently unrelated regions of the body being related may give a clue as to the location of some components. Assuming that their knowledge of anatomy is small, it is left to the osteopathic physician to draw the conclusions necessary to begin treatment

8. Determining the two points is obviously critical to the outcome and this process of selection needs to be very clear—other than the supraorbital point described below

9. For the purpose of proceeding in a logical fashion, the point that is more sensitive is designated as the "primary." To put this in more easily understood language for the patient, the primary point is addressed as the "first point." Both you and the patient can consider the other point, which is found on the other extreme, as the "end point." Table 52C.1 provides examples of primary and end points

10. Determine a muscular, fascial, and/or neurological pathway between the primary sensitive point and the end point. The line may be curved rather than straight. The direction of treatment may be from distal to proximal, medial to lateral, anterior to posterior, or vice versa

11. An understanding of the connection between the two points using knowledge of anatomy is necessary, especially
    (a) Nerve innervation:
        (i) Direct connections (The connection of a point near the antecubital region of the elbow to a point along the middle of the forearm near the wrist-median nerve.)
        (ii) Consider overlap or "watershed regions" of innervation. (The ophthalmic division of the trigeminal nerve travels from the supraorbital notch over the frontal region and to the top of the head.) The greater occipital nerve exits the suboccipital region in the occipital sulcus and travels over the occiput to the top of the head. They overlap in the scalp is near the vertex
    (b) Muscle origins and insertions:
        (i) Typical (A sensitive point may be found at the medial aspect of the clavicle and another found at the mastoid process representing involvement of the sternocleidomastoid muscle.)
        (ii) Overlap (The location of a sensitive point on the superior anterior chest may involve intercostals muscles, pectoralis major, and/or pectoralis minor.)
        (iii) Contiguity (The tensor fascia lata and iliotibial band actually form a continuity for two possible tender points located, respectively, at the greater trochanter and the fibular head. If a terminal point was actually found near the lateral malleolus instead of the fibular head, then there might be a tensor fascia lata, iliotibial band, peroneal muscle connection.)
    (c) Fascia:
        (i) Specialized (Interosseous ligaments are actually specialized fascia connecting the radius and ulna in

TABLE 52C.1

Primary Points, End Points, Connections, and Clinical Conditions

Primary Point	Endpoint	Connection	Clinical Condition
(a) Supraorbital notch	Suboccipital region	Frontalis-occipitalis muscles Trigeminal-greater occipital nerves (Fig. 52C.1)	Tension Headache Chronic daily headache Migraine headache
(b) Superior medial scapular border	Base of occiput	Levator scapula (Fig. 52C.2)	Cervicalgia
(c) Greater trochanter of femur	Fibular head	Iliotibial band (Fig. 52C.3)	Hip pain Knee pain
(d) Sternum at second rib	Coracoid process	Pectoralis minor (Fig. 52C.4)	Chest pain
(e) Gluteal region	Greater trochanter popliteal region	Piriformis muscle (Fig. 52C.5) Sciatic nerve (Figure 52C.6)	Hip pain Sciatica
(f) Xiphoid process	Pubic ramus	Rectus abdominus (Fig. 52C.7)	Abdominal pain nausea
(g) Antecubital region	Wrist	Median nerve (Fig. 52C.8)	Carpal tunnel syndrome Double crush syndrome

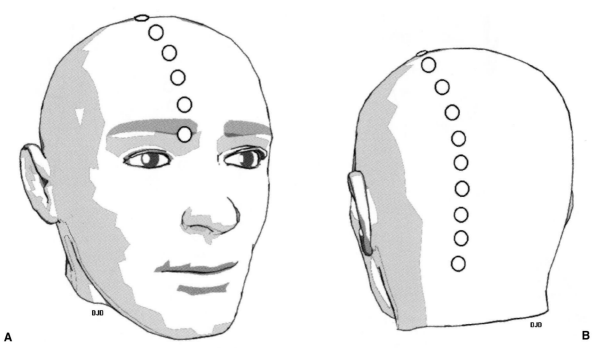

A   B

Figure 52C-1 Primary point: supraorbital notch; endpoint: suboccipital region; connection: frontalis-occipitalis muscles **(A)**, trigeminal-greater occipital nerves **(B)**.

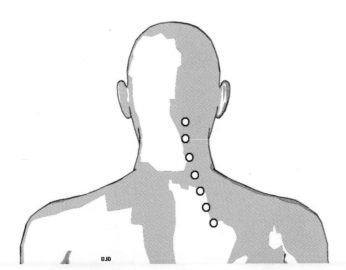

Figure 52C-2 Primary point: superior medial scapular border; endpoint: base of occiput; connection: levator scapula.

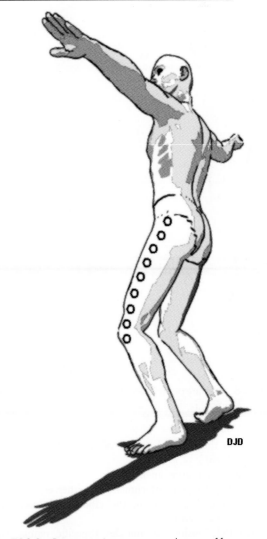

the arm, and the fibula and tibia in the leg. Consider their involvement if a pattern appears to overly their locations.)

(ii) Septums (Even though it is mostly muscular, the diaphragm has fascial components including the central tendon and crus of the diaphragm. It supports and separates. Points found around the lower costal cartilage, the 12th rib, and T10-12 and may represent a diaphragmatic involvement.)

(iii) Overlaps (The common thoracolumbar fascia in the back acts as an attachment for muscles such as the latissimus dorsi and overlaps muscles such as the quadratus lumborum, iliocostalis, and other erector spinae muscles.) Points may be found anywhere within the region and may extend to the lateral edge of the 12th rib (quadratus lumborum) or even

Figure 52C-3 Primary point: greater trochanter of femur; endpoint: fibular head; connection: iliotibial band.

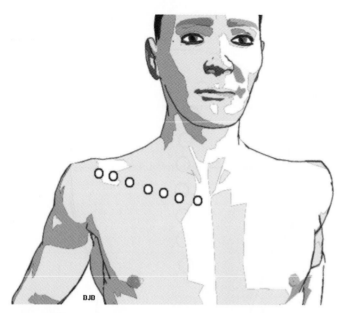

Figure 52C-4 Primary point: sternum at second rib; endpoint: coracoid process; connection: pectoralis minor.

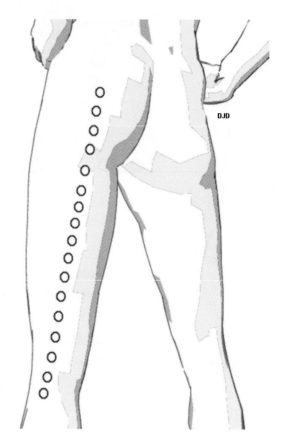

Figure 52C-6 Primary point: gluteal region; endpoint: popliteal region; connection: sciatic nerve.

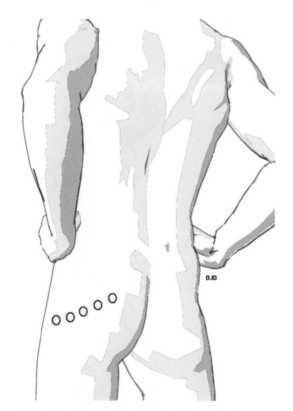

Figure 52C-5 Primary point: gluteal region; endpoint: greater trochanter; connection: piriformis muscle.

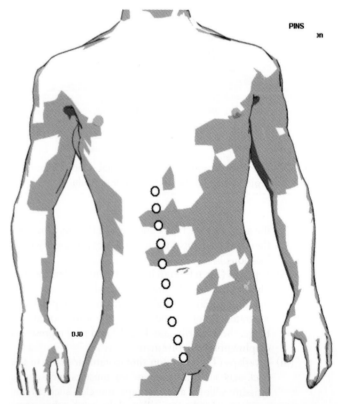

Figure 52C-7 Primary point: xiphoid process; endpoint: pubic ramus; connection: rectus abdominus.

to the bicipital groove of the humerus (latissimus dorsi).)

(d) Ligamentous attachments:
   (i) Typical (The attachments of either end of the collateral ligaments in the elbow and knee can be considered.)
   (ii) Relationships to muscles (Specific points can be found on the superior or lateral C7 spinous process,

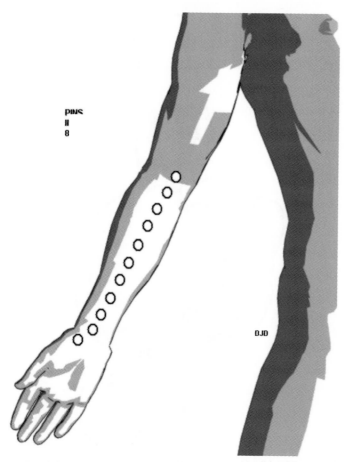

PINS
II
8

Figure 52C-8 Primary point: antecubital region; endpoint: wrist; connection: median nerve.

overall nutrition to the surrounding tissue. It should also be noted that the sympathetic nerves travel with and modify the constriction of the arteries such as occurs in Raynaud's syndrome and complex regional pain syndromes.)

(ii) Veins (The superficial veins often travel with structures such as the nerves. However, care should be taken when addressing vascular structures with PINS or inhibition as there are the possibilities of thrombi and/or phlebitis.)

12. Press both the primary point and the end point simultaneously using the pad region of a finger on each hand (Fig. 52C.9). (Again, for the sake of simplicity, identify the primary point as the "first point" for the patient.) The pressure exerted is a few ounces. It should be enough to elicit the patient's symptoms and should be applied equally on both points. The patient may experience a mild to moderate increase in sensitivity initially. Also, note the soft tissue response to the initial pressure:

(a) Acute dysfunctions may be more sensitive than chronic ones. A muscle that has been hypertonic will usually be more sensitive to pressure than the same muscle on the contralateral side

(b) Chronic hypertonic muscles will usually be larger than those on the contralateral side:

(i) Larger muscles do not necessarily indicate dysfunction. Asymmetric use, where there is preference with one side being used more, will result in the dominant side becoming typically larger. An enlarged muscle does not necessarily mean that there is a dysfunction

and the base of the occiput may represent spinalis muscles or the nuchal ligament.)

(iii) Relationships to nerves (The flexor retinaculum and palmar aponeurosis of the hand are related to the median nerve in the forearm. These, in turn, are related to attachments with at least four (pisiform, hamate, scaphoid, and trapezium) of the retinaculum as well.)

(e) Bones (They and their components should be considered as connective tissue as well.):

(i) Construction of joints (Joint capsules connect two or more bones. At the elbow and the knee, the capsules are stronger and reinforced on their medial and lateral surfaces by collateral ligaments. The anterior and posterior surfaces are relatively weaker and may tighten or loosen in one extreme of motion or the other. Points may occur in the middle of the capsule and at the bony attachments.)

(ii) Lever action (Muscle tendons and ligaments attach to bony prominences. Because of the forces placed upon them, they enlarge into tubercles, trochanters, and other processes. Points located at tendinous insertions may theoretically also represent a contribution from the bony attachments.)

(f) Vascular (They and their components should be considered as connective tissue as well.):

(i) Arteries (Some large arteries travel long distances within the extremities and are responsible for the

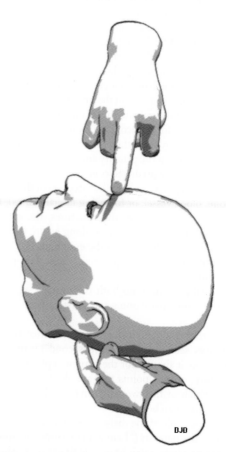

Figure 52C-9 Press both the primary point and end point simultaneously using the pad region of a finger on each hand.

(ii) Whether dysfunctional or not, frequently used muscles or ones in chronic dysfunction may not be quite so sensitive to pressure. This may be due to the chronicity of usage and histological alterations

(a) Both sides can be simultaneously dysfunctional. One side may be more symptomatic than the other. The more dysfunctional tissue should be treated first and then the other is reexamined, and then treated as well, if necessary

(b) A firmer muscle is probably in greater dysfunction

13. Exert the same amount of pressure on both the primary and end points:

(a) Patients may assume that the point that a more sensitive location is being pressed harder. They should be reassured that the reason for the asymmetry is the greater dysfunction or hyperactivity of the involved tissue

(b) Patients may direct the practitioner that they can tolerate greater pressure. This does not accelerate the treatment. It is not necessary to increase the amount of pressure and may even be counterproductive

(c) Pain or tenderness may not be the only sensations experienced due to the applied pressure. The patient may report other sensations. They can occur alone or in combination with pain

14. Maintain constant pressure on the location of the end point throughout the treatment. Initiate pressure on the point with greater sensitivity (primary point). Request that the patient report what they are feeling. When inhibition is utilized properly, any increase in sensitivity at a sensitive point will most probably be transient. There is also a typical rapid decrease in sensitivity as the tissue accommodates to the irritation of the inhibition. Ultimately, it may totally disappear. The duration can vary from several seconds to minutes

15. Maintain contact with the primary point for 20 to 30 seconds before seeking any subsequent points:

(a) One finger remains on the primary point and another finger of the same hand is used to locate a "secondary point." If the middle finger is on the primary point, then the index finger is used to palpate the secondary point (Fig. 52C.10)

(b) The search for a secondary point begins approximately 2 to 3 cm away from the primary point along an imaginary line connecting the primary and end points. This will typically follow the predicted course of an anatomical structure (innervating nerve, along the direction of the muscle fibers, bone, blood vessel, or following fascial planes). Because of the variable nature of the structures, the actual location of a secondary point may be along an arc that occurs 2 to 3 cm into the direction of the endpoint

(c) Identify the secondary point as "the second point" for the patient

16. Exert equal pressure onto both the primary and the secondary points while maintaining the constant pressure on the end point

17. Request that the patient determine which of the two points (primary vs. secondary or "first vs. second") is more sensitive:

(a) To make it simpler for the patient, a phrase such as, "I am pressing on two points that are close together. Please tell me which of the two, the "first" or the "second" is more sensitive," can be used

(b) Give example of the dialogue—what does the practitioner say to the patient? ("I am going to press on another point, close to where my right middle finger is pressing now, and I want you, etc.) If the second point is more or equally sensitive as compared to the first:

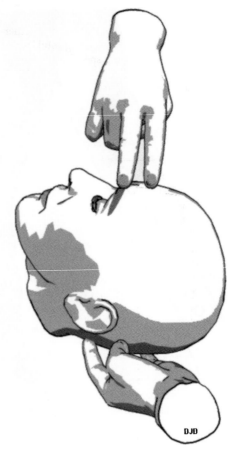

Figure 52C-10 One finger remains on the primary point. Use another finger of the same hand to locate a "secondary point." If the middle finger is on the primary point, then use the index finger to palpate the secondary point.

(i) Relieve the pressure from the first (primary) point and then remove it entirely

(ii) Maintain constant pressure on the new, second (secondary) sensitive point for an additional 20 to 30 seconds

(iii) It is not necessary to wait for the sensitivity at any point to be completely abated before moving on to the next point. It is more important that each subsequent point is more sensitive than the prior one.

(iv) There can be both increased tension and sensitivity in the new secondary point. With practice, the "secondary" points can be located by palpatory sense of tension alone. A return to a lower level of sensitivity and response baseline usually occurs after a few seconds. The amount of time depends on the soft tissue response

(c) Certain points may require further inhibition before progress can be made. After doing so, a new secondary point may be located where previously there was less sensitivity. If the original or a subsequent "first point" persists as the more sensitive of the two points:

(v) Maintain pressure at the location of the primary point for an additional 20 to 30 seconds; and/or

(vi) Move the finger that was locating the secondary point more laterally or medially from the connecting line. A located new secondary point should have at least the same sensitivity, if not more, as the primary point. (The anatomical structure, whether muscle, nerve, or fascia, which is being inhibited, may have slight variations in the specific course in this individual.)

    (vii) Once a secondary point, that is equally or more sensitive, is located, relieve pressure from the primary point and maintain on the new secondary point as described above

    (viii) The secondary point then becomes the new "first" point in the continuing sequence of treatment toward the endpoint

18. Inhibit the endpoint with constant pressure with a finger of the other hand throughout. The patient will often forget that this point is being treated. As the anchor for the dysfunctional tissue, continuous treatment is necessary. It may lose sensitivity during the course of treatment

19. Repeat the process until an ultimate "second" point is located 2 cm from the end point

20. Once the two final points have been treated with inhibition, determine the amount of dysfunction that persists, especially at the endpoint location. It may have become significantly reduced or may disappear totally

21. All of the intervening points are part of the dysfunction. This is the reason that there can be persistence of symptoms when the area of the primary point (chief complaint) is treated by another method. It is not so much that it is not a part of the problem but rather one component in a "reverberating circuit."

22. Occasionally, pressure on one of the intervening points between the primary and end points results in a recurrence of the chief complaint, radiation of symptoms from this point toward the endpoint, the primary point or both. This is actually a good indication of the continuity of the dysfunction and the need for this thorough treatment

23. Another modality of treatment can be used if the dysfunction, including the endpoint, remains persistent. The endpoint and overall dysfunction may now be easier to treat than previously. FPR, strain-counterstrain, muscle energy, balanced ligamentous tension techniques, or some other modality may be used. The use of HVLA that was difficult to perform before may now be easier. Guidelines for determining the choice include:

    (a) The persistence of the dysfunction or related components after treatment

    (b) The ability of the practitioner to perform other modalities of treatment

    (c) The need or capability of the patient to tolerate additional treatment

24. The conclusion of manipulative treatment for the session should be based on the findings for the individual. It should not be based solely on the patient's subjective complaints. Overtreatment can cause as many problems as undertreatment

25. Patients may limit types of treatment based on prior experience or misconceptions. They may have had a reaction to previous treatments or they may have had no previous difficulties but have developed a dislike for a particular modality (i.e., "popping" secondary to HVLA). Attempting to coerce a patient to allow certain forms of treatment would be counterproductive to the therapeutic relationship. In many locales, it could be considered illegal as well (i.e., battery)

26. The somatic dysfunction is always reassessed

27. Despite a relatively comfortable treatment, there may be a posttreatment reaction. The patient should be informed that some treatment reactions can include transient soreness, aches, and fatigue. In some patients who are prone to bruising, or when there are certain other predisposing factors (i.e., medication), ecchymoses may occur. If excessive pressure has been used, it can also occur. Generally, all such side effects resolve in 24 to 48 hours

Possible Mechanism of Action. One of the important components of that distinguishes inhibitory contact from a stimulatory one is the use of a low level, but constant, amount of pressure applied to a dysfunctional tissue. A contact of this type may initiate accommodation or habituation over time even though the initial effect may be irritating. The patient may be acutely sensitive at first with complaints of increased pain, sensitivity, pressure, or some other sensation. These reactions decrease and may disappear altogether as the system adapts (35). Part of this reduction in awareness may be from the screening mechanisms provided by the reticular formation. The body accommodates to other stimuli, such as the relative nonawareness of body contact with eyeglasses, tight belts, stiff clothing, uncomfortable shoes, as well as constant background auditory and visual stimuli. This sensory filtering process may also involve the spinal cord acting as a mediator or as a "brake" when sensory overload (36) occurs. Some stimuli remain relatively subliminal if not of sufficient quality, duration, or quantity.

Some effects may include pressure or contact as a counterirritant. Instead of actually inhibiting they act as stimulation to the neighboring tissue, thus reducing the sensitivity of the original tender point. Scratching in the region of an itch would be one such example. Rapid conducting large nerve afferents gate transmission in the dorsal horn of the spinal cord with collateral fibers in the substanstia gelatinosa or adjacent interneurons inhibiting the transmission of pain to the central nervous system via the spinothalamic tract (37).

Relative ischemia has also been proposed as a theory. Muscle maintained in prolonged contraction produces metabolites and waste products from the local tissue damage (38). Impaired circulation also occurs concomitantly with hyperemia and congestion. Some of the substances also have vasoactive effects, which theoretically address tissue injury. Trophic and fibrotic changes may occur if the injury persists. Normally, the overlying skin shows a brief blanching followed by redness. This typically fades when normal but may persist when the tissue is damaged for a prolonged time. It appears that the use of therapeutic pressure may add temporarily to the ischemia. This does not initially make intuitive sense when considering the amount of nutrient deprivation. However, the increased ischemia may reduce the capacity of the nociceptive receptors to process information. Hyperemia may also occur once this pressure is removed, resulting in the flushing of the waste products from the location.

A muscle in dysfunction may appear to be in its neutral position but may still be hypertonic. Further stretch from the relatively shortened length increases activity of the muscle spindle mechanisms and will result in a reflexive and prolonged contraction. This is a means of protection (39,40–42). Slow stretching of the type applied during inhibition introduces a gentle stretch while allowing the resetting of the stretch receptors (43). Only a small amount of the tissue may be challenged without upsetting the whole structure. Once the small, localized component is overwhelmed, any affected adjacent area can subsequently be inhibited with similar results. Inhibition in general, and **PINS** in particular, may be very effective methods to deal with a series of irritated pieces. The osteopathic physician may treat the entire dysfunction by progressively treating all of the involved elements.

The Golgi tendon organ is a sensory mechanism that becomes relatively stretched during muscular contraction where the overall length of the muscle does not change. When a critical amount of tension occurs, increased Golgi tendon organ activity brings about reflex relaxation of the muscle as a whole. An inhibitory interneuron between the afferent nerve ending in the spinal cord and the alpha motorneuron bring about sudden, almost complete muscular relaxation. The pressure from an osteopathic physician's fingers may create an initial stretch that results in transient contraction. This is then followed by resultant relaxation (44).

Contraindications and Side Effects

There appear to be few contraindications and side effects with the use of **PINS**. Pressure should not be exerted onto localized inflammations, abscesses, or infections as the integrity of the skin or walled infections may be compromised.

SUMMARY

PINS represents a unique variant of the more traditional approach to using inhibition as well as a means of discovering the ways in which dysfunction occurs and is maintained. It can be used solely or in combination with other methods of osteopathic manipulation. The effect of other treatment modalities can be enhanced by the use of **PINS**.

Using **PINS** does require an investment of time. When it appears that other typical interventions are of limited success with recalcitrant dysfunctions, alternative means must be used. However, when this occurs, the time necessary to perform **PINS** would be worth the effort.

REFERENCES

1. Dowling DJ. Progressive inhibition of neuromuscular structures (PINS) technique, *JAOA* 100(5):285–286,289–298.
2. *Glossary of Osteopathic Terminology*. Chicago: AOA Yearbook and Directory of Osteopathic Physicians, 1998.
3. Dowling DJ, Scariati PD. Neurophysiology relevant to osteopathic principles and practice. In: DiGiovanna E, Schiowitz S, eds. *An Osteopathic Approach to Diagnosis and Treatment*. 2nd Ed. Philadelphia, PA: Lippincott-Raven, 1997:33.
4. Ehrenfeuchter WC. Soft tissue techniques. In: Ward RC, ed. *Foundations for Osteopathic Medicine*. Baltimore, MD: Williams & Wilkins, 1997:781–794.
5. Robbins SL, Cotran RS, Kumar V. *Pathologic Basis of Disease*. 3rd Ed. Philadelphia, PA: W.B. Saunders Co., 1984:40.
6. Still AT. *Autobiography of A.T. Still*. Revised ed. Kirksville, Missouri: Published by the author, 1908:32.
7. Still AT. *The Philosophy and Mechanical Principles of Osteopathy*. Kansas City, MD: Hudson-Kimberly Pub. Co., 1902:101.
8. Goetz EW. *A Manual of Osteopathy*. 2nd Ed. Cincinnati, Ohio, 1905.
9. Tasker DD. *Principles of Osteopathy*. 4th Ed. Los Angeles: Bireley & Elson Printing Co., 1916:354–370.
10. Jones LH. *Strain and Counterstrain*. Newark, OH: American Academy of Osteopathy, 1981.
11. Jones LH, Kusenose R, Goering E. *Jones Strain-Counterstrain*. Boise, Idaho: Jones Strain-Counterstrain Company, 1995.
12. Glover JC, Yates HA. Strain and counterstrain techniques. In: Ward RC, ed. *Foundations for Osteopathic Medicine*. Baltimore, MD: Williams & Wilkins, 1997:809–818.
13. Schiowitz S. In: DiGiovanna E, Schiowitz S, eds. *An Osteopathic Approach to Diagnosis and Treatment*. 2nd Ed. Philadelphia, PA: Lippincott-Raven, 1997:91.
14. Van Buskirk VL. A manipulative technique of Andrew Taylor Still as reported by Charles Hazzard, DO, in 1905. *JAOA* 96(10):597–602.
15. Hazzard C. *The Practice and Applied Therapeutics of Osteopathy*, 1905.
16. Johnston WL. Functional technique: an indirect method. In: Ward RC, ed. *Foundations for Osteopathic Medicine*. Baltimore, MD: Williams & Wilkins, 1997:795–808.
17. Dowling DJ. Myofascial release techniques. In: DiGiovanna E, Schiowitz S, eds. *An Osteopathic Approach to Diagnosis and Treatment*. 2nd Ed. Philadelphia, PA: Lippincott-Raven, 1997:381–383.
18. Chila AG. Fascial-ligamentous release: an indirect approach. In: Ward RC, ed. *Foundations for Osteopathic Medicine*. Baltimore, MD: Williams & Wilkins, 1997:819–830.
19. Ward RC. Integrated neuromusculoskeletal release and myofascial release: an introduction to diagnosis and treatment. In: Ward RC, ed. *Foundations for Osteopathic Medicine*. Baltimore, MD: Williams & Wilkins, 1997:846–849.
20. Typaldos S. Introducing the fascial distortion model. *Am Acad Osteopath J* 1994;4(2).
21. Chaitow L. *Neuro-muscular Technique*. Wellingborough, Northamtonshire, England: Thorsons Publishers Ltd, 1980.
22. Chaitow L. *Modern Neuromuscular Techniques*. New York, NY: Churchill Livingstone, 1996.
23. Owens C. *An Endocrine Interpretation of Chapman's Reflexes*. 2nd Ed. Chattanooga, TN, Chattanooga Printing and Engraving Co., 1937.
24. Cyriax J. *Text-book of Orthopaedic Medicine Volume II: Treatment by Manipulation and Massage*. 6th Ed. New York: Harper & Row, 1959.
25. Travell JG, Simmons DG. *Myofascial Pain and Dysfunction: The Trigger Point Manual: The Upper Extremities*. Vol I. Baltimore, MD: Williams & Wilkins, 1983.
26. Chaitlow L. *Osteopathic Self-Treatment*. Wellingborough, England: Thorsons Publishing Group, 1990:105–119.
27. Kenyon J. *Acupressure Techniques: A Self Help Guide*. Rochester, Vermont: Healing Arts Press, 1988.
28. Cerney JV. *Acupuncture Without Needles*. West Nyack, New York, NY: Parker Publishing Company, Inc., 1974.
29. Shultz W. *Shiatsu: Japanese Finger Pressure Therapy*. New York, NY: Bell Publishing Company, 1976.
30. Weil A. *Spontaneous Healing*. New York, NY: Ballantine Books, 1995.
31. The Burton Goldberg Group. *Alternative Medicine: The Definitive Guide*. Puyallup, Washington: Future Medicine Publishing, Inc., 1994:106–108.
32. Prudden B. *Pain Erasure: The Bonnie Prudden Way*. New York, NY: Ballantine Books, 1980.
33. The Burton Goldberg Group. *Alternative Medicine: The Definitive Guide*. Puyallup, Washington: Future Medicine Publishing, Inc., 1994:102–103.
34. Dowling DJ. S.T.A.R.: a more viable alternative descriptor system of somatic dysfunction. *AAO J* 1998;8(2):34–37.
35. Bailey HW. Some problems in making osteopathic spinal manipulative therapy appropriate and specific. *JAOA* 1976;75:486–499.
36. Patterson MM. A model mechanism for spinal segmental facilitation. *JAOA* 1976;76:62–72.
37. Ganong WF. *Review of Medical Physiology*. Los Altos, CA: Lange, 1995:130–131.
38. Stoddard A. *Manual of Osteopathic Practice*. London: Hutchinson Medical Publications, 1969:238.
39. Buzzell KA. The potential disruptive influence of somatic input. *The Physiological Basis of Osteopathic Medicine*. The Postgraduate Institute of Osteopathic Medicine and Surgery, New York, NY: Insight Publishing Company, 1967:39–51.
40. Ganong WF. *Review of Medical Physiology*. Los Altos, CA: Lange, 1995:113–117.
41. Becker RF. The gamma system and its relation to the development and maintenance of muscle tone. In: 1976 *Year Book of the American Academy of Osteopathy*. Colorado Springs, CO: American Academy of Osteopathy, 1976:26–40.
42. Korr IM. Proprioceptors and somatic dysfunction. In: 1976 *Year Book of the American Academy of Osteopathy*. Colorado Springs, CO: American Academy of Osteopathy, 1976:41–50.
43. Korr IM. Proprioceptors and somatic dysfunction. *JAOA* 74:638–650 reprinted in *The Collected Papers of Irvin M. Korr*. Colorado Springs, CO: American Academy of Osteopathy, 1979:200–207.
44. Ganong WF. *Review of Medical Physiology*. Los Altos, CA: Lange, 1995:1178.

52D | Functional Technique

WILLIAM L. JOHNSTON (1921–2003)

KEY CONCEPT

In this section, emphasis is placed on input (physician) palpated and evaluated at the segmental level. The sense of ease (compliance) and bind (increasing palpable resistance) is used to interpret the motion input. Opposite asymmetries (above and below) a segmental level is referred to as *mirror-image motion asymmetry*. Effective treatment is accomplished through the delivery of a smooth torsion arc of therapeutic motion. The component of visceral influence is recognized through the concepts of lack of accord and linkage. Both provide information directly relevant to treatment.

MAJOR PUBLICATIONS

- Johnston WL, Friedman HD. *Functional Methods*. 1st Ed. Indianapolis, IN: American Academy of Osteopathy, 1994.
- Beal MC, ed. *1998 Yearbook, Scientific Contributions of William L. Johnston, DO, FAAO*. Indianapolis, IN: American Academy of Osteopathy.
- Johnston WL, Friedman HD, Eland DC. *Functional Methods*. 2nd Ed. Indianapolis, IN: American Academy of Osteopathy, 2005.

HISTORICAL PERSPECTIVES

To engage the term *functional technique*, one needs to sense the stimulus driving its initial development in the early 1950s. Within the osteopathic discipline, there was a growing recognition that *motor function* had a broader conceptual framework than just bony relationships, with their structural configuration relatively confined to joints, and to concepts for motion of one bone on the bone below. To open up this conceptual model, it was necessary to give increasing attention to the physiologic aspects and clinical manifestations of motor control. For a mobile system, specific directions of regional motion tests were becoming effective in delineating positive diagnostic signs of dysfunctional behaviors, both regional and segmental. Within these broader functional parameters, motion tests would supply promising tools for application in clinical practice and osteopathic research.

To engage the term *indirect*, as a method of manipulation, one needs to refer back to the early 1900s. In the history of osteopathy, information derived from palpatory examination had led to the development of a classification for methods of manipulation. Development of the terms *direct*, and *indirect*, gave recognition to the specific directions of motion forces used in osteopathic manipulative procedures. A brief look at 100 years of professional history indicates a significant struggle regarding the issue of terminology. The controversy involves two areas:

1. Verbalizing palpatory findings in the musculoskeletal system
2. Conceptualizing models for palpable findings, for example: the use of bony malposition at a joint, to depict a local area of segmental dysfunction (referred to in the past as a *lesion*, the *Still lesion*, or *osteopathic lesion*)

Difficulties with terminology create problems for communication about the clinical signs of musculoskeletal dysfunctions. To describe a direct manipulative technique for segmental dysfunction, initial concepts of somatic dysfunction focused on joint restriction and direct forces to encounter and overcome restriction; this fit the layperson's concept of "putting the bone back in place." Other techniques did not directly encounter the restriction yet still overcame restricted movement. Such manipulative procedures did not fit the concept of the direct method. They did use motion and maneuvers in the opposite direction of the restriction effectively, however, and were given the term *indirect*. Owing to the fact that they seem to defy positional relationships and joint concepts, indirect methods are often set aside. Since they do not fit with those earlier models of thought, they continue to present a special challenge for instruction.

Several early osteopathic practitioners expressed these issues. Edythe F. Ashmore, a faculty member at the American College of Osteopathy in Kirksville, Missouri, wrote the first textbook on the mechanics of osteopathy in 1915. She stated:

> There are two methods commonly employed by osteopathists in the correction of lesions the older of which is the traction method, the later the direct method or thrust.* Those who employ the traction method secure the relaxation of the tissues about the articulation by what has been termed exaggeration of the lesion, a motion in the direction of the forcible movement which produced the lesion, as if its purpose were to increase the deformity. The exaggeration is held, traction made upon the joint, replacement initiated and then completed by reversal of the forces.†

The direct method consists in the application of a precisely directed force toward a bony prominence during the process of putting the articulation or lesion through the spinal movement, which is the reversal of that which produced the lesion.

> *The term "direct" is preferred for the reason that the imitators of osteopathy have given the word "thrust" an objectionable meaning of harshness.
> †This method is the more difficult of the two and for the instruction of students does not find favor with the author (1).

Ashmore's footnotes about terminology and instructional problems are particularly illuminating. The limited concepts implied by the expressions *exaggerating the lesion* and *reversal of that* [movement] *which produced the lesion* remained in use for many years. The direction of restricted movement was even then becoming a determinant for methods of manipulative technique and their classification as direct and indirect.

Carl P. McConnell, D.O., was another osteopathic pioneer who actively contributed to osteopathic literature from 1905 to 1938. He commented:

> So, striving to get the bones in normal position, per se, or perhaps to keep them in position, is simply hopeless. In this regard, the bony item is simply an idol, and a similar idol could be made of the muscles, and so forth (2).

McConnell also wrote:

> Precision of method follows definiteness of diagnosis. It is evident that there are many ways of applying the same mechanical principles. But ease and effectiveness should be the goal of operative activity. In adjusting lesions it is obvious that a method which retraces the path of the lesion with a minimum of irritation is highly desirable (3).

McConnell's orientation was still on *the path of the lesion*, but this was tempered by a growing discomfort with using bony position or any single anatomic structure as the key to conceptualizing about areas of musculoskeletal dysfunction.

By 1923, in *Principles and Practice of Osteopathy*, C. Harrison Downing (4) went a step further in describing restriction at a lesioned segment. He referred to the fact that, when testing a physiologic motion, the lesioned segment becomes more restricted going in one direction. He added that the restriction decreases in the opposite direction and *apparently disappears*. Keeping his motion testing procedure as a frame of reference, Downing provided palpatory information about the restriction *decreasing*, in a direction opposite to the direction of restricted motion. These new facts sometimes supported the concepts centered on the joint and bony description of malposition, and sometimes did not.

By 1949, Howard A. Lippincott reported on the osteopathic technique of William G. Sutherland as follows:

> The articulation is carried in the direction of the lesion, exaggerating the lesion position as far as is necessary to cause the tension of the weakened elements of the ligamentous structure to be equal to or slightly in excess of the tension of those that were not strained. This is the point of balanced tension. When the tension is properly balanced, the respiratory or muscular cooperation of the patient is employed to overcome the resistance of the defense mechanism of the body to the release of the lesion (5).

This described an indirect method of treatment, but the anatomic construct was more *ligamentous*. The *point of balanced tension* (also referred to as *the point of balanced ligamentous tension*) became the significant phrase used to describe techniques where the physician palpated throughout the procedure and continually adjusted treatment to the changing tissue tensions. Descriptive terminology still relied mainly on a positional orientation to express this important feedback of palpable information during motion. *Balance and hold* became another phrase to describe indirect techniques, but this phrase fails to point out the continued balancing carried out by the physician in response to the tissues changing.

In the early 1940s at the Chicago College of Osteopathy, indirect diagnostic skills were a part of students' formal training. This involved instructing students regarding the diagnosis of directions of motion that would initially relax the tissues, and their application in combined techniques. In Boston, by 1944, some very prominent physician teachers in the New England area had already been applying indirect methods extensively in their practices; however, the difficulty in communicating these skills was still a problem.

In the 1940s, the Academy of Applied Osteopathy (now known as the American Academy of Osteopathy) initiated a national program of education to improve the clinical skills of physicians, for those proficiencies in practice that can be achieved with continual application of Still's principles. This was done through the implementation of postgraduate instruction. Harold Hoover was a part of this effort. His classification of direct and indirect manipulative methods included the following:

1. Direct technique: the method of moving one bone or segment of the articular lesion directly to a normal relationship with its neighbor. This is accomplished against the resistance of tissues and fluids maintaining the abnormal relationship.
2. Indirect technique: the method of moving one bone or segment slightly in the direction away from the direction of correction until the resistance of holding tissues and fluids is partially overcome and the tensions are bilaterally balanced, then allowing the released ligaments and muscles themselves to aid in pulling the part toward normal. Other body forces, including that of respiration, may be employed (6).

Hoover's experiences with both of these methods of manipulation were beginning to channel his major interest toward the indirect (7). Recognizing a functional model, he was reporting on his use of palpatory tests, palpable findings, and manipulative procedures, especially those of the clinically effective indirect method. He often introduced his functional approaches in seminars. His presentation in New England in 1951 initiated an era of development in the New England Academy of Osteopathy. Biannual study sessions, led by Charles Bowles, resulted in a series of three publications entitled *A Functional Orientation for Technic*.

In his initial report, Bowles wrote:

> This was not the birth of a new entity in osteopathy, but simply a new type of measuring stick for evaluating the Still lesion as a process of aberrated function ... our functional investigation had become formalized by using the pattern of a demand-response transaction, instituting motion demands (which could be named) with a motive hand, down to, and through a given segment, while assessing the motion response of this given segment through a palpatory listening hand. To best understand, follow, and control this demand-response transaction therapeutically at a segmental level, certain specific insights seem necessary, namely:

1. An understanding of typical motion demands and a system of annotation that makes them easily communicable between operators
2. An understanding of responses that allows an accurate reporting and a useful evaluation of the specific demand-response transaction taking place currently under the fingertips of the palpating or "listening hand" during manipulation
3. An understanding of criteria for lesioned and nonlesioned performance, that is, in terms of functional adequacy

Thus, the significant functional information about vertebral motion or restriction is not so much that there is motion or restriction, but rather how these motions and restrictions change, and under what circumstances, and in response to what demands.

It is the response information that eventually guides functional technic (8).

It should be noted that these comments by Bowles are in contrast to guides based on anatomic *concepts*, and bony, muscular, or ligamentous relations.

By 1961, Lippincott was expressing educational concerns similar to those of Ashmore. He reported student confusion, as well as practice trends, that were leading him to analyze and clarify the various methods of correcting lesions. In *Basic Principles of Osteopathic Technique*, he reported:

> It is evident that Dr. Still treated his patients carefully, with due consideration for the delicacy and the welfare of the tissues beneath his fingers. It is also evident that he imparted to the students who

came under his supervision this wholesome respect for the tissues, the structures, and their functioning. Then, after the turn of the century, it became popular with many of the vigorous and enthusiastic young doctors to treat with vigor and enthusiasm. They developed techniques that would produce a "pop" regardless of the force required to produce it. This gave them a sense of accomplishment but it also gave osteopathy a reputation for being rough, painful, and even dangerous, a stigma that still persists among the uninformed. Within a decade or two the trend turned back toward more careful and intelligent, but perhaps less spectacular methods. The result is a wealth of technical procedures representing varied approaches to the correction of osteopathic lesions. It is a decided advantage for the physician to have at his command a variety of methods whereby he can meet the needs of each individual patient (9).

During the 1960s and 1970s, the steadfastness of positional concepts continued to be reflected in the development of new techniques. In 1964, Lawrence H. Jones published his original article, "Spontaneous Release by Positioning," introducing the technique for manipulative treatment called *strain/counterstrain*. Dr. Jones questioned:

Is the muscular tension arranged so as to splint this joint, to prevent it from moving back into its eccentric position? No! The muscular tension resists any position away from the extreme position in which the lesioning occurred. Even the severest lesions will readily tolerate being returned to the position in which lesion formation originally occurred, and only to this position. When the joint is returned to this position (indirect), the muscles promptly and gratefully relax (10).

Since 1969, and possibly starting during the Bowles initiative in New England in 1955, interest has grown in relation to motor function, with a focus on the application of motion tests and palpable findings for descriptive clinical research. A test pattern of passive gross motions evolved with standards relevant to the six elementary directions of the body's movement (Figs. 52D.1 and 52D.2). These motions are as follows:

- Flexion/extension
- Side bending

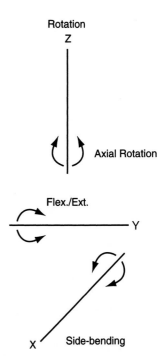

Figure 52D-2 Coordinate system to illustrate directions of movement about axes used to describe rotary motion tests. (From Johnston WL. Segmental definition, part I: a focal point for diagnosis of somatic dysfunction. *JAOA* 1988;88:99–105, with permission.)

- Rotation
- Translation from side to side
- Translation anteriorly/posteriorly
- Translation cephalad/caudad (traction/compression)

This test pattern allows implementation of an organized diagnostic process for describing the motor characteristics of neuromusculoskeletal dysfunctions. Investigations (11) using this test pattern have been advancing our knowledge about functional aspects of both regional and segmental somatic dysfunction, as follows:

1. Passive gross motion tests provide a means to attain baseline palpatory information in medical problem solving for a mobile system:

   Examining *regional* motor performance (12)
   Locating *segmental* motor defects (13,14)
   Characterizing *the specifics of a segment's motor dysfunction* as a basis for designing manipulative interventions to address somatic dysfunction (15–17)

2. Segmental somatic dysfunction is a complete asymmetry of its elementary motion functions: three rotary, three straight-line translatory, and respiratory (18). (Respiratory was the seventh function, and takes under consideration the demands of inhalation and exhalation on motor function.) Palpable recordable cues evident in response to these motion tests provide seven possible descriptors for the motion characteristics of each motor defect.

3. A fundamental unit of segmental somatic dysfunction (16,19) consists of a three-segment complex, as illustrated in Figure 52D.3. A central asymmetric segment is the primary defect. Mirror-image (opposing) motion asymmetries are present at the adjacent segments, above and below. (These are secondary and adaptive, implying a basis in somatosomatic reflex activity.)

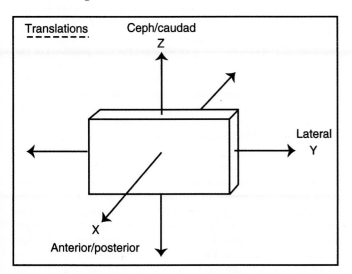

Figure 52D-1 Coordinate system to illustrate straight-line directions of movement used to describe translatory motion tests. (From Johnston WL. Segmental definition, part I: a focal point for diagnosis of somatic dysfunction. *JAOA* 1988;88:99–105, with permission.)

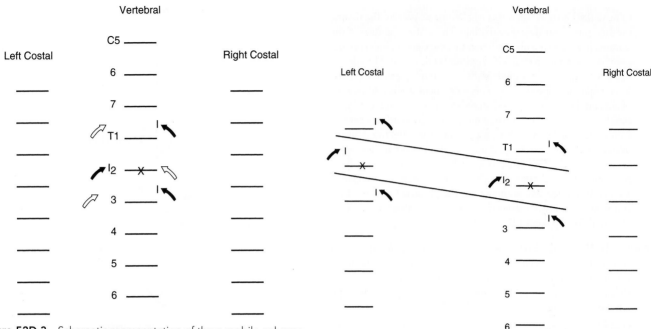

Figure 52D-3 Schematic representation of three mobile columns in thoracic region, with a three-segment unit of dysfunction in vertebral column. *X*, location of primary functional defect at T2, with resistance to shoulder/trunk rotation to right (*short, solid arrow, with bar representing sense of resistance*). In adjacent T1 and T3 segments, mirror-image resistance to left rotation is secondary (*short, solid arrows with bars*). Longer, open arrows without bars at each level represent sense of compliance with motion and a greater range of motion in directions opposite to directions of limited mobility. (From Johnston WL. Somatic manifestations in renal disease: a clinical research study. *JAOA* 1987;87:22–35, with permission.)

Figure 52D-4 Schematic representation of two primary motor asymmetries at T2 spinal level, indicated by *X* in vertebral and adjacent left costal columns. *Arrows with bars* at T2 spinal level indicate resistance in both columns to right rotation of shoulders/trunk. Secondary mirror-image asymmetries of restricted motor function are indicated at T1 and T3 spinal levels by *bars on arrows* for left rotation that is (again) present in both columns.

4. A different organizational principle operates when primary defects are identified at a midline vertebra and an adjacent rib at the same spinal level with *identical* motion asymmetries; this contrasts with the *opposing* asymmetries presented by mirror images (20). An example is illustrated in Figure 52D.4 at T2 and left rib 2. Accompanying this primary defect at the T2 level, note that there still are secondary mirror-image asymmetries at the adjacent segments above and below in both the midline vertebral and left costal columns. Clinical research (21) has supported the premise that visceral afferents contribute to this characteristic configuration of two segmental units, vertebra and rib, *linked* in similar primary motion asymmetries at the same spinal level.

This preceding historical perspective puts one in mind of the classic tale of the blind men and the elephant, with each man describing the elephant according to the part being touched. From clinical palpatory experience, asymmetry (*A*) of joint position, restriction (*R*) of motion, and tissue texture changes (*T*) are expressed in the mnemonic acronym ART. Tenderness (T) has recently been added to the acronym, making it TART, with the first "T" representing tenderness. Each of the last three has emerged as a palpable sign of segmental somatic dysfunction, where motor function is asymmetric and its manifestations are present in structure, motion, and tissue. The functional characteristics of motor asymmetry emerge primarily from motion tests. These characteristics provide detailed descriptors to implement differential diagnosis and also establish basis for the classification of methods of manipulation as direct and indirect.

FUNCTIONAL TECHNIQUE

The term *functional technique* refers to osteopathic manipulative procedures that apply palpatory information gained from tests for motor function, although the term is often applied inappropriately as a general synonym for *indirect*. To be specific, in functional manipulative procedures, the palpable information regarding all six degrees of freedom and respiration is used to address the dysfunctional aspects of segmental behavior. Passive gross motion testing identifies motion symmetry/asymmetry at an individual mobile segment. If you can, temporarily set aside the interpretation of palpatory information about mobility in a format for static concepts of joint position—for example, a posterior transverse process. Instead, criteria for determining a mobile segment's behavior and its resistance to or compliance with opposing directions of specifically induced passive *regional* motion tests are applied. The demonstration in Figure 52D.5 illustrates a single axial motion test introduced through the shoulders and trunk in rotation to the right. With the patient seated and arms folded, right rotation of shoulders and trunk is introduced by the physician's right hand at the patient's right elbow. The fingers of the left hand monitor bilaterally the *immediate* response of paravertebral tissues overlying T6 transverse processes. To compare for response to rotation left, the operator stands to the left and the hand positions are reversed. Finding asymmetric behavior at T6, one can report resistance encountered at T6, for example, during shoulder trunk rotation right. (The test and the criterion are explicit, and the finding becomes clear in relation to the test used to elicit it, thereby attending to scientific method for first-order reporting.) This is in contrast to applying *local*, pressure prone at T6, encountering increased resistance to pressure on the left versus the right, and then reporting a posterior

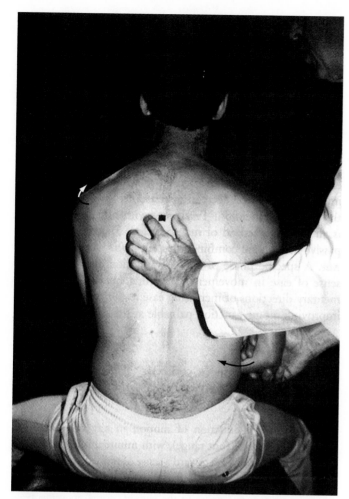

Figure 52D-5 Single axial motion test of shoulders and trunk in rotation to right. (From Johnston WL. Segmental definition, part I: a focal point for diagnosis of somatic dysfunction. *JAOA* 1988;88:99–105, with permission.)

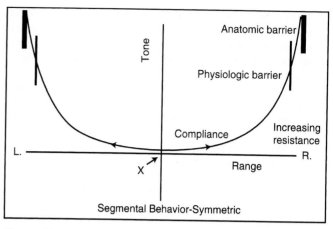

Figure 52D-6 Symmetric response to motion at a nonlesioned thoracic segment where only axial rotation is represented. Shown are equal initial compliance to right (*R*) and left (*L*), and then increasing resistance toward an equidistant final anatomic end point. (From Johnston WL. Segmental definition, part I: a focal point for diagnosis of somatic dysfunction. *JAOA* 1988;88:99–105, with permission.)

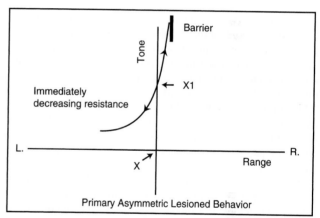

Figure 52D-7 Asymmetric behavior at a dysfunctional (lesioned) segment. (From Johnston WL. Segmental definition, part I: a focal point for diagnosis of somatic dysfunction. *JAOA* 1988;88:99–105, with permission.)

left transverse process, with limited rotation to the right of T6 on T7 within the concept of a joint.

As illustrated in Figure 52D.6 for symmetric behavior, the initial resting level of minimal muscle tone or tension at point X reflects the natural palpable resistance that the operator's fingertips sense as they lightly contact tissues overlying the bony segment at rest. Point X also illustrates there is palpable symmetry in a segment's initial compliance to move right and left with no rise on the tone scale at the initiation of movement. Indicated also is the normally increasing resistance to range as motion approaches a physiologic and an anatomic barrier.

Start with a compression test. The compression test is the application of pressure through the fingers to sense any *increased* tissue tension at one segment compared with adjacent segments. Even at rest, a compression test of a *dysfunctional* segment will register the local increased resistance of that segment's deep musculature; this can be illustrated as an elevation to X1 on a tone scale (Fig. 52D.7). The fingertips mark the site of the increased resistance to pressure.

The segment's tissue tension in the marked area changes *immediately* on initiation of each passive motion test. Palpatory cues reflect the immediately increasing resistance to pressure in one direction (in this example, to the right), while in the opposing direction they reflect an immediate sense of decreasing resistance to

pressure (i.e., a decreasing tension with increasing ease of motion). These palpable changes provide an indicator of asymmetric motor function, to monitor not only during diagnosis to guide accuracy, but also during treatment to guide efficacy in the return to symmetric motor function. Treatment with functional technique is a distinctive application of an indirect method of manipulation. Well-defined directions of passive motion are combined *in their initial stages of increasing ease*. A particular phase of active respiration also increases this sense of ease in movement. As the responses to each precise elementary direction of increasing ease are summed up, the reduced tissue tension signals a rapidly improving motor function palpable at the fingertips.

Guidelines

Certain procedural aspects of functional technique help to ensure success in the application of an indirect method of manipulation for segmental dysfunction (22):

1. The initial introduction of motion in any one elementary direction is small (not range), with minimal forces applied.

2. Motion directions are toward a sense of *immediately increasing ease*. This response manifests a decreasing sense of resistance to pressure at fingers monitoring the tense dysfunctional segment (at the same time, motions are away from the opposing direction in which increasing resistance is encountered).

3. Single elements of rotary and translatory directions are combined, effecting the control of an eventual smooth torsion arc for body movement. The order of introduction of these elements is not important.

4. The final step of the functional procedure involves request for a specific direction of active respiration, whichever direction (inhalation or exhalation) contributes further to the increasing ease. For example, if inhalation, the request is for the subject to take a deep breath *slowly* and hold it briefly.

5. This respiratory interval, adding to a continuous feedback of decreasing resistance, allows the operator to fine-tune the combination of translatory and rotary directions. The objective is to reach a sense of release of tissue tension at the fingertips, which are continually monitoring response at the dysfunctional segment.

6. The release of restraint in the motor mechanism allows a return to midline resting, unobstructed by any sense of the resistance previously encountered in the return direction.

A successful outcome is signaled by a sensed release of the segmental tissues' holding forces, which then allows a free return to a resting position, and a new tissue tone at rest. The segment's new functional symmetry is evident in the responses to further motion retesting. Increased resistance in response to directions previously limited is no longer encountered.

Examples of applying this functional method of palpatory diagnosis and manipulative treatment are presented under "Examples of Functional Technique" later in this chapter. To memorize any technique for use as a manipulative procedure, without recreating each of the steps outlined above, this would be inappropriate and probably clinically ineffective. Bowles (23) stated, "It is … the response information that eventually guides functional technic." Therefore, at a mobile segment, focus attention on the following:

1. The criteria for symmetric and asymmetric motor function
2. The orientation of motion testing to the palpable findings of bony and tissue tension expressed at a dysfunctional mobile segment
3. The way that response at your fingertips, to each direction of motion test, guides not only diagnosis but also the development of each individual manipulative procedure

Conceptual Basis

The following phrases reveal the static positional concepts that emerged during osteopathy's early professional history:

Describing the lesion as a bone out of place
Exaggerating the lesion position
Retracing the path of the lesion
Noting the position in which the lesion occurred
Stacking positions to balance the tension

Bowles' comments about demand/response transactions and the motor coordination necessary for each bone to be in the right place at the right time during demands for body movement strongly indicate that he was moving beyond static positional concepts. His conceptual bias for motor function called for the recognition of a mobile system and mobile segments, patterned

to act in concert with one another. Each mobile segment is a bone with articular surfaces for movement and adnexal tissues under motor control; together, they respond to precise functional demands to:

1. Maintain postural position
2. Carry out active movements
3. Allow passive movement

For Bowles, functional diagnosis and technique were "unique in accuracy and universal in nontraumatic application" (24).

Currently there is widespread recognition, but still limited understanding, of the neural control of these motor dynamics. In 1978, Stein (25) reviewed principles emerging from studies of the properties of interneurons and their application to the organization of the body's motor patterns. Fundamental concepts of command neurons and pattern generators furnished a baseline for continuing research in this field. This growing knowledge about neural networks and motor control systems has been reviewed by Getting (26). Atsuta et al.'s research presents an ongoing example (27). In areas where motion tests detect signs of segmental motor asymmetry, somatic proprioceptive and nociceptive afferents (sensory impulses) acting through feedback loops effect adaptive changes in motor patterns. These changes are palpable as a three-segment unit of segmental dysfunction, which describes a basic unit of defective and adapted function.

During functional technique, the release of holding forces (using minimal force) and the return to motor symmetry have been expressed as follows (28):

> At the moment when the release of resistance forces is sensed, the response (conceptually) appears to be the result of a matching in movement function, in which the local segmental control becomes appropriate to the current, overall movement—a matching of adequacy in physiologic response to specific motion demand. The return to local controlled compliance of the mobile segment within the whole complex movement restores the opportunity for adequate part-to-whole functional relations of this segment within the mobile system.
>
> Basic knowledge about proprioceptor and nociceptor stimuli as a source of reflex communication from somatic tissues to other somatic tissues is well established (29). Even at rest, in response to only gravity and positional demands, the palpable findings of bony irregularity and increased resistance of muscular tissue to pressure at dysfunctional segments reflect ongoing stimulation of proprioceptor sensors. During movement, these palpable cues to the traffic on afferent pathways are highly erratic, since in some directions of ease they decrease whereas in opposing directions of resistance they increase.

The sheer immediacy of the changes palpated during motion testing and treatment suggests the moment-to-moment afferent monitoring by numerous muscle spindle stretch receptors and the resulting efferent control of muscle contraction/relaxation as a physiologic basis for interpreting the response to osteopathic manipulation being reported here (28).

At vertebral levels where segmental motion asymmetry is present, the physical stress of daily demands for movement and positioning accounts for a major increase in somatic sensory afferent impulses reaching the spinal cord (30). A concept of *afferent reduction* has application where the palpable sense of decreasing resistance, monitored throughout a functional manipulative procedure, successfully restores symmetric motor function.

EXAMPLES OF FUNCTIONAL TECHNIQUE

Thoracic, Lumbar, and Sacral Regions: Seated

The method described in the following example of functional technique (17) is applicable in the thoracic, lumbar, or sacral spinal regions.

Findings

This patient has a dysfunctional T6 segment, locally resisting regional rotation of shoulders and trunk to the right. Additional findings on shoulder/trunk rotation tests indicate that the increasing *ease* in rotation left at T6 is accompanied by *resistance* to rotation left at T5 and T7. Other rotary motion tests reveal initial increasing ease at T6 to side bending left and to extension, and to initial *inhalation* on respiratory testing. These directions are resisted at T5 and T7. In the next test (Fig. 52D.8A), the physician initiates right side bending of the trunk with moderate caudally directed force through the right hand, which is on the patient's right shoulder. The fingers of the physician's left hand monitor the response at T6. In the second test (Fig. 52D.8B), trunk flexion and extension are initiated, being careful not to introduce translatory aspects of movement (e.g., the patient is maintained in midline of the intersection of midcoronal and sagittal planes). Slightly relaxed slumping supported by the physician's left arm initiates flexion. Reversal of this rotary direction (about the *y*-axis of Fig. 52D.2) initiates extension. The physician's right fingers compare responses to these opposing directions of motion.

Position

The patient is in the seated position. As indicated in Figure 52D.9, the physician's left arm is over the left shoulder and under the right shoulder of the patient to allow easy introduction of side bending left and rotation left in the following functional application of an indirect method of manipulation.

Treatment Procedure

1. Hold the patient to provide control in side bending left, rotation left, and extension in a smooth torsional arc. Each of these directions will begin to diminish the local tissue resistance being monitored at T6 during the manipulative procedure.
2. Using slight shifting of postural forces to control movement of the patient's body, three translatory tests can be completed. In Figure 52D.10A, with patient's hips relatively fixed by sitting position, a slight shift in the physician's body weight to the right and then to the left allows comparison of response of T6 to lateral translations of the patient's trunk. In Figure 52D.10B, a slight shift in the physician's weight controls patient's shoulders and trunk, relative to the pelvis, to initiate anterior and then posterior translation motions for testing response at T6. In Figure 52D.10C, for testing cephalad/caudad directions, the physician initiates slight lifting cephalad through the patient's shoulders and trunk, and then caudad by applying mild body compression; the segment's responses to opposing directions are monitored by the physician's right hand.

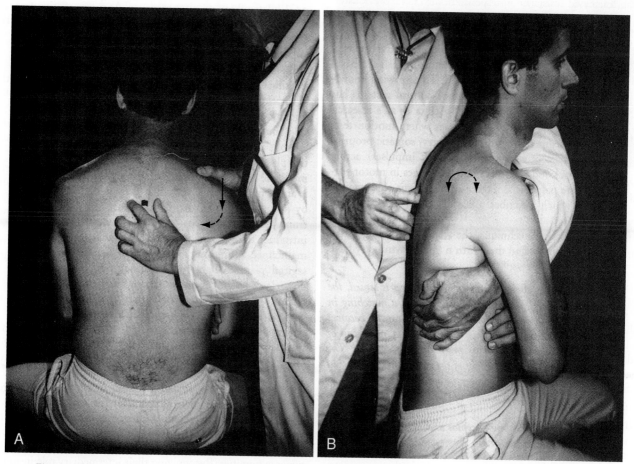

Figure 52D-8 Additional rotary motion tests. **A.** Physician initiates right side bending of trunk. **B.** Trunk flexion and extension. (From Johnston WL. Segmental definition, part II: application of an indirect method in osteopathic manipulative treatment. *JAOA* 1988;88:211–217, with permission.)

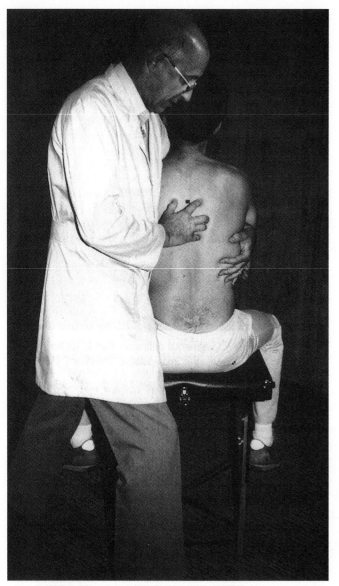

Figure 52D-9 Positioning of patient and physician to facilitate initial introduction of combined three rotary components toward a sense of increasing compliance (ease) in extension, left side bending, and left rotation. (From Johnston WL. Segmental definition, part II: application of an indirect method in osteopathic manipulative treatment. *JAOA* 1988;88:211–217, with permission.)

In this example, movements are added with increasing ease in translations to the left, anterior, and cephalad. Testing had indicated increasing resistance in each opposing translatory direction. Initial introduction of each appropriate direction is more important than extent of range in any one direction alone.

3. The final component is to direct a slow inhalation by the patient. The additional element of increasing ease promotes an eventual release of the holding tensions at the dysfunctional segment. The release allows return to a central resting position without encountering the previous resistance in these opposing directions.
4. Following successful release, retesting confirms a return to compliance and symmetry in response throughout the T5-7 area.

Cervical Region

In this example, the cervical region is examined initially in the seated position, followed by treatment in the supine position.

Findings
The first cervical vertebra (atlas) is limited in head and neck rotation left.

Diagnostic Procedure
Position No. 1
The patient is seated; the practitioner stands behind the patient.

1. With the left hand, contact the frontal-parietal region, palm frontal, with fingerpads at the right, thumb at the left
2. For the rotation test, introduce motion with the left hand. The right hand monitors for restricted motion response to the rotation left, with the third fingerpad of the right hand at the right, thumb at the left, and overlying the facet processes. (Hand placements are reversed to monitor the associated limitations in rotation right at occiput and at C2.)

Position No. 2
The patient is supine; the physician sits at the head of the table as shown in Figure 52D.11.

Positioning of the physician's arms with elbows supported on the knees provides comfortable support of the patient's occiput in the palms of the physician, who then monitors response to introduced motion. The third fingertips overlie cervical articular facets at C1 bilaterally to monitor response. As rotary motion tests continue, C1 responds with initial increasing ease in side bending right and flexion. During respiration, exhalation is easier.

Treatment Procedure
1. (the patient is supine) To small amounts of each of the three directions of rotary ease, add translatory components (of the head in relation to the trunk) in straight-line directions of increasing ease to the left, posterior, and caudal approximation. (Translatory testing in this example has indicated increasing resistance in each opposing direction.)
2. The increasing ease accumulating at C1 during the initial introduction of these six specific elements of motion is enhanced during a directed exhalation
3. The smooth torsion pathway for final release of tissue tension allows an easy return to a central resting position
4. Reexamination in the seated position should reveal a return to symmetry in response to head/neck rotation tests including the occiput, C1, and C2

Costal Region

When diagnosing the motor functions of ribs, it is significant to recognize that their elementary function is respiratory. Ribs also function, however, within the context of routine gross body movements that involve the thoracic spine and cage. Therefore, rib function is examined with the patient in the seated position with fingertip contact over the rib angle to monitor a rib's response to the spinal test pattern of elementary passive gross movements (rotations and translations), as well as active respiration. In principle, costal mobile units also function in association with movement of the upper extremities. Recognizing their intermediary role in so much of the body's movement suggests that costal dysfunctions may show more complex characteristics of motor asymmetry because they have one major motor function (inspiratory/expiratory)

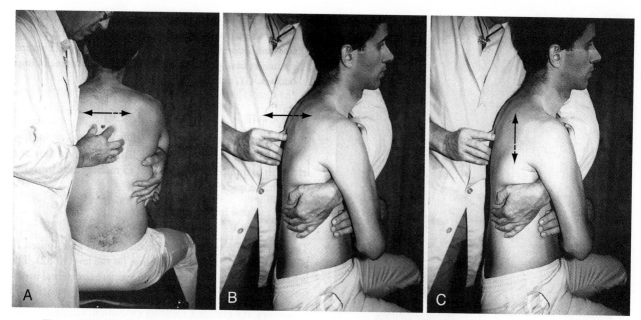

Figure 52D-10 Translatory motion tests. **A.** Patient in sitting position for comparison of response of T6 to lateral translations of trunk. **B.** Shift in physician's weight initiates anterior and then posterior motion testing at T6. **C.** Testing cephalad/caudad directions. (From Johnston WL. Segmental definition, part II: application of an indirect method in osteopathic manipulative treatment. *JAOA* 1988;88:211–217, with permission.)

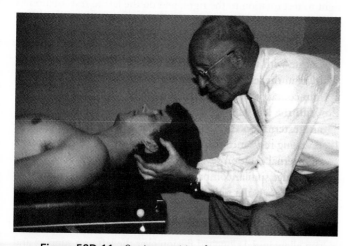

Figure 52D-11 Supine position for cervical technique.

and two subsidiary motor roles active in trunk and appendicular movement.

This complexity becomes evident when the palpatory characteristics of costal motor asymmetries are identified. There appears to be an element of simplicity, however, in the manner in which that asymmetry is organized. The primary movement of the ribs occurs in inhalation and exhalation. It is this respiratory primacy that appears to dictate the remaining characteristics of the total motor asymmetry when a rib becomes dysfunctional.

For example, if a primary costal defect is freer during exhalation and resists inhalation, this respiratory feature distinctively patterns the motor dysfunction of that rib. This becomes apparent when tested through the shoulders and trunk, with the patient seated, and through the ipsilateral arm with the patient in the lateral recumbent position. However, if the dysfunctional rib is freer during inhalation and resists exhalation, then the asymmetric pattern

of this rib's motor function is largely reversed from that of the preceding (exhalation) example.

Ribs are also involved in asymmetric motor function associated with afferent input from visceral disease. This distinctive category of a viscerosomatic component needs consideration separate from the two dysfunctions to be detailed here. They arise more strictly from the physical stresses incurred in this somatic region.

The following two examples illustrate the most common kinds of dysfunction in the rib cage (essentially somatic in origin, rather than visceral). One shows elementary limitation on exhalation; one is limited in inhalation. The predominance of bucket-handle or pump-handle motion during the inspiratory and expiratory function varies throughout the rib cage and is not considered in these examples. Instead, each example is concerned with monitoring a rib's response to specific demands for rotary and translatory aspects of passive motion tests. These are introduced through the shoulders and trunk of the seated patient and through the ipsilateral upper extremity when the patient is in the lateral recumbent position. Each example of treatment has two procedural components, one seated and one side lying.

Findings in Example 1

The right rib 3 resists *exhalation*. It predictably resists shoulder/trunk rotation left and side bending left in the seated position, monitored with the right fingertips overlying the rib angle. Testing adjacent ribs above and below demonstrates mirror-image asymmetries if right rib 3 is the primary functional defect.

Procedure No. 1: Concurrent Diagnosis and Treatment: Through the Trunk

1. Standing at the right of the seated patient, monitor directions of increasing ease of motion with the left fingers (Fig. 52D.12)
2. The right arm is over the patient's right shoulder and under the left to control initiation of motions through shoulders and trunk during side bending and rotation to the right (Fig. 52D.12A)

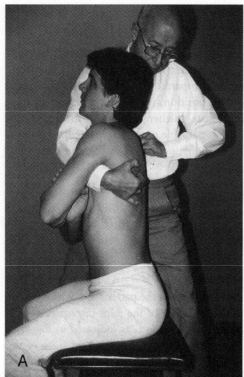

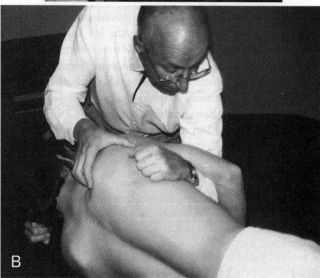

Figure 52D-12 Example 1: Right rib 3 resists exhalation. **A.** In seated position, motions introduced through the shoulder/trunk. **B.** In left side-lying position, motions introduced through the right arm.

3. Tissue tension and limited mobility continue to improve during initial introduction of backward bending and translations to the right and anterior. (They worsen during flexion and translations to the left and posterior.)
4. Direct the patient to inhale slowly and hold the inhalation phase momentarily as directions of motion are carefully combined in a smooth torsion arc of movement. This promotes a release and return to a central resting position
5. Retest shoulder/trunk movements, seated, to assess return to symmetry of these motion components

Procedure No. 2: Concurrent Diagnosis and Treatment: Through the Upper Extremity

1. The patient is in a left lateral recumbent position. Stand in front of the patient with the patient's right upper arm supported just cephalad to the elbow, as shown in Figure 52D.12B, on the physician's left forearm. The patient's right hand hangs toward the floor
2. The right fingers overlie the tissue tension/restriction identified at the rib angle and monitor respiratory motion to confirm continuing resistance to exhalation
3. Palpate for response to motion tests introduced through the patient's right arm. Typical findings include resistance to external rotation (about the long axis of the humerus), abduction, and cephalad movements
4. In the treatment procedure, monitor increasing ease to internal rotation, adduction, and caudad movements during a directed slow inhalation phase of the patient
5. Following a successful release, retest the arm motion components in the side-lying position
6. Following successful release in each of these two treatment components at right rib 3 resisting exhalation, retesting throughout right ribs 2, 3, and 4 confirms return to functional symmetry in this area of the rib cage

Findings in Example 2

Right rib 3 resists *inhalation*. During diagnostic testing, stand on the right to test rotation to the right, and on the left to test rotation to the left. The right rib 3 resisting inhalation predictably resists shoulder/trunk rotation right and side bending right. This is monitored with the left fingertips overlying the rib angle. Testing adjacent ribs above and below demonstrates mirror-image motion asymmetries, if the right rib 3 is the site of the primary dysfunction.

Procedure No. 1: Concurrent Diagnosis and Treatment: Through the Trunk

1. Standing at the left of the seated patient, monitor directions of increasing ease of motion with the right fingers (Fig. 52D.13)
2. The left arm is over the patient's left shoulder and under the right shoulder to control initiation of motions through the shoulders and trunk during side bending left and rotation to the left, as shown in Figure 52D.13A
3. Tissue tension and limited mobility continue to improve as you allow initial slouched flexion over the left arm support and translate to the right and posterior. (They worsen during backward bending and translations to the left and anterior.)
4. Direct the patient to exhale slowly and hold the exhalation phase momentarily as directions of motion are carefully combined in a smooth torsion arc of movement to promote a release and return to a central resting position
5. Retest shoulder/trunk motions in the seated position

Procedure No. 2: Concurrent Diagnosis and Treatment: Through the Upper Extremity

1. The patient is in a left lateral recumbent position. Stand in front of the patient. With the left forearm, support and introduce motion through the patient's right arm, having it relaxed and folded at the elbow as seen in Figure 52D.13B
2. The right fingers overlie the tissue tension/restriction identified at the rib angle and monitor response to respiratory tests to confirm continuing resistance to inhalation
3. Palpate for response to motion tests introduced through the patient's right arm. Typical findings include resistance to internal

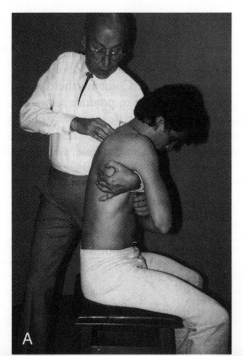

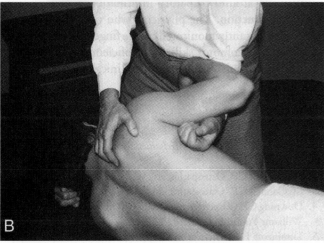

Figure 52D-13 Example 2: Right rib 3 resists inhalation. **A.** In seated position. **B.** In left side-lying position.

rotation (about the long axis of the humerus), adduction, and caudad movements

4. In the treatment procedure, monitor increasing ease to external rotation, abduction, and cephalad movements, during a directed slow exhalation phase of the patient

5. Following release, retest arm motion components in the side-lying position and retest inhalation and exhalation throughout right ribs 2, 3, and 4

Although the description of these two examples of rib technique (exhalation restriction and inhalation restriction) begins with the seated phase followed by the side lying, the order is not necessarily important and can be optional.

The physician's approach in functional technique is important. Evaluate immediately as each direction of motion is introduced. Combine these minor ranges in each direction, as described, to produce a smooth torsion arc of motion during the appropriate final respiratory phase. This complements the continually monitored

response of increasing ease. The palpable tension decreases to a sense of release, and the patient is returned to a resting state. Although these aspects of rib technique are presented as specific directions patterned to inhalation or exhalation restrictions, they should not be applied as if to copy a technique procedure. Rather, test each direction to promote appropriate summation of increasing ease, and monitor decreasing tension throughout each manipulation.

Thoracic Cage: Differentiating Somatic and Visceral Inputs

The spinal cord provides communication pathways that conduct impulses from sensory receptors in both musculoskeletal and visceral tissues. When noxious stimuli are persistent, the afferent bombardment contributes to palpable somatic manifestations of spinal dysfunction. Segmental motion asymmetries develop individuality in their dysfunctional behavior depending on the afferent source, somatic or visceral.

From functional methods in descriptive research, Figure 52D.3 illustrates a three-segment configuration of vertebral motion asymmetries that characterizes somato-somatic reflex activity. The primary dysfunction at the central segment demonstrates a complete asymmetric behavior in response to motion tests introduced through the shoulders and trunk in the seated position; the secondary dysfunctions at adjacent segments display mirror-image (opposing) motion asymmetries. The reflex basis for these secondary mirror images becomes apparent when all three segments return to motion symmetry following successful response to a functional manipulative procedure that addresses only the central (primary) dysfunctional segment.

In Figure 52D.4, the mirror-image phenomenon is still evident. However, this time it accompanies central segments that present a different primary orientation. The primacy relates to a vertebra and one adjacent rib at the same spinal level presenting *identical* motor asymmetries, rather than opposing. The term *linkage* applies to this phenomenon, because both vertebra and rib respond to motion tests in identical fashion, as if they were now linked together as a single mobile unit. This dysfunctional unit's motion asymmetry is typically complete in rotary, translatory, and respiratory tests; secondary mirror images exist at the adjacent coupled segments, as indicated.

Clinical data from interexaminer (31) and longitudinal (32,33) studies with hypertensive subjects, as well as a controlled clinical trial with renal, hypertensive, and normotensive subjects (21) have supported the presence of linkage as a somatic manifestation of visceral disease. The characteristic motion asymmetries at several linkage sites are reproducible and have been reported (20).

Manipulative treatment at a linkage site requires attention to two aspects of the motion behavior disturbed at such a dysfunctional costovertebral level. The segmental locus demonstrates not only asymmetry to spinal motion tests in the seated position induced through the shoulders/trunk, but also in recumbent positions to motion tests introduced through the lower extremities. A manipulative approach to address the former behavior has been detailed for both diagnostic and treatment procedures, seated, in the preceding thoracic section of "Examples of Functional Technique." However, maximum response at a linkage site also demands attention to motion behaviors related to the lower extremities (34). An example of diagnostic and treatment procedures follows.

Findings

Examined in the seated position, the patient has segmental dysfunction at spinal level T5, with linkage to left rib 5, and resistance to inhalation locally (and to exhalation at adjacent segments above and below). There is also resistance to anterior translation, monitored at tissues overlying the transverse processes at T5 and the angle of left rib 5. Under these circumstances, positioning the patient prone (rather than supine) enhances posterior translation and begins to decrease the palpable tension locally, as a first step in a functional procedure (35). The physician now stands at the left of the prone patient, as illustrated in Figure 52D.14. With both legs initially resting on the table, begin with the right leg resting semiflexed. With plantar contacts of your right hand at the patient's right heel, control for the introduction of inversion and eversion motion tests of the whole right limb. Monitoring responses with the left hand in contact at the T5 left linkage site will reveal immediately increasing resistance to *both* directions initiated. Similar testing with the left leg will reveal *asymmetric* behavior; for example, with eversion there is once again resistance, while with inversion there is increasing compliance.

Note: For linked segments in the thoracic region, this characteristic behavior during lower extremity tests is typical, in that responses are asymmetric to tests with the leg ipsilateral to the linked costal component, while resistance is present in both responses to tests with the contralateral leg.

Procedure: Concurrent Diagnosis and Treatment of Costovertebral Linkage

Engage support at the knee for control of the patient's left leg semiflexed as illustrated in Figure 52D.14. Maintaining slight inversion freedom, monitor responses at the T5 linkage site to compare inversion with eversion, flexion with extension and cephalad with caudad directions of the limb. Select and combine initial aspects

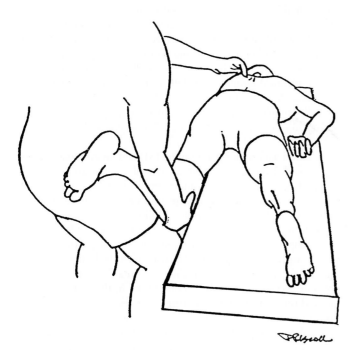

Figure 52D-14 Examination of linkage left site at T5 spinal level leads to treatment, prone, involving specific motion directions introduced through the ipsilateral lower extremity. With appropriate control by right hand support at the left knee, the operator monitors response at the left hand contacting the linked costovertebral segments. (From Johnston WL. Segmental definition, part IV. Updating the differential for somatic and visceral inputs. *JAOA* 2001;5:278–283, with permission.)

of these other elementary directions of increasing ease. In Figure 52D-14, abduction of the limb laterally from the table, flexion, and caudad directions are combined. With the finding of resistance to inhalation, the final decrease in palpable tension is maximized during a slow exhalation phase to release, followed by return of the leg to natural positioning on the table. When successful, repeating the diagnostic tests involved with each leg will reveal a return to symmetry in these aspects of the dysfunctional behavior at T5.

Note: Apart from the linkage phenomenon, as recognized in the costovertebral region, an additional distinctive characteristic of visceral input is now applicable for those spinal levels lacking costal components, that is, in cervical, lumbar, and sacral regions. Our continuing interest in examination of viscerosomatic linkage sites has led to a descriptive study. The following excerpt details that characteristic:

> For example, consider any non-linked dysfunctional vertebral or costal segment that shows increased resistance to the seated test for sidebending right as compared with left, introduced through the shoulders/trunk. In such an instance, an expectation also exists for increased resistance to sidebending right compared with left when introduced through the head/neck. However, segments involved in linkage do not show accord in response to these two apparently similar sidebending tests. Instead, segmental resistance to sidebending *right* through the shoulders/trunk will accompany resistance to sidebending *left* introduced through the head/neck. *This lack of accord serves as a convenient tool for use in differential diagnosis of active visceral influence in any spinal region dysfunction* (34).

Comment: Regarding Somatic Manifestations of Visceral Input

When spinal analysis identifies a site with palpable signs positive for visceral input, the search for the source of the visceral input narrows somewhat, based on the known distribution of visceral afferent pathways via dorsal routes (36,37). Further, the palpable characteristics of the spinal tissue changes presented at a site of visceral input bear directly on the time element involved. When historically connecting possibly relevant incidents of illness, recent/current paravertebral soft tissue changes trend toward aspects of local prominence and congestion. On the contrary, when related illness is longstanding/recurrent, there is a depressed area of the spinal musculature overlying the transverse processes at the vertebral site central to the visceral input. This sparse, deep, horizontal band of markedly increased tissue tension reflects the hypoxia associated with tissues that are subjected to prolonged, concentrated reflex action. In time, this action will be both primary visceral and secondary somatic, since the spinal dysfunction once initiated continues as a focus for motion stress and becomes self-maintaining within continuing demands of the motor system.

Innominate

The patient has an elementary kind of pelvic dysfunction, one with palpatory findings localized to one side of the pelvis, with asymmetric response to motion tests introduced through only the ipsilateral lower extremity (and no resistance encountered with tests introduced through the contralateral limb).

Findings

There is a tissue texture abnormality (TTA) and limited mobility at the left ilium/gluteal region (at the level of S2). There is palpable resistance at the left innominate to external rotation (eversion) of the left lower limb.

Diagnostic Procedure

1. The patient is supine, with the left knee semiflexed and the foot resting on the table; the physician stands at the patient's left
2. Locate with the right hand the area of TTA and limited mobility at the left ilium/gluteal region, at the S2 level, and maintain contact throughout the procedure
3. With the left hand at the patient's left knee, initiate internal and external rotation (moving knee toward right, then left), revealing resistance palpated at the right hand to the initiation of external rotation (eversion)
4. Introduce similar comparison of internal and external rotation tests through the right semiflexed limb, but monitor it at the right hand, revealing left innominate compliance to both directions of the test

Treatment Procedure

1. Position the patient right lateral recumbent. Stand in front, with left hand contact at the innominate, TTA at level S2 (Fig. 52D.15). Direct the patient to shift the pelvis slightly in anterior translation relative to the shoulders. Maintain this positional shift if this direction decreases tension at the S2 level, compared with posterior translation
2. With your right hand supporting the patient's knees, introduce flexion through both legs together to localize action at the S2 sacral level monitored by the left hand
3. Now alter your support to the left leg only (Fig. 52D.15), with the right hand/forearm to monitor (in this example) the increasing ease at your left hand in response to abduction of the limb (vs. adduction), backward bending (vs. flexion), and caudal traction (vs. cephalad). Each of these components is combined during introduction of internal rotation (external rotation is resisted)
4. Direct the patient in inhalation (the direction of ease of the TTA)
5. During the final component of directed inhalation ease, combine these directional elements appropriately to achieve a palpable sense of decreasing tension and then a release by the holding forces. Return the limb to its resting position with the patient in lateral recumbency
6. Reexamining the motion tests supine indicates a return to symmetry of response at the left innominate, with reduced tissue tension of the left gluteal musculature

Variations in the findings from those described for this example simply require application of elementary motion testing procedures at a diagnosed focus of TTA, and restricted mobility, wherever these are evident on pelvic structural examination (35). Specific directions of positioning and motion are then applied in a controlled manner to the pelvic location diagnosed, to ease increasingly the holding forces of restricted motor function.

Appendicular Regions

Note: There is a continuing application of principle here as the physician maintains use of the six elementary motions and respiration as functional tools for testing and reducing specific dysfunction in an appendage.

Findings

In this example, the left knee fails to hyperextend. On examination in the supine position with the physician standing at the left side, the left knee lies slightly raised from the table surface when compared with the right. In this uncomfortable, slightly flexed position, it is tenser to palpation than the right and resists further passively introduced extension. A prominence is palpable at the anteromedial border of the joint interspace (tibiofemoral), indicating the edge of the medial semilunar cartilage.

Position

The patient is supine and the left knee is flexed; stand by the left side of the table.

Procedures: Concurrent Diagnosis and Treatment

1. The right palm spans the patellar area with the thumb following the lateral aspect of the joint interspace. The third finger follows the medial aspect, as indicated in Figure 52D.16. This hand is keyed sharply to the distorted sense of rigid binding resistance where it is most apparent. Keep the contact light enough to appreciate this palpable marker, yet firm enough in grasp to assist in the manipulative procedure
2. The left hand firmly grasps above the left ankle to assist in slowly bringing the knee up into the freer direction of flexion

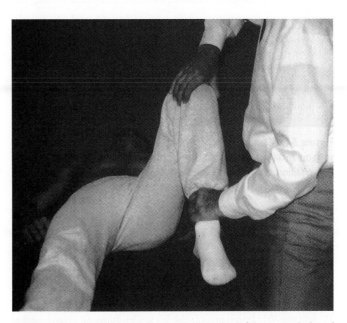

Figure 52D-16 Appendicular example at the left knee. Right hand monitors and supports. Left hand introduces major motions in testing and treatment.

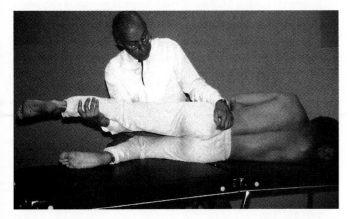

Figure 52D-15 Right lateral recumbent position for left innominate technique.

3. Explore additional directions of motion test for the limb while it is supported in freedom from the table by both hands: these motions address the other rotary aspects, which are found to be freer in medial rotation and abduction. Begin the introduction of these motions with the left hand and monitor response with the right

4. Maintain the initial introduction of rotary components

5. While still monitoring response at the knee, the tests using translatory directions for the limb indicate increasing ease anterior, above the table (binding posterior), increasing ease to the left (compared with right), and cephalad (with binding in caudal traction). The respiratory test indicates easier response to inhalation

6. In the final maneuver, the right-hand contact at the knee guides the lifting support anteriorly to the left, while the left hand controls the amount of each rotary motion in a cephalad direction via the distal tibiofibular contact. There is a proportionately larger amount of flexion introduced, guided by the sense of continuing increasing ease. (This aspect of the knee's template of motion has the greatest range.)

7. Direct the patient to slowly exhale to promote the final release of holding forces. Mobility then allows an easier return into improved extension range as the leg is guided back down onto the table

SUMMARY

The term *functional technique* applies to an indirect method of osteopathic manipulation in which the treatment procedure is organized around palpatory information gained from tests for motor function. By paying attention to the feedback constantly monitored by the fingertips, the physician will experience improved psychomotor skill and proficiency in the use of this treatment method, and in many other clinical procedures as well.

REFERENCES

1. Ashmore EF. *Osteopathic Mechanics*. Kirksville, MO: Journal Printing Co., 1915:72.
2. McConnell CP. Osteopathic art, V. *JAOA* 1935;34:369–374.
3. McConnell CP. Osteopathic studies, IV. *JAOA* 1931;31:206–212.
4. Downing CH. *Principles and Practice of Osteopathy*. Kansas City, MO: Williams Publishing Co., 1923:162.
5. Lippincott HA. The osteopathic technique of Wm. G. Sutherland, D.O. In: Northup TL, ed. *Yearbook of the Academy of Applied Osteopathy*. Ann Arbor, MI: Edwards Brothers Inc., 1949:124.
6. Hoover HV. Fundamentals of technique. In: *Yearbook of the Academy of Applied Osteopathy*. Ann Arbor, MI: Edwards Brothers Inc., 1949:25–41.
7. Hoover HV, Nelson CR. Basic physiologic movements of the spine. In: *Academy of Applied Osteopathy Year Book*. Ann Arbor, MI: Cushing-Malloy Inc., 1950:65.
8. Bowles CH. A functional orientation for technic. In: Page LE, ed. *Yearbook of the Academy of Applied Osteopathy*. Carmel, CA: Academy of Applied Osteopathy; Indianapolis, IN: American Academy of Osteopathy, 1955:177–191.
9. Lippincott HA. Basic principles of osteopathic technique. In: Barnes MW, ed. *Yearbook of the Academy of Applied Osteopathy*. Carmel, CA: Academy of Applied Osteopathy; Indianapolis, IN: American Academy of Osteopathy, 1961:45–48.
10. Jones LH. Spontaneous release by positioning. *DO* 1964;4:109–116.
11. Johnston WL. Interexaminer reliability studies. Spanning a gap in medical research. *JAOA* 1982;81:819–829.
12. Johnston WL. Passive gross motion testing, part 1: its role in physical examination. *JAOA* 1982;81:298–303.
13. Johnston WL, Hill JL. Spinal segmental dysfunction: incidence in cervicothoracic region. *JAOA* 1981;81:67–76.
14. Johnston WL, Kelso AF, Hollandsworth DL, et al. Somatic manifestations in renal disease: a clinical research study. *JAOA* 1987;87:22–35.
15. Kelso AF, Grant RG, Johnston WL. Use of thermograms to support assessment of somatic dysfunction or effects of osteopathic manipulative treatment. *JAOA* 1982;82:182–188.
16. Johnston WL. Segmental definition, part I: a focal point for diagnosis of somatic dysfunction. *JAOA* 1988;88:99–105.
17. Johnston WL. Segmental definition, part II: application of an indirect method in osteopathic manipulative treatment. *JAOA* 1988;88:211–217.
18. Johnston WL. Segmental behavior during motions, 1: a palpatory study of somatic relations. *JAOA* 1972;72:352–361.
19. Johnston WL, Hill JL. Spinal segmental dysfunction: incidence in cervicothoracic region. *JAOA* 1981;81:22–28.
20. Johnston WL. Segmental definition, part III: definitive basis for distinguishing somatic findings of visceral reflex origin. *JAOA* 1988;88:347–353.
21. Johnston WL, Kelso AF, Hollandsworth DL, et al. Somatic manifestations in renal disease: a clinical research study. *JAOA* 1987;87:22–35.
22. Johnston WL, Friedman HD. *Functional Methods: A Manual for Palpatory Skill Development in Osteopathic Examination and Manipulation of Motor Function*. Indianapolis, IN: American Academy of Osteopathy, 1995:44–45.
23. Bowles CH. A functional orientation for technic. In: Page LE, ed. *Yearbook of the Academy of Applied Osteopathy*. Carmel, CA: Academy of Applied Osteopathy, 1955:177–191.
24. Bowles CH. Functional technique: a modern perspective. *JAOA* 1981;80:326–331.
25. Stein PSG. Motor systems, with specific reference to the control of locomotion. *Ann Rev Neurosci*. 1978;1:61–81.
26. Getting PA. Emerging principles governing the operation of neural networks. *Ann Rev Neurosci*. 1989;12:185–204.
27. Atsuta Y, Garcia-Rill E, Skinner RD. Characteristics of electrically induced locomotion in rat in vitro brain stem-spinal cord preparation. *J Neurophysiol*. 1990;64:727–735.
28. Johnston WL. Segmental definition, part II: application of an indirect method in osteopathic manipulative treatment. *JAOA* 1988;88:211–217.
29. Henneman E. Organization of the spinal cord and its reflexes. In: Mountcastle VB, ed. *Medical Physiology*. 14th Ed. Vol 1. St. Louis, MO: CV Mosby, 1980:762–786.
30. Johnston WL. Osteopathic clinical aspects of somatovisceral interaction. In: Patterson MM, Howell JH, eds. *The Central Connection: Somatovisceral/Viscerosomatic Interaction*. Indianapolis, IN: American Academy of Osteopathy, 1992.
31. Johnston WL, Hill JL, Elkiss ML, et al. Identification of stable somatic findings in hypertensive subjects by trained examiners using palpatory examination. *JAOA* 1982;81:830–836.
32. Johnston WL, Kelso AF, Babcock HB. Changes in presence of a segmental dysfunction pattern associated with hypertension, part I: a short-term longitudinal study. *JAOA* 1995;4:243–255.
33. Johnston WL, Kelso AF. Changes in presence of a segmental dysfunction pattern associated with hypertension, part II: a long-term longitudinal study. *JAOA* 1995;5:315–318.
34. Johnston WL, Golden WJ. Segmental definition, part IV: updating the differential for somatic and visceral inputs. *JAOA* 2001;5:278–283.
35. Johnston WL, Friedman HD. *Functional Methods: A Manual for Palpatory Skill Development in Osteopathic Examination and Manipulation of Motor Function*. Indianapolis, IN: The American Academy of Osteopathy, 1995:83–91.
36. Beal MC. Viscerosomatic reflexes: a review. *JAOA* 1985;12:786–801.
37. Johnston WL, Friedman HD. *Functional Methods: A Manual for Palpatory Skill Development in Osteopathic Examination and Manipulation of Motor Function*. Indianapolis, IN: The American Academy of Osteopathy, 1995:135–137.

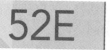

Visceral Manipulation

KENNETH LOSSING

KEY CONCEPT

In this section, emphasis is placed on direct palpation, evaluation, diagnosis, and treatment of viscera. Impaired or altered mobility/motility of the visceral system is reflected in abnormal motion tests showing change in distensibility of attachments or change in normal viscoelasticity. The concomitant consideration is to recognize that visceral and pelvic pathologic processes have spinal effects.

CASE STUDY

A 78-year-old female presented to the office with a history of bronchitis for the last week. She has continued coughing and feeling sick in spite of medical therapy.

Physical Examination:

Vital signs were normal. Pulmonary exam revealed diffuse rhonchi. Structural exam revealed restriction of ribs 1 and 2 on the left and rib 12 bilaterally. The left occiptomastoid suture was restricted. Decreased compliance of the lungs, increased tension in the trachea and bronchus, and congested lymphatics of the lungs, airways, and the thoracic cage were noted.

Diagnosis:

1. Acute bronchitis
2. Somatic dysfunction—thoracic, rib, cranium.

Plan:

The lymphatics of the airways were treated first. The ribs were then treated with balanced ligamentous tension technique. By then, the thoracic compliance had improved a lot and the patient was breathing easier. The lungs were directly treated last, as it was now possible to more accurately palpate their compliance. The lungs were treated by compression and decompression, which resulted in markedly improved compliance and again improved the respiration. The coughing was reduced by significantly within an hour.

INTRODUCTION AND DEFINITION

Direct palpation, evaluation, diagnosis, and treatment of the viscera have existed since the time of Dr. Still. This valuable approach opens the doors to being able to help a wide range of functional disorders. A visceral dysfunction is defined as "impaired or altered mobility or motility of the visceral system and related fascial, neurological, vascular, skeletal, and lymphatic elements." This is reflected in abnormal motion tests, showing a change in the distensibility of the attachments, or a change in their normal viscoelasticity, among other physical findings.

This means we have different aspects/models of a dysfunction, each equally valid:

- Fascial model—tested with motion testing and fascial pull (listening technique)
- Fluid model—arterial and venous blood, interstitial fluids, and lymphatics can be tested with palpation, Doppler ultrasound, or perfusion studies as necessary
- Respiratory model—excursion of tissue with respiration can be tested with palpation, fluoroscopy, or real-time MRI
- Neurological model—tested with palpation and motion testing, or EMG
- Inherent motions model—tested with palpation/sensing
- Temperature changes/energy/emotions—tested with palpation, or thermography

In this chapter, we look at all of these models in connection with the respiratory system, but first a look at history.

HISTORY

Dr. Still developed osteopathy in the late 19th century. He had been trained as a medical doctor, but found that he could treat most diseases by palpating dysfunctional areas, and treating them with his hands. He called this new science Osteopathy, meaning to "begin with the bones." By finding where the bones were not properly aligned and where they were not moving properly, it can guide the physician to the area of the body that needs to be treated, as they reflect where the forces of life are not moving properly. Notice that he "began with the bones," but did not end there. In his writing, he constantly talked about joints, fascia, blood supply, nerves, internal organs, and lymphatic flow. Dr. Still, and his students, treated all of the known medical diseases of the day.

Osteopathic manipulation of the viscera began with Dr. Still. He described treating many different digestive, respiratory, and urogenital complaints (1). For Dr. Still, almost all medical conditions had an osteopathic treatment, in some cases curative, in some cases supportive. Dr. Still left few descriptions of techniques of any kind, but some of his early students, McConnell (2), and Barber (3) did. Dr. Still described few techniques in his writings; the most specific information was in his last book, *Research and Practice*, published in 1911.

There are many principles that we can learn from Dr. Still. For instance, when treating appendicitis, he would treat the colon first, then the spine. In treating colic, he treated the spine first, then the colon. Although he never spoke of his rationale, we can at least assume that there are times to start with the viscera, and times to start with the spine.

A little-known fact is that Dr. Still palpated temperature changes when looking for the dysfunctional areas. In *The lengthening Shadow of Andrew Taylor Still*, (4) Hildreth states that he often observed Dr. Still running his hand along the patients spine, throat, thorax, abdomen and pelvis, looking for areas of heat or a variation in temperature.

One of Dr. Still's earliest students was Carl McConnell. Dr. McConnell graduated from the American School of Osteopathy in

1901 and stayed on as an instructor for some years. Dr. McConnell was very prolific, writing 6 books and over 250 articles. Among this body of literature, he described direct treatment of all of the viscera, except the lungs and the heart. Dr. McConnell wrote over 10 different articles describing various visceral technique principles.

> *"Those who overlook ventral (visceral) technique are practicing a greatly limited osteopathy. In fact, confining osteopathic adjustment to the posterior plane (no matter how fundamental spinal therapy is) means the neglect of essential factors that even enter into vertebral and pelvic pathology. Structural lesions of the chest, abdomen, and pelvis frequently originate primarily within these cavities. Of course these structural changes present concomitant affects in the spine, and vice versa."*
>
> *"There is no organ of the abdomen and pelvis that cannot be influenced by improving the structural and physiological balance through direct adjustment methods."*

Relatedness, 1939. *"One of Dr. Still's most enlightening statements, embryologically, physiologically, biologically, and technically, in my opinion, is as follows; It is only the perfection of the organism and the connected oneness that is the keynote to osteopathic practice. Every part has a duty to perform not only for its own maintenance, but also for the health and harmony of the interrelated whole. This is part of the law of supply and demand, which is absolute through all of nature. It is important to know the exact place that each organ and tissue occupies in its normal position. It is only by knowing the normal we are able to detect the abnormal. Each organ seems to be a creator of its own fluid substances. We must know the nerve and blood supply and the drainage."*

One of Dr. Still's other early students, Sutherland, credited him with the original idea of the cranial concept. Dr. Still often told his students that D.O. stands for "Dig On," encouraging them to expand their view of osteopathy (7). While Dr. Sutherland is most known for his work in the cranial area, he never implied that it should be the only area diagnosed or treated. He gave multiple references to treating the viscera.

> *"When you want to observe the abdominal viscera that may be in ptosis, with the patient supine gently place one hand over or just below the area of interest. This hand is passive; it does nothing. Then place your other hand over it. You use the upper hand for gentle lifts and observation. That gentle application will tell you a great deal about where you are so that you can feel what the tissues can reveal. The lower hand can be permitted to sink into the tissues below, but the upper hand does the lifting in cooperation with the exhalation excursion of the diaphragm."*

Jacques Weischenck, D.O., wrote one of the first textbooks on visceral technique *Traite d'osteopathie Viscerale* in 1982. He described the normal exchange of pressure in the abdomen, visceral dysfunction chains, normal and dysfunctional axis of motion of the organs during respiration, palpatory diagnosis, and manipulative treatment for all of the abdominal viscera. His concept of organs having a normal axis of motion during respiration, which becomes perturbed in a dysfunction, was later tested and proved by two of his students, Georges Finet, D.O., and Christian Williamae, D.O.

The most prolific author, innovator, and teacher of visceral manipulation has been Jean-Pierre Barral. He graduated from the European School of Osteopathy in Maidstone, England, at a time when British Osteopathy consisted of spinal diagnosis and treatment. At the time, most of the early American literature was not easily available. Barral applied the concepts he had learned for the spine in developing visceral approaches. In addition, he came up with the concepts of "general and local listening" to the tissues, manual thermal diagnosis, visceral emotional connections, and visceral motility.

Barral's books (8), energy, enthusiasm, and love of teaching have resulted in visceral manipulation spreading across the world.

THEORETICAL CONSIDERATIONS

> *"Virtually all forms of organ injury start with molecular or structural alterations in cells, a concept first put forth in the nineteenth century by Rudolf Virchow, known as the father of modern pathology. We therefore begin our consideration of pathology with the study of the origins, molecular mechanisms, and structural changes of cell injury. Yet different cells in tissues constantly interact with each other, and an elaborate system of extracellular matrix is necessary for the integrity of organs. Cell-cell and cell-matrix interactions contribute significantly to the response to injury, leading to collectively to tissue and organ injury, which are as important as cell injury in defining the morphologic and clinical patterns of disease."*

Robbins *Pathological Basis of Disease* (9).

In order to understand visceral approaches in osteopathy, we will need to do a short review/update of some basic sciences. Advances in biology, embryology, physics, and physiology over the last 30 years have dramatically changed how we look at the mechanical forces generated, utilized, and distributed during human life.

In the past, it was thought that genetics determined everything. During the 1960s, the German embryologist Blechschmidt (10) questioned this idea. Based on the microscopic dissection of very young embryos, he concluded that mechanical forces generated during embryologic cellular growth interact with the environment to change the way the cell functions and what it develops into. Cellular circulation, metabolism, and waste removal start as soon as there are cells. Differential growth patterns, between the central nervous system, vascular system, the various organ systems, and the musculoskeletal system, cause tension and compression forces to affect the shape and function of the cells.

"It is now known that many cell types express different genes (i.e. perform different functions) in response to even small changes in their mechanical environment." Humphrey and Delance (11).

Until recently, the organelles inside of cells were thought to be floating in the intercellular fluid, as a sort of soup. It turns out that this is not the case. The organelles, cellular membrane, and nucleus are all interconnected by microtubules that act like a cellular skeleton, and microfilaments that give elastic support to the cell (12).

With the recent discovery of integral proteins (intergrins) in the cellular membrane, we now know more about the mechanical links between the cell, the extracellular matrix, and all tissue systems (13). Intergrins mechanically connect the cell membrane with microfilaments, microtubules, the cell nucleus and DNA, with the extracellular matrix, transmitting mechanical forces of tension and compression throughout the whole organism.

Visceral ligaments are viscoelastic (14), that is, they act both like a fluid and like a solid.

Visceral ligaments can respond to a "strain" (compression or tension) biomechanically speaking, with both elastic and plastic properties, depending on the amount of force and the amount of time over which the strain is applied. In an elastic deformation, the tissue returns to its original shape and configuration after the straining force is removed. In a plastic deformation, the original shape and distensibility is altered, with a resulting storage of force. In a visceral dysfunction, the stress in the ligament has a certain amount of force stored (as potential energy or "potency"), in a certain direction, and that tissue has a certain speed that it will respond to. This results in an altered viscoelasticity curve for that ligament. (The viscosity is more, the elasticity is less).

When that force is exactly matched, in force, direction, and speed, the tissue will change, returning to a more normal distensibility. In the process, there is a dissipation of heat, movement of fluid, and a restructuring of the elasticity curve. A dysfunction can be caused by any of or a combination of: trauma, mechanical stress, emotions, chemical imbalances, circulation problems, imbalances in the nervous system, imbalances in circulation of life forces, and hormonal imbalances.

The arteries, veins, nerves, and lymphatic channels to the internal organs all go through the visceral attachments (ligaments). If there is increased mechanical tension in the visceral ligaments, the first fluid vessels to get compressed (compromised) will be the lowest pressure, the lymphatic vessels and veins, leading to a relative edema, with retention of metabolic byproducts. With further increased tension, the artery can become compressed, leading to decreased nutrition, oxygen, and eventual death.

> *"Any occlusion of lymphatic vessels is followed by the abnormal accumulation of interstitial fluid in the affected part, referred to as obstructive lymphedema."*

Robbins Pathologic Basis of Disease (9).

Tension and compression forces are always in relationship with each other. Buckminster Fuller (15) coined the term tensegrity to describe architectural buildings/structures invented in 1948 by Kenneth Snelson. Tension occurs when something is stretched. Integrity is a state of wholeness. So, tensegrity is the balancing of tension and compression forces, attractive and repulsive forces, in a whole structure. When these forces and balanced and relatively evenly distributed, the whole structure is stronger and able to withstand more stress. When the forces are unequally distributed, weakness and strain result. In the human body, we know bones take compressive forces, the connective tissues distribute tension forces, but the viscera also interact with both of these forces. Besides the static forces generated in architecture of buildings, the human frame also has the constantly changing forces of respiration, circulation, physical movement, gravity, digestion, and other factors. Visceral and somatic dysfunctions cause an imbalance in the distribution of tension and compressive forces, weakening the whole structure.

Let us look at what happens during respiration and pulmonary ventilation. The movement of air into and out of the lungs depends on a few basic things: (1) the pressure and volume inverse relationship: as volume increases, the pressure falls and the volume depends on the movement of the diaphragm and ribs, (2) internal and external air pressure, and (3) the compliance of the lungs.

As the ribcage expands during inhalation, the anterior ribcage moves superior (pump handle rib motion), the lateral ribcage moves laterally (bucket handle rib motion), and the respiratory diaphragm descends. The excursion of the diaphragm during normal volume respiration is 1.5 to 4 cm, as measured by CT scan (16), but can go as far as 7 cm. At the same time venous blood flow in the superior vena cava increases, and in the portal vein decreases. This shows a clear respiratory effect on blood circulation. At the same time, the pericardium swings around the attachments for the great vessels, with its inferior border moving 1.5 cm medial and inferior (17). The thoracic contents mechanically are stretched, so the tension increases in the pericardium, pulmonary ligaments, and lung parenchyma, as the negative pressure inside the lungs becomes more negative (8), and the negative pleural pressure becomes more negative. The negative pleural pressure keeps the visceral and parietal pleura in contact, which also increases the mechanical tension to the lung parenchyma. Normal tidal volume is about 500 mL air.

As the thoracic contents expand, along with diaphragmatic contraction, it compresses the abdominal contents. The splenic flexure of the colon descends an average of 1.43 cm and the sigmoid colon descends less, about 0.25 cm. Using fluoroscopy and ultrasound, all of the abdominal viscera have been proved to move in the sagittal, coronal, and frontal planes in specific reproducible motions (7). These movements become perturbed in a visceral dysfunction and can be normalized with treatment.

The lymphatic system of the lungs plays many roles, immune response, disease resistance, and fluid drainage. The lymphatics may become congested due to infection, inflammation, inhalational allergies, and mechanical tension in the surrounding tissues. If the fluid drainage is impaired, the mechanical tension increases, leading to less compliance in the lungs. Only recently has it been discovered that the lymphatic vessels between the valves, called lympangions, contract. These movements are biphasic and palpable (18).

During rest and exercise, the tidal volume changes, depending on demand, but also depending on the functional capacity of the overall structure. For instance, it is easy to understand that if a rib is in dysfunction, it will not move as well, the thorax will not be able to expand as well, and less intrathoracic volume translates into less air inhaled and exhaled. What may not be as immediately evident is the fact that the compliance of the lungs can be impaired by mechanical factors, also reducing tidal volume. A visceral dysfunction of a lung will reflect itself in reduced compliance.

Stretch receptors of the lungs connect via the vagus nerve to the ventral respiratory group of the medulla. Visceral afferent receptors send information to the spine, and also the brain. They are chemosensitive, mechanosensitive, and thermosensitive. The sensory system can be overstimulated leading to a decreased threshold required for stimulation. Osteopathic literature has called this facilitation, very similar to the current medical terminology of peripheral and central sensitization. Whatever the mechanism, and whatever the current terms, the functional result is an associated mechanical tension. In the case of the sympathetics to the lung, facilitation will result in a restricted upper thoracic segment, or segments, between T1 and T6, or rib restrictions in those areas. The parasympathetics can also be irritated. Cranial dysfunction near the jugular foramen can compress the vagus nerve, and there is some reason to think that the parasympathetic nerves can become facilitated also.

Since the time of Hippocrates, there have been clinical associations between problem areas of the body and an increased output of heat in the same area. Hippocrates is said to have put wet mud on a person, to see where it dried first, in an attempt to localize the problem. We know, of course, that often in ankle sprains, the area of the ligament is warmer. What has been less clear is why there are so many small temperature variations in a person's body. Clinical research using temperature recording devices over the 10 years has led to the conclusion that somatic and visceral dysfunctions (functional problems) project heat imbalances, generally warmer, but sometimes cooler, relative to the surrounding area.

To summarize, a visceral dysfunction of the lungs and airways will have related spinal and rib dysfunctions, cranial dysfunctions, neurological dysfunctions, lymphatic other fluid dysfunctions, and temperature imbalances. The art of practice is to find out the most efficient treatment order and the most effective treatment that the body can accept.

INDICATIONS, CONTRAINDICATIONS, AND COMPLICATIONS

The indications for visceral technique can be categorized into the following:

1. Visceral dysfunctions associated with known medical diagnosis. Almost all medical diagnosis of the viscera have a component that is functional, in other words, can be changed. Since the functional component cannot be recognized with lab or radiological test, the only way to find out is to treat it. Generally one to three treatments will reveal if an osteopathic approach is helpful and cost effective
2. Visceral dysfunctions mechanically connected to somatic dysfunction. The viscera are connected to the musculoskeletal system by connective tissue forming functional chains that connect from head to toe, all of the anatomical structures

Contraindications to visceral treatment are abdominal aneurysm, internal bleeding, infections uncontrolled by antibiotics, severe pain induced by palpation or manipulation, and medical indications for emergent medical workup.

PALPATION AND DIAGNOSIS

Palpation of the viscera starts with being able to identify the individual organs. The liver, for instance, is easy to identify and palpate for texture, outline, and size. The lungs, however, present some challenges. How is it possible to palpate through the ribcage to feel a lung? Perhaps not as difficult as one might expect, if one remembers Newton's second law: "For each action, there is a reaction." In this case, doing layer palpation on the thorax will reveal skin, superficial fascia, muscles, ribs, endothoracic fascia, pleura, and finally the lungs. As one compresses deeper, each layer will press back into the hand. At each layer, one can palpate for fascial pulling in the direction of tension, a dysfunction, and motion test for directions of ease and directions of increased tension, a barrier.

EXAMPLES OF TECHNIQUE

When considering any organ, of course it is needed to appreciate all of the functional connections. Here is a brief look at a few of the viscera themselves.

THE MAINSTEM BRONCHUS AND AIRWAYS

The main stem bronchus can be appreciated by tractioning the trachea superiorly to tension, and while maintaining the tension, translate it to the left and the right, noting distance and end feel. If there is no abnormal tension, one should be able to feel the airway distend all the way to the inferior lobes of both lungs. If there is a dysfunction, the distensibility will be less and the "end feel" harder. For instance, if the right airway is in dysfunction, there will be a shorter tracheal translation to the left, and the end feel will be harder. To mobilize the right airway, traction the trachea superiorly to tension while palpating the second and third rib interspace about 2 to 3 cm from the midline. A slight inward tug will be noted. Using the right thenar eminence at that place, compress posteriorly until a slight feeling of tension is appreciated. Have the patient inhale and exhale, drawing the area inferiorly during each exhale, and maintaining tension during the inhale. Typically within about three breaths a release will be felt. Recheck the motion testing parameters.

The Lungs

To evaluate and treat the right lung, place the patient in the left lateral recumbent position. Place the left hand over the lateral chest wall at the level of ribs 3 to 6. Place the right hand over the left hand. Use the right hand to compress and the left hand to palpate. Pay attention to each layer, skin, adipose, superficial fascia, external muscles, ribs, intercostal muscles, endothoracic fascia, parietal pleura, visceral pleura, and the lung. Feel if the lung is being tractioned superior/inferior, anterior/posterior, or medially/laterally. Motion test in these same directions to reconfirm the findings (Figs. 52E.1 and 52E.2). In the plane of the largest restriction, find the direction of ease. Find the midpoint between the restrictive barrier and the physiological barrier in the direction of ease. Stack the middle point of all three planes, and add a slight compression. A change in the viscoelasticity will be felt as the dysfunction resolves. Recheck fascial pull and motion testing. If these are not fully balanced, take the tissues to the largest remaining barrier, and stack the remaining two planes at their

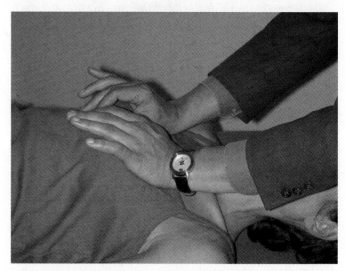

Figure 52E-1 Diagnosis and treatment of bronchi—superior.

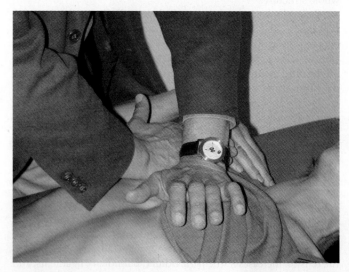

Figure 52E-2 Diagnosis and treatment of bronchi—anterior/posterior.

restrictive barriers. Add a slight compression, and wait for the release. When the motion testing is normalized, compress the lung, and release, noting the ease and speed of the return. Assume this speed, compressing and releasing, until a viscoelasticity shift in the tissue is felt.

CASE STUDIES

Case Study 2

A 45-year-old female presented to the office with a 2-year history of right flank pain subsequent to a motor vehicle accident. During the accident, her trunk was rotated to the right. Her car was struck from behind. Using general and local listening, it was found that the right kidney was in a second degree ptosis (dropped inferior more than a centimeter and externally rotated). The kidney was mobilized. On a follow-up visit one month later, the patient reported all flank pain to be resolved.

Case Study 3

A 7-year-old female presented to the office with a 6-month history of tummy aches and a sensation of acid in her mouth. No other symptoms were present, and her medical history was otherwise normal. Physical exam revealed somatic dysfunction of the left occiptomastoid suture, T6 on the left, and a visceral dysfunction of the gastroesophageal junction. These areas were treated. On a follow-up visit one month later, she reported no tummy arches and no instances of acid taste.

REFERENCES

1. Still AT. *Osteopathy Research and Practice*, Journal Printing, 1910, Seattle, WA: Eastland Press, 1992.
2. McConnell CP. *Selected Writings of Carl Philip McConnell, D.O.* Columbus, OH: Squirrel's Tail Press, 1994.
3. Barber E. *Osteopathy Complete*, 1898.
4. Hildreth A. *The Lengthening Shadow of Andrew Taylor Still*. Kirksville, MI: Simpson Printing, 1942.
5. Sutherland WG. *Teachings in the Science of Osteopathy*. Portland, OR: Rudra Press, 1990.
6. Weischenck J. *Traire D'Osteopathis Viscerale*. Paris: Malione, 1982.
7. Finet G, Williame C. *Treating Visceral Dysfunction*. Portland, OR: Stillness Press, 2000.
8. Barral JP. Visceral Manipulation, 1988; *Visceral Manipulation II*, 1989; *The Thorax*, 1991; *Manual Thermal Evaluation*, 1996. Seattle, WA: Eastland Press.
9. Robbins and Cotran. *Pathological Basis of Disease*. 7th Ed. Philadelphia, PA: Elsevier, 2005.
10. Blechschmidt E. *The Stages of Human Development before Birth*. Philadelphia, PA: W.B. Saunders Company, 1961.
11. Humphrey JD, Delance SL. *An Introduction to Biomechanics*. New York: Springer-Verlag, 2004.
12. Guyton AC, Hall JE. *Textbook of Medical Physiology*. 11th Ed. Philadelphia, PA: Elsevier Saunders, 2006.
13. Oschman J. *Energy Medicine: The Scientific Basis*. London: Churchill Livingston, 2000.
14. Hall S. *Basic Biomechanics*. 4th Ed. New York, NY: McGraw Hill, 2004.
15. Baldwin J. *Bucky Works: Buckminster Fuller's Ideas for Today*. New York, NY: John Wiley and Sons, 1996.
16. Gierada D. *Radiology*. 1995;194:879–884.
17. Fredrickson JO. *J Radiol*. 1995;195:169–175.
18. Chikly B. *Silent Waves*. 2nd Ed. Scottsdale, AZ: International Health and Healing Publishing, 2002.

52F Still Technique

RICHARD L. VAN BUSKIRK

> ## KEY CONCEPT
>
> In this section, emphasis is placed on introduction of a force vector resulting in a smooth arc carried toward the position of tissue compliance. The position is altered while maintaining this force, carrying it toward and through the position of restricted position and motion. Historically, this is described as a redevelopment of a manipulative method developed and used by Andrew Taylor Still.

CASE STUDY

A 47-year-old male presents with a complaint of pain, numbness, and tingling in his right hand and forearm that developed rather suddenly after a fall about 3 months ago. He states that his right hand appears much weaker than it used to be. He is right handed. He also admits that he has some pain in his right neck and dorsal shoulder since the fall. His symptoms have affected his ability to work (he is an accountant and uses computers daily), and over the past week, his sleep is disturbed.

X-rays of his shoulder were unremarkable but those of his neck showed mild C6-7 disc space narrowing and mild spondylotic changes involving C4-6. An electrophysiological study of his brachial plexus demonstrated no abnormalities, including specifically no evidence of conduction slowing across the wrist, eliminating carpal tunnel syndrome. An MRI of the cervical spine demonstrated mild degenerative discs in the lower cervical spine, spondylotic changes, but only a mild stenosis involving the left C5 and C6 foramen.

Past medical history includes being slightly overweight and asthma as a child. He denies any history of diabetes, thyroid disease, peripheral vascular disease, or neurological disease. He does not smoke and limits himself to one glass of wine whenever he and his wife have dinner at a restaurant. Review of systems reveals that he admits to occasional heartburn but only after eating spicy foods.

Physical Examination:

HEENT, GI, GU, Neuro—noncontributory. CV—positive Adson's right. The musculoskeletal examination reveals no tenderness or restriction of motion of the wrist (i.e., scaphoid and lunate bones), the elbow (radial head, medial, and lateral elbow condyles), and the anterior shoulder and clavicle. No joint restrictions are noted in the right arm although there is some tenderness over the coracoid process and proximal medial humerus with restrictions in shoulder anterior and anterior-lateral flexion indicating tightness in the pectoralis minor and major.

Examination of the cervical spine and first ribs identifies the following restrictions: AA is rotated right; C5 ERS right, C6 FRS left, C7 ERS and the right first rib head is superior, tender, noncompliant to compression, and immobile during exhalation. The left first rib head is relatively inferior at rest, tender, noncompliant to compression but immobile during inhalation. Thus, both first ribs are restricted, even though the only nerve compression symptoms are on the right. Spasm and tenderness are noted in the trapezius muscles and rectus capitus posterior superior bilaterally, and the right posterior and medial scalene muscles.

Other spinal segmental restrictions are T1 N SR RL, T3 FRS right, T4 ERS right, T6 ERS right, T10 ERS right, T11 FRS left, L2 FRS right, L3 ERS left, and L4 FRS right. The right innominate is anteriorly rotated and the sacrum shows fascial restrictions at the sacral sulcus and ILA on the left.

ASSESSMENT

1. Acute brachial plexopathy
2. Somatic dysfunction—OA, cervical thoracic, lumbar, sacrum, pelvis, and rib

PLAN

1. OMT to the above areas using Still technique

The restrictions producing the acute brachial plexopathy are most likely due to dysfunctions of the cervical spine or first rib. The possibility that this could represent a carpal tunnel syndrome related to his repetitive computer use has been eliminated as has the remote possibility of it representing a Pancoast's tumor in the lung apex.

HISTORY

The Still technique is a redevelopment of a manipulative method originally developed and used by the founder of osteopathic medicine, Dr. Andrew Taylor Still. The methodology was abstracted from a few quotes by one of Dr. Still's students and colleagues at the American School of Osteopathy, Hazzard, D.O. (4). The first modern statement of this recovered method was published in the *Journal of the American Osteopathic Association* in 1996 (18). Subsequently, a more up-to-date and complete description of the Still Technique and its many applications has been published (19). The attribution of the technique to Dr. Still has been repeatedly confirmed by applying Dr. Still's own quoted applications (ref) as well as being validated by the use of descriptive writings by other students of Dr. Still's students and colleagues (2,4,8,15,16).

The abstracted method of the Still technique had been described by Carl Phillip McConnell, D.O., Ph.D., and later by the author's

friend and mentor, Herb Yates, D.O., F.A.A.O., as "indirect and then direct." Currently, the method includes the following steps:

1. Evaluate the affected tissue and place it in its position of ease
2. Introduce a force vector to the affected tissue from another part of the body. This compression or traction should be less than 5 lb (2 kg)
3. Use the force vector to move the affected tissue initially into a smooth path to its position of ease and then alter the position while maintaining this force toward and through to the position of the restriction of position and movement
4. As the tissue moves through its restriction, a "bump" and/or a click may be felt or heard. Neither is necessary for correction of the somatic dysfunction
5. The region is passively moved back to neutral and retested

It is apparent that the Still technique shares components with a number of other manipulative methods in use in osteopathic medicine today. Its position of ease is comparable to the treatment position of Counterstrain (5). The restricted position through which the tissue is carried is identical to the positioning for muscle energy (3,9,10) and HVLA (3,20).

Still technique has even more in common with Facilitated Positional Release developed by Schiowitz, D.O., F.A.A.O. (11,12), although there are notable differences:

1. Still technique's position of ease is more exaggerated than FPR's "easy neutral."
2. Still technique requires movement of the affected tissue from its ease through the restriction. FPR does not require such movement although frequently its practitioners include a finishing movement into the range of the initial restriction

Among the manipulative techniques that Sutherland, D.O., taught besides cranial osteopathy are those "for the rest of the body." Although there is a range of different methods currently being taught as derived from Sutherland under the term ligamentous articular strain (refs), some are quite similar to the Still technique. Starting with the tissue placed at ease, compressions introduced into the tissue, and then that compressive force and myofascial unwinding are utilized to carry the tissue from ease past restriction. Sutherland himself commented that Dr. Still tended to use a rather more direct approach than what he was accustomed to using since Sutherland felt the tissue's own vitality should carry the tissue into release (ref). As with this and some of the other techniques (i.e., FPR, counterstrain, HVLA), the operating forces are all applied by the physician and the patient remains passive throughout.

Finally, there is the Still-Laughlin technique preserved and taught in the modern era by Edward Stiles, D.O., F.A.A.O. (personal communication; see also Ref. [19]). It is hypothesized that this advanced method was a development by Dr. Still toward the end of his life. It uses much of the same technique as the Still technique, but requires additional identification of the Key dysfunctions or areas of greatest restriction. These are addressed by subsequent stacking of each identified dysfunction into its position of ease on top of those lower in the body and then sequentially using the force vector to unwind the body through each dysfunction. It is an incredibly efficient method but requires a high degree of anatomical knowledge, diagnostic ability, kinesthetic appreciation, and intense concentration. As such, it is not considered a technique that is easily mastered.

The physiological and anatomical mechanisms thought to underlie the Still technique have been extensively discussed elsewhere (17,19). Basically, they are based on the concept that a somatic dysfunction develops and is maintained by a complex inter-action of neural elements, particularly the nociceptor and central nervous system repatterning (memory), myofascial repair mechanisms and elastic memory, and immunological, inflammatory, and vascular changes. The Still technique starts at ease, disarming the neurological protective mechanisms and relaxing the myofascial components. The force vector allows repatterning of the neuro-fascial-vascular complex in the same fashion that trauma originally triggered the somatic dysfunction but in a normalizing direction, freeing the tissue from its restriction.

The Still technique is used successfully to treat virtually all tissues of the body, including the cranium, spine, sacrum, pelvis, limbs, muscles, tendons, ligaments, and viscera. Its efficacy is only limited by the practitioner's knowledge of functional anatomy. As with most manipulative techniques, it is not advisable to use Still technique across recent wounds (surgical or otherwise) or fractures less than 6 weeks old. Since it utilizes minimal force, it is safe to use for patients of all ages.

Diagnostic methods used for the Still technique are similar to those used in determining muscle energy or HVLA diagnoses, although the *Still Technique Manual* (19) does give a number of practical shortcuts. The definitions of rib and sacral dysfunctions used in Still technique are different from those commonly in use (19).

In the case of an acute brachial plexopathy, such as is seen in the aforementioned case study, the primary focus is on the sites of possible restriction to the brachial plexus and as well to the areas of pain. Logically, one would also address and treat the lumbosacral somatic dysfunctions present since failure to do so could result in a recurrence of the cervical, thoracic, rib, and shoulder dysfunctions. However, space constraints preclude further discussion of treatment for the sacrum and pelvic bones.

TECHNIQUES

739.8: Rib Somatic Dysfunction

The superior right first rib dysfunction results in the position of the head of the first rib at ease in a superior position, while the costomanubrial connection will be relatively inferior. Positioning the neck into a flexed and side bent away position from the side of the superior first rib head will place that rib at ease. Its restriction will be with the neck extended and side bent to the same side as the affected first rib:

1. The patient is seated
2. The physician stands either facing or behind the patient
3. Place the monitoring hand so that the index finger is on the affected first rib head
4. Place the operating hand on the top of the patient's head
5. The head and neck are side bent and flexed toward the side opposite the affected first rib (left in this case). This position produces tissue relaxation over the rib head (Fig. 52F.1)
6. Introduce compression through the head in a vector toward the affected rib head
7. While maintaining the compression vector from the top of the patient's head, the patient's head and neck are moved into side bending toward the affected rib. Finally, extension is introduced. Alternately, one can start by carrying the head and neck into extension first and then into side bending toward the side of the elevated first rib. Either sequence may be effective (Fig. 52F.2)

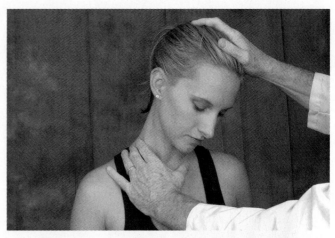

Figure 52F-1   Superior first rib, right, initial position.

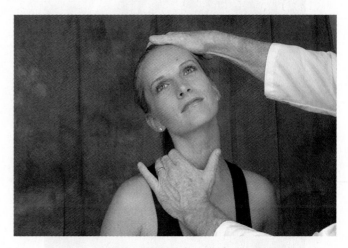

Figure 52F-2   Superior first rib, final position.

8. After release is noted, the head and neck are returned to neutral
9. The dysfunction is reassessed

If a first fib head is inferior, the position of ease will be with the neck side bent toward the side of the inferior rib head and extended down to the rib head. Treatment will carry the neck (and first rib head) into flexion and side bending away from the side of the inferior first rib.

739.2: Thoracic Somatic Dysfunction

Thoracic segmental dysfunctions seen in this case study include vertebrae below T1 or T2. Treatment can be performed in various positions. An example is T3 F RL SL:

1. The patient is seated on a table
2. The physician stands behind the patient
3. The pad of the index finger of the monitoring hand that of the same side as the somatic dysfunction is placed over the prominent transverse process of the affected segment
4. The physician's other arm is placed over the patient's opposite (right) shoulder around the superior chest wall and that hand is placed on the shoulder on the side of the somatic dysfunction (ease). This gives the physician adequate leverage to introduce the necessary flexion or extension, compression, side bending, and rotation

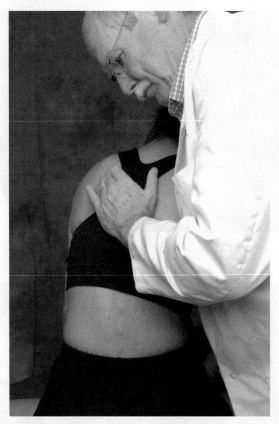

Figure 52F-3   T3 flexed, side bent, and rotated left. Initial position.

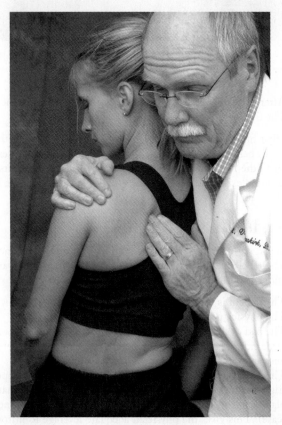

Figure 52F-4   T3 flexed, side bent, and rotated left. Final position.

5. The patient's thorax and spine are then flexed (in this case) and rotated toward the side of the somatic dysfunction (left) and compression introduced (Fig. 52F.3)
6. Once the tissues and transverse process have palpably relaxed, the operating arm simultaneously reduces flexion and rotates the spine through neutral and then into the previously restricted range (right side bending and rotation with extension) (Fig. 52F.4)
7. Compression is reduced and the patient is passively returned to neutral
8. The somatic dysfunction is reassessed

Extended thoracic somatic dysfunctions can be treated with the same method except that the spine is brought to an extended, side bent and rotated toward the side of ease position, the compression force vector is introduced, and the spine and the segment are carried into flexion, side bending and rotation toward the opposite side (restriction). It should be noted that this same method can be used throughout the lumbar spine as well.

REFERENCES

1. Arcasoy SM, Jett JR. Superior pulmonary sulcus tumors and Pancoast's syndrome. *N Engl J Med.* 1997;337:1370–1376.
2. Ashmore EF. *Osteopathic Mechanics.* Kirksville, MO: Journal Printing Company, 1915.
3. Greenman PE. *Principles of Manual Medicine.* 3rd Ed. Baltimore, MD: Lippincott Williams & Wilkins, 2003.
4. Hazzard C. *The Practice and Applied Therapeutics of Osteopathy.* 3rd Revised Ed. Kirksville, MO: Journal Printing Co., 1905.
5. Jones LH. *Strain & Counterstrain.* Newark, OH: American Academy of Osteopathy, 1981.
6. Kuchera M, Kuchera WM. *Osteopathic Principles in Practice.* 2nd Ed. Kirksville, MO: KCOM Press, 1991.
7. Kuchera M, Kuchera WM. *Osteopathic Considerations in Systemic Dysfunction.* Columbus, OH: Greydon Press, 1994.
8. McConnell CP. *The Practice of Osteopathy.* 2nd Ed. The Hammond Press, 1900.
9. Mitchell FL Jr, Mitchell PKG. *The Muscle Energy Manual.* Vols 1,2,3. East Lansing, MI: MET Press, 1995.
10. Mitchell FL Jr, Moran PS, Pruzzo NA. *An Evaluation and Treatment Manual of Osteopathic Muscle Energy Procedures.* Valley Park, MO: Mitchell, Moran, and Pruzzo, Associates, 1979.
11. Schiowitz S. Facilitated positional release. *JAOA.* 1990;90:145–155.
12. Schiowitz S, DiGiovanna EL, Dowling DJ. Facilitated positional release techniques. In: Robert CW, ed. *Foundations for Osteopathic Medicine.* 2nd Ed. Philadelphia, PA: Lippincott Williams & Wilkins, 2003:1017–1025.
13. Speece CR, Crow WT. *Ligamentous Articular Strain.* Seattle, WA: Eastland Press, 2006.
14. Still AT. *Osteopathy, Research & Practice.* Kirksville, MO: Eastland Press, 1910. (Reprinted by Eastland Press, Seattle, WA, 1992.)
15. Sutherland WG. Contributions of thought. In: Sutherland AS, Wales AL, eds. *The Sutherland Cranial Teaching Foundation.* Portland, OR: Ruda Press, 1998.
16. Sutherland WG. *The Cranial Bowl.* USA: Free Press, Co., 1939 (reprinted, 1994).
17. Van Buskirk RL. Nocioceptive reflexes and the somatic dysfunction: a model. *JAOA* 1990;90:792–809.
18. Van Buskirk RL. A manipulative technique of Andrew Taylor Still. *JAOA* 1996;96:597–602.
19. Van Buskirk RL. *The Still Technique Manual.* 2nd Ed. Indianapolis, IN: The American Academy of Osteopathy, 2006.
20. Walton WJ. *Textbook of Osteopathic Diagnosis and Technique Procedures.* Newark, OH: The American Academy of Osteopathy, 1972.

52G | Chapman's Approach

CHRISTIAN FOSSUM, MICHAEL L. KUCHERA, WILLIAM H. DEVINE, AND KENDALL WILSON

KEY CONCEPT

In this section, emphasis is placed on identification of gangliform contractions believed to be fascial congestions resulting from lymph stasis secondary to visceral dysfunction. These contractions are generally deep to the skin and subcutaneous tissue, most often lying on the deep fascia or periosteum. Generally described as neurolymphatic points, vibratory stimulation is utilized for reduction/elimination of the points.

CASE STUDY

A 34-year-old female presented to the office with complaints of gastrointestinal (GI) upset, nausea, and vomiting. The nausea and vomiting started suddenly 7 days ago and has continued "on and off." She was seen in the ED 3 days ago and a diagnosis of early viral gastroenteritis was made. The medicine prescribed had helped the nausea, but the patient continued to have vomiting, fatigue, and weakness. She complained of abdominal pain that was diffuse, sharp, and cramping with eating. She denied fever or chills.

Physical examination revealed a lethargic female with vital signs of $T = 98.0$, $P = 112$, $R = 20$, B/P = 110/80 (normal for the patient was 80+/60). Abdominal examination revealed suprapubic tenderness to palpation. There was no hepatomegaly. Structural exam revealed a tender Chapman's reflex (CR) on the *anterior sternum* consistent with pylorus. The blood sugar was normal at 73 mg/dL. The urine dipstick revealed a high specific gravity of greater than 1.030. The pH was 6.0. There were moderate-large ketones along with 2+ urobilogen and a trace of bilirubin.

Diagnosis:
Vomiting with Dehydration

Plan:
The patient was admitted to the hospital for further workup and rehydration. The patient had a complete workup that included abdominal and pelvic ultrasounds and an upper GI. Other than dehydration, all findings were normal except for "mild swelling of the duodenum" on the UGI, which was reported as a "nonspecific finding." She was treated with IV fluid replacement. The patient was discharged on the third hospital day. Her discharge diagnosis was gastroenteritis with fluid depletion and dehydration.

Her physician continued to treat the patient weekly for headaches using cranial osteopathy. At each of these weekly visits, the patient would report that her GI problem was "getting better." Each time, the CRs on the sternum remained tender—indicating pyloric stenosis (although not always at the same intensity of discomfort as originally noted).

After 11 weeks, the physician performed another regional screen for CR. Again, there was a positive reflex for pyloric stenosis, but also positive reflexes for stomach peristalsis and stomach acidity. The patient finally admitted that she really had not been able to keep much food down since leaving the hospital.

The patient was referred to an osteopathic internist for reevaluation. Endoscopy revealed pyloric valve swelling and constriction necessitating the use of a pediatric endoscope to examine the duodenum. A new diagnosis of prepyloric antral ulcer was made.

In this case, CRs identified the problem almost 3 months *before* the definitive diagnosis was made by endoscopic evaluation. Although the original diagnostic workup was negative, only the CRs consistently pointed to the correct diagnosis 2 months prior to reevaluation. CRs correlate well with her final diagnosis.

DEFINING CRs

The palpable tissue texture phenomenon known as a *Chapman's reflex* has a rich history, appreciating the historical evolution of its definition and integration by different practitioners, and provides a better understanding of how today we locate, interpret, and clinically use this somatic finding. The current definition used by the osteopathic profession defines CRs as "a system of reflex points that present as predictable anterior and posterior fascial tissue texture abnormalities (plaque-like changes or stringiness of the involved tissues) assumed to be reflections of visceral dysfunction or pathology" (ECOP, 2006). This definition encompasses the lymphatic, neuroendocrine, and autonomic response to injury, illness, and disease as palpable and predictable viscerosomatic tissue reflexes found on the anterior and posterior body surface. Historically, definitions of the CR point reflect its structural feel linked to an evolving speculation as to the underlying dysfunction causing it (Table 52G.1).

Several mechanisms for the CR points have been proposed by those who value their use empirically. These include lymphatic abnormalities, fibrositis deposits, inflamed lymph vessels passing over ribs and bones, inflamed nerve endings, and inflamed sympathetic nerve filaments around terminal arterioles (Ketchum, 1943). Thus, it can be seen that lymphatic, neuroendocrine, and autonomic interactions were considered to be a part of CRs from early on.

HISTORICAL BACKGROUND

Early osteopathic medicine emphasized the role of the nervous system and body fluids in health and disease. Somatic dysfunctions of the musculoskeletal system were considered to be anatomical abnormalities obstructing these physiological processes, and through these structure and function considerations, osteopathic manipulation was employed to assist the body's recovery from injuries, illnesses, and disease (Deason, 1940; Hulett, 1922; Still, 1899, 1902, 1910). This was the prevailing philosophy when Frank Chapman (1871 to 1931) enrolled at the American School

TABLE 52G.1

Historical Definitions of CR

Definition	Author
The original description of *Ganglion-formed* became *Gangliform contracted lymphoid tissue nodules*	Frank Chapman, D.O. 1928
"It seemed to me that the lymphatic system had much more profound influence on bodily functions than it had been given credit for … my special plea is on behalf of the lymphatic aspects of disease, which I regard of paramount importance whether they originated in bony lesions, infections, toxins, or other cause."	Frank Chapman, D.O. 1937
"A Chapman lesion is the result of a lymph stasis in the viscus. This lymph stasis is responsible for the dysfunction of the organ. Both the lymph stasis and the resultant dysfunction are reflexly responsible for the Chapman lesion, due, in part, to nerve impulse and also to a chemical reaction of the lymphoid tissue in which the lesion is found"	Charles Owens, D.O. 1944
"I believe that it is an autonomic nerve reflex, and that the lesion or nodule is a granulation tissue reaction"	H.L. Samblanet, D.O. 1944

of Osteopathy in Kirksville, Missouri. After graduating in 1899, he returned to Galesburg, Illinois, where he practiced until his death (Samblanet, 1944). In 1901, Chapman had a patient with severe adenitis whose response to osteopathic treatment directed to the spine was slow. He noticed that the groin glands and those on the medial side of the thighs were indurated and painful, and he decided to gently manipulate these glands and nothing else. When the patient returned, his improvement was such that he confined the treatment solely to the manipulation of these indurated areas. This observation led Chapman to a more detailed study of the lymphatic system and its role in health and disease (Lippincott, 1946). Building on his osteopathic knowledge, which at that time lacked a detailed discourse on the lymphatic system, Chapman came across *Mechanical Vibratory Stimulation* published by Maurice F. Pilgrim, M.D., in 1901. This seminal text emphasized the capacity for mechanical stimulation of reflex centers to influence body fluids and lymphatic drainage, thereby affecting a variety of physiological functions such as respiration, digestion, secretion, excretion, and muscular metabolism (Pilgrim, 1903; Lippincott, 1946). Though Pilgrim's method of treatment differed from Chapman's, it was likely to have provided him with the inspiration that eventually led to the conception of *lymphatic* or *CRs*.

Encouraged by positive clinical outcomes, Chapman diligently began making observations and case records. He mapped the congested lymphatic areas that he found in consistent locations close to the body surface and, believing that they bore a physiological relation to the lymphatic and nervous system, referred to them as *neurolymphatic points*. By the late 1920s, Chapman located over 200 centers on the body surface and established their association with the visceral and endocrine glands (Lippincott, 1946). He published his observations and the first chart in his 1929 text *Lymphatic reflexes: a specific method of osteopathic diagnosis and treatment* (Chapman, 1929).

Charles Owens, D.O., was Chapman's brother-in-law and classmate at the American School of Osteopathy. He had little involvement in the development of the CR system until close to Chapman's death. Owens asked Chapman's clinical opinion on an encumbering dizziness that was troubling him. He was intrigued by the manner in which Chapman diagnosed and relieved the ailment. Owens encouraged Chapman to chart the specific reflex lesion areas for the wider use by the osteopathic profession, a task completed shortly before Chapman's death (Samblanet, 1944). The

concept of the CRs was introduced to the osteopathic community in an article penned by Owens (1930):

"In this connection, I am glad to draw attention to the conclusions of an osteopathic physician, Dr. Frank Chapman of Galesburg, IL. As a result of years of research and study, Dr. Chapman advances the idea that in addition to the well-known spinal and sympathetic nervous system, with its controlling nerve centers, there lies within this same system an independent group of gangliform centers which control the activities of the lymphatic system in its relation to the viscera of the body, the knowledge of which enables the practitioner to determine with the utmost precision and accuracy the exact state of the various organs of the body.... That this information will be received with profound interest by that portion of the profession who have given much attention to the spleen and lymph flow in their practices, goes without saying… That the ability to be able to tell his patient, for example, by the condition of one of these lymphatic centers, that he has a markedly disturbed condition of the hydrochloric secretions of the stomach; or, that the muscular action of the stomach is retarded by the state of another of these same centers, or, that he has a highly acid condition of the blood, due to a stenosis of the pyloric orifice holding the contents of the stomach against normal ejection until, by the continued accumulation of hydrochloric acid, the pylorus is compelled to open and permit some of the stomach content to pass, and do all this by these centers in place of having to resort to test meals, x-rays, etc., is hard to believe."

After Chapman's death, Owens continued developing the system and organized several postgraduate teaching seminars. Owens recognized CRs as viscerosomatic tissue reflexes and believed them to be a result of a lymph stasis in the viscus, which he hypothesized was the cause of the organ dysfunction. He proposed the causative factor to be pelvic girdle somatic dysfunctions interfering with the blood and nerve supply to the gonads, triggering a cascade of endocrine responses. Owens named this cascade the *pelvic-thyroid* (with adrenals) *syndrome* (Owens, 1937, 1943)—later renamed the *pelvic-thyroid-adrenal*, or *PTA syndrome* (Arbuckle, 1947). The thyroid was central to this syndrome and its involvement was considered to result in a widespread metabolic disturbance causing incomplete oxidation in cells, body fluids to move slowly, and lymphatic engorgement leading to retention of toxins. The area of least resistance in the body would develop a local lymph stasis through nerve impulses and chemical reactions of the lymphoid tissue (Owens believed acetylcholine to be involved), and would result in a positive corresponding CR point on the body surface (Owens, 1940). As a treatment approach, addressing CRs was proposed to deal directly with the disturbed body metabolism through the autonomic nervous system, the lymphatic system and the endocrine glands, and the treatment would help normalize endocrine secretions, augment flow of body fluids, and release inhibited trophic (nutritional) centers.

Paul E. Kimberly, D.O., F.A.A.O., first organized CRs into a course for the profession, but it was never offered. In the late 1970s, Kimberly integrated CRs into osteopathic physical examination teachings during his tenure at the Kirksville College of Osteopathic Medicine. Based on the apparent correlation with the tissue texture changes occurring at the anatomic sites where the cutaneous vascular-lymphatic bundle exited together with the anterior and lateral cutaneous nerves (Figs. 52G.1 and 52G.2), and like Chapman and Owens, he used the term *neurolymphatic points* to describe them but presented them to his students as viscerosomatic reflexes related to the facilitated segment concept work of faculty colleagues, Korr and Denslow.

Subsequently, other osteopathic educators tended to describe the reflexes as more highly correlated with the sympathetic nervous system rather than the lymphatic system, indicating that this treatment influences visceral function by acting on some part of a reflex arc (Patriquin, 1992). In the previous edition of the *Foundations* text, Patriquin expresses some discomfort with his earlier attempt at defining these points as being sympathetically mediated findings in and of themselves (Patriquin, 2003). Other authors have classified CRs as part of the palpatory findings in a viscerosomatic reflex level involvement, pointing to the consistency in both the location of the CRs and of the sympathetic innervation of the dysfunctional organ (Kuchera and Kuchera, 1994). In the opinion of one of the authors (MLK), defining a tissue texture abnormality as a CR without the evidence of other concomitant visceral or viscerosomatic findings may be less reliable.

LOCATING AND PALPATING CRs

CRs are manifested by gangliform contractions, which are believed to be congestions within fascia due to lymph stasis secondary to visceral dysfunction (Capobianco, 2004). The types of visceral dysfunction believed to cause positive CRs are inflammation, spasm, or distention of the viscera (Wilson, 2006). The reflexes are located deep to the skin and subcutaneous areolar tissue, most often lying on the deep fascia or periosteum (Patriquin, 1997, 2003). It is mostly found in specific locations with a size varying from a "BB" pellet to a pea, or from a pinhead to an almond, and have certain recognizable palpatory characteristics (Capobianco, 2004; Patriquin, 2003; Samblanet, 1944). Owens described them as follows (Owens, 1943):

- Gangliform
- Edematous
- Ridge-like or ropy
- Fibrospongy
- Shotty

The technique best used for palpation might depend on the location of the CR points (e.g., see Table 52G.2). For instance, in cases where the points are located on the transverse processes of vertebrae, there might be contracted muscles overlying the Chapman's point. Remember that its location in many cases is in the deep fascia or periosteum, and it may be necessary to first relax the overlying muscle to effectively treat the CR point (Hinckley-Chapman and Owens, 1932; Owens, 1943). The patient usually feels tenderness ranging from slightly painful to almost unbearably painful. There may however be a few patients who show no tenderness response to even firm digital pressure, although the CR point is palpable (Owens, 1943). It is unknown if this is related to the visceral dysfunction being in early or chronic stages, if the patient's pain threshold is very high, or if it is just a coincidental finding with no bearing at all. Historically, it has been proposed that the intensity of pain denotes the relative amount of involvement of the related organ, and the complete lack of pain denotes a process of long duration and very marked involvement (Brown, 1949). It has also been suggested that the absence of tenderness in the point might indicate abnormal hypofunction of the associated organ (Mitchell, 1974). For a CR point to be positive, both the anterior and the posterior CR should be present (Lippincott, 1946). It is generally recommended to initially use the anterior CR for diagnostic purposes as their consistency in location and the fact that they are more widespread than the posterior CR points. This eliminates the confusion as to which organ is involved (Brown, 1949). Once a positive anterior CR has been established,

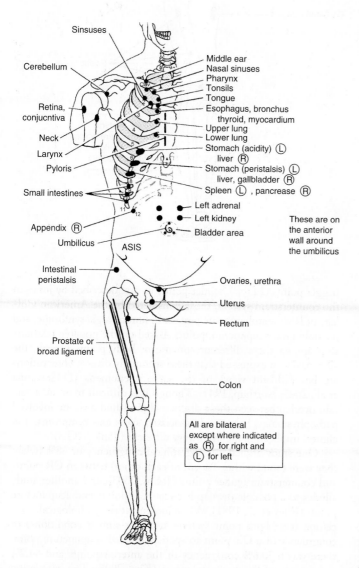

Figure 52G-1   Anterior CR points.

Figure 52G-2   Posterior Chapman points.

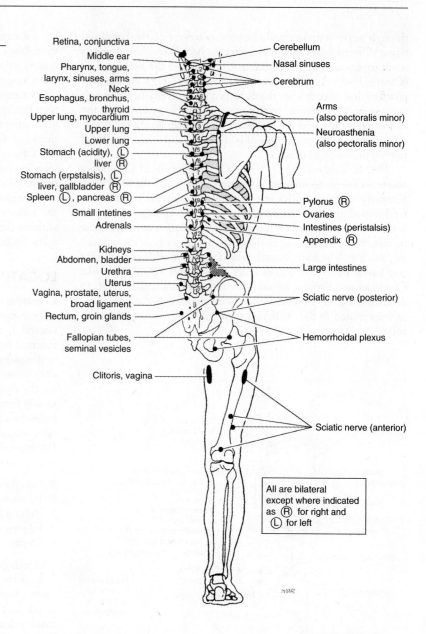

its diagnosis is confirmed through the presence of a posterior CR (Lippincott, 1946).

When examining for CRs, the use of the chart to know the specified location of each CR point together with well-developed tactile skills to discriminate the findings from either normal or other abnormalities, combined with the patient's presenting complaint and medical history, will typically yield best results.

SIMILARITIES AND DIFFERENCES BETWEEN OTHER PALPABLY SIMILAR POINTS

Palpable tissue texture changes appearing in the myofascial tissues have long been described and mapped—in the case of acupuncture points, for thousands of years. Their clinical use, interpretation, and even their names are often dependent upon the perspective of the health care provider who finds and groups them together based on the perception of a commonality. Yet between grouping systems (and even within some systems), there are significant differences that distinguish that set of somatic body points from the others.

Osteopathic physicians should attempt to differentiate between various tissue texture abnormalities, including CRs, myofascial

trigger points (MTrP), tender points as first described by Jones in the counterstrain system, those considered by the American College of Rheumatology to be present in fibromyalgia syndrome, and possibly even acupuncture points. Based on the possible relationship among these different somatic or body point systems, the view has been expressed that these seemingly diverse observations are but different views of the same phenomena (DiGiovanna et al., 2005; Northup, 1941). Though it is difficult to argue a certain overlap between these discrete clinical findings, the involved pathophysiology, pattern of associated signs and symptoms, and clinical implication are often very different (Table 52G.3).

One study argued a topographical congruency of 68% (when they were found within 1.5 cm of each other) between CR points and counterstrain tender points (Johns, 2003), and another study alludes to a possible overlap between CR points and acupuncture points (Riley et al., 1981). When looking at the pathological association (e.g., both point systems used for similar conditions) or congruency of a CR point to spatially related acupuncture point, there was a 20.6% congruency of the anterior points and 44.2% congruency of the posterior points (Kim, 2008). The correlation between MTrP and acupuncture points has also been investigated.

TABLE 52G.2

Examples of Palpatory Techniques for Various CR Points

CR Point	Palpatory Technique
Broad ligament (female) and prostate (male)	Deep kneading pressure with lift (should be longitudinal), fingers flexed toward palm of hand
Colon	
Ovarian	Deep pressure with longitudinal rotary movement
Kidneys	Gentle rotary movement
Adrenals	Deep firm rotary movement
Duodenum	Deep firm rotary movement
Stomach	Gentle but firm rotary movement
Spleen	Firm rotary movement
Small intestine	Firm rotary movement
Eye	Gentle but firm rotary movement
Ear	Gentle but firm rotary movement
Throat, nasal, bronchial, pharynx, larynx,	Gentle rotary movement
Esophagus, tongue	Firm rotary movement
Upper and lower lung	Deep firm rotary movement
Arms	Deep firm rotary movement
Neuritis of the upper limb	Deep firm rotary movement (sometimes steady pressure)
Cerebellar	Firm but gently rotary movement
Cerebral	Gentle rotary movement
Heart	Firm gentle rotary movement
Neurasthenia	Firm deep rotary movement
Atonic constipation	Deep firm rotary movement
Appendix	Gentle rotary movement
Urethral	Deep but gentle rotary movement
Cystitis	Deep but gentle rotary movement
Sciatic–neuritis	Firm and deep rotary movement
Wry neck	Firm rotary movement
Thyroid	Deep rotary movement
Gallbladder and liver	Firm but gentle rotary movement

Source: Adapted from Owens (1943)

Palpation should be directed and titrated to reach the tissue depth and location where the tissue texture change resides. Examples using the more diagnostically suited anterior points are as follows:

- Intercostal Sites (including sinus, bronchus, stomach): finger pad directed posterosuperiorly along undersurface of the rib searching with a deep, firm rotatory movement (examine adjacent sites using a little longitudinal glide along the undersurface of the rib rather than a poking or prodding motion)
- Anterior Point Chart: Tip of floating rib (example appendix): Deep but gentle rotator stimulation at tip of rib using finger pad
- Anterior Point Chart: Abdominal wall (including kidney, bladder): Compress with finger pad through subcutaneous fat and tissues until reaching the deepest layer of the abdominal wall and there use a deep, firm, rotatory motion
- Anterior Point Chart: Pelvis (including ovary and uterus): Use deep, firm, rotatory movement approximating the periosteal level of the pelvic bone
- Anterior Point Chart: Iliotibial band region (including colon and prostate): Deep kneading pressure with lift (should be longitudinal), fingers flexed toward palm of hand; finger pads should compress medially approximating the periosteal level of the lateral femur
- Posterior Point Chart (Paraspinal): Deep firm rotatory pressure midway between transverse processes of the vertebral segment involved and the segment below; lateral distance from the spinous process is about halfway to the tip of the transverse process ipsilateral to the side of the involved organ. Tissue characteristics will involve more bogginess than the anterior points.

Source: Adapted from Kuchera MA. A pragmatic interpretation of Chapman reflexes. *AM Acad osteopath*. 2008.

TABLE 52G.3

CR Points, MTrP and Tender Points

	Location	Palpatory Quality	Pain Characteristics	Association	Classic Treatment
Chapman reflex	Located in soft-tissue structures: subcutaneous tissue, fascia, muscle, ligament, and perichondral or periosteal tissue. Mostly in deep fascia or periosteum.	Granular feel of tissues overlying the CR. The CR itself is gangliaform, contracted, edematous, ridge-like or ropy, fibrospongy, or shotty. Varying in size from a pinhead to that of an almond	Tenderness ranging from slightly painful to almost unbearable. It is well localized under the finger and has an almost sharp quality. No pain radiation.	Viscerosomatic tissue reflex with definite relationship to viscus or gland; pattern of associated somatic dysfunction includes somatic dysfunction in related collateral ganglion, paraspinal tissues (same facilitated segment) and perhaps cranial or sacral referral site of viscus	Rotary stimulation for 20–60 s
MTrP	Central MTrP in fibers in the midportion of muscle. Attachment MTrP in the myotendinous junction. Depth varies with muscles	Distinct nodules (contraction knots) at the MTrP felt in the muscle and a rope-like indulation (taut band)	Localized pain in taut band of muscle with referred pain to a characteristic distant region based on myofascial referral maps	Local pathophysiology in the muscle exhibiting the MTrP. May cause motion restriction in associated joints; often stimulation of point causes taut band twitch	Injection, dry needling, ischemic compression, postisometric relaxation (MET), spray and stretch, counterstrain
Tender point	Typically located in tendinous attachments, in the belly of a muscle, or in the ligaments associated with a joint dysfunction	Discrete, small, tense, and edematous, about the size of a fingertip	Exquisitely tender, very localized with no pain radiation. Typically at least four times as tender as the adjacent tissues	Specific muscle or joint somatic dysfunction	Counterstrain

One study looked at the overlap (positive correlation was when the points were found within 3 cm of each other) between MTrP and acupuncture pain points (Ah Shu), showing a 71% correlation based on spatial orientation of points and pain patterns (Melzack et al., 1977). The results of these studies should be interpreted with caution as the definition of correlation or congruency differs between the authors (e.g., 1.5 to 3 cm).

It should be noted that MTrP have the ability to create altered neural, autonomic, vascular, and lymphatic changes as well, and a number of MTrP with viscerosomatic and somatovisceral reflex activity have been reported in the literature (McPartland, 2004; Travell and Simons, 1999). Several MTrP linked to GI, cardiac, and genitourinary dysfunctions are identical to or in close proximity to the sites of CRs from these organs. Treatment of MTrP now embraces use of multiple interventions from dry needling to osteopathic treatment modalities such as muscle energy and counterstrain. Travell and Simons reported treatment of an MTrP located in the lower anterior chest wall (diagrammatically consistent with the pattern of palpatory findings that might be recorded by an osteopathic physician who found celiac ganglion and stomach CR dysfunction). In treating this point, the following was reported: "Pain, which previously had responded to medical therapy for a duodenal ulcer, became unresponsive and persisted until MTrP in the abdominal musculature were found and inactivated" (Travell and Simons, 1999).

The system now called *Applied Kinesiology* was developed in the 1960s by chiropractor George Goodheart who initially based his system upon applying the muscle testing of physical therapists Kendall and Kendall to the location of Chapman's "neurolymphatic" points. Later, this system added Bennett's points for vascular function and has since expanded to include acupuncture meridians (Kendall and Kendall, 1971; Walther et al., 1988).

A given point in a given system does not need to "read a book" to know where it should or could be; it simply exists. This means that a number of these existing points end up in multiple systems. Their clinical use and interpretation—along with their names—are often dependent upon the perspective of their discoverer. The evolution of CRs is no different. The points were grouped by an osteopathic practitioner reasoning from anatomy and physiology to see their somatic relationship to underlying visceral or systemic dysfunction. Their clinical diagnostic and therapeutic use is still based upon physicians applying them within the major osteopathic models of care and weighing the risk to benefit ratio of doing so.

DIAGNOSTIC UTILITY

Many osteopathic physicians use CRs as part of a screening or comprehensive osteopathic physical examination, contributing to the differential diagnosis and implying dysfunction of an organ system rather than as a therapeutic intervention (Patriquin, 2003). This said, because many modalities can be used to directly treat these points, it is important to perform a complete or focused diagnostic screen prior to any use of physical therapy or preparatory OMT (such as soft-tissue massage) that might temporarily reduce their sensitivity or tissue texture characteristics. One of the authors (KW) has formulated two principles when it comes to using CRs as a diagnostic tool: (1) a nontender CR, *by itself*, indicates nothing. *Never* make a diagnosis based solely on a nontender CR, and (2) *Never* ignore or trivialize a tender CR unless you have a good explanation for the findings. (This is especially true of a persistently tender reflex.)

From a diagnostic perspective and particularly in the hospital, they are more likely to be used selectively, as in the 30- or 45-seconds CR screening examinations (Figs. 52G.3 and 52G.4),

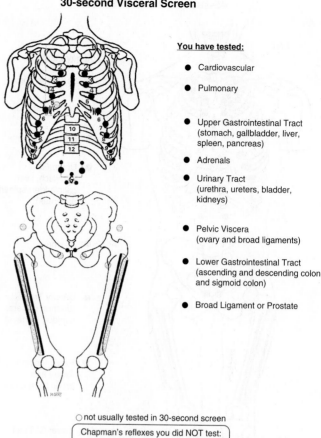

30-second Visceral Screen

You have tested:

- Cardiovascular
- Pulmonary
- Upper Gastrointestinal Tract (stomach, gallbladder, liver, spleen, pancreas)
- Adrenals
- Urinary Tract (urethra, ureters, bladder, kidneys)
- Pelvic Viscera (ovary and broad ligaments)
- Lower Gastrointestinal Tract (ascending and descending colon and sigmoid colon)
- Broad Ligament or Prostate

○ not usually tested in 30-second screen

Chapman's reflexes you did NOT test:		
URI (But you could--see chart marked ENT)		
Cerebellum	Tongue	Thyroid
Middle ear	Neck	Upper limb

Figure 52G-3   30 second visceral screen.

which is a time-effective screen that focuses on selected organ systems and in conjunction with other findings in the history and physical examination of the patient. The following case study illustrates the use of CRs in establishing a diagnosis.

Case Study

A 13-year-old female is admitted to the pediatric floor of an osteopathic teaching hospital for complaints of severe lower abdominal/pelvic pain. She is examined and is found to be tender in the RLQ and midline pelvis. Urinalysis is normal. In this age group, the three most likely diagnoses to consider (in no particular order) are as follows: (1) Appendicitis, (2) Cystitis, and (3) Ovarian cysts.

CRs showed bilateral tender reflexes on the anterior/medial pubic bones near the pubic symphysis and unilateral posterior CRs at T9-10 on the right side only. No other positive CRs were found in that region of the body (particularly those associated with the right kidney, urinary bladder, or appendix):

- Preoperative diagnosis (without the use of CRs): Appendicitis versus right ovarian cyst (50/50 probability)
- Preoperative diagnosis (with the use of CRs): Problem with right ovary involving the entire ovary—both the medial and the lateral halves
- Postoperative diagnosis: Massive right ovarian cyst obliterating the entire right ovary

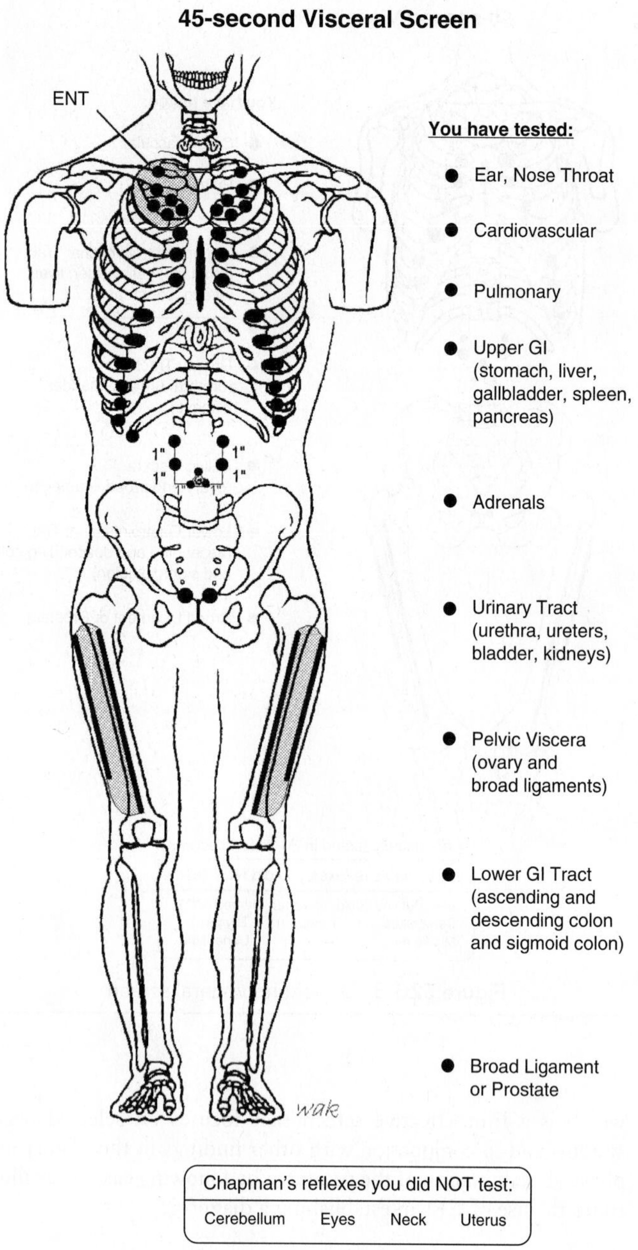

45-second Visceral Screen

You have tested:

- Ear, Nose Throat
- Cardiovascular
- Pulmonary
- Upper GI (stomach, liver, gallbladder, spleen, pancreas)
- Adrenals
- Urinary Tract (urethra, ureters, bladder, kidneys)
- Pelvic Viscera (ovary and broad ligaments)
- Lower GI Tract (ascending and descending colon and sigmoid colon)
- Broad Ligament or Prostate

Chapman's reflexes you did NOT test:			
Cerebellum	Eyes	Neck	Uterus

Figure 52G-4 45 second visceral screen.

The operation performed was a right oophrectomy and right salpingectomy. This case also serves to illustrate the *high degree of specificity* that can be obtained in diagnosing visceral pathology in certain internal organs. It also illustrates the most common use of CRs by osteopathic physicians in the present day—as a *differentiator* when the physician has narrowed the differential diagnosis to two or three possible conditions.

The preoperative prediction of right ovarian involvement was based on the fact that all of the patient's discomfort and tenderness to palpation was to the right of midline in the lower abdominal/pelvic region. As mentioned above, there were bilateral tender Chapman's points on the anterior medial pubis although unilateral posterior CRs on the right. With paired organs where only one organ is dysfunctional, but the dysfunctional organ is associated with a marked degree of pathology, the physician may occasionally encounter a bilateral Chapman response (especially with the anterior points).

Additional palpatory information to help in the differential diagnosis would include tight, tender superior mesenteric ganglion site (not present when the pubic ramus point is secondary to AL5 counterstrain point) and somatic dysfunction (especially ERS_R at T10 or T11).

The use of CRs has also been used to augment other forms of osteopathic patient evaluation. Visceral dysfunctions in terms of *mobility* and *motility* are usually detected through the careful palpatory evaluation of the body cavities. Because of the depth and partial inaccessibility of some structures, it is not uncommon to have an approximate diagnosis where the presence (and relative severity grading of >1) of CRs can help to specifically determine the structure with dysfunction, or differentiate in terms of relevance between two or more diagnosed dysfunctions.

Example

The spinal region of T5-9 had increased sudomotor activity. There was increased tension in the paravertebral muscles and motion restrictions indicating a single type II (extended, rotated, and side bent right) segment within the otherwise type I (side bent left and rotated right) group curve in this region. These findings led to the conclusion that the somatic dysfunction was secondary to viscerosomatic reflex activity. With the patient supine and doing a local listening technique to the abdominal tissue, the palpating hand was drawn toward the upper right abdominal quadrant. Palpation into the quadrant below the border of the ribs revealed tension and tenderness around the liver, gallbladder, lesser omentum, and the hepatic flexure of the colon. Testing the elasticity of the fascial-ligamentous structures as well as the movement of the structures on their sliding surfaces indicated visceral dysfunctions involving the lesser omentum, liver, and gallbladder. Proceeding to using CRs, the physician found positive points for both the liver and the gallbladder, and the CR point to the gallbladder was significantly more positive than the liver CR, leading the physician to conclude that the visceral dysfunction responsible for the viscerosomatic reflex activity was the gallbladder.

INTEGRATING CRs IN THE CLINICAL SETTING

Incorporation of CRs does not constitute a stand-alone approach. Its diagnostic and therapeutic usefulness depends on its integration with a more comprehensive osteopathic management strategy. The lymphatic system should be addressed by removing obstructions to lymph return and techniques to augment lymph flow. Somatic dysfunctions of the thorax and the pelvis should be treated to reduce autonomic interference caused by segmental facilitation. Respiratory efficiency should be restored by addressing rib cage mechanics and muscles of respiration. The patient's overall energy expenditure should be reduced by improving overall biomechanical and postural function. Addressing these factors together with CRs is a useful tool in improving musculoskeletal and systemic function as well as reducing the patient's overall allostatic load.

In the original teachings of CRs, the following points were emphasized when using this system for diagnosis and treatment (Owens, 1943):

- Know the exact anatomical location of each CR and its clinical significance
- Do not overtreat the CR: 15 to 30 or 30 to 60 seconds is enough time for each center
- Sequence your treatment
  - Address biomechanical dysfunctions of the pelvic girdle first
  - Treat the CR comprising the pelvic-thyroid-adrenal syndrome (PTA syndrome)

- Treat the CR corresponding with organs of elimination to reduce load placed on the body from the overall osteopathic treatment of the case at hand
  - Treat the specifically involved CR
- Do not forget assessment and treatment of the lymphatic system, especially involved regions of impaired lymphatic drainage
- Articulatory treatment to the axial spine and ribs to reduce normalize sympathetic activity
- After reestablishing the "endocrine" balance through CR, other somatic dysfunctions can be treated

It is important to keep in mind that this recommendation was made in the 1930s and 1940s, and even though the general principles might still be applicable today, the evolution of osteopathic treatment models has allowed for its reinterpretation. Excessive manipulative intervention is recognized as a potential body stressor: procedures employed prior to the use of CR treatment should be administered judiciously, specifically and with restraint (Mitchell, 1974). The algorithm in Figure 52G.5 serves to illustrate how CRs could be integrated in a clinical setting.

SPECIFIC TREATMENT USING CRs

There are several possible approaches commonly employed to treat patients using the CRs (Table 52G.4):

1. The original recommendation by Chapman was to start with the anterior points and then proceed to the posterior ones. He stated that treating the anterior points first would greatly aid in the treatment of the posterior points. Chapman's original protocol warned against excessive pressure and he wrote that gentler means rather than forceful pressure would result in quicker relaxation (Chapman, 1928)
2. If the points are too sensitive to be palpated and treated, myofascial release of the tissue around the gangliform area can help drainage be more comfortably established, which in turn can make it possible to treat the point directly (Lippincott, 1946)
3. If the anterior points were too sensitive to treat, OMT to the soft tissues posteriorly often decreases or even totally dissipates the related anterior points; the residual change then only needing minimal treatment. For this reason, however, use of preparatory soft-tissue methods that temporally negate the presence of the anterior points for diagnosis should be avoided (Kuchera, 1994)

PATTERNS OF CRs IN CLINICAL CONDITIONS

After having completed the osteopathic evaluation of the patient, the physician will typically sequence their osteopathic manipulative treatment based on the pattern of dysfunctions present in the

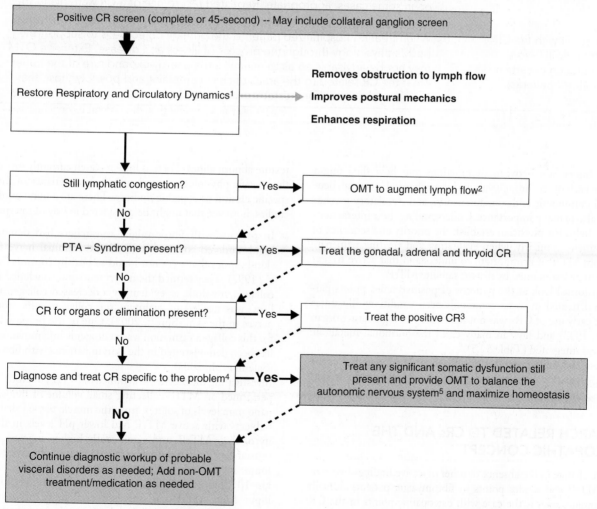

Algorithm for Integrated Chapman's Reflexes Treatment

Positive CR screen (complete or 45-second) -- May include collateral ganglion screen

Restore Respiratory and Circulatory Dynamics[1]
→ Removes obstruction to lymph flow
Improves postural mechanics
Enhances respiration

Still lymphatic congestion? — Yes → OMT to augment lymph flow[2]
No ↓
PTA – Syndrome present? — Yes → Treat the gonadal, adrenal and thryoid CR
No ↓
CR for organs or elimination present? — Yes → Treat the positive CR[3]
No ↓
Diagnose and treat CR specific to the problem[4] — Yes → Treat any significant somatic dysfunction still present and provide OMT to balance the autonomic nervous system[5] and maximize homeostasis
No ↓
Continue diagnostic workup of probable visceral disorders as needed; Add non-OMT treatment/medication as needed

Figure 52G-5 Algorithm for integrated CRs treatment.

TABLE 52G.4

Troubleshooting with CRs

Problem	Possible Solution
The CR is too painful to treat.	Treat the myofascial tissues overlying and surrounding the CR with gentle direct or indirect myofascial release. This may help the local drainage of the tissues reducing the sensitivity of the CR. Somatic dysfunctions if present, in segmentally related areas may also be treated to influence the reflex arc involved in the CR and thereby the sensitivity of the CR this includes considering treating the related CR on the other side of the body).
There is minimal change in the CR in response to its treatment.	Verify that the tissue texture change is a clinically significant CRand not a different type of somatic change.Both the anterior and the posterior for any given structure along with other clues of visceral and viscerosomatic reflex activity should be present for it to be a positive CR. If they are both present, but still little response in the CR to treatment, evaluate for contributing factors, such as somatic dysfunctions in areas segmentally related to the CR, impaired lymphatic drainage of the area or region where the CR is found.
The effect of the CR treatment is short lived.	When treating CR, the sequencing of the treatment can be important. The overall biomechanical and postural pattern of somatic dysfunction should ideally be treated first, together with OMT strategies to improve respiratory and circulatory dynamics. Then the PTA syndrome may have to be addressed specifically with CR before attending to the CR correlated with the presenting complaint. Recall that in viscerosomatic reflexes, the pathophysiology lies in the visceral component. Treatment of the somatic end of the reflex may not alone be either adequate or, in some cases, appropriate. Repeated recurrence of a CR warrants further diagnostic or therapeutic action with respect to the underlying visceral cause.
The patient with the CR is extremely ill (also a consideration in certain hospitalized patients).	When treating hospitalized patients, the primary objective is to support the body's physiology through the process of illness and disease. Extensive OTM may not be advisable so as to minimize the energy expenditure of the patient. Treat the CR related to the areas of chief complaint and possibly those that impede the normal homeostatic processes.

patient. Interaction between dysfunctions and how they might influence each other through various biomechanical, postural, neurological (autonomic and somatosensory), and circulatory mechanisms is also of major importance. Understanding these interactions typically helps the physician establish the priority and sequence of the treatment. Similarly, when evaluating and treating pain patterns from MTrP, it is important to understand that active trigger points can be maintained by distant satellite MTrP.

A historical look at the patterns of positive reflex points palpated and treated in some commonly seen conditions illustrates how the early use of CRs was not focused on a single target organ (Owens, 1943) and how in many cases the hormonal-metabolic model was integrated (Table 52.5).

These and similar patterns of CRs should be integrated in the overall osteopathic management of the patient rather than used as a stand-alone method of treatment.

RESEARCH RELATED TO CRs AND THE OSTEOPATHIC CONCEPT

Palpable change in the absence of other objective findings had rendered MTrP and tender points in fibromyalgia patients difficult to instantiate; such is the case with osteopathic points in the CR and counterstrain systems. Nonetheless, there is a growing body of evidence demonstrating a possible basis for such identifiable tissue texture abnormalities. There is little research currently investigating the specific physiological or chemical characteristics of these very specific clinical osteopathic findings. There are a number of related studies, however, that might be considered in way of interpretation:

- In patients with fibromyalgia, researchers had demonstrated highly ordered collagen cuffs around terminal nerve fibers in skin biopsies that were not found in healthy controls (Sprott et al., 1997). They termed them *microscars* and concluded that this collagen crosslink, as evident by a decreased collagen metabolism, was needed to maintain the collagen cuffs around the nerves in the skin (Sprott, 2003). One of the proposed reasons for this collagen formation was neurogenic inflammation, which has been demonstrated in the skin in patients with fibromyalgia (Salemi et al., 2003)

- Investigating the biochemical milieu of MTrP, microdialysis was performed on MTrP collecting small volume of fluids, at subnanogram levels of solutes, from the muscle tissue (Shah, 2008). Subjects with active MTrP had lower pH levels in the vicinity of their MTrP, and significantly higher concentrations of substance P, calcitonin gene–related peptide, bradykinin, serotonin, norepinephrine, tumor necrosis factor-α, and Interleukin-1β (Shah et al., 2005). Furthermore, continuous nociceptive input from MTrP can increase excitability of dorsal horn neurons, linking the peripheral nociceptive events to central sensitization (Mense, 2008)

TABLE 52G.5

Examples of Patterns of CRs in Clinical Conditions

Condition	CRs Involved
Asthma, hay fever and sinusitis	In hay fever and sinusitis, the sinus CR will be positive. In asthma, the bronchial CR will be positive. The duodenal CR is also invariably present in cases of sinusitis, asthma, common colds, influenza, sore throat, and tonsillitis.. Treat gonadal and thyroid CR for endocrine balance. Treatment may place a load on organs of elimination: diagnose and treat CR of spleen, liver, and kidney in preparation for this; CR for colon and small intestines are therefore also relevant.
Allergy	Treat the whole PTA syndrome. Invariably, the adrenal CR will be involved. For food allergies, check the pancreas CR. In cases where patient regurgitates food, the pyloric CR will be involved.
Diabetes	PTA syndrome, adrenals, pancreas, and duodenum CR are consistently involved. In addition, look for stomach, colon, and kidney CR.
Eyes	In all eye affections, the sinus CR will be involved. In eye strain and conjunctivitis, consider additional examination of liver, small intestines, stomach, and bladder CR.
Digestive disturbances	If present, CR of the gonads, thyroid, and adrenals should be treated first. Then, special attention is given to the entire digestive tract, CR of the stomach, duodenum, pancreas, small intestines, colon, and liver as well as to organs of elimination, kidneys, spleen, and colon. Mesenteric releases may support treatment.
Inflammatory arthitides	Address the PTA syndrome that is invariably present. CR of the pancreas and duodenum are often present, as well as other digestive and eliminative organs. Reestablishing proper lymphatic drainage in conjunction with CR is very important in these cases.
Headaches	If caused by menstrual or menopausal symptoms, treatment to the uterine and ovarian CR may give relief. In blinding, dizzy headache, treatment of the duodenal CR may support the treatment. Often in cases of vertigo, steady pressure to the cerebellar CR may give relief.

- Local tissue findings such as tenderness, edema, and vasodilatation in areas seemingly unrelated to the primary site of dysfunction or injury may be due to neurogenic inflammation where neuropeptides are released from the peripheral terminals of nerves following repeated depolarization. This is referred to as the *axon reflex*. The stimulation of a C-fiber branch due to tissue injury and inflammation can result in depolarization and antidromic activity in other branches unrelated to site of injury or inflammation, releasing neuropeptides into noninflamed or injured tissue (Van Griensven, 2005, Willard, 2008). This may help to explain why tissue texture abnormalities and tenderness can be found in areas that are seemingly unrelated to the actual problem

- Other anatomically localizable, noninflammatory changes in the soft tissues that are thought to be reflexly associated with somatic dysfunctions in the axial spine have also been described. Such tissue texture phenomena are referred to as *irritation zones* and represent small (0.5 to 1.0 cm), painful soft-tissue functional abnormalities that are painful to palpation (Dvorak et al., 2008)

Even though each of the findings abovemight not be able to be universally linked to CRs, MTrP, counterstrain tender points or other such groupings, these and other studies provide a rationale to better understand the relationship between peripheral tissue events, the nervous system, and dysfunction. Reliability when palpating the counterstrain, CRs, and MTrP have in a few studies been found to be moderate to good (Hsieh et al., 2000; McPartland and Goodridge, 1997; Washington et al., 2003), and using palpation of tissue texture abnormalities coupled with pain provocation and the patient's medical history could be considered reliable in detecting the presence of such abnormalities.

Research demonstrating the effectiveness of using CRs on clinical conditions is limited. One study of hypertensive subjects investigated the effect of treating the posterior CRs for the adrenals. This group of subjects demonstrated a decrease in serum aldosterone levels lasting 36 hours after treatment (Mannino, 1979). Another study reported that combining CR treatment and soft-tissue techniques resulted in a significant improvement in forced vital capacity from first pretreatment to last posttreatment in a group of 30 asymptomatic subjects, 5 of which reported a past history of asthma or bronchitis (Lines et al., 1990).

In order to hypothesize how CRs work, it is necessary to consider its potential for modulating autonomic nervous system activity (and its integrated action with the somatomotor and neuroendocrine immune system) and augmenting lymph flow. Though it is not direct evidence for the clinical benefits of CR, it has been proposed that manual techniques stimulating fluid flow can assist repair processes and homeostatic controls in different tissues, which partly explains some of the various effects of manual approaches (Lederman, 2005). In a rat model, using a fluorescent probe placed in the lower extremity, intermittent pressure to the ventral thorax of the animal increased the uptake of lymph in the tissues peripheral to area in which the technique was applied (Dery et al., 2000). Using dogs, it was possible to establish that the thoracic and abdominal lymphatic pump techniques produced net increases in the thoracic duct flow (Knott et al., 2005). Other studies also using a dog model confirmed the net increases in the thoracic duct flow in response to lymphatic pump techniques (Downey et al., 2008; Hodges et al., 2007) and in addition, one of those studies reported a significant increase in the leukocyte count in samples taken from the catheterized thoracic duct, supporting the notion that such techniques can enhance an individual's immune response (Hodges et al., 2007).

The stimulation of somatic structures has been shown to influence autonomic function in many experimental studies using a variety of animal models (Sato et al., 1997). Though caution should be exercised when extrapolating such results to humans and clinical conditions, these observations from animal experiments are an indication of somatosympathetic or somatoautonomic interaction. There are studies in the manual medicine literature providing evidence for sympathetic responses from techniques addressing the spinal zygapophyseal joints. Specific sympathetic nervous system changes reported after articulatory techniques had been applied to the cervical and the lumbar spine include alterations in sudomotor function, cutaneous vasomotor changes, and changes in cardiac and respiratory functions (Chiu and Wright, 1996; McGuiness et al., 1997; Perry and Green, 2008; Petersen et al., 1993; Slater et al., 1994; Sterling et al., 2001; Vicenzino et al., 1994, 1998; Wright and Vicenzino, 1995). Sympathoexcitatory effects following manual spinal therapy have also been reported with the mechanical hypoalgesic effect of such intervention in both asymptomatic and symptomatic human subjects, indicating an activation of the descending pain inhibitory systems from the periaqueductal gray region (Hoeger Bement and Sluka, 2008, Perry and Green, 2008), effects that also has been reported in animal studies (Skyba et al., 2003). Using suboccipital inhibition, a soft-tissue technique applied to the myofascial tissues of the upper cervical spine, and digital strain plethysmography recording changes in the pulse contour, it was concluded that the OMT resulted in favorable autonomic changes in the form of sympathetic dampening (Purdy, et al., 1996). A recent study demonstrated the ability of OMT to influence sympathovagal balance in asymptomatic subjects, reporting that it shifted from the sympathetic to the parasympathetic nervous system in response to myofascial release in the cervical region (Henley et al., 2008).

Even though this is not direct evidence for either the mechanisms of action or the clinical effects of CRs, this information illustrates the potential of OMT to influence the lymphatic system as well as the sympathetic and the parasympathetic nervous system. Much more research is needed to confirm the potential role of CRs in modulating such activity as well as the clinical benefits of the treatment for patients with a variety of conditions.

SUMMARY

CRs have a long tradition in the osteopathic profession as a diagnostic and therapeutic tool. The evidence base for their use as a valuable diagnostic tool has grown considerably from their original empirical and anecdotal descriptions and is currently the focus of numerous interexaminer and correlative studies. Nonetheless, despite being linked to specific visceral or systemic conditions,

there is a lack of research as to what they precisely represent as a tissue texture abnormality. Their somatotopic organization is very predictable and consistent, and it is hypothesized that the lymphatic, the autonomic, and the neuroendocrine immune systems are involved in the mediation of the reflexes and the therapeutic action from treating these reflexes. Their use should be integrated in the overall osteopathic evaluation and management of the patient, which is integral to the success of applying these reflexes in treatment.

References

Arbuckle BE. Chapman's reflexes charts and notes. *The Selected Writings of Beryl E Arbuckle, D.O. F.A.C.O.P.* Colorado, CO: American Academy of Osteopathy. Plenum Publishing Corp., 1997:256–264.

Capobianco JD. The neuroendocrine-immune complex illustrated in the work of Dr Frank Chapman. *J Am Acad Osteopath* 2004;14(1).

Chiu TW, Wright A. To compare the effects of different rates of application of a cervical mobilisation technique on sympathetic outflow to the upper limb in normal subjects. *Man Ther* 1996;1:198–203.

Deason WJ. Body fluids—the original osteopathic concept: the influences behind Dr. Still's theories as revealed in his writings and interviews. *The Osteopathic Profession.* Part I April 1940;7(7):9–11, 43–46, Part 2 May 1940;7(8):20–23, 43–45.

Dery MA, Yonuschot G, Winterson BJ. The effects of manually applied intermittent pulsation pressure to rat ventral thorax on lymph transport. *Lymphology* 2000;33(2):58–61.

DiGiovanna EL, Schiowitz S, Dowling D. *An Osteopathic Approach to Diagnosis and Treatment.* 3rd Ed. Philadelphia, PA: Lippincott Williams & Wilkins, 2005.

Downey HF, Durgam P, Williams AG Jr, et al. Lymph flow in the thoracic duct of conscious dogs during lymphatic pump treatment, exercise, and expansion of extracellular fluid volume. *Lymphat Res Biol* 2008;6(1):3–13.

Dvorak J, Dvorak V, Gilliar W, et al. *Musculoskeletal Manual Medicine.* New York, NY: Thieme, 2008.

ECOP. *Glossary of Osteopathic Terminology.* Educational Council on Osteopathic Principles, AOA, 2006.

Henley CE, Ivins D, Mills M, et al. Osteopathic manipulative treatment and its relationship to autonomic nervous system activity as demonstrated by heart rate variability: a repeated measures study. *Osteopath Med Prim Care* 2008;2:7.

Hoeger Bement K, Sluka KA. Pain: perception and mechanisms. In: Magee DJ, Zachazewski JE, Quillen WS, eds. *Scientific Foundations and Principles and Practice in Musculoskeletal Rehabilitation.* St. Louis, MO: Saunders Elsevier, 2008:217–237.

Hodge LM, King HH, Williams AG Jr, et al. Abdominal lymphatic pump treatment increases leukocyte count and flux in thoracic duct lymph. *Lymphat Res Biol* 2007;5(2):127–133.

Hsieh CY, Hong CZ, Adams AH, et al. Interexaminer reliability of the palpation of trigger points in the trunk and lower limb muscles. *Arch Phys Med Rehabil* 2000;81:258–264.

Hulett GD. *Hulett's Principles.* Chicago: A.T. Still Research Institute, 1922.

Johns PR. *Comparative analysis of the topographical locations of Chapman's reflex points and Jones's strain-counterstrain tender points.* Thesis, Master Degree, Unitec New Zealand, Carrington, Auckland, New Zealand, 2003.

Kendall OT, Kendall FP. *Muscle Testing and Function.* Baltimore, MD: Williams and Wilkins, 1971.

Ketcham AD. *Introduction to Lessons on Chapman Technic.* Kirksville, MI: William L. Johnston Collection, Still National Osteopathic Museum, Typed: ca. 1943:136pp.

Kim OB. Comparative analysis of the topographical locations of acupuncture points and Chapman's reflex points. This paper is posted at coda, An Institutional Repository for the New Zealand ITP Sector. http://www.coda.ac.nz/unitec hs di/2. Accessed 02.02.2009.

Knott EM, Tune JD, Stoll ST, et al. Increased lymphatic flow in the thoracic duct during manipulative intervention *J Am Osteopath Assoc* 2005;105(10):447–456.

Kuchera ML, Kuchera WA. *Osteopathic Considerations in Systemic Dysfunction.* 2nd Ed. Columbus, OH: Greyden Press, 1994.

Kuchera MA. A pragmatic interpretation of Chapman's reflexes. *Am Acad Osteopath* 2008.

Lederman E. *The Science and Practice of Manual Therapy.* 2nd Ed. Edinburgh: Elsevier Churchill Livingstone, 2005.

Lines DH, McMilan AJ, Spehr GJ. Effects of soft tissue technique and Chapman's neurolymphatic reflex stimulation on respiratory function. *J Aust Chiropr Assoc* 1990;20(1):17–22.

Lippincott R. Chaoman's reflexes. *The Osteopathic Profession* 1946:18–22.

Mannino JR. The application of neurological reflexes to the treatment of hypertension. *J Am Osteopath Assoc* 1978;79:225–231.

McGuiness JM, Vicenzino B, Wright A. Influence of a cervical mobilisation technique on respiratory and cardiovascular function. *Man Ther* 1997; 2:216–220.

McPartland JM. Travell trigger points—molecular and osteopathic perspectives. *J Am Osteopath Assoc* 2004;104(6):244–249.

McPartland JM, Goodridge JP. Counterstrain diagnostics and traditional osteopathic examination of the cervical spine compared. *J Bodywork Mov Ther* 1997;1(3):173–178.

Melzack R, Stillwell DM, Fox EJ. Trigger points and acupuncture points for pain: Correlations and implications. *Pain* 1977;3:3–23.

Mense S. Peripheral and central mechanisms of musculoskeletal pain. In: Castro-Lopes J, Raja S, Schmelz M, eds. *Pain 2008: An Updated Review.* Seattle, WA: International Association for the Study of Pain, 2008:55–62.

Owens C. The endocrine glands, the hormones and the osteopathic lesion. *J Am Osteopath Assoc* 1930:421–422.

Owens C. Endocrine concept of disease—an analysis of chemical and anatomical factors in body ailments. *The Osteopathic Profession,* 1935.

Owens C. *An Endocrine Interpretation of Chapman's Reflexes.* Reprint Academy of Applied Osteopathy, Carmel 1963 (1st edition 1937 by the author).

Owens C. *Mechanical Manipulation and Reflexes in the Treatment of Disease.* Self-published, 1940.

Owens C. *Chapman's Reflexes Subseries: 7 Folders.* Kirksville, MI: William L. Johnston Collection, Still National Osteopathic Museum.

Patriquin DA. Viscerosomatic reflexes. In Patterson MM, Howell JN, eds. 1989 International Symposium: *The Central Connection: Somatovisceral/Viscerosomatic Interaction* (pp.). Athens, OH: American Academy of Osteopathy University Classics, Ltd, 1989:4–18.

Patriquin D. Chapman's reflexes. In: Ward RC, ed. *Foundations for Osteopathic Medicine.* 2nd Ed. Baltimore, MD: Lippincott Williams & Wilkins, 2003.

Perry J, Green A. An investigation into the effects of a unilaterally applied lumbar mobilisation technique on peripheral sympathetic nervous system activity in the lower limbs *Man Ther* 2008;13:492–499.

Petersen N, Vicenzino B, Wright A. The effects of a cervical mobilisation technique on sympathetic outflow to the upper limb in normal subjects. *Physiother Theory Pract* 1993;9:149–156.

Pilgrim MF. *Mechanical Vibratory Stimulation.* New York City, NY: Lawrence Press, 1903.

Purdy WR, Frank JJ, Oliver B. Suboccipital dermatomyotomic stimulation and digital blood flow. *J Am Osteopath Assoc* 1996;96(5):285–289.

Riley JN, Mitchell FL Jr, Bensky D. Thai manual medicine as reprinted in Wat Pho Epigraphies: preliminary comparisons. *Med Anthropol* 1981;5(2):155–194.

Salemi S, Rethage J, Wollina U, et al. Detection of Interleukin 1β (IL-1β), IL-6, and Tumor Necrosis Factor-α in skin of patients with fibromyalgia. *J Rheumatol* 2003;30:146–150.

Samblanet HL. An interpretation of Chapman's reflexes. *The Forum of Osteopathy,* 1944.

Sato A, Sato Y, Schmidt RF. The impact of somatosensory input on autonomic functions. *Rev Physiol Biochem Pharmacol.* 1997;130:1–328.

Shah JP, Danoff JV, Desai MJ, et al. Biochemicals associated with pain and inflammation are elevated in sites near to and remote from active myofascial trigger points. *Arch Phys Med Rehabil.* 2008;89(1):16–23.

Shah JP, Gilliams EA. Uncovering the biochemical milieu of myofascial trigger points using in vivo microdialysis: an application of muscle pain concepts to myofascial pain syndrome. *J Bodyw Mov Ther.* 2008;12(4): 371–384.

Shah JP, Phillips TM, Danoff JV, et al. An in vivo microanalytical technique for measuring the local biochemical milieu of human skeletal muscle. J Appl Physiol. 2005 Nov;99(5):1977–1984.

Skyba DA, Radhakrishnan R, Rohlwing JJ, et al. Joint manipulation reduces hyperalgesia by activation of monoamine receptors but not opioid or GABA receptors in the spinal cord. *Pain.* 2003;106(1–2):159–168.

Slater H, Vicenzino B, Wright A. 'Sympathetic Slump': the effects of a novel manual therapy technique on peripheral sympathetic nervous system function. *J Man Manipulative Ther.* 1994;2:156–162.

Sprott H. Muscles and peripheral abnormalities in fibromyalgia. In: Wallace DJ, Clauw DJ. *Fibromyalgia and Other Central Pain Syndromes.* Philadelphia, PA: Lippincott Williams & Wilkins, 2005:101–114.

Sterling M, Jull G, Wright A. Cervical mobilisation: concurrent effects on pain, sympathetic nervous system activity and motor activity. *Man Ther.* 2001;6:72–81.

Still AT. *Philosophy of Osteopathy.* Kirksville, MO: The Journal Printing Company Ltd, 1899.

Still AT. *The Mechanical Principles and Philosophy of Osteopathy.* Kirksville, MO: The Journal Printing Company Ltd, 1902.

Still AT. *Osteopathy: Research and Practice.* Kirksville, MO: The Journal Printing Company Ltd, 1910.

Van Griensven H. *Pain in Practice.* Edinburgh: Butterworth and Heineman Elsevier, 2005

Vicenzino B, Cartwright T, Collins D, et al. Cardiovascular and respiratory changes produced by the lateral glide mobilisation of the cervical spine. *Man Ther.* 1998a;3(2):67–71.

Vicenzino B, Collins D, Benson H, et al. An investigation of the interrelationship between manipulative therapy-induced hypoalgesia and sympathoexcitation. *J Manipulative Physiol Ther.* 1998b;21:448–453.

Vicenzino B, Collins D, Wright A. "Sudomotor changes induced by neural mobilisation techniques in asymptomatic subjects". *J Man Manipulative Ther.* 1994;2:66–74.

Walther DS, Gavin DM, Goodheart G. *Applied Kinesiology: A Synopsis.* Pueblo, CO: Systems DC, 1988.

Washington K, Mosiello R, Venditto M, et al. Presence of Chapman reflex points in hospitalized patients with pneumonia. *J Am Osteopath Assoc.* 2003;103:479–483.

Willard F. Basic mechanisms of pain. In: Audette JF, Bailey A, eds. *Integrative Pain Medicine.* Totowa, NJ: Humana Press, 2008:19–62.

Wilson K. Written *Case Studies Presented at Chapman's Think Tank Retreat.* Glendale: Arizona College of Osteopathic Medicine, 2006.

Wright A, Vicenzino B. Cervical mobilisation techniques, sympathetic nervous system effects and their relationship to analgesia. In: Shacklock M, ed. *Moving in on Pain.* Conference Proceedings, Adelaide, Australia. Sydney: Butterworth-Heinemann, 1995:164–173.

52H Fulford Percussion

RAJIV L. YADAVA

KEY CONCEPT

In this section, emphasis is placed on synchronization of palpatory diagnostic interpretation with the application of an external percussion device. This device, the percussion vibrator, amplifies what is normally done through the hands alone and thus can increase the amount of energy delivered to the tissues. The energy state in the dysfunction field must be matched to properly release it. Intrinsic to this approach is the incorporation of thought derived from Andrew Taylor Still's expression of "mind, matter, motion."

CASE STUDY

A 21 y/o F presents to the office with a complaint of right leg discomfort for the past month. She has an "achiness" of her right leg that radiates into her lateral ankle. She remembers standing on the rung of a ladder for some time to clean her windows. There is no other history of trauma. Past medical/surgical history is negative. She has been using Arnica Montana for relief, but the discomfort returns.

Physical Examination:

T-98.8, P-72, R-12, B/P 110/70, Ht-64," Wt-120#; HEENT/CV/Pulmonary/Abdomen/GU-noncontributory. Neurological exam is intact. Structural exam reveals level landmarks, normal AP curves, no lateral curves. There is tenderness to palpation along the lateral aspect of the right calf. Lateral malleolar motion appears sluggish. There is tension in the interosseous membrane.

Diagnosis:

Somatic dysfunction of the lower extremity—ankle, calf.

Plan:

Treatment of the subtle motion restriction with the percussion hammer (see Example 1 at the end of the chapter).

Definition

It is an osteopathic manipulative technique developed by Robert C. Fulford, D.O., involving the use of an instrument referred to as a percussor. The percussor utilizes a specific application of a mechanical vibratory percussive force to treat somatic dysfunction. This modality is distinct from other massage, vibration, or oscillatory approaches. The use of the percussor is coupled with the operator's palpatory feedback before and during the treatment.

When other physicians used the percussor in a modified way Dr. Fulford would quietly disapprove of it. Although he never addressed these individuals directly or publicly, he felt that they never really understood the philosophy and principles he was teaching and so they would change the way it was used to accommodate their lack of understanding.

History and Philosophy

To understand the philosophy of Dr. Fulford's percussion, it is helpful to have an understanding of the history behind his development of it. Dr. Fulford faced many obstacles in his life, but what he

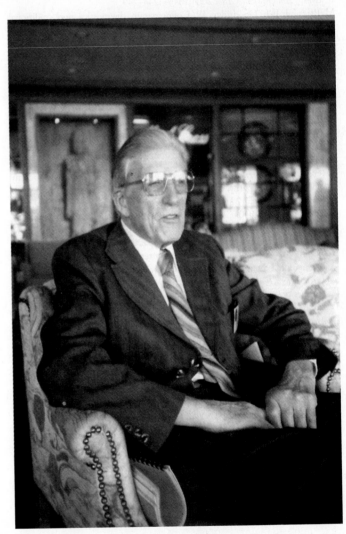

Dr. Robert C. Fulford at the 1985 A.A.O. Convention Colorado Springs, Colorado. Courtesy of Dr. E. Sara Saxton D.O.

learned from the difficulties shaped his understanding and future. He could not attend medical school in 1929 due to the depression. This forced him to work at Union Carbide where he developed an appreciation for subtle motion and the impact it could have on the purity of oxygen produced. There he found that a slight mechanical turn of a dial would be the difference between getting impure oxygen or pure oxygen. In 1936, he was denied admission to medical school. In 1937, he had an injury that awakened an old desire for becoming a physician. He obtained admission to Kansas City College of Osteopathic Medicine and became fascinated with Dr. A.T. Still's Philosophy of Osteopathy. He developed an interest in metaphysics, spirituality of all religious philosophies, astrology, yoga, esoteric teachings, and many natural healing arts of the world. He was well read and knowledgeable in these areas. This broadmindedness, grounded in medical science and an understanding of osteopathic anatomy, allowed him to "read between the lines," so to speak, as he studied the Osteopathy of Dr. A.T. Still.

In his junior year at Kansas City College, he became interested in Dr. Harold Saxson Burr's energy work. Dr. Burr, an anatomist at Yale School of Medicine, published over 90 papers and raised interest among his colleagues many of whom became leaders in science. Through his readings of Dr. Burr's experiments of measuring energy fields, Dr. Fulford believed that these fields provided a blueprint for all living things. Dr. Fulford considered these fields diagnostic for mental as well as physical conditions.

In 1941, WWII resulted in increased hours of work due to a number of physicians having to leave the area for the war efforts. In addition to this, Dr. Fulford noticed that there was considerably more tension among the patient population after the war began. Patients were more challenging to treat. A thought from the past occurred to him when he worked for Union Carbide. His superintendent would say that where possible let a motor do the work for you. After he experimented with various vibrators without acceptable results, the Foredom Vibrator Flyer arrived in the mail in the 1940s by chance and was found to fulfill his needs allowing the manipulative procedures to be performed more easily and effectively after its use. He would say that many instances in his life he found that what he needed was provided to him spontaneously as it were.

Dr. Fulford originally met Dr. Sutherland in 1939 as a student. His first course with Dr. Sutherland was in 1942 as his interest again turned to the energy field. He describes the impact Dr. Sutherland had on his thinking at Des Moines College in 1949. "It was a most important day of my life when I had an opportunity to sit in the classroom of Des Moines College back in 1949. Dr. Sutherland was teaching his cranial concept. His ideas were heavily charged with energy and they soon began to work in me like some powerful force."

Dr. Fulford was convinced Dr. Sutherland was aware of the energy fields.

According to Dr. Fulford, his understanding of cranial osteopathy as taught to him by Dr. Sutherland was different than what was taught after Dr. Sutherland's death. He stated the first week of cranial osteopathy was about anatomy. The second week was taught by Dr. Sutherland himself where Dr. Sutherland would draw a house on the board with all the windows out and floating in the ocean. According to Dr. Fulford, this house symbolized the human body and the ocean with its many waves representing the primary respiratory mechanism (PRM) (universal energy). Dr. Fulford further states this does not correspond with the commentaries of Dr. Sutherland's recordings. In regard to PRM, primary is the universal life force expressed as mind, energy, and breath, the breath being the first principal in the cerebral spinal fluid (CSF). Respiratory is a rhythmic motion of mind energy, fine energies of the CSF, as they motivate and manifest life. Mechanism is a process, conscious or unconscious where a result of accomplishment is produced, in this case, where the sensory motor energies relate sensation, experiences and expression in the world of matter.

Dr. Fulford appreciated two other basic principals from Dr. Sutherland in addition to the ones he drew on the blackboard (the house with wavy lines). One was that as osteopathic physicians we should stay close to our maker and the other is the importance of breath in life and healing. Dr. Fulford was spiritual. He mentioned the use of meditation or "running the energies through the body," and breathing exercises. He credited a breathing exercise with keeping his body alive for as long as he did.

He would say there are many people who are claiming to do cranial work with little or no knowledge of the theory behind the PRM. "They know the mechanics of how (PRM) works but little about how consciousness is part of a successful treatment." His description of Dr. Sutherland treating is as follows, "It was of interest to watch Dr. Sutherland treat. He sat on a stool, his back straight as a rod and his shoulders level and balanced. The arms extended and appeared as though they were weightless. His eyes were closed; whether he was in a meditative or contemplative state no one will ever know. Then after a few minutes his hands and arms would fly out into space as though they were suddenly given a push outward."

It was confusing for some to hear Dr. Fulford downplay the cranial rhythmic impulse (CRI). He did acknowledge rhythms but did not focus on any particular rate. To him, a still point or a fulcrum was not a particular place but a state of being in which everything is centered.

Additionally regarding Dr. Sutherland's writings, Dr. Fulford has stated, "In Dr. Sutherland's writings he stresses the mechanics as part of the cranial concept, as an engineer would and thus he could be understood. But he himself went beyond that in his findings and touch. That was his secret that he could not teach. He tried to leave us his secret when he gave us the phrase, "thinking and knowing fingers...."

Quoting Dr. Sutherland, "seeing, feeling, thinking finger... fingers that endeavor to get away from the sensation of physical touch wherein you have knowing touch....by knowing I mean not information gained by the physical sense but a knowledge that comes from getting as far as one can from the physical sense" (27).

Just as Dr. Fulford says of Dr. Sutherland that he could not teach directly of what he knew of osteopathy, Dr. Sutherland states the same of Dr. Still. "Dr. Still could not speak of all the things he understood about the living human body. We were not ready to hear him. If you read between the lines in his 'Philosophy of Osteopathy' you will see that this is so."

Around 1949 to 1950, Dr. Fulford along with a number of other DOs left to study with Dr. Beryl E. Arbuckle, D.O. The reason being was the impressive results she was obtaining. Dr. Fulford said that her treatment of children would cause an autonomic response in just a few minutes resulting in perspiration. She would then move to the next child lying on an adjacent table and do the same through several tables in a row. She originally met Dr. Sutherland in 1942 and was one of Dr. Sutherland's early trainers for osteopathy in the cranial field. Also, she was one of the few physicians who Dr. Sutherland allowed to treat him. Having done well over 250 dissections of fetal cadavers at the Philadelphia College of Osteopathy, she felt that the dural stress bands and bony buttresses should be given more importance before moving on to nonbony and nonmembranous aspects of cranial osteopathy that Dr. Sutherland was evolving toward at the time. It was not that she did not appreciate the fluid anatomy, but she felt that we must understand what could be verified physically with anatomy before moving on to fluid, potency, and the breath of life aspects of cranial osteopathy Dr. Sutherland was teaching.

Dr. Arbuckle's influence on Dr. Fulford could be seen by the way he firmly put his hands on the cranium. One could also see the use of Dr. Arbuckle's craniometric points in Dr. Fulford's percussion work as well. Dr. Sutherland's communications of the nonphysical aspect of osteopathy, with its mental, emotional, and spiritual implications could be observed and felt on the patients Dr. Fulford would treat as the fluid forces would move with great vigor under his hands, a phenomenon unique among his peers. Dr. Koss states, "Many osteopaths do not realize the power that this humble, feeble-looking man had....the power he generated was, to say the least, incredible."

It is interesting to note that according to Dr. Fulford, the CRI with its rates, and amplitude was not a focus with Dr. Arbuckle or, for that matter, with Dr. Sutherland while he was living. These individuals were more focused on the source of the phenomena manifesting as the rate, rhythm, and amplitude.

After 1950, Dr. Fulford met Randolph Stone, D.O. He said, "Dr. Stone and I were good friends." Both these men had great interest in matters of spirituality beyond the boundaries of any particular religion. Dr. Stone developed Polarity Therapy from his influences of the ancient Ayurvedic Medicine of India. Dr. Fulford knew it to be more involved than those who utilize it today. Many believe Dr. Fulford's understanding and appreciation of polarity with regard to diagnosis and treatment was from Dr. Stone, but Dr. Fulford, himself, credits Baron Karl von Riechenbach (1778 to 1869) with that.

Riechenbach was a chemist, naturalist, geologist, metallurgist, and industrialist known for his discoveries of chemical products extracted from tar. He spent his last years researching the energy field, which he called the odic force.

The number of influences and contacts Dr. Fulford had would be too numerous to name and describe in this short essay. It would be safe to say that he had an almost childlike enthusiasm for knowledge of truth in all matters concerning the understanding osteopathic medicine and healing. Nothing would be overlooked until it was examined by him and then accepted or discarded.

Diagnosis

Dr. Fulford would say that it takes the mind of a physician to understand osteopathy. He felt that without the osteopathic understanding of the interrelationship between structure and function, an accurate diagnosis could not be forthcoming.

Both the history and the examination were important for Dr. Fulford's diagnosis. In fact, diagnosis was considered to be a more important subject than treatment. It was a holistic view of diagnosis and treatment that included the physical as well as the mental and emotional levels of the patient. Another unique feature of Dr. Fulford's diagnosis on the physical level was how much importance was given to the extremities, abdomen, and anterior chest wall as opposed to being primarily restricted, at least by habit of mind, to the spine and cranium for any particular complaint. The breath was also important in diagnosis and not just the breath of the thorax but of the whole body from head to toe. Physical as well as subtle breath was important to him.

Dr. Fulford considered trauma to be an important part of the history intake. First would be birth trauma, which would be reflected in the breath of the individual and greatly influenced by the first breath the individual took as an infant. Second would be physical trauma, especially early in life, and third would be psychological trauma especially early in life. Most of his diagnosis was complete in his mind after getting the history from the patient. As a result, the physical exam served to reassure the patient that he acknowledged their area of complaint.

During the physical examination, the dysfunction was understood to be the area where the "life force is not flowing." The examination would begin in the foot and ankles and continue to the knees, hips and pelvis, abdomen, diaphragm, rib cage, upper extremity, shoulder joint, lumbar, thoracic, cervical vertebrae, and the cranium. The exam would consist of finding restrictions of motion within the joints. One's attention was directed to the subtle motions of the area being examined and looking for the lack of motion there. This is different than gross motion where light touch is not an important factor. Here, we are using a light touch to appreciate the presence or absence of a "life force" or underlying motion.

Mechanism of Action

There are probably multiple explanations of the mechanism of action using the percussion vibrator as Dr. Fulford has instructed. Note that the percussion vibrator simply acts as an amplifying device for what the operator initiates with his hands.

Dr. Fulford added and changed many techniques of treatment over the years as he evolved. Many of these techniques would "just come to him," like a gift, out of nowhere. The diagnosis and treatment of Dr. Fulford relies on the bioelectric properties of fascia and bone. When mechanical energy is absorbed into the body, there is a distortion within this bioelectrical matrix creating a higher energetic state within the fascia and bone. This distortion can be palpated as a subtle motion restriction, a depression, or elevation along the tissues of the body. These restrictions can be very subtle and so the physician's level of skill will determine how much they will appreciate under their palpating hands. Dr. Fulford would say that "When you can feel the placement of a single hair under 18 sheets of paper you are ready to do the cranial work." This higher energy state within the tissue needs to be matched with an equal quantum of energy in order to release to a more normal state of structure and function. This may take time as the cells within the tissues take time to redeposit themselves after partial or full release of this potential energy. Tissues are always being turned over and their chemical components redeposited. The epithelial cells of the gut last about 5 days, but those of the main body of the gut last about 120 days. The epidermis of the skin is recycled every 2 weeks. The liver has a turnover time of 300 to 500 days. The entire human skeleton is replaced every 10 years. The manner in which the tissues are redeposited could be influenced at least in part by the bioelectric field present.

It is also believed that mental/emotional trauma can be absorbed into the memory of the tissue through this bioelectric phenomena described. Thoughts and emotions are known to influence the health and well being of individuals.

The percussion vibrator amplifies what is normally done through the hands alone and thus can increase the amount of energy delivered to the tissues. As mentioned the energy state in the dysfunction field must be matched to properly release it. High-impact physical trauma, great psychological trauma and stress can produce and maintain these dysfunction fields with high-energy states. As a practical matter, if 100 ft-lb of force is absorbed into the tissues, the operator cannot apply that much physical force to release it. One must rely on the bioelectric mechanism of the tissues to address this situation. The operator's intention and attention is amplified with the percussion vibrator and will assist in the release. Dr. Fulford would say empathically that "Thoughts are things," and "Energy follows thought." Following the release of these high energetic states, the body areas can return to having a more normal rhythm, or fluctuation of fluids, through the area and thus, healing can begin.

A cursory description of a practical demonstration would be as follows: The percussion vibrator is placed on one side of the body part being treated. The other side is monitored by the other hand usually on the opposite side of that body part. With the skillful application of the percussor hand and the monitoring hand, there will be a resonant wave of energy created between the two. This force will resonate with the dysfunction field between the hands. In order to get this resonating wave, the speed, direction, pressure, and placement of the percussing hand will vary depending on the area being addressed and the dysfunctional field present. The resonating force will be present until there is a release, relaxation, and flow of the life force through the area. It is believed that the energy within the resonant wave will match the energy within the dysfunctional field before a release occurs. One's thought and intention for the patient's well being will be key in releasing the most difficult of dysfunctional areas. Dr. Fulford states, "The work of healing will be greatly assisted by tremendous stimulation of the love nature.... We must be sure to pursue genuine healing. Far too often, healing is thought of as relieving stressful symptoms, so we are not bothered by them. As a result, the effort to heal frequently becomes little more than an attack on what is wrong or painful. The healing potential is tapped primarily by learning to identify with the health and using the resources of health to enrich the consciousness and heal the distress as we build up greater health while that which is unhealthy fades away."

A true understanding of this can be gained when one has a background in osteopathic medical training, experience, and help from a qualified, experienced instructor.

Use and Response of Fulford Percussion

When used with discrimination, the Fulford percussion vibrator can be used on almost all patients. The Fulford percussor can be utilized for any osteopathic dysfunction, but it is with resistant dysfunctions that its usefulness can be most appreciated. Difficult dysfunctions will respond with less treatment time. Because of the enhanced tissue response and release, there is a greater chance of rebound symptoms to occur. Treatment frequency may need to be reduced. This, of course, will depend on the skill of the operator using the percussor. Contraindications would include an area where one would choose to release less tissue such as postsurgical cardiac, abdominal, or orthopedic patients within the last 6 months, prosthetic devices such as heart valves and hip replacements. The use of Fulford's percussion vibrator is generally not advised in the lumbar, sacral, and lower abdomen areas of pregnant patients. Acutely painful areas should never be addressed directly with the percussor.

Technique

Example One

Subtle motion restriction is found in the right ankle joint involving the talus, distal fibula, and tibia (Fig. 52H.1). Percussor speed is adjusted to the lower end because of the areas relative decrease in soft tissue mass. The placement of the percussor is over the lateral malleolus. Pressure and aim is adjusted for maximum response between the percussing hand and the monitoring hand on the opposite side (over the medial malleolus). The response one is looking for is a process of interchange of the life force between the hands. This response will continue until there is a release and the tissue is relaxed. One will be able to experience the life force flow through the area again.

Example Two

A restriction in the subtle motion of the left femoral head was found (Fig. 52H.2). The percussor will be placed over the right greater trochanter and the monitoring hand over the left greater

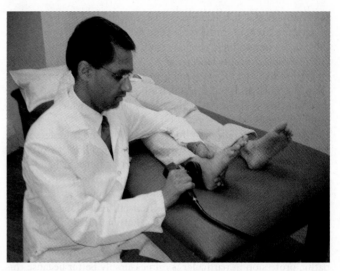

Figure 52H-1 Treatment of ankle.

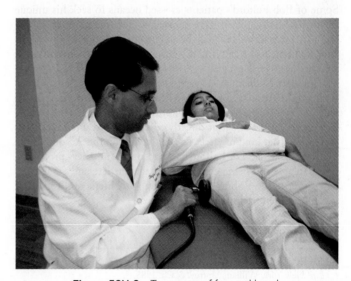

Figure 52H-2 Treatment of femoral head.

trochanter. This is due to concept of polarity that Dr. Fulford used in diagnosis and treatment. In regard to the pelvis, percussion on the right side clinically allows more efficient release even if the restriction is on the opposite side, as in this case, at the left femoral head. This is particularly true when release of the entire pelvis is desired. Percussion speed would be relatively high due to the relative increase in soft tissue in the area. Again, once the release is achieved, one should be able to appreciate the flow of energy through the pelvis at the end of the treatment.

SUMMARY

This chapter offers a glimpse of Dr. Fulford's percussion. It is not intended to provide a substitute for appropriate training, both didactic and practical under credible guidance, and is meant for those with a complete osteopathic education and not for any other purpose.

As a profession, there is much to be gained from those with great clinical results regardless of whether we have theoretical model to support it at that time or ever. The clinical experience shapes and develops the art over time. The osteopathic profession can choose to divide itself among differences or inherit the richness of diversity brought to the table from great minds. The proof is in the consistency of their clinical results as observed by many who witnessed those events repeatedly.

Dr. Still states, "…we should treat with respect and reverence all truths, great and small.....each truth or division as we see it, can only be made known to us by the self-evident fact, which this truth is able to demonstrate by its action."

No description of Dr. Fulford's work would be complete without mention of the love he would say was required to properly carry out diagnosis and treatment. The care and love he had for the patient's welfare came across in every encounter with his patients. It was reflected in his behavior with friends, as well as those from which he would prefer to distance himself. His professional and personal life was living testimony to that embracing principle of love seldom experienced in a life.

Dr. Eschtruth said of him, "Medicine in general, and the osteopathic profession in particular is immeasurably better because this selfless, humble man from southern Ohio who spent his life teaching others his unique way to reach the still point in his patients. Some of Bob Fulford's patients crossed oceans to seek his unique treatment. Bob Fulford gave himself as few others have in the medical profession. He will be sorely missed, but his presence will continue to be felt and his teachings will live on and grow forever."

The late William E. Wyatt, DO, FAAO was a popular presenter at the Annual Convocation Program of the American Academy of Osteopathy. In a striking moment, he stopped in the middle of a presentation to speak directly to Dr. Fulford. He asked "Do you know what kind of effect you are having on the Academy?"

The influence Dr. Fulford has had on the medical profession is undeniable and being enjoyed by us all. The late and great baseball player Jackie Robinson said it simply," A life is not important except in the impact it has on other lives."

SUGGESTED READING

Becker RO, Seldon G. *The Body Electric: Electromagnetism and the Foundation of Life*. New York: William Morrow & Co, 1985.

Blood SD. *AAO Newsletter*, April 2005.

Burr HS. Blue print for immortality. Saffron Walden: CW Daniel, Health Information, 1/12/05. Health Information Center at the Cleveland Clinic, 4/10/08. <http://clevelandclinic.org/health/health-info/docs/2600/2613.asp?index=9821>.

Dolson AL. Acupuncture from a pathologist's perspective: linking physical to energetic. *Med Acupunct*. 1998;10(1).

Eschtruth P. Robert C. Fulford succumbs. *Cranial Lett*. 1997;50(3).

Fulford RC. Personal communication, June 24, 1997.

Fulford RC. Presentations during courses from 1987–1997.

Fulford RC. *Dr. Fulford's Touch of Life, the Healing Power of the Natural Life Force*. New York: Pocket Books, 1996.

Fulford RC. *Are We on the Path? The Collected Works of Robert C. Fulford, D.O.* Indianapolis, IN: The Cranial Academy, Inc., 2003.

Goodman H. *Dr. Arbuckle's Influence on Dr. Fulford*. St. Louis, MD: AAO Presentation, 1999.

Hameroff S. The neuron doctrine is an insult to neurons. *Behav Brain Sci*. 22:838–839.

Ho M-W. *The Rainbow and the Worm—the Physics of the Organism*. 2nd ed. Singapore: World Scientific Essays, 1998.

Ho M-W. *Organism and Psyche in a Participatory Universe*. Institute of Science in Society, 1998. ISIS, 4/24/08. <http://www.i-sis.org.uk./organis.php>

Ho M-W. *Quantum Jazz*. Institute of Science in Society, 10/16/06. ISIS, 4/24/08. http://www.i-sis.org.uk./QuantumJazz.php

Ho M-W. *Strong Medicine for Cell Biology*. Institute of Science in Society, 10/28/04. ISIS, 4/20/08. <http://www-i-sis.org.uk/SMFCB.php>

Ho M-W. *Positive Electricity Zaps Through Water Chains*. Institute of Science in Society, 10/27/05. ISIS, 4/24/08. <http://www.i-sis.org.uk./PEZTWC.php>

Ho M-W. Quantum coherence and conscious experiences. *Kybernetes*. 1997;26:265–276.

Ho M-W. The acupuncture system and the liquid crystalline collagen fibres of the connective tissue. *Am J Chin Med* 1998;26:251–263.

Ho M-W. *The Importance of Cell Water*. Institute of Science in Society, 10/13/04. ISIS, 4/20/08. <http://www-i-sis.org.uk/TIOCW.php>

Ho M-W. *Collagen Water Structure Revealed*. Institute of Science in Society, 10/23/06. ISIS, 4/20/08. <http://www.i-sis.org.uk/Collagenwaterstructurerevealed.php>

Ho M-W. *New Age of Water: Liquid Crystalline Water at the Interface*. Institute of Science in Society, 3/31/08. ISIS, 4/20/08. <http://www.isis.org.ik/liquidCrystallineWater.php>

Koss R. Robert C. Fulford succumbs. *Cranial Lett*. 1997;50(3).

Still AT. *Autobiography of A.T. Still*. Indianapolis, IN: American Academy of Osteopathy, 2005.

Still AT. *The Philosophy and Mechanical Principles of Osteopathy*. Kansas City, MO: Hudson-Kimberly Publishing Company, 1902.

Still AT. *Osteopathy Research and Practice*. Kirksville, MO: The Journal Printing Company, 1910.

Sutherland WG. *Contributions of Thought, The Collected Writings of William Garner Sutherland, D.O.* 2nd Ed. Portland, OR: Rudra Press, 1998.

Sutherland WG, Sutherland A. Personal letter from William and Adah Sutherland to Walter Russell, January 7, 1947.

Wade N. Your body is younger than you think. *The New York Times*, August 2, 2005.

Approach to Osteopathic Patient Management

53

Elderly Patient with Dementia

BRUCE P. BATES AND MARILYN R. GUGLIUCCI

KEY CONCEPTS

- Nonreversible causes of dementia can be classified into four basic categories: (1) degenerative, (2) vascular—previously referred to a multi-infarct, (3) trauma, and (4) infections.
- Standard medical evaluation tends to miss some of the most prevalent health issues experienced by older adults; these tend to include the five I's of geriatrics: (1) impaired homeostasis, (2) incompetence or intellectual impairment, (3) iatrogenesis, (4) immobility, and (5) incontinence.
- Dementia is difficult to diagnose due to the quandary of a potential multifactorial cause.
- There are no pharmacologic agents that can cure dementia; however, medications may be helpful in slowing the progression of the disease.
- The overall goal in older adult patient care is to maximize the patient's residual functional capacity to meet patient-centered goals for care for an optimal quality of life.
- The field of geriatrics and the care of older adult patients are well suited to incorporating the osteopathic approach to patient care.

CASE VIGNETTE

CHIEF COMPLAINT

Mr. S, a 77-year-old white male, is brought to the office by his daughter for a second opinion due to her concerns regarding his walking and his mood and behavior changes.

History of Present Illness:

The daughter, who usually lives out of state, notes that Mr. S has had a gradual progression of difficulty walking and he is getting "just mean." The daughter is concerned that he will really hurt himself some day if he falls. He is using a cane at her request, but he is adamant that he doesn't need it.

She is unsure of the onset of his instability since she lives out of state, but relates that he has had memory difficulties for years and was on donnepizil for this. His wife had cared for him until her recent passing due to a stroke. The daughter admits that her father had trouble walking for some time and maybe for years, but it has been particularly worrisome to her since he was placed on Carbidopa/Levadopa for Parkinson disease a few months ago. He has declined since then without the stabilizing influence of his wife.

The patient denies any difficulty and states that he uses the cane only because the daughter insists. Mr. S stated that he is forced to use a cane by "those people who are trying to put me away" and wishes "they would stop their incessant talking because they just confuse me." He is unable to identify who "they" are but claims he sees them "when they want to be seen." The daughter states that this pattern has been progressive over the last 3 to 4 months. Mr. S has not actually fallen but admits that he is slowed down by what he feels is arthritis. The daughter is also concerned about his driving due to slow reaction times from apparent stiffness. Mr. S refuses to give up the car keys and states "they want to take my car away, how am I suppose to get around?" He has been increasingly frustrated, short tempered, and easily agitated, which he attributed to

daughter's nagging, but the daughter believes his agitation and "weird thoughts" are due to the passing of his wife. She notes that he makes accusations about people taking things from him and talks to people who are not there. He no longer enjoys walking or caring for the dog. He now bathes infrequently and won't accept assistance to clean the house.

Mr. S feels he is being slowed up by stiffness, which he believes could be arthritis from his early life of physical labor. He believes his children want him out of the way and want him in a nursing home.

Past Medical History:

Hypertension at age 45, dyslipidemia at age 45, osteoarthritis at age 70, Alzheimer dementia at age 75, Parkinson disease at age 76.

Past Surgical History:

Appendectomy at age 22; left total knee replacement, osteoarthritis at age 68.

Social History:

He is an ex-smoker (quit 20 years ago) but smoked a pack a day from age 15 until then a 42 pack-yr history; alcohol consumption—couple of beers on the weekend while watching sports; no illicit drugs; married 50 years; two adult children—living and well. Daughter lives in another state 4 hours away, the son lives overseas and is estranged from the family. Mr. S has been relatively socially isolated due to his illness and his wife's illness. He has not resumed previous activities (no longer does maple sugaring or read books) or previous involvement (Rotary Club).

Family History:

He is the youngest of four siblings. A sister is deceased from renal failure and diabetes at age 84. Still living are a brother aged 83 and a sister aged 80. Both have high blood pressure and live independently. His father died at age 90 in a car accident and his mother died at age 87 from a cause unknown to him.

Current Medications:

Metoprolol: 50 mg PO BID
Simvistatin: 40 mg PO qhs
OTC: Naproxyn sodium 222 mg PO once or twice a day for knee or back pain (average 5 pills/wk)
Chondroitin sulfate from the health food store—dose unknown
Donnepizil: 10 mg PO qhs
Carbidopa/Levodopa: 10/100 PO TID

Immunizations:

Flu vaccine last fall. Pneumococcal vaccine 2 years ago. Last PPD or tetanus unknown.

REVIEW OF SYSTEMS

Head:

Denies headaches, no change in vision, hearing, smell, or taste. He wears bifocals with a new prescription nearly a year ago. He denies syncope, near syncope, or dizziness.

Heart:

Denies chest pain or palpitations. He has no cardiac history except as noted in past history without claudication, angina, or history of MI.

Lungs:

He denies shortness of breath, wheezing, coughing, dyspnea on exertion or orthopnea. No history of occupational exposure or TB.

GI:

Denies food intolerance, dysphasia, odynophagia, acid reflux, appetite changes, nausea, vomiting, diarrhea, constipation, changes in character of bowel movements or weight loss; although the daughter believes he looks thinner (Box 53.1).

GU:

Denies frequency of urination, hematuria, or dysuria. He admits to nocturia 1 to 2 per night. He states his stiffness makes him unable to get to the bathroom when he needs to, which causes him to wet himself at times.

Musculoskeletal:

He admits to a general stiffness usually without pain. He takes Naproxen occasionally for what he says is arthritis in his back and left knee. He believes this has caused a slowness of ambulation with gait changes. He denies tics, twitches, convulsions, paresthesias, or paralysis.

Psychiatric History:

He has had no psychiatric evaluations or hospitalizations. He claims to be satisfied with his life if people would just leave him alone. He denies feeling sad hopeless or worthless. He denies suicidal or homicidal ideation but jokes that he might change his mind if they keep pushing him. Despite reporting seeing people who are not there, he denies delusions, hallucinations, anxiety, or depression. The daughter reports social withdrawal, a short temper, and accusatory language and notes her father gets easily agitated and has difficulty with daily routines. He is not compliant with usual daily routines or medications since his wife died.

Activities of Daily Life:

The daughter reports that he dresses himself but would put on the same clothes day after day if she did not lay out the clothes for him. Likewise he feeds himself but only after she prepares the

---

Nutritional Health Checklist

Perform the following Nutritional Health Risk Questionnaire. Circle the score for "yes" responses and add up the total of circled scores at the bottom.

	Yes
Do you have an illness or condition that makes you change the kind and/or amount of food you eat?	2
Do you eat fewer than two meals per day?	3
Do you eat few fruits, vegetables or milk products?	2
Do you have three or more drinks of beer, liquor, or wine almost every day?	2
Do you have tooth or mouth problems that make it hard for you to eat?	2
Are there times when you cannot afford to buy the food you need?	4
Do you eat alone most of the time?	1
Do you take three or more different prescribed or over-the-counter drugs per day?	1
Have lost or gained 10 or more pounds in the last six months without wanting to?	2
Are there times when you are physically unable to shop, cook, and/or feed yourself?	2

Total score

Score interpretation

0–2:	Low nutritional risk
3–5:	Moderate nutritional risk
6 or more:	High nutritional risk

Additional nutritional questions:

How would you describe your current appetite? _____ Good _____ Poor _____ Variable
For how long? _____ Details:

Population Medicine (Richard Glickman-Simon, MD)—Tufts University School of Medicine, 2007

meals and sets them up. He ambulates with a cane as previously noted. He toilets himself, but the daughter notes occasional urinary incontinence and his underwear is sometimes soiled as if he does not clean himself well. He frequently has to be reminded to shower and at those times the daughter is afraid he will fall but he refuses her help or to use the shower chair.

Instrumental Activities of Daily Life:

Mr. S is able to answer a phone but does not dial it or look up numbers. He does no shopping or housework. The daughter shops, prepares meals, and handles his finances for him which her mother had done for the past 2 or 3 years. Mr. S needs assistance with travel and is unable to plan a trip or describe how to get form his house to places with which he was previously familiar yet he insists he can drive.

PHYSICAL EXAM

Vital signs:

BP: 119/72; pulse: 64; respiration: 14; O_2 Sat: 95%.

General:

Mr. S is alert, well hydrated, and well nourished although there are signs of recent weight loss as his clothes are ill fitting. He looks his stated age. He is in no acute distress, but he is obviously displeased at being at the doctor's office.

HEENT:

Head is atraumatic and normocephalic. Facies have a paucity of expression. Pupils are equal and reactive to light. Funduscopic exam reveals no papilledema, AV nicking, exudates, or hemorrhages. Pharynx is without erythema or masses. There is no evidence of cervical or submandibular lymphadenopathy. The thyroid is palpated without tenderness masses or nodularity.

Heart:

The heart is regular without murmur, gallop, or rub. The point of maximum impulse is in the left fifth intercostals space. No jugular venous distention or carotid bruit is appreciated.

Lungs:

The lungs are clear to auscultation and percussion with good respiratory excursion.

Abdomen:

The abdomen is flat and soft without hepatosplenomegaly, masses, tenderness rigidity, or rebound. Bowel sounds are auscultated. A lower right quadrant scar is present compatible with his history of appendectomy.

Extremities:

There is no evidence of digital clubbing, ulceration, or cyanosis. The left knee has a well-healed scar consistent with previous arthroplasty. Degenerative changes of both knees are evident. Dorsalis pedis and tibialis posterior pulses are present. The knees are slightly flexed at rest, as are the hips. He sits comfortably on the exam table, uses his arms to rise to the standing position, and sways slightly upon rising. He uses a cane to walk and has a slight hesitation upon initiation of walking and steps are unequal. He prefers to stand with a widened stance. His attempts to turn are noted to be irregular and discontinuous and he plops into the chair when asked to sit down.

Neurologic:

Deep tendon reflexes are +2/4 at knee, elbow, and forearm but 0/4 at the Achilles bilaterally. Strength is 5/5 proximal and distal in upper and lower extremities. Cranial nerves II to XII are intact. Facies are flat without droop. Speech is articulate but slow. No tremor or cog wheeling is noted, but joint stiffness is noted on range of motion testing and handwriting is particularly small. No clonus is noted and Babinski Reflex Test (Adams, 2000, pp. 19–23) is physiologic.

Psychiatric:

He is oriented to place and person but believes it is 10 years ago and that it is Fall when it is actually Winter. He is able to spell "WORLD" forward but not backward. He recalls 3/3 objects immediately but only 1 of 3 after 5 minutes despite cues. He follows a two-step command but has trouble with a three-step command. He refuses to draw a clock. He writes a three-word sentence that is difficult to read due to its small size. Patient is cordial and responds to questions although he is not happy about being in the physician's office. He believes his daughter wants him declared incompetent to prevent his driving and to place him in a nursing home. He relates that he has heard voices telling him she wants him "put away."

Structural Exam:

There is slight flexion posturing of the knees and hips with a generalized increase in paraspinal muscle tone in the thoracic and lumbar areas. There is flattening of the lumbar lordosis and a mild accentuation of the dorsal kyphosis. Periarticular changes of the knees and fingers are present.

DIFFERENTIAL DIAGNOSIS

The medical evaluation of older adults differs from standard medical evaluation in three general ways: "(1) it focuses on older individuals with complex issues; (2) it emphasizes functional status and quality of life; and (3) it frequently takes advantage of an interdisciplinary team of providers." Quite often standard medical evaluation will tend to miss some of the most prevalent health issues experienced by older adults. These include the *five I's of geriatrics*: (1) *impaired homeostasis*—otherwise referred to as homeostenosis; (2) *incompetence or intellectual impairment*; (3) *iatrogenesis*; (4) *immobility*; and (5) *incontinence* (Wagner et al., 1996). Unfortunately, these conditions are often considered to be the "giants" in geriatrics because they consume much of the physician's time. The geriatric assessment effectively addresses these as well as other areas of older adult care in order to prevent disease and disability while successfully providing care interventions.

It is fitting to review these "giants" in relation to Mr. S and within the context of the osteopathic approach. Questions that may come to mind for the physician as the geriatric assessment is taking place and the geriatric giants are being considered include.

Impaired Homeostasis

Does he have evidence that his situation is due to *homeostenosis*? Has there been a change that has interfered with the body's inherent capacity to self-regulate? Is the loss of his caregiver support evidence that a social homeostasis has been lost?

Incompetence or Intellectual Impairment

Does his mental status exam suggest that he may have *intellectual impairment*? If so, it is important to determine in what realms and to what degree. Is the impairment quantifiable? Is it from a

Competency Evaluation

Due to psychiatric illness, mental retardation, delirium, or dementia, older adult patients may in some situations be incapable of making decisions that safeguard their own self-interests. Although the MMSE provides useful information regarding a patient's global cognitive function, it is important to assess, by way of an interview, his or her competency in at least two areas: medical and financial decision-making. Following are questions to consider in the evaluation of a person's competency to make decisions directly affecting their health and financial security:

- Is the patient aware they have a mental illness (as listed above)?
- Does the patient understand the nature of the proposed treatment?
- Does the patient understand the need for treatment and the implications of refusing treatment?
- Does the mental illness interfere with judgment and reasoning so much that it accounts for refusal of treatment?
- Does the patient have knowledge of their current assets?
- Does the patient have knowledge of their monthly expenses and bills?
- Does the patient know where their assets are located and being managed?
- Can the patient complete simple calculations?
- Is the person's judgment so affected that his or her finances would be in jeopardy?

TABLE 53.1

DSM-IV Diagnostic Criteria for Dementia

A	The development of multiple cognitive deficits manifested by both:
	1. Memory impairment (impaired ability to learn new information or to recall previously learned information)
	2. One (or more) of the following cognitive disturbances: a. Aphasia (Language disturbances) b. Apraxia (impaired ability to carry out motor abilities despite intact motor function) c. Agnosia (failure to recognize or identify objects despite intact sensory function) d. Disturbance in executive function (i.e., planning, organization, sequencing, abstracting)
B	The sequencing deficits in criteria A1 and A2 each cause significant impairment in social or occupational functioning and represent a significant decline from a previous level of functioning
C	The course is characterized by a gradual onset and continuing cognitive decline

Source: Ward RC, Hruby RJ, Jerome JA, et al. *Foundations for Osteopathic Medicine.* Philadelphia, PA: American Osteopathic Association, Lippincott Williams & Wilkins, 2002. Adapted from the Diagnostic and Statistical Manual of Mental Disorders—DSM IV. 4th Ed. American Psychiatric Association: Washington DC, 1994.

---

metabolic, vascular, psychiatric or other source, or perhaps a combination? Physicians may determine capacity to function, use cognition, perform activities of daily living (ADLs), or meet executive abilities such as planning insight and judgment, but it is the courts that decide competence. Therefore, physicians need to be aware of how the courts referred to and define *incompetence*. Box 53.2 presents questions to consider in the evaluation of a person's competency to make decisions directly affecting their health and financial security.

Iatrogenesis

Is there a possibility of *iatrogenesis*? Has a previous diagnosis been in error? Has a treatment been instituted or not instituted that has created or exacerbated the current situation? Has treatment been started that is based on a symptom and rather than a cause? Is there a possibility of polypharmacy with drug/drug interactions?

Immobility

Is Mr. S's apparent *immobility* his central and most important problem? Does this put him at risk for a cascade of disasters as his daughter fears? Although it is the chief complaint, is immobility the root cause or the symptom of something significant?

Incontinence

Finally, Mr. S has an *incontinence* problem. Is it a physical problem (is his bodily system intact), is it caused by decreased cognitive function, or is it a physical function issue (he has difficulty moving to the bathroom)? Perhaps it is not an intrinsic problem unto itself but rather it is the manifestation of another problem.

This patient's history and physical exam are strongly suggestive of dementia, and although it was not the presenting complaint,

his cognitive function has the greatest clinical implication for his long-term health. The physician must determine if there are diagnostic criteria for dementia. The DSM-IV R lists criteria for the diagnosis of dementia (Table 53.1). Concerning Mr. S, one need to only apply the findings of short-term and long-term memory, with the patient's functional capacity in ADLs to recognize that our patient has a cognitive loss that meets the diagnostic criteria for dementia.

The differential diagnosis of dementia can be divided into two broad classifications—those that are reversible (Box 53.3) and

---

Potential Reversible Causes for the Dementia

Neoplasm
Autoimmune (lupus, arthritis, multiple sclerosis)
Metabolic disorders
Drugs/medications
Toxins (ETOH, heavy metals, organic poisons)
Nutritional disorders
Infections
Psychiatric disorders (depression, delirium, psychosis)
Other
Normal pressure hydrocephalus

Source: Kane R, Ouslander J, Abrass I. *Essentials of Clinical Geriatrics.* 5th Ed. New York, NY: McGraw Hill, 2004:130.

those that are not. The first responsibility for the physician is to distinguish between these two categories, and much of the workup is aimed at precisely this distinction. Failure to find reversible causes, if they exist, results in unnecessary treatment and stresses for the patient and the family.

The initial workup for reversible dementias always begins with a thorough history and physical examination. As with many conditions the history is central to the diagnosis and as osteopathic physicians, it is the functional consequences of the disturbance that should be investigated and documented for its impacts on the patient and the patient's support system. The physical exam should emphasize the neurologic and cardiovascular systems. Because the definitive diagnosis of dementia can only be proven by tissue sample from a brain biopsy, the diagnosis is one of exclusion. One must evaluate the patient for other reasonable causes of the diagnosis and when that fails, the physician is left with the likely diagnosis of dementia. Likewise, it is the constellation of signs and symptoms of the whole person that steers the physician to the conclusion of the type of dementia once the determination that a dementia exists is made.

The laboratory and imaging evaluations may include:

A. Blood studies
   Complete blood count (CBC)
   Comprehensive metabolic profile
      Glucose
      Renal functions—BUN, creatinine
      Electrolytes—sodium, potassium, chloride
      Liver functions—AST, ALT
      Calcium and phosphorus
   Thyroid-stimulating hormone (TSH)
   Vitamin B_{12} and folate
   Serologic test for syphilis
B. Radiographic studies
   Computerized tomography (CT) or magnetic resonance imaging (MRI) of the brain
   Selected patients may need autoimmune studies and neuropsychological testing.

It is also important to quantify the degree of the dementia to assist with the diagnosis and to provide a baseline for future assessments to determine the effectiveness of interventions. This could include a test for cognition such as the SLUMS, the Folstein Mini Mental Status Exam, or the Clox test. It could include a test for depression such as the Geriatric Depression Scale. A functional assessment of his ADLs is also useful and can be accomplished with such tests as the ADLs Scale or the Instrumental ADL (IADL) Scale. Many of these tests are easy to administer and can be done in the office by trained paramedical personnel.

Nonreversible causes of dementia can be classified in a number of different ways. The Agency for Health Care Policy and Research lists four basic categories: (1) degenerative, (2) vascular—previously referred to a multi-infarct, (3) trauma, and (4) infections (Costa et al., 1996). There is considerable overlap and some patients may have a mixture.

AD is known to account for approximately 50% of the dementias, vascular (previously called multi-infarct) dementia accounts for another 25%. Fifteen percent of dementias are caused by irreversible central nervous system (CNS) disorders such as Pick disease, Huntington chorea, inoperable brain tumors, and Parkinson disease. The remaining 10% result from treatable causes such as the effects of various drugs, brain tumors, vitamin B_{12} or folate deficiencies, depression, thyroid disturbances, and CNS infection.

Dementia with Lewy bodies accounts for up to 20% to 25% of dementia cases listed above. Age at onset is typically greater than 60 (Galvin et al., 2008).

In some cases, causes of dementia may overlap. That is the case for Alzheimer dementia and Parkinson disease. When the patient has dementia with detailed hallucination, Parkinsonian signs, and alterations in alertness and attention, one might suspect dementia with Lewy bodies (Table 53.2).

Vascular dementias are predominately caused by circulatory interruption to the brain. Often they are related to infarcts (strokes). They can be progressive as the patient experiences recurrent infarcts and hence were previously referred to as multi-infarct dementias. Many of these strokes happen at the subcortical level and are too small to cause permanent residual neurologic deficits in the motor or sensory systems. The key characteristic that distinguishes a classic vascular dementia is the typical stepwise decline. Unlike Alzheimer disease (AD) that usually shows a steady downward course, vascular dementias show a new decline with each new vascular insult followed by a period of stability and then another decline with the next event.

Mr. S presents with a past history of Parkinson disease and Alzheimer dementia with a recent decline in cognition that is slowly getting worse over the previous few months and has been exacerbated since the death of his wife. In treating the whole person, consideration must be given to his previous diagnosis of AD, the recent initiation of anti-Parkinson drugs, and the loss of his primary caregiver whose support may have masked the true seriousness of his cognitive loss.

The physician is left with the quandary of a potential multifactorial cause for his current presentation. This is especially true when one remembers that the body is an integrated sum of its parts and that care of the presenting disease must include considerations by the physician for not only the patient's physical body, but also his emotional, social, and spiritual health. The challenge is that there are no algorithms for such considerations, which calls upon the skill of the physician to consider these factors at every stage of the diagnostic and treatment process. The differential diagnosis of subacute, progressive cognitive decline, and gait and behavioral changes in a 77-year-old man with a history of hypertension, dyslipidemia, AD, and Parkinson disease can be viewed in Table 53.3.

In considering the whole context of Mr. S presentation, the Parkinson disease diagnosis can be confirmed as illustrated by his handwriting, his gait, and his paucity of facial expressions among other characteristics. However, the fact that his dementia was exacerbated by the initiation of anti-Parkinson medication and the presence of delusions and psychotic overlay suggests a Lewy body dementia. Lewy bodies are rounded eosinophilic intracytoplasmic neuronal inclusions that contain the protein α-synuclein; they are characteristic of dementia with Lewy bodies and of Parkinson disease. In dementia with Lewy bodies, Lewy bodies occur in the cerebral cortex and other areas of the brain. In Parkinson disease, Lewy bodies occur in selected subcortical structures, most notably the substantia nigra. Dementia with Lewy bodies, Parkinson disease, and AD overlap considerably. For example, patients who have Parkinson disease may develop dementia with Lewy bodies; patients who have AD may have a modest number of Lewy bodies, and patients who have dementia with Lewy bodies may have neuritic plaques and neurofibrillary tangles. Further research is needed to clarify the relationships among these disorders (Aarsland et al., 2004; Hurtig et al., 2000; Merdes et al., 2003; Tsuboi and Dickson, 2005).

However, in the case of Mr. S, AD is unlikely to be accompanied by the level of psychotic symptoms displayed by Mr. S. Pseudodementia in the form of depression may also be considered,

TABLE 53.2

Diagnosing Lewy Body Dementia

Symptom/Area of Deficit	Dementia with Lewy Bodies	Parkinson Disease Dementia
Diagnostic criteria	**Probable =** • Dementia plus 2 Core • Dementia plus 1 Core 1 Suggestive **Possible =** • Dementia plus 1 Core • Dementia plus 1 Suggestive	**Probable =** • Parkinson's, Dementia plus 2 Core **Possible =** • Parkinson's, Dementia plus 1 Core
Dementia	Required	Required
1. Memory impairment	X	Core
2. Language impairment	X	Core
3. Visuospatial function impairment	Usually prominent	Core
4. Executive function impairment	Usually prominent	Core
Parkinsonism	Core (can occur around the same time OR after dementia)	PD diagnosis required (usually years before dementia)
Fluctuating cognition	Core	X
1. Reduced attention	Usually prominent	Core
2. Excessive daytime sleepiness	X	Supportive
Visual hallucinations	Core	Supportive
Severe neuroleptic sensitivity	Suggestive	X
REM sleep behavior disorder	Suggestive	X
Changes in personality and mood		Supportive
1. Depression	Supportive	X
2. Anxiety	X	X
Delusions	Supportive	Supportive
Apathy	X	Supportive
Hallucinations in other modalities	Supportive	X
Severe autonomic dysfunction	Supportive	X
Repeated falls and syncope	Supportive	X
Transient, unexplained loss of consciousness	Supportive	X

X = Common symptom not required for diagnosis. Galvin JE, Boeve BF, Duda JE, et al. Current Issues in Lewy Body Dementia Diagnosis, Treatment and Research, Report sponsored by The Carmen Foundation, Lewy Body Dementia Association, Inc., 2008:7.

but his presentation is not convincing for depression based on the DSM criteria for depression or his depression test score. Vascular dementia usually has a more abrupt onset with a gradual stepwise decline as more vascular events occur and impact brain function.

OSTEOPATHIC PATIENT MANAGEMENT

The osteopathic approach to patient care, first described in the 19th century, dovetails well with the much newer field of geriatric medicine that stresses the care of the individual as much as the care of the disease state. This symbiotic relationship is paramount in older adult healthcare. The physician is tasked with helping the patient achieve maximal residual functions. It cannot be stressed enough that the majority of older adults age successfully; they are survivors. Nationally, approximately 5% require institutional care (AHCA, 2007), leaving 95% of older adults to be cared for in the community with an increasingly limited number of physicians trained in geriatrics. Unfortunately, it is the 5% who consume much of the health

care dollars and physicians' time and limited resources (Flowers et al., AARP, 2003). Despite this, it is the physician's responsibility to work with older adult patients and their caregivers to facilitate successful aging well before the onset of a health crisis. Implementing preventive activities at younger ages includes primary and secondary disease prevention and health promotion activities such as proper nutrition, physical exercises, cognitive exercises, and the careful exploration of psychosocial dimensions. These activities can be implemented with patients of all ages and health conditions. Suffice to say, it is never too late to make changes to augment health.

The overall goal is to maximize the patient's residual functional capacity to meet patient-centered goals for care for an optimal quality of life. A variety of measures are useful for the well being of patients with dementia and their families. These interventions range from the assessment and potential alteration of the physical living environment, to education on the use of specific strategies of care to providing information and counseling services or referrals. It is important to remember that this can only be done with the

TABLE 53.3

Differential Diagnosis Chart

Differential Diagnosis	Consideration
Vascular	Vascular dementia
Inflammatory	Unlikely
Neoplasia	Unlikely
Degenerative	Alzheimer dementia
	Lewy body dementia
	Picks disease
Iatrogenic idiopathic	Adverse medication effect
Congenital	Unlikely
Autoimmune	Unlikely
Trauma/toxins	Unlikely
Endocrine/metabolic	Hypothyroidism
Psychologic	Depression, delirium

Source: Ward RC, Hruby RJ, Jerome JA, et al. *Foundations for Osteopathic Medicine*. Philadelphia, PA: American Osteopathic Association, Lippincott Williams & Wilkins, 2002.
Adapted from the Diagnostic and Statistical Manual of Mental Disorders—DSM IV. 4th Ed. Washington DC: American Psychiatric Association, 1994.

Caregiver and Patient Resources

A. Alzheimer's Association. Warning signs for Alzheimer's disease. http://www.alz.org/alzheimers_disease_symptoms_of_alzheimers.asp
B. Eldercare Locator - 800-677-1116 http://www.aoa.gov/elderpage/locator.html
C. Lewy Body Dementia Web site (http://www.lbda.org) Resources:
  1. Introduction to Lewy Body Dementia Web address: http://www.lbda.org/feature/1942/an-introduction-to-lewy-body-dementia.htm
  2. Understanding Lewy Body Dementia: 10 Things You Should Know. pdf file accessed through http://www.lbda.org
  3. Facts about Lewy Body Dementia Pamphlet. http://www.lbda.org/feature/1925/facts-about-lbd-brochure.htm
  4. Lewy Body Digest—Newsletter. http://www.lbda.org/category/3477/newsletter.htm
D. National Agencies on Aging (N4A) is the leading voice on aging issues for Area Agencies on Aging. Access this site to find a local Agency on Aging to assist with finding services and answers on older adult resources. http://www.n4a.org/

involvement of a multiprofessional team and it is the physician's duty to recognize the need and to provide avenues to the appropriate resources when possible. The management of patients is best done in the least restrictive environment possible. The preparation for changes in level of care must always be anticipated, as dementia is a progressive disease. The support for the family and caregivers is crucial to this effort. Guilt, feelings of being overwhelmed and underprepared are common. The physician should proactively assess the family for signs of physical, emotional, and financial stresses that will impact the care of the patient and thus advocate for strategies that minimize those stresses. Services, such as those from Area Agencies on Aging, the Alzheimer's Association or Lewy Body Dementia Association may be of value (Box 53.4). Local agency and chapters can be found via a web search or in local phonebooks.

Biomechanical Model

While there are no biomechanical changes specific to the diagnosis of dementia, we are aware of certain prevailing tendencies for the older adult population. It should also be emphasized that many healthy older adults often practiced good health habits in their younger years. If the osteopathic physician is to see the results of healthy aging, then the interventions such as immunizations, smoking cessation, lipid management, calcium and vitamin D supplementation, and exercising the mind and body must begin well in advance of the diagnosis of disease. A good health foundation gives older adults a stronger base to call upon.

Regardless of past health practices, older adults tend to experience alterations in biomechanical functions such as an increased incidence of protein crosslinking in the soft tissues and a loss of elastin that leads to a generalized stiffening and slowness of reaction. There is a loss of subcutaneous fat and subcutaneous tissues making the patient vulnerable to trauma and ecchymoses, Bony joints are subject to the development of degenerative conditions such as arthritis due to longevity and wear and tear. Thus, TART—tissue texture abnormality, asymmetry, restriction of motion,

tenderness—(Mosier and Kohara, 2007) findings must be interpreted in the context of usual aging. We can expect that the older adult will have tissue texture abnormalities based on elastin loss and changes in tone and turgor. We will find there is usually asymmetry and motion restrictions in the absence of trauma. Tenderness can be a useful guide to the onset of new conditions for considerations. The older adult patient loses height while preserving span due to the loss of hydration in the intervertebral discs and the prevalence of osteoporosis. The *typical* older adult will demonstrate a "flexion posture." Thus, the knees and hips may not extend as far and forward bending at the lumbar spine may be restricted. There is typically flattening of the usual lumbar lordosis and accenting of the dorsal kyphosis and or cervical lordosis. Cranial sutures calcify with age and cranial motion abnormalities and their interpretation can be difficult to detect in older adults.

Osteopathic manipulative treatment (OMT) can be applied in cases where there is degenerative neurologic disease especially in which dopaminergic synapses in the corpus stratum deteriorate leading to tremor, bradykinesis, and muscular rigidity. Muscle energy techniques are thought to be especially helpful in treating these patients. The author usually avoids thrust and impulse techniques because of the risk of osteopenia in many geriatric patients. A combination of manipulation, physical therapy, and strength training, especially in the earlier phases of dementia of the Lewy bodies type, may improve head and neck posture, increase stride length, increase hip, knee and ankle flexion, increase foot lift from floor, decrease incidence of falls, decrease depression, thereby improving quality of life (DiGiovanna and Rowante, 2005).

Respiratory Circulatory Model

Vascular dementia may be caused by macrotrauma such as in a stroke, but it can also be caused by the changes in blood flow brought on by aging. Arteries may narrow, slowing capillary flow. This may affect the intrinsic function of the brain; the failure to clear the waste also may assist in the accumulation of waste products, and toxic β-amyloid creating a chemical imbalance of the neuronal ability to function (Center for Dementia Research, NIH Report, 2001).

Many clinicians and researchers have observed lifestyle factors in the onset and progression of dementia. We know that exercise and nutrition play a large role in healthy aging in general, and this seems to be true for dementia prevention as well. The activities reduce concomitant risk factors such as obesity, elevated lipid levels, and high blood pressure. Pursuing intellectual activities (exercise for the mind) and active social contacts are contributors to healthy aging (Snowdon, 2003). Epidemiologic studies show that higher level of physical activities reduces cognitive decline. Animal studies show that activity increases capillary formation in the brain. Although a fair amount of research has been conducted, more trials are needed to expand our knowledge.

Neurological Model

Dementia results from a confluence of numerous influences. Some such as Parkinsonian dementia and Alzheimer dementia are rooted in genetic, environmental, and systemic factors that then lead to the accumulation of abnormal proteins or reduced oxygen flow to tissues and resulting toxic processes. These toxic processes then lead to the manifestations that we can observe. These early symptoms depend on the area of the brain affected but can include tremor, memory loss, executive functions losses of planning insight and judgment, gait and movement disorders, hallucinations, delusions, and rigidity.

Alzheimer researchers have uncovered the apoE gene on chromosome 19 that is believed responsible for some cases of familial AD as it produces a protein referred to as apolipoprotein E. But this connection is incomplete and does not account for all cases. The two hallmarks for AD are the plaques and neurofibrillatory tangles found in brain tissue. Plaque formation involves the production and deposition of β-amyloid plaques. Tau is the protein that is the chief component of the tangles. These tangles are commonly found in the frontotemporal dementias such as those associated with Parkinson disease and may be a cause of dementia. These hypotheses warrant aggressive ongoing research.

Scientists do not yet fully understand what causes AD or other dementias. Age is the most important known risk factor. For example, the number of people with AD doubles every 5 years beyond age 65 (Launer et al., 1999). Some researchers have implicated a low-grade chronic inflammation as an inciting factor. Others have targeted the metabolic processes that produce free radicals that cause oxidative damage on cellular mitochondria. These damaged mitochondria then cause malfunctions of the cellular functions including neurotransmitter production and receptivity. Since the brain has a high rate of metabolism, it may be especially susceptibility to this oxidative damage.

A strong component of the care of patients with dementia is pharmacological therapy that addresses the neurological pathology and sequelea of the condition. The pharmacotherapeutics fall into three broad categories: drugs that (1) enhance cognition and function, (2) treat coexisting depression, and (3) treat complications of dementia. None of the medications in these categories cure the disease but may slow the progression of the disease thereby adding functional months to the patient's quality of life. They may also be useful in managing comorbid conditions associated with the dementia. For medications that enhance cognition, currently available medications include the cholinesterase inhibitors such as Donnepezil (Aricept), Rivastigmine (Exelon), and Galatamine (Razadyne). These drugs work by slowing down the action of acetylcholinesterase to maintain higher levels of the acetylcholine neurotransmitter in the brain.

The newest agent is Memantine (Nemenda) that affects another neurotransmitter, glutamine. Like the cholinesterase inhibitors, this agent will not stop or reverse the dementia. It may be necessary to use these agents in combination (Qaseem et al., 2008).

As with all medications, there are risks and benefits, and drug treatment should be instituted with the mantra of "start low, go slow, but go." Low dosages are instituted and gradually adjusted upward, slowly but deliberately. Consequently, repeated assessments and adjustments of medication over time are needed. The astute physician must recognize and counsel the patient and family on these risks and benefits. For many patients and their families, an ethical struggle may eventually ensue around the discontinuation of medications when they no longer serve to meet a patient-centered goal related to the quality of life.

In considering which pharmacologic agents to institute, one must also consider which agents the patient may already be taking that can exacerbate the symptoms or are incompatible with those planned to be instituted. Reversible causes of dementia may include iatrogenically prescribed medications and other treatments. Mr. S should stop his anti-Parkinson medication as it can exacerbate the psychoses of dementia with Lewy bodies. Antipsychotic medications may be instituted with caution. He probably should continue on donnepizil.

Behavioral Model

In a society with fewer extended families, the psychosocial aspects of the dementias can be paramount in care management. In terms of the whole patient, the cultural and spiritual foundations of the patient and the family of caregivers will influence the care decisions and the context in which they are suggested by the physician and the manner in which they are accepted by the patient and caregivers. Autonomy is prized as an ethical precept and should be honored when possible in the patient with capacity. As dementias progress, practitioners must increasingly rely on secondary sources of information to determine values and wishes of the patient. It is therefore important to try to determine these preferences as early in the disease process as possible.

The psychosocial elements of dementia range from the emotional response to the diagnosis to stressors from coping with the ongoing management of the individual, to honoring the individual's beliefs and values. Honoring the patient's previous stated wishes may cause dissonance among caregivers who want to honor those wishes but find it difficult to do so. Role reversal as offspring assumes care for their parents is stressful. Practical matters of advanced directives, aggressiveness of interventions, preferences for religious support, and guardianships or power of attorney should be discussed early on in the management. Since the "mind is robbed before the body," patients and their families may experience a divide between the apparent abilities of the older adult and the actual abilities. Issues of alone time, driving, and financial management may become obstacles and create a dynamic tension in the patient and in intrafamily relationships (Family Caregiver Alliance, 2009).

The osteopathic philosophy makes very clear the distinction between treating disease in patients and treating patients who have disease (Still, 1892). It is the latter that must dominate our osteopathic approach. Clarity of goals of care, honoring the culture and belief systems of families and individuals, providing support systems for patients and families must all be sought. Care must be tailored to the needs of the individual and families, not institutions. For the physician, the issue involves more than just managing the dementia; it is imperative to help the patient make the most of their remaining years (Rabin, 2000).

Most patients with dementia express the desire to remain in their homes. Caregivers often have considerable guilt and feelings of inadequacies when this is no longer possible. Geriatric practitioners would support the home environment as the best place for ongoing care. As the patient loses ADL skills, the concerns about safety, provision of care, and the need for continual supervision may become overwhelming. Home health agencies can be of assistance but are often limited as to length and depth of service availability. To further compound care for older adults with dementia, financial outlay for care can be considerable, regardless of the skill and availability of such care, it is often difficult to secure even for those with the means to pay out of pocket.

A study conducted in 2006 (Buhr et al., 2006) cited the caregiver reasons for placement of older adult loved ones in nursing homes. These included (a) the need for skilled care (65%), (b) the caregiver's health (49%), (c) dementia-related behaviors (46%), and (4) the need for more assistance (23%). Behaviors are often the last straw for decision makers. These include socially inappropriate behaviors, agitation, delusions, wandering, and incontinence. In an earlier study (Magaziner et al., 2007), the prevalence of dementia in Maryland nursing homes—a state with similar admissions to nursing homes elsewhere in the United States—was 48.2% with an upper bound estimate at 54.5%. Prevalence was highest in smaller (<50 beds) facilities (65.5%) as compared with those with a higher number (200+) of beds (39.6%). Percentages were also higher in urban versus rural areas (50.0% vs. 39.1%). Of note is that dementia-related admissions represent high percentages of all nursing home admissions.

Metabolic Energy Model

The single most identifying characteristic of the aging process is a narrowing of the homeostatic window. As we age, processes come into play that impact the individual's response to physical, biologic, or psychologic insults. This has been called homeostenosis. The ability of the body to self-regulate and to marshal resources to heal is challenged in older adults. For example, the cardiac reserves are lessened as cardiac output diminishes and the heart is less responsive to a catecholamine stimulus. Similarly, the endocrine system is less responsive to the stimulating hormones. There may be reduced receptor responsiveness to endogenous and exogenous stimuli, the immune response may be blunted, and osmoreceptors are less sensitive to changes in fluid and electrolytes. With less ability for older adults to tolerate physiologic stress, the line between health and wellness narrows. Further, a person with dementia may find it difficult to marshal the psychological and social resources to cope with illness. This homeostenosis makes older adults prone to a cascade of disasters. An example of this could be: dementia leads to less mobility, the immobility leads to instability, the instability leads to a fall, the fall leads to a fracture, the fracture leads to more immobility that leads to respiratory stasis and atelectasis, which leads to pneumonia, and so forth. However, it must be stressed that this characteristic of aging does not apply universally. Individuals age individually; meaning that aging itself is not a disease and individuals must be approached individually.

Diet has been an area of interesting research as well with attention to antioxidants and folate. Individual studies have been promising but inconclusive when reviewed as a whole. Mega doses of vitamin B and the use of herbal medications and antioxidants have been proposed. Gingko biloba has been the leading herbal promoted for memory improvement. Vitamin E has been likewise had its advocates. Anti-inflammatory medications such as ibuprofen have been recommended for their anti-inflammatory abilities. Despite the fervor of some, none of these has proven more effective than a balanced diet and exercise of the mind and body (Engelhart et al., 2002; Gray et al., 2008; Heyn et al., 2004; Mazza et al., 2006).

Additional resources on dementia of the Lewy body type may be found in Box 53.5: Lewy body dementia resources for physicians.

The key principles of managing dementia can be found in Box 53.6.

Lewy Body Dementia Resources for Physicians

1. For Emergency Room Physicians: Treating LBD Psychosis. Developed in consultation with LBDA's Scientific Advisory Council. http://www.lbda.org/go/er
2. Current Issues in Lewy Body Dementia: Diagnosis, Treatment, and Research (May 2008) by Galvin et al. PDF found on home page at: http://www.lbda.org/
3. Physician's Reference List of Lewy Body Resources—updated 2008. PDF found on home page at: http://www.lbda.org/
4. Message to Physicians Treating Lewy Body Dementia—PDF found on home page at: http://www.lbda.org/

Principles in Managing Dementia

I. Optimize function
   Investigate and treat reversible and comorbid medical conditions
   Avoid unnecessary medications especially anticholernergic and sedating medications
   Provide appropriate assistive devices such as walkers, hearing aids, eyeglasses
   Modify the environment such as widening doors, the addition of grab bars, ramps, elevated toilet seats and the removal of scatter rugs
   Prepare patient and family for changes in location and time to adapt to new placements
   Emphasize nutrition and exercise
II. Identify and manage complications
   Behavioral disorders
   Depression
   Loss of insight and judgment (wandering, driving, planning)
   Psychoses
   Incontinence
   Team based care with nursing, occupational and physical therapists, social work, home health agencies and others
III. Information management for patient and family
   Nature of disease with regular updates of progression and prognosis
   Social service agency resources such as the Alzheimer's Association
   Advanced directives
   Respite service options
IV. Family/caregiver counseling
   Identify supportive services
   Identify and resolve family conflicts
   Handle feelings of guilt anger and despair
   Legal concerns
   Financial concerns
   Ethical concerns
   End of life care

Source: Modified from Kane R, Ouslander J, Abrass I. *Essentials of Clinical Geriatrics*. 5th Ed. New York, NY: McGraw Hill, 2004:141.

SUMMARY

The treatment of an older adult with dementia begins with a history and physical to determine the degree of progression of the condition. Applying the osteopathic practices and principles including evaluating for predisposing dysfunction of the entire body is a part of the physical examination. The diagnosis includes considerations of two broad classifications of dementia—those that are reversible and those that are not. The physician must distinguish between these two categories, which is accomplished by and large by the history, physical, and lab results. Treatment is directed to the identified dementia and must include considerations of the patient as a whole person. OMT may be utilized when appropriate to improve head-and-neck posture, increase stride length, increase hip, knee and ankle flexion, increase foot lift from floor, decrease incidence of falls, decrease depression, thereby improving quality of life. The environment must also be considered in the case of dementia diagnosis and a determination of ways of modifying the environment to improve the overall health or at least quality of life is essential.

REFERENCES

1. Aarsland D, Ballard CG, Halliday G. Are Parkinson's disease with dementia and dementia with Lewy bodies the same entity? *J Geriatr Psychiatry Neurol* 2004;17:137–145.
2. Adams A. *Neurology in Primary Care*. F.A. Davis Co., 2000.
3. American Geriatrics Society (AGS). Areas of Basic Competency for the Care of Older Patients for Medical and Osteopathic Schools. 1998. Available at: http://www.americangeriatrics.org/education/competency.shtml. Accessed February 2009.
4. American Geriatrics Society (AGS), 2006. Available at: http://www.americangeriatrics.org/news/ags_fact_sheet.shtml. Accessed January 2009.
5. American Health Care Association (AHCA). Trends in Nursing Facility Characteristics. Reimbursement and Research Department. Available at: http://www.ahcancal.org/research_data/trends_statistics/Documents/trends_nursing_facilities_characteristics_Dec2007.pdf
6. Buhr GT, Kuchibhatia M, Clipp EC. Caregivers' reasons for nursing home placement: clues for improving discussions with families prior to the transition. *Gerontologist* 2006;46(1):52–61.
7. Center for Dementia Research Alzheimer's Disease Fact Sheet; NIH Publication No. 01–3431; September 2001. Available at: http://cdr.rfmh.org/pages/infopage.html. Accessed March 2009.
8. Costa PT, Williams TF, Somerfield M, et al. (Guideline Panel). Recognition and initial assessment of Alzheimer's disease and related dementias. Clinical Practice Guideline No. 19. AHCPR Publication No. 97-0702. Rockville, MD: Agency for Health Care Policy and Research (AHCPR), November 1996.
9. DiGiovanna EL, Rowante M. Neurological considerations. In: DiGiovanna EL, Schiowitz S, Dowling DJ. *An Osteopathic Approach to Diagnosis and Treatment*. 3rd Ed. Philadelphia, PA: Lippincott Williams & Wilkins, 2005.
10. Engelhart MJ, Geerlings MI, Ruitenberg A, et al. Diet and risk of dementia: does fat matter? *Neurology* 2002;59:1915–1921.
11. Family Caregiver Alliance Dementia—Is This Dementia and What Does It Mean? Montgomery St, Ste 1100, San Francisco, CA. Available at: http://www.caregiver.org/caregiver/jsp/content_node.jsp?nodeid=569. Accessed March 2009.
12. Flowers L, Cool RJ, Melvin ME. AARP, Public Policy Institute, AARP, 601 E Street, NW, Washington DC, Pub ID: D17984, 2003.
13. Galvin JE, Boeve BF, Duda JE, et al. Current Issues in Lewy Body Dementia Diagnosis, Treatment and Research. Report Sponsored by The Carmen Foundation, Lewy Body Dementia Association, Inc., 2008.
14. Gawande A. The way we age now. *A. Annals of Medicine: The New Yorker*, 2007. Available at: http://www.newyorker.com/reporting/2007/04/30/070430fa_fact_gawande/. Accessed November 2008.
15. Gray SL, Anderson ML, Crane PK, et al. Antioxidant vitamin supplement use and risk of dementia or Alzheimer's disease in older adults. *J Am Geriatr Soc* 2008;56(2):291–295.
16. Heyn P, Abreu BC, Ottenbacher KJ. The effects of exercise training on elderly persons with cognitive impairment and dementia: a meta-analysis. *Arch Phys Med Rehabil* 2004;85:1694–1704.
17. Hurtig HI, Trojanowski JQ, Galvin J, et al. Alpha-synuclein cortical Lewy bodies correlate with dementia in Parkinson's disease. *Neurology* 2000;54:1916–1921.
18. Kane R, Ouslander J, Abrass I. *Essentials of Clinical Geriatrics*. 5th Ed. New York, NY: McGraw Hill, 2004.
19. Launer LJ, Andersen K, Dewey ME, et al. EURODEM Incidence Research Group and Work Groups. Rates and risk factors for dementia and Alzheimer's disease. *Neurology* 1999;52:78.
20. Lee M, Wilkerson L, Reuben DB, et al. Development and validation of a geriatric knowledge test for medical students. *J Am Geriatr Soc* 2004; 52:983–988.
21. Magaziner J, German P, Itkin Zimmerman S, et al. The prevalence of dementia in a statewide sample of new nursing home admissions aged 65 and older. *Gerontologist* 2007;40:663–672.
22. Mazza M, Capuano A, Bria P, et al. A comparison in the treatment of Alzheimer's dementia in a randomized placebo-controlled double-blind study. *Eur J Neurol* 2006;13:981–985 [PMID: 16930364].
23. Merdes AR, Hansen LA, Jeste DV, et al. Influence of Alzheimer pathology on clinical diagnostic accuracy in dementia with Lewy bodies. *Neurology* 2003;60:1586–1590.
24. Mosier AD, Kohara D. *Osteopathic Medicine Recall*. Baltimore, MD: Lippincott Williams & Wilkins, 2007.
25. Rabin B. Social networks and dementia. *Lancet* 2000;356(9233):76–77.
26. Snowdon DA. Healthy aging and dementia: findings from the nun study. *Ann Intern Med* 2003;139:450–454.
27. Still AT. *The Philosophy and Mechanical Principles of Osteopathy*. Kansas City, MO: Hudson-Kimberly, 1892.
28. Tsuboi Y, Dickson DW. Dementia with Lewy bodies and Parkinson's disease with dementia: are they different? *Parkinsonism Relat Disord* 2005;11:S47–S51.
29. Qaseem A, Snow V, Cross JT Jr, et al. the Joint American College of Physicians/American Academy of Family Physicians Panel on Dementia. Current pharmacologic treatment of dementia: a clinical practice guideline from the American College of Physicians and the American Academy of Family Physicians. 2008;148:5:370–378.
30. Wagner EH, Austin BT, Von Korff M. Organizing care for patients with chronic illness. *Milbank Q* 1996;74:511–544.
31. Ward RC, Hruby RJ, Jerome JA, et al. *Foundations for Osteopathic Medicine*. Philadelphia, PA: American Osteopathic Association, Lippincott Williams & Wilkins, 2002.

54

Uncontrolled Asthma

MARY ANNE MORELLI HASKELL AND JESUS SANCHEZ, JR

KEY CONCEPTS

- Asthma is an obstructive pulmonary disease with an inflammatory component.
- The dynamic balance between sympathetic and parasympathetic influences in the lung is distorted in asthma.
- Aspects of anatomical and physiological immaturity in young children with asthma result in vulnerability for respiratory muscle fatigue, inefficiency of diaphragmatic mechanics, and ineffectiveness of tissue recoil.
- There are biomechanical, respiratory-circulatory, metabolic, and neurological influences that need to be considered in the management of the child with asthma.
- Osteopathic manipulative medicine used in conjunction with standard care may improve the severity of asthma symptoms and decrease the need for pharmaceutical management.

CASE VIGNETTE

CHIEF COMPLAINT

A 10-year-old female patient with a history of asthma was brought from school to the clinic by her mother. This patient was well known to the clinic, as she has been seen two to three times per week for her symptoms. She has often been sent to the clinic during school hours.

History of Present Illness:

The patient has been noted to be noncompliant with her medications. On this particular visit, the patient ran out of her albuterol measured dose inhaler (MDI) and was having an asthma attack. The clinic staff approached the patient in a somewhat dismissive manner, stating that the patient was only trying to get out of school.

Past Medical History:

Positive for recurrent upper respiratory tract infections with exacerbation of wheezing and cough. The patient has been hospitalized four times in her lifetime because of asthma exacerbations, but she has never been ventilated. Her last hospitalization was 2 years ago. She has also had numerous emergency room visits because of her asthma. As an infant, she had reflux and recurrent ear infections.

Past Surgical History:

Positive for tympanoplasty and ventilation tubes at 8 months of age and 2 years.

Family History:

Father is 36 with anxiety/depressive disorder and hypertension. Mother is 34 with irritable bowel syndrome. Both parents smoked until 2 years ago. One elder sister with scoliosis, two younger sisters in good health except for ear infections as infants.

Social History:

The patient lives at home with her parents and three sisters. The family is economically challenged and there is some concern about regarding her and her family's ability to comprehend and comply with medical instructions regarding her asthma therapy.

Medications

Albuterol MDI—two puffs q.i.d.
Beclomethasone inhaler—two puffs q4-6h as needed

Immunizations

Up-to-date

REVIEW OF SYSTEMS

General:

She admits to fatigue but denies fever, chills, and sweats.

HEENT:

She denies headache, visual changes, she admits to nasal congestion but denies sneezing and sore throat.

Lungs:

She admits to "trouble breathing" and feeling "chest tightness" and "out of breath." She admits to cough, which is nonproductive. She admits to wheezing.

Cardiovascular:

She denies weakness.

GI:

She denies nausea, vomiting, stomach pain, diarrhea, burning chest pain

Orthopedic:

She denies myalgias and arthralgias

PHYSICAL EXAM

Vital signs:

HR: 98 beats/min, RR: 24 breaths/min, BP: 180/90 mm Hg, and pulse oximetry O_2 saturation: 93% while breathing room air. The patient was afebrile and blood pressure was 120/88.

General:

She appears mildly ill and has occasional paroxysm of coughing.

HEENT:

Normal.

Heart:

Heart rate is regular. No murmur or gallop is auscultated.

Lungs:

Diffuse bilateral expiratory wheezing with full breath sounds. Moderate accessory respiratory muscle use with respiration without paradoxical thoracoabdominal breathing was noted.

Abdomen:

Soft and nontender without hepatospenomegaly. Bowel sounds are normal.

Orthopedic/Structural Exam:

There is a mild right thoracic scoliosis present with forward bending, which is 50% reducible with passive sidebending. The pelvis is rotated right. The lumbosacral junction is sidebent right. The thoracolumbar junction is sidebent right and rotated left. Expiratory motion of the upper ribs on the right is decreased and overall there is decreased rib compliance and reduced excursion during the exhalation phase of respiration especially involving ribs three to five with bilateral paraspinal muscle spasm at these levels. C7-T1 is sidebent and rotated to the left. There is compression of the cranial base and occipito-mastoid area on the right.

DIFFERENTIAL DIAGNOSIS

The differential diagnosis of diffuse expiratory wheezes, moderate accessory respiratory muscle use, increased pulse rate, and decreased oxygen saturation level in a patient with known asthma supports the working diagnosis of an acute exacerbation of asthma. The staff was immediately notified to begin a nebulized albuterol treatment.

Asthma is the most common chronic disease of children and adolescents. The most common symptoms include wheezing, shortness of breath, chest tightness, and cough (Barrios, 2006; Colice, 2004). Asthma symptoms may be exacerbated by cold, exercise, infection, medications such as aspirin and NSAIDS, and allergens. Although the precise etiology is still unclear, asthma involves hypersensitivity of the bronchi and lower airways to allergens, cold, or other irritants including pollution. The resulting inflammation, bronchospasm, and mucous plugging lead to intermittent airway obstruction and difficulties in breathing. In severe cases, death may result (Barrios, 2006; Eder, 2006). The severity of asthma should never be underestimated.

Asthma can be thought of as an obstructive respiratory process. In addition to high-pitched diffuse wheezes, it may present with night time cough or prolonged expiratory phase of respiration.

Asthma is classified by severity of symptoms and management is based upon this classification. Mild intermittent asthma occurs when symptoms present 2 or fewer days per week or 2 nights per month; mild persistent asthma presents more than 2 days per week or more than 2 nights per month but less than once daily; moderate persistent asthma presents daily nightly; and severe persistent asthma occurs continually during the day and frequently at night.

Exploring the natural history of asthma has raised awareness of the variability within the disease continuum (Barrios, 2006). Asthma commonly begins in infancy; as one study found, 5% of infants had at least one physician encounter for reported wheezing within the first year of life (Reed, 2006). During the age range from infancy into adolescence, intrinsic asthma appears to be associated with exposure to respiratory infections, such as Respiratory Syncytial Virus. Asthma, which is termed "allergic or extrinsic,"

has been found to develop most often during the second decade of life with some persistence into adulthood (Barrios, 2006). Persistent symptoms of asthma more often occur in children with atopy (Carroll, 2008; Reed, 1999; Sears, 2008; Singh, 2006). Although different criteria have been used to diagnosis asthma over the past thirty years, the incidence of asthma appears to have increased over the last two decades (CDC, 2008), and external factors such as environmental pollutants may have contributed. There is a greater incidence of asthma in children who are minorities, of low socio-economic status, or live with people who smoke.

A number of factors may precipitate an asthma attack, including:

- Emotional stress including anxiety, fear, anger, and suppressed feelings
- Exercise
- Gastroesophageal reflux
- Inhaled and ingested allergens (e.g., animal dander, food allergies, house dust, mold, pollens, spores, chemicals, food additives)
- Inhaled irritants (e.g., tobacco, smoke, air pollution, aerosol sprays, strong odors)
- Medication (e.g., aspirin, NSAIDs, beta-blockers)
- Poor diet and mucogenic foods (e.g., dairy products)
- Viral respiratory infections especially sinusitis
- Weather changes (including wind and changes in temperature and humidity)

Anecdotally, some osteopathic physicians suspect that mechanical injuries can precipitate an asthma attack. One group has found that injuries to the head or sacral regions may precipitate an asthma attack (Frymann et al., *personal communication*, 2009).

Asthma as a disease has been characterized by intermittent airway obstruction, also termed reversible airway obstruction. It is proposed to consist primarily of two major components, bronchospasm and inflammation. Bronchial smooth muscle is innervated by the vagus nerve (CNX) and vasovagal reflexes can cause bronchoconstriction. This may be the mechanism involved in the reported association between gastroesophageal reflux and asthma (Kase, 2009; Yoshida, 2009). In asthma, bronchial spasm and increased bronchial secretions can be caused by overactivity of the bronchial branches of the vagus nerve. Actions of the sympathetic nerves innervating the bronchi are diminished and the normal equilibrium with the vagus nerve is disturbed. On a cellular level, many changes can take place. The first component is bronchospasm or hyperresponsive bronchial smooth muscle, which is mediated through β-adrenergic receptors and interlukin-13 that act directly on bronchial smooth muscle and epithelium to elicit hyperreactivity. The second component is the inflammatory mechanism leading to edema of the airways. Two principal immune mechanisms linked to the inflammatory process involve the T helper cells, of which secrete multiple cytokines and interleukins, and the hypersensitivity pathway as mediated by IgE produced by the B cells, which leads to activation and degranulation of mast cells, basophils, eosinophils, and other airway cells (Colice, 2004). This in turn leads to the well-known process of histamine release and the subsequent inflammatory response.

Gross pathologic features consist of overinflation of the lung through a process known as "air trapping," especially in individuals who expire in status asthmaticus. Other features are the mucus plugs, composed of mucus, serum proteins, inflammatory cells and debris, occluding the medium and small-sized bronchi and bronchioles. In fact, bronchiectasis has been described as a complication in 15% to 20% of asthmatic patients. Microscopic pathologic features include both goblet cell hyperplasia and submucosal gland hypertrophy. One study reported that there may be up to a three-fold

TABLE 54.1

Asthma Management Recommendations National Asthma Education and Prevention Program

	<5 Years Age	>5 Years Age
Mild intermittent asthma: 2 or less days per week and 2 or less nights per month	Treat as needed only, not daily	Treat as needed only
Mild-persistent asthma: for >2 d/wk but less than once daily, and >2 nights per month	Daily low-dose inhaled corticosteroid, OR cromolyn or leukotriene receptor antagonist	Daily low-dose inhaled corticosteroid, OR nedocrmil and sustained release theophylline.
Moderate-persistent asthma: daily and 1 night per week	<5 years age; low-dose inhaled corticosteroid + long-acting inhaled beta-2 agonist; OR medium-dose inhaled corticosteroid only; medium-dose inhaled corticosteroid + long-acting inhaled beta-2 agonist in recurring severe exacerbations	>5 years: low-to-medium-dose inhaled corticosteroid + long-acting inhaled beta-2 agonist; increase corticosteroid and add long-acting inhaled beta-2 agonist in recurring severe exacerbations
Severe-persistent asthma: continuous or repeatedly during the day and frequent at night	High-dose inhaled corticosteroid + long-acting inhaled beta-2 agonist; oral *corticosteroid* PRN	High-dose inhaled corticosteroid + long-acting inhaled beta-2 agonist; oral *corticosteroid* PRN

Source: Adopted from Key clinical activities for quality asthma care: recommendations of the National Asthma Education and Prevention Program. *MMWR Recomm Rep* 2003;52(RR-6):1–8.

increase of both goblet and mucin cells in asthmatic patients versus controls (Ordonez, 2001).

Repetitive episodes of inflammation lead to a production of matrix proteins and growth factors that in turn can potentially cause airway remodeling. This may include the theory that frequent damage to the epithelium and subsequent repair also contribute to remodeling. It is also thought that remodeling, with increased muscle mass, mucosal edema and reduced elasticity, may lead to decreased efficacy of bronchodilators (Barrios, 2006).

Although wheezing is a characteristic breath sound in asthma, it may not be heard in the most severe cases in which all breath sounds will be markedly reduced. In a patient with suspected asthma exacerbation, look for the following signs and symptoms when examining the patient: use of accessory muscles of respiration, posturing to enhance respiratory muscle mechanics, flaring of the nostrils, a prolonged exhalation phase of breathing, increased heart rate, or acrocyanosis. In addition to the ausculated wheezes, this patient shows moderate accessory muscle use and a slightly increased heart rate.

Based upon this patient's history and physical examination, she appears to have mild persistent asthma; her symptoms are reportedly occurring greater than two times per week but she does not appear to have night-time symptoms. The guidelines for asthma management and prevention from the National Asthma Education and Prevention Program recommend pharmaceutical treatment specific for the severity of the asthma. According to these guidelines, this child is probably not receiving optimal medical therapy and her medication regiment should be adjusted. (Table 54.1.) There is evidence that chronic use of short-acting beta-2 agonists such as albuterol does not provide clinical benefit and may in fact worsen symptoms in patients with mild asthma. Short-acting beta-2 agonists should be reserved for rescue therapy during symptom exacerbation rather than regular control (Walters, 2003). Corticosteroids are effective in controlling asthma in children although there is some evidence that chronic inhaled corticosteroid use may impair growth rate (Pauwels, 2003; Sharek, 1999).

OSTEOPATHIC PATIENT MANAGEMENT

Biomechanical Model

There are key anatomic considerations (Allen and D'Alonzo, 1993) when utilizing osteopathic manipulative treatment (OMT) in asthmatic patients (Box 54.1). Depending upon the degree of accessory muscle involvement needed during labored breathing, the muscles engaged in respiration can extend from the cranial base to the pelvis. The thoracic cage is the center of all this activity. It houses some of the most important organs in the human body, namely, the heart, lungs, and great vessels. The thorax is one of the most intricate and dynamic regions of the body, with an orchestrated movement of over 146 joints (Kuchera and Kuchera, 1994; Moore and Dally, 1999).

Factors That Affect Breathing Difficulties

From an osteopathic perspective, the following areas may contribute to or exacerbate the patient's breathing difficulties.

1. Upper thoracic vertebrae, ribs, sternum
2. T1-6 because of sympathetic innervation to the lungs
3. Occipitoatlantal junction and the course of the vagus nerve that supplies parasympathetic input to the pulmonary tree
4. Accessory muscles of respiration
5. Anterior cervical fascia
6. Thoracic diaphragm (The diaphragm is enervated by the phrenic nerve from the cervical plexus (C3-5), and its mobility is influenced by the lower six ribs, L1-2 and the sternum.)
7. Chapman's reflexes for the lungs, sinuses, and adrenal glands
8. The cranial-sacral mechanism
9. T10-L2 and the lower ribs

Figure 54-1 Dissection of term infant, right lateral view. The ribs 1 through 9 have been removed as has the right lateral abdominal wall to reveal the dome of the diaphragm draping the superior surface of the liver. The zone of apposition lies between the dome of the diaphragm and its inferior attachment and represents the length of inferior excursion possible during inhalation. (Used with permission from Willard & Carreiro Collection.)

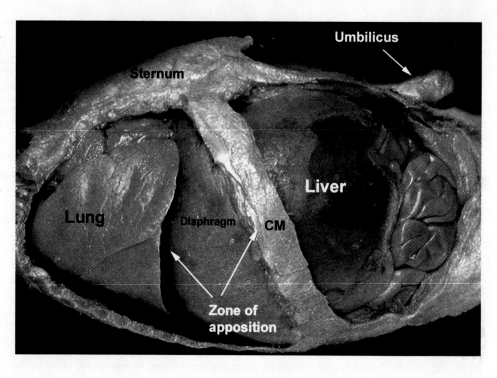

The child with asthma suffers from an obstructive respiratory disease. The amount of effort needed to maintain normal air movement through the bronchioles is increased, as is the work of breathing. This can have significant consequences in the pediatric population. First, infants are at risk for muscle fatigue and respiratory failure due to immaturity of acetylcholinesterase and increased contraction and relaxation times of muscles (Panitch, 1993). There is also evidence that the immature innervation patterns in respiratory muscles of children more than 3 years old result in uncoordinated and random contraction sequences that become exacerbated during times of increased demand (Haddad and Perez Fontain, 1996).

Second, when compared with adults, the mechanical effectiveness of the diaphragm and rib cage is compromised in children less than ten years old. This is because the rib cage is more flexible and laterally splayed, and the dome of the diaphragm is flatter than in an adult (Figs. 54.1 and 54.2). As a result, diaphragm excursion is shallower, intrathoracic respiratory pressures are less negative, and there is less tissue recoil during exhalation (Oppenshaw et al., 1984). During times of increased demand, children will compensate by increasing the rate and decreasing the depth of respiration.

In all children, the increased workload of breathing increases oxygen demand and cellular waste production, which alter pH and change the cellular milieu. This may be a contributing stress on the cardiopulmonary system. Optimizing mechanical function of the structures involved with breathing may help to decrease the overall workload placed on the child's cardiopulmonary system.

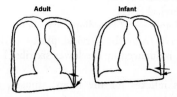

Figure 54-2 Schematic diagram comparing zone of apposition in the infant with that of the adult. The flattened diaphragm and widened thoracic cage contribute to the decreased zone.

Breathing is the only subconscious vital function that can be raised to a conscious level. Proper breathing helps the nervous system relax, while shallow, spasmodic breathing signals alarm. In the older child, breathing exercises may help strengthen peripheral and accessory muscles that aid breathing. Since asthma is an air-trapping disease, exercises that facilitate exhalation may be useful. In older children yoga, tai chi, and noncontact martial arts that integrate breathing with movement can be fun and health promoting. Exercise has been shown to improve breathing function.

RESPIRATORY-CIRCULATORY MODEL

The primary muscle of respiration is the diaphragm. With the average respiratory rate between 10 to 18 breaths/min, the diaphragm will move approximately 14,400 times in a day. The role of the diaphragm goes beyond mere movement as it is intimately connected to the cardiac and pulmonary pleura above and the hepatic and gastric pleura below. The movement of the diaphragm not only changes the intrathoracic and intra-abdominal pressures but also alters the circulation and lymphatic flow in these respective cavities (Moore and Dalley, 1999). Fluid movement through the vena caval system is dependent upon effective diaphragmatic excursion. Lymphatic fluids and deoxygenated blood reenter the cardiac system through the pressure changes generated by the diaphragm and respiratory muscles. Extravascular fluids in the abdominal compartment are absorbed by lymphatic lacunae situated on the abdominal surface of the diaphragm in response to mechanical changes in the diaphragmatic fascia (Schmid-Schonbein, 1990; Shinohara et al., 2003). To some extent, the removal of cellular waste products, the maintenance of tissue pH, and the reentry of fluids into the circulatory cycle are influenced by diaphragmatic function.

Neurologic Model

An important consideration in children with asthma is the perpetually dynamic interplay between the autonomic (sympathetic and parasympathetic) nervous system. The sympathetic nerve fibers of the lungs arise from the sympathetic chain ganglion at the level of T1-6.

The parasympathetic fibers travel within the vagus nerve as it exits the jugular foramen of the cranial vault and makes its way down the cervical region and through the thoracic inlet where it then splays onto the lungs. Smooth muscle fibers traveling from the intrapulmonary bronchial tree to the alveolar duct are innervated by sympathetic, parasympathetic, and primary afferent fibers. Parasympathetic input maintains dynamic tone during quiet breathing. Changes in autonomic activity or inflammation will alter the tone of the smooth muscle.

Somatovisceral reflexes associated with asthma have been found in the paraspinal muscles between T1 and T6 in adults (Beal and Morlock, 1984). The osteopathic physician may attempt to influence sympathetic activity by treating the upper thoracic area, and parasympathetic activity by addressing somatic dysfunction in the cervical region, including the craniocervical junction and cranial base. Dr. A.T. Still reportedly had great success relieving asthma and hay fever. He attributed his success to correcting spinal somatic dysfunctions, especially of the third and fourth thoracic vertebrae, that may represent a viscera-somatic reflex as well as being two of the spinal segments, which provide sympathetic innervation to the lungs.

Many authors have described the role of afferent drive on the neuroendocrine immune system and inflammatory diseases (Ganong, 1988; Gold and Goodwin, 1988; Ricci, 1989; Seeman et al., 1997; Willard et al., 1997). Arguably, somatic dysfunction increases afferent drive. Asthma, which has a strong inflammatory component, appears to be exacerbated by stress, endocrine changes, and immunity The bronchodilators, corticosteroids, and anticholinergics used to treat asthma do so by influencing neuronal control and inflammatory mechanisms in the lower airways. Medications such as leukotriene inhibitors and mast cell stabilizers are used to control related allergy symptoms. OMT used in conjunction with these medications may help to reduce the necessary dosage of medication required to control symptoms.

Behavioral Model

Focusing on the patient as a "whole" is a simplified view of the principles and philosophy of osteopathic medicine. Still M.D., D.O., founded osteopathic medicine in 1874 and during this time established the tenets of the body's own inherent capacity for health and well being, the importance and interrelationship between structure and function, the removal of impediments to the optimal flow of the body's fluids and nerve function, and the concept that the body is an integrated unit (Seffinger, 2003). To achieve this, one must look at a patient collectively and evaluate their physical, mental, emotional, and spiritual state. Additionally, in today's world, the clinician must also consider psychosocioeconomic implications that patients face. In fact, numerous studies have mentioned the significant impact of emotional triggers and poor outcomes in asthmatic individuals with inadequate support systems and insufficient self-care. Two systemic reviews reported improvements in some asthma parameters after self-management education and family therapy (Panton and Barley, 2005; Wolf et al., 2002). The national and global difficulty in providing accessible health care for impoverished patients is a concern of all health care providers. Even if patients were able to receive the necessary medications, their response to these medications is dependent on multifactorial elements ranging from genetics to the environment. In short, one has to approach the patient as an individual and treat the person, not the disease.

Metabolic Energy Model

The importance of a fresh, whole food diet cannot be overemphasized. Just as structure is foundational, so is the food that builds our structure. It is important to avoid processed, devitalized food. Many food colorings, sulfites, preservatives, and other food modifiers cause asthma and allergic reactions. For instance, "modified wheat starch," a thickener used in many processed foods, is "modified" by six different chemicals all of which can trigger asthma and allergic reactions in susceptible individuals. Empirically, some physicians find that asthmatic children benefit from the avoidance of foods such as milk, ice cream, excess cheese and processed flour, sugar, and corn syrup sweeteners. There is some evidence that asthmatics are more likely to have antioxidant imbalances (Nadeem et al., 2008), so adequate vitamin C with bioflavonoid and a B vitamins may be beneficial. Intravenous magnesium has been shown to have a positive effect on respiratory function and hospital stays in children with asthma (Mohammad and Goodacre, 2007). Patients with asthma with a high dietary intake of magnesium have better lung function and a reduction in wheezing (Bede et al., 2008). Encouraging breastfeeding exclusively in the first 3 months of life decreases the incidence of developing reactive airway disease (Scholtens et al., 2009).

Although inhaled corticosteroids are far safer than systemic steroids, some of the inhaled steroid is swallowed and passes through the gastrointestinal (GI) tract. Esophageal candidiasis is most commonly reported (Aun, 2009; Nielsen, 2007), but swallowed steroids may also adversely affect the normal flora of the intestine. Some physicians believe these types of medications can play a role in "leaky gut" syndrome, which in turn may contribute to allergic issues that are already present.

Patient Outcome

OMT may provide some benefit to an asthmatic patient. First, by using myofascial release and balanced ligamentous tension to address thoracic cage and diaphragm impediments, one can restore optimal diaphragmatic motion for that patient. Rib raising techniques may help to mobilize the thoracic cage as well as stimulate the sympathetic chain ganglion and alter sympathetic outflow to the visceral organs. Soft tissue techniques such as paraspinal inhibition of the cervical region and a suboccipital release may influence parasympathetic input to the lungs. Osteopathy in the cranial field may be effective in patients who have suffered a hard fall with mechanical injuries to the head or sacrum that have triggered an asthma attack (Centers et al., 2003). The goal of using OMT in the treatment of a child with asthma is to optimize the dynamic balance between parasympathetic and sympathetic input to the pulmonary system, remove mechanical restrictions that adversely affect respiratory mechanics, decrease the workload of breathing, and facilitate the child's ability to function normally.

SUMMARY

Given its multifactorial nature, asthma is difficult to treat and requires a comprehensive evaluation on the part of the clinician. A multifaceted approach, including diet, allergen prevention, medication, and alternative modalities such as OMT, may work synergistically to control the symptoms of an asthmatic patient and potentially modify the severity (Hondras et al., 2006; NAEPP, 1997; NIH, 2005; Rowane and Rowane, 1999). In a randomized controlled trial, Guiney et al. (2005) reported a statistically significant improvement in peak expiratory flow measures in asthmatic children after treatment with OMT. Bockenhauer et al. (2002) compared OMT to sham treatment in a pilot study of adults with chronic asthma using a crossover design. Upper thoracic and lower thoracic forced respiratory excursion was statistically increased after osteopathic manipulative procedures compared with sham procedures although there were no significant changes in peak expiratory flow rates.

It has been the experience of this author that osteopathic modalities applied to asthmatic patients prior to and during the administration of medication contribute to an improvement in symptoms.

REFERENCES

Allen TW, D'Alonzo GE, Investigating the role of osteopathic manipulation in the treatment of asthma. *J Am Osteopath Assoc* 1993;93:654–656, 659.

Barrios R, Kheradmand F, Batts L, et al. Asthma: pathology and pathophysiology. *Arch Pathol Lab Med* 2006;130:447–451.

Beal MC, Morlock JW, Somatic dysfunction associated with pulmonary disease. *J Am Osteopath Assoc* 1984;84:179–183.

Bede O, Nagy D, Suranyi A, et al. Effects of magnesium supplementation on the glutathione redox system in atopic asthmatic children. Inflamm Res 2008;57:279–286.

Bockenhauer SE, Julliard KN, Lo KS, et al. Quantifiable effects of osteopathic manipulative techniques on patients with chronic asthma. *J Am Osteopath Assoc* 2002;102:371–375.

Carroll KN, Hartert TV. The impact of respiratory viral infection on wheezing illnesses and asthma exacerbations. *Immunol Allergy Clin N Am* 2008;28: 539–561, viii.

Center for Disease Control, National Surveillance for Asthma. Available at: www.cdc.gov/mmwr, date accessed Feb 4, 2008.

Centers S, Morelli MA, Seffinger, et al. Osteopathic philosophy. In: *Foundations of Osteopathic Medicine*. 2nd Ed. 2003:305–337.

Colice G. Asthma severity categorization methods. *Clin Med Res* 2004;3:155–163.

Eder W, Ege M, Von Mutius E. The asthma epidemic. *N Engl J Med* 2006;355:2226–2235.

Ganong W. The stress response—a dynamic overview. *Hosp Prac* 1988;23:155–171.

Gold P, Goodwin F. Clinical and biochemical manifestations of stress: part I. *N Engl J Med* 1988;319:348–353.

Global Initiative for Asthma. A Pocket Guide for Physicians and Nurses. *Global Strategy for Asthma Management and Prevention*. NHLBI/WHO; 2005. NIH Publication No. 02–3659.

Guiney PA, Chou R, Vianna A, et al. Effects of osteopathic manipulative treatment on pediatric patients with asthma: a randomized controlled trial. *J Am Osteopath Assoc* 2005;105:7–12.

Haddad GG, Perez Fontain JJ. Development of the respiratory system. In: Behrman RE, Kliegman RM, Jenson HB, eds. *Nelson's Textbook of Pediatrics*. Philadelphia, PA: WB Saunders, 1996.

Hondras MA, Linde K, Jones AP. Manual therapy for asthma. Cochrane database of systematic reviews. *Cochrane Libr* 2006:4.

Kase JS, Pici M, Visintainer P. Risks for common medical conditions experienced by former preterm infants during toddler years. *J Perinat Med* 2009;37:103–108.

Kuchera ML, Kuchera WA. *Osteopathic Considerations in Systemic Dysfunction*. Rev. 2nd Ed. 1994:33–56.

Mohammed S, Goodacre S. Intravenous and nebulised magnesium sulphate for acute asthma: systematic review and meta-analysis. *Emerg Med J* 2007;24:823–830.

Moore KL, Dalley AF. *Clinically Oriented Anatomy*. 4th Ed. 1999:60–171.

Nadeem A, Masood A, Siddiqui N. Oxidant—antioxidant imbalance in asthma: scientific evidence, epidemiological data and possible therapeutic options. *Ther Adv Respir Dis* 2008;2:215–235.

National Asthma Education and Prevention Program, Expert Panel Report 2. *Guidelines for the Diagnosis and Management of Asthma*. Washington, DC: Dept of Health and Human Services, 1997. NIH Publication No. 97–4051.

Openshaw P, Edwards S, Helms P. Changes in rib cage geometry in childhood. *Thorax* 1984;39:624.

Ordonez CL, Khashayar R, Wong HH, et al. Mild and moderate asthma is associated with airway goblet cell hyperplasia and abnormalities in mucin gene expression. *Am J Respir Crit Care Med* 2001;163:517–523.

Panitch HB, Wolfson MR, Shaffer TH. Epithelial modulation of preterm airway smooth muscle contraction. *J Appl Physiol* 1993;74:1437.

Panton J, Barley EA. Family therapy for asthma in children. *Cochrane Database Syst Rev* 2005:2.

Pauwels RA, Pedersen S, Busse WW, et al. Early intervention with budesonide in mild persistent asthma: a randomised, double-blind trial. *Lancet* 2003;361:1071–1076.

Reed CE. The natural history of asthma in adults: the problem of irreversibility. *J Allergy Clin Immunol* 1999;103:539–547 Issue 2. Art. No.: CD001002. DOI: 10.1002/14561858.CD001002.pub2.

Reed C. The natural history of asthma. *J Allergy Clin Immunol* 2006;118: 543–550.

Rowane WA, Rowane MP. An osteopathic approach to asthma. *J Am Osteopath Assoc* 1999;99:259–264.

Schmid-Schonbein GW. Microlymphatics and lymph flow [review, 288 refs]. *Physiol Rev* 1990;70:987–1028.

Scholtens S, Wijga AH, Brunekreef B, et al. Breast feeding, parental allergy and asthma in children followed for 8 years. The PIAMA birth cohort study. *Thorax* 2009;64:604–609.

Sears MR. Epidemiology of asthma exacerbations. *J Allergy Clin Immunol* 2008;122:662–668.

Seeman TE, Singer BH, Rowe JW, et al. Price of adaptation-allosteric load and its health consequences. *Arch Intern Med* 1997;157:2259–2268.

Seffinger MA, King HH, Ward RC, et al. Osteopathic philosophy. In: *Foundations of Osteopathic Medicine*. 2nd Ed. 2003:1–17.

Sharek PJ, Bergman DA, Ducharme F. Beclomethasone for asthma in children: effects on linear growth. *Cochrane Database Syst Rev* 1999;3.

Shinohara H, Kominami R, Taniguchi Y, et al. The distribution and morphology of lymphatic vessels on the peritoneal surface of the adult human diaphragm, as revealed by an ink-absorption method. *Okajimas Folia Anat Jpn* 2003;79:175–183.

Singh AM, Buse WW. Asthma exacerbations-2: aetiology. *Thorax* 2006;61: 809–816.

Walters EH, Walters J, Gibson P, et al. Inhaled short acting beta2-agonist use in chronic asthma: regular versus as needed treatment. *Cochrane Database Syst Rev* 2003;1.

Weiss ST, Litonjua AA, et al. Overview of the Pharmacogenetics of Asthma Treatment. *Pharmacogenomics J* 2006;6:311–326.

Willard FH, Mokler DJ, Morgane PJ. Neuroendocrine-immune system and homeostasis. In: Ward RC, ed. *Foundations for Osteopathic Medicine*. Baltimore, MD: Williams & Wilkins, 1997:107–135.

Wolf FM, Guevara JP, Grum CM, et al. Educational interventions for asthma in children. *Cochrane Database Syst Rev* 2002;4.

Yoshida Y, Kameda M, Nishikido T, et al. Very short gastroesophageal acid reflux during the upright position could be associated with asthma in children. *Allergol Int* 2009;58:395–401.

Adult with Chronic Cardiovascular Disease

BRIAN KAUFMAN

KEY CONCEPTS

- Heart failure is a clinical syndrome characterized by fluid overload.
- Fatigue and dyspnea are characteristic symptoms of heart failure.
- Heart failure can be both acute and chronic.
- Patients with both acute and chronic heart failure exhibit changes in the musculoskeletal system.
- These musculoskeletal changes can be divided into five distinct pathophysiologic models, which provide an osteopathic interpretation of heart failure.
- The osteopathic physician can utilize these models to plan a rationale for treatment of patients with heart failure that includes both pharmacologic and osteopathic manipulation.
- There are biologic and physiologic data to support this approach.

CASE VIGNETTE

CHIEF COMPLAINT

A 79-year-old female comes to the office complaining of shortness of breath and worsening fatigue for 1 week.

History of Present Illness:

W.S. has a complicated medical history, which is significant for known coronary artery disease (CAD), ischemic cardiomyopathy with an ejection fraction of 45%, previous episodes of congestive heart failure (CHF), hypertension, hypercholesterolemia, diabetes mellitus (DM) type 2, and osteoporosis.

The patient reports that over the last week she's had increasing fatigue and worsening shortness of breath from some baseline symptoms which have exacerbated in the last 24 hours and she is now having shortness of breath at rest. The patient reports a nonproductive cough and wheezing and has noticed increased lower extremity swelling over the past week. She reports that last night she slept in a recliner in order to breath and experienced episodes of chest pressure last night which improved transiently with nitroglycerin.

Prior to this recent episode, the patient has been feeling depressed due the recent loss of her husband. The patient also admits that she has recently been eating some very salty foods and also admits that she has recently missed some dosages of her medications.

Past Medical History:

CAD diagnosed in 1998 after non-ST elevation myocardial infarction (MI). Mild mitral regurgitation and mild aortic stenosis by echocardiogram (ECHO) done last year. Ejection fraction 45% with moderate diastolic dysfunction. CHF. DM type 2. Hyperlipidemia.

Past Surgical History:

Appendectomy in 1960. Total abdominal hysterectomy with bilateral Salpingo oopherectomy in 1980. Coronary artery bypass graft (CABG) in 1998 with left leg vein harvesting. Left knee arthroscopy in 2002.

Allergies:

No known drug allergies. ACE inhibitor caused cough.

Medications:

Carvedilol: 12.5 mg twice daily. Valsartan: 320 mg daily. Aspirin: 81 mg daily. Furosemide: 40 mg daily. Amlodipine: 10 mg daily. Atorvastatin: 10 mg daily. Calcium: 600 mg and Vitamin: D 600 IU taken twice daily. Metformin: 1,000 mg twice daily.

Social History:

Patient is a retired schoolteacher. Patient lives alone in an assisted living complex. Patient's husband is recently deceased. Patient has two grown children nearby who are active in her life.

Family History:

Father deceased at age 57 of MI. Mother deceased at age 80 of old age. Two siblings with cardiac disease. No family history of diabetes, cancer, or blood disorders.

REVIEW OF SYSTEMS

General:

No constitutional symptoms of fever, chills, night sweats. Admits to fatigue and approximately 12-lb weight gain over the last 2 weeks.

Head:

Denies headache.

Eyes:

Denies diplopia, change in vision, eye pain.

ENT:

Denies change in hearing, earache or tinnitus. No sinus tenderness or nasal discharge. No voice changes, hoarseness, or sore throat.

Neck:

No neck stiffness, tenderness, swelling, or masses.

Cardiovascular:

Admits to chest pressure, shortness of breath, and dyspnea on exertion. Three pillow orthopnea. Denies palpitations.

Respiratory:

Admits to nonproductive cough and wheeze. Denies hemoptysis or pleuritic chest pain.

GI:

Admits to decreased appetite, some abdominal fullness. Denies heartburn, abdominal pain, nausea, vomiting, diarrhea, rectal bleeding, change in bowel habits. No change in stool color or caliber.

GU:

No dysuria, polyuria, urinary retention or incontinence. No increased frequency. No blood in urine.

CNS:

No disturbance of smell, dizziness, vertigo, weakness, convulsions, gait disturbance, or involuntary movement.

Extremity:

Admits to recent worsening lower extremity swelling. Denies cyanosis.

Vascular:

No history of claudication but recent complaints of exertional leg pains.

Integument:

No rashes, change in moles, pigmentation, or pruritus noted by the patient.

Endocrine:

No increased hunger, thirst, urination. No hot or cold intolerance.

Hematology:

No history of bleeding or clotting disorders. No active bleeding.

Musculoskeletal:

No significant joint pains, muscle aches, deformities.

Psychiatric:

No mood swings or crying spells, No changes in sleep, personality or memory, No suicidal or homicidal ideation.

PHYSICAL EXAM

Vital Signs:

Temp: 99°F, BP: 150/88 in right arm, pulse: 104 bpm, RR: 22 and shallow. Height: 63 in, Weight: 149 lb.

General:

Patient was alert, attentive, and oriented. She appeared extremely deconditioned.

Head:

Normocephalic and atraumatic.

Eyes:

PERRLA, EOMI, sclera was anicteric, and no xanthelasma was appreciated.

ENT:

Bilateral tympanic membranes were normal. Pharynx was clear without erythema or exudate.

Neck:

Neck was supple, trachea was midline, no carotid bruit was appreciated, and neck veins were slightly distended at 45 degrees.

Cardiovascular:

Faint S1 and prominent S2, rhythm was regular, rate was 104, 2/6 systolic ejection murmur at the RUSB without radiation is appreciated, S3 gallop is appreciated.

Pulmonary:

Decreased air entry bilaterally with normal quality of breath sounds and bilateral crackles midway up lower lung fields and wheezes throughout.

Abdomen:

Abdomen slightly distended but soft, nontender, without guarding or rigidity. Positive Hepatojugular reflux was elicited.

Extremities:

Extremities revealed muscle atrophy and 2 + pitting edema on right, 3+ on left. Bilateral cyanotic appearing feet

Osteopathic/Musculoskeletal:
Cranial:

OA Extended rotated left and sidebent right. Suboccipital tissues were boggy.

Cervical:

C2 is rotated right, C5 is extended rotated and sidebent to the left.

Thoracic:

Increased kyphosis. T1is in a neutral position rotated to the right and sidebent to the left, T3 and T4 are both extended, rotated and sidebent to the left. Skin was warm and boggy, yet with a ropey texture underneath in this region. T12 is flexed, rotated, and sidebent to the right. Sternum inferiorly distracted. Decreased diaphragmatic excursion bilaterally.

Ribs:

Bilateral ribs 10 to 12 have an inhalation dysfunction.

Lumbar:

Psoas hypertonicity on right. Slightly increased lumbar lordosis. Sacrum: Increased nutation

Pelvis:

Right anteriorly rotated innominate.

UE:

left elevated clavicle, internally rotated humerus.

LE:

Right internally rotated femur. Right femoral triangle congestion. Left externally rotated femur with femoral triangle congestion.

DIFFERENTIAL DIAGNOSIS

W.S. is a 79-year-old patient with multiple chronic medical problems presenting with acute or chronic dyspnea, cough,

The American College of Cardiology/American Heart Association College of Cardiology Guidelines for Initial Evaluation of Heart Failure

- History and physical
- CBC
- Chemistry profile
- Calcium
- Magnesium
- Lipid profile
- LFT
- TSH
- UA
- Cardiac enzymes and BNP
- Oxygen saturation level and ABG if needed
- EKG
- CXR
- ECHO, if indicated

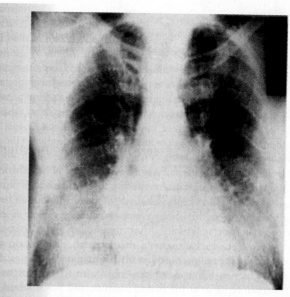

Figure 55-1   Typical heart failure CXR.

wheezing, lower extremity edema, and worsening fatigue. She also admits to several episodes of chest pressure. Although this is a complicated case, the patient's complaints can be categorized into those that are potentially life threatening and those related to her chronic disease. This constellation of symptoms suggests the following possible diagnoses: exacerbation of CHF, first episode of exacerbation of chronic obstructive pulmonary disease, acute bronchitis with exacerbation of chronic CHF, pneumonia, and acute ischemic heart disease.

To help narrow our differential and arrive at an accurate diagnosis, it is reasonable to check basic laboratory studies. The American College of Cardiology/American Heart Association College of Cardiology guidelines for initial evaluation of heart failure (Box 55.1) recommend a thorough history and physical examination, including assessment of volume status (Hunt, 2005). Recommended labs include complete blood count (CBC), chemistry profile including calcium and magnesium, lipid profile, liver function test (LFT), thyroid-stimulating hormone (TSH), and urinalysis (UA). Other tests include cardiac enzymes to evaluate cardiac ischemia, and a beta naturetic peptide (BNP) level to corroborate suspicions of CHF. Liver function studies (LFT) should be considered in this patient, given her abdominal complaints.

In terms of diagnostic imaging and functional testing, a hemoglobin oxygen saturation level is used to evaluate the patient's oxygenation status and if this is abnormal, arterial blood gas (ABG) analysis is a reasonable next step. An electrocardiogram (EKG) is included to evaluate for acute changes consistent with cardiac ischemia. If possible, the EKG should be compared with a previous EKG to evaluate for changes. A chest x-ray (CXR) (Fig. 55.1) can provide evidence of lung infiltrates or findings suggestive of CHF such as vascular prominence, Kerley B lines, bilateral alveolar infiltrates, or bilateral pleural effusions.

Once we have decided on the most likely diagnosis, corroborative tests that are not in the current ACC/AHA guidelines may be used to confirm it such as impedance cardiography, which can be used to evaluate increased thoracic fluid in CHF. The ACC/AHA guidelines do recommend an ECHO to assess left ventricular (LV) function and look for the presence of critical valvular disease.

Ultimately making an accurate diagnosis is a combination of pattern recognition, test results, and clinical judgment.

In this case, the following laboratory and diagnostic test results were obtained:

Na±: 130 mmol/L
K±: 3.0 mmol/L
Bun/Cr: 66/2.4mg/dL
Magnesium: 1.9 mg/dL
Troponin: I 1.5 ng/mL
BNP: 10,000 pg/mL
AST/ALT: 90/120u/L
TSH: 1.25 mlU/L
UA: specific gravity of 1.030, PH of 5.5, no cells or casts seen.
Oxygen saturation: 87% on room air
EKG: Sinus rhythm at 105 bpm. Left bundle branch block pattern. No changes compared with previous EKG from 1 year ago
CXR: Cardiomegaly noted. Cephalization of vessels noted. Bilateral infiltrates. Small bilateral pleural effusions
ECHO: Ejection fraction 45%. Moderate diastolic dysfunction. No critical valvular disease
Impedance cardiogram: Increased thoracic fluid content. Decreased cardiac index. Increased systemic vascular resistance

In summary, we have a 79-year-old female with previous history of CAD, ischemic heart disease with ischemic cardiomyopathy, moderate diastolic dysfunction, previous episodes of CHF who complains of progressive dyspnea, fatigue, chest pressure, increased nitrate use, and a recent history of dietary indiscretion and depression.

Physical examination revealed findings consistent with CHF exacerbation, including:

- Past medical history—CAD, CHF, ischemic cardiomyopathy, and diastolic dysfunction
- Review of systems—progressive dyspnea, fatigue, chest pressure, increased nitrate use, dietary indiscretion, and depression
- Physical exam—tachypnea, shallow breathing, increased jugular venous distension, S3 gallop, pulmonary crackles and wheezes,

positive hepatojugular reflex, LE edema, somatic dysfunction at T3/4, decreased diaphragmatic excursion and thoracic compliance, hyperkyphosis, and femoral triangle congestion

These findings are consistent with the increased respiratory rate and shallow breathing. There was jugular vein distension which is evidence of right heart failure. There was an S3 gallop present on cardiac exam, and crackles and wheezes appreciated on pulmonary exam. Abdomen revealed some minimal distension but more significant was the positive hepatojugular reflux which is consistent with right heart failure. There was significant lower extremity edema which is also consistent with heart failure although could also be a side effect of Amlodipine (1).

There are no musculoskeletal findings specific to heart failure; however, this patient had somatic dysfunctions that have been associated with cardiovascular disease (108,109,110) such as the changes at occipital atlantal joint, C2, and the thoracic area (warm, boggy region at T3/4 region). Additionally, the changes in thoracic compliance, decreased diaphragmatic excursion, changes at the lumbar, sacrum, and pelvis while not specific for either heart disease or cardiac disease are common in patients with pulmonary and cardiovascular disease and could have been impacting W.S.'s presentation. Congestion in the femoral triangle could be seen in any condition of increased lower extremity edema as is this case.

Our patient's troponin and BNP are both elevated, which is evidence of acute cardiac ischemia. This is consistent with the patient's complaints of chest pressure that responded to nitrate use. It should be noted, however, that often in cases such as this, it may initially be unclear whether an acute ischemic event has triggered an exacerbation of heart failure or an exacerbation of heart failure has triggered acute cardiac ischemia. Furthermore, this patient has significantly decreased renal function and the elevated troponin level may a decrease in clearance of troponins from the blood, rather than cardiac ischemia.

The hyponatremia (sodium 130) seen in this patient may be from diuretic use, pulmonary pathology, or pain. It could also result from increased ADH secretion and the absorption of free water (2). Her UA showed a specific gravity of 1.030, which indicates increased ADH secretion. This could be from intravascular depletion (dehydration) or decreased effective circulating volume (fluid overload states). Given the other presenting complaints, historical features, physical examination findings, laboratory and radiological features of this case the latter scenario is more likely.

This patient has renal failure. This patient's baseline creatinine was 1.1 and baseline creatinine clearance was approximately 45 mL/min. When she arrived at the hospital, her creatinine clearance had decreased to approximately 20 mL/min. Although this is a complicated topic on its own, we can explain this by a combination of factors.

In heart failure, there is a decrease in effective circulating volume. This is due to decreased cardiac output. This causes a decrease in renal blood flow. In addition, this patient is on a diuretic agent (furosemide) which may have contributed to intravascular depletion and decreased renal blood flow. She is also taking an Angiotensin 2 receptor blocker. Angiotensin 2 constricts the efferent arteriole in the kidney and acts to increase filtration by raising intraglomerular pressure. Angiotensin 2 receptor blockers remove the ability to constrict the efferent arteriole and effectively reduce intraglomerular pressure and glomerular filtration. Although there may be other factors to

account for the renal findings, there is sufficient evidence that these factors are all prerenal and would act to reduce renal blood flows. The rise in serum creatinine indicates a decrease in glomerular filtration rate. (2). Hyponatremia, renal failure, increased specific gravity in UA, and elevated BNP in a patient who appears to be clinically volume overloaded helps support the diagnosis of heart failure. The diagnosis is further supported by the patient's CXR and echocardiographic findings both of which are consistent with the cardiomyopathy and impedance cardiography results.

HOSPITAL COURSE

The patient was admitted to the hospital and placed on a telemetry unit. The Heart Failure Society of America and the European Society of Cardiology have published guidelines on managing acute decompensated heart failure as well as other topics related to heart failure management (3,4). Our patient was started on nitrates to decrease preload and help decrease pulmonary pressures. Intravenous diuretic treatment was instituted to remove fluid from this patient. We used supplemental oxygen, which was effective at raising oxygen saturation levels. If this had not helped, we could have used noninvasive ventilation methods (CPAP and BiPAP), which is sometimes useful in heart failure exacerbations (5). The patient underwent musculoskeletal and osteopathic evaluation. Osteopathic diagnosis and treatment was instituted as an adjunct to medical treatment (6). Patient underwent serial cardiac enzyme testing, which showed a trend of decreasing enzyme levels. Fluid inputs and outputs were tracked and patient underwent daily weight testing. Patient had an excellent diuresis and over the course of 3 days she lost 5 lb of weight. Patient showed good improvement in oxygen levels and symptoms. She was able to be removed from supplemental oxygen. Because of patient's renal failure, her angiotensin receptor blocker was held. Additionally, because of renal failure, her metformin was also held during her hospitalization (7). Over the next 3 days, patient had normalization of her renal function, sodium level, and the remainder of her electrolytes. Serial electrocardiograms showed no changes. W.S. underwent repeat ECHO and results were obtained as earlier (8). The patient was eventually restarted on her regular medications. In addition, she received counseling from social work while in the hospital and was started on an antidepressant. This patient was discharged to her home at the assisted living with outpatient follow up arranged with her primary care physician. Visiting nurse was arranged to monitor patient at home and do serial weight and vital sign checks (9,10). The patient was referred to a supervised cardiac rehabilitation center to begin a comprehensive rehabilitation course (8). As an outpatient, W.S. continued to receive osteopathic evaluation and manipulative treatment as an adjunct to her medical management.

OSTEOPATHIC PATIENT MANAGEMENT

The case described above is primarily a case on CHF, but the principles that underlie the models of musculoskeletal medicine can apply to many different cardiovascular patients. For the purposes of illustration and brevity, we will focus on this patient and the topic of heart failure for the remainder of the chapter. This is not meant to be an in-depth discussion and review of the topic of heart failure for there are many excellent articles and texts which cover this topic, but the purpose of this chapter is to view this topic through the osteopathic lens. The attempt was to focus in on those aspects of heart failure which relate to musculoskeletal medicine and the osteopathic perspective.

The five pathophysiologic models for musculoskeletal medicine are as follows:

1. Biomechanical model
2. Respiratory—circulatory model
3. Neurologic model
4. Metabolic—energy model
5. Behavioral model

Throughout the remainder of this chapter, we will look at the principles illustrated by this case in each of these pathophysiologic models. By understanding these principles, we can not only understand the role of musculoskeletal medicine in this patient but also construct a rationale for the role of osteopathic treatment to assist in the restoration of homeostasis in this and other patients with cardiovascular disease. At all times, attempts will be made to cite biological, physiologic, pathophysiologic, and clinical data to support an osteopathic approach; however, it should be noted that there are few randomized clinical trials that have examined this subject and fewer that meet the rigor of the current practices of evidenced based medicine. Because of this, most times we must rely on biological and pathophysiologic plausibility to support our approach.

BIOMECHANICAL MODEL

When there is a change in structure, functional changes follow. This is one of the basic osteopathic tenets. Structural changes can lead to changes in physiology and lead to pathology (11).

The heart and associated vascular system are essential for life. The heart is a muscular structure that resides in the mediastinum. It is encased in the pericardium that is anchored to the thoracic diaphragm below and that blends and encases the great vessels above. The left ventricle pumps blood into the systemic circulation via the aorta, which in turn transmits blood into branching vessels. The arterial system accepts blood via the aorta and distributes it throughout the body (Fig. 55.2). The circulatory system provides nourishment and oxygen for the cells and via the venous system provides a waste removal and blood return system (12). The structural model would view those elements that provide support and stability to our system. Structural elements are those of bone, muscle, fascia, and all connective tissues. Alterations in these can affect cardiovascular function. An extreme example is the effect of a pronounced kyphoscoliosis on cardiopulmonary function (13). Less obvious examples are the effect of small alterations in posture affecting the efficiency of the body's ability to regulate venous return to the heart and lymphatic flow to return into the systemic circulation (14). Yet another example is the development of compartment syndrome in an extremity after a trauma (15).

The heart undergoes remodeling and structural changes after MI and heart failure. These occur through neurohumoral activation as well as other processes. Besides the biochemical and biological changes that occur, there are structural alterations in the geometry and architecture that are deleterious. Dilation of the LV, thinning of its wall, change in shape of the left ventricle from an elliptical to a more spherical shape, and mitral valve incompetence can all occur. These changes create mechanical factors which worsen function. The change to a more spherical configuration creates an increase in end diastolic wall stress and dilation will result in

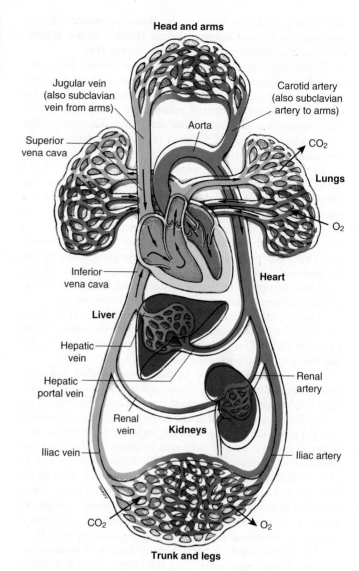

Figure 55-2 Schematic diagram of heart and vascular system and pressure changes with portal circulation.

increased LV work and oxygen usage. There is a cascade of events which result in biochemical and other biophysical changes in the myocardium (16).

The venous and lymphatic systems are low pressure systems and as such are much more susceptible to structural changes (17). The venous system is assisted by muscular contractions to assist in the return blood from the periphery into the abdomen. Once in the abdomen, diaphragmatic contractions and pressure differentials created by diaphragmatic contractions help return venous blood to the right atrium where it is then propelled by cardiac contraction to the lungs (18).

The lymphatic system is also a low pressure system and depends on several factors for return into the systemic circulation. The lymphatics have an intrinsic contraction that occurs at a rate of approximately every 6 seconds (19). The walls of the lymphatic vessels are anchored firmly by filaments (19). Motion of the extremity or structural deformity of the vessel will create pressure changes in the lymph vessel and help draw extravascular proteins and fluids into the lymphatic system and help propulsion. Muscular contraction also assists in propulsion away from the extremities. Valves help prevent back flow. Once in the abdomen, pressure changes generated by the diaphragm will draw lymph into the cisterna chyli and eventually into the systemic circulation (18).

The changes in skeletal muscle tone and volume found in a deconditioned state, combined with decreased physical activity and immobility, can compromise musculoskeletal forces needed to assist in venous and lymphatic return from the periphery. Thoracic mechanics and diaphragmatic action will also greatly influence fluid movement, and if altered can lead to stasis and edema formation (20).

In this patient's surgical history, we note that she has had a CABG which required a midline sternotomy and rib retraction. This can alter the motion of the ribs post sternotomy (21). Recent research suggests that fascia has active contractile properties (22). CABG requires cutting through the pericardium which may change the fascial relations in the mediastinum and fascial attachments both superiorly (investing fascia of the great vessels up into the neck as the pretracheal fascia and eventually to the cranial base [23]) and inferiorly (connection to the central tendon of the diaphragm), although I know of no studies demonstrating this.

The patient's bypass vessels were harvested from her left lower leg. This often predisposes patients to the development of lower extremity edema. Our patient had worse pitting edema on the left and this is a likely contributing factor (24).

The somatic dysfunction in this patient's pelvis and lower extremities is also impacting venous and lymphatic drainage (20). This is evidenced by the increased congestion in the femoral triangle which serves as a drainage point for the lower extremities into the pelvis (25). As we work our way into the systemic circulation, drainage is further hampered by decreased diaphragmatic excursion and decreased rib motion. This decreases the range of the pressure differentials generated with each breath. Adding to this there is somatic dysfunction at the thoracic-lumbar junction and an increased kyphosis which also can decrease pressure changes and pumping action of the thoracoabdominal cylinder. Lastly, there is somatic dysfunction at the T1-rib 1/manubrium complex (14).

The thoracic duct, or left lymphatic duct, is a vascular structure which transmits lymph from the cisterna chyli and returns it into the systemic circulation. The thoracic duct must exit and then reenter this ring as it pierces sibson fascia twice to join at the union of the left Internal jugular and Subclavian veins at which point the lymph reenters the systemic circulation (26,27). Drainage from the right half of the thorax and right upper extremity occurs through the right lymphatic duct, which reenters the circulation at the junction of the right subclavian vein and internal jugular vein (27,28). In the setting of a fluid overload state, these factors will further impede efficient return of lymph into the systemic circulation.

After informed consent was discussed and signed, this patient underwent osteopathic treatment at the hospital bedside. Gentle osteopathic technique was utilized throughout her treatment course. This was a combination of balanced ligamentous tension technique, myofascial release, and some articulatory techniques.

Our goals were to improve range of motion of joints, tissue texture and help improve musculoskeletal structural relationships to assist the body in restoring homeostasis.

RESPIRATORY-CIRCULATORY MODEL

The respiratory-circulatory model is a way of viewing the movement of fluids throughout the body and the maintenance of the intracellular and extracellular environments. From the macroscopic perspective, we look at the movement of blood and lymph throughout the body. From a microscopic view, we can focus on the exchange of oxygen and nutrients and removal of metabolic waste products at a cellular level. There are many scenarios where macrocirculation appears intact, yet at the microscopic level the needs of the end tissues and cells are not met (29). If there is inadequate end tissue oxygen levels, the cells shift from aerobic to anaerobic metabolism (30). This causes the production of lactic acid. If there is inadequate drainage from these regions, there is accumulation of lactic acid. In some cases this is a local phenomenon, but in severe cases can be systemic. These severe cases can occur in heart failure, acute cardiac ischemia as well as other pathophysiologic states such as sepsis (31). Proper tissue functioning depends on adequate supply and removal. As already stated, efficient venous and lymphatic drainage from the extremities requires musculoskeletal assistance. Muscle tone, immobility, and fascial relationships influence this. Neurologic tone influences vascular smooth muscle diameter which influences both arterial inflow and venous and lymphatic outflow from tissues. Increased sympathetic tone raises blood pressure which can promote movement of fluids into the third spaces and inhibits drainage. It can also increase heart rate, contractility, and respiratory rate, which is an adaptive response to restore homeostasis by providing more flow through the system.

Thoracic cage mechanics and diaphragmatic action is important in moving lymph and venous blood from the abdomen and thorax back into circulation (18). The thoracic diaphragm acts as the "heart" of the lymphatic and venous system and as such contributes to preload. It anchors the heart within the pericardium and flattens the spinal curves with each contraction. Estimating 12 breaths per minute yields 17,280 breaths per day. Each healthy diaphragmatic contraction causes a profound change in pressure differentials in our bodies. This contributes to preload, draws air into our lungs, assists in lymphatic flow, flattens the spinal curves, and may contribute to passive diffusion processes throughout the body (18).

Heart failure is characterized by fluid overload. Fluid overload states are characterized by the movement of body fluids from the intravascular space to the extravascular space. Pulmonary edema is a frequent and potentially life-threatening consequence of decompensated heart failure. This occurs when there is an acute rise in the pulmonary capillary pressure, which overwhelms the ability of the pulmonary lymphatic system to drain the excess fluid (32).

The lymphatic system removes the products of inflammation and relieves congestion. Lymphatic system is under autonomic nervous system control, specifically the sympathetic system which produces vasoconstriction and impairs lymph drainage. The Peripheral Lymphatic Ducts contain valves which help move the lymph in one direction (Fig. 55.3). The Lymphatic system utilizes mechanical advantage as much as possible and as such lymphatic vessels travel with the arteries and are usually contained in a sheath. With each pulse bringing arterial blood to the extremities, the lymphatics get a mechanical boost back to the central circulation. Once in the central circulation, lymphatic flow is assisted by the diaphragm creating both pressure differentials and directly influencing the cysterna chyli (18).

Our patient had pleural effusions documented by CXR and peripheral edema. She also had some mild abdominal complaints and some abdominal distension on examination and elevated liver function enzymes in her blood testing. This pattern is consistent with abdominal third spacing and passive hepatic congestion although we did not confirm this with any studies.

In viewing our patient from this respiratory—circulatory perspective, we can see evidence of many of the above concepts.

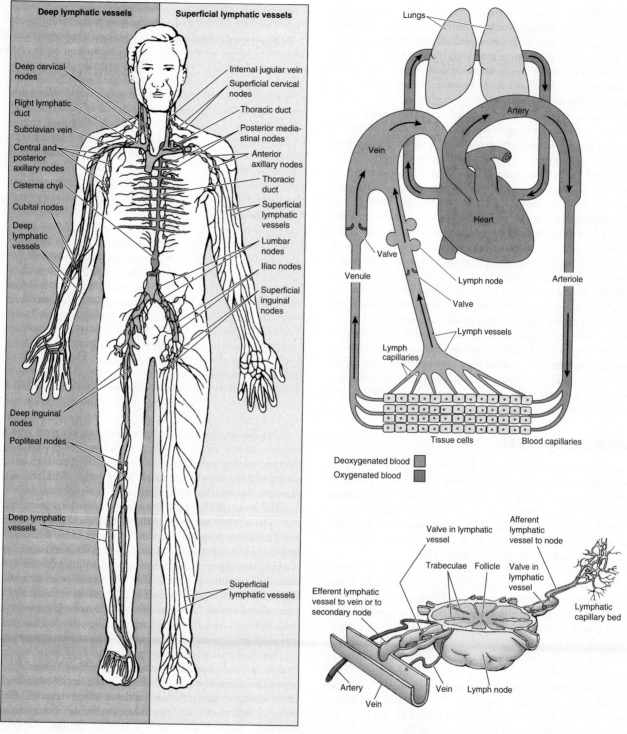

Figure 55-3 Lymphatics.

This patient had a cardiomyopathy with depressed ejection fraction and diastolic dysfunction which makes her more susceptible to fluid balance disturbances. This patient was taking rapid shallow breaths with poor diaphragmatic and thoracic excursion. Additionally, her thoracic mechanics were compromised by poor compliance and an increased kyphosis. This resulted in decreased thoracoabdominal pressure changes. She was quite deconditioned and along with increased lumbar lordosis and sacral nutation had limited musculoskeletal efficiency. She had increased sympathetic activity as evidenced by increased blood pressure, heart rate, respiratory rate, and cyanotic appearing feet. This is also evidence of vasoconstriction that would affect fluid flow throughout the body.

One of the principles of osteopathic medicine is the ability of the body to self-regulate (11). It is the osteopathic physician's job to assist the body in this capacity. There are no adequate randomized controlled trials (RCT) addressing heart failure with OMT; however, by appreciating the factors that influenced this patient's clinical state, we used plausible ways to improve this patient's physiology using an osteopathic approach.

In terms of the respiratory-circulatory model, we looked to augment the pharmacologic and respiratory treatments that were initiated. Our goals were to augment venous and lymphatic drainage to assist in the ability to reabsorb fluids that had been third spaced. This improves the removal of metabolic wastes and as end tissue pressures are decreased, helps improve oxygen delivery and may improve delivery of medications.

Once the patient had stabilized, we addressed peripheral drainage by using myofascial release to improve the mechanics at the T1/rib 1/manubrium. This was done to optimize thoracic duct drainage. We then used a gentle lymph pump to induce drainage (14,33). We used balanced ligamentous tension (BLT) and rib raising to the rib cage, thorax, and lumbar spine to improve compliance, pliability, and decrease the spinal curvature (18). We redomed the diaphragm to improve efficiency of the thoracoabdominal-pelvic cylinder in order to improve flow through the central circulation (14). The goal of this was to increase pressure changes throughout the thoracoabdominal-pelvic cylinder. Lastly, lymphatic pump techniques were employed to assist drainage from the peripheral tissues. As we were mobilizing fluids from extravascular spaces and augmenting return into the systemic circulation, we were careful not to overload the patient at any point and paid careful attention to physiologic parameters (18).

In summary, the respiratory-circulatory model deals with fluid movement. Our patient had fluid overload. We used a combination of diuretics (furosemide), preload reduction (nitrates), and OMT to help restore more physiologic somatic relationships to facilitate venous and lymphatic drainage and help the body mobilize and ultimately remove excess fluids.

NEUROLOGIC MODEL

The cardiovascular system is under constant influence from the nervous system. The autonomic nervous system regulates heart rate, force of cardiac contraction, vascular tone, and blood pressure. The preferred homeostatic state of the cardiovascular system is under parasympathetic dominance. In decompensated heart failure and many chronic cases of heart failure, there are increased levels of catecholamines and hypersympathetatonia (34).

Under states of increased sympathetic tone, the body experiences increased heart rate (chronotropy), increased force of contraction (ionotropy), vasoconstriction, and elevated blood pressure. This in turn leads to increased myocardial oxygen demand. This is coupled with decreased coronary blood flow (CBF) from vasoconstriction and decreased time of diastole and this can lead to cardiac ischemia. Sympathetic and parasympathetic considerations are outlined in Table 55.1.

Under conditions of increased sympathetic tone, the myocardium undergoes a remodeling process (35). There is a prolonged healing time and decreased angiogenesis (36). This has been well recognized after both cardiac ischemia and in the setting of heart failure. This is the heart's attempt to restore homeostasis and occurs through several mechanisms including genetic transduction and protein synthesis. Unfortunately, under the influence of a hypersympathetic state and other neurohumoral influences, the body produces changes that are ineffective and inefficient (35). There are other pathologic structural changes that occur in the myocardium under these conditions which were discussed in the preceding section. This is part of the basis of providing beta blockade and has been shown to modify the remodeling process and improve survival (37–41). Also, adding ACE inhibitors or Angiotensin receptor blockers has also been found to prevent and reverse some of the pathologic remodeling that occurs and also improves mortality (42–46).

TABLE 55.1	
Neurologic Model Considerations	
Sympathetic	• Increased catecholamines • increased chronotropy/ionotropy • increased BP • Increased oxygen demand • Decreased CBF • Decreased time for diastole • Cardiac remodeling • Impaired Lymph drainage • Typical VSR
Parasympathetic	• Vagal • Decreased ionotropy (in some cases increased) • decreased chronotropy • Decreased BP • Increased CBF • Improved lymph drainage • Myocardial stabilizing • C1/2 segments No typical musculoskeletal reflex activity

Our patient had LV dysfunction/cardiomyopathy from her ischemic heart disease and resultant heart failure. This is a common remodeling pattern. On presentation, she had signs of hypersympathetic tone with elevated heart rate, blood pressure, and vasoconstriction (cool extremities).

The sympathetic outflow to the heart is from spinal levels T1-6 (47). The outflow nerves relay through the middle cervical ganglia and the stellate ganglion. They then join up with the cardiac plexus and ultimately synapse on and innervate the myocardium. Nerves carrying nociceptive information are called Nociceptors and travel with the sympathetic nerves. Cardiac nociceptors are very sensitive to ischemia and inflammation (36). Afferent nerves from both visceral and somatic structures synapse in the spinal cord onto the same lamina and facilitate viscerosomatic reflex somatic dysfunctions (48,49).

Viscerosomatic reflexes or segmental facilitation is characterized by warmth, muscle spasm, tenderness, and moisture. These are explained by the physiologic processes of vasodilation, reflex stimulation of alpha motoneurons in the deep back musculature, activation of the inflammatory cascade and inflammatory mediators such as substance P. These are the basic findings that characterize somatic dysfunctions. Several studies have been performed that demonstrate this and that has bearing in our patient (50,51).

In 1983, Cox et al. published a paper entitled "Palpable musculoskeletal findings in CAD: results of a double-blind study." During this study, 97 patients who were having cardiac symptoms had a blinded musculoskeletal assessment for somatic dysfunction. All patients went on for cardiac catheterization. The authors concluded that there was a high correlation of changes at T4 in patients with significant cardiac disease in the men and women (52).

Nicholas published a similar study in the *British Medical Journal* in 1985 entitled "A somatic component to myocardial infarction." The authors concluded there was a significantly higher incidence of somatic dysfunction confined almost entirely to the upper for thoracic levels in patients experiencing MI. The authors then went on to conduct a 3-year follow-up published in the *British Medical Journal* in 1991 whereby they reassessed patients who had had MI in the previous study after 3 years post-MI. They found a significant decrease in palpable somatic dysfunctions in these patients who had survived and were treated (53,54).

A study whereby dogs were subjected to induced myocardial ischemia demonstrated increased muscle tension and texture from T2-5 on the left and increased amplitude on EMG on T4 and T5 during myocardial ischemia. This again demonstrates this well-known phenomenon of this viscerosomatic interaction. Interestingly, the same experiment conducted after sympathectomy failed to demonstrate these somatic changes reinforcing the pathway of viscerosomatic reflexes propagating through the sympathetic nervous system (55).

Although it has been written about in the osteopathic literature, and there are experimental data examining somatovisceral reflex activity, there are no studies that have investigated the impact of somatic dysfunction and in particular somatovisceral reflexes on the development or worsening of visceral dysfunction. This is, however, an in intriguing concept that bears further study (56,57).

Our patient had changes in her upper thoracic region that correlate with cardiovascular viscerosomatic reflexes. In addition to the findings of acute viscerosomatic reflexes, such as the warmth and boggy tissue texture, she was found to have had an underlying ropey texture associated with more chronic somatic reflexes. Perhaps these findings may be contributing to her pathology by acting as a somatovisceral stimulus. Treatment was directed to this area; however, any acute viscerosoamatic reflexes were treated with extreme care because of the potential to induce somatovisceral input on an already pathologic area (18). During outpatient follow-up, we focused on this region to reduce the long-term potential of somatovisceral reflexes to influence her cardiac physiology.

Parasympathetic outflow occurs through the right and left vagus nerves. The vagus nerve exits through the jugular foramen at the occipitomastoid suture and enters the cardiac plexus (58). Parasympathetic activity slows the heart rate and lowers the blood pressure and has a myocardial stabilizing effect that is antiarrhythmic. In the decompensated heart, such as a patient with heart failure, increased parasympathetic activity can increase ionotropy by moving the cardiac physiology to a more favorable portion of the Frank-Starling curve (59).

There are well-described "vagal reflexes" in the osteopathic literature that tend to involve the C2 segment. These have been described by osteopaths in both cardiac and pulmonary conditions (18,50). Along with the C2 segment, the occipital atlantal junction and occipitomastoid are areas that have been written about in osteopathic literature that tend to influence autonomic tone (60). Some experimental animal data have shown that vagal afferent activity is mediated through the C1 and C2 spinal segments (61,62). There is evidence that vagal cardiac afferent activity is inhibitory and decreased muscular spasms and affected response to cardiac sympathetic generated by introducing noxious cardiac stimulation (63–65).

Our patient did have changes at C2, which may indicate that there are changes in vagal tone. If treating C2 and the other areas of vagal outflow (jugular foramen, occipital mastoid suture, occipital atlantal joints) could change the autonomic balance toward a parasympathetic predominating state, then this could have a positive influence on our patient.

In addition to the above changes that take place, there are endocrine changes in the decompensated heart failure patient. There is a cascade of events that lead to heart failure. Our patient admits to eating salty foods and skipping some of her medications. This is quite common for heart failure patients (66). With increased salt load, there is increased retention of fluids. With increased fluids, there is increased pressure in the vasculature. There is a decrease in the effective circulating volume sensed by the kidneys. This leads to activation of the renin-angiotensin-aldosterone system, which attempts to preserve fluid volume by salt and fluid reabsorption. ADH secretion from the hypothalamus acts to reabsorb free water and can contribute to the development of hyponatremia. These changes can lead to heart failure, peripheral edema, and lymphatic stasis.

In summary, along with appropriate medical treatment (beta-blockade and ACE inhibition) to improve neurohumoral balance and prevent or reverse cardiac remodeling, we also utilize osteopathic treatment. Our osteopathic treatment goals were to identify somatic dysfunction that may have contributed to our patient's pathology and defacilitate viscerosomatic reflexes to assist her body help restore parasympathetic dominance to the autonomic nervous system.

METABOLIC ENERGY MODEL

Fatigue and dyspnea are common complaints in heart failure patients. These were our patient's presenting complaints. Exercise capacity is the ability to perform activity or endurance of an individual. Exercise intolerance is when an individual is not able to exercise to the expected level and is a concomitant feature of heart failure (67).

Exercise capacity depends on the ability of the cardiovascular system to deliver oxygen to exercising skeletal muscle and the ability of that muscle to extract oxygen from the blood and is based on cardiovascular dynamics, the ability of pulmonary gas exchange, and skeletal muscle metabolism (68). Peak exercise capacity is defined as the maximum of this capacity and maximal oxygen uptake (VO_{2max}) has a strong linear correlation with cardiac output and skeletal muscle blood flow (67).

Heart failure patients have a reduced capacity to increase cardiac output with even mild exertion (67). Several factors may contribute to the inability of heart failure patients to have sufficient response to exercise (Box 55.2). There is downregulation of beta receptors in the setting of chronically elevated catecholamine levels, and this results in a reduced ionotropic and chronotropic response (69,70). There is an increase in diastolic dysfunction that may impair cardiac output. There is a demonstrated, abnormal increase

---

Changes Occurring in Heart Failure

- **Downregulation of beta receptors**
- **Increased diastolic dysfunction**
- **Increased wedge pressure**
- **Impaired pulmonary diffusion**
- **Muscle changes**
- **Myocyte apoptosis**
- **Reduced capillary density**
- **change from fatigue resistant to fatiguable**
- **change to anaerobic activity and increased lactic acid**
- **enhanced ergoreceptors and mechanoreceptors**
- **Diaphragm change from type 2 to type 1 fibers**

in pulmonary wedge pressure that can exacerbate pulmonary congestion causing dyspnea and limiting exercise capacity. There can be impaired pulmonary diffusion even in the absence of pulmonary congestion.

Previously, it was thought that poor exercise capacity was due to depressed cardiac output and decreased oxygen delivery and that treatment with positive ionotropes would improve symptoms and exercise capacity. Several studies investigated the impact of ionotropes and vasodilators on exercise tolerance and found that although there were measurable increases in both cardiac output and peripheral blood flow, which would also increase oxygen delivery to exercising muscles, there were no significant increases in exercise capacity (71). The researchers were able to demonstrate that these interventions had limited impact on maximal oxygen consumption (VO_{2max}) and concluded that this may have been from decreased oxygen extraction by the muscle. Subsequently, it became recognized that there were intrinsic skeletal muscle changes, which were present in heart failure patients that had a substantial role in exercise tolerance. This became known as the muscle hypothesis (72).

There are several contributing factors in the development of skeletal muscle abnormalities. Physical deconditioning and inactivity is thought to be one factor. Another factor may be chronic hypoperfusion of skeletal muscle secondary to an inadequate response to exercise and a shift from aerobic to anaerobic metabolism (73).

There are several abnormalities that have been found in skeletal muscle of heart failure patients. Myocyte apoptosis has been identified and correlates with the degree of limitation in exercise capacity (74). Capillary density is reduced in heart failure patients compared with controls and has an inverse relationship with oxygen consumption (75). Biochemical abnormalities have been found that include changes in the types of muscle fibers from fatigue resistant to more fatigue able types of fibers (76). Other studies have found lower intracellular pH, indicating increased lactic acid buildup secondary to anaerobic metabolism, evidence of more rapid depletion and, less efficient utilization of high-energy phosphates both in the presence of preserved blood flow (77).

Functional abnormalities have been found in patient with heart failure. There has been demonstrated enhancement of ergoreceptors and metaboreceptors which may partially explain the increased ventilatory response and dyspnea in heart failure (78–80). Respiratory muscles undergo the above changes in heart failure patients and may also be contributing to the symptom complex by early fatigue (81). The diaphragm undergoes change from type 2 (fast twitch, glycolytic, fatigue susceptible) fibers to type 1 (slow twitch, oxidative, fatigue resistant) fibers, which is thought to be from the increased work of breathing and are similar to changes that occur with endurance training (82).

Exercise training and cardiac rehabilitation have been studied and have been shown to have many benefits: Improved peak VO_2, improved muscle energetics, more efficient oxygen utilization, and improved symptoms of fatigue and dyspnea (83,84). Reduced sympathetic tone and increased vagal tone at rest, decreased systemic vascular resistance, reduced neurohumoral activity, and decreased levels of angiotensin, aldosterone, and BNP have also been demonstrated (85–88). Reversal of skeletal muscle abnormalities such as mitochondrial density and a shift from type 2 to type 1 muscle fibers are seen (89).

Improvements in VO_{2peak} can be seen and this translates to improved symptoms, exercise capacity, ability to perform activities of daily living and maintain independence. Also, improvement in NYHA class and 6-minute walk distance as well as reduction in hospitalization rates has been shown (90–93).

One meta-analysis concluded there was reduced mortality and rate of hospitalization in patients who participated in a supervised program for 8 weeks at 2 years of follow up (94).

Exercise training has a class 1 recommendation from the ACC/AHA for heart failure patients with reduced systolic function (8).

W.S. had a stiffened thorax to palpation. She was also very deconditioned and we could reasonably assume that her respiratory muscles were weakened. Because of these changes, the work of breathing and oxygen utilization would be expected to be increased.

One of the tenets of osteopathic medicine is the reciprocal nature of structure and function (11). Many of the above changes in cardiac and skeletal muscle function show this relationship. This is illustrated clearly by the diaphragm which changes structure on the microscopic level to accommodate functional changes on a macroscopic level.

There are no studies looking at the impact of osteopathic manipulation on energy utilization or documenting changes in the structure of skeletal, respiratory, or diaphragmatic muscle or the types of biophysical and biochemical changes listed previously in heart failure patients; however, by evaluating and treating somatic dysfunctions we addressed our patients structure in the expectation the there would be a positive change in her function and functional status.

Our patient had complaints of both dyspnea and fatigue at baseline that were exacerbated at presentation. Once her acute symptoms were treated and she had clinical improvement, she was appropriately referred for a supervised cardiac rehabilitation program. She continued to undergo outpatient osteopathic diagnosis and treatment with a goal of reducing the work of breathing by improved pulmonary and chest wall compliance and improving her overall functional status by improved musculoskeletal relationships and decreased somatic dysfunction severity.

BEHAVIORAL MODEL

In osteopathic medicine, we are trained to look at the person as a whole. One of the basic tenets of osteopathic medicine is that the person is a unity of body, mind, and spirit (11). When we review the history of this patient, it is important to note some of the behavioral aspects that have a direct impact on this patient's life and well-being. She has recently lost her spouse of many years. Our patient reports that she has been feeling depressed because of a recent change in her living arrangement after the death of her husband. She had gone from living independently with her spouse to living interdependently alone in an assisted living apartment. She has been grieving these losses. This could be having a large impact in her immediate and long-term health. She admits to eating foods that she knows are deleterious for her. Additionally, she is skipping her medications at times. These two factors alone could precipitate her present condition and are in a large part resulting not from medical but more behavioral factors. This underscores the importance of addressing these concerns.

It has long been suspected that there is an increase in the incidence of depression in patients with heart failure (95,96). There have been several studies looking at this relationship. And it is becoming clear that not only is depression common in heart failure patients but that it is associated with increased mortality and rehospitalization (97,98). The findings of depression and social isolation worsen mortality (99). Anxiety, although also common in this population, has had conflicting data in regard to whether it is associated with increased mortality (99).

A recently published trial looked at treating heart failure patients with Sertraline for a period of 12 weeks. All patients in the trial received nursing intervention and one arm of the trial received Sertraline (100,101). The trial showed no significant difference in patients treated with the antidepressant versus patients who had just nursing intervention. Although the study was not powered to look at hospitalization rates, there was a trend toward decreased hospitalization rates in the treatment group (101). Another interesting observation was that most of the patients benefited from nursing intervention. The author notes that this was a powerful intervention for these patients and may have blunted the response to medication (100). This may indicate that nursing intervention could be a preferred treatment for these patients. Additionally, the author believes that part of the reason antidepressants may help in heart failure is the restoration of normal autonomic function which may improve immune and inflammatory factors (100).

There are not many controlled trials looking at the treatment of mood disorders with manipulation. The studies that have been performed do not readily translate to the typical heart failure patients.

One small trial looked at treating premenopausal women with depression with osteopathic manipulation. The patients were randomized to either a control group, which received a structural examination; or a treatment group, which received OMT. Both groups received Paxil and psychotherapy weekly for 8 weeks. At the end of the study, there was a significant difference in favor of the treatment group. This was a small pilot study and it is unclear whether the results of this would translate to a larger population group (102). Additionally, this was a study done in pre-menopausal women, few of whom are typical heart failure patients.

Patients with fibromyalgia frequently have concomitant depression. A small study looked at treating patients with fibromyalgia with osteopathic treatment alone or in combination with medication. There was a noted improvement in depression in the patients treated with manipulation and medicine (103). Again, this does not easily translate to our patient's population.

Neither of the above studies found any somatic dysfunction pattern that was "typical" for the patient with depression. Despite the lack of applicable randomized control trials, these studies do offer some evidence in favor of osteopathic manipulation as an intervention for patients with depression. The etiology of this benefit is less clear.

One possible explanation may be found in the concept of Allostatic load. The term Allostatic loadwas coined by Dr. Bruce McEwen and refers to the physiological costs of chronic exposure to neuroendocrine immune stress responses. It is used to explain how frequent activation of the body's stress response, an essential tool

for managing acute threats, can in fact damage the body in the long run through activation of the hypothalamic-pituitary axis (104). The nervous system integrates information from the somatic, visceral, and psychological sources, and these can summate to achieve a stress response (Fig. 55.4). It is possible that by treating underlying somatic dysfunction we might decrease the overall allostatic load to our patients (105–107).

In our patient's case, it was important to discuss her living arrangement. It is important that this patient realize the implications of her actions on both her short-term and long-term health. W.S. received social work evaluation during her hospitalization and then outpatient follow-up from visiting nurse services and social work after she returned home. Additionally, as she believed that she was depressed and still grieving her losses, she was given the option of pharmacologic treatment, which she chose to begin. An antidepressant was started during her hospitalization and followed as an outpatient.

W.S. was receiving osteopathic treatment in hospital as part of a comprehensive plan of acute management for heart failure, and this was also continued after her hospitalization. Over time, this patient's mood did improve and she demonstrated a renewed interest in her health and well-being.

In osteopathic medicine, we are trained to look at the person as a whole. One of the basic tenets of osteopathic medicine is that the person is a unity of body, mind, and spirit (11). This is demonstrated in the connection between depression, anxiety, social isolation, and outcomes in heart failure referenced above. One intervention we can offer as physicians is to recognize the connection between heart failure and depression and take corrective steps in order to address this. Frequent outpatient physician visits, visiting nurse services, counseling, or mobilization of support services may provide improved care. Another intervention may be to include osteopathic diagnosis and treatment in our approach to these patients. Our goals would be to treat the somatic dysfunction we find with the possible goals of decreasing any somatic contribution to the overall allostatic load.

To summarize, there is an established connection between heart failure and depression. This has been demonstrated in several studies and should be in our minds when evaluating patients with either acute or chronic heart failure. It is reasonable to institute appropriate interventions in the belief that these will positively impact our patients' health and although no large RCTs demonstrate this, we have some cursory evidence and pathophysiologic rationale to include osteopathic treatment as a possible intervention in this patient population.

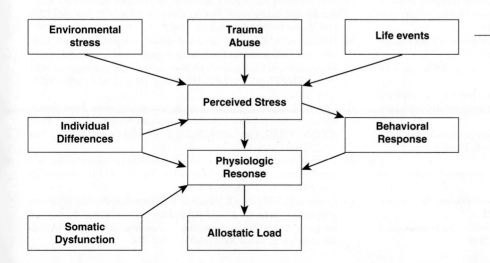

Figure 55-4 Allostatic load.

SUMMARY

Heart failure is a complicated diagnosis, which has many causes that can lead to changes in the structure of the heart and vasculature (remodeling), neurohumoral changes, and endocrinologic changes throughout the body. There are changes in the skeletal muscle that have a large contribution to two of the hallmark symptoms of heart failure: dyspnea and fatigue. There are medications that have been shown to improve mortality and morbidity and decrease hospitalization rates (8). Despite the available medical treatments, there are patients who will remain symptomatic and we must look at other impacting factors. There is a recognized correlation with depression, which should be recognized, evaluated, and will need to be treated in some patients. Lastly, although no sufficient RCTs have been conducted to examine the role of osteopathic medicine in heart failure, there are supporting data in the form of physiologic and pathophysiologic plausibility for the use of adjunctive osteopathic diagnosis and treatments.

W.S. showed many classic findings and complaints consistent with heart failure and has served to illustrate the principles in the evaluation and treatment of heart failure patients.

REFERENCES

1. Amlodipine: Drug information. Adverse reactions. In: Rose BD, ed. *UpTo-Date*. Waltham, MA: UpToDate, 2008.
2. Brenner: *Brenner and Rector's The Kidney*. 8th Ed.
3. Adams, KF, Lindenfeld J, Arnold JM, et al. HFSA 2006 comprehensive heart failure practice guideline *J Card Fail* 2006;12:e1–e119.
4. Nieminen MS, et al. Executive summary of the guidelines on the diagnosis and treatment of acute heart failure: the Task Force on Acute Heart Failure of the European Society of Cardiology. *Eur Heart J* 2005;26(4):384–416; epub Jan 28, 2005.
5. Masip J, Roque M, Sanchez B, et al. Noninvasive ventilation in acute cardiogenic pulmonary edema: systematic review and meta-analysis. *JAMA* 2005;294(24):3124–3130.
6. Fitzgerald M, Stiles E. *Osteopathic Hospital's Solution to DRG's May Be OMT*. In The D.O. November 1984:97–101.
7. Metformin: Drug information—contraindications In: Rose BD, ed. *UpTo-Date*. Waltham, MA: UpToDate, 2008.
8. Hunt SA, Abraham, WT, Chin, MH, et al. ACC/AHA 2005 Guideline Update for the Diagnosis and Management of Chronic Heart Failure in the Adult: a report of the American College of Cardiology/American Heart Association Task Force on Practice Guidelines (Writing Committee to Update the 2001 Guidelines for the Evaluation and Management of Heart Failure): developed in collaboration with the American College of Chest Physicians and the International Society for Heart and Lung Transplantation: endorsed by the Heart Rhythm Society. *Circulation* 2005;112:e154.
9. Young B. A "basket of care" for heart failure patients managing at home: evaluating a community-based nursing intervention from a patient's perspective. *Can J Cardiovasc Nurs* 2008;18(4):10–19.
10. Staples P. The nature of telephone nursing interventions in a heart failure clinic setting. *Can J Cardiovasc Nurs* 2008;18(4):27–33.
11. Ward RC, et al. *Foundations For Osteopathic Medicine*. Baltimore, MD: William & Wilkins, 1997:4–6.
12. Rosse, C. *Hollinshead's Textbook of Anatomy*. The Thorax, the pericardium, the heart, the great vessels. Philadelphia, PA: Lippincott-Raven publishers, 1997:70–82.
13. Essentials of physical medicine and rehabilitation: musculoskeletal disorders, pain, and rehabilitation/ [edited by] Walter R. Frontera, Julie K. Silver, Thomas D. Rizzo Jr—2nd Ed.
14. Zink JG. Respiratory and Circulatory care: the conceptual model. *Osteopath Ann* 1977;108–112.
15. Browner. Compartment Syndromes. In: *Skeletal Trauma: Basic Science, Management, and Reconstruction*. 3rd Ed; chap 12.
16. Mann D. Mechanisms and models in heart failure: the biomechanical model and beyond. *Circulation* 2005;111:2837–2849.
17. Ward RC, et al. *Foundations For Osteopathic Medicine*. 1st Ed. Baltimore, MD: William & Wilkins, 1997:945–946.
18. Ward RC, et al. *Foundations For Osteopathic Medicine*. 2nd Ed. Baltimore, MD: William & Wilkins, 2003: 1115–1135; chapter 71. Ettlinger, H.
19. DeTurk W. et al. Cardiovascular and pulmonary physical therapy: an evidence-based approach. 2004;671–674.
20. Ward RC, et al. *Foundations For Osteopathic Medicine*. 1st Ed. Baltimore, MD: William & Wilkins, 1997:942–946.
21. Kenyon CM, Pedley TJ, Higenbottam TW. Adaptive modeling of the human rib cage in median sternotomy. *J Appl Physiol* 1991;70(5):2287–2302.
22. Schleip R. active fascial contractility: fascia is able to contract and relax in a smooth muscle like manner and thereby influence biomechanical behavior. *Acta Physiologica Congr* (Abstract number: PW06P-6).
23. Ward RC, et al. *Foundations for Osteopathic Medicine*. 2nd Ed. Baltimore, MD: William & Wilkins, 2003:373; chap 25.
24. Massie BM. Heart failure: pathophysiology and diagnosis. In: *Goldman: Cecil Medicine*. 23rd Ed.
25. Rosse C. The Free lower limb. In: *Hollinshead's Textbook of Anatomy*. Lippincott-Raven publishers, 1997:354.
26. Ward RC, et al. *Foundations for Osteopathic Medicine*. 2nd Ed. Baltimore, MD: William & Wilkins, 2003:1063; chapter 68.
27. *Gray's Anatomy*. 38th Ed. 1609–1611.
28. Rosse C. The thorax, the pericardium, the heart, the great vessels. In: *Hollinshead's Textbook of Anatomy*. Lippincott-Raven publishers, 1997:715
29. Hotchkiss RS. Reevaluation of the role of cellular hypoxia and bioenergetic failure in sepsis. *JAMA* 1992;267:1503.
30. Marino P. *The ICU Book*. 2nd Ed. 188.
31. *Harrison's Principles of Internal Medicine*. 16th Ed. 266.
32. *Harrison's Principles of Internal Medicine*. 16th Ed. 204.
33. Knott M, et al. Increased lymphatic flow in the thoracic duct during manipulative intervention. *J Am Osteopath Assoc* 2005;105(10):447–456.
34. Francis GS, Benedict C, Johnstone DE, et al. Comparison of neuroendocrine activation in patients with left ventricular dysfunction with and without congestive heart failure. a substudy of the Studies of Left Ventricular Dysfunction (SOLVD). *Circulation* 1990;82(5):1724–1729.
35. *Harrison's Principles of Internal Medicine*. 16th Ed. 1364–1366.
36. Ward RC, et al. *Foundations for Osteopathic Medicine*. 2nd Ed. Baltimore, MD: William & Wilkins, 2003:1125; chap 71.
37. Doughty RN, Whalley GA, Gamble G, et al. Left ventricular remodeling with carvedilol in patients with congestive heart failure due to ischemic heart disease. Australia-New Zealand Heart Failure Research Collaborative Group. *J Am Coll Cardiol* 1997;29(5):1060–1066.
38. Groenning BA, Nilsson JC, Sondergaard L, et al. Antiremodeling effects on the left ventricle during beta-blockade with metoprolol in the treatment of chronic heart failure. *J Am Coll Cardiol* 2000;;36(7):2072–2080.
39. Bellenger NG, Rajappan K, Rahman SL, et al. Effects of carvedilol on left ventricular remodelling in chronic stable heart failure: a cardiovascular magnetic resonance study. *Heart* 2004;90(7):760–764.
40. Effect of metoprolol CR/XL in chronic heart failure: metoprolol CR/XL Randomised Intervention Trial in Congestive Heart Failure (MERIT-HF). *Lancet* 1999;353(9169):2001–2007.
41. Hjalmarson A. Effects of controlled-release metoprolol on total mortality, hospitalizations, and well-being in patients with heart failure: the Metoprolol CR/XL Randomized Intervention Trial in congestive heart failure (MERIT-HF). MERIT-HF Study Group. *JAMA* 2000;283(10):1295–1302.
42. Effects of enalapril on mortality in severe congestive heart failure. Results of the Cooperative North Scandinavian Enalapril Survival Study (CONSENSUS). The CONSENSUS Trial Study Group. *N Engl J Med* 1987;316(23):1429–1435.
43. Effect of enalapril on survival in patients with reduced left ventricular ejection fractions and congestive heart failure. The SOLVD Investigators. *N Engl J Med* 1991;325(5):293–302.
44. Granger CB, McMurray JJ, Yusuf S, et al. Effects of candesartan in patients with chronic heart failure and reduced left-ventricular systolic function intolerant to angiotensin-converting-enzyme inhibitors: the CHARM-Alternative trial. *Lancet* 2003;362(9386):772–776.

45. Erhardt L, MacLean A, Ilgenfritz J, et al. Fosinopril attenuates clinical deterioration and improves exercise tolerance in patients with heart failure. Fosinopril Efficacy/Safety Trial (FEST) Study Group. *Eur Heart J* 1995;16(12):1892–1899.

46. Pfeffer MA, McMurray JJ, Velazquez EJ, et al. Valsartan, captopril, or both in myocardial infarction complicated by heart failure, left ventricular dysfunction, or both. *N Engl J Med* 2003;349(20):1893–1906; epub Nov 10, 2003.

47. Rosse, C. The thorax, the pericardium, the heart, the great vessels. *Hollinshead's Textbook of Anatomy.* Lippincott-Raven publishers, 1997:481–484.

48. Ward RC, et al. *Foundations for Osteopathic Medicine.* 1st Ed. Baltimore, MD: William & Wilkins, 1997, 137–150.

49. Van Buskirk RL. Nociceptive reflexes and the somatic dysfunction: a model. *J Am Osteopath Assoc* 1990;90:792–809.

50. Beal MC. Palpatory testing for somatic dysfunction in patients with cardiovascular disease. *J Am Osteopath Assoc* 1983;82(11):822–831.

51. Sato A. Reflex modulation of visceral functions by somatic afferent activity. In: Patterson MM, Howell JN, eds. *The Central Connection: Somatovisceral/Viscerosomatic Interaction. 1989 International Symposium.* Athens, OH: American Academy of Osteopathy, 1989:53–76.

52. Cox JM, et al. Palpable musculoskeletal findings in coronary artery disease: results of a double blind study. *J Am Osteopath Assoc* 1983;82(11): 832–836.

53. Nicholas AS, DeBias DA, Ehrenfeuchter W, et al. A somatic component to myocardial infarction. *Br Med J (Clin Res Ed)* 1985;291:13–17.

54. Nicholas AS, et al. Somatic component to myocardial infarction: three year follow up. *BMJ* 1991;302(6792):1581.

55. Gwirtz P. Viscerosomatic interaction induced by myocardial ischemia in conscious dogs. *Appl Physiol* 2007;103:511–517.

56. Ward RC, et al. *Foundations for Osteopathic Medicine.* 2nd Ed. Baltimore, MD: William & Wilkins, 2003: 121–134; chap 7. Paterson, M. Wurster, R., H.

57. Ward RC, et al. *Foundations for Osteopathic Medicine.* 2nd Ed. Baltimore, MD: William & Wilkins, 2003:138–154; chap 8. Willard, F.

58. Rosse, C. *Hollinshead's Textbook of Anatomy.* Lippincott-Raven publishers, 1997;481–484.

59. Braunwald E. et al. *Heart Disease: A Textbook of Cardiovascular Medicine.* 6th Ed. W.B. Saunders company, 2001:660–694; chap. 22.

60. Magoun, H. *Osteopathy in the Cranial Field.* 3rd Ed. 108–115, 268.

61. Ding X. C2 spinal cord stimulation induces dynorphin release from rat T4 spinal cord: potential modulation of myocardial ischemia-sensitive neurons. *Am J Physiol Regul Integr Comp Physiol* 2008;295(5):R1519–R1528.

62. Qin C. Responses and afferent pathways of C1-C2 spinal neurons to cervical and thoracic esophageal stimulation in rats. *J Neurophysiol* 2004;91: 2227–2235.

63. Jou CJ. Afferent pathways for cardiac-somatic motor reflexes in rats. *Am J Physiol Regul Integr Comp Physiol* 2001;281:R2096–R2102.

64. XiaoHui Ding 2008. Modulation of cardiac ischemia-sensitive afferent neuron signaling by preemptive C2 spinal cord stimulation: effect on substance P release from rat spinal cord. *Am J Physiol Regul Integr Comp Physiol* 294:R93–R101.

65. Ammons WS. Vagal afferent inhibition of spinothalamic cell responses to sympathetic afferents and bradykinin in the monkey. *Circ Res* 53:603–612; copyright © 1983 by American Heart Association

66. Van der Wal MH, et al. Non-compliance in patients with heart failure; how can we manage it? *Eur J Heart Fail* 2005;7(1):5–17.

67. Reddy HK, Weber KT, Janicki JS. Hemodynamic, ventilatory and metabolic effects of light isometric exercise in patients with chronic heart failure. *J Am Coll Cardiol* 1988;12(2):353–358.

68. Pina I. Exercise capacity and VO$_2$ in heart failure. In: Rose BD, ed. *UpToDate.* Waltham, MA: UpToDate, 2008.

69. Colucci WS. In vivo studies of myocardial beta-adrenergic receptor pharmacology in patients with congestive heart failure. *Circulation* 1990;82(2 suppl):I44–I51.

70. Bristow MR, Minobe WA, Raynolds MV, et al. Reduced beta 1 receptor messenger RNA abundance in the failing human heart. *J Clin Invest* 1993;92(6):2737–2745.

71. Wilson JR, Martin JL, Ferraro N. Impaired skeletal muscle nutritive flow during exercise in patients with congestive heart failure: role of cardiac pump dysfunction as determined by the effect of dobutamine. *Am J Cardiol* 1984;53(9):1308–1315.

72. Clark AL Poole-Wilson PA; Coats AJ. Exercise limitation in chronic heart failure: central role of the periphery. *J Am Coll Cardiol* 1996;28(5): 1092–1102.

73. Belardinelli R, Barstow TJ, Nguyen P, et al. Skeletal muscle oxygenation and oxygen uptake kinetics following constant work rate exercise in chronic congestive heart failure. *Am J Cardiol* 1997;80(10):1319–1324.

74. Vescovo G, Volterrani M, Zennaro R, et al. Apoptosis in the skeletal muscle of patients with heart failure: investigation of clinical and biochemical changes. *Heart* 2000;84(4):431–437.

75. Duscha BD, Kraus WE, Keteyian SJ, et al. Capillary density of skeletal muscle: a contributing mechanism for exercise intolerance in class II-III chronic heart failure independent of other peripheral alterations. *J Am Coll Cardiol* 1999;33(7):1956–1963.

76. Mancini DM, Coyle E, Coggan A, et al. Contribution of intrinsic skeletal muscle changes to 31P NMR skeletal muscle metabolic abnormalities in patients with chronic heart failure. *Circulation* 1989;80(5): 1338–1346.

77. Massie B, Conway M, Yonge R, et al. Skeletal muscle metabolism in patients with congestive heart failure: relation to clinical severity and blood flow. *Circulation* 1987;76(5):1009–1019.

78. Chua TP, Ponikowski PP, Harrington D, et al. Contribution of peripheral chemoreceptors to ventilation and the effects of their suppression on exercise tolerance in chronic heart failure. *Heart* 1996;76(6):483–489.

79. Piotr P. Muscle ergoreceptor overactivity reflects deterioration in clinical status and cardiorespiratory reflex control in chronic heart failure. *Circulation* 2001;104:2324–2330.

80. Piepoli M. Contribution of muscle afferents to the hemodynamic, autonomic and ventilatory responses to exercise in patients with chronic heart failure. *Circulation* 1996;93:940–952.

81. Meyer FJ, Borst MM, Zugck C, et al. Respiratory muscle dysfunction in congestive heart failure: clinical correlation and prognostic significance. *Circulation* 2001;103(17):2153–2158.

82. Tikunov B, Levine S, Mancini D. Chronic congestive heart failure elicits adaptations of endurance exercise in diaphragmatic muscle. *Circulation* 1997;95(4):910–916.

83. Belardinelli R, Georgiou D, Cianci G, et al. Effects of exercise training on left ventricular filling at rest and during exercise in patients with ischemic cardiomyopathy and severe left ventricular systolic dysfunction. *Am Heart J* 1996;132(1 pt 1):61–70.

84. McKelvie RS, Teo KK, McCartney N, et al. Effects of exercise training in patients with congestive heart failure: a critical review. *J Am Coll Cardiol* 1995;25(3):789–796.

85. Coats AJ. Exercise rehabilitation in chronic heart failure. *J Am Coll Cardiol* 1993;22(4 suppl A):172A–177A.

86. Liu JL, Irvine S, Reid IA, et al. Chronic exercise reduces sympathetic nerve activity in rabbits with pacing-induced heart failure: a role for angiotensin II. *Circulation* 2000;102(15):1854–1862.

86. Braith RW, Welsch MA, Feigenbaum MS, et al. Neuroendocrine activation in heart failure is modified by endurance exercise training. *J Am Coll Cardiol* 1999;34(4):1170–1175.

88. Passino C, Severino S, Poletti R, et al. Aerobic training decreases B-type natriuretic peptide expression and adrenergic activation in patients with heart failure. *J Am Coll Cardiol* 2006;47(9):1835–1839; epub Apr 19, 2006.

89. Hambrecht R, Fiehn E, Yu J, et al. Effects of endurance training on mitochondrial ultrastructure and fiber type distribution in skeletal muscle of patients with stable chronic heart failure. *J Am Coll Cardiol* 1997;29(5): 1067–1073.

90. Tyni-Lenne R, Gordon A, Jansson E, et al. Skeletal muscle endurance training improves peripheral oxidative capacity, exercise tolerance, and health-related quality of life in women with chronic congestive heart failure secondary to either ischemic cardiomyopathy or idiopathic dilated cardiomyopathy. *Am J Cardiol* 1997;80(8):1025–1029.

91. Sullivan MJ, Higginbotham MB, Cobb FR. Exercise training in patients with severe left ventricular dysfunction. Hemodynamic and metabolic effects. *Circulation* 1988;78(3):506–515.

92. Hambrecht R. Physical training in patients with stable chronic heart failure: effects on cardiorespiratory fitness and ultrastructural abnormalities of leg muscles. *J Am Coll Cardiol* 1995;25(6):1239–1249.

93. Meyer K. Effects of exercise training and activity restriction on 6-minute walking test performance in patients with chronic heart failure. *H SO Am Heart J* 1997;133(4):447–453.

94. Piepoli MF. Exercise training meta-analysis of trials in patients with chronic heart failure. *BMJ* 2004;328:189–195.

95. Jiang W. Relationship of depression to increased risk of mortality and rehospitalization in patients with congestive heart failure. *Arch Intern Med* 2001;161 (15):1849–1856.

96. Williams SA. Depression and risk of heart failure among the elderly: a prospective community-based study. *Psychosom Med* 2002;64:6–12.

97. Jiang, W. Relationship between depressive symptoms and long term mortality in patients with heart failure. *Am Heart J* 2007;154(1):102–108.

98. Rutledge T, et al. Depression in heart failure a meta analytic review of prevalence, intervention effects and associations with clinical outcomes. *J Am Coll Cardiolo* 2006;48(8):1527–1537.

99. Friedmann E. Relationship of depression, anxiety, and social isolation to chronic heart failure outpatient mortality. *Am Heart J* 2006;152(5):940.e1–940.e8.

100. Heartwire. SADHART-CHF: Nurse intervention impresses for depression in heart failure, SSRI doesn't. September 23, 2008;Steve Stiles.

101. O'Connor CM. Safety and efficacy of sertraline for depression in patients with congestive heart failure (SADHART-CHF). Heart Failure Society of America 2008 Scientific Meeting. Toronto, ON: Late Breaking Clinical Trials I. September 22, 2008.

102. Plotkin BJ. Adjunctive osteopathic manipulative treatment in women with depression: a pilot study. *J Am Osteopath Assoc* 2001;101(9):517–523.

103. Gamber RG. Osteopathic manipulative treatment in conjunction with medication relieves pain associated with fibromyalgia syndrome: results of a randomized clinical pilot project. *J Am Osteopath Assoc* 2002;102(6):321–325.

104. Rijk OBG. *The Metabolic Syndrome, Depression, and Cardiovascular Disease: Interrelated Conditions that Share Pathophysiologic Mechanisms Medical Clinics of North America.* Vol 90, No 4 (July 2006). Copyright © 2006 W. B. Saunders Company.

105. Karlamangla AS. Allostatic load as a predictor of functional decline MacArthur studies of successful aging. *J Clin Epidemiol* 2002;55(7):696–710.

106. Logan JG. Allostasis and allostatic load: expanding the discourse on stress and cardiovascular disease. *J Clin Nurs* 2008;17(7B):201–208.

107. Ward RC, et al. *Foundations for Osteopathic Medicine.* 2nd Ed. Baltimore, MD: William & Wilkins, 2003:138–154; chap 8. Willard, F.

108. Beal MC, Kleiber GE. Somatic dysfunction as a predictor of coronary artery disease. *J Am Osteopath Assoc* 1985a;85:70–75.

109. Beal MC. Viscerosomatic reflexes: a review. *J Am Osteopath Assoc* 1985b;85:786–801.

110. Cox JM, Gorbis S, Dick L, et al. Palpable musculoskeletal findings in coronary artery disease: Results of a double blind study. *J Am Osteopath Assoc* 1983;832–836.

56

Adult with Chronic Pain and Depression

MICHAEL L. KUCHERA AND JOHN JEROME

KEY CONCEPTS

■ Chronic pain and depression are intimately linked, physiologically and psychologically, and can become part of a vicious interdependent cycle.
■ Osteopathic philosophy provides several perspectives within which to view this chronic pain–depression cycle.
■ Helping a patient to cope with his or her pain can break that cycle and influence his or her life in many ways.

CASE VIGNETTE

Chuck, a 45-year-old farmhand, was seen in the clinic with back pain.

Chief Complaint:

Chronic back pain for 3 years. This discomfort, present on his right side, was described as deep, nagging, and constant, with periods of acute exacerbation into the right hip, groin, and down the back of the leg to just above the knee. Full symptoms would occur with prolonged walking or standing and would persist for several weeks. The patient was unable to lift more than 25 pounds (11 kg) without aggravating his symptoms. His back took several hours to fully relax after lying down, even on "good" days.

History of Present Illness:

Pain onset had first occurred while the patient carried a small bale of hay in front of his body. He had stepped in an unseen pothole, stumbled, and fell. The next day, he noticed full symptoms, which persisted as recurring episodes for several months. Between and during episodes, he achieved only partial relief with ibuprofen (800 mg/d). Physical therapy reportedly aggravated his pain.

During the next 3 years, the patient visited several physicians, visits that were prompted by three to four substantial recurrences of pain radiation per year. Negative results from electromyographic, magnetic resonance imaging, and radiographic studies—coupled with negative results from tests of reflex changes and nonspecific, nonradicular patterns of muscle weakness—during these 3 years left the patient with no specific diagnosis beyond "low back pain with recurrent lumbosacral sprain." He was unable to work on the farm and said that he had the impression that physicians believed he was "malingering," or "lazy." He was depressed because he thought his family also shared these beliefs, and he became concerned about his marriage.

PHYSICAL EXAMINATION

Clinical findings revealed a slim white man who denied smoking or illicit drug use. Review of his nonmusculoskeletal systems was noncontributory. Results of deep tendon reflexes, pathologic reflexes, straight leg-raising testing, Chapman's viscerosomatic reflex screen, and Lloyd test were all negative. The result for a Trendelenburg test (a test to determine any weakness of hip abductors) of the right leg was questionable. Somatic dysfunction included reduced lumbar lordosis, left iliacus tender point, right sacral shear, and tenderness over the right iliolumbar ligament and posterior sacroiliac ligament,

as well as tenderness and hypertonicity in the right piriformis muscle. Flexion tests and measurements of iliac crest height along with very mild scoliotic spinal curves suggested a possible "short leg syndrome." The common compensatory pattern noted by Zink and Lawson was violated by the lumbopelvic junction, and the pelvic floor was tight.

The patient was informed that this constellation of somatic dysfunction could cause chronic low back pain (LBP) that often responded favorably to osteopathic manipulative treatment (OMT).

DIFFERENTIAL DIAGNOSIS

Depression

Depression occurs in roughly 50% of chronic pain patients (56–58). Pain severity is strongly associated with depressed mood (59, 60). Depression worsens suffering (54) (55) by interfering with social and occupational functioning (29, 30) and decreases activity levels (31, 32). Finally, depression predicts negative treatment outcome, disability (33), and increased use of medical services (34). Early treatment of depression avoids excessive diagnostic procedures and multiple surgeries (35).

Chuck depression appears more situational (i.e., dysthymic disorder) and secondary to his pain as there is irritability, sadness, lack of interest in enjoyed activities, fear of movement and reinjury by heavy farm work. In contrast, more severe clinical depression (i.e., major depressive disorder) would occur most of the day, every day with weight change of more than 5% of body weight in a month, insomnia or hypersomnia, fatigue, irritability, difficulties with concentration, and reoccurrent suicidal ideation (39). Remember, pain alone is not usually a sufficient condition for the development of depression (40, 41). Specific perpetuating factors that predict depression secondary to pain are (41–44):

1. Reduction in activity
2. Interference with life activities
3. Decreased sense of quality of life
4. Work interference

All these factors appear present in Chuck case.

Family and Spouse Response

Research has consistently shown that the spouse of the chronic pain patient can exert powerful effects on the way the patient copes with their pain (15). Much of the research focuses on the spouse reactions to their partners in pain.

Chronic LBP drastically changes the roles and relationships in families. The impact is particularly great for the spouses (45, 46) leading to more negative interactions (47–49) which we see in this case. Actually, the spouses are themselves also at greater risk of depression (50), loneliness (49), distress (50, 51), and marital discord (52, 53). Marital discord means less communicating, commitment, sexual frequency (50, 51), and more negative interactions (47). Spouse perceptions that appear critical (i.e., "lazy") and that are hostile or punishing further add to negative thinking and depression on the patients part (52, 53). On the flip side, when pain patients are satisfied with the response of their spouse, then pain and depression are less likely. Spousal support may help to mitigate negative thinking.

Chronic Pain

Persistent nonmalignant pain is not a single entity. It has many different causes and manifestations, each with varied characteristics and names. In an osteopathic approach, a complete patient history and physical examination are used to reveal any previously unidentified pain generator or underlying cause for persistent pain. In addition, osteopathic physicians need to understand the individual's unique response to pain and will therefore screen patients for signs of depression or other significant nonsomatic links contributing to pain. Based on such patient histories and examinations, osteopathic practitioners can develop individualized osteopathic prescriptions to address their findings, with the mutually beneficial goals of decreasing biomechanical, biochemical, and psychological stressors, removing barriers to self-healing, self-regulating mechanisms, and empowering patients themselves to reduce the impact of persistent pain on quality of life.

Figure 56.1 shows an osteopathic algorithm for management of patients with chronic or recurrent pain. An OMM approach that integrates palpatory diagnosis and OMT provides balance for patients with persistent nonmalignant pain seeking both state-of-the-art interventions and individualized patient-centered care. The various osteopathic models offer strategies to both decrease pain and to enhance physiologic function. In this fashion, the osteopathic perspective offers two major recognized advantages: an expanded differential of potentially treatable etiologies and an individualized, patient-centered pain prescription based on the application of osteopathic principles.

Osteopathic Patient Management

In addition to providing appropriate strategies for management of pain, an osteopathic management algorithm (such as the one shown in Fig 56.1) incorporates the five common osteopathic models of care to identify and address a variety of host factors directed toward the underlying cause, secondary signs and symptoms, and the tangible and persistent impact of both in patients. These models also provide a framework for the patient education needed to foster compliance built on an understanding of complex interrelationships among many different factors. Each osteopathic prescription seeks to discover and incorporate those factors needed to address a patient's unique response to pain. The emphasis in treating patients who have persistent nonmalignant pain should be on improving function, decreasing peripheral nociception and central facilitation, and empowering individuals to move forward in resuming their normal activities of daily living.

The five most commonly applied osteopathic models include:

1. Biomechanical
2. Respiratory-circulatory
3. Neurologic
4. Metabolic-energy
5. Behavioral

Each was considered in this case history and two models in particular, biopsychosocial and postural/biomechanical, were found to be most specifically involved in this case. The other three models could easily have been involved as well and are therefore also discussed below.

Biomechanical Model

Significant and distinctive contributions to the evidence base surrounding LBP management commonly stem from application of the postural/biomechanical model. One such contribution lies in the identification of six somatic diagnoses commonly found in chronic back pain patients—the so-called dirty half-dozen. Using a structure-function approach, Greenman examined 183 patients who had persistent LBP for an average of 31 months. With osteopathic palpation, he identified three or more of six common diagnoses of somatic dysfunction in 50% of this cohort. Treatment with OMT to eliminate the identified somatic dysfunctions resulted in nearly 75% of the dysfunctional group returning to work or to their other activities of daily living (37).

Chuck benefited from the osteopathic clinician's recognition of both the mechanism of injury and its potential relationship to at least three of this dirty half-dozen nonphysiological (traumatic) somatic dysfunctions documented in the literature. He also benefited from the capability of the DO to deliver effective OMT to return function to the region itself and to prepare the rest of the body to accept the associated postural and biomechanical change that would inevitably follow.

The beneficial role for manual modes of therapy, including OMT, in removing somatic dysfunction (the "manipulable lesion") has been documented for patients with acute, subacute, and chronic LBP (33–36). In patients with LBP, spinal manipulations generally—and OMT specifically—produce physiologic effects similar to efficacious prescription nonsteroidal anti-inflammatory drugs, and has the potential to create effects more beneficial than either physical therapy or home back exercises (13, 36). Beneficial long-term functional outcomes for manual therapy have also been demonstrated in patients with chronic LBP (38). In fact, based on a review of the literature, Mein postulated that patient populations with subacute (secondary) and chronic (tertiary) LBP would benefit most from manipulative care, rather than from more costly behavioral modification, functional restoration, and chronic pain management programs. Why live with and learn to cope with pain if it is possible to remove somatic dysfunction?

In the postural/biomechanical model, OMT is applied primarily to remove somatic dysfunctions and their objective manifestations of tenderness, asymmetry, ROM alteration, and tissue texture change. That said, identifying and addressing the "key lesions" (or primary somatic dysfunctions) becomes the goal of the model. For example, postural imbalance and compensatory somatic dysfunction above the sacral shear was a real, albeit secondary, consequence in Chuck case. Even in the absence of significant LBP, it would therefore not have been uncommon for other patients like Chuck to be seen repetitively for other somatic symptoms (such as headache, midthoracic back ache, and knee pain) or even somato-visceral symptoms (such as irritable bowel syndrome) that would benefit transiently from the more limited use of the postural/biomechanical model.

Obviously, without specific palpatory examination for sacral, innominate, and pubic shears, they will be overlooked; pubic

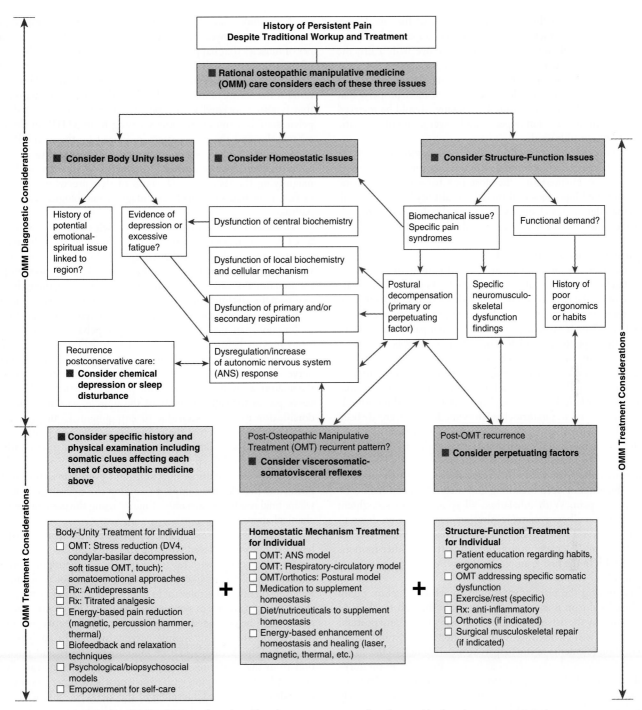

Figure 56-1 Osteopathic algorithm for management of patients with chronic or recurrent pain.

dysfunction (in the front of the pelvis) was present in 76% of Greenman dirty half-dozen causes of chronic LBP! Shears or compression at the pubic symphysis are common dysfunctions that can happen in the peripartum period, after a fall, and after a missed step (40); pubic dysfunction restricting pelvic motion anteriorly causes the two sacroiliac joints to overwork and therefore be painful. Likewise, dysfunction of one sacroiliac joint due to nonphysiologic pelvic shear forces greatly increases functional demand on the other sacroiliac joint and its stabilizing ligaments (40). In this frequently encountered scenario, a unilateral sacral dysfunction is overlooked because the associated pain is located in the overused sacroiliac joint rather than the dysfunctional one.

Failing to make a diagnosis of the key somatic dysfunctions or being misled by pain to concentrate treatment on secondary or compensatory sites constitute two significant elements in the postural/biomechanical model that the physician can rectify. Undiagnosed, key somatic dysfunctions—particularly "nonphysiologic dysfunctions" (e.g., traumatically induced pelvic shears)—might inadvertently result in several years of persistent pain (either locally or at distant sites linked through compensatory mechanisms) or the development of latent myofascial trigger points (MTrPs) that recur whenever they are stressed. If the sacral shear had been overlooked in Chuck case, his apparent "short leg syndrome" might have been recognized as another of the "dirty half-dozen" and treated with a heel or shoe lift on the short leg side to level his sacral base. Unfortunately for Chuck, regardless of the impact initially on restoring balance, alignment, and function above with a lift, the long-term effect of such a strategy would be to increase the shear forces on the sacroiliac joints thereby increasing the patient's symptoms. The diagnosis of "short leg syndrome" (or more properly that of sacral base unleveling requiring lift therapy) should be reserved until—at a minimum—lumbopelvic and lower extremity somatic dysfunctions are addressed.

Reduction or alleviation of pain is one of the greatest benefits of applying the postural/biomechanical model, as was demonstrated in Chuck case. Furthermore, the close link between this somatic model and the biopsychosocial model has already been discussed. The remainder of this chapter will discuss the three other models that were considered or that were secondarily involved.

Respiratory-Circulatory Model

Note that mentally or emotionally stressed patients with chronic pain often breathe more shallowly and rapidly. As pain and stress are relieved, often the patient will be seen and heard to sigh deeply and switch their respiration over to a slower, deeper, and more effective respiration. This, in turn, helps to maintain that pain reduction. To this end, the respiratory-circulatory model has been applied by osteopathic physicians in managing chronic pain patient. One goal is to reduce pain and edema by removing local metabolic waste products such as substance P, histamine, kinins, and certain interleukins that add to the allostatic load. This and the link between the postural-biomechanical and respiratory-circulatory models have already been discussed in the chapters of this text associated with each topic.

In western medicine, focusing on the breath (as in Lamaze) has been an effective method for pain and stress reduction. The ancient Chinese used their own version of a respiratory-circulatory model—the combination of deep breathing and meditation—to help control arthritis pain. With inhalation, all spinal curves straighten; with exhalation all exaggerate; respiration creates motion down to the cellular level. This mental-spiritual focus can be linked with the act of breathing to create motion or to link it with other motions as in Tai Chi. In the first example, the key is motion; in the second, motion is key.

Maximizing the respiratory system to act as a suction pump to reduce local pain is accomplished not only through mechanical intervention by the osteopathic physician using OMT and postural strategies but also by teaching the patient how to link mind, spirit, and emotion (elements in the biopsychosocial model) to the structures most commonly thought of as being part of the respiratory-circulatory model. Again, regardless of the underlying mechanisms involved, the respiratory-circulatory model goals can be effectively applied in the chronic pain patient.

Neurological Model

Although there were only weak neurological signs in Chuck case, those objective findings present—and others—could certainly have been several more prominent. In similar cases possessing stronger neurological symptoms, either patient or physician might become fixated upon a pathologically linked neurological diagnosis such as radiculopathy; even when diagnostic tests or treatment trials fail to confirm the link between the anatomical site and the pain. In this same fashion—and even in the absence of neurological findings—often the concomitant finding of degenerative changes in the lumbar spine or that of a incidental bulging disc eventually prove to be only incidental; in the meantime, their diagnosis and ineffective treatment consume tremendous fiscal, emotional, and temporal resources.

A common example of this is seen in the constellation of pain in the back and lower extremity coupled with weakness of a number of muscles that happen to share the L5 nerve root as the source of their innervation. Travell and Simons have given the moniker "failed laminectomy syndrome" to the practice of surgical intervention for the constellation of back pain with lower extremity referral that is also associated with a positive Trendelenburg test due to pelvic stabilizer muscle weakness arising from MTrPs in the glutei muscles and the pain pattern produced by these MTrPs and stress on overworked posterior sacroiliac ligaments. Missing such a biomechanical cause can lead to unnecessary surgery while also magnifying the risk-to-benefit ratio of that procedure, which is, in fact, indicated in a small percentage of neurological cases with pathology.

Another true neurological finding such as sciatica secondary to Chuck sacral shear somatic dysfunction could easily have been present and would have further complicated the case presentation. Pelvic shears often disrupt muscle balance both related to their pelvic attachments and to the body's compensation for these disruptive somatic dysfunctions. Piriformis hypertonicity is commonly with sacral shears because of its sacral attachments. Such piriformis dysfunction can manifest with posterior pelvis and thigh pain, rarely moving below the knee, secondary to MTrPs or mechanical pressure upon—or even entrapment of—a portion of the sciatic nerve. In the 11% (Caucasian) to 33% (Asian) individuals with the anatomic variation in which the peroneal portion of the sciatic nerve passes through the body of the muscle, weakness of ankle dorsiflexion might be seen due to entrapment. Counterstrain or even procaine injection of the piriformis muscle may provide temporary relief from sciatica, referred pain, or even a mild footdrop, but will recur until the pelvic shear is corrected. One of the authors (MLK) has seen multiple injections and even transaction of the piriformis muscle in attempts to employ the neurological model where final resolution was only obtained using the postural/biomechanical approach.

Lastly, it was interesting in Chuck case to note that his irritable bowel symptoms resolved with the correction of the somatic dysfunctions associated with his traumatic and compensatory somatic dysfunctions. Patients like Chuck will often withhold information that they do not feel is relevant to their chronic pain only to remark about the coincidence of symptom resolution. This common occurrence might be explained through the interaction between somatic dysfunction and the autonomic nervous system. In applying this model to Chuck case, sacral or innominate shears and nociception from the piriformis might all be expected to increase sacral afferent load; overlapping with parasympathetic innervation to the left half of his colon. Unleveling of the sacral base in sacral shear cases typically leads to compensatory scoliotic curves often with a compensatory postural crossover at the thoracolumbar junction, segmental facilitation affecting the sympathetic innervation of the colon. Irritable bowel syndrome is considered as a functional manifestation of dysautonomia or autonomic imbalance between the parasympathetic and the sympathetic systems—leading to alternating diarrhea and constipation. This is further magnified by segmental facilitation that acts like a "neurological lens" for both biopsychosocial model stressors and increased nociceptive afferent load from biomechanical pain generators.

This case may have benefited from the palpation of collateral ganglia and Chapman's points associated with the area of the postural crossover (T11-L2). Such a rapid screening examination could have revealed tissue texture changes and tenderness consistent with colon dysfunction; this is empirically noted in perhaps 80% of irritable bowel cases. After a careful history, such additional somatic clues discovered during the osteopathic structural examination and interpreted through an application of the neurological/autonomic model often prompts the DO to ask additional and more pointed questions. While in Chuck case, the condition appeared to be somatovisceral in nature, but one of the authors (MLK) has seen frequent instances where somatic dysfunction, even in the piriformis, has been perpetuated by visceral pathology through a viscerosomatic reflex.

The neuroendocrine/immune connection is another important component of the neurological model. Stress from pain, inability to accomplish desired tasks, marital discord, and depression all are capable of creating effects beyond central nervous system facilitation, in fact. The hypothalamic-pituitary adrenal axis is affected by the chronic pain state. The resultant increases in cortisol influence interleukin and other components of the immune system. This may impact overall health. Seeman and McEwan have described these relations in terms of allostatic load (61).

Behavioral Model

Over 80% of all physician visits are for complaints of pain. Pain patients are five times more likely to utilize health care services (54–56). Chuck, a 45-year-old farm hand, with chronic LBP represents what is recognized today as the major cause of absenteeism and disability in every industrialized society (59). Like Chuck, those who develop chronic pain will use more than 80% of all health care dollars for back pain.

The behavioral model of chronic pain emphasizes pain as a multidimensional (i.e., mind, body, spirit) phenomenon expressed as interactions among somatosensory inputs, cognitive and behavioral processes, emotions, and various adaptive/ maladaptive coping strategies (57, 58). Chronic pain is punctuated by high incidence, high relapse, and low rate of recovery (Kuchera M.).

Osteopathic physicians treating chronic back pain often encounter returning symptoms. Sometimes, these patients are thought to be exaggerating, "lazy," or malingering when they fail to make expected progress following initial treatments (27) (28). Patients like Chuck who has had pain for 3 years are particularly frustrating to health care providers trying to identify pain generators, somatic dysfunction, and a return to optimal function and health.

"Secondary gain," "malingering," "psychogenic pain," "lazy," "nonorganic," etc. concepts are often invoked as possible explanations for relapse particularly when it is clear that the pain is now adding attention, possible injury compensation, avoidance of work, decreased physical activity/responsibility (16–19).

When all the psychosocial factors are examined, secondary gains are rare (20–22) and the secondary costs (20) are great. In Chuck's case, loss of job, probable financial instability, and the family and physician questioning his intent create tremendous chronic stress affecting immune, neurologic, endocrine, and musculoskeletal systems. Couple this with shame or guilt for not being able to work and not living up to family expectations, perhaps anger for not being believed, and the sheer burden of persistent nociception, and it is clear that secondary losses outweigh any value added by pain. Given any chance of hope, Chuck, like most chronic pain patients, will strive to regain health and function. The art of managing the doctor/patient relationship is essential to success in this case.

Negative attitudes and beliefs by the family physician toward Chuck can greatly expand fear of pain and avoidance of movement and activity (9–12). Osteopathic practitioners know motion is the basic function of life (ECOP). There is strong evidence for chronic back pain that staying active, continuing normal activities, and returning to work as soon as possible leads to faster recovery and lowers rates of disability. In fact, a belief by the physician that there is psychogenic pain ("lazy" or "malingering") leads to no practical diagnosis, is dualistic (i.e., mind vs. body) and counterproductive. Counterproductive means we have challenged Chuck integrity and truthfulness (1,2); contributed to family disruption (7); set the stage for social isolation and withdrawal (13) and; encouraged hypervigilance, negative thinking, and fear (3,4) resulting in avoidance of activity and movement (5,6) as seen in this case. Depression would be the likely result.

CASE CONTINUED

OMT given to the patient consisted of applying the springing, direct method articular technique to the right sacral shear, counterstrain to the iliacus and piriformis tender points, and indirect balanced ligamentous tension to the thoracolumbar and sacral regions. Fascial patterns were treated with high-velocity low-amplitude techniques aimed toward symmetry, and abdominal and pelvic diaphragms were treated with indirect and direct myofascial release, respectively.

Post-OMT iliac crest heights and flexion measurements were normal. The patient left with instructions to drink lots of fluid, switch to acetaminophen as needed, avoid jumping or lifting until his next visit, and return in 1 week for follow-up examination.

At 1-week follow-up, the patient noted that both his acute and nagging pains had been relieved for nearly 4 days, but mild nagging pain had since recurred. A recurrence of sacral shear (approximately 40% of original) and piriformis muscle dysfunction were also noted and re-treated with OMT. Two weeks later, the patient returned with no symptoms and no recurrence of pain. He also noted in passing that what had been diagnosed as irritable bowel syndrome had "coincidentally" disappeared. He was instructed to make an appointment for 1 month later, but to cancel the appointment if he remained symptom-free. He phoned 1 month later, reporting that he was without pain and able to function normally at home.

FOLLOW-UP

Depression must be considered a comorbid condition if Chuck's pain returns, without appreciable presence of somatic dysfunction or reinjury, and in association with continued tension in his marriage, sadness, fear of movement; or failure to return to work. In this case, the osteopathic physician must reassure Chuck and his wife that depression is common and it is normal to feel depressed under the stress of chronic pain and all the trouble it causes. The old saying, "Pain sets in a still joint and depression sets in a still person" applies here.

Remember, a patient's depression does not invalidate somatic dysfunction, pain, or suffering, nor does it imply the pain is "not real," or that being depressed is a personal weakness. Concepts such as sensitization, neuroplasticity, neuromodulation, kindling, wind-up, supersystem, dysregulation, etc. provide cogent hypothesis to explain the clinical spectrum of chronic LBP.

The simple message to Chuck is, "I believe you…I know that you have pain…the pain is real. The pain occurs in your body and for that we will do …, etc." "You also have a reaction to the pain that has affected your function, family and quality of life. For that we will do…, etc."

CHRONIC PAIN CAN REQUIRE CHRONIC CARE

Expect relapse. Effectively managing the biopsychosocial component (25–28) for Chuck and his spouse requires the following:

- Establishing trust and rapport. Address fears. Rule out malingering and communicate this clearly to the patient and family. Define pain generators, mechanisms, and rationale for targeted individualized treatment
- Expect something back. Expect compliance in treatment and recognize specific goals and endpoints to treatment
- Provide logistic and psychosocial support. Advocate, document, and reinforce Chuck pain self-management strategies and active problem-solving efforts
- Confront secondary gain. Lay out clearly the cost to benefit to risk of secondary gain. Dispel illusions. "No 'pot of gold' at the end of a disabling rainbow…Cut your losses and live a meaningful life in spite of pain, if necessary"
- Ignore "exaggeration" and "pain talk" without being judgmental or condescending. Reinforce positive, ignore negative.
- Set goals of decreasing pain, restoring a functional role in the family and return to normal work activities as soon as possible.
- If relapse, discuss and address patient's fears, gather more biopsychosocial information, and recommit to self-management goals of pain control (i.e., not cure) and functional improvement (i.e., not 100% recovery)
- Educate the family. Chuck family also needs education and support to help him and the treatment team achieve specific goals, rather than being an unintended obstacle to rehabilitation. Chuck spouse may be depressed and need treatment. Routinely evaluate the family every few visits and actively engage them in planning treatment. Therapy groups for patients and spouses have also proven very helpful in reducing depression and interpersonal sensitivity

SUMMARY

When osteopathic models are actively integrated and applied to create a treatment plan for a patient with chronic pain, the result is a personalized, effective care plan typically combining nonpharmacological treatment strategies with appropriate types and levels of pharmacotherapy. Placing the patient at the center of the program and including patient education in a comprehensive treatment plan helps to improve quality of life and to break the vicious cycle resulting from pathophysiological mechanisms of persistent pain.

REFERENCES

1. Kuchera ML. Applying osteopathic principles for treatment of patients with chronic pain. *J Am Osteopath Assoc* 107(11 suppl 6):ES28–ES38
2. Waddell G. *The Back Pain Revolution*. 2nd Ed. London, UK: Churchill Livingstone, 2004.
3. Vlaeyen JWS, de Jong J, Geilen M, et al. The treatment of fear of movement/(re)injury in chronic low back pain: further evidence on the effectiveness of exposure in vivo. *Clin J Pain* 2002;18:251–261.
4. Asmundson GJG, Vlaeyen JWS, Crombez G. Understanding and Treating Fear of Pain. Oxford, UK: Oxford University Press, 2004.
5. Geisser ME, Hang AJ, Theisen ME. Activity avoidance and function in persons with chronic back pain. *J Occup Rehab* 2000;10:215–227.
6. Goubert L, Crombez G, vanDamme S, et al. Confirmatory factor analysis of the Tampa Scale for Kinesiophobia: invariant two-factor model across low back pain patients and fibromyalgia patients. *Clin J Pain* 2004;20:103–110.
7. Gallagher RM. The complex relationship between pain and depression. In: Arnoff GM, Giamberardino M, et al., eds. *Current Review of Pain*. Vol 3, No 1. World Institute of Pain, 1991:24–41.
8. Linton SJ, Vlaeyen JW, Ostelo RW. The back pain beliefs of health care providers: are we fear-avoidant? *J Occup Rehabil* 2002;12:223–232.
9. Rainville J, Bagnall D, Phalan L. Health care providers' attitudes and beliefs about functional impairments and chronic back pain. *Clin J Pain* 1995;11:287–295.
10. Houben RM, Ostelo RW, Vlaeyen JW, et al. Health care providers' orientations towards common low back pain predict perceived harmfulness of physical activities and recommendation regarding return to normal activity. *Eur J Pain* 2005;9:173–183.
11. Coudeyre E, Rannou F, Baron G, et al. General practitioners' fear-avoidance beliefs influence their management of patients with low back pain. *Pain* 2006;124:330–337.
12. Bishop A, Foster NE, Thomas E, et al. How does the self-reported clinical management of patients with low back pain relate to the attitudes and beliefs of health practitioners? A survey of UK general practitioners and physiotherapists. *Pain* 2007;135:187–195.
13. Craig KD, Prkachin KM. Social modeling influences on sensory decision theory and psychophysiological indexes of pain. *J Person Social Psychol* 1978;36:805–815.
14. Elliott AM, Smith BH, Hannaford PC, et al. The course of chronic pain in the community: results of a 4-year follow-up study. *Pain* 2002;99 (1–2):299–307.
15. Stanton DF, Dutes J-C. Chronic pain and the chronic pain syndrome: the usefulness of manipulation and behavioral interventions. *Phys Med Rehab Clin N Am* 1996;7:863–875.
16. Fishbain DA, Rosomoff HL, Cutler RB, et al. Secondary gain concept: a review of the scientific evidence. *Clin J Pain Mar* 1995;11(1):6–21.
17. Dersh J, Polatin PB, Leeman G, et al. The management of secondary gain and loss in medicolegal settings: strengths and weaknesses *J Occup Rehabil* 2004;14(4):267–279.
18. von Egmond JJ. The multiple meanings of secondary gain. *Am J Psychoanal* 2003;63(2):137–147.
19. Gatchel RJ, Adams L, Polatin PB, et al. Secondary loss and pain-associated disability: theoretical overview and treatment implications. *J Occup Rehabil* 2002;12(2):99–110.
20. Fishbain DA. Secondary gain concept: definition problems and its abuse in medical practice. *Am Pain Soc J* 1994;3(4):264–273.
21. Leeman G, Polatin PB, Gatchel RJ, et al. Managing secondary gain in patients with pain-associated disability: a clinical perspective. *J Workers Compens* 2000;9(4):25–43.
22. Ferrari R, Kwan O. The no-fault flavor of disability syndromes. *Med Hypotheses* 2001;56(1):77–84.
23. Coleman MT, Newton KS. Supporting self-management in patients with chronic illness. *Am Fam Physician* 2005;72:1503–1510.
24. Leeman G, Polatin P, Gatchel R, et al. Managing secondary gain in patients with pain-associated disability: a clinical perspective. *J Workers Compens* 2000;9:25–44.
25. Mayer TG, Gatchel RJ. *Functional Restoration for Spinal disorders: The Sports Medicine Approach*. Philadelphia, PA: Lea & Febiger, 1988.
26. Rogers R. *Clinical Assessment of Malingering and Deception*. 2nd Ed. New York, NY: Guilford Press, 1997.
27. Aronoff GM, Livengood JM. Pain: psychiatric aspects of impairment and disability. *Curr Pain Headache Rep* 2003;7(2):105–115.
28. Ensalada LH. The importance of illness behavior in disability management. *Occup Med* 2000;15(4):739–754, iv.
29. Wells KB, et al. *Am J Psychiatry* 1988;145:976–981.
30. Doan BD, Wadden NP. *Pain* 1989;36:75–84.
31. Dworkin RH, et al. *Pain* 1986;24:343–353.
32. Haythornthwaite J, et al. *Pain* 1991;46:177–184.
33. Gallagher RM, et al. *Pain* 1989;39:55–68.
34. Van Houdenhove B, Onghena P. In: Robertson MM, Datona CLE, eds. *Depression and Physical Illness*. Chichester, UK: Wiley 1997, pp. 465–497.
35. Long DM. In: Dubner R, et al. eds. *Proceedings of the Vth World Congress on Pain*. Amsterdam, The Netherlands: Elsevier, 1088:244–247.
36. France RD, et al. *Pain* 1987;28:39–44.
37. von Knorring L. In: Dubner R, et al., eds. *Proceedings of the vth World Congress on Pain*. Amsterdam, The Netherlands: Elsevier, 1988:276–285.
38. France RDR, Krishnan KRR. *Pain* 1985;21:49–55.

39. Worz PD. Pain in depression—depression in Pain. Int Assoc. for the Study of Pain. *Pain Clin Update* 2003;XI(5):1–4.
40. Rudy T, et al. *Pain* 1988;35:129–140.
41. Fishbain DA, et al. *Clin J Pain* 1997;13:116–137.
42. Leino P, Magni M. *Pain* 1993;53:89–94.
43. Von Korff M, et al. *Pain* 1993;55:251–258.
44. Von Korff M, et al. *Pain* 1988;32:173–183.
45. Sullivan MJ, Thorn B, Haythornthwaite JA, et al. Theoretical perspectives on the relation between catastrophizing and pain. *Clin J Pain* 2001;17: 52–64.
46. Jensen MP, Turner JA, Romano JM, et al. Coping with chronic pain: a critical review of the literature. *Pain* 1991;47:249–283.
47. Wells KB, et al. *Am J Psychiatry* 1988; 145:976–981.
48. Doan B, Wadden NP. *Pain* 1989;36:75–84
49. Dworkin RH, et al. *Pain* 1986;24:343–353.
50. Haythornthwaite J, et al. *Pain* 1991; 46:177–184.
51. Gallagher RM, et al. *Pain* 1989;39:55–68.
52. Van Houdenhove B, Onghena P. In: Robertson MM, Katona CLE. eds. *Depression and Physical Illness*. Chichester, UK: Wiley, 1997:465–497.
53. Long DM. In: Dubner R, et al. eds. *Proceedings of the Vth World congress on Pain*. Amsterdam, The Netherlands: Elsevier, 1988:244–247.
54. Woodwell DA. National Ambulatory Medical survey: 1998 Summary Advanced Data from Vital and Health Statistics No. 315. National Center for Health Statistics. Hyattsville, MO, 2000.
55. Kerns RD, Otis J, Rosenberg R, et al. Veterans' reports of pain and associations with ratings of health, health-risk behaviors, affective distress, and use of the healthcare system. *J Rehabil Res Dev* 2003;40(5):371–379.
56. Becker N, Bondegaard-Thompson A, Olsen AK, et al. Pain epidemiology and health related quality of life in chronic non-malignant pain patients referred to a Danish multidisciplinary pain center. *Pain* 1997;73(3):339–400.
57. Gatchel RJ. *Clinical Essentials of Pain Management*. Washington, DC: American Psychological Association, 2005.
58. Turk DC, Monarch ES. Biopsychosocial perspective on chronic pain. In: Turk DC, Gatchel RJ, eds. *Psychological Approaches to Pain Management: A Practitioners Handbook*. 2nd Ed. New York, NY: Guilford, 2002.
59. Waddell G. *The Back Pain Revolution*. London, UK: Churchill Livingstone, 1998.
60. Lacey-Cannella DJ, Lobell M, Glass P, et al. Factors associated with depressed mood in chronic pain patients: the role of interpersonal coping skills. *J Pain* 2007;8(3):256–262.
61. Seeman TE, Singer BH, Rowe JW, et al. Price of adaptation-allosteric load and its health consequences. *Arch Intern Med* 1997;157:2259–2268.

57

Dizziness

HARRIET H. SHAW AND MICHAEL B. SHAW

KEY CONCEPTS

- Balance depends on the intricate interaction of **sensory input** (vestibular, visual, and proprioceptive), **central processing** (vestibular nuclear complex and cerebellum), and **motor response** (eyes and postural muscles).
- Disturbance in the cervical proprioceptive input to the vestibular nuclear complex and cerebellum is suggested as a cause for dizziness without hearing loss (cervicogenic vertigo), following neck injury.
- Benign paroxysmal positional vertigo, a common and well-described form of vertigo, is most effectively treated with particle repositioning maneuvers, aimed at the return of displaced otoconia to the vestibule.
- Looking for the root cause is paramount, since dizziness is a symptom that can be associated with a multitude of conditions and diseases.
- Vestibular sedating drugs such as meclinzine and diazepam impair the process of central compensation by decreasing sensory input. These drugs should be avoided in most cases of dizziness, or limited to a short course.
- Because of its effect on proprioceptive input and its ability to help patients stay more active, osteopathic manipulative treatment has an important role in the treatment of many forms of dizziness.

CASE VIGNETTE

CC:

HH is a 72-year-old male who presents to an outpatient clinic complaining of dizziness.

HPI:

The patient reports a sensation of whirling and unsteadiness, which occurs daily, lasting several seconds to 2 hours. It began 1 month ago shortly following a motor vehicle accident in which he was driving, stopped at a red light, and struck from behind by a car going 35 miles/h. Even though he was wearing a seat belt, he experienced rapid flexion and extension of his neck, with subsequent neck pain that was diagnosed as cervical strain. Head and neck movement can bring on or aggravate the dizziness.

Current Medications:

Chlorothiazide 500 mg daily for control of hypertension; ibuprofen 200 mg b.i.d. to t.i.d. when needed for joint pain and stiffness.

Allergies:

None known to medications, inhalants, or food.

Past Medical/Surgical History:

The patient had right medial menisectomy 20 years ago. Currently, he has Type II diabetes controlled with diet and exercise, mild osteoarthritis of the knees, and hypertension controlled with medication, diet, and exercise.

Environmental and Social History:

The patient denies smoking, admits to drinking four to five beers a week, and denies use of recreational drugs. He is a retired engineer, married with grown children.

Family History:

Two younger siblings are living with no apparent health problems. Mother had hypertension and died at age 92 of a myocardial infarction. Father died of colon cancer at age 80. There is no family history of vertigo or neurologic diseases.

Review of Systems:

Eyes—The patient's vision is corrected with glasses. He reports no blurred vision, double vision, or eye pain. ENT—He has dizziness as noted in chief complaint, but denies hearing loss, tinnitus, earaches, sore throat, rhinorrhea, and epistaxis. Cardiovascular—The patient was diagnosed with hypertension 5 years ago. He denies chest pain, fainting, shortness of breath, irregular heartbeats, and palpitations; reports no extremity edema. Respiratory—He denies difficulty breathing, wheezing, and cough. Gastrointestinal—He also denies nausea and vomiting, abdominal pain, diarrhea, and constipation. The patient had a normal colonoscopy 1 year ago. Genitourinary—The patient has no complaint of dysuria, hesitancy, or frequency. His last prostate exam, 6 months ago, revealed mild hypertrophy with no masses. Musculoskeletal—The patient complains of neck pain and stiffness worse on the right side in the upper neck. Ibuprofen offers some relief. He has bilateral knee pain with prolonged standing, also helped by ibuprofen. He denies muscle weakness. Neurological—The patient has vertigo as noted, but denies tremors, seizures, headaches, numbness, or tingling in the extremities. He has had no difficulty with gait other than the unsteadiness associated with his dizziness. He denies memory loss, difficulty with speech or coordination. Psychological—The patient denies anxiety, unwarranted sense of panic or depression. He reports no disturbance of sleep. Endocrine—He denies fatigue, skin and hair changes, and intolerance to heat or cold. Hematologic/lymphatic—He reports no abnormal swelling, bruising or bleeding; denies fatigue and feeling faint.

Vital Signs:

Temperature, 98.6°F; pulse, 74; respirations, 14/min; BP, 130/74 with no significant change from supine to upright; height, 6'1"; weight, 204 lb.

Physical Exam:

The patient is well nourished, appearing stated age, and is alert and communicative. He walks with a normal gait.

Head:

Head is normocephalic without signs of trauma. Pupils are equal and reactive to light and accommodation; conjunctiva is clear. Fundoscopic exam is normal. With the patient looking straight ahead (seated on a swivel stool), nystagmus is noted during rotation of the body.

ENT:

ENT exam is within normal limits. Mild, high frequency, bilateral hearing loss, appropriate to patient age, is identified. There are no bruits ausculted over the carotids and no lymphadenopathy or masses are noted in the neck.

Heart:

Heart has a regular rate and rhythm with no murmurs ausculted.

Lungs:

Lungs are clear to auscultation.

Abdomen:

Bowel sounds are heard in all four quadrants and the abdomen is soft and nontender with no masses palpated. Liver edge is not palpated or percussed below the costal margin.

Neurologic:

Neurologic exam reveals cranial nerves II to XII to be intact, deep tendon reflexes to be equally responsive bilaterally in upper and lower extremities. No atrophy, spasticity, clonus or tremors are noted. The patient is able to perform finger-to-nose, heel-to-shin, and Rhomberg tests. Sensation and two-point discrimination are intact.

Musculoskeletal/Structural:

Findings include tenderness and hypertonicity in the suboccipital area and right upper cervical muscles; left temporal internally rotated, right sphenobasilar side-bending rotation, OA is flexed sidebent left and rotated right, C3 is flexed sidebent and rotated to the left, the right scapula is superior when compared with the left, there is tenderness at the insertion of the right levator scapula, the lumbar paraspinal muscles are hypertonic on the right, and the talus is biomechanically anterior to the tibia on the right.

DISCUSSION

Dizziness is used by patients to describe a variety of symptoms including lightheadedness, feeling faint, weak or unsteady, as well as the sensation that the room is spinning. Giddiness is described as the feeling that one's head in spinning. Vertigo is the sensation of movement, usually spinning, rotating, or whirling, associated with dysfunction in the vestibular system. Disequilibrium, imbalance or unsteadiness, only occurs when walking or standing and may or may not be accompanied by vertigo.

The complaint of dizziness is a common one in the primary care and emergency department settings. It may be due to disease in almost any of the body systems and often presents a perplexing challenge for diagnosis and treatment. Severe dizziness can be disabling, but seldom represents a life-threatening condition. Accurate history and physical will often differentiate dizziness-like symptoms that are related to anemia, cardiac irregularities, orthostatic hypotension, transient ischemic attacks, and stroke. The association with vascular headaches may identify dizziness as a component of migraine. Neurologic signs could suggest a central nervous system lesion and require imagining for further diagnosis. Dizziness is identified in the *Physicians' Desk Reference* as a side effect to numerous prescription drugs, so an accurate drug history in relation to the patient's symptoms may indicate a pharmacologic cause. Lightheadedness, giddiness, faintness can be associated with hyperventilation, anxiety, and panic disorder, making a history of phobias, apprehension, worry, and insomnia helpful in diagnosis.

The assessment of vertigo depends on an understanding of the body's systems of balance. Dysfunction in any of the components can cause a patient to complain of dizziness or vertigo. Certain conditions or dysfunctions have warranted specific names and are associated with distinct presentations. Of these, labyrinthitis, BPPV, Meniere disease, acoustic neuroma, and cervicogenic vertigo will be discussed. Familiarity with the pertinent anatomy and physiology is important in interpreting any presentation of dizziness.

RELEVANT FUNCTIONAL ANATOMY AND PHYSIOLOGY

Balance is a whole-body experience that depends on the interaction of and processing of information from multiple sources. There are three primary sensory inputs to the balance system—vestibular (inner ear), visual, and proprioceptive. Central processing of balance-related information takes place in the vestibular nuclear complex and cerebellum. Motor output, primarily to the eyes and postural muscle, helps the body react to balance issues. (Fig. 57.1)

Vestibular System

The vestibular system consists of the bony and membranous labyrinth, including its blood and nerve supply. The complex, which is housed in the temporal bones bilaterally, consists of the cochlea (responsible for hearing), the semicircular canals, and a central chamber or vestibule. (Fig. 57.2) The bony portion contains perilymphatic fluid (somewhat like cerebral spinal fluid), in which the membranous structures are suspended. The membranous labyrinth contains endolymphatic fluid (similar to intracellular fluid) and specialized sensory hair cells, responsible for the neural firing of the labyrinth. (Fig. 57.3)

The semicircular canals are three in number, each having a widened end called the "ampulla." The sensory hair cells are located in the ampullae and are sensitive to rotational movement of the head. The semicircular canals are oriented perpendicular to each other, similar to the floor and two adjacent walls of a rectangular room. Pairing of the bilateral structures, in mirror image fashion, allows detection of motion in any direction. Their arrangement corresponds closely to the pulling directions of the extraocular muscles. Information from the semicircular canals helps the eyes remain still in space as the head moves, making clear vision possible.

Figure 57-1 Sensorimotor integration for balance—sensory input, central processing, and motor output.

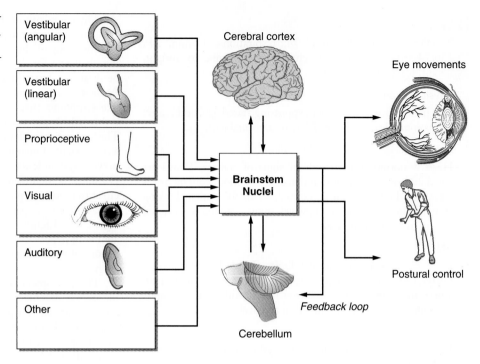

Figure 57-2 Vestibular complex housed in temporal bones.

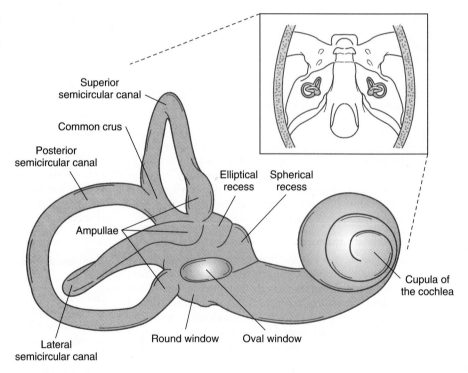

The utricle and saccule are sensory organs of the membranous labyrinth. They are located in the vestibule and contain calcium carbonate crystals called otoconia, in addition to sensory hair cells. Their arrangement (the saccule is vertical while the utricle is horizontal) along with the mass of the otoconia make these otolithic organs sensitive to gravity and linear acceleration (Fig. 57.4).

Afferent signals from the labyrinth are carried by the vestibular nerve, which courses along with the cochlear nerve, facial nerve, and labyrinthine artery, through the internal auditory canal of the petrous portion of the temporal bone. The vestibular nerve enters the brain stem at the pontomedullary junction, and its information goes to the cerebellum and vestibular nuclear complex.

Arterial blood supply to the labyrinth is from the vertebral basilar system. The labyrinthine artery usually is a branch of the anterior inferior cerebellar artery, but may be a direct branch from the basilar. Its branches supply the cochlea, semicircular canals, utricle, saccule, ampulla, and vestibular nerve. There is no collateral circulation, making the labyrinth very susceptible to ischemia and disruption of blood flow.

Visual and Proprioceptive Systems

Visual information is processed along with that from the vestibular system and all the proprioceptors of the body to determine position

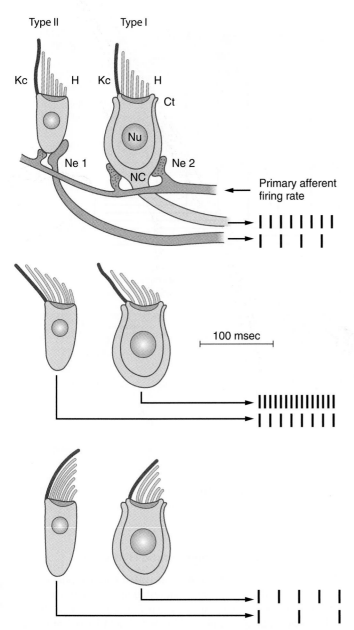

Figure 57-3 Specialized, sensory hair cells of the membranous labyrinth are deflected during head movement.

brain stem and cerebellum depends on symmetrical, accurate, and consistent information from its sensory sources. It can, however, compensate for some missing information by using information from the other sources. Generally, compensation is possible if two of the three sources are functioning properly, even though this may require some adaptation over time.

Vestibuloocular Reflex

Using information from the semicircular canals and otoliths (saccule and utricle), the vestibuloocular reflex (VOR) provides clear vision during head motion. Motor impulses to the extraocular eye muscles generate eye movement compensatory to head movement.

Vestibulospinal Reflex

Functioning to stabilize the body and prevent falling, the vestibulospinal reflex (VSR) is more complex than the VOR. Motor impulses are sent to skeletal muscles, in response to information reaching the vestibular nuclear complex and cerebellum. This information is then used to carry out strategies to maintain upright posture. These may include a number of complex interactions such as stepping forward, flexing the ankles, grabbing a stable object.

Vestibulocollic Reflex

Vestibulocollic reflex (VCR) acts to stabilize the neck in response to vestibular output. This reflex could explain the neck pain sometimes experienced with diseases of the inner ear—viscerosomatic reflex.

Cervico-ocular Reflex

Stimuli from neck ligaments, muscles, and joints cause a responsive movement of the eyes. This cervico-ocular reflex (COR) interacts with the VOR. Normally, the gain of the COR is very low.

Differential Diagnosis

Cervicogenic Vertigo

Many people have reported symptoms of dizziness, unsteadiness, and imbalance following neck injury, especially with whiplash-associated disorder (WAD). The symptoms are concurrent with neck pain and stiffness, and made worse by neck movement. There is no accompanying hearing loss or tinnitus, but nausea may occur. Disturbance in the cervical proprioceptive input to the vestibular nuclear complex and cerebellum has been suggested as the probable cause. De Jong and De Jong (1) produced ataxia and nystagmus by injection of local anesthetic into the neck. Studies based on posturography data showed patients with cervicobrachial pain had poorer postural control than normal subjects (2). Prolonged contraction of the posterior cervical muscles, bilaterally, can alter balance control (3). Montfoort et al. (4) observed increased COR gain in patients with WAD, seemingly linked to reduced neck mobility, and offering a possible explanation for the vertigo reported by these patients.

Various studies have shown different types of manual manipulation to be successful in improving symptoms of dizziness (5–7). In addition, numerous case reports over the years in the osteopathic literature discuss the success osteopathic manipulation in treating dizziness and vertigo. Still, controversy remains as to whether cervicogenic vertigo is a distinct diagnosis. Brandt and Bronstein (9)

in space. Proprioceptive input from postural muscles, related fascia, joints, and ligaments is all interpreted, but information from the ankles and neck is especially important in balance control.

Central Processing

The vestibular nuclear complex (four major and seven minor nuclei) in the pons and medulla is the primary processor of the information from the above sources. It provides fast and direct connection between incoming information and motor output response. The cerebellum is the adaptive processor, acting as a modulator and monitor. Fine tuning and adjustments to the system are done in the cerebellum. Regulation of the various reflexes responsible for balance occurs due to interaction between the vestibular nuclear complex and the cerebellum. The balance function of the

Figure 57-4 Otolithic membrane in the utricle and saccule is embedded with calcium carbonate crystals. Linear acceleration or change with respect to gravity causes the membrane to shift and trigger underlying hair cells.

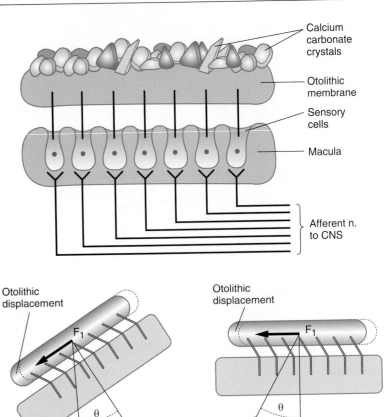

in their summary article on cervical vertigo note that vertigo can be accompanied by cervical pain, associated with head injury, whiplash injury or cervical spinal disease, and be dramatically improved with physiotherapy. Still the mechanism is yet to be proved. They conclude, "If cervical vertigo exists, appropriate management is the same as that for the cervical pain syndrome and that management should not be denied any patient."

Acute Labyrinthitis

Inflammation or infection of the inner ear may occur alone or in combination with a viral, or less commonly, a bacterial infection. In acute labyrinthitis, the patient complains of sudden onset of severe vertigo. It is accompanied by hearing loss, tinnitus, nausea, and vomiting. Nystagmus is present. The acute episode lasts 24 to 48 hours. The condition slowly resolves with several days of disequilibrium and motion-induced vertigo, followed by slow improvement over several weeks.

Benign Paroxysmal Positional Vertigo

Thought to be caused by debris in the endolymph of the posterior semicircular canal, BPPV presents with episodic vertigo brought on by changes in head position. Commonly, patients report rolling over in bed or rapid neck extension precipitates symptoms. The episodes last 30 seconds to 2 minutes, and will subside even if the offending position is maintained. There is no associated hearing loss or tinnitus, but rotatory nystagmus accompanies the vertigo. Performing the Dix-Hallpike positioning test—a rapid change from sitting to lying, with head hanging turned toward affected side—brings on vertigo and nystagmus, which then subsides after

holding the position for 10 to 40 seconds. (Fig. 57.5) BPPV is self-limiting and responds to vestibular exercises and particle repositioning maneuver (Fig. 57.6).

Meniere Disease (Endolymphatic Hydrops)

A disorder of the inner ear with increased endolymphatic pressure, Meniere disease can cause devastating vestibular symptoms and hearing loss. Patients initially experience pressure in the ear, reduced hearing, and tinnitus. This is followed by severe vertigo with nausea and vomiting. Severe symptoms can last 30 minutes to 24 hours. Intensity of symptoms diminishes over several days time. Unsteadiness may persist for weeks. Hearing loss and tinnitus may gradually improve, or sensorineural loss may be permanent. As the disease progresses, attacks continue with continuation of hearing loss, but the severity of vertigo may decrease. Although salt restriction and diuretics have been used as treatment, there is no indication of their effectiveness. Betahistin has been used with some effectiveness (10). Other vestibular suppressants should only be used during the acute attack, not on a chronic basis. Many patients require psychological support in coping with the ramifications of the disease.

Acoustic Neuroma (Vestibular Schwannoma)

Schwannoma of the eighth cranial nerve causes unilateral sensorineural hearing loss and tinnitus. Vertigo, when it occurs, is not an early symptom and is usually short lived, replaced by a sense of imbalance or disequilibrium. Suspicion of acoustic neuroma should be followed up with an MRI of the internal auditory canal with gadolinium contrast.

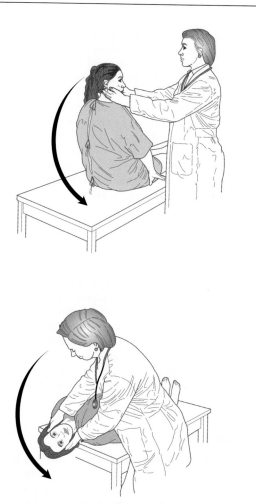

Figure 57-5 Dix-Hallpike maneuver for detecting BPPV.

Osteopathic Patient Management

As dizziness is a symptom that can be associated with a multitude of conditions and diseases, looking for the root cause is paramount. Somatic dysfunction may be present in any of these cases as an associated finding or, as some suggest, a significant etiologic factor. Somatic manifestations of vestibular disease could appear in the cervical area by way of shared neural reflex pathways (VSR, VCR).

Certainly, any identified underlying cause of dizziness needs to be treated. Often, a cause is not identified or available treatment is only symptomatic. Addressing the management from a multifaceted approach is usually the most successful.

Biomechanical Model

Trauma seems to play a role in some types of dizziness. Patients with WAD frequently complain of dizziness (11). Lockhart (12) reported on two cases of Meniere syndrome resulting from multiple traumatic brain injury. Treleaven et al. (13) showed WAD patients with dizziness showed significant error in returning their head to natural posture (joint position error), compared to controls and WAD patients without dizziness.

OMT to normalize proprioceptive input, improve range of motion, promote venous and lymphatic circulation, and balance neurologic reflexes makes sense in the management of patients with balance disorders.

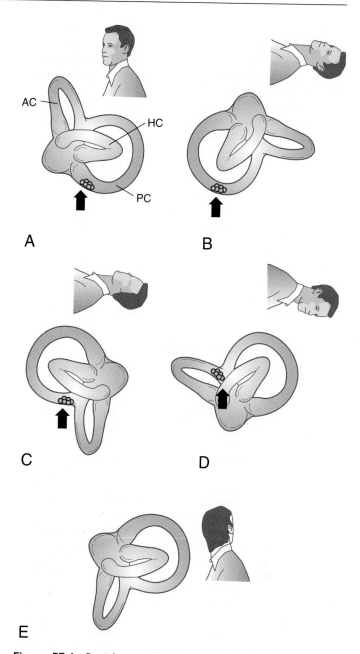

Figure 57-6 Particle repositioning treatment for BPPV may be performed by physician and taught to patients.

Proprioceptors in the neck supply important information to the balance system of the central nervous system. Inappropriate signals due to cervical somatic dysfunction may be responsible for some forms of dizziness or exacerbation of dizziness due to other causes. Recent studies demonstrate decreased range of motion in the cervical spine causes increased activity in the CVR (4) and may partially explain the improvement in dizziness reported with manual manipulation (5–8,14).

Other areas of the body also provide proprioceptive input to help regulate balance and must respond when postural adjustments need to be made. Somatic dysfunction in any of these areas, particularly the feet and ankles, may impact balance and the individual's ability to compensate for imbalance. Range of motion in the extremities is important for balance rehabilitation training. OMT to improve extremity motion can be beneficial in rehabilitation for those patients suffering from dizziness.

Magoun (15) states, "vertigo often follows trauma to the ear or the neck." Considering the location of the paired labyrinth organs on the petrous portions of the temporal bones bilaterally, and the importance of coordinated input from the two sides, dysfunction of the temporal bone may be responsible for disturbance of equilibrium. For those skilled in the cranial approach, gently realigning the temporal bones to their proper orientation and motion will normalize the inner ear mechanisms.

BPPV is a common and well-described form of vertigo, most effectively treated with particle repositioning maneuvers (16). The goal of the maneuvers is the return of displaced otoconia to the vestibule. Vestibular sedating drugs such as meclizine and diazepam are not effective and usually not recommended for these patients. Lower extremity strength, range of motion, and coordination have important roles in the rehabilitation of vertiginous conditions. Good structural diagnosis can help direct appropriate musculoskeletal treatment and home exercises. OMT for somatic dysfunction in the neck, cranium, and extremities can offer relief to many patients suffering from dizziness. For those with cervicogenic vertigo, resolution of involved somatic dysfunction is the treatment of choice.

Respiratory-Circulatory Model

Congestion in the middle and inner ear, while not a major recognized cause of vertigo, is a component to some diseases (e.g., Meniere's) and may be associated with lightheadedness and imbalance. OMT aimed at improving venous and lymphatic circulation from the head and neck may offer symptomatic relief in those cases.

The vestibular system is particularly susceptible to vascular compromise. Awareness of postures and maneuvers that may impede blood flow through the vertebrobasilar system is important in patient education and when applying any type of manipulation. Avoidance of hyperextended positions of the upper cervical spine is recommended. If venous or lymphatic congestion is believed to be involved in the symptomatology, osteopathic techniques that promote venous and lymphatic drainage from the head may offer relief. Diuretics and salt restriction diets have been used with varying success in the treatment of Meniere's in an attempt to decrease the inner ear fluid volume. Although the endolymphatic space of the labyrinth does not directly communicate with the subarachnoid space, fluid movement in the inner ear may be augmented by cranial movement. Cranial treatment to improve cranial bone motion has been used with some success to reduce the symptoms of Meniere disease.

Neurologic Model

When one aspect of the sensory input to the brain stem and cerebellum balance system is absent or dysfunctioning, the brain compensates by using information from the other systems. The more disinformation or lack of information, the more difficult is the compensation process. Rehabilitating patients with vertigo and balance disorders includes retraining the coordination of eye movement with head, neck, and body movements through exercises. Enhancing the intact sensory inputs may entail sharpening proprioceptive input from the neck or extremities through exercises, encouraging activities and OMT. Manipulative techniques contributing to a decrease in afferent load (e.g., counterstrain, indirect myofascial) could help balance the involved neural reflexes. Corrective lens, when needed, can improve the accuracy of sensory input from the eyes. Dural tension around the internal auditory meatus has been suggested to impair proper function of the nerves coursing there (vestibular, cochlear, and facial). Osteopathy in the

cranial field addresses bony relationships and dural tensions in the head, thereby impacting function of the vestibular nerve. Relieving tension in the upper cervical spine and around the jugular foramen (occipitomastoid suture) may reduce symptoms of nausea and vomiting by effecting vagal tone. Medication use must be carefully considered, as vestibular sedatives, such as meclizine, impair the process of central compensation by decreasing the sensory input. If needed to control severe dizziness, these drugs should be limited to a short course (usually two to three doses.) Anticholinergic (e.g., scopolamine) and antidopaminergic (e.g., prochlorperazine) drugs may also offer some relief. Combination therapy can be beneficial when a single drug regimen fails. Again, the sedating effects can be counterproductive to rehabilitation

Metabolic-Energy Model

Postural considerations are especially important in the management of dizziness and balance disorders. Evaluation and treatment of postural imbalance from the standpoint of sacral base unlevelness, muscle tone problems, or postural strains can play an integral part in the resolution of dizziness and unsteadiness.

Drugs with potential for ototoxicity must be considered as a cause of vertigo. A few drugs such as the aminoglycoside antibiotics and some antineoplastic drugs cause irreversible damage. Others such as aspirin, when stopped, will result in resolution of symptoms.

Behavioral Model

Patients with dizziness who succumb to a sedentary life style have much worse outcomes. Encouraging activity, in spite of symptoms, is very important. Persistent vertigo can be very disruptive to a patient's life, and many patients become frustrated, even depressed. Psychological support may be critical. Some antidepressant medications have dizziness as a side effect, so pharmacologic treatment must be carefully monitored. Psychological disorders may also manifest symptoms of dizziness. It is the second most common symptom reported by people with panic disorder.

Discussion

Since dizziness is used to describe a variety of sensations and may result from a variety of problems, approach to a patient complaining of dizziness must start with an in-depth history. Description of the patient's sensation must be specific as to whether it is disorientation, a sense of moving, being off-balance, difficulty walking, impending faint, lightheadedness, motion sickness, panic, trouble focusing, or spinning. History of present illness should include the timing and nature of the first episode and subsequent episodes. What are the frequency and duration of the spells and when was the last spell? Precipitating factors and associated symptoms need to be considered. Other contributory information is found in medication history, allergic history, family history, social history, and review of systems.

Appreciation of the sensorineural integration involved in balance helps in diagnosis and treatment of dizziness. Always consider the three major components in achieving good balance—sensing the environment, central processing of information, and musculoskeletal response. Also consider the three dominant sensory inputs to this system—vestibular (inner ear), visual, somatosensory (joint proprioception). Comprehensive history and understanding of the involved anatomy and physiology will make the evaluation and treatment of patients with dizziness much more satisfying.

Patient Education: Self-treatment of Dizziness

- These exercises can be best done with the help of an assistant
- If on initial attempt of these exercises the response is too severe to continue, the prescribed medication may be used
- Refer to the diagrams below while reading these instructions

Identification of Problem Ear

The first step in the self treatment of dizziness is to identify the side of the poorly functioning ear. This is done as follows:

1. Identify the position on a firm bed where you can lie back without hitting anything.
2. Identify where your shoulders will lie when you lie back in the bed.
3. Place a midsized pillow on the bed where your shoulders will land when you lie back in the bed.
4. Position yourself in the bed as above.
5. Lower yourself with your shoulders contacting the pillow and your head contacting the bed and your head turned to the left.
6. Remain in that position for 2 minutes, and record your feelings.
7. Repeat the above maneuver; however, this time turn your head to the right.
8. Again remain in that position for 2 minutes and record your feelings.
9. Identify the side your head is turned to, which produced the most uncomfortable feelings whether they be dizziness, anxiety, or fear.
10. Record this side that produced the most uncomfortable feelings.

Treatment of the dizziness

1. Sit on the bed positioned as above and with the pillow positioned as above.
2. Turn your head 45 degrees.
   a. If your head turned to the right produced the most uncomfortable feelings, turn to the right in No. 3.
   b. If your head turned to the left produced the most uncomfortable feelings, turn to the left in No. 3.
3. Rapidly lie down in the bed turning your head to the above position, with your shoulders positioned on the pillow and your head touching the bed.
4. Remain in that position for 1 minute.
5. Turn your head 90 degrees toward the opposite side (45 degree angle but to the other side) without raising your head.
6. Remain in that position for 1 minute.
7. Turn your head 90 degrees further in the direction you are presently turned (so you will be looking down at an angle), and move your body as necessary.
8. Hold this position for 1 minute.
9. Sit up in this manner:
   a. keep facing the direction your head was turned
   b. hang feet off the bed
   c. place your chin on your chest throughout the sitting up motion
10. Remain in that sitting position for 1 minute.
11. Do not lie flat for 24 hours. A semirecumbent position is best (recliner position).
12. Assume normal activity after 24 hours.

REFERENCES

1. De Jong P, De Jong M, Cohen B, et al. Ataxia and nystagmus induced by injection of local anesthetic in the neck. *Ann Neurol* 1977;1:240–246.
2. Karlberg M, Persson L, Magnusson M. Impaired postural control in patients with cervicobrachial pain. *Acta Otolaryngol Suppl* 1995;520(2):440–442.
3. Schieppati M, Nardone A, Schmid M. Neck muscle fatigue affects postural control in man. *Neuroscience* 2003;121:277–285.
4. Montfoort I, VanDerGeest J, Slijper H, et al. Adaptation of the cervico- and vestibulo-ocular reflex in whiplash injury patients. *J Neurotrauma* 2008;25(6):687–693.
5. Reid S, Rivett D. Manual therapy treatment of cervicogenic dizziness: a systematic review. *Man Ther* 2005;10(1):4–13.
6. Galm R, Rittmeister M, Schmitt E. Vertigo in patients with cervical spine dysfunction. *Eur Spine J* 1998;7(1):55–58.
7. Malmstrom EM, Karlberg M, Melander A, et al. Cervicogenic dizziness-musculoskeletal findings before and after treatment and long-term outcome. *Disabil Rehabil* 2007;29(15):1193–1205.
8. Heikkila H, Johansson M, Wenngren B. Effects of acupuncture, cervical manipulation and NSAID therapy on dizziness and impaired head repositioning of suspected cervical origin: a pilot study. *Man Ther* 2000;5(3):151–157.
9. Brandt T, Bronstein A. Cervical vertigo. *J Neurol Neurosurg Psychiatry* 2001;71(1):8–12.
10. Meyer E. Treatment of Meniere's disease with betahistin-dimesilate—a double blind, placebo controlled study. *Laryngol Rhinol Otol* 1985;64:269.
11. Spritzer W, Skovron M, Salmi L, et al. Scientific monograph of the Quebec Task Force on Whiplash-Associated Disorders; redefining "whiplash" and its management. *Spine* 1995;20:2S–73S.
12. Lockhart W. Meniere's syndrome resulting from multiple traumatic brain injury: two case studies. *Am Acad Osteopath J* 1999;9(3):21–24.
13. Treleaven J, Jull G, Sterling M. Dizziness and unsteadiness following whiplash injury: characteristic features and relationship with cervical joint position error. *J Rehab Med* 2003;35(1):36–43.
14. Williams N. Prevalence and treatment of dizziness. *Lett Br J Gen Pract* 1998;48(431):1344.
15. Magoun H. The temporal bone: trouble maker in the head. *J Am Osteopath Assoc* 1974;73:825–835.
16. Brooks J, Abidin M. Repositioning maneuver for benign paroxysmal positional vertigo (BPPV). *J Am Osteopath Assoc* 1997;97(5):277–279.

FURTHER READING

Furman JM, Cass SP. *Balance Disorders: A Case-Study Approach*. Philadelphia, PA: F.A. Davis, 1996.
Herdman S. *Vestibular Rehabilitation*. 2nd Ed. Philadelphia, PA: F.A. Davis, 2000.
Goebel JA. *Practical Management of the Dizzy Patient*. Philadelphia, PA: Lippincott Williams & Wilkins, 2001.

58

Child with Ear Pain

KAREN M. STEELE AND MIRIAM V. MILLS

KEY CONCEPTS

- Pediatric ear pain can be caused by diseases and processes both within the ear structure, and referred to the ear from distant structures.
- Structural, environmental, genetic, ethnic, and other factors predispose some children to be "otitis-prone."
- Osteopathic manipulative treatment (OMT) has been shown clinically to be complementary to routine medical care of pediatric ear pain, including acute otitis media.
- Suggested OMT protocols include the treatment of biomechanical, respiratory-circulatory, neurological, biopsychosocial, and metabolic aspects of the pediatric patient.
- The OMT of children differs from that of the adult.

CASE VIGNETTE

DW is a 2-year-old Native American female with a history of three prior ear infections in the last 12 months, who presents with irritability, pulling at her right ear and fever to 102°F for the past day. Her appetite and usual activity level are decreased. She had a mild upper respiratory infection the previous week, which was getting better until these symptoms presented. Her most recent ear infection, which responded to azithromycin, was 2 months prior, and was followed by documented normal tympanograms.

Past Medical History:

Her first ear infection was at 6 months of age, soon after she began attending day care. She has had no other serious illnesses or hospitalizations.

Birth History:

She was delivered via assisted suction extraction to a primigravida mother. She breast fed only for a week, due to poor suck, and required several formula changes during her first few months because of frequent vomiting. Also during her first few months, she had episodes of unexplained irritability lasting up to three hours, usually in the evening, which resolved by four months of age.

Developmental History:

Her development has been appropriate for age. Immunizations are up to date.

Allergies:

She has no known allergies to medications or food.

Social History:

She lives at home with her mother who is single and works at the day care center where the child attends. Mother smokes, but states she doesn't smoke around the child.

Family History:

There are no contributory inherited diseases, except that the mother has a history of frequent ear infections as a child, requiring placement of ventilation tubes.

REVIEW OF SYSTEMS

General:

The child's mother states that "she just hasn't been herself." She is more irritable than usual and having trouble sleeping.

Respiratory:

She has been congested for about a week with alternating stuffy and runny nose. There has been no coughing, wheezing, or blueness about the lips or fingers.

Gastrointestinal:

Her appetite has been decreased since she became congested although she is taking fluids appropriately. There has been no diarrhea.

PHYSICAL EXAMINATION

Vital Signs:

Temperature 102°F, respirations 30, pulse 105

General:

The child is well hydrated but seems in obvious pain.

HEENT:

There is no evidence of tenderness with movement of her pinna or palpation over her jaw or face. Her right tympanic membrane (TM) is dull and inflamed, with a fluid level of yellow pus visualized behind the TM. The left TM is retracted but pearly, and neither TM moves. There is minimal white-yellow nasal drainage, and her throat shows mild redness, but no exudates. Her 2-year molars are erupting. Neck is supple, with mild anterior cervical lymphadenopathy.

Lungs:

Chest is clear to auscultation, and breathing is unlabored.

Heart:

Heart is normal sinus rhythm without murmur or gallop.

Abdomen:

Abdomen is soft and without organomegaly or masses.

Musculoskeletal:

Extremities show no cyanosis, clubbing, or edema, and pulses are normal.

Neurological:

Neurological exam is intact for cranial nerves (CN), strength, reflexes, and sensation.

Osteopathic Structural Examination:

There is compression of the cranial base with right temporal bone internally rotated and compression of the occipitomastoid suture on the right. There is suboccipital muscular tension and the occipitoatlantal joint is extended. The thoracic inlet is rotated right and the abdominal diaphragm is rotated left, with lower ribs held in exhalation. The pelvis shows compression of the right sacroiliac area.

Laboratory

Rapid strep test is negative.

DIFFERENTIAL DIAGNOSIS

The causes of ear pain in children are more numerous than many would imagine. Ear pain can arise from the ear structures themselves (*primary etiology*), including the external, middle, or inner components, or from a nonotogenic origin (*secondary, or referred otalgia*), usually resulting from the complex sensory afferent innervation of the ear, which also provides innervation to a wide variety of other structures, many noncontiguous to the ear. While otitis media is reported to be one of the most common reasons that children visit their physicians (Wetmore, 2007), the actual frequency of this diagnosis as a cause of otalgia may range from as low as 11% (Ijaduola, 1985) to 46% (Ingvarsson, 1982). Secondary causes of otalgia are seen in 22% (Ijaduola) to 44% (Ingvarsson) of children and in as many as 50% of adults (Shah and Blevins, 2003).

Primary Otalgia

Primary otalgia can arise from the external ear (otitis externa or mastoiditis) or middle ear (otitis media). Inner ear disease usually does not result in otalgia, due to the nature of its innervation. (See discussion of neurological model in pediatric ear pain.)

Otitis Externa

External ear pain is usually from one of two causes: otitis externa or a foreign body in the ear. Otitis externa can be subdivided into six distinct subgroups: (1) acute diffuse bacterial (swimmer's ear), (2) acute localized (furunculosis), (3) chronic, (4) eczematous, (5) nectrotizing, and (6) fungal (Bruderly and Bojrab, 1996). All of these causes can give rise to exquisite ear pain, and treatment is based on the underlying cause. The primary cause of swimmer's ear is a rise in the normal acidic pH of the external auditory canal (EAC), which allows for overgrowth of pathogenic bacteria. Furunculosis is usually secondary to trauma of pilosebaceous units in the superior posterior EAC with bacterial overgrowth. Chronic otitis externa is a thickening of the skin of the EAC from chronic low-grade inflammation, leading to narrowing of the EAC with dryness, itching, cracking, and pain of the skin of the EAC. Eczematous otitis externa encompasses those dermatological conditions that predispose the EAC to inflammation. Nectrotizing otitis externa is potentially life threatening, and consists of an invasive bacterial infection of components of the external ear and adjacent structures, usually in an immune-compromised patient. Funtally, fungal otitis externa, which is from a fungal infection of the skin of the external ear, accounts for approximately 10% of otitis externa in the United States.

Foreign bodies in the EAC in children are commonly seen in the primary care clinic and emergency department. Most can be removed under direct visualization and without general anesthesia (Ologe et al., 2007). Impacted cerumen has also been associated with pediatric ear pain. Impacted cerumen may need a few days of softening with an over-the-counter agent prior to in-office removal with a curette. While there is no osteopathic manipulative treatment (OMT) generally indicated in the treatment of otitis externa and foreign bodies in the middle ear, the reader may be interested in a dissertation by Andrew Taylor Still in his *Philosophy of Osteopathy* (1899) regarding the significance of ear wax in diseases of the head and neck. In it, Dr. Still hypothesizes how ear wax production may be influenced by blood flow to the external ear canal, which is regulated by autonomic innervation, and how impairment of blood or lymph flow to and from the canal could be related to underlying somatic dysfunction.

Mastoiditis

Mastoiditis is a rare, but serious, complication of bacterial acute otitis media (AOM). Since the mastoid air space is continuous with the middle ear through the aditus ad antrum mastoideum, infection in the middle ear can spread to the mastoid air cells. Likewise, medical treatment of the AOM generally also treats any infection in the mastoid air space. The incidence of mastoiditis and other intracranial complications of AOM has been approximately 0.24% since the advent of routine antibiotic use in the 1960s. Recently, however, the incidence has been increasing due to emergence of resistant bacterial strains (Wetmore, 2007). Optimum treatment of mastoiditis requires early detection and prompt antimicrobial treatment. Complications of acute mastoidits include periosteitis, acute mastoid osteitis, and intracranial infection.

The addition of OMT in the treatment of mastoiditis should be limited to treatment designed to improve functioning of the lymphatic system, and no direct treatment of the head and neck should be performed until the mastoid infection is under control. Such a treatment could include myofascial release of the thoracic inlet and abdominal diaphragm, and rib raising (respiratory-circulatory model).

Barotrauma

Barotrauma is due to rapidly changing pressures against the TM that cannot be adequately accommodated, leading to ear pain (Bluestone and Klein, 2001; Buchanan et al., 1999). This is most commonly seen in descent when flying in airplanes, when the dysfunctional eustachian tube (ET) is not able to open spontaneously or with yawning or swallowing, to equilibrate the relative negative middle ear pressure. Crying commonly opens the ET, via pull of the tensor veli palatini muscle. Persistent barotitis may result in high negative middle ear pressures and development of effusion. Interestingly, when middle ear effusion (MEE) is present, barotitis is less likely (Bluestone and Klein). Pretreatment before flying with decongestants has been recommended, although some literature indicates its usefulness is limited (Buchanan et al., 1999).

If the parent has been trained in the Galbreath mandibular drainage, doing this procedure during descent when flying in an airplane may assist the child in equilibrating the middle ear pressure, and hence reduce the pain. Treatment of the underlying ET dysfunction is the recommended means of preventing barotitis. Anatomical and functional changes during maturation of the cranial base and ET make barotitis less likely as the child ages. (For a discussion of the rationale for osteopathic treatment to improve ET functioning, please see "The Cranial Base and the Eustachian Tube.").

Otitis Media

Of all of the causes of pain originating from the middle ear, otitis media is by far the most common. AOM is the inflammation or infection of the air-filled middle ear space. It is a significant worldwide problem commonly affecting children between six and 18 months, and is the most frequent reason for childhood illness visits to a physician in the United States (Bluestone and Klein, 2001). The middle ear is an air-filled space that transmits sound vibrations from the TM to the inner ear, where sound is recognized. AOM is usually accompanied by development of fluid (effusion) in the middle ear during the inflammatory process. When the middle ear space is filled with fluid, the ability of the TM to vibrate and transmit sound is impaired. In 70% of children, this fluid persists for 2 weeks after the onset of middle ear infection, and in 40% of children, fluid is still present at 1 month (Bluestone and Klein). Persistent MEE is the sequela of AOM for which there is as yet no widely accepted medical treatment supported by the literature.

The cost of providing care for this prevalent disease is staggering. The annual medical and surgical cost for the treatment of otitis media was estimated to be $5.3 billion in 1998 (Bondy et al., 2000). This estimate did not include social costs, such as lost workdays of caregivers and the costs for speech therapists and learning assistance. A 2001 report in the *Journal of Managed Care Pharmacy* estimated the cost of one episode of AOM to be $483 and the cost for treatment of recurrent AOM including treatment with antibiotics and the eventual insertion of tympanostomy tubes to be $3,683 (Pill, 2005). This cost is borne not only by families of the child, but also society.

Certain children have been described as more "otitis prone." This is thought to be related to age (<3 years old), male gender, family history of ear infections, presence of older siblings or smokers in the home, not being breast fed, and attendance in day care (Bluestone and Klein, 2001; Wetmore, 2007). Children who have their first ear infection before 6 months old tend to have recurrent infections. Racial differences in incidence of otitis may be related to variations in cranial base morphology (see Biomechanical considerations; cranial base). Children in developing countries, children with poor nutrition, and those in lower socioeconomic groups also have more severe and persistent episodes (Lasisi 2007). Pacifier use has been documented to be associated with more episodes of otitis, as well as prone sleep position (Rovers et al., 2008; Sexton, 2008; Tully et al., 1995). The seasonal incidence of otitis follows the increased frequency of upper respiratory infections in general.

The diagnosis and management of uncomplicated AOM in children from two months through 12 years of age was clarified in 2004 by the publication of a Clinical Practice Guideline from the American Academy of Pediatrics (AAP) and the American Academy of Family Physicians (American Academy of Pediatrics Subcommittee on Management of Acute Otitis Media). This guideline states that diagnosis of AOM requires: (1) a history of acute onset of signs and symptoms (e.g., fever, irritability, ear pulling), (2) the presence of middle-ear effusion (confirmed by decreased mobility of the TM), and (3) signs and symptoms of middle-ear inflammation. These three requirements are further defined in that document. The usual treatment for AOM is antimicrobial, although it is recognized that some portion of these infections are viral in origin. Criteria for initial antibacterial treatment versus observation are stratified by age (<6 months, 6 months to 2 years, and >2 years), diagnostic certainty, illness severity, and assurance of follow-up. These protocols give a structured approach to antibiotic

use, with recommendations for "wait and see prescription" or "safety net antibiotic prescription" for children who are not acutely ill. This protocol has substantially reduced the unnecessary use of antibiotics in children (Spiro et al., 2006). The management recommendations in this Clinical Practice Guideline are not to be applied to children with recurrent AOM within 30 days of antibiotic treatment or otitis media with effusion (OME), or children with any underlying condition that may alter the natural course of AOM, such as cleft palate, genetic conditions, immunodeficiencies, and presence of cochlear implants. In cases of chronic MEE, which is often associated with recurrent AOM, there are similar guidelines suggesting when to consider a surgical approach and when not (AAP Clinical Practice Guideline: Otitis Media With Effusion, 2004; Maw et al., 1999). Antibiotic treatment has been shown to be more beneficial in children aged less than 2 years with bilateral AOM, and in those with both AOM and otorrhea (Rovers et al., 2006).

AOM becomes recurrent in about one third of children (Prellner et al., 1991). Consequently, one third of children are receiving frequent treatments with antimicrobials, leading to drug sensitivities and reactions and antimicrobial resistance, as well as significant cost. When recurrent infection leads to persistent middle ear fluid of 3 months or more duration, and hearing loss is documented, surgery is recommended to drain the middle ear of the fluid (American Academy of Pediatrics Clinical Practice Guideline: Otitis Media With Effusion, 2004). The recommended surgery performed for this reason is tympanostomy with tube placement, which has become the most common surgery performed in children in the United States beyond the newborn period, second only to newborn circumcision (Paradise et al., 2001). Evaluation of long-term benefits and sequelae of this procedure on children younger than age three with asymptomatic MEE is calling to question whether three months wait for spontaneous resolution of documented MEE before surgery is sufficient (Paradise et al., 2007).

It is known that the greatest risk of developing AOM is after a viral upper respiratory infection. Therefore, prevention of the initial viral infection is one means of preventing a secondary bacterial AOM. Clinical trials have generally shown improvement in recurrence rates of AOM in children immunized for influenza (Belshe et al., 1998; Clements et al., 1995; Hoberman et al., 2003), and the Centers for Disease Control now recommends immunization of healthy children at age six months for influenza and annually thereafter. Also recommended are immunizations for *Haemophilus influenzae* type b and pneumococcal vaccine beginning at age two months. (Center for Disease Control, 2008) Prolonged antibiotic prophylaxis was once a common practice, but its effect is small and the practice is now discouraged because of the risk of developing antibiotic-resistant bacteria (Wetmore, 2007).

While there are no recommendations for any complementary or alternative treatments for AOM in the 2004 Guidelines "based on limited or controversial data" (American Academy of Pediatrics Subcommittee on Management of Acute Otitis Media, 2004), osteopathic physicians have long reported favorable clinical outcomes in children treated with OMT in addition to standard medical care. In 1928, Galbreath reported on application of manipulation to the jaw for the treatment of "catarrh" (congestion) of the ear in the *Journal of the American Osteopathic Association*. Various case reports and practice guidelines advocating the use of OMT for the treatment of otitis media have been published in the osteopathic literature since that time (Bezilla, 1997; Carreiro, 2003; Centers et al., 2003; Frymann, 1998; Heatherington, 1995; Magoun 1996; Pintal and Kurtz, 1989). There are two clinical studies in the literature, which were published after the period of review of articles utilized for the 2004 Clinical Practice Guidelines and which demonstrate improved outcomes in children with recurrent AOM who receive OMT in addition to standard medical care (Degenhardt and Kuchera, 2006; Mills et al., 2003).

Miriam Mills, M.D., and others published a clinical trial in 2003 on 57 subjects, reporting on the efficacy of OMT as adjunctive treatment in recurrent AOM. This was a prospective, randomized, blinded, controlled, multicenter clinical trial with two study groups: standard care plus OMT and standard care alone. Those subjects who received standard care plus OMT for otitis media demonstrated the following significant findings in comparison to standard medical care alone at 6-month follow-up:

1. Fewer episodes of AOM ($p = 0.04$)
2. Fewer ENT surgeries ($p = 0.03$)
3. More surgery-free months ($p = 0.01$)
4. More normal tympanograms over 6 months ($p = 0.02$)

The Mills study demonstrated a significant improvement in clinical outcomes in children with recurrent AOM and persistent MEE who were treated with OMT in addition to their standard medical care, as compared to children receiving standard care only for treatment of recurrent AOM.

Degenhardt and Kuchera (2006) administered OMT weekly for 3 weeks to eight children, ages 7 to 35 months, with a history of recurrent otitis media, and then followed these subjects for 1 year. Their results showed that five subjects (62.5%) had no recurrence of symptoms during the year follow-up, one had a bulging TM, one had four episodes of otitis media, and one had surgery after AOM recurrence at 6 weeks post treatment. In addition to reduction of recurrence of otitis media, OMT has also been observed to provide immediate improvement in middle ear functioning in children as measured by tympanograms before and immediately after OMT (Carreiro, 2003).

OMT in children with AOM is directed toward structural impediments to optimum functioning (biomechanical model); improvement of middle ear drainage (respiratory-circulatory model); reduction of compression neuropathies affecting functioning of the oropharynx and upper gastrointestinal system and causing pain (neurological model); improvement of the environment in which the child lives (biopsychosocial model); and reducing the stress of infection and hearing impairment so the child can exist in his or her environment with greater functionality and contentment (bioenergetic model). (For a discussion of specific osteopathic techniques for each of these goals, please see the discussion of each model below.)

Secondary Otalgia

Ijaduaola (1985) describes the most common causes of secondary otalgia in children as tonsillitis (21% of all otalgia), foreign body in the pharynx (5%), and foreign body in the nose (2%). Ingvarsson (1982) describes that in children, ear pain not specifically involving infection of the ear is still often associated with upper respiratory congestion, and may be related to the discomfort of swallowing, nasal obstruction, fever, teething, or moderate hearing loss. The aphorism that "more things are missed by not looking than by not knowing" rightly applies in the evaluation of otalgia (Leung et al., 2000). The myriad of pathologies that can present with pain in the ear are complex and occasionally sublime, ranging from ectopic facial hair in the oropharynx (Papay et al., 1989) to fibromyalgia (Goldenberg, 1987; LeLiever, 1990) from ascariasis (LaGrone, 1977) to thyroiditis (Slatosky et al., 2000), and from eccrine spiradenoma (Nadig et al., 2004) to subdural hematoma (Zaidat and Ubogu, 2002). Even Munchausen syndrome in a 13-year-old boy has been reported to present as ear pain (Leung et al., 2000). When

a child with ear pain has a normal exam of the TM, the practitioner must take into consideration the neuroanatomy of the extensive sensory innervation of the ear arising from six nerve roots, which share common neuronal pathways with many other structures in the head, neck, and thorax.

Ingvarsson (1982) emphasizes that otitis media is both overlooked and overdiagnosed. In general, young children may not verbalize or localize pain very accurately, and will frequently point to the ear when experiencing teething pain, if they have experienced ear pain in the past. If a complete examination of the external and middle ear structures, and careful history relating to hearing and balance functions do not point to an etiology relating to the ear structures themselves, it is important to consider the more common etiologies of referred pain, with particular attention to the more rare but insidious presentations of malignancy. A complete head and neck exam should include the nose and nasal cavities, oral cavity, pharynx (particularly teeth and tonsils), the temporomandibular joint, and the nasopharynx and larynx, which may require fiberoptic endoscopy. Dental appliances should be removed if possible to allow for a complete examination, keeping in mind that the appliances themselves may be causing nerve irritation resulting in referred pain. Radiologic imaging may be necessary to rule out abscess or tumor (Teitelbaum et al., 2004).

Relevant features of the history and physical findings will be highlighted in each descriptive section of the following more common etiologies. The following discussion will focus more on children, but the relative frequency of similar presentations in adults will be mentioned.

Sinusitis

Acute sinusitis is the fifth most common diagnosis for which antibiotics are prescribed (Fagnan, 1998). The diagnosis is based in the patient's history of a biphasic illness ("double sickening"), purulent rhinorrhea often associated with fever which first clears and then returns, maxillary toothache, pain on leaning forward, and pain with a unilateral prominence. The symptoms overlap with simple upper respiratory infections, of which young children have an average of six to eight a year. The duration of the illness is a helpful clue. Foreign bodies should be ruled out with examination of the anterior nasopharynx, and adenoid hypertrophy can be excluded with a lateral neck radiograph. Otherwise, radiologic imaging is not considered necessary for diagnosis and can be misleading in children, as they commonly have asymmetric sinus development. A basic evaluation of ocular and neurologic function is necessary to rule out potential complications. OMT is often helpful in relieving the symptoms and enhancing recovery by balancing the autonomic stimulation to the area (neurologic model), stimulating lymph drainage (respiratory-circulatory model), and alleviating the underlying predisposing structural components (biomechanical model).

Pharyngitis and Infections of Other Proximal Structures

Pharyngitis, aphthous ulcers, stomatitis, gingivitis, glossitis, and sialadenitis (inflammation of a salivary gland, which may be associated with obstruction of the duct or infection), including parotiditis (particularly mumps) may also present as otalgia. Older children and adults may also present with abdominal pain or headache. Chronic tonsillitis may be associated with debris within the tonsillar crypts called tonsillitis. Children account for one third of all episodes of peritonsillar abscesses, and it is usually due to group A β-hemolytic *streptococcus*, and is associated with fever, dysphagia, and voice change. Although it is not likely to present with otalgia as an isolated symptom, it must be suspected to be found, especially in a nonverbal child, and may require surgical drainage. It must be differentiated from neoplasia, which will more likely present with fleshy, granular, or pale tissue (Wetmore, 2007). OMT for infections of the pharynx is used to improve lymphatic circulation and respiratory chest wall excursion (respiratory-circulatory model); reduce pain by relieving compression on CNs exiting the cranial base, especially the Vagus nerve (neurologic model); and reduce the muscle spasm of the upper cervical area that exacerbates pain and reduces mobility (biomechanical model). However, direct treatment to the infected areas of the head and upper neck area should not be performed until the infection is under control with medical management.

Viral infections of the mouth include rhinovirus, coxsackievirus, mononucleosis, herpangina, herpes simplex gingivostomatitis, herpes zoster, measles, mumps, and aphthous ulcers. Human papillomavirus may present as painless papillomatous lesions on the soft palate or uvula, and occasionally may undergo malignant transformation. Given the venereal component of this virus, its presence in a child might suggest sexual abuse. Herpes zoster may be accompanied by vesicles on the auricle, but intense otalgia may present weeks before they erupt. When this is associated with facial nerve palsy, it is called Ramsay Hunt syndrome, and may also involve hearing loss and vertigo. The ear pain may persist for weeks after the vesicles resolve. When facial paralysis is associated with vesicle eruption, the facial palsy is more likely to persist (Bluestone et al., 2003; Leung et al., 2000; Shah and Blevins, 2003; Wetmore, 1997). While viral upper respiratory infections are usually self-limited, OMT is useful to reduce inflammation of the tissues that may contribute to pain by promoting lymph and venous sinus drainage (respiratory-circulatory model) and relieving pressure on the associated nerves and ganglia (neurologic model).

Bacterial infections of the mouth such as gingivitis are sometimes associated with poor hygiene, poor nutrition, or immunosuppression. Ludwig angina refers to an acute bacterial infection of the floor of the mouth, associated with submandibular fullness, drooling, and voice change, and may progress without treatment to airway compromise. Parotiditis can be bacterial, as can infection of the submandibular glands, but are also associated with systemic symptoms rather than solely otalgia, and frank pus may be expressed from the associated salivary duct. *Streptococcus pneumoniae* and *Staphylococcus aureus* are usually implicated. Recurrent parotiditis may indicate an underlying collagen vascular disease (Charlett and Coatesworth, 2007; Wetmore, 1997).

Yeast infections in the mouth are common in infants and may be related to recent antibiotics in the child or mother of a nursing baby. It is obvious by inspection of the mouth and cheeks for whitish patches. Medical treatment is simple, and response is usually rapid.

Dental Problems, Including Temporomandibular Joint Dysfunction

Pain from tooth eruption, caries, impacted teeth, gingivitis, and periapical infections may all be referred to the ear, and can usually be diagnosed by thorough visual inspection of the mouth. Carious teeth may be associated with sensitivity to hot or cold temperatures, which may persist after the evoking stimulus is removed. Caries are initially seen as a white spot of the tooth, which changes to a brown color as cavitation progresses. Abscess presents with more systemic symptoms and swelling. Trauma to the mouth and teeth is common in children, who tend to run with things in their mouths and fall down, often unnoticed by a parent. Tooth eruption as an etiology of otalgia is more common in children than is temporomandibular

joint dysfunction (TMD), but the latter is not uncommon, and should be considered in children who have intermittent unilateral otalgia of three or four days' duration and whose exam and ear functioning are normal. Shah and Blevins (2003) noted that as many as 48% of patients with TMD presented with otalgia.

TMD is characterized by temporomandibular joint (TMJ) tenderness on palpation, restricted motion of the jaw, which is frequently accompanied by "clicking," and is often unilateral, more pronounced in the morning, and aggravated by chewing or biting. The ear pain may be related to nerve irritation, muscle spasm, or degenerative changes in the joint. The pain can be elicited by palpating preauricularly, intraotically (with fingers pushing forward), or orally, palpating along the last molar, where the pterygoids connect the maxilla to the mandible. It may be exacerbated by a pillow that is too high (Zenian, 2001). In children, the pain is usually due to muscle spasm and is often seen with a history of recent orthodontic treatment. Other causes of TMD include bruxism, dental malocclusion, jaw clenching, excessive gum chewing, and trauma, Lyme disease, and connective tissue disorders such as juvenile rheumatoid arthritis (Pertes, 1998).

Menner (2003) suggests that TMD is underdiagnosed because it may present with a somewhat abnormal-looking TM. Furthermore, chronic dislocation, ankylosis related to connective tissue diseases, and neoplasia must be considered in refractory cases and require more aggressive intervention (Kramer and Kramer, 1985; Leung et al., 2000; Shah and Blevins, 2003).

TMD often responds to OMT, especially when it relates to orthodontic treatment. In a child with a clear-cut recent history of minor head trauma involving the temporal bone such as a whiplash or fall on the chin, a brief trial of OMT might be warranted and may clear the symptoms completely. The OMT for TMD secondary to dental intervention or head trauma is specific for the somatic dysfunction found and commonly requires treatment of the head using osteopathy in the cranial field (OCF) techniques. Examination and treatment of the child's entire body is necessary following trauma in order to remove somatic dysfunction in areas distant to the head that are causing strain and impaired functioning of the TMD (biomechanical model).

Gastroesophageal Reflux

Children presenting with otalgia secondary to gastroesophageal reflux may be fretful and irritable. Irritation of the respiratory epithelium of the larynx and pharynx by gastric acid stimulates CN IX and X. Other symptoms may include hoarseness, dysphagia, a sensation of a lump in the throat, chronic cough, or overt intermittent wheezing. It can occur in the absence of typical symptoms of gastroesophageal reflux such as heartburn and regurgitation. Direct irritation of the opening of the ET can cause swelling and contribute to middle ear pathology, and an association between recurrent AOM and GER has been suggested (Wetmore, 2007). Endoscopy may demonstrate evidence of inflammation, and pH monitoring is considered the gold standard for diagnosis. It has been shown that in 60% to 90% of children with OME, gastric pepsin can be found in middle ear fluid (Crapko et al., 2007; Tasker et al., 2002). This in itself may be a cause of ear pain (Gibson and Cochran, 1994) as well as a contributor to recurrent middle ear infection.

Compression of the cranial base is a common osteopathic finding seen in children with GERD. From the osteopathic perspective, this compression leads to impingement of the Vagus nerve resulting in ineffective closure of the lower esophageal sphincter and reflux of stomach contents (Sergueef, 2007). OMT is often helpful in reducing the severity of the reflux, using the whole-body approach. Impaired gastric emptying may occur from spasm of the abdominal diaphragm, and can be treated with indirect and direct myofascial techniques (biomechanical model). Soft tissue techniques to the upper cervical area reduce impingement of cervical nerves 3 to 5 innervating the diaphragm, and occipital decompression techniques reduce compression on the Vagus nerve as it exits the jugular foramen, resulting in improved lower esophageal sphincter functioning and reduction of pain mediated via the Vagus nerve (neurologic model).

Headaches and Other Cervicofacial Pain Syndromes

Migraine headaches, which are considered to be related to neurogenic inflammation with secondary cerebrovascular changes (Pertes, 1998), are usually characterized by a throbbing or pounding, often unilateral headache, accompanied by nausea, vomiting, and photophobia, with an aura frequently preceding the headache. Otalgia may be a nondominant symptom (Leung et al., 2001). Tension headaches may be either episodic or chronic, and may trigger migraine-type symptoms. Boes et al. (1998) describe two cases of paryxysmal hemicrania manifested solely by otalgia with a sensation of external acoustic meatus obstruction. Trigeminal neuralgia and glossopharyngeal neuralgia may refer primarily to the ear, and has been found on occasion to be associated with multiple sclerosis and Charcot-Marie-Tooth neuropathy (Manzoni and Torelli, 2005). OMT of migraine headaches is commonly provided between headache episodes and is designed to reduce the intracranial strains that contribute to the frequency and intensity of the headaches. Relief of pressure on the involved intracranial ganglia with OCF is often helpful (Magoun, 1996). (neurologic model).

Yount (2004) reviews atypical earaches and otomandibular symptoms, with reference to Travell's trigger points (Simons et al., 1999) and emphasizes how central sensitization incorporates several different sources of pain (undiagnosed pain, "piggy-back" pains, frequent recurrent pains, and chronic pains) to induce anatomical, neurochemical, and physiological changes in the nervous system that may confound accurate diagnosis. Forward head posture, especially when accompanied by forward shoulder position, has been associated with development of trigger points, or with occipital neuralgia (Pertes, 1998). The areas that frequently refer pain to the ear include the lateral pterygoid, the deep masseter, the clavicular sternocleidomastoid, the medial pterygoid, and the suboccipital muscles. OMT targeted to dysfunctions of the head and neck area, and postural treatment and education are commonly helpful (biomechanical model). OMT without postural realignment and reeducation will generally not provide long-term relief.

Thyroiditis

Thyroiditis, including chronic lymphocytic thyroiditis (also known as Hashimoto thyroiditis), may present with ear pain before a goiter is noticed. Symptoms of hyper- or hypothyroidism may not predominate initially. It is seen more commonly in adults, but is the most common cause of sporadic goiter in children, and its incidence is rising. Subacute granulomatous thyroiditis is more commonly associated with pain, which may be referred (Slatoksy et al., 2000).

Regarding benign space occupying lesions, one series of patients with acoustic neuromas found that 4.2% presented with ear pain (Charlett and Coatesworth, 2007). Branchial cleft cysts, dermoid cysts, and thyroglossal duct cysts may present with ear pain, and usually make their presence known in the first decade of life. A case report of cervical spine meningioma presenting as otalgia, but was associated with progressive neurological deficits over a prolonged time, has also been described, though not in children (Danish and Zager, 2005). Stretching of the dura by a nonneoplastic

lesions, such as a subdural hematoma, may also trigger otalgia (Zaidat and Ubogu, 2002; Charlett and Coatesworth, 2007), and a case of heparin-induced thrombocytopenia involving near total occlusion of the internal jugular and subclavian veins, secondary to placement of a hemodialysis catheter, has also been described (Marinella, 2007). Determining the exact location of the pain may give an indication to the site of the disease (see neurological model considerations in pediatric ear pain).

Diagnosis

The diagnosis in this case is AOM, either from a viral or bacterial etiology. This child demonstrates an increased susceptibility to ear infections due to numerous factors:

1. Age and ethnicity-related anatomical and physiological functioning of the middle ear and auditory or ET (biomechanical model)
2. A history of stress on the fetal head during delivery (biomechanical model)
3. Exposure to other children at day care and exposure to passive cigarette smoke at home (biopsychosocial model)
4. Presence of somatic dysfunction of the head, neck, and torso impairing clearing of the middle ear (respiratory-circulatory model)
5. Presence of somatic dysfunction of the cranial base, causing pain in the head area, and compression of CNs controlling the feeding process leading to autonomic dysfunction (neurological model)

Osteopathic Patient Management

DW has a history of feeding difficulties and presumed colic, which would lead the osteopathic physician to conclude that the somatic dysfunction diagnosed today has been present since birth, and has contributed to feeding disorders and a longstanding impairment of middle ear functioning. In addition to standard medical care of this child, the addition of OMT to her care is provided with the goal of hastening recovery and reducing the chance of recurrence of middle ear infection

Dr. Viola Frymann (1998) wisely notes that "…the identification of otitis media … is only the beginning. A comprehensive diagnosis of the child who suffers from the disease is essential if the etiologic factors… are to be recognized and addressed." The following discussion will review the biomechanical factors affecting middle ear function and dysfunction, and the appropriate use of OMT in the treatment of middle ear disease in children.

Biomechanical model

The Cranial Base and the Eustachian Tube

Middle ear disease has long been considered to be related to ET dysfunction (Bluestone et al., 2003). Under normal conditions, the ET fluctuates between a patent and closed position. Middle ear pressure is equilibrated with atmospheric pressure through the periodic openings of the ET that occur with swallowing and other activities. In children, middle ear pressures are slightly negative compared to adults (Bluestone and Klein 1996), and most children, even those without middle ear disease, have difficulty in maintaining appropriate pressures. The ability to maintain appropriate pressures appears to be related to the stiffness of the ET. The fact that the tube is relatively pliable in children is thought to be responsible for the increased incidence of middle ear disease in this age group (Bylander, 1980; Bylander and Tjernstrom, 1983). Deficits in ET function impede normal drainage to the nasopharynx (Takahashi et al., 1989) and create a negative pressure within the middle ear as compared to atmospheric pressure. The resulting negative pressure may promote insufflation, aspiration, or reflux of nasopharyngeal secretions into the middle ear.

Within the biomechanical model, ET dysfunction is thought to be influenced by mechanical dysfunctions of the cranial base or the surrounding tissues. The child's cranial base and ET differ anatomically and physiologically from those of the adult in ways that make them more vulnerable to otitis media. At birth, the temporal bone is in three parts: the squamous portion, the petrous portion, and the tympanic ring, joined by cartilage (Carreiro, 2003). The ET travels through the petrous portion of the temporal bone, emerging into a cartilaginous sheath, closely adherent to the base of the skull, nestled between the greater wing of the sphenoid and the petrous portion of the temporal bone, emerging into the posterior pharynx at the posterior edge of the medial pterygoid plate of the sphenoid. The juncture, between the osseous and the cartilaginous portions, resembles two "truncated cones," narrower than both portions of the adjacent tube. The tube is lined with pseudostratified columnar epithelium of the ciliated type, continuous with the lining of the tympanic cavity and nasopharynx at each end. It is also tethered at each end by fibrous attachments, at the posterior end extending into the osseous portion by approximately 3 mm, and at the anteromedial end, the cartilage protrudes into the nasopharynx with fibrous bands attaching it to a tubercle on the posterior edge of the medial pterygoid plate (Bluestone et al., 2003).

It is noteworthy that the timing of the decline in frequency of ear infections, about 6 years of age, seems to coincide with the maturation of the cranial base and adjacent structures (Carreiro, 2003). The relationship of the tube to other contiguous structures, particularly the tensor veli palatini, the levator veli palatini, and the saplingopharyngeous muscles, and the difference between the characteristics of the cartilage between children and adults, may contribute to biomechanical forces acting upon the ET in young children (Carreiro, 2003). The medial bundle of the tensor veli palatini muscle lies immediately adjacent to the lateral membranous wall of the ET, and when contracted, opens the tube. This muscle curves around the hamulus of the medial pterygoid plate of the sphenoid and attaches to the posterior margin of the hard palate. In children with cleft palate, its function is less than optimal. In infants, the angle of this muscle to the tube is more acute placing it closer to the middle ear. When contracted, the tensor veli palatini may actually distort the ET rather than effectively open it (Bluestone et al., 2003). Spasm of this muscle, which is comparatively large compared to the tube in infants, may conversely cause the tube to be patulous, leaving it vulnerable to influx of pharyngeal organisms. Carreiro (2003) also suggests a possible contribution of the medial pterygoid muscle, which is comparatively bulkier in the infant, to extrinsic compression on the ET in contraction. Figures 58.1 to 58.3 demonstrate the relationship of these structures.

Figure 58-1 Photograph showing location of ET between petrous portion of the temporal bone and the basisphenoid. (Used with permission, Willard and Carreiro Collection.)

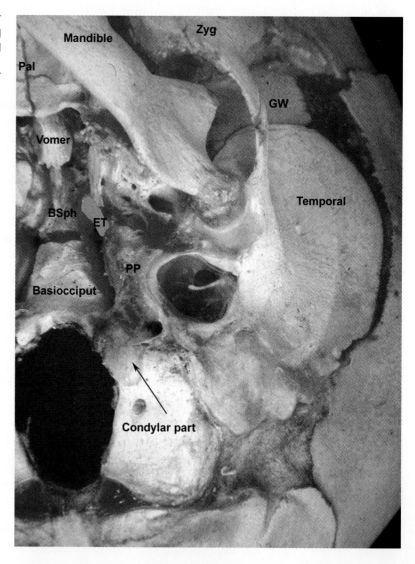

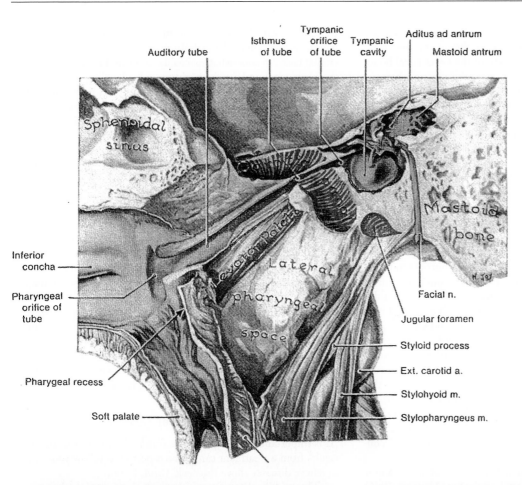

Auditory tube

Isthmus of tube

Tympanic orifice of tube

Tympanic cavity

Aditus ad antrum

Mastoid antrum

Sphenoidal sinus

Mastoid bone

Inferior concha

Pharyngeal orifice of tube

Lateral pharyngeal space

Facial n.

Jugular foramen

Styloid process

Ext. carotid a.

Stylohyoid m.

Stylopharyngeus m.

Pharygeal recess

Soft palate

Figure 58-2 Interior view of relationship of ET to adjacent structures in the adult. (Used by permission, Ward RC, Ed. *Foundations for Osteopathic Medicine.* 2nd Ed. Philadelphia, PA: Lippincott Williams & Wilkins, 2003.)

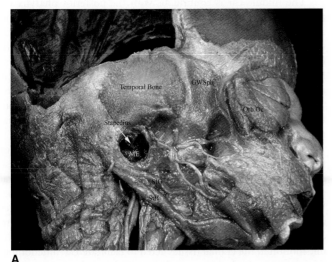

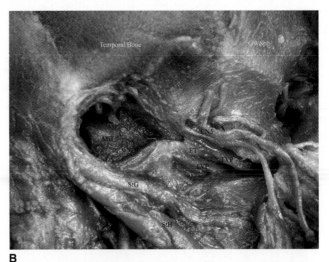

A

B

Figure 58-3 A. Lateral view of neonatal dissection. The mandible and zygoma bones have been cut and the muscles of mastication removed. The TM has collapsed, revealing the middle ear (ME) and malleus. The styloglossus (StG) and stylohoid (StH), orbicularis oculii (ORbOc), mandibular branch of the trigeminal (V3) and greater wing of the sphenoid (GWSph) are labeled. (Used with permission, Willard & Carreiro Collection.) **B.** Close-up of area indicated by the *arrow* in **(A).** The lateral aspect of the temporal bone has been drilled away to reveal the ET surrounded by the tensor veli palatine (TVP) and levator veli palatini (LVP) muscles. Note the relative size of the muscles as compared to the ET. The middle ear (ME), styloglossus (StG), stylohoid (StH), greater wing of the sphenoid (GWSph), and ophthalmic branch of the trigeminal nerve (V3) are labeled. (Used with permission, Willard & Carreiro Collection.)

Other differences between the adult and the pediatric ET include the fact that the infant's tube is more compliant (and therefore more floppy), smaller in diameter, and shorter in length. There is also a difference in the relationship of the ET as it enters the posterior pharyngeal wall. In the infant, the cartilaginous tube lies at a 10 to 30 degree angle from the horizontal in relation to the osseous portion, although in adults, it is increased to 45 to 50 degrees (Bluestone and Klein, 2001; Carreiro, 2003). At the same time, the posterior pharyngeal tissues are relatively more anterior and superior in the child. These differences are due to changes in the shape of the cranial base and the growth of the lower facial bones. The smaller angulation may act to narrow the junction between the two components of the ET, while the position of the posterior pharynx may narrow the orifice of the tube.

The articulation between the temporal and sphenoid changes angle at the point that the ET emerges from the temporal bone. The biomechanical model suggests that via its myofascial structures, neck and jaw movements may contribute to passive pumping actions on the ET, "milking" it and helping clear it of secretions.

Twin studies suggest a genetic component to ET dysfunction, which may be related to anatomy as well as physiology (Caselbrandt et al., 1999). Skull base configuration is also implicated in explaining the clustering of otitis in certain families (Bluestone et al., 2003) and in individuals with skull base malformations such as Down Syndrome, Apert syndrome, Crouzon syndrome, Treacher Collins syndrome, Hurler-Hunter syndrome, and Turner syndrome (Bluestone et al. 2003; Wetmore, 2007). There is a difference in frequency of ear infections racially, with decreased incidence described by some in African Americans and Chinese, and increased in Native American, Canadian, and Alaskan Native children. Doyle (1977) suggested that significant differences among various racial groups in the length, width, and angle of the tube may affect a predilection to otitis. Bluestone (2003) suggests that the relative size of the nasopharynx at the proximal end of the ET may also play a role in a predilection to otitis, in that it has been reported that children with a relatively small nasopharynx, measured radiographically, had a higher incidence of otitis than children with larger dimensions.

According to Sutherland's model, the base of the cranium undergoes rhythmic changes that can be palpated (Magoun, 1996). This phasic change is basic to the concept of OCF. Understanding this model allows the osteopathic practitioner to predict the potential effects of palpated strains on middle ear functioning. According to this model, the cranial base and temporal bone are vulnerable to both compressive and tensile mechanical stress. Furthermore, tissue strains of the cranial base and the contiguous soft tissue may influence ET function, as well as potentially all structures above, below, or penetrating the cranial base (Magoun, 1996). For most children, the process of birth is the most profound force their head experiences (Fig. 58.4).

Carreiro has hypothesized that mechanical strains may contribute to edema of the tissues surrounding the ET (Carriero, 2003). This in turn may influence intravascular fluid exchange in the middle ear, drainage of the tube, and fluid flow through its lymphatic and venous channels. In the newborn, the structures of the cranial base are somewhat malleable, allowing for passage through the birth canal and for the rapid growth (doubling in size) of the head in the first year of life. This same malleability makes the cranial base vulnerable to compression or distortion during delivery.

Pilot studies suggest that osteopathic manipulative medicine, and specifically OCF, may be relevant in treating patients with otitis media and serous otitis media (Degenhardt, 2006; Mills, 2003). Figure 58.2 shows a child receiving OMT in the form of OCF, for treatment of AOM, with the parent nearby.

Using chart analysis, Carreiro (2003) describes somatic dysfunction of the vault often associated with biomechanical strains in the cranial base and venous sinus system. She hypothesizes that the vault findings are probably secondary and recommends normalizing the base mechanics first. Magoun (1996) describes a number of techniques that may be used in infants and children to facilitate function of the ET and the surrounding tissues.. These techniques are used to promote more physiologic functioning of lymph, blood, and nerves in the head. While there have been rare reports of serious adverse events in children treated with high-velocity thrust chiropractic spinal manipulation (Ernst, 2003), the gentle techniques recommended for OMT in children (Bezilla, 1997) have been shown to be well tolerated by children, with few side effects and no serious adverse events reported (Hayes and Bezilla, 2006).

Respiratory-circulatory Model

"It is important to have perfect drainage, for without it, the good results from a treatment cannot be expected to follow your efforts to relieve diseases above the neck" (Still, 1899).

The middle ear is continuous with the posterior pharynx via the ET, and with the mastoid air cells via the narrow aditus and antrum. Ideally, it is filled only with air and serves to transmit sound waves from the TM to the fenestra vestibuli and the eighth CN. Because of various factors, primarily associated with ET dysfunction, the middle ear may become filled with fluid. If the fluid is not drained naturally, surgery may be considered. OMT may provide a means of facilitating the natural drainage of the middle ear, thereby potentially averting recurrence of infection, antimicrobial resistance, and even surgery (Mills, 2003).

The body has many natural mechanisms to ensure drainage of the middle ear, so that an air-filled space can be maintained. These include a dense lymphatic and venous network, and the natural pumping mechanisms associated with sucking and swallowing. William Sutherland, D.O. (Magoun, 1996), described another mechanism, a rhythmic motion in the tissues of the cranium occurring 10 to 14 times/min. He hypothesized that this rhythmic motion in the cranial tissues acted to facilitate ET functioning. Some osteopaths have reported an association between impairments in this "cranial rhythmic motion" and otitis media (Degenhardt and Kuchera, 1994; Frymann, 1966; Mills, 2003). Within the respiratory-circulatory model, chewing, crying, and sucking influence venous and lymphatic structures in the head and neck facilitating tissue perfusion and drainage. In addition, neck movements are thought to provide intermittent tensile forces on the ET and surrounding structures influencing fluid movement through the low pressure circulatory system.

The respiratory circulatory model recognizes that breathing and crying alter intrathoracic pressures and contribute to fluid drainage from the head and neck. Within the concept of this model, crawling and walking may affect the circulatory system by generating intermittent tensions on the abdominal diaphragm and

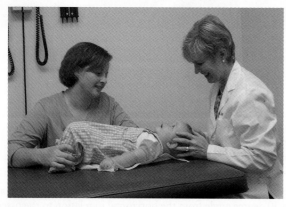

Figure 58-4 Child receiving osteopathic manipulative treatment for AOM with parent nearby, utilizing OCF technique.

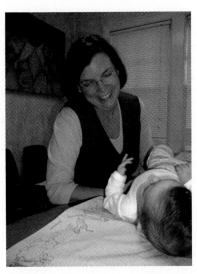

Figure 58-5 Child receiving OMT of the pelvis to assist with function of middle ear drainage.

lower ribs via the myofascial attachments of the iliocostalis and the crura of the diaphragm. Figure 58.3 demonstrates a child receiving OMT for treatment of pelvic somatic dysfunction, with the goal of improving function of the respiratory-circulatory system and indirectly influencing middle ear drainage (Fig. 58.5).

Neurological Model

An appreciation of the complex sensory innervations of the structures surrounding the ear, and the interaction of these same nerves with other, sometimes more distant structures, may facilitate understanding of the many potentially confusing possible etiologies of otalgia. The ear structures are provided sensory innervation by CNs V, VII, IX, and X, and by cervical nerves 2 and 3.

It is important to keep in mind that there is considerable variability among individuals. Though here is no role of the CN VIII in carrying pain fibers from the inner ear, resulting in the observation that significant inner ear pathology can develop without otalgia, sensation mediated by this nerve can be felt by the patient as a "fullness" in the ear, such as is seen in Menieire disease (Shah and Blevins, 2003). Clinically, areas innervated by CN IX may refer an intense pain deep in the ear. There is no evidence of referral of pain from ear pathology to the distal structures (Scarbrough et al. 2003).

These complex interrelationships are the result of embryologic development, stemming from the otic vesicle coming to lie between the branchial arches 1, 2, 3, and 4, giving rise to CN V, VII, IX, and X, respectively (Scarbrough et al., 2003). The autonomic nerve supply to the upper respiratory tract including the middle ear and sinuses consists of parasympathetic stimulation via the CN VII and sympathetic stimulation via T1-4. Figure 58.4 graphically displays the autonomic nerve supply to the upper respiratory tract.

It is useful to be aware of the location and pathways of these nerves and their ganglia, as somatic dysfunction along the way may contribute to otalgia, and relief of those strain patterns might benefit the patient, even if no underlying cause is found for the ear pain.

There are complex immunohistochemical changes associated with ear pain that may contribute to the pathophysiology of otitis media. Nagaraj and Linthicum (1998) described the presence of

catecholaminergic nerve fibers in the human middle ear mucus membrane that may play an important role in the pathogenesis of MEE. Animal studies of the role of substance P in osteoclastogenesis, a common finding in otitis media, and the effect of capsaicin pretreatment on the neurogenic inflammatory component of otitis media offer a tantalizing suggestion into further applications of this area of research in humans (Basak et al., 2005; Sohn, 2005). Caye-Thomasen (2004) describes depletion of mucosal substance P in AOM in rats. In humans, Teodorczyk-Ineyan (2006) has shown that spinal manipulation may reduce inflammatory cytokines but not substance P production in normal subjects. This finding suggests a potential objective marker for monitoring the downregulation of inflammatory responses to manipulation. Whether these findings can explain the improvement of pain in patients receiving manual medicine techniques remains to be determined.

The fact that our case child had a difficult delivery and problems sucking does not surprise the osteopathically oriented physician. The history of colic and spitting up may be related to the patient's somatic dysfunction. Frymann's classic study of 1,250 newborns correlated specific areas of somatic dysfunction on osteopathic examination with distinct symptomatology in the newborn nursery (Frymann, 1966). Carreiro (2003) postulates that babies with compression dysfunction at the cranial base may also develop symptoms as they start to develop head control, adding more muscle tension to an area already irritated, thereby exacerbating preexisting somatic dysfunction.

It is the experience of osteopathic practitioners worldwide, and over many years' observation, that there is an association between recurrent AOM and a difficult or rapid delivery (Carreiro, 2003; Sergueef, 2007; Sorrel, 2004; Woods, 1976). These same authors also report that children with recurrent AOM are often firstborn and frequently have a concomitant history of colic, dacryostenosis, feeding difficulties, or gastroesophageal reflux in the newborn period. As with our patient, there is an association between otitis media and gastroesophageal reflux (Caruso, 2006), which is thought to be either a vagal-vagal reflex or have an inflammatory component. From an osteopathic perspective, gastrointestinal motility and function of the gastroesophageal junction may be influenced by somatic dysfunction in the cranial base via vagal input or thoracolumbar somatic dysfunction influencing the diaphragmatic contribution to the gastroesophageal sphincter. Bluestone (2003) reports that children who are "otitis-prone" also have more episodes of bronchopulmonary, gastrointestinal, and urinary tract infections, as well as more visits to the orthopedic clinic than control subjects. This might lead one to suggest that somatic dysfunction may be a common denominator of these problems.

Metabolic Energy Model

Good nutrition is a staple of good health. Children, who are undernourished or poorly nourished, may be at greater risk for infectious diseases such as otitis media and less able to respond to therapy. Nutritional supplements have gained favor in some communities, as has an emphasis on eating organic and locally grown foods. For example, "glyconutrients," which are reported to have some benefit on immune function (Axford, 1997; Murray, 2006), have enjoyed increased usage in recent years.

Treatment and Outcome

Following the current guidelines for treatment of AOM (American Academy of Pediatrics Subcommittee on Management of Acute

Otitis Media, 2004), DW was treated with ibuprofen to achieve pain control and given a prescription for amoxicillin-clavulanate, to be filled if DW's symptoms were not resolved in 48 hours. She was also treated with OMT, consisting of Galbreath mandibular drainage, temporal decompression, occipitomastoid decompression, myofascial release of the upper cervical musculature, thoracic outlet and abdominal diaphragm, and rib-raising techniques. DW tolerated the procedure very well. Mother was advised to quit smoking, and was taught to do the Galbreath mandibular drainage, rib raising, and lymphatic pump techniques and advised to do them twice daily until recheck. At recheck two weeks later, the ear examination was normal and tympanograms were normal.

Behavioral Model

Environmental and Complementary Measures for Middle Ear Disease

As previously discussed, socioeconomic and environmental factors have been shown to influence the occurrence of otitis media. For children who are unable to control their surroundings, it falls to the physician to encourage healthy habits in the family that might reduce the risk of recurrence. Taking into account the particulars of the patient and his or her home situation, the physician needs to consider breast feeding, discouraging pacifier use and bottle feeding when supine, avoidance of exposure to smoke and other environmental toxins and allergens, avoiding crowded settings and early child care (Bluestone et al., 2003), and teaching hand washing, and avoidance of sharing drinks. The physician also needs to consider the role of comorbidities such as gastroesophageal reflux, which predispose to recurrent otitis media. It is helpful to educate the parent to not mix bottles of milk for prolonged room-temperature storage (as in a diaper bag), not store pacifiers in airtight containers, or bottles with nipples attached in the refrigerator, and not reuse unconsumed formula after a particular feeding, not only because of possible yeast infection, but also bacterial contamination. Parents should also be informed that the Center for Disease Control (CDC) now recommends administration of pneumococcal, *Haemophilus influenzae* type b, and influenza vaccines in infants and children, which have been shown to reduce the incidence and transmission of respiratory disease, and its secondary AOM (CDC, 2008).

Considering that at least 10% of patients have tried at least one or more forms of alternative/complementary medicine before presenting for consultation, it is useful for physicians to inquire regarding their use (Eisenberg et al., 1993; Kemper, 1996). Physicians should be aware of preventative strategies that may have limited benefit such as the use of the xylitol gum or syrup, and probiotic bacterial replacement (Wetmore, 2007). Various herbal and homeopathic remedies and nutritional supplements have been suggested as alternative or complementary to traditional medical approaches (Bluestone and Kline, 2001). A double-blind study comparing naturopathic herbal extract ear drops to anesthetic ear drops, with or without amoxicillin (Sarrell et al., 2003) showed a mild but statistically significant benefit with ear drops, particularly the naturopathic remedy. (Need to add detail re: what study was comparing.) Kemper (1996) has also reported, but does not specifically recommend, herbal teas including those containing Echinacea, goldenseal, and licorice root. Chamomile, hops, and passion flower are sometimes used because of their sedation effect. Homeopathy has been shown to reduce otalgia associated with AOM at 2.4 times faster than placebo, and without complications (Frei and Thurneysen, 2001). Common homeopathic remedies used for children with ear pain include Aconite, Belladonna,

Chamomilla, Ferrum phosphoricum, and Pulsatilla (Kemper, *The Holistic Pediatrician*, 1996; Morgan, 1992; Schmidt, 1990). A combination remedy called "ABC," contains Aconite, Belladonna, and Chamomilla, and is commonly recommended for children. Physicians need to be aware that some parents may choose to treat their children without prior examination by a health care professional. For the sake of the child, it is very important that the physician maintain a relationship with these parents and not alienate them. Physicians should educate parents as to the warning signs of worsening infection, sepsis, meningitis, and other serious complications of untreated infection. The practitioner should also be aware that a systematic review of serious adverse effects of unconventional therapies for children and adolescents revealed the greatest number of adverse events to occur secondary to herbal medicines (Ernst, 2003).

Parents often feel helpless when their child is ill. This can exacerbate their anxiety and influence their response to the sick child and perhaps even the child's perception of their own illness. Interventions that empower the parent without risk to the child may prove beneficial to both on many levels. It is sometimes comforting to apply mild heat to the outer ear, in the form of warm washcloth, heating pad, or hair dryer. A common folk remedy for otalgia is warmed sweet oil, garlic oil, mineral oil, or olive oil instilled in the ear canal. There is no evidence of efficacy but these pose no threat to the child as long as the ear drum is intact.

In addition, parents may also be taught simple osteopathic techniques such as lymphatic pump, rib raising, or the Galbreath mandibular drainage technique, which can be administered at the first signs of an upper respiratory tract infection. Schmidt's classic study of 100 patients with upper, middle, and pararespiratory illnesses, in which 63%, who were treated within day 1 of their illness, compared with 34%, who received OMT >2 days after onset of symptoms, showed more rapid resolution of symptoms, fewer complications, and fewer recurrences in the early-treated group (1990). Given that busy medical practices (and busy parent schedules) may not accommodate same-day appointments for patients with very early respiratory symptoms, the possibility of involving parents early in the child's illness may prove beneficial.

Notes on Treating Children with OMT

Treating children with OMT presents some unique challenges, but the practitioner should not be daunted, as the benefits can be enormously rewarding. Children are not just small adults. Their bodies are more flexible, more resilient, and less complex than adults. Their somatic dysfunction is easier to fix, and doing so can be life changing. Parents can be taught many activities of daily living that can improve somatic dysfunction in children. The normal squirming of a child, though it may be distracting to the practitioner, may actually help in the treatment. Treating children takes flexibility and time to develop trust, using positions familiar to the child, face-on first, such as with changing a diaper, or allowing the child to sit in the parent's lap. Toys, books, and frequent changes in position are often necessary to keep the child engaged. In some children, particularly two-year olds, brief gentle restraint may be necessary during the treatment.

CONCLUSION

The treatment of a child with ear pain begins with a history and physical to determine the cause of the pain. Working within the osteopathic paradigm, an evaluation for predisposing dysfunction of the entire body is a part of the physical examination. The diagnosis includes consideration of the anatomical and functional differences in the child's head and neck, as compared to the adult. Treatment is directed to the identified cause of the pain, as well as removing predisposing factors in the child's body with the use of OMT, when appropriate. Factors in the environment that are modifiable are addressed to improve the overall health of the child.

REFERENCES

Al-Sheikhli ARJ. Pain in the ear—with special reference to referred pain. *J Laryngol Otol* 1980;94:1433–1440.

American Academy of Pediatrics Clinical Practice Guideline: Otitis Media With Effusion. *Pediatrics* 2004;113(5):1412–1429.

American Academy of Pediatrics Subcommittee on Management of Acute Otitis Media. Diagnosis and management of acute otitis media. *Pediatrics* 2004;113(5):1451–1465.

Axford J. Glycobiology and medicine: an introduction. *J R Soc Med* 1997;90:260–264.

Basak S, Dikicioglu E, Turkutanit S, et al. Early and late effects of capsaicin pretreatment in otitis media with effusion. *Otol Neurotol* 2005;26(3):344–350.

Belshe RB, Mendelman PM, Treanor J, et al. The efficacy of live attenuated, cold-adapted, trivalent, intranasal influenzavirus vaccine in children. *N Engl J Med* 1998;338(20):1405–1412.

Bezilla TA. Acute otitis media: an osteopathic approach. *J POMA* 1997; December:8–12.

Bluestone CD, Klein JO. *Otitis Media in Infants and Children.* 3rd Ed. WB Saunders Co., 2001.

Bluestone CD, Stool SE, Alper CM, et al. *Pediatric Otolaryngology.* Vol 1. 3rd Ed. Philadelphia, PA: Saunders, Elsevier Science, 2003.

Boes CJ, Swanson JW, Dodick DW. Chronic paroxysmal hemicrania presenting as otalgia with a sensation of external acoustic meatus obstruction: two cases and a pathophysiologic hypothesis. *Headache* 1998;38:787–791.

Bondy J, Berman S, Glazner J, et al. Direct expenditures related to otitis media diagnoses: extrapolations from a pediatric medicaid cohort. *Pediatrics* 2000;105(6):e72.

Bruderly, TE, Bojrab DI. Otitis externa. *J Osteopath Coll Ophthalmol Otorhinolaryngol* 1996;8(1):101–107.

Buchanan J, Hoagland J, Fischer, PR. Pseudoephedrine and air travel-associated ear pain in children. *Arch Pediatr Adolesc Med* 1999;153(5):466–468.

Carreiro JA. An *Osteopathic Approach to Children.* Edinburgh: Churchill Livingstone. Elsevier Science Limited, 2003.

Casselbrandt ML, Mandel EM, Fall PA, et al. The heritability of otitis media: a Twin and Triplet Study. *JAMA* 1999;282(22):2125–2130.

Caye-Thomasen P, Schmidt PT, Hermansson A, et al. Depletion of mucosal substance P in acute otitis media. *Acta ototolaryngol* 2004;124:794–797.

Center for Disease Control. US government recommended immunization schedule for persons aged 0–6 years. 2008, available at: http://www.cdc.gov/vaccines/recs/schedules/downloads/child/2008/08_0–6yrs_schedule_pr.pdf. (last accessed 05–08–08).

Centers S, Morelli MA, Vallad-Hix C, et al. General pediatrics. In: Ward R, ed. *Foundations for Osteopathic Medicine.* 2nd Ed. Lippincott Williams & Wilkins, 2003:315–316.

Charlett SD, Coatesworth AP. Referred otalgia: a structured approach to diagnosis and treatment. *Int J Clin Pract* 2007;61(6):1015–1021.

Clements DA, Langdon L, Bland C, et al. Influenza a vaccine decreases the incidence of otitis media in 6- to 30-month-old children in day care. *Arch Pediatr Adolesc Med* 1995;149:1113–1117.

Crapko M, Kerschner JE, Syring M, et al. Role of extra-esophageal reflux in chronic otitis media with effusion. *Laryngoscope* 2007;117:1419–1423.

Danish SF, Zager EL. Cervical spine meningioma presenting as otalgia: case report. *Neurosurgery* 2005;56(3):e621.

Degenhardt BF, Kuchera ML. The prevalence of cranial dysfunction in children with a history of otitis media from kindergarten to third grade. *J Am Osteopathic Assoc* 1994;September:10.

Degenhardt BJ, Kuchera ML. Osteopathic evaluation and manipulative treatment in reducing the morbidity of otitis media: a pilot study. *J Am Osteopath Assoc* 2006:106(6);327–334.

Doyle WJ. A functional anatomic description of Eustachian tube vector relations in four ethnic populations: and osteologic study. Ph.D. dissertation. University of Pittsburgh, Pittsburgh, PA 1977.

Eisenberg DM, Kessler RC, Foster C, et al. Unconventional medicine in the United State: prevalence, costs, and patterns of use. *New Engl J Med* 1993;328:246–252.

Ernst E. Serious adverse effects of unconventional therapies for children and adolescents: a systematic review of recent evidence. *Eur J Pediatr* 2003;162:72–80.

Eyman RK, Grossman HJ, Chaney RH, et al. The life expectancy of profoundly handicapped people with mental retardation. *N Engl J Med* 1990;323(9):584–589.

Fagnan LJ. Acute sinusitis: a cost-effective approach to diagnosis and treatment. *Am Fam Phys* 1998;58(8):1795–802, 805–806.

Frei H, Thurneysen A. Homeopathy in acute otitis media in children: treatment effect or spontaneous resolution? *Br Homeopath J* 2001;90:180–182.

Frymann VM. Relation of disturbance of craniosacral mechanism to symptomatology of the newborn: study of 1250 infants. *J Am Osteopath Assoc* 1966;65:1059–1075.

Frymann VM. *The Collected Papers of viola M. Frymann, DO: Legacy of Osteopathy to Children.* American Academy of Osteopathy, 1998.

Galbreath WO. Chronic catarrhal otitis media. *J Am Osteopath Assoc* 1928;April:639.

Gibson WS, Cochran W. Otalgia in infants and children—a manifestation of gastroesophageal reflux. *Int J Pediatr Otorhinolaryngol* 1994;28:213–218.

Goldenberg DL, Fibromyalgia syndrome: an emerging but controversial condition. *JAMA* 1987;257(20):2782–2787.

Hayes NM, Bezilla TA. Incidence of iatrogenesis associated with osteopathic manipulative treatment of pediatric patients. *J Am Osteopath Assoc* 2006;106(10):605–608.

Heatherington JS. Manipulation of the eustachian tube. *AAO J* 1995; (Winter):27–28.

Hoberman A, Greenberg DP, Paradise JL, et al. Effectiveness of inactivated influenza vaccine in preventing acute otitis media in young children. *JAMA* 2003;290(12):1608–1616.

Ijaduola TG. Acute otalgia in Nigerian children. *Trop Geogr Med* 1985;37(4):343–344.

Ingvarsson L. Acute otalgia in children—findings and diagnosis. *Acta Paediatr Scan* 1982;71:705–710.

Kemper KJ. Seven herbs every pediatrician should know. *Contemp Pediatr* 1996;13(12):79–93.

Kemper KJ. *The Holistic Pediatrician.* New York, NY: HarperCollins, 1996.

Kramer II, Kramer CM. The phantom earache: temporomandibular joint dysfunction in children. *Am J Dis Child* 1985;139:943–945.

LaGrone DH. Unusual cause of earache [Letters to the Editor]. *South Med J* 1984;77(4):538.

Lasisi AO, Olaniyan FA, Muibi SA, et al. Clinical and demographic risk factors associated with chronic suppurative otitis media. *Int J Pediatr Otorhinolaryngol* 2007;71:1549–1554.

LeLiever WC, Nonotologic otalgia [Letter]. *JAMA* 1990;260(17):2302.

Leung AKC, Fong JHS, Leong AG. Otalgia in children. *J Natl Med Assoc* 2000;92:254–260.

Magoun HI. *Osteopathy in the Cranial Field.* 3rd Ed. Kirksville, MO: Journal Printing Co., 1996.

Manzoni GC, Torelli P. Epidemiology of typical and atypical craniofacial neuralgias. *Neurolog Sci* 2005;S65–S67.

Marinella MA. Heparin-induced thrombocytopenia presenting as otalgia [Letters to the Editor]. *South Med J* 2007;100(10):1057.

Maw R, Wilks J, Harbey I, et al. Early surgery compared with watchful waiting for glue ear and effect on language development in preschool children: a randomized trial. *Lancet* 1999;353:960–963.

Menner AL. Top 10 clinical misjudgments in ear disorders. In: *A Pocket Guide to the Ear.* New York, NY: Thieme, 2003.

Mills MV, Henley CE, Barnes LLB, et al. The use of osteopathic manipulative treatment as adjuvant therapy in children with recurrent acute otitis media. *Arch Pediatr Adolesc Med* 2003;157:861–866.

Morgan LW. *Homeopathy and Your Child.* Rochester, VT: Healing Arts Press, 1992.

Murray RK. *Harper's Illustrate Biochemistry*. 27th Ed. Lange Medical Books/McGraw-Hill, 2006.

Nadig SK, Alderdice JM, Adair RA, et al. Eccrine spiradenoma: an unusual presentation with otalgia. *Otolaryngology-Head and Neck Surgery.* 2004(Feb):278.

Nagaraj BS, Linthicum FH. Autonomic innervation of the human middle ear: an immunohistochemical study. *American Journal of Otolaryngology* 1998; 19(2):75–82.

Ologe FE, Dunmade AD, Afolabi OA. Aural foreign bodies in children. *The Indian Journal of Pediatrics.* 2007; 74(8):755–758.

Papay FA, Levine HL, Schiavone WA. Facial fuzz and funny findings: Facial hair causing otalgia and oropharyngeal pain. *Cleve Clin J Med* 1989 May; 56(3):273–276.

Paradise JL, Feldman HM, Campbell TF, et al. Effect of Early or Delayed Insertion of Tympanostomy tubes for Persistent Otitis Media on Developmental Outcomes at the Age of Three Years. *N Engl J Med* 2001; 344(16);1179–1187.

Paradise JL, Feldman HM, Campbell TF, et al. Tympanostomy tubes and developmental outcomes at 9 to 11 years of age. *N Engl J Med* 2007;56(3): 248–261.

Pertes RA. Differential diagnosis of orofacial pain. *Mt Sinai J* 1998;65: 348–354.

Pill MW. Applications of disease benchmarks and case presentations. *J Manage Care Pharm* 2005;11(1, suppl A):S12–S18.

Pintal WJ, Kurtz ME. An integrated osteopathic approach in acute otitis media. *J Am Osteopath Assoc* 1989;89(9):1139–1141.

Prellner K, Kalm O, Harsten G. The concept of pronicity in otitis media. *Otolaryngolog Clin N Am* 1991;24(4):787–794.

Rovers MM, Glasziou P, Appelman CL, et al. Antibiotics for acute otitis media: a meta-analysis with individual patient data. *Lancet* 2006;368:1429–1435.

Rovers MM, Numans ME, Langenbach E, et al. Is pacifier use a risk factor for acute otitis media? A dynamic cohort study. *Fam Pract* 2008;25:233–236.

Sarrell EM, Cohen HA, Kahan E. Naturopathic treatment for ear pain in children. *Pediatrics* 2003;111:e574–e579.

Scarbrough TJ, Day TA, Williams TE, et al. Referred otalgia in head and neck cancer: a unifying schema. *Am J Clin Oncol* 2003;26(5):e157–e161.

Schmidt MA. *Childhood Ear Infections: What Every Parent and Physician Should Know About Prevention, Home Care, and Alternative Treatment.* Berkeley, CA: North Atlantic Books, 1990.

Schmidt I. Osteopathic manipulative therapy as a primary factor in the management of upper, middle, and pararespiratory infections. *J Am Osteopath Assoc* 1982;81(6):382–88.

Sergueef N. *Cranial Osteopathy for Infants, Children and Adolescents.* Edinburgh, UK: Churchill Livingstone Elsevier, 2007.

Sexton S, Natale R. Risks and benefits of pacifiers. *Am Fam Phys* 2009;79: 681–685.

Shah RK, Blevins NH. Otalgia. *Otolarygololog Clin N Am* 2003;36(6):1137–1151.

Simons DG, Travell JG, Simons LS, *Myofascial Pain and Dysfunction: The trigger Point Manual, Volume 1, Upper Half of Body.* 2nd Ed. Baltimore, MD: Williams & Wilkins, 1999.

Slatosky J, Shipton B, Wahba H. Thyroiditis: differential diagnosis and management. *Am Fam Phys* 2000;61(4):1047–1052, 1054.

Sohn SJ. Substance P upregulates osteoclastogenesis by activating nuclear factor kappa B in osteoclast precursors. *Acta Otolaryngolog* 2005;125(2):130–133.

Sorrel M. *Osteopathic Treatment and Ear Infections.* American Academy of Osteopathy, Reprinted with permission from the author, Margaret Sorrel, DO, FCA. Indianapolis, IN: Moeller Printing, 2004.

Spiro DM, Tay KY, Arnold DH, et al. Wait-and-see prescription for the treatment of acute otitis media. *JAMA* 2006;296(10):1235–1241.

Still AT. *Osteopathy: Research and Practice.* Seattle, WA: Eastland Press, 1910.

Still AT. *Philosophy of Osteopathy.* Kirksville, MO: A. T. Still publisher, 1899.

Tasker A, Dettmar PW, Panetti M, et al. Is gastric reflux a cause of otitis media with effusion in children? *Laryngoscope* 2002;112:1930–1934.

Teitelbaum JE, Deantonis KO, Kahan S. *Pediatric Signs and Symptoms in a Page.* Malden, MA: Blackwell Publishing, 2004.

Teodorczyk-Injeyan JA, Injeyan HS, Ruegg R. Spinal manipulative therapy reduces inflammatory cytokines but not substance P production in normal subjects. *J Manipulative Physiol Ther* 2006;29(1):14–21.

Thoeny HC, Beer KT, Vock P, et al. Ear pain in patients with oropharynx carcinoma: how MRI contributes to the explanation of a prognostic and predictive symptom. *Eur Radiol* 2004;14:2206–2211.

Tully SB, Bar-Haim Y, Bradley RL. Abnormal tympanography after supine bottle feeding. *J Pediatr* 1995;126:S105–S111.

Ward RC, Ed. *Foundations for Osteopathic Medicine.* 2nd Ed. Philadelphia, PA: Lippincott Williams & Wilkins, 2003.

Wetmore RE. *Pediatric Otolaryngology: The Requisites in Pediatrics.* Philadelphia PA: Mosby Elsevier, 2007.

Woods, R. Osteopathic care of neonates and children. *Osteopath Ann* 1976;34(4):512–515.

Yount KA. Atypical earache and otomandibular symptoms. *Pract Pain Manage* 2004;4(6).

Zaidat OO, Ubogu EE. Otalgia as the sole presenting manifestation of subdural hematoma. *Am J Otolaryngol* 2002;23(3):177–180.

Zenian J. Pillow otalgia [letter] *Arch Otolarygolo Head Neck Surg* 2001;127:1288.

59

Difficulty Breathing

WILLIAM FOLEY, HUGH ETTLINGER, GILBERT D'ALONZO, AND JANE CARREIRO

KEY CONCEPTS

- Most acute exacerbations of chronic obstructive pulmonary disease (COPD) are preceded by an infection, either viral or bacterial. The patient typically reports worsening cough and chest congestion, increased sputum production, and dyspnea.
- Obstructive diseases such as COPD require the patients to alter their mechanics of breathing by engaging accessory muscles causing hypertrophy, which alters biomechanics this creates somatic dysfunction.
- Patients with obstructive diseases such as asthma and COPD have restricted movement of the thoracic tissues during the exhalation phase of respiration, potentially reducing local drainage of lymph from the small airways and central lymph drainage through the thoracic duct.
- Bronchospasm and mucous production, the two main pathophysiologic events of asthma and COPD, are mediated through the vagus nerve.
- Smoking cessation is essential for respiratory health.
- Regular osteopathic manipulative treatment visits focused on facilitating normal posture and function may assist in reducing metabolic energy requirements.

CASE VIGNETTE

Chief Complaint:

A 71-year-old man presents to your office with a 3-day history of shortness of breath, fever, wheezing, chest congestion, and a nonproductive cough, requiring more than usual inhaled albuterol to help his breathing.

History of Present Illness:

He inhales tiotropium every morning and fluticasone and salmeterol every 12 hours each day and usually is comfortable from a pulmonary standpoint. He has never required home oxygen therapy. However, over the last few days, his symptoms have worsened and he currently feels out of breath while doing routine activities. He denies chest pain and diaphoresis. Just 3 months ago, he was admitted to the hospital for an exacerbation of his chronic obstructive pulmonary disease (COPD).

Past Medical/Surgical History:

stable angina pectoris, gastroesophageal reflux disease, essential hypertension and a left inguinal herniorrhaphy 20 years ago.

Medications:

tiotropium 1 inhalation daily, salmeterol/fluticasone 250/50 1 inhalation every 12 hours, omeprazole 20 mg daily, amlodipine 10 mg daily, and lisinopril 10 mg daily.

Allergies:

none.

Social History:

100 pack-year history of tobacco use, presently ½ pack of cigarettes each day. He admits to rarely drinking alcohol and he has never used illicit drugs.

Physical Exam:

Vital Signs:

HR: 100 beats/min, RR: 24 breaths/min, BP: 180/90 mm Hg, and pulse oximetry O_2 saturation: 89% while breathing room air

General:

Mildly ill and has frequent paroxysm of coughing. He does not have lower extremity edema.

HEENT:

Normal. There is no thrush.

Heart:

Heart rate tachycardic and cardiac rhythm is regular. No murmur or gallop is auscultated. Jugular vein distension was not found.

Lungs:

Diffuse bilateral expiratory wheezing, decreased breath sounds, and poor air movement. Significant accessory muscle use with respiration without paradoxical thoracoabdominal breathing was noted. Mild lower intercostals space muscle retractions were seen.

Abdomen:

Soft and nontender without hepatospenomegaly. Bowel sounds are normal.

Structural Exam:

Reveals left ilium posterior, left SI restriction, general decrease in side bending, and rotation throughout lumbars with L1-3 flattening of normal lordosis. The thoracic spine has a significantly reduced range of motion during sidebending and rotation especially between T5-10. T10 is in a flexed position, sidebent, and rotated to the right. T5 is in an extended position, sidebent, and rotated to the right. T2 is also extended but sidebent and rotated to the left. There is decreased rib compliance throughout the rib cage with reduced excursion during the exhalation phase of respiration. Chest is barrel shaped. C7 is flexed, sidebent, and rotated to the left. C2 is extended, sidebent, and rotated to the right. The right occipitoatlantal articulation has restricted motion mechanics. The sternocleidomastoid and scalene muscles are tense and hypertrophied bilaterally. Diaphragm excursion is decreased during inhalation by percussion, and there is decreased motion in the lower ribs.

DIFFERENTIAL DIAGNOSIS

The differential diagnosis of dyspnea with hypoxemia for this patient (Box 59.1) includes COPD, bronchiectasis, pulmonary embolism, pneumonia, and congestive heart failure, and it is possible that more than one condition is present.

Any patient presenting with dyspnea must be stabilized from both a respiratory and hemodynamic standpoint before a more thorough history and examination are conducted. This patient uses accessory respiratory muscles at rest, clearly demonstrating that he is working very hard to breathe. The patient was immediately placed on nasal cannula O_2, and pulse oximetry was used to carefully monitor an improvement in oxygenation. The use of O_2 in a patient with COPD should be monitored closely because of the risk of CO_2 retention or hypercapnea. An office electrocardiogram (EKG) was done, which showed sinus tachycardia. The EKG showed low voltage but no ischemic abnormalities. At this point, the patient was transferred by ambulance to the closest emergency department where he was placed on telemetry. The supplemental O_2 via nasal cannula was continued and nebulized bronchodilator therapy was initiated.

The initial work-up for the complaint of dyspnea should include a chest x-ray (posterior-anterior and lateral views), EKG, and several blood studies (arterial blood gas, complete blood count and differential, serum electrolytes, creatinine, and blood urea nitrogen). This initial work-up will determine if the cause is cardiac, pulmonary, metabolic, or due to anemia. With these data, a more focused, in depth work-up can be pursued (Box 59.2).

The patient's chest x-ray revealed hyperinflated lungs without a lung infiltrate (Fig. 59.1). His hemoglobin and hematocrit are normal, but there was leukocytosis (14,000) without band forms. No metabolic derangement was identified. Arterial blood gas results showed normal acid base balance and moderate hypoxemia, without hypercapnia (Fig. 59.2). These results were used to reduce the initial differential diagnosis to the most likely diagnosis of COPD exacerbation.

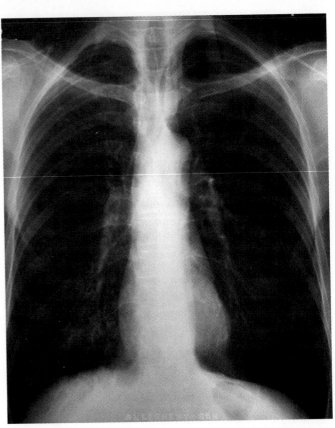

Figure 59-1   COPD. Frontal **(A)** and lateral radiographs show hyperinflation with flattening of the diaphragm **(B)**. In **A,** note the vertical appearance of the heart, which is compressed by the over-inflated lungs.

Differential Diagnosis for Dyspnea with Hypoxemia in an Elderly Male with a History of COPD and Cardiovascular Disease

Exacerbation of COPD
Bronchiectasis
Pulmonary embolism
Pneumonia
Congestive heart failure

Initial Work-up for Patient with Dyspnea and Hypoxemia, Once They are Stabilized

Chest x-ray (posterior-anterior and lateral views)
EKG
Arterial blood gas
Complete blood count with differential
Serum electrolytes
Creatinine
Blood urea nitrogen

Arterial Blood Gas Interpretation Reference			
Normal range: pH 7.35 - 7.45, PaCO₂ 35 - 45 mm Hg, PaO₂ 80 - 100 mm HG, HCO₃ 22 - 26 mEg/L			
Disorder	**pH**	**Primary disturbance**	**Compensation**
Respiratory acidosis	↓	↑PCO₂	↑HCO₃
Respiratory alkalosis	↑	↓PCO₂	↓HCO₃
Metabolic acidosis	↓	↓HCO₃	↓PCO₂
Metabolic alkalosis	↑	↑HCO₃	↑PCO₂

Figure 59-2   Arterial blood gas interpretation.

Medications were begun and included ceftriaxone 1 gm i.v. daily, nebulized ipratropium 0.5 mg, and albuterol 2.5 mg every 6 hours, and methylprednisolone 40 mg i.v. every 6 hours. Supplemental oxygen was continued and an additional albuterol treatment could be given every 2 hours for breathing distress.

Most acute exacerbations of COPD are preceded by an infection, either viral or bacterial. The patient typically reports worsening cough and chest congestion, increased sputum production, and dyspnea. Tachypnea and hypoxemia are common findings. The chest radiograph may show signs of infiltrate (concomitant community-acquired pneumonia or bronchiectasis), and often there are findings consistent with lung hyperinflation (flat diaphragm, hyperlucent lungs, and increased retrosternal air space). Sputum cultures and CT of the chest may be necessary if the clinical picture remains unclear.

COPD patients often have substantial musculosketetal findings on examination, and they can benefit from a carefully planned osteopathic treatment program that involves both pharmacologic and nonpharmacologic interventions.

OSTEOPATHIC PATIENT MANAGEMENT

Biomechanical Model

Breathing is in large part a mechanical process. Changes in intrathoracic pressures involve contraction and relaxation of skeletal musculature that are attached to the spine and bony thorax. These motions, during inspiration and expiration, produce pressure gradients within the thorax and between the thoracic and abdominal cavities. This process is critical for respiration and the movement of fluids throughout the body. A detailed review of these mechanics will offer insight as to how osteopathic treatment may improve the efficiency and effectiveness of breathing for patients that are experiencing an acute exacerbation of COPD. A recent pilot study (Noll et al., 2008) suggests there is a role for osteopathic manipulative treatment (OMT) in the management of COPD patients.

The physical action of producing a negative intrathoracic pressure requires a definable amount of energy, referred to as the work of breathing. Although difficult to quantify, increased work of breathing is clinically relevant, since many pulmonary diseases dramatically alter the work of breathing. An increase in the work of breathing is an important factor in the pathophysiology of all lung diseases (West, 1992). In the pathophysiology of asthma and COPD, patients can progress to respiratory failure due to an inability to maintain adequate ventilation and oxygenation because of respiratory muscle fatigue and eventual exhaustion. Failure of the thoracic pump may be due to severe airflow obstruction and thoracic hyperinflation, both of which develop as a result of obstructive air trapping within the lung. Thoracic hyperinflation places the entire pump at a mechanical disadvantage increasing muscle workload and the potential for muscle fatigue. Any intervention that can improve airflow and reduce hyperinflation will delay the onset of muscle fatigue and respiratory failure.

The mechanical process of breathing involves tissue compliance and recoil. Compliance is the ease with which tissues are stretched during inhalation. Recoil involves the elastic ability of the lung parenchyma to passively contract during exhalation. Respiratory system compliance has at least two components, lung tissue and chest wall, that make up the total thoracic compliance. Lung tissue compliance is reduced in disease processes that are infiltrative or restrictive such as pneumonias or effusions. Lung recoil is affected by the structure of the lung parenchyma. Conditions that destroy or alter the structure of the parenchyma can affect recoil and interfere

with the ability of the lung tissue to expel air. In COPD, the ability of the lung to expel air is compromised. The increased residual volume and decreased O_2 levels damage the delicate alveoli wall. Adjacent alveoli sacs coalesce forming larger tertiary spaces, as a result the surface area of the lung is decreased and there is less area available for gas exchange. This condition is called emphysema (Fig. 59.3). The damage to the parenchyma increases the compliance but decreases the elastic recoil properties of the lung. The subsequent tendency for air trapping increases the workload of both expiratory and inspiratory muscles; expiratory muscles are engaged in an attempt to decrease residual lung volumes, while inspiratory muscles must now work against the increased residual alveoli volume. Consequently, there is an overall increase in the work of breathing.

Obstructive diseases such as COPD require patients to alter their mechanics of breathing by engaging accessory muscles that are not continuously used in a healthy person. The respiratory muscles hypertrophy in response to the increased workload. Muscle hypertrophy alters biomechanics and creates somatic dysfunction. Somatic dysfunction can reduce the compliance of the bony thorax, alter respiratory biomechanics, and further increase the work of breathing. Thus, a vicious cycle is created whereby patients with COPD are compromised in their ability to meet their respiratory demands.

Somatic dysfunction of the thoracic spine and ribs is often found in patients with lung disease (Beal and Morlock, 1984). The shape of the thorax in patients with COPD who have emphysema with hyperinflation (barrel chest) can produce dramatic changes in

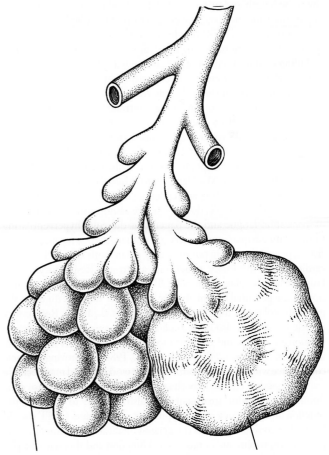

Normal alveoli   Overinflated alveoli (bullae)

Figure 59-3 Schematic diagram depicting normal alveoli and alveoli in COPD.

chest wall compliance, which are obvious on osteopathic structural exam. In addition to the specific dysfunctions noted in association with pulmonary disease, this altered chest wall compliance may contribute to patients' respiratory dysfunction. General osteopathic manipulative techniques may be used to address these thoracic compliance issues, in combination with more specific techniques for individual somatic dysfunctions. Osteopathic treatment to improve the compliance of the thorax may not necessarily directly alter the parenchymal pathology, especially in those with chronic lung disease. However, it should improve the comfort and work of breathing and perhaps exercise tolerance, providing patients with the ability to enhance their functional capacity. Reducing the work of breathing during exercise has been shown to improve exercise tolerance of the chronic lung patient (West, 1995).

As noted, in addition to general changes in compliance of the bony thorax, specific somatic dysfunctions may have an effect on the function of the respiratory mechanism that goes beyond the changes in compliance they invariably produce. The movement of a typical rib during breathing operates in conjunction with the orientation of its costotransverse and costovertebral joints. Rotation of the thoracic vertebrae with somatic dysfunction will not only create resistance to movement but also change the orientation of the costotransverse and costovertebral articulations, further impairing the ability of the muscles for inhalation to move the rib. With rotation of thoracic vertebral units involved in somatic dysfunction, a rib with a predominantly bucket-handle movement might become oriented to move more like a pump-handle movement. Lumbar somatic dysfunction, particularly in the upper lumbar spine, likely alters the length and orientation of the diaphragm crura and could impair their function and the contraction of the diaphragm.

Angus Cathie (1974) has described the movement of the entire spine with respiration. During inhalation all spinal curves straighten, including counternutation of the sacrum with the base moving posteriorly. Reverse movements occur with exhalation. Somatic dysfunction anywhere in the body may adversely affect breathing.

Increases in work of breathing contribute to respiratory muscle fatigue. Respiratory muscle fatigue has been implicated in the pathophysiology of respiratory failure (McKenzie and Bellemare, 1995; Rossi et al., 2002). Obstructive diseases like COPD may produce respiratory muscle fatigue because of the effects of lung hyperinflation (Roussos and Macklem, 1986). Muscular fatigue may be one of the factors contributing to the demise of the patient with respiratory failure. For example, during a severe asthma attack, the muscles of inspiration fatigue and the patient has difficulty hyperventilating to maintain adequate pulmonary gas exchange. As a result, progressive hypercapnia and hypoxemia may occur both of which lead to cardiovascular instability, arrhythmia, and death. Respiratory muscle fatigue may also play a role in COPD and has led to the identification of the potential role of chronic respiratory muscle fatigue in the pathophysiology of lung disease (Grassino et al., 1984). Respiratory muscle fatigue has also been implicated in diverse problems such as pulmonary edema and difficulties weaning patients off mechanical ventilation (Cohen, 1982; Grassino et al., 1984). Improving thoracic compliance will reduce respiratory muscle workload and may decrease the likelihood of fatigue in both acute and chronic lung disease conditions. Osteopathic treatment may also be used to improve the function and efficiency of the respiratory musculature. OMT should be used in conjunction with the general medical management of the patient. Improvements in mechanical function and thoracic compliance may decrease the need for bronchodilators and steroids. As the patient's respiratory function improves, the ability to clear mucous by coughing may also improve, eliminating the need for expectorants and potentially decreasing airway resistance. Incorporating manipulative

treatment into the care of a patient with COPD may allow the physician to decrease the need for pharmaceutical interventions, and the risks and complications associated with the use of these agents.

Respiratory muscles, like all skeletal muscle, operate on the principle of their length-tension relationship. In this relationship, muscles will develop a far stronger contraction at a longer resting tone. Physical changes associated with exacerbations of obstructive lung disease such as a flattened diaphragm (as visualized on x-ray) and hypertonicity of accessory muscles, such as the sternocleidomastoid, represent shortened musculature that have reduced contractile force during increased workload. In the case of chronic obstructive lung disease, the barrel-type changes in the thorax actually prevent respiratory muscles during inspiration from returning to their full resting length during exhalation. Likewise, increased muscle tonicity may prevent the thorax from achieving a position of complete exhalation, contributing to the overall shape change of the thorax. In addition to altering muscle length-tension relationships, increasing the resting tone of the respiratory musculature will alter its blood supply and oxygen delivery/consumption ratio. Muscles receive most of their blood supply during their resting or diastolic phase. The increased tone during contraction increases the pressure within the muscle and shunts blood away via nonnutritive arterioles. This has been demonstrated to occur in the diaphragm (Grassino et al., 1984). It has also been shown that increased demand in an otherwise normal diaphragm will produce oxygen consumption that is in excess of its supply (Grassino et al., 1984). Increasing the resting tone of a muscle will increase its pressure and reduce incoming blood supply, while simultaneously increasing its oxygen demand, further stressing the oxygen delivery/consumption ratio. Muscles that are forced to function anaerobically are as much as 15 times less efficient than those utilizing aerobic metabolism (West, 1991). Fatigued diaphragms have been found to have high levels of lactic acid, indicating a high degree of anaerobic metabolism (Grassino et al., 1984). Increased resting tone of the respiratory musculature during inspiration can be identified during the osteopathic structural exam as increased muscle tone, generalized tenderness, or tissue bogginess. Osteopathic treatment directed toward increasing the length and decreasing the resting tone of respiratory musculature is indicated in the treatment of acute and chronic lung disease. The diaphragm in particular is prone to increases in tone and associated flattening in acute and chronic obstructive disease. If severe enough, the flattening of the diaphragm may reverse the movement of the lower ribs during inspiration, producing paradoxical rib motion. This reduces the transverse diameter of the chest and greatly decreases the efficiency of the entire respiratory mechanism. In osteopathic literature, restoration of the length and vertical orientation of the diaphragm is called doming of the diaphragm. Doming of a flattened diaphragmatic muscle will increase the pressure gradients that are able to be produced between the thoracic and abdominal regions and can help reverse paradoxical rib motion and improve the function of the diaphragm as well as the respiratory mechanism as a whole. Addressing the mechanics of breathing, including the work of breathing, the compliance of the thorax and spine, both specifically and generally, and the function and efficiency of the respiratory musculature will have far-reaching applications in the treatment of acute and chronic respiratory diseases.

Respiratory/Circulatory Model

Traditionally, the osteopathic concept has viewed the cervicothoracic, thoracolumbar, and pelvic diaphragms as working together to maintain pressure gradients in the pelvis, abdomen, and thorax

(Frymann, 1968, Johnson, 1991, 1992; Zink and Lawson, 1979). These gradients aid in fluid movement through the venous and lymphatic systems, often referred to as the low pressure circulatory system. The actions of the diaphragm, and thorax in particular, have a major influence on the function of the lymphatic and venous systems. This is the basis of the "respiratory/circulatory" model. Zink's original model (Zink, 1977) describes the role of respiration, with its action on central venous flow and pressure, as they influence the emptying of the thoracic duct into the junction of the internal jugular and brachiocephalic veins. Studies that have measured the role of respiration on thoracic duct lymph flow demonstrate that 35% to 60% of the total thoracic duct drainage is in response to respiratory movements (Aukland and Reed, 1993; Browse et al., 1971; Dumont, 1975). Thorax motion during respiration has also been shown to be involved in the actual formation of lymph in a variety of areas, including the lungs and abdomen. Lymph formation is a critical step in the overall mechanics of lymphatic circulation, as a small but significant uphill hydrostatic gradient exists that must be overcome in order for fluid to move from the interstitium into the initial lymphatic, a blind, open-ended vessel (Aukland and Reed, 1993). The excursion of the thorax has been shown to be the primary force moving fluid from the pulmonary interstitium into the initial pulmonary lymphatics. The expansion of the pulmonary interstitial tissue, to which the initial lymphatics are tethered by anchoring filaments, increases the volume of the initial lymphatic flow and produces a temporary pressure gradient for filling these small lymphatics. Exhalation then closes the vessel and moves the lymph forward, past the first valve and into the contractile part of the vessel. The respiratory cycle, then, acts as a pump that initiates the process of lymph formation. All initial lymphatics have anchoring filaments and will therefore respond to respiratory movements to the degree which they occur in the area. The initial lymphatics in the abdomen and pelvis, in particular, respond significantly to respiratory excursions. Lymphatic stomata located in the subperitoneal space of the diaphragm are also involved in the absorption of intra-abdominal fluids. Respiratory movements in the diaphragm act to open and close the mesothelial and endothelial cells assisting lymph flow into the collecting lymph vessels (Bettendorf, 1978).

The clinical significance of the respiratory-circulatory concept in pulmonary disease is likely very important and underestimated. Obstructive lung diseases are associated with inflammation of various pulmonary tissues (Fig. 59.4). Asthma and COPD patients have an overall restriction of thoracic movement during the exhalation phase of respiration, reducing both local drainage of lymph from the small airways and central lymph drainage through the thoracic duct. During an obstructive exacerbation, perhaps initiated by lobar pneumonia or acute bronchitis, there is an intrapulmonary inflammatory process produced that will produce an increased demand on the regional lymphatic circulation. The excursion of the thorax, however, is consistently and significantly reduced by the exacerbation. This restriction in movement leads to a reduction in local drainage of exudates, a decrease in the delivery of antigen to regional lymph nodes, and perhaps impairment in both the cellular immunological response and the transport of antibiotics to the affected areas since lung interstitial pressure rises and shunts blood away from the area. Restoring a greater excursion of the thorax will improve the body's ability to move lymph in this situation; specific lymph pump techniques are also indicated.

Neurologic Model

Autonomic nervous system influences are important in a variety of lung diseases. Vagal activity is involved in the bronchospasm and

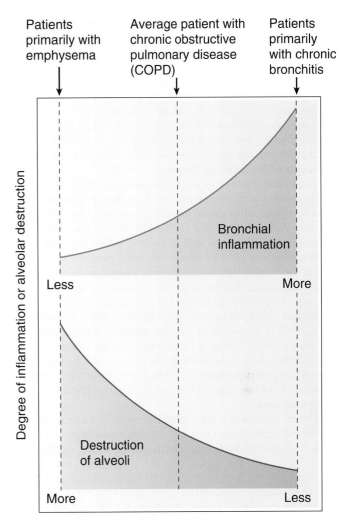

Figure 59-4 The relationship between emphysema and chronic bronchitis. Most patients with COPD have a mixture of bronchial inflammation and alveolar destruction.

mucous production in the pathophysiology of asthma and COPD. C2 somatic dysfunction has been consistently noted in diagnostic studies of pulmonary disease (Beal, 1985). Ipsilateral cranial base dysfunction, in particular the occipitomastoid articulation, is usually involved in reflexes involving the vagus nerve. The sensory ganglion of the vagus nerve lies within the jugular foramen, adjacent to the occipitomastoid suture. Though the cervical findings are reported less frequently than upper thoracic, this may be because the vagus and other parasympathetic nerves will not vasodilate or stimulate sweat glands, producing the associated temperature and skin moisture changes that are among the most common recognizable signs of acute segmental facilitation. It is therefore possible that segments facilitated in areas of parasympathetic innervation are under-recognized. Upper cervical findings in pulmonary disease, especially asthma and COPD, may be the most significant structural findings, due to the pathological effects of segmental facilitation of the vagus nerve in this disease. Perrin Wilson (1946) also notes a consistent finding of right T4-5 and right 4th or 5th rib somatic dysfunctions, another common finding in asthmatic patients. He reported significant improvement in acute asthmatic attacks with OMT of these dysfunctions.

Enhanced vagal tone plays a role in producing bronchospasm and airway secretions (Paggiaro et al., 1989; Szekely and Pataki, 2009). Sensitization or facilitation of the vagus as a result of somatic dysfunction at C2, the occipitomastoid suture or the cranial base may contribute to vagal tone and increase the degree of bronchospasm and secretion. Reducing segmental facilitation may decrease vagal tone and influence bronchospasm. This is turn has the potential to decrease bronchial sensitivity, reduce the need for bronchodilators, and help reduce the severity of an acute attack. Vagal reflex somatic dysfunction should be identified and treated in patients with pulmonary diseases.

A different type of somatic dysfunction is present when pneumonia coexists with the obstructive lung disease. Pneumonia is often accompanied by a local reduction in rib excursion. This dysfunction pattern is described as "barrel chest" in standard physical diagnosis textbooks as well as the osteopathic literature. This phenomenon may be a viscerosomatic reflex carried through visceral afferents, although the dysfunction levels in lower lobe pneumonia are outside the levels of the sympathetic innervation of the lung classically described as T1-5 (Beal and Morlock, 1984; Richardson, 1979; Sato, 1995; Widdicombe, 1991; Wojtarowicz et al., 2003) It is more likely they are produced through the parietal pleura, which carries a local, intercostal innervation. These reflex changes may be involved in the pleuritic chest pain, which often accompanies pneumonia. Treatment of these reflex changes is thought to be important in the overall treatment plan of patients with pneumonia.

Upper thoracic findings associated with pulmonary disease (T1-5, and occasionally T6) are commonly found in patients with acute and chronic bronchitis (Beal and Morlock, 1984). This is consistent with the notion that the primary afferent sensory innervation of the large airways travels via visceral afferent fibers associated with the sympathetic nerves (Cervero, 1985), while the sensory innervation of the small airways (asthma, COPD, lobar pneumonia) travels predominantly via the vagus. While sympathetic outflow may not be as detrimental to pulmonary function as

vagal influence, sympathetic firing may increase the production of the thick, tenacious secretions associated with bronchitis that are difficult to expectorate (Bleecker, 1986). The associated thoracic segmental dysfunction will result in further restriction of the upper thorax and ribs further reducing the ability of the patient to expectorate secretions and should be treated when found.

Costochondritis as well as pectoralis tenderpoints can develop from chronic cough. Osteopathic manipulation to ribs, sternum, thoracic vertebrae, and chest musculature can resolve myofascial and ligamentous articular strains thereby decreasing pain.

Metabolic Energy Model

For COPD patients, physicians need to be acquainted with the metabolic challenges the patient may face. For example, protein-calorie malnutrition is common in severe COPD. High caloric supplements or appetite stimulants can be considered but have not shown long-term benefits. In addition, altered or restricted gait has been shown to increase oxygen demand. Regular OMT visits focused on facilitating normal posture and function may assist in reducing metabolic energy requirements. Once the patient is stable, comprehensive pulmonary rehabilitation should be considered to improve quality of life and exercise capacity. There is a large body of data on the benefits of pulmonary rehabilitation for patients with COPD and other respiratory diseases that you may wish to discuss.

Behavioral Model

Shortness of breath caused by lung disease is a major source of anxiety (Fig. 59.5). Increased sympathetic tone may exacerbate vasoconstriction and bronchial constriction. Stress and anxiety may be higher in patients of lower socioeconomic status. Physicians should have appropriate knowledge of their patients' ability to pay for their medications and meet other financial obligations that impact their health status. Smoking cessation is essential for

Figure 59-5 The cycle of anxiety and COPD symptoms.

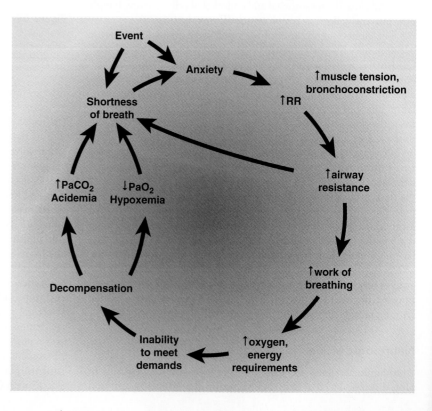

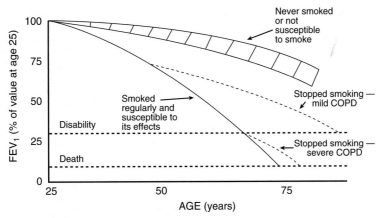

Figure 59-6 Effect of risk factors from smoking on loss of lung function (forced expiratory volume in the first second [FEV1]). Upper curves are derived from subjects who do not smoke or are not susceptible to the effects of smoking. They lose lung function gradually throughout adult life (15 to 30 mL/y). Lower curves show accelerated loss of lung function in subjects who are susceptible to the effects of cigarette smoke. At age 65 years there is respiratory disability because FEV1 has decreased to 25% to 30% of predicted (1 to 1.2 L), and further functional deterioration eventually will cause death because of complications of respiratory insufficiency. If the subject stops smoking, life may be prolonged but a respiratory death still eventually will result. If intervention is initiated earlier in life (age: 40 to 50 years) when COPD is mild, accelerated loss of lung function is reversible and a respiratory death will be prevented. Although this figure illustrates theoretical loss of FEV1 for an adult cigarette smoker, susceptible smokers will lose lung function at different rates, thereby becoming disabled at different ages. (Modified from Fletcher C, Peto R. The natural history of chronic airflow obstruction. *BMJ* 1977;1:1645, with permission.)

all patients and paramount for patients with COPD (Fig. 59.6). The best results are seen when counseling and medication therapy are combined (Sadr et al., 2009). Prevention of infection with the proper the use of vaccines, such as the pneumococcal and influenza vaccines, should be discussed with the patient annually.

PATIENT OUTCOME

The next day the patient had improved. He was now hemodynamically stable. Systemic steroid therapy and nebulized bronchodilator treatments were tapered over a 2-week period. Long-acting anticholinergic and beta-adrenergic inhalers and inhaled corticosteroid therapy was continued and pulmonary rehabilitation was recommended. Rib-raising and diaphragm-doming techniques were continued daily throughout his hospital stay. As he progressed, more focus was given to the cervical and lumbar areas using indirect,

balancing, and soft tissue techniques. The thoracic outlet was also treated to improve lymphatic flow through the thoracic duct. Both thoracic and pedal pumps were initiated and performed two to three times daily. After discharge from the hospital, the patient followed up for monthly OMT to maintain compliance of his thorax.

Suggested protocol for using OMT in the acute stage of a COPD exacerbation: focus the OMT on the ribs, thoracic spine, and diaphragm to reduce mechanical restrictions. Next, incorporate treatments that target the autonomic nervous system (Box 59.3). Start with indirect treatments such as myofascial release, balanced ligamentous tension, osteopathy in the cranial field, and FPR. As the exacerbation improves, more direct techniques such as HVLA and muscle energy are appropriate if no contraindications. A patient with a chronic condition such as COPD may benefit from OMT to prevent further acute exacerbations. The time interval for OMT is individualized and will depend on the patient, but generally speaking follow-up is usually every 1 to 4 months.

Suggested OMT Protocol for Treating Patients with COPD

Adapted from: Noll D, Degenhardt B, Johnson J, et al. Immediate effects of osteopathic manipulative treatment in elderly patients with chronic obstructive pulmonary disease *J Am Osteopath Assoc* 2008;108(5):251–259.

- Soft Tissue to the paraspinal muscles
- Rib raising
- Redoming the abdominal diaphragm (indirect myofascial release)
- Suboccipital decompression
- Thoracic inlet myofascial release
- Pectoral traction
- Thoracic lymphatic pump without activation

REFERENCES

Aukland K, and Reed RK. Interstitial mechanisms in the control of extracellular fluid volume. *Physiol Rev* 1993;73(1).

Beal MC, Morlock JW. Somatic dysfunction associated with pulmonary disease. *J Am Osteopath Assoc* 1984;84:179–183.

Beal MC. Viscerosomatic reflexes: a review. *J Am Osteopath Assoc* 1985;85(12): 53–68.

Bettendorf U. Lymph flow mechanism of the subperitoneal diaphragmatic lymphatics. *Lymphology* 1978;11:111–116

Bleecker ER. Cholinergic and neurogenic mechanisms in obstructive airways disease. *Am J Med* 1986;81:93–102.

Browse NL, et al. Pressure waves and gradients in the canine thoracic duct. *J Physiol* 1971;237:401–413.

Cathie A. Physiologic motions of the spine as related to respiratory activity. In: *American Academy of Osteopathy yearbook.* 1974;59–60.

Cervero F. Visceral nociception: peripheral and central aspects of visceral nociceptive systems. *Philos Trans R Soc Lond B Biol Sci* 1985;308:325–337.

Cohen C, et al. Clinical manifestations of inspiratory muscle fatigue. *Am J Med* 1982;73:308–316.

Dumont AE. The flow capacity of the thoracic duct-venous junction. *Am J Med Sci* 1975;269(3):292–301

Frymann VM. The core-link and the three diaphragms. In: *Year Book of Selected Osteopathic Papers*. Academy of Applied Osteopathy, v. NA, pt. NA, 1968:13–19

Grassino A, et al. Respiratory muscle fatigue and ventilatory failure. *Ann Rev Med* 1984;35:625–647.

Johnson K. An integrated approach for treating the OB patient: treating the five diaphragms of the body, part II. *AAO J Publ Am Acad Osteopath* 1992; 2(pt 1, spr):10–16

Johnson K. An integrated approach for treating the OB patient: treating the five diaphragms of the body, part I. *AAO J Publ Am Acad Osteopath* 1991; 1(pt 4 win):6–9.

Kopp MS, Skrabski A, Szekely A, et al. Chronic stress and social changes: socio-economic determination of chronic stress. *Ann N Y Acad Sci* 2007;1113: 325–338.

McKenzie DK, Bellemare F. Respiratory muscle fatigue. *Adv Exp Med Biol* 1995;384:401–414.

Noll D, Degenhardt B, Johnson J. Immediate effects of osteopathic manipulative treatment in elderly patients with chronic obstructive pulmonary disease. *J Am Osteopath Assoc* 2008;108(5):251–259.

Paggiaro PL, Bacci E, Pulera N, et al. Vagal reflexes and asthma. *Eur Respir J* 1989;suppl 6:502s–507s.

Richardson JB, 1979. Nerve supply to the lungs. *Am. Rev. Respir Dis* 119: 785–802.

Rossi A, Poggi R, Roca J. Physiologic factors predisposing to chronic respiratory failure. *Res Care Clin N Am* 2002;8:379–404.

Roussos C, Macklem, PT. Inspiratory muscle fatigue. *Handbook of Physiology, Section III, The Respiratory System; Volume III, The Mechanics of Breathing; Part II*. MD: American Physiological Society, 1986:521.

Sadr AO, Lindstrom D, Adami J, et al. The efficacy of a smoking cessation programme in patients undergoing elective surgery: a randomised clinical trial. *Anaesthesia* 2009;64:259–265.

Sato A. Somatoviceral reflexes. *J Manipulative Physiol Ther* 1995;18:597–602.

Szekely JI, Pataki A. Recent findings on the pathogenesis of bronchial asthma. Part I. Asthma as a neurohumoral disorder, a pathological vago-vagal axon reflex. *Acta Physiol Hung* 2009;96:1–17.

West JB, ed. *Best and Taylor's Physiologic Basis of Medical Practice*. 12th Ed. Baltimore: MD: Williams & Wilkins, 1991:95–96.

West JB. *Pulmonary Pathophysiology—The Essentials*. 4th Ed. Baltimore, MD: Williams & Wilkins, 1992:74.

West JB. *Respiratory Physiology, the Essentials*. 5th Ed. Baltimore, MD: Williams & Wilkins, 1995.

Widdicombe JG. Neural control of airway vasculature and edema. *Am Rev Respir Dis* 1991;143:S18–S21.

Wilson P. The osteopathic treatment of asthma. J Am Osteopath Assoc 1946;45(11):491–492.

Wojtarowicz A, Podlasz P, Czaja K. Adrenergic and cholinergic innervation of pulmonary tissue in the pig. *Folia Morphol (Warsz)* 2003;62:215–218.

Wright RJ, Subramanian SV, Advancing a multilevel framework for epidemiologic research on asthma disparities. *Chest* 2007;132:757S–769S.

Zink JG. Respiratory and circulatory care: the conceptual model. *Osteopath Ann* 1977; 5(pt 3):108–112.

Zink JG, Lawson WB. Pressure gradients in the osteopathic manipulative management of the obstetric patient. *Osteopath Ann* 1979;7(pt 5): 208–214.

60

Cervicogenic Headache

RAYMOND J. HRUBY, MARCEL P. FRAIX, AND REBECCA E. GIUSTI

KEY CONCEPTS

- Cervicogenic headache (CGH) has a precise clinical definition and a typical presentation.
- The pathophysiology of CGH has been elucidated.
- There is some evidence base for the use of osteopathic manipulative treatment in CGH using the five-model approach.
- Patients with CGH should receive thorough somatic evaluation.

CASE VIGNETTE

A 32-year-old right hand dominant Caucasian female presents to your clinic complaining of episodic headache type pain for the past 2 months. The pain has a pressure-like quality and is located in the bilateral occipital and frontal regions of the head. It lasts for approximately 30 minutes and primarily occurs in the morning. The headaches occur two to three times per week and appear to be more frequent when the patient experiences increased stress at work or lack of sleep. The patient was involved in a motor vehicle accident 3 years prior as a restrained passenger and did sustain a whiplash type of injury. She does not have a history of head trauma and currently denies experiencing photophobia, visual changes, or nausea.

Past Medical History:
Seasonal allergies

Past Surgical History:
Tonsillectomy at age 5 years, wisdom teeth extracted at age 26 years

Family History:
Her mother is 58 years old, and her father is 59 years old with a history of asthma. She has no siblings. There is no family history of migraine headaches.

Social History:
She is single, sexually active in a monogamous relationship for 3 years. She is employed as an administrative assistant. She does not use tobacco and uses coffee and alcohol only occasionally.

Medications:
She takes acetaminophen, two tablets every 2 to 4 hours as needed for pain, uses an antihistamine as needed for seasonal allergies, and takes oral contraceptive pills for birth control.

Allergies:
No history of drug or food allergies

REVIEW OF SYSTEMS
General:
She is in good health, exercises two times per week, and reports no recent change in appetite or weight, no fever or night sweats.

HEENT:
No sore throat or dysphagia, no sinusitis, no auditory changes, tinnitus or vertigo, seasonal allergies

Respiratory:
No cough or dyspnea

Cardiovascular:
No chest pain or palpitations

Nervous:
No sensory changes or motor weakness, no ataxia

Musculoskeletal:
Intermittent neck and upper back pain that occurs with prolonged sitting at work. No joint pain or swelling

PHYSICAL EXAM
Vital Signs:
Temperature 37°C, pulse 82/min and regular, respirations 12/min, blood pressure 128/84

General:
Well-nourished female in no acute distress, alert and oriented to person, place, and time

HEENT:
No signs of trauma, sclera clear, fundoscopic examination demonstrates sharp disc margins without papilledema, visual acuity is 20/20, auditory canals are clear, and tympanic membranes are intact. No nasal drainage is noted and the nasal septum is midline. The oropharynx reveals no exudates or erythema.

Respiratory:
No wheezes, rhonchi, or rales

Cardiovascular:
Regular and without murmurs

Neurological:
Cranial nerves II to XII are grossly intact, motor strength is 5/5, and reflexes are 2+/4+ bilaterally in upper and lower limbs. Sensation is intact to light touch and pinprick, and coordination is intact.

Osteopathic Structural Exam:

Cranial examination reveals restricted movement of the right occipitomastoid suture. The cervical spine demonstrates decreased active and passive ranges of motion in all planes, somewhat worse with right sidebending and rotation. The cervical paravertebral and upper trapezius musculature demonstrate increased tone with mild tenderness to palpation. Specific joint motion restrictions include: OA $R_R S_L$, AA R_R, C2-C3 $ER_L S_L$, T1-3 $R_R S_L$, T4-5 $ER_L S_L$, and a left sacral torsion around the left oblique sacral axis.

DIFFERENTIAL DIAGNOSIS

The differential diagnosis of headache includes the following:

- Cervicogenic headache (CGH)
- Occipital neuralgia
- Migraine and tension-type headache

A particularly difficult diagnostic challenge is distinguishing CGH from migraine without aura and tension-type headache. CGH must also be distinguished from other causes of headache that are more serious and potentially life threatening. These include the following:

- Arteriovenous malformation
- Cerebral aneurysm
- Chiari malformation
- Glaucoma
- Meningitis
- Posterior fossa tumors
- Pseudotumor cerebri
- Epidural, subdural, or subarachnoid hemorrhage
- Vasculitis, such as temporal arteritis
- Vertebral artery dissection

The absence of systemic signs such as fever, chills, etc. rules out infection pathology. Normal vital signs and the absence of neurological signs make tumor, pseudotumor, vertebral artery dissection, atriovenous malformation, vasculitis, and cerebral aneurysm less likely. There are no visual changes but intraocular pressures can be assessed to rule out glaucoma. There are also other causes of head pain that come from cervical pathology, although these are unlikely in this patient because of her age and presentation (Box 60.1).

The most likely differential diagnosis in this patient includes cervicogenic, migraine, or tension-type headache. These three entities are differentiated primarily by patient history. As described below; the most likely diagnosis for this patient is CGH.

Cervical Causes of Headache

A-V malformation
Cervical spondylosis
Greater occipital nerve compression or inflammation
Herniated cervical disc
Rheumatoid arthritis
Trauma
Tumors
Vasculitis
Vertebral artery dissection

OVERVIEW OF CERVICOGENIC HEADACHE

CGH may be defined as pain referred to the head region, typically unilaterally, from cervical musculoskeletal dysfunction. It is characterized by the presence of cervical somatic dysfunction as exhibited by muscle spasm, decreased range of motion, and pain upon digital provocation. It is usually worse with movement and better with rest. It can be associated with tendonitis in any of the cervical muscles, trigger points or tender points in the cervical or head region, and/or inflammation of the cervical spinal joints (1,2).

EPIDEMIOLOGY

Patients of all ages can be affected by this problem, with the mean age being 42.9 years (3). CGH is four times more common in females than males (4) and accounts for 14% to 18% of all chronic and recurrent headaches (5,6). It is a common symptom following neck trauma (54% to 66% of patients with whiplash associated disorder complain of headache). It should be noted that 54.8% of patients seen by pain specialists have CGH or CGH in combination with other types of headache (7). The prevalence of CGH in the general population is estimated to be 0.4% to 2.5% (3).

CGHs often lack a regular pattern. They are often episodic, recurrent, lasting hours to days per episode, and can seriously affect the patient's quality of life (8). Some patients develop CGH after trauma, such as a whiplash injury (9). These headaches often resolve within a year. However, previous traumas or preexisting headache and neck pain may lead to chronic CGH after whiplash injury (10).

The effect of CGH on society is also significant. In a United States survey totaling 13,343 respondents, 9.4% reported missing work more than rarely because of headache, 31% reported that their work level was reduced more than rarely by headache, and 9.2% reported that their work level was reduced more than 50% by headaches during work (11). On average, individuals lost the equivalent of 4.2 d/y because of headache. Subjects with migraine headache were much more likely (57%) to report actual lost workdays because of headache, whereas tension-type and other headache types accounted for a large proportion (64%) of decreased work effectiveness because of headache. Headache type, headache severity, and education level were each independent predictors of workplace impact of headache.

In a 2001 to 2002 random sample telephone survey of over 28,900 American workers, 13% of the total workforce experienced a loss in productive time during a 2-week period due to a common pain condition (12). Headache was the most common pain condition resulting in lost productive time, accounting for a mean loss of 3.5 hours in productive time per week. Among active workers, lost productive time from common pain conditions (i.e., headache, back pain, arthritis) costs an estimated $61.2 billion per year, with $20 billion due to headache. The majority (76.6%) of the lost productive time was not due to an absence from work but was explained by reduced performance while at work.

Risk factors for developing CGH include the following:

- Head or neck traumatic injuries can predispose a patient to CGH symptoms
- Sustained neck postures or movements may precipitate CGH
- Primary or significant compensatory cervical somatic dysfunctions

PATHOPHYSIOLOGY

Cervical somatic dysfunction refers pain to the head and face via the trigeminal nerve (CN V). This same nerve innervates cranial and facial structures, including the cerebral blood vessels and dura mater, and sends its sensory information to the pons in the midbrain and then to the thalamus and somatosensory cortex. The trigeminal nerve also has tracts that descend into the spine. For example, the upper cervical spinal cord contains the Trigeminal Nucleus Caudalis (TNC). The TNC descends as low as C4 and is contiguous with the spinal gray matter in the substantia gelatinosa in lamina II of the dorsal horn.

The first three cervical spinal nerves innervate the zygapophyseal joints, uncovertebral joints, intervertebral discs, cervical muscles and ligaments, the vertebral artery, the cervical spinal dura, the posterior scalp, and even the lower layer of the tentorium cerebelli. Afferent fibers from these structures converge with the TNC within the spinal cord. As a result, pain signals from the neck can be referred to the same receptive field in the thalamus as that of the head and face, giving the patient the sensation that the pain is emanating from the head or face when in fact it is coming from the cervical spine.

Nociceptive stimuli from the C5-7 nerves can also refer pain to the head and face through the TNC since afferent nociceptive information can ascend between 1 and 3 levels before entering the dorsal horn and interacting with interneurons that connect with the TNC.

Nociceptive input originating from cervical structures can therefore be perceived as head pain in the regions innervated by the trigeminal nerve (16,17).

The superior and inferior vagal ganglia lie superior and inferior to the jugular foramina, respectively. The vagus (CN X) is a mixed nerve with motor, sensory, and parasympathetic components. Of interest in CGH is the fact that nociceptive or inflammatory stimuli from the larynx and pharynx, as well as the thoracic and abdominal viscera, are transmitted by the vagus and converge with upper cervical afferents (18). The increased afferent activity converging in the upper cervical region is thought to increase the efferent discharge of cervical spinal motor neurons accounting for the palpable increase in myofascial tissue tension in the upper cervical spine, thus constituting a viscerosomatic reflex. In addition, primary sensory axons from the superior vagal ganglia terminate in the TNC and convey general sensation from the external auditory meatus, external surface of the tympanic membrane and skin of the ear to the trigeminal receptive field in the thalamus. The spinal accessory nerve (CN XI), which sends motor efferents to the trapezius and sternocleidomastoid muscles, also has some sensory afferents that may converge with the TNC (16,17).

With respect to the sympathetic nervous system, sympathetic nerve fibers are dense in the basal region of the occipital dura mater and alongside as well as independent from blood vessels (19). The superior cervical ganglia are positioned anterior to the articular pillars of C2. They have postganglionic fibers that innervate the vasculature, mucous membranes of the head region, including the middle ear, the lacrimal glands, and pupils of the eyes. Their preganglionic cell bodies emanate from the spinal cord at levels T1-4.

Within the peripheral nervous system, a number of structures may be involved with CGH. The greater and lesser occipital nerves originate from roots at C1-3; the medial branches of the dorsal rami of C2 and C3 form the greater occipital nerve and the third occipital nerve. The greater and lesser occipital nerves innervate the posterior scalp. Occipital neuralgia may arise from entrapment or trauma to these nerves, the upper cervical zygapophyseal joints or the C2 spinal root. The suboccipital (C1) nerve innervates the occipitoatlantal joint and may be involved with somatic dysfunction that can refer pain to the occipital region. The AA joint and C2-3 are innervated by the C2 spinal nerve. Neuralgia arising from C2 can result in a deep or dull pain that usually radiates from the occipital to the parietal, temporal, frontal, and periorbital regions. A paroxysmal sharp pain may be superimposed over the constant pain. Lacrimation and conjunctival injection of the eye on the affected side are common associated signs. The third occipital nerve, arising from the dorsal ramus of C3, innervates the joints at C2 and C3. Somatic dysfunction of these joints may be involved in referring pain to the frontotemporal and periorbital regions (17).

TYPICAL PATIENT PRESENTATION

Patients may describe the pain of CGH as moderate to severe in intensity, deep, nonthrobbing, and nonlancinating. Certain precipitating factors may be involved, such as certain neck movements or particular sustained head positions. There may be a history of whiplash or other head or neck injury prior to onset of symptoms. It should be noted, however, that patients frequently have difficulty in identifying factors that precipitate, aggravate, or alleviate their headaches.

In CGH, the location of the head pain may be in the frontal, posterior, or lateral part of the head, at the vertex, or behind the orbit. The pain is typically unilateral, although it may occasionally be bilateral (1). The pain may radiate along the ipsilateral side of the head, to the neck and/or shoulder, and occasionally into the arm (1). There may also be scalp parasthesias or dysesthesia. Other characteristics include headache episodes of varying duration, and lack of response to medications that are usually helpful in alleviating other types of headache. Associated symptoms may include nausea, phonophobia, photophobia, dizziness, ipsilateral blurred vision, difficulties with swallowing, and ipsilateral periorbital edema. Coughing or sneezing may also trigger the pain.

PHYSICAL EXAMINATION OF THE PATIENT WITH HEADACHE

The physical examination of the patient with headache should include vital signs, a screening cardiavascular, neurological and musculoskeletal examination, and a regional evaluation of the head and neck. Normal vital signs help to rule out endocrine, cardiovascular, and infectious processes. The screening neurological examination is used to rule out focal deficits suggesting intracranial mass or event, and peripheral etiology such as peripheral nerve impingement with radiculopathy or spinal cord impingement from a herniated cervical disc.

The screening musculoskeletal exam evaluates large and small joints for systemic inflammatory conditions such as rheumatoid arthritis, which may present with headache. The head and neck areas should be examined for pharyngeal and tonsillar inflammation, glandular hypertrophy and/or tenderness, or lymphadenopathy that would alert the practitioner to internal organic problems that can also be an underlying cause of headache. The carotid arteries should be auscultated for any bruits.

The osteopathic physician should perform a general osteopathic screening exam of the musculoskeletal system, followed by a regional exam and then a segmental exam. The main areas of focus will likely be the head and cervical spine, but as noted above, other body regions may reveal somatic dysfunction deemed to be associated with the patient's CGH symptoms. The reader is referred to Chapters 56, 57, and 58 for further information.

Asymmetry of musculoskeletal structural landmarks, altered quantity or quality of active or passive neck motion, tissue texture abnormalities, and tenderness, lead the practitioner to consider mechanical neck disorder, or somatic dysfunction diagnosis.

It is also possible that somatic dysfunction of more distant body regions, such as the lumbar spine and pelvis, may be contributing factors in the patient with CGH. Restriction of motion of the AA (C1-2) joint is a very common finding in patients with CGH (29). There may be asymmetrical neck and head position in relation to the shoulders. Head pain can often be reproduced by digital pressure over the upper cervical or occipital region on the symptomatic side. Restriction of active and passive neck range of motion, particularly in the upper three cervical joints, is a common finding. There may be neck muscle stiffness and trigger points in the lower cervical or shoulder muscles that refer pain to the ipsilateral head region. Identification of clinically significant somatic dysfunction provides the indication for the use of osteopathic manipulative treatment.

LABORATORY AND RADIOLOGIC FINDINGS

These evaluations are not typically necessary if the history and physical examination is consistent with mild sprain or strain of the neck musculoskeletal tissues. In acute whiplash or other trauma, however, it may be necessary to obtain cervical radiographs to rule out vertebral fracture or dislocation. Patients with chronic mechanical neck pain refractory to osteopathic manipulative treatments and exercise may require further diagnostic imaging to rule out less common causes underlying persistent neck pain. Blood tests for systemic pathology are typically negative, and any cervical disc bulging seen on MRI or CT scan is usually nonspecific (30).

FIVE MODELS FOR APPLYING OMT FOR CGH

The osteopathic physician may organize osteopathic philosophy and principles according to a conceptual framework developed by the Educational Council on Osteopathic Principles (ECOP) (36). ECOP delineated five models for consideration. These models are mechanical, neurologic, respiratory-circulatory, metabolic-nutritional, and biopsychosocial. In the case of CGH, each model allows the osteopathic physician to consider:

- How the elements of the particular model are affecting, or being affected by, the patient's condition by contributing to the overall allostatic load on the patient
- Treatment options applicable to the particular model, including osteopathic manipulative treatment (OMT)
- Preventive measures relative to the specific model

BIOMECHANICAL MODEL

This model deals with factors that alter posture, motion, and gait. This approach includes evaluating altered joint relationships, muscle imbalances, and abnormal fascial tensions. These somatic dysfunctions can cause or contribute to adverse neurologic and circulatory functions. This process, along with the energy demands of the body's attempt to cope with abnormal mechanical stresses, can be part of the allostatic load contributing to CGH. The goal of treatment within this model is the restoration of free motion within the body's musculoskeletal system elements. A wide range of OMT techniques can assist in alleviating these stressors. These OMT techniques include high velocity-low amplitude, muscle energy, and articular and functional techniques, among others.

RESPIRATORY-CIRCULATORY MODEL

This model addresses altered respiratory mechanics that may predispose to congestive changes, decreased lymphatic flow, venous return, and edema formation. These adverse changes can lead to insufficient oxygen and nutrient distribution to tissues, reduced venous and lymphatic return, impaired immune system function, and insufficient removal of metabolic waste products from the body. The treatment goal within this model is to restore the body's ability to adequately move air and fluids throughout its systems. Somatic dysfunctions relative to this model include altered rib cage mechanics and restricted motion of the thoracic diaphragm and other functional diaphragms of the body. Commonly used OMT modalities for this model include osteopathy in the cranial field, myofascial release, and lymphatic pump techniques.

NEUROLOGIC MODEL

The neurologic model deals with the effects of facilitated spinal cord segments and sustained symphaticotonia, resulting in viscerosomatic and somatovisceral reflex phenomena, including the signs and symptoms of CGH. Goals of treatment within this model include restoration of autonomic balance, alleviation of segmental facilitation, decrease in or elimination of abnormal afferent signaling, and relief of pain. Various OMT techniques can be used here, but some modalities that are thought to be especially effective within the neurological model include counterstrain and the treatment of Chapman reflex points.

METABOLIC-ENERGY MODEL

The metabolic-nutritional model takes into consideration such things as dietary deficiencies and excesses, food allergies, the effect of toxins, and any other factors that may affect the self-regulatory and self-healing mechanisms of the body. Treatment goals for this model include promoting energy conservation by balancing the body's energy expenditure and exchange, and enhancing immune system function. In this model, a major emphasis is on such things as nutritional counseling, dietary advice, avoiding obesity, and encouraging exercise.

BEHAVIORAL MODEL

In this model, we consider the psychological and social components of the patient's health status. Some of these components include the patient's spiritual outlook, social support system, ability to cope with stress, and ability to make healthy lifestyle choices. In particular, stress is a well-known cause or contributor to headache, including CGH. Thus, reduction of stress factors can contribute to the ultimate control of CGH in some patients. The treatment goals for this model include optimizing the psychological and social components of the patient's overall health. This might include teaching the patient strategies for stress reduction, helping the patient improve his or her abilities for social interaction, and helping the patient improve his or her spiritual outlook. OMT is not commonly a part of the treatment approach in this model, although some osteopathic physicians advocate the use of OMT to improve autonomic balance for these patients, thus secondarily helping to relieve stress on the body.

BIOLOGICAL BASIS FOR THE USE OF OMT—BEST EVIDENCE

CGH may be related to somatic dysfunction of the OA and AA joints and neck pain most often related to C2-7 somatic dysfunction. Up to 50% of whiplash patients with chronic neck pain and dominant headache symptoms have C2-3 zygapophyseal joint pain that can be abolished with nerve blocks (22,23). Nerve blocks of the greater occipital nerve and lower cervical segments have also abolished headache symptoms, implying that these structures may become sensitized and thus involved in producing CGH (24,25).

Cervical somatic dysfunction has been thought to involve the trigeminal and spinal accessory cranial nerves, which innervate structures in both cervical and head regions. It is theorized that the TNC in the upper cervical spinal cord interacts with upper cervical peripheral afferents and the spinal accessory nerve (CN XI) to account for the bidirectional referral of painful sensations between the neck and the trigeminal receptive sensory fields of the face and head (17).

Muscle hypertonicity in the upper cervical and occipital regions may induce tension transmitted through the myodural connective tissue and elicit head pain. The facet joints between C1 and C2 produce pain in the posterior auricular area in the distribution of the greater occipital nerve. Diseases of the structures innervated by the vagus nerve may produce sensitization of upper cervical spinal segments and predispose the patient to upper cervical somatic dysfunction, leading to CGH (26). Cervicogenic pain has also been abolished with cervical myofascial trigger point and botulinum toxin injections, indicating peripheral sensitization in the soft tissues plays a role in CGH genesis as well. It has also been shown that increased levels of proinflammatory cytokines and nitric oxide are higher in patients with CGH compared with patients with migraine headaches and likely promote hyperalgesia (27). However, the lack of calcitonin gene–related peptide in symptomatic CGH patients indicates that the trigeminovascular system is not activated by this condition as it is in migraine patients (28).

Osteopathic physicians theorize that cervical mobilization and manipulation procedures decrease the afferent stimulus into the spinal cord from cervical joint receptors by relaxing the paraspinal muscles and releasing strain on the connective tissues and joints, thus relieving the pain of CGH. OMT and physical conditioning exercises for moderate to severe pain of any duration are effective for patients of all ages or gender (31–34). Ongoing exercise and physical conditioning programs can be beneficial for long-term prevention and control of symptoms (35).

Although OMT is a highly safe procedure, there are potential risks associated with its use. The primary risk identified in the literature is hyperextension coupled with rotation of the upper cervical spine due to concern regarding potential occlusion of the vertebral artery. Caution should also be exercised with patients with primary or secondary bone, neural or muscular disease as is true in any body region. Commonly accepted contraindications to manual medical treatment of mechanical cervical spine disorders include the following:

- Vertebral or carotid artery dissection
- Acute fracture of cervical vertebra or vertebrae
- Metabolic or neoplastic bone disease in the cervical spine
- Acute trauma to the head or neck without established diagnosis
- Certain primary muscle or joint diseases
- Patient refusal of treatment

Certain clinical conditions do not necessarily contraindicate the use of OMT but do require caution on the part of the osteopathic physician. For example, patients with congenital anomalies, such as those with Down Syndrome, may have deformities of the upper cervical spine that will alter the biomechanics in that region. Caution is also warranted in treating patients with rheumatoid arthritis as there may be laxity of the odontoid ligament and hypermobility of the AA joint.

The benefits of OMT for CGH include decreased pain frequency, intensity, and duration (31); improved ability to perform activities of daily living and work activities; and decreased reliance on analgesic and other medications that can have unwanted side effects and complications. The consensus among most practitioners is that CGH should be treated with a combination of manual treatment, exercise, locally injected and oral medications, stress reduction counseling, and education. Surgery is reserved for refractory conditions.

PHYSICAL MEDICINE AND REHABILITATION PERSPECTIVE

In spite of additional knowledge and experience in managing cervical spine disorders, the physician spine specialist oftentimes still finds the diagnosis of CGH to be quite challenging. Although various anatomical structures, including the cervical spine musculature, nerves, discs, and zygapophyseal joints, have been implicated in the pathophysiology of CGH, there is limited evidence that supports any of these structures as clearly causing CGH. Most research regarding this issue has focused on examining patient symptomology in response to structure-directed treatment, including facet and trigger point injection and cervical diskectomy and fusion. Diagnosing the cause of CHG is also made more challenging by the fact that it is oftentimes difficult to differentiate between cervicogenic, migraine, and tension-type headaches. Given these challenges, it is helpful to use an approach, such as the five conceptual models, that addresses the various structures and pathological processes that may be concomitantly causing CGH.

One reason why it may be difficult to diagnose and define the cause of CHG is that the upper cervical nerve roots innervate many of the structures typically suspected of causing CHG. These nerve roots converge with trigeminal nerve fibers in the upper cervical spinal cord, potentially explaining why nociceptive input from cervical spine structures may cause pain in the head and face. Diagnosis is also difficult due to the fact that there is no diagnostic or clinical finding that is specific for CGH. Historically, radiological abnormalities of the cervical spine have been used as diagnostic criteria for CGH (37). Even though radiographic abnormalities such as cervical spondylosis may be present when evaluating a patient with CGH, there is limited evidence demonstrating that these abnormalities are specific to CGH (38). Additionally, studies examining the cervical MRI studies of patients with CGH failed to demonstrate a difference between control subjects and those with CGH when evaluating for MRI abnormalities such as cervical disc bulging (30). While laboratory results may be abnormal in the presence of systemic disease, such as rheumatoid arthritis, there is also no laboratory marker that is specific for patients with CGH. Some research, however, has demonstrated that proinflammatory mediators may be higher in patients with mechanically induced CGH than those patients with migraine headache (39). Due to the equivocal nature of these diagnostic findings, it is important that the spine specialist perform a detailed history and physical examination when evaluating a patient for CGH. This is helpful in identifying cervical spine disease, including cervical spondylosis and nerve root compression, as well as excluding more serious conditions such as tumor or infection (40). Important components of the clinical evaluation include cervical range of motion, motor and sensory testing, and provocative testing for nerve root compression. Clinical evaluation can also be helpful in differentiating CGH from migraine headache. These are often difficult to discern from one another due to the overlap in diagnostic criteria, including photophobia and nausea. It appears that the most significant criterion in distinguishing CGH from migraine headache is the precipitation of headaches with movement of the neck or application of pressure to the neck (41). Given the fact that the etiology of CGH may be multifaceted and that its diagnosis requires assessment of multiple structures and physiological processes, it again may be useful to use the five conceptual models when evaluating a patient with CGH.

Because of its multifaceted nature, management of CGH often entails a combination of treatments, including osteopathic manipulative medicine (OMM), medication, injections, and surgery. As an expert in spinal disorders, the spine specialist is interested in better understanding the potential pain generating source of CGH, so as to potentially render more effective treatment. One way in which this is accomplished is through the use of cervical injection techniques, which can be helpful in both diagnosing and treating the pain-generating structures causing CGH. These include cervical zygapophyseal joint and medial branch blockade for facet disease, epidural for degenerative disc disease and nerve root compression, and occipital and cervical nerve blockade, and trigger point or botulinum toxin injection for muscle spasm. Although there is limited evidence supporting the efficacy of these techniques, it does appear that patients may experience some degree of pain relief if their CGH is secondary to a well-defined disease process. The idea that CGH may be due to abnormal muscle tension is potentially supported by a study, which found that injection of botulinum toxin into the cervical paraspinal muscles significantly reduced pain and increased cervical range of motion (42). Surgical techniques such as anterior diskectomy and fusion are typically reserved for refractory cases that demonstrate clear cervical spine pathology, including cervical radiculopathy and degenerative disc disease. Some studies have suggested that such surgical techniques are effective in treating CGH when it is associated with specific cervical spine pathology (43). Like much of the research examining the efficacy of injection techniques, however, they are of limited value given their small sample sizes and suboptimal outcome measures. Interestingly, it appears that cervical manipulation is the means of treatment most supported by a reasonable body of literature (44). This includes a randomized controlled trial demonstrating that cervical manipulation utilizing high velocity amplitude technique resulted in reduced CGH intensity and frequency and analgesic use when compared to deep friction massage (45). This is an important point to consider when integrating osteopathic manual medicine into the treatment plan, whether that entails the physician performing OMM or referring a patient to a Neuromusculoskeletal Medicine/OMM specialist.

SUMMARY

CGH is a common medical problem affecting a significant percentage of the population. A holistic, patient-centered approach, consistent with osteopathic philosophy, principles, and practice, provides a strategy for optimal control of this condition in patients. Osteopathic physicians can use the tenets and organizing principles of osteopathic medicine, a five-model approach to patient care, and their distinctive OMT modalities to achieve a high degree of success in helping patients with this condition.

REFERENCES

1. Sjaastad O, Fredriksen TA, Pfaffenrath V. Cervicogenic headache: diagnostic criteria. *Headache* 1998;38:442–445.
2. The international classification of headache disorders: 2nd Ed. *Cephalalgia* 2004;24(suppl 7):114–116.
3. Haldeman S, Dagenais S. Cervicogenic headaches: a critical review. *Spine J* 2001;1(1):31–46.
4. Pöllmann W, Keidel M, Pfaffenrath V. Headache and the cervical spine: a critical review. *Cephalalgia* 1997;17:801–816.
5. Pfaffenrath V, Kaube H. Diagnostics of cervicogenic headache. *Funct Neurol* 1990;5(2):159–64.
6. Nilsson N. The prevalence of cervicogenic headache in a random population sample of 20–59 year olds. *Spine* 1995;20(17):1884–1888.
7. Skovron ML. Epidemiology of whiplash. In: Gunzbrug R, Szpalski M, eds. *Whiplash Injuries: Current Concepts in Prevention, Diagnosis, and Treatment of the Cervical Whiplash Syndrome*. Philadelphia, PA: Lippincott-Raven, 1998.
8. van Suijlekom HA, Lame I, Stomp-van den Berg SG, et al. Quality of life of patients with cervicogenic headache: a comparison with control subjects and patients with migraine or tension-type headache. *Headache* 2003;43:1034–1041.
9. Drottning M, Staff PH, Sjaastad O. Cervicogenic headache after whiplash injury. *Cephalalgia* 1997;17:288–289.
10. Drottning M, Staff PH, Sjaastad O. Cervicogenic headache (CEH) after whiplash injury. *Cephalalgia* 2002;22(3):165–171.
11. Schwartz BS, Stewart WF, Lipton RB. Lost workdays and decreased work effectiveness associated with headache in the workplace. *J Occup Environ Med* 1997;39(4):320–327.
12. Stewart WF, Ricci JA, Chee E, et al. Lost productive time and cost due to common pain conditions in the U.S. workforce. *JAMA* 2003;290:2443–2454.
13. Strandring S, Editor-in-Chief. *Gray's Anatomy*. Philadelphia, PA: Elsevier Churchill Livingstone, 2005.
14. Hack GD, Koritzer RT, Robinson WL, et al. Anatomic relation between the rectus capitis posterior minor muscle and the dura mater. *Spine* 1995;20:2484–2486.
15. Nash L, Nicholson H, Lee ASJ, et al. Configuration of the connective tissue in the posterior atlanto-occipital interspace. *Spine* 2005;30(12):1359–1366.
16. Biondi DM. Cervicogenic headache: mechanisms, evaluation, and treatment strategies. *J Am Osteopath Assoc* 2000;100(9 suppl):S7–S14.
17. Biondi DM. Cervicogenic headache: A review of diagnostic and treatment strategies. *J Am Osteopath Assoc* 2005; 105(4 suppl 2):S16–S22.
18. Foreman RD. Integration of viscerosomatic sensory input at the spinal level. *Prog Brain Res* 2000;122:209–221.
19. Artico M, Cavallotti C. Catecholaminergic and acetylcholine esterase containing nerves of cranial and spinal dura mater in humans and rodents. *Microsc Res Tech* 2001;53(3):212–220.
20. Chikly, B. *Silent Waves: Theory and Practice of Lymph Drainage Therapy*. 1st Ed. Rev. Scottsdale, AZ: I.H.H. Publishing, 2001.
21. Driscoll, B.P. Fascial compartment of the neck. Available at: http://www.utmb.edu/oto/Grand_Rounds_Earlier.dir/Fascial_Compart_Neck_1994.txt. Last accessed February 9, 2008.
22. Lord SM, Barnsley L, Wallis BJ. Third occipital nerve headache: a prevalence study. *J Neurol Neurosurg Psychiatr.* 1994;57(10):1187–1190.
23. Lord SM, Barnsley L, Wallis BJ. Chronic cervical zygapophysial joint pain after whiplash. A placebo-controlled prevalence study. *Spine* 1996;21(15):1737–44.
24. Bovim G, Berg R, Dale LG. Cervicogenic headache: anesthetic blockades of cervical nerves (C2-C5) and facet joint (C2/C3). *Pain* 1992;49(3):315–320.
25. Bovim G, Sand T. Cervicogenic headache, migraine without aura and tension-type headache. Diagnostic blockade of greater occipital and supraorbital nerves. *Pain.* 1992;51(1):43–48.
26. Kuchera ML. Osteopathic principles and practice/osteopathic manipulative treatment considerations in cephalgia. *J Am Osteopath Assoc* 1998; 98(4):S14–S19.
27. Martelletti P, van Suijlekom HA. Cervicogenic headache: practical approaches to therapy. *CNS Drugs* 2004;18(12):793–805.
28. Frese A, Schilgen M, Edvinsson L, et al. Calcitonin gene-related peptide in cervicogenic headache. *Cephalalgia* 2005;25(9):700–703.
29. Hall T, Robinson K. The flexion-rotation test and active cervical mobility—a comparative measurement study in cervicogenic headache. *Man Ther* 2004;9:197–202.

30. Coskun O, Ucler S, Karakurum B, et al. Magnetic resonance imaging of patients with cervicogenic headache. *Cephalalgia* 2003;23(8):842–845.

31. Nilsson N, Christensen HW, Hartvigsen J. The effect of spinal manipulation in the treatment of cervicogenic headache. *J Manipulative Physiol Ther* 1997;20:326–330.

32. Jull GA, Trott P, Potter H, et al. A randomized controlled trial of exercise and manipulative therapy for cervicogenic headache. *Spine* 2002;27: 1835–1843.

33. Jull GA, Stanton WR. Predictors of responsiveness to physiotherapy management of cervicogenic headache. *Cephalalgia* 2005;25:101–108.

34. Bronfort G, Nilsson N, Haas M, et al. Non-invasive physical treatments for chronic/recurrent headache. *Cochrane Database Syst Rev* 2004;(3): CD001878. DOI: 10.1002/14651858.CD001878.pub2.

35. Biondi DM. Physical treatments for headache: a structured review. *Headache* 2005;45(6):738–746.

36. Educational Council on Osteopathic Principles. *Core Curriculum Outline.* Washington, DC: American Association of Colleges of Osteopathic Medicine, 1987.

37. IHS, Headache Classification Committee of the International Headache Society. Classification and diagnostic criteria for headache disorders, cranial neuralgias, and facial pain. *Cephalalgia* 1988;8(suppl 7):1–96.

38. Fredriksen TA, Fougner R, Tangerud A, et al. Cervicogenic headache. Radiological investigations concerning head/neck. *Cephalalgia* 1989;9(2):139–46.

39. Martelletti P, Stirparo G, Giacovazzo M, et al. Proinflammatory cytokines in cervicogenic headache. *Funct Neurol* 1999;14(3):159–62.

40. Nordin M, Carragee EJ, Hogg-Johnson S, et al. Assessment of neck pain and its associated disorders. Results of the Bone and Joint Decade 2000–2010 Task Force on Neck Pain and Its Associated Disorders. *Spine* 2008;33(suppl):S101–S122.

41. Sjaastad O, Bovim G. Cervicogenic headache. The differentiation from common migraine. An overview. *Funct Neurol* 1991;6(2):93–100.

42. Freund BJ, Schwartz M. Treatment of chronic cervical-associated headache with botulinum toxin A: a pilot study. *Headache* 2000;40(3):231–6.

43. Schofferman J, Garges K, Goldthwaite N, et al. Upper cervical anterior diskectomy and fusion improves discogenic cervical headaches *Spine* 2002;27:2240–2244.

44. Haldeman S, Dagenais S. Cervicogenic headaches: a critical review. *Spine J* 2001;1:31–46.

45. Nilsson N, Christensen HW, Hartvigsen J. The effect of spinal manipulation in the treatment of cervicogenic headache. *J Manipul Physiol Ther* 1997;20(5):326–330.

Large Joint Injury in an Athlete

KURT HEINKING, PER GUNNAR BROLINSON, AND THOMAS A. GOODWIN

- Rotator cuff strains can develop as a result of repetitive overuse.
- The kinetic chain associated with shoulder movements extends from the head to the pelvis.
- Somatic dysfunction in any of the tissues associated with the kinetic chain can exacerbate and contribute to shoulder disorders.
- An integrated approach to shoulder pain, including the use of manual medicine, can be effective in decreasing pain, reducing functional disability, and returning the patient to normal activities.

CASE VIGNETTE

Ms. Jones is a 52-year-old Caucasian right-hand dominant high-level recreational tennis player who seeks medical care following an injury to her right shoulder.

CHIEF COMPLAINT

Acute exacerbation of chronic aching pain in her anterior/lateral right shoulder for the past 6 weeks, after participating in the Regional United States Tennis Association (USTA) event.

HISTORY OF PRESENT ILLNESS

The pain has been present for the past 6 weeks. The pain began after participating in the USTA regional event where her team qualified for the State tournament. She noted that the pain began while playing in a doubles match during which she hit multiple overhead strokes in addition to normal serving in the closely contested match. Just prior to the regional event, she purchased a new racquet with all of the "latest technology." She states that that the pain has not improved despite taking one week off from playing, and now she is developing stiffness of the right shoulder. The pain is affecting her in daily activities. She is concerned about the ongoing discomfort as she wants to begin to prepare for the State tournament with her team. She describes her pain as being a constant 5/10 in intensity and having a burning/aching quality. When she attempts to reach overhead, the pain increases to a 7/10 in intensity. The pain radiates to the right medial scapular border and also down the biceps muscle anteriorly. She has difficulty sleeping on her right side night as she develops pain in the region of the deltoid insertion. She notes that she cannot hook her bra or put a sweater on overhead without significant discomfort. She denies having significant neck pain, but does have some stiffness in turning left and right. She denies having numbness or weakness involving her right hand. She denies chest pain, fever, shortness of breath, cough, or stomach upset. She has had shoulder pain on the right side in the past that resolved with home treatment. She has taken naproxen sodium 220 mg twice daily without improvement. She used ice on the shoulder for the first two days, but has not used any ice or heat since then. She has not had any other workup or imaging performed as of this time.

Past Medical History:
Positive for gastroesophageal reflux disease, Hyperlipidemia, and menopause

Past Surgical History:
Appendectomy at age 18, Tonsils and adenoids at age 6

Past Trauma History:
Motor vehicle accident 1982 during which she sustained a minor concussion and whiplash

Family Medical History:
Mother alive (age 75 HTN); type II diabetes; father deceased (cirrhosis of the liver at age 58); siblings, one brother (age 49), healthy

Gynecologic History:
G2 P, 2002; LMP, 2 years ago; last mammogram, 1 year ago—normal; last pap and pelvic, rectal exam 1 year ago—normal

Social History:
Married; husband: Roger, 22 years;, 2 children: Mary—21, healthy and Grace—19, healthy; Denies tobacco use, illicit drug use, occasional alcohol (holidays). Patient is an office manager for a large medical group. She normally plays tennis four to five times weekly during the competitive season and one to two times weekly during the off-season.

Childhood Illnesses:
Chicken pox, possible measles, Mononucleosis at age 18

REVIEW OF SYSTEMS
General:
She denies fever, chills, and malaise

HEENT:
She admits to occasional tension headaches, which have not changed since the onset of the shoulder pain. She denies dizziness.

Cardiovascular:
She denies chest pain, shortness of breath, fatigue.

Pulmonary:

She denies cough, wheeze, and pain with breathing.

Gastrointestinal:

She denies abdominal pain, nausea, vomiting, intolerance to fatty foods, excessive alcohol use, change in stools, and change in appetite.

Musculoskeletal:

She denies pain, swelling and stiffness in other joints, although she does admit to episodes of mid and upper back pain.

Neurological:

She denies weakness, numbness.

Endocrine:

She denies weight change; she admits to occasional hot flashes. She is menopausal.

PHYSICAL EXAMINATION

Vital Signs:

T 97.6, P 78, R 16, BP 140/ 82, height 5′ 6″, weight 148 lb

General:

Alert, oriented, cooperative, neatly groomed, and an excellent historian. She appears younger than her stated age.

Skin:

No rashes, no abnormal-appearing moles, normal hair and nails

HEENT:

PERLA EOMI, Pharynx without erythema, No adenopathy, TM's good cone of light without erythema, no nasal erythema, no sinus tenderness

Cardiovascualar:

RRR without S3 S4 murmur, no clubbing, cyanosis, or peripheral edema. Equal pulses bilaterally

Lungs:

CTA without rales, rhonchi, wheezes

Breast:

No breast masses, nipples everted, no discharge, no axillary adenopathy

Abdomen:

BS × 4 quadrants without rigidity, rebound, guarding, Neg CVA pain, No masses appreciated. No RUQ discomfort on palpation, Negative Murphy sign.

Neurological:

CN's 2 to 12 intact, DTR's 2/4 bilateral, No sensory deficits, 5/5 motor strength bilateral

MUSCULOSKELETAL

Upper Extremities:

Right shoulder: Active abduction full, but with painful arc from 50 degrees to full abduction. Active external rotation limited to 20 degrees secondary to pain. Active and passive adduction, flexion, extension and internal rotation full and pain free. Positive Jobe test (empty/full can), Positive Hawkins sign, Neg Speed's test, Neg Drop arm test, Positive Neer test, Positive A/C tenderness, Neg subscapularis test (lift-off/Napoleon's), Neg labral tests (O'Brien's, Zaslav, Biceps load, Crank etc.), No gross scapular winging although observation of active scapular motion reveals right scapula dyskinetic in early abduction coupled with flexion. Neg Roos test, No cyanosis, clubbing or edema, Pulses equal bilaterally, brisk capillary refill.

Lower Extremities:

Full Hip, Knee, Ankle AROM PROM, Neg Lachman test, Neg joint line pain, Neg Mc Murray's and Apley's; Negative Patellar grind, Neg Hip comp. No cyanosis, clubbing or edema, Pulses equal bilateral, good capillary refill

OSTEOPATHIC STRUCTURAL EXAM

C5 is flexed rotated and sidebent right, T4 is extended sidebent and rotated right, there is an exhalation dysfunction involving rib 10 on right, L1 is flexed rotated and sidebent right, right anterior innominate, left on left sacral torsion, right psoas hypertonic and tight, superior right sternoclavicular joint.

DIFFERENTIAL DIAGNOSIS

Table 61.1 outlines the differential diagnoses for shoulder pain.

WORKUP AND INTERPRETATION

Shoulder x-rays were obtained. These included an AP view, axillary view, scapular y view, and outlet view. The x-rays demonstrated a type II acromion with cystic change at the acromioclavicular joint. The humeral head was without osteoarthritis, fracture, or subluxation. The remainder of the osseous anatomy was normal. An arthrogram of the shoulder was obtained. Again demonstrated is a type II acromion with cystic change at the acromioclavicular joint. Findings also included a full-thickness tear of the supraspinatus tendon with retraction. A small amount of fluid was seen in the subacromial bursa. The humeral head was without osteoarthritis, fracture, or subluxation. The glenoid labrum appeared intact.

Diagnosis

The patient's diagnosis based on the clinical history, examination, and diagnostic imaging was as follows: (1) full-thickness rotator cuff tear with retraction of supraspinatus tendon; (2) type II acromion osteoarthrosis of the acromioclavicular joint; (3) somatic dysfunction: cervical, thoracic, rib, lumbar, sacrum, pelvis, and upper extremity; (4). scapular dyskinesis; (5) kinetic chain dysfunction; and (6) GERD (acid reflux disease)—controlled currently.

Relevant Functional Anatomy

The shoulder complex is a loosely constructed highly mobile complex of bones, muscles, and ligaments. It is designed for increased mobility to the upper extremity with only sufficient stability to provide a proper foundation for muscular function that is vital for the performance of sports or activities of daily living. The shoulder complex includes both static and dynamic stabilizers. The static stabilizers are Glenoid, glenoid labrum, capsule, ligaments (superior glenohumeral, middle glenohumeral, and inferior glenohumeral), joint cohesion, and intra-articular negative pressure.

The dynamic stabilizers are the rotator cuff muscles along with the long head of the biceps. The scapulothoracic stabilizers are the

TABLE 61.1

Differential Diagnosis

Muscular/Tendinous	Osseous	Capsular	Biomechanical	Neurovascular	Referred Pain Pattern
Rotator cuff tendonitis	Osteoarthritis	Shoulder laxity/instability	Impingement syndrome	Thoracic outlet syndrome	Diaphragm, liver, gallbladder
Rotator cuff tear	Humeral stress fracture	Adhesive capsulitis	Scapular dyskinesis	Cervical radiculopathy radiculitis	Pancoast tumor or pulmonary pathology
Subacromial bursitis		Labral tear	Acromio-clavicular dysfunction		
Biceps brachii (long head) tendonitis		Pigmented villonodular synovitis	Somatic dysfunction		
Deltoid muscle strain			Neuromuscular inhibition with abnormal muscle firing patterns		
Trapezius muscle strain					
Rhomboid muscle strain					

rhomboids, trapezius, serratus anterior, and the pectoralis minor muscles (7).

The glenohumeral joint is multiaxial ball and socket synovial joint enclosed by a strong ligamentous capsule. This anatomic design allows for the joint's tremendous mobility, but the unique bony structures sacrifice stability. The capsule is weak anteriorly and inferiorly (inferior glenohumeral ligament complex), allowing for instability or dislocation to commonly occur in that direction. The posterior capsule is commonly tight, which causes anterior translation and elevation of the humeral head. This situation can cause secondary impingement of the rotator cuff (as well as micro-instability perhaps leading to gross instability) (1). Movement of the shoulder requires coordinated movement of the three joints (SC, AC, and GH) and the scapulothoracic articulation. All four of these components work together in a synchronous fashion to allow the extensive range of motion (circumduction). In any given arm position, the scapula aligns itself to allow the glenoid cavity to be in the best position to receive the head of the humerus.

The rotator cuff is critical to the dynamic stability of the glenohumeral joint. The cuff is formed by the confluent tendon of the supraspinatus, infraspinatus, teres minor, and subscapularis. The supraspinatus, infraspinatus, and teres minor insert on the greater tuberosity, whereas the subscapularis inserts on the lesser tuberosity of the humerus. Historically, the supraspinatus has been described as initiating abduction; however, recent evidence suggests that it is functionally more of a glenohumeral joint stabilizer (1). Because of its angle of insertion (70 degrees from the glenoid), the supraspinatus acts as a tensioner, applying a compressive force through the glenohumeral joint. Its synergistic action with the deltoid results in abduction. Without a properly functioning supraspinatus, impingement of the cuff between the humeral head and under surface of the acromion occurs. Over time, this allows the humeral head to glide anteriorly in the glenoid placing strain on the anterior capsule

and ligamentous structures. This microinstability may eventually lead to frank subluxation and/or dislocation.

The teres minor and infraspinatus work synergistically to depress and externally rotate the humeral head. The subscapularis internally rotates and depresses the humeral head. During throwing, the subscapularis and infraspinatus muscles are two of the most important dynamic stabilizers of the glenohumeral joint (1). The teres major functions along with the latisimus to extend internally rotate and adduct the humerus (2).

The majority of the vascular supply to the shoulder is supplied by the axillary artery. The axillary artery passes posterior to the pectoralis minor muscle and becomes the brachial artery at the inferior border of the teres major muscle. Branches from the axillary and brachial arteries supply the structures of the shoulder, arm, forearm, and hand. Some investigators feel that there is a "critical zone" of potentially deficient blood supply to the rotator cuff muscles secondary to the intrinsic vascular anastomotic properties. It is in this critical zone that rotator cuff tears can begin due to the relative avascularity of this region (1). One such example is in the supraspinatus tendon immediately proximal to its insertion on the greater tuberosity of the humerus (1).

Vascular tone and lymphatic flow are determined by the sympathetic nervous system. The sympathetic innervation to the upper extremities arises from the upper thoracic spinal cord (T1-4). The sympathetic ganglia lie anterior to the rib head, in the fascia common to both structures. Nerve roots C5-8 and T1 form the brachial plexus. These nerve roots pass through the intervertebral foramen of the cervical vertebrae and pass between the anterior and the middle scalene muscles. The roots unite to form successive trunks, divisions, cords, and branches. The anterior and the middle scalenes can spasm, applying pressure to the brachial plexus. The thoracic inlet can be considered in both anatomical and functional terms. The anatomic boundaries include the manubrium of the sternum anteriorly, the first thoracic vertebrae posteriorly, and the first rib laterally.

Physiology

Injury to a large joint sets up an inflammatory cascade in the structures involved. The severity, intensity, and location of the inflammation depend upon the mechanism of injury and the structures involved. For the shoulder, many times, the issue is repetitive overuse. Tendonitis and subacromial bursitis occur commonly, as does tendonitis of the long head of the biceps. Because most shoulder problems are soft tissue in nature, pain, tightness, and stiffness with impaired mobility is a concern. Pain is usually due to impingement of the soft tissue structures under the coracoacromial arch. Stiffness and decreased range of motion are multifactorial and can be mediated anatomically, biomechanically, and/or neurologically. Loss of strength may indicate rotator cuff tear but may also be related to the factors described above (5).

Osteopathic Patient Management

Any patient presenting with pain in the shoulder joint complex should receive a thorough osteopathic examination. Osteopathic techniques can be applied to the areas of somatic dysfunction in patients presenting with rotator cuff tear pathology. The models described below of structure-function relationships guide the osteopathic practitioner's approach to diagnosis and treatment. The five structure function models provide a framework for integrating objective and subjective clinical findings with osteopathic structural exam findings.

Biomechanical Model

A kinetic chain is described as a sequencing of individual body segments and joints to accomplish a task. It generally functions from a base of support proximally and then proceeds distally, but this is entirely dependent on the task at hand. Because of the tremendous demands that overhead sporting activities place on the spine and the shoulder joint complex, the ability to recognize kinetic chain disorders related to the upper extremity and their interactions with related components of the musculoskeletal system is important for athletic medical practitioners. Due to the complexity of the anatomic and biomechanical interactions as well as neuromuscular control issues, evaluation and accurate diagnosis are clinically challenging. Disruption of the kinetic chain, if left unidentified, may lead to altered muscle firing patterns resulting in overload to connective tissues (capsular laxity and instability, labral tears), or the joint itself (osteoarthritis, etc.). While the patient may complain of pain due to one traumatic event, the majority of shoulder problems result from repetitive overuse of the osteoarticular system and related neural, soft tissue, and muscular elements. This is especially true in overhead athletes, as they try to transmit the ground reactive force from their pelvis and trunk through their upper extremity. Weakness of the abdominals, gluteus, and scapular stabilizers, with subsequent tightness of the psoas, hamstrings, latissimus dorsi, and upper trapezius, produces the substitution patterns that begin at the myofascial level, which may result in outlet obstruction at the coracoacromial arch. This situation is known as "impingement" (1). Impingement syndrome results in part from suboptimal biomechanical position manifesting grossly as protracted shoulders, weak lower trapezius, and tight upper trapezius. As a result, the glenoid fossa's abnormal position places stress on the anterior stabilizers (both static and dynamic) of the shoulder. Over time,

this abnormal stress leads to loosening of the anterior capsule with subsequent tightening of the posterior capsule. This places stress on not only the joint capsule, but also the glenoid labrum. If left untreated, the asymmetric positioning causes abnormal load on the dynamic stabilizers (the rotator cuff muscles) that may eventually manifest as frank rotator cuff pathology. This situation can be secondary to internal pathology as just discussed or may result from external causes. In the case of scapular dyskinesis of primary origin, abnormal stabilization of the scapula again places the shoulder at a biomechanical disadvantage. This leads to abnormal scapular positioning as discussed above, which may lead to the same pathologic conditions.

Failure to assess the functional biomechanical factors related to the shoulder joint complex may lead to less-than-optimal results. For example, after a patient undergoes surgery for a torn rotator cuff, the mainstay of postoperative care is physical therapy. If the therapist and/or clinician fails to recognize dysfunction in the kinetic chain (scapular dyskinesis, altered muscle firing patterns, etc.) the patient's altered biomechanics will place the shoulder and newly repaired cuff under the same abnormal forces as before and result in a suboptimal outcome.

Impingement is caused by a decrease in the subacromial space and compression of the rotator cuff tendons under the subacromial arch. Tension in the latissimus dorsi causes internal rotation and adduction of the humerus, further causing the greater tuberosity of the humerus to impinge upon the acromion. Weak abdominals cause an increase in the lumbar lordosis, an increase in the thoracic kyphosis, a slumped posture and forward head. The forward head position causes tightness of the scalenes and myofascial strain of the thoracic inlet, clavicles, and shoulders. The clinical biomechanical summation of the above results in a "functional thoracic kyphosis" characterized by rotator cuff impingement resulting from scapular dyskinesis (protracted scapula) and may ultimately lead to rotator cuff muscle fiber failure.

Form follows function. Given enough time, the biomechanical and neuromuscular dysfunctions described above can result in bony and soft tissue changes leading to a painful shoulder syndrome for which the patient seeks medical attention. Functional evaluation of this patient's complaint often reveals that the inciting event is part of a longstanding underlying process of kinetic chain dysfunction.

The key in any patient with somatic dysfunction is the restore normal structural alignment to allow the kinetic chain to function properly (form follows function). In this patient, when considering the biomechanical model, the physician needs to address the flexed lumbar dysfunction and the psoas tension. By treating these, the normal sacral motion should be restored, which will allow the ground reactive force to be efficiently transmitted up the kinetic chain. Osteopathic treatment will also restore functional mobility to the thoracolumbar junction. This will improve diaphragm motion and decrease latisimus tension. Treatment of the upper thoracic dysfunction should correct scapular dyskinesis. The result will be restoration of normal postural alignment and kinetic chain function.

Respiratory/Circulatory Model

Osteopathic manipulation may be used to improve blood flow to the area of injury and remove edema, which may assist in pain reduction and improve mobility. The axillary vein receives tributaries that correspond to the branches of the axillary artery and receives venae comitantes of the brachial artery. The subclavian vein passes over the first rib and below the clavicle, crossing over the anterior scalene muscles insertion on the first rib (3). The left brachiocephalic vein passes posterior to the left sternoclavicular joint then crosses the midline. The right subclavian lymphatic trunk drains into the right lymphatic duct. The left subclavian lymphatic trunk drains into the thoracic duct. Somatic dysfunction affecting the venous system may also affect lymphatic drainage, thereby producing congestion in the upper extremity (4). Fascial restriction of the thoracic inlet and pectoral fascia can also cause lymphatic stasis of the upper extremity.

Improving motion in the lower thoracic region will help the function of the diaphragm from a mechanical prospective. Improving motion in the cervical region will help the function of the diaphragm from a neurologic perspective. Both restore normal diaphragmatic motion, which is the primary driving force to move lymph. This treatment should follow thoracic inlet release, which removes any proximal restrictions to lymphatic flow. In this patient, treatment of the right sternoclavicular restriction will further aid in this process by normalizing fascial tensions of the thoracic inlet. Then, attention is moved distally to remove pectoral and axillary restrictions. Originally, Spencer's technique was described as a lymphatic technique for the upper extremity. Over the years, its clinical utility has broadened and it is often modified to address other musculoskeletal dysfunctions of the upper extremity. It may be used in this case as an adjunctive treatment. Treatment of the distal arm and hand may be necessary as well if indicated.

Additionally, somatic dysfunction involving any of the following structures may affect arterial supply and venous return (4): anterior and middle scalenes, upper thoracic vertebrae, upper ribs, clavicles, and the fascia of the upper extremity.

Neurological Model

Another objective is to normalize neurologic input to the upper extremity. Sympathetic innervation to the shoulder joint complex is mediated through treatment of the T4 dysfunction and the associated ribs. Increased sympathetic tone to the upper extremity can cause vasoconstriction, edema, sensitivity of the nerves, irritability of the muscles, and sweat gland overactivity. OMT in this region can improve those related pathophysiologic findings.

Also peripheral fascial restrictions are removed to limit compression of nerves supplying the region. Tension in the anterior scalenes and the thoracic inlet can compress the neurovascular bundle, impairing nerve transmission and vascular supply to the rotator cuff and scapular stabilizing muscles. Removal of the fascial restrictions and resultant compression to the neurovascular bundle will facilitate axoplasmic flow, enhancing the nerves trophic function.

Metabolic-Energy Model

Efficient transfer of energy in the overhead athlete is vital to performance. While the biomechanical implications of this have been discussed, metabolic processes are also responsible. These manifest grossly in the cardiac, respiratory, neurological, and psychological systems. One analogy is to envision the body as a large machine. The cardiovascular system is the engine that drives the metabolic system. This diverse system has the ability to adapt quickly to changing needs. When needed, the system shifts from the homeostatic life-sustaining mode to supercharged state for athletic activity. This is mediated at the cellular level as cell depolarization that results in measurable changes in cardiac output that enable the athlete to meet the demands placed upon him or her by athletic activity. The "fuel" that drives this system is supplied by the pulmonary system via the gas exchange that occurs at the level of the pulmonary

capillaries. This oxygen-rich blood is transported through the larger pulmonary veins and eventually to the left atrium. This fuel is then supplied to the neuromusculoskeletal system and throughout the rest of the body. Occasionally, these systems function together with perfect harmony and precision. The integration of these processes combined with the influence of psychological factors leads to an efficiently functioning machine that some have referred to as the "quantum athlete." Some believe this balance is responsible for an athlete's "court sense" or "being in the zone." Under these ideal circumstances, there is optimal balance between energy expenditure and energy intake. Disruption in any of these metabolic processes, as in an injured athlete, shifts the balance and leads to an inefficient system (8).

Behavioral Model

An athlete's mood is affected whenever he or she is restricted from practice and competition. Often an athlete's perception of himself or herself is intimately tied to their athletic performance. The effects of an athlete's injury can manifest in many different ways and can impact psychosocial, cultural, behavioral, and spiritual elements. In an affected athlete, this can influence interpersonal relationships, social interactions, school, and/or work performance.

Cognitive learning theory and skills that apply to the athletic setting include self-efficacy, arousal regulation, attentional focus, and mental imagery. During periods of injury, the athlete's ability to access this system is altered, which can have significant psychosocial and emotional impact. For the athlete, this is directly evident by the missed practice and playing time that affects their individual season as well as their teammates. The athlete often feels isolated from the team during treatments and can suffer from a "confidence crisis."

Self-efficacy allows the athlete to actively participate in the rehabilitative process and regain confidence in their ability to get better and return to competitive athletics. Enhanced self-efficacy predicts psychological well-being, adherence to prescribed treatments, and pain-coping mechanisms. Poor self-efficacy produces mood fluctuations, reduction in functional ability, and a feeling of helplessness that frustrates both the patient and the clinician if not understood (9). Enhancing self-efficacy promotes decision-making skills and problem-solving ability through practice and role playing to deal with disease-related issues (10).

INTEGRATIVE TREATMENT APPROACH

As osteopathic physicians, we can use OMT as a powerful treatment tool for musculoskeletal complaints. Application of osteopathic principles is an important component in the treatment of musculoskeletal complaints. As has been discussed previously, restoration of proper function of the shoulder requires reestablishment of normal structure. Barring contraindications, OMT should be performed in all patients with shoulder complaints, as indicated, for this reason. The type of treatment is based on the physician's ability, the patient's response and presentation, the type of dysfunction found, and time limitations of the practice.

While the body has the innate ability to self-heal, adjunctive therapies may be required, most patients will require a comprehensive approach including the appropriate use of other treatment modalities such as medications, injections, physical/occupational therapy, activity modification, dietary changes, occupational changes, and counseling (or emotional support as discussed above) if necessary. In the patient with a full-thickness rotator cuff tear and pain in the shoulder joint complex, the decision between a surgical or conservative approach may not always be straightforward.

Each case should be individualized based on patient desire, activity level, and long-term goals. A patient who wished for nothing more than pain relief would be treated differently than a patient who desired high-level physical activity. A detailed discussion of surgical options is beyond the scope of this chapter. If a surgical approach is elected, the specifics of the procedure should be considered. However, for the patients who undergo surgery, osteopathic treatment is a powerful adjunctive therapy postoperatively.

If conservative treatment is chosen, what should be the chronologic sequence of rehabilitation? Typically, inflammation is reduced with simultaneous improvement in range of motion. Then proprioception, flexibility, and strengthening occur. During these stages of rehabilitation, are different manipulative techniques required?

If conservative treatment is chosen, do the areas of somatic dysfunction need to be removed first, or should exercises be prescribed initially to help alleviate the somatic dysfunction? Where should treatment start? In the involved extremity, at the area of greatest restriction, or at a site distant from the injury?

A major goal in the treatment of acute shoulder pain is to control inflammation. In addition to cryotherapy (icing), systemic therapy with nonsteroidal anti-inflammatory drugs will help resolve swelling and decrease pain. Local anti-inflammatory measures (with corticosteroid medication or NSAIDs) can also be employed. Steroids or NSAIDs may be used topically by iontophoresis and phonophoresis during physical therapy, while subacromial bursal steroid injections may be performed as well. Additionally, some patients may require narcotic analgesic for short-term use. Muscle spasticity may need to be treated with muscle relaxers or benzodiazepines.

Activity modification, work restrictions, and lifestyle change are important aspects of the rehabilitative process. For shoulder injuries, the physician needs to stress relative rest vs. absolute rest. If the patient begins to restrict certain ranges of motion secondary to pain, eventually the shoulder capsule will adapt to this decreased range of motion and a fibrous adhesive capsulitis will result. Many times, Codman pendulum exercises and wall walking exercises are prescribed to maintain mobility. Overhead movements should be modified as they can exacerbate impingement. In the case of fractures, dislocations, and surgeries, shoulder immobilizers are sometimes required for short periods of time.

Outcome Studies for Manual Treatment of the Shoulder

Described below are three randomized, controlled trials that showed promising results for the application of manipulation and physiotherapy in the management of shoulder pain.

The first randomized clinical trial evaluating the effectiveness of shoulder manipulation as an addition to standard care (i.e., nonsteroidal medication) compared with physiotherapy and corticosteroid injection was reported in the *British Medical Journal* by Winter and colleagues 1997 (6). A total of 172 subjects were randomized to receive one of the adjunct therapies after a standard 1-week treatment with anti-inflammatory medication. Results showed that the shoulder girdle dysfunction group that received manipulation had a shorter duration of complaints and fewer reports of treatment failure than those that received physiotherapy.[6]

Berman and coworkers recruited 150 patients with shoulder symptoms and dysfunction of the shoulder girdle from general practices in the Netherlands. The patients were randomly assigned into usual care versus usual care plus manipulative therapy (up to six treatment sessions). At the end of the study period of 12 weeks, 21% of the usual care group and 43% of the intervention group reported full recovery. This significant difference in improvement was also observed at 52 weeks of follow-up.[6]

In a trial by Hay and associates, 207 patients with shoulder pain recruited from primary care clinics in the United Kingdom were randomly divided into a physiotherapy group and a corticosteroid injection group. At 6 months, 60% in the physiotherapy group and 53% in the injection group reported a minimum 50% drop in their disability scores.[6]

Risks and Benefits of Manipulative Treatment for the Shoulder

Complications or adverse events occurring after manipulation of the shoulder have not been reported in the literature (6). None of the clinical trials evaluating this modality have reported any complications or adverse events in patients with shoulder somatic dysfunction.

Risks of increasing shoulder pain, dislocation, and disability may occur if proper diagnosis is not made. For example, if the practitioner manipulates a hypermobile shoulder that is already unstable due to loss of integrity (i.e., tear) of the rotator cuff, labrum, or other primary shoulder structure, a poor outcome may result.

Manual medicine can be used to treat shoulder pain related to somatic dysfunction. Manual procedures can increase motion, strengthen weak muscles, lyse adhesions, and decrease pain. As described above, manipulative therapy for the shoulder girdle in addition to usual care by a general practitioner can accelerate recovery from shoulder symptoms and reduce their severity (6).

REFERENCES

1. DeLee JC, Drez D. Orthopaedic *Sports Medicine Principles and Practice.* Vol 2. 2nd Ed. Philadelphia, PA: Saunders, 2003:1065–1095.
2. DeLee JC, Drez D. *Orthopaedic Sports Medicine Principles and Practice.* Vol 2. 2nd Ed. Philadelphia, PA: Saunders, 2003, 840–850.
3. Moore KL. *Clinically Oriented Anatomy.* 3rd Ed. Baltimore, MD: Williams & Wilkins, 1992:528.
4. Ward RC. *Foundations for Osteopathic Medicine.* 2nd Ed. Lippincott, Williams & Wilkins, 2003:690–704; chap. 47, Upper Extremities.
5. Greenman PE. *Principles of Manual Medicine.* 2nd Ed. Baltimore, MD: Williams & Wilkins, 1996:271–285.
6. Seffinger MA, Hruby RJ, Kuchera WA. *Evidence-Based Manual Medicine Problem Oriented Approach.* Philadelphia, PA: Saunders Elsevier, 2007:221–272.
7. Kalman VR, Sampson MJ, Brolinson PG. The shoulder: common conditionsin chapt 17.3. In: Karageanes SJ, ed. *Principles of Manual Sports Medicine.* Baltimore, MD: Lippincott, Williams & Wilkins, 2005:181–200.
8. Kerger S. exercise principles chpt 10. In: Karageanes SJ, ed. *Principles of Manual Sports Medicine.* Baltimore, MD: Lippincott, Williams & Wilkins, 2005:65–76.
9. Strecher VJ, et al. *Health Educ Q* 1986;13(1):73–92.
10. Allegrante JP, Marks R. *Rheum Dis Clin North Am.* 29(4):747–768.

Multiple Small Joint Diseases in an Elderly Patient

KURT HEINKING, JAMES LIPTON, AND BETH VALASHINAS

KEY CONCEPTS

- Hand pain and stiffness is a common complaint in the elderly patient, and thorough history and physical exam need to be done to rule out an inflammatory condition.
- Chronic hand pain and stiffness can adversely affect daily living activities and contribute to depression and a loss of personal motivation in an otherwise healthy individual.
- An integrated approach to the management of the patient with hand pain and stiffness, including pharmacotherapeutics, osteopathic manipulation, and behavioral modification, can provide relief and improved function.

CASE VIGNETTE

Ms. Anderson is a 62-year-old Caucasian female who seeks medical care for chronic severe worsening hand stiffness and pain.

CHIEF COMPLAINT

A 3-month history of chronic aching pain in bilateral hands with associated morning stiffness lasting over 1 hour, as well as chronic daily headaches for the past year

HISTORY OF PRESENT ILLNESS

The patient denies any recent traumas. The pain has been affecting her in daily activities as well as in employment. Over the past 3 months, Ms. Anderson missed a significant amount of time at work and she lost her job. She worked at a health food store and had a difficult time stocking the shelves. She is concerned about the ongoing discomfort in her hands, as well as having daily headaches. She attributes both of these to a multi-level cervical fusion 6 years ago. Her hand pain is approximately a 7/10 in. intensity with attempting to open jars, or perform repetitive tasks. She describes symmetrical joint stiffness in her hands, worse in the morning upon awakening, often lasting over 1 hour. She further relates difficulty sleeping at night secondary to pain, predominantly in her neck. She notes that she cannot hook her bra, undo buttons, or knit a sweater without significant discomfort. She has taken naproxen sodium 220 mg twice daily with minimal improvement. She used a heating pad for her neck, and "arthritis cream" for her hands, but has not used any ice as therapy. She has not had any other work-up or imaging performed as of this time. She denies having numbness, weakness, or paresthesias involving her hands. She denies chest pain, fever, shortness of breath, cough, or stomach upset.

Past Medical History:

Osteopenia, osteoarthritis cervical spine, knees, hips; GERD (acid reflux disease), chronic daily tension headaches, hyperlipidemia, postmenopausal, last colonoscopy 1-year ago normal.

Past Surgical History:

Cervical fusion C5-7 at age 52, cervical fusion C2-5 at age 54, right knee replacement at age 59, appendectomy at age 18, tonsillectomy and adenoidectomy at age 6, C-section at age 29.

PAST TRAUMA HISTORY: MOTOR VEHICLE ACCIDENT 1982, MINOR CONCUSSION, WHIPLASH INJURY

Family Medical History:

Father deceased secondary to alcohol-induced cirrhosis at age 58, siblings: one brother aged 59, healthy, no family history of rheumatologic disorders other than OA

Gynecologic History:

G2 P 1011, LMP 12 years ago, last mammogram 2 years ago—normal, last pap and pelvic, rectal exam 2 years ago—normal, last DEXA scan 2 years ago osteopenia

Social History:

Widowed—husband John passed 10 years ago, 1 son—Marty 29 healthy, positive tobacco use (1 pk day intermittent for 35 years), denies illicit drug use, occasional alcohol (holidays). Patient was an employee for a large nutrition store. She does not exercise regularly.

CHILDHOOD ILLNESSES: CHICKEN POX AND POSSIBLE MEASLES

Medications:

Alendronate Sodium: 70 mg wk, Atorvastatin Calcium: 40 mg daily, Esomeprazole Magnesium: 40 mg daily, Naproxen Sodium: 220 mg twice daily, Acetaminophen: 500 mg four times daily prn, conjugated estrogens/medroxyprogesterone acetate tablets: 0.625 mg daily

REVIEW OF SYSTEMS

General:

She complains of fatigue and daily tension headaches. She denies fever, chills, change in appetite, or weight change.

Cardiopulmonary:

She denies chest pain, palpitations, and shortness of breath.

Neurological:

She denies numbness, weakness, and paresthesias of the extremities. She further denies any visual changes.

Musculoskeletal:

She admits to neck stiffness, bilateral hand pain and stiffness, daily tension headaches in the suboccipital and frontal region described as a tight sensation. She denies shoulder and hip discomfort and jaw claudication.

PHYSICAL EXAMINATION

Vital Signs:

T: 97.6, P: 78, R: 16, BP: 150/82, height: 5'4", weight: 138 lb.

General:

Alert, oriented, cooperative, affect somewhat flat, and a good historian. She appears her stated age.

HEENT:

PERLA EOMI, normal visual acuity. No xeropthalmia or xerostomia. Pharynx without erythema, no adenopathy, no thyromegaly, TMs good cone of light without erythema, no nasal erythema, no sinus tenderness, no tenderness over the temporal arteries or scalp

Neck:

Supple, no JVD or bruits. Some discomfort noted with full ROM

Skin:

No rashes, no abnormal appearing moles, multiple seborrheic keratoses (back), dry hair and nails. No petechiae, purpura, livedo reticularis, telangiectasias, or evidence of Raynaud phenomenon

Breast:

No breast masses, nipples everted, no discharge, no axillary adenopathy

Cardiovascular:

RRR without S3 S4 murmur, no clubbing, cyanosis, or peripheral edema. Equal pulses bilaterally

Lungs:

CTA without rales, rhonchi, wheezes

Abdomen:

BS × 4 quadrants without rigidity, rebound, guarding, Neg CVA pain, no masses appreciated. No RUQ discomfort on palpation, negative Murphy sign

Neurological:

CNs 2 to 12 intact, DTRs 2/4 bilateral, no sensory deficits, 5/5 motor strength bilateral

Musculoskeletal:

Upper extremities: Active and passive adduction, flexion, extension and internal rotation of the shoulders full and pain free. Slightly decreased full extension of both elbows, but no nodules palpated or frank contractures noted. Tenderness over both lateral and medial epicondyles bilaterally. Tenderness and synovitis noted over the second and third metacarpal phalangeal joints and proximal interphalangeal joints (PIPs) bilaterally, with evidence of underlying bony swelling consistent with Bouchard nodes on multiple PIPs. Several Heberden nodes also noted. No ulnar deviation appreciated. Nails appear brittle with ridges, but no pitting is observed. No cyanosis, clubbing, or edema. Pulses equal bilaterally, brisk capillary refill noted. Negative Tinel and Phalen sign. No thenar atrophy. Normal nail fold capillaroscopy

Lower extremities: Full hip, knee, ankle AROM PROM, negative Lachman test, negative joint line pain, negative Mc Murray and Apley; negative Patellar grind, mild crepitus noted in left knee. Negative hip compression test. Positive Bunion deformity of both great toes with tenderness of the metatarsal phalangeal joints bilaterally, without synovitis. No cyanosis, clubbing, or edema. Mild onychomycosis of the toenails. Pulses equal bilateral, good capillary refill

Osteopathic Structural Exam:

Sphenobasilar compression with a right lateral strain, bilateral occipitomastoid compression. C2 rotated left, occiput rotated right, and sidebent right, T4 ERS right, increased paraspinal muscle tension bilaterally at T10-12 and T12-L3 sidebent left and rotated right, sacrum has a left on left forward torsion, right sternoclavicular joint is superior with fascial restriction bilaterally in the upper extremities, short right leg, ribs 4 and 5 on the right have an inhalation dysfunction, and first rib on the right is elevated.

DIFFERENTIAL DIAGNOSIS

The most common pathophysiological processes that need to be considered in the differentiate diagnosis of bilateral hand pain and stiffness are mechanical, inflammatory, and neurological (Table 62.1).

TABLE 62.1

Differential Diagnosis for Symmetric Hand Stiffness and Pain in an Elderly Patient

Mechanical	a. Extensor tendonitis
	b. Repetitive overuse
	c. Thoracic outlet syndrome
	d. Compartment syndrome
	e. Osteoarthritis of the hands
	f. Cervical Spondylosis Hemochromatosis
Inflammatory	g. Rheumatoid arthritis
	h. Psoriatic arthritis
	i. Calcium Pyrophosphate Dihydrate Deposition Disease (CPPD or Pseudogout)
	j. Systemic Lupus Erythematosus
	k. Seronegative Spondyloarthropathies
	l. Scleroderma
	m. Polymyalgia rheumatica
	n. Polyarticular gout
	o. Bechet syndrome
	p. Reactive arthritis Infectious arthritis
Neurologic	q. Peripheral neuropathy
	r. Bilateral carpal tunnel syndrome
	s. Cervical stenosis/radiculopathy
	t. Syringomyelia/myelopathy

WORKUP AND INTERPRETATION

Cervical spine and bilateral hand x-rays were obtained. The cervical spine films showed A-P, lateral, oblique, and open mouth views were obtained. There is a reversal of the normal cervical lordosis. There is no fracture or subluxation. There is a stable appearing cervical fusion from C2 to C7. Diffuse degenerative changes are seen from C4 to C7. Facet hypertrophy is seen at the C5 to C7 levels. Degenerative changes are seen from C0 to C2 suggesting an arthritic process. No evidence of atlantoaxial instability, but full cervical spine series with flexion and extension views needed to adequately evaluate. Clinical correlation advised.

A-P and lateral views of the hands were obtained. There are no fractures or subluxations appreciated. Periarticular soft-tissue swelling with a fusiform appearance and juxta-articular osteopenia noted in interphalangeal joints. Suggestion of small marginal erosions along second and third metacarpophalangeal joints. Some diffuse joint space narrowing noted. Sclerosis and osteophyte formation predominantly involving distal interphalangeal joints bilaterally, with limited PIP involvement.

DIAGNOSIS

The patient's diagnosis based on the clinical history, examination, and diagnostic imaging was as follows:

1. Rheumatoid arthritis
2. Osteoarthritis of the cervical spine, knees, and hands
3. Somatic dysfunction: cervical, thoracic, rib, lumbar, sacrum, pelvis, and upper extremity, lower extremity
4. Osteopenia
5. Multilevel cervical fusion × 2
6. GERD (acid reflux disease)-controlled currently
7. Hyperlipidemia
8. Tobacco abuse

Relevant Functional Anatomy

In a patient with a bilateral upper extremity complaint, a functional anatomy review should cover the thoracic spine and ribs, the cervical spine, the thoracic inlet, and finally the forearm wrist and hand. This is because from a biomechanical standpoint, each of these areas can produce, intensify, or be related to the symptoms in this patient. Osteopathic manipulative treatment of these anatomic areas may also improve the patient's symptoms; therefore, a prior knowledge of the anatomy is necessary in order to carry out these procedures.

The upper thoracic spine neurologically influences the upper extremity via the sympathetic nervous system. The sympathetic innervation to the upper extremities arises from the upper thoracic spinal cord (segments T1–4). The sympathetic ganglia lie anterior to the rib head, in the fascia common to both structures. Dysfunction in the upper thoracic spine and ribs may increase sympathetic tone to the upper extremity and produce altered motion, nerve dysfunction, and lymphatic and venous congestion (1). Increased sympathetic tone is accompanied by palpatory findings in the upper thoracic/rib area and increased sensitivity to painful stimulus. Restricted motion or position of the ribs, and abnormal position of the costovertebral joints can apply fascial tension to the sympathetic chain ganglia. The upper thoracic spine and ribs are the origin for the scapular stabilizing muscles. These muscles include the rhomboids, serratus anterior, trapezius, and pectoralis minor.

Dysfunction in these muscles alters the position of the scapula, which in turn alters the position of the upper extremity. Triggerpoints in these muscles can refer pain into the upper extremity.

The cervical spine supplies neurologic innervation to the upper extremities. From an anatomic perspective, a smooth cervical lordosis, adequate intervertebral disc height, and patent neuroforamina are desirable. However, with degeneration due to aging, genetic factors, trauma, postural effects and repetitive overuse, the anatomy of the cervical spine may be far from optimal. The cervical vertebrae from C2 to C7 are saddle shaped and contain a specialized set of synovial joints on the lateral surface of the vertebral bodies. These are known as uncovertebral joints (uncinate) or joints of Luschka, and provide stability to the cervical spine. They may also decrease the likelihood of herniated nucleus pulposus in the cervical region. The joints of Luschka are not synovial in nature; thus, inflammatory arthropathies would spare these areas. However, the facet joints and atlantal-axial joint have synovial membrane that could be involved in inflammatory arthropathies. At the base of the skull, the tectoral membrane (occipital-axial ligament) is a strong continuation of the posterior longitudinal ligament that lies immediately behind the body of the axis. The alar ligaments are short, strong bundles of fibrous tissue directed obliquely upward and laterally from either side of the upper part of the odontoid process to the medial aspect of the occipital condyles (2). They are often referred to as the "check" ligaments. The transverse ligament of the atlas is a broad strong triangular ligament arching across the ring of the atlas and firmly anchored on each side to a tubercle in the medial surface of the lateral masses of the atlas. The transverse ligament has two fascicles layered in a crosswise fashion, which gives it a cruciate configuration. The transverse ligament portion of the cruciate ligament complex supports the atlas in rotating about the dens. The anterior surface of the spinal cord lies immediately posterior to the transverse ligament. Rupture of this ligament (or laxity, which may occur with rheumatoid arthritis) creates the possibility of the dens contacting the spinal cord and causing catastrophic neurologic damage. The cervical spinal canal is wider at the atlantoaxial level and narrows maximally at the C6 level. The cervical cord itself is wider from C3 to T2, corresponding to the increase in nerves supplying the upper extremities (2).

In the cervical spine, the discs are thicker anteriorly than posteriorly and are entirely responsible for the normal cervical lordosis. Each disc is situated between the cartilaginous endplates of two vertebrae. Successive layers of these fibers slant in alternate directions so that they cross each other at different angles depending on the intradiscal pressure of the nucleus pulposus. Positions of the cervical spine affect intradiscal pressure. Intradiscal pressure is least in the supine position, and extension of the cervical spine results in the greatest intradiscal pressure (3). After 50 years of age, the nucleus pulposus becomes a fibrocartilaginous mass that has characteristics similar to those of the inner zone of the annulus fibrosis (3).

The thoracic inlet is anatomically defined as the area above the clavicles; between the sternum, the first thoracic segment (T1), and the first rib. The brachial plexus and the subclavian artery travel through this area. The subclavian artery traverses between the first rib and clavicle (a potential site of compression) and then between the anterior and middle scalene muscles. The brachial plexus also travels between the anterior and middle scalene muscles. The thoracic outlet is the area where the neurovascular bundle travels between the clavicle and first rib, exiting between the anterior and middle scalene muscles. The subclavian vein passes over the first rib anterior to the anterior scalene muscle, so it is not involved in compression (2). Moving toward the arm, the subclavian artery becomes the axillary artery at the lateral border of the first rib. The axillary artery passes posterior to the pectoralis minor muscle and becomes the brachial artery at the inferior border of the teres major muscle. Branches from the axillary and brachial arteries supply the structures of the shoulder, arm, forearm, and hand.

Lymphatic compression can also occur, usually due to myofascial restrictions. The major lymph nodes of the upper extremities are found in the fibrofatty connective tissue of the axilla. They are arranged in five groups, four of which lie inferior to the pectoralis minor tendon and one lies superior to it. The thoracic duct is on the left and drains into the brachiocephalic trunk.

The three main peripheral nerves of the upper extremity include the median nerve, the ulnar nerve, and the radial nerve. Understanding the innervation of each and site of potential compression is important. Compression of the median nerve in the carpal tunnel (carpal tunnel syndrome) typically causes sensory symptoms such as night pain, paresthesias, and numbness in the hand in the radial three and one half digits. Symptoms may be referred proximally from the hand toward the forearm and even the elbow and may be reproduced or elicited by Phalen maneuver or Tinel sign. Thenar muscle weakness and atrophy represent advanced disease. Moving down into the hand, the *scaphoid, lunate,* and the *triquetral* bones articulate with the greater and lesser multangular, the capitate, and hamate where motion between these rows of bones is freer in flexion. If bony point tenderness is present in the face of hand trauma, always x-ray the hand, and in particular with respect to the anatomic snuff-box to make sure a navicular fracture is initially evaluated. The first carpometacarpal articulation is cavoconvex, and classified as a saddle-shaped joint. It is freely movable in two planes and rarely subject to dysfunction. The second to fifth carpometacarpal joints are gliding joints. The fifth is the most mobile, then the fourth. The second and third are fairly restricted in motion (4). Patients with arthritis of the wrists and hands can develop bony encroachment or irritation of tendons, blood vessels, and nerves. This may lead to comorbid conditions such as carpal tunnel syndrome in a patient with wrist osteoarthritis, or a de Quervain tenosynovitis in a patient with thumb arthritis and instability of the first carpometacarpal joint.

Motion, Posture, and Biomechanics

The cervical spine is better suited for mobility and is not required to transmit heavy loads. Precise control of head position and unrestricted movement is essential for normal functioning of the special senses. The saddle shape of each cervical vertebra provides mobility and stability. The anterior column composed of the vertebral body, longitudinal ligaments, and intervertebral disc provides some weight-bearing capacity, shock absorption, and a flexible structure. The posterior elements composed of the osseous canal, the zygapophyseal joints, and the erector spinae muscles protect the neural elements, and act as a fulcrum, to guide movement for the functional unit.

Alterations in the degree of curvature in one area of the spine result in reciprocal alterations in curvature in other areas of the spinal column to preserve the orientation of the body over the center of gravity. For example, an increase in lumbar lordosis results in increased cervical lordosis.

Physiology

Small joints, in particular those of the hand, are made up of a number of structures that allow for smooth motion, specificity of function, and strength of purpose. The small joint structure includes articular cartilage, and subchondral bone forming articulating surfaces in an attempt to work in concert with the musculoskeletal system making demands upon joint structure and function as a whole. Normally, articular cartilage is produced, and functioning bone is maintained, through cellular metabolism, circulation, respiration, synthesis, and remodeling. Homeostasis is a physiologic process by the organism to preserve form and function, an effort that declines in effectiveness as the organism ages.

Manifestations of Joint Disease

Joint disease in general can be monoarticular or polyarticular in nature. Monoarticular joint symptoms may be caused by many diseases, including infectious, traumatic, and crystal deposition diseases as well as noninflammatory conditions, such as osteoarthritis or avascular necrosis. Some inflammatory polyarticular diseases may occasionally present with monoarticular symptoms as well, such as early rheumatoid arthritis, psoriatic arthritis, viral arthritis, or reactive arthritis. Monoarticular joint disease by chronology can be transient (intermittent hydrarthrosis), acute (septic arthritis, trauma, gout), or subacute/chronic (pseudogout, neuropathic Charcot, tumor, infectious granuloma, TB, or osteoarthritis) in nature. Polyarticular joint disease in inflammatory arthritis often presents with symmetric, small joint involvement in diseases such as rheumatoid arthritis, SLE, psoriatic arthritis, and viral hepatitis. Polyarticular diseases with acute presentations include infectious arthritides, such as gonococcal, meningococcal, viral, Lyme disease, acute rheumatic fever, and bacterial endocarditis. Inflammatory polyarthritis that may be either acute or chronic in nature includes diseases such as rheumatoid arthritis, juvenile idiopathic arthritis, systemic lupus erythematosus, reactive arthritis, polyarticular gout, psoriatic arthritis, and arthritis associated with sarcoidosis. Noninflammatory polyarticular symptoms commonly arise from osteoarthritis, calcium pyrophosphate deposition disease (CPPD), fibromyalgia, benign hypermobility syndrome, and hemochromatosis (5). In this case, we will focus on both osteoarthritis and rheumatoid arthritis.

Pathophysiology

Osteoarthritis

Osteoarthritis (OA) is a disease process that characteristically includes degeneration of articular cartilage, subchondral sclerosis, hypertrophy of bone at joint margins (osteophytes), and multiple alterations in the synovial membrane as well as the joint capsule itself. There are multifactorial considerations germane to a discussion of the pathogenesis of OA, including biomechanical influences (isolated macrotrauma or repeated microtrauma), genetic alterations, and the relationship to aging, particularly with regard to morphologic changes in cartilage matrix composition and structure.

While aging is considered the most significant risk factor for the development of OA, obesity, mineral deposition, and systemic hormones all impart a higher risk for OA.

Morphologic, biochemical, and metabolic changes occur in OA. In early OA, irregularity of the surface of articular cartilage and changes in proteoglycan distribution occurs, followed by eventual ulceration of cartilage with exposure of bone, resulting in attempts at self-repair. Local repair involves increased chondrocyte concentration, and new bone formation in the form of osteophytes. Biochemical changes vary during the stages of OA, with increased water content of articular cartilage in early OA, and increased collagen and diminished proteoglycan concentrations later in the disease. Early degeneration of cartilage is likely related to matrix metalloproteinases whose enzymes degrade both collagen and proteoglycans (6). The initial stages of OA are thus marked by a complex interplay of multiple factors, including increased cell proliferation and synthesis of matrix proteins, proteinases, growth factors, cytokines, and other inflammatory mediators by chondrocytes. The disease process ultimately affects the joint structure in its entirety, including cartilage, synovium, ligaments, and subchondral bone.

One central problem with osteoarthritis is that an adult articular chondrocyte has limited capacity to regenerate damaged original cartilage matrix architecture. Indeed, an age-related reduction in chondrocyte function has been shown with the end result of morphologic and structural changes in aging articular cartilage, such as thinning of the articular surface, decreased size of matrix proteoglycans, and diminished strength and stiffness of the matrix (6). The chondrocyte may attempt to regenerate the matrix by mimicking early stages of cartilage development, but original cartilage cannot be replicated. Current pharmacological interventions do not include a proven structure-modifying approach. Cartilage tissue engineering (with or without replacement) or gene therapy is a possible approach in the future. Animal models of OA have yet to reproduce the human condition, perhaps in part because they often represent secondary rather than primary OA (7).

Rheumatoid Arthritis

Rheumatoid arthritis is a chronic systemic inflammatory disease characterized predominantly by persistent, symmetric inflammation of multiple joints, although extra-articular manifestations may also occur. It is the most common inflammatory arthritis, affecting approximately 1% of the population. The primary target in RA is the synovium, in which infiltration of mononuclear cells, such as T cells and macrophages, synovial intimal lining hyperplasia and angiogenesis occur. A complex interplay between synoviocytes, T cells, B cells, and inflammatory mediators eventually leads to aggressive cartilage destruction and progressive bony erosions. Untreated, rheumatoid arthritis often leads to progressive joint destruction, disability, and premature death.

Although extensive research has been conducted with regard to the pathogenesis of RA, the exact etiology remains elusive. Roles of multiple inflammatory mediators, including cytokines, chemokines, growth factors, adhesion molecules, and matrix metalloproteinases, have been defined thus far. It is known that these mediators are responsible for both attracting and activating cells in the peripheral blood, in addition to local activation and proliferation of synoviocytes (8). Susceptibility to RA is likely resultant from a combination of environmental and genetic factors. One of the most significant genetic risk factors uncovered thus far involves the class II MCH haplotype of an individual. Certain HLA-DR molecules are more commonly found in patients with RA (e.g., HLA-DR4), and consistency in a particular amino acid sequence in the third hypervariable region of the beta chain of MHC-susceptible alleles has led to the "shared-epitope" hypothesis. This hypothesis postulates that presumed antigen(s) bind to this particular site, resulting in the cascade of inflammation in RA (9).

Rheumatoid arthritis is also closely mimicked by transient arthritic conditions provoked by several microbial pathogens, leading to the consideration of infectious etiologies in the pathogenesis of RA. A role for infection in the development of rheumatoid arthritis has long been postulated, including potential bacterial and viral pathogens, but it has not yet been proven. Other potential antigens include heat-shock proteins, MHC molecules themselves, and certain epitopes within type II collagen (9).

A complex array of constituents in the immune system interact to cause the initiation and perpetuation of inflammation found in RA. Memory T cells, B cells, plasma cells, cytokines, macrophages, vascular endothelium, and rheumatoid factor all play important roles. Just a few of the memory T cells functions include enhanced T cell, macrophage, and antigen-presenting cell activation, while macrophages act as effectors, producing multiple proinflammatory cytokines, such as IL-1, IL-6, TNF, among others. Rheumatoid factors of multiple isotypes form immune complexes that not only fix complement but also activate neutrophils. B cells are also found within the rheumatoid synovium, and although the exact mechanisms involved in pathogenesis are yet unknown, the therapeutic use of rituximab, and a chimeric anti-CD20 (B cell) monoclonal antibody, has produced significant responses in patients with RA. Multiple cytokines exist within the rheumatoid synovium, exhibiting complex roles, including mononuclear cell migration, cell activation, and direct damage to articular cartilage and bone. Tumor necrosis factor-α (TNF-α) is an important proinflammatory cytokine, and TNF-blocking therapies (adalimumab, etanercept, and infliximab) have been successful in the treatment of RA. Newer therapies focused on cytokines currently under investigation or soon to be released include inhibitors for IL-15 and IL-17, and IL-6 blockade, respectively (10).

Osteopathic Patient Management

For any patient presenting with pain in the hands, a thorough osteopathic examination, using the five-point structure function model, is essential. Osteopathic techniques can be applied to the areas of somatic dysfunction in patients presenting with arthritic-type pathology. The models of structure-function relationships described below guide the osteopathic practitioner's approach to diagnosis and treatment. These models provide a framework for integrating objective and subjective clinical findings with osteopathic structural exam findings.

Biomechanical Model

Short leg mechanics can lead to a worsening of a patient's arthritic upper extremity symptoms by adding postural stress to the upper extremity with resultant aches and pains. Vleeming's work can be used to understand the anatomical relationship between sacral base unleveling from short leg mechanics, subsequent iliac crest unleveling, and the postural tension created in the shoulders through the latissimus dorsi muscle via the thoracolumbar fascia. Altered shoulder biomechanics can strain muscles and increase intrinsic pressure on the intra-articular tissues, both of which may exacerbate joint pain.

Another biomechanical consequence of postural imbalance is concomitant changes in the A-P curves. With a forward head position and protracted shoulders, the rotator cuff muscles, levator scapulae, and serratus posterior superior become tight and develop myofascial triggerpoints. Triggerpoints in these muscles refer to the upper extremity (14). Scalene tension can cause neurovascular compression as can elevation of the first rib, narrowing the space between itself and the clavicle. All these factors can biomechanically be related to painful syndromes in the upper extremity, including the hands.

Respiratory/Circulatory Model

Another objective of osteopathic treatment is improvement of local blood flow to the area of arthritis in the hands as well as removal of edema to assist in pain reduction and improve mobility. This is done by addressing the areas of somatic dysfunction that may influence arterial, venous, or lymphatic flow. Our patient has dysfunction in the lower thoracic and thoracolumbar areas, both of which may influence diaphragm function. Improving motion in the lower thoracic region will help the function of the diaphragm from a mechanical prospective. Improving motion in the cervical region may help the function of the diaphragm from a neurologic perspective. Treating both regions will aid in restoring normal diaphragmatic motion, which is the primary driving force to move lymph and venous blood. This treatment should follow thoracic inlet release, which removes any proximal restrictions to lymphatic flow coming from the upper extremities. In the patient described in the case, treatment of the right sternoclavicular restriction will further aid in this process by normalizing fascial tensions of the thoracic inlet. Then, attention can be moved distally to remove pectoral and axillary restrictions, and then on to the elbow, wrist, and hand for the same purpose. Abnormal interosseous membrane tension of the forearm may contribute to lymphatic and venous stasis by altering the mechanics of radius and ulnar and their role in generating intracompartmental pressures. This is especially true in patients who repetitively use their forearms, as their muscles and fascias become tight. Peripheral fascial restrictions in the distal arms may affect the vascular structures traveling through them. Restrictions in the scalene muscles, first rib or thoracic inlet may impede fluid movement through the vascular bundle supplying the upper extremity. Treatment of these areas may improve lymphatic and venous drainage and arterial flow.

Neurological Model

The sacrum is the base of support of the spinal column; unleveling of the sacrum results in adaptive or compensatory curves in the vertebral column. No matter if there is an "S"-shaped or a "C"-shaped adaptive group curve, there will be crossover points of the curve. A crossover point is where the curve changes direction. This vertebral unit is commonly found to have type II dysfunction. These segments can become facilitated and act as an "irritable focus" of neuronal activity (11). If the crossover point is between T1 and T4, as it is in this patient, the upper extremities may be affected. Increased activity in somatic fibers between T1 and T4 can be referred to the upper extremity via a somato-somatic reflex. Dorsal root reflexes may activate primary afferent fibers in the peripheral area served by the upper thorax resulting in the secretion of proinflammatory substances that may exacerbate arthritic symptoms. Increased nociceptive activity at the level of T1–4 has the potential to activate fibers in the adjacent lateral horn. As the sympathetic neurons become facilitated (12), the abnormal sympathetic drive affects vascular tone and peristalsis resulting in venous and lymphatic stasis in the upper extremities. Increased vascular tone can also make muscles stiff and noncompliant. Sympathetic overactivity will alter the secretory activity of sweat glands, and sensitize nocioceptors and mechanoreceptors (13).

One objective of osteopathic management is to normalize neurologic input to the upper extremity. Sympathetic innervation to the upper extremity may be influences through treatment of the upper thoracic and the associated rib dysfunctions. As stated above, increased sympathetic tone to the upper extremity can cause vasoconstriction, edema, sensitivity of the nerves, irritability of the muscles, and sweat gland overactivity. OMT in this region may improve those related pathophysiologic findings.

Peripheral fascial restrictions may affect somatic nerves, in addition to the aforementioned vascular structures. Tension in the anterior scalenes and the thoracic inlet can compress the neurovascular bundle, impairing nerve transmission and vascular supply to the rotator cuff and scapular stabilizing muscles. Removal of the fascial restrictions and resultant compression to the neurovascular bundle will facilitate axoplasmic flow, enhancing the nerves' trophic function. Tension of the pronator teres muscle in the forearm can compress the median nerve (pronator syndrome) producing hand symptoms as well (15). Stiffness of the joints of the hands and elbows can cause overuse of the forearm muscles to make up the motion lost. Stiffness, swelling, enlargement, and ulnar deviation of the digits can affect the small nerves in the hands. If these nerves are already sensitized from spinal facilitation, they will report increased levels of pain.

Metabolic Energy Model

Patients who have painful musculoskeletal conditions can require increased energy expenditure to function when compared to a healthy patient of the same age. Increased oxygen demand can cause fatigue if they have to ambulate a long distance with arthritic knees, hips, ankles, or feet. For those who repetitively use their hands, as in typing, upper extremity stiffness and pain can be problematic. They can become fatigued, make errors, and become frustrated. Both the working environment and the recreational environment may become affected, changing the patient's ability to cope in comparison to their premorbid condition. Osteopathic patient management must address the factors that may contribute to energy demand and production.

If the clinician's objective is to improve the patient's energy flow and metabolic activity, then removing barriers to the proper function of physiological mechanisms is important. Osteopathy in the cranial field recognizes the primary respiratory mechanism as a fundamental component of health (1990). According to Sutherland model (1998), patients who have a significant sphenobasilar synchondrosis compression do not have optimal function of the primary respiratory mechanism and therefore suboptimal recuperative capacity. Compression of the fourth ventricle, a cranial technique, has been hypothesized to assist in the normalization of cerebrospinal fluid flow and other components of the primary respiratory mechanism (16).

Behavioral Model

Small joint disease presents a challenge in accomplishing these tasks subsumed under the concept of activities of daily living (ADLs). For those patients with small joint disease, simple tasks such as opening a jar of pickles can present a constant reminder of declining capabilities. The challenge in caring for these patients is to provide alternative coping skills for the maintenance of spirit. When met with challenges, many people turn to prayer or spirituality to guide and strengthen their efforts to lead meaningful lives in the larger sense and to accomplish ADLs on a much smaller scale. Support groups may be of value, especially if the patient has expressed feelings of isolation with regard to his or her disease. Patient education can assist in the preservation of self-worth, and educational materials for patients with RA may be obtained from the Arthritis Foundation, American College of Rheumatology, and the National Institutes of Health. Encouragement along with the revelation of the many ways in which the patient can rise above the pain and diminished function that can accompany small joint disease can help them to achieve or maintain spiritual and behavioral satisfaction. The goal is to achieve or maintain function at a premorbid level though this may not be possible in the long run. In this fashion, patients with small joint disease with proper treatment can maintain their own self-image in addition to the way they are perceived by society to be functioning as a whole. The osteopathic physician is well placed to provide not only physical and pharmacologic medicine, but also education and emotional support to assist the patient in achievement of shared goals.

Outcomes Studies and Best Evidence for Manual Treatment

Both osteoarthritis and rheumatoid arthritis are common problems and can be chronic disabling conditions. For many patients, conventional therapies are not completely effective and are limited by side effects. This can lead to ongoing pain and frustration. Complementary and alternative medical therapies (CAM) therapies are defined as being outside scientific mainstream medicine. These nonpharmaceutical treatments are generally unproven in efficacy but perceived as safe. The American College of Rheumatology (ACR) believes practitioners should be informed about cam therapies and be able to discuss them knowledgably with patients. Meanwhile, scientific studies are underway to test the efficacy of these modalities. OMT may be considered a CAM therapy by some clinicians, while others feel it is an integral part of osteopathic patient care.

Conservative treatment for patients with hand arthritis (both RA and OA) may include (but is not limited to) the following: medications, diet, heat or cold therapy, physical or occupational therapy, modalities, tens, braces and splints, injections, osteopathic manipulation, chiropractic manipulation, massage therapy, and acupuncture.

Manipulative techniques for upper extremity complaints have been taught in the osteopathic schools' curriculum since its inception. OMT has been shown to be beneficial to decrease pain and increase patient's function in a variety of clinical situations. Manipulative techniques have been employed and studied in the treatment of injuries and osteoarthritis of the fingers and hand (17). Yet, there none or few randomized controlled studies to show that OMT is beneficial for patients with RA or OA of the hands.

There have been a number of studies in the literature reporting that acupuncture is effective in treating rheumatoid arthritis. One such study evaluated acupuncture in the treatment of rheumatic knee pain. As compared to sham treatment, the acupuncture group had improved pain scores for as long as 3 months after treatment (18). More studies assessing the effectiveness of acupuncture for rheumatoid arthritis are needed. There is moderately strong evidence from the above studies to support the use of acupuncture as an adjunctive therapy for osteoarthritis.

A recent meta-analysis (19) of seven studies concluded that chondroitin sulfate may be useful in decreasing pain and improving function in osteoarthritis. Chondroitin sulfate may be useful in the treatment of osteoarthritis. Larger studies are needed to further examine the usefulness of chondroitin sulfate in osteoarthritis.

The application of pulsed electric device (PEMF) stimulation for osteoarthritis is a relatively new area. In two different studies (20,21), chronic knee osteoarthritis was treated with PEMF by way of skin surface electrodes. The treatment was superior to placebo in symptom reduction. The treatment also seemed to be cost effective. PEMF therapy is considered safe but should be avoided in those who are pregnant, with permanent pacemakers, and patients with known cancer.

Integrative Treatment Approach
Osteopathic Manipulation
As Osteopathic physicians, we often make use of Osteopathic Manipulative Treatment (OMT) as a powerful treatment tool for musculoskeletal complaints. OMT is part of the Osteopathic physician's overall treatment armamentarium and the use should follow from the careful consideration of Osteopathic principles and practice used in the evaluation of every patient. The use of OMT is frequently based on the physician's ability, the patient's presentation and responses, and the type of dysfunction found. OMT can be tailored to fit almost any practice model. There are many benefits to osteopathic manipulation. Some of the primary benefits include increased range of motion, decreased pain, improved ADLs, and shortened disability time (quicker return to work). Some secondary benefits include reduced reliance on medications (especially narcotics) and improved postural efficiency (22). In patients with rheumatoid arthritis of the occipitoatlantal and atlantal-axial articulations, caution must be applied to the choice of technique used to treat the somatic dysfunction present. Rheumatoid arthritis of the upper cervical spine is a contradiction to thrust (HVLA)-type manipulation. This is thought to be due to the relative laxity and instability in this region due to the inflammatory process (23). However, it is also to be remembered that for subacute and chronic neck pain, spinal manipulation is more effective when compared with muscle relaxants or the usual medical care. Efficacy was enhanced when combined with other modalities, such as exercise (24).

Pharmacologic Treatment

While the body has the innate ability to self-heal, therapies with pharmacological treatments are often essential in the treatment of an inflammatory arthritis such as RA. Disease-modifying antirheumatic drugs (DMARDs), either alone or in combination, as well as biologic therapies (e.g., TNF-α blockers), and nonsteroidal anti-inflammatory drugs (NSAIDs) are often the cornerstone of treatment therapies. Early and aggressive interventions may result in lower morbidity and mortality, as evidenced by slower radiographic progression, less disability, and fewer surgical interventions (25). In fact, recent studies have suggested that patients on methotrexate combination therapy or TNF inhibitors have less morbidity and mortality from cardiovascular events as well due to diminished systemic inflammation (26,27). Thus, even in the most skilled hands, most patients require a combined approach with the appropriate use of other treatment modalities including medications or local injections of corticosteroids to reduce inflammation.

Physical and Occupational Therapy

The role of physical and occupational therapy is also of great importance, especially in the early treatment of an inflammatory arthritis such as RA, but may also be beneficial in OA as well. Physical therapy is usually considered for issues related to ambulation or predominantly lower extremity dysfunction, while occupational therapy encompasses the upper extremity, focusing on the assessment of functional abilities within home/work environments. Patients should be evaluated for ability to engage in ADLs, ability to ambulate, level of fitness, etc. Treatment modalities may then be fashioned to ensure joint function as well as joint protection, and steps may be taken to potentially prevent contractures or deformities (28). Joint protection interventions have been studied in patients with RA, and home hand exercises have resulted in improved grip strength as well as diminished morning stiffness (29–33). Another study evaluating joint protection and home hand exercises for patients with hand osteoarthritis also showed increased hand strength and global hand function, underscoring the importance of nonpharmacologic interventions in the treatment of both RA and OA (34). Whole-body strength training and gripper exercises have also been shown to improve dynamic and static grip strength while decreasing pain in older patients with hand OA (35). These therapeutic modalities have no side effects, are generally readily acceptable, and can be performed easily, making them useful adjunctive treatments in both of these chronic diseases. Other useful non-pharmacologic interventions include adaptive devices that may be customized to improve independence in daily activities, such as opening jars and car doors, self-care, grooming, and dressing.

Multiple lines of evidence support the case for early intervention in rheumatoid arthritis, as functional health status tends to decline early in the disease, mortality rates rise over the course of the disease, and radiographic changes occur much earlier in the disease process than previously thought. Work disability increases from approximately 25% at 6.4 years to 50% at 20.9 years after onset of disease (36). Mortality rates also rise over the course of the disease, with rates as high as 35% by 20 years (37).

All of these factors have to be taken into consideration, coupled with the need to individualize each case based on patient desire, functional status, and long-term goals. Additionally, due to patient desire, medical conditions and/or other factors, the patient may not be a candidate for certain treatment modalities, such as surgical joint replacement, forcing a conservative approach. More than 70% of patients with RA have some form of hand disability, often crippling hand deformities if the disease has been longstanding (38).

Surgical Intervention

The role of surgical intervention in the treatment of RA remains somewhat controversial, and it should be determined by both the level of pain and the functional status of the individual. Many practitioners will not recommend surgical intervention unless pain disrupts sleep, and true functional gain has to be rigorously assessed as well. Likewise, nonoperative treatments for osteoarthritis should be employed, such as medications, intra-articular steroid injections, hand therapies, and splinting prior to consideration of surgical interventions (39). If a surgical approach is required, the specifics of the procedure should be considered. If two different procedures are being considered, how would each of these different procedures change the duration of healing and required physical therapy postoperatively? How would any or each of these procedures affect the presence of somatic dysfunction in the cervical, thoracic or lumbar spine? Osteopathic treatment can be a helpful adjunctive therapy postoperatively. Postoperative patients who develop cervical spasm, rib restrictions, atelectasis, or sacral malpositioning, for example, may benefit from OMT for relief of cervical, thoracic, lumbar, or sacral somatic dysfunction. Postoperatively, activity modification, work restrictions, and lifestyle change are important aspects to consider to assist patients in their recovery and to enhance the healing process.

Treatment Sequence

A good rule of thumb for the practitioner is to assess how acute the area to be treated actually has become. There are many reflexes active in the body and generally the more normal relationships that can be established distant from an acute area the easier it will be to address that remaining acute area for a response. For example, suppose a patient has an elevated first rib that is causing distal arm pain, but the patient's main complaint is radial head dysfunction felt at the elbow. Advantage can be gained in relaxing to as normal a state the facilitated irritation being generated by the elevated first rib, which can reasonably be expected to increase tone in distal musculature. By following this approach, when it comes time to move the radial head, there may be that much less resistance to movement encountered from muscles attached to the radius. Similarly, with small joint disease, working to release the carpal tunnel from undue pressure via the opponens roll technique may decrease pain perceived distally is the small joints of the fingers (40).

The emotional component to the patient's condition needs to be evaluated and addressed. For example, the patient may not be compliant with therapy due to financial constraints, personal reasons, or other factors. This may result in delayed progress/healing and perhaps a sense of guilt that they are not doing everything they could for their condition.

SUMMARY

In conclusion, it is through the use of multiple modalities that we as osteopathic physicians can provide the most comprehensive and therapeutic treatment strategies for patients with both rheumatoid arthritis and osteoarthritis as it involves small joints of the hands. The combination of state-of-the-art pharmacologic interventions, physical and occupational therapies, and osteopathic principles and practice enable osteopathic physicians to uniquely enhance the lives of individuals affected by these debilitating and potentially devastating diseases.

REFERENCES

1. Nelson KE, Glonek T. *Somatic Dysfunction in Osteopathic Family Practice, ACOFP.* Baltimore MD: Lippincott Williams & Wilkins, Copyright 2007:345–349.
2. Moore KL. *Clinically Oriented Anatomy.* 3rd Ed. Baltimore, MD: Williams & Wilkins; 1992:528.
3. DeLee JC, Drez D. *Orthopaedic Sports Medicine Principles and Practice.* Vol 2, 2nd Ed. Philadelphia, PA: Saunders, Copyright 2003:1065–1095.
4. Fryette HH. *Principles of Osteopathic Technique.* Carmel, California, CA: Academy of Applied Osteopathy, 1954:190–202.
5. Hawkins, RA. Approach to the patient with monoarticular symptoms. *Rheumatology Secrets.* 2nd Ed. 2002:88–100.
6. Cesare PE, Abramson SB. Pathogenesis of osteoarthritis. *Kelley's Textbook of Rheumatology,* 7th Ed. 2004; 1493–1537.
7. Goldring MB, Goldring SR. *J Cell Physiol* 2007;13(3):626–634.
8. Firestein GS. Etiology and pathogenesis of rheumatoid arthritis. *Kelley's Textbook of Rheumatology.* 7th Ed. 2004; 996–1014.
9. Cush JJ, et al. *Rheumatoid Arthritis: Early Diagnosis and Treatment.* 2nd Ed. 2008:13–28.
10. Cush JJ, et al. *Rheumatoid Arthritis: Early Diagnosis and Treatment.* 2nd Ed. 2008:175–180.
11. Korr IM. The facilitated segment: A factor in injury to the body framework (1973). In: *The Collected Papers of Irvin M. Korr.* Colorado Springs, CO: American Academy of Osteopathy, 1979:188–189.
12. Korr IM. The neural basis of the osteopathic lesion (1947). In: *The Collected Papers of Irvin M. Korr.* Colorado Springs, CO: American Academy of Osteopathy, 1979:1120–1127.
13. Ward RC. Foundations for Osteopathic Medicine, Neurophysiologic Mechanisms of Integration and Disintegration. Philadelphia, PA: Lippincott Williams & Wilkins, 2003:129–133, chap 7.
14. Travell JG, Simons DG. *Myofascial Pain and Dysfunction, The Triggerpoint Manual.* Baltimore, MD: Williams and Wilkins, 1983:377–382, 614–618.
15. Pronator syndrome. *Clin Sports Med.* Volume 20(3):531–540.
16. Magoun HI. *Osteopathy in the Cranial Field.* Meridian, Idaho: The Cranial Academy, 1976:110, 336.
17. Tucker WE. Physiotherapy, 1971, Jun 10; 57(6):255–8
18. Berman BM, Singh BB, Lao L, et al. A randomized trial of acupuncture as an adjunctive therapy in osteoarthritis of the knee. *Rheumatology (Oxford)* 1999;38:346–354.
19. Leeb B, et al. A metaanalysis of chondroitin sulfate in the treatment of osteoarthritis. *J Rheumatol* 2000;27:205–211.

20. Zizic TM, Hoffman KC, Holt PA, et al. The treatment of osteoarthritis of the knee with pulsed electrical stimulation. *J Rheumatol* 1995;22(9):1757–1761.

21. Trock DH, Bollet AJ, Markoll R. The effect of pulsed electromagnetic fields in the treatment of osteoarthritis of the knee and cervical spine. Report of randomized, double blind, placebo controlled trials. *J Rheumatol* 1994;21(10):1903–1911.

22. Ward RC. *Foundations for Osteopathic Medicine*. 1st Ed. Efficacy and Complications. Baltimore, MD: Lippincott Williams & Wilkins, 1997:1015–1018, chap 73.

23. Ward RC. *Foundations for Osteopathic Medicine*. 1st Ed. Efficacy and Complications. Baltimore, MD: Lippincott Williams & Wilkins, 1997:1019, chap 73.

24. Seffinger MA, Hruby RJ. illustrator Kuchera WA. Evidence-based manual medicine. In: *Problem Oriented Approach*. Saunders Elsevier, Copyright 2007:221–272.

25. da Silva E, et al. Declining use of orthopedic surgery in patients with rheumatoid arthritis? Results of a long-term, population-based assessment. *Arthritis Rheum* 2003;49:216–220.

26. Choi HK, et al. Methotrexate and mortality in patients with rheumatoid arthritis: a prospective study. *Lancet* 2002;359:1173–1177.

27. Jackobsson LT, et al. Treatment with tumor necrosis factor blockers is associated with a lower incidence of first cardiovascular events in patients with rheumatoid arthritis. *J Rheumatol* 2005;32:1213–1218.

28. Cush JJ, et al. *Rheumatoid Arthritis: Early Diagnosis and Treatment*. 2nd Ed. 2008:99–103.

29. Hammond A, et al. A crossover trial evaluating an educational-behavioral joint protection program for people with rheumatoid arthritis. *Patient Educ Couns* 1999;37:19–32.

30. Hoenig H, et al. A randomized controlled trial of home exercise on the rheumatoid hand. *J Rheumatol* 1993;20:785–789.

31. Hwakes J, et al. Comparison of three physiotherapy regimens for hands with rheumatoid arthritis. *Br Med J (Clin Res Ed)* 1985;291:1016.

32. Shaufler J, et al. "Hand gym" for patients with arthritic hand disabilities: preliminary report. *Arch Phys Med Rehabil* 1978;59:221–226.

33. Castillo BA, et al. Physical activity, cystic erosions, and osteoporosis in rheumatoid arthritis. *Ann Rheum Dis* 1965;24:522–527.

34. Stamm TA, et al. Joint protection and home hand exercises improve hand function in patients with hand osteoarthritis: a randomized controlled trial. *Arth Care Res* 2002;47:44–49.

35. Rogers MW, Wilder FV. The effects of strength training among persons with hand osteoarthritis: a two-year follow-up study. *J Hand Ther* 2007; 20(3):244–249.

36. Wolfe F, Hawley DJ: The long-term outcomes of rheumatoid arthritis: Work disability: a prospective 18 year study of 823 patients. *J Rheumatol* 1998;25(11):2108–2117.

37. Scott DL, et al. Long-term outcome of treating rheumatoid arthritis: results after 20 years. *Lancet* 1987;1(8542):1108.

38. De la Mata lord J, et al. Rheumatoid arthritis: are outcomes better with medical or surgical management? *Orthopedics* 1998;21:1085–1086.

39. Palmieri TJ, et al. Treatment of hand OA in the hand and wrist: non-operative treatment. *Clin Rheum Dis* 1985;11(2):433–445.

40. Sucher BM, Hinrichs BM, Welcher RN, et al. Manipulative treatment of carpal tunnel syndrome: biomechanical and osteopathic intervention to increase the length of the transverse carpal ligament: part 2. Effect of sex differences and manipulative "priming". *J Am Osteopath Assoc* 2005;105(3):135–143.

41. Vleeming A, Pool-Goudzwaard AL, Stoeckart R, et al. The posterior layer of the thoracolumbar fascia: its function in load transfer from spine to legs. *Spine* 1995:753–758.

42. Sutherland WG. *Contributions of Thought*. Portland, OR: Rudra Press, 1998.

43. Sutherland WG. *Teachings in the Science of Osteopathy*. Portland, OR: Rudra Press, 1990.

63

Lower Extremity Swelling in Pregnancy

MELICIEN TETTAMBEL

KEY CONCEPTS

- Swollen legs are a common condition of pregnancy and are often related to the physiologic hypervolemia of pregnancy.
- A woman's body undergoes many biomechanical adaptations as her pregnancy progresses; these may adversely impact the low-pressure systems of the body resulting in passive venous congestion.
- While passive venous congestion is often a contributing factor in swollen legs during pregnancy, other causes must be ruled out.
- Addressing tissue strains and compensatory postural adaptations to pregnancy may help alleviate passive tissue congestion and improve symptoms associated with peripheral edema.

CASE VIGNETTE

Diane, a 26-year-old primigravid female, is seen for her prenatal care visit, complaining of swelling of both lower extremities. She is 29 weeks pregnant, and to date, has not had any other problems in her prenatal course.

Chief Complaint:

Swelling of lower extremities

History of Present Illness:

She reports that the swelling in her legs usually resolves by morning; but gradually increases throughout the day. Shoes become tight and uncomfortable as well. She denies trauma to the lower extremities or pelvis.

Past Medical History:

Noncontributory

Past Surgical History:

Negative

REVIEW OF SYSTEMS

She denies headache, dizziness, and nausea. She denies blurred and double vision. She denies high blood pressure. She admits to occasional acid reflux. She denies diarrhea and constipation. She denies change in tolerance to temperature. She admits to mild fatigue. She denies pain, burning, weakness, and paresthesias.

PHYSICAL EXAMINATION

Vital Signs:

Blood pressure: 116/62, heart rate: 68 and regular, weight: 146 lb (increased by 3 lb from last month's visit). Urine dipstick indicates absence of glucose, protein, and nitrite.

Cardiovascular:

Heart has a regular rhythm without murmur or gallop; all pulses are intact.

Lungs:

Clear to auscultation and percussion

Abdomen:

Gravid abdomen, no tenderness to palpation, no venous distention

OB/GYN:

Fundal height consistent with gestational age, fetal heart tones located in lower right quadrant with rate of 146

Extremities:

No tenderness on palpation of lower extremities. Mild, nonpitting edema appreciated in both lower extremities, no edema in the upper extremities, and pulses are regular and intact. There is no venous distension and no signs of trauma are noted.

Neurological:

Deep tendon reflexes +2/4 bilaterally symmetrical and equal in all extremities, sensory and motor are grossly intact.

Musculoskeletal:

Gait and posture are unremarkable for this stage of pregnancy. There is a slight increase of lumbar lordosis and anterior pelvic tilt, but there is no tenderness to palpation of muscles of lumbar spine and pelvis.

Osteopathic Structural Exam:

Lumbosacral junction is rotated to the left, and thoracolumbar junction is also rotated to the left. The right innominate is rotated anteriorly and the right pubic tubercle is inferior and tender to light palpation. The left quadratus lumborum is hypertonic and ribs 10 to 12 on the left are inferior compared with those on the right. There is restricted movement in exhalation of the lower ribs 6 to 12 bilaterally. The thoracic kyphosis is somewhat flattened, and there is tension in the cervical muscles bilaterally extending from the cervicothoracic junction to the suboccipital area. The cervicothoracic junction is rotated right, the occiput is sidebent right and rotated left, and C2 is rotated right. There is mild restriction at the left occipitomastoid area.

DIFFERENTIAL DIAGNOSIS OF LOWER EXTREMITY EDEMA

Complaints of swelling of the face, hands and, especially, the legs and feet are common in pregnancy. This chapter describes the causes of lower extremity swelling in pregnancy from osteopathic and obstetric points of view. There are standard recommended guidelines for "routine" prenatal visits that are utilized by most obstetrical care providers (1–5). These guidelines identify potential problems of fetal growth and development, as well as maternal well-being. Baseline information such as maternal age, first day of last normal menstrual period, number of pregnancies and their outcomes, maternal weight, employment activity, past and present family and medical history is recorded. At each prenatal care visit, the following information is recorded: gestational age, weight, blood pressure, fundal height, fetal heart tones, and urine dipstick detection of glucose, protein, and maternal urine nitrites. Patient concerns are recorded with related care plans or screening tests. Next follow-up visit is also documented.

In the second and third trimesters of pregnancy, women are concerned about weight gain, fetal activity, fatigue, and edema. During this time, swelling may be the result of salt and fluid retention, hormonal changes, alteration of cardiovascular, lymphatic and renal dynamics; and/or musculoskeletal changes to accommodate an enlarging uterus.

Eighty percent of pregnant women report swelling of the legs and feet in pregnancy (6). There are a variety of causes from benign physiologic changes to serious medical problems. Box 63.1 lists some of the most usual differential diagnoses. Each of these potential causes will be discussed within the framework of the case presented at the beginning of this chapter.

Varicosities

Varicose veins, also known as varicosities, occur when a valve in the blood vessel wall weakens, causing stagnation of blood flow. Venous circulation slows as the venous walls dilate and distend. Just below the skin, the vein may swell into a small balloon-like structure. Leg veins are most commonly affected as they are working against gravity especially with prolonged standing. Pregnancy is a major contributing factor in the development of varicose veins as the enlarging uterus puts additional valvular pressure on veins of the pelvis resulting in hemorrhoids and varicosities of the vulva. The increasing weight of the expanding uterus also puts pressure on the inferior vena cava. Veins in the legs are most commonly affected by additional gravitational challenges to supply circulation to the lower half of the body.

Varicose veins are most commonly seen in women in North America and Western Europe where people may have more sedentary

---

lives and utilize modes of transportation rather than walking long distances. Varicose veins are less common in the Mediterranean, South America, and India; and even more uncommon in the Far East and Africa, where obesity is not prevalent (7,8). The development of varicose veins may also be due to a history of phlebitis, type of physical activity, or genetics (familial dominant, x-linked) (9). Parous women have a higher incidence of varicose veins compared with nulliparous women and multiparous women have the highest risk (10). Previous pregnancy with resultant weight gain, and fascial and ligamentous laxity may have further tilted the pelvic bowl with its contents in a more anterior position. Tissue changes, postural changes, and maternal age, in conjunction with weight changes, all may contribute to varicosities. Though varicosities often manifest in pregnancy, they may regress until the next pregnancy. Furthermore, there is no direct correlation between the severity of varicosities and the severity of the patient's symptoms.

The development of varicose veins during pregnancy may be influenced by the combination of high cardiac output and an increase in the hormone progesterone that relaxes the muscular walls of the blood vessel. It is hypothesized that estrogen and progesterone receptors on saphenous veins may provoke venous dilation and valve failure in pregnancy (11).

The most common symptoms of varicose veins are swelling, pain, night cramps, numbness, tingling, and heavy aching legs. The skin around visible venous distention may itch, throb, or feel like it is burning. Legs appear unsightly. Symptoms tend to worsen after long periods of standing and with each subsequent pregnancy. For some women, however, varicose veins and swelling may cause little or no discomfort.

On physical exam, pulses are intact, and neurological exam is unremarkable, and there may or may not be tenderness to palpation of the area of venous distention.

PASSIVE VENOUS CONGESTION

The same process responsible for varicose veins in the lower extremities can in turn lead to venous insufficiency. Impeded circulation causes blood to pool in the legs, forcing fluid from the intravascular space into the extravascular tissues of the feet and ankles. Leg edema affects up to 80% of pregnant women and should not be considered a sign of pregnancy-induced hypertension or preeclampsia (12). Chronic venous insufficiency may lead to varicose eczema, with brown or purplish discoloration of the skin. Over time, skin ulcers may develop (13).

Preeclampsia

Preeclampsia is a condition specific to pregnancy. Pregnant women with a blood pressure of 140/90 after the 20th week of pregnancy should be evaluated for preeclampsia (14). The obstetrical literature defines preeclampsia as an elevation in blood pressure of 140/90 mm Hg after 20 weeks of pregnancy, with or without proteinuria or edema (15). There is reduced organ perfusion secondary to vasospasm and vascular endothelial activation resulting in elevated blood pressure and proteinuria of greater than 300 mg per 24 hours. Urine dipstick testing may register +1 proteinuria (30 mL/dL). Patients may have gradual or rapid onset of edema of the extremities. They may also complain of rapid weight gain of up to 2 lb on a prenatal care visit. On clinical exam, the edema may be mild or pitting. There is no cyanosis of the lower extremities. Pulses are equal and intact.

Differential Diagnoses of Swelling of Lower Extremity in Pregnancy

Varicosities
Passive vascular congestion
Preeclampsia
Lymphedema
Thrombophlebitis
Deep vein thrombosis
Cellulitis
Urinary tract changes in pregnancy
Somatic dysfunction

Lymphedema

Lymphedema may be a lifelong condition that results from disruption of the lymphatic system. It can be classified as either primary or secondary. Primary lymphedema is an inherited disorder from prenatal developmental abnormalities of the lymph vessels. In females, it may first present during their late teens or early twenties, and become worse with pregnancy. Symptoms usually persist postpartum (16). The secondary form is acquired and may be the result of prolonged venous insufficiency, increased weight, obesity, and/or trauma to the lymphatic capillaries. In addition to biomechanical injury, burns and cicatrix formation may cause chronic edema and subcutaneous fibrosis. On clinical exam, often only one extremity is swollen although both legs may be affected. The patient does not complain of pain, and while neither tenderness nor pitting edema is elicited on examination, the leg feels rubbery to palpation. Ulceration and stasis dermatitis are absent (17).

Thrombophlebitis and Deep Vein Thrombosis

Potential complications associated with varicose veins and resultant edema are thrombophlebitis and venous thrombosis. Thrombophlebitis is inflammation of the vein, due to trauma (10,13,18). The patient may complain of throbbing of her legs with weight bearing although she is able to ambulate independently. On examination, the traumatized area is warm, mild erythematous and tender to light palpation. Sometimes, there is a bruise over the traumatized area. The pulses of the leg are intact.

A venous thrombus is a clot in the vein. The clot may occur in a superficial vein or in a deeper vein. If there is obstruction in a deep vein, a clot may migrate to the lung and cause a pulmonary embolism, which could be fatal. On physical exam, there is tenderness to manual compression of the vein or the muscles of the calf with pitting edema. In advanced cases, with deep vein involvement, the patient may have difficulty walking or bearing weight. On inspection of the leg, the calf circumference may be three or more centimeters greater than the unaffected leg. There may be low-grade fever. If pain is elicited with dorsiflexion of the foot, the extremity feels cold and pulseless or appears cyanotic; duplex sonography and D-dimer studies should be obtained to confirm a diagnosis of deep venous thrombosis. Treatment with anticoagulants should be initiated as soon as possible (13).

Cellulitis

Cellulitis usually occurs as a result of lower extremity trauma with secondary acute superficial staphylococcal or streptococcal skin infection. Common causes of cellulitis include cuts from shaving legs or abrasions that may develop into inflammation or pustules. Pregnant diabetic patients are at increased risk of developing cellulites. Patients complain of mild edema and erythema with tenderness on palpation. There is no difficulty with weight bearing or ambulation. Fever may or may not be present. On clinical examination, red streaks on the legs along the path of trauma, laceration, or abrasion may be present (9).

Urinary Tract Infection

Hypervolemia occurs in pregnancy to protect the mother, as well as the fetus, against negative effects of compromised venous return in the supine and erect positions. However, as the circulatory system delivers nourishment to the expanding uterus, pressure is placed upon the renal system. The renal calyces, ureters, and bladder all experience changes in shape and function. Glomerular filtration rate increases in pregnancy. The calyces and ureters become dilated, usually the right ureter more than the left (19). The left ureter may be cushioned by the sigmoid colon. The uterus also undergoes dextrorotation as it enlarges. Additional pressure is placed upon the right ovarian vein complex near the ureter. Ureteral dilation causes urinary stasis, which may lead to urinary tract infection. The bladder also becomes compressed by the uterus. Complete emptying during urination may be prohibited. Urinary stasis with some retention may also result. Urinary tract infection is one of the most common bacterial infections in pregnancy. In addition to complaints of changes in frequency, amount, pressure, or pain with urination, pregnant women may also report a puffiness of the lower extremities. Urinalysis, with urine culture, confirms the diagnosis of infection, which influenced the mild edema of the legs.

Somatic Dysfunction

During the course of pregnancy, maternal posture and gait change to accommodate the shifting center of gravity. Gait is steadied by increased separation the feet and legs while in standing position. As lumbar lordosis increases, the pelvic bowl tilts forward, and weight is put on areas of the posterior leg and pubic region. As previously mentioned, the expanding uterus puts pressure on the boney skeleton and structures contained within the pelvis. Vascular congestion of the organs and lower extremities results to cause edema constipation, bladder pressure, varicosities, and hemorrhoids. There is also concomitant drag on muscles fascias and ligaments. Weight gain, gravitational, pressure of the uterus, and increasing anterior-posterior spinal curves all present challenges to comfortable respiration in the pregnant patient.

OSTEOPATHIC PATIENT MANAGEMENT

Biomechanical Model

It is understood that the body may have a variety of areas of somatic dysfunction that may impact edema, such as the cervical spine and the thoracic outlet. Weight and postural strain of pregnancy may be addressed through the osteopathic biomechanical treatment model. Abnormalities of gait, unlevel sacral base, accentuated spinal curvature in either the lateral or anterior-posterior planes should be addressed to reduce musculoskeletal fatigue and circulatory congestion. Bony and ligamentous restrictions of the hips and lower extremities are reduced to remove circulatory impediments within the pelvic floor. The patient may also experience greater ease in ambulation to help with venous return of the lower extremities. Reduction of lumbar lordosis and anterior pelvic bowl tilt may assist in lifting the uterus off the veins of the lower extremities. Diuresis may also ensue when the uterus and related ligamentous-visceral strains are reduced in the area around the bladder.

Attention to body regions below the respiratory diaphragm will be given through utilization of the respiratory/circulatory model. Osteopathic manipulative treatment may attempt to resolve restrictions of the respiratory and pelvic diaphragms to improve respiration. Circulation of fluids within the abdominal-pelvic cavity may become more efficient with improved respiratory effort. Myofascial treatment of the anterior abdominal-pelvic wall addresses strains of the subcutaneous and deeper fascias that also contain lymphatic tissue. Edema of the legs due to lymphatic congestion may respond to osteopathic techniques to increase lymphatic drainage after somatic dysfunction of the pelvis has been addressed. Diuresis may also ensue when the uterus and related ligamentous-visceral strains are reduced in the area around the bladder. Visceral treatment of the uterus is applied to "center" the uterus and to reduce congestion and compression of other pelvic organs and related vasculature.

Respiratory/Circulatory Model

Within the respiratory-circulatory model of structure and function the inability to breathe deeply due to restriction of motion of the respiratory diaphragm, rib cage, and cervical fascias increases fatigue and vascular congestion; both which may aggravate edema. The enlarging uterus may also compress the vena cava when the patient lies in a supine position for a period of time. In this position, there is edema due to delay of venous return of the lower body. When the patient lies on her left side, the uterus is displaced, facilitating diuresis and decreasing swelling of the lower extremities.

On palpatory musculoskeletal examination, the following should be evaluated: respiratory diaphragm motion restrictions, leg length discrepancy, compression of lumbosacral junction, physiologic motion of the sacrum; strains of the pubic symphysis, pelvic diaphragm, hip joints, fibular heads, ankles, feet; and tissue texture changes of anterior abdominal wall, groin, and lower extremities. Scars on abdomen, pelvis, and lower extremities may constitute fascial restrictions or tissue texture changes. Note any lymphatic congestion or circulatory comprise resulting in edema. Palpate temperature changes with tissue texture changes locally and regionally throughout the musculoskeletal system which may suggest autonomic imbalance that could influence body fluid dynamics of cardiovascular circulation or renal function (Box 63.2).

Incorporation of adjunctive integrative treatment may be beneficial within the bioenergetic treatment model as well. Compression stockings have been used to control edema; however, the result is also temporary and transient. Bamigboye and Smyth reviewed the 2006 updated Cochrane database regarding treatment of edema in pregnant women and found that compression stockings often were no more effective than elevation of the feet for 30 minutes (20).

Neurological Model

The neurological model of osteopathic treatment recognizes the dynamic balance between the parasympathetic and sympathetic nervous systems and the potentially disruptive influences of nociception and biomechanical strain on those systems.

Osteopathic manipulative treatment of the thoracolumbar junction is performed to correct diaphragm and lower rib dysfunction that may interfere with balanced autonomic nerve activity to the kidneys and urine output. Treatment of the sacrum may

---

Areas of Somatic Dysfunction in Patients with Lower Extremity Edema

Cervical spine
Thoracic outlet
Lumbar spine
Sacrum
Boney pelvis
Ligaments of pelvis
Uterus
Pubic symphysis
Abdominal and pelvic fascias
Hip joints
Lower extremity

---

influence parasympathetic activity to the vascular and structures of the renal and urinary systems.

Metabolic Energy Model

Consideration of the metabolic energy model of osteopathic care entails evaluation of the patient's ability to maintain balance between energy production and expenditure during pregnancy to reduce edema of her lower extremities. Discussion about avoidance of tight or restrictive clothing about the waist that may reduce venous return from the lower half of the body should occur. The patient should be advised to wear comfortable shoes that would not challenge her gait or aggravate her already increased lumbar lordosis.

Behavioral Model

The biopsychosocial social model of osteopathic treatment considerations of pregnant patients with swelling of the lower extremity may include evaluation of patient environment and work activities. Prolonged sitting or standing may aggravate edema. Low-impact exercises and frequent walks throughout the day will help the patient to improve vascular and lymphatic circulation. Intake of water, rather than caffeine or carbonated beverages, may increase hydration and elimination of metabolic waste that may contribute to edema. Additionally, an exercise program may help the patient to avoid gaining large amounts of weight that may further tax her musculoskeletal system, and changing posture during her pregnancy. Physical activity provides beneficial stressors such as improved respiration and circulation to accommodate visceral and other structural changes from both anatomical and physiological perspectives.

CONTRAINDICATIONS TO OSTEOPATHIC MANIPULATIVE TREATMENT

There are some contraindications to osteopathic manipulative treatment of edema in pregnancy. Patients with unstable blood pressure and deep vein thrombosis should be evaluated, treated, and stabilized. Fetal health should be established. Assessment of risk factors for preterm labor should also be performed.

INTEGRATIVE TREATMENT CONSIDERATIONS

In addition to osteopathic treatment, other recommendations may be offered to the pregnant patient to relieve swelling of the lower extremities.

Advice pertaining to rest or exercise depends upon a medical condition related to the pregnancy. If the patient has preeclampsia or venous insufficiency, rest or elevation of the legs is recommended. When the patient rests on her left side, the uterus is displaced from the aorta and inferior vena cava to facilitate venous return and diuresis. "Water weight" is also reduced. Varicosities are also temporarily reduced. Exercise, especially walking, may enhance circulation of blood and lymph to relieve dependent edema. Exercise in moderation also controls weight gain in pregnancy. Ladies with lymph edema have additional challenge of increased pregnancy weight on their extremities. Those who cannot exercise have derived benefit from hydrotherapy, or water aerobics (21,22).

Studies of manual massage-reflexology treatments addressing the lymph glands around the feet and ankles did not result in significant reduction of edema in third trimester patients; however, in these small study group populations, there seemed to be a pattern of symptom relief from the patients' view points (21–23).

Some women have requested diuretics to relieve edema or abdominal bloating associated with their menstrual periods. During the course of their pregnancies, they may again request diuretics to reduce edema of their extremities. However, diuretics are not indicated as they do not mobilize extracellular fluids that have extravasated into the legs. These extrarenal fluid factors can override the kidneys' usual function. The "pregnant" kidney continues to retain sodium and water despite expanded blood, plasma, and extracellular fluid volumes. The kidney's modulation of total body sodium and water during pregnancy is not completely understood. Cardiac output cannot provide the major influence on the ability of the kidney to regulate sodium and water balance (24). Pregnancy is a hypercoagulable state. Diuretic-induced acute or chronic depletion of the plasma volume can lead to placental hypoperfusion and preeclampsia (25). Fluid restriction has not been found to reduce edema as the "normal" kidney can retain excessive amounts of sodium and water when cardiac output is low or high. Therefore, the integrity of arterial circulation is an important factor in body fluid composition and volume regulation.

OPPORTUNITIES FOR RESEARCH

For clinical research, pregnancy constitutes a "special population" because of risk of adverse reaction to the mother or to the unborn fetus. Presently, there are studies being conducted on the effects of osteopathic treatment on pregnant women at the University of North Texas Health Science Center-Osteopathic Research Center (26). There are no recent published studies regarding osteopathic treatment of lower extremity swelling in pregnancy. However, the aim of osteopathic treatment principles is to reduce edema through application of basic scientific principles pertaining to the understanding and attempted management of changes of body fluid volume in pregnancy. Combination of increased fluid intake and retention causes elevation in total body water content during high estrogen states (i.e. pregnancy). Some of this excess water resides in plasma, leading to plasma volume expansion. Regulatory mechanisms to maintain optimal body fluid volume involve reflexes within blood vessels and the brain that act to modify rates of fluid intake and output (27). Osteopathic treatment effectiveness incorporating fluid and fascial techniques to reduce edema could be investigated to understand arterial and venous function within the musculoskeletal system and to pelvic viscera (28,29).

CASE VIGNETTE (CONTINUED)

Diane was diagnosed with mild passive venous congestion. She was evaluated for somatic dysfunction in the above-mentioned areas and treated with a variety of manual osteopathic techniques. She was advised to continue walking and to wear comfortable clothing. Evaluation of complaints of edema was performed at each prenatal visit, along with her weight, blood pressure, and urine dipstick testing for proteinuria. During the third trimester of pregnancy, Diane was also advised to rest frequently, on her left side, with her legs elevated for at least 30 minutes. Her blood pressure remained stable. She reported that she felt less "puffy" after her osteopathic treatments, which were coordinated with her prenatal visits. She also continued to take short walks in the afternoon, and sometimes in the early evening. At 39 weeks of gestation, she delivered a healthy baby girl without complication. During her postpartum visit 6 weeks later, she had no complaint of swelling of her legs. On exam, no edema was detected. She returned to her usual duties as wife and mother. She also continued to walk outside and lost 15 lb. An osteopathic treatment was performed to mobilize the pelvis and related structures, as well as the lower extremities so that Diane could comfortably maintain her busy schedule. She was advised to monitor herself for any signs of edema or bloating that might be associated with return of her menstrual periods, and to return as needed for further osteopathic care.

REFERENCES

1. American College of Obstetricians and Gynecologists. *Standards for Obstetric-Gynecologic Services*. 7th Ed. Washington, DC: Public Health Services, Department of Health and Human Services, 1989.
2. US Public Health Service Expert Panel on the Content of Prenatal Care. *Caring for Our Future: The Content of Prenatal Care*. Washington, DC: Public Health Services, Dept. of Health and Human Services, 1989.
3. Kirkham C, Harris S, Grzybowski S. Evidence-based prenatal care: Part I. General prenatal care and counseling issues. *Am Fam Physician* 2005;71(7):1307–1316.
4. Institute for Clinical Systems Improvement. Knowledge resources. Routine prenatal care. Accessed online February 25, 2008 at http://wwwicsi.org/knowledge/detail.asp?catID=29&item ID=191
5. Prenatal Care Guidelines. Accessed online February 25, 2008 at http://www.wellmark.com/e_businessprovider/pdf/PRENATAL_Health_Maintenance.pdf
6. Smith A. Pre-eclampsia. *Prim Care* 1993;20:655–664.
7. Carr SC. Current management of varicose veins. *Clin Obstet Gynecol* 2006;49(2):414–426.
8. Criquiui MH. The San Diego Population Study. Chronic venous disease in ethnically diverse population. *Am J Epidemiol* 2003;158:448–456.
9. Florence JA. Varicose veins. In: Domino FJ, ed. *5-minute Clinical Consult*. 16th Ed. Philadelphia, PA: Lippincott Williams Wilkins, 2007. Accessed online February 26, 2008 at http://online.statref.com/document.aspx?fxid=31&docid=956
10. Beebe-Dimmer JL, Pfeifer JR, Engle JS, et al. The epidemiology of chronic venous insufficiency and varicose veins. *Ann Epidemiol* 2005;15(3):178–184.
11. Mashiah A, Berman V, Thole HH. Estrogen and progesterone receptors in normal and varicose saphenous veins. *Cardiovasc Surg* 1999;7(3):327–331.
12. Mohaupt MG. Edema in pregnancy—trivial? *Ther Umsch* 2004;61(11):687–690.
13. Campbell B. Clinical review: varicose veins and their management. *BMJ* 2006;333:287–292.
14. ACOG Practice Bulletin #33: Diagnosis and Management of Pre-eclampsia and Eclampsia, January 2002.
15. Cunningham FG, Hauth J, Leveno K, et al. *Williams' Obstetrics*. 22nd ed. New York, McGraw-Hill, 2005:769–780.
16. Reid T. Pregnancy and lymph edema. Lymphatic Research Foundation, 2006. Accessed online February 26, 2008 at www.Lymphnotes.com
17. Tiwari A, et al. Differential diagnosis, investigation, and current treatment of lower limb lymph edema. *Arch Surg* 2003;138(2):152–161.
18. Stansby G. Women, pregnancy, and varicose veins. *Lancet* 2000;355(9210):117–118.
19. Schulman A, Herlinger H. Urinary tract dilatation in pregnancy. *Br J Radiol* 1975;48:638.
20. Bamigboye AA, Smyth R. Interventions for varicose veins and leg oedema in pregnancy: reviews. *Cochrane Pregnancy and Childbirth Group Trials Register*, November 2006.
21. Bamigboye AA, Hofmeyer GJ. Interventions for leg edema and varicosities in pregnancy. What evidence? *Eur J Obstet Gynecol Reprod Biol* 2006;129(1):3–8.

22. Kent T, Gregor J, Deardorff L et al. Edema of pregnancy: a comparison of water aerobics and static immersion. *Obstet Gynecol* 1991;94:726–729.

23. Mollart L. Single-blind trial addressing the differential effects of two reflexology techniques versus rest, on ankle and foot oedema in late pregnancy. *Complement Ther Nurs Midwifery* 2003;9(4):203–208.

24. Bekheirnia MR, Schrier RW. Pathophysiology of water and sodium retention: edematous states with normal kidney function. *Curr Opin Pharmacol* 2006;6(2):202–207.

25. Huynh-Do U, Frey FJ. Potential dangers of diuretics. *Ther Umschau* 2000;57(6):408–411.

26. Hensel K. Osteopathic manipulative medicine in pregnancy: physiologic and clinical effects. NCCAM ClinicalTrials.govidentifier:NCT 00426244.

27. Schrier RW. Decreased effective blood volume in edematous disorders: what does this mean? *J Am Soc Nephrol* 2007;18(7):2028–2031.

28. Stachenfeld N. Impact of physical activity during pregnancy and postpartum on chronic disease risk. *Roundtable Consensus Statement—Medicine and Science in Sports and Exercise*, 2006:989–1006. Accessed online June 9, 2008 at www.acsm-msse.org

29. Welsch MA, Alomari M, Parish TR, et al. Influence of venous function on exercise tolerance in chronic heart failure. *J Cardiopulm Rehabil* 2002;22(5):321–326.

64

Low Back Pain in Pregnancy

MELICIEN TETTAMBEL

KEY CONCEPTS

- Low back pain is a common condition of pregnancy and may be related to hormonal changes associated with pregnancy; however, other causes should be ruled out.
- A woman's body undergoes many physiologic changes and adaptations as her pregnancy progresses; these may adversely impact her postural stability mechanisms resulting in biomechanical instability and pain.
- Passive venous congestion in the vertebral vessels may contribute to low back pain during pregnancy.
- Addressing tissue strains and compensatory postural adaptations to pregnancy may help improve postural stability mechanisms and back pain.

CASE VIGNETTE

Barbara is a 26-year-old pregnant patient at 35 weeks' gestation.

Chief Complaint:

Low back pain that sometimes radiates into her posterior legs, just above her knees.

History of Present Illness:

She has had this pain since the fourth month of her pregnancy, and it is gradually getting worse. She is considering taking early maternity leave. Her back pain is aggravated by lifting children and. sometimes, by rising from a chair. Relief is obtained by resting in bed, sitting with her feet propped up in a recliner-chair, or with a prolonged warm shower.

Past Medical History:

She has a history of endometriosis, which was confirmed with laparoscopy a few years ago

Past Obstetrical History:

Her first baby was delivered by cesarean section, after an arduous labor, 3 years ago.

Past Surgical History:

Cesarean section as described above

Family History:

Noncontributory

Social History:

She is employed as a child care attendant for 3 year olds at a day care center.

REVIEW OF SYSTEMS

General:

She is well hydrated, alert, and uncomfortable.

Obstetrical:

To date, there have been no complications during this pregnancy. She has gained 20 lb, which is similar to her previous pregnancy.

Gastrointestinal:

Denies nausea, vomiting, and changes in bowel.

Neurological:

Denies weakness and tingling in the arms and legs. The pain does not radiate. There have been no changes in bladder function.

Musculoskeletal:

There is joint swelling. She admits to feeling stiff in her back but denies other joint stiffness or pain.

PHYSICAL EXAMINATION

Vital Signs:

Temperature: 37°C, Pulse: 88/min and regular, respirations: 20/min, blood pressure: 124/80

General:

Well hydrated in no acute distress

Obstetrical:

Obstetrical exam reveals no abnormalities; active fetus in vertex position, no contractions, mild swelling of all extremities.

Neurovascular:

Unremarkable, DTRs are intact and symmetrical. There is no weakness. Negative straight leg raise.

Musculoskeletal:

No joint swelling, erythema, or tenderness is noted. There is no tenderness to percussion of the vertebral spinous processes.

Osteopathic Structural Exam:

There is an increased lumbar lordosis with anterior pelvic tilt and unlevel sacral base. The psoas muscles are hypertonic bilaterally. There are no lateral spinal curves. Tissue texture of the lumbar spine is congested but also mildly taut. There is tenderness to palpation of the lumbosacral junction and right sacroiliac joint. Patient has a waddling gait due to change in center of gravity to accommodate enlarging uterus. On examination of anterior pelvis, a small infraumbilical scar and a transverse scar above the pubes are noted. Increased fascial tension is noted about the lower scar.

DIFFERENTIAL DIAGNOSIS OF BACK PIAN IN PREGNANCY

Approximately, two thirds of pregnant women complain of low back pain during pregnancy (1,2). Pain may start as early as the first trimester, when levels of the hormone relaxin are most elevated, or worsen during the course of pregnancy, causing fatigue, sleep changes, and interference with work or activities of daily living (3,4). Cause of the back pain may be anatomical, biomechanical, traumatic, or psychoemotional. Contributing factors, osteopathic diagnosis and treatment, as well as other methods of treatment will be presented and discussed within the context of a case presentation.

Overview of Low Back Pain in Pregnancy

Low back pain rates have been found to increase in young gravidas: women with advanced maternal age (1,5), woman with a history of back pain during previous pregnancy, and woman with an increasing number of previous births (either vaginally or operatively). There is no consistent relationship reported regarding height, weight, maternal weight gain, or weight of the fetus (6). Low back pain may also occur postpartum. However, back pain beyond pregnancy will be further discussed in another chapter about pelvic pain.

In addition to changes in maternal weight and posture in pregnancy, there can be a variety of factors contributing to low back pain in pregnancy (Table 64.1). Biomechanical instability is the most prevalent cause, as the enlarging gravid uterus and accompanying compensatory lordosis of the lumbar spine contribute to musculoskeletal strain. The psoas muscles may become shortened with lordosis, aggravating back pain (7). It is interesting to note that there is much discussion about lumbar lordosis and low back pain in pregnancy, but there is little discussion about low back pain in pregnant women who have scoliosis. Two hundred sixty seven women with adolescent idiopathic scoliosis, treated either surgically or with bracing, did not appear to have more or worse low back pain in pregnancy than matched control subjects who did not have scoliosis (8). It was also observed that the scoliotic curve did not seem to increase as a result of childbearing.

Pelvic rotation about a fulcrum at the second sacral segment increases as the lordosis increases. Center of gravity is shifted anteriorly, producing additional strain on lumbar spine and sacroiliac joints. As the sacroiliac joints become increasingly lax under the hormonal influence of relaxin during pregnancy, even more strain is placed on the low back and pelvis (9). It has been reported that pregnant women who were most incapacitated by low back pain had highest levels of relaxin (10–12). Not all were obese or had multifetal gestations. Weight gain during pregnancy is usual; however, in combination with ligamentous laxity, a 20% weight increase may increase force on a joint by as much as 100% (3,7,8).

The additional hormonal influences of estrogen and relaxin cause the pubic symphysis to widen. This widening normally is less than 10 mm (13,14) and begins during the 10th to 12th week of pregnancy. Relaxin levels begin to decline again until the 17th week (11). Palpation of the pubic symphysis may refer pain to the low back. Osteitis pubis is characterized by resorption of the pubic bones, followed by spontaneous reossifiction. In later pregnancy, there is a gradual onset of pubic symphysis pain; however, there can be rapid progression over the course of a few days to excruciating pain radiating down the medial aspect of the thighs. Walking or lower leg motion aggravates the pain. Because of pain due to weight bearing with altered gait, the muscles and ligaments become involved in the pain mechanism (15).

TABLE 64.1

Causes of Low Back Pain in Pregnancy

Cause	Examples
Mechanical	Spinal facet Spondylolisthesis Leg-length inequality Congenital disorders (e.g., scoliosis, anatomical structural variants) Increased weight Multifetal gestation Trauma Discogenic Spinal curves Ligamentous laxity Somatic dysfunction
Nonmechanical— Viscerogenic	Urinary tract changes Bowel function changes Endometriosis Pelvic infection Labor
Nonmechanical—Vascular	Compression of great vessels Venous plexopathy Thrombosis Placental location
Metabolic	Osteoporosis Osteonecrosis
Psychoemotional	Seeking disability Depression

Neuropathies of Pregnancy

Peripheral nerves are susceptible to injury in the pregnant woman by compression, traction, and ischemia. Soft tissue edema is common during pregnancy, and also contributes to the weight-bearing factor on biomechanics of prolonged standing or sitting. Additionally, the uterus puts pressure on neighboring pelvic organs, ligaments, lumbosacral plexus, and lower limb peripheral nerves. Compression neuropathy is most common in anatomic locations where excessive pressure can occur. An example is meralgia paresthetica, or compression of the lateral femoral cutaneous nerve. The lateral femoral cutaneous nerve is a sensory nerve supplying sensation to the waist band area and down into the anterolateral thigh. It arises at the level of the third lumbar vertebra and travels toward the pelvis to pass slightly medial and inferior to the anterior superior iliac spine; then exiting the pelvis beneath the inguinal ligament. Injury to this nerve can result in burning, pain, or numbness along the course of innervation, causing what is known as meralgia paresthetica syndrome (16). Pregnancy along, with obesity, diabetes mellitus, trauma, belt pressure, and anatomic variations are risk factors for this syndrome (17). An anatomical variation is bisection of the inguinal ligament by the lateral femoral cutaneous nerve. Augmented lumbar lordosis of pregnancy may also contribute compressive forces on this nerve. Cesarean delivery may also lead to meralgia paresthetica from a wide incision, stretching of tissues around the incision, or surgical retractor equipment; although the prevalence does not substantially vary with method of delivery (18,19). In subsequent pregnancies, nerve irritation may recur with physiologic and postural changes.

Lumbosacral Plexopathies

Lumbosacral plexopathies may result from prolonged standing, sitting, or squatting. Proximal or distal lower limb weakness can occur. Plexus-associated foot drop can be the result of compression of the peroneal division of the sciatic nerve in the pelvis. The common peroneal nerve can also become compressed at the fibular head (20).

Unlike the above anatomical changes discussed as predisposing factors for low back pain, true lumbar disc herniation is rare. LaBan has written extensively about this problem and reported that about 1 in 10,000 cases of lumbosacral pain in pregnancy are herniated lumbar discs (21–23). Previous sciatica may become aggravated in subsequent pregnancy. Surgery for low back pain is generally contraindicated unless a herniated disk fails to respond to conservative treatment or produces bowel or bladder incontinence. Most patients will respond to conservative treatment until the baby is born. At times, cesarean section delivery may be offered to avoid increased pressure on the nerve root during delivery.

There are additional sites and causes of nerve compression; however, many occur in the labor and delivery process. Therefore, they will not be discussed in this chapter.

Spondylolisthesis

Spondylolisthesis is a condition where one vertebral body (usually in the lumbar spine) appears anteriorly displaced to the one just below. This most commonly occurs from L5 slipped forward from S1. This may be secondary to a defect in the pars interarticulares (24). Degenerative spondylolisthesis is most common at the L4-5 level. This condition is more prevalent in females than males in general. It has not been determined why this condition most commonly occurs at L4-5 level. Sanderson and Fraser (25) reported that women who had children had a significantly higher incidence of spondylolisthesis at this level than nulliparous women. In women with previous spondylosis, it has been thought that this slip may progress; however, there may be no increase in back symptoms or an increase in segmental slip in subsequently pregnant patients.

There are additional sites and causes of nerve compression; however, many occur in the labor and delivery process. Therefore, they will not be discussed in this chapter.

Hip Pain of Pregnancy

Pregnancy-related hip pain can present with progressive symptoms and lead to disability. Conditions of the low back and pelvic girdle can present with pain in the hip. Likewise, intra-articular hip pathology can refer pain to the back and pelvis, and can be misdiagnosed as pelvic instability. With the pelvis and lower spine maintained in a stable position, to differentiate intra-articular hip pathology from referred pain, hip range of motion must be assessed to rule out referred pain (14). Antalgic gait in a pregnant woman should raise the question of the possibility of transient osteoporosis of the hip or osteonecrosis of the femoral head.

A rare condition, usually occurring with weight bearing in the third trimester of pregnancy, is transient osteoporosis of the hip (26,27). Etiology of this condition is unknown. It is characterized by pain and limitation of hip motion. The pain may be of sudden or insidious onset. Weightbearing exaggerates the pain, causing the patient to require a wheelchair or bed rest. This diagnosis is made by x-ray, MRI, or pelvic sonogram, not by palpatory physical exam (28). X-ray, with appropriate shielding, is helpful to establish that the osteoporosis is associated with the current pregnancy and not related to osteoporosis antecedent to the pregnancy. Failure to diagnose this condition can result in fracture (29). Surgical intervention then becomes necessary.

Avascular necrosis of the femoral head has been reported in pregnant women without any previous or additional risk factors (30). Proposed theories of pathogenesis include higher adrenocorticoid metabolism combined with weight gain as well as elevated levels of estrogen and progesterone in conjunction with increased joint pressure and strain (31). Symptoms typically occur in the third trimester, with increased weightbearing in the hip, pelvis, or groin. Symptoms of osteonecrosis usually begin in the third trimester with pain deep in the groin. Pain radiates to the knee, thigh, or back. Pain with range-of-motion testing of the hip may differentiate this from pain felt in the pubic symphysis or sacroiliac joint. Treatment consists of decreased weightbearing by using a walker or crutches to allow revascularization of the femoral head (32).

Vascular Causes of Low Back Pain in Pregnancy

Abnormalities or changes of the lumbar epidural venous plexus may give rise to symptoms mimicking nerve root compression. Gormus, Paksoy, et al. (33,34), noted that epidural veins were enlarged in patients with inferior vena caval thrombosis or obstruction just below the renal vein orifices in pregnant women. They presented with radicular syndromes or back pain. Vascular studies confirmed deep vein thrombosis Pain resolved with medical treatment or delivery.

Posterior location of the placenta has been noted on pelvic obstetrical sonography in nonlaboring women who have complained of low back pain during pregnancy. Musculoskeletal exam usually is unremarkable. Fetal activity does not influence the pain. Possible explanation for this pain may be that pain insidiously occurs as the enlarging uterus strains the vascular bed to which the placenta is attached (35). If the patient has sustained some kind of physical trauma, such as a fall or motor vehicle accident, she may experience low back pain in conjunction with uterine activity that may be associated with placental abruption (36). Vaginal bleeding may also occur. She and her fetus should be evaluated as soon as possible to prepare her for an emergent operative delivery, which will resolve the back pain.

Organic Causes of Back Pain in Pregnancy

In women with upper urinary tract infections, pyelonephritis may present as lumbar pain in pregnancy (37). The pain may be dull and persistent. Fever or chills may also accompany the pain. Urinalysis indicates the possibility of infection; urine culture identifies the offending organism (usually *Escherichia coli*). If the back pain is colicky in nature, and there is tenderness of the costovertebral angle on palpation, nephrolithiasis may be present. Urinary tract infection may or may not accompany the process of attempting to pass the stone (38). Most stones are calcium oxalate (39). Ninety percent of gravidas with nephrolithiasis present with back pain. The possibility of preterm labor must also be considered as complication of infection, or result of irritation of the sympathetic nervous system on uterine activity.

Other obstetrical conditions can present as low back pain. Ectopic pregnancy (in the first trimester) with bleeding or impending rupture causes peritoneal irritation as blood may collect in the cul de sac. Threatened or impending spontaneous abortion may manifest as back pain if the uterus is retroverted. Ovarian cyst or concomitant pelvic infection may cause back pain due to pressure within the pelvic cavity, stretching of previously formed adhesions, or collection of fluid in the cul de sac. A posterior uterine fibroid may put pressure on the pelvis and hypogastric plexus as the pregnant uterus is growing out of the pelvis and into the abdomen. Some patients experience low back pain as a sign of labor. As labor progresses, pain may become more intense as the fetal head enters the pelvic outlet, or if the maternal pelvis is trying to accommodate a fetal presenting part that is putting excessive pressure on maternal pelvis and soft tissues during the labor or delivery process.

Evaluation and Treatment Plans

The pregnant patient who develops low back pain will usually also describe low anterior or posterior pelvic pain. Pain can be aggravated by activity and most often relieved by lying down, sitting, or using a supportive device. Occasionally, the pain may radiate down to one or both buttocks and into the posterior thighs to the knees. Sciatica has pain distribution all the way down the posterior leg to the heel, along the distribution of the nerve root. Meralgia paresthetica, likewise, causes burning and numbness along the course of the lateral femoral cutaneous nerve. She does not correlate this type of pain with fetal activity (1,3,9).

Further questioning may reveal what factors improve or aggravate pain. These factors may be physical or psychological, and affect the patient's ability to perform her usual activities of daily living. Inquiries about stress, or changes in sleep, diet, or working conditions may provide opportunities to explore what remedies, if any, the patient may have tried in her pursuit to obtain relief.

The physical examination of the pregnant woman should begin with an obstetrical evaluation to evaluate maternal and fetal health. Regarding maternal well-being, the physician should ascertain whether complaints of low back pain are related to urinary dysfunction, colon dysfunction, or "early warning" signs of uterine dysfunction that may precipitate labor.

The neuromusculoskeletal examination should include observation, palpation, range of motion, muscle imbalances, leg-length inequality, deep tendon reflexes, posture, station, gait, and degree of lumbar lordosis. There may be spasms of the paraspinous muscles. Tenderness may be elicited over the sacroiliac joints. Sacroiliac compression tests, bimanual compression over the iliac crests; FABER and Patrick tests all may elicit sacroiliac pain. The hip joint and pubic symphysis should also be evaluated. Segmental motion of the lumbar spine should be noted. Lumbosacral mechanics can be evaluated according to the various motion tests discussed elsewhere in this book, regarding diagnosis of somatic dysfunction of this area of the spine. It would be interesting to note whether osteopathic physicians diagnosed a greater frequency of sacral torsion or unilateral sacral flexion (shear) somatic dysfunction in pregnant patients.

Osteopathic Patient Management
Biomechanical Model

As previously described, biomechanical instability is the most prevalent cause of back pain in pregnant women. Our patient had an anterior pelvic tilt, unleveled sacral base, dysfunction at the sacroiliac and lumbosacral areas, hypertonic psoas muscles, and signs of somatic dysfunction in the paralumbar tissues. Any and all of these findings could be causing or contributing to her chief complaint. While many of these areas of somatic dysfunction probably represent postural adaptations to pregnancy, the resulting biomechanical changes will stress and potentially strain the involved joints and myofascial structures. This produces tissue irritation, inflammation, and pain that may present as back or pelvic pain (62).

Respiratory/Circulatory Model

The gravid uterus tends to put pressure on neighboring organs in the abdomen and pelvis, altering function. Decreased fluid intake, in conjunction with altered, usually slowed, bowel function may lead to constipation. Back pain can occur as result of colonic distention and pressure, or from straining efforts of the patient to empty the bowels. Our patient has somatic dysfunction involving the sacrum and pelvis, which affect the pelvic diaphragm. Within the respiratory/circulatory model of structure function, the pelvic diaphragm is thought to play an important role in venous and lymphatic drainage from the pelvic organs including the gravid uterus. In this patient, we would be concerned that her pelvic and sacral dysfunction may contribute to venous stasis and congestion in the pelvic tissues and uterus. Distension of the uterine veins and pelvic tissues has been shown to produce pelvic and back pain (59–61).

Neurological Model

Several studies have described an association between a history of trauma or previous pain presentation and the occurrence of low back pain during pregnancy (5,6,43,44). In one study, women with pelvic girdle pain revealed a history of previous low back pain or trauma of the back or pelvis. Women who complained of double-sided sacroiliac pain had previous low back pain or trauma to the back and pelvis. Most of the women who reported low back pain also had history of hypermobility before and during pregnancy. These findings suggest the presence of sensitization or low-level spinal facilitation that may predispose a patient to developing pain as the pregnancy progresses. Our patient has a history of endometriosis, a painful pelvic condition that may have sensitized neurons in the lower lumbar cord.

Low back pain as a predictor of depression in pregnancy has also been studied. Gutke investigated the possible association of lumbopelvic pain, pelvic girdle pain, and postpartum depression (40). Pregnant women were given a musculoskeletal exam of the lumbar spine and pelvis, completed a pain drawing, and were evaluated according to the Edinburgh Postnatal Depression Scale. Postpartum depressive symptoms were three times more prevalent in women having lumbopelvic pain than those without. Field attempted to correlate low back pain with mood states and biochemistry in pregnancy. Relationships were noted between back pain and urinary cortisol and epinephrine. Pain and increased levels of cortisol and epinephrine measured in second and third trimester pregnancy were present in women who were angry or depressed (41). In a study of 412 primigravidas, patients recorded low back pain or pelvic girdle pain early in pregnancy and again at 36 weeks' gestation. They were followed at 3 months and again at 1 year after delivery. Those reporting pelvic girdle pain in pregnancy were less mobile and often required ambulatory assistance. They also required treatment for depression. No association was found between obstetric factors and pelvic girdle pain (42). The association between pain and depression is a chicken and egg conundrum. On one hand, pain has been shown to alter the hypothalamic-pituitary-adrenal axis resulting in increased cortisol and symptoms of depression. Alternatively, clinical depression is associated with lowered tolerance for nociception, a heightened perception of pain, and increased risk for developing chronic pain.

Metabolic-Energy Model

There is great physiologic stress associated with pregnancy, and while the female body has developed to meet these demands, they extract a cost. The overall metabolic energy needed for daily activities increases significantly during pregnancy. Nutritional intake is being used for both mother and child. The metabolic building blocks for strong bones, brain, and muscles come from maternal food intake and maternal stores. Pregnant women should be counseled in dietary and nutritional matters to best meet their own metabolic needs and those of their growing child. Normal physical demands and activities may be more difficult and fatiguing for the pregnant woman. Many pregnant women complain of increased fatigue during the latter stages of pregnancy and physicians need to make appropriate recommendations regarding workload, sleep requirements, and other activities.

Behavioral Model

Osteopathy also encompasses the behavioral approach to patient care. History, reviewed from perspective of the interrelationship of structure and function, also aids in development of a treatment plan. Wang et al. (1) reported that 95% of 640 patients informed their prenatal care providers about loss of sleep and inability to perform routine activities because of low back pain. However, 25% of the care providers recommended adjunctive care for biomechanical problems. Other investigators linked patient complaints with physical examination and devised a classification of back in pregnancy (6,43,44). In addition to a history of previous pain patterns, the aforementioned studies also reported an association between various biopsychosocial factors and back pain in pregnancy. In one study, women with pelvic girdle syndrome were more likely to report multiparity higher weight, higher level of self-reported stress, and lower job satisfaction. They also had higher postpregnancy weight and body mass index. Women with pubic pain, or symphysiolysis, were more likely to be multiparous, overweight, and smokers. Women with one-sided sacroiliac pain had a prior negative obstetrical delivery experience. This group also had vocational training or professional education that contributed to stress levels. Women who complained of double-sided sacroiliac pain were also multiparous, and had poorer spousal relationships and less job satisfaction than the previously mentioned groups. In all four groups, there was no correlation with menarche or use of oral contraceptives (estrogen).

Osteopathic Manipulative Treatment

A variety of osteopathic manipulative treatment approaches to low back pain in pregnant patients can address the many factors that cause pain. Muscle energy techniques focus on addressing muscle imbalances. High-velocity low-amplitude approaches have been utilized to relieve joint restrictions. Although there is only a single case report published concerning complications of direct manipulation in the pregnant patient (63), osteopathic practitioners have expressed their reasons for avoiding certain kinds of techniques in pregnant women. Some prefer to treat soft tissues and balance ligaments because they are mildly edematous from hormonal influences, have increased laxity; both influences that tend to contribute to the pain of neurovascular entrapment. Others prefer to relieve joint restrictions with more direct approaches other than thrust by incorporating patient's weight or posture to mobilize skeletal dysfunctions. Pregnant patients present interesting challenges to those who perform osteopathic treatment while positioning the patient comfortably without compromising her fetus. An enlarged uterus may preclude the patient from being treated in a prone position or lying supine for a prolonged period of time. Technique selection often depends upon the patient's ability to lie or sit comfortably for a period of time while being treated.

It is important to establish the etiology of low back pain in order to develop and execute a treatment plan that may consist of medication or manipulation or both. Box 64.1 lists contraindications

---

Contraindications to Osteopathic Manipulative Treatment of Low Back Pain in Pregnancy

- **Undiagnosed vaginal bleeding**
- **Ectopic pregnancy**
- **Placental abruption**
- **Untreated deep vein thrombosis**
- **Elevated maternal blood pressure**
- **Preterm labor**
- **Unstable maternal vital signs**
- **Fetal distress**

---

to manipulative treatment in pregnant patients. From an obstetrical perspective, manipulative treatment should not be performed on pregnant patients with low back pain who have undiagnosed vaginal bleeding, ectopic pregnancy, placental abruption, uncontrolled elevated blood pressure, untreated deep vein thrombosis, unstable vital signs after sustaining physical trauma, preterm labor. These conditions may require aggressive medical or surgical treatment. Maternal health and fetal health are assessed before somatic dysfunction is to be addressed.

Additional Treatment Considerations

Currently, there are no studies to determine whether low back pain can be prevented in pregnancy. Risk factors have been previously discussed. Exercise and weight control before pregnancy have been recommended, but they do not prevent or determine who will have low back pain in pregnancy. Some investigators report that prenatal care providers are aware of back pain, but do not consistently offer treatment or have specific recommendations for relief, other than rest (1). This may be due to the fact that some back pain is expected to occur during the course of pregnancy and that it almost always resolves in the postpartum period. Most commonly, activity modification with periods of rest with feet elevation is advised. Elevated feet with flexed hips reduce lumbar lordosis and ease muscle spasm in acute pain. An exercise program, following a period of rest, may increase muscle strength and abdominal tone to reduce low back pain symptoms. There are a variety of published American and Canadian guidelines pertaining to exercising before and after pregnancy (45–48). Both the American and the Canadian guidelines caution against activities with high risk of falling or abdominal trauma. The guidelines also include specific warning signs to discontinue exercising, such as incompetent cervix, vaginal bleeding, history of preterm labor, or extreme shortness of breath. Exercise in normal temperature pool water has been shown to reduce back pain in pregnant women due to buoyancy unloading joint pressure (2). However, immersion in a warm whirlpool or hot tub can produce maternal hyperthermia. Elevated maternal body temperature can cause deleterious fetal effects in the first trimester of pregnancy, the time of fetal neural tube closure and organogenesis.

Orthoses may be able to temporarily relieve back pain. A trochanteric belt, if comfortable for the patient with lumbar lordosis, may reduce anterior pelvic tilt while stretching psoas muscles (2). A belt that supports the sacroiliac joints may reduce pelvic joint laxity (49). A pilot study evaluating the use of maternity back supports found a reduction in pain scores in a small population (50). In addition to osteopathic treatment to reduce sacral base unleveling, a heel lift may help maintain lumbosacral stability or reduce lumbar lordosis (51). Acetaminophen can be added for pain relief since antiprostaglandins such as aspirin and NSAIDs are relatively contraindicated in pregnancy. Narcotics are not indicated as first-line pharmacotherapy.

Physical therapy modalities may be limited or contraindicated when the energy produced by the modality may adversely affect the developing fetus. In a recent review by Batavia (52), pregnancy has been cited as a contraindication to therapeutic ultrasound and superficial heat. Heat may produce maternal hyperthermia; therefore, precaution should be taken with application of hot packs to the low back and abdomen. Diathermy is also contraindicated due to the effect of deep heat and exposure to electromagnetic fields (53).

There are no recent data available in the medical literature regarding the use of lumbar traction during pregnancy. However, lumbar traction belts may cause excessive pressure on the abdomen and aggravate pelvic ligament laxity (54).

Because electrical current effects on the fetus are not yet fully understood, electrical stimulation should not be applied to the low back, abdomen, or pelvis. On the other hand, the electrical current of transcutaneous nerve stimulation (TNS) has been used safely during pregnancy, labor, and delivery for pain control. In a meta-analysis of six randomized placebo controlled trials, TNS provided some relief of back pain (55).

Acupuncture for pain relief has been studied in the last trimester of pregnancy. No maternal or fetal adverse effects have been reported in three studies (56–58). In all three studies, women receiving acupuncture completed either questionnaires or visual analog scales to report decrease in pain at rest, increased energy, and positive emotions to complete activities of daily living. The study by Guerreiro (57) indicated that those who received acupuncture also utilized less acetaminophen for pain

CASE VIGNETTE (CONTINUED)

Barbara's low back pain is a result of normal biomechanical changes of pregnancy: increased lumbar lordosis, weight gain, and ligamentous laxity due to hormonal influence. Bending and lifting aggravate the pain, as well as uterine pressure on scar tissue from endometriosis and previous surgery. Rest, exercise, and osteopathic treatment to stabilize musculoskeletal imbalance, joint laxity, and postural changes would be helpful to relieve pain during pregnancy. Hydrotherapy, acupuncture, possibly orthotics, and acetaminophen may provide additional relief before delivery. Barbara would also appreciate family and social support as she prepares to welcome a new baby into the family.

REFERENCES

1. Wang SM, Dezinno P, Maranets I, et al: Low back pain during pregnancy: Prevalence, risk factors, and outcomes. *Obstet Gynecol* 2004;104:65–70.
2. Pennick VE, Young G. Interventions for preventing and treating pelvic and back pain in pregnancy [update of Cochrane Database Syst Rev. 2002; (1); CD001139; PMID: 11869592]. *Cochrane Database Syst Rev* 2007;(2): CD001139.
3. Borg-Stein J, Dugan S, Gruber J. Musculoskeletal aspects of pregnancy. *Am J Physical Med Rehabil* 2005;84(3):180–192.
4. Carlson HL, Carlson NL, Pasternak BA, et al: Understanding and managing the back pain of pregnancy. *Curr Womens Health Rep* 2003;3:65–71.
5. Mogren IM. BMI, pain and hyper-mobility are determinants of long-term outcome for women with low back pain and pelvic pain during pregnancy. *Eur Spine J* 2006;15(7):1093–1102.
6. Mogren IM, Pohjanen AI. Low back pain and pelvic pain during pregnancy: prevalence and risk factors. *Spine* 2005;30(8):983–991.
7. Tettambel M. Obstetrics. In Ward RC, ed. *Foundations for Osteopathic Medicine*. 2nd Ed. Lippincott Williams & Wilkins, Philadelphia, PA: 2003:450–451.
8. Danielsson AJ, Nachemson AL. Childbearing, curve progression, and sexual function in women 22 years after treatment for adolescent idioapthic scoliosis: a case-control study. *Spine* 2001;26(13):1449–1456.
9. Ritchie JR. Orthopedic considerations during pregnancy. *Clin Obstet Gynecol* 2003;46:456–466.
10. Weiss M, Nagelschmidt M, Struck H. Relaxin and collagen metabolism. *Horm Metab Res* 1979;11:408–410.
11. Kristiansson P, Svardsudd K, von Schoultz B. Serum relaxin, symphyseal pain and back pain during pregnancy. *Am J Obstet Gynecol* 1996;175:1342–1347.
12. MacLennan, AH, Nicolson R, Green RC, et al. Serum relaxin and pelvic pain of pregnancy. *Lancet* 1986;2:243–245.
13. Owens K, Pearson A, Mason G. Symphysis pubis dysfunction: a cause of significant obstetric morbidity. *Eur J Obstet Gynecol Reprod Biol* 2002;105:143–146.
14. Young J. Relaxation of the pelvic joints in pregnancy: pelvic arthropathy of pregnancy. *J Obstet Gynecol Br Empire* 1940;47:493.
15. Kubitz RL, Goodlin RC. Symptomatic separation of the pubic symphysis. *South Med J* 1946;79:578–580.
16. Weinreb JC, et al. Prevalence of lumbosacral intervertebral lumbosacral intervertebral disk abnormalities on MR images in pregnant and asymptomatic nonpregnant women. *Radiology* 1989;170:125–128.
17. Van Stobbe AM, Bohnen AM, Bernsen RM, et al. Incidence rates and determinants in meralgia paresthetica in general practice. *J Neurol* 2004;251:294–297.
18. Wong CA, Scavone BM, Dugan S, et al. Incidence of postpartum lumbosacral spine and lower extremity nerve injuries. *Obstet Gynecol* 2003; 101:279–288.
19. Redick LF. Maternal perinatal nerve palsies. *Postgrad Obstet Gynecol* 1992;12:1–5.
20. Aminoff MJ. Neurological disorders and pregnancy. *Obstet Gynecol* 1978;132:325–335.
21. LaBan MM, Perrin JC, Latimer FR. Pregnancy and the herniated lumbar disc. *Arch Phys Med Rehabil* 1983;64:319–321.
22. LaBan MM, Viola S, Williams DA, et al. Magnetic resonance imaging of the lumbar herniated disc in pregnancy. *Am J Phys Med Rehabil* 1995;74: 59–61.
23. LaBan MM, Rapp NS, von Deyen P, et al. The lumbar herniated disk of pregnancy: A report of six cases identified by magnetic resonance imaging. *Arch Phys Med Rehabil* 1995;76:476–479.
24. Saraste H. Spondylolysis and pregnancy: a risk analysis. *Acta Obstet Gynecol Scand* 1986;65:727–729.
25. Sanderson PL, Fraser RD. The influence of pregnancy on the development of degenerative spondylolisthesis. *J Bone Joint Surg Br* 1996;78:951–954.
26. Bloem JL. Transient osteoporosis of the hip. MR imaging. *Radiology* 1988;167:753–755.
27. Takatori Y, Kokubo T, Ninomiya S, et al. Transient osteoporosis of the hip. Magnetic resonance imaging. *Clin Orthop* 1991;271:190–194.
28. Pellici PM, Zolla-Pazner S, Rabhan WN, Wilson PD. Osteonecrosis of the femoral head associated with pregnancy. Report of three cases. *Clin Orthop* 1984185:49–63.
29. Lausten GS. Osteonecrosis of the femoral head during pregnancy. *Arch Orthop Trauma Surg* 1991;110:214–215.
30. Van den Veyver I, Vanderheyden J, Krauss E, et al. Aseptic necrosis of the femoral head associated with pregnancy. A case report. *Eur J Obstet Gynecol Reprod Biol* 1990;36:167–173.
31. Cheng N, et al. Pregnancy and post-pregnancy avascular necrosis of the femoral head. *Arch Orthop Trauma Surg* 1982;100:199–210.
32. Hungerford DS, Lennox DW. The importance of increased interosseous pressure in the development of osteonecrosis of the femoral head. Implications for treatment. *Orthop Clin North Am* 1985;16:635–654.
33. Gormus N, Ustun ME, Paksoy Y, et al. Acute thrombosis of inferior vena cava in a pregnant woman presenting with sciatica: a case report. *Ann Vasc Srug* 2005;19(1):120–122.
34. Paksoy Y, Gormus N. Epidural venous plexus enlargements presenting with radiculopathy and back pain in patients with inferior vena cava obstruction or occlusion. *Spine* 2004;29(21):2419–2424.

35. Berg G, Hammar M, et al: Low back pain during pregnancy. *Obstet Gynecol* 1988;71:71–78.

36. ABRUPTION

37. Williams OB, Urinary Tract changes in pregnancy, p. 137.

38. Butler EL, Cox SM, Eberts E, et al. Symptomatic nephrolithiasis complicating pregnancy. *Obstet Gyn* 2000;96:753–760.

39. Lewis DF, Robichaux AG, Jaekle RK, et al. Urolithiasis in pregnancy: diagnosis, management, and pregnancy outcome. *J Reprod Med* 2003;48:28–35.

40. Gutke A, Josefsson A, Oberg B. Pelvic girdle pain and lumbar pain in relation to postpartum depressive symptoms. *Spine* 2007;32(13):1430–1436.

41. Field T. Stability of mood states and biochemistry across pregnancy. *Infant Behav Develop* 2006;29(2):262–267.

42. Haugland KS, Rasmussen S, Daltveit AK. Group intervention for women with pelvic girdle pain in pregnancy. A randomized controlled trial. *Acta Obstet Gynecol Scand* 2006;85(11):1320–1326.

43. Albert HB, Godskesen M, Korsholm L, et al. Risk factors in developing pregnancy-related pelvic girdle pain. Acta Obstet Gynecol Scand 2006;85(5):539–544.

44. Gutke A, Ostgarrd HC, Oberg B. Pelvic girdle pain and lumbar pain in pregnancy: a cohort study of the consequences in terms of health and functioning. *Spine* 2006;31(5):E149–E155.

45. American College of Sports Medicine. *ACSM'S Guidelines for Exercise Testing And Prescription*. 6th Ed. Philadelphia, PA: Lippincott Williams & Wilkins, 2000.

46. American College of Obstetrics and Gynecology. Exercise during pregnancy and the postnatal period. *Clin J Obstet Gynecol* 203;46:496–499.

47. American College of Obstetricians and Gynecologists (ACOG). *Exercise During Pregnancy and the Postnatal Period*. Washington, DC, 1985.

48. Davies GAL, Wolfe LA, Mottola MF, et al. Joint SOGC/CSEP Clinical Practice Guideline: exercise in pregnancy and the postpartum period. *Can J Appl Physiol* 2003;28:329–341.

49. Mens JMA, Damen L, Snijders CJ, et al. The mechanical effect of a pelvic belt in patients with pregnancy-related pelvic pain. *Clin Biomech* 2006;21(2):122–127.

50. Carr CA. Use of a maternity support binder for relief of pregnancy-related back pain. *J Obstet Gynecol Neonatal Nurs* 2003;32:495–502.

51. Kuchera ML, Kappler RE. Considerations of posture and group curves. In: Ward RC, ed. *Foundations for Osteopathic Medicine*. 2nd Ed. Philadelphia, PA: Lippincott Williams & Wilkins, 2003: 588–589.

52. Batavia M. Contraindications for superficial heat and therapeutic ultrasound: Do sources agree? *Arch Phys Med Rehabil* 2004;85:1006–1010.

53. Cameron MH. *Physical Agents in Rehabilitation*. St. Louis, MO: Saunders, 2003.

54. Jellema P, van Tulder MW, van Poppel M, et al. Lumbar supports for the prevention and treatment of low back pain: a systematic review within the framework of the Cochrane Back Review Group. *Spine* 2001;26: 377–386.

55. Howell CJ. Transcutaneous nerve stimulation (TNS) in labor. In: Keirse MJNC, Renfew MJ, Neilson JP, et al., eds. *Pregnancy and Childbirth Module: The Cochrane Database of Systematic Reviews, The Cochrane Collaboration, Issue 2*. Oxford Update Software, 1995.

56. Lund I, Lundeberg T, Lonnberg L, et al. Decrease of pregnant women's pelvic pain after acupuncture: a randomized controlled single-blind study. *Acta Obstet Gynecol Scan* 2006;85(1):12–19.

57. Guerreiro da Silva JB, Nakamura MU, Cordeiro JA,. Acupuncture for low back pain in pregnancy—a prospective, quasi-randomized, controlled study. *Acupunct Med* 2004;22(2):60–67.

58. Kvorning N, Holmberg C, Grennert L, et al. Acupuncture relieves pelvic and low back pain in late pregnancy. *Acta Obstet Gynecol Scan* 2004;83(3): 246–250.

59. Beard RW, Reginald PW, Wadsworth J. Clinical features of women with chronic lower abdominal pain and pelvic congestion. *Br J Obstet Gynaecol* 1988;95:153–161.

60. Beard RW, Highman JH, Pearce S, et al. Diagnosis of pelvic varicosities in women with chronic pelvic pain. *Lancet* 1984;2:946–949.

61. Gupta A, McCarthy S,. Pelvic varices as a cause for pelvic pain: MRI appearance. *Magn Reson Imaging* 1994;12:679–681.

62. Simons DG, Travell JG. Myofascial origins of low back pain. 3. Pelvic and lower extremity muscles. *Postgrad Med* 1983;73:99–105, 108.

63. Schmitz A, Lutterbey G, von EL, von FM, et al. Pathological cervical fracture after spinal manipulation in a pregnant patient. *J Manipulative Physiol Ther* 2005;28:633–636.

65

Adult with Myalgias

MICHAEL WIETING AND WILLIAM FOLEY

KEY CONCEPTS

- The differential diagnosis of myalgia can be extensive, encompassing common, easily diagnosed, and less well recognized clinical conditions.
- The chief complaint in fibromyalgia is a condition encompassing chronic, relapsing, diffuse aching pain, and tenderness, which can be intermittent and nondermatomal.
- Other features of fibromyalgia include hyperesthesia, allodynia, severe fatigue, insomnia, depression, anxiety, cognitive difficulty (specifically, issues with motivation, concentration, and organization), exercise intolerance, and nonrestorative sleep.
- Approximately 2% of United States and Canadian citizens have fibromyalgia.
- Current theories include atypical sensory processing in the central nervous system (i.e., central sensitization), dysfunction of skeletal muscle nociception, and dysfunction of the hypothalamic-pituitary-adrenal axis.
- Treatment for fibromyalgia should include OMT, patient education, and aerobic exercise.

CASE VIGNETTE

A 31-year-old woman reports muscle pain "all over my body" with the most intense pain in the neck, back, shoulders, and thighs. The pain started 2 years ago in her low back after a minor car accident. The back pain at that time was mild and plain x-rays were negative. Since then, the pain has gradually spread to her entire body and has become a constant ache that waxes and wanes in intensity. Over-the-counter medications such as ibuprofen and acetaminophen have been somewhat helpful but only on a temporary basis. She has not used narcotics since they made her nauseated when she took them after a previous surgery.

She describes her pain as a 6/10 currently but that it can range from 4 to 8 on a scale of 1 to 10. About a year ago, she completed 6 weeks of physical therapy that she feels was beneficial, but she did not keep up with her prescribed home exercises due to excessive pain. She reports no known tick or other insect exposure or bite. Her biggest complaint is that she can no longer work due to the pain and that she is having a hard time caring for her two small children. She feels like "a prisoner to her pain." Six months after the car accident, she began experiencing new fatigue, insomnia, and abdominal bloating; she denies abdominal pain, diarrhea, or constipation. Her fatigue is now most pronounced after increased or sustained activity. She can feel exhausted after simple events such as going to the mall or cleaning the house. At night, she falls asleep easily but awakens two to three times per night and finds it difficult to fall back asleep.

Past Medical History:

Her past medical history is significant only for seasonal allergies.

Past Surgical History:

Positive for uncomplicated Cesarean sections x 2

Medications:

She is currently taking loratadine 10 mg as need for her allergies and a daily multivitamin.

Allergies:

She has no known drug allergies.

Social History:

She does not smoke or use illicit drugs. She drinks one glass of wine daily. She reports that she is happily married for 6 years.

REVIEW OF SYSTEMS

She reports no fevers or recent weight loss.

HEENT:

Her vision and hearing are normal.

Cardiovascular:

She has no chest pain, palpitations, or shortness of breath.

Lungs:

She denies shortness of breath, wheezing, and cough.

Gastrointestinal:

She denies stomach pain, nausea, vomiting, diarrhea, and change in stools. She admits to bloating.

Skin:

She has no skin rash.

Musculoskeletal:

She denies joint swelling and joint pain although she admits to muscle pain as described above.

Neurological:

She denies paresthesias, weakness, loss of consciousness, tics, twitches, and seizures.

Psychiatric:

She complains of difficulty with concentration, organization of tasks, motivation, and a shortened attention span. She has progressively had more depression as a result of her condition and reports feeling hopeless at times.

Endocrine:

She denies chills, fever, and weight change. She admits to fatigue and sleeping difficulties as previously described.

PHYSICAL EXAMINATION

Vital Signs:

In the office, her heart rate is 68 beats per minute, respiratory rate is 16 beats per minute, blood pressure is 112/70, and she is afebrile.

General:

She appears in no acute distress.

Eyes:

Extraocular muscles are intact and pupils are equally round and reactive to light.

ENT:

Her oral mucosa is moist. Her neck is supple with no lymphadenopathy or thyromegaly.

Cardiovascular:

Her heart has a regular rate and rhythm without murmurs and the lungs are bilaterally clear to auscultation.

Lungs:

Breath sounds are full and clear to auscultation.

Abdomen:

The abdomen is soft and nontender.

Skin:

She has no rash.

Neurological:

Reflexes are +2 and equal in both the upper and lower extremities. Sensation is intact to light touch and pin prick. Muscle strength is 5/5 globally.

Musculoskeletal/Structural:

She has no muscle atrophy or spinous process tenderness. There are no joint effusions or tenderness. No synovitis is palpable. Multiple tender points are present in the anterior neck at the C5–7 intertransverse spaces, at the insertions of the suboccipital muscles, in the upper midtrapezius bilaterally, in the supraspinatus above the medial scapular spine, just distal to the lateral epicondyles, at the upper outer quadrant of the buttocks, and posterior to the greater trochanter prominences. The cervical, thoracic, and lumbar paraspinal muscles are tender and hypertonic. The occipital-atlantial junction is extended sidebent right and rotated left. There is a sphenobasilar synchondrosis compression, the atlantial-axial junction is rotated right, the thoracolumbar junction is sidebent left and rotated right and the lumbosacral junction is sidebent right and rotated left, the right innominate is rotated posteriorly, and there is bilateral sacroiliac restriction. Both shoulders are protracted.

DIFFERENTIAL DIAGNOSIS

Diffuse myalgia associated with fatigue is a common complaint in the primary care setting. The differential diagnosis of myalgia can be extensive, encompassing common easily diagnosed and less well recognized clinical conditions, some of which can present with similar manifestations and can coexist with fibromyalgia. Careful history taking and methodical physical examination assist in narrowing down the possibilities. The differential (Table 65.1) includes most commonly, bursitis, tendonitis or synovitis, hypothyroidism. Somewhat less common but deserving of consideration are infectious conditions such as Lyme disease and hepatitis C and inflammatory conditions such as polymyalgia rheumatica, polymyositis, dermatomyositis, rheumatoid arthritis, systemic lupus erythematosis, and scleroderma.

Degenerative/structural problems such as cervical stenosis may present as myalgias, but the patient will also typically have neck pain associated with dysesthesia, numbness, and, if involving the central canal, myelopathic symptoms of extremity spasm, bowel and bladder dysfunction, unsteady gait, lower limb weakness and numbness, abnormal reflexes, muscle atrophy, and decreased muscle tone. Certain metabolic processes can be associated with myalgias, the most common being thyroid disease and vitamin B_{12} deficiency and, rarely, as well as toxicities or side effects of some lipid-lowering agents, and antiviral medications. Frequent concomitant conditions that need to be considered are depression, chronic fatigue, fibromyalgia, and myofascial pain.

The presence of fatigue, insomnia, or other constitutional symptoms in a patient with diffuse myalgia tends to focus the differential on systemic or chronic conditions. Often, lab work (such as complete blood count [CBC], liver and kidney functions, creatinine phosphokinase [CPK], erythrocyte sedimentation rate [ESR], C-reactive protein [CRP], and thyroid functions) may be needed to rule out diffuse or systemic pathology.

In this case, the patient's pain and constitutional symptoms seem to be temporally related to a motor vehicle accident suggesting myofascial pain as a result of trauma rather than a systemic condition. However, some inflammatory diseases such as rheumatoid arthritis and systemic lupus erythematosus can initially present in similar fashion with myalgia as the initial complaint followed by fatigue and other systemic signs. Consequently, a careful review of all systems and laboratory studies is necessary to determine the diagnosis. Also, myofascial disease can coexist with other disorders of defined structural pathology, such as rheumatoid arthritis, fibromyalgia, and chronic fatigue syndrome, which are considered diagnoses of exclusion, necessitating that other causes of diffuse muscle pain be first ruled out.

Workup and Interpretation

This patient's chronic and diffuse clinical temporal profile helps to rule out most infectious processes; however, an elevated white blood cell count could indicate chronic infection or an inflammatory disease. Elevated CRP and/or an ESR are also indicators of inflammation. If either is elevated, further studies would be necessary to identify the etiology of the inflammation. Elevated CPK levels suggest an inflammation of muscle. Liver and renal function tests can be elevated in hepatitis C, myositis, lupus, rheumatoid arthritis, and other autoimmune diseases. Thyroid disease can present with muscle pain or weakness, depression, fatigue, and insomnia; a thyroid-stimulating hormone (TSH) level is usually sufficient to rule out this as a cause.

Other tests that could be considered in the workup of diffuse myalgia include vitamin B_{12} level, hepatitis C screen, and a Lyme titer. Vitamin B_{12} deficiency would be high on the differential if the patient had undergone small bowel resection, was malnourished, had a history of excessive alcohol intake, or followed a diet low in B vitamins. Generally, this information can be obtained from the history and, unless there is suspicion, lab testing is not necessary. In the same way, a hepatitis C screen should be performed if hepatitis C is suspected or there is a history of blood transfusion, multiple sexual contacts, intravenous drug use, or a prior accidental needle stick. Screening for

TABLE 65.1

Differential Diagnosis of Myalgias

Mechanical/Degenerative Conditions

Bursitis	Involves Only One Joint or Limb
Tendonitis or synovitis	Usually has a single focus and is associated with tendon motion
Cervical stenosis	Neck pain associated with dysesthesia, numbness, and, if involving the central canal, myelopathic symptoms of extremity spasm, bowel and bladder dysfunction, unsteady gait, lower limb weakness and numbness, abnormal reflexes, muscle atrophy, and decreased muscle tone

Infectious Conditions

Lyme disease	A characteristic erythema migrans, usually only one to two joints are involved, one of which is often the knee and associated neuropathy and nephropathy and frequent facial nerve involvement
Hepatitis C	Need characteristic lab findings

Inflammatory Conditions

Polymyalgia rheumatica	Features symmetric, proximal weakness, normal CPK, neuropathic pain, and hyperesthesia
Polymyositis and dermatomyositis	Present with severe, symmetric proximal weakness, and high CPK
Rheumatoid arthritis:	Morning stiffness that may last for several hours, joint swelling and pain, symmetric polyarthritis, joint warmth and effusion, multiple elevated serum immune complexes, and complement consumption
Systemic lupus erythematosis	Characteristic malar or discoid rash, vasculitis, lymphadenopathy, thrombocytopenia, and nephritis associated dark urine and peripheral edema along with elevated ANA
Scleroderma	Features skin and multiorgan fibrosis

Metabolic Processes

Hypothyroidism	Can be assessed via a TSH level
Thyroid disease	Can be assessed with imaging
Vitamin B_{12} deficiency	A simple blood test can measure B_{12}
Toxicities or side effects of some lipid-lowering agents	This is a diagnosis based upon clinical presentation and exclusion of other etiologies
Toxicities or side effects antiviral medications	This is a diagnosis based upon clinical presentation and exclusion of other etiologies

Lyme disease should be performed if the patient has a history of tick bite, a characteristic rash, or reported migratory joint pains. There was no objective muscle weakness found in this patient; however, if weakness of unknown etiology were present after initial workup or if there were concern for possible radiculopathy, myopathy, or nerve entrapment, an electrodiagnostic study should be performed. If any of these tests are abnormal, then a muscle biopsy or further testing for immunologic or other systemic disorders may be warranted.

CASE VIGNETTE (CONTINUED)

Labs performed during the initial visit with this patient included a CBC, renal and liver functions, CRP, ESR, CPK), and TSH levels. The initial lab work was negative. This patient was diagnosed with fibromyalgia. The history and physical exam, in conjunction with lab results, indicate her pain is likely myofascial in origin.

Diagnosis

The three most common causes for myofascial pain are myofascial pain syndrome, chronic fatigue syndrome, and fibromyalgia. Fibromyalgia is differentiated from myofascial pain syndrome in that it usually has multiple tender points in predictable bilateral locations, chronic widespread pain, a 10:1 ratio prevalence in females, fatigue, and sleep disturbance while myofascial pain syndrome has trigger points, more regionalized pain, a 1:1 ratio of males and females, and rarely has systemic features.

Fibromyalgia may be distinguished from chronic fatigue syndrome by virtue of the fact that chronic fatigue syndrome is usually preceded by a viral illness, which is not the case with fibromyalgia. Fatigue, a characteristic of both diseases, is usually of more than 6 months' duration but is, in chronic fatigue syndrome, also associated with at least 4 of the following: decreased memory or concentration, sore throat, tender cervical or axillary nodes, multijoint pain, new headache, postexertion malaise, nonrestorative sleep, and muscle pain. Fibromyalgia is a chronic syndrome, predominantly in women, that is marked by generalized chronic pain, multiple well-defined tender points, fatigue, and sleep disturbance.

The chief complaint in fibromyalgia is a condition encompassing chronic, relapsing, diffuse aching pain, not just tenderness, that can be intermittent and nondermatomal. Patients may complain of hyperesthesia and allodynia. The pain presents, often bilaterally, in muscles and muscle tendon junctions especially in the neck, shoulders, second ribs, elbows, hips, buttocks, and knees. Other features of fibromyalgia include severe fatigue, insomnia, depression, anxiety, cognitive difficulty (specifically, issues with motivation, concentration, and organization), exercise intolerance and nonrestorative sleep. Fibromyalgia patients may have concomitant migraine headaches, temporomandibular joint disorder, urinary frequency, paresthesias in the hands and feet, or irritable bowel syndrome.

Approximately 2% of United States and Canadian citizens have fibromyalgia. On a typical day, a primary care physician may see several patients with this diagnosis. The etiology of fibromyalgia is unknown. To date, no pathology has been found in the muscles of fibromyalgia patients. Current theories include atypical sensory processing in the central nervous system (i.e., central sensitization) and dysfunction of skeletal muscle nociception and the hypothalamic-pituitary-adrenal axis. Psychosocial factors seem to play a large role in the development of the disease; in fact, disability is most common in persons with jobs involving physical labor, who have poor coping strategies, who feel helpless, and who are involved in litigation (Winfield, 2006).

Osteopathic Patient Management
Biomechanical Model
This patient has a large number of somatic dysfunctions that likely contribute to biomechanical stress and increased nociception. Since 2 years have passed after the proposed inciting insult, treating the original somatic dysfunction in the low back will likely not be sufficient due to local and central sensitization. It is important to treat all areas of somatic dysfunction initially in this patient, concentrating on the areas of greatest functional compromise. Decreasing biomechanical stress is key in avoiding continued local and central sensitization. Aerobic exercise should focus on stretching and strengthening the musculature and combating deconditioning. Core strengthening is beneficial in treating deconditioned abdominals and paraspinal muscles that are either weak or inordinately tight.

Respiratory/Circulatory Model
Somatic dysfunction can alter the musculoskeletal system's contribution to tissue perfusion. The venous and lymphatic systems are low-pressure circulatory systems dependent upon external forces for proper function. Pain may result in muscle splinting and altered movement mechanics in the thoracic tissues and respiratory muscles. Altered tissue tone and restrictions can directly impede tissue perfusion. Resolution of somatic dysfunction may improve circulation to injured or damaged muscles and nerves.

Neurological Model
Recent clinical investigations have suggested that fibromyalgia is a central sensitivity syndrome and that it has a neurophysiologic base. Many researchers now feel that risk factors for developing fibromyalgia include vulnerability issues (such as being female, low self-efficacy, history of adverse experiences) occurring while the brain was developing and persistent stress or distress, in terms of anxiety, poor coping skills, and personality disorders, all of which

may negatively impact long-term prognosis. It is felt that patients with fibromyalgia have a generalized decreased pain perception threshold, excess excitatory (nociceptive) neurotransmitters (as examples, substance P and glutamate, which concentrate in the insula of the brain), low levels of inhibitory neurotransmitters (such as serotonin and norepinephrine), enhanced temporal summation of pain, altered endogenous opioid analgesic activity, and dopamine dysregulation. (Winfield, JB. "Fibromyalgia" eMedicine, 2009)

In treating fibromyalgia, it is important to remember that this is not a localized condition. Treating myofascial trigger points may help in the short term but have not been shown to be effective in long-term treatment of fibromyalgia. An osteopathic treatment approach should address the whole patient. Empathetic listening and acknowledgment of the legitimacy of the patient's pain, assessing possible perpetuating or concomitant factors, relaxation training, activity pacing, and exercise are useful initial strategies that can be supplemented with other approaches as needed. In this patient, pain started locally in the back and then spread. If the original injury to the back does not resolve, it may continue to send acute nociceptive signals to the spinal cord, which in turn sends signals to the brain. Chronically sustained insults to a nerve can lead to local sensitization and phenomena known as "facilitation" and "wind-up," where short-term potentiation of pain signals occurs that is associated with repeated C-fiber stimulation (Gary, 2002). Afferent pain signals from hypersensitive spinal nerves can affect related muscles and joints. Hyperesthesia, allodynia, and pain may then result in innervated structures. Hypersensitive proprioceptors can also cause structural alterations that lead to somatic dysfunctions, such as ligamentous articular strains, muscle spasm, fascial strains, and myofascial trigger points, all of which may lead to increased or sustained pain. The central nervous system's response to prolonged painful stimulation is known as central sensitization, a long-term potentiation of pain signals associated with NMDA receptor activation and with the induction of specific genes. Chronic nerve impingement can lead to dorsal horn sensitization of its nerve roots. When central sensitization occurs, it can affect two segments above and below the innervating site. Therefore, multiple spinal levels can become painful and dysfunctional, as is seen in this patient. As a result, pain from a local injury can appear to spread to other regions of the body. Nociceptive signals from the spinal cord can be consolidated in the brain causing further sensitization in the central nervous system. In this patient, central sensitization may account for her depression, fatigue, insomnia, and cognitive impairment.

The patient was treated pharmacologically with duloxetine and later pregabalin. Duloxetine, a serotonin and norepinephrine-reuptake inhibitor and antidepressant, has shown encouraging results in fibromyalgia studies (Arnold et al., 2007). Pregabalin, an anticonvulsant, is the only FDA-approved drug for fibromyalgia. Recent studies show statistically greater improvement in pain, fatigue, sleep, and quality of life (Crofford et al., 2005). Both act on the central nervous system and are likely able to lessen fibromyalgia symptoms by modulating neurotransmitters and affecting central sensitization. The literature does not support the effectiveness of nonsteroid anti-inflammatory drugs or steroids for the disease, but they can be useful in management of coexisting inflammatory processes. Beta blockers, increased fluid intake, NMDA receptor antagonists under supervision, analgesics, anxiolytics and hypnotics, muscle relaxants, and the selective estrogen receptor modulator raloxifene are desirable, to name a few. Tricyclic antidepressants have shown benefit with pain and sleep. When using this class of medication, it should be remembered that nortryptilene has a lesser side effect profile (i.e., dry mouth, constipation, fluid retention, weight gain, and decreased concentration). Botulinum neurotoxin, produced by the anaerobic bacterium *Clostridium botulinum*, is one of several neurotoxins with similar effects on human tissue—it has been shown to inhibit release of neurotransmitters involved in pain transmission (such as substance P and glutamate) in animal studies; it also reduces signs of pain, local edema, and appears to act only upon motor nerve endings, thereby sparing sensory nerve fibers. Botulinum toxin also secondarily appears to affect improved blood flow and to release nerve fibers under compression by abnormally contracting muscle via its presynaptic inhibition of release of acetylcholine.

Metabolic Energy Model

Finally, it is important to consider the metabolic energy model when planning long-term treatment for a patient with fibromyalgia. Diet (especially addressing potential 25-hydroxyvitamin D deficiency), graded aerobic exercise, lifestyle modifications, and decreased somatic dysfunction load are all important in decreasing or eliminating future exacerbations of fibromyalgia.

Behavioral Model

Psychological components are often prominent in fibromyalgia. Not only does the patient report depression but also the worry and anxiety about her family and work. While this may be partially emotional, somatic dysfunctions may contribute to the sensitization of the brain's emotional center, that is, the limbic system. Gold and Goodwin (1988a,b) first reported depression and other "psychological" symptoms in patients with chronic pain. Since that time, the association between depression and pain has become widespread (Robinson et al., 2009). Recent evidence suggests in patients with fibromyalgia, pain may also adversely affect overall health via its contribution to allostatic load (Martinez-Lavin and Vargas, 2009).

CASE VIGNETTE (CONTINUED)

PATIENT OUTCOME

Information about fibromyalgia was provided to the patient through patient-physician discussion and patient handouts from the American Pain Society. OMT was performed starting on the first visit. Initially, gentle techniques including myofascial release, balanced ligamentous tension, and cranial osteopathy were performed due to the patient's sensitivity even to light touch. As she progressed with treatments, other techniques were added. She was also started on an exercise program that consisted of gradually increasing aerobic workouts to reach a goal of 30 minutes of daily exercise. Most authorities agree on the value of patient education and aerobic exercise. Education should be centered on reassurance that the illness is real and that fibromyalgia is neither progressive nor life threatening.

The patient returned every 4 weeks for reevaluation and OMT. At each visit, continued aerobic exercise was encouraged and medications were titrated as needed. Counseling to improve diet and decrease stress was provided at each visit.

From the osteopathic perspective, it is important for the patient to be as healthy as possible in order to heal. This would include modifications in diet, habits, exercise, and stress. In the case of this patient, diet was not an issue but she did start a weekly meditation and yoga class. In other patients, discussion of whole foods, proper water intake, and smoking cessation may need to be addressed. For some patients, referral to a nutritionist or psychologist may be helpful.

By the fifth treatment, the patient was 75% improved. Follow-up visits were increased to every 3 months where she has been stable for 3 years. While her fibromyalgia has not completely resolved, she is now able to do work, take care of her family, and is not restricted by her disease.

SUMMARY

Using the osteopathic models of patient management, the physician can approach the patient with fibromyalgia from a whole person perspective, addressing all the various factors that may contribute to this multifaceted condition.

SUGGESTED READINGS

Arnold LM, Goldenberg DL, Stanford SB, et. al. Gabapentin in the treatment of fibromyalgia: a randomized, double-blind, placebo-controlled, multicenter trial. *Arthritis Rheum* 2007;56(4):1336–1344.

Berman BM, Ezzo J, Hadhazy V, et al. Is acupuncture effective in the treatment of fibromyalgia? *J Fam Pract* 1999;48(3):213–218.

Busch A, Schachter CL, Peloso PM, et al. Exercise for treating fibromyalgia syndrome. *Cochrane Database Syst Rev (Online)* 2002;(3).

Crofford LJ, Rowbotham MC, Mease PJ, et al. Pregabalin for the treatment of fibromyalgia syndrome: results of a randomized, double-blind, placebo-controlled trial. *Arthritis Rheum* 2005;52(4):1264–1273.

Gamber RG, Shores JH, Russo DP, et al. Osteopathic manipulative treatment in conjunction with medication relieves pain associated with fibromyalgia syndrome: results of a randomized clinical pilot project. *J Am Osteopath Assoc* 2002;102(6):321–325.

Gary J. Neural basis of pain. In: Ballantyne J, et al., eds. *Massachusetts General Hospital Handbook of Pain Management*. 2nd Ed. Baltimore, MD: Lippincott Williams & Wilkins, 2002:12.

Gold P, Goodwin F. Clinical and biochemical manifestations of stress: Part I. *NEJM* 1988a;319:348–353.

Gold P, Goodwin F. Clinical and biochemical manifestations of depression: Part II. *NEJM* 1988b;319:413–420.

Goldenberg D, Mayskiy M, Mossey C, et al. A randomized, double-blind crossover trial of fluoxetine and amitriptyline in the treatment of fibromyalgia. *Arthritis Rheum* 1996;39(11):1852–1859.

Gowans SE, de Hueck A. Effectiveness of exercise in management of fibromyalgia. *Curr Opin Rheumatol* 2004;16(2):138–142.

Martinez-Lavin M, Vargas A. Complex adaptive systems allostasis in fibromyalgia. *Rheum Dis Clin North Am* 2009;35:285–298.

Robinson MJ, Edwards SE, Iyengar S, et al. Depression and pain. *Front Biosci* 2009;14:5031–5051.

Winfield JB. XIII fibromyalgia: 15 rheumatology. In: Dale DC, Federman DD, eds. *ACP Medicine Online*. New York, NY: WebMD Inc., 2006; *Curr Opin Rheumatol* 2007;19(2):111–117.

66

Acute Neck Pain

MICHAEL SEFFINGER, JESUS SANCHEZ, AND MARCEL FRAIX

KEY CONCEPTS

- The osteopathic approach to patients with neck pain begins with a thorough history and physical exam, including an osteopathic palpatory exam of the neuromusculoskeletal system.
- Differential diagnosis utilizes a structure-function approach in determining whether the pain is due to local pathology, spinal somatic dysfunction of the cervical or upper thoracic region, localized manifestation of a systemic pathophysiologic process, or referred pain from intern organ disease.
- Osteopathic treatment plan includes judicious application of osteopathic manipulative treatment to alleviate somatic dysfunction and improve biomechanical, neurological, metabolic, respiratory/circulatory, and behavioral functions.
- Neck pain due to whiplash-associated disorder is a common cause of neck pain in middle-age adults and is considered to involve the whole person, not just the cervical spine.

CASE STUDY

Chief Complaint: Neck Pain

HPI:

A 45-year-old female presents to the ambulatory clinic with a complaint of acute neck pain that began after a motor vehicle accident (MVA) 3 days ago; she requests a note to stay off work. Three days ago, she was sitting in her car at a stoplight in her compact car when it was hit from behind by a pickup truck going about 35 mph. She was wearing her seat belt, hit her head against the headrest, but had no loss of consciousness; however, she did complain of neck pain after she stepped out of her car. She was looking up to the right into her rear view mirror at the time of impact. She was seen in an emergency room (ER) later that day where a cervical spine x-ray series showed no fractures or dislocations, but loss of cervical lordosis was noted. She was discharged home the same day with a soft cervical collar and given a prescription for an analgesic for pain, a narcotic for severe pain, and a muscle relaxant for muscle spasms.

She still has neck stiffness and pain, 8/10, better laying supine, worse when sitting up. It lasts throughout the day and is dulled a little by the analgesics. The neck collar gives her some relief. She has no other medical problems. Currently, she is taking the medications given to her at the ER, which provide some relief, although they make her drowsy and she has been sleeping several times throughout the day. The pain radiates to her shoulders and head. It is constant with intermittent sharp and shooting radiating pain to her shoulders and head.

PMH:

She has no major medical problems, no hospitalizations.

PSHx:

None to date.

MEDS:

Ibuprofen 800 mg tid prn pain; hydrocodone/acetaminophen 500 mg one every 4 hours prn severe pain; carsiprodol one every 6 hours prn muscle spasms.

ALL:

She has no allergies to medications.

SOC Hx:

She works as a secretary at a business office, types, files and answers phones 8 hours a day, 5 days a week. She is divorced, is sole caregiver for her elderly and frail mother, has two grown children and one grandchild. She denies smoking, drinks a glass of wine with dinner nightly, and denies illicit drug use.

REVIEW OF SYSTEMS

General:

She denies recent weight loss or gain, fevers, night sweats, or travel.

Cardiovascular:

She denies chest pain, shortness of breath, orthopnea, dyspnea on exertion.

Respiratory:

She denies history of tuberculosis, asthma, cough, phlegm, difficulty breathing.

HEENT:

She denies visual, hearing, smell, taste, or phonation problems; no drainage or infections.

GI:

She has nausea but no emesis; decreased appetite; constipation; no hematochezia, melana, or hematemesis. She has no history of abdominal pain or distention. No history of ulcers, hepatitis, gallstones, pancreatitis, or colitis.

Neurological:

She gets intermittent dizziness that resolves spontaneously; no history of seizures, stroke or weakness; she does have chronic low back pain.

OB/GYN:

She is G2P2. Her last menstrual period was 2 weeks ago, normal flow and regular. She has not been sexually active in the past 2 years. She states that her last pap and breast exams were normal 6 months ago.

Psychiatric:

She denies fatigue, but has had nightmares since the accident. She is anxious, fearing she will not be able to continue her job or take care of her mother. However, she denies a history of anxiety or psychiatric illness or hospitalization. She denies bipolar disease, depression, or schizophrenia. She is frustrated that the narcotics and muscle relaxers make her unable to function. She would like to have another alternative to help her deal with the pain that will allow her to still carry out her responsibilities at home and at work.

Hematological:

She denies history of anemia or bleeding dyscrasias. She sustained a bruise from the seat belt across her neck, but has no history of easy bruising.

Endocrine:

She denies heat or cold intolerance; no polydypsia, polyphagia, polyuria.

MSK:

She denies skin lesions or rashes; no swollen joints, hands, or feet; constant bilateral frontal vice-like headaches and low back pain since the accident, with radiation to the left buttocks. She has a history of low back pain treated by a series of visits to chiropractors, osteopathic physicians, and physical therapists off and on for over 10 years since she fell skiing when she was 18. She was told she had scoliosis and a short left leg for which she wore a ¼ in. lift for 10 years, but stopped using it for the past 17 years. She has not had disabling back or neck pain since then, though on occasion gets a headache or low back pain that resolves with a nonsteroidal anti-inflammatory medication, some stretching exercises for the neck and low back, and a couple of days of rest from strenuous activities.

PHYSICAL EXAM

Vital signs:

Height: 5'6", weight: 150, BP: 150/88 mm Hg, R: 18 breaths/minute, P: 86 beats/minute, T: 98.6F.

General:

Although somewhat low energy and anxious in appearance, she is well nourished, well developed, and in obvious pain and discomfort in the seated position with a soft cervical collar around her neck.

Integument:

There is a mild abrasion over the left upper shoulder where the seatbelt was with slight ecchymosis. No ecchymosis in the other extremities, chest, or abdomen.

HEENT:

There are no contusions, lacerations, erythema, discharge, or swelling. Pupils are equal, round, reactive to light and accommodation, and external ocular muscles are intact (PERRLA, EOMI). There is no thyromegaly or tenderness. No lymphadenopathy.

Heart:

Has a regular rhythm without murmurs; no carotid or vertebral bruits.

Lungs:

Are clear to auscultation with equal breath sounds bilaterally.

Abdomen:

The abdomen is flat; there are bowel sounds present in all four quadrants, nondistended, tympanic, no masses, no hepatosplenomegaly or tenderness. No suprapubic tenderness.

Extremities:

No swelling, full ROM of the joints, pulses full and capillary refill less than 2 seconds in upper and lower extremities.

Neurologic exam:

Alert and oriented to person, place, and time. Gait is normal. Muscle strength is 5+/5+ in all muscles in upper and lower extremities. CN II to XII are grossly intact. Deep tendon reflexes are 2+/4+ bilaterally, symmetric in the upper and lower extremities. Babinski's test elicits bilateral downward going toes. There are no cerebellar or sensory deficits. Straight leg raise is negative bilaterally to 90 degrees. Cognitive exam (mini mental status exam) is negative. Spurling's maneuver for the cervical spine is negative for eliciting radiating pain.

Osteopathic/musculoskeletal exam:

Static tests for symmetry of anatomical landmarks: In the standing postural assessment, her head is held anterior to the gravitational line, with loss of cervical lordosis, decreased thoracic kyphosis and lumbar lordosis; the left shoulder is elevated; the left tip of scapula is superior; there is a thoracic scoliosis T5-11 convex right, apex at T8; there is a lumbar scoliosis L1-5, convex left with apex at L3; the left PSIS landmark is lower than the right; the left iliac crest is about 1 cm lower than the right; there is a short left leg approximately ¼ inch; and the left ASIS is inferior.

Motion tests reveal:

Positive standing and seated flexion tests on the left; the sacrum has decreased motion in both flexion and extension and feels compressed into L5; inherent sacral motion is diminished; L1-5 are rotated left sidebent right in neutral and the sacrum is also rotating to the left; T5-11 are neutral rotated right sidebent left; T3 is extended, rotated, and sidebent right with boggy, edematous, and tender paraspinal soft tissues at that level; T1 and T2 are extended rotated left sidebent left; there are myofascial restrictions of the thoracic inlet; the left first rib is restricted during exhalation; right ribs 3 to 6 are restricted during inhalation; left ribs 6 to 12 are restricted in exhalation; the left diaphragm is restricted during exhalation; there is decreased cervical range of motion bilaterally, especially flexion, extension, and sidebending; the occipitoatlantal (OA) articulation is extended sidebent left rotated right; the atlantoaxial (AA) articulation is rotated right; cranial motion is diminished in amplitude bilaterally with little movement palpable.

Palpation reveals:

Tender anterior cervical muscles; there are bilateral cervical spasms from C3 to C7 making it difficult to assess segmental restrictions; trigger points are present in the trapezius and pectoralis muscles bilaterally; there is a tender L5-S1 interspinous ligament; and Jones' tenderpoints are found at the left LPL5, right LC1, right AC1, and right PC2.

ASSESSMENT

1. Neck Pain ICD-9: 723.1
2. Whiplash-Associated Disorder (WAD) ICD-9: 847.1

3. Somatic Dysfunction ICD-9: cranium (739.0), cervical (739.1), thoracic (739.2), lumbar (739.3), sacrum (739.4), pelvis (739.5), lower extremity(739.6), and ribs (739.8)
4. Abrasion ICD-9: 911
5. Anxiety ICD-9: 300.4
6. Contusion ICD-9: 923.0
7. Dizziness ICD-9: 780.4
8. Muscle spasms ICD-9: 729.1
9. Nausea ICD-9: 787.02
10. Scoliosis, idiopathic ICD-9: 737.30
11. Short leg ICD-9: 755.32

DIFFERENTIAL DIAGNOSIS

Differential diagnosis utilizes a structure-function approach in determining whether the pain is due to local pathology, spinal somatic dysfunction of the cervical or upper thoracic region, localized manifestation of a systemic pathophysiologic process, or referred pain from intern organ disease. Since local neck pain generators may be located in the muscles, fascia, ligaments and joint capsules, periosteum, intervertebral discs, arteries, glands, organs, esophagus, trachea, lung and dura, all pathologic processes affecting these structures should be considered as possible causes of her pain. These include degenerative, infectious, inflammatory, neoplastic, congenital diseases, fractures, dislocations, spinal cord and peripheral nerve injuries, and vascular diseases, including arterial dissection. Differential diagnoses of acute neck pain from local pathology are listed in Table 66.1 along with characteristics and diagnostic tests used to confirm each.

In the patient above, gross fracture and dislocation are not likely, but possible, even in light of a negative initial cervical spine x-ray series (1). The upper cervical somatic dysfunction is symptomatic and likely related to her recent accident, but she has underlying dysfunction in all body regions related to her short leg and scoliosis. Her neck pain could be an exacerbation of her already dysfunctional back and spine.

It is unlikely she has a disease process radiating pain to the neck as her history and physical do not support this theory, so a myocardial infarction, pancoast lung tumor, esophageal or tracheal tumor or inflammation, thyroiditis or tumor, pulmonary embolus, collapsed lung, pleurisy, vertebral artery dissection, carotid artery dissection, tuberculosis, cancer of the mediastinum or neck or cervical lymphadenopathy are less likely and can be removed from the differential at this time; however, if her course of recovery does not follow a pattern consistent with a primary musculoskeletal injury, these occult sources of pain might be investigated further.

An underlying metabolic disease, such as osteoarthritis, rheumatoid arthritis, rheumatoid-related conditions, like dermatomyositis, temporal arteritis, Lyme's disease and fibromyalgia, goiter or thyroiditis, infection of the soft tissues, that is, cellulitis, the cervical discs or lymph channels (lymphangitis), or diet-related calcium or potassium deficits are not likely as there is no support for these conditions in the history and physical.

Neurological conditions that cause neck pain need to be considered, such as cervical radiculitis, atypical facial pain, trigeminal and glossopharyngeal neuralgia, reflex sympathetic dystrophy, neurogenic inflammation, but these are less common causes and are unlikely given the history of a recent whiplash injury just before the onset of her pain.

Neck pain from somatic dysfunction that is mechanical in origin is typically amenable to osteopathic manipulative treatment (OMT) and not only involves the cervical region but also is accompanied by dysfunction in the upper back, ribs, head, and upper extremities (2). It is characterized by the presence of muscle

TABLE 66.1

Differential Diagnosis of Neck Pain from Local Pathology

Diagnosis	Characteristics	Tests
Acute pharyngitis	Erythematous pharynx; exudates	Strep screen
Carotid aneurysm dissection	Tender carotid, bruit on auscultation	Carotid US, angiogram
Carotidynia	Tender carotid	Carotid US
Cervical fracture	Muscle splinting, history of trauma	Cervical spine x-rays
Dental disease	Teeth and/or gingival pain, tenderness, swelling	Dental x-rays
Lymphadenitis	Enlarged, tender lymph nodes	CBC, ESR
Meningitis	Nuchal ligament rigidity, fever, malaise	Spinal tap
Myositis	Very tender muscles	CBC, ESR
Peritonsillar abscess	Tonsil protruding anteriorly and/or medially	Aspiration
Spinal cord injury	Neurologic deficits below neck; if C3-5: diaphragm paralysis	MRI C-spine
Submandibular gland disease	Tender, mass palpable	US, CT
Temporomandibular joint syndrome	Tender TMJ, deviation of jaw upon opening, decreased movement	CT
Thyroiditis	Palpable thyroid, may be tender	TSH, T4, T3
Torticollis	Contracture of SCM muscle	Cervical x-rays
Tumor of tongue	Palpable mass	MRI
Vertebral artery dissection	Ophthalmologic and neurologic deficits	US, MRI angiogram

spasm, decreased range of motion, as well as a reduction in the quality of motion; there is pain with movement that improves with rest; and there is no organic pathology that could radiate pain to the region or cause viscerosomatic reflexes (2).

The incidence of motor vehicle collisions and WAD has increased in western nations over the past 30 years (3). Neck pain is the most frequently reported complaint in connection with whiplash (acceleration/deceleration); however, as is the case with low back pain, neck pain in general runs an episodic course and the most significant risk factor predictive of future episodes of neck pain is a previous history of neck pain (3). The Quebec Task Force on WAD defined whiplash as "an acceleration-deceleration mechanism of energy transferred to the neck that results in soft tissue injury that may lead to a variety of clinical manifestations including neck pain and its associated symptoms" (4). That task force also coined the term "WAD" to describe the clinical entities related to the injury, and to distinguish them from the injury mechanism. Though people mostly associate whiplash injury with neck symptoms, osteopathic physicians have long advocated for the perspective of whiplash as a total body, or total person, injury (5–10). Indeed, along with neck pain, patients also complain of a variety of WAD, including headache, cognitive disturbances, vertigo, visual disturbances, jaw pain, low back pain, and/or interscapular pain (11,12).

Cervical spine "whiplash" or acceleration/deceleration injury is a mechanism of injury, not a type or extent of injury. There are conflicting theories of the mechanism of the cervical spine component of the injury:

■ One is that the body propels forward with the head relatively stationary, followed by hyperextension, which then is followed by hyperflexion of the neck while the head recoils forward (after hitting the headrest), the damage being rapid tissue stretch secondary to traction, hyperextension, and hyperflexion
■ Another theory proposes that compression and concomitant torques at the level of C1 and C7, with a flexion torque at C1 and an extension torque at C7, cause ligamentous and myofascial sprain (13)

Probably both occur, with hyperextension causing the greatest insult. With hyperextension, if there is no head rest support for the head, the motion far exceeds the physiologic barrier and anterior neck soft tissues can be stretched, strained, and ruptured. However, cervical response is not so simple; it is modified by impact force, awareness and direction (14):

■ The greater the weight and speed (force) of the impacting vehicle, the more force is transmitted to the people in the car being hit
■ If the person is aware of the impact, muscles will contract in preparation for the collision, stabilizing the spine and diminishing the strain and stretch on the myofascial tissues; an unaware person's muscles and connective tissue would stretch before contracting, likely causing more damage
■ Direction of impact affects the muscles that will be activated in response to the force, and those that will likely be injured by stretch and strain forces (14)

The patient described above has WAD and somatic dysfunction in several body regions. The dizziness and nausea are likely secondary to the cervical somatic dysfunction as it affects equilibrium and neural afferents involved in the sensation of nausea (CN X). Muscle spasms and tenderpoints are also related to the WAD and associated somatic dysfunctions. The contusion and abrasion is most likely caused by the seat belt restraint. The underlying short leg and scoliosis are chronic problems and, although not directly related to her complaint of neck pain, likely have a significant role in the decreased resilience of the cervical spine to the whiplash motion effect.

OSTEOPATHIC PATIENT MANAGEMENT

Biomechanical Model

The entire postural mechanism needs to be considered even though the patient's primary complaints are in the neck and upper body regions (5–9). The motion present in the cervical spine is determined by the unique cervical spine articular anatomy (see Chapter on Cervical Region Anatomy) and dynamic interaction of the various muscles attached to the cervical spine that are coordinated in function during head, neck, thoracic, rib and upper extremity movements (14). The thoracic spine anchors the origins of muscles that stabilize and extend the cervical spine, such as the splenius cervicus and semispinalis capitus. These are not the muscles often injured in WAD; rather, the muscles most commonly injured, hypertonic, or tender upon palpation include the sternocleidomastoid, splenius capitus, and trapezius (14).

Assessing the mechanics of any injury is helpful in making a diagnosis and developing a management plan. Mechanical aspects of a whiplash-associated injury affect the degree of injury, treatment options, and prognosis. For example:

■ Bracing the hands against the steering wheel reduces anterior translation of the body, thereby reducing cervical injury but increasing the probability of soft tissue injury to the shoulders, ribs, and thoracic region
■ The presence of a headrest on top of the driver's seat reduces the chance of hyperextension and reduces the chance of cervical injury (15)

The body is a unit mechanism and all parts are deranged in a whiplash injury (7–9). The prevertebral fascia of the anterior neck is continuous with the mediastinum, which is continuous with the crura of the diaphragm surrounding the psoas major muscle. Thus, hyperextension can lead to strains in fascial patterns and dysfunctions in the thorax, abdomen, pelvis, and even the lower extremities (9). Comorbidities, in this case, scoliosis and short leg, will decrease the patient's adaptability to the sprained and strained upper body myofascial and ligamentous structures; osteoarthritis, rheumatoid arthritis, and similar soft tissue or joint inflammatory diseases can alter the tissue responses to the acceleration/deceleration injury. In many cases, sacral dysfunctions may prevent the patient from recovering in spite of OMT provided to the cervical and thoracic regions (5).

Pelvic somatic dysfunction occurs most commonly associated with the driver planting the foot on the brake in anticipation of, or in attempt to avoid, the accident, causing ilial rotations and superior pubic shears. The paravertebral muscles of the spine and the latissimus dorsi attach to the iliac crests. Movements of the spine and shoulder girdle operate against the resistance of the stabilized ileum. Patients may exhibit pain and decreased range of motion secondary to sacral and ilial dysfunction. Look for iliopsoas strains, strain or sprain of the hip, knee, foot, and ankle. Hip and pelvic fractures are quite common if the patient's foot was planted at the time of impact. Sacral dysfunction disturbs the body's balance and homeostatic mechanism—thus hindering the healing process (5). During cervical hyperextension and hyperflexion, the continuity of various muscular, ligamentous, and dural attachments causes the sacrum to be forcibly lifted and dislodged from its floating position between the ilia (5). Craniosacral restriction may be accompanied by gross lumbosacral and sacroiliac dysfunctions. Becker recommends diagnosing and restoring the primary respiratory (i.e., craniosacral) mechanism before addressing the interaction between the pelvis and the sacrum (5).

Whiplash injury occurs simultaneously in the cervical and thoracic regions (6). The continuity of the cervical, thoracic, and lumbar spine that is provided by the ligamentous attachments and paravertebral musculature, along with somatosomatic reflexes, transmits the acute cervical strain to the thoracic and lumbar regions. A significant thoracic extended dysfunction is produced in taller patients, often in the region of the top of the seat. Also, rotation and lateral forces are introduced into the spine. Lastly, the intimate relationship of the thoracic and cervical spine with the shoulder girdle makes it especially susceptible to injury. Usually, the occiput and the sacrum have the same dysfunctions. Asymmetric traction by muscles that attach to the cranium can result in torsions and sidebending or rotary dysfunctions; the temporal bones are especially vulnerable to these forces (7). Strain patterns are usually present if the patient has struck any object (7). The patient described above has decreased palpable cranial and sacral motion likely because of sphenobasilar compression as well as lumbosacral compression.

An osteopathic approach to this patient would entail helping her to improve her posture, short leg and scoliosis, as well as to evaluate and improve joint motion with OMT and exercises.

For patients with WAD, even in the 1960s and 1970s, osteopathic physicians advocated for adjunctive therapies in addition to OMT for somatic dysfunctions of the thoracic, lumbar, and sacral areas, and any obvious dysfunctions of the cranial and cervical spine (6–8):

- Acupuncture
- Adequate nutritional support
- Appropriate exercise
- Cervical traction
- Gentler forms of manipulation such as myofascial release and muscle energy (i.e., isometric resistance) techniques
- Heat and cold applications
- Help the patient to effectively address emotional difficulties such as anxiety and depression often associated with WAD
- Muscle relaxants
- Preventative measures including public education regarding whiplash injury, and the use of seatbelts and appropriately adjusted head restraints while driving
- Treatment of myofascial trigger points with ice massage or ethyl chloride spray and stretch
- Ultrasound
- Various types of neck collars in the acute phase
- Vitamin therapy.

Current evidence-based recommendations emphasize OMT to relieve somatic dysfunction and individualized exercises for rehabilitation (2,16); cervical collars are still used in the first few days up to a couple of weeks, but evidence has shown that patients who use a soft or firm cervical collar have no measurable benefit in improvement when compared to patients who receive general medical care only (17).

Respiratory/Circulatory Model

In the respiratory/circulatory model, evaluating and treating patients with neck pain considers the possible respiratory and circulatory relationships involved in the cause as well as in the treatment.

As is common with patients suffering from neck pain, the above described patient exhibits not only cervical, but also thoracic, lumbar, and sacral spinal somatic dysfunctions as well; costal and diaphragmatic dysfunctions are also present. Respiratory movements are compromised not only at the level of the diaphragm, but also in the costal cage and spine. Proper respiratory motion and optimal function relies on normal spinal and costal cage mechanics. The diaphragm attaches to ribs 6 to 10, and to the upper three lumbar vertebrae. Dysfunctions in these joints render the diaphragm less effective. The phrenic nerve, which emanates from cervical spinal nerves C3-5, controls diaphragm contraction. Optimal lymph drainage also requires normal costal cage mobility that enables alternating intrathoracic pressure differentials with each breath so that the passive lymphatic channels return lymph from below the diaphragm to the heart via the thoracic duct. Cervical and cranial lymphatics drain into the subclavian veins en route to return to the central circulation via the heart. Cervical somatic dysfunction involving the scalene muscles and anterior cervical fascia can compromise the supraclavicular fascia surrounding the thoracic inlet and thoracic duct and right lymphatic duct as they empty their contents into the subclavian veins. The fascial tension can interfere with free flow of the lymphatic drainage, so OMT using, for example, myofascial release, will help restore normal motion mechanics to that vital region. Therefore, in addressing the cervical, costal, upper extremity, thoracic, lumbar, and sacral somatic dysfunctions of the patient, consider the goal of restoring normal lymphatic and venous drainage through improved respiratory mechanics. Relieve tense myofascial components of the supraclavicular, thoracic inlet and outlet, the ribs, and the diaphragm. Maximize cervical lymphatic drainage with soft tissue and lymphatic OMT. Relieve somatic dysfunction along the entire spine, including the sacrum and pelvis. The patient may benefit from a shoe lift to relieve strain at the lumbosacral junction due to the unlevel sacral base. Improving sacral motion improves the primary respiratory mechanism function through the core link to the occiput via the spinal dura.

The vertebral artery traverses the cervical spine within a foramen in each vertebra but makes three 90-degree turns at the C1-occipital joint before entering the foramen magnum to provide blood to the base of the brain and cerebellum via the basilar arteries. Due to the vulnerability of this artery to dissection and occlusion resulting in stroke (cerebral vascular accident and subsequent central nervous system deficits), cervical spine HVLA procedures, especially those that require extension and rotation at the upper cervical spine to correct somatic dysfunctions, need to be performed with great caution and skill. It is impossible to predict whether a manual procedure will cause vertebral artery compromise; however, if prior to manipulation of the upper cervical spine, the patient complains of vertigo, has nystagmus, or syncope upon rotation of the head, these could be signs of vertebral artery compromise. If these symptoms or signs are present, performing the HVLA procedure is not recommended. Rather, place the patient's head back on the treatment table and reassess for vertebral artery compromise (auscultate for bruit, and obtain imaging with ultrasound and/or magnetic resonance or computerized axial angiograms to rule out dissection or occlusion). The American Osteopathic Association supports the use of HVLA for cervical somatic dysfunction. This position paper reviews the literature related to this topic as well and is highly recommended reading.

Somatic dysfunction in the upper thoracic spine and cervical spine is thought to affect blood flow to the cranium as the sympathetic cervical chain ganglia are situated just anterior to the cervical vertebra bodies. Louisa Burns, D.O., demonstrated the effects on cranial blood flow and ears, nose, and throat diseases from

Comorbid Conditions that are Found Associated Most Commonly in Patients with Neck Pain Include

- Autonomic failure (49)
- Cardiovascular disease (35,36)
- Concentration problems (50)
- Digestive system disease (36,41)
- Dizziness (50)
- Headaches (39,41)
- Low back pain (36,39,41)
- Nausea (50)
- Occipitoatlantal osteoarthritis (51)
- Orthostatic hypotension (49)
- Shoulder pain (36–40, 45, 52–55)
- TMJ syndrome (56)
- Trapezius muscle ischemia (57)

experimentally induced thoracic and cervical somatic dysfunction in animal models (31). Johnston and Kelso later documented a somatic dysfunction pattern of C6, T2, T6 in patients with hypertension (32). In a large retrospective chart review from osteopathic physicians across America in the 1950s, the most common somatic dysfunction related to cardiac symptomatology was OA dysfunction (33). More recently, much other comorbidity have been found in association with neck pain (Box 66.1).

Neurological Model

The patient has dizziness from her WAD and somatic dysfunctions. Understanding the upper cervical spine anatomy provides clues to the relationship of the somatic dysfunction found on physical exam and her symptoms. Dizziness is a symptom that occurs when there is disequilibrium. Equilibrium depends on normal vestibular function. The eyes and neck movement are coordinated via the tectospinal tract to maintain balance and equilibrium. The temporal bones house the vestibular apparatus that consists of three semicircular canals in three different planes with endolymphatic fluid and cilia that enable us to maintain a sense of where we are in relation to our environment. The posterior suboccipital muscles level the head to the horizon and keep the temporal bones level so we feel balanced. Thus, cervical somatic dysfunction interferes with head position, temporal bone levels, and eye-neck coordination, disturbing equilibrium function. Correcting the cervical somatic dysfunction with OMT should relieve the sense of dizziness if indeed this is the cause of the troublesome symptom. Dizziness could also be a symptom of vertebral artery dissection or occlusion, so the astute osteopathic physician should be aware of this possibility, especially if there are other central neurologic signs of deficit or dysfunction.

The patient also has nausea. Peripherally induced nausea sensation is transmitted to the brain most commonly via the vagus nerve afferents. The inferior nodosal (vagal) ganglia is situated immediately outside the cranial cavity as the vagus nerve exits the jugular foramen between the occiput and temporal bones, before the nerve enters the carotid sheath along with the jugular vein and carotid artery. Osteopathic clinicians believe the vagus nerve is vulnerable to the effects of somatic dysfunction in that vicinity and vice versa; if there is increased vagus nerve activity, that is, from thoracic or abdominal visceral inflammation, the surrounding somatic structures are affected and show signs of somatic dysfunction in the upper cervical spinal joints and surrounding soft tissues. Treatment

of the cervical somatic dysfunction with OMT is also intended to restore normal vagal activity and function, including relieving sensation of nausea that is caused by the cervical somatic dysfunction.

The relationship between cervical somatic dysfunction and symptoms of dizziness and nausea, and their abolishment by OMT, are anecdotal (expert clinical experience) and await animal or human laboratory studies and prospective randomized clinical trials to prove cause and effect. The current trend in osteopathic manual medicine practice, as exemplified by recent articles by osteopathic clinicians, favors treatment of somatic dysfunction not only in the cervical region, but throughout the body for patients with symptoms of dizziness and nausea (18,19).

The patient has pain and tenderpoints in the cervical as well as pelvic regions. They are likely due to the WAD. However, WAD is not the only cause of acute neck pain. In the United States, almost 85% of neck pain may be attributed to chronic stresses and strains or acute or repetitive neck injuries (20). In general, somatic dysfunction involving the OA and AA joints usually causes head pain primarily with neck pain secondarily, and somatic dysfunction of C2-7 joints causes neck pain primarily with head pain and/or shoulder pain secondarily (21,22). Cervical facet pain is typically a unilateral, dull aching pain with occasional referral into the occipital or trapezial region, depending on the facet joint involved. C1 and C2 zygapophyseal joints refer pain to the cranium, whereas C3-7 refer pain to the trapezium and interscapular regions (20). The pain referral zones for facet pain overlap both myofascial and disc pain patterns making it difficult to ascertain the exact level of the pain generator. In some patients, neck and head pain are associated with trigeminal nerve activity, either from dental-facial problems, activation of the cervical branches of the trigeminal nerve or influence of the trigeminal nerve on the thalamic pain receptor field in the brain (23).

With WAD, myofascial tenderpoints are commonly found in the trapezius, scalene, semispinalis cervicis, semispinalis capitis, and multifidus (10); the semispinalis capitis muscle seems to be most likely to develop a painful trigger point (24). In some patients, neck and head pain are associated with trigeminal nerve activity, either from dental-facial problems, activation of the cervical branches of the trigeminal nerve, or influence of the trigeminal nerve on the thalamic pain receptor field in the brain (23).

The most reliable physical examination tests for patients complaining of neck pain are the patient's response to digital pressure on bone or muscle, as is used with assessing for strain/counterstrain tenderpoints; tests for regional range of motion; and Spurling's maneuver for cervical radiculopathy (extension, sidebending, and rotation at the cervical spinal level of suspected spinal nerve root compression, combined with axial compression to limit the size of the intervertebral foramen, to see if pain radiates to the arm in a dermatomal distribution related to the spinal nerve being assessed) (25).

Systematic reviews of randomized clinical trials have shown that manipulation plus exercise is beneficial for acute and chronic mechanical neck disorders with or without accompanying pain radiation to the head (16). In a multisite randomized clinical trial comparing the effectiveness of OMT with intramuscular non-steroidal anti-inflammatory medication (ketorolac tromethamine) for patients with acute neck pain seen in the emergency department, the OMT group had significantly reduced pain intensity and equivalent efficacy at relieving pain assessed at 1 hour post treatment (26). All patients received an initial structural exam. Fifty-eight patients were enrolled and met inclusion criteria if they had somatic dysfunction with no history or evidence of underlying organic disease. More than half of the patients in each group had neck pain as a result of a motor vehicle collision. Osteopathic physicians palpated the cervical region to assess patients for tissue texture changes, joint restrictions, and areas of tenderness. OMT performed at the discretion of each physician with no set protocol included isolated or a combination of HVLA thrust, muscle energy, and/or soft tissue techniques. Intervention with OMT lasted less than 5 minutes (26).

Autonomic effects can accompany cervical somatic dysfunction. Sympathetic innervation to the head and neck regions is derived from preganglionic fibers arising from the lateral horn of the spinal cord from T1 to T6. These fibers proceed cephalad to the sympathetic chain to enter the cervical ganglia and synapse with the postganglionic fibers. The inferior cervical ganglia lie at the superior border of the first ribs, anterior to C7. The inferior cervical ganglia send branches to the heart. The middle cervical ganglia are at the level of the transverse process of C6. The middle cervical ganglia send fibers to the thyroid gland and also to the heart. The superior cervical ganglia are at the level of the AA joint. The superior cervical ganglion postganglionic fibers accompany the internal carotid and ophthalmic arteries into the orbit, and to the glands of the head and face. Postganglionic fibers accompany the vertebral arteries and enter the skull to supply the vestibular portion of the ear, some cranial nerves, and the pharynx. Additionally, the cervical vertebra bodies and intervertebral discs are entirely surrounded by a network of interlacing nerve fibers (27). The anterior longitudinal ligament (ALL) receives bilateral contributions from the medioventral small branches of the sympathetic trunk forming a plexus of nerves throughout all levels. The posterior longitudinal ligament (PLL) likewise receives bilateral contributions from the sinuvertebral nerves that form a nerve plexus throughout all levels. There, nerve plexus of both the ALL and the PLL meet through the rami communicantes (27). Sympathetic symptoms can occur as a result of stimulation of the peripheral nerves as they pierce the soft tissue, stimulation of the sensory elements of C1 and C2, simultaneous compression of the nerve route in its foraminal passage or compression of the vertebral artery. Sympathetic symptoms include the following:

- Aural: tinnitus, deafness
- Ocular: blurred vision, retrobulbar pain, and a pupil that dilates when the head is turned and returns to a neutral midline position
- Vestibular: postural dizziness or vertigo

This patient exhibits signs of central and peripheral sensitization, or facilitation. OMT would be helpful in decreasing the irritability of the nervous system. It has been demonstrated that cervical spine manipulation alters cortical somatosensory processing and sensorimotor integration; the primary muscle afferents (probably Ia) are the most likely mediators of these effects (28). Resetting of the muscle spindle afferents with muscle energy OMT increases range of motion in cervical spinal joints (29). In randomized clinical trials, cervical spine manipulation and mobilization provide at least short-term benefits for patients with acute neck pain and headaches (17).

For this patient, OMT was directed at removing any impingement upon peripheral or central nervous structures, with cervical traction and indirect OMT procedures in the acute phase of recovery; tenderpoints were treated with strain/counterstrain; medications or other adjunct therapies may be needed to modulate neurological function depending on the patient's response to OMT. Thoracic manipulation has an analgesic effect in patients with mechanical neck pain (30). OMT for somatic dysfunction in other body regions, especially the thoracic spine and upper ribs, will help relieve the pain and dysfunction of the cervical spine.

Relieving somatic dysfunction with OMT to the rest of the body will decrease the somatic burden, relieve pain, and reduce the allopathic load. This will contribute significantly to the restoration of normal neurological function.

Metabolic Energy Model

The physiologic and metabolic mechanisms, set into motion due to internal or external factors, that are interpreted by the human body as pain are very complex and have yet to be completely elucidated. What is known is that irritation of the tissues through trauma, repetitive/overuse injury patterns, structural abnormalities, infection, degenerative and systemic disease can lead to the process of nociception and eventually a facilitated spinal cord segment. The inflammatory cascade can lead to a relentless positive-feedback cycle where inflammation can increase the pain that then potentiates the inflammation further (34). As inflammation and harmful metabolites begin to accumulate, structural changes in the affected tissue begin to occur and can ultimately lead to ischemia of the tissue (34). If the metabolic and physiologic alternations are not modified and persist for an extended period of time, long-term structural changes occur in the muscles, tendons, or joints and lead to limited functionality and eventual disability. The goal of soft tissue OMT is in part to relieve muscle spasms and assist the lymphatic system in clearing local toxic metabolites.

Some patients present with acute neck pain related to pharyngitis or peritonisillar abscess. Thus, even though there is evidence of somatic dysfunction on palpatory exam, the osteopathic physician should also assess the status of the internal organs capable of causing pain in the cervical region. OMT for somatic dysfunction related to infection or inflammation is directed at improving venous and lymphatic drainage, as in the respiratory-circulatory model. Using antibiotics as an adjunctive therapy is warranted when a bacterial pathogen is identified or highly likely based on the physical exam and course of the signs and symptoms over time.

There are patients with acute neck pain from thyroiditis who need further management with radiation, medication and/or surgery. In these patients, OMT was employed in the earlier part of the 20th century when no other treatment was available, and may be adjunctive in helping to improve lymphatic drainage even today, but in America OMT is not the standard treatment for this condition in the 21st century. Similarly, neck pain from metastatic cancer in the lymph glands or cervical structures, or primary carcinomas in the cervical region, are not treated directly with OMT. Patients may benefit from OMT to other body regions with the goal of reducing somatic dysfunction burden and relaxing the nervous system during and after definitive diagnosis and treatment with biopsy, radiation, chemotherapy and/or surgery.

For this patient, addressing metabolic-energy expenditure goals entails applying OMT to relieve muscle spasm and restore normal and efficient spinal motion to decrease the burden of poor posture and motion mechanics on energy expenditure. Additionally, ensure proper nutrition using wholesome foods and eliminate fast and fried foods, help the patient to restore normal sleep cycles, and encourage regular exercise. Remove infectious agents and decrease inflammation if present. Restore normal endocrine function if needed.

Behavioral Model

The patient typifies the most common scenario seen in osteopathic primary care practice. Patients with neck pain range in age from the first through the tenth decades (35–38). However, most patients with neck pain related to motor vehicle collisions are between the ages of 20–40 (15). Although neck pain occurs in children and adults of all ages and genders, neck pain is most commonly reported by middle-age females, especially those who experience WAD (37). In the general population, peak incidence of neck pain is between ages 30 and 59 (35,39). Age and gender standardized annual incidence is 14.6%; however, only less than 1% develop disabling neck pain, so most patients continue to work (35). The point prevalence of neck pain is 8% to 24%. The lifetime prevalence is 71% (35–37,40). Fifty-four percent of a general population surveyed have experienced neck pain within a 6 month period (41,42).

Neck pain is a chronic, episodic condition characterized by persistent, recurrent, or fluctuating pain and disability (35). Only about one third of patients with neck pain experience complete resolution (35). About one half of patients with an acute episode have persistent neck pain at 12 months (39). After whiplash injury, neck pain along with headache persists for up to 2 years in 29% to 90% of patients (depending on the study) and neck pain alone can persist at 10 years in 74% of patients (43). Drivers who have sustained a whiplash injury have a nearly three-fold risk of neck or shoulder pain 7 years after the collision (44). Even 17 years after a MVA, 55% still experience neck pain (11).

Neck pain is one of the most common complaints of patients seen by primary care practitioners worldwide (45). Mechanical neck disorder is the most common cause of neck pain (20). Second only to low back pain, neck pain is one of the most common reasons for which patients seek manual medical treatment. Neck pain is the most frequently reported symptom in connection with whiplash injury (43). Neck pain can result from 66% to 82% of rear end collisions and 56% of side impact collisions (43). Seventy percent of patients with neck pain after rear-end traffic collisions are female drivers (15). For female drivers involved in collisions, neck pain likelihood increases as head restraint height decreases below the head's center of gravity (15). Reported neck pain decreases for older female drivers, drivers in less severe crashes, and female drivers in heavier cars (15).

Neck pain accounts for substantial medical consumption, absenteeism from work, and disability (46). Medical disability can be temporary, but in about 10% of patients, permanent medical disability occurs. Permanent medical disability occurs in about 10% of patients involved in rear-end motor vehicle collisions (43). Although 79% may return to work within 1 month, 6% are unable to return to work at 1 year (43). A higher severity of pain at onset and a history of previous attacks seem to be associated with a worse prognosis; however, localization (radiation to the arms/neurologic signs) and radiographic findings (degenerative changes in the discs and joints) are not associated with a worse prognosis (47). Work-related risk factors for neck pain are listed in Box 66.2. (Compare with non–work-related risk factors in Box 66.3 and risk factors for radicular neck pain in Box 66.4.)

Based on data obtained from the Work Loss Data Institute's report on "Disorders of the neck and upper back," the 2008 edition of the National Guidelines Clearinghouse (http://www.ngc.gov/summary/summary.aspx?doc_id=12675&nbr=006563&string=neck+AND+pain) recommends up to 4 weeks of manual therapy, which includes OMT by osteopathic physicians, for workers with job-related acute neck pain not due to damaged tissue injury, that is, neck muscle strain, or whiplash as a mechanism of injury, with no radicular signs or symptoms (48). Initial management recommendations are for muscle relaxants for spasm for the first couple of days up to 1 week, with manual therapy beginning after day 3 at the earliest. After 2 weeks of manual therapy, the guideline

---

Work-Related Risk Factors for Neck Pain Include

- Hand-arm vibration (58)
- High and low skill (59)
- High quantitative job demands (59)
- Low job control (59)
- Low job satisfaction (59)
- Low social (coworker) support (59)
- Neck flexion (>20 degrees) (59)
- Sitting at work >95% of the time (59)
- Sustained arm postures (58)
- Twisting or bending of the trunk (58)
- Use of arm force (58)
- Workplace design not conducive to efficient cervical motion and function (58)

Non–Work-Related Risk Factors for Neck Pain Include

- Cycling (39)
- Poor ergonomics with driving (60)
- Female (39,60)
- History of motor vehicle collision (61)
- Older age (39)
- Previous low back pain (39)
- Previous neck injury (39,62)
- Psychological distress (39,55)
- Static postures (children) (63)
- Unemployed (39)
- Very slow or very rapid arm motion speed (64)

Characteristics of Patients with Radicular Neck Pain Include

- Dental-facial problems (65)
- Duration of work with a hand above shoulder level (66)
- Female (66)
- Mental stress (66)
- Middle age (66)
- Other musculoskeletal problems (66)
- Overweight (66)
- Smoking (66,67)

---

recommends switching from passive to active manual modalities. In the case of OMT, this would mean using more of the muscle energy–type procedures in which the patient is actively involved in the treatment. Contraindications and cautions regarding use of OMT for patients with acute neck pain are listed in Box 66.5.

Osteopathic primary care physicians are likely to see many patients with neck pain caused by somatic dysfunction and amenable to OMT. Neck pain from strain or sprain of the paraspinal soft tissues accounts for the greatest number of primary care visits to an outpatient clinic or ER of all musculoskeletal non–skin laceration soft tissue injuries (68). Neck somatic dysfunction was the most commonly reported somatic dysfunction in patients seen by 10 osteopathic practitioners board certified in neuromusculoskeletal medicine and osteopathic manipulative medicine over a 6-month period (69). Somatic dysfunction in the upper back, low back, and

Contraindications and Cautions Regarding OMT for Somatic Dysfunction in Patients with Acute Neck Pain

Care must be taken in the patient with an unstable cervical spine. Contraindications to HVLA OMT to the cervical spine include the following:

- A history of acute trauma before an assessment for any damage to the anatomy of the region and diagnosis of the origin of the pain
- Acute cervical herniated nucleus pulposus
- Acute cervical vertebra fracture or dislocation
- Carotid or vertebral artery dissection
- Ligamentous laxity
- Metabolic or neoplastic bone disease
- Patient refusal
- Primary muscle or joint disease in the cervical spine

shoulder can also predispose a person to develop cervical somatic dysfunction and pain. Thoracic somatic dysfunction is a significant predictor of neck-shoulder pain and hand weakness symptoms (30,70–72). This further supports the osteopathic approach to the patient with acute neck pain, which includes assessment and treatment of not only the cervical spine but also the entire musculoskeletal system as an integrated dynamic functional unit.

The human body functions as a unit and typically will respond to trauma, injury, or disease as a unit. This includes the psychological, behavioral, and social response that a person may have to pain and somatic dysfunction. Uncontrolled pain can lead to decreased functional capacity, which then increases the psychological burden of the patient and can lead to increased anxiety, stress, and depression. The increased psychological burden can impair the body's ability to heal and can further exacerbate the pain experienced by the patient. Therefore, it becomes vital for the osteopathic physician to evaluate the patient for comorbidities and mitigating factors that may impede a healthy recovery for the patient. Certainly, anxiety plays a role in this patient's neck pain, but she has no history of chronic anxiety or other psychiatric condition; her nightmares are related to her anxiety and probably disrupting her sleep patterns, which, along with the muscle spasms, increases her fatigue. She is not an active sports type person and has a sedentary lifestyle, so her muscles likely lack good tone. Her posture is normally not efficient and does not lend itself to compensation or adaptation to injuries such as she sustained recently.

Better psychological health and greater social support predicted a better outcome in primary care and general population samples with initial neck pain, whereas passive coping predicted a worse outcome (73). Economically, manual therapy (i.e., spinal mobilization) has been more effective and less costly for treating mechanical neck pain than physiotherapy modalities or care by a general practitioner who doesn't use manipulation (74).

For patients with neck pain, the osteopathic approach of treating the whole patient and not just the symptoms will help maximize the patient's restorative health potential. Applying the behavioral perspective to this patient, treat her anxiety, work with her to improve her sleep habits, dietary choices and habits, encourage nonsedentary lifestyle, improve posture and exercise habits, and encourage her to stop repetitive work behaviors that aggravate her condition. In patients who are athletes, help them to modify sports or other activities. If there is alcohol, tobacco and/or drug abuse as part of the clinical picture, encourage and help the patient to eliminate these addictions and abuses as part of the management plan.

Specialist Referral

The patient would be referred to the physician spine or pain management specialist for further evaluation and management if her neck pain did not improve or progressively worsened in spite of appropriate conservative treatments. If there is progressive or persistent loss of motor or sensory function, or altered sensorium or brain function, certainly neurological and surgical referrals are indicated. However, it is less clear if there is only limb parasthesias or radicular pain, which may be indicative of cervical nerve root compression. Nevertheless, it is helpful to utilize screening protocols, such as the Canadian C-spine rules, for patients with a low risk of cervical spine fracture and CT imaging for high risk patients with blunt trauma to the neck (75). In conjunction with the history and physical examination, electromyography (EMG) is relatively sensitive and specific for diagnosing cervical nerve root compression. Often, a neurologist or physiatrist is called upon to utilize the EMG to distinguish neck pain that is radicular versus nonradicular in nature. This distinction, along with an assessment for somatic dysfunction and relevant imaging studies, aids in more clearly identifying the cause of a patient's neck pain and instituting the appropriate treatment.

In general, it appears that the physical examination is more predictive of "ruling out" than "ruling in" a structural lesion, especially when assessing for neurological compression or significant pathology, such as cervical spine instability (75). Although MRI imaging is helpful in identifying cervical degenerative changes, these changes are common in asymptomatic subjects and research has failed to demonstrate a correlation between degenerative changes and neck pain symptoms. Similarly, there is no strong evidence supporting the validity of cervical discography or facet joint injections in diagnosing disc or facet pain, respectively, as the primary cause of neck pain (75). Evidence supports the use of provocative maneuvers, such as Spurling's test or contralateral rotation of the head with arm extension, when evaluating for cervical radiculopathy (76,77). Other physical examination components that should be incorporated include motor strength and sensory testing and cervical spine range-of-motion evaluation. There is some evidence suggesting that patients with chronic neck pain secondary to WAD have decreased cervical spine range of motion when compared to control subjects (78).

After completing the clinical and diagnostic evaluation and excluding significant pathology, including cervical spine instability or an infectious, neoplastic, or inflammatory process, the physician spine or pain management specialist utilizes a variety of modalities to treat neck pain, including medication, physical therapy, interventional procedures, manual medicine, and referral for surgical consultation. If a patient's neck pain is nonradicular and mechanical in nature, a multitherapeutic approach that incorporates medication, exercise therapy, and manual medicine is a reasonable approach. There is some evidence supporting exercise therapy, either alone or in combination with spinal manipulation, as being positively associated with short-term (6 to 13 weeks) reduction in chronic or recurrent neck pain when compared to spinal manipulation alone or usual care (17). Using one's skills as an osteopathic physician is sensible since the evidence supports the use of manual medicine in the treatment of neck pain. Cervical spine manipulation is more effective in reducing neck pain than muscle relaxants or usual care and at least provides short-term benefits for patients with acute neck pain. Furthermore, it appears that the benefits of manual medicine are enhanced when combined with exercise therapy and ergonomic adjustments (2). There is no evidence supporting the use of epidural or intra-articular corticosteroid injections in the treatment of nonradicular neck pain (79). In contrast, patients with neck pain secondary to nerve root compression do have short-term improvement of cervical radicular symptoms with epidural or selective nerve root corticosteroid injections (79). This, however, has not been shown to decrease the overall rate of surgery in patients with significant cervical radiculopathy (79). The long-term outcomes of treating cervical radiculopathy surgically when compared to nonoperative treatment have not been studied. Regardless, both anterior cervical discectomy with fusion and cervical disc arthroplasty seem to offer rapid and substantial relief of pain and impairment in patients with true cervical radiculopathy (79). As with the clinical evaluation, it is imperative to make the distinction between radicular and nonradicular neck pain when implementing treatment. In doing so, the physician specialist improves the likelihood of successfully treating a patient's neck pain, whether that entails treating radicular pain with injections or mechanical pain with a multimodal approach, including of medication, exercise and physical therapy, and manual medicine.

SUMMARY

In summary, the osteopathic approach to the patient with acute neck pain begins with a thorough history and physical examination, including an osteopathic structural examination of the musculoskeletal system. The differential diagnosis considers potential etiologies from local pathology, somatic dysfunction in the cervical as well as other body regions, systemic pathophysiology with cervical manifestations, and referred pain from organs in the vicinity of the cervical region, that is, lungs and heart. Associated comorbidities are also assessed and treated as appropriate. One of the most common causes of neck pain is a history of whiplash-type injury. However, though this type of injury affects the cervical spine, its effects are not limited to the cervical region. Understanding the total body response to a traumatic event such as a motor vehicle collision helps to elucidate the application of osteopathic principles in practice. Osteopathic treatment utilizes a health-oriented, patient-centered approach, focusing on improving structure-function interrelationships. This entails applying OMT to alleviate somatic dysfunction and maximize biomechanical, neurological, metabolic, respiratory/circulatory, and behavioral functions. Patient education, individualized exercise prescription, and close follow-up are important components of the management plan. Referral to a spine or pain specialist is indicated if the patient's pain and/or dysfunction does not improve or progressively worsens with conservative measures.

REFERENCES

1. Greenbaum J, Walters N, Levy PD. An evidenced-based approach to radiographic assessment of cervical spine injuries in the emergency department. *J Emerg Med* 2009;(1):64–71. Epub 2008 Sep 10.
2. Seffinger MA, Hruby RJ. Mechanical neck and upper back pain. In: *Evidence-based Manual Medicine: a Problem Oriented Approach.* Philadelphia, PA: Saunders/Elsevier, 2007.
3. Holm LW, Carroll LJ, Cassidy JD. The burden and determinants of neck pain in whiplash-associated disorders after traffic collisions. Results of the bone and joint decade 2000–2010 task force on neck pain and its associated disorders. *Spine* 33(4S):S39–S51.
4. Spitzer WO, Skovron ML, Salmi LR, et al. Scientific monograph of the Quebec Task Force on whiplash-associated disorders: redefining "whiplash" and its management. *Spine* 1995;20:1S–73S.
5. Becker RE. Whiplash injuries. *Academy of Applied Osteopathy Yearbook.* Indianapolis: American Academy of Osteopathy, 1958:65–69; 1961:90–98.
6. Heilig D. Whiplash mechanics of injury: management of cervical and dorsal involvement. *J Am Osteopath Assoc* 1963;63:113–120.
7. Magoun HI. Whiplash injury: a greater lesion complex. *J Am Osteopath Assoc* 1964;63:524–535.
8. Harakal JH. An osteopathically-integrated approach to the whiplash complex. *J Am Osteopath Assoc* 1975;74:941–956.
9. Cisler TA. Whiplash as a total-body injury. *J Am Osteopath Assoc* 1994;94(2):145–148.
10. Nadler S, Cooke P. Myofascial pain in whiplash injuries: diagnosis and treatment. *Spine St Art Rev* 1998;12(2):357–376.
11. Bunkertorp L, Nordholm L, Carlsson J. A descriptive analysis of disorders in patients 17 years following motor vehicle accidents. *Eur Spine J* 2002;11:227–234.
12. Ferrari R, Russell AS, Carroll LJ, et al. A re-examination of the whiplash associated disorders (WAD) as a systemic illness. *Ann Rheum Dis* 2005;64(9):1337–1342; [Epub 2005 Feb 24].
13. Panjabi MM, Pearson AM, Ito S, et al. Cervical spine curvature during simulated whiplash. *Clin Biomech* 2004;19:1–9.
14. Kumar S, Ferrari R, Narayan Y. Kinematic and electromyographic response to whiplash loading in low-velocity whiplash impacts—a review. *Clin Biomech (Bristol, Avon)* 2005;20(4):343–56; [Epub 2005 Jan 12].
15. Chapline JF, Ferguson SA, Lillis RP, et al. Neck pain and head restraint position relative to the driver's head in rear-end collisions. *Accid Anal Prev* 2000;32(2):287–97.
16. Gross A, Miller J, D'Sylva J, et al. Manipulation or mobilisation for neck pain. *Cochrane Database Syst Rev* 2010;(1):CD004249.
17. Hurwitz EL, Carragee EJ, van der Velde G. Treatment of neck pain: noninvasive interventions. Results of the Bone and Joint Decade 2000–2010 Task Force on Neck Pain and its Associated Disorders. *Spine* 2008;33(4S):S123–S152.
18. Fraix M. Osteopathic manual medicine for vertigo: review of the literature, case report and future research. *AAO J* 2009;19(2):25–29.
19. Batchelor K, Gamber R. Migraine and OMT. *AAO J* 2008;18(1):30–33.
20. Narayan P, Haid RW. Treatment of degenerative cervical disc disease. *Neurol Clin* 2001;19(1):217–229.
21. Lord SM, Barnsley L, Wallis BJ, et al. Chronic cervical zygapophysial joint pain after whiplash: a placebo-controlled prevalence study. *Spine* 1996;21(15):1737–1745.
22. Speldewinde GC, Bashford GM, Davidson IR. Diagnostic cervical zygapophyseal joint blocks for chronic cervical pain. *Med J Aust* 2001;174(4):174–176.
23. Friedman MH, Nelson AJ Jr. Head and neck pain review: traditional and new perspectives. *J Orthop Sports Phys Ther* 1996;24(4):268–278.
24. Ettlin T, Schuster C, Stoffel R, et al. A distinct pattern of myofascial findings in patients after whiplash injury. *Arch Phys Med Rehabil* 2008;89(7):1290–3. Epub 2008 Jun 13.
25. Seffinger MA, Najm WI, Mishra SI, et al. Reliability of spinal palpation for diagnosis of neck or back pain: a systematic review of the literature. *Spine* 2004;29(19):413–425.
26. McReynolds TM, Sheridan BJ. Intramuscular ketorolac versus osteopathic manipulative treatment in the management of acute neck pain in the emergency department: a randomized clinical trial. *J Am Osteopath Assoc* 2005;105(2):57–68.
27. Groen G, Balget B, Drukker J. Nerve and nerve plexuses of the human vertebral column. *Am J Anat* 1990;188:282–296.
28. Haavik-Taylor H, Murphy B. Cervical spine manipulation alters sensorimotor integration: a somatosensory evoked potential study. *Clin Neurophysiol* 2007;118:391–402.
29. Burns DK, Wells MR. Gross range of motion in the cervical spine: the effects of osteopathic muscle energy technique in asymptomatic subjects. *J Am Osteopath Assoc* 2006;106(3):137–42.
30. Cleland JA, Childs JD, McRae M, et al. Immediate effects of thoracic manipulation in patients with neck pain: a randomized controlled trial. *Man Ther* 2005;10:127–135.
31. Burns L. *Pathogenesis of Visceral Disease Following Vertebral Lesions.* Chicago: The American Osteopathic Association, 1948.
32. Kelso AF, Johnston WL. The status of a C6-T2-T6 (CT) pattern of segmental somatic dysfunction in research subjects after 3–7 years. *J Am Osteopath Assoc* 1989;89(10):1356.
33. Burns L and Treat CL. Incidence of certain etiologic factors in cardiac disorders. *J Am Osteopath Assoc* 1953;52:369–372.

34. Howell JN, Willard F. Nociception: new understandings and their possible relation to somatic dysfunction and its treatment. *Ohio Res Clin Rev* 2005;15.

35. Côté P, Cassidy JD, Carroll LJ, et al. The annual incidence and course of neck pain in the general population: a population-based cohort study. *Pain* 2004;112(3):267–273.

36. Hartvigsen J, Christensen K, Frederiksen H. Back and neck pain exhibit many common features in old age: a population-based study of 4,486 Danish twins 70–102 years of age. *Spine* 2004;29(5):576–580.

37. Walker-Bone K, Reading I, Coggon D, et al. The anatomical pattern and determinants of pain in the neck and upper limbs: an epidemiologic study. *Pain* 2004;109(1–2):45–51.

38. Ståhl M, Mikkelsson M, Kautiainen H, et al. Neck pain in adolescence: a 4-year follow-up of pain-free preadolescents. *Pain* 2004;110(1–2):427–431.

39. Hill J, Lewis M, Papageorgiou AC, et al. Predicting persistent neck pain: a 1-year follow-up of a population cohort. *Spine* 2004;29(15):1648–1654.

40. Vogt MT, Simonsick EM, Harris TB, et al. Neck and shoulder pain in 70- to 79-year-old men and women: findings from the Health, Aging and Body Composition Study. *Spine J* 2003;3(6):435–441.

41. Côté P, Cassidy JD, Carroll L. Is a lifetime history of neck injury in a traffic collision associated with prevalent neck pain, headache and depressive symptomatology? *Accid Anal Prev* 2000;32(2):151–159.

42. Côté P, Cassidy JD, Carroll L. The factors associated with neck pain and its related disability in the Saskatchewan population. *Spine* 2000;25(9):1109–1117.

43. Bilkey WJ. Manual medicine approach to the cervical spine and whiplash injury. *Phys Med Rehabil Clin N Am* 1996;7(4):749–759.

44. Berglund A, Alfredsson L, Cassidy JD, et al. The association between exposure to a rear-end collision and future neck or shoulder pain: a cohort study. *J Clin Epidemiol* 2000;53(11):1089–1094.

45. Bot SD, van der Waal JM, Terwee CB, et al. Incidence and prevalence of complaints of the neck and upper extremity in general practice. *Ann Rheum Dis* 2005;64(1):118–123.

46. Borghouts JA, Koes BW, Vondeling H, et al. Cost-of-illness of neck pain in The Netherlands in 1996. *Pain* 1999;80(3):629–636.

47. Borghouts JA, Koes BW, Bouter LM. The clinical course and prognostic factors of non-specific neck pain: a systematic review. *Pain* 1998;77(1):1–13.

48. Work Loss Data Institute. *Disorders of the Neck and Upper Back.* National Guidelines Clearinghouse, 2008. Available at: http://www.ngc.gov/summary/summary.aspx?doc_id=12675&nbr=006563&string=neck+AND+pain; accessed February 15, 2010.

49. Bleasdale-Barr KM, Mathias CJ. Neck and other muscle pains in autonomic failure: their association with orthostatic hypotension. *J R Soc Med* 1998;91(7):355–359.

50. Hoving JL, Koes BW, De Vet HC, et al. Manual therapy, physical therapy or continued care by the general practitioner for patients with neck pain: short-term results from a pragmatic randomized trial. *Ann Intern Med* 2002;136:713–722.

51. Zapletal J, Hekster RE, Straver JS, et al. Relationship between atlanto-odontoid osteoarthritis and idiopathic suboccipital neck pain. *Neuroradiology* 1996;38(1):62–65.

52. Andersen JH, Kaergaard A, Mikkelsen S, et al. Risk factors in the onset of neck/shoulder pain in a prospective study of workers in industrial and service companies. *Occup Environ Med* 2003;60:649–654.

53. Borg K, Hensing G, Alexanderson K. Risk factors for disability pension over 11 years in a cohort of young persons initially sick-listed with low back, neck, or shoulder diagnoses. *Scand J Public Health* 2004;32(4):272–278.

54. Grooten WJ, Wiktorin C, Norrman L, et al. Seeking care for neck/shoulder pain: a prospective study of work-related risk factors in a healthy population. *J Occup Environ Med* 2004;46(2):138–146.

55. Siivola SM, Levoska S, Latvala K, et al. Predictive factors for neck and shoulder pain: a longitudinal study in young adults. *Spine* 2004;29(15):1662–1669.

56. Ciancaglini R, Testa M, Radaelli G. Association of neck pain with symptoms of temporomandibular dysfunction in the general adult population. *Scand J Rehabil Med* 1999;31(1):17–22.

57. Larsson R, Oberg PA, Larsson SE. Changes of trapezius muscle blood flow and electromyography in chronic neck pain due to trapezius myalgia. *Pain* 1999;79(1):45–50.

58. Ariëns GA, van Mechelen W, Bongers PM, et al. Physical risk factors for neck pain. *Scand J Work Environ Health* 2000;26(1):7–19.

59. Ariëns GA, Bongers PM, Douwes M, et al. Are neck flexion, neck rotation, and sitting at work risk factors for neck pain? Results of a prospective cohort study. *Occup Environ Med* 2001;58(3):200–207.

60. Krause N, Ragland DR, Greiner BA, et al. Physical workload and ergonomic factors associated with prevalence of back and neck pain in urban transit operators. *Spine* 1997;22(18):2117–2127.

61. Bunketorp L, Stener-Victorin E, Carlsson J. Neck pain and disability following motor vehicle accidents-a cohort study. *Eur Spine J* 2005;14(1):84–89.

62. Guez M, Hildingsson C, Stegmayr B, et al. Chronic neck pain of traumatic and non-traumatic origin: a population-based study. *Acta Orthop Scand* 2003;74(5):576–579.

63. Murphy S. Buckle P, Stubbs D. Classroom posture and self-reported back and neck pain in schoolchildren. *Appl Ergon* 2004;35(2):113–120.

64. Lauren H, Luoto S, Alaranta H, et al. Arm motion speed and risk of neck pain: a preliminary communication. *Spine* 1997;22(18):2094–2099.

65. Friedman MH, Nelson AJ Jr. Head and neck pain review: traditional and new perspectives. *J Orthop Sports Phys Ther* 1996;24(4):268–278.

66. Viikari-Juntura E, Martikainen R, Luukkonen R, et al. Longitudinal study on work related and individual risk factors affecting radiating neck pain. *Occup Environ Med* 2001;58(5):345–352.

67. Hogg-Johnson S, van der Velde G, Carroll LJ et al. The burden and determinants of neck pain in the general population. Results of the Bone and Joint Decade 2000–2010 Task Force on Neck Pain and its Associated Disorders. *Spine* 2008;33(4S):S39–S51.

68. United States National Health Survey, 1999–2000, reported Sept. 2004; Ambulatory Care Visits to Practitioner Offices, Hospital Outpatient Departments, and Emergency Departments.

69. Sleszynski SL, Glonek T. Outpatient osteopathic SOAP note form: preliminary results in osteopathic outcomes-based research. *J Am Osteopath Assoc* 2005;105(4):181–205.

70. Norlander S, Gustavsson BA, Lindell J, et al. Reduced mobility in the cervico-thoracic motion segment—a risk factor for musculoskeletal neck-shoulder pain: a two-year prospective follow-up study. *Scand J Rehabil Med* 1997;29(3):167–174.

71. Norlander S, Aste-Norlander U, Nordgren B, et al. Mobility in the cervico-thoracic motion segment: an indicative factor of musculo-skeletal neck-shoulder pain. *Scand J Rehabil Med* 1996;28(4):183–192.

72. Norlander S, Nordgren B. Clinical symptoms related to musculoskeletal neck-shoulder pain and mobility in the cervico-thoracic spine. *Scand J Rehabil Med* 1998;30(4):243–251.

73. Caroll LJ, Hogg-Johnson S, van der Velde G. Course and prognostic factors for neck pain in the general population: Results of the Bone and Joint Decade 2000–2010 Task Force on Neck Pain and its Associated Disorders. *Spine* 2008;33(45):S75–S82.

74. Korthalis-de Bos IBC, Hoving J, van Tulder MW, et al. Cost effectiveness of physiotherapy, manual therapy and general practitioner care for neck pain: economic evaluation alongside a randomized controlled trial. *BMJ* 2003;326:911–914.

75. Nordin M, Carragee EJ, Hogg-Johnson S, et al. Assessment of neck pain and its associated disorders. Results of the Bone and Joint Decade 2000–2010 Task Force on Neck Pain and Its Associated Disorders. *Spine* 2008;33(suppl):S101–S122.

76. Rubinstein S, Pool JJ, van Tulder M, et al. A systematic review of the diagnostic accuracy of provocative tests of the neck for diagnosing cervical radiculopathy. *Eur Spine J* 2007;16:307–319.

77. Wainner RS, Fritz JM, Irrgang JJ, et al. Reliability and diagnostic accuracy of the clinical examination and patient self-report measures for cervical radiculopathy. *Spine* 2003;28:52–62.

78. Puglisi F, Ridi R, Cecchi F, et al. Segmental vertebral motion in the assessment of neck range of motion in whiplash patients. *Int J Legal Med* 2004;118:235–239.

79. Carragee EJ, Hurwitz EL, Cheng I, et al. Treatment of neck pain: injections and surgical interventions. Results of the Bone and Joint Decade 2000–2010 Task Force on Neck Pain and its Associated Disorders. *Spine* 2008;33(suppl):S153–S169.

67

Rhinosinusitis

MICHAEL B. SHAW AND HARRIET H. SHAW

KEY CONCEPTS

- Inflammation of the nasal and paranasal mucosa may be caused by bacterial or viral infection; fungal or allergic conditions. The most common bacterial pathogens involved in acute sinusitis in adults are *Streptococcus pneumoniae*, *Haemophilus Influenzae*, and *Moraxella catarrhalis*.
- Obstruction of the sinus drainage pathways and decreased mucociliary transport lead to stagnation of mucus in the sinuses, predisposing to sinusitis. Swelling and inflammation are common causes of obstruction.
- Osteopathic manipulative treatment, as a means to improve venous and lymphatic circulation, can play a major role in the treatment of sinusitis. Improving venous and lymphatic circulation from the head and neck to decrease the congestion and inflammation of the nasal mucosa would be expected to facilitate the sinus drainage pathways.
- Unopposed sympathetic stimulation leads to vasoconstriction and drying of the nasal mucosa. Sympathetic preganglionic fibers to the sinuses arise from T1-4 cord level, synapsing in the superior cervical ganglion (C2-3). Facilitation due to somatic dysfunction in the upper thoracic and cervical spine may, thereby, affect the health of the mucosa.
- Some over-the-counter antihistamines, often used for upper respiratory infections, can dry mucus and decrease ciliary effectiveness. Patients should be cautioned about their role in the development of acute sinusitis.
- Start nonantibiotic therapy initially for patients with low probability of bacterial infection.
- Consider antibiotic therapy in patients with high probability of bacterial sinusitis, severe symptoms, or when nonantibiotic therapy fails.

CASE VIGNETTE

CHIEF COMPLAINT

JP is a 42-year-old female accountant who presents to the family practice clinic complaining of headache, fever, and scratchy throat.

History of Present Illness

The last 4 days she has had a full feeling in her face, pressure behind her eyes, nasal congestion, sensitivity of her nose, pain in her upper teeth, and fatigue. At times, she is sensitive to light and sounds and has decreased sense of smell. A week earlier, she had a "cold" for which she took an over-the-counter "cold and sinus" preparation. She has a history of similar symptoms 2 to 3 years ago, treated with antibiotics with a prolonged recovery.

Current Medications

Over-the-counter cold and sinus preparation, but no other medications

Allergy

None known to medication, inhalants, or foods

Past Medical History

Patient was hospitalized for uncomplicated vaginal delivery at age 29. She had a tonsillectomy at age 5, for which she was not hospitalized. She has had no other surgery. Her most recent mammogram was 18 months ago and reported normal.

Environmental and Social History

She smokes ½ pack cigarettes per day and has an occasional glass of wine. She is married with one child. Two dogs also live in the house. She works part-time as dental hygienist.

Family History

Both parents are living. Father has hypertension. Mother is healthy. One female and one male sibling are both healthy. No family history of diabetes, asthma, stroke, or heart disease (other than father's hypertension).

REVIEW OF SYSTEMS

Eyes:
No visual disturbance noted, but in the spring has watery, itchy eyes.

ENT:
As noted in chief complaint.

Cardiovascular:
Denies chest pain, syncope, shortness of breath, and extremity edema.

Respiratory:
Has occasional morning cough, gets "colds" several times a year, denies difficulty breathing.

Gastrointestinal:
Denies nausea, vomiting, food intolerance, diarrhea, constipation, or changes in bowel habits.

Genitourinary:
P1G1, denies hematuria, frequency, urgency, pelvic pain.

Musculoskeletal:
Complains of frequent neck and upper back stiffness and aching, denies weakness, muscle cramping, or other areas of back pain.

Neurological:

Denies vertigo, unsteadiness, numbness, or tingling or radiating pain.

Psychiatric:

Denies signs of depression, reports normal sleep, denies hallucinations or alterations in consciousness.

Endocrine:

Denies intolerance to heat and cold, rashes or changes in skin and hair.

Hematologic/Lymphatic:

Denies swelling and abnormal bruising.

VITAL SIGNS

Temperature: 101.6°F; pulse: 90; respirations: 14/min; BP: 134/80; height: 5'6" weight: 140 lb

PHYSICAL EXAM

General:

Patient appears stated age and in no acute distress, but fatigued.

Skin:

Skin color is normal.

Eyes:

Conjunctiva appears clear. Pupils are equal and reactive to light and fundoscopic evaluation is normal.

ENT:

Examination reveals erythema and generalized congestion of the nasal mucosa. Pustular drainage is noted and there is a mild to moderate septal deviation caudally to the left. Posterior pharynx is inflamed with pustular drainage evident. Tympanic membranes are dull with questionable cone of light, but have adequate response to insufflation. Thyroid is not enlarged.

Musculoskeletal/Structural:

Tenderness is palpated in the upper cervical area, upper thoracic area, and in the right supraclavicular area. Motion changes are noted at T2, upper right ribs and C2, consistent with T2 FSR_L, rib 1 inhalation somatic dysfunction, and C2 FSR_R. Tenderness associated with slight nodularity is palpated anteriorly in the first intercostal space on the right and posteriorly between the spinous and the transverse process of C2 on the right. The suboccipital tissues are hypertonic and tender. There is decreased amplitude of the cranial rhythmic impulse, but the rate is normal. Tenderness is noted over the bridge of the nose and over the maxillae and zygomae. Percussion over the maxilla intensifies the tenderness.

Hematological:

There is no lymphadenopathy is palpated in the cervical or supraclavicular areas.

Respiratory:

Lungs are clear to auscultation.

Cardiovascular:

Heart has regular rhythm with rate of 90 bpm. There are no murmurs and no extremity edema is noted. Nail beds and digits appear normal.

Abdomen:

Bowel sounds are ausculted in all four quadrants. Abdomen is soft and nontender. No organomegaly is noted.

Neurological:

Patient is oriented in time and place and responds appropriately to questions. Cranial nerves II to XII are intact. Deep tendon reflexes of upper and lower extremities are equal and moderate bilaterally. Sensation is intact.

ANATOMICAL CONSIDERATIONS

Nose and Paranasal Sinuses Airflow

The nose, being an organ of respiration and olfaction, functions to filter, humidify, and regulate the temperature of inspired air. The superior, middle, and inferior turbinates or conchae are elevations on the lateral nasal walls. Heavily endowed with blood vessels, they help in the temperature control of the inspired air. The nose also serves as a filter for particulate matter in the air. Much of the smoke, dust, pollens, bacteria, and viruses are trapped and removed before the air enters the lungs. The nasal septum and the turbinates create an air flow pattern in the nose that maximizes the air-conditioning function of the nose and paranasal sinuses. The paranasal sinuses in the maxillary, frontal, sphenoid, and ethmoid bones are air-filled cells and extensions of the nasal cavities. They serve similar functions to that of the nose. Regardless of the temperature of outside air, the temperature of inspired air is changed to approximate body temperature during its passage through the nose and sinuses. Similar changes are made in moisture content of inspired air so that it reaches the trachea at almost ambient humidity.

MUCOCILIARY TRANSPORT IN THE UPPER RESPIRATORY SYSTEM

The nasal cavity and paranasal sinuses are covered by pseudostratified, columnar, ciliated epithelium, as is the rest of the respiratory system, including the middle ear and auditory tube. Goblet cells and submucosal glands contribute a mucus blanket that covers and protects the epithelium. This mucus film has two layers. The cilia beat within the inner, serous (sol phase) layer. The outer, more viscous (gel phase) layer is moved by the synchronized ciliary action. (Fig. 67.1). The process is called mucociliary transport (or mucociliary clearance).

Secretions from the paranasal sinuses pass into the nasal cavity through the various ostia or openings in the sinuses. There are two basic drainage patterns for the sinuses. The anterior ethmoid, frontal and maxillary sinuses are part of the anterior pattern draining to the ostiomeatal unit under the middle turbinate. The posterior ethmoid and sphenoid sinuses are in the posterior pattern draining to the sphenoethmoid recess (Fig. 67.2). To appreciate the importance of efficient mucociliary transport, note that the ostiomeatal unit is located superior to much of the maxillary sinus, making it necessary to actively move the mucous blanket "uphill" for effective drainage. This nondependent drainage situation exists with the sphenoid and in some instances with the ethmoid sinuses, as well. The outer layer of mucous traps particulate matter, moving it through the sinus ostia into the nasal cavity, where mucus is transported into the nasopharynx and swallowed. Mucociliary transport actively collects and concentrates particulate matter, moving it out of the sinuses. Pathogens may be incorporated into the cells of the mucosa or destroyed by lysozymes and secretory immunoglobulin A within the mucus.

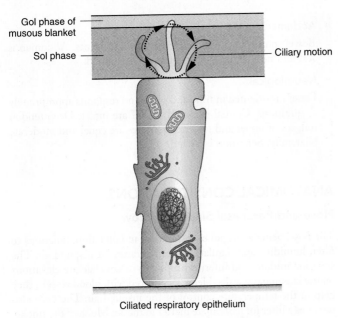

Figure 67-1 Ciliated respiratory epithelium.

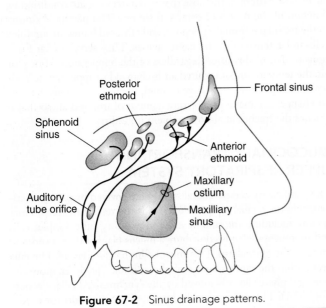

Figure 67-2 Sinus drainage patterns.

The viscosity of the mucus plays a role in the efficiency of the process. The architecture of the nose and the sinus ostia influence these mucus flow patterns. The way cilia are controlled and coordinated to power this process is only partly understood. Ciliary beat frequency may be influenced by primitive neurologic control, may be genetically determined, or may be an interactive phenomenon depending on the physical nature of the particulates. It is known that healthy functioning of this upper respiratory system depends on unimpaired nasal airflow and optimal mucociliary transport. Factors that disturb these body mechanisms lead to disease processes.

NERVOUS SYSTEM RELEVANT TO NOSE AND PARANASAL SINUSES

The autonomic nervous system (ANS) plays a crucial role in the physiologic function of the nose and paranasal sinuses (Loehrl,

2005; Sarin et al., 2006). Proper balance of the sympathetic and parasympathetic systems, and appropriate response of the sensory nerves are necessary for optimal function. It follows that disease of the nose and paranasal sinuses results when these factors are dysfunctional and poorly balanced. The nervous system of the nose also interfaces with the immune system especially in the face of inflammation (Lacroix, 2003).

Parasympathetic supply to the nose originates from the superior salivary nucleus. Its preganglionic fibers form part of the superficial greater petrosal nerve, which joins the deep petrosal nerve, forming the nerve of the ptergyoid canal (vidian nerve). After passing through the ptergyoid canal, the fibers synapse in the sphenopalatine ganglion (Fig. 67.3). The sphenopalatine ganglion is suspended in the pterygopalatine fossa, bordered by the pterygoid process, maxilla, palatine bone, and floor of the sphenoid. The parasympathetic postganglionic nerves modulate their effect by integrating inhibitory and stimulatory channels. Postganglionic fibers are distributed to the nasal mucosa from the sphenopalatine ganglion along with the sensory and sympathetic fibers.

The action of the parasympathetic nervous system on the upper respiratory mucosa is stimulation of the glandular epithelium with production of mucous, rich in glycoproteins, lactoferrin, lysozmes, secretory leukoprotease inhibitor, neural endopeptidase, and secretory IgA. There is a parasympathetic effect of vasodilation, although of much less significance than the glandular effect (Sarin et al., 2006) Several neuropeptides, including vasoactive intestinal peptide, neuropeptide Y, nitric oxide (NO), enkephalin and somatostatin, are associated with the nasal parasympathetic system (Lacroix, 2003). Nitric oxide is thought to be an activator of ciliary beat frequency, but its role is variable and still poorly understood (Landis, 2003).

Sympathetic fibers to the head arise from the upper thoracic segments of the cord (T1-3). Preganglionic fibers ascend from there to the superior cervical ganglion, located in the upper cervical area, where they synapse. Postganglionic fibers from the superior cervical ganglion join the internal carotid plexus, becoming part of the deep petrosal nerve and the nerve of the ptergyoid canal (see Fig. 67.3). Sympathetic supply to the nose and paranasal sinuses passes (without synapsing) through the sphenopalatine ganglion in the pterygopalatine fossa. They continue with the parasympathetic fibers to the nose and sinuses.

The sympathetic nervous system acts in the nose to produce vasoconstriction and increased nasal airway patency. Norepinephrine is the primary neurotransmitter of the sympathetic system in the nose. Interaction and balance between these systems is complex, intricate, and only partially understood. It is quite clear, however, that the ANS plays a major role in regulating nasal airflow, and at least some role in mucociliary transport mechanisms (Sarin et al., 2006).

Afferent nerves, supplying the nose and derived from the olfactory nerve and ophthalmic and maxillary branches of cranial nerve V, provide protective reflexes. For example, exposing the nasal mucosa to mechanical irritation, allergens, or cold air elicits a response of sneezing, coughing, apnea, or avoidance behavior. This occurs through an axonal reflex. These afferent nerves also recruit systemic autonomic reflexes and mediate vascular, glandular, and inflammatory defenses. Stimulation of these afferent nerves also leads to the release of neuropeptides such as calcitonin gene–related peptide, gastrin-releasing peptide, substance P, and neurokinin A. Increase in these sensory neuropeptides along with reduction of their catabolism leads to the process of neurogenic inflammation (Lacroix, 2003). Symptoms resulting from nasal neurogenic inflammation are those common to rhinosinusitis—nasal

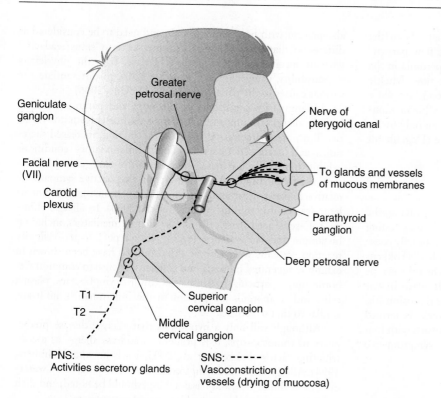

Figure 67-3 Autonomic nerve supply to upper respiratory tract.

obstruction, rhinorrhea, and headache. Interestingly, similar symptoms accompany migraine and may also implicate neuropeptides in the causal relationship (Bellamy et al., 2006).

LYMPHATIC SYSTEM RELEVANT TO THE HEAD AND NECK

The lymphatic system of the neck consists of numerous lymph nodes connected by lymphatic channels, eventually ending in the thoracic and right lymphatic ducts. The thoracic duct receives drainage from the left side of the head and neck, while the right lymphatic duct drains the right side. Each empties independently into the junction of the internal jugular and subclavian veins on their respective side of the body (Fig. 67.4). Significant individual variability exists in these drainage sites.

Cervical lymph nodes are generally divided into the following groups—submandibular, submental, superficial cervical, deep cervical, and paratracheal. The submandibular and submental nodes are intimately connected with the superficial fascia covering the digastric and mylohyoid muscles. The superficial cervical nodes lie along the external jugular vein and on the external surface of the sternocleidomastoid muscle. The paratracheal nodes are irregularly located, and, as do all the aforementioned groups of nodes, drain into the deep cervical lymph nodes. These prominent, deep nodes form a chain embedded in the connective tissue of the carotid sheath around the internal jugular vein (Fig. 67.5).

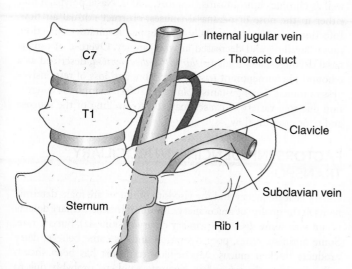

Figure 67-4 Skeletal structures in relationship to thoracic duct termination.

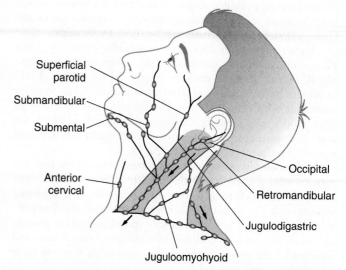

Figure 67-5 Superficial cervical lymph nodes. (From Moore, KL. *Clinically Oriented Anatomy.* 2nd Ed. Baltimore, MD: Williams & Wilkins, 1985; with permission.)

The intimate association of the lymphatic channels to the myofascial structures in the neck makes lymphatic flow particularly susceptible to changes in myofascial tone. Hypertonia in the cervical myofascial tissues can impede lymphatic flow. Muscle movement improves lymphatic circulation. Autonomic influence on lymphatic contractility suggests a role for osteopathic manipulative techniques to improve lymphatic circulation not only for its impact on muscle tone but also on autonomic tone (Degenhardt and Kuchera, 1996).

RHINOSINUSITIS

Acute rhinosinusitis is an inflammatory process involving the mucus membranes of the paranasal sinuses and nasal cavity lasting no longer than four weeks. Since rhinitis and sinusitis usually coexist, "rhinosinusitis" is the current preferred terminology (Fokkens et al., 2005). Chronic rhinosinusitis is diagnosed when the symptoms of sinusitis are present for 12 weeks or more. It differs in histopathology, prognosis, and management from acute rhinosinusitis. Rhinosinusitis lasting between four and twelve weeks is termed subacute. Some patients develop recurrent acute sinusitis with four or more acute episodes annually, interspersed with symptom-free intervals.

DIAGNOSIS

Patients who have had a recent upper respiratory infection and develop nasal obstruction, periorbital pain, and purulent rhinorrhea are suspect for acute rhinosinusitis. Other symptoms often present include olfactory disturbance, fever, maxillary toothache, fatigue, cough, and facial pressure made worse by bending over. The headache (or face pain) is usually described as pressure-like and dull. Engorgement of the nasal mucosa, which occurs during sleeping, causes sinus-related pain to be worse in the morning, improving after the patient is upright for a time.

Examination of the nose may reveal a deviated septum, inflamed nasal mucosa, and pus in the nasal cavity. Nasal polyps may be present especially if inflammation has been chronically present. The posterior oropharynx may demonstrate signs of postnasal drainage such as a lateral red streak, obvious drainage, or the cobblestone appearance of lymphoid hyperplasia. Although transillumination of the sinuses is a valuable diagnostic tool for some practitioners, it has been found to be unreliable for definitive diagnosis (Otten and Grote, 1989). Facial tenderness may be elicited with palpation.

Acute rhinosinusitis does not warrant radiographic diagnosis. Plain film radiographs, ultrasonography, computerized tomography (CT), and magnetic resonant imaging of the sinuses should be avoided in the diagnosis of acute rhinosinusitis and reserved for patients at risk for complications. Radiographs and CTs have high false-positive rates for acute rhinosinusitis, and radiography is not cost-effective compared to the use of clinical criteria with indicated treatment regimens (Fokkens et al., 2005).

Serious complications of acute bacterial sinusitis are rare, but patients who also present with ophthalmic or neurologic signs and symptoms need to be worked up in more depth and referred appropriately. Local extension of infection includes orbital or periorbital cellulitis and osteitis. Infectious spread beyond the paranasal sinuses may occur in the forms of meningitis, brain abscess, and infection of the venous sinuses. CT is appropriate if any of these complications are suspected.

Differentiating viral from bacterial rhinosinusitis is difficult except by way of sinus puncture, which is reserved for research use. Trigeminal neuralgia, migraine, dental abscess, and neoplasm may also present with head and face pain and need to be considered as differential diagnoses. Many patients use the term "sinus headache" without specific diagnosis of sinus disease. It is the physician's responsibility, using clinical diagnostic skills, to differentiate the various causes of the patient's headache (Levine, 2006).

Inflammatory conditions in the nose and paranasal sinuses include allergic rhinitis and nonallergic rhinitis (vasomotor rhinitis). Both are characterized by nasal obstruction, increased secretions, and decreased olfaction. These inflammatory conditions exhibit hyper-reactive nasal mucosa, with exaggerated neural response to all stimuli. ANS dysfunction (hypoactive sympathetic relative to parasympathetic tone) has been demonstrated in nonallergic/vasomotor rhinitis (Jaradeh et al., 2000). In allergic rhinitis, IgE-sensitized mast cells release allergic mediators, including histamine and leukotrienes, leading to a type I hypersensitivity reaction. Patients with chronic rhinosinusitis have been shown to exhibit exaggerated humoral and cellular response to common airborne fungi, particularly Alternaria. (Shin) Lymphocytes, plasma cells, and eosinophils are present in the inflammatory infiltrate, similar to that of asthma.

Although still only a hypothesis that allergic disease predisposes to rhinosinusitis, it is prudent to address allergy as a contributing factor (Fokkens et al., 2005; Karlsson and Holmberg, 1994). Allergic signs and symptoms, such as sneezing, itchy, watery eyes, clear rhinorrhea, and nasal itching, should be noted, and their treatment considered as part of integrated patient care.

When evaluating a patient with rhinosinusitis, attention needs to be paid to the factors that decrease airway patency and limit air flow, and those that decrease the effectiveness of mucociliary transport. Treatment can then be directed toward the specific factors influencing each patient's problem.

FACTORS INFLUENCING AIRWAY PATENCY

Anatomic structures can compromise airway patency. Typically seen are deviated nasal septum, turbinate hypertrophy, and collapsed nasal valve. Various types of neural dysfunction are associated with upper airway disorders. Recent evidence suggests that hypoactive sympathetic influence leads to increased nasal airway resistance (Loehrl, 2007). Vasodilatation, due to increased activity of sensory neuropeptides, occurs in patients with hyperactive nasal mucosa characteristic of allergic and nonallergic rhinitis, as well as chronic rhinosinusitis (Lacroix, 2003). Nasal polyps, found either in the nose or paranasal sinuses, obstruct normal air flow. Infectious processes, especially viral upper respiratory infection, causes swelling and decreased airway patency. Overuse of topical nasal decongestants leads to *rhinitis medicamentosa*, described as a rebound phenomenon of nasal congestion, and loss of responsiveness to topical decongestants (Lin et al., 2004). Lymphatic congestion due to a variety of causes may add to swelling of the mucosa and poor nasal air flow.

FACTORS INFLUENCING MUCOCILIARY TRANSPORT

Ciliary beat frequency and the viscosity of mucus are main determinants in the quality of mucociliary clearance. Intrinsic ciliary defects occur with some diseases (primary ciliary dyskinesia), but are rare. Some antihistamines, poor hydration and, as some believe, dairy products thicken mucus. Mucociliary transport has been shown to be significantly reduced in cigarette smokers, probably due to decreased number of cilia or changes in the mucus (Cole et al., 1986; Mahakit and Pumhirun, 1995). Inflammatory conditions of the nose, sinuses, and airways (allergic and nonallergic rhinitis, rhinosinusitis, and brochiectasis) are also associated with decreased mucociliary clearance (Schuhl, 1995; Stanley et al., 1985). Cystic fibrosis, a hereditary disease that produces thick, abundant respiratory secretions, is accompanied by significant slowing of nasal mucociliary transport (Armengot et al., 1997). Slowed transport has been noted with chronic infection and in diabetics.

INTEGRATED TREATMENT APPROACH

Figure 67.6 presents a treatment algorithm for rhinosinusitis. Most patients with acute bacterial rhinosinusitis improve without antibiotics. For patients having symptoms more than seven days and those with more severe symptoms, consider antibiotic therapy with a narrow spectrum agent (Fokkens et al., 2005; Hickner et al., 2001). For those patients who require antibiotics for rhinosinusitis, amoxicillin or trimethoprim/sulfamethoxazole are considered first-line antibiotics for the common pathogens—*Streptococcus pneumoniae* and *Haemophilus influenzae*. Alternatives such as doxycycline and azithromycin should only be used for patients allergic to both first-line drugs. Initial course of antibiotic treatment should be 10 to 14 days (except if using azithromycin). In the case of partial resolution, extend antibiotic therapy to a total of three weeks.

Patient education regarding the incidence of antibiotic-resistant infections is important, whether or not prescribing antibiotic therapy. Patient information is available online at www.cdc.gov/drugresistance/community.

Since many cases of acute rhinosinusitis are due to viral infections and do not require antibiotics, treatment that is symptomatic and encourages inherent healing mechanisms should be considered. Of the nonpharmacologic therapies, none have been thoroughly studied and their effectiveness is unknown. Considering the underlying pathophysiologic process can direct decision making about recommending these therapies.

Promoting mucociliary clearance is essential to the overall treatment of rhinosinusitis and prevention of complications. Patients may be instructed to drink warm, clear fluids in order to hydrate the mucous membranes, and refrain from drinking milk. Saline nasal irrigation may relieve symptoms and is a low-cost option. Decreasing nasal inflammation improves airway patency. Identification of allergic symptoms in the patient history suggests the need to address allergy treatment of some kind. Perennial allergy symptoms may warrant allergy testing and immunotherapy. Avoidance of allergens or irritants can be difficult, but patient education is essential and often needs to be ongoing. Smoking cessation and avoidance of second-hand smoke and other chemical irritants are

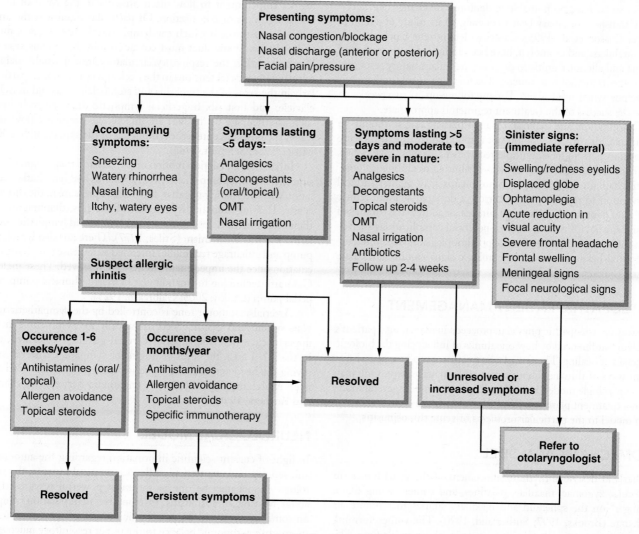

Figure 67-6 Sinusitis algorithm.

important for reducing inflammation and improving health of the mucus membranes. Osteopathic manipulative treatment (OMT) offers a nonpharmacologic approach to rhinosinusitis.

Many nonantibiotic pharmacologic agents are available and often used in the treatment of rhinosinusitis. Current knowledge indicating the role of sympathetic hypoactivity in nasal vasodilatation would suggest the use of sympathomimetics (phenylephrine) and alpha-receptor agonists (oxymetaazoline, naphazoline) as decongestants. Decongesting the nasal mucosa improves air flow and allows for better mucociliary transport and clearing of contaminants from the sinuses.

Nasal steroids, although more often used in chronic rhinosinusitis and in patients with polyps, are intended to decrease the inflammatory response thereby improving airway patency and mucociliary transport. They may be more effective if used after a nasal decongestant, so as to reach more of the nasal mucosal surface. Antihistamines make sense in the face of seasonal allergic rhinitis. Since many patients have already used over-the-counter antihistamines to treat the symptoms of an upper respiratory infection, overdrying of the mucosa and thickening of the mucus may have occurred. Most of the nonsedating antihistamines are not as apt to cause mucosal drying, but caution needs to be taken to assess whether antihistamines present a deterrent to good mucociliary transport. Guaifenesin has been associated with improvement of the symptoms of nasal congestion and thickened nasal secretions. Studies so far have been unable to demonstrate changes in mucociliary transport or ciliary beat frequency, so its mode of action is unclear (Sisson et al., 1995). Cysteinyl leukotriene blockers, such as montelukast and cromolyn, have been indicated in treatment of asthma and allergic rhinitis to decrease the inflammatory response. These agents are not recommended as first-line agents and are not efficacious when used alone. Patient follow-up in two weeks to assess the success of the treatment regimen is appropriate.

Consultation and referral to an otolaryngologist should be considered for patients who do not respond to treatment of acute rhinosinusitis, who have multiple recurrences, or who have polyps or other nasal structural problems contributing to chronic rhinosinusitis. Patients with chronic rhinosinusitis may require surgical intervention to remove polyps, correct a deviated septum, reduce the size of hypertrophied nasal turbinates, or address the patency of the sinus ostia. Of course, signs of potential complications such as periorbital edema, double vision, opthalmoplegia, severe, unrelenting frontal headache, or focal neurologic signs require immediate referral (Fokkens et al., 2005).

OSTEOPATHIC PATIENT MANAGEMENT

The way an osteopathic physician proceeds in managing a patient's problem is influenced by how one thinks of influencing the biologic processes of healing. The five, classic treatment models suggest different ways of thinking about osteopathic management. One may focus on a single model or, as often happens, combine several models in a treatment plan. It is helpful to identify the contributions of each model to the particular problems of acute rhinosinusitis.

BIOMECHANICAL MODEL

Sutherland describes rhythmic movement of the facial bones (in particular zygomae, maxillae, palatines, and vomer) acting like a "plunger" on the sphenoid and maxillary sinuses to promote air exchange (Brooks, 1997; Sutherland, 1990). The vomer, forming part of the nasal septum, is important in directing air flow. The location of the sphenopalatine ganglion, as noted above, surrounded

by the palatine, sphenoid, and maxillary bones, puts it at risk for mechanical compromise if there is history of facial trauma. Many patients with nasal and sinus congestion have tenderness over the area of the ethmoid notch of the frontal bone, and respond to release of compression in that area (Cairro, 2003). Attention to the possibility of dysfunction in the cranial base and facial bones should be part of the evaluation of any patient with rhinosinusitis. Manipulative treatment specific to any identified cranial dysfunction is part of addressing the biomechanical issues of both acute and chronic rhinosinusitis. There are also mechanical considerations in the obstruction of venous and lymphatic flow from the head and neck.

RESPIRATORY/CIRCULATORY MODEL

Lymphatic and venous circulations are vital to reducing swelling in any part of the body and the tissues of the upper respiratory system are no exception. Removing metabolic waste products and inflammatory mediators that have accumulated in the tissues is another function of the lymphatic system. It has already been noted that the neuropeptides released from the sensory nerves, when stimulated, in the nasal and paranasal mucosa explain some of the symptoms of rhinosinusitis. OMT focused on removing impediments to venous and lymphatic circulation and stimulating flow when appropriate would aid in decreasing swelling and inflammation in the nasal region. Impediment to flow often presents in the form of myofascial tightness or constriction. Of particular interest is the anatomical area through which the lymph vessels, the thoracic duct, and right lymphatic duct must course to join the venous system. Working within the respiratory/circulatory model would include releasing myofascial tensions in the neck and upper thorax, particularly in the areas of the trapezius and sternocleidomastoid muscles, clavicle, and first rib. Superficial lymphatic drainage techniques such as effleurage to the face are directed at lymphatic flow as it leaves the nose and enters the lymphatics of the skin (Chikly, 2005; Moser, 1953; Schmidt, 1982).

Inhalation/exhalation motion of the ribs and diaphragm excursion also create a pump-like action for venous and lymphatic circulation with alternating negative and positive pressure in the thoracic cavity. Treating somatic dysfunction of the ribs, diaphragm, and their attachments helps promote good venous and lymphatic circulation *via* this mechanism (Stiles, 1977). There are also lymphatic pump and effleurage techniques intended to increase lymphatic circulation once the impediments to flow are removed. These include Galbraith technique for mandibular drainage, thoracic pump, and pedal pump (Chikly, 2005; Galbreath, 1925).

Arterial vasomotor tone is controlled by the sympathetic nervous system and is influenced somatically by dysfunction in the upper neck, where the superior cervical ganglion is located, and in the T1-3 area, the level of origin for sympathetic nerves supplying the head and neck. Lymphatic contractility in the head and neck is also mediated by these sympathetic nerves (Degenhardt and Kuchera, 1996).

NEUROLOGICAL MODEL

In light of current scientific information regarding the autonomic and sensory nervous system's influence on nasal mucosa, the neurologic model may be one of the most powerful ways to think about treating rhinosinusitis. Osteopathic manipulation's impact on somatovisceral and viscerosomatic reflexes offers a mechanism to improve autonomic balance to the upper respiratory mucosa. If, for instance, somatic dysfunction in the upper thoracic or upper cervical area is inhibiting sympathetic tone or if parasympathetic tone is being facilitated by dysfunction in the sphenoid and palatine areas, the nasal muscosa would be congested and/or produce excessive mucus. Removing the somatic dysfunction allows better balance to be achieved in the autonomic system and nasal mucosa to function more normally. Irritation of the sensory nerves in the nose and sinuses clearly adds to neurogenic inflammation by way of antidromic stimulation and release of neuropeptides (Loehrl, 2005; Sarin et al., 2006). Addressing factors, such as pain and mechanical irritation, which excessively stimulate those reflexes in the nose, can offer an opportunity to reduce inflammation of the nasal mucosa (Lacroix, 2003).

METABOLIC ENERGY MODEL

Fatigue is a complaint that often accompanies rhinosinusitis. Working from a bioenergetic perspective, the physician would consider the impact of somatic dysfunction on body efficiency and energy expenditure. Though not totally explained, there seems to be therapeutic effect related to the energetic interaction of hands-on treatment of various kinds. An awareness of how osteopathic manipulation may impact the patient's feeling of well-being as well as their ability to function more efficiently is consistent with the bioenergic model.

BEHAVIORAL MODEL

From an osteopathic point of view, educating patients as to behaviors that assist the body's innate healing can go hand in hand with OMT. Encouraging lifestyle modifications such as smoking cessation, allergen avoidance, adequate hydration, efficient breathing, and stress relief are important aspects in the treatment of rhinosinusitis. Informing patients relative to the appropriate use of all pharmacologic agents and symptomatic treatment options will improve patient compliance and satisfaction.

Palpation and identification of the structural and biomechanical dysfunctions associated with their problem can give patients confidence and trust in the treating physician. Patients with chronic rhinosinusitis often experience frustration and difficulty with treatment options. The ability to give them symptomatic relief with manipulative techniques relieves some of the anxiety and stress that accompanies any chronic disease.

DISCUSSION OF RELEVANT STUDIES

The osteopathic literature is replete with case reports and descriptions of the use of OMT to treat upper respiratory conditions including sinusitis. In the 1930s, articles in "The Osteopathic Profession" describe osteopathic manipulative approaches to address lymphatic drainage, normalize circulation, and balance viscerasomatic relationships for patients with sinusitis (Deason, 1935; Schoelles, 1937). L.M. Bush, D.O., at the 1942 American Osteopathic Association meeting in Chicago presented, "How the 'Old Doctor' treated nose and throat conditions," stressing "correction of spinal lesions and lesions of the clavicle" (Bush, 1942). In each of the following decades, case reports, promoting the use of OMT for sinusitis, appear in the literature. Shrum et al. (2001) describe the integration of pharmacologic agents and OMT (occipitoatlantal decompression, rib raising, lymphatic pump, myofascial release to the cervical, thoracic and lumbar areas, and mandibular drainage technique) into the treatment of sinusitis in children. Opinions expressed in letters to the editor of the *Journal of the American Osteopathic Association* in recent years have advocated the use of OMT in the treatment of sinusitis (Abend, 1999; Dudley, 1998).

The physiologic studies of Sato and Schmidt have shown that various types of mechanical, thermal, and chemical stimulation of the skin, muscles, and joints at various spinal levels produce reflex responses in visceral organs (Sato, 1989) That somatic afferent nerve stimulation can reflexively regulate various visceral functions, gives credence to the practice of relieving somatic dysfunction in the upper thoracic and cervical spine to improve function of the upper respiratory mucosa. Beal (1985), reviewed the specific somatic manifestations of visceral disease. Correlation of palpatory findings with visceral diagnoses suggests that an osteopathic structural examination makes a valuable contribution to clinical diagnosis.

Data gathered by the survey responses of 955 osteopathic physicians indicated that 2.49% of the respondents used OMT to treat sinusitis (Johnson and Krutz, 2002). When students were surveyed regarding which conditions they anticipated using OMT as part of their treatment plan, 20% included sinusitis (Chamberlain, 2003). A report on use of OMT in the emergency department suggests that symptoms of sinusitis (as well as several other complaints) could be ameliorated or eliminated with OMT (Paul, 1996).

Experience, coupled with anatomic and physiologic principles, strongly suggests that diagnosing and treating sinusitis, like so many other patient conditions, can be enhanced by the practice of osteopathic principles. This includes patient education and preventative care, musculoskeletal considerations for venous and lymphatic drainage and autonomic balance, use of other medical interventions that acknowledge the patient's self-healing mechanisms and respect their psychosocial milieu.

REFERENCES

Abend DS. Letters: revisiting the role of osteopathic manipulation in primary care. *J Am Osteopath Assoc* 1999;99(2):88–89.

Armengot M, Excribano A, Carda C, et al. Nasal mucociliary transport and ciliary ultrastructure in cystic fibrosis: a comparative study with healthy volunteers. *Int J Pediatr Otorhinolaryngol* 1997;40:27–44.

Beal MC. Viscerosomatic reflexes: a review. *J Am Osteopath Assoc* 1985;85(12):786/53–801/68.

Bellamy JL, Cady RK, Durham PL. Salivary levels of CGRP and VIP in rhinosinusitis and migraine patients. *Am Headache Soc* 2006;46:24–33.

Brooks RE. *Life in Motion: The Osteopathic Vision of Rollin E. Becker, D.O.* Portland, OR: Rudra Press, 1997.

Bush LM. How the old doctor treated nose and throat conditions. *Selected papers from the sections of Technic and Manipulative Therapy, American Osteopathic Association,* 1942:3–5.

Cairro J. *An Osteopathic Approach to Children.* Livingston, NJ: Churchill, 2003.

Chamberlain NR, Yates HA. A prospective study of osteopathic medical students' attitudes toward use of osteopathic manipulative treatment in caring for patients. *J Am Osteopath Assoc* 2003;103(10):470–478.

Chikly BJ. Manual techniques addressing the lymphatic system: origins and development. *J Am Osteopath Assoc* 2005;105(10):457–464.

Cole PJ, Greenstone MA, MacWilliam L, et al. Effect of cigarette smoking on nasal mucociliary clearance and ciliary beat frequency. *Thorax* 1986;41:519–523.

Deason WJ. Specific circulatory results: in the field of Otolaryngology conditions. *Osteopath Prof* 1935;2(9):7–11, 44, 46, 48.

Degenhardt BF, Kuchera ML. Update on osteopathic medical concepts and the lymphatic system. *J Am Osteopath Assoc* 1996;96(2):97–100.

Dudley G. Sinusitis supplement missing osteopathic component. *J Am Osteopath Assoc* 1998;98:539–540.

Fokkens W, Bachert C, Clement P, et al. EAACI position paper of rhinosinusitis and nasal polyps. *Allergy* 2005;60:583–601.

Galbreath W. Manipulative structural adjustive treatment in middle ear deafness. *J Am Osteopath Assoc* 1925;24:741.

Hickner JM, et al. Principles of appropriate antibiotic use for acute rhinosinusitis in adults: background. *Ann Intern Med* 2001;134(6):498–505.

Jaradeh S, Smith T, Torrico L, et al. Autonomic nervous system evaluation of patients with vasomotor rhinitis. *Laryngoscope* 2000;110:1828–1831.

Johnson SM, Kurtz ME. Conditions and diagnosis for which osteopathic primary care physicians and specialists use osteopathic manipulative treatment. *J Am Osteopath Assoc* 2002;102(10):527–532, 537–540, 565, 566.

Karlsson G, Holmberg K. Does allergic rhinitis predispose to sinusitis? *Acta Otolaryngol Suppl* 1994;515:26–28.

Lacroix JS. Chronic rhinosinusitis and neuropeptides. *Swiss Med Wkly* 2003;113, 560–562.

Landis BN, Beghetti M, Morel DR, et al. Somato-sympathetic vasoconstriction to intranasal fluid administration with consecutive decrease in nasal nitric oxide. *Scand Physiol Soc* 2003;177:507–515.

Levine HL, Setzen M, Cady RK, et al. An otolaryngology, neurology, allergy, and primary care consensus on diagnosis and treatment of sinus headache. *Otolaryngology* 2006;134:516–523.

Lin C, Cheng P, Fang SC. Mucosal changes in rhinitis medicamentosa. *Dep Otolaryngol Natl Cheng King Univ Hosp* 2004;113:147–151.

Loehrl TA. Autonomic function and dysfunction of the nose and sinuses. *Otolaryngol Clin N Am* 2005;1155–1161.

Loehrl TA. Autonomic dysfunction, allergy and the upper airway. *Curr Opin Otolaryngol Head Neck Surg* 2007;15:264–267.

Mahakit P, Pumhirun PA. A preliminary study of nasal mucociliary clearance in smokers, sinusitis and allergic rhinitis patients. *Asian Pac J Allergy Immunol* 1995;13:119–121.

Moser RJ. Sinusitis, the effective osteopathic manipulative procedures in the management thereof. *Yearb Acad Appl Osteopath* 1953;15–16.

Otten FW, Grote JJ. The diagnostic value of transillumination of maxillary sinusitis in children. *Int J Pediatr Otorhinolaryngol* 1989;18:9–11.

Paul F, Buser B. Osteopathic manipulative treatment applications for the emergency department patient. *J Am Osteopath Assoc* 1996;96(7):403–409.

Sarin S, Sanico A, Togias A, et al. The role of the nervous system in rhinitis. *J Allergy Clin Immunol* 2006;118:999–1014.

Sato A. Reflex modulation of visceral functions by somatic afferent activity. The central connection: somatovisceral/viscerosomatic interaction. *Am Acad Osteopath Symp* 1989:53–72.

Schmidt IC. Osteopathic manipulative therapy as a primary factor in the management of upper, middle, and pararespiratory infections. *J Am Osteopath Assoc* 1982;81(6):382/83–388/89.

Schoelles GJ. Treatment of Sinusitis: a technique for normalizing circulation in acute cases. *Osteopath Prof* 1937;4(7):11–13.

Schuhl JF. Nasal mucociliary clearance in personal rhinitis. *J Allergy Clin Immunol* 1995;5(6):333–336.

Shin SH, Ponikau JU, Sherris DA, et al. Chronic rhinosinusitis: an enhanced immune response to ubiquitous airborne fungi. *J Allergy Clin Immunol* 2004;114(6):1369–1375.

Shrum KM, Grogg SE, Barton P, et al. Sinusitis in children: the importance of diagnosis and treatment. *J Am Osteopath Assoc* 2001;101(5):S8–S13.

Sisson JH, Yonkers AJ, Waldman RH. Effects of guaifenesin on nasal mucociliary clearance and ciliary beat frequency in healthy volunteers. *Chest* 1995;107:747–751.

Stanley PJ, Wilson R, Greenstone MA, et al. Abnormal nasal mucociliary clearance in patients with rhinitis and its relationship to concomitant chest disease. *Br J Dis Chest* 1985;79:77–82.

Stiles EG. Osteopathic manipulation in a hospital environment. *Yearb Am Acad Osteopath* 1977;17–32.

Sutherland WG. *Teachings in the Science of Osteopathy.* 1st Ed. Portland, OR: Rudra Press, 1990.

68

Abdominal Pain

PETER ADLER-MICHAELSON AND MICHAEL A. SEFFINGER

KEY CONCEPTS

- Osteopathic evaluation of the patient with abdominal pain considers five different domains that involve the musculoskeletal system: posture and motion, respiration and circulation, metabolic functions, neurological functions, and behavioral aspects.
- Differential diagnosis of abdominal pain entails consideration of possible etiologies based on the history and physical using an anatomical, pathophysiological approach.
- The osteopathic evaluation and treatment of abdominal pain considers the effects of somatovisceral and viscerosomatic reflexes, as well as somatosomatic and viscerovisero reflexes.
- Somatic dysfunction may be a primary cause or a secondary finding in patients with abdominal pain and gastrointestinal dysfunction
- Osteopathic management of patients with abdominal pain utilizes five models of osteopathic patient care
- Osteopathic manipulative treatment is used as an adjunct in the prevention and treatment of postoperative ileus and atelectasis which often occurs after abdominal surgery for treatment of acute abdominal pathology.

CASE VIGNETTE

PATIENT PRESENTATION

Chief Complaint:

Right lower quadrant (RLQ) abdominal pain.

History of Chief Complaint:

Janequa is a 28-year-old African American female who presents to the emergency department (ED) on a weekend with increasingly painful RLQ abdominal pain over the past 8 hours. It is accompanied by slight nausea, but no vomiting. The doctor on call for her primary care physician recommended she go to the ED for evaluation. She was brought by car from home. Onset was initially 3 weeks prior, with fluctuating pain daily since then, but usually tolerable. The pain intensity ranged from 2 to 5/10, but today it rose to an 8 on a scale of 10 (8/10) after lifting groceries out of the trunk of her car. The pain initially began after she traveled to Brazil for a week. She carried heavy luggage to and from the airport, and felt a pull in her right side when yanking it off the conveyer belt. The pain is constant now but had previously varied throughout the day depending on her activities. It is dull in nature, but does not have a cramping, off and on, quality. The pain has been in the RLQ without radiation since onset. Food does not make it worse. Medications such as aspirin, ibuprofen, and acetaminophen have not helped. It is worse with standing up after bending over while lifting over twenty pounds. The pain seems to be least when she is lying on her side in the fetal (knee to chest) position. There is no change in the pain with application of heat or cold. Her menstruation has been regular, normal in amount without clots, and neither exacerbates nor ameliorates the pain. Her pain is such that she cannot tolerate vacuuming, reaching into the cupboard over the kitchen counter, or sexual intercourse. She had right flank pain for 2 days 4 months ago when she passed a kidney stone.

Past Medical History:

No hospitalizations. She denies having any medical illnesses and takes no prescription medications, other than her oral contraceptives. No history of sickle cell disease, ulcer disease, gallstones, cholecystitis, gastritis, colitis, appendicitis, tuberculosis, diabetes, or lupus erythematosis.

Past Surgical History:

She reports no surgeries in the past.

Family History:

Her mother is 54, had cholelithiasis and cholecystectomy, multiple kidney stones through the years, but no renal failure. Father is 56 and has hypertension and diabetes. Two brothers, 34 and 32, and her sister, 26, are well.

Social History:

The patient is an executive secretary, newly married with no children, working long hours but enjoys her work. She does not smoke and denies any illicit drug use. She rarely drinks alcohol. She is not active in sports. She recently traveled to South America with her husband on her honeymoon.

Allergies:

She denies any allergies to known medications.

Medications:

No prescription medications; multivitamins, herbal products from a friend who sells them to her for weight maintenance, unknown contents.

REVIEW OF SYSTEMS

General:

She normally sleeps well but has been sleeping poorly due to this pain. She is very health conscious and has exercised regularly before this pain started. She describes her nutrition as excellent. She denies fevers, chills, night sweats, recent weight loss or gain, although she feels not as hungry when the pain intensity increases.

Skin:

No history of rashes, moles, scaling.

HEENT:

No history of head trauma, changes in hearing, vision, smell, taste, or swallowing. No sore throat or swollen neck glands.

Cardiovascular:

No history of chest pain, shortness of breath, palpitations, congestive heart failure.

Respiratory:

No history of cough, phlegm, wheezing, or pneumonia.

Gastrointestinal:

She has had slight nausea, but no vomiting, diarrhea, constipation, hematemesis, melena, or hematochezia; no history of gastroesophageal reflux disease; no increased flatulence or bloating; she has normal daily bowel movements with no change in the color of her stool. No history of intolerance to fatty or fried foods.

Gynecological:

G0P0, she is sexually active, has unprotected intercourse with a single partner, has not missed any periods which have been regular and not heavier or lighter than normal; intercourse had not been painful for her prior to the onset of pain, but is now.

Genitourinary:

Has had a kidney stone, passed without sequelae 4 months ago, no recent hematuria, dysuria, or change in color of urine.

Neurological:

No history of seizures or stroke; no weakness, spasms, ticks, or problems with coordination.

Hematological:

No history of anemia, no sickle cell anemia or trait; any hemorrhage or abnormal bleeding diathesis.

Musculoskeletal:

No history of fractures, dislocations; had a sprained right ankle playing tennis 8 years ago; she gets occasional low back pain which resolves spontaneously with stretching. She denies joint pains or swelling.

PHYSICAL EXAM

Vital signs:

Pulse supine: 100/min; seated: 108. BP supine: 120/72 mm Hg; seated: 124/70. T: 37.5°C., R: 16/min, height: 5'8", weight: 145 lb.

General:

This is a well-developed, well-nourished female in moderate distress due to her abdominal pain, laying comfortably on her right side with knees flexed to chest.

HEENT:

Pupils are equal, round, and reactive to light and accommodation; external ocular muscles are intact; no skin lesions; mucous membranes slight dry otherwise oral exam normal; neck was supple; no bruits; no enlarged lymph nodes are present.

Heart:

Slight tachycardia, with regular rhythm; no extra sounds, murmurs, or rubs.

Lungs:

Clear to auscultation in all fields.

Abdomen:

No scars were present; no asymmetry to inspection; bowel sounds normal in all quadrants; moderate RLQ discomfort to palpation which is nonradiating; no masses or abnormal pulsations are palpated; no rebound tenderness is elicited. There is no guarding or costovertebral tenderness.

Pelvic exam:

Normal external and internal anatomy; no masses palpated; slight referral of pain to the RLQ on bimanual examination; no discharge or unusual odor noted, no cervical motion tenderness.

Breasts:

No masses, erythema, asymmetries, or discharge.

Rectal Exam:

tone is normal; no masses present; stool is brown, soft, no gross blood, and Guaiac test is negative for occult blood.

Extremities:

Normal range of motion all joints; no swelling is present; no pain is elicited on motion testing; no skin lesions are present; and pulses are present and normal to all extremities; capillary refill is less than 2 seconds in fingertips, nail polish occludes visualization of nail beds.

Neurological:

CN II to XII grossly intact; no sensory or motor abnormalities present; DTRs are 2+/4+ in biceps, triceps, brachioradialis, patellar, and Achilles tendons bilaterally. Babinski's tests elicit plantar flexion bilaterally.

Osteopathic Structural Exam:

Patient is examined in the standing, seated, prone, and supine positions for evidence of structural landmark asymmetries, altered range or quality of motion, tissue texture abnormalities, tenderness, or temperature variations.

Gait:

Gait is not antalgic but her left lower extremity is slightly externally rotated.

Postural Landmarks:

The right shoulder is inferior to the left; the head is held forward of the gravitational line; thoracic kyphosis is diminished as is the lumbar lordosis; the right anterior superior iliac spine is superior, right posterior superior iliac spine is inferior; the right leg appears shorter by 3 mm with the patient supine.

Active Motion:

Trunk sidebending left is restricted. There are positive right standing and seated flexion tests; in the prone position, with the patient backward bending, there is a right rotated sacrum on a left oblique axis and L5 is flexed, rotated left, and sidebent left (L/R sacral torsion).

Passive and Inherent Motion:

There is an externally rotated right temporal bone; C2-3 is flexed, rotated left, sidebent left (F R$_L$S$_L$); T1 is extended, rotated right, sidebent right (ER$_R$S$_R$); T5 is extended, rotated right, sidebent right (ER$_R$S$_R$); T6 is extended, rotated left, sidebent left (ER$_L$S$_L$); L1 is flexed, rotated right, sidebent right (FR$_R$S$_R$); there is poor compliance of the sacrum to posterior-anterior pressure at L5-S1 (positive spring test); the right thoracic diaphragm is restricted in inhalation; her axial fascial pattern is rotated left in at the craniocervical junction, rotated right at the cervicothoracic junction, rotated right at the thoracolumbar junction and rotated left at the lumbosacral junction (L/R/R/L) there is restricted internal rotation of the left femur.

Soft Tissue Palpation:

There are no abnormal temperature variations over the abdomen or back regions; the superior mesenteric ganglion area is tender to palpation; the right psoas is hypertonic and shortened, and there is a positive right counterstrain tender point for the psoas muscle (see also Chapter 49); a positive left piriformis tender point (see also Chapter 49); there were no Chapman's points palpable at the stomach, liver, small intestine, large intestine, kidneys, and appendix sites. (see also Chapter 52G:)

DIFFERENTIAL DIAGNOSES

Regardless of the region of the abdomen in which the patient states she has pain, since the visceral afferents diverge several segments within the spinal cord, the pain is not always an accurate indicator of the precise location of a visceral pathology. The differential diagnosis of subacute RLQ abdominal pain without bowel changes in a female of child-bearing age includes infectious, inflammatory, metabolic, and mechanical pathology. As an Osteopathic Emergency Physician, the first priority is to rule out a life-threatening illness. For example, an ectopic pregnancy is a true medical/surgical emergency where the patient could bleed profusely from a ruptured fallopian tube and die within minutes, before definitive care can be delivered. The patient must be quickly evaluated and any necessary treatment measures begun immediately. Given this patient's presentation, several emergency conditions need to be ruled out. Ectopic pregnancy, appendicitis, infection, internal bleeding, hydronephrosis, hepatitis, pancreatitis, ruptured diverticula, perforated bowel and bowel obstruction are at the top of the list. Possible urgent conditions also include pregnancy, placenta previa if pregnant, salpingitis, ovarian cyst, endometriosis, tumor, kidney stone/infection, cystitis, and colonic inflammation.

OSTEOPATHIC PATIENT MANAGEMENT

Biomechanical Model

In the ED, whether there is or is not any signs of somatic dysfunction, it is imperative to first distinguish whether a patient with abdominal pain has pathophysiology requiring solely medical management or will require surgical management as well. If there is somatic dysfunction present, as in this patient's case, the osteopathic physician should determine if it is a primary musculoskeletal disorder or secondary to internal organ pathophysiology. If the somatic dysfunction is determined to NOT be primarily of

musculoskeletal origin, such as is found in the case of viscerosomatic dysfunction, osteopathic manipulative treatment (OMT) may not be the primary treatment for the patient. However, the osteopathic physician should consider whether osteopathic evaluation or treatment using OMT could help to diagnose or treat the condition better, as an adjunct to the primary treatment, which may be medical and/or surgical. If the patient has a surgical abdomen, meaning her abdomen would require life-saving surgery and is typically firm and tender, her soma should display signs of guarding and protecting an obstructed or inflamed internal organ. Related Chapman's reflex points should be positive. Another consideration is whether osteopathic principles or OMT could assist in making the patient a better operative candidate. Can osteopathic principles or OMT assist the patient to better handle the postoperative phase? Can osteopathic principles or OMT assist the patient in the recovery phase? Conversely, if the somatic dysfunction is determined to be primarily of musculoskeletal origin and there is no evidence of internal organ pathophysiology, as in this patient's case, then OMT would be the treatment of choice for her problem. Muscle energy treatment using isometric contraction against a controlled resistance, followed by relaxation and passive stretching to lengthen the psoas would be effective. Alleviation of the spinal somatic dysfunctions with high-velocity low-amplitude (HVLA), muscle energy, or other OMT procedures would also be beneficial.

The normal fascial patterns in a healthy patient are either L/R/L/R or R/L/R/L/ pattern at the transition zones. Her fascial pattern would indicate especially a loss of compensation and therefore a problem in the thoracolumbar region. The pattern of somatic dysfunctions of the ipsilateral respiratory diaphragm and psoas muscle with the contralateral piriformis muscle is a very common pattern with psoas syndrome.

The Thomas Test (7) involves flexing one hip joint at a time in the supine patient, whose legs from the midfemurs distally are off the end of the table, and comparing the distance of separation of the extended thigh from the table. For example, with a tight, hypertonic, and shortened psoas muscle on the right, the right leg will be pulled away from the table further upon flexion of the left hip joint compared to the contralateral test. This is seen as a screening test only and is not specific for the psoas, as other conditions (i.e., hip joint capsule restrictions) can influence this test as well. Sometimes with a very flexible patient the Thomas test will be normal despite a psoas dysfunction being present. However, in the patient with a normal hip joint, a positive test is a good indicator of psoas hypertonicity. The counterstrain tender points for the psoas and iliacus muscles provide further evidence of a primary psoas dysfunction/spasm. The points are palpated and the findings compared left with right. In the case of this patient, both the Thomas test and the counterstrain tender point for the right psoas muscle were positive, indicating a somatic dysfunction of the right psoas muscle.

The psoas muscles are attached to the vertebral bodies and the anterior surface of the transverse processes of the lumbar vertebra. They pass along the superior border of the true pelvis, are joined by the iliacus muscles, pass over the superior ramus of the pubes, and then turn posteriorly to insert on the lesser trochanter of each femur via common tendons.

Psoas syndrome is usually initiated when a person assumes any number of positions that shorten the origin and insertion of the psoas muscle for a significant length of time and then gets up quickly, suddenly lengthening the origin and insertion, and attempts to assume normal upright activity. The initial positions that might bring about this syndrome include sitting in a soft easy chair or recliner, bending over from the waist for a long period of time, working at a desk, or weeding in the garden. Psoas syndrome can also be precipitated by overuse, such as doing sit-ups with the lower extremities fully extended. Apparently, each of these situations creates a neuromuscular imbalance that results in psoas muscle hypertonicity. The subsequent formation of somatic dysfunction then affects the psoas muscle and the lumbar spine. Once a patient realizes that he or she has been in one of these positions, the possibility of initiating a psoas syndrome can usually be avoided if he or she *slowly* returns to a neutral postural position.

The physician must be aware that there are organic causes for psoas tension or spasm, and if suspected, these must be ruled out by history and/or physical examination and special tests. These include:

> Femoral bursitis
> Arthritis of the hip
> Diverticulosis of the colon
> Ureteral calculi
> Prostatitis
> Cancer of the descending or sigmoid colon
> Salpingitis
> Psoas abscess

The key somatic dysfunction initiating or perpetuating psoas syndrome is believed to be a type II (nonneutral) somatic dysfunction (F Rx Sx) usually occurring in the L1 or L2 vertebral unit, where "x" is the side of side-bending of the somatic dysfunction. If this key somatic dysfunction remains, the patient's symptoms may progress to full-blown psoas syndrome. Osteopathic structural exam findings indicative of this syndrome include:

- The key, nonneutral (type II) somatic dysfunction at L1 or L2
- Sacral somatic dysfunction on an oblique axis, usually to the side of lumbar side-bending
- Pelvic shift to the opposite side of the greatest psoas spasm
- Hypertonicity of the piriformis muscle contralateral to the side of greatest psoas spasm
- Sciatic nerve irritation on the side of the piriformis spasm
- Gluteal muscular and posterior thigh pain that does not go past the knee, on the side of the piriformis muscle spasm

Manipulative treatment is preceded by ruling out psoas involvement caused by one of the organic etiologies previously listed. Effective treatment of the "key" somatic dysfunction (usually found at L1 or L2) is essential for the patient's comfort and for effective, long-lasting effects of manipulative treatment, regardless of the administration of other indicated medicines, chemotherapy, radiation, or surgery. Removing somatic dysfunction, wherever it occurs in the body, reduces afferent load to the spinal cord from secondary somatic sources and lessens the segmental activity of the primary facilitated spinal cord segments. This makes the patient more comfortable and supports the body's homeostatic and defense mechanisms, thus hastening recovery.

An iliopsoas or psoas somatic dysfunction with hypertonicity and muscle shortening present for a long enough period of time can create a posterior position of the ipsilateral innominate. This is likely due presumably to the superior pull from the muscle leading to a compensatory shift of the innominate to ease tension within the muscle. This often leads to a functional (not anatomic) shortening of the ipsilateral leg, as is demonstrated by this patient.

The L5, sacrum, and innominate dysfunctions are likely compensatory to the initial psoas dysfunction (8).

The C-spine (C3-5) somatic dysfunction is likely related to her diaphragm somatic dysfunction via somatosomatic reflexes. (see also Chapter 13) The temporal bone somatic dysfunction is likely secondary to the cervical and sacral somatic dysfunctions. The "normal" Chapman's points for the foregoing organs lend

further weight to the hypothesis that the internal organs are not primarily involved in her case but rather secondarily altered. (see also Chapter 52G)

Respiratory-Circulatory Model

This patient's respiratory and circulatory functions seem to be intact. On exam, her resting pulse and respiratory rates are slightly elevated and her mucous membranes are slightly dry. This raises the possibility of her being volume depleted, but her blood pressure was within normal limits, and she was not dizzy upon standing. If she was volume depleted, that is, dehydrated, her blood pressure would drop more than 15 mm Hg, and/or pulse rate rise, more than 15 beats per minute, respectively, upon sitting from the supine position. But since her blood pressure is stable, her elevated heart and respiratory rates, and dry membranes, are therefore likely due to pain and anxiety as opposed to hemorrhage. She may have an ectopic pregnancy causing these signs, and the urine pregnancy test will help to rule that out.

An air embolism is typically discovered on plain upright abdominal x-ray under the diaphragm. Although causing some pain and bloating, the intensity of this pain is lancinating if the air transects fascial planes, that is, through the abdominal wall or fascia of the diaphragm, which is contiguous with the pericardium and fascia of the mediastinum. On occasion, air can enter the vaginal canal and find its way through the uterus, fallopian tubes, and into the abdominal cavity. A perforated intestine from ruptured diverticula, cancer, and inflammatory bowel disease can also cause air embolism, but there is no evidence in her history or physical exam to support this.

The color of the stool is another important finding when assessing a patient with abdominal pain. A finding of bright red blood makes us think of processes nearer to the anus, for example, hemorrhoids. While a finding of black tarry stool makes us think more of upper gastrointestinal (GI) processes, for example, a stomach or duodenal ulcer with bleeding. A normal color does not rule out GI bleeding. A Guaiac test is a test for occult blood in the stool. The test is done at the bedside following a rectal exam. If the stool is negative for gross blood and the Guaiac test is negative for occult blood, we can be fairly sure that there is no process present involving bleeding from the bowels. The normal vascular exam of the abdomen and lower extremities ruled out aortic aneurysm as well as other vascular problems or bleeding abnormalities in this patient.

An intravenous (IV) line was started with normal saline (NS) at 125 cc/h, as she was kept "n.p.o." (*Latin*—nil per os—nothing by mouth); oxygen was started per nasal canula at 2 L/min, which could have been titrated upward as needed in case of shortness of breath, and a heart monitor was attached to her chest to continually assess whether her heart maintained its normal sinus rhythm or required further interventions due to an arrhythmia, for example. Blood was drawn; urine was obtained and sent to the lab.

Recall that the patient's resting pulse and respiratory rate are slightly elevated and her mucous membranes are somewhat dry, which is likely due to anxiety, given her negative lab and radiological studies. If this patient did have tachycardia due to blood loss or dehydration, she would need greater amounts of IV fluids, usually NS or lactated Ringers solution (5). Starting oxygen and attaching an EKG monitor are standard measures in the ED to support and monitor the patient (6).

Neurological Model

An appreciation of the neuroanatomy of nociception is helpful in discerning the cause of acute abdominal pain. Both somatic (peripheral nervous system) and visceral (autonomic nervous system) innervations are involved. Visceral afferents transmit noxious stimuli, such as stretch, distention, inflammation, and ischemia, to the central nervous system (CNS). However, other tissue-destroying processes, such as is found with some intra-abdominal tumors or cancerous growths, or cutting and burning during surgery, cannot be perceived via these visceral afferent nerves and are thus not perceived as pain by the patient.

In the abdomen, the sympathetic component is contributed by the thoracic, lumbar, and pelvic splanchnic nerves, and the parasympathetic by the paired vagus nerves arising from the tenth cranial nuclei of the brainstem and the sacral splanchnic nerves arising from S2-S4 spinal segments (see also Chapter 10). The sympathetic cell bodies are in the intermediolateral cell columns of spinal segments T1-L2 with axons traversing through the ventral roots to the paravertebral ganglia. These paired chains of interconnected ganglia lie along each side of the spinal cord just anterior to the heads of the ribs like a string of pearls. The fibers from the paravertebral sympathetic chain ganglia converge anteriorly to form the sympathetic prevertebral or collateral ganglia: the greater splanchnic nerves from segments T5-9 form the celiac plexus; the lesser splanchnic nerves from segments T10-11 form the superior mesenteric plexus and the least splanchnic nerves from segments T12-L2 form the inferior mesenteric plexus. Postganglionic fibers innervate their target organs.

The parasympathetic innervation structure is more streamlined. Long, preganglionic axons from the vagus nerves extend through the prevertebral ganglia as they pass directly to the viscera. Their short, postganglionic fibers form part of the network in the visceral wall called the enteric nervous system. Both the sympathetic and the parasympathetic nerves exert their effects through the enteric nervous system. This network of fibers is composed of two layers. The outer myenteric (Auerbach) plexus controls GI motility. The inner plexus (Meissner) controls GI secretion and local blood flow. Perception of nociceptive stimuli results in alterations in gut function mediated at this level. For example, marked reduction in gut motility—ileus—commonly occurs in peritonitis via viscerovisceral reflexes.

Specific aspects of this anatomy explain why visceral pain is initially perceived as vague in location and quality. (see also Chapter 10) It is generally described as aching in nature, rather than sharp or intense, and is perceived as originating in the one of three midline regions versus a discrete unilateral location. This relates partly to the paucity of visceral afferents compared with the large number of somatic afferents originating in skin and musculoskeletal structures. Equally important is that the transmission of visceral pain occurs via slow nonmyelinated C fibers versus the fast-conducting A-δ fibers that transmit somatic pain.

Finally, the initial location of pain as regional versus specific relates to the embryologic development of abdominal viscera as midline structures with midline neurovascular supply. They divide into foregut (T5-9), midgut (T10-11), and hindgut (T11-L2) areas. Foregut structures include the distal esophagus, stomach, and the proximal duodenum, as well as the liver, biliary tree, and pancreas. Midgut structures include the small intestine, appendix, ascending colon, and proximal two third of the transverse colon. The hindgut includes the distal third of the transverse colon, the descending colon, and the rectosigmoid. They are loosely associated with the celiac, superior mesenteric, and inferior mesenteric ganglia, respectively. Thus, in general, pain from structures innervated at these levels will be perceived as occurring in the epigastric, periumbilical, or hypogastric midline areas, respectively.

The somatic component of acute abdominal pain is caused by the parietal peritonitis that occurs adjacent to the involved viscera as inflammation progresses. Also referred to as the "percutaneous

reflex of Morley," it is conducted by A-δ fibers following the associated dermatome to unilateral spinal segments, which results in the localization and increasing intensity of acute abdominal pain, as well as the increased muscle tone of the abdominal wall associated with guarding and rebound tenderness.

The third component of acute abdominal pain, known as referred pain, is a clear example of how structure determines function. Referred pain is defined as discomfort occurring in a site distant from the diseased viscus. The explanation of referred pain lies in the intricacies of the neuroanatomy previously described. The spinothalamic tract is largely nondiscriminatory for visceral versus somatic pain. Because somatic nervous input far exceeds visceral, the CNS is "fooled" and perceives the pain as originating partly in the peripheral structures innervated by the same spinal segments as the diseased viscus. For example, the pain initiated by gallbladder inflammation (T7-8 visceral afferent innervation) is perceived as occurring in the right subscapular area (T7-8 somatic afferent innervation).

In a similar manner, visceral afferents synapse on interneurons in the spinal cord that stimulate somatic efferent neurons at the same level. This local reflex activity is referred to as a viscerosomatic reflex. It results in somatosensory changes palpable in a paraspinal location as tissue tenderness, asymmetry, range-of-motion restriction, and tissue texture changes. The finding of specific somatic dysfunction in a patient with acute abdominal pain can provide useful information as to the origin of the pain. The paraspinal location should direct one to consider organs known to have sympathetic innervation at the same level, resulting from the fact that visceral afferents that trigger viscerosomatic reflexes predictably follow the sympathetic efferent pathways. (see also Chapter 39)

With this discussion of nociceptive anatomy as a backdrop, consider the more clinical aspects of our patient with acute abdominal pain. The patient does not show signs of peritoneal inflammation or an acute abdomen and her vital signs are stable. The onset of the pain began shortly after strenuous physical activity and was associated with decreased ability to perform activities that required her to extend her hip and trunk. The pain intensity gradually increased over a period of weeks, as opposed to pain from an obstructed viscous or acute inflammatory process which typically has a more rapid progression of pain intensity.

With the patient supine, the sensitivity of the connective tissues surrounding the collateral sympathetic ganglia can be assessed gently palpating the abdomen overlying these areas. Assessment involves determining increased subjective sensitivity as well as tissue texture changes in these regions. Positive results will lead to further assessment of structures related to the altered ganglion. In this patient, a tender and noncompliant superior mesenteric ganglion area can be a sign of visceral pathology involving, for example, the small intestine or proximal half of the large intestine, or a kidney; or it can mean an increased afferent input to the segments T10-11 from another somatic structure, for example, the lower extremity or the respiratory diaphragm. In this patient, the decreased mobility of the right kidney compared to the left side (which can also be in part due to the respiratory diaphragm somatic dysfunction on the right) could be the explanation of the tissue texture changes felt around the superior mesenteric ganglion (3).

A common neurologic problem causing superficial abdominal pain is shingles (herpes zoster), which are vesicular, painful lesions along a cutaneous peripheral nerve, usually the intercostal nerve in the intercostal space, resulting from prior infection as a child (varicella zoster, aka "chicken pox"). However, her skin had no lesions so this possibility is highly unlikely.

Certainly, lower thoracic or upper lumbar spinal disease could cause nerve irritation, inflammation, and radiation of pain into the lower abdomen. Although there was spinal somatic dysfunction, there was no history of trauma, cancer, or metastasis, and disc herniation is not common in this patient's age group, so these are least likely possibilities.

While the diagnostics to rule out emergent and urgent processes are ongoing, treatment involves primarily pain management, as well as OMT modalities. OMT to relieve pain is most efficacious when there are palpable signs of somatic dysfunction related to the pain, that is, muscle spasm, fascial restrictions, tissue congestion, or tenderness. Often, visceral OMT relieves pain related to tissue congestion, strain-counterstrain OMT relieves tenderpoints and myofascial, articulatory procedures or muscle energy OMT releases muscle spasms and connective tissue restrictions; HVLA may be used for restricted joint motion refractory to less forceful methods. For paraspinal muscle spasms and Chapman's reflex nodules, inhibition (sustained digital pressure with a slight circular motion) OMT is helpful.

An extremely important issue is whether or not to give analgesic (pain) medication to the patient pending lab and imaging studies as well as while awaiting consultations. Theoretically, if the patient receives a strong analgesic, they will no longer be able to respond appropriately to the assessment, and we will get confusing results from our examination. The patient is asking for medications for her pain. Current practice guidelines recommend using short-acting narcotic analgesics to control the patient's pain while undergoing laboratory and radiographic procedures and waiting for consultants to come to perform their evaluations (4).

Metabolic Energy Model

Four of the most common causes of acute abdominal pain that warrant surgical intervention include acute appendicitis, acute cholecystitis, diverticulitis, and small bowel obstruction. In each of these diseases, inflammation and infection are the result of obstruction of normal function of a hollow viscus or duct structure. The obstruction results in luminal distention, stasis of organ contents, which causes back pressure against the organ walls. Because venous and lymphatic drainage are passive, low-pressure networks, the increasing back pressure prevents proper drainage of these tissues, resulting in organ wall edema. This progresses to arterial obstruction and ischemia. Ischemia leads to wall gangrene, perforation, and peritonitis.

Because the GI tract is colonized with varying levels and types of bacteria, the stasis described above causes bacterial overgrowth. Transmural infection of the compromised viscus results and contributes to the peritonitis caused by gangrene and perforation. Bacterial liberation of endotoxins and the release of inflammatory mediators result in the systemic septic response. Inflammation and infection increase metabolic processes, elicit release of interleukins and other cytokines with subsequent generation of fever. Fatigue ensues. Left untreated, the systemic inflammatory response syndrome of multiple organ failure occurs with high levels of comorbidity and mortality.

In considering metabolic pathophysiology as the source of her abdominal pain, recall that she had nausea, but she did not have any other signs of GI or genitourinary system dysfunctions, including vomiting, oral or rectal bleeding, bloating, or fevers. She has a history of a kidney stone, and it is possible she has one again with associated muscle spasm related to a viscerosomatic reflex. An abdominal (kidney-urinary-bladder, or "KUB") x-ray would identify a calcium stone if present in a kidney or ureter; however, the absence of costovertebral tenderness argues against kidney stone or infection. A urine test is an inexpensive means by which hematuria could be detected if there is a ureteral stone, kidney or bladder inflammation, infection or hemorrhage. Although she has had regular menstruation

cycles and flow, a urine pregnancy test will help confirm she is not indeed pregnant and rule out ectopic pregnancy. If necessary an abdominal ultrasound would detect swelling, enlargement, cysts or masses in the liver, spleen, pancreas, intestines, kidneys, ovaries, fallopian tubes or uterus as would an abdominal or pelvic CT.

Although she is afebrile, this does not necessarily rule out an intra-abdominal infection and/or inflammation or other noninfectious pathology. Typically, intra-abdominal inflammation causes inflammation of the peritoneal lining of the intra-abdominal wall. As there was no rebound abdominal tenderness on physical exam, which is a fairly reliable sign of peritonitis, this possibility is unlikely. In this patient, the absence of rebound tenderness and palpable masses and the presence of normal bowel sounds make it less likely that she has a significant intra-abdominal pathology. A computerized tomography scan would help to rule out masses or abnormal anatomy from other pathophysiological processes.

The right ovary and/or fallopian tube could be inflamed, obstructed, or cystic and cause pain without causing a fever, so these pathologies are possible given her symptoms. The physical exam, including lack of Chapman's reflexes, did not localize a pathologic pelvic structure, though pain was felt in the RLQ during the pelvic bimanual exam.

The decision as to which lab tests to order is often a difficult one. Ideally, this is based upon having a solid differential diagnosis in mind. Lab test results should not be seen as a definitive "rule-out" but rather as another piece in the larger puzzle of the entire presentation of the patient. For example, with a normal complete blood count (CBC) and "normal" abdominal ultrasound studies, one might be inclined to rule out appendicitis in this case (1). That would be unwise as some cases of appendicitis have been found in spite of negative laboratory and radiographic tests. Similarly, with normal liver function studies and normal abdominal ultrasound exam, you might be inclined to rule out gall bladder disease. Keep in mind, however, that although the false-negative rate of abdominal ultrasound for detection of gallstones is less than 5%, sole reliance on this modality may miss a diagnosis of small stones or disease that could cause abdominal pain and require surgical treatment (2). A urine drug screen test is also helpful as the patient may not divulge use of illicit drugs during the history.

The results are back from the laboratory and radiology departments. Blood tests: CBC with differential is within normal limits, as are the electrolytes, amylase, lipase, liver function studies, and blood urea nitrogen: creatinine ratio; Urinalysis is negative for white blood cells, red blood cells, or nitrates. Drug screen is negative. Guaiac test is negative for occult blood. Urine and serum pregnancy tests are negative. Review of the abdominal x-ray series shows no free air, calcifications, or other pathology. Ultrasound study of the abdomen shows no pathology, and abdominopelvic CT study shows no free fluid, no masses, no abnormal visceral or vascular structures. Thus, a hemorrhagic problem, anemia, electrolyte abnormality, illicit drug use, pregnancy, urinary obstruction, renal failure, urinary tract infection, intra-abdominal, or intra-pelvic pathology were ruled out. If any of these test results are positive or equivocal (unable to discern positive vs. negative test), general surgical and/or gynecological consults would be ordered for opinions from their perspective as well as management beyond the ED in case the patient requires hospital admission or ambulatory care follow up with a surgical specialist.

Behavioral Model

Behavioral issues such as anxiety or depression, drug abuse, especially opiates, may all cause abdominal pain. A urine drug screen would help determine if drug abuse is a potential cause of her pain. Anxiety and depression are possible in her situation, but less likely to cause such severe abdominal pain as she expresses. With somatic dysfunction in so many regions of the body, and constant pain, as well as being newly wed, anxiety is certainly part of the problem, and there may be underlying depression that was not admitted to in the history.

CASE VIGNETTE (CONTINUED)

The patient was treated with myofascial release (MFR) technique for the thorax and respiratory diaphragm; counterstrain, muscle energy technique (MET) and Still techniques for the right psoas; visceral techniques for the superior mesenteric ganglion and right kidney; counterstrain, MET for the left piriformis hypertonicity; MFR for the left pelvic floor; MFR, MET, and HVLA techniques for the right innominate; MFR, MET, and Still techniques for the sacrum. The patient tolerated the OMM treatment very well and reported a reduction of symptoms of about one-half, from 8/10 to about 4/10. She did not feel a need for medications at that point.

Final Diagnoses

The work-up for medical or surgical pathology was negative. The final diagnoses were as follows:

Somatic dysfunctions of the lower extremities, abdomen, costal cage, pelvis, lumbar spine, thoracic spine, cervical spine, and cranial regions. (ICD-9: 739.6, 739.9, 739.8, 739.5, 739.3, 739.2, 739.1, 739)

The primary source of her abdominal pain was attributed to a psoas spasm.

Disposition of the Patient

Based upon the negative work-up, negative consultation results, and excellent response of the patient to the OMM treatment, the decision was made to discharge the patient home with follow-up with a local osteopathic physician specializing in NMM/OMM or skilled in using OMT. The patient was instructed to return to the ED or to her regular family doctor if the symptoms did not improve, worsen or, if they resolved from this treatment but returned again.

Further Treatment Modality Options

Treatment emphasizing self-help techniques for the patient will allow the patient to be an active part of her own return to homeostasis. Muscle-energy techniques for the psoas and piriformis muscles can be easily learned and applied several times daily for a faster and better result. (see also Chapter 46) MFR for the respiratory diaphragm and superior mesenteric ganglion can likewise be learned and applied regularly. (see also Chapter 47)

REFERENCES

1. Brunicardi CF, ed. *Schwartz's Principles of Surgery*. 9th Ed. New York, NY: McGraw-Hill, 2010; chap. 30.
2. Chintapalli KN, Ghiatas AA, Chopra S, et al. Sonographic findings in cases of missed gallstones. *J Clin Ultrasound* 1999;27(3):117–121.
3. Patterson MM, Howell JN, eds. *The Central Connection: Somatovisceral/Viscerosomatic Interaction*. Indianapolis, IN: American Academy of Osteopathy, 1992.
4. Decosterd I, Hugli O, Tamchès E, et al. Oligoanalgesia in the emergency department: Short-term beneficial effects of an education program on acute pain. *Ann Emerg Med* 2007;50(4):462–471.
5. American College of Surgeons. *Advanced Trauma Life Support Manual*. Chicago, IL, 2004.
6. American Heart Association. *Advanced Cardiac Life Support Program Manual*. Dallas, TX, 2006:7–10.
7. Kuchera WA. Lumbar region. In: Ward RC, exec. ed. *Foundations for Osteopathic Medicine*. 2nd Ed. Philadelphia, PA: Lippincott Williams & Wilkins, 2003:743.
8. Kappler RE. Role of psoas mechanism in low-back complaints. *J Am Osteopath Assoc* 1973;72:794.

69

Acute Low Back Pain

MARCEL P. FRAIX AND MICHAEL A. SEFFINGER

KEY CONCEPTS

- Osteopathic considerations for the patient with low back pain (LBP) entail assessing and treating biomechanical, respiratory-circulatory, metabolic-energy, neurologic, and behavioral aspects of the clinical condition.
- Differential diagnosis utilizes a structure-function approach in determining whether the pain is due to spinal or pelvic musculoskeletal somatic dysfunction, localized manifestation of a systemic pathophysiologic process, or referred from internal organ disease.
- Most causes of LBP are musculoskeletal and amenable to osteopathic manipulative treatment.
- Evidence-based literature and expert consensus guidelines support the utilization of OMT for patients with acute, subacute, and chronic back pain.
- The AOA House of Delegates passed a resolution accepting an evidence-based practice guideline recommending utilization of OMT for patients with LBP.

CASE VIGNETTE

Chief Complaint:

Low back pain (LBP)

History of Chief Complaint:

A 52-year-old male presents to the ambulatory clinic complaining of persistent LBP for the past 3 weeks. The pain started a few days after he hurt his left knee playing tennis. His knee pain has improved and he is no longer limping, but now he is experiencing dull, achy constant pain in the area of his low back, primarily on the right side. The pain is exacerbated with prolonged sitting and lifting more than 25 lb. It seems to get better with rest and lying down, although he does admit to having difficulty with finding a comfortable position when sleeping and prefers to lie on his side with his knees bent. The pain is sometimes sharp and radiates to the right posterior thigh, but not past the knee or into the foot. In the past, he had LBP that did radiate to the lateral foot, causing an intermittent numbness sensation, but it resolved after a week or so with decreased physical activity and stretching. He has also contended with dull and aching back pain periodically throughout the years that also resolved spontaneously after a couple of days. Over-the-counter nonsteroidal anti-inflammatory drugs (NSAIDs) offer some relief and reduce his current acute LBP from 8/10 to 4/10 in intensity. He is usually relatively active and enjoys playing tennis and golf on the weekends. He denies any problems with bowel or bladder function but has not been able to play for the past three weeks.

Past Medical History:

Hypercholesterolemia, seasonal allergies, left tibial stress fracture at age 35 while training to run a marathon; right rotator cuff tendonitis. No hospitalizations. Last physical was 10 months ago. He had a normal baseline prostate evaluation, PSA test, and colonoscopy at age 50. No history of rheumatoid arthritis, direct trauma to the low back, or motor vehicle accidents.

Past Surgical History:

Appendectomy at age 16

Social History:

Employed as a software engineer; nonsmoker; occasionally has a glass of wine or beer with dinner; lives at home with his wife and two children aged 16 and 14 who are all well.

Medications:

Atorvastatin 10 mg daily for hypercholesterolemia, loratidine 20 mg daily as needed for allergic rhinitis, naproxen 500 mg, 1 tablet every 12 hours as needed for pain.

Allergies:

Penicillin causes hives.

REVIEW OF SYSTEMS

General:

No fever or weight loss; mild fatigue

Skin:

No rashes or eczema.

HEENT:

No history of head trauma, recent changes in vision, smell, taste, hearing, or swallowing.

Cardiovascular:

No chest pain at rest or with exertion; no palpitations; no cyanosis or peripheral edema.

Respiratory:

No cough, shortness of breath, dyspnea; has history of exercise-induced and allergic asthma for which he used to use an inhaler as needed but has not needed it for several months; no history of pneumonia or tuberculosis.

Gastrointestinal:

No nausea or vomiting, loss of appetite or abdominal pain; no bloody stools; no diarrhea or constipation; no history of hepatitis, ulcer, diverticulosis, or gallstones.

Genitourinary:

No hematuria, dysuria, incontinence, but he does note that his urinary stream is not as strong as usual; no history of hernia;

sexual relations have diminished for past three weeks due to LBP.

Endocrine:

No polydypsia, polyphagia, polyuria. No heat or cold intolerance.

Musculoskeletal:

Mild left knee pain; sharp right-sided LBP; history of intermittent LBP that is usually dull and aching in nature; occasional right shoulder pain that is exacerbated with playing tennis.

Neurological:

No history of sciatica neuralgia; no muscle weakness in his upper or lower limbs; no muscle cramping or spasm; no persistent loss of sensation in his feet; occasional headaches characterized by a sensation of bilateral squeezing (tightness) which resolve with rest; no history of seizures or stroke.

Hematologic:

No history of anemia, blood dyscrasias, or bleeding tendencies.

Psychiatric:

No history of depression, anxiety, mania, hallucinations, or hospitalizations.

PHYSICAL EXAM

Vital signs:

Height: 5´10˝, weight: 170 lb, BP: 135/80, P: 86, R:14, T: 98.8°F

General:

Alert and in mild distress due to LBP; appearance is well kept, unable to get comfortable sitting on the treatment table; appears well dressed, clean and groomed.

Integument:

No erythema or increased warmth in lumbar region; no trophic changes in bilateral lower limbs; no malar or other rashes.

HEENT:

Head is atraumatic, normocephalic; pupils equal, round, reactive to light and accommodation; CN II to XII are grossly intact; external auditory canals are patent and tympanic membranes are intact with good cone of light; nasal mucosa is slightly erythematous and edematous; no sinus pressure tenderness to palpation or percussion; pharynx not injected, no tonsillar hypertrophy, no erythema or exudates.

Hematologic/Lymphatics:

No lymphadenopathy or peripheral edema.

Cardiovascular:

Heart has a regular rhythm; no murmurs; lower limbs nonedematous; dorsalis pedis and posterior tibial pulses are palpable bilaterally; no carotid bruits; no abdominal bruits or masses.

Respiratory:

Lungs are clear to auscultation bilaterally; no wheezes or rhonchi in the airways; no prolongation of exhalation.

Gastrointestinal:

Abdomen is nondistended and bowel sounds are auscultated in all four quadrants without bruits; abdomen is tympanic to percussion, soft, nontender to palpation without rebound tenderness or masses. Normal rectal sphincter tone on digital exam; guaiac stool test is negative for blood.

Genitourinary:

Prostate is firm, nontender, and small without nodules. No inguinal hernia.

Neurological:

Full motor strength present in bilateral upper and lower extremities; sensation diminished to light touch and pinprick over dorsal surface of right foot, with remainder of sensory exam normal in upper and lower limbs; muscle stretch reflexes: bilateral patellar and left Achilles 2+/4+; right Achilles 1+/4+; Babinski tests elicit down going toes bilaterally; straight leg raise tests elicit mild increase in LBP and tingling sensation but no pain in posterior legs or feet at 80 degrees; bilateral lower limb proprioception intact (negative Romberg test); normal heel and toe walking.

Musculoskeletal:

Mildly antalgic gait with decreased loading of left lower limb; increased right-sided lumbar paravertebral muscle tension with moderate tenderness lateral to L5 spinous process, decreased lumbar spine flexion (30 degree) and extension (10 degree), moderate pain with lumbar spine extension and left side-bending; limited range of motion of squat test; negative FABERE test bilateral hip joints; medial joint line tenderness of left knee with 5° deficit in extension, negative drawer test, and mild pain with McMurray's test; no effusion of left or right knee; right bicipital tendon tender to palpation, negative Yergason test; there is a right positive Thomas test for iliopsoas tension.

Osteopathic Structural Exam:

Patient is evaluated in the standing, seated, supine, and prone positions.

Cranial:

Normocephalic, atraumatic cranium, asymmetrical motion posterior quadrants, primary respiratory mechanism at 8 cycles per minute, restriction of the right occipitomastoid suture.

Cervical:

increased cervical lordosis with head anterior to gravitational line; OA extended, sidebent right, rotated left; C2 rotated right.

Thoracic:

Decreased thoracic kyphosis; T1 Extended Rotated right, Sidebent right; palpable deep right paraspinal muscle tension (intertransversarii, rotatores, multifidi) at T4-5 extending out to the 4th intercostal space laterally that binds even more with passive cervical right sidebending using the head as a lever in the seated position during exhalation; T8-10 Neutral Sidebent left, rotated right; T12-L2 Neutral Sidebent right, rotated left; tenderness of right 12th posterior thoracic counterstrain point.

Costal:

Exhalation restriction of right 1st rib, inhalation restriction of right 12th rib and thoracic diaphragm.

Lumbar:

Decreased lumbar lordosis; L5 Flexed rotated right, Sidebent right; tenderness of 5th posterior lumbar and right piriformis counterstrain points, and in the area overlying the right iliolumbar ligament;

Pelvis:

Positive left standing flexion test; ASIS, PSIS, and pubic tubercles are level;

Sacrum:

Positive left seated flexion test; left sacral torsion on a right oblique axis and positive (poor/decreased) lumbar spring test.

Lower Extremities:

No gross leg length discrepancy; tenderness of left medial meniscus counterstrain tenderpoint; ankle decreased quality and range in passive dorsiflexion.

Upper Extremity:

Right scapula inferior; full range of motion present in bilaterally upper extremities.

ASSESSMENT

LBP (lumbago)

Somatic dysfunctions in the following regions: cranial (739.0); cervical (739.1), thoracic (739.2) with (viscerosomatic reflex at T4-5 related to asthma); lumbar (739.3); sacral (739.4); lower extremities (739.6); costal cage (739.8)

Left medial meniscus injury

History of hypercholesterolemia

Allergic rhinitis

Asthma

Right bicipital tendonitis

PLAN

This patient has acute LBP (<6 weeks' duration) due to somatic dysfunction that is amenable to osteopathic manipulative treatment (OMT). A review of the scientific literature supports this diagnosis and management plan (1–3). Osteopathic manipulative medicine (OMM) methods that can be used to address his somatic dysfunctions include soft tissue, articulatory, muscle energy, strain-counterstrain, high-velocity/low-amplitude (HVLA), osteopathy in the cranial field and myofascial release procedures. Lumbar spine range of motion and strengthening exercises, such as the commonly prescribed knee-to-chest and pelvic tilt exercises, 3 cycles of 10 repetitions, once or twice daily, often aid recovery and rehabilitation (1). Patient-specific exercise prescriptions based on the physical exam findings and goals of treatment are most beneficial (1,4,5). Physical therapy referral for abdominal, lumbar, and pelvic muscle stabilization exercises and training may be useful if progress is slow with self-directed home exercises (6).

The American Osteopathic Association recommended parameters for frequency of application of OMT for patients with acute somatic dysfunction are one to three times per week for 2 weeks, followed by two to three times per week for 2 weeks, then one to two times per week thereafter, up to 6 weeks (5). If symptoms and signs are continually improving, OMT should be continued. If symptoms and signs are not improving, or worsening, reassessment of the diagnosis and a new management plan should be initiated (5). However, this is only a guideline, for at each visit, the osteopathic physician should determine the frequency and duration of OMT based on the patient's response to previous treatments, prescribed exercises and ergonomics and current assessment of the clinical condition (5).

For patients with acute LBP who do not improve with self-care options, spinal manipulation is the best evidence recommendation (6). Patients should be educated to stay active and use proper ergonomics (6) (i.e., to pick up something to the side, do not bend over to the side, twisting the lumbar spine, with extended knees, which puts significant strain and stress on the low back; instead, face the object, bend the knees, keep the back extended and lift the object close to the body). Both acetaminophen and NSAIDs have demonstrated benefit as first-line medications for short term pain relief (6).

National evidence-based practice recommendations for patients with subacute (6 to 12 weeks after onset) or chronic LBP (more than 3 months after onset) include spinal manipulation; intensive interdisciplinary rehabilitation; exercise therapy; acupuncture; massage therapy; yoga; cognitive-behavioral therapy; or progressive relaxation (6).

It is not recommended that physicians obtain radiological or laboratory evaluation routinely on patients with nonspecific (anatomical pathophysiology undefined) acute LBP (6). This includes patients with somatic dysfunction and no symptoms or signs of radiculopathy below the knee or evidence of organic or spinal pathology. It is recommended to obtain radiological evaluation (e.g., lumbar spine x-rays, A-P and lateral views, MRI, CT) if the LBP persists beyond 6 weeks, which is the average time frame of resolution of acute symptoms, or if there are signs of radiculopathy, or severe or progressive neurological deficits (6). Diagnostic imaging is also indicated when serious underlying conditions are suspected on the basis of the history and physical examination (6). Electromyograms and Nerve Conduction Studies (EMG/NCS) are useful if radiculopathy distal to the knee occurs. Refer patients with radiculopathy below the knee to a pain management specialist for epidural steroid injections or a surgeon for potential definitive intervention is appropriate (6). Assess for symptoms and signs of severe or progressive neurological deficits (i.e., bowel or bladder incontinence or change in lower limb muscle strength and sensation) at each office visit. Refer to a spine surgeon if there are signs of severe or progressive neurological deficits (6).

DIFFERENTIAL DIAGNOSIS

A patient's LBP can be defined as either acute or chronic. In general, acute LBP is self-limiting, and if it lasts longer than 3 months, it can be classified as chronic in nature (6). While this is a broad generalization, it can be a helpful one, since the diagnosis, prognosis, and treatment of acute versus chronic LBP differ from one another. It is important to keep in mind, however, that up to one third of patients presenting with LBP will have a recurrent, episodic clinical course over their lifetime (7).

This patient presents a clinical example of a patient with acute LBP, although he has had episodes of back pain with and without radiculopathy in the past. He currently has no symptoms of pain radiating past his knee, but the physical exam did find dermatome-specific signs of decreased sensation in his foot. This could be residual from previous injury or part of the current clinical picture. Since other neurological tests, including lower extremity motor, sensory and reflex exams, were within normal parameters, continued follow-up exams at each visit to document improvement, stability, or progression of this sensory deficit is indicated. EMG/NCS and diagnostic imaging would assist in the diagnosis if the deficit persists or progresses.

In developing a differential diagnosis, it is helpful to characterize the patient's LBP as localized or referred. Localized pathophysiology can be categorized as mechanical or nonmechanical. Even though it is often times not possible to define the exact etiology of LBP, up to 97% of LBP is mechanical in nature (8). Mechanical etiologies can cause pain in the low back region, or the pain may radiate to one or both legs or feet, that is, cause radiculopathy. LBP that is accompanied with radicular symptoms is usually indicative of nerve root irritation or compression. Patients who are experiencing radicular symptoms typically report pain that is "burning" or "shooting" in nature and travels into the leg and below the knee. On the other hand, nonradicular mechanical LBP tends to be characterized as "aching" or throbbing" in nature and may radiate into the gluteal or upper thigh region, but not usually below the knee. There are also nonmechanical causes of LBP. These include infections, inflammation, and cancer. Psychological issues may also play a significant role (6). Lastly, LBP may be referred from another site. This type of pain can be visceral or retroperitoneal in origin and although rare, it should not be missed, as it may be indicative of a serious disease process, such as gastrointestinal or renal disease or abdominal aortic aneurysm. Tables 69.1 and 69.2 categorize the differential diagnosis for LBP and provide a means by which the osteopathic physician can stratify it.

As can be discerned from Tables 69.1 and 69.2, the patient does not have history or physical findings of any of the pathological conditions listed; however, the history and physical do support the diagnosis of somatic dysfunction. Thus, the osteopathic physician

TABLE 69.1

Differential Diagnosis of LBP

	Characteristics	Labs/imaging
Localized LBP—Mechanical without Radiation Below the Knee		
Nonspecific–muscular and ligamentous injury	Localized to low back and buttocks Better with lying down and change of position Worse with activity Cyclic in nature Intact neurological function	Typically none
Somatic dysfunction	Asymmetry of structural position Altered range of motion Tissue texture abnormalities Tenderness Resolves with OMT	Typically none
Degenerative disc disease	Localized to low back and buttocks Better with lying down and change of position Worse with prolonged standing or sitting Chronic > acute	Lumbar films: A/P and lateral views MRI
Degenerative joint disease—facet arthropathy	Localized to low back and buttocks Better with lying down and change of position Worse with spinal extension Chronic > acute	Lumbar films: A/P and lateral views MRI
Fracture: Vertebral Spondylolysis	Acute > chronic Compression fracture: history of osteoporosis or trauma Pars interarticularis fracture: new-onset LBP in athletically active adolescent or history of trauma	Lumbar films: A/P, lateral and oblique views CT
Localized LBP-mechanical with pain radiation below the knee		
Radiculopathy	Leg pain that radiates below the knee Pain with dermatomal distribution Neurological function may be impaired: Lower extremity weakness Diminished reflexes	MRI

Spinal stenosis	Bilateral lower limb pain
	Neurogenic claudication
	Neurological function may be impaired:
	    Lower extremity weakness
	    Diminished reflexes
		MRI

Cauda equina syndrome	Impaired neurological function:
	    Saddle anesthesia
	    Lower extremity weakness
	    Diminished reflexes
	    Urinary retention
		MRI

(continued)

TABLE 69.1	(Continued)		
Localized LBP—nonmechanical			
Infection:	Pain at rest or night		CBC, Blood cultures MRI
Osteomyelitis	Fever		
Discitis	Recent skin infection or UTI or IVDA		
Neoplasm:	Pain at rest or night		MRI, CT, PSA, alkaline phosphatase
Primary: osteosarcoma, osteoid osteoma	Weight loss		
Metastatic: prostrate, breast, lung, kidney			
Multiple myeloma			
Inflammation:	Significant morning stiffness		Lumbar and pelvic films
Spondyloarthropathy—ankylosing spondylitis reactive arthritis (Reiter disease)	Sacroiliac pain		CBC, ESR, CRP, HLA-B27, Rh factor
Rheumatoid arthritis	Uveitis		
	Urethritis		
	Joint pain and swelling		
Referred LBP			
Gastrointestinal disease:	Abdominal pain, tenderness, distention		Abdominal films, US, CT
Inflammatory bowel disease			CBC, amylase/lipase
Diverticulitis	Hematochezia		
Pancreatitis			
Renal Disease:	Abdominal pain		US, CT
Nephrolithiasis Pyelonephritis	Hematuria		UA
Gynecological:	Pelvic pain		US
Endometriosis	Cyclical in nature		
Menstrual	Dysmenorrhea		
Vascular:	"Ripping" or "tearing"-like abdominal pain		US, CT
Abdominal aortic aneurysm	Pulsatile abdominal mass		
Psychological:	Disproportionate pain		Typically none
Somatoform disorder			
Malingering			
Central sensitization/chronic pain syndrome			

A/P, anterior/posterior; CBC, complete blood count; CRP, C-reactive protein; CT, computerized tomography; ESR, erythrocyte sedimentation rate; HLA-B27, Human leukocyte antigen-B27; IVDA, intravenous drug abuse; MRI, magnetic resonance imaging; OMT, osteopathic manipulative treatment; PSA, prostatic specific antigen; Rh, rheumatoid; UA, urinalysis; US, ultrasound; UTI, urinary tract infection.

can be confident in making that diagnosis and provide appropriate OMT as part of the management plan.

OSTEOPATHIC PATIENT MANAGEMENT

Biomechanical Model

As stated above, the majority of LBP is mechanical in origin. In general, mechanical LBP is improved with rest and exacerbated with activity. Although the etiology of mechanical LBP can at times be identified, such as with degenerative disc and joint disease, the vast majority of the time it is not. In the setting of a poorly defined etiology, it is thought that injury of muscular and ligamentous structures plays an important role. It likely involves injury of muscle fibers at the musculotendinous junction that is precipitated by physical activity. The musculature of the lumbar spine can be classified as being anterior or posterior. The anterior musculature comprises the abdominal and iliopsoas muscles. Abdominal muscles include the rectus abdominis, external and internal oblique, and transverses abdominis muscles. These muscles act in concert with one another to produce flexion of the lumbar spine. While it is unlikely that they are a source for LBP, these muscles are very important in providing core stability and are of benefit to strengthen in patients with LBP. Iliopsoas is located deep within the abdomen and pelvis, originating along the lateral aspects of the lumbar vertebrae and intervertebral discs and the iliac fossa and inserting on the lesser trochanter of the femur. It is the primary flexor of the hip

TABLE 69.2

Structure/Function Model of Differential Diagnosis of LBP

	Red Flags: Spinal Pathology (Mechanical)	Somatic Dysfunction (Mechanical, amenable to OMT)	LBP Work-related (Behavioral)	LBP radiating below knee (Neurological)	Inflammatory Disorder (Metabolic)
History	• Age of presentation <20 or onset >55 • Violent trauma, e.g., fall from height, MVA • Constant, progressive, nonmechanical pain • Thoracic pain • Past history of carcinoma • Systemic corticosteroids • Drug abuse • HIV • Difficulty with micturition • Fecal incontinence	• Aged 20–55 • Pain may be in lumbar and sacral spine, buttocks and thighs; does not radiate below knee • Mechanical in nature • Lifting and twisting • Pain varies with physical activity and time	• Postural stress • Whole-body vibration • Monotonous work • Lack of personal control • Low job satisfaction • Smoking	• Unilateral leg pain > back pain • Pain generally radiates to foot or toes • Numbness and paresthesias in the same dermatome distribution	• Gradual onset • Marked morning stiffness • Family history
Physical	• Systemically unwell • Weight loss • Persisting severe restriction of lumbar flexion • Structural deformity • Loss of anal sphincter tone • Saddle anesthesia around the anus, perineum or genital • Widespread (>one nerve root) or progressive motor weakness in the legs or gait disturbance	• Patient well • Lumbosacral spine and/or pelvis somatic dysfunction present	• Low physical fitness • Inadequate trunk strength	• Nerve root irritation signs • Reduced SLR which reproduces leg pain • Motor, sensory or reflex change is limited to one nerve root	• Iritis, skin rashes (psoriasis), colitis, urethra discharge • Persisting limitation of spinal movements in all directions • Peripheral joint involvement
Lab and x-ray	• X-ray: look for vertebral collapse or bone destruction • CT or MRI: look for cauda equina compression	• Nondiagnostic	• Nondiagnostic	• Nondiagnostic or MRI: look for disc herniation with compression of peripheral nerve root	• Nondiagnostic or blood tests: look for Rh factor or seronegative arthropathy; ESR > 25 • X-ray shows evidence of arthritis
Course	• If pain not resolved in 6 wk, an ESR and x-ray should be considered	• Prognosis good • 90% recover from acute attack in 6 wk; but most recur throughout life • Manipulation and exercise provide pain relief, improved mobility and may shorten course	• Usually resolves within 6 wk • Responsive to manipulation and exercise, and use of proper posture and ergonomics • Potential for prolonged recovery if there is secondary gain involved	• Prognosis reasonable • 50% recover from acute attack within 6 wk	• Usually resolves with anti-inflammatory medication • Episodic

joint and can act as a lumbar flexor when the hips are fixed. Because it is a postural muscle, it is prone to shortening in the absence of activity. This leads to decreased hip extension and increased lumbar lordosis and anterior pelvic tilt, which may predispose a patient to develop lumbar and pelvic somatic dysfunction and LBP. The posterior muscles are subdivided into superficial, intermediate, and deep layers. The superficial layer comprises the lumbodorsal fascia. This expansive layer of connective tissue provides stability for the thoracolumbar and pelvic regions, as well continuity with the upper limb via its connection with the latissimus dorsi muscle. The intermediate layer consists of the iliocostalis, longissimus, and spinalis muscles. These erector spinae muscles function bilaterally to produce extension and unilaterally to produce sidebending of the lumbar spine. The deep layer consists of those muscles responsible for localized vertebral movement, including lateral flexion (sidebending) with contralateral rotation. They include the multifidi, rotators, and intertransversarii muscles. The deep layer also contains the quadratus lumborum muscle, which connects the pelvis to the spine and produces lumbar extension when contracting bilaterally. If it undergoes overuse due to deconditioning of the erector spinae muscles, it can be a potential source of LBP.

Just as injury to muscle fibers can cause mechanical LBP, so too can injury to ligamentous structures. Like muscle injury, ligamentous injury is characterized by pain that can be either dull and aching or sharp in nature. Two of the most important ligaments are the anterior and posterior longitudinal ligaments, which traverse the respective surfaces of the vertebral bodies and intervertebral discs. They provide stability and respectively prevent hyperextension and hyperflexion of the spine. The posterior longitudinal ligament is of particular interest due to its location within the spinal canal. Its position helps prevent posterior displacement of the intervertebral disc. Because it is richly innervated with nociceptors, it can be a source for LBP (9). It can also succumb to different disease processes, such as ossification, which can cause other disorders of the spine, including spinal stenosis. Like the posterior longitudinal ligament, the ligamentum flavum, which connects the laminae of adjacent vertebrae, is susceptible to ossification. However, since it contains few nociceptors, it is not considered to be an important pain generator.

Because the precise anatomical source of mechanical LBP is not identifiable in the majority of patients, the physical examination is often times used to exclude serious underlying pathology and confirm the diagnosis. In the absence of well-defined spinal pathology and with signs of TART indicative of somatic dysfunction, osteopathic physicians consider somatic dysfunction as the cause of the LBP if its alleviation with OMT relieves the pain and restores normal function.

In addition to assessing the lumbar region for tissue texture changes, asymmetry, increased or decreased range of motion and tenderness, the physical examination should include an assessment of gait and posture, neurological function of the lower limbs, and appropriate provocative tests, such as the straight leg raise and FABERE (hip flexion, abduction, external rotation, and extension) tests. Abdominal and rectal examinations may also be indicated if intra-abdominal or pelvic pathology are suspected. With the continuity that exists between the lower limbs and pelvis and lumbar spine, it is useful to perform an evaluation of gait, as it may give insight into the etiology of the patient's LBP. For example, a patient with a radiculopathy affecting the 5th lumbar nerve root may have weakness of his ankle dorsiflexors that is demonstrated high steppage by gait. Although it is almost always normal in patients with nonradiating mechanical LBP, a neurological examination is essential when assessing any patient with LBP. It involves assessing motor strength and sensation for the L1 to L5 myotomes

and dermatomes, as well as the Achilles and patellar muscle stretch reflexes. The straight leg raising test, as well as other nerve stretching maneuvers (e.g., flexing the knee and passively dorsiflexing the ipsilateral ankle, or squeezing the ipsilateral calf along the midline course of the sciatic nerve), is useful for assessing sciatic nerve inflammation or irritation.

Somatic Dysfunction

Since up to 70% of mechanical LBP may be due to somatic dysfunction, performing an osteopathic structural examination can be quite useful (1). As with other regions of the body, lumbar somatic dysfunction is characterized by asymmetry of structural position, altered range of motion, and palpable tissue texture abnormalities and/or tenderness. There are three primary anatomic sites of somatic dysfunction in the lumbo-sacral-pelvic region that can cause LBP and are amenable to treatment with OMM. Surrounding soft tissues, e.g., lumbar myofascial paraspinal tissues and lumbosacral-pelvic ligaments, are often treated along with the specific lumbar, sacral, or pelvic joint somatic dysfunctions. Box 69.1 lists the soft tissue elements often addressed with OMT, and Table 69.3 lists the three types of somatic dysfunction commonly associated with LBP and the types of segmental somatic dysfunction that are typically found with each one.

As with all osteopathic structural examinations, evaluation of the lumbar spine for segmental somatic dysfunction requires proficiency in palpating the appropriate anatomical landmarks and performing a regional and segmental examination.

From a biomechanical perspective, treatment of LBP seeks to address somatic dysfunction and restore posture and balance so as to allow the musculoskeletal system to operate more efficiently and with less pain. This entails not only addressing lumbar somatic dysfunction, but somatic dysfunction elsewhere in the body, particularly the spine, pelvis, and lower extremities. Because the spine works a functional unit, treating somatic dysfunction that exists in the thoracic and cervical spine will ideally allow for restoration of normal spinal motion. Likewise, the aim of treating lower extremity somatic dysfunction is to improve posture and balance and allow the body to more efficiently cope with the forces of gravity during sitting, standing, and ambulation. Certain anatomic structures that are known to cause or exacerbate LBP should be taken into account when formulating an osteopathic treatment plan. These structures, which are amenable to manipulation, include the lumbar intervertebral joints, myofascial paraspinal soft tissues, sacroiliac joints and iliosacral joints, and lumbosacral and lumbopelvic ligaments.

Muscles, Fascia, and Ligaments (Soft Tissues) Commonly Associated with Lumbosacral Somatic Dysfunctions in Patients with LBP

Superficial layer:
- Lumbodorsal fascia

Intermediate layer:
- Erector spinae

Deep layer:
- Multifidi
- Rotatores
- Intertransversarii
- Pelvic Diaphragm
- Quadratus lumborum

Lower extremities:
- "Hamstrings"
- Piriformis
- Psoas-Iliacus
- Gluteal muscles

Ligaments:
- Interspinous
- Iliolumbar
- Sacroiliac
- Sacrotuberous

TABLE 69.3

Somatic Dysfunctions Associated with LBP

Lumbar Vertebral Joint Somatic Dysfunctions	Lumbosacral—Pelvic (Sacroiliac) Dysfunctions	Ilium—Pelvic (Iliosacral and Pubic) Dysfunctions
Type I: • Neutral, sidebent left or right *Type II:* • Flexed or Extended, rotated and sidebent right or left	• Sacral Torsion (L/L; L/R; R/L; R/R) • Bilateral or Unilateral Sacral Flexion or Extension • Lumbosacral joint compression • Unlevel sacral base due to anatomic short leg	• Superior or inferior ilial shear • Anterior or posterior rotated ilium • Inflared or outflared ilium • Superior or inferior pubic symphysis shear

Soft tissue and myofascial techniques such as lumbar prone pressure with counter leverage and lumbosacral decompression can be used to address increased tension of the lumbar paraspinal musculature and lack of compliance in the tissues surrounding the lumbosacral junction. Sidelying lumbar articulatory or HVLA technique is useful for treating lumbar segmental dysfunction at L5. With respect to pelvic dysfunction, muscle energy technique can be used to treat sacral torsions and counterstrain technique for piriformis somatic dysfunction. Care should also be taken to address somatic dysfunction outside of the lumbar and pelvis regions. This may entail treating dysfunction at the atlantooccipital (OA) joint with HVLA and decompression of the OA joint, as well as treating knee or ankle somatic dysfunction with counterstrain technique. This again will allow the osteopathic physician to address somatic dysfunction that may have predisposed the patient to develop LBP and be interfering with structural balance.

Degenerative Disc and Joint Disease

Spondylosis is a term that is used to describe degenerative changes of the spine, including degenerative disc and joint disease. It tends to affect the lumbar spine in particular due to its mobile nature and load bearing responsibilities. There are five lumbar vertebrae, each of which is separated by an intervertebral disc. Each vertebra consists of a body and vertebral arch. The vertebral arch is further composed of a pair of pedicles and laminae and supports a number of additional structures, including the inferior and superior articular processes, transverse processes, and spinous process. It forms the intervertebral foramen, through which the spinal nerves exit, and helps protect the spinal by cord by forming part of the spinal canal. The vertebrae articulate with one another via the fibrocartilaginous intervertebral disc and synovial facet joints, which exist on the inferior and superior articular processes. The disc consists of an outer fibrocartilaginous ring, the annulus fibrosis, and inner gelatinous mass, the nucleus pulposus. It acts as a dampening mechanism for forces transmitted along the vertebral column, while simultaneously allowing for movement between the individual vertebrae. Disease or injury to any of these structures can potentially lead to instability of the lumbar spine and LBP. While injuries such as fracture of the vertebral body or arch tend to result in acute LBP, spondylosis tends to be associated with chronic LBP. In general, it is a natural part of the aging process and by 49 years of age, 60% of women and 80% of men have osteophytes and other changes indicative of spondylosis (10). As with acute LBP due to muscular and ligamentous injury, back pain due to degenerative changes is difficult to localize and symptoms and signs tend to be nonspecific. Additionally, radiological findings, both on MRI and plain films, must be interpreted with caution, since there is poor correlation between radiographic degenerative changes and LBP. For example, disc herniation on lumbar MRI is a common finding in asymptomatic patients (11,12).

Piriformis Syndrome

Although it is not part of the musculature or ligamentous structures of the lumbar spine, the piriformis muscle should be a consideration in the differential diagnosis of LBP due to the fact that pain associated with its dysfunction can be interpreted as low back in origin. Typically, piriformis syndrome–type pain is characterized by aching pain in the gluteal region, especially at the attachment sites of the piriformis muscle. Patients complain of increasing pain after sitting for longer than 15 to 20 minutes. Additionally, because of the close proximity of the piriformis muscle to the sciatic nerve, patients can report parasthesias that radiate down the posterior aspect of the thigh. Having an appreciation for the anatomy of the piriformis muscle, as well as its surrounding structures, is helpful in understanding the possible pathophysiology behind piriformis syndrome and physical examination findings. The piriformis muscle originates on the anterior surface of the sacrum and passes through the sciatic notch before inserting on the upper aspect of the greater trochanter. It is innervated by the first and second sacral nerves and primarily acts as an external rotator of the hip joint. With the hip flexed to 90 degrees, it acts as an abductor of the hip. It is an important structure since all neurovascular structures that exit from the pelvis via the greater sciatic notch do so either inferior or superior to the piriformis muscle. This includes the inferior and superior gluteal nerve and artery and pudendal and sciatic nerves. Even though the mechanism of sciatica or radicular type pain in piriformis syndrome is not completely understood, it is thought that the sciatic nerve may become impinged or compressed by the piriformis muscle. This may be secondary to trauma, such as falling on the buttock, or overuse, both of which can result in inflammation of surrounding tissues and spasm of the piriformis muscle. Additionally, in some patients, the sciatic nerve may pierce the piriformis muscle, rendering the sciatic nerve more susceptible to entrapment and injury. Regardless of the etiology, piriformis syndrome is usually characterized by tenderness in the region of the greater sciatic foramen. Provocative maneuvers that evaluate for piriformis syndrome attempt to induce radicular-type pain by either active contraction of the piriformis muscle in resistance or passively stretching it (13). The straight leg raise test may be positive in piriformis syndrome, but is nonspecific since it does not localize where the nerve is compressed and is typically more indicative of nerve root compression. In the supine position, a patient may exhibit external rotation of the affected lower limb and range of motion testing may reveal decreased internal rotation of the affected side. The sacrum is typically rotated anteriorly toward the ipsilateral side on a contralateral oblique axis, resulting in compensatory rotation of the lower lumbar vertebrae in the opposite direction (14).

Sacroiliac Joint Pain

Although the sacrum and sacroiliac joints are technically part of the pelvis, they warrant mention here since pain due to dysfunction of these structures can be difficult to distinguish from pain originating in the lumbar spine. In fact, the prevalence of sacroiliac joint pain, as established on the basis of clinical evaluation, varies from 15% to 30% in patients with LBP (15). The sacrum is a triangular-shaped bone that is formed from the fusion of five sacral vertebrae. It articulates with the ilium bones at the sacroiliac joints and fifth lumbar vertebra via the last lumbar intervertebral disc and facet joints. The sacroiliac joints are L-shaped synovial joints that are stabilized by a combination of bony structure and strong ligamentous structures, including the anterior and posterior sacroiliac and sacrotuberous ligaments. As with the lumbar spine, injury, inflammation, degeneration, and somatic dysfunction of the sacroiliac joints can result in LBP. Like mechanical LBP, sacroiliac pain can also be nonspecific and refer to a variety of places, including the low back, buttock, groin, and lower extremity (16). The International Association for the Study of Pain suggests incorporating at least three selective sacroiliac joint stress tests in order to more clearly diagnose sacroiliac pain. These provocative tests include compression, distraction, thigh thrust, Gaenslen test, and Patrick sign. Lastly, performing a pelvic regional and segmental examination is useful in diagnosing sacroiliac and iliosacral somatic dysfunction that may be responsible for a patient's LBP and amenable to treatment with OMM.

Coccydynia

Coccydynia or pain associated with the coccyx (tailbone). The coccyx is located at the terminal end of the spinal column and is specifically attached at the distal sacrum. It usually consists of three to five segments that may or may not be fused. Pain in this area is uncommon. The complaint of pain may follow from sacral trauma (falls onto the buttocks, post childbirth, severe cases of whiplash). Pain is made worse with sitting or having pressure applied to this area and is reduced or relieved with standing or the reduction of pressure to the coccyx. Treatments used to relieve the symptoms depend upon the knowledge base of the practitioner and include OMT in an attempt to reposition the coccyx to its normal position by using either direct or indirect MFR or an assessment and treatment of the sacrum and pelvis to correct any associated dysfunctions. Strain/Counterstrain, balanced ligamentous tension, or a direct pressure applied to the sacrococcygeal ligaments to relieve strains that might be present can be effective. Other techniques utilized include hot packs, ultrasound (US), sitz baths or towels, acupuncture, and injections into the ganglion impar. Strategies used to reduce the pain include the use of pillows or "donuts" to minimize the pressure against the coccyx and also the reduction of time spent in the seated position.

Psoas Syndrome

A chronic psoas spasm can create a persistent strain across the lumbosacral junction and impede resolution of lumbosacral somatic dysfunction in spite of OMT and exercises directed at the L-S region. Treatment of the psoas by relieving the thoracolumbar junction and upper lumbar somatic dysfunction and stretching a hypertonic psoas muscle facilitates resolution of a long-standing lumbosacral somatic dysfunction. Commonly, the L1 or L2 vertebra is flexed and rotated to the side of the shortened, hypertonic psoas muscle. In the patient above, the thoracolumbar junction has two type I curves, one superior and the other inferior, to the thoracolumbar junction. This indicates a long-term somatic dysfunction in that region, as type I group dysfunctions are often compensatory changes to a longstanding type II segmental dysfunction. Treating the type I spinal somatic dysfunctions with OMT as well as stretching the tight psoas muscle would be a reasonable approach in this patient.

Short Leg Syndrome and LBP

Patients with anatomic short leg syndrome often have sacral base unleveling and sacroiliac and lumbosacral joint dysfunction and pain. (See chapters 41 and 42 for more information regarding anatomic short leg diagnosis and treatment with lift therapy). OMT combined with lift therapy has been shown to relieve LBP in many of these patients (17–19).

Respiratory/Circulatory Model

From a respiratory/circulatory perspective, maximizing oxygenation and delivery of nutrients facilitate the recovery of tissues that may have been injured or compromised in a patient with LBP. Therefore, patients may benefit from OMM that addresses somatic dysfunction of the thoracic diaphragm and pelvic diaphragms and costal cage. The upper lumbar vertebral bodies serve as the sites of insertion for the diaphragm. The diaphragm is most efficient when the lumbar spine is in its natural lordosis in the seated or standing positions. An important goal of osteopathic management therefore is to restore lumbar lordosis to maximize diaphragmatic function. As important as the thoracolumbar junction is to diaphragmatic activity, similarly, normal lumbosacral mechanics are key for pelvic diaphragm function. With each breath, the sacrum should be able to oscillate in its articulation with the ilia. The second sacral segment serves as the attachment of the spinal dura, which is also attached firmly to C1, C2, and the occiput at the foramen magnum. Thus, somatic dysfunction of the lumbosacral spine and sacroiliac joints has an effect upon mechanics in distal spinal segments as well as in the cranium through this "core link" of spinal dura. (see chapter 48). Primary respiratory mechanism motions at the sacrum as well as the occiput are compromised by lumbosacral somatic dysfunction. Evaluating and treating the sacral and occipital somatic dysfunctions using balanced ligamentous tension and osteopathy in the cranial field techniques will improve the motions related to the primary respiratory mechanism and the natural respiratory mobility of the sacrum.

In addition to receiving OMM, patients can benefit from regular cardiovascular exercise. There is evidence supporting the fact that patients with acute, nonspecific LBP who stay active have reduced pain and improvement in function compared to patients who receive bed rest (23).

Neurological Model

Neurogenic LBP is characterized by involvement of the nerve roots, cauda equina, or spinal cord. Symptoms include unilateral or bilateral radiation of pain or parasthesias distal to the knee, or muscle weakness, which may include loss of bowel and bladder sphincter control in the case of cauda equine syndrome. It is far less common than mechanical LBP and comprises approximately

5% to 15% of LBP cases. Because it usually involves compression of a neural structure, it is typically associated with demonstrable pathology, including disc herniation or spondylosis. The two most common types of neurogenic LBP are lumbar radiculopathy and spinal stenosis. The prevalence of lumbar radiculopathy is approximately 3% to 5%, with L5 and S1 radiculopathies comprising 90% of all lumbosacral radiculopathies (20). Unlike mechanical LBP, in which pain is mediated by the anterior and posterior rami of the spinal nerves or sinuvertebral nerves, radicular pain is mediated by the proximal spinal nerves. Radicular pain also differs from mechanical LBP in that the symptoms and signs are more specific and tend to point to a diagnosis of lumbar radiculopathy. Patients describe radicular pain as "burning" or "shooting" in nature and traveling into the leg and foot, sometimes following a dermatomal distribution. Neural tension signs, such as the straight leg test, are helpful in determining if there is compression of a lumbar nerve root. The supine straight leg test has a sensitivity of 91% and specificity of 26%, indicating that when it is negative, a diagnosis of lumbar radiculopathy can be reasonably excluded (21). Because spinal pathology is often present, MRI of the lumbar spine is useful. MRI has been shown to have a sensitivity of 83% and specificity of 78% when assessing for compromise of a neural structure in the lumbar spine (22). However, due to the fact that it is common to find abnormalities such as bulging or protruding discs in asymptomatic patients, it is important to correlate imaging findings with the history and physical examination. A detailed neurologic examination is imperative not only to establish a diagnosis, but to also evaluate for serious findings that may warrant immediate intervention. These can include saddle anesthesia, bladder or bowel dysfunction, or progressive neurological deficits in the lower limbs. These findings must also be kept in mind when evaluating a patient with lumbar spinal stenosis, which is usually the result of spondylosis. Symptomatic lumbar spinal stenosis is characterized by neurogenic claudication, which is defined as aching pain in the lower limbs that is precipitated by walking or standing and alleviated with rest and flexion of the trunk. Somatic dysfunction is often times present in patients with neurogenic LBP. It may be primary in nature or secondary to compression of lumbar spine nerve roots. In secondary somatic dysfunction, nerve root irritation and its associated spinal pathology may be causing spinal facilitation, which in turn leads to maintenance of the somatic dysfunction.

The neurological model takes into consideration the integration of central, peripheral, and autonomic nervous systems and how they may be impacted by somatic dysfunction. Since mechanical LBP is often due to somatic dysfunction, it improves with OMT. This, however, does not mean that neurogenic or nonmechanical LBP cannot be helped with OMT. In these situations, it can be helpful in addressing facilitated segments that are due to nonmechanical pathology. OMT can be helpful in providing information regarding the source of the referred pain. Addressing somatic dysfunction in these cases will ideally lead to a reduction in mechanical stress and the nociceptive input associated with it. This in turn will potentially decrease peripheral sensitization and will in turn lead to decreased spinal facilitation and subsequent improvement in lumbar segmental motion. Also, with decreased pain, the patient may perceive less stress and achieve more balanced function of the autonomic nervous system and neuroendocrine immune network. The body will have a decrease in neuroendocrine activation of the hypothalamic-adrenal axis, resulting in decreased cortisol production and sympathetic tone which will restore autonomic balance. The allostatic load will be diminished, leading to a restoration of homeostasis.

Metabolic-Energy Model

The metabolic, energy expenditure and exchange perspective entails maximizing internal organ functions to support recovery from somatic dysfunction or pathological conditions causing or related to the LBP. Using analgesic medications such as NSAIDs to modulate the pain impulses facilitates healing by decreasing inflammation and allowing the patient to stay active and continue normal daily activities. Bed rest beyond three days is not recommended for patients with acute LBP as muscles begin to atrophy and weaken, impeding healing and recovery of normal function. Rheumatologic conditions are primarily managed with medications, though osteopathic manipulation may have an adjunctive role (30). An inflamed joint, such as the sacroiliac joint (sacroiliitis) found in patients with ankylosing spondylitis, should not be manipulated with direct action OMT as this will aggravate the condition. However, OMT designed to improve lymphatic drainage of swollen joints without moving the joint, and nociceptor "afferent reduction" techniques such as functional, balanced ligamentous tension, and strain-counterstrain may be helpful.

Behavioral Model

The patient evaluated has somatic dysfunction from mechanical LBP. LBP is one of the most common complaints in the outpatient clinic. With a lifetime prevalence of 49% to 70%, most adults will experience an episode of LBP at some point in their life (24). LBP is the third most commonly reported symptom, the second most frequent cause of worker absenteeism, and the most costly ailment of working-age adults in the United States (7). It causes more disability among working-age adults than any other disability and is the most common ailment of working-age adults in the United States (7). Some of the largest components of direct costs include physical therapy, inpatient care, pharmacy, and primary care (25). The economic burden of LBP, both in terms of direct and indirect costs, is great. The combined direct and indirect costs due to LBP are estimated to be $50 billion (26). Incorporating OMM may allow the osteopathic physician to more efficiently manage patients with LBP and therefore reduce direct costs. It may also help patients return to work earlier and experience a greater sense of satisfaction with their treatment (1).

LBP affects males and females of all ages, disabling those in the 35 to 54 years of age, and also is found in 30% to 50% of teenagers aged 13 to 18 (1,7). Risk factors for the development of acute LBP include increasing age, demanding physical activity (bending, twisting, and lifting movements and prolonged standing), and psychological factors (work dissatisfaction or monotonous work) (1,7). The strongest known predictor of a future episode of LBP is the history of previous episodes (7). Fortunately, the majority of acute back pain cases resolve within 6 weeks, but one third may continue to have intermittent, episodic recurrences (7). When LBP becomes chronic in nature, typically lasting longer than 6 months in duration, certain risk factors may have a more important role. These include a prior episode of LBP, poor job satisfaction, smoking, and poor coping skills. Comorbid conditions are commonly found in chronic LBP patients, and psychological factors play a greater role than anatomical pathology in predicting persistent LBP (7,27).

Age is an important consideration when evaluating a patient with LBP. For example, the patient's age in and of itself leads the physician toward a particular diagnosis. Because of the anatomical differences in the adolescent and adult spine, each is susceptible to different spinal pathologies. The adolescent spine is still growing and its primary and secondary centers of ossification remain active, and in the setting of trauma or significant physical activity, this can predispose the adolescent to such spinal disorders as spondylolysis and spondylolisthesis, which can be a significant cause of LBP and instability. On the contrary, an adult spine has a higher likelihood of having spondylosis which may or may not be related to the LBP. Females over 60 years old, as are those who are postmenopausal, are more prone to osteoporosis-related vertebral fractures as a cause of acute LBP.

The behavioral model also addresses the psychological status of a patient and how health may be affected by stress and environmental and socioeconomic factors. It is particularly important to consider in patients with LBP. Systematic review has found psychological and occupational factors to have the highest reliability among prognostic factors with LBP (28). These factors are important to consider in patients with acute LBP, as they may predispose a patient to the development of chronic LBP. There is also strong evidence demonstrating that expectation of recovery is a predictor of work outcome in patients with nonspecific LBP (29). Therefore, it is important to not only understand the life stressors and job satisfaction of patients, but also their expectations and goals with respect to recovering from LBP. Encouraging and assisting the patient in restricting abuse of tobacco and alcohol, engaging in regular exercises, and maintaining normal body weight range will aid in restoration of normal low back neuromusculoskeletal function.

PATIENT OUTCOME

After receiving OMT, the patient noted a reduction in his LBP. He was able to walk and sit without pain and no longer required the use of NSAIDs for pain relief. He was also able to once again sleep comfortably on his back and the right lower limb numbness had nearly resolved.

Treatment focused on resolving somatic dysfunction and addressing postural decompensation. Attention was given to restoring postural balance by correcting thoracic, lumbar, and sacral somatic dysfunctions. The patient's sacral torsion and hypertonic piriformis muscle were treated. Physical therapy aimed at restoring the flexibility and strength of the psoas, erector spinae, and abdominal musculature facilitated restoration of the patient's lumbar lordosis and he reported diminished tenderness in the area of the iliolumbar ligament.

An MRI of the lumbar spine showed a 2-mm broad based protrusion of the L5-S1 disc with mild right-sided neuroforamenal stenosis at L5. EMG and nerve conduction studies were normal. Spinal somatic dysfunction improved with OMT, indicating no persistent viscerosomatic reflexes.

Treatment also addressed somatic dysfunction of the thoracic diaphragm and 12th rib, as well as surrounding structures connecting the costal cage with the pelvis, including quadratus lumborum. This assisted in resolving somatic dysfunction within close proximity to the lumbar region. At the same time, it also helped maximize respiratory and circulatory function and improve the delivery of oxygen and nutrients to and removal of metabolic wastes from the area.

Finally, stressors and ergonomic factors were considered in order to speed recovery and prevent future episodes of LBP.

SPECIALIST REFERRAL

LBP is one of the most common reasons for a visit to the primary care physician's office. However, even more so than the primary care physician, the spine or pain management specialist routinely evaluates and manages patients with LBP. Fortunately, 90% of acute LBP and 50% of LBP with radicular symptoms resolve within 6 and 4 weeks, respectively (1). It is typically the patient who does not experience a resolution of his or her LBP who is referred to the physician specialist for further evaluation and management. Regardless of whether it is acute or chronic in nature, diagnosis of LBP is oftentimes complex and requires thorough knowledge of the functional anatomy of the lumbar region and pathophysiology of LBP. This must be integrated with an understanding of the risk factors associated with developing LBP and prognostic factors for recovering from it. For example, the overall health and well-being of a patient are important predictors of back pain (31). Additionally, the risk of developing LBP is approximately double for those with a history of LBP, indicating that it may be less likely to spontaneously resolve and more recurrent in nature than once thought (32). Therefore, when performing an evaluation, the physician specialist must not only have an appreciation for the complex etiology of LBP, but also the overall patient and his or her experiences with it.

When evaluating the patient with LBP, one of the most important factors to consider is age. Because certain age groups are more prone to develop certain lumbar spine pathology than others, it is helpful to stratify a patient by age in order to simplify the potential causes of the LBP and eliminate more serious conditions, such as fracture, tumor, or infection. This may be particularly true given the fact that a clear diagnosis of LBP cannot be determined in 85% of patients, given the poor association between symptoms, pathologic changes, and imaging results (33). Although the focus of this chapter is on the evaluation and management of LBP in the adult population, it is important to be able to recognize the primary causes of LBP in the adolescent patient, especially those actively involved in athletics. Unlike adults, it appears that adolescents, particularly those below the age of twelve, have an identifiable cause for their LBP 45% to 50% of the time (34). This is especially true for lumbar spondylolysis, which accounts for 47% of LBP in adolescent athletes versus 5% in adult athletes (35). When evaluating an adolescent, it is therefore important to have a high index of suspicion for an identifiable cause of LBP and low threshold for ordering diagnostic imaging studies, including plain films, CT, and MRI.

As with the adolescent patient, it is also useful for the physician spine or pain management specialist to identify as best possible the anatomical structure responsible for an adult patient's LBP. This can be quite challenging due to the number of structures that can be involved, including lumbar spine musculature, nerves, discs, and zygapophysial joints. Like other regions of the spine, evaluation should begin with a history and physical examination. This includes defining the duration, location, and quality of the LBP, as well as the factors that alleviate and exacerbate it. As mentioned before, it is valuable to gain an overall sense of the patient, their psychological health, and how they are functioning with their pain, since these influence their prognosis for recovery.

As mentioned in the differential diagnosis section, when characterizing pain, it can be particularly helpful to distinguish it as being either mechanical or neuropathic in nature. Mechanical LBP is caused by involvement of the lumbar vertebrae, discs, joints, and myofascial structures, including muscles and ligaments. It is dull and aching in nature, exacerbated with prolonged standing or sitting, and alleviated with rest. It is also typically associated with lumbar spondylosis and degenerative disease. In contrast, neuropathic pain is shooting and stabbing in nature, radiates into the lower limb and foot, and is indicative of lumbar nerve root irritation or compression. This characterization can be useful, since neuropathic or radicular pain may have a more definable cause, such as a disc herniation, and requires different treatment (36). When performing the physical examination, the physician can evaluate for lumbar nerve root compression by performing a provocative maneuver such as the straight leg raise test. In fact, in a systematic review, the straight leg raise test was found to be one of the most sensitive tests for radiculopathy (37). Other important components of the physical examination include motor strength and sensory testing and lumbar spine range of motion. The osteopathic structural exam evaluates for asymmetry of structural position, altered range of motion, and tissue texture abnormalities or tenderness.

Although it is beyond the scope of this chapter, it is also essential to evaluate the hip and sacroiliac joints, since pain in the low back can be referred from these neighboring structures. After performing a history and physical examination, diagnostic studies may be indicated to further aid in the diagnosis of LBP. The utility of MRI imaging is limited by the high prevalence of lumbar degenerative changes in adults without LBP. Research has shown that approximately 30% of adults without LBP have evidence of a protruded disc and over 50% have bulging or degenerative discs (38). If the clinical picture is consistent with lumbar spinal stenosis, however, MRI of the lumbar spine can be useful in evaluating for spinal canal narrowing. In general, spinal imaging is typically only indicated if certain conditions are suspected, including fracture, neoplasm, infection, and cauda equina syndrome. Other studies, including lumbar discography and facet injections and electromyography (EMG), can potentially be useful in confirming a diagnosis in patients suspected of having involvement of specific anatomical structures, such as the intervertebral disc or nerve root. Lumbar provocation discography is potentially a useful tool in evaluating chronic lumbar discogenic pain (39). EMG can be used to assess the physiological status of the nerves innervating the lower limbs and diagnose lumbar radiculopathy. In addition to the history and physical examination, it can be helpful in distinguishing LBP that is radicular versus nonradicular in nature. This distinction, along with an assessment for somatic dysfunction and relevant imaging studies, aids in more clearly identifying the cause of a patient's LBP and instituting appropriate treatment.

After completing clinical and diagnostic evaluation and excluding significant pathology, including cervical spine instability or an infectious, neoplastic, or inflammatory process, the physician spine or pain management specialist utilizes a variety of modalities to treat LBP, including medication, physical therapy, interventional procedures, manipulative medicine, and referral for surgical consultation. When addressing chronic LBP that is nonradicular in nature, a multidisciplinary plan that combines pharmacologic and nonpharmacologic therapy is reasonable. Nonpharmacologic therapies with evidence of moderate efficacy for chronic or subacute LBP include cognitive-behavioral therapy, exercise, spinal manipulation, and interdisciplinary rehabilitation (40). Because of compelling evidence supporting its use in the treatment of LBP, OMM should be part of most LBP treatment plans (2). This may entail the physician performing OMM or referring the patient to a neuromusculoskeletal medicine specialist. Meta-analysis of clinical trials examining the efficacy of OMM in the treatment of LBP has demonstrated decreased pain and use of medications when compared to standard medical care (2). Patients with LBP that is radicular in nature may benefit from lumbar epidural steroid injection. Systematic reviews have demonstrated level II-1 evidence for lumbar transforminal injections providing short-term relief and level II-2 for long-term improvement in the management of lumbar radicular pain (41). There is however no evidence supporting the use of these injections in nonspecific LBP. Likewise, there is no strong evidence supporting the use of injections or radiofrequency

denervation in the treatment of facet-mediated pain. If conservative treatment and interventional procedures fail, referral to a surgical specialist can be considered. This is especially true if the source of the patient's LBP is clear. For example, in patients with lumbar radiculopathy, surgery can reduce pain and improve function, and in those with disc herniation, it can facilitate a quicker return of function. A favorable outcome appears to far less likely in those patients with chronic LBP and common lumbar degenerative changes who undergo surgical intervention (42). Ultimately, it is helpful for the physician to employ specific treatment if the etiology of a patient's LBP is clear and a multidisciplinary approach that incorporates OMM if it is there is evidence of somatic dysfunction.

In July 2009, the American Osteopathic Association House of Delegates passed a resolution in support of submitting a profession-wide interdisciplinary Guideline for Utilization of OMT for patients with LBP. The guideline was based upon a systematic review and meta-analysis of randomized clinical trials of osteopathic manipulation for patients with LBP (2), as well as two other clinical practice guidelines developed by interdisciplinary groups of physicians for treatment of patients with LBP developed by the U.S. Department of Defense and Veteran's Administration in 1999 (43), and the American College of Physicians and American Pain Society in 2007 (6). The AOA's evidence-based guideline recommending that osteopathic physicians utilize OMT to treat somatic dysfunction found in patients with LBP is posted on the AOA's web site, and an abstract is available at the Agency for Healthcare Research and Quality National Guidelines Clearinghouse web site (wwww.ngc.gov) (44).

REFERENCES

1. Seffinger M, Hruby R. *Evidence-Based Manual Medicine: A Problem-Oriented Approach.* Philadelphia, PA: Saunders/Elsevier, 2007.
2. Licciardone JC, Brimhall AK, King LN. Osteopathic manipulative treatment for low back pain: a systematic review and meta-analysis of randomized controlled trials. *BMC Musculoskelet Disord* 2005;6:43.
3. AOA Guidelines For Osteopathic Manipulative Treatment For Patients With Low Back Pain, accessed January 2010. Chicago, IL: American Osteopathic Association.
4. Greenman PE. *Principles of Manual Medicine.* 3rd Ed. Philadelphia, PA: Lippincott Williams & Wilkins, 2003.
5. American Osteopathic Association. *Protocols for Osteopathic Manipulative Treatment.* Chicago, IL. Accessed from the AOA January 2010.
6. Chou R, Qaseem A, Snow V, et al. Diagnosis and treatment of low back pain: a joint clinical practice guideline from the American College of Physicians and the American Pain Society. *Ann Int Med* 2007;147: 478–491.
7. Hurwitz EL, Shekelle PG. Epidemiology of low back syndromes. In Morris CE, ed. *Low Back Syndromes: Integrated Clinical Management.* New York, NY: McGraw-Hill Publishers, 2006.
8. Deyo R, Weinstein J. Low back pain. *N Engl J Med* 2001;344:363–370.
9. Groen GJ, Baljet B, Drukker J. Nerves and nerve plexuses of the human vertebral column. *Am J Anat* 1990;188:282–296.
10. Devereaux M. Low back pain. *Med Clin North Am* 2009;93(2):477–501.
11. Jensen M, Brant-Zawadzki M, Obuchowski N, et al. Magnetic resonance imaging of the lumbar spine in people without back pain. *N Engl J Med* 1994;331:69–73.
12. Boden S, Davis D, Dina T, et al. Abnormal magnetic resonance scans of the lumbar spine in asymptomatic subjects: a prospective investigation. *J Bone Joint Surg Am* 1990;72:403–408.
13. Papadopoulos E, Khan K. Piriformis syndrome and low back pain: a new classification and review of the literature. *Orthop Clin North Am* 2004;35(1).
14. Boyajian-O'Neill L, McClain R, Coleman M, et al. Diagnosis and Management of Piriformis Syndrome: An Osteopathic Approach. *J Am Osteopath Assoc* 2008;108:657–664.

15. Szadek K, van der Wurff P, van Tulder M, et al. Diagnostic validity of criteria for sacroiliac joint pain: a systematic review. *J Pain* 2009;10(4):354–368.

16. Slipman C, Jackson H, Lipetz J, et al. Sacroiliac joint pain referral zones. *Arch Phys Med Rehabil* 2000;81:334–338.

17. Hoffman KS, Hoffman LL. Effects of adding sacral base leveling to osteopathic manipulative treatment of low back pain: a pilot study. *J Am Osteopath Assoc* 1994;94:217–226.

18. Lipton JA, et al. Lift Treatment in Naval Special Warfare (NSW) Personnel: A Retrospective Study. *Am Acad Osteopath J* 2000;(spring):31–37.

19. Lipton JA, Flowers-Johnson J, Bunnell MT, et al. The use of heel lifts and custom orthotics in reducing self-reported chronic musculoskeletal pain scores. *Am Acad Osteopath J* 2009;19(1):15–17,19–20.

20. Tarulli A, Raynor E. Lumbosacral radiculopathy. *Neurol Clin* 2007;25(2):387–405.

21. Deville L, van der Windt D, Dzaferagic A, et al. The test of Lasegue: systematic review of the accuracy in diagnosing herniated discs. *Spine* 2000;25:1140–1147.

22. Boos N, Rieder R, Schade V, et al. 1995 Volvo Award in clinical sciences. The diagnostic accuracy of magnetic resonance imaging, work perception, and psychosocial factors in identifying symptomatic disc herniations. *Spine* 1995;20:2613–2625.

23. Hagen K, Hilde G, Jamtveldt G, et al. Bed rest for acute low back pain and sciatica. *Cochrane Database Syst Rev* 2004;(4):CD001254.

24. Koes B, Van Tulder M, Thomas S. Diagnosis and treatment of low back pain. *BMJ* 2006;332:1430–1433.

25. Dagenais S, Caro J, Haldeman S. A systematic review of low back pain cost of illness studies in the United States and internationally. *Spine J* 2008;8:8–20.

26. National Research Council and the Institute of Medicine. Panel on Musculoskeletal Disorders and the Workplace, Commission on Behavioral and Social Sciences and Education. Washington, DC: National Academy Press, 2001.

27. Pincus T, Burton A, Vogel S, et al. A systematic review of psychological factors as predictors of chronicity/disability in prospective cohorts of low back pain. *Spine* 2002;27:E109–E120.

28. Melloh M, Elfering A, Egli Presland C. Identification of prognostic factors for chronicity in patients with low back pain: a review of screening instruments. *Int Orthop.* 2009;33(2):301–313.

29. Iles R, Davidson M, Taylor N. Psychosocial predictors of failure to return to work in non-chronic non-specific low back pain: a systematic review. *Occup Environ Med* 2008;65(8):507–517.

30. Fiechtner JJ, Brodeur RR. Manual and manipulation techniques for rheumatic disease. *Rheum Dis Clin North Am* 2000;26:83–96.

31. Kopec J, Sayre E, Esdaile J. Predictors of back pain in a general population cohort. *Spine* 2004;29:70–77.

32. Hestbaek L. Low back pain: what is the long-term course? A review of studies of general patient populations. *Eur Spine J* 2003;12(2):149–165.

33. Deyo R, Cherkin D, Conrad D, et al. Cost, controversy, crisis: low back pain and the health of the public. *Annu Rev Public Health* 1992;12:141–155.

34. Burton A, Clarke R, McClune T. The natural history of low back pain in adolescents. *Spine* 1996;21:323–2328.

35. Bono C. Current concepts review: low-back pain in athletes. *J Bone Joint Surg* 2004;86-A:382–396.

36. Freynhagen R, Baron R, Gockel U, et al. Pain DETECT: a new screening questionnaire to identify neuropathic components in patients with back pain. *Curr Med Res Opin* 2006;22:1911–1920.

37. Rubinstein S, van Tulder M. A best-evidence review of diagnostic procedures for neck and low-back pain. *Best Pract Res Clin Rheumatol* 2008;22:471–482.

38. Jarvik JG, Deyo RA. Diagnostic evaluation of low back pain with emphasis on imaging. *Ann Intern Med* 2002;137:586–597.

39. Manchikanti L, Glaser SE, Wolfer LR. Systematic review of lumbar discography as a diagnostic test for chronic low back pain. *Pain Physician* 2009;12(3):541–559.

40. Chou R, Huffman LH. Non-pharmacologic therapies for acute and chronic low back pain: a review of the evidence for an American Pain Society/American College of Physicians clinical practice guideline. *Ann Int Med* 2007;147(7):492–504.

41. Buenaventura RM, Datta S, Abdi S. Systematic review of therapeutic lumbar transforaminal epidural steroid injections. *Pain Physician* 2009;12(1):233–251.

42. Cohen SP, Argoff CE, Carragee EJ. Management of low back pain. *BMJ* 2008;337.

43. Guideline Working Group, Veterans Health Administration, Department of Veterans Affairs, and Health Affairs, Department of Defense: Low Back Pain or Sciatica in the Primary Care Setting. Evidence-Based Clinical Practice. Office of Quality and Performance. Publication 10Q-CPG/LBP-99. Washington, DC: Veterans Health Administration and Department of Defense. November 1999.

44. AOA Low Back Pain Clinical Practice Guidelines. Available at: http://www.do-online.org/pdf/AOALowBackPainClinicalPracticeGuidelines.pdf, accessed January 15, 2010. Chicago, IL: American Osteopathic Association.

PART

V

Approaches to Osteopathic Medical Research

70

Foundations of Osteopathic Medical Research

MICHAEL M. PATTERSON

KEY CONCEPTS

- The osteopathic profession has supported research since its inception. It founded a research institute in the early 1900s, and while its research efforts have at times been small, it has produced a wide range of research in both the basic and clinical sciences.
- The osteopathic profession is entering an era of globalization of osteopathic research that promises to produce a wider variety of projects not only in the United States but also in several other countries with viable osteopathic movements. In addition, collaboration with other manual medicine professions promises to further expand the profession's research reach.
- Osteopathic research must be defined by the meaning of the research to osteopathic principles and practice. It is up to the investigator to define his/her research as osteopathically relevant by understanding osteopathic medicine sufficiently to make the connections between the research and osteopathic medicine.
- It is important to make every attempt to familiarize scientists coming into the profession's schools with osteopathic philosophy and practice, and for them to make the intellectually honest attempt to understand the profession. This will allow the profession's scientists to orient their research to topics important to the profession.
- The difference between a technique study and a treatment study is a very important distinction. In a technique study, the same thing is done to each patient, whereas in a treatment study, the physician treats what is found and uses the modality best suited to the patient.
- The study question or hypothesis dictates the design of the study, and hence must be clear and concise. The design flows from the question, not the other way around.
- The use of a sham control group in manual medicine studies must be carefully thought out. Improper use of a sham control can seriously weaken the study and may result in no significant outcomes. It must be realized that a sham using touch is actually a form of treatment, and is never neutral, so the comparison is one treatment against another treatment.

DEVELOPMENT OF RESEARCH IN THE OSTEOPATHIC MEDICAL PROFESSION

Early Research (1874 to 1939)

Research began in the osteopathic profession before the formal inception of the profession itself. A.T. Still was a true researcher, practicing observation, questioning his observations, trying new ways of thinking, and refining his hypotheses about his practice. He did not do what would now be regarded as organized research, but in fact, he did research at the basic level in a way that is still at the basis of almost all medical research. He observed, studied, questioned, and constructed testable hypotheses. The ideas and philosophy that have become the osteopathic profession and that undergird much of the research in the profession today came out of his questioning.

Soon after Still founded the first school in Kirksville in 1892, his students began to do formal research into the concepts he espoused. At first, these research endeavors were mainly devoted to inquiries into the anomalies that became known as the "osteopathic lesion," which is now called somatic dysfunction. Skiagraphy, a crude form of x-ray, was used before 1900 to try to find evidence of the structural abnormalities attributed to the osteopathic lesion. Soon after, animal models were used to determine the actual physiologic effects of the palpatory findings that made up the "lesion" (1). In 1906, the American Osteopathic Association (AOA) formed a research center, the A.T. Still Postgraduate College of Osteopathy, and called for donations to fund it. The name was changed to the A.T. Still Research Institute in 1909, and about $16,000 was raised to support its efforts. It was not until about 1913, when the Institute opened in a dedicated building in Chicago, that research under Wilborn J. Deason began. Funding continued to be a problem even after Louisa Burns was appointed Director, and the Institute struggled to meet its modest needs, despite calls from the AOA for more research and support. Over the ensuing years, Burns produced a body of work investigating the effects of spinal "lesions" in a rabbit model. The results of her studies indicated that artificially produced strains of specific vertebral segments produced a somewhat reproducible constellation of changes in function of organs and tissues innervated from the area of strain. These changes were later substantiated by Wilbur Cole using various neural stains (2). Burns published four books (3–6), a collected work (7), and several reports from the Institute that, unfortunately, are not widely available today but that contain much of value to the modern researcher. She continued her work until the early 1950s.

During the first third of the 1900s, research in the profession was encouraged at several osteopathic schools (8). This research included studies on basic neural and physiologic mechanisms underlying somatic dysfunction and the effects of osteopathic treatment on symptoms and immune function. Much of this research would only be considered suggestive by today's standards, but formed the basis for lines of study produced later within the profession.

The Second Period of Research (1940–1969)

In 1938, J.S. Denslow began a path of inquiry that would lead to a program of research that literally defined the modern research era in the profession. He became convinced that to bring increased credibility to the profession, research based on the latest research standards and published in highly recognized journals would have to be done. This research would have to show the basic mechanisms underlying the osteopathic lesion (9). He received training from internationally known biomedical scientists, including Ralph Gerard, and began a program of studies aimed at understanding the characteristics of muscle activity in relation to palpatory diagnosis. Joined by I.M. Korr in 1945, and by several others at Kirksville, they expounded the concept of the facilitated segment (10–12). This conceptual framework was to dominate much of the osteopathic thinking about the basis for palpation and treatment to the present day.

During the 1950s and 1960s, the research base of the profession did not expand greatly. The Bureau of Research, founded by the AOA in 1939 to fund research projects, supported fledgling efforts at several schools, but except for the Denslow/Korr project, no research efforts of a full project nature were begun. Several studies, such as those on joint mechanics (e.g., Beckwith), were published (13), but in general, research in the profession progressed slowly during this time. After World War II, the profession was busy training a flood of returning soldiers and adjusting to the new postwar world.

However, in the late 1950s, a threat to the life to the profession emerged. Culminating in the merger of the California Osteopathic and Medical Associations in 1962, the danger that the profession would be eradicated by takeover was very real. The years from 1960 to 1969 were years of uncertainty about the profession's future. However, determined that it would not be taken over, the profession rallied. In 1969, a new osteopathic school was founded in Pontiac, Michigan, as the first of 10 new schools founded between 1969 and 1980. The threat of death by merger was over, and the profession began a period of expansion and organizational prosperity unparalleled in its history.

Unfortunately, it was during this period of uncertainty and threat that the profession missed out on the tremendous expansion of biomedical research facilities and effort that resulted from World War II. The expansion of the National Institutes of Health (NIH), with its emphasis on biomedical research and its funding of new laboratories and programs, fueled an explosive growth of the biomedical research community in the United States. The osteopathic profession was unable to take advantage of this early expansion. By the time new schools with university bases were established in the 1970s, this first wave of biomedical research expansion was over.

The Third Period of Research (1970–2000)

With the founding of new schools and expansion of the five original schools remaining after the California merger (Kirksville, Chicago, Kansas City, Philadelphia, and Des Moines), the profession finally achieved a base for producing increased amounts of research. The schools began to hire more research-trained faculty, and the political arms of the profession began to more actively encourage research endeavors. The AOA began actively promoting research through the Bureau of Research and the annual Research Conference. Awards were established to honor research productivity, such as the Louisa Burns Award (1969), the Gutensohn/Denslow Award (1984), and the Korr Award (1999). Student research efforts were recognized as vital and began to be encouraged more actively with, for example, the establishment of the

Burnett Osteopathic Student Research Award and more recently, the Student Osteopathic History and Identity Essay Award. More importantly, the basis of research programs was established at many of the new schools and rejuvenated at some of the original schools, especially at Kirksville, where, beginning in 1970, Denslow and Korr oversaw the hiring of faculty specifically for research efforts. The Michigan State University College of Osteopathic Medicine formed a Department of Biomechanics specifically devoted to osteopathic research. Many of the other schools began to provide funds from their operating budgets to seed research programs and encouraged faculty and students to engage in research projects. In the early 1970s, NIH funding was awarded for the first time in many years for research in an osteopathic school.

In the years of the 1970s and 1980s, funding for research at osteopathic institutions from sources outside the profession itself grew tremendously, with many NIH and other grants being awarded. With encouragement from the Bureau of Research and individual schools, several osteopathic students undertook joint DO, PhD studies designed to further careers as clinician researchers. Many of these students have entered successful research appointments at osteopathic or other institutions.

Also in the decade of the 1990s, research requirements were instituted in many osteopathic residency programs. These requirements were aimed at familiarizing the residents with research methods and thinking, and have been expanding into some of the Osteopathic Postgraduate Training Institutes within the profession.

Thus, in the beginning of the 21st century, the amount of research being accomplished in the osteopathic profession was at an all-time high. However, a step was missing.

The Fourth Period of Research (2001–2007)

The research efforts in the profession by 2000 were both at an all-time high and increasing rapidly as research efforts at schools and at hospitals reached maturity and gained recognition. However, the profession lacked another element that had characterized many research efforts sponsored by the NIH. In the 1980s and 1990s, the NIH had sponsored a series of centers of excellence as foci for directed research efforts around the nation. The research efforts of the osteopathic profession had not yet matured sufficiently to support such an endeavor. By about 1997, several organizations in the profession, including the Louisa Burns Research Committee of the American Academy of Osteopathy (AAO), the AOA Bureau of Research, the American Association of Colleges of Osteopathic Medicine, and others, were beginning to discuss the formation of such a center. By 1999, it had become evident that NIH funding for such a center would probably not be available and that the profession would have to commit funds from its own resources. By 2000, funds had been secured for this enterprise, and requests for a center were sent to the Osteopathic Medical Schools. Five schools responded with plans for developing a center for osteopathic research. The award, announced at the AOA Research Conference in October 2001, went to the College of Osteopathic Medicine at the University of North Texas Health Science Center. The Texas school had been building its research infrastructure for several years and had a solid research record. The development of a center sponsored by the profession itself and devoted to research in manipulative medicine is the logical next step in the development of a mature research enterprise in the osteopathic profession. This center has now become a coordinating and centralizing force in developing mature research efforts into the fundamental questions facing the profession. It is attracting national funding and fostering collaboration within the osteopathic research community.

Another successful research center has appeared at the A.T. Still University in Kirksville. This center, funded mainly by internal funds, has sponsored several successful research efforts and recently published the outline of a large, multicenter trial of the effects of osteopathic manipulative treatment (OMT) on pneumonia in the elderly, the MPOSE study (14). This study has now been completed and results are being evaluated.

The Fifth Period of Research (2008 Onward)

The profession is now entering a fifth period of research development. This period is characterized by increased participation in research funding by osteopathic foundations and by the entry into the research arena of international players and other manual medicine professions. The Columbus Osteopathic Heritage Foundation has for several years been providing grants and endowments to various osteopathic schools and other organizations. It and other osteopathic foundations are now taking a major role in evolving plans for more organized and multicenter research programs. This centralizing effort along with the research centers that were developed over the fourth period will greatly enhance the ability of the profession to actively pursue research vital to the osteopathic profession.

Over several years, research has quietly expanded to osteopathic movements around the world. In the past 20 years, osteopathy has literally exploded in Europe and even Russia and Japan, to name a few of the prominent countries. Now many of these osteopathic movements are developing research programs that are adding to the fund of osteopathic research knowledge. Much of this research effort is directed to the core aspects of osteopathic practice, since most of the osteopathic movements outside the United States are manipulative only schools; their practitioners are not licensed to practice the full scope of medicine, but only manipulative treatment.

A third characteristic of the dawning fifth period is increased multidisciplinary cooperation. In March 2008, an international and interdisciplinary symposium was held in Texas under the auspices of the Texas Osteopathic Research Center. Funded by the NIH, various osteopathic foundations and the funding organizations for the Chiropractic, Massage Therapy and Physical Therapy professions, this conference represented a breakthrough in interprofessional cooperation. Scientists and clinicians from the United States and several foreign countries met to discuss data bearing on manual therapy and treatment, and the latest findings on somatovisceral interactions. There will be a book published on the conference. This spirit of increasing globalization and interdisciplinary cooperation between various manual medicine professions is a necessary part of increased understanding of the efficacy and mechanisms of OMT.

Thus, the next phase of research development in the osteopathic profession has begun. This chapter will provide information on the basics for conceptualizing research on topics germane to osteopathic medicine and some of the challenges faced by investigators designing research in these topics.

WHAT IS OSTEOPATHIC RESEARCH AND WHO DOES IT?

A definition for osteopathic research has eluded politicians and osteopathic researchers since its inception. Why would this question be asked? It is often asked in regard to whether a research project should be funded by an osteopathic funding agency, such as the AOA Bureau of Research. It may be asked to determine whether research should be included in osteopathic publications. It can be a condition for whether students are to be included in a research project. Whether research is "osteopathic" or not has both political and practical implications. In this regard, several definitions of osteopathic research have been put forward at various times.

Research Under Osteopathic Auspices

Perhaps the broadest definition is that osteopathic research is any research done under osteopathic auspices. This definition implies that any research, basic or clinical, no matter what the subject matter, is osteopathic when performed at an osteopathic institution or under the control of an osteopathic institution. Under this rubric, research on any topic could be considered osteopathic. This is obviously too broad.

Research on Topics of Special Interest to the Profession

Some topics in biomedicine have historically been of greater interest to the osteopathic profession than others. For example, the actions of the nervous system in controlling various autonomic functions and the effects of manipulative treatment on immune function have been topics of investigation for many years. At times, efforts have been made to define lists of such topics as the ones that define osteopathic research. The problem here is that new avenues of inquiry are constantly being found that apply to the clinical and theoretical topics of the profession, and no one list can be devised that will cover or predict them all.

Research on Osteopathic Manipulative Treatment

Definitions of osteopathic research have at times been restricted to those studies attempting to determine efficacy or value of osteopathic treatment. This approach leaves out the entire area of mechanism inquiry that seeks to explain the basis of treatment efficacy. Obviously, this is too narrow a view. In addition, research into mechanisms of action and underlying process is becoming increasingly emphasized by the NIH.

Any Research into Biologic Mechanisms, Because Osteopathy Is Holistic, Therefore Encompasses Everything

Although ecumenical, this is not a definition because it says nothing. It would assume that there are no basic theoretical underpinnings to the osteopathic philosophy or practice that have or should be identified, thus that there is no definition of osteopathic medicine. If this were so, there would be little basis for the profession to exist.

A New Definition of Osteopathic Research

Attempts to define *a priori* the scope or type of research that is considered osteopathic seem doomed to failure. However, perhaps there is one way to determine whether research is osteopathic: To require the investigator to explain how the hypothesis and expected findings of their research would be relevant to the theory, mechanisms, or practice of osteopathic medicine. That is, investigators must have sufficient understanding of the basic principles of osteopathic medicine to explain how the interpretation of their data would impact osteopathic medicine. They must know enough about the perspectives of the profession, its theoretical basis, and/or its clinical practice to coherently build bridges from their studies to the profession. If they cannot do that, then, although their data may be interesting, important, and even cutting edge, it is not osteopathic. Perhaps someone else can build those bridges, but until that happens, it is not osteopathic research.

It is of great value to have physician researchers and PhD researchers who expend the time and intellectual energy to understand the profession's theoretical and clinical perspectives, because the results of any study must be interpreted within some context. If the context is that of osteopathic medicine, the data are much more likely to be correctly used in understanding the profession's basic questions.

Thus, anyone can do osteopathic research, provided that they make the intellectual effort to become familiar with the profession's clinical, theoretical, and/or historical experience. Otherwise, they are doing interesting research that must be interpreted by others to be useful to the osteopathic profession. The burden of proof that research is osteopathic lies with the investigator.

HOW DO RESEARCHERS BECOME AWARE OF THE THEORY OR CLINICAL ASPECTS OF THE PROFESSION?

Although trained osteopathic physicians can be expected to be familiar with the background necessary to relate research findings to their profession, such is not the case with many basic scientists (including many currently at osteopathic institutions) or researchers outside the profession. Cultivating basic scientists who understand the clinical tenets of the profession and training basic scientists to gain such understanding pays off in increased theory building and data interpretation. One excellent way to begin the process of understanding osteopathic principles and practice is to ask PhD and other non-DO faculty to attend OMT courses. Experience in learning and receiving manipulative treatment is also an enlightening experience. However, researchers are trained to investigate new areas of knowledge and to ask questions of those areas. Basic scientists and others within the profession can easily access books and journals relevant to their osteopathic understanding. This book is a good start in that journey. A second source is the *Journal of the American Osteopathic Association*, where reviews, original research articles, and case studies are available. Other sources, such as Still's *Autobiography* (15) or his *Osteopathy Research and Practice* (16), are useful. Other books, such as Northup's books on the profession (17) and research (2), are useful in helping the basic scientist understand the profession.

As much as the researcher must be expected to find and read materials pertinent to his or her understanding, so must those knowledgeable in the profession be willing to help promote the necessary understanding. Osteopathic physicians and students must be willing to discuss their beliefs and clinical observations with often skeptical scientists. The experience of the 1989 AAO symposium (18) is illustrative of this point. Several internationally known basic scientists were assembled for 2 days of discussion prior to the symposium itself. They questioned the attending osteopathic physicians about the experiences of the profession and consented to having OMT. Rather than being antagonistic to the largely anecdotal clinical observations, they were uniformly supportive and excited by them. Several altered their prepared talks to reflect their new understanding and have maintained active contact with the profession since. In fact, one is actively training DO students in his laboratories. A similar although more limited experience occurred at the 2008 International Symposium between scientists and clinicians. Active and open communication about ideas most often leads to exciting opportunities. Thus, the development of basic scientists who understand the osteopathic profession is a two-way street.

Although much has been accomplished in this area, the cadre of trained clinical and basic science investigators must be expanded to those who understand the principles and clinical experiences of osteopathy so that they can frame their research questions in the light of osteopathic clinical experience and theory. Without this understanding, data will not be examined from the perspective of osteopathic treatment and insight.

ETHICAL CONSIDERATIONS IN OSTEOPATHIC RESEARCH

Human Subjects Protection

Since the end of World War II, there has been a growing understanding of the problems associated with the ethical considerations of research on both human and animal subjects. The horrible experiments performed by physicians on prisoners in the Nazi concentration camps sparked reforms and regulations to control human medical experimentation. Coming out of the Nuremberg Trials and codified in the 1964 Declaration of Helsinki, these regulations have been the subject of continuing review, refinement, and discussion since then (19–21). The researcher who contemplates doing research in osteopathic topics must be aware of and abide by the current human subject regulations. Not only is this the law, but it is the moral and just thing to do. In fact, no reputable journal will publish results of a human study without evidence that applicable human subject guidelines have been scrupulously followed.

The novice investigator must be familiar with not only the principles of ethical treatment of subjects, but also with the procedures in effect in the institution where the research will be done. In the event that a private physician wishes to conduct human subject research in a private office, the research must first be approved by an appropriate human subjects review board, usually known as the institutional review board (IRB). The IRB is a governmentally sanctioned body whose members are appointed by the institutional executive in charge of research and the President or CEO of the institution, and must include individuals with specific interests, including a person who has no other affiliation with the institution.

INSTITUTIONAL REVIEW BOARD AUTHORITY

The IRB has the authority to deny or approve any research proposal involving human subjects. The main purpose of the IRB is to protect the safety of the subjects. It can stop ongoing research if it deems protection not sufficient or uncovers problems in the research. When applications for research are submitted to the IRB, the application can receive expedited review if certain conditions are met, such as that the research uses only data collected in the normal course of office practice and that are not identified with a patient. However, it is not up to the investigator to determine whether the research is exempt, can have expedited review, or must undergo full review. Case reports and retrospective reviews of cases (see discussion below) seen in the routine office practice do not generally need IRB approval unless the patient is identified or if written permission is given prior to release of any information.

MAJOR INSTITUTIONAL REVIEW BOARD CONSIDERATIONS

The major factors in human subject research include:

- Informed consent
- Confidentiality statements
- Risk

- Absence of coercion
- How subjects will be obtained and paid for service

One of the cornerstones of human subject protection is the principle of informed consent. This idea holds that the subject be informed of the study fully and completely and be able to give free consent to participation. If the subject is a minor, incapable of giving consent due to mental or other disability, or a prisoner, special and specific protections are specified.

The principle of subject confidentiality is another vital concern. The subject's confidentiality is to be protected and not divulged without the subject's written consent. Thus, medical and research data are considered private matters when linked to an identifiable subject. Data are usually coded in such a way that they cannot be linked to a particular patient, and great care must be taken that no such link can be inferred. The recently enacted HIPAA standards must be followed to protect patient privacy and confidentiality. (See http://www.hhs.gov/ocr/hipaa/ for more information on HIPAA.)

Risk to the patient is another factor in human research. Risk to a patient runs from essentially nonexistent to grave. If the risk is anything but incidental, the subject must be fully informed of that risk and have every option to decline participation. The risk must also be justified by potential gain, perhaps not to the individual subject, but to the field. This assessment is difficult to make, and the investigator must therefore justify the study well.

Absence of coercion is a complex topic that is often debated in study design. Is providing a monetary incentive to a subject for time taken by the study coercion? Is the investigator using force of personality or doctor–patient relationship to coerce the subject to enter the study? These questions are difficult to quantify, and the committee and investigator must consider them carefully.

IRBs are usually in existence in osteopathic medical schools and in many hospitals. Each IRB is allowed operating discretion within established NIH guidelines as to how it reviews protocols. Some IRBs meet on a regular basis and others are on call. The potential investigator is responsible for finding the protocols used by the appropriate IRB and fully following these regulations.

It cannot be overemphasized how important it is to be cognizant of current guidelines for human subject protection and to fully adhere to them. (For current and full information, including downloadable human subjects research guidelines, go the NIH web site at: *http://ohsr.od.nih.gov.*)

Animal Protection

No less important in research on human subjects is the protection of subjects in animal research. As is evident from the media, animal rights have become a volatile issue in much of the world. Some of the emotion surrounding animal rights obviously stems from the fact that animals cannot give informed consent or judge risk in a study. In addition, by its nature, animal research often ends in the subject's death. For these and other reasons, some groups use violence to attempt to stop animal research.

Not unlike human subject protection, a well-defined, protective structure has been implemented by the NIH and other groups, such as the American Association for Assessment and Accreditation of Laboratory Animal Care (AAALAC), have promulgated guidelines and rules for the proper use of animals in research studies. The Animal Care and Use Committee (ACUC), a governmentally mandated body, enforces these rules at research institutions. Like the IRB, the ACUC has the authority to shut down research not in compliance with applicable regulations and must approve all animal research prior to its start. The osteopathic researcher

who wishes to use animals in research must first successfully seek ACUC approval. As with the IRB, each ACUC has latitude in its procedures about which the investigator must be informed. Again, as with human research, the investigator must be meticulous in following animal care and use guidelines: first and foremost, for moral and ethical reasons but also because humanely treated and well cared for animal subjects provide more reliable information. (For more information on animal care and use guidelines, visit the NIH Office of Animal Care and Use site at http://oacu.od.nih.gov/.) Another useful site is the American Association for Laboratory Animal Science site at *www.aalas.org* or the AAALAC site at *www.aaalac.org.*

Applying for Institutional Review Board or Animal Care and Use Committee Approval

The process for applying for research approval for either human or animal research is determined by each committee. Some committees meet monthly or more often; others meet on call. However, at the least, each protocol submitted for IRB or ACUC approval will have to contain the following elements:

- Background literature review
- Justification for the project
- Hypothesis to be tested
- Complete description of the methods to be used
  - Evidence that animals will be legally obtained and humanely housed
  - Evidence that precautions will be taken to minimize any necessary pain or suffering
  - Evidence that other alternatives to animal use are not available
  - Data to be collected
  - Statistical methods for analysis
  - Any pilot data available

These items represent a fair amount of work that must be done prior to submitting a protocol for review. It also means that the investigator will find it necessary to think through the studies prior to getting approval. The appropriate approvals are also necessary before funds are awarded for the proposed research from government agencies.

TYPES OF RESEARCH IN OSTEOPATHIC MEDICINE

Basic Science

Within the purview of osteopathic research, there are several valid types of studies. Perhaps the most basic is research that flows from basic science studies. This research includes studies designed to define the basic functions of the body and mind, and explain how they interact with the environment. These studies are mainstream biomedical research. An increased understanding of the human organism and its function is invaluable in validating osteopathic practice. The osteopathic profession must therefore nurture the basic sciences, but the links between basic research and osteopathic philosophy and practice must be made.

Basic Research in Other Institutions and Professions

Basic science has been performed for many years in most biomedical facilities and research institutes. Most basic research relevant to the osteopathic profession is done not in the educational institutions of the profession but in other biomedical settings. The amount of research that can be supported directly by the profession is small compared with the amount of such research performed around the world. The total amount of funding available from within the osteopathic profession for support of its research programs is less per year than the annual budgets of many individual laboratories outside the profession. This suggests two things. First, maximal use must be made of data from laboratories outside the profession. Osteopathic researchers and clinicians must cultivate interactions with biochemical researchers at other institutions who can supply data and interpretations. Second, the limited resources of the profession must be put into research endeavors that provide the greatest return in explaining osteopathic experience and theory. This requires, as stated above, that investigators within the osteopathic profession understand the unique and defining concepts of osteopathy within which to interpret their findings. Without this understanding, the investigator is unable to interpret the findings in ways that are useful to the profession, and a large part of the research investment is lost.

The use of data from laboratories outside the profession is certainly a very useful and fruitful endeavor. We have made use of this mechanism in proposing mechanisms for the facilitated segment (22). However, care must be taken in using data generated in studies not specifically designed to answer the question to which the data are now being applied. Unless the limitations and specifics of the data are well known, implications can easily be made that are beyond the scope of the data and hence potentially misleading. It is important to realize these limitations, but to use data and sources from outside the profession whenever possible. Such was the case when the AAO commissioned two international symposia held in 1989 and 1992, which resulted in proceedings publications (18,23) that have been very useful in informing the profession of possible mechanisms for clinical phenomena and the results of manipulative treatment.

Integrative Model Building: Integrating Basic Science and Clinical Observation

A second type of research activity necessary within the profession is the integration of basic science knowledge and clinical observation. This endeavor is extremely valuable and potentially dangerous. A recent article by Van Buskirk (24) illustrates such research. In this article, Van Buskirk builds a theoretical model of somatic dysfunction based on nociceptive input. He marshals an impressive array of basic science data and synthesizes it in a unique way from his clinical understandings and observations. The result is a well-grounded look at one of the central concepts of the osteopathic philosophy of health and disease. This is the valuable aspect of the article.

The dangerous part is that the model will be taken as fact. Van Buskirk goes to great lengths to point out that the model seems to be explanatory but still needs to be subjected to rigorous research verification and clinical observation before it can be accepted as proven. Unfortunately, the pioneering models that came out of the research of Korr and Denslow (11,25) suffered from being taken as factual explanation rather than as models in need of experimental verification. Once a model has been accepted as truth, the perceived need for further research or theory is impeded or stopped, and the model becomes accepted as truth. This can be disastrous if the model is then shown to be erroneous or incomplete because there are then no alternatives to take its place. Integrative model building provides much needed direction for both basic and clinical research but must not be taken at face value without verification and experimental testing.

Thus, the osteopathic profession must continually examine its theories and subject its explanations to close scrutiny. The vast body of clinical evidence demonstrates that the precepts of the osteopathic profession are sound. However, often the profession embraces explanations that are not solidly research based. The result is theory taken for fact with further exploration of alternative theory or factual basis effectively stymied.

Synthesis and Meta-Analysis Research

Two types of scholarly activities that can be of immense benefit to any area are the synthesis review and the meta-analysis. Synthesis papers are efforts to review and critically analyze an area or field of study. In this type of work, the author would select a topic area for analysis and review all available work in that area. Although the review is in itself important, a synthesis then analyzes the work that has been done and attempts to find common themes, areas of agreement or disagreement, and then builds a hypothesis as to what the accumulated knowledge of the area is saying. This type of paper can often point to why seeming contradictions between studies exist, what studies should be done to finalize questions in the field, and so forth. Early in my career, we did such a synthesis for the field of spinal cord learning (26). The insights from that activity directed spinal cord plasticity research for many years—not only in our laboratories, but in other laboratories (27). Often, a good synthesis of an area will open the area for more intensive study and can be an impetus for real advances in an area that was seemingly uninteresting or filled with conflicting data.

The meta-analysis is another useful tool for research. This analysis attempts to accumulate all studies in a field that are deemed sufficiently rigorous and determine the combined power of the results. In this way, by statistically combining smaller studies that are not particularly convincing by themselves, it is often possible to achieve sufficient statistical or analytical power to have confidence in the phenomenon being investigated. Such an analysis was done on the area of spinal manipulation for low back pain and resulted in acceptance of that modality as effective treatment for acute low back pain (28). An analysis of spinal palpatory procedure validity and reliability is currently under way at the Center for Complementary and Alternative Medicine at the University of California Irvine College of Medicine, and is sponsored by the trust fund acquired by that school when the California College of Osteopathic Medicine became the University of California Irvine College of Medicine in 1962. More information on procedures of meta-analysis can be found in many statistical texts (29).

Qualitative Studies in Osteopathy

Valuable information can often be gathered by means of surveys and interviews. Such studies, although not experimental, are often the only way to find trends in populations, practice distributions, or to gather the collected thought of experts in a field. Often, surveys seem simple and easy to perform. The investigator must only write down a few questions on a topic and send them out to some selected individuals and wait for the returns. Such simplicity is illusory. Good surveys must be well planned and executed. The topic must be carefully framed and the questions prepared with precision. Pitfalls in the use of surveys include poorly framed questions, problems in determining to whom the survey should be sent, poor return rates, and others (29). Prior to instituting a survey, an investigator must consult texts and/or experts in survey design and procedure. Within the osteopathic profession, Johnson and Kurtz (30–32) have performed several surveys addressing such issues as student interests and the use of manipulative treatment. These studies have provided a baseline for the use of osteopathic manipulation in the profession and are invaluable in charting future direction within the profession. These surveys are excellent examples of well-done and analyzed survey studies.

Another instrument that can provide valuable information is the collection and analysis of expert interviews or writings of often long-departed authors. These methods also often seem deceptively simple. In fact, as with surveys, interviews with experts require extensive preparation and careful planning. Both directed and open-ended questions may be asked and answers recorded for later transcription, or the expert may be asked to write on predetermined topics. In any event, the answers must be carefully analyzed for content and other information. The analysis of writings by departed authors can be valuable in translating what may now seem to be arcane jargon into terms understandable in today's terminology. For example, why did Still put so much emphasis on the fasciae of the body? What did he mean by such terms as "fluids of life?" To understand these ideas in the way in which Still did, it would be necessary to find the meaning of those terms in the late 1800s, as well as to look at the context in which he used them. Various means of content analysis are available to help in such a task (34). Both interview analysis and writing analysis can be of great value to osteopathic understanding. A particularly good example of such work can be found in Jane Stark's (35) recent book, *Still's Fascia*. This book came out of a particularly comprehensive thesis done by Stark for her Canadian osteopathic degree and analyzes Still's ideas on fascia in light of his background and his times.

Epidemiology and Outcome Studies

Epidemiologic studies have not been widely used in the osteopathic profession. It should be noted, however, that there are some very important epidemiologic topics awaiting study. Because epidemiology refers to the study of patterns of health and disease and what influences these patterns, those influences on health and loss of health that are of particular interest to osteopathic medicine should be subjected to such studies. One of the most important such study would be the incidence and natural history of somatic dysfunction in normal populations and various subpopulations with defined illness. As with most studies, epidemiologic studies of this entity would require careful planning and execution. However, it could reveal very important information on the potential uses for manipulative treatment modalities. The interested investigator can find more information in such references as *Medical Epidemiology* (35).

Outcome studies are a very important type of research that bridges both epidemiology and at times, experimental studies. In the usual such study, outcome measures are taken or reviewed for patient populations, and the outcomes of one type of treatment outcome, cost, patient satisfaction, and so on are reported. Outcome studies usually require large patient populations to gain sufficient data to be meaningful.

Research on Manipulation

As one of the key elements of osteopathic care, manipulative treatment should be the subject of increasing amounts of research in the profession. In research aimed at investigating the usefulness of manipulative treatment, there is much confusion about proper research methodology. However, the researcher approaching osteopathic manipulation as an independent variable must decide which of the following is to be evaluated: a treatment or manipulative technique, OMT, or osteopathic health care.

Depending on the aspect of manipulation to be studied, different experimental designs will be employed. Too often, investigators fail to distinguish between these three entities and hence have difficulty determining the correct experimental design for their study.

MANIPULATIVE TECHNIQUES

One of the most illustrative studies of manipulative technique is the Irvine study, performed by Buerger and colleagues (36,37) at the School of Medicine at the University of California, Irvine, in the late 1970s and early 1980s. They wished to determine the effects of a single lateral recumbent roll (high-velocity/low-amplitude thrust) on low back pain. The study was elegantly designed and executed, with a result that showed an immediate effect of the lateral recumbent roll on certain measured variables; simply positioning the patient for a lateral recumbent roll and omitting the thrust did not provide the same changes. After a few weeks, however, no differences between the experimental and control groups remained, probably the result of the nature of the presenting complaint, which has a natural history of relief in a few weeks. Nonetheless, an immediate effect of the thrust was seen. The point missed by many readers was that the investigation was not of OMT but of a treatment technique.

THE IRVINE STUDY COMPARED WITH CLINICAL TRIALS OF MEDICAL INTERVENTIONS

In many ways, the Irvine study was similar to drug studies. One specific manipulative technique was used on each patient in the experimental group (and not in the control group), the patients were blinded to whether they received manipulation, and measurable variables were used. In the typical drug trial, the specific effects of a certain chemical compound on the course of a specific set of symptoms are studied. The design of the study controls for other factors that might cause a change in the outcome. This is a legitimate model for the study of a specific technique within manipulative treatment. If the intent of the study is to determine the effect of a specific and repeatable manipulation, the research design should emulate the design of a drug trial, including attempts to blind the patient to whether the technique was delivered. Such studies are useful in instances where there may be reason to suspect that a specific manipulative technique would change a particular condition. Great care must be taken to control for the actual presenting complaint, whether the patient has knowledge of manipulation, and the actual delivery of the technique to make certain that it is given in the same way to each patient.

Such studies can be useful as long as it is recognized that the study's purpose is to evaluate the effect of a specific, single, or small group of physical manipulations on a specific condition. Another recent example of this design was published by Wells et al. (38), who looked at the effects of a set of standard manipulative techniques on gait parameters of patients with Parkinson disease. They found that the standardized techniques produced increased performance in various aspects of gait in these individuals. Such designs, performed correctly, give information on the effects of a technique on some aspect of patient function.

STUDIES OF MANIPULATIVE TREATMENT

This type of research is used to study the effects of OMT on one or more measurable patient parameters. The research design and the goals are somewhat different from those used in technique studies. Korr (39) has elegantly reviewed these differences. Osteopathic theory and practice holds that the full treatment of an individual by an osteopathic physician entails an interaction between the physician and the patient that is not static but dynamic, changing from treatment to treatment and instant to instant as the treatment progresses. The physician responds to the dynamic changes in the patient's function; the patient responds to the attitudes and touch of the physician. The treatment is not a prearranged set of movements and thrusts given to each patient, but an ongoing stimulus/response synergism between the physician and patient, with the patient's response guiding the actions of the physician.

In this case, the manipulation cannot be predetermined or prescribed by the research protocol but must "go with the flow" in response to the reactions of both physician and patient. The manipulative treatment is properly a "black box." The physician/patient interaction determines what manipulative treatment is performed. The physician is free to do what is deemed best for the interaction. Because one of the basic axioms of osteopathy is that each person responds differently to stress and treatment, this freedom of interaction cannot be removed from the physician without changing the research to a technique investigation. To investigate manipulative treatment rather than a manipulative technique, manipulative treatment must be used.

The recent study on the effects of osteopathic treatment on low back pain by Andersson et al. (40), comparing manipulation with standard of care is a case in point. In this study, treating osteopathic physicians were allowed to use any manipulative techniques necessary for the patient. The study found that there were no differences in outcomes but that the group treated with manipulation required less medication and physical therapy. In this study, unlike in a technique study, the physician chose the treatment that was indicated for the patient.

Technique Versus Manipulative Treatment

Once the difference between these two basic types of research on manipulation is realized, many of the other problems associated with investigating manipulation can be much more easily resolved. Both types of research are valuable and valid. Research on techniques gives information on specific techniques; research on treatment gives information on what the osteopathic physician does in practice. Both are necessary and essential for the future of the profession. Their differences must be recognized and appreciated for appropriate studies to be designed.

Subtypes of Manipulative Treatment

Within the general types of research on manipulative treatment, there can be several subtypes. One aims at the effect of manipulative treatment in general on some aspect of a disease or body function. This could be called the nonspecific design. It is done to improve body function without identifying specific somatic dysfunction in patients with some clinical presenting complaint. The treating physician provides a general manipulative treatment without specifying areas of somatic dysfunction or specific areas to be addressed. By contrast, in specific treatment designs, the physician applies manipulative treatment to specific somatic dysfunction as defined by palpatory diagnosis and documented with such signs as asymmetric motion, tissue texture changes, and so forth. This type of treatment is designed to restore function or ameliorate functional difficulties and may or may not be related to actual presenting complaints (the patient may not be aware of some somatic dysfunction). In each of these study types, appropriate data on what is done must be collected, and specific measures of outcome must be made.

Effectiveness Studies

A third type of study incorporates either of the first two: the effectiveness study, in which manipulative treatment is given to alleviate a specific presenting complaint. The patient is selected for a particular complaint, such as low back pain; the treating physician gives appropriate manipulative treatment. The effect of the treatment on the complaint (e.g., low back pain) is measured. This study type may or may not require the delineation of somatic dysfunction during treatment. Efficacy studies are the most usual in the literature because the measure of results is the most straightforward.

Functional Outcomes of Manipulative Treatment

In the fourth design subtype, the functional outcome design, the effect of manipulative treatment on general physiologic function is assessed. In the philosophy of the osteopathic profession, the origin of disease is believed to be some loss of normal function in the body that then allows for the development of clinical symptoms. This type of study is accomplished on clinically disease-free subjects with somatic dysfunction who are addressed with specific treatment. Measures of outcome are such things as immune system function, tolerance to stress, general activities of daily living assessments (in older subjects), and other measures of normal function that assess general health and function.

Presumably, such studies would find increases in the functional ability or capacity of treated subjects.

TOTAL OSTEOPATHIC CARE STUDIES

Another general study design takes into account the total care given by the osteopathic physician; it is not limited to manipulative treatment. This study type assesses the health status of patients given care by osteopathic physicians and presumably, but not necessarily, includes manipulative treatment over the course of care. Such studies are longitudinal or cross-sectional in nature and include as data such things as disease episodes and measures of total body function and activities of daily living. If the osteopathic philosophy of health is taken seriously, there is a heavy component of preventive care that would include periodic manipulative treatment to correct somatic dysfunction as it occurs. Such care should prevent a least some of the acute disease episodes seen in nonmanipulated subjects. A study of this kind would be expensive and long term, and could be approached in various ways. Research of this type could show whether the application of osteopathic principles to health care is differentiated from disease care. Practitioners applying total osteopathic care to their patients would be used to determine if their outcomes in terms of patient health were different from physicians not using osteopathic care. Obviously, there would be many potentially confounding factors that would have to be analyzed. Interesting results, such as cost/benefit ratios, quality-of-life issues, and others, could be addressed.

DESIGNING AND CONDUCTING OSTEOPATHIC RESEARCH

Understanding the basics of what type of study is to be done is an important step in beginning osteopathic research. Realizing the importance of ethical considerations and data confidentiality is vital. The next steps in a research project are also vital. These steps can be characterized as follows:

1. Observation
2. Literature search

3. Hypothesis building
4. Study design
5. Data collection
6. Data analysis
7. Discussion of results
8. Writing and publication

These steps are all necessary and important in the conduct of research in any field. We will briefly discuss each.

Observation

Virtually all biomedical research stems from clinical observation. The clinician observes patients and their response to illness and treatment. He or she often conducts impromptu "experiments" to see if there is any effect on a patient's outcome. Such observations are valuable, but rarely conclusive. Observations are usually subject to too many uncertainties, called biases, to lead to definitive conclusions about what actually occurred or whether there was really an effect of a certain treatment on a condition. The realization over many years that observation by itself was rarely useful in establishing reliable cause and effect relationships in fact led to the art of research design. However, observation is the beginning point for investigation. The investigator should begin with observation of his or her practice. What is of special interest to the investigator? One of the most important aspects of doing research is to pick a topic that piques the interest. Once that is accomplished, the basis of a research project is laid. A prime example of observation being the basis for a lifetime of research is that of Lawrence H. Jones (41). He made the observation of a patient with severe muscle spasm that was relieved by placing the patient into an extremely awkward position to alleviate the pain. Instead of dismissing the result as spurious or inconsequential, Jones pursued the observation and developed the area of strain/counterstrain.

Literature Search

The next step in developing a research project is the literature search. This is a very important step and one that is often either slighted or done without sufficient diligence. The first steps in a literature search are to examine texts and other reference works easily available. Do they show that the problem interesting the investigator has already been thoroughly researched? Is there an abundance of literature already available? Or does a preliminary search reveal little or no information? Texts and reference books are called secondary literature because they report second hand on research articles (primary literature). Hopefully, something will easily be found in the secondary literature that will lead to primary research articles or even reviews of the topic.

The search for information will almost invariably lead to the primary literature; to journals in which research findings are presented. The search for primary literature can be greatly simplified by using one of the many computer resources now available. The National Library of Medicine (NLM) has the largest compilation of medical literature in the world. This resource is available to anyone with World Wide Web access. The "search engines" for the NLM database may be accessed free through services like PUBMED or by fee-for-service engines, such as PaperChase. These search engines make searching the many millions of articles in MEDLINE and its associated databases easy and fast. However, the search must be done with some skill in selecting appropriate search terms or author names, or the result may be a return of thousands of often irrelevant articles. Hopefully, the search will be productive in producing several articles and papers on the topic at hand. The investigator may then proceed to acquire the articles through libraries or by ordering them online, and begin to read about what is known about his or her topic.

The search can be both a time-consuming and strenuous task. In osteopathic medicine, there is only one journal included in the NLM databanks: the *Journal of the American Osteopathic Association* (*JAOA*). Because the NLM Medline database only goes back to 1966, it is also important to review articles in earlier issues of the JAOA (as it often is for other journals). This can now be done by searching the online JAOA database at *www.jaoa.org*. The investigator may have to actually go to a library with holdings of the journal and search back issues, or ask the librarian to review an index of the journal for relevant topics. In addition, other osteopathic source materials should be searched. The AAO has an important collection of osteopathic articles in its Yearbook collection and has now released a CD-ROM with its bibliography in searchable form. This listing should be included in any search. Other osteopathic collections, such as the *Osteopathic Annals* (no longer published), are also valuable sources of information.

Many public libraries have access to many search engines and can assist in locating materials. University libraries usually have electronic access to full-text research journal archives that are very useful. When using any database, it is advisable to keep careful records of articles read and what was in each. A computer database program, such as Reference Manager or Endnote *(www.isiresearchsoft.com)*, is excellent for this purpose, and such programs also allow easy construction of bibliographies when writing papers. In fact, the Endnote program is one of the most useful writing tools in a researchers toolbox.

What should be looked for during a literature search? Obviously, the primary goal is to find articles and information on the topic of interest. What has been found about the topic? What research or observations have already been made? It is also important to find how others have looked at the area. If research has been done, how was it done, and what measures did the investigators use in the studies? What techniques and research designs were used? If other research has been done, it is best to find how it was done, what pitfalls were encountered, and how they were overcome.

Thus, the literature review is a vital and often very poorly done part of any study. Careful literature review will often save the investigator much work and even embarrassment. It is not good to find, after doing a study, that someone else has already done it or one similar.

The literature search allows the investigator to go to the next step of research design: the formation of the research hypothesis.

The Hypothesis

One of the most important aspects of designing any research project, be it quantitative or qualitative, experimental or observational, is forming the hypothesis. The hypothesis is the statement of the question being asked by the study. The hypothesis must be clear and concise. It must state exactly what the research is to investigate. Most beginning researchers try to make the hypothesis too complex or design a hypothesis that is simply not testable. For example, the hypothesis "osteopathic treatment is good for headaches" is not a good hypothesis. Although we would like to think that the statement is true, can we test it? The answer is "no." What is "osteopathic treatment?" What does "good" mean? What type of headache is to be studied? A good experimental hypothesis is simple, precise, and well defined.

The Hypothesis Dictates the Study Design

The hypothesis also will dictate the design of the study to be done. Too often, an investigator produces an imprecise hypothesis and then has difficulty designing the appropriate study because the actual question and its implications are not clear. If the hypothesis is clear and simple, the design of the study will not only be much more evident, but it will be defensible to others. For example, in the Irvine study referenced (42), the hypothesis was simple and straightforward: "What is the effect of a lateral recumbent roll thrust on measures of well-defined, acute low back pain?" This hypothesis defined the study as a technique study on a well-defined problem, acute low back pain (which was very precisely specified).

Thus, the hypothesis, not a preconceived notion of design, must dictate the study design. Too often, it is assumed that one type of study design is the only one appropriate for some type of research, such as manipulative medicine, when in actuality, the design flows from the question being asked. If the investigator has the question clearly in mind, the research design can be chosen and refined to reflect that question, not some other question that is not being asked.

Once the hypothesis is determined, it is usually converted to the "null hypothesis." The null hypothesis simply states the negative of the experimental hypothesis. Thus, if the experimental hypothesis was that "a lateral recumbent thrust will have an effect on acute low back pain," the null hypothesis would be that "a lateral recumbent thrust will have no effect on acute low back pain." The null hypothesis can be disproved by a study showing an effect, but a study showing no effect does not necessarily prove that no effect exists. Rather, it shows only that an effect was not observed in the present study. Thus, the null hypothesis is the preferred statement with the intent of the study to disprove it. In fact, many study designs provide both null and experimental hypotheses.

Study Design

The design of a research project is vital to the success and value of that project. In osteopathic research, there are many types of studies that can be done, as outlined above in this chapter. Once the investigator has chosen the topic of the study and has at least stated the hypothesis, if not completely refined it, the choice of research designs must be made. Is the research to be observational, epidemiologic, descriptive, or experimental? Each of these types of research has particular requirement for design components (29,33,34,43). The investigator must consult with experienced clinical research designers for appropriate help.

In the area of research on manipulative techniques or treatment, the most usual type of study is either a descriptive or experimental study. In descriptive studies, patients are simply treated, and the results of the treatment are reported.

CASE STUDIES

CASE REPORT

A case study is the report of a single, supposedly unique case, or of a unique treatment of a case. In case studies, a patient's history is given, the treatment is described, and the results are reported. The case study was the staple for medical research many years ago, but is now only infrequently used. Many medical journals will no longer publish case studies except under the most stringent circumstances. Case studies are useful as observations leading to more complete studies, but rarely stand on their own. The limitations of case studies include poor recording of findings, incomplete history and physical reporting, and in many cases, unconfirmed diagnosis. If the investigator believes that a case is sufficiently unique to warrant publication, a very complete literature review must be done prior to attempted publication to ensure that no such findings have been previously reported. Kaprow and Sandhouse (43) recently reported on the treatment of a case by osteopathic manipulation, an example of a relatively unique treatment of an uncommon complaint.

CASE SERIES: RETROSPECTIVE

Case series are of two types. The first is the retrospective case series. In this design, the investigator searches the office files for all cases of a similar type and attempts, through reviewing the cases, to find commonalities in symptoms, treatment, or outcomes that warrant publication. The retrospective case series brings together similar cases to add credibility to a unique or new clinical entity or treatment regime. The retrospective case series may add weight to an argument that a new or unrecognized clinical syndrome is emerging, or that a new treatment technique is effective, but suffers the same problems as the single case study; the data are usually not uniform and diagnoses may be lacking. In addition, there is little assurance in a retrospective case series that all patients of the targeted type have been included; it is possible that only selected cases have been reported, making the results seem more beneficial than is actually the case.

CASE SERIES: PROSPECTIVE

Prospective case series studies are usually done after the realization that some treatment has a greater impact than thought or can be used on some unique condition. In this study type, nothing new is introduced, but only usual and standard practices may be used in a different manner. However, the means of identifying prospective patients, the data to be collected, and the methods of treatment are clearly specified in advance. All patients who meet the predefined criteria are treated and the data recorded uniformly. Thus, there is some assurance that the patients actually had the specified condition and the data gathered are uniform.

In most cases, case series do not have to be approved by an IRB unless a new treatment is being tried or data not usually collected in the course of practice are being collected. Although somewhat more indicative of effect, the prospective case series fall short of providing convincing arguments for effectiveness, because there is no comparison with other treatments or subjects.

OTHER OBSERVATIONAL STUDY DESIGNS

As mentioned above, various other types of designs, such as interview, epidemiologic, survey, and outcomes designs, are useful for many aspects of osteopathic research and can bring powerful and useful data to bear on such questions as:

- How do the attitudes of osteopathic students toward the profession change over their training?
- How satisfied are the patients of osteopathic physicians?
- What did statements of pioneers in the profession mean?
- How do patients of osteopathic physicians choose their doctors?
- What is the incidence of somatic dysfunction in the normal population?

These and many other questions are awaiting well-planned studies and would produce information valuable for planning the future of the profession.

Experimental Design

The proof of cause-and-effect relationships is very difficult. Humans are very good at recognizing what seem to be correlations between two events, a trait that has undoubtedly been honed over thousands of years. The rustle of grass on a dark night correlates well with the approach of a tiger intent on finding a meal and quickly becomes a signal for retreat to a safe cave. However, the rustle does not cause the cat to eat the unwary human. The human (and other animal) nervous systems are well adapted to recognizing correlation, but poorly designed to establish cause and effect. The art (and some would say, science) of experimental design has been developed to find ways to be able to assign cause-and-effect relationships in all areas of science.

Medical science is one of the most difficult areas in which to assign cause-and-effect relationships. The human organism is very complex, and what may seem like cause-and-effect relationships may be nothing more than random variation in function or disease state, or even the patient's own perception of how they are feeling. For example, the drug Laetrile was for years thought to produce good results for advanced cancer patients, but was finally shown to be useless and perhaps harmful (44). Patients and doctors alike thought that there was a cause-effect relationship between cancer outcomes and Laetrile therapy (that Laetrile cured cancer); in fact, there was neither a cause-effect relationship, nor even a decent correlation.

In experimental studies, a treatment group of some sort is compared with a control group. Ideally, the experimental and control groups differ in only one way; the treatment is given to the experimental group and not to the control group. Although this seems a simple task at first, in reality it is very difficult, especially in medical areas. As the complexity of this task unfolds, remember that when designing a research project, there is no such thing as the perfect design. Research designs always mean making compromises and choices that open the results to other interpretations. The problem is not that the design is not perfect; the problem is in not recognizing the imperfections and dealing with them.

Types of Experimental Designs

Experimental designs for osteopathic research can take several forms, depending on the question being asked. These include:

- Between-subject designs
- Within-subject designs
- Crossover designs
- Variations

The hallmark of an experimental design is the comparison of the treated or experimental group of patients with a group receiving no, or some other, treatment. The experimental study is always prospective, that is, it is planned in advance and must always be approved by an IRB.

BETWEEN-SUBJECT DESIGNS

The simplest experimental design is that comparing a treated group with a historical control. Historical controls would be patients from the practice or from other practices who had received some other form of treatment than the one being investigated. This design is con-

sidered to be weak in its ability to define cause-effect relationships. It is only one step above the prospective case series design, because the control subjects may or may not be comparable to the experimental subjects. However, in some cases, such as very severe disease states or when it is considered unethical to withhold a putative treatment, it may be the only way to attempt to determine the effect of a new or altered treatment regimen.

The most usual of the experimental designs is the two or more group direct comparison design. In this study design, patients fitting the criteria for inclusion in the study are randomly assigned to one group or the other. If the design is an experimental and control group design, the subjects in the experimental group receive the treatment and the subjects in the control group receive either no treatment or some alternative (perhaps community standard) treatment. The results of the two groups are then compared on one or more measures.

Independent and Dependent Variables

The treatment given to the experimental group is the "independent variable," and the measures taken to judge results in both groups are the "dependent variables." Thus, in a study comparing the lateral recumbent thrust, such as the Irvine study, the independent variable was the thrust given to the experimental group, but not the control group. The dependent variables included straight leg raising and judgment of pain before and after the treatment. One of the hardest aspects of research on OMT is finding good dependent variables or measures of results.

Random Assignment to Groups

In experimental studies, it is very important that the two groups of patients be as much alike as possible. For example, if some systematic difference between the groups existed at the beginning of the study, such as the mean age of the experimental group being 24 and the control group being 56, a better result in the experimental group may well be due not to the treatment provided, but to the superior health of the younger patients. The comparability of the groups is usually achieved by "random assignment" of the patients to the groups. The patients are assigned to the groups completely at random, so that neither the investigator's bias nor other factors will result in patients in one group being different in any systematic way from the other group. There are many ways to do random assignment (44), but it is vital that it be done; how it is to be done must be specified prior to the study. Randomization can be as simple as flipping a coin to determine the group a patient is assigned to, but more reliable means are available, such as random number tables in books or on computers.

Blinding

One of the most important aspects of experimental research is the principle of blinding. It is well known that even the most honest investigator can unwittingly affect the results of a study by judging the results of a treated patient as better than an untreated patient. This often slight and unconscious bias or systematic error has often resulted in faulty and unreliable results from an otherwise well-designed study. To preclude this type of error, it is almost always necessary to make sure that the person measuring the outcome of a treatment does not know whether the patient received the experimental treatment (independent variable) or not. If the observer is blind to the patient's group, the study is called a single-blind study. If the patient is also blinded to the treatment given, the study is a double-blind study. At times, it is also desirable to have others in the study blind to patient group. However, at the absolute least, the observer must be blind to the patient's treatment status. If blinding of this sort cannot be shown or is not feasible, the study has a very serious problem that almost always will make the results suspect. This subject will be further discussed in the section "Special Considerations in Osteopathic Clinical Research".

WITHIN-SUBJECT AND CROSSOVER DESIGNS

The research types reviewed above include mainly those that use planned comparisons between experimental and control groups, or long-term determinations of health status that are then compared with the general population. Many variations on these study types exist. Another group of study types should receive careful attention when the effects of manipulative techniques or treatment are studied. These designs are within-subject designs; they essentially use the same subject as both the control and the experimental group. Keating et al. (45) have summarized this type of design in some detail.

The within-subject study usually involves following a patient for a period of time to determine the baseline symptoms and whether they are fairly stable or changing in some fairly predictable fashion. After the baseline measurement, treatment is introduced and the measurements continued. The measured variables can be compared before and after treatment to see if the treatment had an effect. The baseline measurement period will vary among several subjects, allowing the treatment to be introduced at different times, ensuring that there was no peculiar effect of time on treatment intervention. This is known as the variable baseline, within-subject study design. Frymann (46) used this design type in her study of the effects of osteopathic care of children with neurologic and developmental deficits.

Crossover designs usually use experimental and control groups, but after the control group has finished, these patients are "crossed over" to receive the experimental treatment. Crossing over sometimes satisfies objections that the control group will not get the benefit of a supposedly effective treatment. This design is useful if the illness or disease being studied is not particularly severe and can wait to receive the experimental treatment.

Crossover and within-subject studies are not especially effective if the measurements and symptoms are not fairly stable for a period of time that can be used as the control condition. In addition, there is some problem with establishing whether the manipulative intervention actually did cause any change in the symptoms being measured. However, these designs allow treatment for every subject in the study, whereas the control group does not receive treatment in traditional experimental and control group studies.

The study designs considered here have many variations that must be considered before final design elements are determined. Some of the major issues in design of osteopathic research are considered below in the "Special Considerations" section of this chapter. The investigator is also urged to consult design experts and/or reference texts (29,33).

Data Collection

The actual work of doing the study comes only after careful planning, written statement of the study, and IRB approval. It is absolutely necessary to do the preliminary steps carefully and completely, or the study will almost certainly be useless due to problems of design, execution, or data collection. The entire procedure of the study design must be written out so that all those involved in the study will fully understand every step. When writing or reviewing a clinical study protocol, I do not consider the design to be complete until the informed reader of the protocol will know from reading the document what happens to the patient all the way through the study.

Data collection is the actual performance of the study. The patients are recruited, assigned to groups, treated (or not), and measurements performed. The data are collected by the appropriate study participant, including measures of somatic dysfunction, functional tests, laboratory results, and so forth. All data must be kept confidential until the study is over (unless it is agreed to look at preliminary data earlier). The study group should meet frequently during the study itself to discuss any problems or concerns. Data analysis is the next step.

Data Analysis

Once data collection has been completed, the task of data analysis begins. Data from most studies must be subjected to some form of statistical analysis as a help in decision making. At most, statistical analysis is a way to help the investigator make informed decisions about the meaning of the data. Statistical tests are of three basic types: descriptive statistics, nonparametric statistics, and parametric statistics.

Descriptive statistics give information about the basic attributes of the collected data, such as the mean, median, and standard deviation. These numbers tell the investigator how each group performed on the dependent variables used. However, to obtain information about whether there might be a difference between the performance means of the experimental and control groups, some form of nonparametric or parametric statistical tests is used. The decisions about whether the independent variable caused a change in the experimental group's responses (dependent variables) rely on the results of tests of significance.

Statistical tests to determine differences between group data rely on the assumption that the experimental or independent variable caused a change in the experimental group that resulted in an actual difference being created between the groups, as measured by the dependent variable(s). According to this view, if the measure was the distance moved by the leg in a straight leg raising test, both groups would have the same average movement prior to treatment, but the treated group would have more movement after treatment. Thus, the treated group would now be a different group or population, as measured by straight leg raising tests. The treatment changed them from what they were before to a group able to perform straight leg raising to a greater level.

Several things determine how well the statistical test is able to indicate this difference. Two of the most powerful of these are the amount of variability in the initial measurements of the groups and the number of subjects in each group (subject numbers are discussed below, under Power). If all subjects initially had exactly the same movement distances, then a very small increase in all the treated subjects would be detected by the statistical test as a significant effect. However, if there was a great deal of variability among the subjects, then a much larger average increase due to the treatment would be necessary before the statistical test could predict that the treatment had produced an effect. Thus, variability is best kept as small as possible between subjects in any study.

Parametric statistical tests, such as the t-test or analysis of variance, make some assumptions about the distributions of the data and the population of subjects, in effect relying on the data to have a "normal" or bell-shaped distribution. If the data do not have roughly such a distribution, it is best to use nonparametric statistics, such as the Mann-Whitney test, to determine whether the results of the study show a difference due to the independent variable (47).

Many fairly simple computer programs are now available to help with statistical analysis. Such programs as KaleidaGraph (*www.synergy.com*), Instat (*www.graphpad.com*), GB Stat (*www. gbstat.com*), the SPSS packages (such as SYSTAT at *www.spss science.com/SYSTAT*), and others are available for both Apple and IBM-compatible computers (see also, e.g., *http://ebook.stat.ucla. edu/*,). However, statistical assistance should be sought to avoid mistakes in analysis.

STATISTICAL SIGNIFICANCE

Tests for differences between groups provide an estimate of whether differences in the dependent measures seen between the groups after the study can be relied on to have actually been produced by the independent variable, or whether the differences are more likely to have been the result of random or chance fluctuations. The reliability of the difference is called the significance of the test, or the level of statistical significance. By tradition, and some logic, the usual standard value that must be reached for a difference between the experimental and the control groups to be considered significant is $p = 0.05$. This is the so-called p value, and is a measure that takes into account the variability of the data and the numbers of subjects in the study, among other things. The p value is essentially an estimate of the probability that the study would show a difference as great as or greater than the observed difference purely by chance.

Thus, a p value equal to 0.05 means that only one time in 20 or 5 in 100 would a difference as great or greater than that observed happen by chance alone, if the experimental variable actually had no effect. Thus, p values greater than 0.05 are considered probably due to chance fluctuations in measurement or to weak effects of the experimental variable. If the p value is 0.05 or less, it is assumed that the chances of finding the observed differences by chance are so small that the differences can be accepted as due to the experimental variable.

It is a mistake, however, to assume that if the data show a p value "approaching" 0.05 (e.g., $p = 0.056$), the data are "almost" significant. In many cases, the addition of extra subjects or other refinements of the study produce no more significant results. If the data are close to significance, consider ways to redo the study with less variable data or stronger treatment.

The investigator must generally consult with a biostatistician before finalizing a study design. The statistician will give advice on what data can be successfully analyzed and how the data can best be collected. In addition, due to the number of different statistical tests available, the methods of analysis should be specified before the study is undertaken.

Discussion of Results

Once the data are analyzed, the investigator can undertake a discussion of the results and the study. The results must be considered in light of the background of the study, the results themselves, and the interpretation of those results by the investigator.

Data are only data; they are nothing until interpreted. The results of any study can be looked at in various ways. Consider what happened in the Irvine study. Osteopathic physicians looked at the data and basically said that the study was not important because the independent variable, the thrust, was not osteopathic treatment or spinal manipulation, but only a thrust. Allopathic physicians

viewed the results as insignificant because the thrust and nonthrust groups showed no differences 3 weeks later. However, immediately after the technique, there was a significant difference. Presumably, the thrust patients would have been able to return to work sooner, an important difference to an insurance company paying for time off work. Thus, if the study had been correctly interpreted as a technique study and the immediate effects recognized as important, the study would have made more of an impact.

The discussion or interpretation of the data is where the investigator can state his or her opinion of the outcomes, link them to other data, and interpret them for the osteopathic profession. The discussion should not be too grandiose, claiming that the study had proven everything in the universe (unless it really has), but the investigator should legitimately link the study to the areas of interest and suggest to the reader how the data are important. This is another reason that a good literature review is necessary; without that background, the investigator will not be able to properly interpret the results.

Writing and Publication

If it is not documented, it did not happen. This statement is true for data gathering, observations during a study, orders given for participants of a study, and for publication of the results of a study. If a study is done but not published, it did not happen. It is vital to write a report of a study and publish it in some format. There are numerous books available for the novice scientific writer (47). However, the investigator can follow basically the same format as that given above in the design of a study for writing a scientific paper.

The parts of a research paper, although varying to some extent, are basically:

- Abstract
- Introduction
- Methods
- Results
- Discussion
- Conclusions (sometimes not included)
- References

The abstract of any paper should present a concise and informative overview of the paper. Where the idea came from should be stated; this can be an overview of the literature review or observations that led to the idea for the study. The major methods should be given along with the major findings. The import of these findings finishes the abstract. Such statements as "The results are found below" or "The results will be discussed" are inappropriate. The abstract is the only thing that many people will read, so it must immediately tell the reader why they should look at the rest of the paper. Seeing it as unimportant, many writers dash off an abstract although it is a very important part of the paper.

The introduction is basically the background of the study. It gives an overview of the literature and other information about why the study was conceived. It provides the reader with the rationale for the hypothesis of the study. In fact, the introduction can be conceived of as a funnel with the hypothesis being at the bottom, small end. The introduction starts from the big picture overview and comes down to the hypothesis. The reader can see immediately why the hypothesis makes sense, given the background. Of course, some reports, such as case histories, have no hypothesis, but nonetheless, should have the background presented in the introduction.

The methods section is a fully detailed report of the procedures, tests, manipulative procedures, subject selection criteria, and so forth of the study. The methods section should allow a reader knowledgeable in the field to reproduce the study. The methods section should present sufficient detail that the reader can make judgments about the validity and usefulness of the study results.

The results section presents the actual data from the study and the analyses of the data. It gives tables and graphics to clearly show the reader the outcomes of the study. Graphs should be presented in formats that clearly show differences, data trends, and group data descriptions. Most graphs showing group data should show error bars so that the reader can see the amount of variability within the data (29,48). As with statistical analysis programs, there are several computer programs available to help with graphic presentations, such as KaleidaGraph (*www.synergy.com*), GraphPad (*www.graphpad.com*), GB Stat (*www.gbstat.com*), and Microsoft Excel. One of the most common errors in presenting data in a paper is to have graphics that are misleading, confusing, or not readily interpretable.

As stated earlier, the discussion section is where the author can express his or her opinions on the outcomes of the study. It is often helpful to begin the discussion section with a bullet recap of the major results. This helps both the writer and the reader to focus on the important aspects of the data. The discussion allows the author a place to express opinions about the meaning of the data and interpret it for the reader. Of course, the reader does not have to agree with the writer's interpretations.

The reference section should list the sources consulted by the author. All references that are cited in the text or that contributed to the ideas in the article should be cited. It is a serious ethical problem to use the material of others and not give attribution to them. Plagiarism is poorly looked on. It is a good idea to be inclusive rather than exclusive in referencing others' work.

The beginning and even the seasoned author can get help in writing articles by consulting the instructions for authors given in most medical journals. The only osteopathic journal fully indexed in the Index Medicus library is the *Journal of the American Osteopathic Association* (JAOA). It publishes full instructions to authors on the internet at the *JAOA* web site, *www.jaoa.org*. Other invaluable sources of information on writing style is the *Publication Manual of the American Psychological Association* (49) and the *AMA Manual of Style: A Guide for Authors and Editors, 10* (50). These invaluable books give not only style guidelines but also information on presenting graphics, writing theses, plagiarism, and much more.

When considering a journal for publication of an article, first choice should be given to journals indexed in the Index Medicus or similar worldwide listings. The target audience should be identified and the chosen journal should target that audience. The journal should be peer reviewed to insure quality of the articles published.

If the study is not sufficient for stand-alone publication, the author should consider presenting the data at a medical or scientific meeting from which abstracts are published. This provides a public reference of the work. The AOA research conference held each year in conjunction with the AOA convention is such a venue. The abstracts of the scientific presentations are published in the *JAOA* and indexed in the world literature.

SPECIAL CONSIDERATIONS IN OSTEOPATHIC CLINICAL RESEARCH

In the sections on research design, several ideas were introduced that require discussion in terms of osteopathic research questions. The areas that are of special interest to the design of osteopathic studies are:

- The "gold standard" for medical research
- The question being asked
- Blinding
- Control groups
- Patient populations
- Pilot studies and statistical power
- Inclusion/exclusion criteria
- Dependent variables

The "Gold Standard" for Clinical Research

The randomized, double-blind, placebo-controlled study has evolved as the "gold standard" for clinical research studies. This design was developed in the 1940s and 1950s as the appropriate design to test the effects of drug treatments. The major elements of this particular design are:

- Randomization of subjects into the treatment groups (or arms)
- Blinding of subjects, drug givers, and data collectors as to treatment given
- Provision to the control subjects of a "placebo" or inactive substance that is indistinguishable from the active drug

This design was developed to answer a very specific question in drug therapy. For practical purposes, the question or experimental hypothesis to be answered is, "What is the effect of this drug on the natural course of a disease process in the human unaware of what drug is given?"

The random assignment of subjects to the experimental or control group hopefully ensures that the experimental and control groups (or more groups if, e.g., a group given neither drug nor placebo is used) have the same characteristics to begin the study. The blinding of the patient to what is being received (active drug or inactive substance) will hopefully ensure that the patients in the experimental group do not feel better simply because they are getting an active drug. In other words, the psychological aspects of the treatment should be equal for the two groups. Blinding the drug giver and caregivers as to which group the patient is in hopefully insures that the treated patients do not get subtle cues that they are being given an active substance; blinding the data gatherers ensures that bias is not introduced by knowing the patients receiving the active drug. Thus, for the question being asked, this design is a good one. Unfortunately, studies of manipulative treatment are not always amenable to this design and may often ask different questions. Thus, we must examine briefly what affects the interpretation of clinical trials.

Validity and Bias

The validity of a study is simply how strongly we can believe that the results are a reflection of what is actually the case. Did the manipulative technique really cause the observed change or was some other mechanism at work? Will the technique work with other patients, or was the result limited to the patients being studied? Many factors can influence how results can be interpreted, and these factors are called biases.

The definition of bias in a research study is basically anything that could interfere with the correct interpretation of the results of the study. If the study asks about the effect of a technique on low back pain, then measuring the pain differently in experimental and control groups would constitute a bias that would invalidate the results. There are many forms of bias that affect the validity of a study.

External Validity

Simply put, an external bias is something that interferes with the generalization of the results of a study from the patients in the study to other patients (32). If an experimenter wanted to have an externally valid study of the effects of a manipulative technique on asthma in the general population, the study group would be chosen not from a hospitalized population but from the whole group of people with asthma. If the asthma study patients were all hospitalized, the effects of a manipulative technique might well be different than if the technique were performed on patients with a less severe form of the disease. The study would not be externally valid because it would not be generalizable to the whole population of asthma sufferers. Of course, if the intent of the study were to study the effects of manipulative interventions on asthma in hospitalized patients, it would be externally valid. Thus, it is very important to frame the hypothesis with knowledge of whom the subjects will be and to whom the data will be generalized. Many things can affect external validity, including the lack of proper control procedures, improper selection of patients, and the simple length of time the patient is in the study (symptoms may change over time even without treatment).

Biases that threaten the external validity of a study are often fairly easily seen and recognized. For the example above, the bias of using only hospitalized patients as subjects obviously limits the results to that population of patients. Other problems of generalizability are not so obvious. For this reason, the investigator must keep records of the patients and be able to define at least the demographics of the patients so that the reader will be able to judge which population the results are most likely to be applicable to.

Internal Validity

Much more serious are the threats to internal validity. These biases are often very subtle and can make statements about the actual meaning of results difficult if not impossible. A nonblinded observer who takes data in a study and who knows whether or not the subject was treated is an obvious source of bias that will almost surely make interpretation of between-group differences impossible. Other sources of biases threatening internal validity include (32):

- Inappropriate control groups
- Measures that do not accurately determine the response being studied
- Objectivity in the measures being used
- Small numbers of patients in the groups
- Initial differences between experimental and control groups
- Random fluctuations in the course of a disease process
- Regression of symptoms to the mean

Thus, the investigator must pay close attention to issues affecting the internal validity of the study design and would be well advised to consult an experienced clinical trials designer on the issue.

DESIGN OF OSTEOPATHIC CLINICAL TRIALS

Blinding

As noted above, the design of clinical trials of osteopathic manipulation is more complex and may ask different questions than drug trials. Obviously, the person providing the treatment cannot be blinded to whether manipulation is given or not. In some cases, the patient can be blinded to treatment condition, as in the Irvine study. None of the patients included in the study had any experience with manipulative treatment, and results showed that there was no difference between the groups as to their recognition of whether manipulation had been given or not. Blinding was done for the data gatherers, so the study can be considered a blinded trial with

the exception of the treating physician. Although patient blinding is possible in cases of technique studies like the Irvine study, it is not as likely in studies of full treatment effects. In addition, it is difficult to find large numbers of patients in most osteopathic practices who are completely naïve to manipulation. Thus, the question of patient blinding is one that must be examined for each study and dealt with as the study and situation allow. The consequences of not blinding the patients to treatment are considered under the section on control groups, below. In any event, it is imperative to have the data collectors blinded as to group assignment.

Population Selection

In most cases, studies of manipulative treatment will use patients from the investigators' practices. The study design should include recording the demographics of the patients so that there will be a basis to generalize from the study population to other patients. It is obvious that the patients coming to an osteopathic practice are not a random sample of the general population, but a highly self-selected group that may be motivated to seek osteopathic care. Thus, caution must be taken when generalizing results of manipulative trials to the general population, and this bias must be taken into account.

Control Groups

One of the most contentious issues in osteopathic research design is the issue of appropriate control groups. The idea of the control group stems from the necessity of having some way to compare the active treatment with some baseline. As mentioned above, historical controls are sometimes used, but are far from ideal. Historical controls may differ widely from the contemporary study group in many aspects, so give only an impression of effects. Historical controls are used only as a last resort.

The "gold standard" control is the placebo control. Defined above, the placebo control is designed to mask from the patient the knowledge of whether the active drug or the inactive substance is being given. Such a control is meant to take the psychological effects of the patient's knowledge on the interaction between drug and disease natural history out of the therapeutic picture. It has been widely assumed that the simple knowledge of treatment had about a 30% effect on the patients response to the treatment (the "placebo effect") (49). Thus, according to the commonly held view, the simple psychological effect of knowing that a treatment was being given could alleviate symptoms by a large amount. Thus, the placebo control is designed to keep the placebo effect from entering into the difference a drug would make in the course of a disease.

Significant questions are being raised about the placebo as an effective control condition (51–55). For example, is the "placebo effect" really as robust as has been assumed? Is factoring out the psychological effect giving a true picture of the actual effect of a drug or treatment on the course of a disease, or is the placebo control consistently causing an underestimation of the total effect of drug plus knowledge? It is now well known that an individual's psychological status has real and measurable effects on their physiologic processes (see Chapter 8). Is the placebo the best control for treatment studies? The placebo's sister control group, the sham control, is often used in studies of manipulative treatments and techniques. With a sham control, some type of "hands-on" experience is given to the patient so that the physiologic and psychological effects of placing the hands on the patient are equal in the treatment and control groups. The Irvine study is a good example of a sham treatment control. Because the question being asked was regarding the effectiveness of the thrust alone, a sham was appropriate.

However, what if the question being asked is of the effect of the osteopathic treatment as a total treatment effect? Is it then not appropriate to test the total treatment, including the effect of hands-on and patient knowledge, against giving the patient no treatment? The question being asked determines the control group. If the question is to test the totality of the treatment effect against no treatment, and treatment includes the effect of putting hands on the patient, then the appropriate control is a patient receiving only rest during the treatment time. It may also be appropriate to use the musculoskeletal examination as the "sham" in such cases. Here, both groups would receive the structural examination, but the control group would then rest while the manipulative treatment was given to experimental group. Blinding of the subjects to treatment group in many cases is simply impossible, thus leaving the concept of a "placebo" group as a moot point.

Another control often used in manipulation studies is the "community standard" control in which, for example, low back pain is treated manipulatively in the experimental group, but by drugs, physical therapy, and counseling in the control group. This type of active control group is asking yet another question: Is the effect of manipulation equal to or better than standard care? The recent Andersson study (40) on manipulative treatment for low back pain is a good example of this type of control group. Because of the ethical considerations of giving no care to a patient in a "do nothing" control group, the active or community standard of care control may be the only way some conditions can be examined.

Thus, the osteopathic researcher must carefully determine the actual intent of the experimental question prior to determining the appropriate control group. The myth of the "gold standard" must not be forced onto research designs for manipulation. If the question of the study is whether the manipulative treatment is better than nothing, a rest or nothing control is appropriate. If the question is whether the manipulation is better than community standard care, the appropriate control is the active community standard treatment. If the question is whether the manipulation is better than simply placing hands on the patient, probably the best control is the examination-only control.

Thus, careful consideration of what is being asked will determine the appropriate control group, not a preconceived notion of what a control should be.

Study Size and Power

Studies on the effects of manipulative treatment are in their infancy. It is difficult for an individual investigator to procure sufficient subjects for a large study. In fact, it is now becoming increasingly evident that many studies have not been sufficiently large for their results to be reliable. The term for the probability that a study contains sufficient subjects for an effect to be accurately found if, in fact, there is an effect of the independent variable, is called "power." The measure of the power of a study is called power analysis (56). The probability that the statistical analysis of a clinical trial will show a significant p value is remarkably large if the number of subjects in the study is small. In a study with few subjects, one subject's large change in findings may result in a significant effect, although the effect is not general. In this case, a "type I" error will result; the experimental hypothesis that there is a treatment effect will be accepted although no such effect is present. Thus, power analysis gives an estimate of the number of subjects required in a study to be reasonably sure that if there is an effect it will be found. Power

calculations can be made with relatively simple formulas found in standard books (55) or on the internet (e.g., *http://ebook.stat.ucla.edu/calculator/powercalc/*).

Pilot Versus Full Studies

Thus, the Andersson study (40), although well done with about 178 patients, is most likely still lacking sufficient patient numbers to fulfill power requirements. Studies not meeting standard power requirements must be termed "pilot studies," and their results should be viewed with caution. Pilot studies are very useful in giving indications of what effects may be valuable to further study and in providing data on the amount of variability inherent in outcome measures; therefore, they are very valuable. Studies that meet the required numbers of subjects indicated by power calculations are considered full-scale studies and, other things equal, are more reliable than studies with fewer subjects.

Dropouts

The problem of dropouts can be acute in any clinical study. In studies of manipulation, the investigator must account for patients not finishing the study. This is important because of the potential for causing imbalances between the experimental and the control groups. For example, if all the patients with more severe disease dropped out of the experimental group but stayed in the control group, the results would be inaccurate or biased toward a larger effect in the experimental group. The usual practice is to try to determine the cause of the patient's failure to finish the study and to carefully examine the drop-outs for commonalities that could affect study results.

Inclusion and Exclusion Criteria

The issue of inclusion/exclusion criteria is also difficult in many studies of manipulative treatment. The inclusion criteria are those things that make the patient eligible for the study, such as low back pain. However, the inclusion criteria must be well specified and measurable prior to the study. In the example of low back pain, the type, duration, and other factors should be carefully delineated. An area that needs special attention in inclusion criteria is that of a well-defined diagnosis. Often, studies of manipulation do not have well-defined structural diagnoses that can be justified and defended to the greater medical community, which results in poor acceptance of the study.

Exclusion criteria are those factors that exclude a patient from a study. These can be age, pregnancy, drug use, and so forth. Exclusion criteria must also be clearly specified in the study design. It had been standard practice to exclude women from many drug studies because of the danger of pregnancy. This practice resulted in a lack of information on the effects of drugs on females (poor external validity), and the effects were often different than the effects on males. It is now unacceptable to simply exclude females; if a study does so, explicit reasons must be given.

Dependent Variables: Selecting Appropriate Measures

The best measures to determine if a manipulative procedure had an effect are often difficult to decide. These measures are known as the dependent variables because their values are supposedly dependent on the experimental treatment. In studies of the efficacy of a manipulative technique or a manipulative treatment on the outcome of a specific disease process, the measures are presumably some aspect of the disease process or of the natural course of the symptoms. In assessing the contributions of manipulative treatment to resolution of somatic dysfunction or to the maintenance of health, the task of defining sensitive dependent variables becomes more difficult. Some dependent measures include measures of immune system function, studies of the activities of daily living, episodes of loss of health (for long-term studies), and other measures of body function, including reports of feelings of well-being and comfort.

One of the problems in many studies of manipulative treatment is the use of purely subjective, dependent variables in the study. Typically in these cases, an examiner performs a musculoskeletal examination of a patient and records the somatic dysfunction found. The treating physician typically repeats the examination and treats the findings for experimental subjects and simply does nothing for control subjects. The blinded examiner then performs a second examination and reports differences between the two examinations. The problems inherent in this design are mainly a lack of any knowledge of the reliability of the examiner. How much do the findings vary between examinations (repeat reliability) and how do the examinations of the two examiners correlate (interexaminer reliability)? These are significant issues that must be acknowledged in such a study.

The answer to such issues is to use dependent variables that are not dependent on the subjective examination of either a blinded examiner or the treating physician. Such measures can be instrumented measures, such as Doppler blood flow, respiratory volumes, and so on.

Whatever the dependent variable or variables, the measures of manipulative treatment results should include an evaluation of whether the treating physician determined that the treatment given actually did what it was designed to do. Sometimes, the manipulation fails to accomplish the desired immediate outcome in restoring range of motion or proper muscle relaxation. These facts must be recorded and used in analysis of the outcome of the treatment so that unsuccessful treatments can be looked at separately from those judged to achieve the desired end points. This will help reduce the variability of the data.

Another problem in choosing dependent variables is the temptation to simply measure everything available and hope to find a few that change. This may be a good strategy for a preliminary exploration of a treatment technique, but holds many pitfalls. In fact, this is sometimes called "oh heck" research design: Oh heck, let's do this and see what happens!

Given enough measures, the probability that one or a few will show significant changes is very high. In fact, if 20 dependent measures are chosen for measurement, expect that one will show a significant outcome by chance (when no effect actually exists). Thus, special statistical tests must be used when several measures are studied to guard against chance significant results. It is best to design a study with a few dependent variables that have either been shown to be affected by the independent variable, or to have good reason for suspecting that they may be so affected.

Characteristics of Well-Designed and Pitfalls of Poorly Designed Osteopathic Research

Good osteopathic research will have the characteristics of any well-designed clinical study. These characteristics include:

- A complete and well-documented literature search
- A well-defined working hypothesis
- Research design is logical and fits the hypothesis
- Complete and well-documented methodology
- Statistical methods and data processing procedures defined in advance
- Power calculations completed
- Well-defined inclusion and exclusion criteria
- Both objective and subjective dependent variables
- Adequate statistic and logistic support
- IRB approval obtained

These characteristics of a well-designed osteopathic trial should lead to reliable and believable data.

On the other hand, some of the pitfalls, especially for novice investigators, include the converse of the above, but also some perhaps less-obvious points when planning and conducting research:

- Planning is incomplete and not well documented
- Protocols are not rigorously followed
- Record keeping is not complete
- Time for study completion is underestimated
- Patients cannot be recruited in sufficient numbers
- Study is too complex
- Too many dependent variables

Many of these areas have been covered earlier in the chapter. However, some deserve brief mention here. As a study is carried out, it is very important for the investigator to make sure the protocols are followed at every step. If a mistake is made, it must be noted and any problem corrected. Mistakes will be made in any protocol; difficulties arise if the mistakes are not acknowledged.

Many investigators underestimate the time needed to complete a study. At times, patients cannot be recruited readily or replacement patients must be sought. These things can add significantly to the time required for study completion. A careful investigator plans extra time into the study design. It is good to offer a bonus to key personnel for subject recruitment and for help with the protocol.

As stated in the hypothesis section, a simple study is often the best one. A study with too many hypotheses to be tested or too many dependent variables or measures can become uncontrollable and even impossible to analyze. It is often better to perform several small, well-designed studies that together paint a picture, than one large, complex study that is not interpretable.

SUMMARY

Clinical research in osteopathic medicine is at the cutting edge of research design technology. The uncertainties surrounding controls, dependent variable measures, and interpretation of results makes it a difficult and challenging field. Well-designed studies that make a small contribution to understanding the mechanisms and efficacy of manipulative treatment, such as are now coming out in the osteopathic literature, will eventually paint a compelling and fascinating picture of this treatment modality. The profession must take full advantage of the fifth period of osteopathic research to strengthen its foundation in the coming years. By the results of research the profession will prosper.

REFERENCES

1. Smith WA. Skiagraphy and the circulation. *J Osteopath* 1899;5(8):365–384.
2. Northup GW, ed. *Osteopathic Research: Growth and Development.* Chicago, IL: American Osteopathic Association, 1987.
3. Burns L. *The Nerve Centers.* Vol II. Cincinnati, OH: Monfort and Company, 1911.
4. Burns L. *Basic Principles.* Vol I. Los Angeles, CA: The Occident Printery, 1907.

5. Burns L. *The Physiology of Consciousness*. Vol III. Cincinnati, OH: Monfort and Company, 1911.

6. Burns L. *Cells of the Blood*. Vol IV. A. T. Still Research Institute, Chicago, IL, 1931.

7. Burns L, ed. *Pathogenesis of Visceral Disease Following Vertebral Lesions*. Chicago, IL: American Osteopathic Association, 1948.

8. Kelso AF, Townsend AA. The status and future of osteopathic research. In: Northup GW, ed. *Osteopathic Research: Growth and Development*. Chicago, IL: American Osteopathic Association, 1987:93–117.

9. Denslow JS. *The Early Years of Research at the Kirksville College of Osteopathic Medicine*. Kirksville, MO: Kirksville College of Osteopathic Medicine Press, 1982.

10. Denslow JS, Korr IM, Krems AD. Quantitative studies of chronic facilitation in human motoneuron pools. *Am J Physiol* 1947;105(2):229–238.

11. Korr IM. The neural basis of the osteopathic lesion. *J Am Osteopath Assoc* 1947;46:191–198.

12. Korr IM. The emerging concept of the osteopathic lesion. *J Am Osteopath Assoc* 1948;November:1–8.

13. Beckwith CG. Thoracic vertebral mechanics. *J Am Osteopath Assoc* 1944;43:436–439.

14. Noll DR, Degenhardt BF, Fossum C, et al. Clinical and research protocol for osteopathic manipulative treatment of elderly patients with pneumonia. *J Am Osteopath Assoc* 2008;108:508–516.

15. Still AT. *Autobiography of A. T. Still*. Kirksville, MO: A. T. Still, 1897.

16. Still AT. *Osteopathy Research and Practice*. Kirksville, MO: The Pioneer Press, 1910.

17. Northup GW. *Osteopathic Medicine: An American Reformation*. Chicago, IL: American Osteopathic Association, 1966.

18. Patterson MM, Howell JN, eds. *The Central Connection: Somatovisceral Viscerosomatic Interaction*. Indianapolis, IN: American Academy of Osteopathy, 1992.

19. Enserink M. Helsinki's new clinical rules: Fewer placebos, more disclosure. *Science* 2000;290(20 October):418–419.

20. Emanuel EJ, Wendler D, Grady C. What makes clinical research ethical? *JAMA* 2000;283(20):2701–2711.

21. Taylor TE. Increased supervision of clinical research at home and abroad. *J Am Osteopath Assoc* 2001;101(12):696–698.

22. Patterson MM, Steinmetz JE. Long-lasting alterations of spinal reflexes: a potential basis for somatic dysfunction. *J Am Osteopath Assoc* 1986;2:38–42.

23. Willard FW, Patterson MM, eds. *Nociception and the Neuroendocrine-Immune Connection*. Indianapolis, IN: American Academy of Osteopathy, 1994.

24. Van Buskirk RL. Nociceptive reflexes and the somatic dysfunction: a model. *J Am Osteopath Assoc* 1990;90(9):792–794.

25. Denslow JS, Korr IM, Krems AD. Quantitative studies of chronic facilitation in human motoneuron pools. *Am J Physiol* 1947:229–238.

26. Patterson MM. Mechanisms of classical conditioning and fixation in spinal mammals. *Adv Psychobiol* 1976;3:381–436.

27. Patterson MM, Grau JW, eds. *Spinal Cord Plasticity*. Boston, MA: Kluwer Academic Publishers, 2001.

28. Shekelle PG, Adams AH, Chassin MR, et al. Spinal manipulation for low-back pain. *Ann Intern Med* 1992;117(7):590–598.

29. Dawson B, Trapp RG. *Basic and Clinical Biostatistics*. 3rd Ed. New York, NY: Lang Medical Books/McGraw-Hill, 2001.

30. Johnson SM, Bordinat D. Professional identity: key to the future of the osteopathic medical profession in the United States. *J Am Osteopath Assoc* 1998;98(6):325–331.

31. Johnson SM, Kurtz ME. Diminished use of osteopathic manipulative treatment and its impact on the uniqueness of the osteopathic profession. *Acad Med* 2001;76(8):821–828.

32. Johnson SM, Kurtz ME, Kurtz JC. Variables influencing the use of osteopathic manipulative treatment in family. *J Am Osteopath Assoc* 1997;97(2):80–87.

33. Trochim WMK. *The Research Methods Knowledge Base*. 2nd Ed. Cincinnati, OH: Atomic Dog Publishing, 2001.

34. Greenberg RS. *Medical Epidemiology*. 2nd Ed. New York, NY: Appleton & Lange, 1966.

35. Stark, J. *Still's Fascia*. Pahl, Germany: Jolandos, 2007

36. Buerger AA. A controlled trial of rotational manipulation in low back pain. *Man Med* 1980;2:17–26.

37. Hoehler F, Tobis J, Buerger AA. Spinal manipulation for low back pain. *JAMA* 1981;245(18):1835–1838.

38. Wells MR, Giantinoto S, D'Agate D, et al. Standard osteopathic manipulative treatment acutely improves gait performance in patients with Parkinson's disease. *J Am Osteopath Assoc* 1999;99(2):92–98.

39. Korr IM. Osteopathic medicine: the profession's role in society. *J Am Osteopath Assoc* 1990;90(9):824–832.

40. Andersson GBJ, Lucente T, Davis A, et al. A comparison of osteopathic spinal manipulation with standard care for patients with low back pain. *N Engl J Med* 1999;341(19):1426–1431.

41. Jones LH. *Jones Strain-Counterstrain*. Boise, ID: Jones Strain-Counterstrain, 1995. (Available from the American Academy of Osteopathy, Indianapolis, IN.)

42. Hulley SB, Cummings SR. *Designing Clinical Research: An Epidemiologic Approach*. Baltimore, MD: Williams & Wilkins, 1988.

43. Kaprow MG, Sandhouse M. Refractory torticollis after a fall. *J Am Osteopath Assoc* 2000;100(3):148–150.

44. Pocock SJ. *Clinical Trials: A Practical Approach*. New York, NY: John Wiley and Sons, 1983.

45. Keating JC, Seville J, Meeder WC, et al. Intrasubject experimental designs in osteopathic medicine: Applications in clinical practice. *J Am Osteopath Assoc* 1985;85:192–203.

46. Frymann VM, Carney RE, Springall P. Effect of osteopathic medical management on neurologic development in children. *J Am Osteopath Assoc* 1992;92(6):729–744.

47. Daniel WW. *Biostatistics: A Foundation for Analysis in the Health Sciences*. New York, NY: John Wiley and Sons, 1999.

48. Byrne DW. *Publishing Your Medical Research Paper: What They Don't Teach You in Medical School*. 2nd Ed. Baltimore, MD: Williams & Wilkins, 1998.

49. *Publication Manual of the American Psychological Association*. 5th Ed. Washington, DC: American Psychological Association, 2001.

50. *AMA Manual of Style: A Guide for Authors and Editors*. 10th Ed. New York, NY: Oxford Press, 2007.

51. Beecher HK. The powerful placebo. *JAMA* 1955;159(17):1602–1606.

52. Hrobjartsson A, Gotzsche PC. Is the placebo powerless? An analysis of clinical trials comparing placebo with no treatment. *N Engl J Med* 2001;344(21):1594–1602.

53. Kiene H. A critique of the double-blind clinical trial. *Altern Ther Health Med* 1996;2(1):74–80.

54. Al-Khatib SM, Kaliff RM, Hasselblad V, et al. Placebo controls in short-term clinical trials of hypertension. *Science* 2001;292(15 June):2013–2015.

55. Kienle GS, Kiene H. Placebo effect and placebo concept: A critical methodological and conceptual analysis of reports on the magnitude of the placebo effect. *Altern Ther Health Med* 1996;2(6):39–54.

56. Murphy KR, Myors B. *Statistical Power Analysis*. Mahwah, NJ: Lawrence Erlbaum Associates, 1998.

71

Research Priorities in Osteopathic Medicine

BRIAN F. DEGENHARDT AND SCOTT T. STOLL

KEY CONCEPTS

- There is a societal expectation and responsibility within the medical professions for clinicians to provide the best level of patient care based on current knowledge, not to be blinded by or become complacent with current practice outcomes, but to advance the practice of medicine to levels previously unimaginable.
- Although there is a trend in the biomedical research community toward reductionistic science, the osteopathic profession is uniquely positioned to perform research that integrates the principles underlying osteopathic medicine with a cost-effective distribution of its health care services worldwide.
- Researchers and research advocates representing the various constituencies within the profession need the mandate and resources to convene, to inform/educate members of constituency research initiatives, to coordinate goals and resources, to update research priorities, and to assess profession-wide research activities.
- Meaningful research comes from the burning desire to know and understand something better, not from the enthusiasm to "prove" that something works.
- Current evidence has repetitively demonstrated a therapeutic effect from human touch.
- When designing osteopathic manipulative medicine clinical trials, special consideration must be given during the study design phase to the control and/or placebo cohorts (touch vs. no-touch control), the blinding of osteopathic manipulative treatment (OMT) providers, and the selection and training of the OMT techniques that will be used in the study.

INTRODUCTION

Underlying the inception, establishment, and success of the osteopathic profession is its membership's desire to improve patient health. In the 20th century, the level of training of osteopathic physicians and the service provided by those physicians succeeded in placing osteopathic medicine clearly within the biomedical community, a community challenged with the dual responsibility of providing the best level of care based on current knowledge and advancing that knowledge to levels previously unimaginable. The osteopathic profession was established in the late 1800s in response to limitations in the practice of medicine at that time (1) and promoted many concepts that have been accepted in the 20th century (2). As the 21st century unfolds, the questions and challenges that the osteopathic profession needs to address are numerous and predominately relate to how its membership will continue to contribute to the practice of medicine. Will D.O.s recognize their responsibility and opportunity to become leaders in advancing patient care in both practice and research within the health care professions? Will they see health care research as a key component of patient care? Will they have the vision and fortitude to contribute to health care through research? Will training institutions prioritize education that promotes not only health care services but research activities as well? This chapter is intended to provide perspectives to compel profession constituencies to assertively answer these questions.

To establish a strong foundation for meaningful research priorities within the osteopathic profession, the term osteopathic needs to be used more precisely. When the profession transitioned from labeling itself "osteopathy" to "osteopathic medicine," the act of changing a noun to an adjective created a problem: osteopathic was suddenly used to modify a variety of nouns in an attempt to illustrate distinctiveness. For instance, osteopathic

began modifying research to try to make a distinction between "osteopathic" research and other forms of research, like "allopathic" or biomedical research. Linking osteopathic to research can be confusing and divisive within the scientific community, both within and outside the profession. Is not the goal of osteopathic research to pursue fundamental knowledge about the nature and behavior of living systems and to use that knowledge to extend healthy life while reducing the burdens of illness and disability? Wouldn't another goal of osteopathic research be to develop, maintain, and renew through the highest level of scientific integrity our capacity to prevent disease? While these are clearly osteopathic goals, these are also the explicit goals and mission of the National Institutes of Health (3). It is critical that members of the osteopathic profession who feel it is important to link osteopathic to research remember that a substantial amount of the research that has been identified by the profession as osteopathic was developed, performed, and interpreted by investigators who know nothing about osteopathic principles and practices.

Science and research are intended to be blind to labels. All scientists and clinicians should be united in the pursuit of an evidence base that leads to improved efficiency and quality in the provision of health care. The osteopathic profession, as a recognized member of the biomedical community, needs to fully engage in its dual responsibility of providing the best level of care based on current knowledge and of aggressively advancing that knowledge. The future contributions of the osteopathic profession will and should be judged on the merits of D.O.s within the scientific community in addition to the profession's provision of unique health care services. Osteopathic should be accurately linked to the practice of medicine that promotes patient-centered health care and to professionals who are willing to evaluate scientific outcomes through a set of standards or osteopathic principles that help discern what best supports the individual's, family's, and community's natural health potential. Further, as the practice of osteopathic medicine benefits from general biomedical research, it should be expected that the profession's scientific contributions will be incorporated into all appropriate levels of the health care system, as intended at the inception of the osteopathic medical profession. The profession's distinctiveness is not through labels that sustain isolation. It is through the complete participation in the biomedical community in ways that are unique and visionary that the true potential of osteopathic principles and practice will become evident.

While there has been an ongoing desire and attempt by the osteopathic profession to contribute to the scientific basis of health care (4–12), some report that the degree and quality of such research has been limited (5,12–14). Some may argue that the profession's resources in the last century have primarily been directed toward training D.O.s (15). As a result, there have been limited resources available to perform credible research. Others may argue that the resources that were available were not used effectively. While recent trends indicate a new level of commitment and success in research by the profession (14), it is clear that without a sustained concerted set of research priorities, a strategic plan that constituencies within the profession can own and consistently engage in, and a broad-based leadership to drive the strategic plan, the influence of the osteopathic profession on the provision of health care will wane and the potential of the application of osteopathic principles to health care will never be realized.

VISIONS OF MEDICAL RESEARCH IN THE 21ST CENTURY

In this era of globalization, it is important to appreciate that science and health care are global activities. As a result, there are personal, family, community, regional, and global considerations that need to be considered as the profession develops its research priorities. Beginning at the national level, in the past decade, two groups of U.S. experts independently convened a series of meetings to determine the major opportunities and gaps within medical research. One group consisted of over 300 nationally recognized leaders and researchers within the health care industry who advised the NIH regarding the future of that Institute's medical research (16). The other group became known as the Osteopathic Research Task Force (ORT), created and supported by key osteopathic educational, research, and professional organizations (13,17) to help foster cooperation and collaboration across the profession in order to enhance the quality and quantity of research evaluating the unique aspects of health care provided by osteopathic physicians. The conclusions from both groups provide a good context for developing research priorities within the osteopathic profession.

The group of experts convened by the director of the NIH recognized the "daunting challenge" of understanding the complexity of life (16). They noted that no single center within the NIH could address the many areas and issues that need to be studied to better understand these complexities. Therefore, the experts developed a set of research priorities, called the roadmap, which was intended to define the Institute's research direction. This group proposed that "progress in medicine requires a quantitative understanding of the many interconnected networks of molecules that comprise our cells and tissues, their interactions, and their regulation." They concluded that it is necessary to more precisely know the combination of molecular events that lead to disease in order to advance medicine. Therefore, they emphasized the need for cellular and molecular/genomic research, heralding

the expected level of influence nanomedicine will have in the future of health care (18).

The ORT, the second group of experts, consisted of representatives from the following organizations: the American Academy of Osteopathy; the American Association of Colleges of Osteopathic Medicine (AACOM); the American Osteopathic Association (AOA); the American College of Osteopathic Family Physicians; the Association of Directors and Medical Educators; the American Osteopathic Hospital Association; the Council of Osteopathic Student Government Presidents; the International Federation of Manual/Musculoskeletal Medicine; the Osteopathic Research Centers at the A.T. Still University's Kirksville College of Osteopathic Medicine, the Philadelphia College of Osteopathic Medicine and the University of North Texas Health Science Center; the National Undergraduate Fellows Academy; and the Postgraduate American Academy of Osteopathy. The ORT identified the lack of a unified, profession-wide research plan to advance the practice of medicine within an osteopathic context. Because within the profession there are limited resources available to support research activities and because there is a significantly better record in obtaining outside funding for basic science research (5,14), the ORT recommended continued support for the AOA directive that the profession make a concerted effort to prioritize research in osteopathic manipulative medicine (OMM) (4,8): "the application of osteopathic philosophy, structural diagnosis and the use of osteopathic manipulative treatment (OMT) in the diagnosis and management of the patient" (19). This consortium of experts produced a white paper consisting of an assessment of the current status of OMM research and a well-organized set of priorities/specific aims with strategies to advance OMM research and a profession-wide culture of research over a 5-year period (20). The ORT identified six domains of deficiencies or challenges within the profession that keep osteopathic medicine from having a scientifically based impact on the current practice of medicine (Table 71.1).

These domains are in research activities, funding and resources, research training, infrastructure, health policy issues, and leadership. The ORT White Paper Summary outlines priorities/specific aims and strategies promoted by the ORT for each domain and suggests potential organizations that seem appropriate to take responsibility for the various strategies based on the organization's representatives at that time.

The ORT White Paper is a significant contribution to the direction of research within the osteopathic profession. It offers a vision created by a broad-based collective from numerous constituencies and so represents the insight of the profession as a whole while challenging the profession to actively participate in fulfilling its research responsibility. Many of the specific aims and strategies of the white paper are related to the fundamentals of creating the infrastructure needed to be able to significantly contribute to the medical evidence base. While some progress has been made in certain domains of the white paper, most of the framework and details of the document are still pertinent as we head into the second decade of the 21st century.

To appreciate the role of the osteopathic profession within the scientific community, it is helpful to compare the NIH roadmap with the ORT White Paper. By doing so, research priorities for osteopathic medicine begin to take shape.

The conclusions presented in the NIH roadmap have significant implications worldwide. First, this vision of medical research is dependent on highly advanced technology, where outcomes will be generalized to establish protocols that create consistent standards for the treatment of patient populations. However, these outcomes may de-emphasize, minimize, or even ignore the individualized

> **TABLE 71.1**
>
> ## Challenges Facing the Osteopathic Profession in the OMM Research Arena
>
> | Domain of Deficiency | Examples of Challenges |
> |---|---|
> | Funding and Resources | Lack of adequate money to fund pilot projects. |
> | Research Activities | Insufficient number of OMM research studies underway. |
> | | Inadequate interactions between basic and clinical scientists. |
> | | Inadequate vehicles for disseminating research results. |
> | | Inadequate supply of trained researchers. |
> | | Lack of accountability for researchers. |
> | | Non-OMM DO specialists question OMM research relevance to their practices. |
> | | No universally available central data pool on previous research studies. |
> | Research Training | Insufficient opportunities for research training in OMM. |
> | | No broadly adopted and assessed research objectives/competencies. |
> | | No NIH-supported osteopathic medical scientist training program. |
> | | No identified mechanism to train and support mid career physician scientists. |
> | | No dedicated pool of money for timely resident and student research. |
> | Infrastructure | No commitment from most colleges of osteopathic medicine to foster a culture of research. |
> | Health Policy | General paucity of evidence-based medicine to justify reimbursement. |
> | | Evidence base that does exist not recorded or disseminated to impact stakeholders and health policy decision makers. |
> | | Poor communication between OMM researchers, OMM research-oriented committees and organizations, and the AOA leadership. |
> | Leadership | Unclear OMM research priorities cause lack of cohesiveness in OMM research. |
> | | No broad-based team given formal recognized authority to serve as the strategic leader of OMM research efforts. |

biopsychosocial aspects of health and disease, important factors in the provision of osteopathic health care. Second, because of the highly advanced technological resources needed to engage in this kind of research, the number of researchers able to participate is significantly limited. Third, the sophisticated instrumentation and networks required to translate medical advances from this roadmap into health care practices may not be available or affordable in all regions of the world, increasing disparities in health care services worldwide.

Conversely, the ORT supported previous AOA directives (4,8) to focus on research in the area of OMM in order to fill the research void in this area and best utilize profession resources in a concerted effort. This decision has significant global implications. By rigorously evaluating the application of osteopathic philosophy, structural diagnosis, and the use of OMT, positive outcomes from this research can impact society on biological and psychosocial levels on the individual, family, and community levels. Successful outcomes would likely be cost effective and easily distributed since OMM is not linked to expensive or extensive technology.

Although some may see these two research directions as opposing, it serves the osteopathic profession better to see them as complementary. While the NIH roadmap will lead to an expansion

of reductionistic science, the National Center for Complementary and Alternative Medicine (NCCAM), a center within the NIH, demonstrates the Institute's recognition that high-quality research in more holistic and integrative approaches deserves support as well. In 2006 (21), 2007 (22), and 2008 (23), NCCAM supported 318, 306, and 275 projects, respectively, of which 100, 87, and 92 were new projects for each year. The NCCAM budget, while only a fraction of the total annual NIH budget (just over $20 billion for the past 3 years [24]), still provides the largest resource of funding for research in complementary medicine practices like OMT. For instance, the total costs for NCCAM projects were $97.3 million in 2006, $100.2 million in 2007, and $97.6 million in 2008 (24). Studies that relate to manual therapies are outlined in Table 71.2.

While many factors can be considered when interpreting the extent of federally funded research in osteopathic manipulation, the osteopathic profession has had some success in obtaining NIH funding. As the primary profession that recognizes the value of incorporating both complementary/holistic and medical approaches into patient care, there is a need, and thus an opportunity, for the osteopathic profession to perform and support research that investigates the principles underlying the integrative nature of osteopathic medical care.

TABLE 71.2

NIH Funding of Manual Therapies: 2006 to 2008

Year	Funding Type and ID	Title	Primary Investigator	Location
2006–2008	R01 AT000123	Z Joint Changes in Low Back Pain Following Adjusting	Cramer, Gregory D	National University of Health Sciences
2006	R01 AT000370	Massaging Preterm Infants Enhances Growth	Field, Tiffany M	University of Miami Medical School FL
2006	R01 AT002689	Massage Benefits in HIV+ Children: Mechanisms of Action	Shor-Posner, Gail	University of Miami Medical School FL
2006–2008	R01 AT001927	Effect of Massage on Chronic Low Back Pain	Cherkin, Daniel C	Center for Health Studies
2006–2008	R21 AT001872	Effects of Massage on Immune System of Preterm Infants	Ang, Jocelyn Y	Wayne State University MI
2007–2008	R21 AT002303-02	Treatment Efficacy of OMT for Carpal Tunnel Syndrome	Stoll, Scott T	University of North Texas Health Science Center
2006–2007	R21 AT002560-02	Therapeutic Massage for Generalized Anxiety Disorder	Sherman, Karen J	Center for Health Studies
2006–2008	R21 AT002750-02	Craniosacral Therapy in Migraine Feasibility Study	Mann, J Douglas	University of North Carolina Chapel Hill
2006–2008	R21 AT002324–03	Dose-Response of Manipulation for Chronic Headache	Haas, Mitchell	Western States Chiropractic College
2006	R21 AT002751-02	A Model for the Mechanism of Action of Massage	Rapaport, Mark H	Cedars-Sinai Medical Center
2007	U01 AT001908-02	Dose-Response/Efficacy of Manipulation for Chronic Low Back Pain	Haas, Mitchell	Western States Chiropractic College
2006–2008	U19 AT002023-03	Mechanisms of OMM	Smith, Michael L	University of North Texas Health Science Center
2007–2008	K23 AT003304–02	OMM in Pregnancy: Physiologic and Clinical Effects	Hensel, Kendi Lee	University of North Texas Health Science Center
2007–2008	K24 AT002422-03	Midcareer Investigator Award in CAM-Osteopathic Medicine	Licciardone, John C	University of North Texas Health Science Center
2007–2008	R25 AT003580-01A1	Expanding Evidence-Based Medicine and Research Across the Palmer College of Chiropractic	Choate, Christine M	Palmer College of Chiropractic
2006–2008	R25 AT003579-02	Curriculum and Faculty Development in Evidence-Based Medicine	Laird, Stephen D	A.T. Still University of Health Sciences
2007	R25 AT002877–01A2	Competencies in Research in Manual Medicine and CAM	Cruser, Des Anges	University of North Texas Health Science Center
2006–2008	K30 AT000977	Chiropractic Clinical Research Curriculum	Meeker, William C	Palmer College of Chiropractic
2007–2008	F31 AT002666	Biomechanics of Spinal Manipulation Using a Cat Model	Ianuzzi, Allyson	State University New York Stony Brook

RESEARCH DOMAINS AND STRATEGIES IN OSTEOPATHIC MEDICINE

Many of the current and future research priorities of osteopathic medicine are consistent with those outlined in the ORT White Paper. Consequently, many of the research priorities described in this chapter will be presented with headings crossreferencing the domains and strategies of the white paper. Additional comments on certain specific aims and strategies will not be presented because the description in the white paper is self-explanatory.

Research Leadership

Research leadership requires the ability to direct or facilitate meaningful research activities, a vision to identify pertinent areas of research for society, and the ability to disseminate research outcomes to effect health care policy and the daily practice of medicine. Research leadership in the osteopathic profession has been fulfilled for years by the AOA board, bureaus, and councils (5,7,8,25). The AOA leadership has often been burdened by challenges within the research arena beyond the scope of their typical responsibilities as a membership organization. Alternatively, numerous organizations within the profession have a research arm or committee, but their success has been limited due to time, isolation, and limited resources. Better coordination of the current research-oriented leadership within the various organizations of the profession is critical for success of the osteopathic research enterprise. Although listed as the sixth domain within the white paper, expanding, empowering, and coordinating research leadership must be the first priority of the osteopathic profession. This is vital to the establishment of a productive infrastructure that is required for the profession to become competitive for NIH funding and to be able to produce the quality research needed to impact medical practice and health policy.

An example of insightful, collective leadership was the promotion of osteopathic research centers (ORCs) within the profession (13,17). While only one center at the University of North Texas has been funded thus far, this support has resulted in very positive outcomes (26). Five of the six NCCAM-funded investigational grants to the profession (Table 71.3) were granted to the ORC. Building on the outcomes from one of the R21 grants, in 2009 an R01 was also received by Hodges to study the "mechanisms of lymphatic pump enhancement of immune function." The ORC has also received seven funded grants from the AOA since 2006 (Table 71.3).

The center funding from many constituencies within the profession has helped the ORC build the needed infrastructure to become a successful contributor to the biomedical community while minimizing the financial burden on any one entity. The original intent of this directive was to establish a consortium of several centers strategically placed throughout the profession (17). Due to the success of the first funded ORC and the lessons learned from it, funding other ORCs is warranted to further promote the establishment of a successful, profession-wide research infrastructure.

The ORT served an important and unprecedented leadership role for a few years, coordinating the Osteopathic Collaborative Clinical Trials Initiative Conferences (OCCTICs), helping the profession establish an ORC, and developing the white paper. After the ORC was established, the ORT no longer had a clear mandate and disbanded. As a result, the momentum created by the integration of organization leadership diminished and many of the initiatives outlined in the white paper have not been addressed. It is critical to appreciate that the ORT was not designed to take over any of the current committees or organizations that support research but provided a venue where these constituencies came together, became educated about the activities occurring outside of their immediate focus, and coordinated and strategically planned a vision as articulated in the white paper. For the vision to be achieved, ongoing communication, coordination, timely assessment of successes and failures, and subsequent refinement and updating of the strategic plan is critical. The ORT or a similar body needs to be re-established and supported in the long term for the profession to be able to actively and progressively contribute to the general scientific community.

In addition to the ORT, a greater level of commitment to research must come from other entities. An organization, such as the AACOM, should take a leadership role in advancing the annual reporting of research activities, which could be used to benchmark success and refine strategic planning. Accrediting bodies within the AOA need to demonstrate leadership by emphasizing to colleges and hospitals the importance of promoting and participating in research. If the profession truly agrees that it has the dual responsibility of providing the best level of medical care based on current knowledge while advancing that knowledge, the AOA needs to give accrediting bodies the directive and authority to assess an institution's progress in research activities. Such leadership is necessary because without invigorating research at osteopathic colleges and associated research centers, institutes, or medical facilities, the profession will not succeed in fulfilling its research goals and societal responsibility to improve health care (14,27). Description of the ways in which the colleges can lead in research will be discussed later as specific research priorities are presented. As for practicing physicians, they need to see the value of and join a practice-based research network and support research financially through their alma mater and/or the profession. Future DOs must take the initiative to become involved in research activities, encourage curricular content toward critical thinking, research methodologies, and evidence-based medicine, and consider pursuing secondary degrees in order to expand their clinical research options. Thus, it should be clear that leadership which supports research priorities needs to be shared at all levels of the profession.

OMM Research Activities

Challenges and Opportunities Facing Current Researchers

While the number of practicing DOs is increasing (28), few have adequate training to develop and conduct quality research. In addition, across the biomedical community, the number of clinical researchers is diminishing (29,30). Consequently to deal with the current deficit, it is critical to increase the collaboration between physicians and scientists both within the profession and without.

Each osteopathic medical school has a cohort of basic scientists who can serve as a pool of potential collaborators for OMM research. These basic scientists usually come into the profession with little to no understanding of osteopathic principles or of how their talents could be used to generate meaningful research in the osteopathic practice of medicine. A standardized introductory program highlighting osteopathic principles, practices, and models of research needs to be developed and provided to all professors entering the profession, with modifications at the college level to highlight research opportunities unique to that institution. Productive lines of OMM research have been established between clinicians and basic scientists whose skills appear quite unrelated to OMM (31–36). However, both senior and novice clinical and basic science faculty must be open-minded and think innovatively to create

TABLE 71.3

Grants Awarded by the AOA: Years 2006 to 2009

AOA Grants 2006

Grant Number	Principal Investigator	Grant Title	Affiliation	Term of Grant
06-04-545	Donald R. Noll, D.O.	Testing Thoracic Lymphatic Pump Techniques for Reducing Lung Volume in Persons With COPD	ATSU/KCOM	1 y
06-11-547	Lisa H. Hodge, Ph.D	Lymphatic Pump Manipulation: Effects on Lower Respiratory Tract Infection and Immunity	UNTHSC/TCOM	2 y
06-11-549	Kendi L. Hensel, D.O.	OMM in Pregnancy: Physiologic and Clinical Effects	UNTHSC/TCOM	2 y
06-04-550	Brian F. Degenhardt, D.O.	Investigation of Inflammatory Markers for Effects of OMT on Subjects with Low Back Pain	ATSU/KCOM	1 y

1 year, 09/01/2006-08/31/2007

2 years, 09/01/2006-08/31/2008

AOA Grants 2007

Grant Number	Principal Investigator	Grant Title	Affiliation	Term of Grant
07-05-554	Richard Hallgren, Ph.D	Development of a Standardized Protocol for Collecting EMG Data From Suboccipital Muscles in Head and Neck Pain Patients	MSUCOM	1 y
07-41-557	Michael L. Kuchera, D.O.	Documenting Mechanics and Mechanisms in Pedal Pump OMT	PCOM	1 y
07-04-561	Vineet Singh, Ph.D	Changes in Gene Expression Resulting From Osteopathic Manipulation	ATSU/KCOM	1 y
07-06-562	Richard T. Jermyn, D.O.	Effect of OMT on the Use of Opioid and Analgesic Medication for Chronic Low Back Pain	UMDNJ/SOM	2 y

1 year = 09/01/2007-08/31/2008

2 years = 09/01/2007-08/31/2009

AOA Grants 2008

Grant Number	Principal Investigator	Grant Title	Affiliation	Term of Grant
08-08-563	Richard L. Williams, III, Ph.D, M.S., B.S.	Extension of the Virtual Haptic Back for Advanced Palpatory Diagnosis With Motion Testing	OSU-COM	2 y
08-11-569	Rita M. Patterson, PhD	Functional Hand Kinematics	UNTHSC/TCOM	1 y
08-11-570	Shrawan Kumar, Ph.D, D.Sc, FRSC	Reliability and Validity of Therapeutic Spinal Mobilizer and Measurement of Spinal Segmental Stiffness/Compliance in Healthy People and Toward the Development of a Three Segment	UNTHSC/TCOM	2 y

(continued)

TABLE 71.3 *(Continued)*

| 08-21-572 | Paul R. Standley, Ph.D | In Vitro Modeling of Myofascial Release: Fibroblast Cytokine Regulation of Muscle Contractility | UA | 2 y |
| 08-11-573 | Lisa Hodge, Ph.D | The Effects of Lymphatic Pump Manipulation on Tumor Development and Metastasis | UNTHSC/TCOM | 2 y |

1 year = 09/01/2008-08/31/2009
2 years = 09/01/2008-08/31/2010

AOA Grants 2009

Grant Number	Principal Investigator	Grant Title	Affiliation	Term of Grant
09-12-580	Kristie Grove Bridges, B.S., Ph.D	Salivary Alpha-Amylase as a Biomarker of the Response to OMT	WVSOM	1 y
09-05-581	Joseph Vorro, B.S., M.A., Ph.D	Interexaminer Reliability, Validity, and Outcomes Study of OMT for Patients With Cervical Somatic Dysfunction Using Three Dimensional Kinematics	MSUCOM	2 y
09-05-586	Richard Hallgren, Ph.D	Use of EMG Data to Investigate the Functional Role of Rectus Capitis Posterior Minor Muscles	MSUCOM	1 y
09-10-591	Michael L. Kuchera, D.O.	High-Tech/High-Touch Translational Care for Multiple Sclerosis: Integrating OMT, Periodic Acceleration Therapy and Therapeutic Magnetic Resonance With IsoPUMP Maximal Effort Exercise	PCOM	2 y
09-05-592	Jacek Cholewicki, Ph.D	The Effect of Osteopathic Manual Therapy on Postural Control in Patients With Low Back Pain	MSUCOM	2 y
09-11-594	Xiangrong Shi, Ph.D	Cranial Osteopathy and Cerebral Tissue Oxygenation	UNTHSC/TCOM	1 y
09-04-597	Neil J. Sargentini, Ph.D	New Rat Model for Pain, Relief by Manual Therapy, and Gene Expression Studies	ATSU/KCOM	2 y
09-04-598	Brian F. Degenhardt, D.O.	Determining the Clinical Value of Positional Asymmetry Tests of the Pelvis – Phase I	ATSU/KCOM	1 y
09-38-599	John C. Licciardone, D.O., M.S., MBA	Mechanisms of Action of OMT for Chronic Low Back Pain	ORC	2 y
09-43-605	Mary Goldman, D.O.	OMT in Chronic Obstructive Pulmonary Disease, Short Term Effects in Hospitalized Patients	GRMC	2 y

1 year = 09/01/2009-08/31/2010
2 years = 09/01/2009-08/31/2011

these associations. The administration and department chairs at each college need to take a leadership role in facilitating these collaborations and in identifying, recruiting, and nurturing clinicians and basic scientists who are willing to participate in these interdisciplinary research teams. Critical for success in fostering these collaborations are college administrators who can provide routine encouragement to the interdisciplinary research teams with meaningful incentives, such as additional research support (technicians, computers), as collaborations become established.

Supporting collaboration with scientists outside of osteopathic colleges requires a different strategy. First, it is important to know what type of researcher or what type of skill set is needed for a particular line of research in OMM. There are disciplines, such as engineering, biomechanics, motor control, neurobehavioral sciences, and pain management, that have overlapping areas of interest with OMM, but associations with researchers in these fields have not been adequately pursued. Osteopathic colleges that exist within large universities with significant research infrastructures have the opportunity to create collaborations with experts from the other colleges within their institution to advance OMM research. Establishing these collaborations will only occur if leadership and initiative comes from the osteopathic profession to create a research question/vision that is meaningful and provocative to these researchers. Resources must be given to key osteopathic personnel, particularly research-trained DOs and PhDs, who can identify external researchers whose skills seem ideal to perform collaborative research within an osteopathic context. Further, the osteopathic researchers must routinely monitor the activities of potential collaborators so that the research direction and instrumentation within those labs are clearly understood. Such knowledge will allow the osteopathic researcher to develop meaningful research questions linking the independent lab's areas of interest to research questions that overlap with osteopathic principles. Then through interactions set up at routine meetings, conferences, or special invitation luncheons, a quality presentation of the research idea can be given and hopefully a productive collaboration initiated.

Limiting the profession's success in promoting research is its lack of awareness of the current DOs participating in research. A profession-wide survey of DOs involved in research activities would be useful to identify the current pool of clinical researchers. The profession could then develop programming to promote dialogue between those researchers. In addition, an underutilized research resource is DOs trained in non-AOA sanctioned residencies and practice in the general biomedical community. These physicians are likely to have the background and connections to facilitate research relationships between the osteopathic profession and other disciplines within the biomedical community. Therefore, these DOs need to be identified, and the profession needs to nurture positive relationships with them. In an era where the number of graduating DOs is dramatically increasing while the number of DO residencies is not, the AOA needs to develop policies that strengthen their relationship with MD trained DOs instead of isolating them.

In previous studies in OMM, osteopathic medical students, predoctoral fellows, residents, and board-certified OMT specialist physicians have participated as treatment providers. Different studies have found positive and negative results from each respective skill level of OMT provider (37–40). A case can be made that if students or residents (relative OMT novices) can have a positive clinical effect within a research study then the osteopathic profession's contention that all DOs have the requisite skills at graduation to help their patients with OMT is supported. Yet achieving positive outcomes in clinical efficacy studies may be more risky when using novice practitioners. The more experienced osteopathic

researchers and research centers in the US utilize board-certified OMT specialists almost exclusively in the provision of OMT for their research trials. At this very early stage of OMT research, treatment protocols and providers should be selected to maximize the likelihood of finding a treatment effect if one actually exists.

Considering the substantial paucity of board-certified OMT specialists, even if OMT provided by these specialists is proven efficacious, the information has limited practical utility since there are only a few providers in practice to make the treatments available to the public. Consequently, if OMT is found to be effective when administered by board-certified providers, a task that should be more likely than with less trained individuals based on face validity, subsequent research should be undertaken to determine whether generalists or physicians-in-training can attain similar results.

Although the current research environment within the profession recommends against the use of student researchers as treatment providers in clinical efficacy studies, there are research projects appropriate for student participation. One area of research ripe for student participation involves investigating the baseline palpatory skills of osteopathic medical students and determining the impact of current training programs on those skills. This area of research is also ideal for establishing interdisciplinary collaborations.

Regardless of the skill level of the OMT provider, all treatment providers should undergo repetitive training (certification) in the specific diagnostic skills, OMT techniques, and any other protocol parameters associated with a particular trial. Such training adds significantly to the perceived and actual validity of the provided OMT.

Over the past several years, the Osteopathic Heritage Foundation (OHF) has been instrumental in supporting current researchers within the profession by establishing endowments that provide resources to augment research programs showing productivity (41). This format has been successful in the general clinical research arena and their establishment within the osteopathic profession demonstrates insightful leadership. Such support needs to continue.

Types of Research: Defining a Meaningful Research Portfolio

A critical goal for research leadership is to create a research portfolio that prioritizes and strategizes research for a period of time (5 year blocks) to optimize utilization of resources and outcomes. This section is offered to help individual researchers, funders, and reviewers have a framework from which to develop personal research and to determine funding priorities.

While not specifically outlined in the ORT White Paper, one purpose of the initial OCCTIC meetings was to prioritize specific areas of research. Much debate ensued over the topics and types of research that should be initiated first, such as clinical efficacy versus mechanistic studies or studies on musculoskeletal conditions versus systemic diseases. This debate continues today.

Clinical Efficacy Versus Mechanistic Research

Generally speaking, clinical efficacy research involves exploring whether or not a particular clinical intervention is beneficial. In contrast, mechanistic research focuses on how a particular clinical intervention is beneficial. Most biomedical research progresses from mechanistic toward clinical research. For example, scientists must first understand the mechanisms by which the body controls blood sugar levels before they can develop treatments for diabetes. Potential treatments based on these mechanisms are then evaluated for safety and optimal dosing in Phase 1 clinical trials, for feasibility and effect size in Phase 2 clinical trials, and for efficacy and possibly cost effectiveness in Phase 3 clinical trials. An understanding of the underlying physiological and pathophysiological mechanisms is extremely powerful in the development of effective novel clinical interventions. For this reason (and others), the vast majority of research resources in the United States over the last century have been awarded to scientists exploring biological mechanisms. The underlying principle for this approach is that this wealth of knowledge on mechanisms will eventually translate into applied breakthroughs in clinical care. This principle has been reconfirmed in the NIH roadmap.

This sequence of first mechanistic and then clinical research is turned upside down in areas where systems of health care have been practiced for hundreds (if not thousands) of years, are broadly accepted, and are in popular use. These areas include OMT as well as other traditional treatment methods, such as acupuncture, Ayurvedic medicine, and the use of botanicals. Since these traditional treatment methods have weathered the test of time, they are generally accepted as safe especially when they do not prevent the use of modern treatments clearly known to have efficacy. Osteopathic clinical researchers often favor efficacy studies since they do not have the constraint of mechanistic research superseding efficacy research in order of priority and because efficacy studies give them the opportunity to "prove" that OMT works.

There are many factors to consider when choosing between clinical efficacy and mechanistic research. Mechanistic research has in its favor its relative low cost, a defined facility for performing the research (a lab), and the potential for variable control. Efficacy research typically costs more, is more difficult and time consuming, and is perceived as less scientifically rigorous due to the high intrinsic variability within human subjects and the inability to control many significant variables. Even though efficacy research may lack in practicality, it has the potential of being more relevant to health care.

What is most important, no matter which kind of research is chosen, is to develop a research question with a good basis or rationale for why the hypothesis could be true. In the case of current clinical research within OMM, developing research questions is simple since little research has been performed to narrow the field of questions. Yet it can be difficult to have a good basis for the hypothesis when most claims of the efficacy of OMT have been anecdotal and when the parameters for the condition being treated as well as the intervention being performed are poorly defined. Meaningful research does not come from the enthusiasm to "prove" something works but from the burning desire to know and understand something better. Too often, osteopathic research is performed and little is learned because too many assumptions were made in the design of the study. In the back of every researcher's mind must be the concern that time is short and resources are limited. Poor motives and poor study designs result in poor outcomes as well as wasted time and resources. The availability of time will be gained when small but sequential steps in knowledge are made when answering a question.

This fundamental in science of making small but sequential steps in knowledge challenges clinicians and researchers to observe phenomena thoroughly first so that appropriate questions, rationale, and designs for research can arise from these observations. An observational study design has the potential of identifying what might be efficacious for a specific condition. Based on sound observations, a well-controlled, competitive clinical efficacy study can be developed and the likelihood of achieving meaningful outcomes can be optimized. As a patient-focused profession that promotes optimizing intrinsic health for each individual, establishing well-designed and coordinated procedures to observe characteristics, conditions, and treatment outcomes could and should drive the research agenda, whether it is in clinical efficacy or mechanistic studies.

Musculoskeletal Versus Systemic Disease

OMM was built upon the reports of treatment success for systemic diseases. Yet for decades, the practice of OMM has been directed more toward musculoskeletal diseases. Musculoskeletal disease as an OMM research focus has in its favor the high incidence of musculoskeletal diseases and pain in the general population and the high costs of care for these problems. Low back pain alone has health care costs of over $100 billion annually in the United States (42). The efficacy of OMT for purely musculoskeletal conditions also has in its favor more easily understandable and defensible theoretical mechanisms of action. It is relatively easy to understand how the application of manually guided forces may affect and align elements of the musculoskeletal system with known discrete elastic, plastic, viscous, and colloidal properties. It is more challenging to suggest that these forces could improve conditions like irritable bowel disease, improve pulmonary function to fight pneumonia, or resolve recurrent ear infections.

However, only the osteopathic profession has the history, incentive, and potential capability to conduct clinical research into the use of manually applied, body-based treatment of systemic diseases. While research on manually applied, body-based treatment of systemic diseases could be seen as an opportunity, there needs to be an open and critical assessment of the training students and recent DOs have received in OMM in order to determine if current osteopathic physicians have adequate training to treat systemic diseases with OMT. Regarding manual diagnostic and therapeutic skills, members of the profession can talk about legacy and licensure, but what are we able to validly report on capability? For visceral diseases, how much training do our students receive in diagnosing the musculoskeletal manifestations of visceral diseases or treating them with OMT? How much training do students receive in the hospital setting treating systemic illnesses? How many cases do students report that they used OMT as part of the care for common visceral diseases? Over the past 30 years, the number of curricular hours in OMM within osteopathic colleges has diminished by 50%. How much confidence does or should the profession currently have regarding the efficacy of OMT? As a result of the dramatic changes in OMM training, are the current therapeutic outcomes from OMT representative of the model itself or of the current training standards? This change in training further emphasizes the need to perform observational studies, as described in the previous section, so that a reasonable assessment of the current therapeutic nature of OMT can be made.

Special Considerations in OMT Clinical Trials
Placebo

Literature on the use of placebo control in clinical trials is amazingly complex and nuanced, and it is beyond the scope of this chapter to provide a review of placebo literature. However, there is active and valid debate within the osteopathic research community as to whether OMT clinical research should even utilize placebo control due to its nuanced complexity. On the one hand, the use of placebo control is so ingrained in the medical research culture that clinical trials lacking this design component are summarily rejected. On the other hand, placebo control in OMT clinical trials is so fundamentally misunderstood that the use of a placebo practically ensures misinterpretation of the associated results.

Central to this debate is an understanding of how a placebo intervention is selected for use in an OMT clinical trial. Theoretically, subjects in the placebo arm of a clinical trial should experience everything identically to the subjects in the OMT arm with one notable exception; they do not receive the active ingredient inherent in OMT. The specific placebo selected depends on what one hypothesizes is the active ingredient in OMT for a particular trial. In order of increasing specificity, the active ingredient in OMT could include physician time and attention, therapeutic touch, nonspecific musculoskeletal mobilization (jostling), and/or reversal of specific somatic dysfunctions. If the research question is to determine whether the difference a DO makes includes all of these potential mechanisms (effects) of OMT, then a placebo should be selected that includes none of these clinical interactions (e.g., an educational brochure). It is rational to promote that placebo interventions could include: (1) a DO simply spending extra time with the patient (without physical contact) to test effect of OMT versus touch, jostling, and somatic dysfunctions reversal; (2) a DO providing light touch (without movement or intent to treat) to test effect of OMT versus jostling and somatic dysfunctions reversal; or (3) a DO providing nonspecific musculoskeletal mobilizations (without the physician intending to produce a therapeutic treatment) to test the effect of OMT versus somatic dysfunctions reversal alone. Yet most NIH reviewers and clinicians do not understand that OMT may actually positively impact health through a combination of these potential mechanisms. Evidence indicates that touch itself is therapeutic (43), and so by its very nature, cannot be considered as a placebo but as an alternative yet overlapping form of treatment. Consequently, research designed to compare OMT to a light-touch group is not an adequate placebo design. A no-touch control is required in manual medicine research. A design without a no-treatment, light touch control group will likely require a larger number of subjects than commonly predicted in order to demonstrate efficacy because the touch, nonmanipulation group will have therapeutic results representing a portion of the therapeutic effects of the OMT intervention.

This understanding explains the results of many placebo-controlled manual therapy clinical trials where the touch-only placebo intervention produces results that fall between the results of the OMT group and those of the no-treat controls (39,40). Since the term placebo is so ubiquitously associated with a sham, fake, or false treatment, the interpretation that OMT produces results comparable to placebo is the most common and possibly most misleading conclusion. Since placebo controls are standard and customary in clinical research but are oversimplified and misunderstood, placebos should be used properly within OMM clinical efficacy studies but interpreted and discussed cautiously and insightfully in OMT clinical trial grant applications and publications.

Blinding

It is commonly accepted that a Phase 3 clinical trial must be double blind. This expectation is another significant hurdle for OMT clinical trial research. Simply defined, double blind means that both the patient and the doctor (provider) are blind to research intervention group assignments, so neither the patient nor their doctor knows which treatment group the patient is in. This is a fundamental design element in double-blind studies because knowledge of group assignment by anyone involved in care or data collection has the potential to bias results. However, it is impossible for certain therapeutic interventions to be administered without the provider knowing that a given treatment is the real treatment and not the placebo. This predicament exists for clinical research on surgical interventions, exercise prescriptions, therapeutic ultrasound, and, of course, OMT. In fact, clinical trials of medications or nutraceuticals represent some of the few types of interventions that can truly be double blind by the above definition.

In OMT research, the goal is to blind everyone possible. Although the actual OMT provider must be unblinded, the patient, all other clinical personnel (nurses, therapists, front office staff, etc.), the clinical trial coordinators, the data entry staff, and the principal investigator(s) should be kept blind. Further, if the presence or severity of somatic dysfunction is used as a clinical outcome measure, then an osteopathic physician other than the OMT provider should perform all pre- and post-OMT palpatory assessments of somatic dysfunction. Although this addition greatly increases the complexity and cost of an OMT clinical trial, it is the only way to eliminate the potential for bias from the unblinded OMT provider.

OMT Technique Selection

For many clinical conditions, an OMT prescription will include a variety of techniques intended to address different elements of the disease pathophysiology and will be selectively tailored in response to a given patient's palpated specific somatic dysfunction. According to osteopathic principles and practices, an osteopathic researcher would likely hypothesize that the greatest therapeutic effect would occur when OMT is utilized in this individualized, pragmatic, and holistic fashion. On the surface, this method seems inconsistent with best research practices, which dictate that interventions in clinical research trials must be standardized. However, on closer examination and with a better understanding of OMT, it becomes apparent that a somewhat individualized approach using multiple techniques in multiple body regions is most appropriate and even critically necessary for quality OMT research at this stage of its development.

Using research that investigated OMT in the treatment of pneumonia as an example, most clinicians who regularly use OMT for this condition would advocate a whole-body treatment that included different techniques to (1) improve the biomechanics and mobility of the rib cage (bellows), (2) normalize autonomic nervous function, (3) remove diaphragmatic impediments to fluid flow, (4) minimize the overall body burden of somatic dysfunction, and (5) enhance lymphatic circulation and immune function (44). This kind of treatment protocol would be performed in a clinical trial by having the treatment providers repetitively trained and certified to accurately and consistently provide this constellation of techniques, individualized to each given patient's specific somatic dysfunction. In addition to specifying the time allowed and expected for OMT, these providers should be given latitude, based on their training and clinical judgment, in order to provide an additional 5 minutes of treatment for any additional OMT necessary to enhance the patient's health and recovery. Critics of this methodology argue that, in the end, regardless of how positive the clinical outcome, this kind of trial is valueless as nothing can be known about which techniques caused the improvements.

Proponents of this multifaceted OMT design emphasize that until it has been proven that OMT is actually effective, there is no reason to design a trial with methodology focused on underlying mechanisms. With so very little definitive OMT clinical trial research completed at this time, the highest research priority at present is to design trials that first determine whether OMT, under even the most ideal circumstances, can have a positive clinical effect. Once this has been determined, research efforts and resources can be directed to those elements of OMT that contribute the most to the positive effect.

Interpreting Results

There are two fundamental types of research errors, Type 1 and Type 2, which should be considered when interpreting study results. An example of a Type 1 error in the context of OMT pneumonia research would be to conclude that OMT helps pneumonia patients when it actually does not. A Type 1 error is the most common research error due, in part, to investigator biases and the incentives associated with positive research findings and publications. An example of a Type 2 error in OMT pneumonia research would be to conclude that OMT does not help pneumonia patients when it actually does. The osteopathic profession must make it a priority to be particularly careful not to make Type 2 errors. Out of confusion regarding the true research question and a misguided perception that the above described OMT technique selection is insufficiently standardized (unscientific), osteopathic researchers tend to address important clinical questions with overly restrictive OMT research protocols. Consequently, early investigations into important questions regarding the clinical efficacy of OMT have ended with negative results (possibly Type 2 errors). Negative results (erroneous or otherwise) significantly reduce future funding opportunities and investigator interest. Nothing could be more detrimental to our quest for truth regarding the effects of OMT than this kind of Type 2 error generated by well-meaning, misguided osteopathic researchers. Both types of errors need to be considered when designing a study and interpreting the results.

Improving Research Sophistication

Maturing OMM research sophistication from pilot studies through large, multicenter trials is critical to establish a successful research enterprise and expand the current OMM evidence base to a level consistent with current scientific standards. More and more, clinical studies are reporting on sample sizes in the thousands and tens of thousands of subjects instead of tens or hundreds. To achieve this level of sophistication, collaboration throughout the profession is essential. Young, enthusiastic researchers with a promising area of research must be given adequate support and resources to generate sound pilot data from which these larger studies can be developed. Research teams need to use well-designed studies and perform multicenter studies within the profession, including especially the smaller or younger osteopathic schools or colleges who may not have the expertise or resources to develop and oversee such rigorous study designs but who can, with mentorship, establish productive data collection sites and develop skills necessary to build a productive research infrastructure.

Conferences

Conferences designed to support the osteopathic research community are an important issue to consider. Currently, there are numerous society and professional conferences within the general biomedical community, where leading researchers present the outcomes of their investigations. These conferences are a fundamental part of the scientific establishment and are invaluable in helping all researchers refine and create methodologies that will withstand critical peer evaluation. These meetings are also instrumental in identifying researchers with similar interests and establishing relationships that could lead to fruitful collaborations. The profession should be cautious and not develop alternative scientific conferences, thinking that OMM research requires methods or outcome measures that are different from the general biomedical community. Instead, the osteopathic profession should encourage researchers in osteopathic principles or practices to identify the best research-oriented society and its associated conference that fits their area of interest and should help them regularly attend and present their work at these premier research conferences.

During the past 10 years, there have been two conferences that focus on research sponsored by the osteopathic profession, the AOA

Annual Scientific Conference and the OCCTIC. While there is a long history to the AOA Annual Scientific Conference, its format has varied, and its outcomes/participation has been quite variable. OCCTIC, coordinated initially by the ORT and most recently by the ORC, has had success in developing programs for research training and in coordinating research priorities and strategies in OMM research. The last OCCTIC in 2008 was quite successful as an interdisciplinary research conference focusing on manual therapies. The planning committee for that conference recognized that the osteopathic profession is positioned to be a leader and facilitator for establishing and continuing such a conference. At that OCCTIC meeting, which focused on somatovisceral interactions, osteopathic physicians, chiropractors, physical therapists, massage therapists, and basic scientists were in attendance. The conference was sponsored by all the professions in attendance and by the NIH through NCCAM. A book of proceedings from this conference will be in press soon (45). While osteopathic medicine has a historical claim of rejuvenating the field of manipulative medicine, D.O.s represent just one of many disciplines that utilize the hands as part of their therapeutic armamentarium. Providing the leadership to advance the understanding of the therapeutic potential of palpation should be considered an important goal and responsibility of the profession.

Previous interdisciplinary research-oriented conferences have been sponsored by the American Academy of Osteopathy over the past two decades and have been very well received by both clinicians and scientists. Each resulted in a book of conference proceedings (46,47). Unfortunately, outcomes have been limited due to a lack of regular interactions between the attendees. Sustaining such venues on a regular basis, perhaps on a triennial basis, would be quite fruitful for the profession.

To develop a productive research conference format and schedule, stakeholders must be supported in order to develop a coordinated, invigorated, novel, and fiscally responsible conference schedule. This leadership is also needed to create a 5- to 10-year integrated conference plan that will provide the necessary education and exposure to advance the profession's research infrastructure.

OMM RESEARCH FUNDING AND RESOURCE ALLOCATION

Currently, there is funding for OMM research from the AOA through the Osteopathic Research and Development Fund (ORDF) and from several specialty societies, such as the American Academy of Osteopathy, the Cranial Academy Foundation, and several osteopathic foundations like the OHFs. Expanding and coordinating these funding resources is vital for the success of research within the profession. As a result of the ORT White Paper, one goal has already been achieved. The OHFs provided matching funds in 2009 with the annual AOA funding for grants. As a result (Table 71.3), the number of funded grants has doubled and the scope of the grants has increased in comparison to recent years. It is projected that these matching funds will improve the design and outcomes of these studies and the subsequent potential for funding from federal sources.

Personal experience has shown that a successful NCCAM grant application requires an experienced research team, good pilot data, and an outcome that will have a clear impact on medical knowledge and care. Unfortunately, it is not always apparent to reviewers how or why osteopathic practices would improve medical knowledge and practice. Consequently, it is critical for the AOA to continue to expand the funding of pilot studies so that the potential influence of osteopathic practice on medical care can be shown. Further, as a result of the grants being critically reviewed and screened through the strategic priorities and portfolio established within the AOA, funded grants should be better prepared to successfully compete at the NIH level.

While coordination of funds is having a positive impact on the profession's research efforts, the financial infrastructure for supporting research is weak. The ORDF, established in the 1980s to support research through AOA membership dues, is not receiving new funds and is, thus, greatly influenced by stock market forces. For example, within the past 10 years when the market was low, funding of grants was suspended for 2 years until the market improved. Each member of the profession should have an invested interest in sustaining a successful research enterprise. In order to support the ORDF, reinitiating and sustaining dues allocation for research must remain an ongoing priority.

Expanding the resources available for research needs to go beyond the AOA to include the schools, colleges, and universities where DOs are trained. Each institution must take a leadership role and seriously consider its fiscal responsibility as a center of higher learning, with the goal of promoting scholarly activity and expanding the knowledge base of the practice of medicine, while not focusing solely on the granting of diplomas and the revenue it brings to the institution. Establishing or expanding internal funds for pilot projects, especially ones that help provide experience to future clinicians and interdisciplinary teams, would greatly improve the chances of this profession having an impact on the health care industry in this century.

Promoting dual-degree programs, especially ones that foster research and promote clinical research careers, also needs to be prioritized throughout the profession's training programs. While many colleges offer dual degrees, enrollment in those programs must be encouraged. As numerous allied health professions increase the rigor of their programs and grant higher levels of degrees (48), there is also a greater need to advance the level of physician training. Earmarking institutional scholarships as well as seeking external funding and fellowships to support the development of future osteopathic clinical researchers is a critical investment for the profession.

Meetings that coordinate priorities and strategies between the profession's successful research teams and research leaders, like the ORT, are important and require a funding stream of support. Providing resources to maintain an interdisciplinary research conference in manual therapies should be considered as well. And finally, a funding strategy that includes many stakeholders within the profession needs to be developed to achieve success.

OMM RESEARCH TRAINING

While the focus of the ORT's recommendation in the white paper was on OMM research, it seems more appropriate when discussing this domain to maintain a broader focus, including aspects of research topics associated with OMM without being limited solely to those topics.

The focal point for research training lies primarily with the colleges of osteopathic medicine and begins in the selection process of applicants to DO programs. In a supporting role, AACOM can help disseminate the research opportunities for potential students within the colleges, but the pipeline for identifying and nurturing students through dual-degree programs and providing various research experiences throughout the medical school experience clearly lies within the purview of the colleges. While it is common that the colleges harness the excitement and idealism of youth to encourage students to become good clinicians and lifelong learners, students also need to be given the opportunity throughout their medical education to observe the nature and behavior of living

systems (30,49,50) through the eyes of a clinician researcher and to experience the excitement of asking new questions and finding answers that will advance health and the practice of medicine. Clinical activities, like behaviors, are difficult to change once they have been established. Preliminary data suggest that the sooner research activities are initiated within the educational experience, the more interested the students will be in participating in such activities (30,49,50). Consequently, clinician researchers must be grown in order for a profession-wide culture of research to be developed, where clinicians will be driven to sustain proven health care practices and develop new ones that extend healthy life while reducing the burdens of illness and disability.

Even though several specialty colleges recommend or require residents to engage in research activities, meaningful outcomes from those activities have been quite limited (51). A new paradigm should be considered that coordinates residents in the same research project, either at the same time or over time, in order to generate more meaningful training experiences and outcomes that will have value within the scientific community. This type of programming would require longitudinal and possibly multicenter mentorship and coordination. Developing such programs within specialty colleges or Osteopathic Post-graduate Training Institutions should be considered. One of the profession's research centers/institutes could assist in this endeavor by providing the consultative services necessary to ensure projects are rigorously designed and support the implementation and interpretation of results.

SUMMARY

For many within this profession, much of the information presented in this chapter will seem very familiar. In fact, some of these priorities were identified and reported decades ago (5). Herein lies the greatest issue facing the profession regarding research: priorities are supposed to be important and aggressively addressed. There is an urgency to have them accomplished or incorporated into routine activities and expectations. Certainly, there are challenges and finite resources that must be considered as the profession engages its research priorities. It is a daunting challenge to better understand the complexity of life, but with a clear and unified vision, good coordination of available resources and responsibilities, and adequate accountability, this profession can become a leader in the advancement of health care in both practice and research. The outcomes from the ORT demonstrate the potential of having a unified vision and profession-wide coordination. By reconstituting and expanding a forum where leading researchers and research advocates can meet to inform each other of independent research activities and initiatives; to confirm, update, and advance profession-wide research priorities; and to coordinate resources and action plans, the profession will establish the infrastructure needed to become a productive member of the research community. A key constituent within the profession that needs to take on a leadership role in achieving research priorities is the colleges of osteopathic medicine. A greater level of commitment and participation is needed from each of the colleges for success to be achieved.

As the direction of research at the NIH becomes more technologically driven in molecular, submolecular, and genomic arenas, the osteopathic profession has the opportunity to remain true to its legacy by focusing on research in medical care that is broadly applicable, holistic, and patient centered. Successful outcomes in holistic, patient-centered research will have the potential of influencing public health policy not just nationally, but globally due to the minimal level of technology needed to implement OMM approaches. Further, funding for research in osteopathic medicine is currently available through NCCAM at an unprecedented level. The successes over the past several years in obtaining NIH funding illustrate the opportunities and possibilities available to the profession, while highlighting the deficiency within the profession in generating fundable research proposals. The profession needs to have the foresight to invest in its present and future members by establishing an infrastructure dedicated to expanding the evidence base for osteopathic medical care. This infrastructure can be quickly built by facilitating interdisciplinary collaborations between basic and clinical scientists, both within and outside the profession. Concurrently, facets within the profession must relinquish the posturing of the past that isolates us from the greater biomedical community and is divisive within the profession itself.

While the membership of the profession needs to understand the importance of research and participate in research activities in general, we must also recognize that our resources should be used to promote research that is important to osteopathic principles since the level of potential funding is limited compared to other areas of biomedical research. While all scientists and clinicians should be united in the pursuit of an evidence base that leads to improved efficiency and quality in the provision of health care, special interests do enter into this process. Therefore, it is critical that all osteopathic physicians have training in research methodologies and critical thinking in order to discern strong versus weak research and to remain true to the profession's founding principles by advocating for health care approaches that prioritize and promote intrinsic health for every individual.

There truly is an important role for the osteopathic profession and its principles in modern scientific activity. Society waits to see if and how the osteopathic profession chooses to fulfill its dual responsibility of providing the best level of care based on current knowledge while advancing that knowledge to levels previously unimaginable.

REFERENCES

1. Still AT. *Autobiography of Andrew T. Still.* Rev Ed. Kirksville, MO: Andrew T. Still, 1908.
2. Sirica CM, ed. *Current Challenges to MDs and DOs: Proceedings of a Conference Sponsored by the Josiah Macy, Jr. Foundation.* New York, NY: Josiah Macy, Jr. Foundation, 1996.
3. NIH Mission. National Institutes of Health Web site. Available at: http://www.nih.gov/about/index.html#mission. Reviewed August 17, 2009. Accessed August 19, 2009.
4. Rivers DW. AOA initiatives in research. *J Am Osteopath Assoc* 1987;87:753–754.
5. D'Alonzo GE. Clinical research in osteopathic medicine. *J Am Osteopath Assoc* 1987;87:440–445.
6. Allen TW. Osteopathic research: where have we been and where are we going? *J Am Osteopath Assoc* 1991;91:122.
7. Sorg RJ, Shaw HA. Osteopathic research priorities. *J Am Osteopath Assoc* 1985;85:736–738.
8. McGill SL, Retz KC. Research programs of the AOA and their role in osteopathic medical education. *J Am Osteopath Assoc* 1998;98:627–631.
9. Rose RC, Prozialeck WC. Productivity outcomes for recent grants and fellowships awarded by the American Osteopathic Association Bureau of Research. *J Am Osteopath Assoc* 2003;103:435–440.
10. Northup GW. An adventure in excellence. 1962. *J Am Osteopath Assoc* 2001;101:726–730.
11. Gevitz N. 'Parallel and distinctive': the philosophic pathway for reform in osteopathic medical education. *J Am Osteopath Assoc* 1994;94:328–332.
12. Patterson MM. Osteopathic research: challenges of the future. In: Ward RC, ed. *Foundations for Osteopathic Medicine.* 2nd Ed. Philadelphia, PA: Lippincott Williams & Wilkins, 2003:1219–1228.
13. Rodgers FJ, Dyer MJ. Adopting research. *J Am Osteopath Assoc* 2000;100:234–237.
14. Guillory VJ, Sharp G. Research at US colleges of osteopathic medicine: a decade of growth. *J Am Osteopath Assoc* 2003;103:176–181.
15. Papa FJ. Research secures the future of osteopathic medicine: Part 1. Research–foundation for faculty development, institutional recognition. *J Am Osteopath Assoc* 1993;93:606–610.
16. Overview of the NIH Roadmap. National Institutes of Health Web site. Available at: http://www.nihroadmap.nih.gov/overview.asp. Reviewed September 11, 2008. Accessed August 19, 2009.
17. Rubin B, Rose R. AOA Bureau of research provides retrospective on 2000 Research Conference. *J Am Osteopath Assoc* 2001;101:154–155.
18. NIH Roadmap for Medical Research. National Institutes of Health Web site. Available at: http://www.nihroadmap.nih.gov/. Reviewed August 12, 2009. Accessed August 19, 2009.
19. Educational Council on Osteopathic Principles. Glossary of Osteopathic Terminology. Available at: http://www.osteopathic.org/pdf/sir_collegegloss.pdf. Updated August 15, 2006. Accessed August 19, 2009.
20. Research Synergy Conclave. Osteopathic manipulative medicine research: a 21st century vision. Available at: www.aacom.org/InfoFor/researchers/Documents/synergy-white-paper.doc. Published September, 2003. Accessed August 19, 2009.
21. NCCAM-Funded Research for FY 2006. National Center for Complementary and Alternative Medicine Web site. http://nccam.nih.gov/research/extramural/awards/2006/. Updated May 27, 2009. Accessed August 19, 2009.
22. NCCAM-Funded Research for FY 2007. National Center for Complementary and Alternative Medicine Web site. http://nccam.nih.gov/research/extramural/awards/2007/. Updated May 27, 2009. Accessed August 19, 2009.
23. NCCAM-Funded Research for FY 2008. National center for Complementary And Alternative Medicine Web site. Available at: http://nccam.nih.gov/research/extramural/awards/2008/. Updated May 27, 2009. Accessed August 19, 2009.
24. Research Portfolio Online Reporting Tool (RePORT). National Institutes of Health Web site. Available at: http://www.report.nih.gov/. Updated August 11, 2009. Accessed August 19, 2009.
25. Retz KC. Research programs of the AOA and their role in osteopathic medical education. *J Am Osteopath Assoc* 1992;92:1418, 1425–1429.
26. Stoll ST, McCormick J, Degenhardt BF, et al. The National Osteopathic Research Center at the University of North Texas Health Science Center: inception, growth, and future. *Acad Med* 2009;84:737–743.
27. Papa F. Research secures the future of osteopathic medicine: Part 2. Readdressing the function and structure of colleges of osteopathic medicine. *J Am Osteopath Assoc* 1993;93:701–706.
28. Levitan T. AACOM projections for growth through 2012: results of a 2007 survey of US Colleges of Osteopathic Medicine. *J Am Osteopath Assoc* 2008;108:116–120.
29. Hiatt H, Sutton J. The nation's changing needs for biomedical and behavioral scientists. *Acad Med* 2000;75:778–779.
30. Pheley AM, Lois H, Strobl J. Interests in research electives among osteopathic medical students. *J Am Osteopath Assoc* 2006;106:667–670.
31. Nelson KE, Sergueef N, Glonek T. Recording the rate of the cranial rhythmic impulse. *J Am Osteopath Assoc* 2006;106:337–341.
32. Licciardone JC, Nelson KE, Glonek T, et al. Osteopathic manipulative treatment of somatic dysfunction among patients in the family practice clinic setting: a retrospective analysis. *J Am Osteopath Assoc* 2005;105:537–544.
33. Darmani NA, Izzo AA, Degenhardt B, et al. Involvement of the cannabimimetic compound, N-palmitoyl-ethanolamine, in inflammatory and neuropathic conditions: review of the available pre-clinical data, and first human studies. *Neuropharmacology* 2005;48:1154–1163.
34. Noll DR, Degenhardt BF, Stuart MK, et al. The effect of osteopathic manipulative treatment on immune response to the influenza vaccine in nursing home residents: a pilot study. *Altern Ther Health Med* 2004;10:74–76.
35. Hodge LM, King HH, Williams AG, et al. Abdominal lymphatic pump treatment increases leukocyte count and flux in thoracic duct lymph. *Lymphat Res Biol* 2007;5:127–134.
36. Knott EM, Tune JD, Stoll ST, et al. Increased lymphatic flow in the thoracic duct during manipulative intervention. *J Am Osteopath Assoc* 2005;105:447–456.

37. Licciardone JC, Brimhall AK, King LN. Osteopathic manipulative treatment for low back pain: a systematic review and meta-analysis of randomized controlled trials. *BMC Musculoskelet Disord.* 2005;6:43. Available at: http://www.biomedcentral.com/1471-2474/6/43. Published August 4, 2005. Accessed August 21, 2009.

38. Andersson GB, Lucente T, Davis AM, et al. A comparison of osteopathic spinal manipulation with standard care for patients with low back pain. *N Engl J Med* 1999;341:1426–1431.

39. Licciardone JC, Stoll ST, Fulda KG, et al. Osteopathic manipulative treatment for chronic low back pain: a randomized controlled trial. *Spine* 2003;28:1355–1362.

40. Degenhardt BF, Johnson JC, Noll DR, et al. Adjunctive manual treatment for older adults hospitalized with community-acquired pneumonia. Presented at: Infectious Diseases Society of America 46th Annual Meeting, Washington, DC, October 25–28, 2008.

41. Funding Priorities: Funding Search. Osteopathic Heritage Foundations Web site. Available at: http://www.osteopathicheritage.org/FundingPriorities/fundingawards. Accessed August 21, 2009.

42. Freburger JK, Holmes GM, Agans RP, et al. The rising prevalence of chronic low back pain. *Arch Intern Med* 2009;169:251–258.

43. Touch Research Institute Web site. Available at: http://www6.miami.edu/touch-research/. Updated February 2008. Accessed August 21, 2009.

44. Noll DR, Degenhardt BF, Fossum C, et al. Clinical and research protocol for osteopathic manipulative treatment of elderly patients with pneumonia. *J Am Osteopath Assoc* 2008;108:508–516.

45. King HH, Janig W, Patterson MM, eds. *The Science and Clinical Application of Manual Therapy.* Maryland Heights, MO: Elsevier, In press; Oct, 2010.

46. Patterson MM, Howell JN, eds. *The Central Connection: Somatovisceral/Viscerosomatic Interaction. Proceedings of the 1989 International Symposium.* Indianapolis, IN: American Academy of Osteopathy, 1992.

47. Willard FH, Patterson MM, eds. *Nociception and the Neuroendocrine-Immune Connection: Proceedings of the 1992 International Symposium.* Indianapolis, IN: American Academy of Osteopathy, 1994.

48. Montoya ID, Kimball OM. A marketing clinical doctorate programs. *J Allied Health* 2007;36:107–112.

49. Solomon SS, Tom SC, Pichert J, et al. Impact of medical student research in the development of physician-scientists. *J Invest Med* 2003;51:149–156.

50. Licciardone JC, Fulda KG, Smith-Barbaro P. Rating interest in clinical research among osteopathic medical students. *J Am Osteopath Assoc* 2002;102:410–412.

51. Smith-Barbaro P, Fulda KG, Coleridge ST. A divisional approach to enhancing research among osteopathic family practice residents. *J Am Osteopath Assoc* 2004;104:177–179.

Development and Support of Osteopathic Medical Research

HOLLIS H. KING

KEY CONCEPTS

- The focus of osteopathic research is more than manual medicine and osteopathic manipulative treatment. The osteopathic medical philosophy, described elsewhere, provides the underpinning for the research done, which addresses the unique and distinctive elements brought to the health care arena by osteopathic physicians.
- Evidence-based osteopathic research has a history as old as the osteopathic profession itself. Published osteopathic research was comparable to any research done in a particular era and included several large-scale projects. Highlights of over a hundred years of osteopathic research are described and development of the osteopathic terminology based on the research is described.
- Clinical trials utilizing osteopathic manipulative medicine have been accomplished and are being developed. The focus on the need for clinical trials research resulted in the establishment of the Osteopathic Research Center.
- Principles of developing uniquely osteopathic research are based on traditional basic and clinical science design models. Due to limited resources and availability of trained researchers, a number of unique adaptations have been required to accomplish the osteopathic research agenda. Resources for research grant development and writing, "grantsmanship," and collaboration development are presented.
- Uniquely osteopathic research has not received extensive federal funding such as from NIH. Funding from these sources has increased in the last 10 to 15 years but remains a very small proportion of biomedical research in the United States. Osteopathic research has been funded primarily by osteopathic foundations and institutions.

UNIQUELY OSTEOPATHIC RESEARCH

The focus of this chapter is clinical research done and documented from a uniquely osteopathic perspective. Many faculty members at colleges of osteopathic medicine (COMs) have produced significant research studies in areas not directly related to osteopathic principles and practice (OPP), osteopathic manipulative medicine (OMM), and osteopathic manipulative treatment (OMT). Examples of this is the work at Michigan State University College of Osteopathic Medicine done by Justin McCormick, Ph.D., in cancer research (3,4); by Andres Amalfitano, D.O., in genetics research (5,6); and at the University of North Texas Health Science Center (UNTHSC), Texas College of Osteopathic Medicine by Albert O-Yurvati, D.O., in cardiovascular function (7,8). At these and other COMs, the presence of the basic and clinical scientists like Drs. McCormick, Amalfitano, and O-Yurvati has helped to create a research environment in which uniquely osteopathic research is more likely to be carried out and at a higher level of quality.

The development of OMM-related research is enhanced in institutions that have faculty who are experienced and well-funded basic and clinical science researchers in areas other than OMM-related research. The influence and collegiality created by interactions with active researchers enhance the atmosphere likely to lead to higher quality research in both the clinical and basic science arenas. As discussed later, the collaboration between researchers is often central to furthering the research capability of the collaborators. This is particularly true for osteopathic clinicians who forge collaborations with basic scientists whose areas of research can be related to OPP/OMM/OMT, which has been a key to the development of osteopathic research.

The American Osteopathic Association (AOA) has a long history of promoting and supporting osteopathic research. Crucial to the current state of osteopathic research was the establishment

of the AOA Research Task Force, which published two guiding documents that facilitated the establishment of, and guidance for, the Osteopathic Research Center (ORC) (9,10). In the 2005 AOA Research Task Force Report, *Research Strategic Direction for the American Osteopathic Association* (9), the statement is made, "The Task Force recognizes the value of areas of biomedical research. However, the recommendation is that the AOA focuses its research funding exclusively on those areas of research that investigate the unique aspects of osteopathic medicine with an emphasis on OMM. The breadth of this research focus may include but is not limited to:

- Mechanisms of action of OMM
- Clinical efficacy of OMM
- Interrater and intrarater reliability of palpatory assessment
- Osteopathic physician and patient interactions
- Cost-effectiveness of osteopathic health care
- Methods of teaching palpation and OMM

Based on the prominence of the members and groups represented by the AOA Research Task Force, also more commonly referred to as the Osteopathic Research Task Force (ORT), this is the most authoritative guide given to date as to the nature of uniquely osteopathic research, and for the sake of discussion comprises the topics that are the focus of this chapter. These topics have all received research scrutiny in the past but are now receiving priority as new OMM-related research projects are planned.

The increased emphasis on and urgency to produce uniquely osteopathic research by the osteopathic medical profession was articulated in the National OMM Research Synergy White Paper, *Osteopathic Manipulative Medicine Research: A 21st Century Vision* (10), where it is stated, "In this era of modern health care, insurers, policy makers and consumers are interested in evidence-based medicine. Therefore, it is of paramount importance for physicians to document, through well-designed and well-executed research studies, which specific aspects of the clinical care they provide to patients are proven to be beneficial. This is particularly true in osteopathic medicine. Instead of saying, 'we know it works because patients get better,' the profession must channel its resources to determine through scientific research studies whether osteopathic manipulative medicine (OMM) does indeed improve patient outcomes in a broad range of specific situations. The profession must also elucidate the mechanisms by which this unique, hands-on approach to patient care works."

In an era of increasing costs for health care, insurance companies and other third-party payers are demanding evidence of health benefit for OMM, as reimbursement requests for these services are submitted by osteopathic physicians. As described later, this financially driven imperative is gradually receiving empirically based answers. However, there exist other reasons to generate this research, including clarifying the distinctiveness of osteopathic medicine, demonstrating the value of osteopathic medical care as well as the financial reimbursement for OMM services.

Another compelling reason to generate the evidence base for OMM is the very confidence with which OPP/OMM/OMT are taught in the first 2 years of osteopathic medical curricula and perception of OMM by rank and file osteopathic physicians. Osteopathic medical students (OMSs) are entering their medical training with a generally higher awareness of, and in many cases experience in, research. From the author's experience in teaching at the OMS-I and OMS-II levels, there are more questions being asked by students about the research underpinnings for OMM/OMT. Further, when quality evidence-based OMM research is presented, there is a much greater attentiveness to and practice of the OMM/OMT lessons by the students.

Furthermore, based on discussions at AOA conventions and the AOA House of Delegates with a wide geographic and professional diversity of osteopathic physicians, as more uniquely osteopathic research is published, the application of OMM/OMT increases in clinical practice. Discussion at coding and reimbursement seminars at the AOA and American College of Osteopathic Family Physicians (ACOFP) conventions and the American Academy of Osteopathy (AAO) convocation also suggest a trend toward increased likelihood of reimbursement based on citation of evidence for OMM/OMT benefit, although the greatest success in obtaining reimbursement is based on dealing with the complicated, detailed and diverse rules for claim submission. This informed observation is shared by many who are involved in OMM-related clinical research and is based on input and requests from osteopathic physicians who want to do more OMM but are constrained by reimbursement issues based on insurance and managed care panels who cite the lack of research support for the medical necessity for OMM services.

DEVELOPING OSTEOPATHIC RESEARCH: A HISTORICAL PERSPECTIVE

From Still Through Korr—Studies and Funding

The heuristic value of Andrew Taylor Still's osteopathic philosophy, principles, and practice has never been in doubt. That is, Still's philosophy and teaching were the source of ideas for the generation of research hypotheses. A careful examination of early osteopathic research suggests that it was comparable to medical research performed by others of that era. Just as with allopathic medical and basic scientific research, there were shortcomings in comparison to today's standards, such as adequate definition of procedures and utilization of control groups.

In the early days, osteopathic research was largely observational and the question was how those receiving osteopathic medical care fared in their health as compared with those receiving care by allopathic physicians. Examples of some of these studies had relatively large sample sizes and comparison groups. In 1911, Whiting (11) reported on the impact of OMT on labor and delivery outcomes. She reported data for a sample size of 223 women in which 198 received OMT and 98 did not. The outcome was that the labor times for the women receiving OMT were dramatically shorter. At the Still Research Institute (funded by the AOA at that time) also in the area of OMT and obstetrics, S.V. Robuck reported in 1933 a chart analysis of 13,816 women who received OMT during pregnancy and found the maternal mortality rate to be much lower, with only one-third as much of the maternal mortality reported in "government bulletins." (12) While caution is advised in the interpretation of the data (13), Smith (14) reported an observational study with 110,120 influenza patients in 1918 to 1919 who received OMT and suffered a much lower mortality rate than the general population. While such studies may have lacked the rigor of modern research design, they were certainly at or above the standards of the day and are cited here to make the point that large-scale studies have been carried out in osteopathic research from the beginning of the profession.

Other aspects of modern day research emphases are seen in very early osteopathic research. The current "bench to bedside" model of translational research was pioneered in the work of Louisa Burns, D.O., who developed an animal model, primarily rabbits, for exploration of the impact of OMT on visceral function (15,16).

Still's teaching that OMT had an impact on the whole body, visceral physiology as well as the musculoskeletal system, was the heart of this early translational research. Dr. Burns also described the impact of OMT on humans and its effect on heart rate and blood pressure (15). Dr. Burns' work is still highly regarded for its contribution to the establishment of credibility for OMT and distinguished research awards bear her name. However, Wilbur V. Cole, D.O. (17), who worked with Louisa Burns in the 1940s, acknowledged the difficulty Dr. Burns had in describing the "boney lesion" in operationally defined terms that are now routine through the application of technology (18).

If the early work of Burns, Cole, and others initiated and maintained a research consciousness in the osteopathic medical profession, the work of John Stedman Denslow, DO, and Irvin M. Korr, Ph.D., marked the beginning of the modern renaissance of osteopathic research. In the 1940s, technology had advanced and after World War II was affordable so that the research laboratory at the Kirksville College of Osteopathic Medicine (KCOM) was able to produce significant research describing the concept of the "osteopathic lesion," which we now know as "somatic dysfunction" (19–23). In their work, the Kirksville group forged an early pattern of research article submission to journals outside the osteopathic profession, which is a goal reiterated in the present day as a way to "spread the word and findings" of uniquely osteopathic research to the medical/scientific community as a whole.

The funding for the Kirksville group's research was primarily from the AOA, the A.T. Still Osteopathic Foundation and the KCOM. However, as early as 1958, federal funding came from the Public Health Service and Office of Naval Research (23,24). Through the 1960s and 1970s, funding initially came from the National Institutes of Health (25,26). Then when formed, came from the National Institutes of Neurological Diseases and Stroke (27,28). Current research funding trends mirror the pattern started in the late 1950s and early 1960s but with different proportions and significant support added from foundations supportive of osteopathic medicine.

From Korr to the Osteopathic Research Center

The work of William L. Johnston, D.O. and Myron C. Beal, D.O., at Michigan State University College of Osteopathic Medicine, and Albert F. Kelso, Ph.D., at the Chicago College of Osteopathic Medicine, together and individually, kept up the momentum of OMM-related research through the 1980s and 1990s. A review of the annual AOA Research Conferences proceedings in the *Journal of the American Osteopathic Association* during this period showed that these individuals provided the leadership for the conferences themselves as well as leadership to develop and define a number of the terms now at the center of osteopathic terminology such as TART (Tissue texture changes, Asymmetry, Restriction, Tenderness) and somatic dysfunction.

The importance of interrater and intrarater reliability of palpatory assessment was the hallmark work of these researchers (29–32). Review and development of the somato–visceral interactions was also a great contribution (33,34). They also lead in research on the impact of OMM on systemic disorders (35–38). Perusal of their published papers reveals that the funding for their research was primarily from the AOA along with some financial support from their respective institutions. Given the breadth of their work, it is hard to imagine what could have been done had foundation and government funding been available.

CONSOLIDATING RESOURCES: OSTEOPATHIC RESEARCH CENTER

Since the late 1990s, the osteopathic medical profession began to deal with the need for more and higher quality osteopathic research. The ORT was constituted and was composed of representatives from AOA, AAO, American Association of Colleges of Osteopathic Medicine (AACOM), the American College of Osteopathic Family Physicians (ACOFP), and American Osteopathic Foundation (AOF). The ORT supported and convened a research conference titled Osteopathic Collaborative Clinical Trials Initiative Conference (OCCTIC). The first OCCTIC was in 1999, and through discussions carried on at subsequent OCCTIC meetings, the decision to establish a national ORC was made in 2001 (2). Through a competitive application process, the ORC was placed on the campus of the UNTHSC, Texas College of Osteopathic Medicine.

The mission of the ORC is "Fostering nationwide collaborative OMM research." The ORC, in collaboration with key members of the ORT, has conducted a number of "Focused Research Forums." Bringing together researchers and funders in "focused" discussions have resulted in specific research projects described below. In this way, the creation and existence of the ORC have significantly forwarded the research agenda of the osteopathic medical profession.

In addition to the ORC, the osteopathic medical profession is fortunate to have other research organizations that have received significant external funding. One of these, the A.T. Research Institute, is located on the campus of the A.T. Still University in Kirksville, MO. The A.T. Still Research Institute is actively involved in OMM-related research, especially in the area of interrater and intrarater reliability of palpatory assessment. It also served as the Clinical Trial Coordinating Center (CTCC) for the Multi-Center Osteopathic Pneumonia Study in the Elderly (MOPSE). The A.T. Still Research Institute has received external funding from the Osteopathic Heritage Foundation (OHF) and NIH National Center for Complementary and Alternative Medicine (NIH-NCCAM) and internally from A.T. Still University.

Multi-Center Osteopathic Pneumonia Study in the Elderly

The MOPSE project is a prototype for what is hoped will be a number of multicenter clinical trials based on the application of OMM/OMT with a specific disorder or subject population. Through a process of several Focused Research Forum meetings, the consensus was developed that the osteopathic treatment of pneumonia in the elderly was the strongest area in which OMM/OMT could be expected to have impact when examined by a multicentered clinical trial.

The focused research forum reviewed the research literature and clinical experience with the treatment of pneumonia. There were the experiences of the 1918 to 1919 influenza pandemic (14) and two preliminary clinical trials that showed benefit of OMT as adjuvant treatment in cases of pneumonia in elderly hospitalized patients (39,40). Donald Noll, D.O., was selected by the CTCC to be the principle investigator and a grant proposal was assembled and submitted in September 2002. The MOPSE study was funded at $1,504,871 for a 2-year study by the OHF and a number of other osteopathic-supportive foundations, with funding coordination by the Foundation for Osteopathic Health Services (FOHS). Five clinical sites were determined and included hospitals in Kirksville, MO; Stratford, NJ; Columbus, OH; Mount Clemens, MI; and Fort Worth, TX.

For MOPSE, the ORC provided oversight on behalf of the funders and the A.T. Still Research Institute served as the CTCC, selecting the principle investigator, providing direction for conduct of the study, and making multiple site visits to train the treatment providers and audit charts for the results. The MOPSE study is registered on ClinicalTrials.gov and had an active Data and Safety Monitoring Board (DSMB). One of the initial challenges was to obtain Institutional Review Board (IRB) approvals at each of the involved hospitals, and all approvals were acquired.

One other challenge encountered during MOPSE was the difficulty recruiting subjects at all the sites. This was indeed one of the "lessons learned" as far as estimating numbers of subjects and timetables for study completion. The nature of treatment for pneumonia changed from the time the initial OMM/pneumonia studies were conducted and in 2005 when MOPSE was in full progress, with fewer patients admitted to hospitals for pneumonia. Consequently, a 1-year extension to complete MOPSE was carried out by the investigators and their institutions to ensure that an acceptable number of patients were enrolled. The direct and indirect financial contributions by these institutions increased the total cost for MOPSE, and additional foundation funding was provided to engage a clinical trial organization to consult regarding data analysis and publication submission.

At the time of submission of this chapter, the MOPSE data had been locked, analyzed, and a primary paper and a protocol paper were developed by the MOPSE Publication Committee and primary investigators. Discussions pertaining to the osteopathic contribution to treatment of an avian flu possibility prompted development and submission of the MOPSE OMT treatment protocol for publication (41,42). Also at the time of completion of this chapter, the primary MOPSE study manuscript was under review by a high impact journal that the MOPSE Publication Committee determined would provide the greatest distribution for the findings. Discussions are underway for a larger clinical trial proposal to be submitted to NIH. Such a trial, if positive and with a significantly larger number of subjects, would have the potential to impact the standard of practice for the treatment of pneumonia in the hospitalized elderly.

Research Projects Developed by the Focused Research Forum Process

Otitis Media

To date, the MOPSE study constitutes the largest multisite prospective clinical trial in the osteopathic medical profession. Previous studies with tens of thousands of subjects were retrospective observational studies (12,14). Once the MOPSE study was underway, another set of focused research forums were hosted by the ORC on the topic of OMT for the treatment of otitis media. It was felt by osteopathic research leaders to have high clinical research potential based on published literature and clinical practice (43–46).

A six-site multicenter clinical trial proposal was developed through the focused research forum process and submitted to osteopathic-supportive foundations as the Multi-Center Osteopathic Otitis Media Study (MOMS). However, MOMS was not funded by the osteopathic foundations due in part to considerations brought to light with lessons learned from the MOPSE study. However, a reduced scope, two-site clinical trial proposal titled Osteopathic Otitis Media Research Study (OOMRS) was submitted to the AAO's Louisa Burns Osteopathic Research Committee (LBORC) and was funded with $100,000 for 2 years.

At the time of submission of this chapter, OOMRS was in its second year of recruitment of subjects. This trial is registered on ClinicalTrials.gov (48), has an active DSMB, and has oversight by AAO-LBORC. If results are positive, the data collected will constitute the basis for submission of a grant proposal at the R21 award level probably to the NIH-NCCAM.

Cervical Spine Manipulation: Safety and Efficacy

Utilizing the focused research forum process, the ORC responded to requests from the AOA Council on Scientific Affairs to examine the AOA Position Paper on Osteopathic Manipulative Treatment of the Cervical Spine, based on some reports of neurological damage and even death from cervical spine manipulation (49,50). The ORC convened a "blue ribbon" panel of researchers in 2006 and again in 2007. Reports of these focused research forums were made to the AOA Council of Scientific Affairs in 2006 and to the AOA Bureau of Scientific Affairs in 2007 (51). The AOA House of Delegates accepted the reports and recommended funding of a clinical trial on the efficacy of OMT for neck pain. At the time of this writing, there have been no grant applications submitted to the AOA Council of Research on this topic.

Concerns about cervical spine manipulation resulted in some professional liability insurance companies to temporarily curtail issuing policies to osteopathic physicians who did OMT on more than 25% of their patients. Negotiations with these insurance companies by the AOA were successful in resolving these concerns. The ORC reports (51) pointed out that the preponderance of reported and litigated instances of adverse events from cervical spine manipulation involved providers not trained in or licensed to practice osteopathic medicine.

Observational Studies on the Effects of Osteopathic Medicine

This initiative has grown out of interest by leaders of osteopathic-supportive foundations, primarily the OHF and FOHS. Using the precedent of the cervical spine manipulation focused research forum process, there have been five meetings of a panel of OMM research and foundation leaders held during meetings of the AOA, AAO, and OCCTIC research conferences to discuss the best approach to this concept.

Identified as the "Practice Based Research Network (PBRN)," a plan is in development that includes the potential recruitment of several hundred physicians who will systematically record standardized data on a number of their patients over a multiple-year period. A professional clinical trials consulting company has provided a proposal to the panel of osteopathic researchers. In the author's opinion, this would be the most appropriate direction to take in osteopathic research. This direction toward an observational study reflects a maturing process in the sophistication and focusing of research resources within the osteopathic medical profession and is a logical continuation of the ORT consultations begun in the late 1990s.

Status of OMM Research

The foregoing discussion of specific OMM-related research projects, planned and partially completed, represents application of many of the research development procedures discussed subsequently. Also, while not exhaustive, the studies cited are good examples of the progress of OMM research from professional beginnings to the present. The *Synergy* (10) document and ORT-guided collaborative efforts have produced results as discussed in the foregoing sections. Further progress is dependent to some degree on the actualization of the potential of the ORC and other research centers as well as support of OMM-related research in COMs and postdoctoral training. Some of the channels by which research has been developed are discussed next and may provide some insight to the reader as to ways to accomplish uniquely osteopathic research.

DEVELOPMENT OF OSTEOPATHIC RESEARCH "FROM THE GROUND UP"

As reviewed above, the osteopathic medical profession has embraced research from its beginning and has produced a relatively large body of research, given the size and resources available within the profession. The research history recounted above often reflected the interests of the researcher as well as the resources available to support a given research idea.

By the time of the work of Denslow and Korr, there were certain topics that were deemed priorities for research, such as the experimental delineation of the "osteopathic lesion" now termed somatic dysfunction. Gradually, OMM-related research priorities have been developed and appear to have been influenced by perceived needs such as delineated above (9,10). Chapter 71 gives a fuller discussion.

It is hoped that the series of discussions in this "Research" section of the *Foundations for Osteopathic Research, 3e*, will constitute a solid basis for understanding that will enable the reader to appreciate from where the osteopathic profession has come and where it needs to go with regard to OMM research. One of the oft elucidated clinical dictums given to OMSs is to "think osteopathically." This phrase is well understood to mean that considerations of a holistic body-mind-spirit, as well as structure-function relationships, are integrated into the thought process of an osteopathic medical clinician/practitioner. In an effort to apply similar logic to the research endeavor, basic clinical research principles are presented next.

Principles of Research—An Osteopathic Adaptation

The realization by the ORT and other key researchers and research funders that a research consciousness needed to be developed within the osteopathic profession was the motivation behind the mission statement adopted by the ORC, "Fostering nationwide collaborative OMM research." There have been a number of efforts to present research skills training opportunities to OMM faculties and particularly to students and residents.

Comprehensive programs have been provided at the AOA Research Conference at the 2005 AOA Convention, featuring a half day devoted to "Clinical Research Training Program: Designing Residency Research." Again at the Research Conference at the 2006 AOA Convention, there were featured presentations on "Osteopathic Research—Training at our Colleges," and "Getting Published: What You Need to Know about Reporting Research in Biomedical Journals." In 2006, at the OCCTIC-VII program, "Developing Excellence in Osteopathic Research" held in Birmingham, AL, there were panels and presentations on the development of research ideas into viable research projects. The program for OCCTIC-VIII in Colorado Springs was completely devoted to the development of research and was titled "Research Opportunities in Osteopathic Manipulation: Training Our Residents and Undergraduates Now! (ROOM TO RUN)." There have been other similar programs offered at state and society meetings and more are planned as the numbers of osteopathic clinical researchers who can provide training grow and the quality of OMM research attracts more students and residents to consider a research career or becoming involved in active OMM clinical research.

The essence of these research skills training programs centers on several main issues:

- Types of research
- Defining a research question
- Assessing resources for a project
- Biostatistical and design issues
- Mentors and collaborators
- Grant writing and "grantsmanship"
- Pilot studies
- Leveraging pilot studies into larger projects and grants
- Conducting a clinical trial—IRB and research coordinators

Types of Research

From the perspective of evidenced-based medicine, there is a hierarchy of the types of research in an ascending order as to the strength of the evidence for a particular subject. The generally accepted order is (52) (a) expert opinion, (b) case reports or series, (c) case-control studies, (d) cohort studies, (e) randomized controlled trial, and (f) systematic review, with systematic review being the strongest form of evidence.

While there have been many systematic reviews of various forms of treatment of musculoskeletal disorders, there has been only one done on OMT (53). This systematic review was supportive of the benefit of OMT for low back pain.

Defining a Research Question

Essential to defining a research question is knowledge of the area under consideration. Skill at doing a literature search is essential. Databases related to OMM are described in some detail in Chapter 74. Researchers who have published in a particular area are also valuable resources for the novice researcher as well for some-one who may not be very familiar with a particular topic but is interested in exploring research possibilities.

Assessing Resources for a Project

In all the OMM research training workshops mentioned above, the point has been made that the project must be conceived and carried out within the limits of available resources. This includes funding for subject compensation, treatment providers, research coordinators, and technical assistance. Also included in the resource availability considerations are the clinics from which subjects would be recruited, to determine whether or not there will be an appropriate number of subjects, and if the investigators have the time and assistance to recruit and consent the subjects. These considerations are essential for planning successful research and are based on recent experience at the ORC, as each item has been a source of challenge in one or more of the OMM research projects completed or currently under way.

Biostatistical and Design Issues

No matter the design of the project, training in and the availability of experienced biostatistical consultation are crucial to address the myriad of questions regarding outcome measures. For example, questions regarding "before and after" or "serial measures," whether or not you are doing a "prospective" or "retrospective" study, are issues that impact the kind of statistical analysis that can be used. Since some statistical tests are "stronger" than others, this becomes a critical matter for which expert guidance is needed.

Mentors and Collaborators

One element of the ROOM TO RUN conference of OCCTIC was the opportunity to make contact with mentors and collaborators. For the young investigators, students, and residents, the contact with a mentor or senior collaborator is most helpful, if not necessary to begin the process of OMM-related research. Most COMs have basic scientists on faculty who are willing to mentor, but OMM mentorship from a clinician may be harder to find. The ORC has limited time resources to provide mentorship but has consulted on many questions of research design and networked to build research collaborations, the essence of its mission statement. This topic of mentorship is of nearly universal interest in the world of biomedical research and has received much consideration (54).

One means of locating a collaborator, especially if you have an idea about a biomarker or outcome measure for the effects of OMM/OMT, is the Computer Retrieval of Information on Scientific Projects datebase (55). Another resource is the National Science Foundation Web site (56). At the 2007 AACOM Annual Meeting, an excellent panel titled "Collaboration on a Shoestring Budget or None at All" dealt with the collaboration issue in several presentations and is another fine resource to access (57).

Grant Writing and "Grantsmanship"

The NIH form SF424 (R&R) is necessary for electronic submissions to most NIH award programs (58). This electronic format is based on form PHS 398, which is the basic format for most external research grant applications to foundations and state and federal agencies that do not require electronic grant submissions (59). Familiarity with these forms helps to focus the writing process, as a research proposal is formulated. Some COMs have a grants management office that can assist in the writing process, but the purpose of the present discussion is to encourage the reader to integrate this aspect of "research work" into their awareness and training.

The process of "grantsmanship" includes getting to know the agency, institute, or foundation to which you would likely submit a grant proposal. What have they funded? What are the submission guidelines? Who do you know that was successful in a grant submission to the entity you are considering and can tell you the types of issues to be covered? In most grant submission processes, the investigator will receive feedback from reviewers on their particular submission, and this feedback should help guide future submissions.

With regard to grant writing, NIH-NCCAM has provided a grant writing workshop that dealt with all these issues and will remain posted substantially beyond publication of this book (60). An agenda, outline, and some content of this grant writing workshop are also available online (61).

Two other valuable resources for research with an OMM perspective are the *Manual of Basic Tools for Research in Osteopathic Manipulative Medicine* (62) published by the ORC and the *AOA Research Handbook* published by the AOA (63). These two publications provide detailed guidance on research conduct and grant development.

In a broader context, but with application for OMM researchers contemplating submission to NIH, there have been several articles and reviews that give further insight, based on experience, about the grant application process (64–66). As more and more foundations and agencies pattern their grant application process after NIH's, these articles may be very helpful in any context.

Pilot Studies

Prototypical of government and foundation funded pilot projects is the NIH R21 "Exploratory" grant mechanism. The R21 mechanism for a clinical trial typically allows for 2 years of support and requires a proposal with a number of subjects at 60 or more, with active intervention, sham intervention, and no-treat control group. What researchers have found is that to be competitive for an R21, there must be considerable "preliminary data" to suggest that there is efficacy to the intervention to be studied. This requirement is usually met by intramural seed grants funded by a researcher's institution or sometimes by the AOA, AAO or, in some cases, by an osteopathic-supportive foundation. Only a few COMs have allocated the resources for pilot studies, but when they have, as described below, there is often reward in funding at the higher levels afforded by foundations and governmental agencies.

Leveraging Pilot Studies into Larger Projects and Grants

This consideration is an amplification of the pilot study discussion, but mention of this concept is placed here to emphasize its importance in the research planning process. Specifics are discussed subsequently and illustrated in citations of student and resident research projects that have been published in peer-reviewed journals and, in some cases, leveraged into larger research projects.

Conducting a Clinical Trial—IRB and Research Coordinators

As the osteopathic medical profession progresses in its OMM-related research endeavors, appreciation of the complexity and infrastructure needed for the completion of successful studies has revealed what has been a part of every clinical trial done in the last 20 or more years. IRB requirements for the protection of the public have become a major consideration and require considerable preparation and often a back-and-forth process between research team and IRB to obtain final approval for a project.

Research coordinators often are skilled at the IRB review process and are of invaluable assistance as a part of the research team in this respect. The recruitment and consent of subjects are an increasingly complex process as the consent form approved by the IRB can be lengthy and requires careful presentation to a prospective subject.

Even to experienced researchers, the IRB approval and subject recruitment issues can be challenging. For newer researchers, it will be helpful to become as familiar as possible with these aspects of the research process.

In depth consideration of several of these research issues is made in Chapter 74. Some overlap in content may be fruitful in stressing crucial themes and skills necessary to carry out successful OMM-related research

Osteopathic Applications of Research Development Principles

Research Done During Residency Training

Virtually every medical resident trained in the United States has had to fulfill a requirement to do a research or scholarly activity project. It is difficult to do a full-fledged clinical trial while completing residency requirements, but certain fruitful lines of research pertaining to OMM/OMT have began during residency training.

In the last 10 years, several clinical studies completed during residency have reached publication. Three noteworthy studies were carried through to publication by the resident. An emergency medicine resident at St. Barnabus Hospital in Bronx, NY, published findings that OMT in the emergency department benefited acute ankle injuries (67). At the Michigan Hospital and Medical Center, Detroit, MI, a family practice resident published findings suggestive of benefit of OMT in reducing length of hospitalization for patients with pancreatitis (68). At the Kirksville College of Osteopathic Medicine (KCOM, now the A.T. Still University), an OMM resident published findings on the nature of the musculoskeletal system of a newborn from the cranial manipulation perspective (69). At the Osteopathic Medical Center of Texas in Fort Worth, an OMM resident joined with a mentor to publish an elucidation of the impact of OMT as a credible intervention. Active OMT intervention is perceived as more credible than sham OMT (70).

All of these published studies have been cited in subsequent studies and have provided the basis for trials of related disorders using OMT. All of these publications were preceded by poster or abstract presentations and received some financial support from the institutions in which the residency program operated.

Research Done During Medical Student Training

There is a wide variety of research backgrounds found in each year's new group of OMSs. Some matriculate with extensive research backgrounds including having multiple publications. A number of student research projects develop from ideas of mentors who have already published in a certain area and are initially presented as abstracts at research conferences. An example is the study on the impact of the CV4 maneuver on autonomic nervous system balance during paced breathing done by students and their mentors at the Western University of Health Sciences (71). Another example of student-involved research initially presented as a poster/abstract is a study carried out at the University of Medicine and Dentistry New Jersey School of Osteopathic Medicine, which found that the use of certain OMT technique may have benefit in the treatment of acute otitis media (72).

Student-involved studies can be of sufficient merit to be published in a peer-reviewed journal. A student at the New York College of Osteopathic Medicine worked with a mentor on a research project that demonstrated the patency of certain cranial sutures well into advanced age and offered an explanation based on the activity of neck muscles and the masticatory process (73). This was an exceptional study involving a student. Most student-involved research of this caliber has been done in dual-degree programs.

Research Done in Dual-Degree Programs

Several COMs have dual DO/PhD programs. The typical process is for the student to take the first 2 years of medical curriculum and then the next 2 years are devoted to the PhD work, usually in one of the basic sciences. Upon completion of the PhD, the student then completes the last 2 years of medical training and proceeds to residency training.

Two outstanding publications involving OMM were done by students in the dual DO/PhD program at the UNTHSC, Texas College of Osteopathic Medicine and in the Integrative Physiology Department of the Graduate School of Biomedical Science. Empirical demonstration that the lymphatic pump technique actually does increase lymphatic flow was done on instrumented conscious dogs (74). The second significant study documented the autonomic nervous system impact of the cranial manipulation maneuver known as the CV4 (75). Both of these studies have spawned a number of related research projects, some of which are noted below.

Most DO/PhD dissertation projects are in some area of basic science not directly related to OMM, but it is hoped that as the benefits of OMM/OMT are further documented, there will be an expansion in many basic science labs to include OMM related projects. At the UNTHSC, there is a dual-degree program in the OMM Department where the PhD is in "Osteopathic Manipulative Medicine Research and Education." Currently, there are two students in this program. One student, already an osteopathic physician in the OMM Department and staff of the ORC, received a K23 grant award from the NCCAM to study "Osteopathic Manipulative Medicine in Pregnancy: Physiological and Clinical Effects." This study is an example of leveraging of previous pilot work into an NIH-NCCAM grant award. Preliminary data for this K23 included research had been published (76,77) and had been presented at a research conference (78).

Based in part on the Knott et al. (74) work, another DO/PhD student became involved with research on the impact of OMT on the immune system. These studies are being carried out in the laboratory of the OHF Basic Science Chair holder of the ORC who is one of the faculty in the Molecular Biology and Immunology Department at UNTHSC (75). This exciting work has been funded in part by a U19 Developmental Center grant awarded to the ORC and in part by a grant awarded by the AOA. An initial publication demonstrated that the lymphatic pump treatment increased the leukocyte count and flux in the thoracic duct lymph in dogs (80). Further research by this DO/PhD student using a rat model showed that lymphatic pump treatment enhanced immunity and reduced pulmonary disease during experimental pneumonia infection (81). More recent work from this lab showed that the leukocytes came from gut-associated lymphoid tissue as they travel to the thoracic duct upon application of the lymphatic pump treatment (82).

A number of DO/MS students, primarily in the Pre-Doctoral Fellowship program in the OMM Department at UNTHSC-TCOM, have produced Master's degree theses and abstracts that have provided pilot data for research grants and explored research topics that otherwise might never be considered. Central to an NCCAM R21 grant submission that was awarded to an investigator at the ORC on "Treatment Efficacy of OMT for Carpal Tunnel Syndrome," were two master's theses that generated the preliminary data showing the OMT benefits for reducing pain and improving nerve conduction. These two Master's degree theses results were best accessed by the citations to research conference abstracts (83,84).

One topic that started with student and master's thesis research is showing the effects of OMM on physiologic functions such as heart rate variability (HRV). A student project (85) was completed almost simultaneously with a master's thesis (86), both showing improvement in HRV after OMT. Interest in this topic has been high, as a research project related to OMT and HRV did not show any differences between OMT and Sham OMT (87) but suggested that the trend may produce significance, had the sample size been larger.

Other ideas that were explored at the student and master's thesis level of research were the impact of OMT on postoperative nausea and vomiting (88), the immediate effects of splenic pump on blood cell counts (89), and the role of OMT in the treatment of fibromyalgia syndrome (90). All of these studies reported insignificant results, but that is beside the point. What is significant is that these studies were carried out in the first place. It is at this very preliminary phase of research that ideas are explored, and the published report, abstract, or poster may point the way to a better design or deter further study as likely unfruitful.

The fact is that a number of studies do not produce significant results and that these results are published is a healthy sign. Not only does this speak to the integrity of the research effort but it also shows the research energy and high quality of effort put forth by osteopathic students, residents, and physicians who are involved in OMM research. Some level of preliminary data are always required for NIH, federal government funding agency, or foundation research grant submission. Research "from the ground up" is the status for a profession that has received relatively little external funding compared to allopathic institutions. This discussion is intended to give the reader at every level of research background, medical student through experienced researcher, a fuller idea of how OMM research has been synergistic and often interactive.

Model for Support of Student and Resident Research Projects

These studies are cited as representative of efforts made through the osteopathic profession to promote research by undergraduate OMSs, residents, and dual-degree students. Perhaps the largest program for support of such research is that of the Center for Osteopathic Research and Education (CORE) located in the state of Ohio, with administrative offices at the Ohio University College of Osteopathic Medicine (91) The research support to students and residents located in Ohio is very strong and well staffed and serves as a model to be emulated. The CORE program is funded by Ohio University, the participating training hospitals, and the Osteopathic Heritage Foundation.

While not all states have enough osteopathic physicians and institutions to replicate the Ohio CORE program, it is a fine model to replicate if only in certain pieces by another state or consortium of states through the respective Osteopathic Post-Graduate Training Institutes.

Clinician and Basic Science Collaboration

The model set by Denslow and Korr, Johnston and Kelso, and others is still a benchmark to be emulated by researchers in the present time. It has not been easy to garner collaboration between OMM clinical researchers and basic scientists who come out of traditional academic settings and whose interests and dissertation work may not relate directly to OMM or any other aspect of musculoskeletal disease. However, this goal is a high priority for OMM research, especially in the mechanisms of actions for OMM and impact of OMM on systemic disorders.

When such collaborations are forged, good results come about. Certain examples already cited are the mechanism of action research on lymphatic flow (74) and impact of OMM on immune system processes (80–82). Concurrent with other collaborations going on at Michigan State University College of Osteopathic Medicine at the time, two neuroscientists collaborated with an OMM clinician to demonstrate experimentally induced cranial bone motion in cats (92).

More recent basic scientist-clinician collaborations have been forged at the New York College of Osteopathic Medicine with work on the impact of OMT on Parkinson disease (93) and the effect of muscle energy technique on cervical spine range of motion (94). At Midwestern University Chicago College of Osteopathic Medicine, a series of studies were carried out by a basic scientist-clinician team, which established a possible means by which cranial bone motion could be measured (95,96) and then related such motion to the physiologic process known as the Traube-Hering-Mayer phenomenon (97).

Funded by the Osteopathic Heritage Foundation, a team of basic scientist-clinician researchers at the Ohio University College of Osteopathic Medicine have measured the beneficial effects of OMT on Achilles tendinitis (98) and plantar fasciitis (99) and developed a virtual reality program, which has been added to the medical student curriculum to train medical students in osteopathic palpatory diagnosis (100). At the A.T. Still Research Institute in Kirksville, MO, a basic scientist-clinician team showed the effect of OMT on altering pain biomarkers (101). As part of a Developmental Center Grant (U19 Award) from NCCAM, work was carried out, first at the Midwestern University Arizona College of Osteopathic Medicine and then at the University of Arizona Medical School in Phoenix, showing the impact of simulated OMT on tissue fibroblasts in vitro. This exciting work on human fibroblast showed significant changes in cytokine production (102).

Some of these promising basic scientist-clinician collaborations continue, but it is hoped that more will be developed. This will be made more likely as more OMM-related research is generated at all levels.

FINANCIAL SUPPORT FOR OSTEOPATHIC RESEARCH

U.S. funding of biomedical research in 2003 was 94.3 billion USD (103), and in 2008 alone, the research departments at allopathic academic medical centers averaged 85 million USD (104). The total research for all the COMs in 2004 was 101.3 million USD (105). These figures are for all research funding and suggest that there is much more research taking place at COMs than might have been imagined; however, it was necessary to lump all the COMs together to achieve a figure that could rival just one allopathic academic medical center.

With regard to NIH funding alone, the *JAOA* reported that combined NIH funding to all COMs in 2004 ranked 163rd among funding totals provided by the NIH to the top 500 research institutions (106). The *JAOA* article (105) went on to report that the largest COM research funding in 2004 was almost 32 million USD at the UNTHSC/Texas College of Osteopathic Medicine.

In the context of these figures for all biomedical research, even in osteopathic institutions, the funding amounts for OMM-related research are very small by comparison. There is no one source that keeps records of OMM-related research funding, and indeed from review of lists of funding, it is not always possible to tell from a project title whether or not the research pertained to OMM in any way.

In preparation for this chapter, contact was made with the AOA Department of Quality and Research and a list of all research projects funded by the AOA was requested. AOA staff was very cooperative, and a list of all research funding from 1989 to 2007 was provided. These were projects reviewed by the AOA Council on Research and recommended for funding and approved by the AOA Board of Trustees. The funding amounts reported varied from year to year and came primarily from the Osteopathic Research Development Fund (ORDF), which was originally accumulated from contributions from osteopathic physicians. The corpus of the ORDF is approximately 7 million USD and annual funding depends on the performance of investments in this fund. The total research funding from 1989 to 2007 was $3,276,363, with no funding provided from 2002 to 2006 because of investment portfolio decreases.

From a close review of the titles of the projects funded by the AOA, the amount awarded to OMM-related topics was $2,667,062. This amount was 81.4% of all the funds awarded to research by the AOA. It is worthy to note that the membership organization of the osteopathic medical profession does indeed invest the majority of its research funding into OMM-related projects. Most of the research funds since the beginning of OMM-related research have come from sources internal to the osteopathic profession, that is, the AOA, AAO/LBORC, COMs, and osteopathic-supportive foundations.

The current major funding provider for projects and programs supporting osteopathic medical research is the Columbus, Ohio-based Osteopathic Heritage Foundation, oft mentioned in the foregoing discussions. Data published on the OHF Web site document a number of the awards provided since 2000 (107). The total amount awarded during this period to support osteopathic research such as the Ohio CORE program, specific OMM-related research projects, capital research investments, endowed research chairs, and programs such as the ORC was nearly $30 million. To those involved in the development of quality research that provides the evidence base for OMM, the contribution of the OHF has been the capstone and central to the recent progress reported above (105,108). One objective of this Foundation, in accord with the ORT strategic plan (105,108), is to provide the necessary support to enable the ORC and future possible regional ORCs to become self-sustaining with external funding. In light of the leveling off of NIH research funding and reductions in certain areas, it has become an even more difficult task to obtain external funding, which makes the contributions of this Foundation much more significant.

The FOHS and a consortium of osteopathic-supportive foundations have contributed significantly to the MOPSE study and other projects. FOHS leadership is involved in support of OCCTIC and in projects such as the osteopathic observational research project.

By the time of the publication of this edition of the *Foundations for Osteopathic Medicine* book, there may be additional data on OMM-related research funding. There are other entities that need to be cited for their significant contributions to OMM research funding. AACOM and AOF as well as the AOA continue to provide infrastructure funding to the ORC. Securing the funds to support OMM-related research is an ongoing process. The comments in this section are an attempt to describe the history and current status of funding support for OMM research, which is in part an outgrowth of the realization by the osteopathic profession of the need to establish the evidence base for OMM (10,105,108).

ACKNOWLEDGEMENTS

In preparation of this chapter, extensive review and confirmation of accuracy of financial data were made by Richard A. Vincent, President, Osteopathic Heritage Foundation, and Sharon McGill, Director of American Osteopathic Association Department of Quality and Research.

REFERENCES

1. Patterson MM. Osteopathic research: the future. In: Ward RC, ed. *Foundations for Osteopathic Medicine.* Baltimore, MD: Lippincott Williams & Wilkins, 1997:1115–1124.

2. Patterson MM. Foundations for osteopathic medical research. In: Ward RC, ed. *Foundations for Osteopathic Medicine.* 2nd Ed. Baltimore, MD: Lippincott Williams & Wilkins, 2003:1167–1187.

3. Lito P, Mets BD, Kleff S, et al. Evidence that sprouty 2 is necessary for sarcoma formation by H-Ras oncogene-transformed human fibroblasts. *J Biological Chem* 2008;283(4):2002–2009.

4. Wang Y, Woodgate R, McManus TP, et al. Evidence that in xeroderma pigmentosum variant cells, which lack DNA polymerase eta, DNA polymerase iota causes the very high frequency and unique spectrum of UV-induced mutations. *Cancer Res* 2007;67(7):3018–3026.

5. Appledorn DM, Kiang A, McBride A, et al. Wild-type adenoviruses from groups A-F evoke unique innate immune responses, of which HAd3 and SAd23 are partially complement dependent. *Gene Ther* 2008;15(12): 885–901.

6. Xu F. Serra D. Amalfitano A. Applications of adenoviral vector-mediated gene transfer in cardiovascular research. *Methods Mol Med* 2006;129: 209–239.

7. Formes KJ, Wray DW, O-Yurvati AH, et al. Sympathetic cardiac influence and arterial blood pressure instability. *Auton Neurosci* 2005;118(1–2): 116–124.

8. O-Yurvati AH. Pyruvate-enhanced cardioplegia preserves myocardial HSP 70 and endothelial NOS in a porcine model of cardiopulmonary bypass. Poster and abstract presented March 28, 2008 at Research Appreciation Day, University of North Texas Health Science Center. Supported by Osteopathic Heritage Foundation grant #02-18-522.

9. AOA Research Task Force Report. *Research Strategic Direction for the American Osteopathic Association.* January 2005.

10. National OMM Research Synergy White Paper. *Osteopathic Manipulative Medicine Research: A 21ˢᵗ Century Vision.* Available at: http://www.aacom. org/InfoFor/researchers/Pages/ default.aspx. Accessed August 15, 2008.

11. Whiting LM. Can length of labor be shortened by osteopathic treatment? *J Am Osteopath Assoc* 1911;11:917–921.

12. Jones M. Osteopathy and obstetrical mortality and stillbirth and infant mortality: symposium on osteopathy in obstetrics chaired by S.V. Robuck, DO. *J Am Osteopath Assoc* 1933;33:350–353.

13. D'Alonzo GE. Influenza epidemic or pandemic? time to roll up sleeves, vaccinate patients, and hone osteopathic manipulative skills [Editorial]. *J Am Osteopath Assoc* 2004;104(9):370–371.

14. Smith RK. One hundred thousand cases of influenza with a death rate of one-fortieth of that officially reported under conventional medical treatment. *J Am Osteopath Assoc* 1920;20:172–175. Reprinted in: *J Am Osteopath Assoc* 2000;100:320–323.

15. Burns L. Viscero-sensory and somato-visceral spinal reflexes. *J Am Osteopath Assoc* 1907;7:51–60.

16. Burns L. The immediate effects of boney lesions. *J Am Osteopath Assoc* 1910;9:469–475.

17. Cole WV. Louisa Burns memorial lecture. *J Am Osteopath Assoc* 1970; 69:1005–1017.

18. Kawchuk GN, Fauvel OR, Dmowski J. Ultrasonic indentation (UI): a procedure for the non-invasive quantification of force-displacement properties of the lumbar spine. *J Manipulative Physiol Ther* 2001;24(3):149–156.

19. Denslow JS, Hassett CC. The central excitatory state associated with postural abnormalities. *J Neurolphysiol* 1942;5:393–402.

20. Korr IM. The neural basis of the osteopathic lesion. *J Am Osteopath Assoc* 1947;47:191–198.

21. Denslow JS, Korr IM, Krems AD. Quantitative studies of chronic facilitation in human motoneuron pools. *Am J Physiol* 1947;105:229–238.

22. Korr IM, Thomas PE. The automatic recording of electrical skin resistance patterns on the human trunk. *EEG Clin Neurophysiol* 1951;3:361–368.

23. Thomas PE, Korr IM. Relationship between sweat gland activity and electrical resistance of the skin. *J Neural Transm* 1958;17:77–96.

24. Korr IM, Wright HM, Thomas PE. Effects of experimental myofascial insults on cutaneous patterns of sympathic activity in man. *J Neural Transm* 1962;23:330–355.

25. Neural and spinal components of disease: progress in the application of "thermography." *J Am Osteopath Assoc* 1965;64:918–921.

26. Korr IM, Appletauer GSL. The time-course of axonal proteins to muscle. *Exper Neurol* 1974;43:452–463.

27. Appletauer GSL, Korr IM. Axonal delivery of soluble, insoluble and electrophoretic fractions of neuronal proteins to muscle. *Exper Neurol* 1975;46:132–146.

28. Appletauer GSL, Korr IM. Axonal migration of some particle-bound proteins in the hypoglossal nerve and their failure t enter the styloglossus muscle. *J Am Osteopath Assoc* 1978;77:479–481.

29. Johnston WL. Interexaminer reliability studies; spanning a gap in medical research. Louisa Burns Memorial Lecture. *J Am Osteopath Assoc* 1982;81(2):43–53.

30. Johnston WL, Elkiss ML, Marino RV. Passive gross motion testing Part II: a study of interexaminer agreement. *J Am Osteopath Assoc* 1982;81(5):65–69.

31. Johnston WL, Beal MC, Blum GA. Passive gross motion testing Part III: examiner agreement on selected subjects. *J Am Osteopath Assoc* 1982;81(5):70–74.

32. Johnston WL, Kelso AF, Beal MC, et al. Standardization of the hospital record for osteopathic structural examination. *J Am Osteopath Assoc* 1996;96(9):529–536.

33. Beal MC. Viscerosomatic reflexes: a review. *J Am Osteopath Assoc* 1985; 85(7):786–801.

34. Johnston, WL. Osteopathic clinical aspects of somatovisceral interaction. In: Patterson MM, Howell JN, eds. *The central connection: somatovisceral/ viscerosomatic interaction.* Indianapolis, IN: American Academy of Osteopathy, 1989.

35. Beal MC, Kleiber GE. Somatic dysfunction as a predictor of coronary artery disease. *J Am Osteopath Assoc* 1985;85(5):302–307.

36. Kelso AF, Grant RG, Johnston WL. Use of thermograms to support assessment of somatic dysfunction or effects of osteopathic manipulative treatment: a preliminary report. *J Am Osteopath Assoc* 1982;82(3):59–65.

37. Johnston WL, Kelso AF, Hollandsworth DL. Somatic manifestations in renal disease: a clinical research study. *J Am Osteopath Assoc* 1987;87(1): 61–74.

38. Johnston WL, Kelso AF. Changes in presence of a segmental dysfunction pattern associated with hypertension: Part II. A long-term longitudinal study. *J Am Osteopath Assoc* 1995;95(5):315–318.

39. Noll DR, Shores J, Bryman PN, et al. Adjunctive osteopathic manipulative treatment in the elderly hospitalized with pneumonia: a pilot study. *J Am Osteopath Assoc* 1999;99(3):143–143.

40. Noll DR, Shores J, Gamber RG, et al. Benefits of osteopathic manipulative treatment for hospitalized elderly patients with pneumonia. *J Am Osteopath Assoc* 2000;100(12):776–782.

41. Degenhardt BF. OMT in the Treatment of Pneumonia. In: King HH, ed. *Building Excellence in Osteopathic Research: Proceedings of OCCTIC-VII.* March 2006, Birmingham, AL. Available at: http://www.hsc.unt.edu/ ORC/. Accessed August 31, 2008.

42. Noll DR, Degenhardt BF, Fossum C, et al. Clinical and research protocol for osteopathic manipulative treatment of elderly patients with pneumonia. *J Am Osteopath Assoc* 2008;108:508–516.

43. Mills MV, Henley CE, Barnes LLB, et al. The use of osteopathic manipulative treatment as adjuvant therapy in children with recurrent acute otitis media. *Arch Pediatrics Adol Med* 2003;157:861–866.

44. Steele K, Kukulka G, Ikner C. Effect of Osteopathic manipulative treatment (OMT) on childhood otitis media outcomes. *J Am Osteopath Assoc* 1997;97:484.

45. Degenhardt BF, Kuchera ML. Efficacy of osteopathic evaluation and manipulative treatment in reducing the morbidity of otitis media in children. *J Am Osteopath Assoc* 1994;94:673.

46. Degenhardt BF, Kuchera ML. The Prevalence of Cranial Dysfunction in Children with a History of Otitis Media from Kindergarten to Third Grade. *J Amer Osteopath Assoc* 1994;94:754.

47. Blood H. Infections of the Ear, Nose and Throat. *Osteopathic Annals* 1978;6:465–469.

48. Osteopathic Otitis Media Research Study. Available at: http://clinicaltrials.gov/ct2/results?term= otitis+media. Accessed August 25, 2005.

49. Haldeman S, Kohlbeck FJ, McGregor M. Stroke, cerebral artery dissection, and cervical spine manipulation therapy. *J Neurol* 2002;249:1098–1104.

50. Haldeman S, Kohlbeck FJ, McGregor M. Unpredictability of cerebrovascular ischemia associated with cervical spine manipulation therapy. *Spine* 2002;27:49–55.

51. Reports to the AOA Council of Scientific Affairs (2006) and Bureau of Scientific Affairs (2007) are available on ORC website http://www.hsc.unt.edu/ORC/

52. Straus SE, Richardson WS, Glasziou P, Haynes RB. *Evidence based medicine.* 3rd Ed. London: UK: Churchill Livingstone, 2005.

53. Licciardone JC, Brimhall AK, King LN. Osteopathic manipulative treatment for low back pain: a systematic review and meta-analysis of randomized controlled trials. *BMC Musculoskelet Disord* 2005;6:43. Available at: http:www.biomedcentral.com/1471-2474/6/43. Accessed July 3, 2008.

54. Detsky AS, Baerlocher MO. Academic mentoring—how to give it and how to get it. *JAMA* 2007;297(19):2134–2136.

55. http:// crisp.cit.nih.gov/. Accessed September 3, 2008.

56. http://www.nsf.gov/awardsearch/. Accessed September 3, 2008.

57. http://www.aacom.org/events/annualmtg/past/2007aacom/Pages/aacom2007reports. aspx #wednesday. Accessed September 3, 2008.

58. http://era.nih.gov/ElectronicReceipt/. Accessed September 3, 2008.

59. http://grants.nih.gov/grants/funding/phs398/phs398.html. Accessed September 3, 2008.

60. http://videocast.nih.gov/PastEvents.asp?c=1. Accessed September 3, 2008.

61. http://nccam.nih.gov/news/2007/110707.htm. Accessed September 3, 2008.

62. http://www.hsc.unt.edu/ORC/Documents/ResearchManual.pdf. Accessed August 15, 2008.

63. AOA Research Handbook. http://www.osteopathic.org/pdf/res_hndbk.pdf. Accessed September 3, 2008.

64. Berg KM, Gill TM, Brown AF, et al. Demystifying the NIH grant application process. *J Gen Intern Med* 2007;22(11):1587–1595.

65. Horner RD. Demystifying the NIH grant application process: the rest of the story. *J Gen Intern Med* 2007;22(11):1628–1629.

66. Agarwal R, Chertow GM, Mehta RL. Strategies for successful patient oriented research: why did I (not) get funded. *Clin J Am Soc Nephrol* 2006;1:340–343.

67. Eisenhart AW, Gaeta TJ, Yens DP. Osteopathic treatment in the emergency department for patients with acute ankle injuries. *J Am Osteopath Assoc* 2003;103(9):417–421.

68. Radjieski JM, Lumley MA, Cantieri MS. Effect of osteopathic treatment on length of stay for pancreatitis: a randomized pilot study. *J Am Osteopath Assoc*1998;98(5):264–272.

69. Allen DM. Observations from normal newborn osteopathic evaluations. In: King HH, Ed. *Proceedings of international research conference: Osteopathy in Pediatrics at the Osteopathic Center for Children in San Diego, CA 2002.* Indianapolis, IN: American Academy of Osteopathy, 2005:99–106.

70. Licciardone JC, Russo DP. Blinding protocols, treatment credibility, and expectancy: methodologic issues in clinical trials of osteopathic manipulative treatment. *J Am Osteopath Assoc* 2006;106:457–463.

71. Ananyev DA, Rodriguez C Jr, Mercado R, et al. CV4 alters autonomic balance during paced breathing [abstract]. *J Am Osteopath Assoc* 2008;108(8):415.

72. Torres JW, Mason DC, Kaari J. Osteopathic manipulative medicine in the treatment of acute otitis media symptoms [abstract]. *J Am Osteopath Assoc* 2008;108(8):416.

73. Sabini RC, Elkowitz DE. Significance of differences in patency among cranial sutures. *J Am Osteopath Assoc* 2006;106:600–604.

74. Knott, EM, Tune, JD, Stoll, ST, et al. Increased lymphatic flow in the thoracic duct during manipulative intervention. *J Am Osteopath Assoc* 2005;105:447–456.

75. Cutler MJ, Holland SH, Stupski BA, et al. Cranial manipulatioin can alter sleep latency and sympathetic nerve activity in humans: a pilot study. *J Altern Comp Med* 2005;11(1):103–108.

76. King HH, Tettambel MA, Lockwood MD, et al. Osteopathic manipulative treatment in prenatal care: A retrospective case control design study. *J Am Osteopath Assoc* 2003;103(12):577–582.

77. Licciardone JC, Buchanan S, Hensel KL, et al. Osteopathic manipulative treatment of back pain and related symptoms during pregnancy: a randomized controlled trial. *Am J Obstet Gyn* 2010;202:43.e1–8.

78. Licciardone JC. A Pilot Clinical Trial of Osteopathic Manipulative Treatment in Pregnancy. Presented at OCCTIC-VII in Birmingham, AL March 27, 2006.

79. Lisa Hodge, PhD accessed August 28, 2008 http://www.hsc.unt.edu/ORC/team.htm.

80. Hodge LM, King HH, Williams AG, Simecka JW, Stoll ST, Downey HF. Abdominal lymphatic pump treatment increases leukocyte count and flux in thoracic duct lymph. *Lymphat Res Biol* 2007;5(2):127–132.

81. Huff JB, Schander A, Stoll ST, et al. Lymphatic pump treatment enhances immunity and reduces pulmonary disease during experimental pneumonia infection [abstract]. *J Am Osteopath Assoc* 2008;108(8):447.

82. Schander A, Bearden MK, Huff JB, et al. Lymphatic pump treatment mobilizes leukocytes from the gut associated lymphoid tissue into thoracic duct lymph [abstract]. *J Am Osteopath Assoc* 2008;108(8):441.

83. Meyer P, Stoll ST, Cruser d, et al. Improving symptoms, pain, functioning, and strength for persons with carpal tunnel syndrome [abstract]. *J Am Osteopath Assoc* 2006;106(8):486.

84. White HD, Stoll ST, Cruser d, et al. Osteopathic manipulative medicine for carpal tunnel syndrome; changes in nerve conduction [abstract]. *J Am Osteopath Assoc* 2006;106(8):473.

85. Guinn K, Seffinger MA, Ali H, et al. Validation of transcutaneous laser Doppler flowmeter in measuring autonomic balance [abstract]. *J Am Osteopath Assoc* 2006;106(8):475–476.

86. Giles P, Hensel K, Smith M. The effects of upper cervical spine manipulation on cardiac autonomic control. Poster presented at OCCTIC-VIII Colorado Springs, March 23, 2007.

87. Henley CE, Ivins D, Mills M, et al. Osteopathic manipulation and its relationship to autonomic nervous system activity as demonstrated by heart rate variability; a repeated measures study. *Osteopath Med Prim Care* 2008, 2:7. Available at: http://www.om-pc.com/content/2/1/7.

88. Schrick-Senasac S, King HH. Osteopathic Manipulative treatment for postoperative nausea and vomiting [abstract]. *J Am Osteopath Assoc* 2008;108(8):413.

89. Harpenau CM, Inoue A, Johnson JC, et al. The immediate effects of the splenic pump technique on blood cell counts in normal adults [abstract]. *J Am Osteopath Assoc* 2006;106(8):474.

90. Yahnert JL, Hartman RJ, Steward PE, et al. The role of osteopathic manipulative treatment in the treatment of fibromyalgia syndrome [abstract]. *J Am Osteopath Assoc* 2006;106(8):472.

91. http://www.ohiocore.org/research/CRONews.htm. Accessed August 28, 2008.

92. Adams T, Heisey RS, Smith MC, et al. Parietal bone mobility in the anesthetized cat. *J Am Osteopath Assoc* 1992(5);92:599–604.

93. Wells MR, Giantinoto S, D'Agate D, et al. Standard osteopathic manipulative treatment acutely improves gait performance in patients with Parkinson's disease. *J Am Osteopath Assoc* 1999;99(2):92–100.

94. Burns DK, Wells MR. Gross range of motion in the cervical spine: the effects of osteopathic muscle energy technique in asymptomatic subjects. *J Am Osteopath Assoc* 2006;106:137–142.

95. Sergueef N, Nelson KE, Glonek T. The effect of cranial manipulation upon the Traube Hering Meyer oscillation. *Altern Therap Health Med* 2002;8:74–76.

96. Nelson KE, Sergueef N, Glonek T. Cranial manipulation induces sequential changes in blood flow velocity on demand. *Amer Acad Osteopath J* 2004;14:15–17.

97. Nelson KE, Sergueef N, Glonek T. Recording the rate of the cranial rhythmic impulse. *J Am Osteopath Assoc* 2006;106:337–341.

98. Howell JN, Cabell KS, Chila AG, et al. Stretch reflex and Hoffmann Reflex responses to osteopathic manipulative treatment in subjects with Achilles tendinitis. *J Am Osteopath Assoc* 2006;106(9):537–545.

99. Wynne MM, Burns JM, Eland DC, et al. Effect of counterstrain on stretch reflexes, Hoffmann Reflexes, and clinical outcomes in subjects with plantar fasciitis. *J Am Osteopath Assoc* 2006;106(9):547–556.

100. Howell JN, Conatser RR, Williams RL, et al. Palpatory diagnosis training on the Virtual Haptic Back: performance improvement and user evaluations. *J Am Osteopath Assoc* 2008;108:29–36.

101. Degenhardt BF, Darmani NA, Johnson JC, et al. Role of osteopathic manipulative treatment in altering pain biomarkers: a pilot study. *J Am Osteopath Assoc* 2007;107(9):387–400.

102. Meltzer KR, Standley PR. Modeled repetitive motion strain and indirect osteopathic manipulative techniques in regulation of human fibroblast proliferation and interleukin secretion. *J Am Osteopath Assoc* 2007;107:527–536.

103. Moses H, Dorsey ER, Matheson DHM, et al. Financial anatomy of biomedical research. *JAMA* 2005;294(11):1333–1342.

104. Heinig SJ, Krakower JY, Dickler HB, et al. Sustaining the engine of U.S. biomedical discovery. *N Eng J Med* 2007;357(10):1042–1047.

105. Clearfield MB, Smith-Barbaro P, Guillory, et al. Research funding at colleges of osteopathic medicine: 15 years of growth. *J Am Osteopath Assoc* 2007;107(11):469–478.

106. NIH awards to all institutions by rank, fiscal year 2004, rank 1 to 500 page. National Institutes of Health Web site. Available at: http://www.grants.nih.gov/grants/award/trend/rnk04all1to500.htm. Accessed May 17, 2007.

107. Osteopathic Heritage Foundation. http://www.osteopathicheritage.org/funding.htm. Accessed September 3, 2008.

108. Clearfield MB, Smith-Barbaro P, Guillory, et al. How can we keep research growing at colleges of osteopathic medicine? [editorial]. *J Am Osteopath Assoc* 2007;107(11):463–465.

73

Biobehavioral Research

JOHN A. JEROME, BRIAN H. FORESMAN, AND GILBERT E. D'ALONZO

KEY CONCEPTS

- Biobehavioral mechanisms alter health and disease through three basic pathways: physiologic responses to stress that lead to disease, behavioral choices that increase or decrease health risk, and behavioral reactions to disease that alter surveillance activities or adherence with medical interventions.
- The major behavioral factors that have been studied and shown to have clear associations with health and disease include diet, exercise, sleep, cigarette smoking, tobacco use, alcohol use, and prevention of excessive sun exposure.
- Placebos are also a biobehavioral mechanism that must be addressed in most forms of research. Behavioral research strategies must consider the effects of race, direct suggestion, patient belief in the treatment, trust in the physician, genetic variation, environmental effects, and nonspecific cause–effect relationships with placebos.
- As with other types of research, the biobehavioral research process begins with the acquisition of measurement data and the development of a hypothesis about the mechanisms involved with the processes under consideration. Selection of the study design, subjects, and analysis methods to be used constitute the major components of the process and lead to a systematic analysis of the data.
- Biobehavioral research and evidence-based knowledge will provide effective and proven treatment strategies and render valuable insight into the impact of osteopathic principles and practice. Major topics in biobehavioral measurement and research will likely focus on behaviors leading to the development of somatic dysfunction, behaviors resulting from somatic dysfunction, quality-of-life (QOL) issues, the effects of pain on function, and relationships between somatic dysfunction, and patient self-managing of self-defeating behaviors.

INTRODUCTION

Biobehavioral research involves the investigation of behaviors on the maintenance of health and the development of disease. The onset of disease is a complex phenomenon that incorporates the tissue pathology (musculoskeletal abnormalities), psychosocial and behavioral response to that physical insult, and the environmental factors that maintain or reinforce that disability (even after the initial cause has been resolved). A large portion of the measurable variance in an individual response to any disease outcome is accounted for by the individual's unique behavior and emotional response to the stress of the illness (1). In fact, the majority of today's health woes—obesity, cancer, and anxiety disorders to heart disease, hypertension, and adult-onset diabetes—are actually relatively new "diseases of civilization" brought on by our behavioral choices and mind-body interactions. Although the concepts that the mind influences disease processes have long been a part of osteopathic medicine, research strategies to describe the mechanisms of disease modification through biobehavioral interactions have only recently become a part of evidence-based medicine.

Our current understanding of biobehavioral interactions suggests that these processes are a complex interplay between psychologic, physiologic, environmental, and behavioral factors that influence health and disease (2). Behavioral mechanisms can alter the musculoskeletal, immune, neurologic, and endocrine systems, directly and indirectly, thereby influencing such medical illnesses as cancer and cardiovascular disease. Diet, exercise, drugs, alcohol, and tobacco use, along with a variety of other behaviors, modify disease progression and/or disease risk. Finally, behaviors directly related to seeking or avoiding medical care can have important consequences on prevention, early detection, and adherence with medical regimens. Thus, the implication is that biobehavioral

factors may significantly affect health care and health maintenance through a variety of direct and indirect mechanisms (2), and these effects should be addressed in osteopathic research and clinical practice (3–5).

BIOBEHAVIORAL MECHANISMS IN HEALTH

Behavioral components of the mind-body interaction manifest in cognitive processes, emotions, and/or physical behaviors. The study of cognitive processes (e.g., language acquisition, reading, emotional appraisal, memory, attention, mental models or representations, learning and cognition, problem solving, ascribing meaning, abstraction, and action) primarily focuses on acquisition, understanding, retention, and processing of information. However, under most circumstances, thoughts, emotions, and cognitive processes must transmit information, be translated into motor actions, or have identifiable physiologic responses before a behavior can be identified. It is for these reasons that many consider mental phenomena to be a special form of physical phenomena (i.e., biobehavioral) and therefore inseparable from physiologic processes.

Biobehavioral factors exert their influence through three defined pathways, which are illustrated in Figure 73.1 (2,6). In the first of these pathways, *cognition and emotional reactions* are creating physiologic alterations that contribute to the pathophysiology of the disease. An example is the classical stress response (described in Chapters 17 and 18) that is associated with increases in blood pressure and heart rate displayed as part of global sympathetic arousal. Chronic arousal creates dysregulation. These sympathetic alterations can, in turn, contribute directly to the development of cardiac disease and sudden death. Excessive or unwanted stress that creates inescapable demands, whether induced by external events or internal mental processes, can create a sense of powerlessness and alter

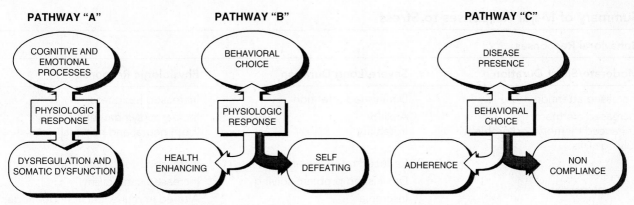

Figure 73-1   Common biobehavioral pathways in health and disease.

neural and hormonal responses, leading to enhanced vulnerability to infection and inappropriate response to disease (i.e., viral infections, wound healing, and cancer).

The second pathway for biobehavioral interactions involves *behaviors* in response to illnesses that are associated with increasing or minimizing health risk. These particular behaviors are referred to as "high-risk" or "health-enhancing" behaviors. Examples of health-enhancing behaviors include diet and exercise (due to their ability to minimize the development cardiovascular disease and cancer). Tobacco use and alcohol abuse are examples of high-risk behaviors typically associated with adverse effects that frequently lead to emphysema, lung cancer, and cardiovascular disease. Other examples include drug use and high-risk sexual activity. Each of these activities conveys a risk or benefit to an alteration of the underlying physiology and/or exposure.

The third and final pathway involves behaviors that occur in response to the *possibility* that a disease is present. For self-managing individuals, these behaviors lead to early detection include ongoing surveillance (i.e., retained breast examinations, sigmoidoscopy, etc.), recognition of symptoms, and the decision to actively participate in medical care or follow-up care. If a disease or a symptom is identified and a medical regimen is prescribed, adherence with the medical regimen (or lack thereof) is a behavior that can affect the outcome of the disease process. On the other hand, high-risk behaviors can lead to the sudden discontinuation of medications or their erratic administration that can only hinder the effectiveness of standard evidence-based medical regimens; such behaviors may also create secondary adverse consequences.

There are many situations under which this theoretic disease development pathway would be applicable to biobehavioral research and might offer distinct advantages in understanding the relevant pathophysiologic relationships. The consideration of such pathways is in keeping with known stress responses of the somatic musculature. This theoretic framework is also consistent with the biologic and behavioral responses of individuals with acute and chronic pain.

Disease Development (Pathway "A")

The major biobehavioral interactions on disease development that have been studied involve the effects of stress on health or illness. Because of the vast scope of data involving stress, physiologic response, and behavioral issues, our intent is to discuss the learned mechanisms wherein stress responses affect selected diseases and how these variables can be measured and researched.

From an evolutionary standpoint, most neural events can be considered to develop and have been selected by evolutionary process associated with species survival (2). In this viewpoint, stress responses and other emotional patterns are hardwired into the central nervous system (CNS) and modified by learning and experience. Thus, content and environmental conditions give rise to particular responses that can modify the emotional or cognitive response. Essentially, our bodies "learn" about the external correlates of internal responses much like a baby learns that food and eating extinguish the uncomfortable response later labeled as hunger. This process of "learning" can be significantly affected by the intensity and chronicity of the stress response under which the learning occurred. Less intense and intermittent stressors allow more complex and appropriate coping strategies to be learned; whereas more severe and prolonged stressors may cause a conditioned biobehavioral response that is less adaptable. In this sense, learning may be either adaptive or maladaptive and may affect predisposition to disease.

CARDIOVASCULAR DISEASE

Previous research has shown that stress, whether physical or emotional, perceived or real, often results in characteristic physiologic and behavior responses (Table 73.1). The physiologic and behavioral correlates may trigger acute, disease-related events and alter the pathophysiology of the disorders (7). Acute cardiovascular events, such as ischemic episodes, heart attacks, arterial occlusion, and arrhythmias, have been shown to occur with anxiety, bereavement, and anger (3,8,9). Similar effects are also seen with strong positive emotions associated with desirable events (e.g., weddings). Several mechanisms have been proposed to account for these responses, including alteration of sympathetic-parasympathetic balance, activation of platelets, alterations of intravascular flow dynamics, and changes of endothelial function (10,11).

Within these hardwired responses, maladaptive behaviors may lead to secondary physiologic responses that may have additional adverse consequences. For example, when assessing cardiovascular responses, physiologic reactivity is measured by the magnitude and the duration of the particular response. Studies have shown that increased cardiac reactivity may be a direct index of the underlying predisposition toward developing cardiovascular disorders or may reflect the activity of mediators of cardiovascular risk (12). In several studies, exaggerated blood pressure responses identified individuals at risk for developing hypertension and atherosclerosis

TABLE 73.1

Summary of Major Responses to Stress

Behavioral Responses

Moderate/Short Duration	Severe/Long Duration	Physiologic Response
Increased attention	Diminished attention	Increased heart rate
Increased alertness	Anxiety	Increased sympathetic activity (both neural and humoral)
Enhanced memory and problem-solving skills	Irritability	
	Reduced retention and recall	Increased blood pressure
	Diminished problem solving	Increased catabolism
	Insomnia	Altered immune function (dependent on the duration and intensity of the stressor)

(13–15). Similarly, other behaviors may have adverse affects on serum lipid composition, silent ischemia oxidative damage (9,16) (such as that seen with smoking), personality styles (e.g., type A), and altered coping mechanisms (17). Through the use of biobehavioral research approaches, cardiovascular researchers are now beginning to enhance our understanding of the statistical relationships between the cognitions, emotions, and behaviors in the development and progression of cardiovascular disease (6,9).

IMMUNE FUNCTION AND INFECTIOUS DISORDERS

Immunologic activity has also been shown to be altered by behavioral responses; the impact on disease development is described in the Basic Sciences Section of this book. Some of the difficulty in making assessments regarding immune function involves the variability of the stressors and the dynamic nature of the immune system. For instance, natural killer cells have a different response to acute and chronic stress exposures (18), and these responses are also subject to circadian variations. Changes in latent viral activity, lymphocyte proliferation, and natural killer cell activity have all been demonstrated in response to stress (19–21). These changes in immune function and cell numbers may also occur with physical stress, such as severe exercise (22). Several immunologic responses may also promote facilitating responses. The activation of inflammatory mediators, such as interleukin-6 and proinflammatory cytokines, may alter neural processes to enhance aspects of the CNS stress response (23).

Behaviors can have a more direct effect on the development of disease by altering bodily functions associated with disease risk (24). Perhaps the most classic example involves human immunodeficiency virus (HIV) disease. The transmission of HIV typically occurs during sexual activity, intravenous drug use, or through other forms of direct contact with bodily fluids. An attenuation of these behaviors or the addition of protective measures can result in substantial decreases in the risk of acquiring HIV. Conversely, increases in risky behaviors or the occurrence of impulse behaviors, as can occur with individuals with certain types of mental health problems (25) or during drug and alcohol use (26,27), can change routine behaviors of the individual and increase the risk of acquiring

HIV. In this setting, stress or drug use may initiate impulsive behaviors or may inhibit intentions to avoid the risky behaviors (28) leading to impaired judgment, a lack of attention to details, or in some instances, disregarding the potential consequences of their actions (29).

SLEEP AND CIRCADIAN BIOLOGY

Sleep and sleep wake activities also constitute a major biobehavioral mechanism that may lend themselves to biobehavioral research. Sleep deprivation and sleep fragmentation result in excessive daytime sleepiness, chronic fatigue, and other symptoms. Many of the symptoms are measurable and distinguishable from depression, and they may have some of the same adverse consequences on medical adherence as depression does (30). More recently, studies have suggested that alterations of sleep wake schedule may contribute to the development of disease. In one recent study, Bursztyn et al. (31) assessed daytime napping in an older patient cohort (n = 455). The findings suggested that an afternoon nap appeared to be an independent predictor of mortality with a risk odds ratio of 2.1. In a separate study using self-administered questionnaires on health status and lifestyle (32), the investigators identified that significantly longer and shorter sleep times, compared with 7 to 8 hours, were associated with increases in total mortality in men. In addition, female users of sleeping pills and those with self-reported poor sleep quality also shared an increased risk of mortality independent of sleep duration. Similar findings have been noted by others (33) and were noted to be unaffected by later arousal times. However, a recent review of the literature on shift work, an extreme form of late risers, suggested there is an overall increase in cardiovascular risk of 40%. These data suggest that disrupted sleep or significantly altered sleep schedules may have adverse effects on medical outcomes through measurable biobehavioral interactions.

PAIN SYNDROMES

Specific diseases need not be the only focus of biobehavioral investigations. Major symptoms, and specifically chronic pain, may benefit from a biobehavioral approach to investigations (34–36). In a review from an NIH-sponsored workshop, the current status and major directions for biobehavioral pain research were outlined. Pain was identified as a subjective experience that could only be quantified through behavior (37), and there are many measurable behavioral responses to chronic pain that impacted treatment and recovery. Consistent with the NIH initiative, investigators demonstrated that biobehavioral models offer significant insight into the mechanisms active in chronic pain (38,39). Several studies suggest that dysfunctional information processing occurs, accentuating the perception of pain, and reinforcing the concept that learning plays a significant role in pain syndromes (38,40). Such mechanisms may also be actively involved in the disability associated with several disorders (e.g., osteoarthritis and cardiac pain) (5,41), and research in this area may have a significant impact in our understanding of the neurophysiology of somatic dysfunction (42).

Disease Risk (Pathway "B")

Several behaviors exert their primary effect by modifying disease risk or factors associated with disease risk. The major behavioral factors within this category that are also supported by substantial data include diet, exercise, sleep, cigarette smoking, tobacco use, alcohol use, and the prevention of excessive sun exposure. In general, modifications of diet, exercise, sleep, and relaxation constitute factors associated with a protective influence over physiologic sources of risks. They also function in an indirect manner by minimizing the effects of stress and enhancing coping mechanisms. Smoking, excessive alcohol consumption, and drug abuse typically fall into the category of health-impairing behaviors that directly influence disease processes and have secondary effects on mood and other behaviors. Physical behaviors (e.g., exercise, aerobics, and other types of physical exertion) often exert a protective influence and therefore fall in the category of health-enhancing behaviors. The consequences of these physical behaviors may directly or indirectly affect pain syndromes, medical interventions, and the natural history of disease. For example, an individual attempting to undergo a weight control regimen without substantial lifestyle changes that include increases in activity may experience difficulty in achieving and maintaining weight loss (43,44).

In general, the preponderance of data demonstrating association between diet and disease outcomes is found in the cardiovascular literature. Weight gain, obesity, excessive salt consumption, and fat or cholesterol intake are major contributors in the development of coronary artery disease, hypertension, and stroke. Interventions directed at weight loss and weight maintenance have engendered some success when the interventions were maintained (45) and when the interventions target specific ethnic or socioeconomic groups (46). These interventions recognize that adherence and cultural affects were an important part of an effective regimen.

The role of dietary influence on cancer risk is more speculative than the data regarding cardiovascular disease. For example, there appears to be an association between fat/fiber content in the diet and the mammography profile associated with breast cancer (47) or recurrence of breast cancer among women with estrogen receptor–positive tumors (48). Whether patients can effectively alter their fat intake and weight has also been studied by investigators. Several studies have shown that diet can be effectively modified (49), secondarily leading to an increase in consumption of healthier food (50). These programs appear to be more effective when there is good research evidence to support the dietary changes and the individuals are aware of the evidence (51).

Exercise appears to exert beneficial effects by reducing stress and increasing caloric consumption. The increasing caloric consumption is important in designing effective weight management programs. There are data to suggest that routine exercise programs reduce the relative risk of developing cancer (52) through either a reduction in sedentary activities or weight loss (53). Exercise also appears to be an effective coping strategy for stress (22). These effects may be related to alterations in mood and a reduction in perceived stress that occurs with routine exercise (54). The latter of these effects may relate more specifically to an attenuation of physiologic reactivity. Unfortunately, for many individuals, increasing stress reduces the amount of physical activity undertaken (55). Reduction of stress and an improvement in the physiologic adaptability have also been cited as possible mechanisms by which exercise could exert its effect in cancer.

Our knowledge of the effects of tobacco use dates back to the early 1960s. Since that time, extensive data have demonstrated the adverse health consequences of cigarette smoking and tobacco use. The habitual use of tobacco relates to physiologic responses to nicotine (e.g., sense of well-being, arousal, and appetite suppression) and the avoidance of or the relief from withdrawal (56). Smoking contributes to the development of atherosclerosis, coronary artery disease, hypertension, stroke, emphysema, bronchitis, and several malignancies through recognized physiologic mechanisms (57). Even secondhand smoke may carry some of the habituating and cardiovascular responses related to nicotine exposure (58). In this regard, prevention may be a more effective strategy for limiting cigarette smoking and its adverse health consequences (59). However, in individuals who smoke, stress appears to be a significant contributor to the amount and frequency of tobacco use (55), as well as to relapse after smoking cessation. Thus, the combination of stress and tobacco use is a self-reinforcing behavioral pattern that is complicated by nicotine addiction. Behavioral strategies designed to alter tobacco use must address these interactive behaviors to be effective (60).

Understanding the issues and relevant research on the health consequences of sun exposure is illustrative of the complexity of some biobehavioral interactions. Ultraviolet (UV) radiation in sunlight has been linked to the development of basal-cell cancers, squamous-cell cancers, and melanomas (61–63). For basal-cell and squamous-cell cancers, the risk parallels cumulative lifetime UV exposure. Routine use of avoidance measures or sunscreen can substantially decrease the risk of skin cancer. Unfortunately, despite increased awareness and research evidence on skin cancer, there has been little change in individual behavior. One reason is the belief that sun tanning makes an individual look healthier and that exposure to the sun is healthy (64). This persistence of irrational beliefs and behaviors underlies these high-risk behaviors. Solid research and education is the foundation for changing behavior. For the osteopathic physician, healthy lifestyle changes and the formation of adaptive daily habits form the cornerstone of the restoration and maintenance of health.

Disease-Related Biobehavioral Activities (Pathway "C")

The final general mechanism relating behavior with disease involves behaviors that occur when illness is present, suspected, or where there is grave risk of illness. Many factors influence individual behaviors under the threat of severe pathology. When significant illnesses are suspected or where there is the potential for illness, the perception of "harm" (e.g., fear), and the potential impact (e.g., loss of function) may significantly alter the coping response of the individual. Socioeconomic factors, issues involved with physician support or confidence, the perception of risk, and emotional reaction of the individual all significantly affect surveillance efforts (65,66). Health beliefs, perceptions of risk, and generalized anxiety regarding disease or illness greatly contribute to avoidance on the part of the patient (65,67). Consistent with these concepts, Lerman et al. (67) reported heightened anxiety about developing breast cancer in association with intrusive thoughts and demonstrated some relationship with adherence (68). Similar findings were noted in women undergoing genetic counseling for breast cancer (69). However, the distress associated with disease risk does not have a consistent effect on surveillance activities (70). These findings have also been noted in screening for HIV. Studies have linked the associated anxiety with undergoing screening and failure to follow-up for test results. In general, stress, emotional responses, and past stress coping behaviors are often the best predictors (71) of adherence.

A variety of behaviors related to the presence of illness may arise. Two major behavioral mechanisms affect outcomes in individuals with existing disease. The first of these mechanisms relates to adherence. Medical regimens are rarely effective when patients are nonadherent. However, nonadherence may arise from many sources, including inadequate understanding (72), forgetfulness, confusion, health beliefs, personal (naïve) theories of illness, and cost (73). There are few reliable predictors of adherence; however, high-quality communication, patient supervision, social support, and the recognition measurement and management of underlying impairments, especially depression (30), all contribute to improving adherence (30,73).

PLACEBO AS A BIOBEHAVIORAL MECHANISM

Improvement of a condition during clinical trials or treatment can be attributable to one of three causes: natural history, specific effects of the intervention, and nonspecific effects of intervention. The latter of the three causes is typically termed a "placebo effect" (74). If this effect were to be represented in graphic form with the spectrum of intervention along the horizontal axis and clinical improvement along the vertical axis, the placebo effect would be represented by gradual improvement in the clinical condition. The perceived drug effect would be represented by a more significant clinical improvement over the same course of treatment. The difference between the placebo and perceived drug effect would then be considered the active drug effect (75). Because of the possibility that new interventions could show improvement simply due to a placebo effect, this has typically been cited as a major reason for including a placebo control in most biobehavioral research studies.

Measurable factors that need to be included in the design of a study and have been shown to affect the placebo response include race, direct suggestion, belief in the treatment, trust in the physician, genetic variation, environmental effects, and nonspecific cause-effect relationships all interact creating a placebo effect. Environmental effects include personal interactions (e.g., the doctor-patient interaction), perceptions based on relevant previous experiences, and the influence of the setting (76). Each of these must be considered when planning research protocols, especially in light of the potential for interactions between the researcher, an examiner, or an intervention. The importance of such effects has recently been reviewed with regard to cardiovascular disease (75) and pain treatment (74). Some major mechanisms that have been proposed to explain the placebo effect include decreased anxiety, altered expectations, learning or classical conditioning, and endogenous opium release (74–76). In each of these mechanisms, there appears to be interaction between the behavioral aspects of the

individual and the placebo, resulting in a biologic improvement. However, in a recent review of over 130 clinical trials, Hrobjartsson and Gotzsche (77) concluded that there is little evidence to support the contention that placebos have powerful clinical effects. In their review, the authors concluded that placebos had no significant effects in most studies with measurable *objective* variables or simple binary outcomes. However, placebo effects were noted in trials involving continuous measurements of *subjective* outcomes and those trials involving the treatment of pain. In addition, there was a greater likelihood of identifying a placebo effect when the experimental and control group sizes were relatively small.

Placebos can generally be categorized into pharmacologic, physical, or psychological (77). For the purpose of investigating manipulative interventions, an appropriate placebo control is both essential and difficult to achieve. For individuals who previously have undergone manipulative interventions, there is an element of learning on the part of the subject that may allow them to differentiate a placebo from an active intervention. Even when naive individuals can be used, the physical component of touching a patient or subject has an active component known as an active placebo that creates difficulty in designing clinical trials. In some instances, as has occurred with studies investigating antidepressant therapy (78), the placebo effect has a measurable physiologic effect that must be considered in the interpretation and the research paradigm.

OVERVIEW OF THE BIOBEHAVIORAL RESEARCH PROCESS

The biobehavioral research process can be broken down into arbitrary steps beginning with the development of a research question and ending with a written report of the research findings (Table 73.2) (79). The choices involved in the process are not unique to biobehavioral research but have some methodological considerations that should be understood by all researchers. Decisions made about the methodologies employed and measurements obtained will significantly affect the value and validity of any research (80). Overall, the primary goal of the medical researcher and clinician is to provide greater understanding of the relationship between biologic processes and behavior and to communicate those results effectively to both the professional and lay readership.

Osteopathic medicine is being challenged to provide evidence of efficacy for osteopathic manipulative treatment. The evidence-based outcomes important to third-party payers, clinical professionals, and patients all involve biobehavioral aspects that must be incorporated into any research design. Further, solid experimental research will need to prove that osteopathic treatment is less costly than other alternatives, or that it is an effective alternative with objective measurable outcome improvement. Improvement means restoring function, quality of life (QOL), and a lessening of symptoms. In treatment settings, using biobehavioral measures and research may provide a more effective treatment paradigm and may render valuable insight into the impact of osteopathic principles and practice.

Basic Research Paradigms

The essence of a *descriptive research* design is to identify the characteristics of a system or an intervention applied, in this context, to a patient or subject. Often, comparisons include intensity, magnitude, frequency, or duration of a characteristic (e.g., symptom or clinical finding) across different phases of the treatment or across time. Such research paradigms do not routinely give mechanistic insight.

TABLE 73.2

Steps in Research Design and Implementation

Process Steps	Considerations
1. Develop the hypothesis and the components of the hypothesis	Is there sufficient published or preliminary data to develop a hypothesis?
	Is the hypothesis consistent with the available data?
	Is the hypothesis testable?
	Has the hypothesis been tested before?
	Would testing the hypothesis add to the current body of scientific knowledge?
	Refine the hypothesis
2. Determine the methods necessary for testing the hypothesis	Determine the biologic and behavioral effects pertinent to the hypothesis
	Determine the most optimal method for measuring the processes. Under some circumstances, this may require that methods be developed and validated before performing the research
	Determine the conditions for the assessment
3. Determine the research design that can be employed	Determining the necessary comparisons
	Assess the need for blinding and placebos
	Determine the subject-selection process
	Perform a power analysis
4. Perform the project and analyze the results	Identify unforeseen problems with the methods or study design
	Modify the processes to improve the study
5. Evaluate the hypothesis in light of the results and the limitations of the study	What were the major findings of the study?
	How do the data support or refute the hypothesis?
	Are these data consistent with prior investigations?
6. Identify the major findings of the research that verify previous findings and those that add new information.	What are the implications of the study and how generalizable are the results?
	What were the limitations of the study and how do they affect the conclusions?
7. Communicate the results.	Determine the most appropriate venue for presentation of the study
	Identify areas for future investigation

Source: From Delahanty DL, Dougall AL, Schmitz L, et al. Time course of natural killer cell activity and lymphocyte proliferation in response to two acute stressors in healthy men. *Health Psychol* 1996;15:48–55, with permission.

Hypothesis-driven research proposes that a certain intervention or perturbation will yield a specific result on the basis of prior knowledge of the system, disease, or condition being studied. The research hypothesis is based on an understanding of an active mechanism(s) and is designed to assess how a particular intervention exerts a specific effect. For example, a researcher might propose using a drug that affects a specific enzyme known to be the cause of a particular disease using an outcome measure pertinent to that disease. In this setting, the goal is to see whether there are differences in the groups that can be accounted for by the treatment delivered.

In any research, the selection of subjects and other factors may affect the outcome or validity of the study. Some research designs use *random selection* of subjects while others may use a highly selected population or matched samples to minimize the variance and increase the likelihood of finding a significant effect. Other factors that need to be considered include the effect of preexisting conditions (covariants), the blinding of researcher and/or subjects, effect size, the power of the study (i.e., a determination of the number of subjects needed to have a valid study), and the utility of the outcome measures. Nonetheless, hypothesis-driven research is critical in developing new knowledge about cause and effect, and it is the backbone of good osteopathic medicine.

Basic research paradigms are illustrated in Figure 73.2.

Starting the Research Process

Before a hypothesis may be developed, the researcher must review or be knowledgeable about the current body of scientific knowledge related to the research question. Occasionally, a paucity of

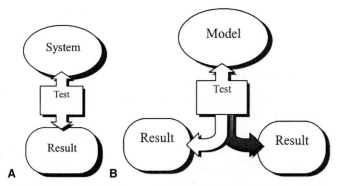

Figure 73-2 Basic research paradigms. **A.** Descriptive research. Descriptive research typically involves identifying the frequency of occurrence and/or characteristics of a system, condition, or population under specified conditions across time. **B.** Hypothesis-driven research. Hypothesis-driven research uses known data about a system, condition, or population to generate a mechanistic model of interaction. Using this model, predictions about the behavior of the system or *causal* relationships between variables are generated. Testing conditions and measurements are then selected to determine the predictive validity of the model.

data exists sufficient so that a mechanistic hypothesis cannot be developed. In that circumstance, the initial research may be descriptive rather than mechanistic, but should be directed toward developing a sufficient body of knowledge to advance to mechanistic investigations.

The research process begins with a question in the form of hypothesis about the mechanism of an effect (81). In general, the hypotheses should center around testing mechanisms as opposed to descriptive research or, "what happens if …," as discussed above. This simple understanding of the difference between these two approaches is difficult for many individuals. In descriptive research, a system is studied under a given test condition to determine the effect or the impact. This style of research is most appropriate for situations where basic background information or assessments are needed before a more precise experimental model of mechanisms can be undertaken. Hypothesis-driven research will typically formulate a research question that may have two or more potential outcomes, depending on the mechanism that is active and the design that is being employed for the research. The researcher then chooses conditions and measurements that allow the clearest delineation between the potential outcomes.

Depending on the type of biobehavioral research employed, major interactions between biology and behavior must be addressed. In simplest form, these interactions may be summarized as behavior affecting the physiologic response, a physiologic response affecting a behavior, or behaviors arising in relation to a disease process. The relationship that is hypothesized constitutes a possible cause-and-effect relationship and how to measure the constructs around variables and which the research plan will be initiated.

To observe the cause-and-effect relationship, the exact behavioral and physiologic variables that are involved need to be specified. In addition, the conditions under which these measured variables interact must also be specified in significant detail. The research model selected must include controls for the confounding effects found in the interaction between the variables being studied and the behavioral/biologic measurements. Essentially, specifying the specific conditions, behaviors, and biologic processes that are involved is necessary to limit outside interactions or

variance within the measurements, determine cause and effect, and not jeopardize the validity of the study. There are six factors that may jeopardize validity, confound the results, and decrease the validity of any conclusions.

Selection into Groups

Groups formed for experimental reasons, with a specific illness, seeking medical care, and willing to participate in a hypothesis-driven design where they may receive a sham or no treatment do not represent the universe of patients with that particular illness. We know, for example, that chronic pain patients who are enrolled in multidisciplinary pain clinics are a very unique group of self-selected patients with whom results do not generalize to the overall chronic pain population (40).

Intent to Treat

There is a natural loss of subjects during a study from the beginning to the end. The dropout rates are critical, but of particular importance is the question of, "who were the people who dropped out and why?" For example, they may have dropped out because the treatment was actually detrimental; if those scores were included, it would have substantially altered the conclusion. Scores not collected often cause a "type II" or false-positive statistical conclusion.

Multiple Treatment Interference

The effects of *prior* treatments are usually not erasable when multiple treatments are applied to the same person. Such is the case with manipulative treatment.

Maturation

Internal cognitive/emotional processes operating during the experiment, including learning, getting tired, unintended reinforcement or punishment for certain behaviors, and so on, affect future scores.

Instrumentation

Any change in the measuring instruments or in an observer's use of the instruments or scoring methods produces changes in the obtained measurement over time and confounds results.

Measurement Variance

This is the most common factor invalidating research results. Most patients are treated and selected into the treatment groups by *extreme* scores to begin with. For example, they may have high pain scores, severe impairment in range of motion, or activities of daily living, mood, on so forth. Because they were selected on an extreme of a bell-shaped curve, they will show subsequent test scores that are improved simply as a function of moving from the tail of the curve toward the mean average, which is a statistical artifact in measuring. In other words, if you take the worst of the worst and measure them at that point and do anything to them and remeasure in the future, some will have better scores on retesting and will have moved toward the average by chance.

For these reasons, the exact specifications for the behaviors to be studied and the methods for the measurement of intensity, frequency, and duration of symptoms are especially important in biobehavioral research. These characteristics of each behavioral measurement are important variables that must be quantified for the study design. Under some circumstances, the characteristics may either be dependent or independent variables, as determined by the specific interaction that is being identified in the design of the study and how the variable is quantified and measured.

Qualitative Measurements

Measurements of behavior may be either quantitative or qualitative. Quantitative measurements typically convert the behavior to a categorical or numeric scale. The major benefit of using numeric measurements is that they are more amenable to statistical analysis. Categorical scales may be used to place subjects or behaviors into particular categories on the basis of specific characteristics. Under some circumstances, categorical scales may be based on qualitative or subjective assessments. Thus, the investigators should consider that qualitative tools requiring subjective interpretation may be affected by examiner bias, and need to be applied in a uniform fashion to obtain reliable numeric results. Qualitative measurements are typically based on the assessment of particular characteristics that allow them to be placed in discrete categories or transformed into a numeric scale. Quantitative measurements should not be assumed to be better than qualitative assessments. The caveat that is best followed is to choose the most appropriate measurement tool for the physiologic and behavioral components given the study participants and situation under investigation. Frequently, the researcher may benefit from the work of other investigators and use known, standardized tools that have established validity and reliability. Some standardized tools may be used to obtain self-reporting of the data. In many instances, these tools can be easily administered, completed, and scored in a standardized fashion. There are many standardized measurement instruments available, but they should be carefully selected to address the specific needs of the research.

Quantitative Measurements

Measurement of behavior requires that we employ a quantification system to reliably describe and identify characteristics of behavior in the context being studied. The spectrum of potential behaviors that may be studied in biobehavioral research is exceptionally broad and ranges from physical behaviors that may be objectively quantified to particular thoughts, or thought patterns that must be indirectly inferred. The assessment of subjective constructs may be further complicated by languages, dialects, cultures, age, socioeconomic status, gender, race, and other situational considerations. Previous experience or familiarity with many interventions or measurements may alter the conditions for a research project, complicating or invalidating the results. For example, a subject's familiarity with osteopathic interventions may invalidate a research design using a placebo control because the patient is able to identify therapeutic intervention and is not blinded to the study's designed placebo control.

Biobehavioral Measurement Data

The basic data resulting from any measurements are a series of numbers. These numbers represent the numerical value of some biobehavioral characteristic, and the measurements are often obtained from one or more groups of individuals. We can seldom make much sense out of these numbers if we leave them in their raw form. For that reason, we use *statistical procedures* to answer questions we have raised about the basic data. We want to put some kind of order into our numbers. We can graph the numbers, look at percentiles, rank order numbers, and see how group patterns are made clearer by sorting the raw data into frequency distributions and looking at the mean average. The arithmetic *mean* is simply the result of adding up all the measures and dividing by the number of measures. We can look at the *mode*, which is defined as the score that occurs most frequently, and the *median*, which is a label for the point at which 50% of scores fall below and 50% of the scores fall

above. We can look at how individuals and groups vary and deviate from the mean score for each raw score obtained. This is called the *variance*. You find the variance by subtracting the mean average from each raw score, squaring that number, then dividing by the total number of scores. Find the square root of the variance, and you have the *standard deviation*. It is from the *mean and standard deviation that all further statistical techniques evolve*.

The simple goal of statistical techniques is to answer the question of whether the changes in scores obtained would have occurred by chance. In these statistical procedures, we set our *confidence intervals* at usually five times out of a 100 (i.e., 0.05 level). This means that we would be satisfied that the scores obtained would have happened by chance only five times out of a 100. This is a basis for common tests, such as the *t*-test for two groups and *analysis of variance*, for more than two experimental groups. These two tests are commonly used statistical methods in biobehavioral research. Researcher's interest may also rest in the aggregate set of measures rather than on any one single measure considered apart from the others. The logic, algebra, distribution theory, numerical analysis, and computer programs for these types of analyses are all described elegantly and available at most computer and research facilities.

Designing a Study

A wide variety of designs may be employed in biobehavioral research. One of the more common study designs involves *comparisons among groups*. In this setting, there may be two or more or groups wherein the comparison occurs. The specific design chosen will affect the number of independent variables that may be considered and the precision and power of the statistical analysis. Knowledge about the variance of the independent measurements that are being made allows the investigator to determine the number of subjects that will be needed within each group. The process of determining the number of subjects necessary for a particular design is referred to as *power analysis*. Another fundamental type of study design involves the assessment of effects across time or a comparison over time. This type of design paradigm is typically used to assess cumulative effects or gradually developing changes in the system. Designation of members within a group must also be considered by the researcher. Determining whether the population should be limited to a particular gender, race, or age may significantly affect the study design and measurements that may be employed. In some instances, variation in underlying physiology, such as with sleep wake cycles and circadian biology, may affect the time of the day, the time of the month, and the time of the year the study or component of the study may be performed. These possible confounding variables can be controlled by the design of the study and by the predetermined statistical analysis.

Statistical Analysis

Although the statistical analysis is performed after the actual study has been completed (or at least partially completed), the statistics to be employed must be determined before the study is implemented. In some instances, significant biobehavioral differences found among groups require additional separation to determine exactly which group is different. This additional data analysis procedure is referred to as a post hoc analysis, is only employed if the main effect studied was significant. The goal of the post hoc analysis is to detail exactly what specific factors account for the overall differences found in the main study. Occasionally, researchers employ other statistical identifying techniques in identifying subgroups with significant differences when the main effect model *failed* to show significance. This process is used when the subgroup analyses were planned as part of the original research proposal and appropriate accommodations for the small group size were undertaken. Once all statistics are completed, a judgment is made about whether the research results confirm or refutes the initial hypothesis.

Generally, the results of the research study, if well designed, should be fairly clear. The statistical analyses should show whether changes found in the measured biobehavioral variables were significant or not. If the analyses confirmed the initial hypothesis, then the investigator should undertake the process of analyzing the results in light of other investigations. Comparing differences in techniques, the selected populations, and limitations in methodology is a valuable exercise in analyzing the results of the study. The investigator should then assess the implications or generalizability of the research findings. Elements of the study or the theoretical framework on which the study is based that were unclear or undefined can then be identified for future investigation. Once all these elements have been completed, the study and analyses should be communicated to the appropriate scientific audience. Under most circumstances, this occurs in the form of a peer-reviewed publication in a scientific journal and adds to the evidence-based knowledge, which is the bedrock of osteopathic practice.

OPPORTUNITIES FOR OSTEOPATHIC RESEARCHERS

Biobehavioral interactions present the osteopathic researcher a somewhat novel and rich environment for the development of investigations. Despite the variety of investigations that could be undertaken, a review of the literature demonstrates paucity of studies addressing biobehavioral mechanisms or effects in osteopathic principles and practice. Major topics in this area will likely focus on behaviors leading to the development of somatic dysfunction, behaviors resulting from somatic dysfunction, QOL effects of pain, and relationships between locomotor function, somatic dysfunction, and subsequent behavior (82).

Manipulative intervention (83), alone or in combination, may have as much affect on subsequent behaviors as other types of medical intervention, and should not be ignored when considering a biobehavioral research paradigm. For instance, the improvement in locomotor function or a decrement in pain resulting from manipulative intervention could result in substantial behavioral adjustments or improvements in QOL that may not be immediately apparent without biobehavioral research. In this regard, considering a biobehavioral research approach would enhance the ability to detect improvements related to the manipulative intervention and may give additional insights into the true treatment effects of osteopathic principles and practice.

The biobehavioral approach will require clear and creative research designs directed more toward behavioral outcomes rather than physiologic measurements or end point assessments, as is commonly done. In this regard, all major types of biobehavioral designs should be considered, including those associated with *chronic illness*, not commonly the focus of osteopathic research. Avoidance or development of emotional issues (e.g., depression), QOL, and changes in behavioral responses to chronic illness in relationship to osteopathic principles and practice represent investigations potentially adhering to the third pathway described above. This type of investigation may be less concerned with the direct effects of the disease process and more directly interested in the secondary effects on the behavior of patients (when adherence with medical regimens and tolerance of side effects are improved). Quantifying

these relationships or the effect on QOL becomes the major issue in developing a biobehavioral research design and might even include developing a specific osteopathic QOL instrument. Other types of investigations could focus on the interrelationship between somatic dysfunction or manipulative interventions and cognitive performance, health status, or other neurobehavioral manifestations. From these investigations, one could inquire about other biophysiologic relationships and whether somatic dysfunction could serve additional diagnostic roles yet to be determined, or answers to questions not previously envisioned. The field of biobehavioral research is wide open for future osteopathic research to develop the evidence-based foundations for the uniqueness of the osteopathic approach.

SUMMARY

Biobehavioral interactions are a complex interplay between genetic, physiologic, environmental, and behavioral factors that have been shown to influence health and disease through many different pathways. Three major pathways for the effects of behavior to manifest on health and disease are ripe for research. Some types of disorders manifest these interactions more directly than others; but in each case, we find that behavior alters the physiologic "landscape," and physiologic alterations result in significant behavioral accommodations that affect health and disease outcomes. Thus, physiologic phenomena are inseparable from their behavioral counterparts and must be considered as part of the process wherein disease develops. For the osteopathic researcher, biobehavioral interactions and research may play a significant role in advancing our understanding of our patients, improving treatment regimens, and advancing the evidence-based understanding of osteopathic principles in medicine.

REFERENCES

1. Spiegel D. Healing words: emotional expression and disease outcome. *JAMA* 1999;281:1328–1329.
2. Baum A, Posluszny DM. Health psychology: mapping biobehavioral contributions to health and illness. *Annu Rev Psychol* 1999;50:137–163.
3. Ahern DK, Gorkin L, Anderson JL, et al. Biobehavioral variables and mortality or cardiac arrest in the Cardiac Arrhythmia Pilot Study (CAPS). *Am J Cardiol* 1990;66:59–62.
4. Andersen BL, Kiecolt-Glaser JK, Glaser R. A biobehavioral model of cancer stress and disease course. *Am Psychol* 1994;49:389–404.
5. Dekker J, Boot B, van der Woude LH, et al. Pain and disability in osteoarthritis: a review of biobehavioral mechanisms. *J Behav Med* 1992;15:189–214.
6. Krantz DS, Grunberg NE, Baum A. Health psychology. *Annu Rev Psychol* 1985;36:349–383.
7. Kop WJ, Verdino RJ, Gottdiener JS, et al. Changes in heart rate and heart rate variability before ambulatory ischemic events. *J Am Coll Cardiol* 2001;38:742–749.
8. Carney RM, McMahon RP, Freedland KE, et al. Reproducibility of mental stress-induced myocardial ischemia in the psychophysiological Investigations of myocardial ischemia (PIMI). *Psychosom Med* 1998;60:64–70.
9. Wielgosz AT, Nolan RP. Biobehavioral factors in the context of ischemic cardiovascular diseases. *J Psychosom Res* 2000;48:339–345.
10. Hasser EM, Moffitt JA. Regulation of sympathetic nervous system function after cardiovascular deconditioning. *Ann N Y Acad Sci* 2001;940:454–468.
11. Sitruk-Ware R. Progestins and cardiovascular risk markers. *Steroids* 2000; 65:651–658.
12. Matthews KA, Woodall KL, Stoney CM. Changes in and stability of cardiovascular responses to behavioral stress: results from a four-year longitudinal study of children. *Child Dev* 1990;61:1134–1144.
13. Kamarck T, Jennings JR. Biobehavioral factors in sudden cardiac death. *Psychol Bull* 1991;109:42–75.

14. Manuck SB, Henry JP, Anderson DE, et al. Biobehavioral mechanisms in coronary artery disease: chronic stress. *Circulation* 1987;76:II58–II63.

15. Matthews KA, Woodall KL, Allen MT. Cardiovascular reactivity to stress predicts future blood pressure status. *Hypertension* 1993;22:479–485.

16. Knox SS. Biobehavioral mechanisms in lipid metabolism and atherosclerosis: an overview. *Metabolism* 1993;42:1–2.

17. Helmers KF, Krantz DS, Merz CN, et al. Defensive hostility: relationship to multiple markers of cardiac ischemia in patients with coronary disease. *Health Psychol* 1995;14:202–209.

18. Delahanty DL, Dougall AL, Schmitz JB, et al. Time course of natural killer cell activity and lymphocyte proliferation in response to two acute stressors in healthy men. *Health Psychol* 1996;15:48–55.

19. Andersen BL, Farrar WB, Golden-Kreutz D, et al. Stress and immune responses after surgical treatment for regional breast cancer [comments]. *J Natl Cancer Inst* 1998;90:30–36.

20. Benschop RJ, Geenen R, Mills PJ, et al. Cardiovascular and immune responses to acute psychological stress in young and old women: a meta-analysis. *Psychosom Med* 1998;60:290–296.

21. Pariante CM, Carpiniello B, Orru MG, et al. Chronic caregiving stress alters peripheral blood immune parameters: The role of age and severity of stress. *Psychother Psychosom* 1997;66:199–207.

22. Perna FM, Schneiderman N, LaPerriere A. Psychological stress, exercise and immunity. *Int J Sports Med* 1997;18(suppl 1):S78–S83.

23. Goujon E, Laye S, Parnet P, et al. Regulation of cytokine gene expression in the central nervous system by glucocorticoids: mechanisms and functional consequences. *Psychoneuroendocrinology* 1997;22(suppl 1):S75–S80.

24. Catalan J, Beevor A, Cassidy L, et al. Women and HIV infection: Investigation of its psychosocial consequences. *J Psychosom Res* 1996;41:39–47.

25. Cohen JI. Stress and mental health: a biobehavioral perspective. *Issues Mental Health Nurs* 2000;21:185–202.

26. Booth RE, Kwiatkowski CF, Chitwood DD. Sex-related HIV risk behaviors: differential risks among injection drug users, crack smokers, and injection drug users who smoke crack. *Drug Alcohol Depend* 2000;58:219–226.

27. Denison ME, Paredes A, Booth JB. Alcohol and cocaine interactions and aggressive behaviors. *Recent Dev Alcohol* 1997;13:283–303.

28. Fishbein M. Changing behavior to prevent STDs/AIDS. *Int J Gynaecol Obstet* 1998;63(suppl 1):S175–S181.

29. Dingle GA, Oei TP. Is alcohol a cofactor of HIV and AIDS? Evidence from immunological and behavioral studies. *Psychol Bull* 1997;122:56–71.

30. Ciechanowski PS, Katon WJ, Russo JE. Depression and diabetes: Impact of depressive symptoms on adherence, function, and costs. *Arch Intern Med* 2000;160:3278–3285.

31. Bursztyn M, Ginsberg G, Hammerman-Rozenberg R, et al. The siesta in the elderly: Risk factor for mortality? [comments] *Arch Intern Med* 1999;159:1582–1586.

32. Kojima M, Wakai K, Kawamura T, et al. Sleep patterns and total mortality: a 12-year follow-up study in Japan. *J Epidemiol* 2000;10:87–93.

33. Gale C, Martyn C. Larks and owls and health, wealth, and wisdom. *BMJ* 1998;317:1675–1677.

34. Keefe FJ, Jacobs M, Underwood-Gordon L. Biobehavioral pain research: A multi-institute assessment of cross-cutting issues and research needs. *Clin J Pain* 1997;13:91–103.

35. Morley S, Eccleston C, Williams A. Systematic review and meta-analysis of randomized controlled trials of cognitive behavioral therapy for chronic pain in adults, excluding headache. *Pain* 1999;80:1–13.

36. Turk D. *Handbook of Pain Assessment*. New York NY: The Guilford Press, 2001.

37. Fordyce WE. *Behavioral Methods for Chronic Pain and Illness*. St. Louis, MO: Mosby, 1976.

38. Gerber WD, Schoenen J. Biobehavioral correlates in migraine: the role of hypersensitivity and information-processing dysfunction. *Cephalalgia* 1998;18(suppl 21):5–11.

39. Naliboff BD, Munakata J, Chang L, et al. Toward a biobehavioral model of visceral hypersensitivity in irritable bowel syndrome. *J Psychosom Res* 1998;45:485–492.

40. Jerome J. Transmission or transformation? Information processing theory of chronic human pain. *Am Pain Soc J* 1993;2:160–171.

41. Feuerstein M, Beattie P. Biobehavioral factors affecting pain and disability in low back pain: Mechanisms and assessment. *Phys Ther* 1995;75:267–280.

42. Foresman BH. *Master's Thesis/Ph.D. Diss.*, Fort Worth: University of North Texas, 2001.

43. Katahn M, McMinn MR. Obesity. A biobehavioral point of view. *Ann NY Acad Sci* 1990;602:189–204.

44. Owens JF, Matthews KA, Wing RR, et al. Physical activity and cardiovascular risk: a cross-sectional study of middle-aged premenopausal women. *Prev Med* 1990;19:147–157.

45. Metz JA, Kris-Etherton PM, Morris CD, et al. Dietary compliance and cardiovascular risk reduction with a prepared meal plan compared with a self-selected diet [comments]. *Am J Clin Nutr* 1997;66:373–385.

46. Fitzgibbon ML, Stolley MR, Avellone ME, et al. Involving parents in cancer risk reduction: A program for Hispanic American families. *Health Psychol* 1996;15:413–422.

47. Nordevang E, Azavedo E, Svane G, et al. Dietary habits and mammographic patterns in patients with breast cancer. *Breast Cancer Res Treat* 1993;26:207–215.

48. Holm LE, Nordevang E, Hjalmar ML, et al. Treatment failure and dietary habits in women with breast cancer. *J Natl Cancer Inst* 1993;85:32–36.

49. Heber D, Ashley JM, McCarthy WJ, et al. Assessment of adherence to a low-fat diet for breast cancer prevention. *Prev Med* 1992;21:218–227.

50. Atwood JR, Aickin M, Giordano L, et al. The effectiveness of adherence intervention in a colon cancer prevention field trial. *Prev Med* 1992;21:637–653.

51. Patterson RE, Kristal AR, White E. Do beliefs, knowledge, and perceived norms about diet and cancer predict dietary change? *Am J Public Health* 1996;86:1394–1400.

52. Drake DA. A longitudinal study of physical activity and breast cancer prediction. *Cancer Nurs* 2001;24:371–377.

53. Shephard RJ. Exercise and cancer: linkages with obesity? *Crit Rev Food Sci Nutr* 1996;36:321–339.

54. Anshel M. Coping styles among adolescent competitive athletes. *J Soc Psychol* 1996;136:311–323.

55. Steptoe A, Wardle J, Pollard TM, et al. Stress, social support and health-related behavior: a study of smoking, alcohol consumption and physical exercise. *J Psychosom Res* 1996;41:171–180.

56. Kassel JD. Smoking and attention: a review and reformulation of the stimulus-filter hypothesis. *Clin Psychol Rev* 1997;17:451–478.

57. Girdler SS, Jamner LD, Jarvik M, et al. Smoking status and nicotine administration differentially modify hemodynamic stress reactivity in men and women. *Psychosom Med* 1997;59:294–306.

58. Hausberg M, Mark AL, Winniford MD, et al. Sympathetic and vascular effects of short-term passive smoke exposure in healthy nonsmokers. *Circulation* 1997;96:282–287.

59. Eckhardt L, Woodruff SI, Elder JP. Related effectiveness of continued, lapsed, and delayed smoking prevention intervention in senior high school students. *Am J Health Promot* 1997;11:418–421.

60. Brandon TH. Behavioral tobacco cessation treatments: yesterday's news or tomorrow's headlines? *J Clin Oncol* 2001;19:64S–68S.

61. Katsambas A, Nicolaidou E. Cutaneous malignant melanoma and sun exposure. Recent developments in epidemiology. *Arch Dermatol* 1996;132:444–450.

62. Marks R. An overview of skin cancers. Incidence and causation. *Cancer* 1995;75:607–612.

63. Strom SS, Yamamura Y. Epidemiology of nonmelanoma skin cancer. *Clin Plast Surg* 1997;24:627–636.

64. Baum A, Cohen L. Successful behavioral interventions to prevent cancer: the example of skin cancer. *Annu Rev Public Health* 1998;19:319–333.

65. Aiken LS, West SG, Woodward CK, et al. Health beliefs and compliance with mammography-screening recommendations in asymptomatic women. *Health Psychol* 1994;13:122–129.

66. Calle EE, Flanders WD, Thun MJ, et al. Demographic predictors of mammography and pap smear screening in U.S. women. *Am J Public Health* 1993;83:53–60.

67. Lerman C, Daly M, Sands C, et al. Mammography adherence and psychological distress among women at risk for breast cancer. *J Natl Cancer Inst* 1993;85:1074–1080.

68. Lerman C, Schwartz M. Adherence and psychological adjustment among women at high risk for breast cancer. *Breast Cancer Res Treat* 1993;28:145–155.

69. Lloyd S, Watson M, Waites B, et al. Familial breast cancer: a controlled study of risk perception, psychological morbidity and health beliefs in women attending for genetic counseling. *Br J Cancer* 1996;74:482–487.

70. Epstein SA, Lin TH, Audrain J, et al. High-Risk Breast Cancer Consortium. Excessive breast self-examination among first-degree relatives of newly diagnosed breast cancer patients. *Psychosomatics* 1997;38:253–261.

71. Ickovics JR, Morrill AC, Beren SE, et al. Limited effects of HIV counseling and testing for women: a prospective study of behavioral and psychological consequences. *JAMA* 1994;272:443–448.

72. Hussey LC, Gilliland K. Compliance, low literacy, and locus of control. *Nurs Clin North Am* 1989;24:605–611.

73. Cameron C. Patient compliance: recognition of factors involved and suggestions for promoting compliance with therapeutic regimens. *J Adv Nurs* 1996;24:244–250.

74. Turner JA, Deyo RA, Loeser JD, et al. The importance of placebo effects in pain treatment and research [comments]. *JAMA* 1994;271:1609–1614.

75. Bienenfeld L, Frishman W, Glasser SP. The placebo effect in cardiovascular disease. *Am Heart J* 1996;132:1207–1221.

76. Weiner M, Weiner GJ. The kinetics and dynamics of responses to placebo. *Clin Pharmacol Ther* 1996;60:247–254.

77. Hrobjartsson A, Gotzsche PC. Is the placebo powerless? An analysis of clinical trials comparing placebo with no treatment [comments] [erratum appears in *N Engl J Med* 2001;345(4):304]. *N Engl J Med* 2001;344:1594–1602.

78. Salamone JD. A critique of recent studies on placebo effects of antidepressants: Importance of research on active placebos. *Psychopharmacology (Berl)* 2000;152:1–6.

79. Cherulnick PD. *Methods for Behavioral Research: A Systematic Approach.* Thousand Oaks, CA: Sage Publications, 2001.

80. Corcoran K, Fischer J. *Measure for Clinical Practice.* New York, NY: The Free Press, 2000.

81. Jerome J. Theory leads: statistics follow. *Am Pain Soc J* 1995;4:274–276.

82. Hallas B, Lehman S, Bosak A, et al. Establishment of behavioral parameters for the evaluation of osteopathic treatment principles in a rat model of arthritis [comments]. *J Am Osteopath Assoc* 1997;97:207–214.

83. Northup GW. Time to reemphasize OMT as stress reliever. *J Am Osteopath Assoc* 1990;90:681.

The Future of Osteopathic Medical Research

MICHAEL M. PATTERSON

KEY CONCEPTS

- The profession has a long history of research, but faces an uncertain future as it tries to realign research priorities to new health care realities. Shifts in federal research funding may make the profession even more reliant on its own resources for initial research development.

- The osteopathic teaching institutions, especially the COMs, must lead the way in developing organized research efforts. While a number of the schools are or have developed the necessary infrastructure to support at least modest research programs, several have not and have no plans to do so. Research is vital to good teaching faculty, and must be encouraged, not discouraged.

- The faculty at osteopathic institutions need to understand the philosophy and practice of osteopathic medicine and to design research studies that will bear on the questions that come from osteopathic clinical practice and philosophy. Research done in osteopathic institutions that has no bearing on the issues of osteopathic medicine, while good research does little to further the osteopathic profession.

- Osteopathic students need to be better informed about the history of osteopathic research, the opportunities for osteopathic research, and research training. There is a proposed curriculum for schools to follow in training students in basic research principles, but it needs to be put into practice more fully. Several initiatives have been taken to provide interested students with research information and training, and some grant funds are being made available for student research by foundations and individual schools.

- The profession has developed its first research center and must continue to support it as well as develop other national research efforts. Osteopathic foundations who have a mission to support and broaden osteopathy are increasingly stepping up to fund major research efforts. Foundation support is often the only way for researchers to reach the level necessary to apply for further NIH funding.

- The development of collaborative efforts is vital to large-scale clinical trials. The Osteopathic Research Center (ORC) is organized to do such efforts as shown by the MPOSE study. Other such trials must be organized. The Osteopathic Postgraduate Training Institute organizations and confederations of solo practitioners can gather data from practice that can be useful in illuminating the practice efficacy of osteopathic medicine.

- There is a great potential for increased research collaboration with foreign osteopathic movements. Osteopathic schools in England, Germany, Italy, and elsewhere are beginning research efforts that will produce valuable information, especially if aided by U. S. osteopathic institutions.

- Designing studies of osteopathic manipulative therapy is a difficult task. The question being asked must be very clear and the study designed to answer the question being asked. The use of sham controls is especially difficult as any "sham" in manipulative medicine is actually a form of treatment and hence should be evaluated against no treatment to assess the actual effect of the "sham." To assume that a sham treatment has no effect and hence can be thought of as neutral is simply not acceptable. The use of a sham contrast control is actually comparing one form of treatment with another.

- It is tempting to say that all research that can be done is important and no area should be singled out above others. However, some suggestions can be made as to areas that may be most valuable in determining the usefulness and value of osteopathic theory and practice.

- The philosophical basis of osteopathy medicine should be used to drive the main research programs of the profession.

INTRODUCTION

In his 1962 Andrew Taylor memorial lecture, Northup (1) stated, "we are on the precipice of either our greatest success or ultimate defeat. This success or failure depends not on the policy of organized medicine, but on the decisions and integrity of organized osteopathy."

These words were spoken at the darkest hour in the history of the osteopathic profession. There was a real question about the continued survival of the profession as an organization. The California merger had occurred and pressure was mounting to turn even more of the profession over to allopathic control. One of the

profession's six schools had been lost, and about 10% of its members had been granted an M.D. degree in California. Indeed, the decisions and integrity of the leaders, as well as the rank-and-file members, would decide its fate.

Over the next few years, the decisions of the profession and its leaders led to a revival and rebuilding of both the physical plant and the organization of osteopathic medicine. The profession's members responded to the challenges and supported a renaissance of unprecedented proportions. Between 1969 and 1996, 13 new schools were founded, about half university based. Today, the profession is growing at an unprecedented rate and enjoys support from the government and private sectors. It now has 28 open osteopathic schools, including the branch campuses, with several more scheduled to open in the next 2 to 3 years.

However, today the osteopathic profession faces a future still filled with unknown and unpredictable forces that will shape and challenge it in many ways. It is increasingly challenged to show that the claims it makes for its unique philosophy and practice are beneficial to the patients it serves. Government and third-party insurance carriers mandate that the outcomes of health care be used as evidence of the quality of service. Osteopathic physicians who utilize manipulative treatment are finding it increasingly difficult to attract reimbursement for these services as government tries to cut health care costs. The existence of osteopathy as a unique and separate profession rests on its ability to continually demonstrate that its practices are efficacious and its theories are sound. The overriding challenge for the profession is to show through well-conducted research that the services it provides are both efficacious and cost effective and to show a logical rationale for manipulative treatment.

Meeting these challenges is not a simple task or one to be taken for granted. To achieve this goal, all components of the profession must to take an active role. These institutions include:

- Educational institutions
- Osteopathic foundations
- Hospitals
- Affiliated societies
- Individual physicians in practice

However, the greatest challenge now facing the profession is that of building its research base to support and expand its claims of efficacious and unique practice. Without demonstrable substantiation of its claims to a unique role in health care, the osteopathic profession risks its existence.

It is not that data do not exist to show that the osteopathic profession has made unique contributions to health care and that its philosophy is sound. Research began in the profession with its inception and has continued since. Louisa Burns performed studies showing viscerosomatic and somatovisceral interactions long before the medical world recognized their importance. The research from the Kirksville group in the 1940s and 1950s, data from the Chicago College and other osteopathic schools, and papers published in the *Journal of the American Osteopathic Association (JAOA)* over the years show that the osteopathic contribution to health care is substantial. However, further substantiating the unique contributions and emerging quality of osteopathic care requires new and innovative ways to measure health and clinical outcomes, as well as the development of new and innovative research techniques. The art of clinical research is a relatively new endeavor, and its practices are just now developing to the point of being able to show the unique features of osteopathic medicine.

This chapter summarizes the present state of research in the profession, the opportunities and challenges ahead, and the areas critical to understanding the unique role of osteopathic medicine in human health and disease.

OSTEOPATHIC RESEARCH: 2008

Late in 2008, the research efforts of the osteopathic profession are set to enter their fifth era. The fourth era began in 2001 with the founding of the first osteopathic research center at North Texas State Health Science Center College of Osteopathic Medicine (see Chapter 70 for a summary of these eras). Since 1970, the profession's research had been expanding as new schools, many university based, began to mature and begin research programs. Recent developments in the building of research programs have been evident throughout the profession. Research programs at the Texas COM had been strongly fostered for many years, allowing that school the infrastructure to support a research center. At about the same time, the founding school at Kirksville pledged several hundred thousand dollars in internal funding for expansion of its already successful research programs, with the funds to go preferentially to research directed to the elucidation of osteopathic principles and practice. Several other schools have pledged funding for basic and clinical research and have established mechanisms for active research. Unfortunately, some of the newer schools have not built active research efforts into their plans.

While the academic research base of the profession has been growing and maturing, other efforts were being made to foster research among osteopathic physicians. Some of the specialty colleges have had some form of research requirement in their programs for several years. This requirement has fostered an understanding of the research process in students that was not given during undergraduate training. More recently, some of the Osteopathic Postgraduate Training Institutes (OPTIs) have instituted research training in their programs. Although only beginning, these efforts to train more practitioners in the art and process of research are another way to increase not only the development of research programs but also an appreciation of its importance.

Other organizations of the profession have begun to take a more active role in research development and support. The AOA has, since 1951, had the Bureau of Research to promote and support research development. This group has taken an increasingly active role not only in granting research funds, but also in developing new programs. It now supports the training of osteopathic students in D.O./Ph.D. programs. Such combined degree programs are also available at several of the university-based COMs. The bureau also sponsored the development of an osteopathic bibliographic database as a joint venture between the Texas and Kirksville COMs. This database, known as OSTMED, was to be the premier repository for references to osteopathic literature that is generally very difficult to find and access. Unfortunately, the funding for the project was not renewed and the database, while still accessible, has not been added to for at least 2 years. On a positive note, the *JAOA* has been placed online and all back issues are either available or their contents can be searched.

The AOA's Louisa Burns research committee has become increasingly active in developing research protocols and initiatives, such as the online SOAP note project and SOAP note forms that may allow collection of large clinical databases in the near future. The American Association of Colleges of Osteopathic Medicine (AACOM) has led the organization and funding efforts for three national meetings to discuss research development, out of which came the osteopathic research center. Leaders within the organizations of the profession, especially the AACOM and the AOA, have increased their contacts with governmental funding agencies in efforts to secure federal funds and recognition for the profession's research efforts.

However, most notable in the dawning of the fifth era of osteopathic research is the increased role of the osteopathic foundations, especially the Columbus, Ohio-based Osteopathic Heritage Foundation. The Heritage Foundation, along with the other osteopathic foundations, has become increasingly active in sponsoring research efforts endowing research chairs, providing infrastructure at schools, and supporting meetings and conferences aimed at furthering the osteopathic research agenda.

The fifth era now emerging is one of expanding the reach and recognition of both osteopathic research and of osteopathic philosophy and practice. In 1989 and 1992, symposia that included internationally known scientists from around the world were held (2,3). These symposia generated publications, but perhaps more importantly, knowledge of osteopathic philosophy and practice in a number of scientists who had never before heard of osteopathic medicine. Several of them continued their interest in the profession and have provided support and even training opportunities for young osteopathic physicians. In early 2008, another international symposium was sponsored by the Texas Osteopathic Research Center, with support from the osteopathic profession, the NIH (NCCAM) and the chiropractic, massage therapy and physical therapy professions. Most importantly, this meeting brought together not only osteopathic scientists interested in somatovisceral interactions, but also scientists and clinicians from the chiropractic, massage therapy and physical therapy professions as well as leading scientists involved in somatovisceral research. The osteopathic profession, in organizing such a unique meeting, demonstrated that it was willing to broaden its scope of interactions to include other manual medicine areas. This effort must be the beginning of the expanded interactions necessary for osteopathic research to tap the resources and information available. In this way, the philosopathy and practice of osteopathy can be increased by using insights and findings from other professions to enhance understanding of osteopathic practice. This expansion of interactions should be the hallmark of the fifth era of osteopathic research efforts.

These and other accomplishments have taken place over the last several years and point to an unprecedented effort to organize and support a profession-wide research effort. Although these efforts have been remarkable in a profession devoted to training practitioners since its founding, they are only the beginning. The increasing interactions between osteopathic researchers and clinicians that hopefully will expand are evidence that the profession has begun to tap larger resources and is a sign of a maturing discipline. However, it is only the beginning of the maturation process. What are the challenges now facing further development of quality research efforts?

INSTITUTIONAL CHALLENGES FOR RESEARCH DEVELOPMENT

Academic Challenges: The Schools

Clearly, some of the teaching institutions of the profession have made great strides in the last 30 years in developing nationally competitive research efforts. As pointed out in the first chapter in this section, the profession's schools were not in a position to take advantage of the immense expansion of biomedical research infrastructure during the 1950s and 1960s. In fact, it was not until the 1980s that a few of the COMs were able to develop sufficiently strong research initiatives that they could attract significant federal funding. In 1974, the first RO1 NIH research grant was awarded to a researcher in an osteopathic institution. Since then, a number of large federal and private grants have been awarded to several of the COMs. The ORC at Texas has emerged as a nationally competitive institution, attracting NIH funding.

The challenge for all the academic institutions now lies in seeing the urgent need to show the efficacy and mechanisms of manipulative treatment. They must provide time for research and provide incentives to their faculty, thus harnessing the expertise of researchers now in place or being brought into the institutions. The institutions that have done this most effectively have made several commitments:

- A stated commitment to an osteopathic research environment
- Internal funding for startup research
- Committed time for research
- Support personnel
- Encouragement to take research risks
- Recognition that research is a long-term commitment that simply cannot be hurried

In any endeavor, experience has shown that one of the best ways to get started on a process of change is to publicly commit to the process. This provides an impetus for planning and goal setting against which the outcomes can be measured. A public announcement shows the commitment and produces expectations that are harder to shirk than if the commitment is private.

Although the announcement of intent is laudable, providing the means to begin the task is necessary. The days of having a good idea and simply going to the NIH or National Science Foundation and asking to be funded are simply gone. Public and private funding sources require demonstrated research capability (pilot data) before funding a project. Therefore, the commitment must be backed up with a dollar support to seed research efforts. The college administration must be willing to provide dollars to insure that researchers are able to do the necessary work on which to base their grant proposals. Often, such seed periods, especially in newer areas of inquiry, take several years before external funding is successfully garnered. In addition, even seasoned investigators at times need infusions of funds to continue between grants, start new research projects, or for unexpected needs. The institution must be capable of meeting these needs.

As important as funds are for the beginning researcher, it is often the lack of committed time that impedes a fledgling research program. If a researcher has sufficient funds to do a project, but the blocks of time are not available, the project will fail or the researcher will lose interest. Unlike such things as committee meetings, patient care, and even teaching, the research endeavor requires large blocks of time on a regular basis. First, the researcher must be allowed time to look into the background of the project, to reflect on the available information, and to synthesize its meaning. This literature review and synthesis means a substantial intellectual effort that cannot be done in 5-minute periods between patients or classes. The investigator must be allowed the free and unencumbered time to become an expert in the field—not only his or her field of training, such as internal medicine or osteopathic principles and practice, but in research design and practice. The administration can relieve the prospective researcher of some committee duties, give lighter teaching or patient care loads, and not expect the faculty member committed to research to attend all administration functions. Of course, the quid pro quo will be research productivity.

There must be support personnel for research efforts. A faculty member pursuing a fledgling research effort must expect to initially do much of the footwork in getting a program under way. However, support is needed in terms of technical help, secretarial backup, and patient scheduling. As a research effort develops, support must be provided for grant writing and grant budget administration, as well as for keeping up on the latest federal, state, and local regulations. It is not logical or financially responsible to expect researchers to spend much of their productive time typing letters or purchase orders, rather than reading the latest literature or doing the actual study. The level of support personnel will be rewarded in exponential gains in research productivity.

The institution must also make it clear that it understands that not all research efforts are successful. Research studies by their very nature are trips into the unknown. The researcher, especially the beginner, will have studies that do not show significant results. The institution must show that its support is not only for successful studies, but also for the effort. Without this understanding, the researcher will not be free to undertake anything but the most mundane and predictable efforts. The institution, by showing that it rewards not only research efforts, but also risk taking in research, will foster a higher level of research endeavor. This can be shown by providing raises commensurate with cutting-edge research projects, granting advancement to those willing to take risks, and publicly acknowledging such activities.

For any research endeavor to be anything but an isolated event, to become a program of research, not an isolated study, the researcher must become committed to continuing over an extended time. No one research study will tell a story about an area. Several studies will begin to weave a tapestry that will answer meaningful questions. Research programs evolve with time and continued effort, not isolated, brief efforts. The institutional commitment to its researchers and research programs must be long term. Only then will a research effort make a meaningful contribution to showing the basis and efficacy of osteopathic medicine.

The academic institutions of the osteopathic profession are beginning to build the bases for the long-term commitments necessary for meaningful research programs. Some have advanced further than others, as evidenced by the founding of the center for osteopathic research at the Texas school. Others are only starting the task and need the encouragement and support of the rest of the profession as they proceed.

Academic Challenges: The Faculty

In Chapter 70 "Foundations of Osteopathic Research," we made the observation that the definition of osteopathic research must come from the investigator and cannot be determined a priori. This means that the researcher, basic scientist, or clinician must become sufficiently familiar with the background and clinical experience of osteopathic medicine that he or she can link the ideas and results of their research to the needs and experiences of the profession. Although data from studies not constructed or performed to test the tenets and clinical observations of the osteopathic profession can be used for that purpose, it is far more efficient and less risky of incorrect interpretation to perform studies stemming directly from questions generated by osteopathic theory and experience.

Basic scientists, both from the biomedical tradition and from the social sciences, have been incorporated into the osteopathic profession in increasing numbers, especially since 1970. Earlier, it had been the usual custom in osteopathic teaching institutions to use D.O.s to teach most of the basic science subjects, as well as the clinical areas. With the explosive growth in numbers of schools in the 1970s and heightened expectations for subject experts in the basic sciences, faculty trained in nonosteopathic settings were increasingly hired. Many of these professors had research backgrounds, as well as backgrounds in their disciplines.

These faculty face difficult challenges in doing research meaningful to the osteopathic profession. Although it is often argued that any research is valuable, the profession's research resources seem best spent on research projects that can be expected to provide information useful in giving answers to the theoretical and clinical underpinnings of osteopathic medicine. Some of the challenges faced by basic science researchers include:

- Lack of knowledge of the history, theory, and basis of osteopathic medicine
- Difficult or impossible access to the literature of the osteopathic profession
- Lack of access to the clinical experience of osteopathic medicine
- Difficulty in understanding the practice or jargon of osteopathic clinicians
- Insecurity of switching from an established research program to an unfamiliar one
- Unwillingness to make the effort to explore an unfamiliar and seemingly out-of-the-mainstream topic

These challenges are severe but surmountable. The osteopathic profession is moving to provide the materials needed to acquaint its basic scientists with its background, theoretical basis, and research data. The Texas bibliographic project, while now dormant, still provides references to much of the early research and philosophical writing of the profession and thus provides greater access to the literature of the profession. With the growth of older books and articles available on the web, it is increasingly easy for scientists to access previously unavailable osteopathic resources. The AAO, as mentioned earlier, has provided its literature bibliography on CD-ROM. Such sources as this book and others now appearing provide the willing basic scientist with useful information.

Despite increased reference availability, ready access to the profession's older research literature is poor. Ways must be found to make those sources more available, not only to basic scientists, but to clinician researchers and students as well. Many of the works of Burns and other early anatomists and physiologists investigating basic mechanisms of manipulation are available in only a few college libraries. This is a continuing challenge to the profession, but may be solved by scanning older literature to be made available on the web.

A basic scientist trained in conventional settings coming into an osteopathic school to teach is faced with the task of teaching in a profession about which he or she usually knows nothing. In this case, the only option is to teach a topic in the same way it was taught elsewhere. The osteopathic profession thinks of itself as a unique entity, implying that the teaching of its students should be somehow different from the experience of other medical students. How can that occur if the basic scientist does not know the basis of the profession? One way is to integrate osteopathic physicians into the teaching of the sciences. Of course, another is to inform the basic scientists of the profession. Clinicians and others knowledgeable of the profession can provide seminars and workshops on osteopathic medicine for their colleagues. Basic scientists can be encouraged to sit in on the osteopathic courses. Clinicians can take basic scientists as shadowers in their practices and discuss the unique aspects of osteopathic medicine with them. Administrators can provide expectations and rewards for basic scientists who show a willingness to avail themselves of opportunities to become knowledgeable about the profession. In general, the profession has not held sufficiently high expectations for its basic scientists nor has it provided good opportunities for them to become familiar with the theory and practice of osteopathic medicine.

A basic scientist coming into the profession with a budding or established research program faces real obstacles in retooling or realigning that program to the needs of osteopathic medicine. Funding may not be as readily available. The switch or realignment may take several years to accomplish. The comfort of a known research enterprise is lost. The schools can help this transition by providing funding for the transition, understanding that productivity may decrease for a time, and finding clinicians to supply information and experience to the investigator. In addition, the expectation should be clear that such a transition will be rewarded in tangible ways. Korr (4–11) has published several articles on the challenges posed by osteopathic theory and practice that can be given to entering faculty.

Although the school and profession can do much to help an investigator realign their research and intellectual efforts toward the questions of osteopathic medicine, there is also an onus on those coming into the profession to make an effort to gain this understanding. Intellectual honesty would seem to demand of a person coming into a profession that knowledge of that profession be acquired. The investigator should have some intellectual curiosity and desire to find out about what it is he or she is getting into. Thus, an investigator may be expected to make efforts to seek out opportunities to become familiar with the backgrounds, theoretical underpinnings, and research basis of the profession. Too often, this does not happen, but should be encouraged. Osteopathic clinicians can be very helpful in this by offering manipulative treatment to their basic science colleagues. Osteopathic students can challenge their basic science professors to investigate the profession. In this way, a healthier interaction can be accomplished.

But what about osteopathic clinician researchers within the profession? They also need help in meeting the challenges of research. They often are not schooled in research methods and skills. They are pressured for time and are expected to provide patient care to generate income, not research studies. These individuals also need to be given the time, resources, and encouragement to pursue the difficult and often discouraging field of research. They need to have the backing of their administrators for time and resources to acquire research skills and protected time for intellectual pursuits. They need to become aware of the long-term nature of a research endeavor. They need collaborations with their basic science colleagues in designing and carrying out osteopathically oriented studies. In short, they have the same needs as do the basic scientists. The D.O. making a transition to research is venturing into unknown and uncertain territory, just as is the basic scientist trained in other institutions. Support and understanding are needed for both groups.

Academic Challenges: The Students

In planning for the long-term health of osteopathically oriented research, the role of the students must be considered. At present, in most osteopathic schools, little attention is given to providing the students with a background in prior research of the profession, let alone in the basics of research design and process relevant to the profession. One of the best ways to increase research power in the profession is to orient its students early in their training to the basic properties and needs for research. Only a small percentage will become researchers, but only a few are needed to make a large difference. If only one student per class aspired to become a full-time researcher in the profession and were provided sufficient support to pursue that goal, the profession would soon have an abundance of trained and functioning researchers in its institutions.

The schools can implement lectures on research background, methodology, and process for all students. For those showing more interest, mentors can be provided to work with the more motivated students to provide initial training, research opportunities, and support. These students can be integrated into ongoing investigations of osteopathic manipulation and technique. There have been some efforts to provide a model research curriculum to all the schools,

and this should be encouraged. Too often, the schools are attracting students with research interests, only to destroy that interest by failing to provide opportunities and training.

In addition, opportunities can be made available for graduate training for students interested in well-recognized laboratories outside the profession. However, it is imperative that such opportunities incorporate aspects of research particularly pertinent to the profession, lest the student be discouraged from building the knowledge bridges to the important issues of the profession. An osteopathic student trained in traditional research institutions who goes into research that does not build on osteopathic principles and practice does little to further the osteopathic profession.

The profession is beginning to take steps to add a research basis to the curriculum. In late 2001, a workshop was held at the Osteopathic Clinical Trials Initiative Conference (OCCTIC) meetings for the purposed of outlining a research curriculum for the years of osteopathic medical training. The results of this meeting have been endorsed by the Educational Council on Osteopathic Principles and made available to the schools. Should the schools adopt these guidelines for research training, a real step forward in producing research-oriented students will have been taken. However, 8 years later, it is not clear that most schools have adopted the guidelines. The recommended research curriculum consists of the following:

By the end of osteopathic medical school years 1 and 2, the student should have the following capabilities:

- History of osteopathic research
- Knowledge of research vocabulary
- Ability to do a literature search
- Knowledge of basic statistics
- Understanding of research problems that are uniquely osteopathic (OMT)
- Awareness of support resources available consistent with level of competency expected

By the end of osteopathic medical school years 3 and 4, the student should have the following capabilities:

- Ability to review and summarize journal articles
- Ability to formulate a research question/hypothesis
- Awareness of support resources available consistent with level of competency expected

By the end of postgraduate years 1 through 3, the student should have the following capabilities:

- Understand the process of design and implementation of a research project
- Ability to critique journal articles
- Ability to write a manuscript suitable for publication or a grant application
- Awareness of support resources available consistent with level of competency expected

One of the additional steps that has been taken by the profession is the establishment of a biannual research training workshop, Room to Run, to be held every other year as the OCCTIC meeting. The first was held in 2007 and provided a premiere experience in osteopathic research training to students at all levels of training. When combined with other research training opportunities, this meeting, if continued regularly, will greatly increase the research capabilities of the younger members of the profession. Another very promising development over the recent years is the growth of the SOAR (Student Osteopathic Association of Research). Most osteopathic schools now have a SOAR chapter that provides opportunities for osteopathic students to discuss research interests and to interact with interested faculty.

Organizational Challenges: Other Osteopathic Institutions

As the profession moves into its fifth research era, it is increasingly evident that the challenges of providing a research basis for osteopathic theory and practice cannot be met by the COMs alone. The establishment of the Center for Osteopathic Research was not an isolated effort of one or more schools. It was an effort spanning several years and with its roots in the early days of the profession with the A. T. Still Research Institute. Several institutions of the profession came together to promote and fund the center's formation, including the AOA, AAO, AACOM, the American College of Osteopathic Family Physicians, and the American Osteopathic Healthcare Association. These and other organizations within the profession have realized the necessity of promoting a research culture in the profession. These institutions, the profession's leaders, and the rank and file of the profession must continue to support (in concept and financially) the development of researchers who understand the osteopathic profession and can apply their skills and intellectual abilities to answering the vital questions posed by this unique philosophy and practice. Without continued support and encouragement from all, a research-friendly atmosphere will not flourish.

There is another vital source of research support now operating in the profession—the various osteopathic foundations, such as the Osteopathic Heritage Foundation of Ohio. These foundations have in the past several years become more involved in actively supporting research projects and symposia. Such support is becoming increasingly vital as a bridge between COM supported pilot research and NIH-supported studies. It is no longer possible to attain NIH major research support without a proven track record of data and research productivity. Often, the only way for a researcher or research team to get to the point of being competitive for NIH funds is to obtain midlevel funding from one of the foundations. The support of several osteopathic foundations has made possible the Multi-Center Osteopathic Pneumonia Study in the Elderly (MOPSE) study, directed by the Texas Osteopathic Research Center. This study was only possible with foundation support.

Collaborative Challenges: Building Research Networks

As the research efforts of the profession mature, clinical trials of the effects and efficacy of osteopathic techniques, osteopathic manipulative treatment, and osteopathic care will move from the pilot study format to full-blown clinical trials. These trials will be expensive and time consuming. A full clinical trial often requires hundreds of subjects and many practitioners. The osteopathic profession is, despite its rapid growth, still a small profession. The conduct of full trials will require collaboration between multiple sites and practitioners. Such collaboration has now been successfully done in the MOPSE study (see above) coordinated by the ORC, which with its mandate to conduct studies on osteopathic manipulative themes, is an appropriate venue for such planning. However, there exist other avenues that can begin the process in preparation for these trials. One such avenue lies in the OPTI networks. These confederations of hospital training sites affiliated with osteopathic colleges provide ready-made resources for pilot studies of collaborative trials. Some OPTIs already have provision for research efforts and research training. The OPTI networks can be valuable testing grounds for collaborative efforts in the next few years. In addition, encouraging practitioners in their office practices to join research networks would lead to more viable clinical trials.

Recent developments in clinical research stimulated by the acquired immunodeficiency syndrome (AIDS) epidemic are also useful models for the osteopathic profession to follow. In the past, there has been little clinical research performed outside major research centers. In response to increasing pressure for clinical data on the AIDS epidemic, there has been an increasing use of smaller neighborhood clinics and solo practitioners to collect data on the disease (Goldstein M, Personal Communication, 1992). It is becoming evident that there is an important role for the practicing physician in collecting data for clinical studies. Studies using this important resource for data collection must be designed to take advantage of the practice of medicine in the office setting so as not to disrupt the daily flow of the practice. However, it is here that the real practice of osteopathic medicine takes place. It is here that there is the best chance to ask such questions as:

- What is the incidence of somatic dysfunction?
- What is its natural course?
- What is the effectiveness of manipulative treatment on it?

The questions of real life in osteopathic medicine can be approached at the office level. Such research must be encouraged. That such research can be accomplished is seen in the recent report from the office of Frymann et al. (12) on the effects of osteopathic care on neurologic development in children. Other office-based studies that include many practitioners would provide important data on the basis for and efficacy of osteopathic care. The recent development by the American Academy of Osteopathy Louisa Burns Research Committee of several data forms may make the collection of office data feasible, especially when they become web based.

Collaborative Challenges: Isolation

The osteopathic profession began in the United States but quickly spread to other countries. Early in the 1900s, osteopathy was established in the United Kingdom; in 1916, an osteopathic school was established there. Currently, there are osteopathic movements in many countries of the world, some nascent, as in Russia, and some well developed, as in the United Kingdom. Although the practitioners of most of these schools are licensed to practice manipulation only, they are valuable resources for research collaboration. In addition, many countries have active allopathic groups who have traditions of manual medicine, and some have become well trained in osteopathic techniques and theory, as is the case in Germany. The International Federation of Manual Medicine, or FIMM, has an active research component. Canadian students of osteopathy, in fact, must complete an extensive research thesis, practically comparable to a U.S. doctoral thesis before becoming certified as diplomats in osteopathy.

The U.S. osteopathic movement has an opportunity to greatly enhance its research efforts by encouraging interactions with these movements. In fact, it may be that, taken together, these organized osteopathic schools outside the United States have more potential for research on efficacy and outcomes than does the U.S. profession. Clearly, there are aspects of osteopathic care that can only be studied in the United States, because only here at present are osteopathic doctors fully licensed physicians; however, technique, reliability, and treatment studies can be collaboratively studied with many other sections of the world osteopathic community. These types of collaboration should not be wasted by isolationism.

CHALLENGES OF RESEARCH DESIGN

The design of osteopathic clinical research faces unique challenges. The design of clinical research is actually in its infancy, beginning only about 60 to 70 years ago. Clinical research grew up around the testing of drug efficacy, and the gold standard design for such studies is the randomized, placebo-controlled, double-blind (RPCDB) study. The two major challenges facing the osteopathic and manipulative medicine communities are as follows:

1. Is the RPCDB methodology appropriate for studies of osteopathic manipulative treatment?
2. What research designs are appropriate for studies of osteopathic manipulative treatment?

These questions cannot be answered in a vacuum. The design of any study should flow from an understanding of the research question and the available research techniques. Parts of this challenge have been examined in Chapter 70: "Foundations for Osteopathic Research," but other aspects will be discussed here.

Shams and Placebos

One of the most interesting issues facing the design of research in osteopathic manipulative treatment or techniques is whether to use placebo or sham controls and, if so, what to use. The use of placebos is well known and documented in clinical research literature (as is the use of sham controls), but these are being called into question (13,14). The placebo treatment was initially developed for research on the effectiveness of drugs, and entails the delivery of a substance that is, from the standpoint of the patient and physician, indistinguishable from the drug being tested. Such a placebo is often in the form of a capsule that is the same color, size, and weight as the capsule containing the drug, but the placebo contains only inert substances. The patient is given either the drug-containing capsule or the inert-substance capsule, not knowing which is being given. The sham is a procedure given to the patient that has been shown or is thought to have no effect on the symptoms being treated. With both placebos and shams, the intent is to keep the patient from knowing whether he or she is receiving an active or inactive drug or procedure. This should keep the expectations of both the experimental and control groups equal and thus allow the effect of the active ingredient or procedure to be seen, independent of patient expectations.

In the case of drug tests or for testing specific manipulative techniques, placebo and sham controls are entirely appropriate. The intent of such studies is to ascertain the effect of the active ingredient alone. They look at the effect of either a certain molecule (or, more precisely, many millions of molecules) on the natural course of something like a bacterial invasion of the body, or of a particular procedure (such as a lateral recumbent roll) on the course of a particular symptom (15). The patient's expectations and conscious processes are not at issue. The use of placebo or sham procedures as control groups against which the drug or procedure groups can be compared gives the researcher a measure of the effectiveness of the drug or technique alone.

Thus, in the design of manipulative technique research, it seems entirely appropriate to use sham treatment control groups. Here, the rationale is to test the effectiveness of a certain specific technique that is administered in the same way to each patient for presumably the same symptom or symptoms. The treating physician has no leeway in how the maneuver is accomplished, and the patients are screened closely so that the symptoms are much the same from patient to patient.

However, at the heart of osteopathic philosophy is the premise that treatment should be aimed at normalization of function by removing the barriers to the body's ability to optimize its function. Once these barriers are removed, the body can regain its optimal function and return to or maintain health. To think that this is

purely a physiologic function and has nothing to do with conscious processes or the mind (i.e., the patient's expectations, desires, beliefs, and will) is to return to a belief in mind/body dualism holding that the mind has nothing to do with physiologic function, and vice versa. It is to deny the most vital part of the whole equation of health and disease: the patients themselves. In addition, the treating physician is a part of the equation. Both the skill and the manner of the treating physician affect the results of the treatment, because both the patient's tactile and mental perceptions of the physician influence how the patient responds to the treatment.

In osteopathic treatment, the treatment is an interaction between patient and physician, each responding to the other throughout the treatment. The osteopathic physician relies on the very effect that is labeled placebo or expectation in drug testing to help with the alteration he or she is attempting to produce—that of normalized function. The patient's expectation is an important and vital factor in OMT; it must not be cast off as some spurious side effect. It is also a real and unusually safe therapeutic tool. There are few deleterious side effects to positive expectations.

In addition, the use of a sham treatment group in which the patient is exposed to a treatment that is considered ineffective presents another real problem for the evaluation of OMT (again, as contrasted to the evaluation of a particular technique). It is assumed that in the sham control group, the treatment of a body area distant from a particular somatic dysfunction does not influence the resolution of a diagnosed dysfunction being treated in the experimental group. Many available data show that the simple act of touching and moving an individual produces real changes in function and response. The act of manipulative treatment involves touching and moving the patient as an integral part of the process. To compare a manipulation group with some sham group that has also received touch and movement may well lead to an underestimation of the effects of manipulative treatment, unless it can be shown that the sham treatment had no effect on the total mind and body function of the patient.

Thus, initial attempts to evaluate the true effectiveness of manipulative treatment (as opposed to techniques) on either the progression of symptoms or on total body function require the use of a control group that either receives some standard medical therapy not requiring manipulation or the use of a totally untreated control group that would simply undergo the natural course of the malfunction being studied. This could be done by simply requiring control subjects to come to the physician's office for diagnostic measurements. To try to factor out the mental process involved in manipulative treatment is to deny much of the actual treatment. It is akin to studying the effectiveness of a drug by giving only a partial dose.

To study the effects of osteopathic manipulation, one must study osteopathic manipulation as it is given, as an interaction between physician and patient, with all components intact and functioning. To factor out any particular component, such as the so-called hands-on effect, and call it an artifact is to underestimate the effect of manipulative treatment and deny that the natural power of cognitive and recuperative processes is a factor in the effects of OMT. It must be understood that unless the sham treatment has been actually shown to have no effect on any aspect of the patient's function, a study contrasting manipulation with a sham is really comparing one form of treatment with another form of treatment.

Once the overall effects of manipulative treatment have been established, studies can be designed to tease apart the various components of the treatment, including the effects of touching the patient, and so forth. However, to try to parse out various aspects of a complex treatment in the absence of demonstrated effects is both inefficient and impractical. The study of OMT must flow from the philosophy of osteopathy and not from some other philosophic orientation.

One example of a study using a sham control was published recently by Yelland et al. (16). They compared the effects of active prolotherapy with similar injections of saline on nonspecific low back pain. The results showed no difference between the irritant prolotherapy-injected group and the saline-injected group. Both groups showed the same reduction in low back pain over the 24-month study. In point of fact, it seems likely that no conclusions can be drawn from the study, because there was no way of ascertaining whether the decreased overall pain levels would have occurred anyway or even if the interventions resulted in less pain decrease over the time of the study than would have occurred had nothing been done. The only conclusion that may be able to be drawn is that irritant injections and saline injections cause no different results, but it may be that neither one did anything for nonspecific low back pain. This study shows the problems of assuming that a treatment is a sham (having no effect) without actually testing it against no treatment.

The investigator designing studies of OMT must determine what is really being asked of the study so that the appropriate contrast control can be used. Using the incorrect control may result in underestimation of the effect of manipulative treatment, although the same control may be the appropriate one for evaluation of a manipulative technique. The decision rests on whether the total response of the individual to the interaction between patient and physician is being evaluated or whether manipulative technique is being studied as a procedure. The challenge here is to actively defend the use of appropriate designs for osteopathic manipulative research, and not to be forced into inappropriate designs by preconceived notions of how research is done.

PRIORITY CHALLENGES: WHAT RESEARCH IS MOST IMPORTANT?

Basic Research

Research on the mechanisms underlying osteopathic practice begins with either the theoretical underpinnings of the profession, or clinical observations of practitioners. As an example, Korr (17) followed both theory and clinical observation when beginning his line of research on transsynaptic delivery of proteins from nerve to muscle tissue. The nurturing of tissues by their nerve supply had long been a theme in osteopathic medicine, but almost ignored in other Western traditions. Clinical observations showed that muscles deprived of nerve supply would degenerate, but those only deprived of nerve activity would only atrophy. Korr's research program was driven by osteopathic clinical and theoretical considerations.

Clearly, some of the vital areas in the traditions and clinical experiences of the profession can lead to distinctive basic research programs. Examples of such areas include:

- The interactions between somatic and visceral structures are vital issues that are receiving attention in laboratories now, but are very underresearched.
- How does the mechanoreceptor input from muscle affect sympathetic outflow?
- How does sympathetic activity affect somatic structure and function?
- How can virus and bacterial activity be influenced by sympathetic activity?
- What is the structure and function of the fasciae of the body?

- How do strains in the somatic structures affect visceral function over time?
- What are the effects of various osteopathic procedures on visceral function?

Certainly one of the most basic questions in the area of osteopathic basic research is the prevalence and incidence of the entity known as somatic dysfunction. This is perhaps one of the most pressing and most difficult questions that remain unanswered in the profession. It actually crosses the bounds of basic and clinical areas.

The list of questions generated by osteopathic theory and clinical experience is almost endless. However, to tap these areas, the researcher must be able to see how they apply to the osteopathic experience.

Clinical Research

As long as is the list of questions in the basic sciences flowing from the osteopathic theory and practice, it is perhaps longer in the clinical arena. Various lists of the most important areas of clinical research have been generated, but consensus has not been reached. Areas that seem to be especially critical, although not prioritized, are included here.

Teaching Techniques in Osteopathic Manipulation

The area of research on educational techniques, although not clinical, would provide important information on how to pass on the techniques and skills of osteopathic medicine. Research into how to best teach palpation, recognition of tissues texture alterations, and so forth, is badly needed.

Inter- and Intraexaminer Reliability Studies

One of the basic unknowns in osteopathic medicine (and manual medicine in general) is how to assess and improve the reliability between the examination skills of practitioners, and indeed, how reliable the same individual is when examining the same patient twice. There are studies available on the reliability between examiners of the same patient (e.g., 17,18), but the studies vary widely in quality and findings. In addition to being an important question in terms of how much value can be placed on palpatory findings, studies on the factors influencing the reliability within and between palpators would help inform the teaching of these skills. This is an area that probably should be a priority in the profession and on which several projects are being mounted.

Outcomes and Cost Effectiveness of Osteopathic Manipulative Treatment

Although seemingly obvious, simple outcome studies that look at what happens to patients, without the use of controls, is needed. One such study is under way at present in Maine (the Maine Osteopathic Outcomes Study, or MOOS), and more may be planned. However, with the amount of data collected by state, federal, and private entities, the numbers of epidemiologically related studies that are now possible are immense. Models for these types of studies must be generated more frequently in the profession.

Comparing Osteopathic Treatment Techniques with Other Forms of Manual Medicine

Many other forms of manual medicine exist. How do treatment techniques generated by the osteopathic profession compare with these? Is a manipulative treatment driven by osteopathic theory more effective than that given by other practitioners of manual medicine? Such questions are not only fascinating, but also vital to understanding the value of osteopathic medicine.

Comparing Different Modalities of Osteopathic Treatment

There are several major treatment modalities used in the profession. How do they compare in outcomes when used on a common disease process? Is a high-velocity/low-amplitude thrust better than a muscle treatment for a sore neck? Comparing one modality with another would produce interesting insights into the potential mechanisms of the different modalities, as well as their efficacy in various conditions.

Effects of Manipulation on a Somatic Dysfunction

Just as the questions of prevalence and incidence of somatic dysfunction are basic to the profession, so are the questions surrounding the actual influence of a manipulative treatment on a well-delineated somatic dysfunction. How do such parameters as chronicity and cause affect the outcome? Although it is assumed that an osteopathic treatment corrects somatic dysfunction, how long does the effect last in chronic cases, and how susceptible is the dysfunction to reoccurrence?

Effects of Manipulation on Diagnosed Disease Entities

This question has been debated for years and is, in fact, a basic question for payment for services. Actually, the list of conditions to target for such research has received much attention. At a recent meeting, several conditions were targeted for special consideration:

- Chronic low back pain
- Headache (type unspecified)
- Asthma
- Otitis media

These conditions have a history of study in and outside the profession, and may be more amenable to tight research designs than many other conditions.

There is a wide range of studies either under way or in planning stages at osteopathic schools and other institutions. All should be encouraged, as each will add to the body of design knowledge about how to do research in osteopathic manipulative treatment. It is likely that a few conditions will have to be selected for full-scale studies due to cost and manpower limitations. Pilot studies will pave the way for selecting those conditions most likely to provide meaningful information on the large-scale effects of osteopathic treatment.

OSTEOPATHIC PHILOSOPHY AND LARGER RESEARCH QUESTIONS

Although these specific areas of research are important, the role of the osteopathic philosophy in shaping even larger questions, and directions of osteopathic research must be mentioned.

Basic to the philosophy and theory of osteopathy is the idea that the body is an integrated functional unit. This unit includes the physical, cognitive, and spiritual aspects of the individual. Indeed, there is a growing body of evidence suggesting positive effects of spiritual interventions, such as prayer, in the healing process (18–23). How these elements interact within the total individual and with the external environment determine the long-term health status of the person. From the beginning of osteopathic medicine, osteopathic practitioners have held that there was an entity that would adversely affect a person's health status. This entity, which could be palpated and specifically treated with manipulation, was first known as the osteopathic lesion and then, more recently, as somatic dysfunction. In the 1940s and 1950s, Denslow, Korr (24), and their colleagues postulated that a major component of the osteopathic lesion was the facilitated segment. The facilitated segment concept arose from the data gathered by these researchers, which showed that, in most individuals, there was no uniform excitability throughout the spinal cord. The areas of hyperexcitability were shown to react more strongly to afferent input, exposing innervated structures, both visceral and somatic, to increased activation. This break in body unity was postulated to lead to early breakdown and malfunction over time—in short, to disease. Clinical disease was, then, a consequence of earlier body dysfunction. Indeed, this was a data-based theory that truly embodied one of Still's basic insights; that clinical disease was a manifestation of body malfunction rather than a primary event.

DETERIORATION OF NORMAL FUNCTION AS A CENTRAL CONCEPT

That clinical disease is a result of earlier deterioration of normal function is central to osteopathic philosophy. It is perhaps best manifest in the treatment of somatic dysfunction, an entity not recognized by most medical practitioners as a clinical entity at all. Why treat it? Because it is the beginning of disease, the start of body breakdown. To treat the root of disease would seem to be more cost effective than waiting until the final breakdown of clinical disease has occurred before beginning treatment.

OTHER ROLES FOR SOMATIC DYSFUNCTION

Given this view, osteopathic research should be aimed at elucidating the relationships between disturbances of body function and health status:

- How does the presence of somatic dysfunction predict the health status of the individual?
- What is the incidence of serious somatic dysfunction and its natural history?
- What environmental and lifestyle attributes seem to contribute to the incidence of somatic dysfunction?
- How does lifestyle contribute to the incidence of somatic dysfunction in old age?
- Flowing from these questions are even larger questions that should be at the forefront of osteopathic thinking.
- What is the contribution of early lifestyle or events that happen to the person and the health status of the individual in old age?
- What regime of manipulative treatment in early life will contribute most to deterring the deterioration of health usually associated with old age?
- More simply, why are some very old people vital and healthy and others completely overtaken by deterioration and disease?
- What role does long-lasting somatic dysfunction play in the presence or absence of vitality in old age?

These questions are complex and not easily answered. The critical point is that at least some research of the profession should take as its starting point body unity and the concept that the start of disease is the deterioration of that functional unity, not a bacterial or viral invasion.

INTEGRATION AND SELF-REGULATION IN HEALTH

These questions suggest several important areas of research for the osteopathic profession. In the basic sciences, increasing attention must be paid to understanding the integration of body systems and what can cause the fine-tuned integration of body function to deteriorate. The capacity of the body to self-regulate (homeostasis) and the limits of that capacity in both the short term and the long term must be better understood. Research aimed at elucidating the fine control and adaptation of body function would be especially useful. Integration of basic science data with data from studies of cognitive function gives a greater understanding of the role of the physician in the health maintenance process. A greater understanding of the effects of afferent input and cognitive function on the immune system, and how manipulative treatment can affect this system, would be useful.

HEALTH BENEFITS OF MANIPULATIVE TREATMENT

Within the clinical research areas, there must be studies of the efficacy of manipulative techniques and manipulative treatment. Measurements of the effects of manipulation on specific disease entities, such as those listed above, need to be carried out to demonstrate that manipulation can be used effectively in treating specific disease processes. To rely on such demonstration studies to show the most significant benefits of manipulation would, however, be unwise. The most beneficial and lasting effects of manipulation and, indeed, of osteopathic care should be searched for in the effects on total functional capacity of individuals and in their long-term health status. The current health care system is preoccupied with the treatment of disease, especially in the chronic degeneration of old age. It is by no means clear that the chronic diseases commonly associated with old age are inevitable. What are the enabling or protective roles of early and continued normal body function in the aging process? Osteopathy is ideally suited by its philosophy and clinical experience to look at the effects of early disruptions of body unity on the deterioration of old age. This is a golden opportunity for osteopathic research.

TOTAL NATURE OF SOMATIC DYSFUNCTION

Clinical research should continue to look at the effects of manipulation on specific disease processes. Such studies can be effectiveness studies, such as the use of manipulative treatment in low back and chronic pain syndromes. These studies could have fairly quick and valuable outcomes for the profession. Other less specific studies, such as the effects of manipulation on sympathetic tone, vasomotor reactivity, and muscle spasticity, contribute to an understanding of the more general effects of manipulation on body function. Studies of the effects of somatic dysfunction and its etiology, prevalence, and contributions to the long-term health of the individual form a solid base for a greater understanding of the fundamental dynamics of health and disease. Investigations of the effects of manipulation on somatic dysfunction and of osteopathic care on old age health status are probably the most important area of study to which the profession can aspire.

SUMMARY

Northup (1) wisely noted that the future of the profession rested in the decisions and integrity of organized osteopathy. Organized osteopathy now must rise to the challenge of mounting and sustaining a research enterprise that will test the central tenets and beliefs of the profession. These studies must be done on the playing fields of the profession, not on those of other professions. The studies must test the profession's questions and assumptions and be interpreted by those knowledgeable in the theories and practices of osteopathic medicine, not by others. The risk of allowing others to do the studies or interpret the results from other points of view is simply unacceptable. The future of the profession now rests as much on its research endeavors as on its teaching and clinical endeavors. The three legs of the profession's stool are equal, and all are vital.

By closely following the basic philosophy of osteopathy and the insights from its years of clinical experience, the research efforts of the profession can truly add to the most beneficial aspects of health care to which osteopathy is fundamentally dedicated: the maintenance of health and optimal function of the total person throughout life.

REFERENCES

1. Northup GW. An adventure in excellence. *J Am Osteopath Assoc* 2001;101(12):726–730.
2. Patterson MM, Howell JN, eds. *The Central Connection: Somatovisceral Viscerosomatic Interaction.* Indianapolis, IN: American Academy of Osteopathy, 1992.
3. Willard F, Patterson MM, eds. Nociception and the Neuroendocrine-Immune Connection. *Proceedings of the 1992 American Academy of Osteopathy International Symposium.* Indianapolis, IN: American Academy of Osteopathy, 1994.
4. Korr IM. Biological basis for the osteopathic concept. In: Beal MC, *1960, and 1963 Academy Yearbooks.* Indianapolis, IN: American Academy of Osteopathy, 1960:129 and 1963:114.
5. Korr IM. Some thoughts on an osteopathic curriculum. *J Am Osteopath Assoc* 1975;74(8):685–688.
6. Korr IM. Biologic process in the context of human uniqueness and diversity. *Osteopath Ann* 1978;6(1):10–13.
7. Korr IM. Osteopathic principles for basic scientists. *J Am Osteopath Assoc* 1987;87(7):513–515.
8. Korr IM. Medical education: the resistance to change. *Advances* 1987;4(2):5–10.
9. Korr IM. Osteopathic principles: a way of life. *DO* 1987;May:25–27.
10. Korr IM. An explication of osteopathic principles. In: Ward RC, ed. *Foundations for Osteopathic Medicine.* Baltimore, MD: Williams & Wilkins, 1997:7–12.
11. Korr IM. Pathways to excellence in clinical research. In: Beal MC, ed. *1994 Yearbook, Louisa Burns, DO Memorial.* Indianapolis, IN: American Academy of Osteopathy, 1994:60.
12. Frymann VM, Carney RE, Springall P. Effect of osteopathic medical management on neurologic development in children. *J Am Osteopath Assoc* 1992;92(6):729–744.
13. Kienle GS, Kiene H. Placebo effect and placebo concept: a critical methodological and conceptual analysis of reports on the magnitude of the placebo effect. *Altern Ther Health Med* 1996;2(6):39–54.
14. Kiene H. A critique of the double-blind clinical trial. *Altern Ther Health Med* 1996;2(1):74–80.
15. Hoehler F, Tobis J, Buerger A. Spinal manipulation for low back pain. *JAMA* 1981;245(18):1835–1838.
16. Yelland, M, Glasziou, PP, Bogduk, N, et al. Prolotherapy injections, saline injections, and exercises for chronic low-back pain: a randomized trial. *Spine* 2004;29(1):9–16.
17. Korr IM, Wilkinson PN, Chornock FW. Axonal delivery of neuroplasmic components to muscle cells. *Science* 1967;155(760):342–345.

18. Beal MC, Patriquin DA. Interexaminer agreement on palpatory diagnosis and patient self-assessment of disability: a pilot study. *J Am Osteopath Assoc* 1995;95(2):97–100, 103–106.

19. Halma KD, Degenhardt BF, Snider KT, et al. Intraobserver reliability of cranial strain patterns as evaluated by osteopathic physicians: a pilot study. *J Am Osteopath Assoc* 2008;108:493–502.

20. Abbot NC, Harkness EF, Stevinson C, et al. Spiritual healing as a therapy for chronic pain: A randomized, clinical trial. *Pain* 2001;91:79–89.

21. Dossey L. The return of prayer. *Altern Ther Health Med* 1997;3(6):10–17.

22. Harris WS, Gowda M, Kolb JW, et al. A randomized, controlled trial of the effects of remote, intercessory prayer on outcomes in patients admitted to the coronary care unit. *Arch Intern Med* 1999;159:2273–2278.

23. Thomson KS. The revival of experiments on prayer. *Am Sci* 1996;84:532–534.

24. Korr IM. The emerging concept of the osteopathic lesion. *J Am Osteopath Assoc* 1948;47:1–8.

The result of many years' work by members of the Educational Council on Osteopathic Principles (ECOP), the *Glossary of Osteopathic Terminology* (Glossary) was first published in the *Journal of the American Osteopathic Association* April 1981 (No. 80, pages 552–567). The appearance of *Foundations for Osteopathic Medicine*, Ward RC (ed.); Williams & Wilkins, Baltimore, MD led to inclusion of the Glossary in the first edition (1997, pp. 1126–1140) and the second edition (2003, pp. 1229–1253).

The revision process for the Glossary is ongoing, conducted by members of the ECOP Glossary Review Committee. Definitions are sought which are uniquely osteopathic in their origin or common word usage. Other considerations include distinctiveness in the osteopathic usage of a common word, and/or importance in describing osteopathic principles, philosophy, and osteopathic manipulative treatment. The Glossary is expected to be useful to students and practitioners of osteopathic medicine, and helpful to authors and other professionals in understanding and making proper use of osteopathic vocabulary. The most current and revised version is available on two websites: American Association of Colleges of Osteopathic Medicine (AACOM) in PDF format at www.aacom.org and the American Osteopathic Association (AOA) at www.osteopathic.org.

The April 2009 glossary review was performed by John Glover, D.O., F.A.A.O., ECOP Chairman, Lisa DeStefano, D.O., William Devine, D.O., Walter Ehrenfeuchter, D.O., F.A.A.O., David Eland, D.O., F.A.A.O., Heather Ferrill, D.O., Tom Fotopoulos, D.O., Eric Gish, D.O., Rebecca Giusti, D.O., John Glover, D.O., F.A.A.O., Laura Griffin, D.O., F.A.A.O., David Harden, D.O., Kurt Heinking, D.O., F.A.A.O., Jan Hendryx, D.O., F.A.A.M.A., Kendi Hensel, D.O., Ph.D., Robert Kappler, D.O., F.A.A.O., Jon Kirsch, D.O., Bradley Klock, D.O., F.A.A.O., William Lemley, D.O., F.A.A.O., David Mason, D.O., F.A.C.O.F.P., William Morris, D.O., Evan Nicholas, D.O., Paul Rennie, D.O., F.A.A.O., Mark Sandhouse, D.O., Harriet Shaw, D.O., Karen Snider, D.O., Melicien Tettambel, D.O., F.A.A.O., Greg Thompson, D.O., Kevin Treffer, D.O.

A

abbreviations (types of osteopathic manipulative treatment):

ART: articulatory treatment
BLT: balanced ligamentous tension treatment
CR: osteopathy in the cranial field
CS: counterstrain treatment
D: direct treatment
DIR: direct treatment
FPR: facilitated positional release treatment
HVLA: high velocity/low amplitude treatment
I: indirect treatment
IND: indirect treatment
INR: integrated neuromusculoskeletal release treatment
LAS: ligamentous articular strain treatment
ME: muscle energy treatment *MFR:* myofascial release treatment
NMM-OMM: neuromusculoskeletal medicine
OCF: osteopathy in the cranial field/cranial treatment
OMTh: osteopathic manipulative therapy (non-US terminology)
OMT: osteopathic manipulative treatment
PINS: progressive inhibition of neuromuscular structures
ST: soft tissue treatment
VIS: visceral manipulative treatment

accessory joint motions: See *secondary joint motion.*
accessory movements: Movements used to potentiate, accentuate, or compensate for an impairment in a physiologic motion (e.g., the movements needed to move a paralyzed limb).
accommodation: A self-reversing and nonpersistent adaptation.
active motion: See *motion, active.*
acute somatic dysfunction: See *somatic dysfunction, acute.*
allopathy: A therapeutic system in which a disease is treated by producing a second condition that is incompatible with or antagonistic to the first *(Stedman's).*
allopath, allopathic physician: 1. A term originated by Samuel Hahnemann, MD, to distinguish homeopaths from physicians practicing traditional/orthodox medicine. 2. In common usage, a general term used to differentiate MDs (medical doctors) from other schools of medicine. See *allopathy, osteopathic physician.*
anatomical barrier: See *barrier (motion barrier).*
angle:
   Ferguson a., See *angle, lumbosacral.*
   lumbolumbar lordotic a., an objective quantification of lumbar lordosis typically determined by measuring the angle between the superior surface of the second lumbar vertebra and the inferior surface of the fifth lumbar vertebra; best measured from a standing lateral x-ray film (Fig. 1).
   lumbosacral a., represents the angle of the lumbosacral junction as measured by the inclination of the superior surface of the first sacral vertebra to the horizontal (this is actually a sacral angle); usually measured from standing lateral x-ray films; also known as Ferguson angle (Fig. 2).
   lumbosacral lordotic a., an objective quantification of lumbar lordosis typically determined by measuring the angle between the superior surface of the second lumbar vertebra and the superior surface of the first sacral segment; best measured from a standing lateral x-ray film (Fig. 3).
anterior component: A positional descriptor used to identify the side of reference when rotation of a vertebra has occurred; in a condition of right rotation, the left side is the anterior component; usually refers to the less prominent transverse process; See also *posterior component.*
anterior compression test: See *ASIS (anterior superior iliac spine) compression test.*

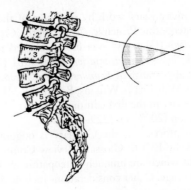

Figure 1 Lumbolumbar angle (L2-L5)

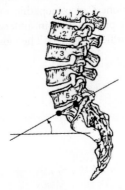

Figure 2 Lumbosacral angle (S1-horizon) (Ferguson's angle).

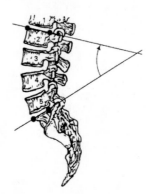

Figure 3 Lumbosacral lordotic angle.

anterior iliac rotation: See *ilium, somatic dysfunction of, anterior (forward) innominate (iliac) rotation.*
anterior nutation, See *nutation.*
anterior rib: See *rib somatic dysfunction, inhalation rib dysfunction.*
ART: See *TART.*
articular pillar: 1. Refers to the columnar arrangement of the articular portions of the cervical vertebrae. 2. Those parts of the lateral arches of the cervical vertebrae that contain a superior and inferior articular facet.
articulation: 1. The place of union or junction between two or more bones of the skeleton. 2. The active or passive process of moving a joint through its permitted anatomic range of motion. See also *osteopathic manipulative treatment, articulatory treatment (ART) system.*

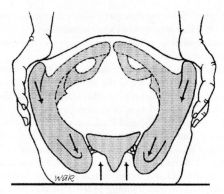

Figure 4 ASIS compression test.

articulatory pop: The sound made when cavitation occurs in a joint. See also *cavitation*.

articulatory technique: See also *technique*. See *osteopathic manipulative treatment, articulatory treatment (ART) system*.

asymmetry: Absence of symmetry of position or motion; dissimilarity in corresponding parts or organs on opposite sides of the body that are normally alike; of particular use when describing position or motion alteration resulting from somatic dysfunction. NB: *This term is part of the TART acronym for an osteopathic somatic dysfunction.*

axis: 1. An imaginary line about which motion occurs. 2. The second cervical vertebra. 3. One component of an axis system.

axis of rib motion: See *rib motion, axis.*

ASIS (anterior superior iliac spine) compression test: 1. A test for lateralization of somatic dysfunction of the sacrum, innominate or pubic symphysis. 2. Application of a force through the ASIS into one of the pelvic axes to assess the mechanics of the pelvis. See also *sacral motion, axis of* (Fig. 4).

axis of sacral motion: See *sacral motion, axis of.*

axoplasmic flow: See *axoplasmic transport.*

axoplasmic transport: The antegrade movement of substances from the nerve cell along the axon toward the terminals, and the retrograde movement from the terminals toward the nerve cell.

B

backward bending: Opposite of forward bending. See *extension.*

backward bending test: 1. This test discriminates between forward and backward sacral torsion/rotation. 2. This test discriminates between unilateral sacral flexion and unilateral sacral extension.

backward torsion: See *sacrum, somatic dysfunctions of, backward torsions.*

balanced ligamentous tension technique: See *osteopathic manipulative treatment, balanced ligamentous tension*. See also *osteopathic manipulative treatment, ligamentous articular strain.*

barrier (motion barrier): The limit to motion; in defining barriers, the palpatory end-feel characteristics are useful (Fig. 5).

    anatomic b., the limit of motion imposed by anatomic structure; the limit of passive motion.

    elastic b., the range between the physiologic and anatomic barrier of motion in which passive ligamentous stretching occurs before tissue disruption.

    pathologic b., a restriction of joint motion associated with pathologic change of tissues (example: osteophytes). See also *barrier, restrictive b.*

    physiologic b., the limit of active motion.

    restrictive b., a functional limit that abnormally diminishes the normal physiologic range.

batwing deformity: See *transitional vertebrae, sacralization.*

bind: Palpable resistance to motion of an articulation or tissue. Synonym: resistance. Antonyms: ease, compliance, resilience.

biomechanics: Mechanical principles applied to the study of biological functions; the application of mechanical laws to living structures; the study and knowledge of biological function from an application of mechanical principles.

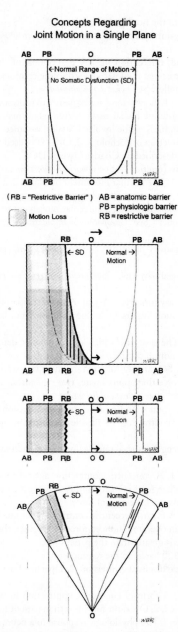

Figure 5 **Somatic dysfunction in a single plane: three methods illustrating the "restrictive barrier" (the restrainer): AB, anatomic barrier; PB, physiologic barrier; RB, restrictive barrier; SD, somatic dysfunction** (From *Foundations for Osteopathic Medicine*, Baltimore, Williams & Wilkins, 1997:484.)

body unity: One of the basic tenets of the osteopathic philosophy; the human being is a dynamic unit of function; See also *osteopathic philosophy.*

bogginess: A tissue texture abnormality characterized principally by a palpable sense of sponginess in the tissue, interpreted as resulting from congestion due to increased fluid content.

bucket handle rib motion: See *rib motion, bucket handle.*

C

caliper rib motion: See *rib motion, caliper rib motion.*

caudad: Toward the tail or inferiorly.

caught in inhalation: See *inhalation rib dysfunction.*

caught in exhalation: See *exhalation rib dysfunction.*

cavitation: The formation of small vapor and gas bubbles within fluid caused by local reduction in pressure. This phenomenon is believed to produce an audible "pop" in certain forms of OMT.

cephalad: Toward the head.

cephalad pubic dysfunction: See *pubic bone, somatic dysfunctions of, superior pubic shear.*

cerebrospinal fluid, fluctuation of: A description of the hypothesized action of cerebrospinal fluid with regard to the craniosacral mechanism. cervicolumbar reflex: See *reflex, cervicolumbar r.*

Chapman reflex: 1. A system of reflex points that present as predictable anterior and posterior fascial tissue texture abnormalities (plaque-like changes or stringiness of the involved tissues) assumed to be reflections of visceral dysfunction or pathology. 2. Originally used by Frank Chapman, DO, and described by Charles Owens, DO.

chronic somatic dysfunction: See *somatic dysfunction, chronic.*

circumduction: 1. The circular movement of a limb. 2. The rotary movement by which a structure is made to describe a cone, the apex of the cone being a fixed point (e.g., the circular movement of the shoulder).

combined technique: See *osteopathic manipulative treatment, combined method.*

common compensatory pattern: See *fascial patterns, common compensatory pattern.*

compensatory fascial patterns: See *fascial patterns, common compensatory pattern.*

complete motor asymmetry: Asymmetry of palpatory responses to all regional motion inputs including rotation, translation and active respiration.

compliance: 1. The ease with which a tissue may be deformed. 2. Direction of ease in motion testing.

compression: 1. Somatic dysfunction in which two structures are forced together. 2. A force that approximates two structures.

conditioned reflex: See *reflex, conditioned r.*

contraction: Shortening and/or development of tension in muscle.

  concentric c., contraction of muscle resulting in approximation of attachments.

  eccentric c., lengthening of muscle during contraction due to an external force.

  isokinetic c., 1. A concentric contraction against resistance in which the angular change of joint motion is at the same rate. 2. The counterforce is less than the patient force.

  isolytic c., 1. A form of eccentric contraction designed to break adhesions using an operator-induced force to lengthen the muscle. 2. The counterforce is greater than the patient force.

  isometric c., 1. Change in the tension of a muscle without approximation of muscle origin and insertion. 2. Operator force equal to patient force.

  isotonic c., 1. A form of concentric contraction in which a constant force is applied. 2. Operator force less than patient force.

contracted muscle: The physiologic response to a neuromuscular excitation. See also *contractured muscle.*

contracture: A condition of fixed high resistance to passive stretch of a muscle, resulting from fibrosis of the tissues supporting the muscles or the joints, or from disorders of the muscle fibers.

  Dupuytren c., shortening, thickening and fibrosis of the palmar fascia, producing a flexion deformity of a finger *(Dorland's).*

contractured muscle: histological change substituting noncontractile tissue for muscle tissue, which prevents the muscle from reaching normal relaxed length. See also *contracted muscle.*

core link: The connection of the spinal dura mater from the occiput at the foramen magnum to the sacrum. It coordinates the synchronous motion of these two structures.

coronal plane: See *plane, frontal.*

costal dysfunction: See *rib, dysfunction.*

counternutation: Posterior movement of the sacral base around a transverse axis in relation to the ilia. See also *nutation.*

counterstrain technique: See *osteopathic manipulative treatment, counterstrain.*

cranial manipulation: See *osteopathic manipulative treatment, cranial manipulation.*

cranial rhythmic impulse (CRI): 1. A palpable, rhythmic fluctuation believed to be synchronous with the primary respiratory mechanism. 2. Term coined by John Woods, DO, and Rachel Woods, DO.

cranial technique: See *osteopathic manipulative treatment, osteopathy in the cranial field.* See also *primary respiratory mechanism.*

craniosacral manipulation: See *osteopathic manipulative treatment, osteopathy in the cranial field.*

craniosacral mechanism: 1. A term used to refer to the anatomical connection between the occiput and the sacrum by the spinal dura mater. 2. A term coined by William G. Sutherland, DO. See also *extension, craniosacral extension and flexion, craniosacral flexion.*

C-SPOMM: Certification Special Proficiency in Osteopathic Manipulative Medicine. Granted by the American Osteopathic Association through the American Osteopathic Board of Special Proficiency in Osteopathic Manipulative Medicine from 1989 through 1999. See also *NMM-OMM.*

creep: The capacity of fascia and other tissue to lengthen when subjected to a constant tension load resulting in less resistance to a second load application.

CV-4: See *osteopathic manipulative treatment, CV-4.*

D

Dalrymple treatment: See *osteopathic manipulative treatment, pedal pump.*

decompensation: A dysfunctional, persistent pattern, in some cases reversible, resulting when homeostatic mechanisms are partially or totally overwhelmed.

depressed rib: See *rib somatic dysfunction, exhalation rib dysfunction.*

dermatome: 1. The area of skin supplied by cutaneous branches from a single spinal nerve. (Neighboring dermatomes may overlap.) 2. Cutis plate; the dorsolateral part of an embryonic somite (Figs. 6 and 7).

diagnostic palpation: See *palpatory diagnosis.*

diagonal axis: See *sacral, oblique axis, diagonal.*

direct method (technique): See *osteopathic manipulative treatment, direct treatment.*

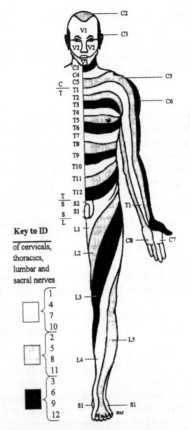

Figure 6 Dermatomal map (anterior). (Modified from Agur AMR, *Grant's Atlas of Anatomy,* 9th ed. Baltimore, Md: Williams & Wilkins; 1991:37).

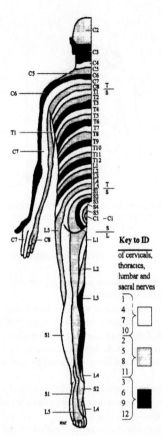

Figure 7 Dermatomal map (posterior). (Modified from Agur AMR, *Grant's Atlas of Anatomy*, 9th ed. Baltimore, Md: Williams & Wilkins; 1991:37).

Key to ID
of cervicals, thoracics, lumbar and sacral nerves

DO: 1. Doctor of Osteopathy (graduate of a school accredited by the American Osteopathic Association). 2. Doctor of Osteopathic Medicine (graduate of a school accredited by the American Osteopathic Association). 3. Diplomate in Osteopathy (The first degree granted by American School of Osteopathy). 4. Diplomate of Osteopathy, a degree granted by some schools of osteopathy outside the United States (not accredited by the American Osteopathic Association).

drag: See *skin drag*.

E

ease: Relative palpable freedom of motion of an articulation or tissue. Synonyms: compliance, resilience. Antonyms: bind, resistance.

easy normal: See *neutral, definition number 2.*

-ed: A suffix describing status, position, or condition (e.g., extended, flexed, rotated, restricted).

effleurage: Stroking movement used to move fluids.

elastic deformation: Any recoverable deformation. See also *plastic deformation.*

elasticity: Ability of a strained body or tissue to recover its original shape after deformation. See also *plasticity and viscosity.*

elevated rib: See *rib somatic dysfunction, inhalation rib dysfunction.* See also *rib motion, exhalation rib restriction.*

end feel: Perceived quality of motion as an anatomic or physiologic restrictive barrier is approached.

enthesitis: 1. Traumatic disease occurring at the insertion of muscles where recurring concentration of muscle stress provokes inflammation with a strong tendency toward fibrosis and calcification *(Stedman's).* 2. Inflammation of the muscular or tendinous attachment to bone *(Dorland's).*

ERS: A descriptor of spinal somatic dysfunction used to denote a combination extended (E), rotated (R), and sidebent (S) vertebral position.

ERS left, somatic dysfunction in which the vertebral unit is extended, rotated and sidebent left; usually preceded by a designation of the vertebral unit(s) involved (e.g., T5 ERS left or T5 ERLSL).

ERS right, somatic dysfunction in which the vertebral unit is extended, rotated and sidebent right; usually preceded by a designation of the vertebral unit(s) involved (e.g., C3-5 ERS right or C3-5 ERRSR).

exaggeration method: See *osteopathic manipulative treatment, exaggeration method.*

exaggeration technique: See *osteopathic manipulative treatment, exaggeration technique.*

exhaled rib: (Archaic) using positional (static) diagnosis. See *rib somatic dysfunction, exhalation rib dysfunction.*

exhalation rib dysfunction: See *rib somatic dysfunction, exhalation rib dysfunction.*

exhalation rib restriction: See *rib motion, exhalation rib restriction.* See also *rib somatic dysfunction, inhalation rib dysfunction.*

exhalation strain: See *rib somatic dysfunction, exhalation rib dysfunction.*

extension: 1. Accepted universal term for backward motion of the spine in a sagittal plane about a transverse axis; in a vertebral unit when the superior part moves backward. 2. In extremities, it is the straightening of a curve or angle (biomechanics). 3. Separation of the ends of a curve in a spinal region; See *extension, regional extension.*

craniosacral e., motion occurring during the cranial rhythmic impulse when the sphenobasilar symphysis descends and sacral base moves anteriorly (Fig. 8).

regional e., historically, the straightening in the sagittal plane of a spinal region; also called Fryette's regional extension (Fig. 9).

sacral e., posterior movement of the base of the sacrum in relation to the ilia (Fig. 10). See also *flexion, sacral flexion.*

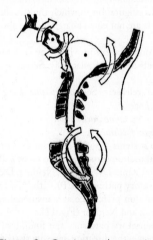

Figure 8 Craniosacral extension.

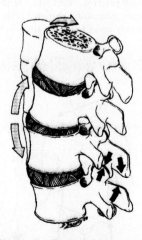

Figure 9 Regional extension.

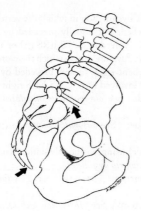

Figure 10 Sacral extension.

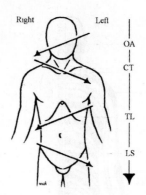

Figure 12 Uncommon compensatory fascial pattern (Zink).

extrinsic corrective forces: Treatment forces external to the patient that may include operator effort, effect of gravity, mechanical tables, etc. See also *intrinsic corrective forces.*

F

FAAO: 1. Fellow of American Academy of Osteopathy. 2. This fellowship is an earned postdoctoral degree conferred by the American Academy of Osteopathy. Those who earn the FAAO degree must have demonstrated their commitment to osteopathic principles and practice through teaching, writing, and professional service, performed at the highest level of professional and ethical standards.

facet asymmetry: Configuration in which the structure, position and/or motion of the facets are not equal bilaterally. See also *facet symmetry and tropism, facet.*

facet symmetry: Configuration in which the structure, position and/or motion of the facets are equal bilaterally. See also *facet asymmetry and symmetry.*

facilitated positional release: See *osteopathic manipulative treatment, facilitated positional release.*

facilitated segment: See *spinal facilitation.*

facilitation: See *spinal facilitation.*

fascial patterns: 1. Systems for classifying and recording the preferred directions of fascial motion throughout the body. 2. Based on the observations of J. Gordon Zink, DO, and W. Neidner, DO.

common compensatory pattern (CCP), the specific finding of alternating fascial motion preference at transitional regions of the body described by Zink and Neidner (Fig. 11).

uncommon compensatory pattern, the finding of alternating fascial motion preference in the direction opposite that of the common compensatory pattern described by Zink and Neidner (Fig. 12).

uncompensated fascial pattern, the finding of fascial preferences that do not demonstrate alternating patterns of findings at transitional regions. Because they occur following stress or trauma, they tend to be symptomatic.

fascial release technique: See *osteopathic manipulative treatment, myofascial release.*

fascial unwinding: See *osteopathic manipulative treatment, fascial unwinding.*

Ferguson angle: See *angle, lumbosacral.*

flexion: 1. Accepted universal term for forward motion of the spine, in its sagittal plane about a transverse axis, where the superior part moves forward. 2. In the extremities, it is the approximation of a curve or angle (biomechanics). 3. Approximation of the ends of a curve in a spinal region; also called Fryette regional flexion. See *flexion, regional flexion.*

craniosacral flexion, motion occurring during the cranial rhythmic impulse, when the sphenobasilar symphysis ascends and the sacral base moves posteriorly. (Fig. 13)

regional f., historically, is the approximation of the ends of a curve in the sagittal plane of the spine; also called Fryette regional flexion. See *flexion.* (Fig. 14)

sacral f., anterior movement of sacral base in relation to the ilia (Fig. 15). See also *extension, sacral extension.*

flexion left: See *sidebending.*

flexion right: See *sidebending.*

flexion tests: Tests for iliosacral or sacroiliac somatic dysfunction.

seated flexion test, a screening test that determines the side of sacroiliac somatic dysfunction (motion of the sacrum on the ilium).

standing flexion test, a screening test that determines the side of iliosacral somatic dysfunction (motion of ilium on the sacrum).

forward bending: Reciprocal of backward bending. See *flexion.*

forward torsions: See *sacrum, somatic dysfunctions of, forward torsions.*

FRS: A descriptor of spinal somatic dysfunction used to denote a combination flexed (F), rotated (R), and sidebent (S) vertebral position.

FRS left, somatic dysfunction in which the vertebral unit is flexed, rotated and sidebent left; usually preceded by a designation of the vertebral unit(s) involved (e.g., T5 FRS left or T5 FRLSL).

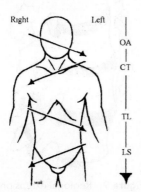

Figure 11 Common compensatory fascial pattern (Zink).

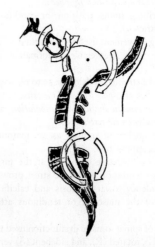

Figure 13 Craniosacral flexion.

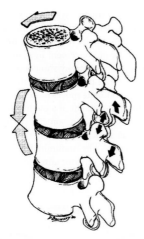

Figure 14 Regional flexion.

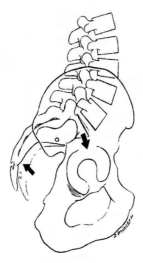

Figure 15 Sacral flexion.

FRS right, somatic dysfunction in which the vertebral unit is flexed, rotated and sidebent right; usually preceded by a designation of the vertebral unit(s) involved (e.g., C3-5 FRS right or C3-5 FRRSR).

frontal plane: See *plane, frontal.*

Fryette laws: See *laws, Fryette.* See *physiologic motion of the spine.*

Fryette principles: See *physiologic motion of the spine.*

Fryette regional extension: See *extension, regional extension.*

Fryette regional flexion: See *flexion, regional flexion.*

FSR: A descriptor of spinal somatic dysfunction used to denote a combination flexed (F), sidebent (S), and rotated (R) vertebral position. See *FRS.*

functional method: See *osteopathic manipulative treatment, functional method.*

functional technique: See *osteopathic manipulative treatment, functional method.*

G

gait: a forward translation of the body's center of gravity by bipedal locomotion. *(DeLisa)*

Galbreath treatment: See *osteopathic manipulative treatment, mandibular drainage.*

gravitational line: Viewing the patient from the side, an imaginary line in a coronal plane which, in the theoretical ideal posture, starts slightly anterior to the lateral malleolus, passes across the lateral condyle of the knee, the greater trochanter, through the lateral head of the humerus at the tip of the shoulder to the external auditory meatus; if this were a plane through the body, it would intersect the middle of the third lumbar vertebra and the anterior one third of the sacrum. It is used to evaluate

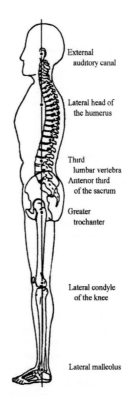

Figure 16 Gravitational line.

the A-P (anterior-posterior) curves of the spine. See also *mid-malleolar line* (Fig. 16).

H

habituation: Decreased physiologic response to repeated stimulation.

health: Adaptive and optimal attainment of physical, mental, emotional, spiritual and environmental well-being.

hepatic pump: See *osteopathic manipulative treatment, hepatic pump.*

high velocity/low amplitude technique (HVLA): See *osteopathic manipulative treatment, high velocity/low amplitude technique (HVLA).*

hip bone: See *innominate.* See also *innominate, somatic dysfunctions of.*

homeostasis: 1. Maintenance of static or constant conditions in the internal environment. 2. The level of well-being of an individual maintained by internal physiologic harmony that is the result of a relatively stable state or equilibrium among the interdependent body functions.

homeostatic mechanism: A system of control activated by negative feedback *(Dorland's).*

Hoover technique: See *osteopathic manipulative treatment, Hoover technique.*

hysteresis: During the loading and unloading of connective tissue, the restoration of the final length of the tissue occurs at a rate and to an extent less than during deformation (loading). These differences represent energy loss in the connective tissue system. This difference in viscoelastic behavior (and energy loss) is known as hysteresis (or "stress-strain"). *(Foundations, 2nd ed, p. 1158).*

hypertonicity: 1. A condition of excessive tone of the skeletal muscles. 2. Increased resistance of muscle to passive stretching.

I

ILA: See *sacrum, inferior lateral angle of.*

ilia: The plural of ilium. See *ilium.*

ilial compression test: See *ASIS compression test.*

ilial rocking test: See *ASIS compression test.*

iliosacral motion: Motion of one innominate (ilium) with respect to the sacrum. Iliosacral motion is part of pelvic motion during the gait cycle.

iliosacral dysfunction: See *innominate somatic dysfunctions.*

ilium: the expansive superior portion of the innominate (hip bone or os coxae).

indirect method: See *osteopathic manipulative treatment, indirect method.*

inferior ilium: See *innominate, somatic dysfunctions of, inferior innominate shear.*

inferior lateral angle (ILA) of the sacrum: See *sacrum, inferior lateral angle.*

inferior pubis: See *pubic bone, somatic dysfunctions of, inferior pubic shear.*

inferior transverse axis: See *sacral motion axis, inferior transverse axis.*

inhalation rib: See *rib somatic dysfunction, inhalation rib dysfunction.*

inhalation rib restriction: See *rib somatic dysfunction, inhalation rib dysfunction.*

inhalation strain: See *rib somatic dysfunction, inhalation rib dysfunction.*

inhibition: See *osteopathic manipulative treatment, inhibitory pressure technique.*

inhibitory pressure technique: See *osteopathic manipulative treatment, inhibitory pressure technique.*

innominate: The os coxae is a large irregular shaped bone that consists of three parts: ilium, ischium and pubis, which meet at the acetabulum, the cup shaped cavity for the head of the femur at the hip (femoroacetabular) joint. Also called the innominate bone or pelvic bone. See also *hip bone.*

innominate rotation: Rotational motion of one innominate bone relative to the sacrum on the inferior transverse axis.

innominate somatic dysfunctions: anterior innominate rotation, a somatic dysfunction in which the anterior superior iliac spine (ASIS) is anterior and inferior to the contralateral landmark. The innominate (os coxae) moves more freely in an anterior and inferior direction, and is restricted from movement in a posterior and superior direction (Fig. 17).

downslipped innominate, See *inferior innominate shear.*

inferior innominate shear, a somatic dysfunction in which the anterior superior iliac spine (ASIS) and posterior superior iliac spines (PSIS) are inferior to the contralateral landmarks. The innominate (os coxae) moves more freely in an inferior direction, and is restricted from movement in a superior direction (Fig. 18).

inflared innominate, a somatic dysfunction of the innominate (os coxae) resulting in medial positioning of the anterior superior iliac spine (ASIS). The innominate moves more freely in a medial direction, and is restricted from movement in a lateral direction (Fig. 19).

outflared innominate, a somatic dysfunction of the innominate (os coxae) resulting in lateral positioning of the anterior superior iliac spine (ASIS). The innominate moves more freely in a lateral direction, and is restricted from movement in a medial direction (Fig. 20).

posterior innominate rotation, a somatic dysfunction in which the anterior superior iliac spine (ASIS) is posterior and superior to the contralateral landmarks. The innominate (os coxae) moves more freely in a posterior and superior direction, and is restricted from movement in an anterior and inferior direction (Fig. 21).

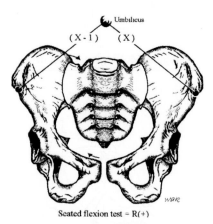

Figure 19 Inflared right innominate.

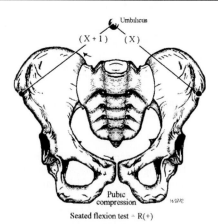

Figure 20 Outflared right innominate.

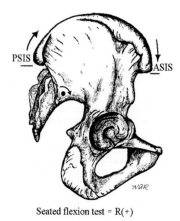

Figure 17 Anterior right innominate. Forced anterior rotation can also result in an inferior pubic shear.

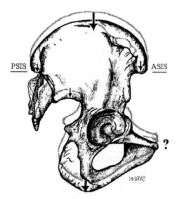

Figure 18 Right inferior innominate shear. This also may or may not result in an inferior pubic shear.

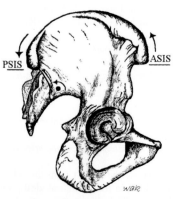

Figure 21 Right posterior innominate. Forced posterior rotation may or may not result in a superior pubic shear.

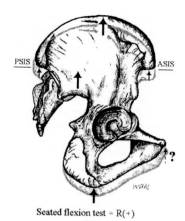

PSIS   ASIS

?

wak

Seated flexion test = R(+)

Figure 22 Right superior innominate shear. This also may or may not result in a superior pubic shear.

superior innominate shear, a somatic dysfunction in which the anterior superior iliac spine (ASIS) and posterior superior iliac spines (PSIS) are superior to the contralateral landmarks. The innominate (os coxae) moves more freely in a superior direction, and is restricted from movement in an inferior direction (Fig. 22).

upslipped innominate, See *superior innominate shear.*

integrated neuromusculoskeletal release: See *osteopathic manipulative treatment, integrated neuromusculoskeletal release.*

intersegmental motion: Designates relative motion taking place between two adjacent vertebral segments or within a vertebral unit that is described as the upper vertebral segment moving on the lower.

intrinsic corrective forces: Voluntary or involuntary forces from within the patient that assist in the manipulative treatment process. See also *extrinsic corrective forces.*

isokinetic exercise: Exercise using a constant speed of movement of the body part.

isolytic contraction: See *contraction, isolytic c.*

isometric contraction: See *contraction, isometric c.*

isotonic contraction: See *contraction, isotonic c.*

J

Jones technique: See *osteopathic manipulative treatment, counterstrain.*

junctional region: See *transitional region.*

K

key lesion: The somatic dysfunction that maintains a total dysfunction pattern including other secondary dysfunctions.

kinesthesia: The sense by which muscular motion, weight, position, etc. are perceived.

kinesthetic: Pertaining to kinesthesia.

kinetics: The body of knowledge that deals with the effects of forces that produce or modify body motion.

klapping: Striking the skin with cupped palms to produce vibrations with the intention of loosening material in the lumen of hollow tubes or sacs within the body, particularly the lungs.

kneading: A soft tissue technique that utilizes an intermittent force applied perpendicular to the long axis of the muscle.

kyphoscoliosis: A spinal curve pattern combining kyphosis and scoliosis. See also *kyphosis.* See also *scoliosis.*

kyphosis: 1. The exaggerated (pathologic) A-P curve of the thoracic spine with concavity anteriorly. 2. Abnormally increased convexity in the curvature of the thoracic spine as viewed from the side *(Dorland's).*

kyphotic: Pertaining to or characterized by kyphosis.

L

lateral flexed vertebral body: See *sidebent.*

lateral flexion: Also called lateroflexion. See *sidebending.*

lateral masses (of the atlas): The most bulky and solid parts of the atlas that support the weight of the head.

lateroflexion: See *sidebending.*

law:

Fryette l., of motion, See *physiologic motion of the spine.*

Head l., when a painful stimulus is applied to a body part of low sensitivity (e.g., viscus) that is in close central connection with a point of higher sensitivity (e.g., soma), the pain is felt at the point of higher sensitivity rather than at the point where the stimulus was applied.

Lovett l., An observed association between the superior and inferior vertebrae, which are paired two by two. The cervical and superior thoracic biomechanics act in a synchronous manner with the lumbar and inferior thoracic biomechanics. For example, if C1 is in a right posterior positional lesion, L5 also moves into a right posterior position. In this case, L5 is the "Lovett partner" of C1. The treatment of L5 helps to stabilize C1 and the skull by changing the lines of gravity (French usage).

Sherrington l., 1. Every posterior spinal nerve root supplies a specific region of the skin, although fibers from adjacent spinal segments may invade such a region. 2. When a muscle receives a nerve impulse to contract, its antagonist receives, simultaneously, an impulse to relax. (These are only two of Sherrington's contributions to neurophysiology; these are the ones most relevant to osteopathic principles.)

Wolff l., every change in form and function of a bone, or in its function alone, is followed by certain definite changes in its internal architecture, and secondary alterations in its external conformations *(Stedman's, 25th ed);* (e.g., bone is laid down along lines of stress).

lesion (osteopathic): See *osteopathic lesion.* See *somatic dysfunction*

ligamentous:

l. **articular strain,** any somatic dysfunction resulting in abnormal ligamentous tension or strain. See also *osteopathic manipulative treatment, ligamentous articular strain technique.*

l. **articular strain technique,** See *osteopathic manipulative treatment, ligamentous articular strain technique.*

l. **strain,** motion and/or positional asymmetry associated with elastic deformation of connective tissue (fascia, ligament, membrane). See *strain and ligamentous articular strain.*

line of gravity: See *gravitational line.*

linkage: See *somatic dysfunction, linkage.*

liver pump: See *osteopathic manipulative treatment, hepatic pump.*

localization: 1. In manipulative technique, the precise positioning of the patient and vector application of forces required to produce a desired result. 2. The reference of a sensation to a particular locality in the body.

longitudinal axis: See *sacral, sacral motion axis, longitudinal axis.*

lordosis: 1. The anterior convexity in the curvature of the lumbar and cervical spine as viewed from the side. The term is used to refer to abnormally increased curvature (hollow back, saddle back, sway back) and to the normal curvature (normal lordosis). *(Dorland's).* 2. Hollow back or saddle back; an abnormal extension deformity; anteroposterior curvature of the spine, generally lumbar with the convexity looking anteriorly *(Stedman's).*

lordotic: Pertaining to or characterized by lordosis.

lumbarization: See *transitional vertebrae, lumbarization.*

lumbolumbar lordotic angle: See *angle, lumbolumbar lordotic.*

lumbosacral angle: See *angle, lumbosacral.*

lumbosacral lordotic angle: See *angle, lumbosacral lordotic.*

lumbosacral spring test: See *spring test.*

lymphatic pumps: See *osteopathic manipulative treatment, lymphatic pump.* See also *osteopathic manipulative treatment, pedal pump.* See also *osteopathic manipulative treatment, thoracic pump.*

lymphatic treatment: Techniques used to optimize function of the lymphatic system. See *osteopathic manipulative treatment, lymphatic pump.* See also *osteopathic manipulative treatment, pedal pump.* See also *osteopathic manipulative treatment, thoracic pump.*

M

mandibular drainage technique: See *osteopathic manipulative treatment, mandibular drainage technique.*

manipulation: Therapeutic application of manual force. See also *technique.* See also *osteopathic manipulative treatment.*

manual medicine: The skillful use of the hands to diagnose and treat structural and functional abnormalities in various tissues and organs throughout the body, including bones, joints, muscles and other soft tissues as an integral part of complete medical care. 1. This term originated from the German *Manuelle Medizin* (manual medicine) and has been used interchangeably with the term manipulation. 2. This term is not identical to manual therapy, which has been used by nonphysician practitioners (e.g., physical therapists).

massage: Therapeutic friction, stroking, and kneading of the body. See also *osteopathic manipulative treatment, soft tissue treatment.*

membranous articular strain: Any cranial somatic dysfunction resulting in abnormal dural membrane tensions.

membranous balance: The ideal physiologic state of harmonious equilibrium in the tension of the dura mater of the brain and spinal cord.

mesenteric lift: See *osteopathic manipulative treatment, mesenteric release technique.*

mesenteric release technique: See *osteopathic manipulative treatment, mesenteric release technique.*

middle transverse axis: See *sacral motion axis, middle transverse axis (postural).*

mid-heel line: A vertical line used as a reference in standing anteroposterior (A-P) x-rays and postural evaluation, passing equidistant between the heels.

mid-gravitational line: See *gravitational line.*

mid-malleolar line: A vertical line passing through the lateral malleolus, used as a point of reference in standing lateral x-rays and postural evaluation. See also *gravitational line.*

mirror-image motion asymmetries: A grouping of primary and secondary sites of somatic dysfunction describing a three-segment complex fundamental to dysfunction in a mobile system. Each adjacent segment, above and below the primary locus, demonstrates opposing asymmetries to that locus. For example, if the primary locus resists rotation right, the segments above and below resist rotation left.

mobile point: In counterstrain, the final position of treatment at which tenderness is no longer elicited by palpation of the tender point. mobile segment: A term in functional methods to describe a bony structure with its articular surfaces and adnexal tissues (neuromuscular and connective) for segmental motion which affects movement, stabilizes position and allows coordinated participation in passive movement.

mobile system: An osteopathic construct associated with functional methods in which the body as a whole is viewed as a centrally integrated system in which all of the individual elements (e.g., mobile segments) have coordinated and specific motion characteristics. See also *functional methods.*

mobile unit: See *mobile segment.*

models of osteopathic care: Five models that articulate how an osteopathic practitioner seeks to influence a patient's physiological processes.

structural model, the goal of the structural model is biomechanical adjustment and the mobilization of joints. This model also seeks to address problems in the myofascial connective tissues, as well as in the bony and soft tissues, to remove restrictive forces and enhance motion. This is accomplished by the use of a wide range of osteopathic manipulative techniques such as high velocity-low amplitude, muscle energy, counterstrain, myofascial release, ligamentous articular techniques and functional techniques.

respiratory-circulatory model, the goal of the respiratory-circulatory model is to improve all of the diaphragm restrictions in the body. Diaphragms are considered to be "transverse restrictors" of motion, venous and lymphatic drainage and cerebrospinal fluid. The techniques used in this model are osteopathy in the cranial field, ligamentous articular strain, myofascial release and lymphatic pump techniques.

metabolic model, the goal of the metabolic model is to enhance the selfregulatory and self-healing mechanisms, to foster energy conservation by balancing the body's energy expenditure and exchange, and to enhance immune system function, endocrine function and organ function. The osteopathic considerations in this area are not manipulative in nature except for the use of lymphatic pump techniques. Nutritional counseling, diet and exercise advice are the most common approaches to balancing the body through this model.

neurologic model, the goal of the neurologic model is to attain autonomic balance and address neural reflex activity, remove facilitated segments, decrease afferent nerve signals and relieve pain. The osteopathic manipulative techniques used to influence this area of patient health include counterstrain and Chapman reflex points.

behavioral model, the goal of this model is to improve the biological, psychological and social components of the health spectrum. This includes emotional balancing and compensatory mechanisms. Reproductive processes and behavioral adaption are also included under this model.

motion: 1. A change of position (rotation and/or translation) with respect to a fixed system; 2. An act or process of a body changing position in terms of direction, course and velocity.

active m., movement produced voluntarily by the patient.

inherent m., spontaneous motion of every cell, organ, system and their component units within the body.

m. barrier, See *barrier (motion barrier).*

passive m., motion induced by the osteopathic practitioner while the patient remains passive or relaxed.

physiologic m., changes in position of body structures within the normal range. See also *physiologic motion of the spine.*

translatory m., motion of a body part along an axis. See also *translation.*

muscle energy technique: See *osteopathic manipulative treatment, muscle energy.*

myofascial release technique: See *osteopathic manipulative treatment, myofascial release.*

myofascial technique: See *osteopathic manipulative treatment, myofascial technique.*

myofascial trigger point: See *trigger point.*

myogenic tonus: 1. Tonic contraction of muscle dependent on some property of the muscle itself or of its intrinsic nerve cells. 2. Contraction of a muscle caused by intrinsic properties of the muscle or by its intrinsic innervation *(Stedman's).*

myotome: 1. All muscles derived from one somite and innervated by one segmental spinal nerve. 2. That part of the somite that develops into skeletal muscle *(Stedman's).*

N

neurotrophicity: See *neurotrophy.*

neurotrophy: The nutrition and maintenance of tissues as regulated by direct innervation.

neutral: 1. The range of sagittal plane spinal positioning in which the first principle of physiologic motion of the spine applies. See also *physiologic motion of the spine.* 2. The point of balance of an articular surface from which all the motions physiologic to that articulation may take place (Fig. 23).

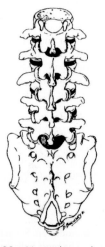

Figure 23 Neutral spinal position.

NMM-OMM: Osteopathic neuromusculoskeletal medicine certification is granted by the American Osteopathic Association through the American Osteopathic Board of Neuromusculoskeletal Medicine. First granted in 1999.

non-neutral: The range of sagittal plane spinal positioning in which the second principle of physiologic motion of the spine applies. See also *extension*. See also *flexion*. See also *physiologic motion of the spine*.

normalization: The therapeutic use of anatomic and physiologic mechanisms to facilitate the body's response toward homeostasis and improved health.

NSR: A descriptor of spinal somatic dysfunction used to denote a combination neutral (N), sidebent (S), and rotated (R) vertebral position; similar descriptors may involve flexed (F) and extended (E) position.

nutation: Nodding forward; anterior movement of the sacral base around a transverse axis in relation to the ilia.

O

oblique axis: See *sacral motion axis, oblique (diagonal)*.

OMM: See *osteopathic manipulative medicine*.

OMTh: See *osteopathic manipulative therapy*.

OMT: See *osteopathic manipulative treatment*.

ONM: See *NMM-OMM*.

OP&P: Osteopathic principles and practice. See also *osteopathic philosophy*. Archaic.

OPP: Osteopathic principles and practice. See also *osteopathic philosophy*.

os coxae: See *innominate*.

osteopath: 1. A person who has achieved the nationally recognized academic and professional standards within her or his country to independently practice diagnosis and treatment based upon the principles of osteopathic philosophy. Individual countries establish the national academic and professional standards for osteopaths practicing within their countries (International usage). 2. Considered by the American Osteopathic Association to be an archaic term when applied to graduates of U.S. schools.

osteopathic lesion (osteopathic lesion complex): Archaic term used to describe somatic dysfunction. See *somatic dysfunction*.

osteopathic manipulative medicine (OMM): The application of osteopathic philosophy, structural diagnosis and use of OMT in the diagnosis and management of the patient.

osteopathic manipulative therapy (OMTh): The therapeutic application of manually guided forces by an osteopath (nonphysician) to improve physiological function and homeostasis that has been altered by somatic dysfunction.

osteopathic manipulative treatment (OMT): The therapeutic application of manually guided forces by an osteopathic physician (U.S. usage) to improve physiologic function and/or support homeostasis that has been altered by somatic dysfunction. OMT employs a variety of techniques including:

active method, technique in which the person voluntarily performs an osteopathic practitioner-directed motion.

articulatory treatment, (Archaic). See *osteopathic manipulative treatment, articulatory treatment system*.

articulatory (ART), a low velocity/moderate to high amplitude technique where a joint is carried through its full motion with the therapeutic goal of increased range of movement. The activating force is either a repetitive springing motion or repetitive concentric movement of the joint through the restrictive barrier.

balanced ligamentous tension (BLT), 1. According to Sutherland's model, all the joints in the body are balanced ligamentous articular mechanisms. The ligaments provide proprioceptive information that guides the muscle response for positioning the joint, and the ligaments themselves guide the motion of the articular components. (*Foundations*) 2. First described in "Osteopathic Technique of William G. Sutherland," that was published in the *1949 Year Book of Academy of Applied Osteopathy*. See also *ligamentous articular strain*.

Chapman reflex, See *Chapman reflex*. combined method, 1. A treatment strategy where the initial movements are indirect; as the technique is completed the movements change to direct forces. 2. A manipulative sequence involving two or more different osteopathic manipulative treatment systems (e.g., Spencer technique combined with muscle energy technique). 3. A concept described by Paul Kimberly, DO.

combined treatment, (Archaic). See *osteopathic manipulative treatment, combined method*.

compression of the fourth ventricle (CV-4), a cranial technique in which the lateral angles of the occipital squama are manually approximated slightly exaggerating the posterior convexity of the occiput and taking the cranium into sustained extension.

counterstrain (CS), 1. A system of diagnosis and treatment that considers the dysfunction to be a continuing, inappropriate strain reflex, which is inhibited by applying a position of mild strain in the direction exactly opposite to that of the reflex; this is accomplished by specific directed positioning about the point of tenderness to achieve the desired therapeutic response. 2. Australian and French use: Jones technique, (correction spontaneous by position), spontaneous release by position. 3. Developed by Lawrence Jones, DO in 1955 (originally "Spontaneous Release by Positioning," later termed "strain-counterstrain").

cranial treatment (CR), See *primary respiratory mechanism*. See *osteopathy in the cranial field*.

CV-4, abbreviation for compression of the fourth ventricle. See *osteopathic manipulative treatment, compression of the fourth ventricle*.

Dalrymple treatment, See *osteopathic manipulative treatment, pedal pump*.

direct method (D/DIR), an osteopathic treatment strategy by which the restrictive barrier is engaged and a final activating force is applied to correct somatic dysfunction.

exaggeration method, an osteopathic treatment strategy by which the dysfunctional component is carried away from the restrictive barrier and beyond the range of voluntary motion to a point of palpably increased tension.

exaggeration technique, an indirect procedure that involves carrying the dysfunctional part away from the restrictive barrier, then applying a high velocity/low amplitude force in the same direction.

facilitated oscillatory release technique (FOR), 1. A technique intended to normalize neuromuscular function by applying a manual oscillatory force, which may be combined with any other ligamentous or myofascial technique. 2. A refinement of a long-standing use of oscillatory force in osteopathic diagnosis and treatment as published in early osteopathic literature. 3. A technique developed by Zachary Comeaux, DO.

facilitated positional release (FPR), a system of indirect myofascial release treatment. The component region of the body is placed into a neutral position, diminishing tissue and joint tension in all planes, and an activating force (compression or torsion) is added. 2. A technique developed by Stanley Schiowitz, DO.

fascial release treatment, See *osteopathic manipulative treatment, myofascial release*.

fascial unwinding, a manual technique involving constant feedback to the osteopathic practitioner who is passively moving a portion of the patient's body in response to the sensation of movement. Its forces are localized using the sensations of ease and bind over wider regions.

functional method, an indirect treatment approach that involves finding the dynamic balance point and one of the following: applying an indirect guiding force, holding the position or adding compression to exaggerate position and allow for spontaneous readjustment. The osteopathic practitioner guides the manipulative procedure while the dysfunctional area is being palpated in order to obtain a continuous feedback of the physiologic response to induced motion. The osteopathic practitioner guides the dysfunctional part so as to create a decreasing sense of tissue resistance (increased compliance).

Galbreath treatment, See *osteopathic manipulative treatment, mandibular drainage*.

hepatic pump, rhythmic compression applied over the liver for purposes of increasing blood flow through the liver and enhancing bile and lymphatic drainage from the liver.

high velocity/low amplitude technique (HVLA), an osteopathic technique employing a rapid, therapeutic force of brief duration that travels a short distance within the anatomic range of motion of a joint, and that engages the restrictive barrier in one or more planes of motion to elicit release of restriction. Also known as thrust technique.

Hoover technique, 1. A form of functional method. 2. Developed by H.V. Hoover, DO. See also *osteopathic manipulative treatment, functional technique.*

indirect method (I/IND), a manipulative technique where the restrictive barrier is disengaged and the dysfunctional body part is moved away from the restrictive barrier until tissue tension is equal in one or all planes and directions.

inhibitory pressure technique, the application of steady pressure to soft tissues to reduce reflex activity and produce relaxation.

integrated neuromusculoskeletal release (INR), a treatment system in which combined procedures are designed to stretch and reflexly release patterned soft tissue and joint-related restrictions. Both direct and indirect methods are used interactively.

Jones technique, See *osteopathic manipulative treatment, counterstrain.*

ligamentous articular strain technique (LAS), 1. A manipulative technique in which the goal of treatment is to balance the tension in opposing ligaments where there is abnormal tension present. 2. A set of myofascial release techniques described by Howard Lippincott, DO, and Rebecca Lippincott, DO. 3. Title of reference work by Conrad Speece, DO, and William Thomas Crow, DO.

liver pump, See *hepatic pump.*

lymphatic pump, 1. A term used to describe the impact of intrathoracic pressure changes on lymphatic flow. This was the name originally given to the thoracic pump technique before the more extensive physiologic effects of the technique were recognized. 2. A term coined by C. Earl Miller, DO.

mandibular drainage technique, soft tissue manipulative technique using passively induced jaw motion to effect increased drainage of middle ear structures via the eustachian tube and lymphatics.

mesenteric release technique (mesenteric lift), technique in which tension is taken off the attachment of the root of the mesentery to the posterior body wall. Simultaneously, the abdominal contents are compressed to enhance venous and lymphatic drainage from the bowel.

muscle energy, a form of osteopathic manipulative diagnosis and treatment in which the patient's muscles are actively used on request, from a precisely controlled position, in a specific direction, and against a distinctly executed physician counterforce. First described in 1948 by Fred Mitchell, Sr, DO.

myofascial release (MFR), a system of diagnosis and treatment first described by Andrew Taylor Still and his early students, which engages continual palpatory feedback to achieve release of myofascial tissues.

direct MFR, a myofascial tissue restrictive barrier is engaged for the myofascial tissues and the tissue is loaded with a constant force until tissue release occurs.

indirect MFR, the dysfunctional tissues are guided along the path of least resistance until free movement is achieved.

myofascial technique, any technique directed at the muscles and fascia. See also *osteopathic manipulative treatment, myofascial release.* See also *osteopathic manipulative treatment, soft tissue technique.*

myotension, a system of diagnosis and treatment that uses muscular contractions and relaxations under resistance of the osteopathic practitioner to relax, strengthen or stretch muscles, or mobilize joints.

Osteopathy in the Cranial Field (OCF), 1. A system of diagnosis and treatment by an osteopathic practitioner using the primary respiratory mechanism and balanced membranous tension. See also *primary respiratory mechanism.* 2. Refers to the system of diagnosis and treatment first described by William G. Sutherland, DO. 3. Title of reference work by Harold Magoun, Sr, DO.

passive method, based on techniques in which the patient refrains from voluntary muscle contraction.

pedal pump, a venous and lymphatic drainage technique applied through the lower extremities; also called the pedal fascial pump or Dalrymple treatment.

percussion vibrator technique, 1. A manipulative technique involving the specific application of mechanical vibratory force to treat somatic dysfunction. 2. An osteopathic manipulative technique developed by Robert Fulford, DO.

positional technique, a direct segmental technique in which a combination of leverage, patient ventilatory movements and a fulcrum are used to achieve mobilization of the dysfunctional segment. May be combined with springing or thrust technique.

progressive inhibition of neuromuscular structures (PINS), 1. A system of diagnosis and treatment in which the osteopathic practitioner locates two related points and sequentially applies inhibitory pressure along a series of related points. 2. Developed by Dennis Dowling, DO.

range of motion technique, active or passive movement of a body part to its physiologic or anatomic limit in any or all planes of motion.

soft tissue (ST), A system of diagnosis and treatment directed toward tissues other than skeletal or arthrodial elements.

soft tissue technique, a direct technique that usually involves lateral stretching, linear stretching, deep pressure, traction and/or separation of muscle origin and insertion while monitoring tissue response and motion changes by palpation. Also called myofascial treatment.

Spencer technique, a series of direct manipulative procedures to prevent or decrease soft tissue restrictions about the shoulder. See also *osteopathic manipulative treatment (OMT), articulatory treatment (ART).*

splenic pump technique, rhythmic compression applied over the spleen for the purpose of enhancing the patient's immune response. See also *osteopathic manipulative treatment (OMT), lymphatic pump.*

spontaneous release by positioning, See *osteopathic manipulative treatment, counterstrain.*

springing technique, a low velocity/moderate amplitude technique where the restrictive barrier is engaged repeatedly to produce an increased freedom of motion. See also *osteopathic manipulative treatment, articulatory treatment system.*

Still technique, 1. Characterized as a specific, nonrepetitive articulatory method that is indirect, then direct. 2. Attributed to A.T. Still. 3. A term coined by Richard Van Buskirk, DO, PhD.

Strain-Counterstrain, 1. An osteopathic system of diagnosis and indirect treatment in which the patient's somatic dysfunction, diagnosed by (an) associated myofascial tenderpoint(s), is treated by using a passive position, resulting in spontaneous tissue release and at least 70% decrease in tenderness. 2. Developed by Lawrence H. Jones, DO, in 1955. See *osteopathic treatments, counterstrain.*

thoracic pump, 1. A technique that consists of intermittent compression of the thoracic cage. 2. Developed by C. Earl Miller, DO.

thrust technique (HVLA), See *osteopathic manipulative treatment, high velocity/low amplitude technique (HVLA).*

toggle technique, short lever technique using compression and shearing forces.

traction technique, a procedure of high or low amplitude in which the parts are stretched or separated along a longitudinal axis with continuous or intermittent force.

v-spread, technique using forces transmitted across the diameter of the skull to accomplish sutural gapping.

ventral techniques, See *osteopathic manipulative treatment, visceral manipulation.*

visceral manipulation (VIS), a system of diagnosis and treatment directed to the viscera to improve physiologic function. Typically, the viscera are moved toward their fascial attachments to a point of fascial balance. Also called ventral techniques.

osteopathic medicine: The preferred term for a complete system of medical care practiced by physicians with an unlimited license that is represented by a philosophy that combines the needs of the patient with the current practice of medicine, surgery and obstetrics. Emphasizes the interrelationship between structure and function, and has an appreciation of the body's ability to heal itself.

osteopathic musculoskeletal evaluation: The osteopathic musculoskeletal evaluation provides information regarding the health of the patient. Utilizing the concepts of body unity, self-regulation and structure-function interrelationships, the osteopathic physician uses data from the musculoskeletal evaluation to assess the patient's status and develop a treatment plan. (AOA House of Delegates)

osteopathic philosophy: a concept of health care supported by expanding scientific knowledge that embraces the concept of the unity of the living organism's structure (anatomy) and function (physiology). Osteopathic philosophy emphasizes the following principles: 1. The human being is a dynamic unit of function. 2. The body possesses self-regulatory mechanisms that are self-healing in nature. 3. Structure and function are interrelated at all levels. 4. Rational treatment is based on these principles.

osteopathic physician: A person with full unlimited medical practice rights who has achieved the nationally recognized academic and professional standards within his or her country to practice diagnosis and treatment based upon the principles of osteopathic philosophy. Individual countries establish the national academic and professional standards for osteopathic physicians practicing within their countries.

osteopathic postural examination: The part of the osteopathic musculoskeletal examination that focuses on the static and dynamic responses of the body to gravity while in the erect position.

osteopathic practitioner: Refers to an osteopath, an osteopathic physician or an allopathic physician who has been trained in osteopathic principles, practices and philosophy.

osteopathic structural examination: The examination of a patient by an osteopathic practitioner with emphasis on the neuromusculoskeletal system including palpatory diagnosis for somatic dysfunction and viscerosomatic change within the context of total patient care. The examination is concerned with finding somatic dysfunction in all parts of the body, and is performed with the patient in multiple positions to provide static and dynamic evaluation.

osteopathy: Archaic usage. No longer a preferred term in the United States. See *Osteopathic Medicine.*

P

palpation: The application of the fingers to the surface of the skin or other tissues, using varying amounts of pressure, to selectively determine the condition of the parts beneath.

palpatory diagnosis: A term used by osteopathic practitioners to denote the process of palpating the patient to evaluate the structure and function of the neuromusculoskeletal and visceral systems.

palpatory skills: Sensory skills used in performing palpatory diagnosis and osteopathic manipulative treatment.

passive method: See *osteopathic manipulative treatment, passive method.*

passive motion: See *motion, passive motion.*

patient cooperation: Voluntary movement by the patient (on instruction from the osteopathic practitioner) to assist in the palpatory diagnosis and treatment process.

pedal pump: See *osteopathic manipulative treatment, pedal pump.*

pelvic bone: See *hip bone.*

pelvic declination (pelvic unleveling): Pelvic rotation about an anterior-posterior (A-P) axis.

pelvic girdle dysfunction: See *pelvic somatic dysfunction.*

pelvic index (PI): Represents a ratio of the measurements determined from postural radiograph: One (y) beginning from a vertical line originating at the sacral promontory to the intersection with the horizontal line from the anteriorsuperior position of the pubic bone. The second measurement (x) is along this same horizontal line. Normal values are age-related and increase in subjects with sagittal plane postural decompensation. Pelvic index (PI) equals x/y (Fig. 24).

pelvic rotation: Movement of the entire pelvis in a relatively horizontal plane about a vertical (longitudinal) axis.

pelvic sideshift: Deviation of the pelvis to the right or left of the central vertical axis as translation occurs along the horizontal (z) axis. Usually observed in the standing position.

pelvic somatic dysfunctions: a group of somatic dysfunctions involving the sacrum and innominates. See *sacral somatic dysfunction and innominate somatic dysfunction.*

pelvic tilt: Pelvic rotation about a transverse (horizontal) axis (forward or backward tilt) or about an anterior-posterior axis (right or left side tilt).

pelvis: Within the context of structural diagnosis, the pelvis is made up of the right and left innominates, (hip bone or os coxae) the sacrum and coccyx.

percussion vibrator technique: See *osteopathic manipulative treatment, percussion vibrator technique.*

pétrissage: Deep kneading or squeezing action to express swelling.

physiologic barrier: See *barrier, physiologic barrier.*

physiologic motion: See *motion, physiologic motion.*

physiologic motion of the spine: The three major principles of physiologic motion are:

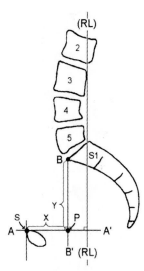

Figure 24 Pelvic index (PI). (Modified from Kuchera WA, Kuchera ML, *Osteopathic Principles in Practice,* Greyden Press, Columbus, OH, 1994:263).

I. When the thoracic and lumbar spine are in a neutral position (easy normal; See *neutral* Fig. 23), the coupled motions of sidebending and rotation for a group of vertebrae are such that sidebending and rotation occur in opposite directions (with rotation occurring toward the convexity) (Fig. 25). See *somatic dysfunction, type I s.d.*

II. When the thoracic and lumbar spine are sufficiently forward or backward bent (non-neutral), the coupled motions of sidebending and rotation in a single vertebral unit occur in the same direction (Fig. 26). See *somatic dysfunction, type II, s.d.*

III. 1. Initiating motion of a vertebral segment in any plane of motion will modify the movement of that segment in other planes of motion. 2. Principles I and II of thoracic and lumbar spinal motion described by Harrison H. Fryette, DO (1918), Principle III was described by C.R. Nelson, DO (1948). See *rotation.* See also *rotation of vertebra.*

plane: A flat surface determined by the position of three points in space. Any of a number of imaginary surfaces passing through the body and dividing it into segments (Fig. 27).

AP plane, See *plane, sagittal plane.*

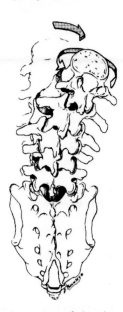

Figure 25 Physiologic motion of the thoracic or lumbar spine resulting from a neutral spinal position (Type I motion).

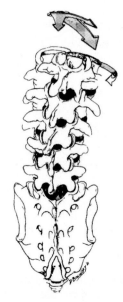

Figure 26 Physiologic motion of the thoracic or lumbar spine resulting from a non-neutral spinal position (Type II motion).

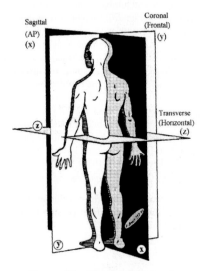

Figure 27 Planes of the body.

coronal plane (frontal plane), a plane passing longitudinally through the body from one side to the other, and dividing the body into anterior and posterior portions.

frontal plane, See *plane, coronal plane.*

horizontal plane, See *plane, transverse plane.*

sagittal plane, a plane passing longitudinally through the body from front to back and dividing it into right and left portions. The median or midsagittal plane divides the body into approximately equal right and left portions.

transverse plane (horizontal plane), a plane passing horizontally through the body perpendicular to the sagittal and frontal planes, dividing the body into upper and lower portions.

plastic deformation: A nonrecoverable deformation. See also *elastic deformation.*

plasticity: Ability to retain a shape attained by deformation. See also *elasticity.* See also *viscosity.*

positional technique: See *osteopathic manipulative treatment, positional technique.*

posterior component: A positional descriptor used to identify the side of reference when rotation of a vertebral segment has occurred. In a condition of right rotation, the right side is the posterior component.

It usually refers to a prominent vertebral transverse process. See also *anterior component.*

posterior nutation: See *counternutation.*

post-isometric relaxation: Immediately following an isometric contraction, the neuromuscular apparatus is in a refractory state during which enhanced passive stretching may be performed. The osteopathic practitioner may take up the myofascial slack during the relaxed refractory period.

postural axis: See *sacral motion axis, postural axis.*

postural balance: A condition of optimal distribution of body mass in relation to gravity.

postural decompensation: Distribution of body mass away from ideal when postural homeostatic mechanisms are overwhelmed. It occurs in all cardinal planes, but is classified by the major plane(s) affected. See *planes of the body.* (Fig. 27)

    coronal plane p. d., causes scoliotic changes.

    horizontal plane p. d., may cause postural changes where part or all of the body rotates to the right or left. When viewed from the right or left sides, alignment appears asymmetrical.

    sagittal plane p. d., causes kyphotic and/or lordotic changes.

postural imbalance: A condition in which ideal body mass distribution is not achieved.

posture: Position of the body. The distribution of body mass in relation to gravity.

primary machinery of life: 1. The neuromusculoskeletal system. A term used to denote that body parts act together to transmit and modify force and motion through which man acts out his life. This integration is achieved via the central nervous system acting in response to continued sensory input from the internal and external environment. 2. A term coined by I.M. Korr, PhD.

primary respiratory mechanism:

1. A conceptual model that describes a process involving five interactive, involuntary functions:

    (1) The inherent motility of the brain and spinal cord.

    (2) Fluctuation of the cerebrospinal fluid.

    (3) Mobility of the intracranial and intraspinal membranes.

    (4) Articular mobility of the cranial bones.

    (5) Mobility of the sacrum between the ilia (pelvic bones) that is interdependent with the motion at the sphenobasilar synchondrosis.

This mechanism refers to the presumed inherent (primordial) driving mechanism of internal respiration as opposed to the cycle of diaphragmatic respiration (inhalation and exhalation). It further refers to the innate interconnected movement of every tissue and structure of the body. Optimal health promotes optimal function and the inherent function of this interdependent movement can be negatively altered by trauma, disease states or other pathology.

2. This mechanism was first described by William G. Sutherland, DO, in 1939 in his self-published volume, "The Cranial Bowl." The mechanism is thought to affect cellular respiration and other body processes. In the original definition, the following descriptions were given:

    primary, because it is directly concerned with the internal tissue respiration of the central nervous system.

    respiratory, because it further concerns the physiological function of the interchange of fluids necessary for normal metabolism and biochemistry, not only of the central nervous system, but also of all body cells.

    mechanism, because all the constituent parts work together as a unit carrying out this fundamental physiology. See also *osteopathic manipulative treatment (OMT), osteopathy in the cranial field.*

prime mover: A muscle primarily responsible for causing a specific joint action.

progressive inhibition of neuromuscular structures (PINS): See *osteopathic manipulative treatment, Progressive Inhibition of Neuromuscular Structures.*

prolotherapy: See *sclerotherapy.*

pronation: In relation to the anatomical position, as applied to the hand, rotation of the forearm in such a way that the palmar surface turns backward (internal rotation) in relationship to the anatomical position. Applied to the foot: a combination of eversion and abduction movements taking place in the tarsal and metatarsal joints, resulting in lowering of the medial margin of the foot. See also *supination.*

prone: Lying face downward *(Dorland's)*.

psoas syndrome: A painful low back condition characterized by hypertonicity of psoas musculature. The syndrome consists of a constellation of typically related signs and symptoms:

typical posture, flexion at the hip and sidebending of the lumbar spine to the side of the most hypertonic psoas muscle.

typical gait, Trendelenburg gait.

typical pain pattern, low back pain frequently accompanied by pain on the lateral aspect of the lower extremity extending no lower than the knee.

typical associated somatic dysfunctions, as a long restrictor muscle, psoas hypertonicity is frequently associated with flexed dysfunctions of the upper lumbars, extended dysfunction of L5, and variable sacral and innominate dysfunctions. Tender points typically are found in the ipsilateral iliacus and contralateral piriformis muscles.

pubic bone, somatic dysfunctions of:

anterior pubic shear, a somatic dysfunction in which one pubic bone is displaced anteriorly with relation to its normal mate.

inferior pubic shear, a somatic dysfunction in which one pubic bone is displaced inferiorly with relation to its normal mate (Fig. 28).

posterior pubic shear, a somatic dysfunction in which one pubic bone is displaced posteriorly with relation to its normal mate.

pubic abduction, See *pubic gapping*.

pubic adduction, See *pubic compression*.

pubic compression (pubic adduction), a somatic dysfunction in which the pubic bones are forced toward each other at the pubic symphysis. This dysfunction is characterized by tenderness to palpation over the pubic symphysis, lack of apparent asymmetry, but associated with restricted motion of the pelvic ring (Fig. 29).

pubic gapping (pubic abduction), a somatic dysfunction in which the pubic bones are pulled away from each other at the pubic symphysis. This dysfunction is frequently seen in women following childbirth (Fig. 30).

superior pubic shear, a somatic dysfunction in which one pubic bone is displaced superiorly with relation to its normal mate (Fig. 31).

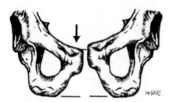

Seated flexion test = R(+)

Figure 28 Right inferior pubic shear.

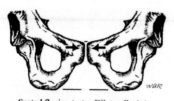

Seated flexion test = Bilaterally (+)
(False negative)

Figure 29 Pubic compression.

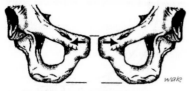

Seated flexion test = Bilaterally (+)
(False negative)

Figure 30 Pubic gapping (pubic abduction).

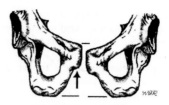

Seated flexion test = R(+)

Figure 31 Right superior pubic shear.

pubic symphysis, somatic dysfunctions of: See *pubic bone, somatic dysfunctions of.*

pump handle rib motion: See *rib motion, pump handle motion.*

R

range of motion technique: See *osteopathic manipulative treatment, range of motion technique.*

reciprocal inhibition: The inhibition of antagonist muscles when the agonist is stimulated. See also *laws, Sherrington's.*

reciprocal tension membrane: The intracranial and spinal dural membrane including the falx cerebri, falx cerebelli, tentorium and spinal dura.

red reflex: See *reflex, red r.*

reflex: An involuntary nervous system response to a sensory input. The sum total of any particular involuntary activity. See also *Chapman reflexes.*

cephalogyric reflex, See *oculocephalogyric r.*

cervicolumbar r., automatic contraction of the lumbar paravertebral muscles in response to contraction of postural muscles in the neck.

conditioned r., one that does not occur naturally in the organism or system, but that is developed by regular association of some physiological function with a related outside event.

myotatic r., tonic contraction of the muscles in response to a stretching force, due to stimulation of muscle receptors (e.g., deep tendon reflex).

oculocephalogyric r., (oculogyric reflex, cephalogyric reflex), automatic movement of the head that leads or accompanies movement of the eyes.

oculogyric r., See *oculocephalogyric r.*

red r., 1. The erythematous biochemical reaction (reactive hyperemia) of the skin in an area that has been stimulated mechanically by friction. The reflex is greater in degree and duration in an area of acute somatic dysfunction as compared to an area of chronic somatic dysfunction. It is a reflection of the segmentally related sympathicotonia commonly observed in the paraspinal area. 2. A red glow reflected from the fundus of the eye when a light is cast upon the retina.

somatosomatic r., localized somatic stimuli producing patterns of reflex response in segmentally related somatic structures.

somatovisceral r., localized somatic stimulation producing patterns of reflex response in segmentally related visceral structures.

viscerosomatic r., localized visceral stimuli producing patterns of reflex response in segmentally related somatic structures.

viscerovisceral r., localized visceral stimuli producing patterns of reflex response in segmentally related visceral structures.

regenerative injection therapy (RIT): See *sclerotherapy.* **region:** 1. An anatomical division of the body defined either by natural, functional or arbitrary boundaries. 2. Body areas for the diagnosis and coding of somatic dysfunction as defined in the International Classification of Diseases (currently ICD-9 CM) using the codes:

739.0 somatic dysfunction, head

739.1 somatic dysfunction, cervical

739.2 somatic dysfunction, thoracic

739.3 somatic dysfunction, lumbar

739.4 somatic dysfunction, sacrum

739.5 somatic dysfunction, pelvis

739.6 somatic dysfunction, lower extremity

739.7 somatic dysfunction, upper extremity

739.8 somatic dysfunction, rib cage

739.9 somatic dysfunction, abdomen/other

See also *transitional region.*

regional extension: See *extension, regional extension.*

regional motor inputs: Motion initiated by an osteopathic practitioner through body contact and vector input that produces a specific response at each segment in the mobile system.

resilience: Property of returning to the former shape or size after mechanical distortion. See also *elasticity.* See also *plasticity.*

respiratory axis of the sacrum: See *sacral motion axis, superior transverse axis.*

respiratory cooperation: An osteopathic practitioner-directed inhalation and/or exhalation by the patient to assist the manipulative treatment process.

restriction: A resistance or impediment to movement. For joint restriction, See *barrier (motion barrier). NB: This term is part of the TART acronym for an osteopathic somatic dysfunction.*

retrolisthesis: Posterior displacement of one vertebra relative to the one immediately below.

rib lesion: (Archaic) See *rib somatic dysfunction.*

rib motion:

    axis of rib motion, an imaginary line through the costotransverse and the costovertebral articulations of the rib.

    anteroposterior rib axis, (Fig. 32) See also *bucket handle rib motion.*

    bucket handle motion, movement of the ribs during respiration such that with inhalation, the lateral aspect of the rib moves cephalad resulting in an increase of transverse diameter of the thorax. This type of rib motion is predominantly found in lower ribs, increasing in motion from the upper to the lower ribs (Fig. 33). See also *rib motion, axis of.* See also *rib motion, pump handle.*

    caliper rib motion, rib motion of ribs 11 and 12 characterized by single joint motion; analogous to internal and external rotation.

    exhalation rib restriction, involves a rib or group of ribs that first stops moving during exhalation. The key rib is the bottom rib in the group. See also *rib somatic dysfunction, inhalation rib dysfunction.*

    inhalation rib restriction, involves a rib or group of ribs that first stops moving during inhalation. The key rib is the top rib in the group. See also *rib somatic dysfunction, exhalation rib dysfunction.*

pump handle motion, movement of the ribs during respiration such that with inhalation the anterior aspect of the rib moves cephalad and causes an increase in the anteroposterior diameter of the thorax. This type of rib motion is found predominantly in the upper ribs, decreasing in motion from the upper to the lower ribs (Fig. 34). See *rib motion, axis of.* See also *rib motion, bucket handle motion.*

transverse rib axis, (Fig. 35) See *rib motion, pump handle rib motion inhalation.* See also *rib motion, inhalation rib restriction.* See also *rib motion, exhalation rib restriction.*

rib somatic dysfunction: A somatic dysfunction in which movement or position of one or several ribs is altered or disrupted. For example, an elevated rib is one held in a position of inhalation such that motion toward inhalation is freer, and motion toward exhalation is restricted. A depressed rib is one held in a position of exhalation such that motion toward exhalation is freer and there is a restriction in inhalation. See also *rib motion, inhalation rib restriction.* See also *rib motion, exhalation rib restriction.*

    exhalation rib dysfunction, 1. Somatic dysfunction characterized by a rib being held in a position of exhalation such that motion toward exhalation is more free and motion toward inhalation is restricted. Synonyms: inhalation rib restriction depressed rib. 2. An anterior rib tender point in counterstrain. See also *rib motion, inhalation rib restriction.*

    inhalation rib dysfunction, a somatic dysfunction characterized by a rib being held in a position of inhalation such that motion toward inhalation is more free and motion toward exhalation is restricted. Synonyms: inhaled rib, anterior rib, elevated rib.

ropiness: A tissue texture abnormality characterized by a cord-like feeling. See also *tissue texture abnormality.*

rotation: Motion about an axis.

    rotation dysfunction of the sacrum, See *sacrum, somatic dysfunctions of.*

    rotation of sacrum, movement of the sacrum about a vertical (y) axis (usually in relation to the innominate bones).

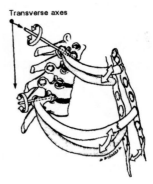

Figure 34 Pump handle rib motion.

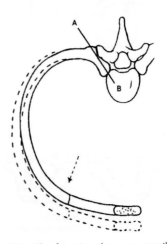

Figure 35 The functional transverse rib axis.

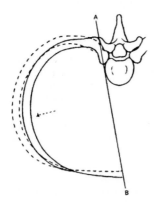

Figure 32 The functional anterior-posterior rib axis.

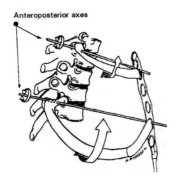

Figure 33 Bucket handle rib motion.

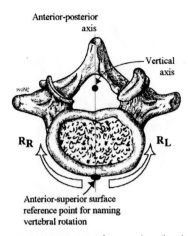

Figure 36 Rotation of a vertebra (lumbar).

rotation of vertebra, movement about the anatomical vertical axis (y axis) of a vertebra; named by the motion of a midpoint on the anterior-superior surface of the vertebral body (Fig. 36).

rule of threes: A method to locate the approximate position of the transverse process (TP) of a thoracic segment by using the location of the spinous process (SP) of that same vertebra. The relationship is as follows:

T1 to T3,	TP is at the same level as tip of the SP
T4 to T6,	TP is one half vertebral level above the tip of the SP
T7 to T9,	TP is one full vertebral level above the tip of the SP
T10,	TP is one full vertebral level above the tip of the SP
T11,	TP is one half vertebral level above the tip of the SP
T12,	TP is at the same level as tip of the SP.

S

sacral base: 1. In osteopathic palpation, the uppermost posterior portion of the sacrum. 2. The most cephalad portion of the first sacral segment (*Gray's Anatomy*).

sacral base anterior: See *sacrum, somatic dysfunctions of, bilateral sacral flexion.*

sacral base declination (unleveling): With the patient in a standing or seated position, any deviation of the sacral base from the horizontal in a coronal plane. Generally, the rotation of the sacrum about an anterior-posterior axis.

sacral base posterior: See *sacrum, somatic dysfunctions of, bilateral sacral flexion.*

sacral base unleveling: See *sacral base declination.*

sacralization: See *transitional vertebrae, sacralization.*

sacral movement axis: Any of the hypothetical axes for motion of the sacrum (Figs. 37 and 38).

anterior-posterior (x) axis, axis formed at the line of intersection of a sagittal and transverse plane.

inferior transverse axis (innominate), 1. The hypothetical functional axis of sacral motion that passes from side to side on a line through the inferior auricular surface of the sacrum and ilia, and represents the axis for movement of the ilia on the sacrum. 2. A term described by Fred Mitchell, Sr, DO (Fig. 37).

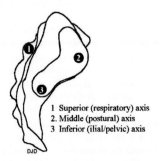

1 Superior (respiratory) axis
2 Middle (postural) axis
3 Inferior (ilial/pelvic) axis

Figure 37 Sacral transverse axes (lateral view).

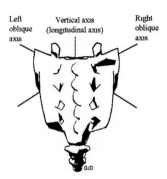

Figure 38 Axes of sacral motion (posterior view).

longitudinal axis, the hypothetical axis formed at the line of intersection of the midsagittal plane and a coronal plane, See *sacral motion axis, vertical (y) axis longitudinal* (Fig. 38).

middle transverse axis (postural), 1. The hypothetical functional axis of sacral nutation/counternutation in the standing position, passing horizontally through the anterior aspect of the sacrum at the level of the second sacral segment. 2. A term described by Fred Mitchell, Sr, DO (Fig. 37).

oblique axis (diagonal), 1. a hypothetical functional axis from the superior area of a sacroiliac articulation to the contralateral inferior sacroiliac articulation. It is designated as right or left relevant to its superior point of origin. 2. A term described by Fred Mitchell, Sr, DO (Fig. 38).

postural axis, See *sacrum, middle transverse axis (postural)* (Fig. 37).

respiratory axis, See *sacrum, superior transverse axis (respiratory)* (Fig. 37).

superior transverse axis (respiratory), 1. The hypothetical transverse axis about which the sacrum moves during the respiratory cycle. It passes from side to side through the articular processes posterior to the point of attachment of the dura at the level of the second sacral segment. Involuntary sacral motion occurs as part of the craniosacral mechanism, and is believed to occur about this axis. 2. A term described by Fred Mitchell, Sr, DO (Fig. 37).

transverse (z) axes, axes formed by intersection of the coronal and transverse planes about which nutation/counternutation occurs (Fig. 37).

vertical (y) axis (longitudinal), the axis formed by the intersection of the sagittal and coronal planes (Fig. 38).

sacral somatic dysfunction: See *sacrum, somatic dysfunctions of.*

sacral sulcus: A depression just medial to the posterior superior iliac spine (PSIS) as a result of the spatial relationship of the PSIS to the dorsal aspect of the sacrum (Figs. 39 and 40).

sacral torsion: 1. A physiologic function occurring in the sacrum during ambulation and forward bending. 2. A sacral somatic dysfunction around an oblique axis in which a torque occurs between the sacrum and

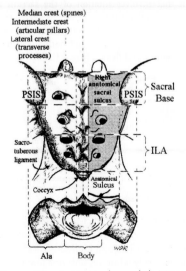

Figure 39 Anatomical sacral divisions.

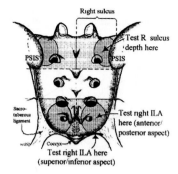

Figure 40 Clinical sacral divisions: sacral sulcus at the base, and inferior lateral angles (ILA).

innominates. The L5 vertebra rotates in the opposite direction of the sacrum. 3. If the L5 does not rotate opposite to the sacrum, L5 is termed maladapted. 4. Other terms for this maladaption include: rotations about an oblique axis, anterior or posterior sacrum and a torsion with a non-compensated L5 (Archaic use). See also *sacrum, somatic dysfunctions of.*

sacroiliac motion: Motion of the sacrum in relationship to the innominate(s) (ilium/ilia).

sacrum, inferior lateral angle (ILA) of: The point on the lateral surface of the sacrum where it curves medially to the body of the fifth sacral vertebrae *(Gray's Anatomy)* (Figs. 39 and 40).

sacrum, somatic dysfunctions of: Any of a group of somatic dysfunctions involving the sacrum. These may be the result of restriction of normal physiologic motion or trauma to the sacrum. See also *TART.*

  anterior sacrum, a positional term based on the Strachan model referring to sacral somatic dysfunction in which the sacral base has rotated anterior and sidebent to the side opposite the rotation. The upper limb (pole) of the SI joint has restricted motion and is named for the side on which forward rotation had occurred. Tissue texture changes are found at the deep sulcus. (The motion characteristics of L5 are not described.) (Fig. 41).

  anterior translated sacrum, a sacral somatic dysfunction in which the entire sacrum has moved anteriorly (forward) between the ilia. Anterior motion is freer, and the posterior motion is restricted (Fig. 42).

  backward torsions, 1. A backward sacral torsion is a physiologic rotation of the sacrum around an oblique axis such that the side of the sacral base contralateral to the named axis rotates posteriorly. L5 rotates in the direction opposite to the rotation of the sacral base. 2. Referred to as non-neutral sacral somatic dysfunctions (Archaic use). 3. A term by Fred Mitchell, Sr, DO, that describes the backward torsion as being nonphysiologic in terms of the walking cycle.

  bilateral sacral extension (sacral base posterior), 1. A sacral somatic dysfunction that involves rotation of the sacrum about a middle transverse axis such that the sacral base has moved posteriorly relative to the pelvic bones. Backward movement of the sacral base is freer, forward movement is restricted and both sulci are shallow. 2. The reverse of bilateral sacral flexion (Fig. 43).

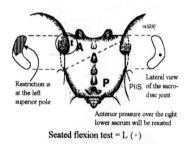

Figure 41 Anterior sacrum left. Motion of L5 is not described. There is tissue texture change (t) over the left sacral base. The superior pole of the left sacroiliac joint is affected and the left sacral base will not move posteriorly when an anterior test pressure is applied over the right lower sacrum.

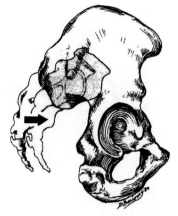

Figure 42 Anterior translated sacrum.

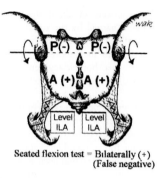

Seated flexion test = Bilaterally (+)
(False negative)

Figure 43 Bilateral sacral extension. (Sacral base posterior)

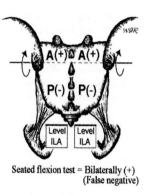

Seated flexion test = Bilaterally (+)
(False negative)

Figure 44 Bilateral sacral flexion. (Sacral base anterior)

  bilateral sacral flexion (sacral base anterior), 1. A sacral somatic dysfunction that involves rotation of the sacrum about a middle transverse axis such that the sacral base has moved anteriorly between the pelvic bones. Forward movement of the sacral base is freer, backward movement is restricted and both sulci are deep. 2. The reverse of bilateral sacral extension (Fig 44).

  forward torsions, 1. Forward torsion is a physiologic rotation of the sacrum around an oblique axis such that the side of the sacral base contralateral to the named axis glides anteriorly and produces a deep sulcus. L5 rotates in the direction opposite to the rotation of the sacral base. 2. Referred to as neutral sacral somatic dysfunctions (Archaic use). 3. A group of somatic dysfunctions described by Fred Mitchell, Sr, DO, based on the motion cycle of walking.

  left on left (forward) sacral torsion, refers to left rotation torsion around a left oblique axis (Fig. 45). See also *sacral torsion.*

  left on right (backward) sacral torsion, refers to left rotation around a right oblique axis. Findings: The left superior sacral sulcus is posterior or shallow, and the right ILA is anterior or deep. There is a positive

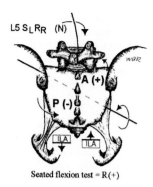

Figure 45 Left on left sacral torsion. (Left on left forward torsion)

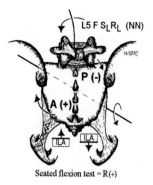

Figure 48 Right on left backward torsion. (Right on left sacral torsion)

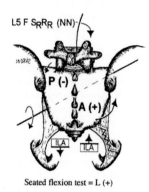

Figure 46 Left on right sacral torsion. (Left on right backward torsion)

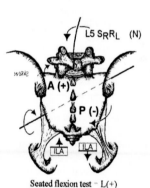

Figure 49 Posterior translated sacrum.

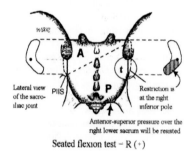

Figure 47 Posterior sacrum right. Motion of L5 is not described. There is tissue texture change (t) over the right sacroiliac joint (SI). The inferior pole of the right SI joint is affected. During motion testing, there is resistance to an anterior/superior test pressure applied over the right lower sacrum.

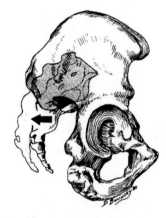

Figure 50 Right on right forward torsion.

seated flexion test on the left. L5 is non-neutral SRRR. Left superior sacral sulcus will be restricted when springing. The lumbosacral spring test is positive, and the sphinx test is positive (Fig. 46). See *sacral torsion*.

posterior sacrum, a positional term based on the Strachan model referring to a sacral somatic dysfunction in which the sacral base has rotated posterior and sidebent to the side opposite to the rotation. The dysfunction is named for the side on which the posterior rotation occurs. The tissue texture changes are found at the lower pole on the side of rotation *(Foundations)*. (The motion characteristics of L5 are not described.) (Fig. 47). right on left (backward) sacral torsion, refers to right rotation on a left oblique axis. Findings: The right superior sacral sulcus is posterior or shallow, and the left ILA is anterior or deep. The seated flexion test is positive on the right. L5 is nonneutral SLRL. The right superior sacral sulcus is restricted when springing. The lumbosacral spring test is positive. The sphinx test is positive (Fig. 48). See *sacral torsion*.

posterior translated sacrum, a sacral somatic dysfunction in which the entire sacrum has moved posteriorly (backward) between the ilia.

Posterior motion is freer, and anterior motion is restricted (Fig. 49). Right on right (forward) torsion, refers to a right rotation about a right oblique axis (Fig. 50). See *sacral torsion*.

rotated dysfunction of the sacrum, a sacral somatic dysfunction in which the sacrum has rotated about an axis approximating the longitudinal (y) axis. Motion is freer in the direction that rotation has occurred, and is restricted in the opposite direction (Fig. 51).

sacral shear, a complex translational motion of the sacrum in its relationship to the innominates. (Sometimes described as a sidebending in one direction and rotation in the opposite direction. Alternatively described as a unilateral movement along the arc of the L-shaped curve of the sacroiliac joint.) See also *sacrum, somatic dysfunctions of, unilateral sacral flexion and sacrum, somatic dysfunctions of, unilateral sacral extension*.

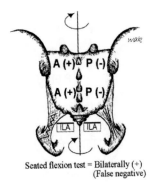

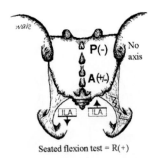

Seated flexion test = Bilaterally (+)
(False negative)

Figure 51 Right rotated dysfunction of the sacrum. (Right rotation about a vertical axis)

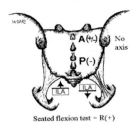

Seated flexion test = R(+)

Figure 52 Right unilateral sacral extension. (Right superior sacral shear)

Seated flexion test = R(+)

Figure 53 Right unilateral sacral flexion. (Right inferior sacral shear)

unilateral sacral extension, a sacral somatic dysfunction described as a superior shear of one side of the sacrum resulting in a shallow (full) sacral sulcus and ipsilateral superior-anterior inferolateral angle of the sacrum (Fig. 52). See *sacrum, somatic dysfunctions of, sacral shear.*

unilateral sacral flexion, a sacral somatic dysfunction described as an inferior shear of one side of the sacrum resulting in a deep sacral sulcus and ipsilateral inferior-posterior inferolateral angle of the sacrum (Fig. 53). See *sacrum, somatic dysfunctions of, sacral shear.*

sagittal plane: See *plane, sagittal plane.*

scan: An intermediate detailed examination of specific body regions that have been identified by findings emerging from the initial examination.

scaphocephaly: Also called scaphoid head or hatchet head, it is a transverse compression of the cranium with a resultant mid-sagittal ridge.

scaphoid head: See also *scaphocephaly.*

sclerotherapy: 1. Treatment involving injection of a proliferant solution at the osseous-ligamentous junction. 2. Treatment involving injection of irritating substances into weakened connective tissue areas such as fascia, varicose veins, hemorrhoids, esophageal varices, or weakened ligaments. The intended body's response to the irritant is fibrous proliferation with shortening/strengthening of the tissues injected.

sclerotome: 1. The pattern of innervation of structures derived from embryonal mesenchyme (joint capsule, ligament and bone). 2. The area of bone innervated by a single spinal segment. 3. The group of mesenchymal cells emerging from the ventromedial part of a mesodermal

somite and migrating toward the notochord. Sclerotomal cells from adjacent somites become merged in intersomatically located masses that are the primordia of the centra of the vertebrae (Fig. 54).

sclerotomal pain: Deep, dull achy pain associated with tissues derived from a common sclerotome (Fig. 54).

scoliosis: 1. Pathological or functional lateral curvature of the spine. 2. An appreciable lateral deviation in the normally straight vertical line of the spine (*Dorland's*) (Fig. 55).

screen: The initial general somatic examination to determine signs of somatic dysfunction in various regions of the body. See also *scan.*

secondary joint motion: Involuntary or passive motion of a joint. Also called accessory joint motion. segment: 1. A portion of a larger body or structure set off by natural or arbitrarily established boundaries, often equated with spinal segment. 2. To describe a single vertebrae or a vertebral segment corresponding to the sites of origin of rootlets of individual spinal nerves. 3. A portion of the spinal cord segmental diagnosis: The final stage of the spinal somatic examination in which the nature of the somatic problem is detailed at a segmental level. See also *scan.* See also *screen.*

segmental dysfunction: Dysfunction in a mobile system located at explicit segmental mobile units. Palpable characteristics of a dysfunctional segment are those associated with somatic dysfunction. (See also *STAR, TART and ART*) Responses to regional motor inputs at the dysfunctional segment support the concepts of complete motor asymmetry and mirrorimage motion asymmetries.

segmental mobile unit: A unit of the human movement system consisting of a bone, with articular surfaces for movement, as well as the adnexal tissues that create movement, allow movement and establish position under motor control.

segmental motion: Movement within a vertebral unit described by displacement of a point at the anterior-superior aspect of the superior vertebral body with respect to the segment below.

sensitization: Hypothetically, a shortlived (minutes or hours) increase in central nervous system (CNS) response to repeated sensory stimulation that generally follows habituation.

shear: An action or force causing or tending to cause two contiguous parts of an articulation to slide relative to each other in a direction parallel to their plane of contact. See also *pubic bone, somatic dysfunctions of.* See also *innominates, somatic dysfunctions of, inferior innominate shear.* See also *innominates, somatic dysfunction of, superior innominate shear.* See also *sacrum, somatic dysfunctions of, sacral shear.*

Sherrington law: See *law, Sherrington.*

sidebending: Movement in a coronal (frontal) plane about an anteriorposterior (x) axis. Also called lateral flexion, lateroflexion, or flexion right (or left).

sidebent: The position of any one or several vertebral bodies after sidebending has occurred (Fig. 56). See also *sidebending.*

skin drag: Sense of resistance to light traction applied to the skin. Related to the degree of moisture and degree of sympathetic nervous system activity.

soft tissue (ST): See *osteopathic manipulative treatment, soft tissue.*

soft tissue technique: See *osteopathic manipulative treatment, soft tissue technique.*

somatic dysfunction: Impaired or altered function of related components of the somatic (body framework) system: skeletal, arthrodial and myofascial structures, and their related vascular, lymphatic, and neural elements. Somatic dysfunction is treatable using osteopathic manipulative treatment. The positional and motion aspects of somatic dysfunction are best described using at least one of three parameters: 1). The position of a body part as determined by palpation and referenced to its adjacent defined structure, 2). The directions in which motion is freer, and 3). The directions in which motion is restricted. See also *TART.* See also *STAR.*

acute s. d., immediate or short-term impairment or altered function of related components of the somatic (body framework) system. Characterized in early stages by vasodilation, edema, tenderness, pain and tissue contraction. Diagnosed by history and palpatory assessment of tenderness, asymmetry of motion and relative position, restriction of motion and tissue texture change (TART). See also *TART.*

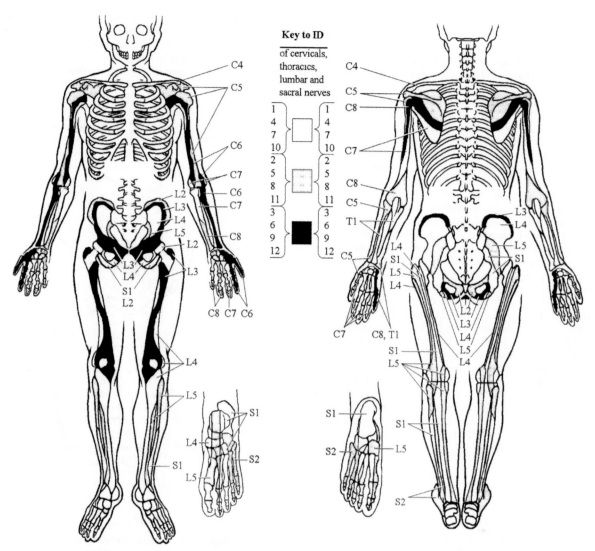

Figure 54 **Anterior and posterior sclerotomal innervations.** (Modified from *Foundations for Osteopathic Medicine*, Ward RC—Ed., Williams & Wilkins; 1997:644).

chronic s. d., impairment or altered function of related components of the somatic (body framework) system. It is characterized by tenderness, itching, fibrosis, paresthesias and tissue contraction. Identified by TART. See also *TART.*

linkage, dysfunctional segmental behavior where a single vertebra and an adjacent rib respond to the same regional motion tests with identical asymmetric behaviors (rather than opposing behaviors). This suggests visceral reflex inputs.

primary s. d., 1. The somatic dysfunction that maintains a total pattern of dysfunction. See also *key lesion.* 2. The initial or first somatic dysfunction to appear temporally.

secondary s. d., somatic dysfunction arising either from mechanical or neurophysiologic response subsequent to or as a consequence of other etiologies.

type I s. d., a group curve of thoracic and/or lumbar vertebrae in which the freedoms of motion are in neutral with sidebending and rotation

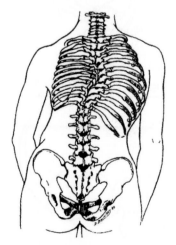

Figure 55 Scoliosis.

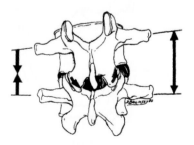

Figure 56 Sidebent.

in opposite directions with maximum rotation at the apex (rotation occurs toward the convexity of the curve) based upon the Principles of Fryette.

type II s. d., thoracic or lumbar somatic dysfunction of a single vertebral unit in which the vertebra is significantly flexed or extended with sidebending and rotation in the same direction (rotation occurs into the concavity of the curve) based upon the Principles of Fryette.

somatogenic: That which is produced by activity, reaction and change originating in the musculoskeletal system.

somatosomatic reflex: See *reflex, somatosomatic r.*

somatovisceral reflex: See *reflex, somatovisceral r.*

spasm: (compare with hypertonicity) a sudden, violent, involuntary contraction of a muscle or group of muscles, attended by pain and interference with function, producing involuntary movement and distortion *(Dorland's).*

Spencer technique: See *osteopathic manipulative treatment, Spencer technique.*

sphenobasilar synchondrosis (symphysis), somatic dysfunctions of: Any of a group of somatic dysfunctions involving primarily the inter-relationship between the basilar portion of the sphenoid (basisphenoid) and the basilar portion of the occiput (basiocciput). The abbreviation, SBS, is often used in reporting the following somatic dysfunctions:

SBS compression, somatic dysfunction in which the basisphenoid and basiocciput are held forced together significantly limiting SBS motion.

SBS extension, sphenoid and occiput have rotated in opposite directions around parallel transverse axes; the basiocciput and basisphenoid are both inferior in SBS extension with a decrease in the dorsal convexity between these two bones (Fig. 57).

SBS flexion, sphenoid and occiput have rotated in opposite directions around parallel transverse axes; the basiocciput and basisphenoid are both superior in SBS extension with an increase in the dorsal convexity between these two bones (Fig. 58). lateral strain, sphenoid and occiput have rotated in the same direction around parallel vertical axes. Lateral strains of the SBS are named for the position of the basisphenoid, right or left (Fig. 59).

sidebending-rotation, sphenoid and occiput have rotated in opposite directions around parallel vertical axes and rotate in the same direction around an A-P axis. SBS sidebending-rotations are named for the convexity, right or left (Fig. 60).

torsion, sphenoid and occiput have rotated in opposite directions around an anterior-posterior (A-P) axis. SBS torsions are named for the high greater wing of the sphenoid, right or left (Fig. 61).

vertical strain, sphenoid and occiput have rotated in the same direction around parallel transverse axes. Vertical strains of the SBS are named for the position of the basisphenoid, superior or inferior (Fig. 62).

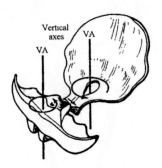

Figure 59 Right lateral strain (SBS).

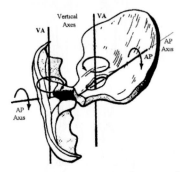

Figure 60 Left sidebending/rotation (SBS).

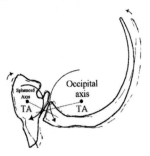

Figure 57 Extension (SBS).

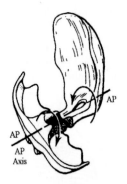

Figure 61 Right torsion (SBS).

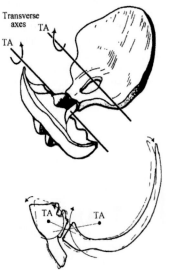

Figure 58 Flexion (SBS).

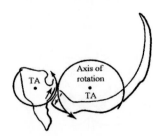

Figure 62 Superior vertical strain (SBS).

spinal facilitation: 1. The maintenance of a pool of neurons (e.g., premotor neurons, motor neurons or preganglionic sympathetic neurons in one or more segments of the spinal cord) in a state of partial or subthreshold excitation; in this state, less afferent stimulation is required to trigger the discharge of impulses. 2. A theory regarding the neurophysiological mechanisms underlying the neuronal activity associated with somatic dysfunction. 3. Facilitation may be due to sustained increase in afferent input, aberrant patterns of afferent input, or changes within the affected neurons themselves or their chemical environment. Once established, facilitation can be sustained by normal central nervous system (CNS) activity.

splenic pump technique: See *osteopathic manipulative treatment, splenic pump technique.*

spontaneous release by positioning: See *osteopathic manipulative treatment, counterstrain.*

sprain: Stretching injuries of ligamentous tissue (compare with strain). First degree: microtrauma; second degree: partial tear; third degree: complete disruption. springing technique: See *osteopathic manipulative treatment, springing technique.* See also *osteopathic manipulative treatment, articulatory treatment system.*

sphinx test: See *backward bending test.*

spring test: 1. A test used to differentiate between backward or forward sacral torsions/rotations. 2. A test used to differentiate bilateral sacral extension and bilateral sacral flexion. 3. A test used to differentiate unilateral sacral extension and unilateral sacral flexion.

S.T.A.R.: A mnemonic for four diagnostic criteria of somatic dysfunction: sensitivity changes, tissue texture abnormality, asymmetry and alteration of the quality and quantity of range of motion.

static contraction: See *contraction, isometric contraction.*

Still, MD, DO: Andrew Taylor. Founder of osteopathy; 1828–1917. First announced the tenets of osteopathy on June 22, 1874, established the American School of Osteopathy in 1892 at Kirksville, MO.

still point: 1. A term used to identify and describe the temporary cessation of the rhythmic motion of the primary respiratory mechanism. It may occur during osteopathic manipulative treatment when a point of balanced membranous or ligamentous tension is achieved. 2. A term used by William G. Sutherland, DO.

Still Technique: See *osteopathic manipulative treatment, Still Technique.*

strain: 1. Stretching injuries of muscle tissue. 2. Distortion with deformation of tissue. See also *ligamentous strain.*

Strachan model: See *sacrum, somatic dysfunctions of, anterior sacrum.* See *sacrum, somatic dysfunctions of, posterior sacrum.*

Strain-Counterstrain: See *osteopathic manipulative treatment, counterstrain.*

stretching: Separation of the origin and insertion of a muscle and/or attachments of fascia and ligaments.

stringiness: A palpable tissue texture abnormality characterized by fine or stringlike myofascial structures.

structural examination: See *osteopathic structural examination.* subluxation: 1. A partial or incomplete dislocation. 2. A term describing an abnormal anatomical position of a joint which exceeds the normal physiologic limit, but does not exceed the joint's anatomical limit.

superior (upslipped) innominate: See *innominate, somatic dysfunctions of, superior innominate shear.*

superior pubic shear: See *pubic bone, somatic dysfunctions of.* See also *symphyseal shear* (Fig. 31).

superior transverse axis: See *sacral motion axis, superior transverse axis (respiratory) and (z) axis.*

supination: 1. Beginning in anatomical position, applied to the hand, the act of turning the palm forward (anteriorly) or upward, performed by lateral external rotation of the forearm. 2. Applied to the foot, it generally applies to movements (adduction and inversion) resulting in raising of the medial margin of the foot, hence of the longitudinal arch. A compound motion of plantar flexion, adduction and inversion. See also *pronation.*

supine: Lying with the face upward *(Dorland's).*

symmetry: The similar arrangement in form and relationships of parts around a common axis, or on each side of a plane of the body *(Dorland's).*

Sutherland fulcrum: A shifting suspension fulcrum of the reciprocal tension membrane located along the straight sinus at the junction of the falx cerebri and tentorium cerebelli. See also *reciprocal tension membrane.* See also *osteopathic manipulative treatment, Osteopathy in the Cranial Field (OCF).*

symphyseal shear: The resultant of an action or force causing or tending to cause the two parts of the symphysis to slide relative to each other in a direction parallel to their plane of contact. It is usually found in an inferior/superior direction but is occasionally found to be in an anterior/posterior direction (Figs. 28 and 31).

T

tapotement: Striking the belly of a muscle with the hypothenar edge of the open hand in rapid succession in an attempt to increase its tone and arterial perfusion.

TART: A mnemonic for four diagnostic criteria of somatic dysfunction: tissue texture abnormality, asymmetry, restriction of motion and tenderness, any one of which must be present for the diagnosis.

technic: See *technique.*

technique: Methods, procedures and details of a mechanical process or surgical operation *(Dorland's).* See also *osteopathic manipulative treatment.*

tenderness: 1. Discomfort or pain elicited by the osteopathic practitioner through palpation. 2. A state of unusual sensitivity to touch or pressure *(Dorland's). NB: This term is part of the TART acronym for an osteopathic somatic dysfunction.*

tender points: 1. Small, hypersensitive points in the myofascial tissues of the body that do not have a pattern of pain radiation. These points are a manifestation of somatic dysfunction and are used as diagnostic criteria and for monitoring treatment. 2. A system of diagnosis and treatment originally described by Lawrence Jones, DO, FAAO. See also *osteopathic manipulative treatment, counterstrain.*

terminal barrier: See *barrier, physiologic b.* thoracic aperture (superior): See *thoracic inlet.*

thoracic outlet: 1. The functional thoracic inlet consists of T1-4 vertebrae, ribs 1 and 2 plus their costicartilages, and the manubrium of the sternum. See *fascial patterns.* 2. The anatomical thoracic inlet consists of T1 vertebra, the first ribs and their costal cartilages, and the superior end of the manubrium.

thoracic pump: See *osteopathic manipulative treatment, thoracic pump.*

thrust technique: See *osteopathic manipulative treatment, thrust technique.* See also *osteopathic manipulative treatment, high velocity/low amplitude technique (HVLA).*

tissue texture abnormality (TTA): A palpable change in tissues from skin to periarticular structures that represents any combination of the following signs: vasodilation, edema, flaccidity, hypertonicity, contracture, fibrosis, as well as the following symptoms: itching, pain, tenderness, paresthesias. Types of TTA's include: bogginess, thickening, stringiness, ropiness, firmness (hardening), increased/decreased temperature and increased/decreased moisture. *NB: This term is part of the TART acronym for an osteopathic somatic dysfunction.*

toggle technique: See *osteopathic manipulative treatment, toggle technique.*

tonus: The slight continuous contraction of muscle, which in skeletal muscles, aids in the maintenance of posture and in the return of blood to the heart *(Dorland's).*

torsion: 1. A motion or state where one end of a part is twisted about a longitudinal axis while the opposite end is held fast or turned in the opposite direction. 2. A physiologic motion pattern about an anteroposterior axis of the sphenobasilar symphysis/synchondrosis. See also *sphenobasilar synchondrosis (symphysis), somatic dysfunctions of, torsion.*

torsion, sacral: See *sacral torsion.* See also *sacrum, somatic dysfunctions of, sacral torsions.*

traction: A linear force acting to draw structures apart.

traction technique: See *osteopathic manipulative treatment, traction technique.*

transitional region: Areas of the axial skeleton where structure changes significantly lead to functional changes; transitional areas commonly include the following:

Figure 63 The pedicle (B) is the key structure from which other vertebral parts can be identified. (Ward RC, Ex. Ed., *Foundations for Osteopathic Medicine,* Second Edition, Lippincott Williams & Wilkins, Philadelphia, 2003:730.)

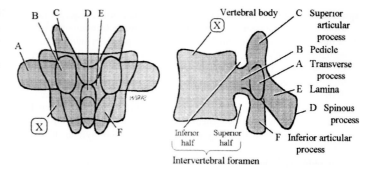

occipitocervical region (OA), typically the OA-AA-C2 region is described.

cervicothoracic region (CT), typically C7-T1.

thoracolumbar region (TL), typically T10-L1.

lumbosacral region (LS), typically L5-S1.

transitional vertebrae: A congenital anomaly of a vertebra in which it develops characteristic(s) of the adjoining structure or region.

    lumbarization, a transitional segment in which the first sacral segment becomes like an additional lumbar vertebra articulating with the second sacral segment.

    sacralization, 1. Incomplete separation and differentiation of the fifth lumbar vertebra (L5) such that it takes on characteristics of a sacral vertebra. 2. When transverse processes of the fifth lumbar (L5) are atypically large, causing pseudoarthrosis with the sacrum and/or ilia(um), referred to as batwing deformity, if bilateral.

translation: Motion along an axis.

translatory motion: See *motion, translatory motion.*

transverse axis of sacrum: See *sacral, sacral movement axis, transverse (z) axis* (Fig. 37).

transverse process: Projects laterally from the region of each pedicle. The pedicle connects the posterior elements to the vertebral body (Fig. 63).

transverse rib axis: See (Fig. 35). See also *rib motion, pump handle rib motion* (Fig. 34).

Traube-Herring-Mayer wave: An oscillation that has been measured in association with blood pressure, heart rate, cardiac contractility, pulmonary blood flow, cerebral blood flow and movement of the cerebrospinal fluid, and peripheral blood flow including venous volume and thermal regulation. This whole-body phenomenon, which exhibits a rate typically slightly less than and independent of respiration, bears a striking resemblance to the primary respiratory mechanism.

Travell trigger point: See *trigger point.*

treatment, active: (Archaic). See *osteopathic manipulative treatment, active method.*

treatment, osteopathic manipulative techniques: See *osteopathic manipulative treatment.*

Trendelenburg test: The patient, with back to the examiner, is told to lift first one foot and then the other. The position and movements of the gluteal fold are watched. When standing on the affected limb the gluteal fold on the sound side falls instead of rising. Seen in poliomyelitis, un-united fracture of the femoral neck, coxa vara and congenital dislocations.

trigger point (myofascial trigger point): 1. A small hypersensitive site that, when stimulated, consistently produces a reflex mechanism that gives rise to referred pain and/or other manifestations in a consistent reference zone that is consistent from person to person. 2. These points were most extensively and systematically documented by Janet Travell, MD, and David Simons, MD. trophic: Pertaining to nutrition, especially in the cellular environment (e.g., trophic function—a nutritional function).

trophicity: 1. A nutritional function or relation. 2. The natural tendency to replenish the body stores that have been depleted.

trophotropic: Concerned with or pertaining to the natural tendency for maintenance and/or restoration of nutritional stores.

-tropic: A word termination denoting turning toward, changing or tendency to change.

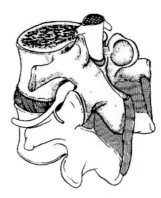

Figure 64 Vertebral unit.

tropism, facet: Unequal size and/or facing of the zygapophyseal joints of a vertebra. See also *facet asymmetry.*

type I somatic dysfunction: See *somatic dysfunction, type I s.d.* See also *physiologic motion of the spine.*

type II somatic dysfunction: See *somatic dysfunction, type II s.d.* See also *physiologic motion of the spine.*

U

uncommon compensatory pattern: See *fascial patterns, uncommon compensatory pattern.*

uncompensated fascial pattern: See *fascial patterns, uncompensated fascial pattern.*

V

v-spread: See *osteopathic manipulative treatment, v-spread.*

velocity: The instantaneous rate of motion in a given direction.

ventral technique: See *osteopathic manipulative treatment, visceral manipulation.*

vertebral unit: Two adjacent vertebrae with their associated intervertebral disk, arthrodial, ligamentous, muscular, vascular, lymphatic and neural elements (Fig. 64).

visceral dysfunction: Impaired or altered mobility or motility of the visceral system and related fascial, neurological, vascular, skeletal and lymphatic elements.

visceral manipulation: See *osteopathic manipulative treatment, visceral manipulation.*

viscerosomatic reflex: See *reflex, viscerosomatic r.* viscerovisceral reflex: See *reflex, viscerovisceral r.*

viscosity: 1. A measurement of the rate of deformation of any material under load. 2. The capability possessed by a solid of yielding continually under stress. See also *elasticity.* See also *plasticity.*

W

weight-bearing line of L3: See *gravitational line* (Fig. 16). Vertical axis: See *sacral motion axis, vertical (y) axis (longitudinal).*

Note: Page numbers followed by b indicate box; those followed by t indicate table. Page numbers in italics indicate figure.